CARDIAC ARRHYTHMIAS

Their Mechanisms, Diagnosis, and Management

SECOND EDITION

William J. Mandel, M.D., F.A.C.C.

Professor of Medicine (Adjunct), University of California, Los Angeles, UCLA School of Medicine; Clinical Director, Electrophysiology, Cedars-Sinai Medical Center, Los Angeles, California

With 66 Contributors

J. B. LIPPINCOTT COMPANY Philadelphia

London • Mexico City • New York • St. Louis • São Paulo • Sydney

Sponsoring Editor: Richard Winters
Manuscript Editor: Helen Ewan
Indexer: Ruth Low
Design Director: Tracy Baldwin
Design Coordinator: Earl Gerhart
Designer: Katharine Nichols
Production Supervisor: Kathleen P. Dunn
Production Coordinator: Susan Hess
Compositor: Progressive Typographers
Printer/Binder: Maple Press

Second Edition

For information write J. B. Lippincott Company, East Washington Square, Philadelphia, Pennsylvania 19105.

6 5 4 3 2 1

Library of Congress Cataloging-in-Publication Data

Cardiac arrhythmias.

Includes bibliographies and index.
1. Arrhythmia. I. Mandel, William J., 1937–
[DNLM: 1. Arrhythmia. WG 330 C2685]
RC685.A65C283 1987 616.1′28 86-7340
ISBN 0-397-50561-2

The authors and publisher have exerted every effort to ensure that drug selection and dosage set forth in this text are in accord with current recommendations and practice at the time of publication. However, in view of ongoing research, changes in government regulations, and the constant flow of information relating to drug therapy and drug reactions, the reader is urged to check the package insert for each drug for any change in indications and dosage and for added warnings and precautions. This is particularly important when the recommended agent is a new or infrequently employed drug.

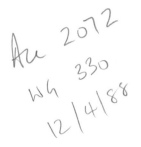

CARDIAC
ARRHYTHMIAS

Contributors

Maurits A. Allessie, M.D., Ph.D. Chapter 7
Professor of Physiology, University of Limburg, Maastricht, The Netherlands

Robert H. Anderson, B.Sc., M.D., M.R.C.Path. Chapter 2
Joseph Levy Professor of Paediatric Cardiac Morphology, Cardiothoracic Institute, London, England

Frits W. H. M. Bär, M.D. Chapter 11
Associate Professor of Cardiology, University of Limburg; Staff Member, Department of Cardiology, Maastricht Hospital, Maastricht, The Netherlands

Robert A. Bauernfeind, M.D. Chapter 10
Associate Professor of Medicine, Virginia Commonwealth University Medical College of Virginia; Director of Electrophysiology, Medical College of Virginia Hospitals, Richmond, Virginia

Anton E. Becker, M.D. Chapter 2
Professor of Pathology, University of Amsterdam, Academic Medical Center, Amsterdam, The Netherlands

Selvyn B. Bleifer, M.D. Chapter 23
Associate Clinical Professor of Medicine, University of California, Los Angeles, UCLA School of Medicine; Director, Department of Cardiology, Brotman Memorial Hospital, Los Angeles, California

Felix I. M. Bonke, M.D., Ph.D. Chapter 7
Professor of Physiology, University of Limburg, Maastricht, The Netherlands

Martin Borggrefe, M.D. Chapter 22
University of Duesseldorf, Medical Hospital of the University of Duesseldorf, Department of Cardiology, Pneumology and Angiology, Duesseldorf, Germany

Günter Breithardt, M.D. Chapter 22
Professor of Medicine, University of Duesseldorf, Medical Hospital of the University of Duesseldorf, Department of Cardiology, Pneumology and Angiology, Duesseldorf, Germany

Christian Cabrol, M.D. Chapter 34
Chief, Department of Cardiovascular Surgery, Hôpital de la Pitie, Paris, France

A. John Camm, M.D., F.R.C.P., F.A.C.C. Chapter 35
Professor of Cardiovascular Medicine, St. Bartholomew's Hospital, London, England

Agustin Castellanos, M.D. Chapter 25
Professor of Medicine, University of Miami School of Medicine; Director, Clinical Electrophysiology, University of Miami/Jackson Memorial Medical Center, Miami, Florida

Howard C. Cohen, M.D., F.A.C.C., F.A.C.C.P. Chapters 15 and 16
Clinical Associate Professor of Medicine, University of Chicago Pritzker School of Medicine; Attending Physician, Michael Reese Hospital and Medical Center, Illinois Masonic Medical Center, Chicago, Illinois

Keith Cohn, M.D. Chapter 19
Clinical Professor of Medicine, University of California, San Francisco, School of Medicine; Co-Director, Division of Cardiology, Pacific Presbyterian Medical Center, San Francisco, California

Paul V. L. Curry, M.D., F.R.C.P. Chapter 8
Lecturer, Consultant Cardiologist, Guy's Hospital, London, England

Mary L. Dohrmann, M.D. Chapter 19
Assistant Clinical Professor of Medicine, University of California, San Francisco, School of Medicine; Director, Cardiology Clinic, San Francisco General Hospital, San Francisco, California

Leonard S. Dreifus, M.D. Chapter 12
Professor of Medicine, Jefferson Medical College of Thomas Jefferson University; Chief, Cardiovascular Division, Lankenau Hospital, Philadelphia, Pennsylvania

Edwin G. Duffin, Jr., Ph.D. Chapter 32
Manager of the Special Devices and Medtronic Fellow, Medtronic, Inc., Minneapolis, Minnesota

Nabil El-Sherif, M.D., F.A.C.C. Chapter 18
Professor of Medicine and Physiology, State University of New York, Downstate Medical Center College of Medicine; Chief, Cardiology Division, SUNY, Downstate Medical Center and Brooklyn Veterans Administration Medical Center, Brooklyn, New York

Jerónimo Farré, M.D. Chapter 11
Director, Coronary Care Unit and Electrophysiology Laboratory, Department of Cardiology, Fundación Jiménez Diaz, Madrid, Spain

Guy Fontaine, M.D., F.A.C.C. Chapter 34
Professor of Medicine, Director, Department of Cardiac Pacing and Clinical Electrophysiology, Hôpital Jean Rostand, Ivry, France

Robert Frank, M.D. Chapter 34
Praticien Hôpitalier, Hôpital Jean Rostand, Ivry, France

Derek A. Fyfe, M.D., Ph.D. Chapter 26
Assistant Professor, Pediatric Cardiology, Medical University of South Carolina College of Medicine, Charleston, South Carolina

David C. Gadsby, M.A., Ph.D. Chapter 3
Associate Professor, Laboratory of Cardiac Physiology, The Rockefeller University, New York, New York

Eli S. Gang, M.D. Chapter 33
Assistant Professor of Medicine, University of California, Los Angeles, UCLA School of Medicine; Staff Cardiologist, Cedars-Sinai Medical Center, Los Angeles, California

Paul C. Gillette, M.D., F.A.C.C. Chapter 26
Professor of Pediatrics, Director of Pediatric Cardiology, Medical University of South Carolina College of Medicine, Charleston, South Carolina

Nora Goldschlager, M.D. Chapter 19
Clinical Professor of Medicine, University of California, San Francisco, School of Medicine; Director, Coronary Care Unit, San Francisco General Hospital, San Francisco, California

Yves Grosgogeat, M.D., F.A.C.C. Chapter 34
Professor of Cardiology, Chief, Department of Cardiology, Hôpital de la Salpetriere, Paris, France

Gérard Guiraudon, M.D. Chapter 34
Professor of Cardiovascular Surgery, University Hospital, London, Ontario, Canada

John M. Herre, M.D. Chapter 10
Assistant Professor of Medicine, University of California, San Francisco, School of Medicine; Director, Electrophysiology Laboratory, Moffitt Hospital, San Francisco, California

Siew Yen Ho, Ph.D. Chapter 2
Senior Lecturer, Paediatric Cardiac Morphology, Cardiothoracic Institute, London, England

Jay L. Jordan, M.D. Chapter 6
Assistant Clinical Professor, University of California, Los Angeles, UCLA School of Medicine; Clinical Co-Director, Outpatient Cardiac Arrhythmias Center, Cedars-Sinai Medical Center, Los Angeles, California

Hrayr S. Karagueuzian, M.S., Ph.D. Chapters 17, 28, and 29
Assistant Professor of Medicine, University of California, Los Angeles, UCLA School of Medicine; Research Scientist, Director, Cardiac Electrophysiology Research, Cedars-Sinai Medical Center, Los Angeles, California

Dennis M. Krikler, M.D., F.R.C.P., F.A.C.C. Chapter 20
Senior Lecturer in Cardiology, Royal Postgraduate Medical School, University of London; Consultant Cardiologist, Hammersmith Hospital, London, England

Richard M. Luceri, M.D. Chapter 25
Assistant Professor of Medicine, University of Miami School of Medicine; Director, Clinical Arrhythmia and Pacemaker Programs, Jackson Memorial Medical Center, Miami, Florida

R. A. Massumi, M.D. Chapters 9 and 14
Adjunct Professor of Medicine (Cardiology), University of California, UCLA School of Medicine; Director, Electrophysiology Laboratory, Sepulveda Veterans Administration Medical Center, Sepulveda, California

Victor A. Medina-Ravell, M.D., F.A.C.C. Chapter 25
Medical Director Fundación COR, Director Cardiac Electrophysiology, Laboratory and Cardiac Pacing Unit—"Dr. Agustin Castellanos", Hospital Central de Valencia, Venezuela; Cardiólogo Especialista I, Departamento Nacional de Enfermedades—Cardiovasculares, Ministerio de Sanidad y Asistencia Social, Caracas, Venezuela; Coordinador Sección de Arritmias-Especialista I, Hospital Central de Valencia, Valencia, Venezuela

Fred Morady, M.D. Chapter 24
Associate Professor Internal Medicine, University of Michigan Medical School; Director, Clinical Cardiac Electrophysiology Laboratory, University of Michigan Medical Center, Ann Arbor, Michigan

Morton M. Mower, M.D. Chapter 36
Assistant Professor of Medicine, Johns Hopkins University School of Medicine; Director of Heart Station, Sinai Hospital of Baltimore, Baltimore, Maryland

Robert J. Myerburg, M.D. Chapter 25
Professor of Medicine and Physiology, Director, Division of Cardiology, University of Miami School of Medicine, University of Miami Medical Center, Miami, Florida

Onkar S. Narula, M.D. Chapter 13
Clinical Professor of Medicine, Division of Cardiology, University of Miami School of Medicine, Cedars Medical Center, Miami, Florida

Daniel S. Oseran, M.D. Chapter 21
Attending Physician, Cedars-Sinai Medical Center, Los Angeles, California

Michael Perelman, M.A., M.B., M.Chir., M.R.C.P. Chapter 20
Research Fellow, Royal Postgraduate Medical Center, Hammersmith Hospital, London, England

C. Thomas Peter, M.D., F.A.C.C., F.A.C.P., F.C.C.P. Chapters 21 and 23
Associate Professor of Medicine, University of California, Los Angeles, UCLA School of Medicine; Director, Section of Electrocardiography and Electrophysiology, Cedars-Sinai Medical Center, Los Angeles, California

Leon Resnekov, M.D., F.R.C.P. Chapter 30
Rawson Professor of Medicine (Cardiology), University of Chicago Pritzker School of Medicine, University of Chicago Medical Center, Chicago, Illinois

Bertrand Ross, M.D., F.A.A.P. Chapter 26
Assistant Professor of Pediatric Cardiology, Director of the Exercise Performance Laboratory, Division of Pediatric Cardiology, Medical University of South Carolina, South Carolina Children's Heart Center, Charleston, South Carolina

Thomas F. Ross, M.D., F.A.C.C. Chapter 5
Cedars-Sinai Medical Center, Los Angeles, California

Edward Rowland, M.B., B.S. Chapter 20
Waring Lecturer, Cardiothoracic Institute; Honorary Senior Registrar, Brompton Hospital, London, England

Melvin M. Scheinman, M.D. Chapter 31
Professor of Medicine, University of California, San Francisco, School of Medicine; Chief, Electrocardiography and Clinical Cardiac Electrophysiology Section, Moffitt Hospital, San Francisco, California

Edward Shapiro, M.D., F.A.C.C. Chapter 1
Clinical Professor of Medicine, Emeritus, University of Southern California School of Medicine; Attending Physician, Cedars-Sinai Medical Center, Los Angeles, California

Mohammad Shenasa, M.D., Ph.D. Chapter 8
Associate Professor of Medicine, Department of Medicine, University of Montreal Faculty of Medicine; Director, Clinical Electrophysiology Laboratory, Sacre-Coeur Hospital, Montreal, Quebec, Canada

Donad H. Singer, M.D. Chapters 15 and 16
Professor of Medicine (Cardiology) and Pharmacology, Director, Reingold ECG Center, Northwestern University Medical School; Attending Physician, Northwestern Memorial Hospital, Chicago, Illinois

Bramah N. Singh, M.D., D.Phil. Chapter 29
Professor of Medicine, Assistant Chief of Cardiology—V.A. Wadsworth Medical Center, Los Angeles, California

Thomas W. Smith, M.D. Chapter 28
Professor of Medicine, Harvard Medical School; Chief, Cardiovascular Division, Brigham and Women's Hospital, Boston, Massachusetts

R.A.J. Spurrell, M.D., B.Sc., F.R.C.P., F.A.C.C. Chapter 35
Consultant in Clinical Cardiology, St. Bartholomew's Hospital, London, England

Borys Surawicz, M.D. Chapter 4
Professor of Medicine, Indiana University School of Medicine, Indianapolis, Indiana

Ashby B. Taylor, M.D. Chapter 26
Associate Professor of Pediatrics, Medical University of South Carolina College of Medicine, Medical University of South Carolina Hospital, Charleston, South Carolina

Albert L. Waldo, M.D. Chapter 27
Professor of Medicine and Walter H. Pritchard Professor of Cardiology, Case Western Reserve University School of Medicine, University Hospitals of Cleveland, Cleveland, Ohio

Yoshio Watanabe, M.D., F.A.C.C. Chapter 12
Professor of Medicine and Director, Cardiovascular Institute, Fujita Gakuen University School of Medicine, Tokyoake, Japan

William J. Welch, M.D. Chapter 10
Assistant Professor of Medicine, Virginia Commonwealth University Medical College of Virginia; Clinical Cardiac Electrophysiologist, Medical College of Virginia Hospital, Richmond, Virginia

Hein J. J. Wellens, M.D. Chapter 11
Professor of Cardiology, University of Limburg; Chairman of the Department of Cardiology, Maastricht Hospital, Maastricht, The Netherlands

Andrew L. Wit, Ph.D. Chapter 3
Professor of Pharmacology, Columbia University College of Physicians and Surgeons, New York, New York

Vicki L. Zeigler, R.N., B.S.N. Chapter 26
Electrophysiology/Pacemaker Nurse, Medical University of South Carolina, South Carolina Children's Heart Center, Charleston, South Carolina

Alexander J. Zinner, III, B.M.E. Chapter 26
Pacemaker Clinic Coordinator, Electrophysiologic Technologist, Medical University of South Carolina, South Carolina Children's Heart Center, Charleston, South Carolina

Douglas P. Zipes, M.D. Chapter 32
Professor of Medicine, Indiana University School of Medicine; Senior Research Associate, Krannert Institute of Cardiology, Indianapolis, Indiana

Preface

The second edition of this textbook on cardiac arrhythmias has come about because of the continued expansion of our knowledge concerning the mechanisms, diagnosis, and management of rhythm disorders in man.

In the time span between these two editions, there has been a significant increase in data concerning cellular electrophysiologic mechanisms of arrhythmias, which can be expected to enhance the understanding and management of clinical arrhythmias. Pharmacologically, the armamentarium of clinically available antiarrhythmic drugs has expanded dramatically. This increase in drug availability has been associated with an increase in basic electrophysiologic–pharmacologic data concerning drug mechanisms. The latter is essential to the clinician in the management of patients with cardiac arrhythmias.

This edition also addresses noninvasive assessment of the propensity for ventricular arrhythmias with the use of late potential recordings, as well as alteration of autonomic tone for assessment of the types and location of AV block.

New therapeutic approaches have been emphasized in this edition, including the use of lasers and other ablation techniques, new modes of pacemaker therapy, and the use of the automatic implantable defibrillator.

An extensive new section has been added on the techniques of general electrophysiologic testing, with a separate chapter on ventricular tachycardia evaluation. A chapter on the evaluation of patients with unexplained syncope has also been added.

Finally, significant changes have been made in the chapters on cardiac surgery for atrial arrhythmias, the WPW syndrome, and ventricular tachycardia.

In total, there has been updating and expansion of the electrophysiologic material in this textbook, so that the clinician with a keen interest in clinical electrophysiology may have a ready reference source of basic and clinical electrophysiologic material.

The editor wishes to acknowledge the important contributions made by his colleagues: Doctors C. Thomas Peter, Eli Gang, Daniel Oseran, and Hrayr Karagueuzian. He would also particularly like to acknowledge the essential contribution of Ms. Brenda Williams, without whose assistance in all areas of preparation this text could not have been completed.

The support of my family, Dede, Stacy, and Jay, was essential to the completion of this manuscript.

Finally, to the staff of J. B. Lippincott Company and, especially, Richard Winters, I am most grateful.

William J. Mandel, M.D.

Preface to First Edition

This textbook has been written to fill a void caused by the rapid growth of knowledge over the past decade in cardiac electrophysiology. This growth has resulted from significant advances in a wide spectrum of areas, including anatomic-electrophysiologic correlations, basic science studies on the mechanisms of arrhythmias, the availability of intracardiac electrogram recordings in humans, and cardiac pharmacology. This text, in addition to discussing these important advances, will review historical aspects of electrophysiology research in an attempt to give the reader a proper perspective of the field.

It is hoped that this textbook will serve as a major reference source for the student of cardiac arrhythmias. The intention of thc authors is to offer a definitive text on all pertinent aspects of cardiac arrhythmias which could be used by physicians and paramedical personnel who deal with the care of patients with significant rhythm disorders.

The editor wishes to gratefully acknowledge the important contributions made by his colleagues Doctors Jay Jordan, C. Thomas Peter, and Steven Halpern. He would also particularly like to acknowledge the essential contribution of Mrs. Bernadette Fluharty, without whose assistance in all areas of preparation this text could not have been completed.

I am deeply grateful to my family, Dede, Stacy, and Jay, for their patience and inspiration during the preparation of this text.

Finally, to the staff of J. B. Lippincott, I am most grateful. Their meticulous attention to all details is appreciated.

William J. Mandel, M.D.

Contents

CARDIAC
ARRHYTHMIAS

1

The Electrocardiogram and the Arrhythmias: Historical Insights

Edward Shapiro

> I compare myself to a scavenger: with my hook in my hand and my pack on my back, I go about the domain of science picking up what I can find.
>
> Francois Magendie[1]

Although the electrocardiograph is without question the Rosetta stone of the arrhythmias, we should not assume that before Einthoven only ignorance existed in the realm of cardiac irregularities. In 1902, James Mackenzie published *The Study of the Pulse,* the compilation of his diligent studies of arterial and venous pulsations by his improved clinical ink-writings polygraph (Fig. 1-1). The reliable tracings of this instrument were used as guides to correct the inexact interpretations of electrocardiograms in the early days of Einthoven and Thomas Lewis. Basically, for the diagnosis of arrhythmias, the electrocardiogram is searched for P and QRS complexes and their relationship to each other. The polygraph's a and v waves gave the same information, not from electrical activation, but from the consequent contraction of the atria and ventricles as reflected in the jugular and radial pulses.

The laddergram we use with profit today to aid the analysis of complex arrhythmias was devised by Engelmann in 1896 to explain tracings inscribed by the polygraph.[2] In 1903, Wenckebach published *Die Arrhythmie, als Ausdruck bestimmter Funktionsstörungen des Herzens,* also based on the ink-writing polygraph. His eponymic phenomenon to explain recurrent dropped beats was discovered in 1899 by using the polygraph to record the radial arteriogram, not the electrocardiogram, as is often assumed.

Just before the electrocardiograph was invented in 1903, the ink-writing polygraph allowed the accurate graphic diagnosis of the following:

1. Sinus arrhythmia
2. Sinus tachycardia and bradycardia
3. Atrial fibrillation
4. First, second, and third degree heart block
5. Wenckebach phenomenon
6. Junctional rhythm
7. Pulsus alternans
8. Paroxysmal atrial tachycardia
9. Atrial tachycardia with block

The polygraph, however, could not clearly distinguish flutter from paroxysmal atrial tachycardia.

Cushny[3] in 1897 observed and described interfer-

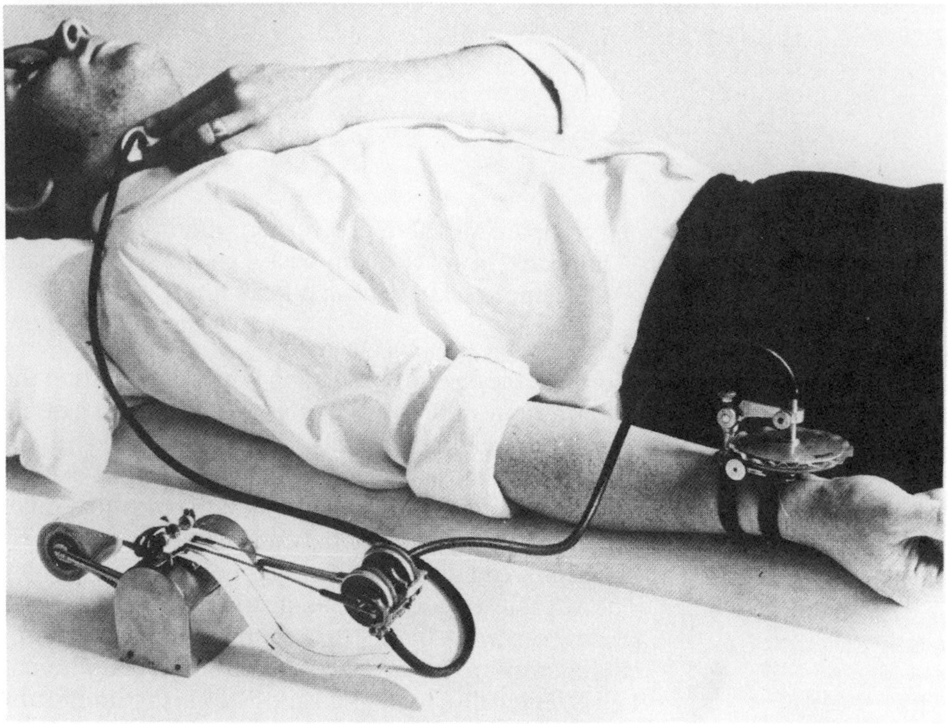

Figure 1-1. *Mackenzie's ink-writing polygraph inscribing the radial arterial and jugular venous pulsations. (Courtesy of the Wellcome Trustees)*

ence-dissociation in myographic tracings of rabbits, cats, and dogs poisoned with digitalis, although the complicated name of the clashing double rhythm was not given to this arrhythmia until 1923 by Mobitz.[4]

Since the electrocardiogram is merely the graphic inscription of electrophysiologic events, it is germane to read what was known of electrophysiology circa 1900, as collated by Wiggers.[5] DuBois-Reymond had recognized that action-currents reflected potential difference between the interior and the exterior of the skeletal muscle cell. As early as 1899, Samojloff, Einthoven's Russian friend, published an estimate of 60 to 80 mV as being 60% of the actual transmembrane potential difference. In 1902, Overton postulated that excitation of the skeletal muscle cell depends on a shift of sodium and potassium ions. He was perplexed that by the age of 70 years a human heart had contracted a quarter of a billion times, yet the ionic balance in the cardiac cell was unchanged. Julius Bernstein went on to write a monograph on the membrane theory. Augustus D. Waller clearly perceived that electrical activity in the heart preceded mechanical contraction.

Marey in 1876[6] had established the existence of the refractory period of cardiac muscle. He invented the term and learned that after the heart contracted, the refractory period lasted longer than that of skeletal muscle or nerve. (This long action potential of cardiac muscle, states Burn,[7] serves "to prevent fibrillation among fibers which are out of phase.") A. J. Carlson[8] first used the terms *absolute* and *relative frequency period.* Both Gaskell (1883) and Engelmann (1897) recognized that conduction in the hearts of warm-blooded animals was myogenic. By 1893, Wilhelm His, Jr. had described the atrioventricular (AV) bundle and logically postulated that it ferried atrioventricular conduction. Purkinje had put his pupil, Palicke, to study the unusual muscle cells seen in the sheep's heart, and by 1845, they had described the fine ramifications of the conduction system. By 1900, Engelmann, Wenckebach, and Bowditch had promulgated the axioms of cardiac muscle, characterizing it by (1) automaticity, (2) a refractory period, (3) an all-or-none reactivity to stimuli of diverse strengths, and (4) the treppe phenomenon after excitation.[5]

Ventricular fibrillation had been first recognized by Erichsen in 1842, and Oskar Langendorff had watched it in his isolated, perfused-heart preparation in 1898. Atrial fibrillation had been studied clinically as early as 1827. Cushny in 1903 learned that poisonous doses of digitalis could provoke ventricular fibrillation. Hering demonstrated in 1900 that excess potassium in the perfusate of the isolated-heart preparation arrested ventricular fibrillation. Following the potassium with Locke's solution reinstituted sinoatrial rhythm. Sidney Ringer proved that calcium ion was needed for cardiac contraction.

Extrasystoles

Because of its very brevity, one may surmise that the detection of the extrasystole would have to await the discovery of the string galvanometer. Nevertheless, in

1876, Marey,[6] the French genius of cardiac physiology, showed that the ventricle was excitable by artificial stimuli during diastole but refractory during systole. Knoll[9] in 1872 delineated the compensatory pause of premature ventricular contractions (PVCs) as equal to twice the original cardiac cycle, but it was Engelmann,[10] working with the frog's heart, who explained that the next atrial impulse falls during the refractory period set up by the PVC, making the ventricle await the next atrial stimulus. Engelmann coined the term *extrasystole* and also demonstrated that atrial extrasystoles reset sinoatrial rhythm. Wenckebach[11] noted atrial extrasystoles in humans, as did Cushny.[12]

Kraus and Nicolai[13] first registered extrasystoles with the electrocardiograph. They explained the premature beat as being caused by the contraction of a single ventricle, later called *hemisystole.* Mackenzie accepted this concept. Lewis[14] quashed this error by simultaneous tracings of the venous pulse and the electrocardiogram, studies that enabled him to become the bridge between Mackenzie and Einthoven. Junctional extrasystoles shown in venous pulse tracings were published by Pan[15] in 1904.

Extrasystoles, considered in Lewis's time to be an active usurpative arrhythmia, are today believed to be forced by the preceding sinoatrial contraction. Despite the frequency of extrasystoles (trillions must have been recorded since Einthoven), Langendorf, Pick, and Winternitz[16] did not enunciate their "rule of bigeminy" until 1955. In 1960, Shinji Kinoshita[17] described the "rule of multiple interectopic sinus impulses." The same phenomenon was espoused by Schamroth and Marriott[18] in 1961; their designation was "concealed bigeminy or trigeminy" caused by concealed ventricular extrasystoles from a focus that was at least semiprotected.

Atrial Fibrillation

Robert Adams, better known by his Adams-Stokes eponym, was probably the first to recognize atrial fibrillation and mark it in 1827 as a sign of mitral stenosis.[19] So common was rheumatic heart disease in England at the time that some 50 years later George Balfour[20] wrote "extremely irregular action (of the heart) is almost pathognomonic of mitral stenosis." (The saintly William Osler, more gifted in refining clinical-pathologic nosology than physiology, called delirium cordis the result of multiple irregularly recurring extrasystoles. For the first time in the eighth edition [1912] of his celebrated textbook, there appears a section titled "Fibrillation of the Heart.")

Meanwhile, Marey[21] in 1863 had published a pulse tracing of atrial fibrillation from a patient with mitral stenosis. Mackenzie[22] conceived the atria to be immobile and paralyzed, allowing the cardiac rhythm to originate in the AV node, because his polygraph could record no jugular pulsations in patients with atrial fibrillation. H. E. Hering[23] in 1903 called the arrhythmia *pulsus irregularis perpetuus.* In 1908, his subsequent article[24] demonstrated the electrocardiograms of two patients with atrial fibrillation. Inexplicably, he declared atrial activity to be invisible on the electrocardiogram. Rothenberger and Winterberg[25] in 1909 first used the term *Vorhofflimmern* (fibrillation of the auricles). In the same year, Thomas Lewis[26] published a brief paper, titled "Auricular Fibrillation: a Common Clinical Condition," in which he labeled the f waves. He emphasized that digitalis slowed the ventricular rate "by enhancing a previously existing auriculo-ventricular heart block." In 1906, Einthoven's paper on the clinical use of the electrocardiograph contained an inscription of atrial fibrillation but without any hints as to the nature or significance of irregularity.[27] Gossage and Braxton Hicks[28] in 1913 first recognized that atrial fibrillation could occur transiently or permanently in normal hearts.

It is remarkable that Engelmann in 1894[29] had theorized that atrial fibrillation was caused by multiple foci in the atria. Nevertheless, Thomas Lewis[30] became convinced that an irregular circus movement caused atrial fibrillation. He reported that he had been influenced by A. G. Mayer's demonstration of a self-perpetuating contraction wave in a ring of jellyfish tissue. In order to clarify the mechanism, David Scherf[31] in 1948 injected aconitine into the head of the sinus node to induce atrial fibrillation that could be reverted by local cooling. Like Engelmann, he was convinced that high-frequency heterotopic foci were responsible for atrial fibrillation, not circus movement, a conviction he had held for 20 years.[32]

In 1951, Prinzmetal[33] and his co-workers used high-speed cinematography, later studied in slow motion, to actually see the fibrillating atria, which they described as being activated by "hetero-rhythmic large and small waves occurring simultaneously at rapid and irregular rates. No circus movement was found."

Finally, the ventricular response to atrial fibrillation was found to be related to exit block by Söderström.[34] The computer was used by Bootsma[35] and co-workers to analyze the R-R intervals, with the conclusion that the random nature of the ventricular rhythm is due to the "effect of randomly spaced atrial impulses of random strength reaching the A-V node from random directions." The arrhythmia that was once well-nigh pathognomonic of mitral stenosis remains a physiologic mystery, despite the computer.

Atrial Flutter

The most eye-catching of all the arrhythmias is atrial flutter. In 1887, MacWilliam[36] saw fluttering atria in a dog with his naked eye. "The application of (faradic) current sets the auricle with a rapid flutter," he wrote. In 1905, William Ritchie[37] first recorded flutter on the ink-polygraph from a patient whose complete heart block fortunately enabled the atrial flutter to be recognized. In 1909, Jolly and Ritchie[38] were fortunate to be able to restudy the same patient, now using the electrocardiograph. However, in 1906 Einthoven[39] had unknowingly recorded atrial flutter with 2:1 block by laying over 1.5 km of wire to connect the galvanometer in his laboratory to the patient bedded in the Academic Hospital in Leiden. In 1913, Thomas Lewis[40] enunciated the criteria for the electrocardiographic diagnosis—the restless, sawtooth baseline and the inverted, regular, identical P waves in leads II and III.

Prinzmetal[41] and group in 1952 pointed out that atrial flutter was often atypical. Peaked P waves in the anterior leads were not always visible, and an isoelectric interval between P waves could sometimes be seen.

Lewis[30] and co-workers in 1921 showed that in flutter a circus movement circled down the right atrium and up the left atrium. This was confirmed in 1947 by Cabrera and Sodi-Pollares,[42] using the Lewis bipolar electrogram method. Rytand's[43] direct exploratory activation-mapping of a human heart exposed for surgical operation was also confirmatory. Wellens,[44] however, could not find a circus movement in an exposed heart, and Prinzmetal's[41] studies showed a normal P wave axis in at least 15% of flutter, raising the question of reentry or circuits involving the right internodal tracts, but not a circus movement.

Vectorcardiographic studies of P loops by the Rosen and Damato groups[45] working in concert did not identify the secret mechanism of common or uncommon atrial flutter in humans.

Supraventricular Tachycardia

Supraventricular tachycardia (SVT) fortunately afflicts the healthy, in whom the sudden acceleration and abrupt termination nearly guarantee an acute awareness in the individual affected or corroboration by an observer. Cotton[46] in 1867 and 1869 described the first few instances of SVT, and by 1888, Bristowe[47] had studied nine patients with SVT, some of whom suffered from serious heart disease. In 1899, Bouveret[48] employed the term *tachycardie essentielle paroxystique* to describe this arrhythmia, and by 1900, Augustus Hoffmann,[49] having amassed 135 cases of SVT, had teutonically composed an entire monograph on *Die paroxysmale Tachycardie.*

Both Gaskell[50] and Engelmann,[10] immured in the myogenic theory of cardiac conduction, early insisted that only the sinoatrial area could act as such a rapid pacemaker, a remarkable insight. However, because Czermak[51] in 1868 had stopped SVT by vagal pressure, and since polyuria was deemed related to the medulla oblongata, the theory of vagal neurosis was not discarded.

Polygraphic pulse tracings by Winternitz[52] in 1886 first established that SVT consisted of a series of atrial extrasystoles. Thus, the soil was tilled for Thomas Lewis[53] to demonstrate in 1909 that SVT could have its origin experimentally and clinically in either the atrium or the AV junction. By 1925, in his epochal third edition of *The Mechanism and Graphic Registration of the Heart Beat,*[54] Lewis had described all the electrocardiographic *Feinschmeckerei* of the expert.

Although Vidella[55] in 1947 first described and named the posttachycardia syndrome, his perceptive observation had to wait 5 years for Mayerson and Clagett[56] to call it to our attention.

Although Lewis believed a circus movement generated atrial fibrillation and flutter, he declined to accept it as the mechanism in SVT, mainly because of the slower rate in the latter and the inability of the small-sized atrium to accommodate a circus wave of needed speed. Both David Scherf[57] (1947) and the Prinzmetal[41] group (1952) accepted the focal atrial origin of SVT.

Of all the atrial arrhythmias, SVT, particularly junctional tachycardia, gives characteristic evidence on the electrocardiogram of a rapidly activating ectopic focus. Evidence is accumulating that the 1928 model of Schmidt and Erlanger[58] for reentry as a mechanism for the genesis of SVT is still valid.

In 1959, Bernard Lown[59] did a great service by emphasizing that paroxysmal atrial tachycardia (PAT) with block was a sign of either digitalis toxicity or was induced by hypokalemia.

Complete Atrioventricular Block

A convulsive fit startles all bystanders and imprints on the memory. It is therefore no wonder that complete heart block is the most ancient arrhythmia to be recognized and that it was already known at a time when the physician was served only by his five senses. When, following the seizure, a remarkable slowness of the pulse was recognized, heart block became evident even to the novice. Gaskell[60] originated the self-explanatory term in 1883, 10 years before the conduction system was discovered.

Morgagni (1761); Spens (1793), Burnett (1825), Adams (1827), Mayo (1838), Gibson (1839), Holbertson (1840), and finally Stokes (1846) all contributed to characterization of the Adams-Stokes syndrome. Huchard[61] first used the double-barreled eponym, calling it Stokes-Adams disease despite his writing "noted first by Adams and then Stokes." Gibson's paper, Arthur Bloomfield[62] wrote, is the most thorough and thoughtful of them all.

Galabin[63] in 1875 published the first graphic record of heart block, an apex cardiogram, which he thought was the result of mitral stenosis. Nevertheless, he suggested that the atria and ventricles contracted independently. Chauveau,[64] although a veterinarian, described a man with heart block, and found he could produce AV dissociation in the horse by stimulating the peripheral end of the cut vagus.

Fortune smiled on Wilhelm His, Jr.[65] in that it is a rare occurrence for the experimenter to reap the clinical harvest of his own researches. He not only described the AV conduction system in 1893, but in 1899 was the first to document a patient with heart block with syncope, presenting polygraph tracings of arterial and venous pulsations.[66] Mackenzie in 1902 did the same. He translated Gaskell's *heart block* into *Herzblock.*

Osler was not able to fit together the pieces of bradycardia, syncope, and the bundle of His, so he persuaded Joseph Erlanger[67] to take physiologic tools to the beside to record the apex impulse (with Marey's cardiograph) and the radial pulse with his own recording sphygmomanometer. Erlanger and Blackman[68] also created chronic heart block with an adjustable clamp in dogs as models for Adams-Stokes attacks. In three dogs, syncope was produced not by asystole but by ventricular tachycardia. Parkinson, Papp, and Evans[69] in 1941 found the same phenomenon in human Adams-Stokes attacks as had Robinson and Bredeck[70] in a single case in 1917.

Einthoven recorded the first electrocardiogram of complete heart block in 1906, and Thomas Lewis obtained one in 1910. Two years later, A. E. Cohn and Lewis[71] published the electrocardiograms and autopsy of a patient who died of complete heart block. Fibrosis of the main bundle and right bundle branch was found. This is an early and unusual verification by autopsy of an electrocardiogram. Hay[72] in 1905 had also published an autopsy showing disease of the AV bundle in a patient with AV block. Unfortunately, arrhythmias other than heart block are not subject to autopsy verification.

Complete heart block, occurring most frequently in senior citizens, had been assumed to be caused mainly by ischemic heart disease, until Yater (1935), Lev (1958), and Lenegre (1963) clarified the nonischemic etiology in favor of purely mechanogenic and degenerative lesions.

Ventricular Tachycardia

Ventricular tachycardia (VT) is an electrocardiographic latecomer. Although VT had been induced by Panum[73] in 1862 by injecting tallow into the coronary arteries, and the mechanism had been theorized upon by Lewis[74] in 1909, an electrocardiographic registration from a patient stricken with myocardial infarction was first published by Robinson and Herrmann[75] in 1921.

The simulation of VT by PAT with aberration is the *cloaca maxima* of confusion in electrocardiology. Adding to the confusion are several items. First, VT is known to occur in normal hearts.[76] Second, the criteria for diagnosis established by Langendorf and Pick[77]—AV dissociation plus capture beats or fusion beats among bizarre ventricular complexes—may have exceptions, as they emphasized. In addition, there is that electrocardiographic *rara avis,* bidirectional VT caused by digitalis intoxication. Some doubt as to the ventricular origin of this rarity is offered by Zimdahl and Kramer,[78] who demonstrated that carotid sinus stimulation obliterated the upward-directed complexes, suggesting that the inhibited focus lay above the bifurcation of the bundle of His.

Lewis[74] in 1909 had noted that coronary artery ligation provoked PVCs and VT. It is astonishing to realize that this genius of cardiology failed to appreciate that he had induced myocardial infarction, the disorder that would eventually kill him after three tries, at age 46, 54, and 64.

Although the term *vulnerable period* is now deeply rooted in our daily coronary care unit lingo, the concept is only a half century old. Louis Katz[79] in 1928 first emphasized the danger of PVCs falling on the T wave. Ashman and David Scherf agreed. Wiggers[80] in 1940 repeated Lewis's experimental causation of VT by coronary artery ligation, which now made clinical sense.

Smirk[81] found that many patients (over 300 by 1969) showed the R-on-T phenomenon. These patients were subject to lethal VT and sudden death, which he had anticipated from his prior animal experiments. He also described the "cardiac ballet," an arrhythmia that appeared chaotic but actually consisted of recurrent multifocal ventricular complexes caused by asynchronous conduction and refractoriness.

It is now generally agreed that VT is created by a short-coupled PVC and is usually identifiable on the coronary care unit monitor.

Ventricular Fibrillation

Ventricular fibrillation (VF) was first described by Erichsen[82] in 1842, induced by a faradic current by Ludwig and Hoffa[83] in 1850, and depicted vividly by MacWilliam in 1887.[36] The label *mouvement fibrillaire* was attached by Vulpian in 1874.[84]

The earliest electrocardiogram of human VF (questioned by some) was published by August Hoffmann[85] in 1912; VF terminated the VT. Since VF in many ways seemed analogous to atrial fibrillation, Lewis[14] proferred his concept of a circus movement. Fast on his heels, DeBoer[86] first provoked VF in the frog ventricle by a single shock late in systole; he also favored reentry as the mechanism of VF. His work was corroborated in 1940 when the concept and naming of the vulnerable period was firmly established by Wiggers and Wegria.[87] They induced VF by a single, localized induction and condenser shock applied during the vulnerable period of ventricular systole. With Moe,[88] in 1941 they found an increased duration of the vulnerable period in premature ventricular beats.

The evolution of ventricular fibrillation from ventricular tachycardia was fortunately presented by a patient during an Adams-Stokes episode. Kerr and Bender[89] in 1922 recorded that quinidine given to a patient with complete heart block induced VT that degenerated to VF. The electrocardiogram of their patient showing VF is the first undisputed example.

Atrioventricular Junctional Rhythm

In 1903, Engelmann[90] experimentally induced junctional rhythm in the frog heart by a ligature that isolated the sinus venosus and caused the atria and ventricles to beat simultaneously. Atrioventricular extrasystoles were described by Hering[91] in 1906. Lewis[92] induced junctional rhythm in the dog's heart by cooling the sulcus terminalis. He published an electrocardiogram of junctional tachycardia in humans in 1909, but gave priority to Belski. Lewis stressed the inverted P waves in leads II and III as a proof of junctional pacemaking.

Parasystole

It was the ingenious idea of Kaufmann and Rothberger[93] in 1919 that an ectopic focus could be protected from suppression by the normal cardiac pacemaker. This led to their defining parasystole in order to explain how certain extrasystoles and tachycardias could maintain autonomy independently of the dominant rhythm. They theorized, in seven papers written over 6 years, that the ectopic center, constantly active and nearly perfectly rhythmic, was protected by a unidirectional block similar to that which is normally present in AV junctional tissue. It was considered an entrance block, to which there is added an exit block, so that the ectopic focus is protected throughout its complete cycle. They clearly described the interectopic interval, the varied coupling time, and the *Schutzblokierung* (protection).

Sick Sinus Syndrome

Sinoatrial (SA) block was described by Mackenzie[94] in 1902 during an epidemic of influenza. At first thought to be a benign vagal phenomenon, SA block is now considered to be part of the sick sinus syndrome. In 1912, Cohn and Lewis[95] reported an instance of Adams-Stokes attack from sudden asystole in a patient subject to paroxysmal atrial fibrillation. In 1916, Samuel Levine[96] described four patients with sinoatrial arrest following paroxysmal atrial fibrillation. By 1951, Pick and colleagues[97] instilled meaning to this phenomenon as expressed in the title of their article, "Depression of Cardiac Pacemakers by Premature Impulses."

However, except for Short's[98] early (1954) and neglected article, titled "The Syndrome of Alternating Bradycardia and Tachycardia," paroxysmal atrial fibrillation, sinus bradycardia, sinoatrial arrest, sinoatrial exit block, and carotid sinus hypersensitivity were all considered unrelated nuisances. When Lown[99] in 1967 recognized that inadequate sinus node function at times appeared after cardioversion for atrial fibrillation, he coined the alliterative term *sick sinus syndrome.* Both Short and Lown recognized that since untampered atrial fibrillation was the natural cure of the sick sinus syndrome, these patients were better off without cardioversion.

In 1968, M. Irene Ferrer[100] popularized the sick sinus syndrome. However, she did not then include the bradycardia-tachycardia syndrome.

The ECG often showed intra-atrial block or a spatial orientation of the P wave different from the usual, suggesting takeover pacemaking not far from the diseased SA node. Posttachycardia bradycardia that shows delayed sinoatrial activation is also significant. Most often, however, the usual electrocardiogram was not diagnostic.

Studies using the Holter monitor, determining the SA nodal recovery time, and the induction of atrial premature depolarizations are useful for theoretical and patient-care problems, as demonstrated by Mandel.[101]

Concealed Conduction

T. W. Engelmann[102] in 1894 sagaciously noted after visual observation of a frog's heart that a blocked atrial contraction was followed by prolonged AV conduction. Erlanger[67] in 1905 noted concealed conduction in his studies on complete heart block. Engelmann and Erlanger postulated that the delayed conduction was caused by incomplete penetration of the junctional tissues causing partial refractoriness. In 1925, Lewis and Master[103] carefully studied incomplete penetration, and Ashman,[104] on this side of the Atlantic, did the same in the turtle heart.

The electrocardiogram was first used in the study of concealed conduction in atrial flutter with 2:1 block showing long and short cycles by Kaufmann and Rothberger[105] in 1927.

The importance of concealed conduction as the key to many arrhythmias, however, was submerged until 1948 when Richard Langendorf[106] published "Concealed A-V Conduction: the Effect of Blocked Impulses on the Formation and Conduction of Subsequent Impulses," with the definition stated in the title. He was truly the Sherlock Holmes of the arrhythmias. Popularization, however, was delayed until 1956, when Katz and Pick[107] further emphasized the mechanism and outlined its details. Soon it was obvious that incomplete penetration could merely delay conduction, speed up conduction, cause block, slow down a pacemaker, or establish QRS aberrancy. Concealed conduction offered explanations for otherwise unexplainable electrical events in the surface electrocardiograms. Experimental evidence of concealed conduction was demonstrated by Hoffman, Cranefield, and Stuckey[108] in 1961 to take place in any part of the conduction system. They truly revealed the concealed impulse.

Söderström[34] pointed out in 1950 that the irregular ventricular response in atrial fibrillation is often owing to concealed conduction, and Moe and Abildskov[109] in 1964 gave more sophisticated evidence to support this.

Reentry

It is now recognized that reentry is not limited to the conduction tissues but can take place in any area of the heart. This concept, so vital to the understanding of the generation of the tachyarrhythmias, was demonstrated by D. Scherf and C. Schookhoff[110] in 1926 by showing that experimental extrasystoles can return in the AV node and again activate the atria. They developed the idea that longitudinal dissociation exists in the AV node, allowing conduction up one half and down the other.

Joseph Erlanger,[58] the American physiologist who later became a Nobel laureate, had studied cardiac conduction in Adams-Stokes disease. He published a graphic model for the reentry mechanism in which he recognized that reentry required both slowed conduction and unidirectional block. Moe[111] first demonstrated dual pathways in the AV node of animals in 1956.

Exit Block

In order to explain why a parasystolic focus did not make its anticipated appearance late in diastole, in 1920, Kaufmann and Rothberger[112] and Singer and Winterberg[113] independently developed the concept of exit block. A conduction disorder involving failure of a cardiac pacemaker of any kind to propagate and depolarize adjoining myocardium, the exit block may be gradual (Wenckebach) or sudden (Mobitz).

Wenckebach and Mobitz Block

The AV block that is progressively lengthened until an atrial complex is not conducted was first seen in the frog's heart by Engelmann[102] in 1894. Wenckebach,[114] Engelmann's pupil, described this complicated arrhythmia in humans in 1899 from an insightful analysis of radial arteriograms and clearly showed that the greatest increase in conduction time occurred in the second complex of the group beats. He also reported that Luciani had observed this phenomenon in the frog heart in 1872. Wenckebach called the pauses in the radial pulse Luciani periods. David Scherf[115] reminds us that in radial and venous pulse tracings sent by a friend to Wenckebach, he found dropped beats without AV hesitation.

In a brilliant but neglected study, John Hay[116] in 1906 published venous and arterial pulse tracings, clarified by laddergrams, that also showed normal atrioventricular conduction followed by absence of ventricular activation. He believed the cause to be "depression of excitability." In 1924, Mobitz[117] found Wenckebach periods (which he called type I) and the block described by Hay in the same patient. The latter arrhythmia he named type II. It soon became apparent that Mobitz type I was a physiologic block and that type II was caused by serious infra-AV nodal disease, as guessed by Wenckebach.[114]

Today, despite Hay's priority and despite Wenckebach's manifold genius, these blocks are called Mobitz I and Mobitz II. So perished a noble eponym.

Ventricular Aberration

That quicksand of electrocardiography, ventricular aberration, was defined first by Thomas Lewis.[118] His famous book illustrates the varieties of aberration from permanent in bundle branch block, to variable in atrial fibrillation and flutter, to the single supraventricular extrasystole. He was acutely aware of the dilemma of deformed ventricular complexes caused by PAT that resembled VT.

However, it remained for Gouaux and Ashman[119] in 1947 to clarify the mechanism of aberration by relating it to the refractory period and cycle length. "Aberration occurs when a short cycle follows a long one because the refractory period varies with cycle length," they wrote. Also stressed was the longer effective refractory period of the right bundle branch. Since then, the Ashman phenomenon has found a secure niche in arrhythmology.

It is of interest and encouragement to remember that aberration was recognized clinically even before experimental verification by Moe and colleagues[120] that the refractory period of the right bundle was longer than that of the left bundle.

Wolff-Parkinson-White Syndrome

Because of inexplicable paroxysmal atrial fibrillation, a young athlete was referred to Paul Dudley White in 1928. The only abnormality that could be found was in the electrocardiogram, which revealed a short PR interval of only 100 msec and an abnormal QRS resembling bundle branch block. Since gymnastic workouts had at times caused the tachycardia, the patient was asked to run up and down four flights of stairs. Unexpectedly, his electrocardiogram reverted to normal, with a PR of 160 msec and a normal QRS at a heart rate of 120. After the patient had rested, his electrocardiogram again became abnormal, and again reverted to normal after an injection of atropine was given. Once, when the tracing was normal, carotid sinus massage induced the abnormality of short PR and long QRS.

Dr. White's search of his files unearthed six similar cases. Puzzled by these unusual electrocardiograms, he carried them with him on a tour of foreign medical centers. In Vienna, the experts dampened White's enthusiasm by interpreting the abnormality as ordinary bundle branch block plus AV nodal rhythm. However, in London, Sir John Parkinson, intrigued sufficiently to search his own files, found five additional instances, which he mailed to White. The report by Wolff, Parkinson, and White[121] in 1930 caused much head scratching and file searching by interested electrocardiographers. In 1915, Frank Wilson had published "a case in which the vagus influenced the form of the ventricular complex of the electrocardiogram," [122] which described the patient's "four distinct rhythms and at least three types of ventricular complexes." Franklin Johnston[123] tells that after reading the WPW article, Wilson went back to his 1915 work and found that his fourth figure was a replica of the new syndrome. Similar earlier examples were found in reports by Wedd in 1921[124] and separately by Bach[125] and Hamburger[126] in 1929.

The theory of an accessory conduction pathway between atria and ventricles bypassing the AV node was postulated independently by Holzmann and Scherf in 1932[127] and by Wolferth and Wood[128] a year later, based on Kent's anatomic discovery in animals published in 1893 and known to anatomists as the bundle of Kent.[129] The theory was confirmed in 1942 by the ingenious work of Butterworth and Poindexter,[130] who transmitted greatly amplified action currents from the SA node to the ventricle of a cat. This electromechanical bypass of the AV node inscribed electrocardiograms resembling the WPW syndrome. By reversing the conduction pathway and sending amplified impulses from the ventricle to the atrium, bursts of tachycardia ascribable to reentry were generated. The explorations by Wilson's group of the hearts of patients with known WPW syndrome pointed to premature activation of the dorsal wall of the ventricle. Fortunate were they that their patients' tracings showed alternating normal and anomalous conduction.[131]

Wood and colleagues[132] in 1943 and Ohnell[133] a year later proved the WPW syndrome by autopsy demonstration of bypass bundles. The Wood paper was based on a tragic case of a young boy who died of tachycardia complicating his WPW syndrome. In 1967 Ferrer[134] found sufficient studies by his own group and others to review the panorama of the basic variants of preexcitation: the classic WPW, the Lown-Ganong-Levine syndrome, and the Mahaim type. The Lenegre[135] group was able to show multiple bypasses in certain patients, sometimes latent and sometimes severally active.

His bundle electrophysiologic studies truly clarified the WPW conundrum (see chapter 13).

Torsade De Pointes

If the WPW syndrome is likened to the Columbus of the arrhythmias because the original 11 cases have generated thousands of investigations into the new world of bypass tracts and reentry, the atypical ventricular tachycardia named torsade de pointes (twisting of the points) by Dessertenne[136] in 1966 may be considered the Cinderella of the arrhythmias. Dessertenne had become interested in the bizarre patterns of ventricular fibrillation inscribed during cardiopulmonary resuscitation. A woman of 80 years, long afflicted with complete heart block, entered his service at the Lariboisiére Hospital because of Adams-Stokes attacks resulting in convulsions. Digitalis was discontinued. Procainamide, isoproterenol, and ephedrin were not helpful. Hydroxyzine hydrochloride, potassium, and propranolol gave only transient surcease. After ventricular asystole left the woman a neurologic cripple, her family took her home to die.

The three-channel electrocardiographic tracings showed the characteristics of torsade de points, which Dessertenne described as "a tachycardia whose frequency is 200 per minute, which displays alteration of the direction of the QRS complexes every 2 seconds, so that they successively point upwards and downwards." In another section, he writes that "the same phenomenon just described, recurring at a frequency of 200 per minute, with the difference that the amplitude of the QRS complexes now varies in a more definitely sinusoidal pattern. The first three torsades are especially interesting. Each lasts for about three seconds. . . . The complexes occurring during the transition between torsades maintain the same frequency. . . . This phenomenon of sinusoidal variation in the amplitude recalls the undulating phase of ventricular fibrillation described by Wiggers in his animal experiments."

Dessertenne sagaciously suggested that "the occurrence of phasic variation in the electrical polarity of the QRS complexes during the arrhythmia could be explained by postulating two ventricular foci, one initiating QRS complexes pointing upwards, the other initiating complexes pointing downwards . . . The transition from one focus to the other generates a torsade de pointes."[137]

Unique as was Dessertenne's report, time soon revealed earlier recognition of torsade without the catchy name. Examples were found in MacWilliam[138] in 1923 and in Schwartz and associates in 1949[139] and 1954,[140] the latter work stressing the association of torsade with bradycardia and prolongation of the QT interval.

Ironic is the appreciation of late that all class 1 antiarrhythmic drugs, so therapeutic in many arrhythmias, can evoke torsade in patients with normal QT interval. And were it not so tragic in a world one third hungry, one might find comic overtones in the instances of lethal torsade caused by liquid-protein reducing diets.[141]

Conclusion

The foregoing pages have exhumed many landmarks in the history of the arrhythmias. Can any conclusions be considered? First and foremost, it is evident that advances were made step by slow step, not by a Vesuvian breakthrough. Second, it is likely that the electrocardiogram, truly the Ariadne thread to the arrhythmias, will maintain its worth and not be a flash by meteor as was the ballistocardiogram.

However, there were a few dissonant voices. P. M. Rautaharju, in a paper excitingly titled "Highways, Byways and Deadends in Electrocardiographic Research," declared "There is too much information in the ECG and VCG for analysis by a human reader." Alan C. Burton[142] concluded: "The science of electrocardiography is not purely empirical, but is based on fundamental experiments and physical laws: However, its enormous usefulness in clinical diagnosis has a basis that is almost empirical. Electrocardiography is like bird-watching, which depends not on theory, but on rules."

References

1. Olmsted, J. M. D.: Claude Bernard, Physiologist, p. 25. New York. Schuman, 1938.
2. Shapiro, E.: Engelmann and his laddergram. Am. J. Cardiol. 39:464, 1977.
3. Cushny, A. R.: On the action of substances of the digitalis series on the circulation in mammals. J. Exp. Med., 2:223, 1897.
4. Mobitz, W.: Zur Frage der atrioventrikularen Autonomie. Die Interferenz Dissoziation. Dtsch. Arch. klin. Med., 141:257, 1923.
5. Wiggers, C. J.: Cardiac physiology of 50 years ago. Circ. Res., 5:121, 1957.
6. Marey, E. J.: Des excitations éléctriques du coeur. In Physiologie Experimentale. Travaux de Laboratorie de M Marey, vol. 2, p. 63. Paris, Masson, 1876.
7. Burn, J. H.: The relation of the autonomic nervous system to cardiac arrhythmias. Prog. Cardiovasc. Dis., 2:334, 1960.
8. Carlson, A. J.: Comparative physiology of the invertebrate heart. VI. The excitability of the heart during the different phases of the heart beat. Am. J. Physiol., 16:67, 1906.
9. Knoll, P.: Ueber die Veränderung des Herzschlages bei reflectorischer Erregnung des vasomotorischen Nervensystems. Wiener Sitzungberichte der deutschen Akadamie der Wissenschafter, 66:195, 1872.
10. Engelmann, T. W.: Ueber den Urspring der Herzbewegung und die physiologischen Eigenschaften der grossen Herznerven des Frosches. Arch. Ges. Physiol., 65:109, 1896–1897.
11. Wenckebach, K. F.: Zur Analyse des unregelmässigen Pulses. Z. klin. Med., 39:293, 1900.
12. Cushny, A. R.: On the interpretation of pulse tracings. J. Exp. Med., 4:327, 1899.
13. Kraus, F., and Nicolai, G. F.: Ueber des Elektrokardiogramm unter normalen und pathologischen Verhältnissen. Berl klin. Wchnschr., 34:1, 1908.
14. Lewis, T.: The Mechanism and Graphic Registration of the Heart Beat, 3rd ed., p. 219. London, Shaw and Sons, 1925.
15. Pan, O.: Klinische Beobachtung über ventrikuläre Extrasystolen ohne kompensatorische Pause. Dtsch. Arch. klin. Med., 98:128, 1903.
16. Langendorf, R., Pick, A., and Winternitz, M.: Mechanisms of intermittent bigeminy. 1 Appearance of ectopic beats dependent upon the length of the ventricular cycle, the "rule of bigeminy." Circulation, 11:422, 1955.
17. Satou, T., Kinoshita, S., Tanabe, Y., et al.: Impulse conductivity in the region surrounding the extrasystolic focus: Wenckebach phenomenon of the coupling intervals, and the "rule of multiples." Saishin-Igaku [Modern Medicine], 15:1865, 1960 (in Japanese).
18. Schamroth, L., and Marriott, H. J. L.: Intermittent ventricular parasystole with observations on its relationship to extrasystolic bigeminy. Am. J. Cardiol., 7:779, 1961.
19. Adams, R.: Cases of diseases of heart accompanied with pathological observations. Dublin Hosp. Rep., 4:353, 1827.
20. Balfour, G.: Clinical Lectures on Diseases of the Heart and Aorta. p. 256. London, Churchill, 1882.
21. Marey, E. J.: Physiologie Mêdicale de la Circulation du Sang. p. 525. Paris, Delahaye, 1863.
22. Mackenzie, J.: The inception of the rhythm of the heart by the ventricle, as the cause of continuous irregularity of the heart. Br. Med. J., 1:529, 1904.
23. Hering, H. E.: Analyse des Pulses irregularis perpetuus. Prager med. Wchnschr., 38:377, 1903.
24. Hering, H. E.: Das Elektrocardiogram des Pulsus irregularis perpetuus. Dtsch. Arch. klin. Med. 94:205, 1908.
25. Rothenberger, C. J., and Winterberg, H.: Vorhofflimmern und Arrhythmia perpetuus. Wien. klin. Wchnschr., 22:839, 1909.
26. Lewis, T.: Auricular fibrillation: a common clinical condition. Br. Med. J., 2:1528, 1909.
27. Einthoven, W.: Le Télécardiogramme. Arch. Internat. Physiol., 4:132, 1906–1907.
28. Gossage, A. M., and Braxton Hicks, J. A.: On auricular fibrillation. Q. J. Med., 6:435, 1913.
29. Engelmann, T. W.: Refractäre Phase and kompensatorische Ruhe in ihrer Bedeutung für den Herzrhythmus. Arch. ges. Physiol., 59:309, 1894–1895.
30. Lewis, T., Drury, A. N., and Iliescu, C. C.: A demonstration of circus movement on clinical fibrillation of the auricles. Heart, 8:361, 1921.

31. Scherf, D., Romano, F. J., and Terranova, R.: Experimental studies on auricular flutter and auricular fibrillation. Am. Heart J., 6:241, 1948.
32. Scherf, D.: Versuche zur Theorie des Vorhofflatterns und Vorhofflimmerns. Z. ges. exp. Med., 61:30, 1928.
33. Prinzmetal, M., Oblath, R., Corday, E., et al.: Auricular fibrillation. J.A.M.A., 146:1275, 1951.
34. Södorström, N.: What is the reason for the ventricular arrhythmia in cases of atrial fibrillation. Am. Heart J., 40:212, 1970.
35. Bootsma, B. K., Hoelen, A. J., Strackee, J., et al.: Analysis of R-R intervals in patients with atrial fibrillation at rest and during exercise. Circulation, 41:783, 1970.
36. MacWilliam, J. A.: Fibrillar contraction of the heart. J. Physiol., 8:296, 1887.
37. Ritchie, W.: Complete heart block with dissociation of the action of the auricles and ventricles. Proc. R. Soc. Edinburgh, 25:1085, 1905.
38. Jolly, W. A., and Ritchie, W. T.: Auricular flutter and fibrillation. Heart, 2:177, 1910–1911.
39. Einthoven, W.: Le Télécardiogramme. Arch. Internat. Physiol., 4:132, 1906–1907, Fig. 32.
40. Lewis, T.: Observations upon a curious and not uncommon form of extreme acceleration of the auricle: "Auricular flutter." Heart, 4:171, 1913.
41. Prinzmetal, M., Corday, E., Brill, C., et al.: The Auricular Arrhythmias, p. 189. Springfield, Ill., Charles C Thomas, 1952.
42. Cabrera, C. E., and Sodi-Pollares, D: Discussion del movimento circular y prueba directa de su existencia en el flutter auricular clinico. Arch. Inst. Cardiol. Mex., 17:850, 1947.
43. Rytand, D.: The circus movement entrapped. Circus wave hypothesis and atrial flutter. Ann. Intern. Med., 65:125, 1966.
44. Wellens, H. J. J., Janse, M. J., Van Dam, R. T., et al.: Epicardial excitation of the atria in a patient with atrial flutter. Br. Heart J., 33:233, 1971.
45. Cohen, S. I., Koh, D., Lau, S. H., et al.: P loops during common and uncommon atrial flutter in man. Br. Heart J., 39:173, 1977.
46. Cotton, P.: Notes and observations upon a case of unusually rapid action of the heart. Br. Med J., 1:629, 1867.
47. Bristowe, J. S.: On recurrent palpitations of extreme rapidity in persons otherwise apparently healthy. Brain, 10:164, 1888.
48. Bouveret, L.: De la tachycardic essentielle paroxystique. Rév. Méd., 9:753, 1889.
49. Hoffmann, A.: Die paroxysmale Tachycardie. Wiesbaden, Bergmann, 1900.
50. Gaskell, W. H.: Observations on the innervation of the heart. Br. Med. J., 2:572, 1882.
51. von Czermak, J. N.: Ueber mechanische Reizung des Vagus bei Menschen. Prager Vierteljahrschrift, 100:30, 1868.
52. Winternitz, W.: Ein Beitrag zu den Motilitätsneurosen des Herzens. Berl. klin. Wchnschr., 20:93, 112, 1883.
53. Lewis, T.: The experimental production of paroxysmal tachycardia and the effect of ligation of the coronary arteries. Heart, 1:98, 1909.
54. Lewis, T.: The Mechanism and Graphic Registration of the Heart Beat. ed. 3, pp. 240–258. London, Shaw and Sons, 1925.
55. Videlia, J. G.: El sindrome electrocardiografico post-tachycardiaco. Rev. Argent. Cardiol., 14:30, 1947.
56. Mayerson, R. M., and Clagett, A. H., Jr.: Transient inversion of T waves after paroxysmal tachycardia. J.A.M.A., 143:193, 1952.
57. Scherf, D.: Studies on auricular tachycardia caused by aconitine administration. Proc. Soc. Exp. Biol. Med., 64:233, 1947.
58. Schmidt, F. O., and Erlanger, J.: Directional differences in the conduction of the impulse through heart muscle and their possible relation to extrasystolic and fibrillary contractions. Am. J. Physiol., 87:326, 1928–1929.
59. Lown, B., Marcus, F., and Levine, H. D.: Digitalis and the atrial tachycardias with block. N. Engl. J. Med., 260:301, 1959.
60. Gaskell, W. H.: On the innervation of the heart, with especial reference to the heart of the tortoise. J. Physiol., 4:43, 1883.
61. Huchard, H.: Maladies du Coeur et des Vaisseaux. p. 255. Paris, Octave Doin, 1889.
62. Bloomfield, A. L.: A Bibliography of Internal Medicine, p. 33. Chicago, University of Chicago Press, 1960.
63. Galabin, A. L.: On the interpretation of cardiographic tracings and the evidence they afford as to the murmurs attendant upon mitral stenosis. Guy's Hosp. Rep., 20:261, 1875.
64. Chauveau, A.: De la dissociation du rhythme auricularie et du rhythme ventriculaire. Rév. Méd., 5:161, 1885.
65. His, W., Jr.: Die Tätigkeit des embryonalen Herzen und deren Bedeutung für die Lehre von der Herzbewegung beim Erwachsenen. Arbeiten aus der medizinischen Klinik zur Leipzig, pp. 14–50, 1893.
66. His, W., Jr.: Ein Fall von Adams-Stokes'scher Krankheit mit ungleichzeitigen Schlagen der Vorhöfe und Herzkammern (Herzblok). Dtsch. Arch. klin. Med., 64:316, 1899.
67. Erlanger, J.: On the physiology of heart block in mammals, with especial reference to the causation of Stokes-Adams disease. J. Exp. Med., 7:676, 1905.
68. Erlanger, J., and Blackman, J. R.: Further studies on the physiology of heart-block in mammals. Heart, 1:117, 1904.
69. Parkinson, J., Papp, C., and Evans, W.: The electrocardiogram of the Stokes-Adams attack. Br. Heart J., 3:171, 1941.
70. Robinson, C. C., and Bredeck, J. F.: Ventricular fibrillation in man with cardiac recovery. Arch. Intern. Med., 20:725, 1917.
71. Cohn, A. E., and Lewis, T.: A description of a case of complete heart-block; including the postmortem examination. Heart, 4:7, 1912–1913.
72. Hay, J.: The pathology of bradycardia. Br. Med. J., 2:1034, 1905.
73. Panum, P. L.: Experimentale Beiträge zur Lehre der Emboli. Arch. Pathol. Anat., 25:308, 1862.
74. Lewis, T.: The experimental production of paroxysmal tachycardia and the effect of ligation of the coronary arteries. Heart, 1:98, 1909.
75. Robinson, G., and Herrmann, G.: Paroxysmal tachycardia of ventricular origin and its relation to coronary occlusion. Heart, 8:59, 1921.
76. Wilson, F. N., Wishart, S. W., Mcloed, A. C., et al.: A clinical type of paroxysmal tachycardia of ventricular origin in which paroxysms are induced by exertion. Am. Heart J., 7:155, 1932.
77. Langendorf, R., and Pick, A.: Differentiation of supraventricular and ventricular tachycardias. Prog. Cardiovasc. Dis., 2:391, 1960.
78. Zimdahl, W. T., and Kramer, L. I.: On the mechanism of paroxysmal tachycardia with rhythmic alteration in the direction of the ventricular complexes. Am. Heart J., 33:244, 1947.
79. Katz, L. N.: The significance of the T wave in the electrogram and the electrocardiogram. Physiol. Rev., 8:447, 1928.
80. Wiggers, C. J., Wegria, R., and Piñera, B.: The effects of myocardial ischemia on the fibrillation threshold—the mechanism of spontaneous ventricular fibrillation following coronary occlusion. Am. J. Physiol., 131:309, 1940.
81. Smirk, F. H.: R waves interrupting T waves. Br. Heart J., 11:23, 1949.
82. Erichsen, J. E.: On the influence of the coronary circulation on the action of the heart. London Med. Gaz., 2:561, 1942.
83. Hoffa, M., and Ludwig, C.: Eine neue Versuche über Herzbewegung. Z. rat., Med., 9:107, 1850.
84. Surawicz, B., and Steffens, T.: Cardiac vulnerability in complex electrocardiography. J. Cardiovasc. Clin., 5(3):160, 1973.
85. Hoffmann, A.: Fibrillation of ventricles at the end of an attack of paroxysmal tachycardia in man. Heart, 3:213, 1912.
86. DeBoer, S.: Die Physiologie und Pharmakologie des Flimmerns. Ergeb. Physiol., 21:1, 1923.
87. Wiggers, C. J., and Wegria, R.: Ventricular fibrillation due to

single localized induction and condenser shocks applied during the vulnerable phase of ventricular systole. Am. J. Physiol., 128:500, 1940.
88. Wegria, R., Moe, G. K., and Wiggers, C. J.: Comparison of the vulnerable period and fibrillation thresholds of normal and idioventricular beats. Am. J. Physiol., 133:651, 1941.
89. Kerr, W. J., and Bender, W. L.: Paroxysmal ventricular fibrillation with cardiac recovery in a case of auricular fibrillation and complete heart block while under quinidine sulfate therapy. Heart, 9:269, 1922.
90. Engelmann, T. W.: Der Versuch von Stannius, seine Folgen und deren Deutung. Arch. Anat. Physiol. (Physiol. Abtheilung), 505, 1903.
91. Hering, H. F., and Rihl, J.: Ueber atrioventriculare Extrasystolen. Z. exp. Pathol. Therap., 2:510, 1906.
92. Lewis, T.: Auricular fibrillation and its relationship to clinical irregularity of the heart. Heart, 1:306, 1909–1910.
93. Kaufmann, R., and Rothberger, C. J.: Beiträge zur Entstehungeweise extrasystolischer Allorhythmien. Z. ges. exp. Med., 7:119, 1919.
94. Mackenzie, J.: The cause of heart irregularity in influenza. Br. Med. J., 2:1411, 1902.
95. Cohn, A. E., and Lewis, T.: Auricular fibrillation and complete heart block. A description of a case of Adams-Stokes syndrome, including the post-mortem examination. Heart, 4:15, 1912–1913.
96. Levine, S.: Observations on sino-auricular heart block. Arch. Intern. Med., 17:153, 1916.
97. Pick, A., Langendorf, R., and Katz, L. N.: Depression of cardiac pacemakers by premature impulses. Am. Heart J., 41:49, 1951.
98. Short, D. S.: The syndrome of alternating bradycardia and tachycardia. Br. Heart J., 16:208, 1954.
99. Lown, B.: Electrical reversion of cardiac arrhythmias. Br. Heart J., 29:469, 1967.
100. Ferrer, M. I.: The sick sinus syndrome in atrial disease. J.A.M.A., 206:645, 1968.
101. Mandel, W. J., Hawakawa, H., Allen, H. N., et al.: Assessment of sinus node function in patients with the sick sinus syndrome. Circulation, 46:761, 1972.
102. Engelmann, T. W.: Beobachten und Versuche am suspendierten Herzen. Pfluegers Arch., 56:149, 1894.
103. Lewis, T., and Master, A. M.: Observations upon conduction in the mammalian heart. A-V conduction. Heart, 12:209, 1925.
104. Ashman, K.: Conductivity in compressed cardiac muscle; supernormal phase in conductivity in compressed auricular muscle in the turtle heart. Am. J. Physiol., 74:140, 1925.
105. Kaufmann, R., and Rothberger, C. J.: Der Uebergang von Kammerallorhythmien in Kammerarrhythmie in klinischen Fällen von Vorhofflattern. Alternan der Reitzleitung. Z. ges. exp. Med., 57:600, 1927.
106. Langendorf, R.: Concealed AV conduction: the effect of blocked impulses on the formation and conduction of subsequent impulses. Am. Heart J., 35:542, 1948.
107. Katz, L. N., and Pick, A.: Clinical Electrocardography. 1. Arrhythmias, p. 540. Philadelphia, Lea & Febiger, 1956.
108. Hoffman, B. F., Cranefield, P. F., and Stuckey, J. H.: Concealed conduction. Circ. Res., 9:194, 1961.
109. Moe, G. K., Abildskov, J. A., and Mendez, C.: An experimental study of concealed conduction. Am. Heart J., 67:338, 1964.
110. Scherf, D., and Shookhoff, C.: Experimentelle Untersuchingen ueber die "Umkehr-Extrasystole." Wien. Arch. inn. Med., 12:50, 1926.
111. Moe, G. K., Preston, G. B., and Burlington, H.: Physiologic evidence for a dual AV transmission system. Circ. Res., 4:357, 1956.
112. Kaufmann, R., and Rothberger, C. J.: Beiträge zur Entstehungeweise extrasystolischer Allorhythmien. 4 Mitteilung. Z. ges. exp. Med., 11:40, 1920.
113. Singer, R., and Winterberg, H.: Extrasystolen als Interferenzerscheinung. Wien. Arch. inn. Med., 1:391, 1920.
114. Wenckebach, K. F.: Zur Analyse des unregelmässigen Pulses. II Ueber den regelmässig intermitterenden Puls. Z. klin. Med., 37:475, 1899.
115. Scherf, D.: A cardiologist remembers. Perspect Biol. Med., 11:615, 1968.
116. Hay, J.: Bradycardia and cardiac arrhythmia produced by depression of certain of the functions of the heart. Lancet, 1:139, 1908.
117. Mobitz, W.: Ueber die unvollständige Störung der Erregungsüberleitung zwischen Vorhof und Kammer des menschlichen Herzens. Z. ges. exp. Med., 41:180, 1924.
118. Lewis, T.: The Mechanism and Graphic Registration of the Heart Beat. ed. 3, pp. 127–133. London, Shaw and Sons, 1925.
119. Gouaux, J. L., and Ashman, R.: Auricular fibrillation with aberration simulating ventricular paroxysmal tachycardia. Am. Heart J., 34:366, 1947.
120. Moe, G. K., Mendez, C., and Han, J.: Aberrant AV impulse propagation in the dog heart: a study of functional bundle branch block. Circ. Res., 16:261, 1965.
121. Wolff, L., Parkinson, J., and White, P. D.: Bundle branch block with short PR interval in healthy young people prone to paroxysmal tachycardia. Am. Heart J., 5:685, 1930.
122. Wilson, F. N.: A case in which the vagus influenced the form of the ventricular complex of the electrocardiogram. Arch. Intern. Med., 16:1008, 1915.
123. Johnston, F. D., and Lepeschkin, E. (eds.): Selected Papers of Dr. Frank N. Wilson. Ann Arbor, Mich., J. W. Edwards, 1954.
124. Wedd, A. M.: Paroxysmal tachycardia with reference to normotropic tachycardia and the role of the intrinsic cardiac nerves. Arch. Intern Med., 27:571, 1921.
125. Bach, F.: Paroxysmal tachycardia of forty-eight years duration and right bundle branch block. Proc. R. Soc. Med., 22:412, 1929.
126. Hamburger, W. W.: Bundle branch block. Four cases of intraventricular block showing interesting and unusual clinical features. Med. Clin. North Am., 13:343, 1929.
127. Holzmann, M., and Scherf, D.: Ueber Electrokardiogramme mit verkwezter Vorhof-Kammer-Distanz und positiven P-Zacken. Ztschr. f. Klin. Med., 121:404, 1932.
128. Wolferth, C. C., and Wood, F. C.: The mechanism of production of short PR intervals and prolonged QRS complexes in patients with presumably undamaged hearts: Hypothesis of an accessory pathway of auriculo-ventricular conduction (bundle of Kent). Am. Heart J., 8:297, 1933.
129. Kent, A. F. S.: Researchers on structure and function of mammalian heart. J. Physiol., 14:233, 1893.
130. Butterworth, J. C., and Poindexter, C. A.: Short PR interval associated with a prolonged QRS complex. A clinical and experimental study. Arch. Intern, Med. 69:437, 1942.
131. Rosenbaum, F. F., Hecht, H. H., Wilson, F. N., and Johnston, F. D.: The potential variations of the thorax and the esophagus in anomalous atrioventricular excitement (Wolff-Parkinson-White syndrome). Am. Heart J., 29:281, 1945.
132. Wood, F. C., Wolferth, C. C., and Geckler, G. D.: Histological demonstration of accessory muscular connections between auricle and ventricle in a case of short PR interval and prolonged QRS complex. Am. Heart J., 25:454, 1943.
133. Ohnell, R. F.: Pre-excitation, a cardiac abnormality. Acta Med. Scan. (Suppl.), 152:74, 1944.
134. Ferrer, M. I.: New concepts relating to the preexcitation syndrome. J.A.M.A., 201:162, 1967.
135. Brechenmacher, C., Laham, J., Iris, L., et al.: Etude histologique des voies anormales de conduction dans un syndrome de Wolff-

Parkinson-White et dans un syndrome de Lown-Ganong-Levine. Arch. Mal. Coeur, 67:507, 1974.
136. Dessertenne, F.: La tachycardie ventriculaire à deux foyers opposés variables. Arch. Mal. Coeur, 59:263, 1966.
137. De Léan, A: Translation of Dessertenne, F. (136), distributed by Editorial Office, Ann. Intern. Med., Philadelphia, Pa., with permission of Dr. André De Léan, Dr. Francois Dessertenne, and J. Ballière, Paris, France, October, 1980.
138. MacWilliam, J. A.: Some applications of physiology to medicine. II. Ventricular fibrillation and sudden death. Br. Med. J., 2:215, 1923.
139. Schwartz, S. P., Orloff, J., and Fox, C.: The prefibrillatory period during established auriculoventricular dissociation, with a note on the phonocardiograms obtained at such times. Am. Heart J., 37:21, 1949.
140. Schwartz, S. P., and Hallinger, L. N.: VI. Observations on the peripheral arterial pulse pressures in the course of transient ventricular fibrillation during established auriculoventricular dissociation. Am. Heart J., 48:390, 1954.
141. Singh, B. N., Gaarder, T. D., Kanagae, T., et al.: Liquid protein diets and torsade de pointes. J.A.M.A., 240:115–119, 1978.
142. Burton, A. C.: Physiology and Biophysics of the Circulation, 2d ed., p. 138. Chicago, Year Book Medical Publishers, 1972.

2

Gross Anatomy and Microscopy of the Conducting System

Robert H. Anderson, Siew Yen Ho, and Anton E. Becker

This work was supported in part by a grant from the British Heart Foundation. We are greatly indebted to our colleagues and collaborators who have been involved in many of the investigations abstracted in this review, notably, James L. Wilkinson, M.D., Kenneth R. Anderson, M.D., Arnold C. G. Wenink, M.D., and Audrey Smith, Ph.D.

Mrs. Christine Anderson helped considerably in compiling the manuscript.

The morphology and microscopy described in this chapter are for the most part an endorsement of the initial descriptions of the conduction system by Tawara[1] and Keith and Flack[2,3] and their refinement by Monckeberg[4] and Koch.[5,6] This fact should not be surprising. The methodology of those early investigations, microscopic study of serial sections, is the same as that used today. Why then should the results of investigation be any different? Indeed, descriptions of the morphology of conduction tissue have been remarkably consistent since its discovery. The disagreements that have developed in recent years have mostly been the result of interpretation of the morphologic findings in the light of electrophysiologic observations,[7,8] the latter themselves rarely being unequivocal.[9] Unfortunately, it is not possible to deduce the function of any cell by looking at it through a microscope.

The Sinus Node

Gross Morphology

Cardiologists were aware of the site of the "ultimum moriens" before its morphologic substrate was described by Keith and Flack.[3] Indeed, Wenckebach[10] gave a colorful description of a cruise off the coast of Scotland where he suggested to Keith that histologic study of the site of "ultimum moriens" may prove fruitful, particularly in view of the findings of Tawara[1] at the atrioventricular junction, which had already been confirmed by Keith.[2] The result of this histologic study was the discovery of the sinus node,[3] subsequently proved to be the cardiac pacemaker by the elegant anatomicoelectrophysiologic correlations of Lewis and colleagues.[11] In their initial publication, Keith and Flack[3] described the lateral position of the node in the terminal groove. This finding was endorsed by Koch,[5] who also described the variable extent of the tail of the node, which continued in the terminal groove toward the orifice of the inferior caval vein (Fig. 2-1). This lateral position of the node has been substantiated by most subsequent investigators.[12–14] The exception was Hudson,[15] who argued that the node was related in horseshoe fashion to the junction of the superior caval vein with the crest of the right atrial appendage. Our findings[16] largely confirm the opinion of those who observed the node in lateral position (Fig. 2-2), although in a minority of cases we found it arranged in horseshoe fashion (Fig. 2-3).

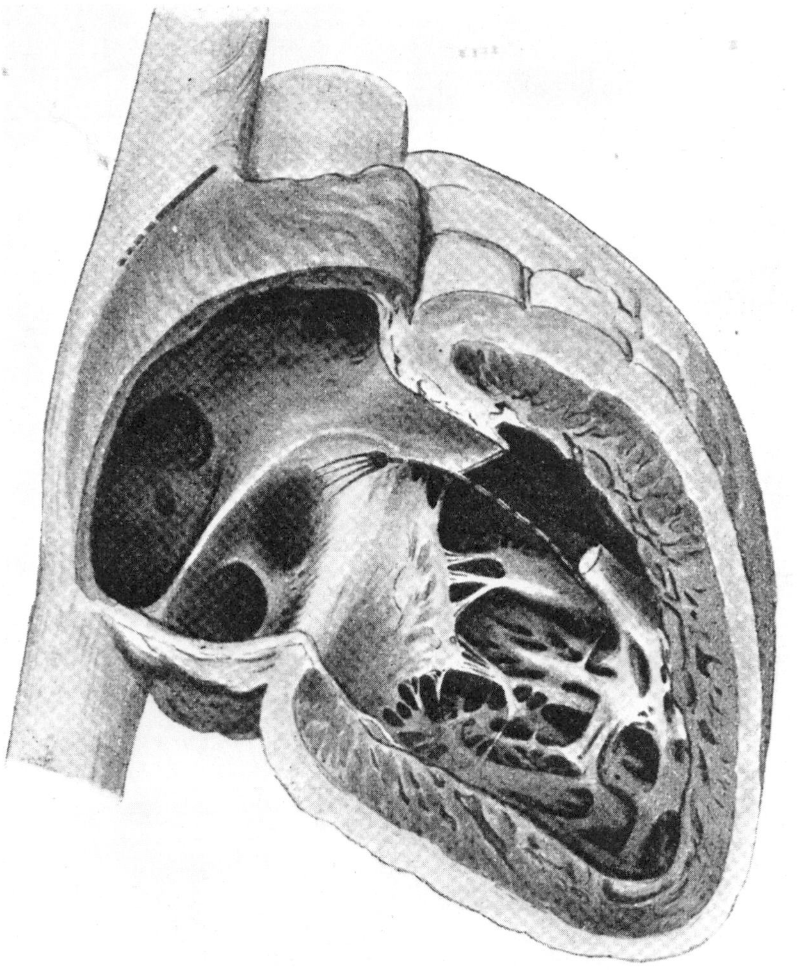

Figure 2-1. *Diagram taken from the publication of Koch showing the position of the sinoatrial node and the relations of the atrioventricular node to the triangle that now bears his name. (Koch, W.: Weitere Mitteilungen über den Sinusknoten des Herzens. Verk. Dtsch. Pathol. Ges., 13:85, 1909)*

As Truex has indicated,[12] the precise shape of the node as seen in sections varies, depending on the plane of section employed. In those at right angles to the terminal groove, the node is seen to form an immediately subepicardial wedge set into the junction of the wall of the superior caval vein with the terminal crest (Fig. 2-4). The wedge of tissue is usually most bulky anteriorly toward the crest of the atrial appendage, and it tends to taper as its tail passes posteriorly toward the inferior caval vein (see Fig. 2-2). Our serial reconstructions have shown a

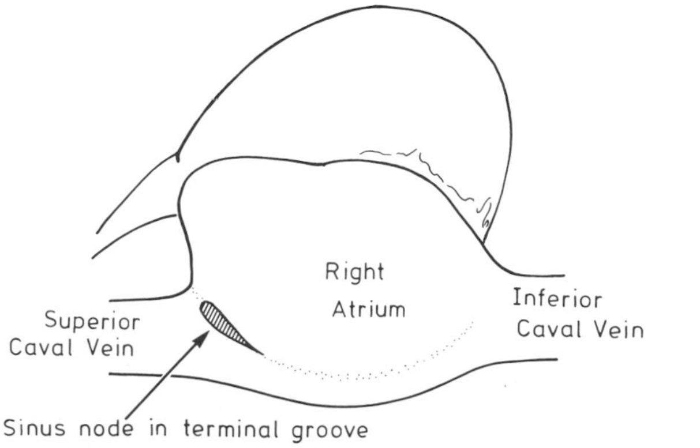

Figure 2-2. *Diagram of the heart in surgical orientation showing the lateral position of the sinus node.*

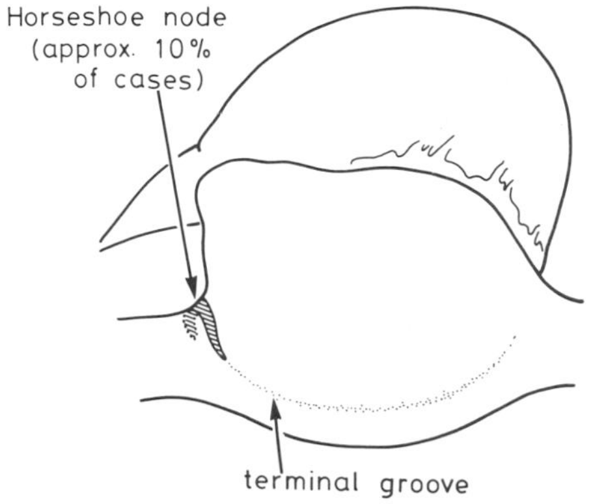

Figure 2-3. *Diagram illustrating the less usual disposition of the sinus node.*

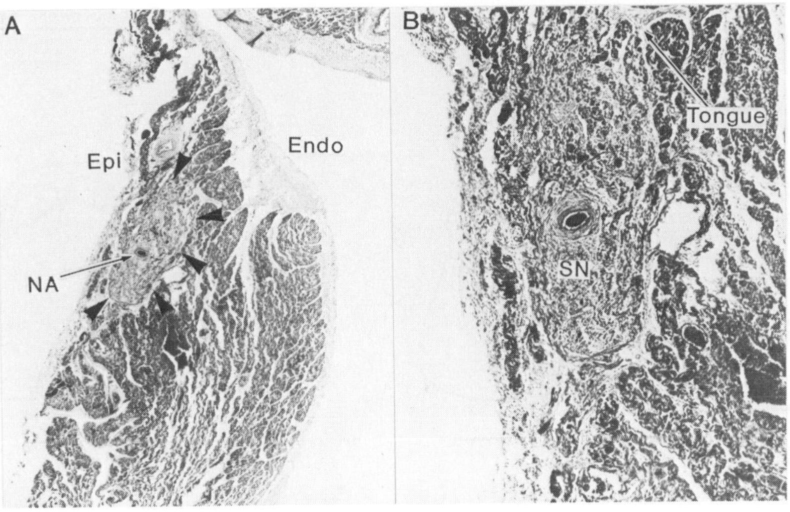

Figure 2-4. *Photomicrographs at low power (A) and enlarged (B) showing the relationships of the sinus node (labeled SN in B; between arrows in A) to the wall of the superior caval vein (SCV), the terminal crest (TC), and the epicardial (Epi) and endocardial (Endo) surfaces of the cavoatrial junction. The node is seen in a section at right angles to its long axis and the terminal groove and is arranged around a prominent nodal artery (NA). B shows a tongue of transitional cells extending into the atrial musculature.*

variable extent of the nodal tissue. In infant hearts it is usual for the tail to be extensive. It is rare to find an extension across the crest of the atrial appendage toward the interatrial band (Fig. 2-5).

The node is usually related to a prominent nodal artery that runs toward the node in the interatrial furrow, originating from the right coronary artery in 55% of cases and from the left coronary artery in the remainder.[14] James[14] has described how, in the human heart, the artery can then run clockwise or counterclockwise around the superior cavoatrial junction. Our serial reconstructions confirm and extend this observation.[16] In some cases arteries enter the node from both sides, forming an arterial circle around the junction (Fig. 2-8*A*). We have also found more variation in the origin of the nodal artery,[17] a feature noted previously by McAlpine.[18] Although the nodal artery arises from either the right or left coronary artery, and usually does so close to their origin (Fig. 2-6), it may also arise laterally from the right artery (Fig. 2-7*A*) or distally from the circumflex artery (Fig. 2-7*B*). These findings have major surgical significance, since they show that the *precise* disposition of the node

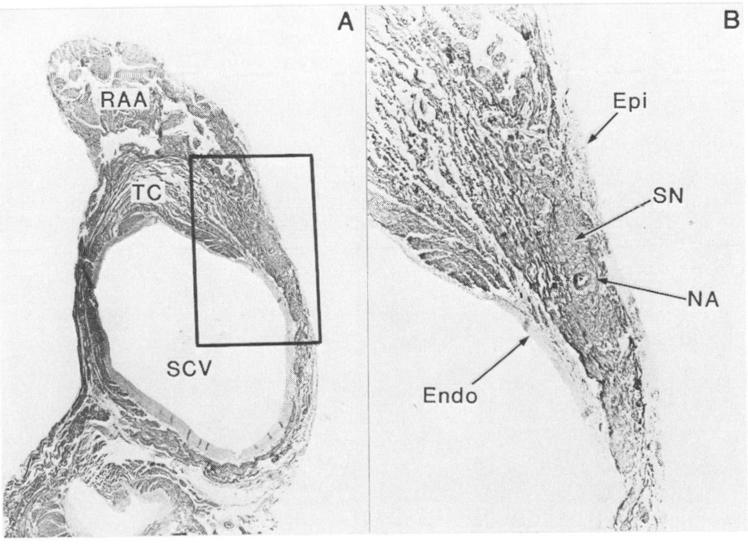

Figure 2-5. *Photomicrographs showing the relationship of the sinus node (SN) to the junction of the superior caval vein (SCV) and right atrial appendage (RAA). A is a low-power view, and B shows the magnified inset. The node is between the terminal crest (TC) and the caval musculature. (Epi, epicardium; Endo, endocardium; NA, nodal artery)*

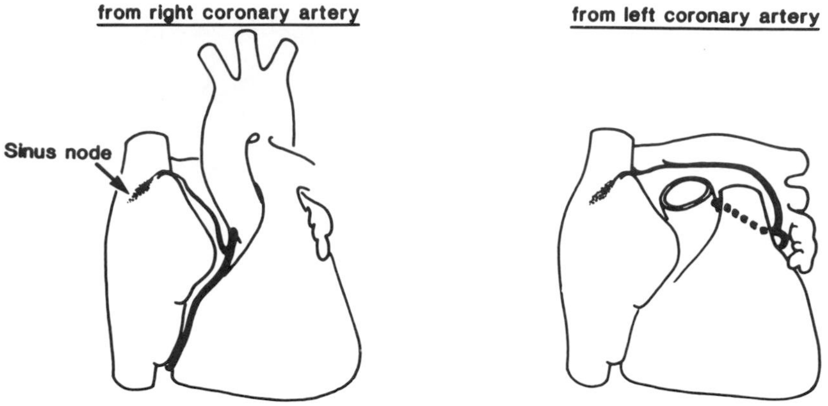

Figure 2-6. *Diagram illustrating the origin of the sinus node artery from the proximal portion of the right or left coronary arteries.*

and its arterial supply cannot be predicted with accuracy. The entire junction between the superior caval vein and the right atrium should be treated as a potential danger area. Care should also be taken to distinguish anomalous routes across the atrial walls. In addition to the variability in the course of the nodal artery, its relation to the nodal tissue is also variable. In only some cases does the artery run completely through the nodal substance. In other hearts it either ramifies within the nodal substance, runs an eccentric course through the node, or is not present as a prominent artery (Fig. 2-8*B*). It is difficult to reconcile these findings with the contention that the sinus node and its artery function as a servomechanism.[19]

Development

Various views have been expressed concerning development of the sinus node. Some hold it to be developed early[20,21]; others hold that it does not become recognizable morphologically until relatively late.[22,23] Some suggest that it is a derivative of the right side of a pair of specialized structures related to the sinus horns[24,25]; others suggest that it is a unilateral structure related to the right sinus horn.[26] Our own investigation[27] has demonstrated that a histologically discrete area can be recognized at the cavoatrial junction in the earliest embryos studied (Fig. 2-9). The position of this area corresponds approximately to the position of the definitive node, being marginally more extensive in the embryo. It does not occupy the entire sinoatrial junction (Fig. 2-10). We recognized such a histologically discrete structure only in relation to the superior caval vein. The area of the left sinus horn was devoid of tissue histologically discrete from the remainder of the atrial tissues. The size of the node relative to atrial tissues is greatest early in development. As the heart grows, the area occupied by sinus nodal tissue decreases relative to the remainder of the atrial bulk. From the earliest stages the nodal cells are set in a matrix of connective tissue. The volume of connective tissue within the node is small in the youngest embryos, but becomes more evident toward term.[27]

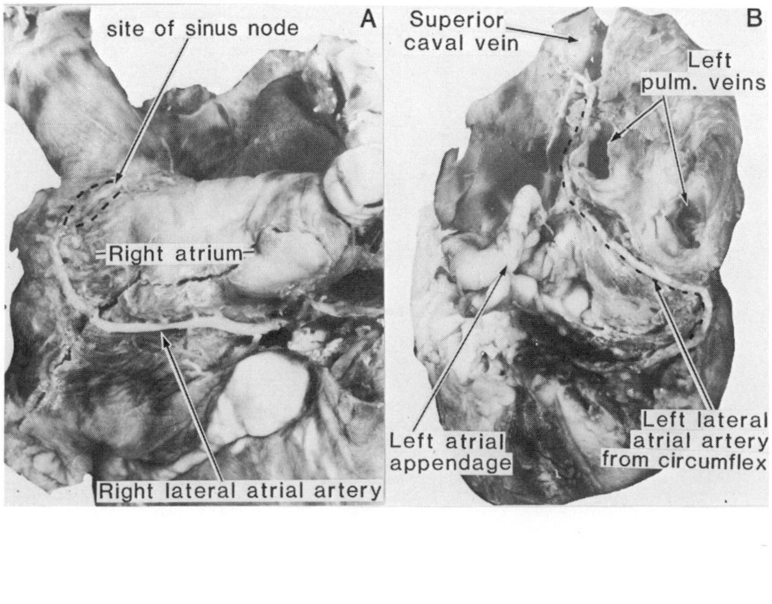

Figure 2-7. *Photographs of two dissected hearts that show the sinus node artery arising from a right lateral artery (A) and a left lateral artery (B).*

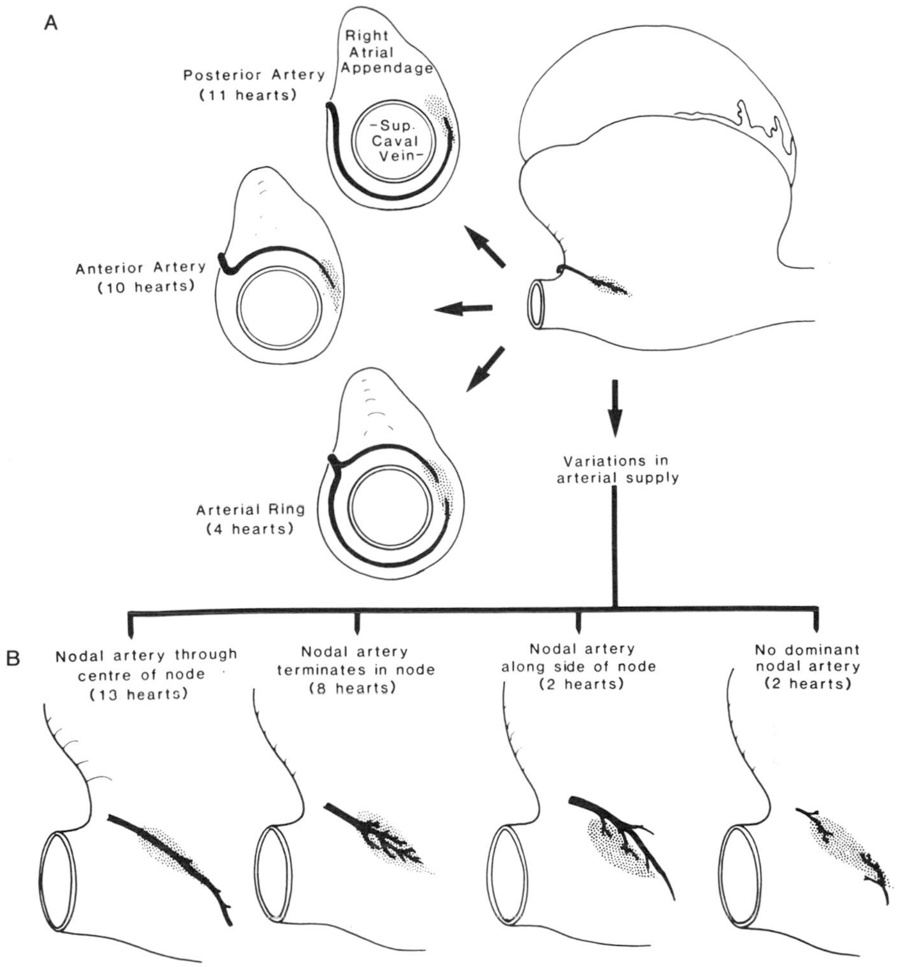

Figure 2-8. *Diagram showing variability in arterial blood supply to the sinus node as reconstructed by serial section techniques.*

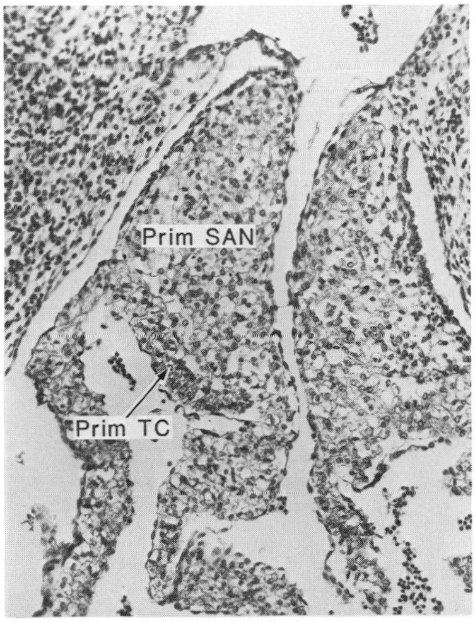

Figure 2-9. *Photomicrograph of the junction of the superior caval vein and right atrium in a 15-mm human fetus. The distinction between the cells that will become the node (Prim SAN) and those which will form the terminal crest (Prim TC) is already evident.*

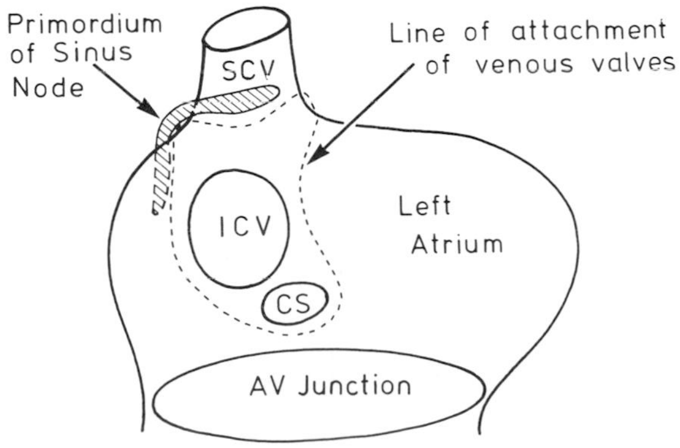

Figure 2-10. *Diagram illustrating the extent of the nodal primordium shown in Figure 2-9. The primordium is related only to the junction of the right atrium with the superior caval vein.*

Microscopy

The cells making up the sinus node are histologically discrete from the cells of the atrial myocardium and can be distinguished at low powers of magnification (see Figs. 2-5 and 2-6). The prominent nodal artery seen in most hearts and the fibrous tissue matrix are other good guides to nodal identification. The nodal cells are smaller than atrial myocardial cells. They are grouped together in interweaving fasciculi, the whole intermingling network of cells being set in the prominent fibrous matrix (see Fig. 2-5*B*). At the nodal surfaces that face the myocardium of the superior caval vein and the terminal crest, junctional zones are found between the nodal cells and the atrial myocardium. In some areas the margin between node and atrial myocardium is discrete (see Fig. 2-5*B*). In other areas, tongues of nodal cells extend for some distance into the atrial myocardium, merging by way of short zones of transitional cells into the myocardial zones. In these interdigitating zones, the overlapping of nodal and atrial cells can be interpreted as the presence of atrial cells within the confines of the node.[14] These zones of interdigitation are most frequently observed on the nodal surface that abuts against the terminal crest, but their precise distribution remains to be quantified. Our experience has mostly been with infant and developing tissues, and we have rarely observed the "large pale" atrial cells described by some as "Purkinje" cells.[14] The function and presence of these cells in the atria is contentious, and the use of the term *Purkinje* to describe them compounds the problem. To quote Truex,[12] "it is recommended that the term Purkinje cell be restricted and applied only to the specific cells of the ventricle which Purkinje described originally. The indiscriminate use of this term for large atrial cells leads not only to semantic problems but also connotes a functional pacemaker property that has never been established."

The true cellular content of the sinus node can best be established by using ultrastructural techniques in well-fixed material controlled by light microscopy. The latter point is essential so that the investigator can be sure he is sampling nodal material. These criteria have thus far been fulfilled only in animal tissues. The careful studies of Tranum-Jensen[28] have shown that the node of the rabbit is composed mostly of typical nodal cells. These

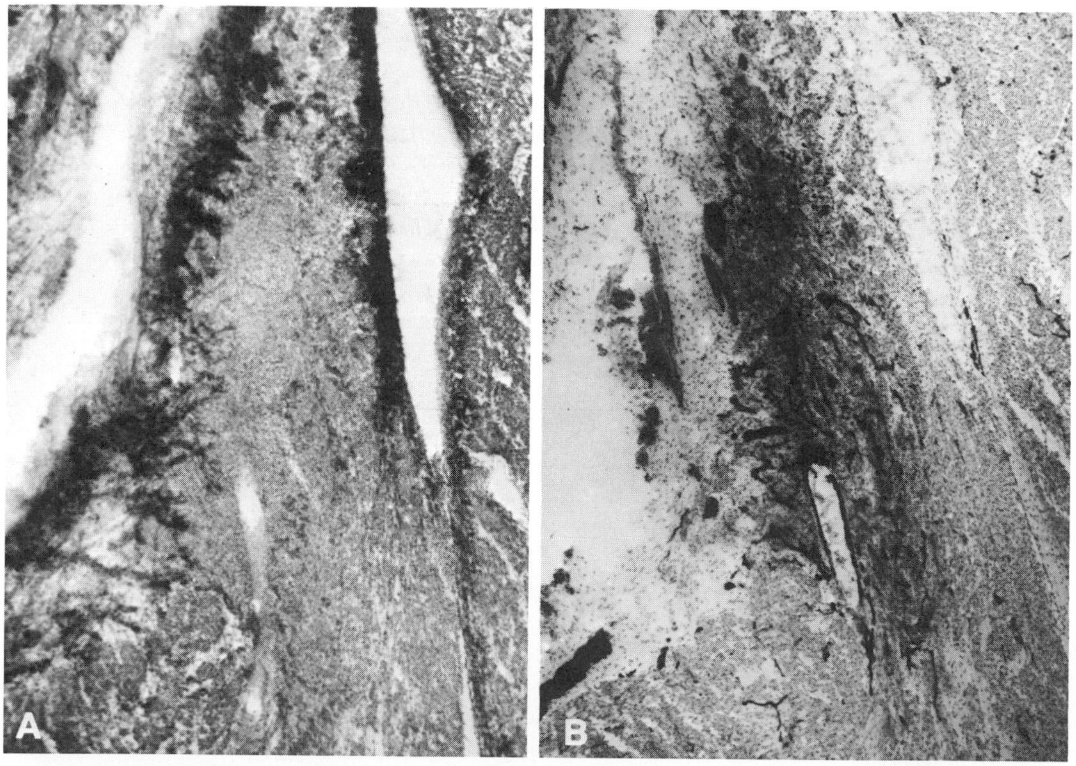

Figure 2-11. *Photomicrographs of the sinus node of a midterm human fetus sectioned at right angles to its long axis (compare with Fig. 2-4). A is stained routinely, and the node can be distinguished from atrial myocardium by its staining characteristics. B shows a section processed to demonstrate cholinesterase activity; the nodal cells themselves are cholinesterase positive and are abundantly supplied by cholinesterase-containing nerves.*

cells are irregular, roughly spindle shaped, and sometimes branching, with thin, tapering ends. They possess poorly developed contractile apparatus and randomly distributed mitochondria. The sarcoplasmic reticulum is less well developed than in the atrial myocardium, and a T-tubule system is lacking. However, as Tranum-Jensen points out, T-tubules are not universally observed in working atrial cardiocytes, and atrial "specialized cells" cannot therefore be defined according to the presence or absence of T-tubules. At the margins of the rabbit node, Tranum-Jensen observed transitional cells that differed from the typical nodal cells by containing more and better-organized myofibrils, together with a higher content of nexus junctions. Regarding the pale cells, or "intercalated clear cells," described in the human sinus node,[29] Tranum-Jensen opined from his own experience that the cells may be artifactual.

Innervation

There is general agreement that in animal species the sinus node can be distinguished from the working myocardium by its abundant supply of both adrenergic and cholinergic nerve fibers (see review by Yamauchi[30]). It is also known that considerable species variation exists in innervation pattern, and so results in animals may not be directly applicable to the human heart. Our studies in the developing human heart have shown an abundant cholinesterase-containing nerve supply that develops early and have also shown that the nodal cells themselves have a high cholinesterase content compared to the atrial myocardium (Fig. 2-11). To the best of our knowledge, evidence concerning the adrenergic innervation of the human heart and its development is at present lacking. In animals there is evidence that development of the adrenergic component lags considerably behind the cholinergic innervation.[31]

Internodal Conduction

Controversy concerning the anatomic substrates for conduction between the sinus and atrioventricular nodes is as old as the history of the conduction system itself. Some investigators[8] have suggested that Wenckebach[10] described an internodal tract. He certainly observed a bundle of myocardial fibers connecting the musculature of the superior caval vein to the muscle of the right atrial appendage, but he did this *before* the discovery of the sinus node. At the time, he believed that this bundle of myocardial fibers might conduct the impulse from the "ultimum moriens" to the atrial myocardium and that its division might result in sinuatrial block. When Keith and Flack[3] described the precise morphology of the sinus node, Wenckebach realized that his bundle could have no significance to sinuatrial block, as has been recounted by Lewis.[32]

The first real suggestion of a histologically discrete pathway between the nodes was made by Thorel.[33,34] He claimed to have traced a tract of "Purkinje" cells running along the terminal crest and connecting the nodes. This suggestion created sufficient interest to be debated at length in a session of the German Pathological Society held in 1910.[35] The consensus of this meeting was that Thorel had not shown unequivocal evidence of a histologically discrete pathway as he claimed. In the opinion of Aschoff,[36] Monckeberg,[37] and Koch,[38] the tissue between the nodes was composed of plain atrial myocardium and did not contain histologically discrete pathways separate from this myocardium. In an attempt to avoid subsequent disagreements, these observers suggested that investigators claiming to demonstrate atrial pathways should show them to be discrete in a fashion analagous to that seen in the atrioventricular conduction tissue axis. Despite this advice, authors such as Condorelli[39] and Franco[40] described atrial pathways using histologic criteria as tenuous as those of Thorel, but their suggestions were not generally accepted. The real impetus to a search for histologically specialized tracts came with the finding that not all cells in the atria had the same electrophysiologic characteristics.[41] Construing this to mean that specialized pathways had been demonstrated unequivocally using electrophysiologic techniques, James[8] stated that the problem to be investigated was not whether pathways existed but where they were. On the basis of subserial and dissection techniques, he described three "specialized pathways" connecting the nodes: anterior, middle, and posterior. As we interpret his writings, it seems that James described the entirety of the atrial septum and the terminal crest as these three specialized pathways.

The outstanding morphologic question concerning "specialized internodal pathways" is therefore remarkably simple. Does the area of the atrial septum and terminal crest contain tracts that have features distinguishing them histologically from other atrial myocardium, or is the myocardium of these areas itself different from the remaining atrial myocardium? No one has ever, to the best of our knowledge, suggested on the basis of morphologic observations that narrow tracts exist in the atrial septum and terminal crest that are in any way comparable with the atrioventricular bundle and bundle branches. The problem of the specialized pathways devolves simply on the criteria for specialization. The major criterion for James[8] was that the three described pathways, comprising the entirety of the atrial septum and the terminal crest, contained a high percentage of "Purkinje" cells, thus differentiating them from the rest of the atrial myocardium. We have already referred to the comments of Truex[12] concerning the nature of these

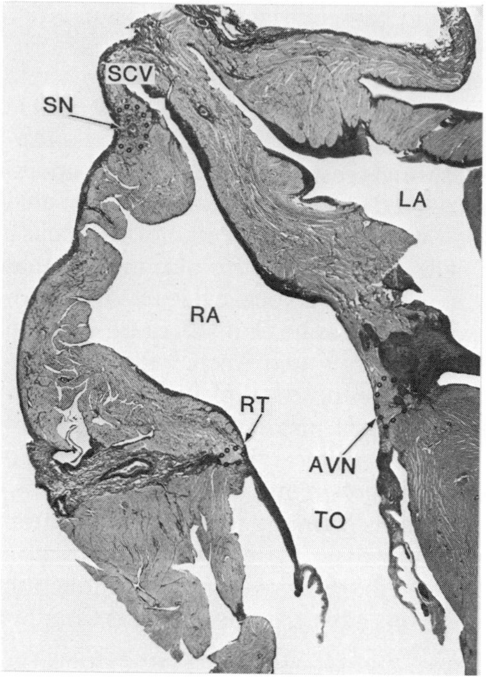

Figure 2-12. *Low-power photomicrograph of a section of the right atrium cut to transect both the sinus (SN) and atrioventricular (AVN) nodes. Both these structures can be easily recognized at low-power magnification. However, the muscle mass connecting the nodes cannot be distinguished by light microscopy from the remainder of the atrial myocardium. The segment of ring tissue (RT) at the lateral insertion of atrial myocardium into the tricuspid orifice (TO) can be recognized.*

so-called Purkinje cells. It is pertinent here to quote also his comments concerning the pathways.[12] He stated that:

> The present intensive search for anatomic evidence to substantiate the presence or absence of the much publicized atrial internodal tracts has been a tedious and time consuming task. Indeed we have looked at innumerable SAN and atrial myocardial cells in many hearts of several mammals, but alas, we have failed to delineate the widely acclaimed specific interatrial pathways. . . . It is concluded that bundles of regular atrial muscle cells are the predominant elements that provide cellular continuity between the SAN and AVN.

More recently, similar conclusions were reached by Lev and Bharati.[42] Chuaqui[43,44] had previously voiced these opinions following an extensive review of the literature and his own stereomicroscopic investigation. Thus, most modern investigators apart from James[45] substantiate the views of the early German researchers. Our own studies, mostly using fetal and infant hearts, are in keeping with this majority viewpoint. The small size of these specimens has enabled us to cut the entirety of the right atrium, including the atrial septum and the terminal crest, in a single block of tissue. In these sections, the sinus and atrioventricular nodes are easily distinguished by their histologic characteristics. They show unequivocal evidence of histologic specialization (Fig. 2-12). The remainder of the atrial tissues (apart from the atrioventricular ring specialized tissue, see below) shows no evidence of morphologic or histochemical specialization. As viewed through the light microscope, the atrial septum and terminal crest are composed solely of plain atrial myocardium. It was rare in our material to find large pale cells resembling so-called Purkinje cells. When present, such cells were also found in the tissues of the right atrial appendage and the left atrium. We therefore strongly endorse the opinions of Aschoff,[36] Monckeberg,[37] Koch,[38] Chuaqui,[43,44] Truex,[12] and Lev and Bharati[42] that there are *no* histologically discrete tracts of specialized conduction tissue extending between the sinus and atrioventricular nodes. The tissue conducting the impulse is best referred to as the *internodal atrial myocardium.* Nonetheless, it must be emphasized that although we are unable to identify histologically "specialized internodal tracts," this does not in itself rule out either preferential conduction of the cardiac impulse through the atrial myocardium or the possibility that cells with different electrophysiologic properties exist within the myocardium. The existence of preferential conduction is well established, but its pattern can be accounted for simply by the geometric arrangement of the muscle bundles of the right atrium[46–48] (Fig. 2-13). The behavior of given cells within the atrial myocardium

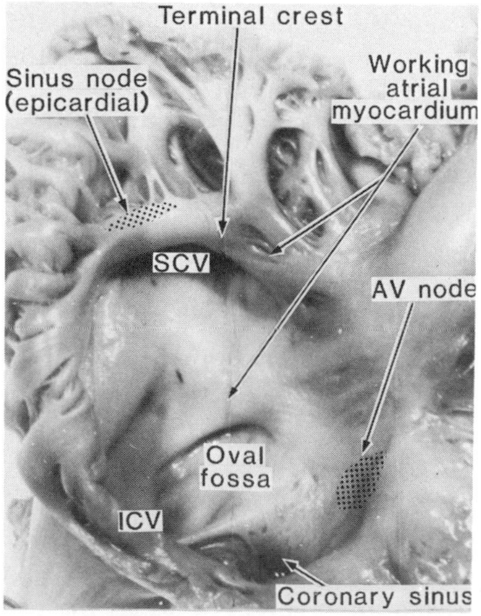

Figure 2-13. *The anatomy of the right atrium is that of a bag of holes. The simple geometric arrangement of the atrial myocardium accounts fully for the preferential conduction that certainly exists between the nodes.*[46]

is a different problem and may have no bearing on conduction within the atrium. The significance of this finding will be resolved only by performing marking experiments and studying the marked tissue with the electron microscope. Those experiments performed thus far have shown that plain atrial myocardial cells are able to produce both "working" and "specialized" action potentials.[49]

The Atrioventricular Junctional Area

The *atrioventricular junctional area* is the area of specialized conduction tissues forming the connection between the atrial and ventricular working myocardium.[50] It can be subdivided into various anatomic zones, namely, the atrioventricular node and its transitional cell zone, the penetrating bundle, and the branching atrioventricular bundle (Fig. 2-14). Opinion is by no means unanimous on the subdivision and extent of the zones of the specialized junctional area and on whether the branching bundle should be considered part of the junctional area.[51] These differences are entirely related to clinical correlations and can be resolved only by extensive anatomicoclinical correlations as yet unperformed.

Gross Morphology

The gross landmarks to the site of the atrial component of the specialized junctional area were well described by Koch.[5,6] He pointed out that the atrioventricular node was to be found toward the apex of a triangle formed by the continuation of the eustachian valve (the tendon of Todaro[52]), the septal attachment of the tricuspid valve, and the orifice of the coronary sinus (see Fig. 2-14). At the apex of this triangle the tendon of Todaro inserts into the central fibrous body. Immediately posterior to this is

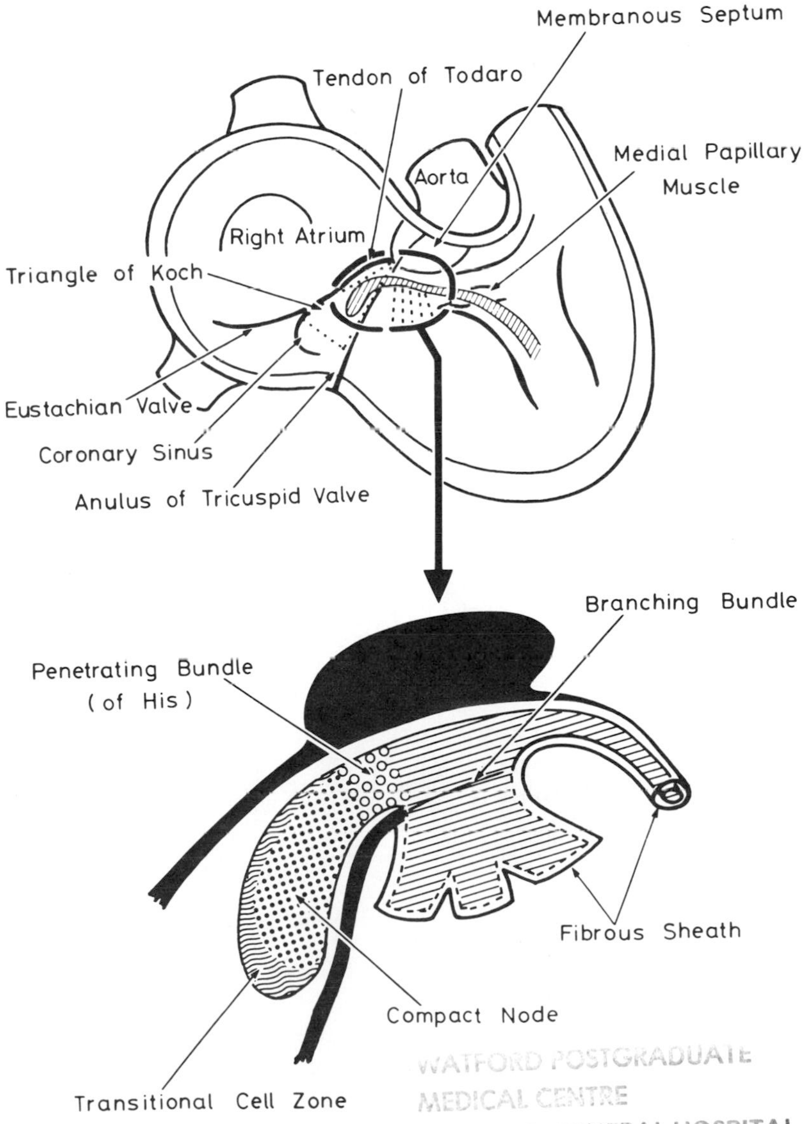

Figure 2-14. *Diagram illustrating the gross landmarks to the atrioventricular junctional area and its cellular components and zones.*

the site of penetration of the atrioventricular bundle. Having passed into the ventricular tissues, the axis branches on the crest of the muscular interventricular septum immediately subjacent to the interventricular component of the membranous septum. The left ventricular specialized tissues are immediately subendocardial on the septal surface of the ventricular outflow tract and cascade immediately beneath the noncoronary aortic leaflet. On the right ventricular side, the right bundle branch extends intramyocardially from the branching bundle. In the normal heart, the medial papillary muscle is an excellent guide to its position. These landmarks are of considerable value as guides to the conduction tissues during surgery, since in most living hearts the triangle of Koch springs into prominence when tension is placed on the eustachian valve. In fixed hearts at least, it is usually possible to see the left bundle branch as it extends down the left ventricular septal surface.

Development

Knowledge of the development of the atrioventricular junctional area aids considerably in the understanding of its subdivision and cellular architecture. Our interpretation of development is based on studies of developing hearts,[53] together with inferences drawn from studies of cases with congenitally complete heart block.[54] At the earliest stage of development, the atrial and ventricular myocardia are continuous all around the atrioventricular junction, with a ring of histologically discrete tissue forming the muscular junction (Fig. 2-15). The ring is particularly well seen in the developing tricuspid orifice. Within the ventricles themselves, the entire subendocardial layer of the trabecular zones of each ventricle is discrete from the compact myoblastic layer. The primordium of the branching bundle is located on the crest of the muscular septum, connecting with the subendocardial networks of both ventricles (Fig. 2-15). When traced posteriorly, this bundle runs an extensive course on the septum developing between the ventricular inlet portions. It bifurcates posteriorly to become continuous to either side with the specialized atrioventricular ring tissues (Fig. 2-16). The branching bundle and the bundle on the inlet septum develop in relation to different zones of the primary heart tube, the branching bundle at the inlet–outlet junction, and the bundle on the inlet septum.[54] In the normal heart, however, the axis is formed as a continuum so that the ventricular bundle branches are connected through the inlet septum to the posterior atrioventricular junction (Fig. 2-16). This is the disposition of conduction tissue before establishment of the definitive atrial septum. This stage, therefore, bears no resemblance to the arrangement in the mature heart; it is highly reminiscent of that seen in hearts with atrioven-

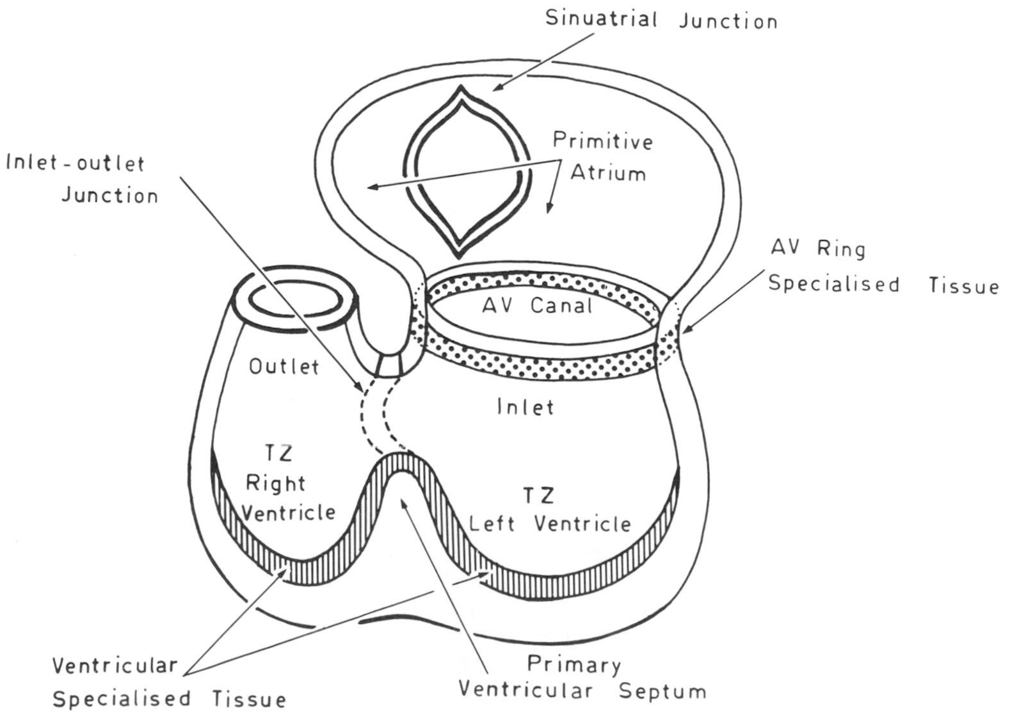

Figure 2-15. *Diagrammatic representation of the presumed disposition of tissues within the primary heart tube immediately following the looping process of the tube and growth of the ventricular trabecular zones (TZ).*

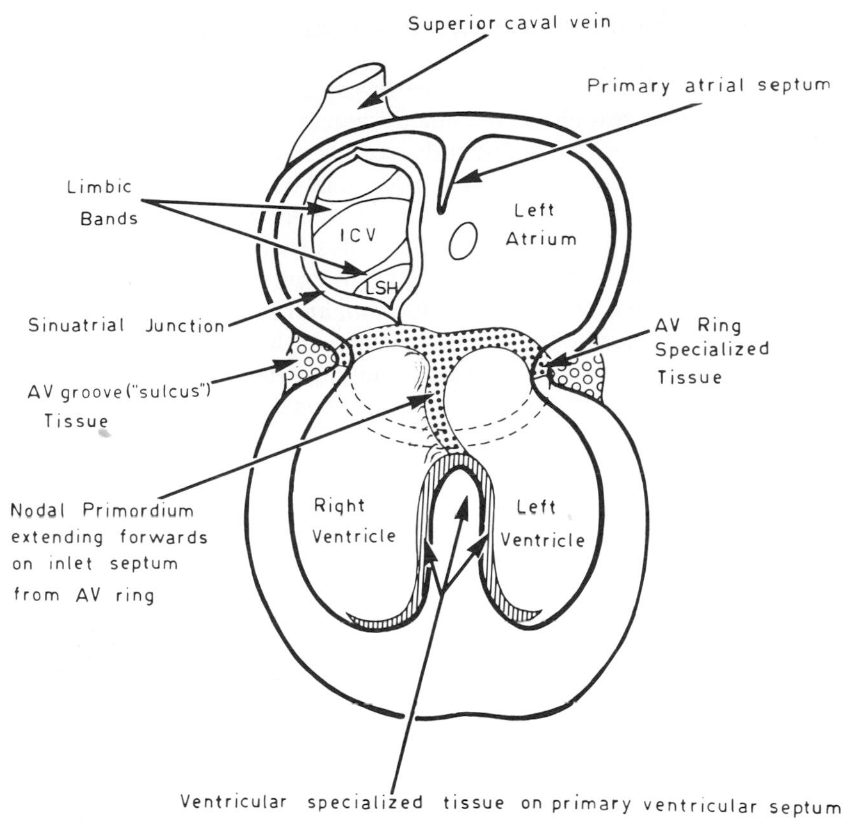

Figure 2-16. *Diagram showing how development of an inlet septum joins together the atrioventricular ring specialized tissue with the ventricular specialized tissues developed on the primary component of the muscular ventricular septum.*

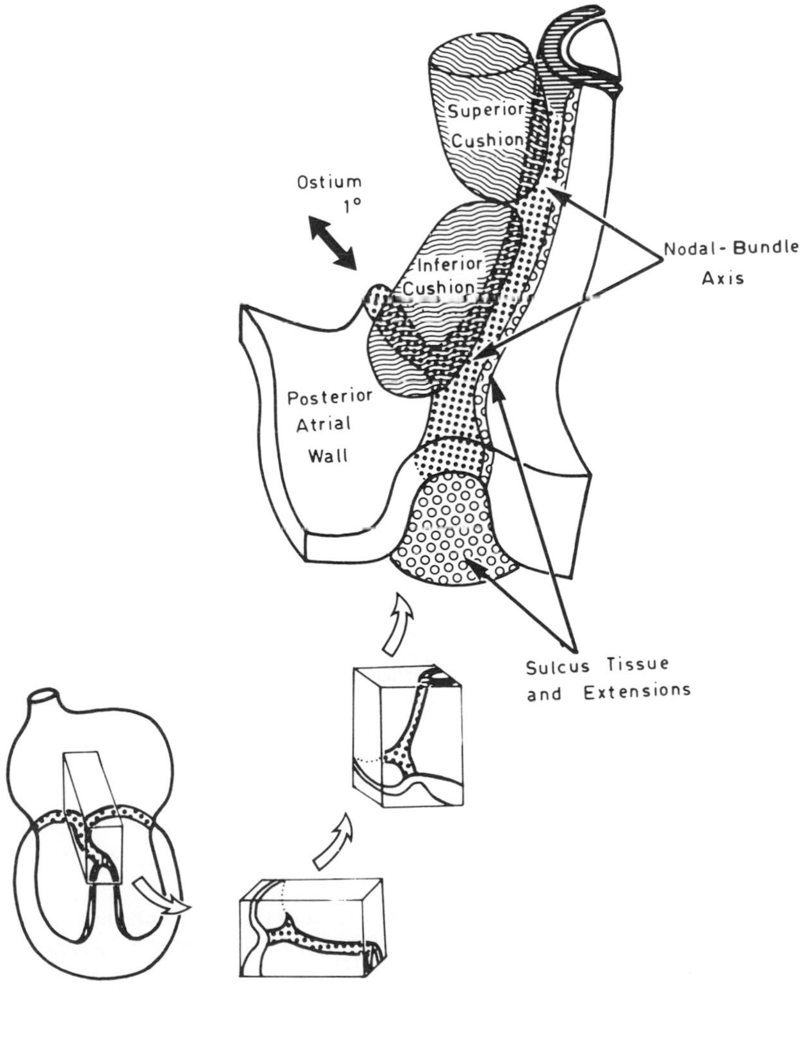

Figure 2-17. *Diagram showing how the bundle of tissue developed on the inlet septum (the nodal-bundle axis) forms the "meat" in a sandwich of the endocardial cushions (inside the heart tube) and the atrioventricular groove (sulcus) tissue (outside the heart tube). The insets show how the diagram is reoriented from the position of Figures 2-15 and 2-16 to correspond to the definitive orientation shown in Fig. 2-14.*

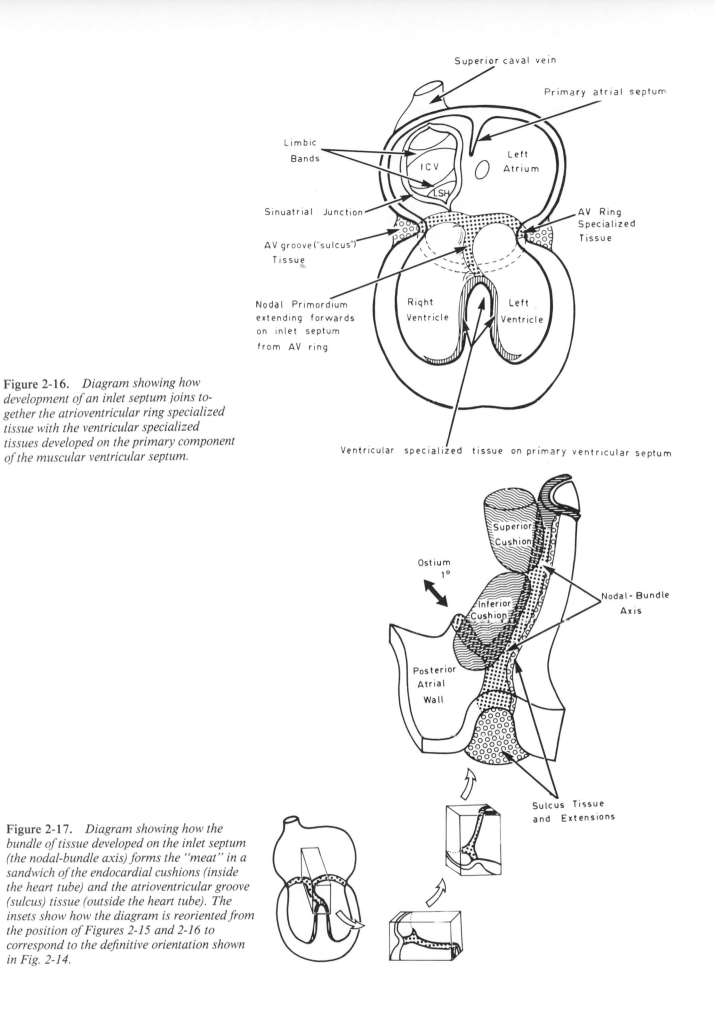

tricular septal defects.[55-57] At this early stage, the endocardial cushions (which are helping to septate the atrioventricular junction) are on the endocardial aspect of the developing conduction tissue axis. Additional tissue, the atrioventricular groove (sulcus) tissue, is present on the epicardial aspect, and extensions from this tissue surround the developing bundles (Fig. 2-17). A "sandwich" is therefore formed of sulcus, conduction, and cushion tissues that persists into the definitive heart. At this stage there is a very long nonbranching bundle extending along the inlet septum, which comes into contact with atrial tissues only at the posterior atrial wall. As the atrial septum forms, the atrial tissues are initially in contact only with the endocardial cushions. These separate the atrial myocardium from the conduction axis running on the inlet septum (Fig. 2-18*A*). With increasing development and growth there is a gradual recession of the endocardial cushions.

This permits the inferior rim of the atrial septum to make contact with the conduction bundle on the inlet septum, converting what had originally been a long nonbranching bundle into the definitive compact atrioven-

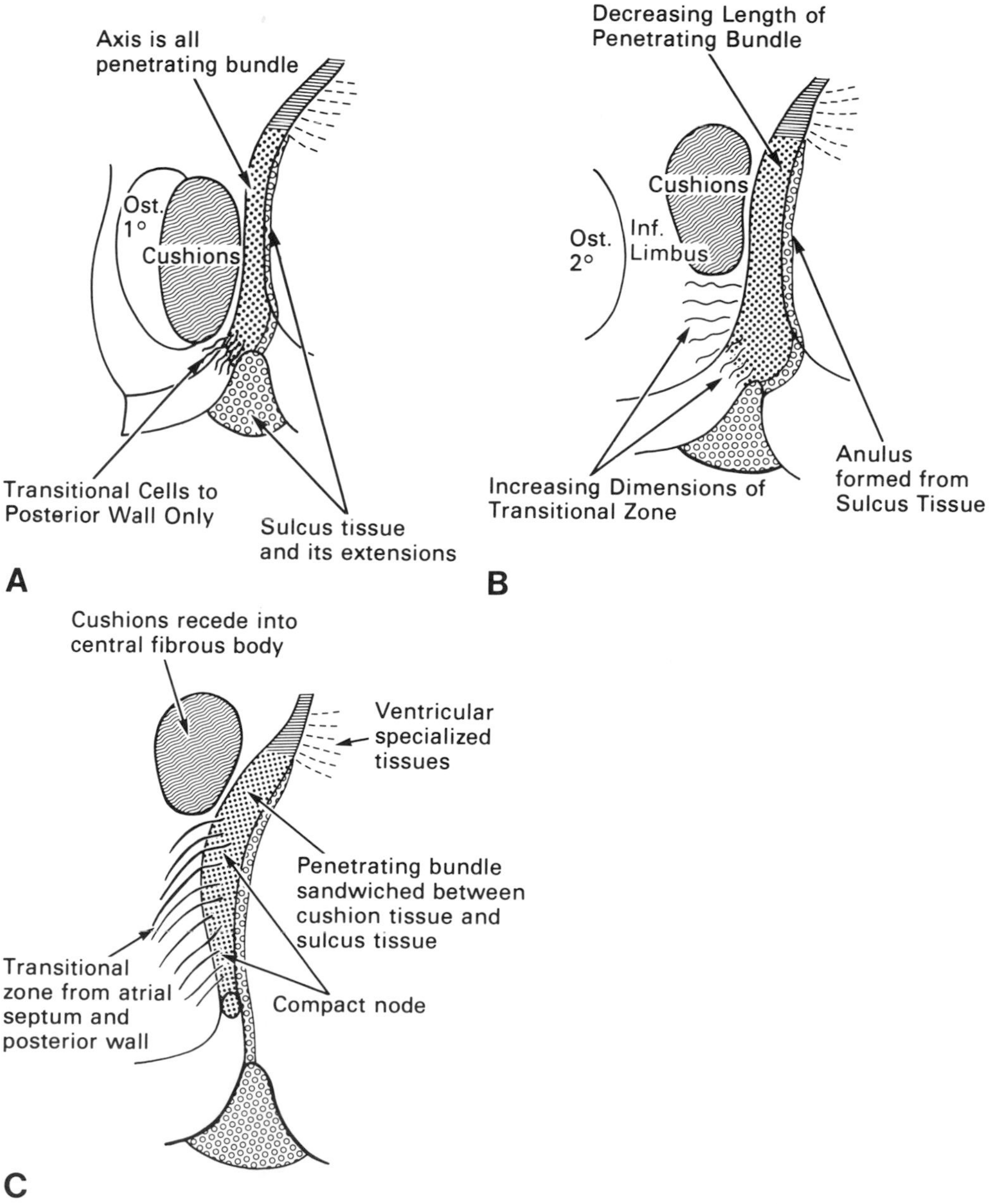

Figure 2-18. *Diagram showing progressive stages (A to C) in conversion of the nodal-bundle axis, initially a penetrating bundle, into the atrioventricular node concomitant with the formation of the definitive atrial septum.*

tricular node (Fig. 2-18*B*). The newly formed node is still in a directly subepicardial position and is separated from the inlet septum and ventricular myocardium by extensions of the adipose tissue of the atrioventricular groove (Fig. 2-18*C*). The compact portion of the definitive node and the penetrating bundle are derived from the same developmental source, which may be termed the *nodal-bundle axis* (Fig. 2-17). The point of division between the node and penetrating bundle depends on the degree of recession of the endocardial cushions. It is the point at which the insulating tissue of the central fibrous body (derived in part from the cushions) comes to separate the atrial myocardium from the nodal-bundle axis. Since the atrial septum grows down onto the conduction tissue axis to form the node, the definitive node is an interatrial structure.[58] In summary, the definitive compact node and bundle are derived from the same developmental source. The transitional zone between them and the atrial tissue has a different origin. The compact node itself in the definitive heart retains its embryologic subepicardial position.

Cellular Architecture and Microscopy

The junctional area is disposed as an axis of conduction tissue carried on the inlet and apical trabecular components of the muscular interventricular septum, which then extends upward into the atrial septum. We will consider its architecture in this fashion, describing its components as it ascends from the ventricle into the atrial myocardium. The *branching bundle* is arranged on the crest of the apical trabecular septum, immediately

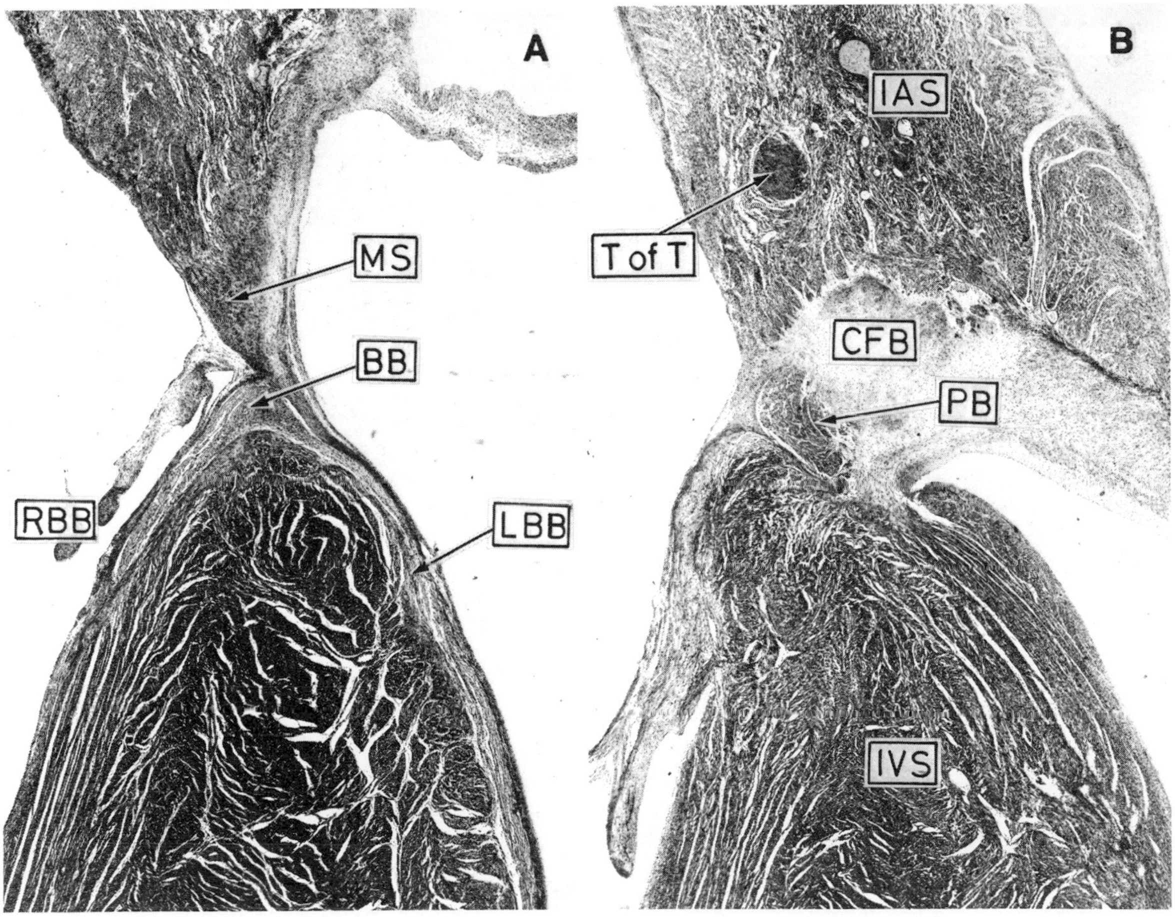

Figure 2-19. *Photomicrographs through the junctional area of the heart of a child illustrated as sectioned from anterior (A) to posterior (Fig. 2-20C). A shows the branching bundle (BB) directly beneath the membranous septum (MS), which in this heart has only an atrioventricular component. The right bundle branch (RBB) is the continuation of the nodal bundle axis (see Figs. 2-16 to 2-18), with the left bundle branch (LBB) fanning out from the axis as a sheet of cells. B shows the penetrating bundle (PB) passing through the central fibrous body (CFB). Note that the tendon of Todaro (T of T) is already striking upward into the atrial septum (IAS). (IVS, interventricular septum)*

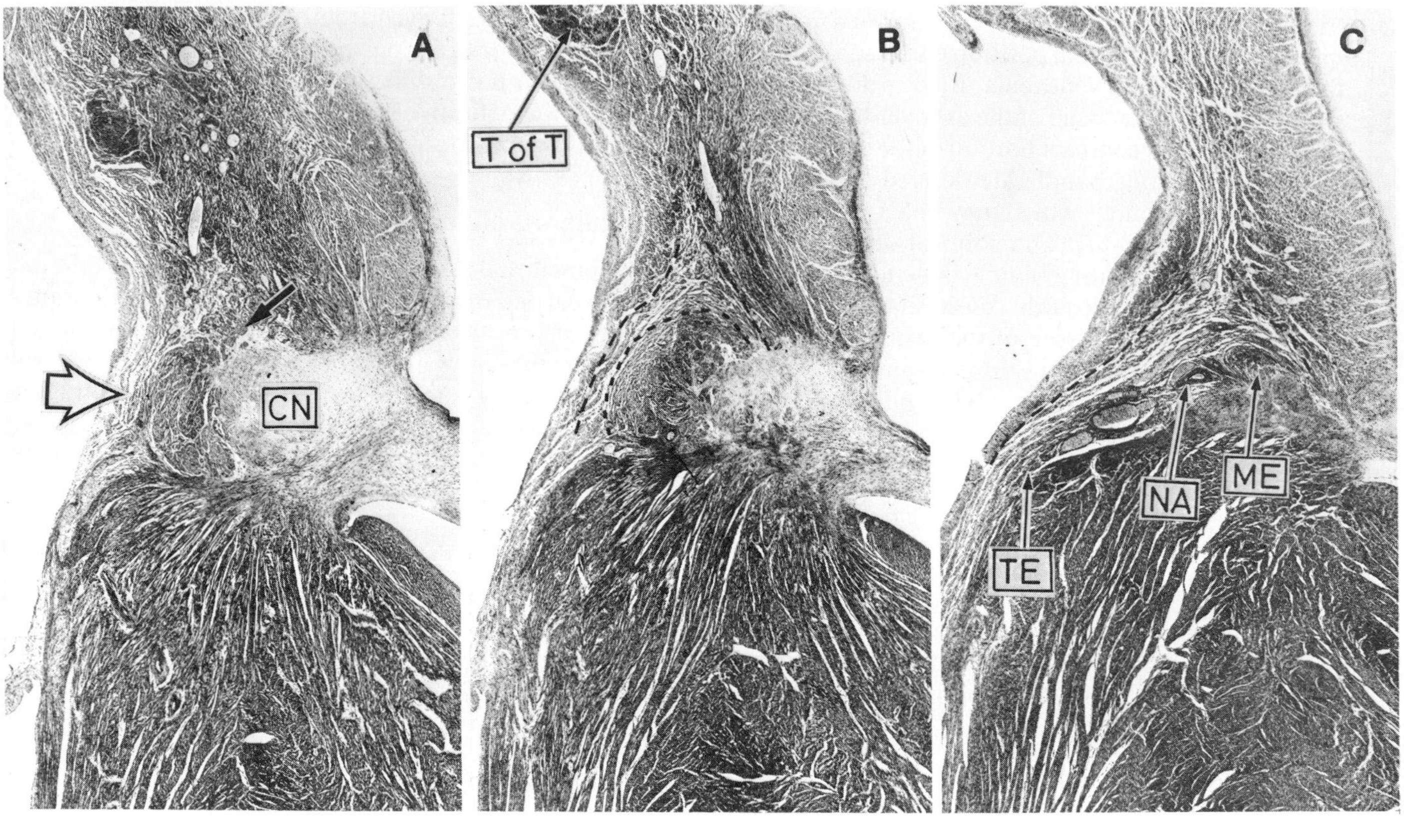

Figure 2-20. *Photomicrographs continuing the series shown in Figure 2-19. A shows the junction between compact node (CN) and penetrating bundle. The axis has passed between the tricuspid anulus fibrosus and the central fibrous body and is now the node because it is making contact with atrial transitional cells, both from the overlay area (open arrow) and the deep part of the septum (closed arrow). B shows the body of the compact node. It is set as a half oval against the anulus fibrosus (within dots), with the transitional cell zone (within dashes) circling the compact zone. Note the tendon of Todaro passing out of the section. C shows the posterior reaches of the junctional area. The compact zone has bifurcated into extensions that pass toward the tricuspid (TE) and mitral (ME) valve attachments. The transitional cell zone surrounds these extensions (within dashes), and the nodal artery (NA) enters between them.*

beneath the membranous septum, in such a way that the right bundle branch is (in terms of its orientation) the anterior continuation of the axis (Fig. 2-19). In contrast, the left bundle branch fibers cascade from the axis as a continuous fan (Fig. 2-20). Massing and James[59] took exception to the earlier suggestion[60] that the right bundle was the *direct* continuation of the nodal-bundle axis. Subsequent studies have confirmed their opinion. Thus in neonatal hearts a "dead-end tract" has been shown to be the direct continuation of the axis,[61] the tract ending blindly within the central fibrous body. We have considered the axis as the *penetrating bundle* proximal to the point of descent of the "first" left bundle branch fiber (Fig. 2-19). Hecht and colleagues[51] divided this zone of the axis, in which it passes from the atrial tissues to the "first" left bundle branch fiber, into two portions—the penetrating bundle and the nonbranching bundle. We have examined some normal hearts in which this arrangement is to be found. However, in most normal hearts the nodal-bundle axis starts to branch as soon as it emerges from the central fibrous body onto the septal crest. The distinction between the *penetrating bundle* and the *compact node* is best made at the point at which the nodal-bundle axis enters the central fibrous body (Fig. 2-20), thereby ceasing to make contact with the atrial myocardium. This point depends on the formation of the central fibrous body (Fig. 2-21). In some hearts the "last" contact is made with the superficial overlay fibers of the right side of the atrial septum. In other hearts it is with the deeper left-sided septal musculature.[50] The atrial portion of the axis can itself be divided into the *compact node* and the *transitional cell zone.* The compact node throughout its length retains a close relationship to the fibrous ring, which forms its baseplate (see

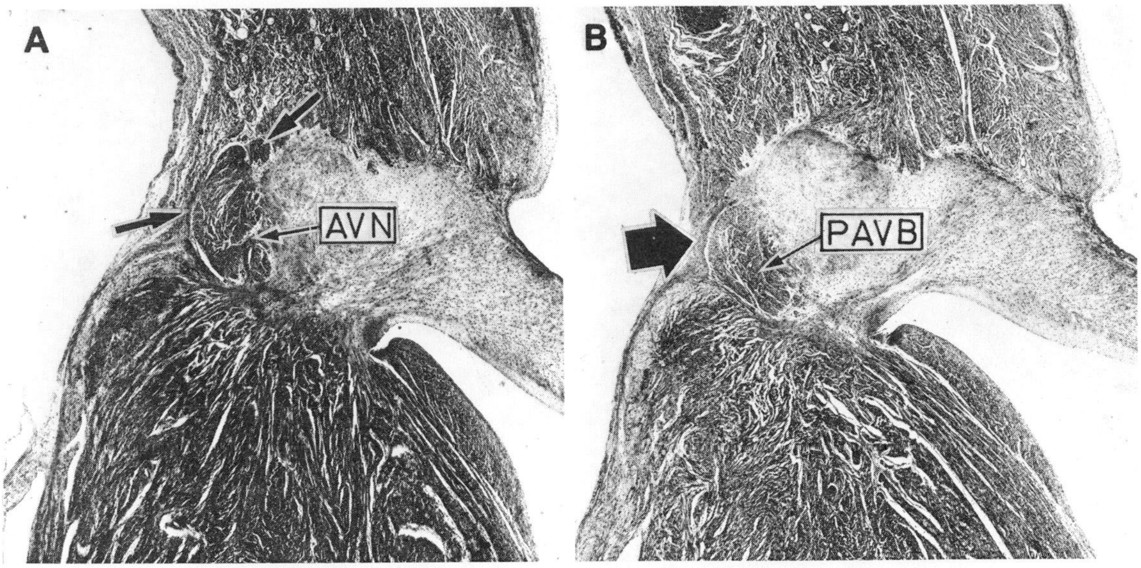

Figure 2-21. *Photomicrographs illustrating the distinction between compact node (AVN) and penetrating bundle (PAVB) in the junctional area illustrated in Figures 2-19 and 2-20. In A, the axis makes contact with atrial tissues (between arrows) and is therefore compact node. In B, the axis, identical in histologic terms, is engulfed in the central fibrous body and is prevented by fibrous tissue (arrow) from making contact with the atrial septum. It is therefore the penetrating bundle.*

Fig. 2-20). It can usually be traced as two extensions that continue along the baseplate, the right extension running toward the tricuspid valve and the left extension toward the mitral valve (see Fig. 2-20). This arrangement of an axis of conduction tissue penetrating the fibrous plane and bifurcating posteriorly was well described and illustrated by Tawara[1] (Fig. 2-22). The transitional cell zone is a diffuse area of atrial muscle interposed between the "working" myocardium and the specialized cells of the compact node. It was termed the *nodal approaches* by Hecht and associates.[51] In most hearts, the transitional cells are most conspicuous posteriorly between the bifurcating extensions of the compact node (see Fig. 2-20*C*), but they also form a half-oval cap for the compact node itself (see Fig. 2-20*B*).

From the standpoint of histology, the cells of the atrial portion of the junctional area are smaller than the working atrial myocardial cells. In the transitional cell zones, the cells are long and attenuated, tending to be separated from each other by fibrous tissue strands. In the compact node itself the cells are more closely packed together and are frequently arranged in interconnecting fasciculi and whorls (Fig. 2-23). In many hearts there is evidence of stratification of the compact node into deep and superficial layers, as previously described by Truex and Smythe.[62] The additional layer of overlying transitional cells then gives the node a trilaminar appearance (Fig. 2-24). As the node becomes the penetrating bundle there is a marginal increase in cell size, but for the most part the cellular architecture is comparable with that seen in

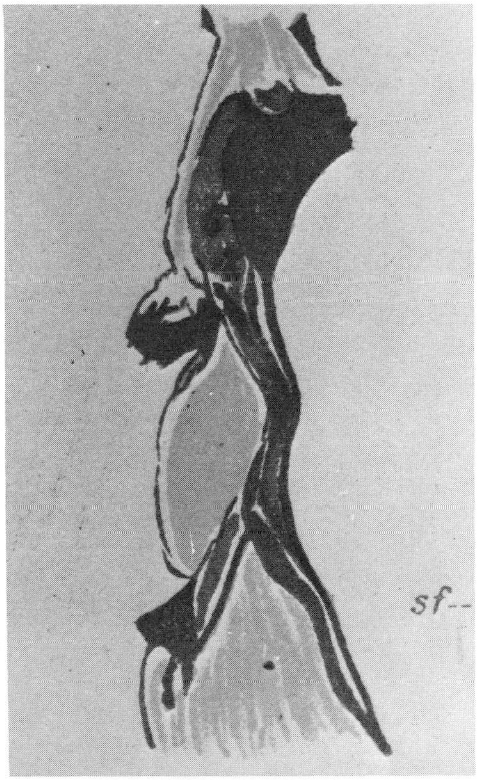

Figure 2-22. *Photograph of the diagram prepared by Tawara to illustrate the atrioventricular node. He shows a nodal-bundle axis of tissue, which in this infantile heart interdigitates with the central fibrous body and has an extension that runs toward the mitral valve. Compare with Figures 2-19 and 2-20. (Tawara, S.: Das Reitzleitungssystem des Saügetierherzens. Jena, Gustav Fischer, 1906)*

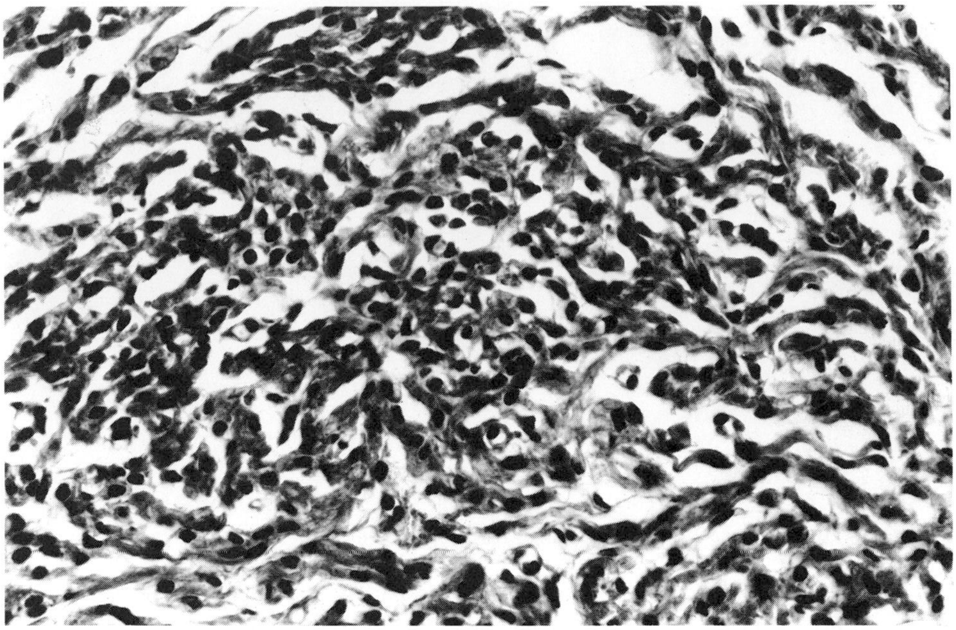

Figure 2-23. *High-power photomicrograph of the cells of the compact node illustrated in Figures 2-19 to 2-21. The cells are small and aggregated into interweaving fasciculi.*

the compact node.[50] It is difficult to differentiate node and penetrating bundle on the basis of histology; for that reason, we prefer a distinction based on architecture, namely, the point at which the axis enters the fibrous body. The cells making up the branching bundle are similar in size to the ventricular myocardial cells. It is rare to observe pale or swollen cells (so-called Purkinje cells) in the specialized junctional area of infants and young children.

Electron Microscopy and Anatomicoelectrophysiologic Correlations

The greater part of our knowledge of the electrophysiology of the junctional area has come from studies of the rabbit heart. Significant differences exist between the architecture of the rabbit junctional area and that of the human, so direct comparisons cannot be made between them. The classic studies of Paes de Carvalho,[63] working in the laboratory of Hoffman,[64] showed that (from an electrophysiologic standpoint) the rabbit junctional area was a trilaminar structure with "AN," "N," and "NH" zones. Some anatomic studies showed little morphologic evidence of such a nodal division.[65] However, combined histologic and histochemical studies demonstrated that the rabbit junctional area was indeed a trilaminar structure. Transitional, mid-nodal, and lower nodal zones were identified, the latter being directly continuous with the atrioventricular bundle.[66] Subsequent anatomicoelectrophysiologic correlative investigations

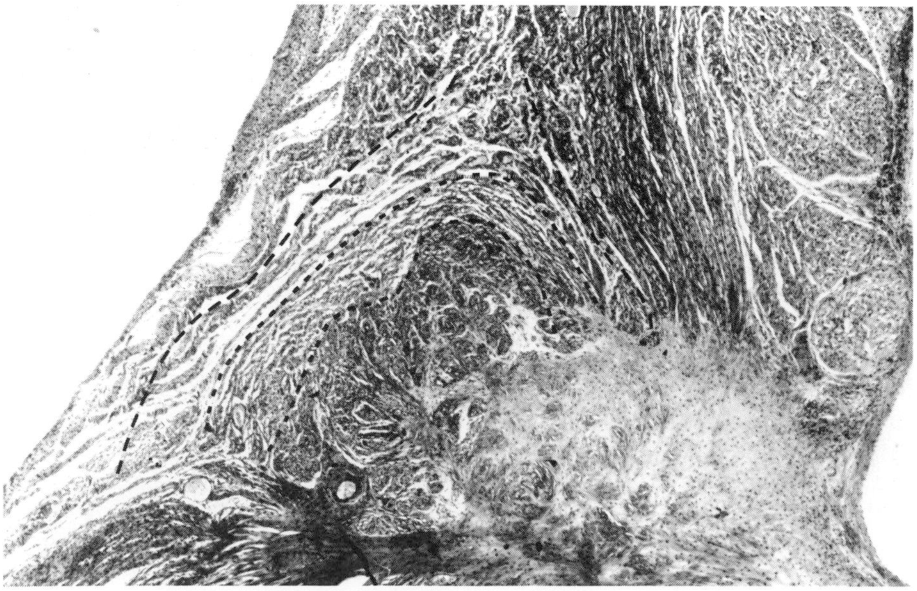

Figure 2-24. *Photomicrograph of the compact node illustrated in Figures 2-19 to 2-21 showing how the compact node itself has two strata (dotted lines), with the transitional cell zone (dashed line) giving the atrial part of the junctional area a trilaminar appearance.*

in the rabbit using a cobalt marking technique[67] showed that the AN potentials were produced in the transitional cell zone and the NH potentials in the anterior part of the lower nodal zone (Fig. 2-25). N potentials were recorded from the small knot of middle nodal cells but were also recorded from cells in the transitional zone. The greater part of nodal delay was produced in the transitional cell area. When comparing these findings with human or canine data, it must be remembered that the entire area of the "compact node" of the rabbit is isolated from the atrial tissues by an extensive collar derived from the central fibrous body. Therefore, in terms of human architecture described above, the whole of the rabbit "node" would be considered to be the penetrating bundle.

The division of the rabbit node into morphologically discrete cellular areas has been confirmed by ultrastructural observations.[28] The cells in the different areas possess a similar ultrastructure, having few myofibrils and randomly arranged mitochondria. In this respect the cells resemble those of the sinus node. The differences between the areas of the rabbit node reside in the arrangement of the cells. The transitional cells are arranged in individual fashion, the upper nodal cells aggregated in a ball, and the lower nodal cells grouped together in cable fashion.[28] Ultrastructural studies of the human node performed with the precision of the study in the rabbit[28] are as yet lacking, largely because of the difficulty of obtaining optimal fixation. Thus, the details of differences between human and animal junctional areas at the ultrastructural level remain unresolved.

Innervation

As with the sinus node, major species differences exist concerning innervation pattern and are considerably magnified in the atrioventricular junction. The rabbit junctional area receives copious innervation from both cholinergic and adrenergic sources.[68] The guinea pig junctional area is profusely innervated with cholinesterase-containing nerves but lacks any adrenergic innervation that can be demonstrated using fluorescence techniques.[68] In humans, although the transitional cell zone of the junctional area has a cholinesterase-positive innervation at midterm development, the ventricular conducting tissues (although themselves cholinesterase positive) are entirely lacking a cholinergic innervation.[53] Existing evidence is such that it cannot be presumed from morphologic studies that the human specialized

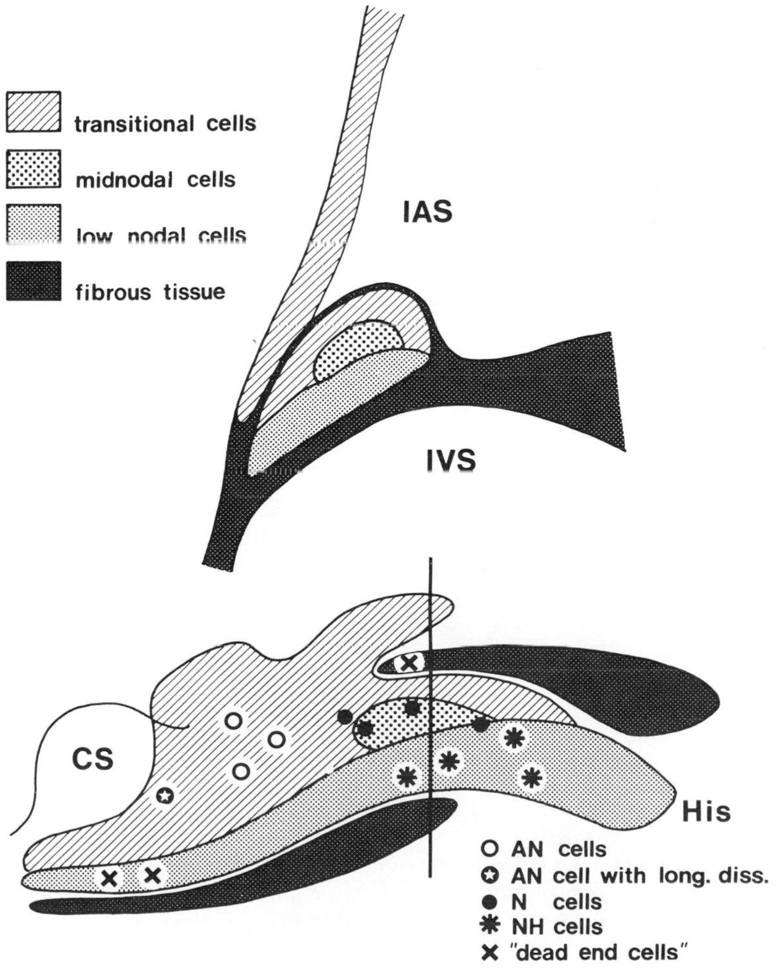

Figure 2-25. *Diagram showing the correlation between action potential configuration and nodal morphology in the rabbit atrioventricular junctional area. (Janse, M. J., Anderson R. H., Van Capelle F., et al.: Electrophysiology and structure of the AV node. In Wellens, H. J. J., Lie K. I., Janse M. J., [eds]: The Conduction System of the Heart—Structure, Function and Clinical Implications. The Hague, Martinus Nijhoff, 1976).*

junctional area receives either a cholinergic or adrenergic innervation. Further morphologic and ultrastructural studies are required to elucidate this problem. Until they are performed, considerable caution is necessary when extrapolating from animal experiments to the human situation. These constraints are equally valid regarding the innervation pattern of the ventricular specialized tissues, which also show marked species variation.[53,66,68]

The Specialized Atrioventricular Ring Tissue

If serial sections are taken of the parietal atrioventricular junctions, then it is the rule in many hearts to find "rests" of histologically specialized tissue sequestrated in the atrial myocardium at its insertion to the junctions.[69] This arrangement is particularly noticeable at the anterolateral quadrant of the right atrioventricular junction. These "rests" are almost certainly the remnants of the more complete ring of specialized tissue present in fetuses, observed initially by Keith and Flack[3] and confirmed by our studies.[53] When seen in mature hearts, these areas of specialized tissue are remarkedly reminiscent of the structures described by Kent in the 19th century[70] and illustrated in subsequent demonstrations.[71] Kent has suffered somewhat in regard to his early work, since the atrioventricular bundle has come to be described with the name of His, while we and others have questioned the propriety of Kent's own eponym. Our concern at the application of Kent's name to the accessory atrioventricular connections, which unequivocally underscore the Wolff-Parkinson-White variant of preexcitation (see below), should not be construed as indicating that we doubt Kent's descriptions. Far from it. As we described in 1974, our observations are very much an endorsement of Kent's illustrations. Where we differ is that we have never observed in normal hearts these "rests" of atrioventricular ring specialized tissue effecting *connections* across the junction. This was the claim made by Kent, and we cannot endorse this statement. But the structures do exist. Nodes of Kent? Yes! Bundles of Kent? Only in exceedingly rare circumstances (see below).

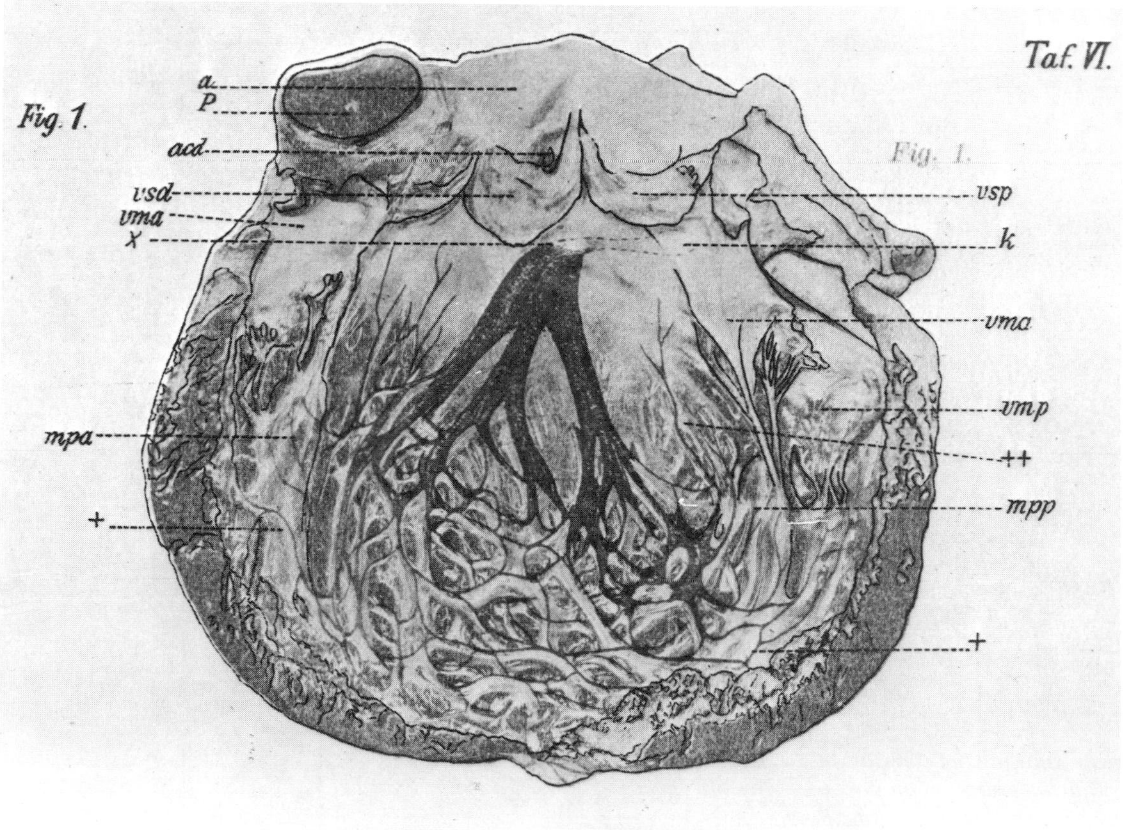

Figure 2-26. *Photomicrograph from the original publication of Tawara, showing the distribution of the left bundle branch in the human heart. (Tawara, S.: Das Reitzleitungs-system des Saügetierherzens. Jena, Gustav Fischer, 1906)*

The Ventricular Specialized Tissues

In light of suggestions concerning the bifascicular nature of the human left bundle branch system and its clinical significance,[72] it is illuminating to study the initial illustrations of the left bundle branch prepared by Tawara[1] (Fig. 2-26). Tawara demonstrated the left bundle branch cascading down the septal surface in fanlike fashion from the branching bundle and ramifying into the left ventricle in some hearts in trifascicular rather than bifascicular fashion. This arrangement has been endorsed by numerous subsequent investigators and was restated by authors such as Rossi[73] and Uhlcy and colleagues[74] in the face of contradictory reports by Rosenbaum.[72] Despite the overwhelming anatomic evidence, the concept of a bifascicular left bundle branch received enthusiastic acceptance by a clinical audience who found that it provided a basis for their electrocardiographic findings. However, recent elegant studies employing serial methods of reconstruction[59,75] have shown unequivocally that the left bundle branch does *not* have a bifascicular structure. Again, our own findings are in keeping with the majority viewpoint (Fig. 2-27). We find that the

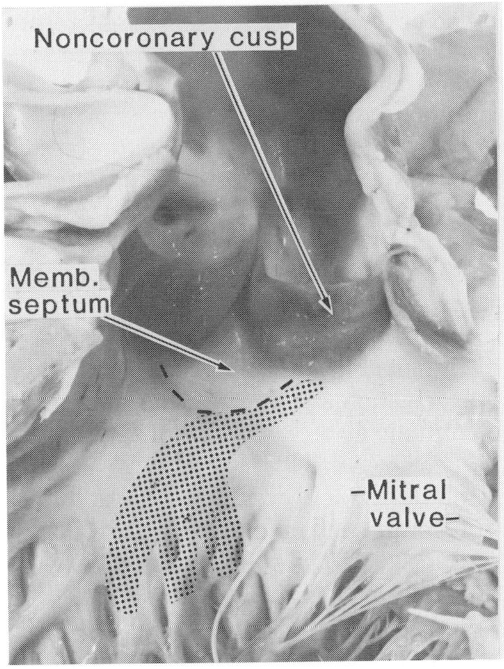

Figure 2-27. *Photograph of a normal human heart illustrating the distribution of the conduction system as viewed from the left ventricle. Compare with Figure 2-26.*

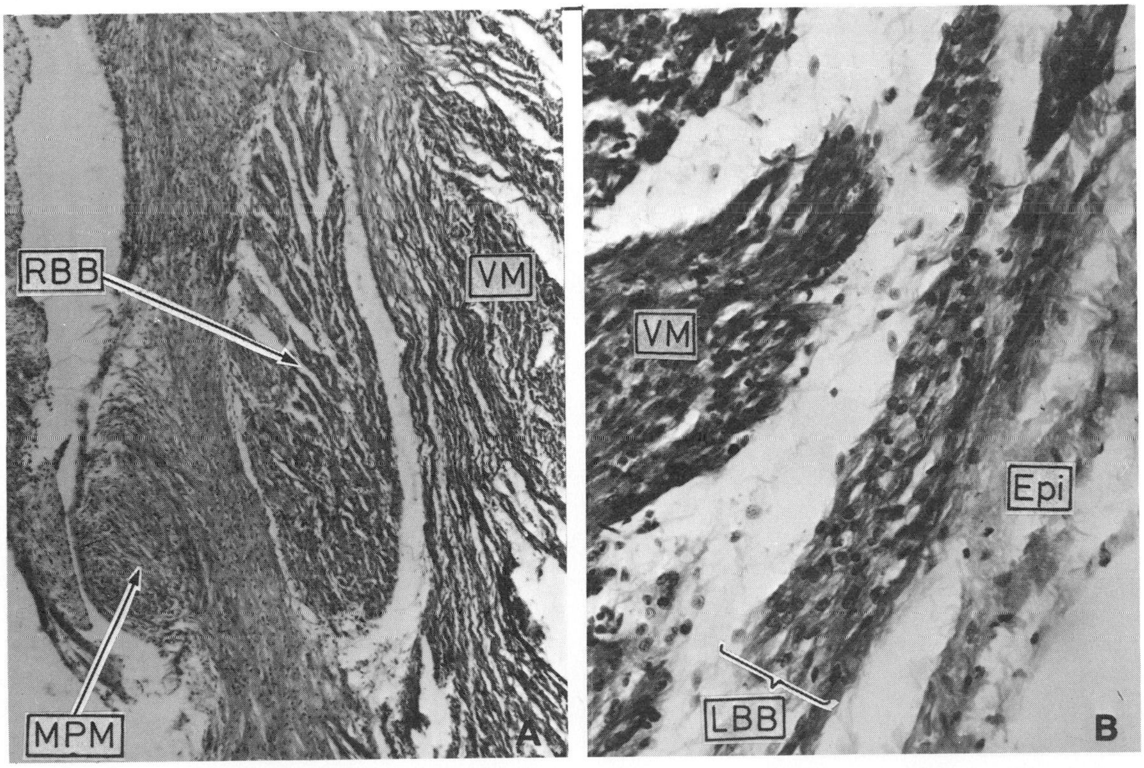

Figure 2-28. *Photomicrographs showing (A) a normal right bundle branch (RBB) and (B) left bundle branch (LBB) in an infant heart. The bundles are discrete from the ventricular myocardium (VM). Their cells are of a size similar to the myocardial cells. (MPM, medial papillary muscle)*

left bundle branch fibers originate as a single sheet from the branching bundle on the crest of the trabecular septum. As it descends, the sheet fans out into three broad divisions—anterior, septal, and posterior (Fig. 2-27). On the smooth part of the septum the left bundle branch is clearly isolated from the ventricular myocardium by a fibrous sheath (Fig. 2-28). The cells of the left bundle can be distinguished from the myocardial cells by their position and staining characteristics. It is rare in our experience with infant and child material for these cells to show "Purkinje" characteristics. When traced peripherally, the cells ramify into the ventricular myocardium. When they lose their aggregation and tissue sheath it becomes difficult to differentiate a specialized cell from an ordinary myocardial cell.

The right bundle branch continues on from the branching bundle in the general direction of the nodal-bundle axis (see Fig. 2-14). It is a thin cordlike structure that usually runs intramyocardially. Its cells frequently cannot be distinguished on cytologic grounds from the "working" myocardium, but the bundle can easily be traced through serial sections because of its aggregation and fibrous sheath (see Fig. 2-28). As with the left bundle, when it breaks up distally it is difficult to trace the terminal ramifications because of the cytologic similarities with myocardium.

Anatomic Substrates of Preexcitation

Ventricular preexcitation is defined as the situation where the ventricles are activated more rapidly than would be anticipated had the impulse been conducted through the normal atrioventricular junctional area.[76] Although some authorities have suggested that the disorder can result from a functional malformation in a normal conduction system,[77] it is more usual to search for discrete anatomic "short circuits" of the junctional area as its explanation. In order to understand the site

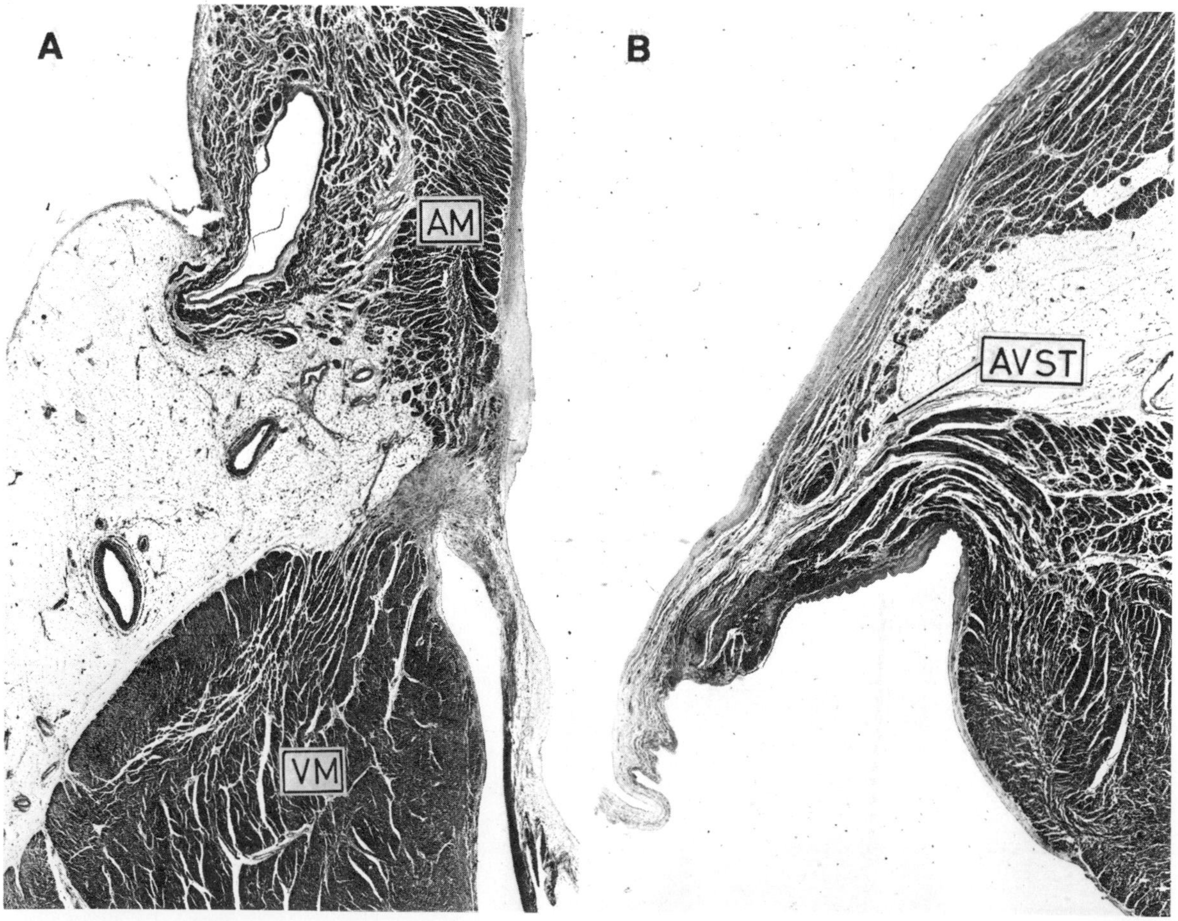

Figure 2-29. *Photomicrographs illustrating the differences between the mitral anulus fibrosus (A) and the tricuspid anulus (B). The mitral anulus separates atrial (AM) and ventricular (VM) myocardial tissues. The tricuspid anulus is less well formed, and the muscular tissues are separated only by the atrioventricular sulcus tissue (AVST).*

and morphology of such substrates, it is necessary to have a thorough knowledge of the disposition of the normal junctional specialized tissues (see above) together with the morphology of the atrioventricular junctional insulating mechanism.

The Atrioventricular Fibrous Rings

In the normal heart, the atrioventricular bundle is believed to be the only muscular structure connecting the atrial and ventricular myocardial tissues, although as James[78] has indicated, studies comparable to those carried out in hearts with ventricular preexcitation are lacking in normal hearts. In hearts with preexcitation, it is mandatory to study the entirety of the atrioventricular junction in any search for accessory muscular atrioventricular connections. As Lev[79] has commented, such studies are exceedingly time consuming. In an attempt to provide some information on this topic, and also on the structure of the fibrous rings themselves, we have conducted subserial sectioning of the atrioventricular muscular junctions in human hearts. It must be emphasized that these studies do *not* provide the precision demanded in hearts with preexcitation.[78] Nevertheless, we believe they provide important information regarding the anatomic substrates for this malformation. In these subserial sections, we never observed any atrioventricular muscular connections outside the specialized junctional area. We did observe that the fibrous ring of the mitral valve was a solid, well-formed collagenous structure that, at all points, separated the atrial and ventricular myocardial tissues in addition to supporting the mitral valve leaflets (Fig. 2-29*A*). In contrast to this, the ring of the tricuspid valve was variably formed even in individual hearts (Fig. 2-30). At some points in each of the hearts studied, segments of collagenous tissue separated atrial and ventricular myocardial segments. At other points in the same hearts the junction was inturned and the collagenous ring supported only the tricuspid leaflets, the atrial and ventricular muscular tissues being separated only by the adipose tissue of the atrioventricular groove (see Fig. 2-29*B*). A similar variability was found in the region of the septum. In the majority of the hearts studied, only the adipose atrioventricular groove tissue separated the posterior reaches of the compact atrioventricular node and the base of the atrial septum from the ventricular septum. Furthermore, when viewed from within the right atrium, the compact node appears as an anterior structure close to the central fibrous body.[80] However, the node is also a directly *subepicardial* structure (Figs. 2-31 and 2-32). This is because the tissue plane of the posterior atrioventricular groove extends beneath the coronary sinus toward the central fibrous body. The artery to the atrioventricular node runs through the plane (Fig. 2-32). One further finding of our study of "normal" hearts is of significance to the anatomy of preexcitation. As discussed above, rests of histologically specialized tissue are found adjacent to the tricuspid valve fibrous ring (Fig. 2-30). These are the remnants of the atrioventricular ring specialized tissue initially illustrated by Kent.[70,71]

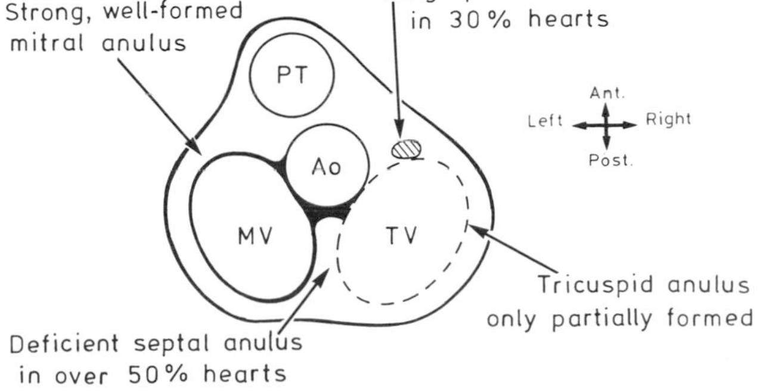

Figure 2-30. *Results obtained from the study of the anulus fibrosus in normal hearts.*

Anatomic Substrates for Preexcitation

The function of the specialized atrioventricular junctional area is to produce delay. In animal hearts the majority of the delay occurs in the transitional cell zones of the area.[67] Some delay is also produced in the atrioventricular bundle and bundle branches, because these structures are isolated from the septal myocardium and the normal impulse must traverse their length before activating the ventricular myocardium. Consequently, there are several possibilities whereby anatomic connections could "short-circuit" all or part of this normal delay. The morphology of these connections has been described previously by several investigators, notably Lev.[79] It is not always easy to correlate anatomic and clinical studies because of the eponyms used to describe the various connections. For example, accessory atrioventricular connections existing outside the specialized junctional area are widely termed *bundles of Kent*. Unfortunately, the connections thus described bear no resemblance to the structures observed by Kent himself,[70,71] which are the remnants of the atrioventricular ring specialized tissue. As Sherf and James have pointed out,[81] because there is no resemblance between these structures and the actual connections, this is an inappropriate eponym. This point is conceded by those who use it in the interests of brevity.[82] The propriety of the eponym has subsequently been debated by ourselves[83] and Sealy.[84] Let us emphasize once more that we do not doubt the existence of the structures illustrated by Kent. Our point is that they bear no resemblance to the accessory atrioventricular connections that, in almost all

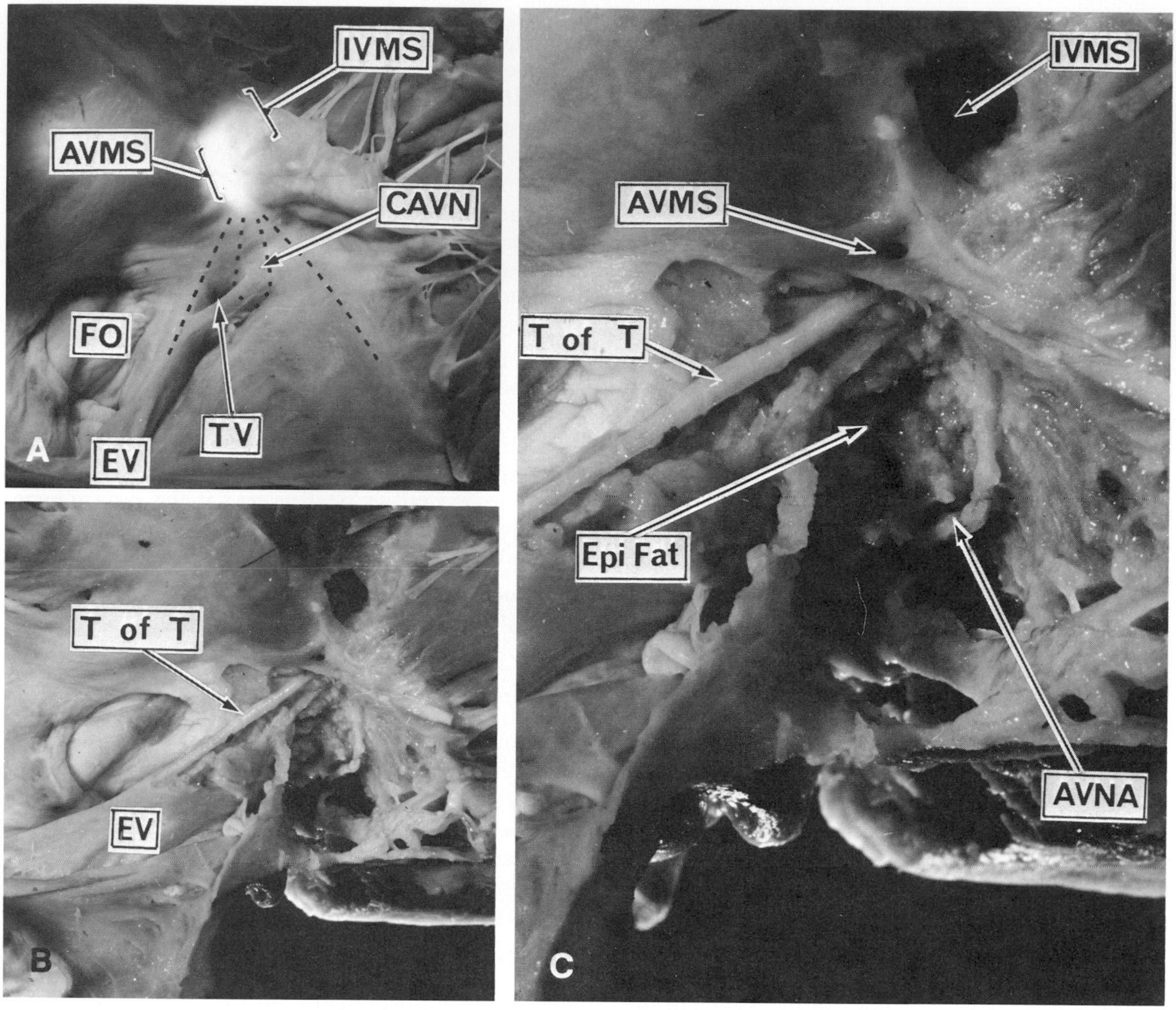

Figure 2-31. *Dissection illustrating the position of the atrioventricular node and its directly subepicardial position.*

cases, are the substrates of preexcitation. The fibers described by Mahaim[85] certainly do short-circuit the junctional area, but can be present throughout the junctional area. For present-day needs it seems desirable to differentiate "Mahaim fibers," which arise from the node, from those arising from the fascicular portion of the conduction axis. Further confusion exists concerning the nodal bypass fibers described as being present in the normal heart by James.[7] These tracts in no way resemble the fiber tract described by Brechenmacher[86] in hearts with short PR–normal QRS syndrome. Yet such syndromes are frequently explained on the basis of so-called James fibers. For all these reasons, we suggested that eponyms be avoided in the nomenclature of preexcitation and that descriptive terms be employed instead.[87] The possibilities for a short-circuit of the junctional area can therefore be considered in terms of accessory atrioventricular connections, accessory nodoventricular connections, accessory fasciculoventricular connections, accessory atriofascicular connections, and, finally, intranodal bypass tracts (Fig. 2-33). Those interested in the historical background of the various eponyms are referred to the excellent review by Burchell.[88]

Accessory Atrioventricular Connections

Accessory atrioventricular connections are pathways that connect the atrial and ventricular myocardial tissues outside the specialized junctional area. Except when the pathways originate in the segments of specialized atrioventricular ring tissue originally described by Kent,[70,71] it is incorrect to refer to these pathways as "Kent bundles." The first accessory atrioventricular

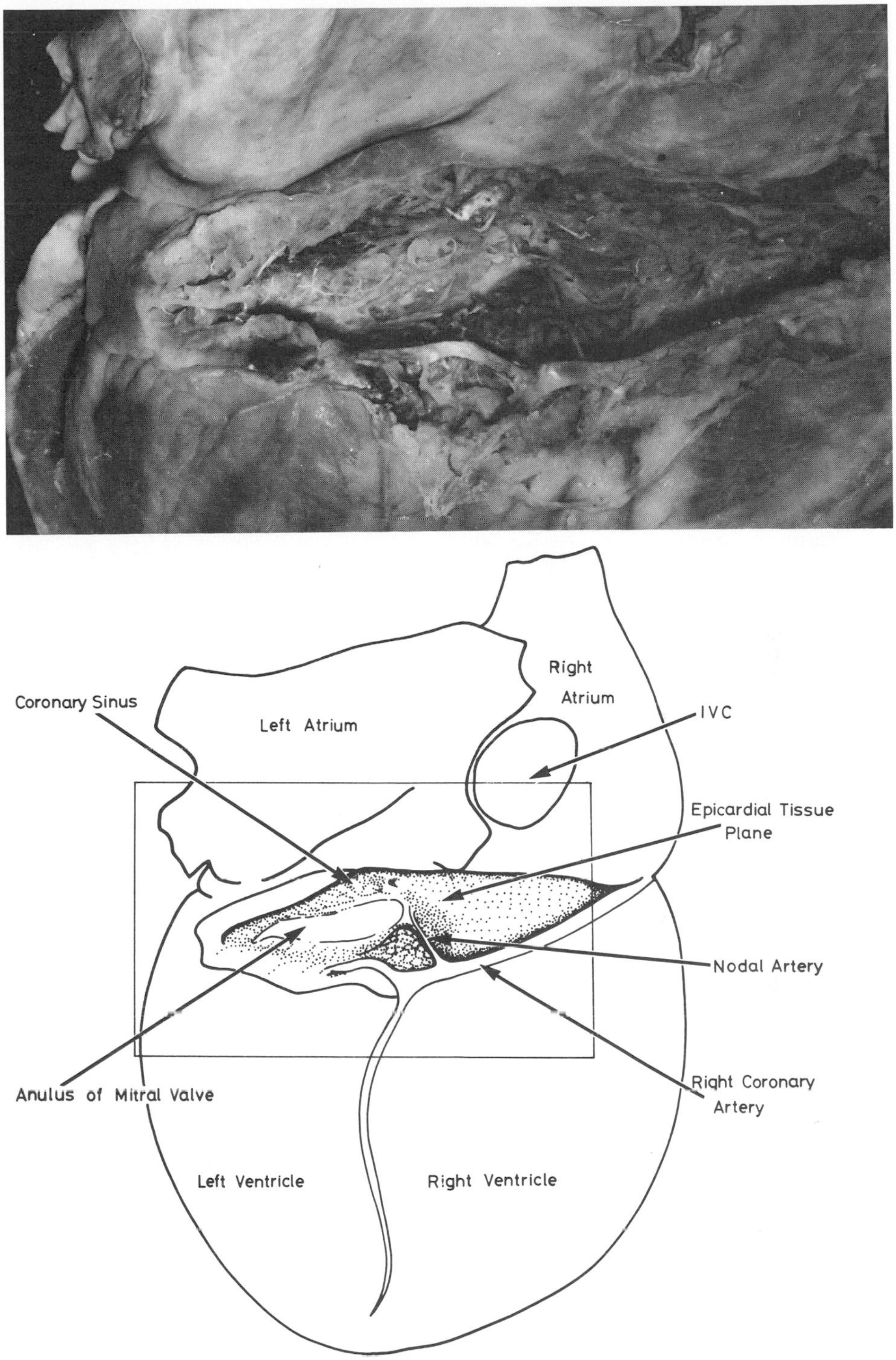

Figure 2-32. *Dissection of a normal human heart, showing how a tissue plane exists beneath the coronary sinus, which extends from the posterior atrioventricular sulcus to the region of the atrioventricular node and the central fibrous body.*

pathway to be demonstrated histologically was that studied by Wood and associates,[89] but the most exemplary demonstration was that given by Ohnell[90] (Fig. 2-34). It is pertinent that nearly all left-sided pathways studied subsequently are very similar to this pathway (Fig. 2-35). Subsequent histologic studies, together with recent electrophysiologic mapping studies such as those of Gallagher and colleagues[91] have demonstrated unequivocally that these pathways are the anatomic substrates for the classic Wolff-Parkinson-White variety of preexcita-

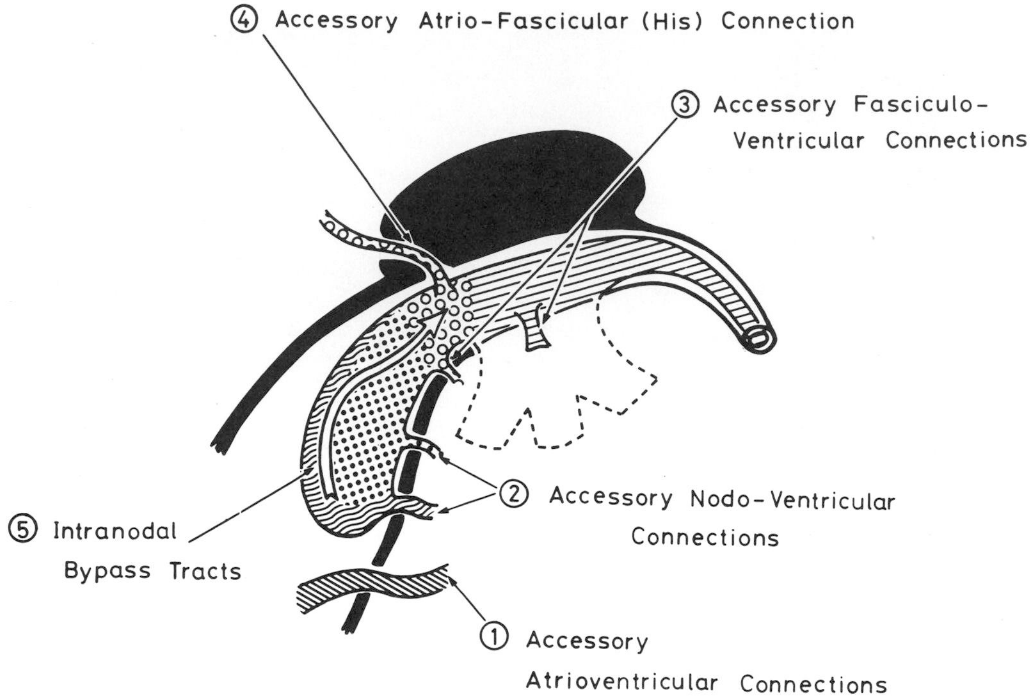

Figure 2-33. *Diagram illustrating the theoretic ways in which accessory anatomic connections could "short-circuit" the delay-producing area of the specialized atrioventricular junctional area (compare with Fig. 2-14).*

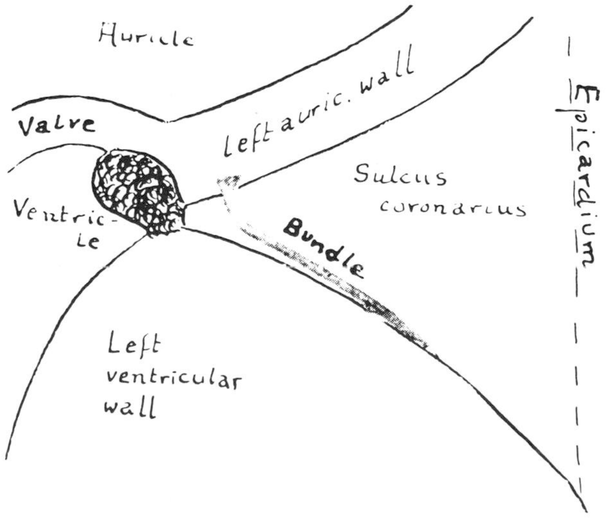

Figure 2-34. *Diagram taken from the thesis of Ohnell demonstrating the epicardial course of a left-sided accessory atrioventricular connection. (Ohnell, R. F.: Pre-excitation: A cardiac abnormality. Acta Med. Scand. [Suppl.], 152, 1944)*

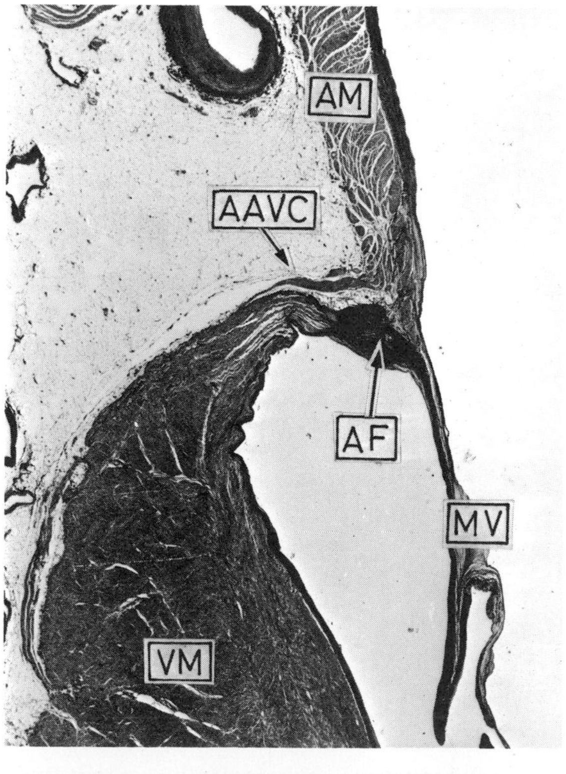

Figure 2-35. *Photomicrograph of a left-side accessory atrioventricular (AAVC) connection from a patient with preexcitation, showing its epicardial course relative to the anulus fibrosus (AF) of the mitral valve (MV). (AM, atrial myocardium; VM, ventricular myocardium)*

tion. It has also been demonstrated in recent years that the pathways can be successfully divided at surgery either by standard surgical techniques[92] or by cryothermy. In this respect, it should also be remembered that it may, on occasion, be necessary to divide the conduction axis itself to cure particular troublesome arrhythmias. This is best done by cryothermy, and a recent ingenious experiment has shown how this can be done without entering the heart.[93] The axis is destroyed as it traverses the central fibrous body by a cryothermy probe introduced through the transverse sinus. Returning to the accessory connections, it is important to understand their architecture and their relations to the fibrous rings. The pathways can exist at any point around the atrioventricular junctions where the atrial tissues are adjacent to ventricular myocardium. In this respect, at least one pathway has been demonstrated extending across the area of fibrous continuity between the mitral and aortic valves.[94] Considered together, they can be divided into left-sided, right-sided, or septal pathways. The lateral pathways do *not* always pass through gaps in the fibrous ring. Left-sided pathways, in the majority of cases, skirt a well-formed fibrous ring on its epicardial aspect (Figs. 2-34 and 2-35). They traverse the fat of the epicardial groove and adhere closely to the fibrous ring. This means that cuts used by the surgeons with intent to divide these pathways probably divide the atrial wall above the connection rather than extirpating the pathway itself (Fig. 2-36). It is almost always necessary to dissect the epicardial aspect of the groove itself in order to avulse the pathway. The position of right-sided pathways is complicated by the absence of a well-formed tricuspid fibrous ring. Thus the pathways are able to pass directly through the adipose tissue dividing atrial and ventricular musculatures, although in addition they may directly traverse the subendocardial tissues, particularly when accompanying an Ebstein's malformation, a frequent association of right-sided preexcitation (Fig. 2-37). Septal pathways are theoretically able to pass across the septal ring at any point from the tricuspid to the mitral side of the septum. The only septal pathway we have identified[95] crossed the ring at the point of origin of the tricuspid valve. Septal pathways are the hardest to divide at surgery.[96] A helpful technique for dividing these pathways may be to dissect in the tissue plane running forward from the posterior atrioventricular sulcus to the node (see Fig. 2-32), entering this space through the right atrial wall.[96] The majority of connections identified histologically have been tiny threads of working myocardium (see Fig. 2-35). In our experience,[95] they have been thicker at their atrial origin and have ramified like the roots of a tree at their ventricular insertion. One of the pathways we studied had its atrial origin in a segment of atrioventricular specialized tissue (see Fig. 2-37). This connection could truly be considered a Kent bundle. The bundle itself was composed of specialized conduction tissue, a finding described by other investigators.[97,98] It is possible that the specialized nature of such connections have electrophysiologic significance. Multiple connections have been identified histologically by several investigators,[89,95,99] and this finding has also been reported on the basis of clinical studies.[100]

Nodoventricular and Fasciculoventricular Connections

The precise structure and morphology of nodoventricular and fasciculoventricular connections (see Fig. 2-33) and their relation to ventricular preexcitation remain to

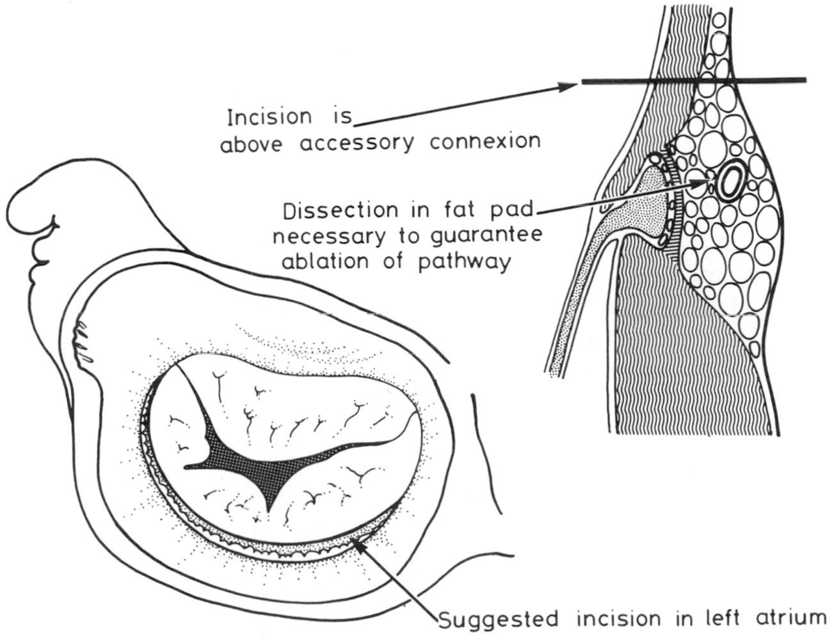

Figure 2-36. *Diagram illustrating the likely site of a surgical incision to divide an accessory pathway. It is unlikely to divide the actual connection.*

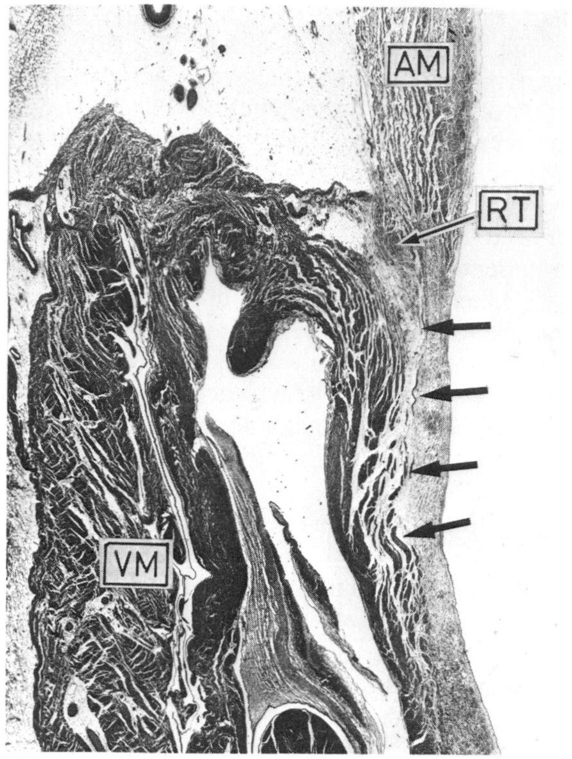

Figure 2-37. *Photomicrograph of a right-sided accessory connection (arrows) from a patient with preexcitation. The connection is directly subendocardial (compare with Fig. 2-36) and originates from a segment of specialized atrioventricular ring tissue (RT).*

be elucidated. During development, the septal fibrous ring is perforated by numerous strands of specialized tissue that pass between the nodal-bundle axis and the crest of the muscular septum. Despite this anatomic continuity, electrophysiologic studies have shown that conduction occurred as though the nodal-bundle axis was totally isolated from the ventricular septal myocardium, as in the definitive heart.[101] At birth the septal fibrous plane is much better developed, but in most hearts it is still possible to trace archipelagos of conduction tissue that pass through the central fibrous body in such a position that the compact node and penetrating bundle are in anatomic continuity with the ventricular tissues (Fig. 2-38). The subsequent fate of these tenuous connections has not, to the best of our knowledge, been studied in a systematic manner in the hearts of children and young adults. Nonetheless, in our experience, direct nodoventricular and fasciculoventricular connections are frequently found in the hearts of "normal" children and young adults (Fig. 2-39). Systematic studies should, in our opinion, be performed in order to establish the "normal" complement of these connections. A relationship between their presence and preexcitation has been strongly suggested in one case by the correlative anatomicoclinical study of Lev and colleagues.[102]

Accessory Atriofascicular Connections

Accessory atriofascicular connections produce preexcitation with a normal QRS complex—the Lown-Ganong-Levine syndrome. Such preexcitation is also explained on the basis of the "James" fiber, but an anatomic distinction must be made between a "James" fiber and an atriofascicular accessory connection (Fig. 2-40). The fibers described by James[7] are a finding in normal hearts. He described them as a gathering together of fibers from the eustachian ridge that passed forward to insert into the junction of the atrioventricular node and bundle. In contrast, atriofascicular connections are fibers that insert directly through the fibrous tissue collar to enter the penetrating atrioventricular bundle. The latter fibers were identified by Brechenmacher[86] in hearts from patients known to have exhibited preexcitation of the short PR–normal QRS variety. The key to distinction of an atriofascicular connection is that it must enter the nodal-bundle axis after the axis has entered the central fibrous body and become the penetrating atrioventricular bundle.

Intradnodal Bypass Trusts

The fibers described by James[7] are best considered as intranodal bypass tracts. They are confined entirely to the atrial component of the specialized junctional area. Since, as James has indicated, they are to be found in normal hearts, it will be difficult from the standpoint of anatomic studies to implicate them as a source of preexcitation. It is likely that any evidence will be circumstantial, such as, for example, the finding of short PR–normal QRS preexcitation in patients without accessory atriofascicular connections. There are numerous additonal possibilities for bypass within the atrial component of the specialized junctional area (Fig. 2-41). There is considerable variation in the normal heart in the architecture of the "last" atrial fiber to make contact with the nodal-bundle axis before it becomes the penetrating bundle.[50] In most hearts this fiber is an atrial overlay transitional fiber. In other hearts the fiber originates deep from the left atrial aspect of the septum. Further variation exists with regard to the morphology of the compact node and its posterior extension. In some hearts the major axis is toward the mitral valve and the left side of the septum. In other hearts the tricuspid extension of the compact node is dominant. Within the node itself, the stratification of the normal node gives multiple possibilities for bypass pathways. These variations and the problem of the substrates for normal PR–short QRS preexcitation will be solved only following extensive studies of "normal" hearts and comparison with those

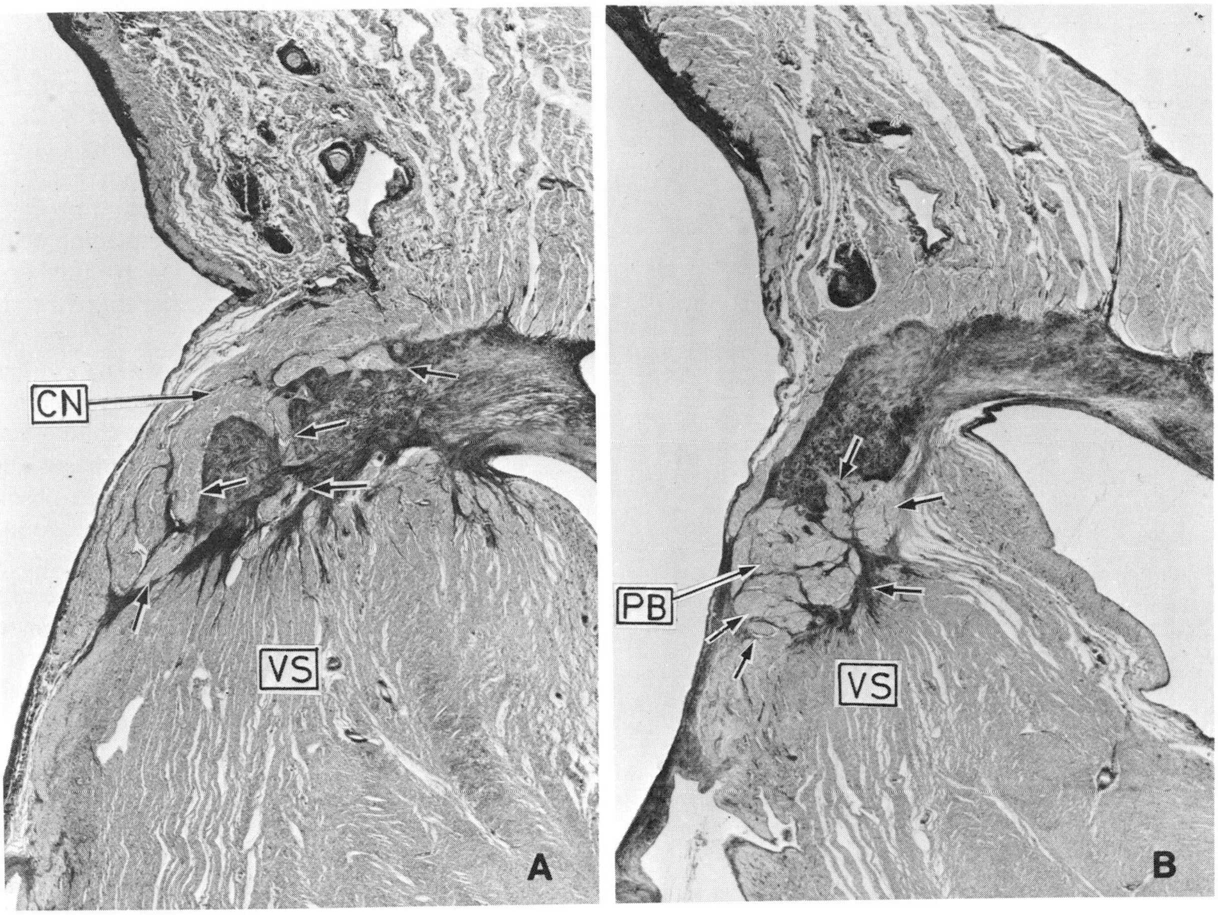

Figure 2-38. *Photomicrograph of a junctional area from a neonate, showing the archipelagos of conduction tissue (arrows) that pass through the anulus fibrosus and connect the compact node (CN) and penetrating bundle (PB) to the crest of the ventricular septum (VS).*

hearts known to have exhibited this form of preexcitation.

Dual Atrioventricular Nodal Pathways and Longitudinal Dissociation

The possible candidates for pathways as intranodal bypass tracts must also be considered as substrates for dual nodal pathways and longitudinal dissociation. In the anatomicoelectrophysiologic studies we performed in the specialized junctional area of the rabbit,[67] an area of longitudinal dissociation was positively identified within the transitional cell zone of the atrioventricular node. In this area the transitional cells themselves were attenuated and separated by strands of connective tissue. Similar cell arrangements are found in the posterior transitional area of the human node. Surprisingly, the grosser alternate pathways we studied in the rabbit node, such as the anterior atrial overlay fibers and the extensive posterior bundlelike prolongation of the lower nodal cells, both proved to be electrophysiologic "dead-end pathways"[67] when examined by anterograde and retrograde stimulation.

Conduction Tissues and Sudden Infant Death Syndrome

The possibility that fatal arrhythmias may be responsible for some of the far too numerous cases of sudden infant death is both reasonable and of preventive significance.[103] However, histologic studies of the conduction system of infants who have died suddenly have done little to help alleviate the problem. Indeed, the contention that surrounds the topic may well have a positively deleterious effect,[104] which is to be regretted greatly. Contention has arisen because some observers[103-106] consider that changes noted in archipelagos of conduction tissue that extend into the central fibrous body of infant hearts (see Fig. 2-38) may play a role in sudden infant death. Others[107-109] question these interpreta-

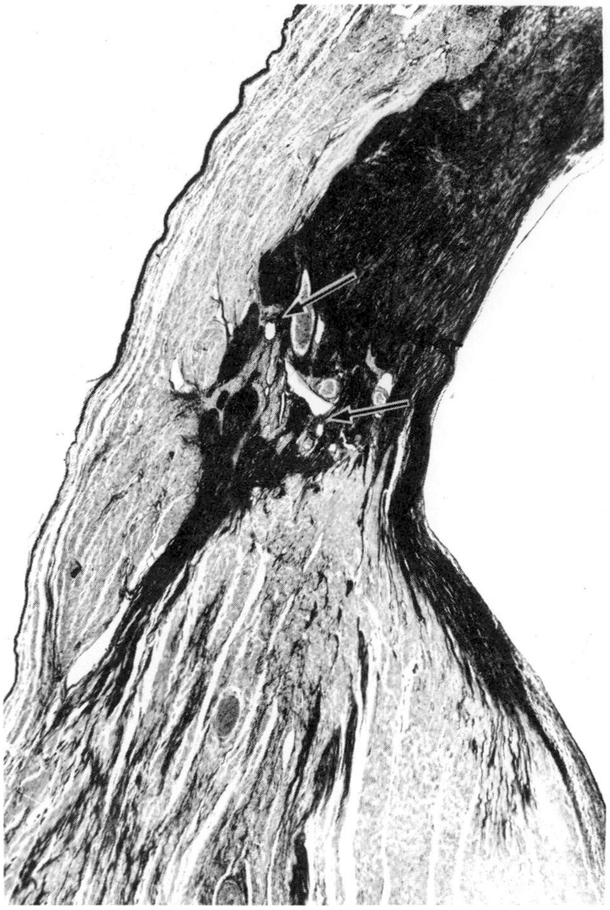

Figure 2-39. *Photomicrograph of a normal adult junctional area, showing persistent archipelagos (arrows) that penetrate the anulus fibrosus when traced in serial sections to form a nodoventricular connection.*

tions, either because they were unable to find the described changes or because they found similar changes in the conduction systems of infants dying of known causes. Lesions in these archipelagos were first implicated as a possible substrate for sudden infant death by James.[103] He described a process of "orderly resorptive degeneration of portions of the undivided His bundle and A-V node" in all hearts he studied, both from infants who died suddenly and from those dying of known causes. Although denying the presence of inflammatory changes, massive necrosis, or hemorrhage, he nonetheless described "a slowly destructive process in which neighbouring fibroblasts were replacing necrotic fibers of the His bundle or A-V node." He further stated that "macrophages were present adjacent to the small foci of necrosis, acting as scavenger cells" and that "those pockets of tissue were in various stages of degeneration and resorption, some with relatively little necrosis and others in which nearly all the fibers had been destroyed and were being removed by macrophages and replaced by fibroblastic invasion." Subsequent observers, ourselves included, were unable to confirm these interpretations,[107-109] since they were unable to identify any necrosis or macrophage aggregation. James, in a subsequent editorial,[104] suggested that these negative reports were adopting a "straw-man approach," since he had intended to indicate that "resorptive degeneration" was a normal developmental process. It is difficult to reread his original account and *not* reach the conclusion that he was observing focal areas of cell death and necrosis. It seems to us, therefore, that the argument centers on whether there is evidence of focal cell death in the infant junctional area. If it is there, the second question is whether it represents a pathologic process. James[103] described such focal necrosis but evidently did not consider it pathologic.[104] Others[107-109] have not observed any evidence of the reported focal necrosis, regarding the appearance of the archipelagos of conduction tissue in the central fibrous body as consistent with normal development of the junctional area.

Aside from this problem, whether any evidence links this process of normal development (or focal necrosis) to arrhythmias must also be considered. James[103] argued that cell death may cause release of intracellular potassium and produce local tissue acidosis, which may affect

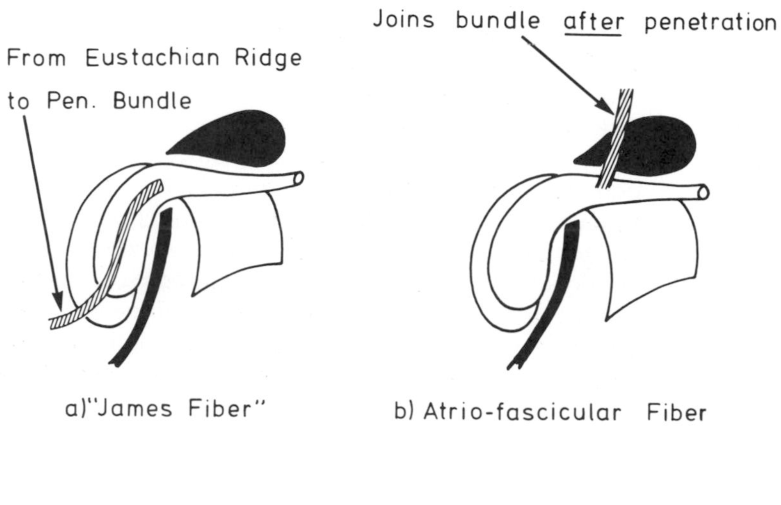

Figure 2-40. *Diagram illustrating the anatomic difference between a "James" fiber[7] and an atriofascicular accessory connection such as described by Brechenmacher.[86]*

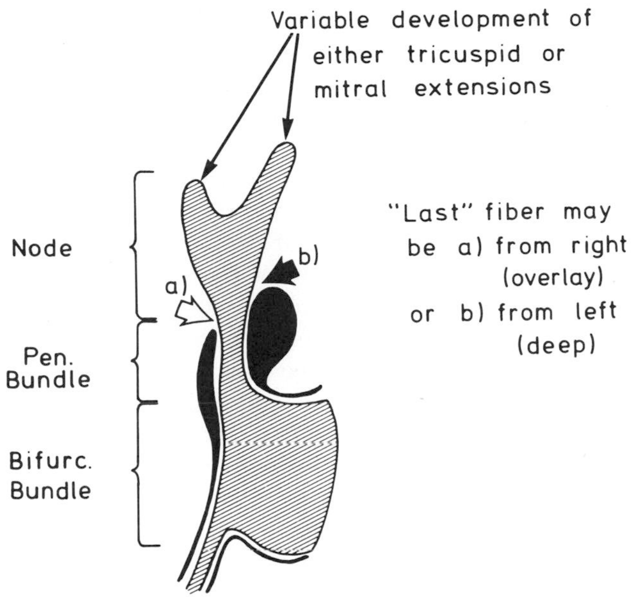

Figure 2-41. *Diagram illustrating some of the possibilities for bypass tracts provided by variations in a normal specialized junctional area.*

function in adjacent surviving tissue. Alternatively, he opined that the degenerating tissue in the archipelagos may become hyperexcitable and give rise to ectopic beats or ectopic rhythm. He also directed attention to the studies of Preston[110] and co-workers, which demonstrated "immaturity" of the junctional area in three different species of young mammals. Extending this, he reasoned that the shaggy, large atrioventricular bundle of the fetus was electrophysiologically unsafe, orderly conduction being better performed by the thin, smooth bundle of the adult.

Our own electrophysiologic studies of the human fetal heart[101] have subsequently demonstrated that the conduction patterns are mature before midterm, despite the fact that the specialized tissue at this stage is in extensive anatomic continuity throughout its length with the ventricular myocardium. Our histologic studies in hearts of infants dying suddenly[108] have demonstrated the archipelagos of conduction tissue extending into the central fibrous body observed by James[103] and others.[105-107,109] We, in keeping with other investigators,[107,109] have not observed the changes described as "resorptive degeneration," be they normal or abnormal. We would wish for antemortem evidence of conduction disorders before suggesting that changes occurring as a normal developmental process may be substrates for sudden death.

Nonetheless, it is not our intention to denigrate the possibility that arrhythmias may be the cause of some sudden deaths in infancy. We have studied hearts from two infants known to have died suddenly in which a gross abnormality was observed in the conduction system. In the first, an accessory connection was observed in the region of the compact node.[108] In the other,[111] we found stenosis of the penetrating bundle, a lesion suggested to be a cause of sudden death in some canine species[112]; but we have no evidence that these anatomic substrates had been the mechanisms of arrhythmia. Only by studying the conduction systems from infants dying suddenly who have had prior electrocardiographic investigation will we discover if these are indeed the substrates for some of these tragic deaths. In this respect we endorse fully the observation of James[103] that it would be regrettable if the interpretations offered by Lie and coworkers[109] discouraged others from investigating the functional aspect of the conduction system in infancy.

Aging Changes in the Conduction Tissues

The process of aging and its effect on the histologic appearances of the conduction tissues have been much neglected. Apart from the studies of Lev and Erickson[113,114] and the investigations on the sinus node and internodal atrial myocardium by Davies and Pomerance,[115] we are unaware of any systematic researches on this important topic. There is a general increase, with aging, in the amount of fibrous tissue present in the conduction tissues. Whether this increase in fibrosis is due to actual increased deposition of fibrous tissue or a decrease in the amount of conduction tissues relative to the heart remains to be established. Several workers[20,103] have shown how the fetal penetrating bundle is a vast structure compared with its adult counterpart. This is equally true of the atrial component of the junctional area and the sinus node. Our studies of fetal tissues show that all these structures are laid down within a matrix of connective tissue, particularly the sinus node (see Fig. 2-11), although James[116] indicated that the fetal sinus node was lacking in fibrous tissue. Our studies show rather that the content of nodal tissue per unit area of node decreases with increasing age.[27] It may well be that the excessive fibrosis reported in aged nodes is a continuation of this process, since very few nodal cells persist in these nodes. Our observations suggest a similar progression in the atrioventricular junctional area,[50] notably on the archipelagos of conduction tissue in the central fibrous body of fetal and infant hearts. In his editorial, James[104] asked what happened to the archipelagos if they were not removed by the "resorptive degeneration." The islands become less evident with increasing growth of the heart, but they continue to protrude into the fibrous body, since we find some of these remnants in the majority of adult and adolescent hearts studied.[117]

The Conduction Tissues in Congenital Heart Disease

It is axiomatic that knowledge of the disposition of the conduction tissues is a prerequisite for any surgeon wishing to correct congenital cardiac malformations. This is as true with regard to the atrial conduction tissues as it is with regard to the atrioventricular bundle. In this section, therefore, we will briefly review the pertinent details of conduction tissue architecture in the more important anomalies.

The Sinus Node and Internodal Atrial Myocardium

During surgery, damage must be avoided not only to the sinus node but also to its nutrient artery. These structures are at risk during incisions into the right atrium as well as during the placement of atrial cannulas. The entire junction of the superior caval vein with the right atrium should be considered a danger area. The area of maximal danger is the part of the terminal groove between the crest of the atrial appendage and the orifice of the inferior caval vein (see Fig. 2-2). The sinus node is directly subepicardial in this position and particularly susceptible to any form of trauma.

The sinus node is likely to be in most danger during operations for complete transposition that redirect the systemic and pulmonary venous returns (Mustard and Senning procedures). Much has been written on the role of the "specialized internodal tracts" in the genesis of postoperative arrhythmias in this condition.[118] Histologic studies are conflicting in this respect. One investigation suggested damage to the tracts as the cause[119]; another pointed to the high incidence of sinus node trauma in patients dying following repair.[120] Our own studies[9,50] and those of others have not demonstrated the narrow tracts of specialized cells presumed by some[118] to exist in the atrial septum and walls. It is self-evident that, following removal of the atrial septum, the impulse will pass either in front of the hole thus created or behind it in the remainder of the atrial myocardium. This premise was borne out by the mapping studies carried out at Great Ormond Street Hospital, London.[121] It seems sensible to avoid incisions across the major muscle bundles such as the terminal crest in the repair procedure. However, even if the crest is cut (as was the policy of Lincoln at the Brompton Hospital, London[122]), if care is taken to avoid the areas of the sinus and atrioventricular nodes, postoperative arrhythmias can be prevented, provided one remembers to take account of those abnormal rhythms that had existed before the operation.[123]

One condition that must be considered when planning an atrial incision is that of juxtaposition of the atrial appendages. This anomaly (a frequent accompaniment of tricuspid atresia and occasionally encountered with transposed great arteries) alters the position of the sinus node. Our results[124] show that the node is unrelated to the juxtaposed right atrial appendage. Instead, it is disposed on the epicardial aspect of the anterior interatrial septum, either at the orifice of the superior caval vein or near the atrioventricular groove (Fig. 2-42). The node is smaller than anticipated for normal hearts.[124]

The Atrioventricular Conduction Tissues

As described in the section on development of the junctional area, formation of the normal node and bundle demands contributions from both the atrial and ventricular tissues. The ventricular component is formed in relation to both the inlet and apical trabecular portions of the muscular interventricular septum. To produce a normal atrioventricular conduction mechanism, it is necessary to have normal formation and alignment of the atrial septum and the inlet and apical trabecular components of the muscular septum (Fig. 2-43). If this alignment does not occur, an anomalous node can be derived from the complete ring of conduction tissue that surrounded the atrioventricular junction during development (Fig. 2-30). These considerations underscore the disposition of the atrioventricular conduction mechanism in those hearts with normally aligned septal struc-

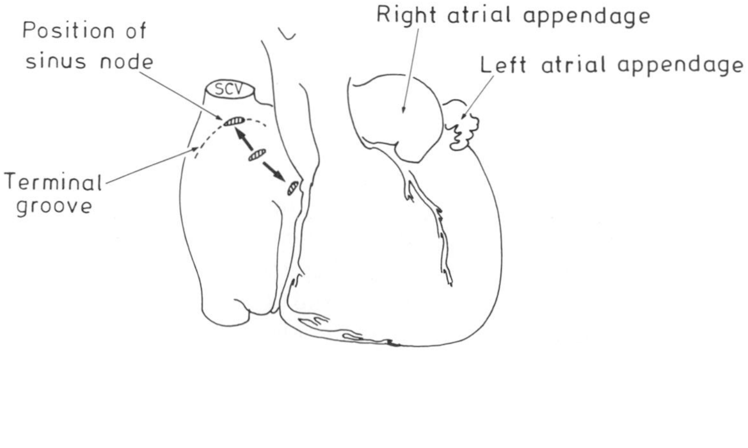

Figure 2-42. *Diagram showing the position of the sinus node in five patients with juxtaposition of the atrial appendages.*

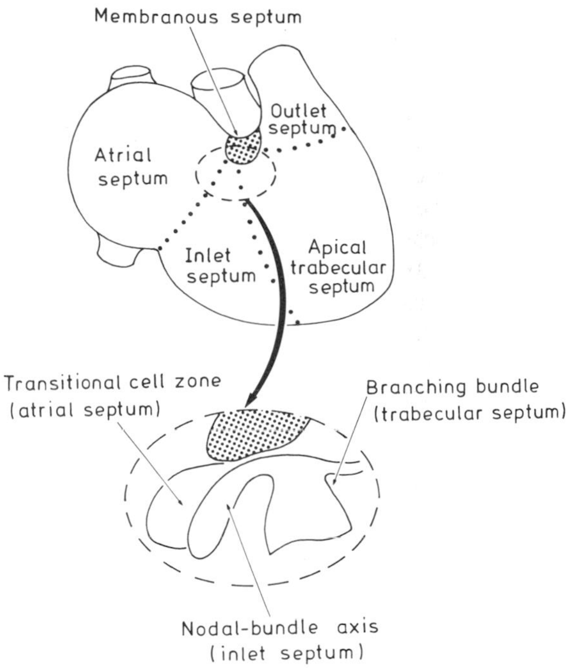

Figure 2-43. *Diagram illustrating how the alignment of the atrial septum, inlet septum, and trabecular septum is necessary for formation of a normal atrioventricular junctional area.*

tures as opposed to those with either septal malalignment or absence of the ventricular inlet septum.

Hearts with Normally Aligned Septal Structures

Hearts with "isolated" ventricular septal defects, Fallot's tetralogy, atrioventricular septal defects, and abnormal ventriculoarterial connections associated with concordant atrioventricular connection all fall into this group. There are minor differences in each subgroup, but in all of them the landmark to the penetrating atrioventricular bundle is the apex of the triangle of Koch, as in the normal heart (see Fig. 2-14). In hearts with atrioventricular septal defects this nodal triangle (not *the* triangle of Koch) is displaced posteriorly by the defect[57] (Fig. 2-44).

In hearts with ventricular septal defects (Fig. 2-45), the disposition of the atrioventricular bundle varies depending on the type of defect present.[126] Most defects result from deficiency of the crest of the muscular ventricular septum in the environs of the membranous septum—so-called membranous defects but better referred to as perimembranous defects. In these defects, all of which have the central fibrous body in their posteroinferior rims and roof, the ventricular conducting tissues are related to the crest of the septum. The atrioventricular bundle penetrates through the fibrous tissue, which is the area of greatest danger. In some the branching bundle sits directly on the septal crest,[126–129] but in most[130]

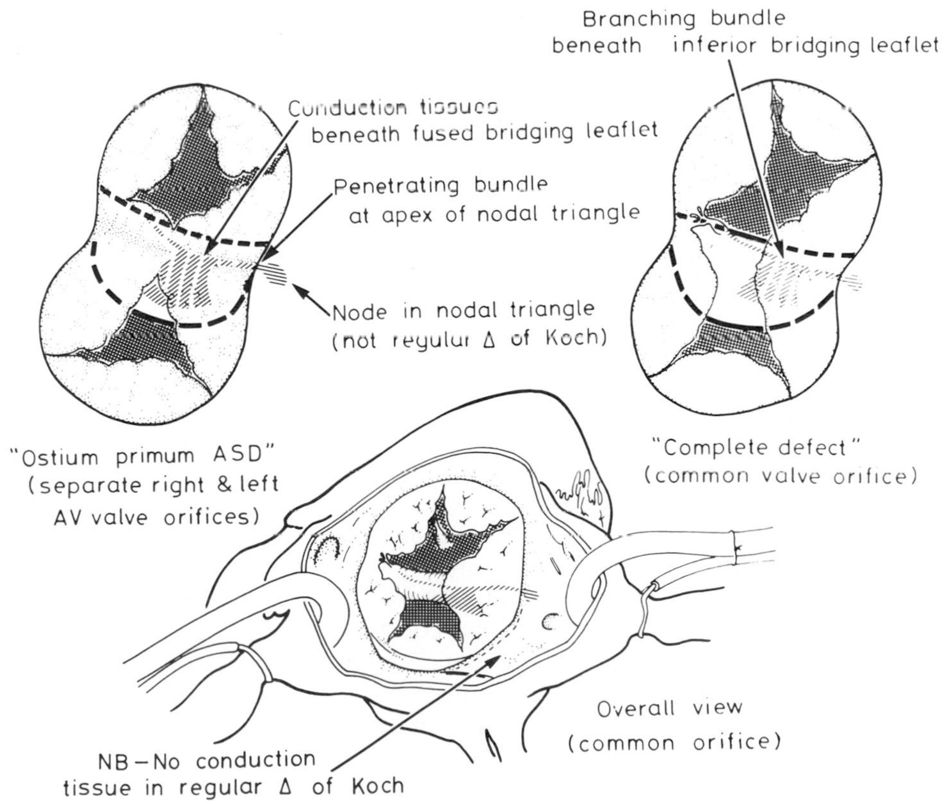

Figure 2-44. *Diagrams illustrating the position of the conducting tissues in hearts with atrioventricular septal defects.*

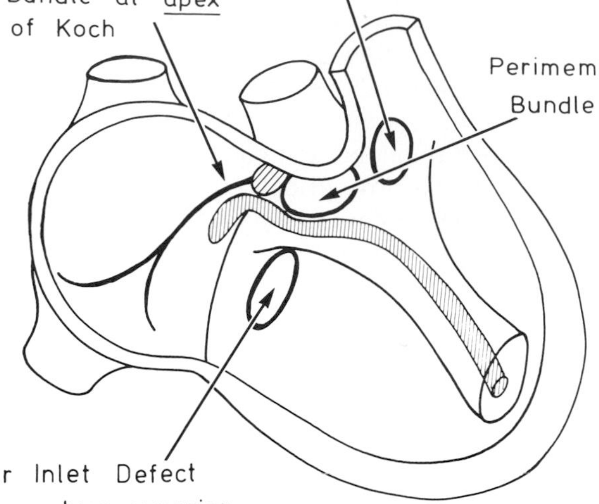

Figure 2-45. *Diagram illustrating the relationship of the ventricular conducting tissues to different types of ventricular septal defects.*

the bundle may be to the left side, as in patients with tetralogy of Fallot (see below). When defects are in the muscular part of the inlet septum, the bundle bears a significantly different relation.[126] The defect is within the inlet septum, thus below and behind the penetrating and branching atrioventricular bundles. Because of this, the superoanterior and anterior quadrants are thosc parts of the defect "at risk" (Fig. 2-45). Such muscular inlet defects can be distinguished from perimembranous inlet defects because of their complete muscular rim. Muscular defects of the outlet septum are remote from the ventricular conducting tissues (Fig. 2-45). However, muscular defects in the apical trabecular septum can be related to the peripheral bundle branches.[129]

In tetralogy of Fallot, the conducting tissue is disposed in a similar fashion to perimembranous defects, and in most cases the branching bundle is to the left side of the septal crest.[131] The septal crest is therefore devoid of conducting tissues, the major danger area being the posteroinferior angle where the penetrating bundle passes through the central fibrous body.[132] In a small number of patients with tetralogy of Fallot,[128,132] the branching bundle can be positioned directly on the septal crest (Fig. 2-46). In these patients, whose condition cannot be distinguished on gross anatomic observations, it would be dangerous to place sutures directly into the septal crest during repair as advocated by Starr and colleagues.[133] When the defect in tetralogy has a muscular posteroinferior rim (as occurs with muscular outlet ventricular septal defects), the ventricular conducting tissues are remote from the defect rim.

The ventricular component of an atrioventricular septal defect can be considered as a large perimembranous inlet defect extending to the crux of the heart (see Fig. 2-44). The disposition of conduction tissue is very similar in the varieties with either separate valve orifices or a common valve.[55-57] The nodal triangle is displaced posteroinferiorly by the septal defect and is not the usual triangle of Koch. The penetrating bundle is found at its apex. Because of the septal deficiency, the atrioventricular node is hypoplastic. The posterior displacement contributes both to the longer nonbranching bundle seen in these hearts and the posteriorly situated left bundle branch. This runs down from the branching bundle, which is positioned along the full length of the crest of the inlet septum. In the anomaly with separate right and left valve orifices ("ostium primum ASD"), the penetrating and branching bundles are directly inferior to the conjoined bridging leaflets.

In hearts with abnormal ventriculoarterial connections but concordant atrioventricular connections, the variability of conduction tissue disposition depends on the type of ventricular septal defect present (*e.g.*, perimembranous or with a muscular posteroinferior rim). These anomalies include complete transposition,[134] double outlet right ventricle with subaortic or subpulmonary defect,[135] and common arterial trunk.[136] The septal crest of the muscular septum is usually devoid of conducting tissues, but exceptions to this rule do occur.[137]

Hearts with Malaligned Septal Structures

The defect typifying this arrangement is congenitally corrected transposition, which is the combination of

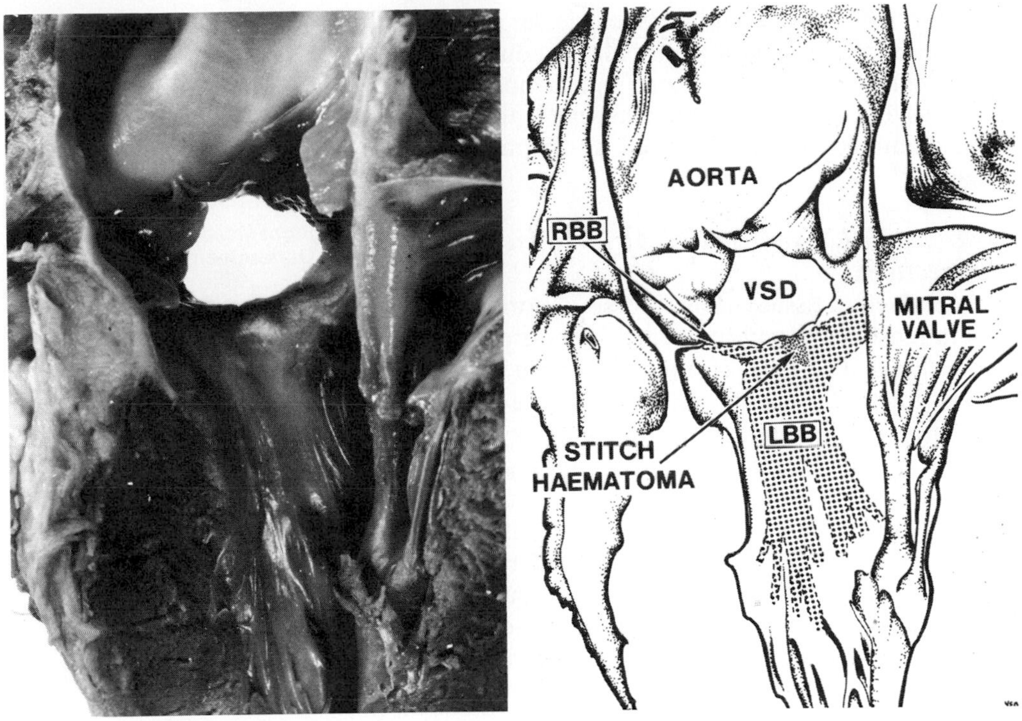

Figure 2-46. *Photograph and drawing illustrating the left aspect of a heart with tetralogy of Fallot, showing the conducting tissues (RBB, LBB) directly astride the crest of the defect (VSD). Placement of stitches directly into the septal crest (stitch hematoma) resulted in this case in traumatic heart block. (Anderson, R., Ho, S. V., Monro J. L., et al.: Coeur, 8:793, 1977)*

atrioventricular discordant and ventriculoarterial connection.[138] When this anomaly exists in persons with normally arranged atria, there is a vital derangement in disposition of the conducting tissue. Because of septal malalignment, the apex of the triangle of Koch is out of line with the inlet component of the muscular septum. The regular atrioventricular node at the apex of the triangle of Koch cannot make contact with the ventricular conduction tissues on the trabecular septum.[139,140] Instead, an anterior atrioventricular node is present, which communicates through a long nonbranching bundle with ventricular conduction tissues. In the presence of a ventricular septal defect,[141] the bundle passes lateral to the pulmonary outflow tract (Fig. 2-47). Others[142] have suggested that the bundle passes between the pulmonary valve and the defect. Anatomic considerations[143] suggest that this apparent difference is related to perspective and interpretation rather than variable disposition of the bundle.

When there is a mirror-image arrangement of the atria in congenitally corrected transposition, all the cases studied thus far[144–146] have had posterior atrioventricular nodes and penetrating bundles. This is probably related to the better alignment of septal structures seen in these hearts. Despite these findings, the possibility must not be discounted that anterior connections may exist in

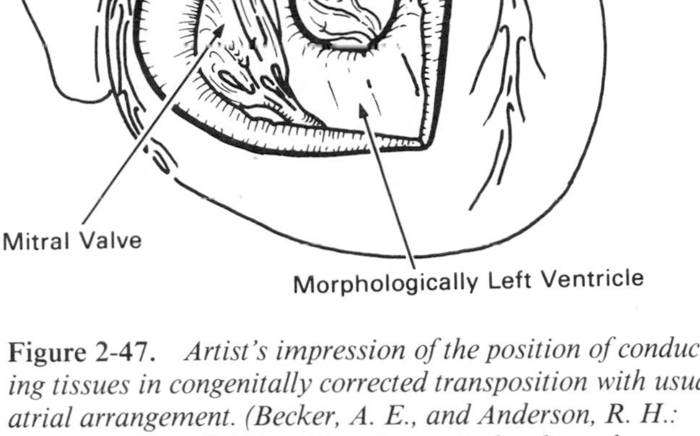

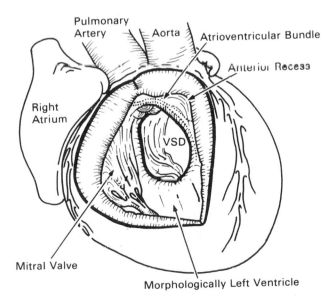

Figure 2-47. *Artist's impression of the position of conducting tissues in congenitally corrected transposition with usual atrial arrangement. (Becker, A. E., and Anderson, R. H.: Anatomy of conditions with atrioventricular discordance. In Anderson, R. H., and Shinebourne, E. A. [eds.]: Paediatric Cardiology, 1977. Edinburgh, Churchill Livingstone, 1978)*

any heart with a discordant atrioventricular connection, or even an entire sling of ventricular conduction tissue connected to both anterior and regular nodes. Such a sling was first observed by Monckeberg[147] and has since been identified by us[148] as well as Bharati and colleagues.[149]

Hearts with Univentricular Atrioventricular Connections

The conduction tissues have a grossly abnormal disposition in most hearts with univentricular atrioventricular connections. The most common example is that with double inlet left ventricle (single ventricle with outlet chamber). The feature of these hearts is lack of a septum extending to the crux. Because of this, the regular node is again unable to make contact with the ventricular conduction tissues, and an anterior node assumes this role.[150,151] In the variety with left-sided rudimentary right ventricle, the disposition of the ventricular conduction tissues is very similar to that seen in congenitally corrected transposition with usually arranged atria (compare Figs. 2-47 and 2-48). In a double inlet left ventricle heart with a right-sided rudimentary right ventricle, any surgery to the dominant ventricle might involve a left-sided incision. If approached in this fashion, the bundle would be seen to pass beneath the defect despite originating from an anterior node (Fig. 2-49). If the surgeon approaches any heart with a double inlet left ventricle through the rudimentary right ventricle, the conduction tissue will always be distant. It will lie on the left ventricular side and beneath the crest of the ventricular septal defect (Fig. 2-50). The key to the abnormal disposition of the conducting tissues is the presence or absence of a septum running to the crux. When a double inlet goes to a solitary and indeterminate ventricle there is no such septum present. An anterior or anterolateral node is therefore the rule.[152,153] In contrast, in a double inlet right ventricle heart with left-sided rudimentary left ventricle, or in hearts with huge ventricular septal defects, a septum or septal remnant does extend to the crux, and a regular connecting node is found in these anomalies.[153,154] Ventricular surgery in classic tricuspid

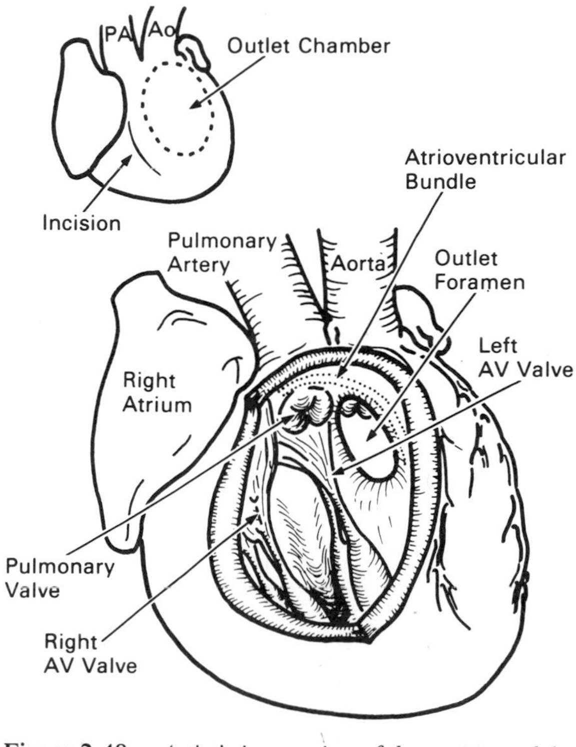

Figure 2-48. *Artist's impression of the position of the conducting tissues in double inlet left ventricle with left-sided rudimentary right ventricle. (Anderson, R. H., Wilkinson, J. L., and Becker, A. E.: The conducting tissues in the univentricular heart. In Van Mierop, L. H. S., Oppenheimer-Decker, A., and Bruins, C. H. L. Ch. [eds.]: Embryology and Tetralogy of the Heart and Great Arteries. The Hague, Leiden University Press, 1978)*

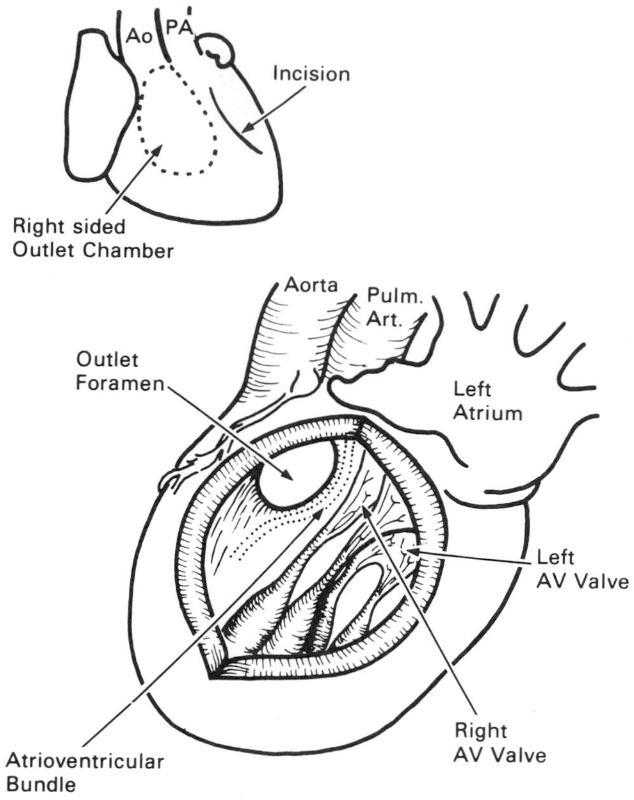

Figure 2-49. *Artist's impression of the position of the conducting tissues in double inlet left ventricle with right-sided rudimentary right ventricle. (Anderson, R. H., Wilkinson, J. L., and Becker, A. E.: The conducting tissues in the univentricular heart. In Van Meirop, L. H. S., Oppenheimer-Decker, A., and Bruins, C. H. L. Ch. [eds.]: Embryology and Tetralogy of the Heart and Great Arteries. The Hague, Leiden University Press, 1978)*

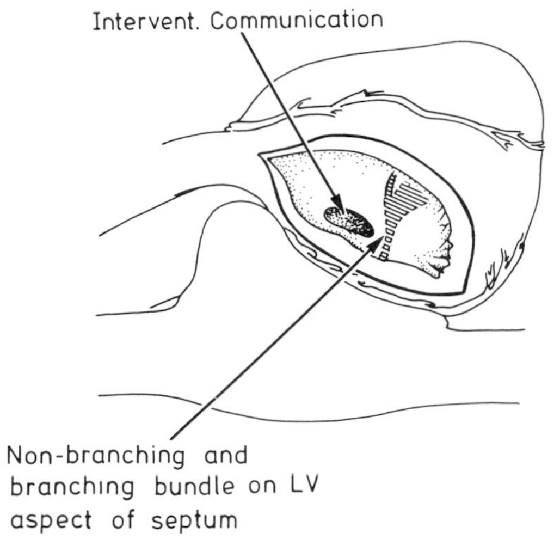

Figure 2-50. *Diagram illustrating the relationship of the conducting tissues to the ventricular septal defect in any form of subventricular connection to a left ventricle.*

atresia is likely to be confined to the rudimentary right ventricle. The conduction tissues are related to the septum exactly as in double inlet left ventricle (see Fig. 2-50). In all these hearts with univentricular atrioventricular connection to a dominant left ventricle, if it is necessary to enlarge the ventricular septal defect, it is always the margin of the apical trabecular septum closest to the left border of the heart that can most safely be excised.

Congenital Heart Block

Lev[155] has divided congenitally complete heart block into two basic varieties, one of which occurs in a congenitally malformed heart and the other in an otherwise normal heart.

Congenital heart block associated with a cardiac malformation is most frequently seen with congenitally corrected transposition and atrioventricular septal defects having separate right and left orifices ("ostium primum ASD"). Although it may be complete at birth, it is more usual for the arrhythmia to be progressive, starting with first degree block and leading to complete block. Our histologic studies[140] suggest that the progression may be related to increasing fibrosis of the atrioventricular bundle, which is situated in a very mobile part of the heart compared to the normal heart. The degree of fibrosis of the ventricular conduction tissues may also be related to known vulnerability to the mildest trauma, block being known to occur during induction of anesthesia or at an initial thoracotomy.[156]

Congenitally complete heart block occurring in an otherwise normal heart can also be divided into various

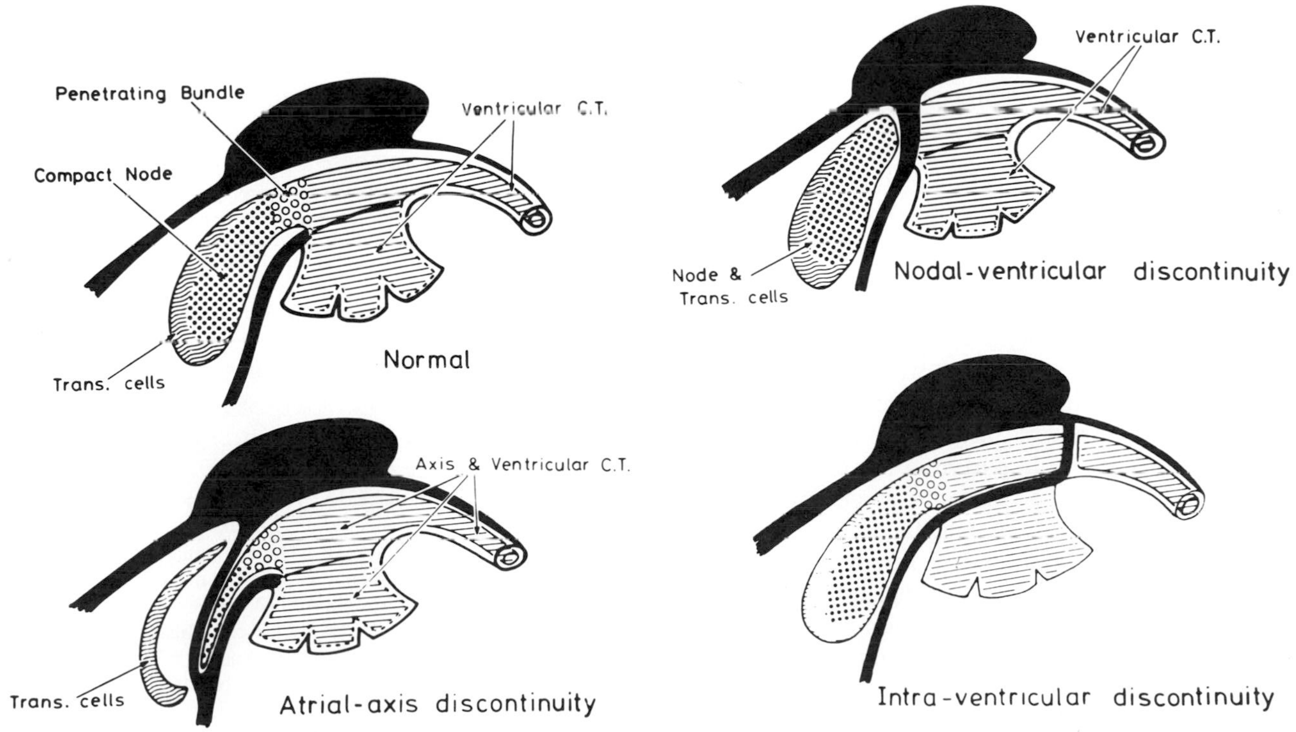

Figure 2-51. *Diagram illustrating the differentiations of complete heart block on histologic findings.*

forms depending on the histology of the junctional area.[157,158] Three types are described. In the first type, discontinuity is found between the atrial tissues and a hypoplastic nodal-bundle axis.[157] In the second type, the atrioventricular node is normally formed but discontinuous from the ventricular specialized tissues[158] (Fig. 2-51). The third type is by far the rarest, existing when the bundle branches are discontinuous from the branching bundle.[159] A recent study pointed to a strong correlation between isolated congenitally complete heart block and anti-RO (SS-A) antibody in maternal serum.[160] Our histologic studies[161] of seven hearts from children whose maternal serum was anti-RO positive shared absence of the atrioventricular node. In its place were fibrous and adipose tissues.

Acquired Diseases of the Conduction System

Many disease processes that affect the heart can involve the normally situated conduction tissues. It is not possible to describe all these processes in the context of this review, but it should be remembered that any disease affecting the endocardium, myocardium, and pericardium may produce functional and anatomic abnormalities in the conduction tissues. The reader is referred to the exhaustive catalogue of these processes given in the book by Davies and co-workers.[162] The most important are coronary artery disease and the effect of aging processes on the ventricular conduction system.

Coronary Artery Disease and Conduction Abnormalities

It is common experience that acute myocardial infarction may become complicated either by bundle branch block or atrioventricular dissociation. The prognostic significance of these findings depends on the localization of the primary infarct. In patients with anteroseptal infarction, the development of bundle branch block carries a grave prognosis, contrasting with its relatively benign course in those with posteroinferior wall infarction. The pathologic substrate of the arrhythmias has been a matter of dispute.[163-168] In part, this is because the conduction tissues are more resistant to ischemia than is the working myocardium, making the interpretation of histologic findings more difficult. Bundle branch block in the setting of an acute myocardial infarction can only rarely be attributed to overt bundle branch necrosis.[166-168] Nonetheless, ischemic changes such as edema and inflammatory cell infiltration present in the direct vicinity of the bundle branches or within the conduction fibers are found in the great majority of patients with electrocardiographic changes. The development of bundle branch block is related to the extent of the infarction rather than actual necrosis of conduction fibers. One might anticipate regression of electrocardiographic changes should the patient survive. It is common in posteroinferior wall infarction to find atrioventricular dissociation in the early phase, which is nearly always reversible. The underlying pathology is quite similar to that described for anteroseptal infarctions.[169]

The frequency of chronic conduction disturbances as a direct result of myocardial infarction has not yet been determined. It is widely accepted that the usual case of atrioventricular dissociation or bundle branch block in the elderly patient is not directly related to coronary artery disease.

Aging Processes in the Ventricular Conduction Tissues

It may be generalized that increasing age is accompanied by increasing fibrosis of the ventricular conduction tissues together with fall-off in the number of conduction fibers present per unit area. The precise nature of these changes is as yet not fully understood. The degenerative changes may affect the penetrating and nonbranching segments of the bundle in their position on the crest of the ventricular septum. Abnormalities at these sites are claimed to be the substrates of so-called Lev's disease.[170,171] Similar changes affecting the more distal portions of the bundle branches themselves, often found with patchy distribution, most likely underlie so-called Lenegre's disease.[172,173] Whether these disease processes form the extreme ends of a spectrum of pathology of the ventricular conduction tissues, or whether they are discrete entities each with its own pathogenesis, has not yet been determined.[174] Progression of the pathologic changes found in these disease entities, whatever their etiology, may result in complete heart block. This so-called idiopathic complete heart block is the most common reason for pacemaker insertion in the elderly.[175]

References

1. Tawara, S.: Das Reizleitungssytem des Saugetierherzens. Jena, Gustav Fischer, 1906.
2. Keith, A., and Flack, M.: The auriculo-ventricular bundle of the human heart. Lancet, 2:359, 1906.
3. Keith, A., and Flack, M.: The form and nature of the muscular connections between the primary divisions of the vertebrate heart. J. Anat. Physiol., 41:172, 1907.
4. Monckeberg, J. G.: Das spezifische Muskelsystem in menschlichen Herzen. Erge. allg. Path. Anat., 19:328, 1921.
5. Koch, W.: Weiter Mitteilungen uber den Sinusknoten der Herzens. Verh. Dtsch. Pathol. Ges., 13:85, 1909.
6. Koch, W.: Der funktionelle Bau des menschlichen Herzens, p. 92. Berlin, Urban v. Schwarzenburg, 1922.
7. James, T. N.: Morphology of the human atrioventricular node,

with remarks pertinent to its electrophysiology. Am. Heart J., 62:756, 1961.
8. James, T. N.: The connecting pathways between the sinus node and the A-V node and between the right and the left atrium in the human heart. Am. Heart J., 66:498, 1963.
9. Janse, M. J., and Anderson, R. H.: Specialized internodal atrial pathways—fact or fiction? Eur. J. Cardiol., 2:117, 1974.
10. Wenckebach, K. F.: Beitrage zur Kenntis der menschlichen Herztatigkeit. Archiv. Anat. Physiol., 2:297, 1906.
11. Lewis, T., Oppenheimer, B. S., and Oppenheimer, A.: Site of origin of the mammalian heart beat: The pacemaker in the dog. Heart, 2:147, 1910.
12. Truex, R. C.: The sinuatrial node and its connections with the atrial tissues. In Wellens, H. J. J., Lie, K. I., and Janse, M. J. (eds.): The Conduction System of the Heart: Structure, Function and Clinical Implications, p. 209. Leiden, H. E. Stenfert Kroese B. V., 1976.
13. Lev, M.: The conduction system. In Gould, S. E. (ed.): Pathology of the Heart and Blood Vessels, 3rd. ed., p. 185. Springfield, Ill., Charles C Thomas, 1968.
14. James, T. N.: Anatomy of the human sinus node. Anat. Rec., 141:109, 1961.
15. Hudson, R. E. B.: Surgical pathology of the conducting system of the heart. Br. Heart J., 29:646, 1967.
16. Anderson, K. R., Ho, S. Y., and Anderson, R. H.: The location and vascular supply of the sinus node in the human heart. Br. Heart J., 41:28, 1979.
17. Busquet, J., Fontan, F., Anderson, R. H., et al.: The surgical significance of the atrial branches of the coronary arteries. Int. J. Cardiol., 6:223, 1984.
18. McAlpine, W. A.: Heart and Coronary Arteries. An Anatomical Atlas for Clinical Diagnosis, Radiological Investigation and Surgical Treatment, p. 154. New York, Springer-Verlag, 1975.
19. James, T. N.: The sinus node as a servomechanism. Circ. Res., 32:307, 1973.
20. Walls, E. W.: The development of the specialized conducting tissue of the human heart. J. Anat., 81:93, 1947.
21. Sanabria, T.: Recherches sur la differenciation du tissu nodal et connecteur du coeur des mammiferes. Arch. Biol. Leige., 47:1, 1936.
22. Shaner, R. F.: The development of the atrioventricular node, bundle of His and sinoatrial node in the calf with a description of a third embryonic nodelike structure. Anat. Rec., 44:85, 1929.
23. Robb, J. S., Kaylor, C. T., and Turman, W. G.: A study of specialized heart tissue at various stages of development of the human fetal heart. Am. J. Med., 5:324, 1948.
24. Patten, B. M.: Development of the sinoventricular conduction system. Univ. Mich. Med. Bull., 22:1, 1956.
25. Heinzberger, C. F. M.: The development of the sinoatrial node in the mouse. Acta Morphol. Neerl. Scand., 12:317, 1974.
26. Van Mierop, L. H. S., and Gessner, I. H.: The morphologic development of the sinoatrial node in the mouse. Am. J. Cardiol. 25:204, 1970.
27. Anderson, R. H., Ho, S. Y., Becker, A. E., and Gosling, J. A.: The development of the sinoatrial node. In Bonke, F. I. M. (ed.): The Sinus Node. Structure, Function and Clinical Relevance, p. 166. The Hague, Martinus Nijhoff, 1978.
28. Tranum-Jensen, J.: The fine structure of the atrial and atrio-ventricular (AV) junctional specialized tissues of the rabbit heart. In Wellens, H. J. J., Lie, K. I., and Janse, M. J. (eds.): Conduction System of the Heart. Structure, Function and Clinical Implications, p. 55. Leiden, H. E. Stenfert Kroese B. V., 1976.
29. James, T. N., Sherf, L., Fine, G., and Morales, A. R.: Comparative ultrastructure of the sinus node in man and dog. Circulation, 34:139, 1966.
30. Yamauchi, A.: Ultrastructure of the innervation of the mammalian heart. In Challice, C. E., and Viragh, S. (eds.): Ultrastructure of the Mammalian Heart, p. 127. New York, Academic Press, 1973.
31. James, T. N.: Cardiac conduction system. Fetal and postnatal development. Am. J. Cardiol., 25:213, 1970.
32. Lewis, T.: The Mechanism and Graphic Registration of the Heart Beat, p. 1. London, Shaw and Sons, 1920.
33. Thorel, C.: Verlaufige Mitteilung uber eine besondere Muskelverbindung zwischen der Cava Superior und dem Hisschen Bundel. Munch. Med. Wochenschr., 56:2159, 1909.
34. Thorel, C.: Uber den Aufbau des Sinusknotens und seine Verbindung mit der Cava superior und den Wenckbachschen bundel. Munch. Med. Wochenschr., 57:186, 1910.
35. German Pathological Society: Bericht uber die Verhandlungen der XIV Tagung der Deutschen pathologischen Gesellschaft in Erlangen vom 4–6 April 1910. Z. all. Path. Path. Anat., 21:433, 1910.
36. Aschoff, L.: Referat uber die Herzstorungen in ihren Beziehungen zu den Spezifischen Muskelsystem des Herzens. Verh. Dtsch. Pathol. Ges., 14:3, 1910.
37. Monckeberg, J. G.: Beitrage zur normalen und pathologischen Anatomie des Herzens. Verh. Dtsch. Pathol. Ges., 14:64, 1910.
38. Koch, W.: Discussion in The German Pathological, Society. Bericht uber die Verhandlungen der XIV Tagung der Deutschen pathologischen Gesellschaft in Erlangen vom 4–6 April 1910. Z. all. Path. Path. Anat., 21:433, 1910.
39. Condorelli, L.: Uber die Bahnen der Reizleitung vom Keithr-Flackschen Knoten zu den Vorhofen. Z. Ges. exp. Med., 68:493, 1929.
40. Franco, P. M.: Recherches sur les faisceaux de connexion auriculaires dans les conditions normales et pathologues. Arch. Mal. Coeur, 44:287, 1951.
41. Paes de Carvalho, A.: Cellular electrophysiology of the atrial specialized tissues. In Paes de Carvalho, A., Mello, W. C., and Hoffman, B. F. (eds.): Specialized Tissues of the Heart, p. 115. Amsterdam, Elsevier, 1961.
42. Lev, M., and Bharati, S.: Lesions of the conduction system and their functional significance. In Sommers, S. C. (ed.): Pathology Annual, 1974, p. 157. New York, Appleton-Century-Crofts, 1974.
43. Chuaqui, B.: Uber die Ausbreitungsbundel des Sinusknoten. Eine kritische analyse der wichtigsten Arbeiten. Virchows Arch. Path. Anat., 355:179, 1972.
44. Chuaqui, B.: Lupenpraparatorische Darstellung der Ausbreitungszuge des Sinusknotens. (Stereomicroscopic demonstration of the extensions of the sinus node). Virchows Arch. Path. Anat., 356:141, 1972.
45. James, T. N.: Sir Thomas Lewis redivivus: From pebbles in a quiet pond to autonomic storms. Br. Heart J., 52:1, 1984.
46. Spach, M. S., Lieberman, M., Scott, J. G., et al.: Excitation sequences of the atrial septum and AV node in isolated hearts of the dog and the rabbit. Circ. Res., 29:156, 1971.
47. Spach, M. S., King, T. D., Barr, R. C., et al.: Electrical potential distribution surrounding the atria during depolarization and repolarization in the dog. Circ. Res., 24:857, 1969.
48. Spach, M. S., and Kootsey, J. M.: The nature of electrical propagation in cardiac muscle. Am. J. Physiol., 244:H-3, 1983.
49. Tranum-Jensen, J., and Janse, M. J.: Fine structural identification of individual cells subjected to microelectrode recording in perfused cardiac preparations. J. Mol. Cell. Cardiol., 14:233, 1982.
50. Becker, A. E., and Anderson, R. H.: Morphology of the human atrioventricular junctional area. In Wellens, H. J. J., Lie, K. I., and Janse, M. J. (eds.): The Conduction System of the Heart. Structure, Function and Clinical Implications, p. 263. Leiden, H. E. Stenfert Kroese B. V., 1976.

51. Hecht, H. H., Kossmann, C. E., Childers, R. W., et al.: Atrioventricular and intraventricular conduction—revised nomenclature and concepts. Am. J. Cardiol., 31:232, 1973.
52. Todaro, F.: Novelle richerche sopra la struttura muscolare delle orecchiette del coure umano e sopra la valvola d'Eustachio. Sperimentale, 16:217, 1865.
53. Anderson, R. H., and Taylor, I. M.: Development of atrioventricular specialized tissue in the human heart. Br. Heart J., 34:1205, 1972.
54. Anderson, R. H., Wenink, A. C. G., Losekoot, T. G., and Becker, A. E.: Congenitally complete heart block. Developmental aspects. Circulation, 56:90, 1977.
55. Lev, M.: The architecture of the conduction system in congenital heart disease. I. Common atrioventricular orifice. Arch. Pathol., 65:174, 1958.
56. Feldt, R. H., DuShane, J. W., and Titus, J. L.: The atrioventricular conduction system in persistent common atrioventricular canal defect: Correlations with electrocardiogram. Circulation, 42:437, 1970.
57. Thiene, G., Wenink, A. C. G., Frescura, C., et al.: The surgical anatomy of the conduction tissues in atrioventricular defects. J. Thorac. Cardiovasc. Surg., 82:928, 1981.
58. Scherf, D., and Cohen, J.: The Atrioventricular Node And Selected Cardiac Arrhythmias, p. 1. New York, Grune & Stratton, 1964.
59. Massing, G. K., and James, T. N.: Anatomical configuration of the His bundle and bundle branches in the human heart. Circulation, 53:609, 1976.
60. Davies, M. J.: The Conduction System of the Heart. London, Butterworths, 1971.
61. Kurosawa, H., and Becker, A. E.: Dead-end tract of the conduction axis. Int. J. Cardiol., 7:13, 1985.
62. Truex, R. C., and Smythe, M. Q.: Reconstruction of the human atrioventricular node. Anat. Rec., 158:11, 1967.
63. Paes de Carvalho, A., De Mello, W. G., and Hoffman, B. F.: Electrophysiological evidence for specialised fiber types in rabbit atrium. Am. J. Physiol. 196:483, 1959.
64. Hoffman, B. F., and Cranefield, P. F.: Electrophysiology of the Heart, p. 48. New York, McGraw Hill, 1960.
65. James, T. N.: Anatomy of the cardiac conduction system in the rabbit. Circ. Res., 20:638, 1967.
66. Anderson, R. H.: Histologic and histochemical evidence concerning the presence of morphologically distinct cellular zones within the rabbit atrioventricular node. Anat. Rec., 173:7, 1972.
67. Anderson, R. H., Janse, M. J., Van Capelle, F. J. L., et al.: A combined morphological and electrophysiological study of the atrioventricular node of the rabbit heart. Circ. Res., 35:909, 1974.
68. Anderson, R. H.: The disposition, morphology and innervation of cardiac specialized tissues in the guinea pig. J. Anat., 111:453, 1972.
69. Anderson, R. H., Davies, M. J., and Becker, A. E.: Atrioventricular ring specialized tissue in the normal heart. Eur. J. Cardiol., 2:219, 1974.
70. Kent, A. F. S.: Researches on the structure and function of the mammalian heart. J. Physiol., 14:233, 1893.
71. Kent, A. F. S.: The right lateral auriculo-ventricular junction of the heart. J. Physiol., 48:22, 1914.
72. Rosenbaum, M. B., Elizari, M. V., and Lazzari, J. O.: The Hemiblocks. Oldsmar, Fl., Tampa Tracings, 1970.
73. Rossi, L.: Histopathology of the conducting system. G. Ital. Cardiol., 2:484, 1972.
74. Uhley, H. N.: The quadrifascicular nature of the peripheral conduction system. In Dreifus, L. S., and Liboff, W. (eds.): Cardiac Arrhythmias, p. 339. New York, Grune & Stratton, 1973.
75. Demoulin, J. C., and Kulbertus, H. E.: Histopathological examination of concept of left hemiblock. Br. Heart J., 34:807, 1972.
76. Durrer, D., Schuilenberg, R. M., and Wells, H. J. J.: Preexcitation revisited. Am. J. Cardiol., 25:690, 1970.
77. Sherf, L., and James, T. N.: A new electrocardographic concept: Synchronized sino-ventricular conduction. Dis. Chest, 55:127, 1969.
78. James, T. N.: Heuristic thoughts on the Wolff-Parkinson-White syndrome. In Schlant, R. C., and Hurst, J. W. (eds.): Advances in Electrophysiology, p. 269. New York, Grune & Stratton, 1972.
79. Lev, M.: The pre-excitation syndrome: Anatomic considerations of anomalous A-V pathways. In Dreifus, L. S., and Koff, W. S. (eds.): Mechanisms and Therapy of Cardiac Arrhythmias, p. 665. New York, Grune & Stratton, 1966.
80. Anderson, R. H., and Becker, A. E.: Anatomy of conducting tissues revisited. Br. Heart J., 40 (Suppl.):2, 1978.
81. Sherf, L., and James, T. N.: Wolff-Parkinson-White Syndrome. Circulation, 43:456, 1971.
82. Durrer, D., and Wellens, H. J.: The Wolff-Parkinson-White syndrome. Eur. J. Cardiol., 1:347, 1974.
83. Anderson, R. H., and Becker, A. E.: Stanley Kent and accessory atrioventricular connexions. J. Thorac. Cardiovasc. Surg., 81:649, 1981.
84. Sealy, W. C.: Reply to: Accessory atrioventricular connections. J. Thorac. Cardiovasc. Surg., 78:311, 1979.
85. Mahaim, I.: Kent's fiber in the A-V paraspecific conduction through the upper connection of the bundle of His-Tawara. Am. Heart J., 33:651, 1947.
86. Brechenmacher, C.: Atrio-His bundle tracts. Br Heart J., 37:853, 1975.
87. Anderson, R. H., Becker, A. E., Brechenmacher, C., et al.: Ventricular preexcitation. A proposed nomenclature for its substrates. Eur. J. Cardiol., 3:27, 1975.
88. Burchell, H. B.: Ventricular Pre-excitation. Historical Overview, in press.
89. Wood, F. C., Wolferth, C. G., and Geckeler, G. D.: Histologic demonstration of accessory muscular connections between auricle and ventricle in a case of short P-R interval and prolonged QRS complex. Am. Heart J., 25:454, 1943.
90. Ohnell, R. F.: Preexcitation, a cardiac abnormality. Acta Med. Scand., 152:1, 1944.
91. Gallagher, J., Svenson, R., Sealy, W. C., and Wallace, A.: The Wolff-Parkinson-White syndrome and the pre-excitation dysrhythmias. Med. Clin. North Am., 60:101, 1976.
92. Sealy, W. C., Wallace, A. G., Ramming, K. P., et al.: An improved operation for the definitive treatment of the Wolff-Parkinson-White syndrome. Ann. Thorac. Surg., 17:107, 1974.
93. Painvin, G. A., Gillette, P. A., Zinner, A., et al.: Epicardial cryoablation of the bundle of His: An experimental study. J. Thorac. Cardiovasc. Surg., 88:273, 1984.
94. Gotlieb, A. I., Chan, M., Palmer, W. H., and Huang, S.-N.: Ventricular preexcitation syndrome. Accessory left atrioventricular connection and rhabdomyomatous myocardial fibers. Arch. Pathol. Lab. Med., 101:486, 1977.
95. Becker, A. E., Anderson, R. H., Durrer, D., and Wellens, H. J. J.: The anatomical substrates of Wolff-Parkinson-White Syndrome: A clinico-pathologic correlation in seven patients. Circulation, 57:870, 1978.
96. Sealy, W. C., and Gallagher, J. J.: The surgical approach to the septal area of the heart based on experience with 45 patients with Kent bundles. J. Thorac. Cardiovasc. Surg., 79:542, 1980.
97. De Villenave, V. H., and Schornagel, H. E.: Voorkomen van een accessoire atrioventriculaire spierbundel by een zuigeling met paroxysmale tachycardia en her Wolff-Parkinson-White syndrome. Maandschrift, Fur Kindergeneesekund. 26:23, 1958.

98. James, T. N., and Puech, P.: De subitaneis mortibus. IX. Type A Wolff-Parkinson-White syndrome. Circulation, 50:1264, 1974.
99. Dreifus, L. S., Wellens, H. J., Watanabe, Y., et al.: Sinus bradycardia and atrial fibrillation associated with the Wolff-Parkinson-White syndrome. Am. J. Cardiol., 38:149, 1976.
100. Denes, P., Amat-y-Leon, F., Wyndham, C., et al.: Electrophysiological demonstration of bilateral anomalous pathways in a patient with Wolff-Parkinson-White syndrome (Type B pre-excitation). Am. J. Cardiol., 37:93, 1976.
101. Janse, M. J., Anderson, R. H., Van Capelle, F. J. L., and Durrer, D.: A combined electrophysiological and anatomical study of the human fetal heart. Am. Heart J., 91:556, 1976.
102. Lev, M., Fox, S. M., Bharati, S., et al.: Mahaim and James fibers as a basis for a unique variety of ventricular pre-excitation. Am. J. Cardiol., 36:880, 1975.
103. James, T. N.: Sudden death in babies: New observations in the heart. Am. J. Cardiol., 22:479, 1968.
104. James, T. N.: Sudden death of babies. Circulation, 53:1, 1976.
105. Anderson, W. R., Edland, J. F., and Schenk, E. A.: Conducting system changes in the sudden infant death syndrome (abstr.). Am. J. Pathol., 59:35a, 1970.
106. Ferris, J. A. J.: Hypoxic changes in conducting tissue of the heart in sudden death in infancy syndrome. Br. Med. J., 2:23, 1973.
107. Valdes-Dapena, M. A., Greene, M., Basavarand, N., et al.: The myocardial conduction system in sudden death in infancy. N. Engl. J. Med., 289:1179, 1973.
108. Anderson, R. H., Bouton, J., Burrow, C. T., Smith, A.: Sudden death in infancy: A study of the cardiac specialized tissue. Br. Med. J., 2:135, 1974.
109. Lie, J. T., Rosenberg, H. S., and Erickson, E. E.: Histopathology of the conduction system in the sudden infant death syndrome. Circulation, 53:3, 1976.
110. Preston, J. B., McFadden, S., and Moe, G. K.: Atrioventricular transmission in young mammals. Am. J. Physiol., 197:236, 1959.
111. Southall, D. P., Vulliamy, D. G., Davies, M. J., et al.: A new look at the neonatal electrocardiogram. Br. Med. J., 2:615, 1976.
112. James, T. N., Robertson, B. T., Waldo, A. L., and Branch, C. E.: De subitaneis mortibus. XV. Hereditary stenosis of His bundle in pug dogs. Circulation, 52:1152, 1975.
113. Lev, M.: Ageing changes in the human sinoatrial node. J. Gerontol., 9:1, 1954.
114. Erickson, E. E., and Lev, M.: Ageing changes in the human AV node, bundle and bundle branches. J. Gerontol., 7:1, 1952.
115. Davies, M. J., and Pomerance, A.: Quantitative study of ageing changes in the human sinoatrial node and internodal tracts. Br. Heart J., 34:150, 1972.
116. James, T. N.: The sinus node. Am. J. Cardiol., 40:965, 1977.
117. Davies, M. J., Anderson, R. H., and Becker, A. E.: The Conduction System of the Heart, p. 306. London, Butterworths, 1983.
118. Angelini, P., and Sandiford, F. M.: Functional correction of transposition of the great arteries: A new approach to avoid postoperative arrhythmias. J. Thorac. Cardiovasc. Surg., 66:87, 1973.
119. Isaacson, R., Titus, J. L., Merideth, J., et al.: Apparent interruption of atrial conduction pathways after surgical repair of transposition of the great arteries. Am. J. Cardiol., 30:533, 1972.
120. El-Said, G., Rosenberg, H. S., Mullins, C. E., et al.: Dysrhythmias after Mustard's operation for transposition of the great arteries. Am. J. Cardiol., 39:526, 1972.
121. Wittig, J. H., De Leval, M. R., and Stark, J.: Intraoperative mapping of atrial activation before, during and after Mustard's operation. J. Thorac. Cardiovasc. Surg., 73:1, 1977.
122. Ullal, R. R., Anderson, R. H., and Lincoln, C.: Mustard's operation modified to avoid dysrhythmias and pulmonary and systemic venous obstruction. J. Thorac. Cardiovasc. Surg., 78:431, 1979.
123. Southall, D. P., Keeton, B. R., Leanage, R., et al.: Cardiac rhythm and conduction before and after Mustard's operation for complete transposition of the great arteries. Br. Heart J., 43:21, 1980.
124. Ho, S. Y., Monro, J. L., and Anderson, R. H.: The disposition of the sinus node in left-sided juxtaposition of the atrial appendage. Br. Heart J., 41:129, 1979.
125. Fontan, F., Choussat, A., Brom, A. G., et al.: Repair of tricuspid atresia — surgical considerations and results. In Anderson, R. H., and Shinebourne, E. A. (eds.): Paediatric Cardiology 1977, p. 567, Edinburgh, Churchill Livingstone, 1978.
126. Truex, R. C., and Bishof, J. K.: Conduction system in human hearts with interventricular septal defects. J. Thorac. Surg., 35:421, 1958.
127. Lev, M.: The architecture of the conduction system in congenital heart disease. III. Ventricular septal defect. Arch. Pathol., 70:529, 1960.
128. Titus, J. L., Daugherty, G. W., and Edwards, J. E.: Anatomy of the atrioventricular conduction system in venticular septal defect. Circulation, 28:72, 1963.
129. Latham, R. A., and Anderson, R. H.: Anatomical variations in atrioventricular conduction system with reference to ventricular septal defects. Br. Heart J., 34:185, 1972.
130. Milo, S., Ho, S. Y., Wilkinson, J. L., and Anderson, R. H.: The surgical anatomy and atrioventricular conduction tissues of hearts with isolated ventricular septal defects. J. Thorac. Cardiovasc. Surg., 79:244, 1980.
131. Lev, M.: The architecture of the conduction system in congenital heart disease II. Tetralogy of Fallot. Arch. Pathol., 67:572, 1959.
132. Anderson, R. H., Monro, J. L., Ho, S. Y., et al.: Les voies de conduction auriculo-ventriculaires dans le tetralogie de Fallot. Coeur, 8:793, 1977.
133. Starr, A., Bonchek, L. I., and Sunderland, C. O.: Total correction of tetralogy of Fallot in infancy. J. Thorac. Cardiovasc. Surg., 65:45, 1973.
134. Bharati, S., and Lev, M.: The conduction system in simple, regular (d-), complete transposition with ventricular septal defect. J. Thorac. Cardiovasc. Surg., 72:194, 1976.
135. Bharati, S., and Lev, M.: The conduction system in double outlet right ventricle with sub-pulmonic ventricular septal defect and related hearts (the Taussig-Bing group). Circulation, 54:459, 1976.
136. Thiene, G., Bortolotti, V., Gallucci, V., et al.: Anatomical study of truncus arteriosus communis with embryological and surgical considerations. Br. Heart J., 38:II-1109, 1976.
137. Lincoln, G., Anderson, R. H., Shinebourne, E. A., et al.: Double outlet right ventricle with l malposition of the aorta. Br. Heart J., 37:453, 1975.
138. Allwork, S. P., Bentall, H. H., Becker, A. E., et al.: Congenitally corrected transposition of the great arteries: Morphologic study of 32 cases. Am. J. Cardiol., 38:910, 1976.
139. Anderson, R. H., Arnold, R., and Wilkinson, J. L.: The conducting system in congenitally corrected transposition. Lancet, 1:1286, 1973.
140. Anderson, R. H., Becker, A. E., Arnold, R., and Wilkinson, J. L.: The conducting tissues in congenitally corrected transposition. Circulation, 50:911, 1974.
141. De Leval, M., Bastos, P., Stark, J., et al.: Surgical technique to reduce the risks of heart block following closure of ventricular septal defect in atrioventricular discordance. J. Thorac. Cardiovasc. Surg., 78:515, 1979.
142. Kupersmith, J., Krongrad, E., Gersony, W. M., and Bowman, F. O.: Electrophysiologic identification of the specialized con-

duction system in corrected transposition of the great arteries. Circulation, 50:795, 1974.

143. Anderson, R. H., Danielson, G. K., Maloney, J. D., and Becker, A. E.: Atrioventricular bundle in corrected transposition. Ann. Thorac. Surg., 26:95, 1978.
144. Dick, M., Van Praagh, R., Rudd, M., et al.: Electrophysiological delineation of the specialised atrioventricular conduction system in two patients with corrected transposition of the great arteries with situs inversus (I,D,D). Circulation, 55:896, 1977.
145. Thiene, G., Nava, A., and Rossi, L.: The conduction system in corrected transposition with situs inversus. Eur. J. Cardiol., 6:57, 1977.
146. Wilkinson, J. L., Smith, A., Lincoln, C., and Anderson, R. H.: The conducting tissues in congenitally corrected transposition with situs inversus. Br. Heart J., 40:41, 1978.
147. Monckeberg, J. G.: Zur Entwicklungsgeschichte des Atrioventrikulsarsystems. Ver. deutsch. Path. Ges., 16:228, 1913.
148. Symons, J. C., Shinebourne, E. A., Joseph, M. C., et al.: Criss-cross heart with congenitally corrected transposition: Report of a case with d-transposed aorta and ventricular preexcitation. Eur. J. Cardiol., 5:493, 1977.
149. Bharati, S., and Lev, M.: The course of the conduction system in dextrocardia. Circulation, 50:163, 1978.
150. Anderson, R. H., Arnold, R., Thaper, M. K., et al.: Cardiac specialized tissues in hearts with an apparently single ventricular chamber. (Double inlet left ventricle.). Am. J. Cardiol., 33:95, 1974.
151. Bharati, S., and Lev, M.: The course of the conduction system in single ventricle with inverted (L) loop and inverted (L) transposition. Circulation, 51:723, 1975.
152. Wilkinson, J. L., Anderson, R. H., Arnold, R., et al.: The conducting tissues in primitive ventricular hearts without an outlet chamber. Circulation, 53:930, 1976.
153. Anderson, R. H., Wilkinson, J. L., and Becker, A. E.: Conducting tissues in the univentricular heart. In Van Mierop, L. H. S., Oppenheimer-Dekker, A., and Bruins, C. L. D. (eds.): Embryology and Teratology of the Heart and the Great Arteries (Boerhaave Course 13), p. 62. The Hague, Leiden University Press, 1978.
154. Wilkinson, J. L., Macartney, F. J., Keeton, B. R., et al.: Morphology and conducting tissue in univentricular hearts of right ventricular type. Herz, 4:151, 1979.
155. Lev, M.: Pathogenesis of congenital atrioventricular block. Progr. Cardiovasc. Dis., 15:145, 1972.
156. El Sayed, H., Cleland, W. P., Bentall, H. H., et al.: Corrected transposition of the great arterial trunks: Surgical treatment of the associated defects. J. Thorac. Cardovasc. Surg., 44:443, 1962.
157. Lev, M., Silverman, J., Fitzmaurice, F. M., et al.: Lack of connection between the atria and the more peripheral conduction system in congenital atrioventricular block. Am. J. Cardiol., 27:481, 1971.
158. Lev, M., Cuadros, H., and Paul, M. H.: Interruption of the atrioventricular bundle with congenital atrioventricular block. Circulation, 43:703, 1971.
159. Husson, G. S., Blackman, M. S., Rogers, M. C., et al.: Familial congenital bundle branch system disease. Am. J. Cardiol., 32:365, 1973.
160. Scott, J. S., Maddison, P. J., Taylor, P. V., et al.: Connective tissue disease, antibodies to ribonucleoprotein, and congenital heart block. N. Engl. J. Med., 4:209, 1983.
161. Ho, S. Y., Anderson, R. H., Scott, J. S., et al.: Congenitally complete heart block (abstr.). Eur. Heart J., 5:I-236, 1984.
162. Davies, M. J., Anderson, R. H., and Becker, A. E.: The Conduction System of the Heart. London, Butterworths, 1983.
163. Blondeau, M., Maurice, P., Reverdy, V., and Lenegre, J.: Troubles de rhythme de la conduction auriculo-ventriculaire dans l'infarctus du myocarde recent. Considerations anatomiques. Arch. Mal. Coeur, 60:1733, 1967.
164. Blondeau, M., Rizzon, P., and Lenègre, J.: Les troubles de la conduction auriculo-ventriculaire dans l'infarctus myocardiaque recent. Il etude anatomique. Arch. Mal. Coeur, 53:1104, 1961.
165. Sutton, R., and Davies, M.: The conduction system in acute myocardial infarction complicated by complete heart block. Circulation, 38:987, 1968.
166. Hunt, D., Lie, J. T., Vohra, J., and Sloman, G.: Histopathology of heart block complicating acute myocardial infarction. Correlation with the His bundle electrogram. Circulation, 48:1252, 1973.
167. Hackel, D. G., and Estes, E. H., Jr.: Pathologic features of atrioventricular and intraventricular conduction disturbances in acute myocardial infarction. Circulation, 43:977, 1971.
168. Hackel, D. B., Wagner, G., Ratliff, N. B., et al.: Anatomic studies of the cardiac conducting system in acute myocardial infarction. Am. Heart J., 83:77, 1972.
169. Becker, A. E., Lie, K. I., and Anderson, R. H.: Bundle branch block in the setting of acute anteroseptal myocardial infarction: a clinico-pathologic investigation. Br. Heart J., 40:773, 1978.
170. Lev, M.: The pathology of complete atrioventricular block. Progr. Cardiovasc. Dis., 6:317, 1964.
171. Lev, M.: Anatomic basis for atrioventricular block. Am. J. Med., 37:742, 1964.
172. Lenègre, J.: Etiology and pathology of bilateral bundle branch block in relation to complete heart block. Progr. Cardiovasc. Dis., 6:409, 1964.
173. Lenègre, J.: Bilateral bundle branch block. Cardiologia (Basel), 46:261, 1966.
174. Davies, M.: Pathology of the Conducting Tissue of the Heart, p. 92. London, Butterworths, 1971.
175. Davies, M.: Pathology of the Conducting Tissues of the Heart, p. 67. London, Butterworths, 1971.

3

Normal and Abnormal Electrical Activity in Cardiac Cells

David C. Gadsby and Andrew L. Wit

Supported in part by U.S. Public Health Service Grant HL-14899

In general, an arrhythmia is any abnormality in the rate, regularity, or site of origin of the cardiac impulse or disturbance in the conduction of that impulse, such that the normal sequence of activation of atria and ventricles is altered.[1] Arrhythmias may thus be said to result from abnormalities of impulse initiation, impulse conduction, or both.[2] Such abnormalities may result from quite small changes in the mechanisms underlying the generation of the normal transmembrane action potential. On the other hand, they may also be caused by more substantial changes resulting in electrical activity with characteristics quite unlike those found in normal cardiac cells.

As discussed throughout this book, cardiac arrhythmias and conduction disturbances may have many different pathologic causes. In the final analysis, however, all arrhythmias and conduction abnormalities result from critical alterations in the electrical activity of myocardial cells. In this chapter we will outline the mechanisms underlying normal activity of cardiac cells and then go on to show how this activity may be changed by disease in such a way as to cause arrhythmias. A more detailed treatment of specific types of arrhythmias, for example, supraventricular tachycardia, ventricular fibrillation, and ischemic arrhythmias, will be found in other chapters of this book.

The Resting and Action Potential of Normal Atrial, Ventricular, and Purkinje Fibers

The normal, regular beating of the heart is accompanied by cyclic changes in the membrane potential of cardiac cells. The use of intracellular microelectrodes has allowed these membrane potential changes to be measured directly, and they have been shown to vary in amplitude and time course as the impulse travels through the heart.[3] The microelectrode technique involves the insertion of a fine glass needle into a cell, so that the membrane potential, that is, the potential difference between the cell interior and the extracellular fluid, may be recorded directly and continuously. A micromanipulator is used to advance the microelectrode until its tip (usually less than 0.1 μm in diameter) pierces the cell membrane. At the moment the microelectrode tip passes from the outside to the inside of the cell, it suddenly records a negative potential difference with respect to a reference electrode placed in the extracellular fluid (Fig. 3-1). Microelectrode studies are usually made on isolated bundles of cardiac fibers mounted in a tissue bath and superfused with warmed, oxygenated solutions. Action potentials may be initiated in such preparations by the application of brief current pulses through electrodes placed on the fiber surface (Fig. 3-1). In the absence of stimulated action potentials, however, the interior of most cardiac cells (except those of the sinus and atrioventricular node, which are discussed separately below) remains 80 to 90 mV negative with respect to the extracellular space.[3] This transmembrane potential during electrical quiescence is referred to as the *resting potential.*

As with many other excitable cells,[4] the resting potential of cardiac cells is largely determined by the concentration gradient for potassium ions across the cell membrane, while the rapid potential change during impulse initiation depends on the concentration gradient for sodium ions.[5,6] These concentration gradients run in opposite directions. The intracellular potassium concentration, $[K^+]_i$, is some 30 times greater than the extracellular concentration, $[K^+]_o$. In Purkinje fibers, for example, $[K^+]_i$ and $[K^+]_o$ are typically 140 to 150 mM and 4 to 5 mM, respectively.[7] The intracellular sodium concentration, $[Na^+]_i$, is much smaller than the extracellular concentration, $[Na^+]_o$; $[Na^+]_i$ and $[Na^+]_o$ are usually about 10 mM and 150 mM, respectively, in Purkinje fibers.[8] During each action potential, a small amount of sodium enters the cell and a small amount of potassium is lost from the cell. We will see later that normal electrical activity depends on the existence of the steep concentration gradients for Na^+ and K^+, and the long-term maintenance of these gradients depends on an active transport mechanism called the sodium pump. This mechanism has been studied extensively, and it is known that the pump is a Mg^{++}-ATPase (adenosine triphosphatase) that is located within the cell membrane and that uses the energy stored in the form of ATP (adenosine triphosphate) to pump sodium ions out of the cell and potassium ions into the cell. These ion movements necessarily involve the expenditure of energy, since they are both normally uphill, that is, against the respective electrochemical potential gradients. The pumped ion movements, however, are probably not equal in the two directions, more than one Na^+ being pumped out for each K^+ pumped in.[9] Thus the sodium pump generates a net outward movement of positive charge, or, in other words, a net outward current across the cell membrane. This pump current is usually quite

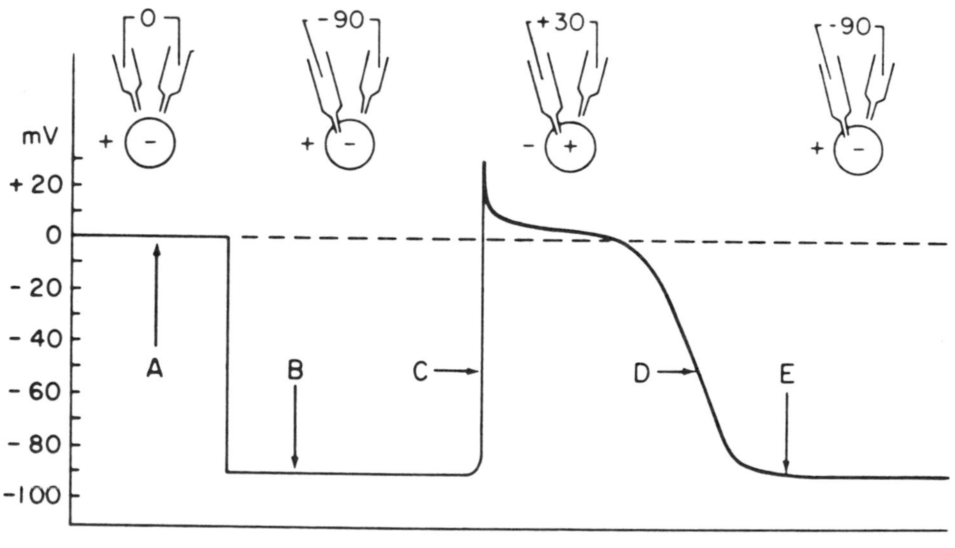

Figure 3-1. *The resting and action potential of a cardiac cell. The upper row of diagrams shows a cell (the circle) and two microelectrodes. In A, both electrodes are in the extracellular space, and there is no potential difference between them. B shows the tip of one microelectrode inside the cell; the potential difference between the inside and outside of the cell, the resting potential, which in this example is −90 mV, is now recorded. C shows the upstroke of the action potential, which occurs when the cell is excited. At the peak of the upstroke the inside of this cell is 30 mV positive with respect to the outside. D represents the final phase of repolarization, which returns membrane potential to its resting level, shown at E. (Cranefield, P. F.: The Conduction of the Cardiac Impulse. Mt. Kisco, N.Y., Futura, 1975; with permission.)*

small, but it may make a significant contribution to membrane potential changes under certain conditions, as will be described later.

The Resting Potential

As already mentioned, the level of the resting potential is predominantly determined by the potassium ion concentration gradient. This is because, at rest, the cell membrane is relatively permeable to potassium ions but relatively impermeable to other ions such as sodium, calcium, or chloride ions. Because of the concentration gradient, potassium ions tend to diffuse out of the cell across the membrane. Electroneutrality cannot be maintained by an outward movement of cellular anions, since these are mainly large polyvalent ions (often associated with cell proteins) to which the cell membrane is impermeable.[10] The outward movement of the positively charged potassium ions therefore causes a net negative charge to build up inside the cell (Fig. 3-2). If the cell membrane were permeable only to potassium ions, then these would continue to diffuse from the cell until the cell interior became sufficiently negative that electrostatic attraction would oppose further, net outward, potassium movement. In this case the inwardly directed

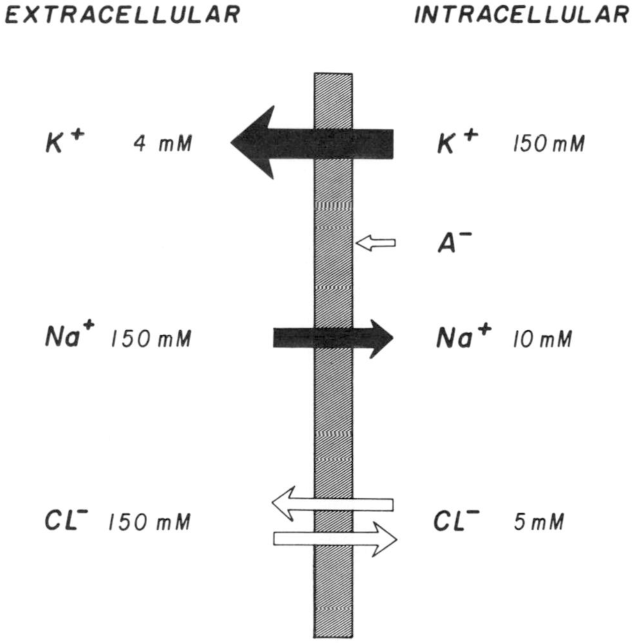

Figure 3-2. *Distribution of ions contributing to the resting potential. Typical concentrations of ions inside and outside the cell are shown. At rest the membrane is highly permeable to K^+ but impermeable to large anions (A^-), and the permeability to Na^+ is low. The permeability to Cl^- is also relatively low, and the distribution of Cl^- is most probably determined by the average value of the membrane potential.*

electrical force exactly counters the outwardly directed force due to the concentration gradient, and net movement of potassium ions ceases: the algebraic sum of these two forces, called the electrochemical potential gradient, is then zero. The intracellular potential at which the net passive flux of potassium ions is zero is called the equilibrium potential for potassium ions, E_K, and its value is given by the Nernst equation[3–5]:

$$E_K = \frac{RT}{F} \ln \frac{[K^+]_o}{[K^+]_i}$$

where R is the gas constant, T is the absolute temperature, F is Faraday's constant, and $[K^+]_o$ and $[K^+]_i$ are the extracellular and intracellular concentrations of potassium ions, respectively (strictly speaking, the ratio of the ion activities should be used in place of the concentration ratio but these two ratios are approximately the same when the internal and external activity coefficients for K^+ are similar). For example, the value of E_K for a Purkinje fiber at 36°C for which $[K^+]_o$ is 4 mM and $[K^+]_i$ is 150 mM would be:

$$E_K = \frac{RT}{F} \ln \frac{4}{150} = 26.6 \ln \frac{4}{150}$$
$$= 61.4 \log \frac{4}{150} = -96.6 \text{ mV}$$

By examining the Nernst equation, we can see that E_K will change by 61.4 mV following a tenfold change in either $[K^+]_o$ or $[K^+]_i$. If the cell membrane were exclusively permeable to K^+, then the cell would behave just like a potassium electrode, and its intracellular potential would change with variations in $[K^+]_o$ and $[K^+]_i$ just as predicted by the Nernst equation. In fact, the membrane potentials of resting Purkinje fibers and atrial and ventricular myocardial fibers are reasonably well approximated by the Nernst relation when $[K^+]_o$ is higher than about 10 mM. At lower values of $[K^+]_o$, however, the resting potentials of these cells are less negative than the potassium equilibrium potential, and this discrepancy increases as $[K^+]_o$ is lowered.[5,11] For instance, the resting potential of Purkinje fibers exposed to a solution containing 4 mM K^+ is a few millivolts less negative than the value of E_K estimated above. The reason for this is that the cell membrane is not exclusively permeable to K^+, as we assumed above, but has a relatively low permeability to Na^+. Since both the electrical gradient and the concentration gradient favor the inward movement of Na^+, a small inward depolarizing current of sodium ions flows across the cell membrane. The depolarization caused by this Na^+ current is negligibly small when $[K^+]_o$ is high and the membrane K^+ conductance, therefore, also high, but it becomes significant when $[K^+]_o$ is low, since membrane K^+ currents also become small under these conditions.

This depolarizing influence of Na^+ is most easily discussed in terms of the Goldman[12] and Hodgkin and Katz[13] "constant field" equation for the resting potential, V_r, of a cell permeable to both K^+ and Na^+,

$$V_r = \frac{RT}{F} \ln \frac{[K^+]_o + P_{Na}/P_K[Na^+]_o}{[K^+]_i + P_{Na}/P_K[Na^+]_i}$$

where P_{Na}/P_K is the ratio of the sodium to the potassium permeability coefficient of the cell membrane. This equation has been shown to approximate well the resting potentials of skeletal muscle fibers and cardiac Purkinje fibers over a wider range of $[K^+]_o$ values than does the Nernst equation, when P_{Na}/P_K is assigned a constant value of about 1/100. In this case, since $[K^+]_i$ is normally much greater than $[Na^+]_i$, the second term in the denominator is sufficiently small that we may neglect it and so rewrite the above equation:

$$V_r = \frac{RT}{F} \ln \frac{[K^+]_o + 0.01\ [Na^+]_o}{[K^+]_i}$$

or, if $[Na^+]_o$ is taken to be 150 mM,

$$V_r = \frac{RT}{F} \ln \frac{[K^+]_o + 1.5}{[K^+]_i}$$

It is immediately clear from this equation that the resting potential, V_r, approximates the K^+ equilibrium potential, E_K, only when $[K^+]_o$ is much greater than 1.5 mM; at low $[K^+]_o$ values the second term in the numerator makes an important contribution. For example, at a $[K^+]_o$ of 1.5 mM, V_r will be less negative than E_K by $61.4 \log (3/1.5) = 61.4 \log 2$ or approximately 18 mV. Note that so far we have talked only in terms of the *relative* permeability of the membrane to potassium and sodium ions without considering the absolute *magnitude* of these permeability coefficients. As the Goldman and Hodgkin and Katz equation shows, the resting potential is sensitive to the ratio of the permeabilities of the ions involved but not to the permeability values themselves. Even if the Na^+ permeability were to be quite substantial, for example, the resting potential would still be determined predominantly by the K^+ concentration gradient as long as the membrane retained a much *higher* permeability to K^+ than to Na^+. The membrane channels through which K ions move to generate the K^+ currents that determine the resting membrane potential are known as inward rectifier K^+ channels. K^+ currents flowing in these channels are strikingly dependent on the size and direction of the electrochemical driving force on K^+, given by $(V_m - E_K)$, the difference between the membrane potential, V_m, and the K^+ equilibrium potential, E_K. The channels are called inward rectifiers because they allow passage of large inward K^+ currents when $(V_m - E_K)$ is large and negative but only very small outward K^+ currents when the driving force is large and positive.[10,11,36]

Changes in the resting potential level may be a primary cause of arrhythmias and conduction disturbances, and we can see already how such changes might come about under pathologic conditions. For example, cardiac disease might result in alterations in the level of either intracellular or extracellular K^+ concentration or both and thereby cause a change in the resting membrane potential. Alternatively, the characteristics of the cell membrane might change in such a way that the relative permeability of the membrane to Na^+ or other ions (such as Ca^{++}) is increased, also resulting in a change in the level of resting potential. We will discuss some of these possibilities in more detail later.

The Depolarization Phases of the Cardiac Action Potential

The electrical impulse that travels through the heart to initiate each heartbeat is called the action potential; it is a propagated wave of transient depolarization during which the intracellular potential of each cell in turn briefly becomes positive and then returns to its initial negative level. The potential changes during the normal cardiac action potential have a characteristic time course that, for convenience, has been subdivided into the following phases[3]: phase 0 is the initial, rapid membrane depolarization; phase 1 consists of rapid but limited repolarization; phase 2 is the "plateau" or prolonged depolarization characteristic of the action potential of cardiac cells; phase 3 is the final rapid repolarization; and phase 4 is the period of diastole.

The intracellular potential becomes positive during the action potential because the excited membrane temporarily becomes more permeable to Na^+ than to K^+, and so the membrane potential transiently approaches the equilibrium potential for sodium ions, E_{Na}. E_{Na} can be estimated by use of the Nernst relation, and for extracellular and intracellular Na^+ concentrations of 150 mM and 10 mM, respectively, it amounts to:

$$E_{Na} = \frac{RT}{F} \ln \frac{[Na^+]_o}{[Na^+]_i} = 26.6 \ln \frac{150}{10}$$
$$= 61.4 \log \frac{150}{10} = +72.2 \text{ mV}$$

The increased Na^+ permeability is not maintained, however, and so the membrane potential does not reach E_{Na} but returns toward its resting level during termination of the action potential.

The permeability changes mentioned above, which cause the depolarization phase of the action potential, result from the opening and closing of special membrane channels or pores through which sodium ions can easily pass. It is believed that the movements of "gates" control the opening and closing of individual channels that can exist in at least three conformations—"closed," "open," and "inactivated." One gate, corresponding to the activation variable "m" in the Hodgkin-Huxley[13] analysis of sodium currents in the membrane of squid giant axons, moves rapidly to open the channel when the membrane is suddenly depolarized by a stimulus. The other gate, corresponding to the inactivation variable "h" in the Hodgkin-Huxley analysis, moves more slowly on depolarization, and its function is to close the channel (Fig. 3-3). Both the steady-state distribution of the gates within the channel population and the speed with which they move into and out of position depend on the level of the membrane potential. Hence, the use of adjectives "time- and voltage-dependent" to describe membrane Na^+ conductance.

If a step depolarization to a positive potential level is suddenly applied to the resting membrane (in a voltage clamp experiment, for example), the activation gates move rapidly to open the sodium channels and then the inactivation gates slowly close them (Fig. 3-3). "Slowly" here means that inactivation takes several milliseconds, while activation occurs in a fraction of a millisecond. The gates remain in these positions until the membrane potential is changed again, and in order to return all the gates to their resting positions the membrane must be fully repolarized to large negative potential levels. If the membrane is repolarized to only small negative potential levels, some of the inactivation gates remain closed and the maximum number of sodium channels available

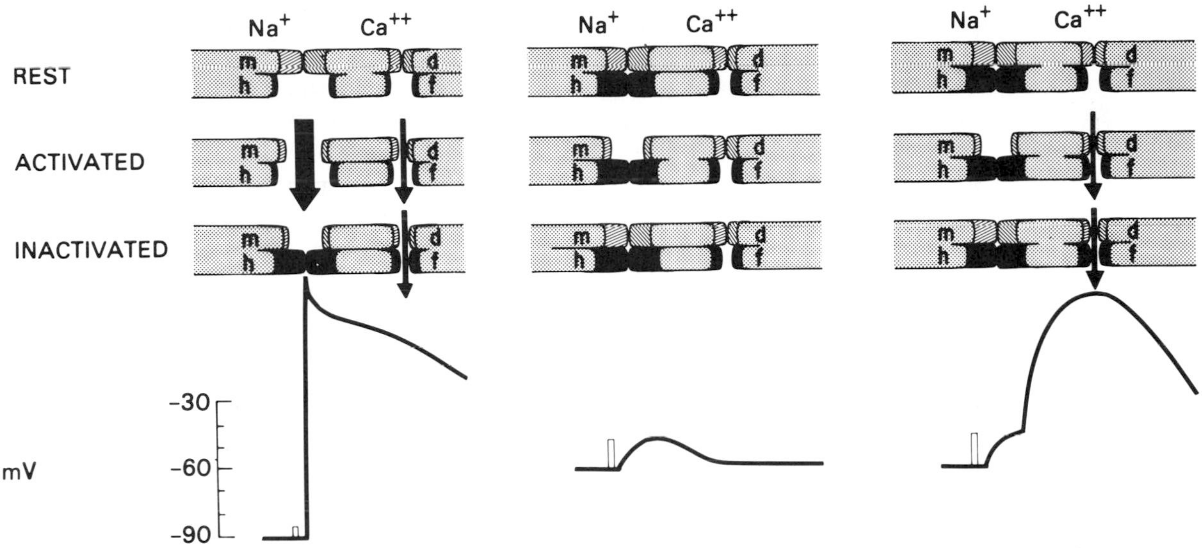

Figure 3-3. *Schematic representation of membrane channels for inward current at the resting potential and during activation and inactivation. The left panel illustrates the sequence of events in a fiber with a normal resting potential of −90 mV. The inactivation gates of the Na^+ channel (h) and the slow Ca^{++}/Na^+ channel (f) are both open at rest. During* activation *(when the cell is excited), the "m" gates of the Na^+ channel open and the resulting inward current of Na ions depolarizes the cell, giving rise to the upstroke of the action potential depicted below. The h gates then close the channel, thereby* inactivating *the Na^+ conductance. During the upstroke of the action potential the membrane potential exceeds the more positive threshold potential of the slow channel; the activation (d) gates of this channel then open, and Ca^{++} and Na^+ flow into the cell, giving rise to the plateau phase of the action potential. The f gates, which* inactivate *the Ca^{++}/Na^+ channel, close much more slowly than the h gates, which inactivate the Na^+ channel. The middle panel shows the behavior of the channels when the resting potential is reduced to below −60 mV. The majority of the inactivation gates of the Na^+ channel remain closed as long as the membrane remains depolarized; when the cell is stimulated, the resulting inward Na^+ current is too small to cause an action potential. The inactivation (f) gates of the slow channel, however, are not closed, and, as shown in the right panel, excitation of the cell sufficient to open the slow channel, permitting the flow of slow inward current, may cause a slow response action potential to occur (Wit, A. L., and Bigger, J. T.: Possible electrophysiological mechanisms for lethal arrhythmias accompanying myocardial ischemia and infarction. Circulation [Suppl.], 51 and 52, III–96, 1975; by permission of the American Heart Association, Inc.)*

to be opened by subsequent depolarization is reduced.[14] (The electrical behavior of cardiac cells in which some Na^+ channels remain inactivated will be discussed later.) The full membrane repolarization at the end of a normal action potential ensures that the sodium channel gates are reset, ready for the next action potential.

The rapid depolarization at the beginning of the action potential is caused by a large inward current of sodium ions flowing into the cell, down their electrochemical potential gradient, through the opened sodium channels.[6,15] However, first the sodium channels must be opened effectively, which requires that a sufficiently large area of membrane be depolarized rapidly enough to a level called the *threshold potential* (Fig. 3-4). This can be achieved experimentally by applying current to the membrane from an outside source through either an extracellular or an intracellular stimulating electrode. More usually, the local circuit currents flowing across the membrane just in front of a propagating action potential serve this same purpose. At the threshold potential, enough sodium channels are opened to give rise to an inward sodium current of sufficient magnitude to cause further membrane depolarization; this in turn

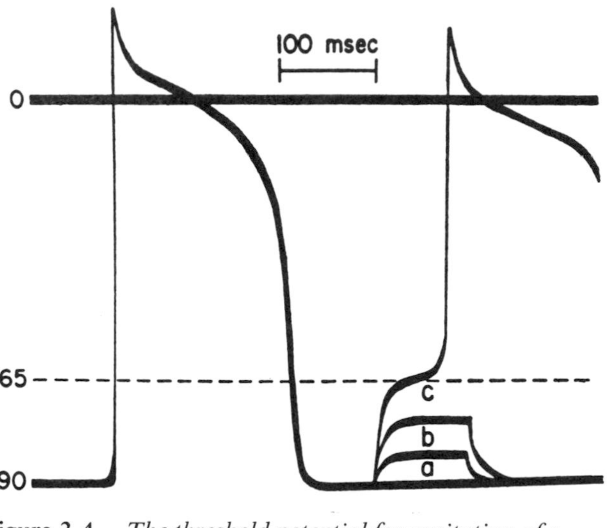

Figure 3-4. *The threshold potential for excitation of a cardiac cell. The action potential shown at the left arises from a resting potential of −90 mV; this occurs when the fiber is excited by a propagating impulse or by any suprathreshold stimulus that rapidly lowers the membrane potential to below the threshold level of −65 mV. At the right, the effects of two subthreshold stimuli and a third threshold stimulus are shown. The subthreshold stimuli (a and b) do not lower the membrane potential to the threshold level, and therefore an action potential is not elicited. The threshold stimulus (c) reduces the membrane potential just to the threshold level from which an action potential then arises. (Hoffman, B. F., and Cranefield, P. F.: Electrophysiology of the Heart. New York, McGraw-Hill, 1960)*

causes a greater number of channels to open, resulting in more inward current, so that the depolarization then becomes self-regenerative. The speed of this regenerative depolarization (or "upstroke" of the action potential) depends on the intensity of the inward sodium current, which itself depends on factors such as the size of the Na^+ electrochemical potential gradient and the fraction of available (or noninactivated) sodium channels. In Purkinje fibers the maximum rate of depolarization during the action potential, referred to as dV/dt_{max} or $\dot{V}_{max}$, reaches about 500 V/sec, and if this were maintained throughout the entire upstroke from −90 mV to +30 mV, the 120 mV excursion would take about 0.25 msec. The maximum rate of depolarization of fibers in ventricular muscle is about 200 V/sec, and in atrial muscle it is between 100 and 200 V/sec.[3] (The depolarization phase of the action potentials in sinus and atrioventricular [AV] nodal cells is quite different from that just described and will be discussed separately below).

Action potentials with such rapid rates of rise are often called *fast responses,* and they propagate rapidly through the heart.[16] In cells with similar membrane capacitance and axial resistance properties, the speed of action potential propagation is largely determined by the magnitude of the inward current flowing during the upstroke of the action potential, which also determines $\dot{V}_{max}$. This is because the local circuit currents that flow through the cells just ahead of the action potentials are larger during faster upstrokes and so can bring the membrane potential of those cells to the threshold level sooner than can smaller currents (Fig. 3-4). Of course, these local currents also flow across the membrane just behind an advancing action potential, but they are unable to excite this membrane because it is refractory.

The prolonged refractory period following excitation of cardiac cells results from the long duration of the action potential and the voltage dependence of the gating of the Na^+ channels. Following the upstroke of the action potential, there is a period of a hundred to several hundred milliseconds during which there is no regenerative electrical response to a second stimulus (Fig. 3-5). This is called the *absolute refractory period,* and it usually covers the plateau (phase 2) of the action potential. As already described, the sodium channels become inactivated and remain closed during such a maintained depolarization. During the repolarization phase of the action potential (phase 3) a progressive removal of inactivation occurs so that a progressively increasing fraction of the sodium channels becomes available again for subsequent activation. Consequently, it is possible to induce only small inward sodium currents by applying a stimulus at the beginning of repolarization, but these currents increase as action potential repolarization proceeds. In-

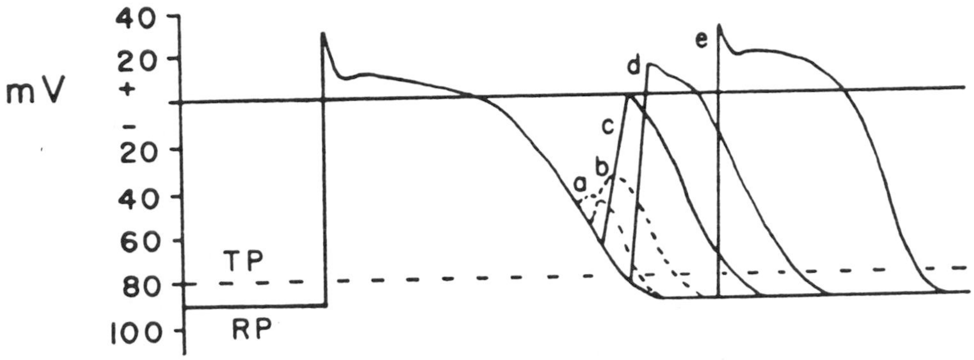

Figure 3-5. *Diagrammatic representation of a normal action potential and of responses elicited by stimuli applied at various stages of repolarization. The amplitude and upstroke velocity of the responses elicited during repolarization are related to the level of the membrane potential from which they arise. The earliest responses (a and b) arise from such low levels of membrane potential that they are too small to propagate (graded or local responses). Response c represents the earliest propagated action potential, but it propagates slowly because of its low upstroke velocity and low amplitude. Response d is elicited just before complete repolarization, and its rate of rise and amplitude are greater than those of c because it arises from a higher membrane potential: however, it still propagates more slowly than normal. Response e is elicited after complete repolarization and therefore has a normal rate of depolarization and amplitude and so propagates rapidly. (Singer, D. H., and Ten Eick, R. E.: Pharmacology of cardiac arrhythmias. Progr. Cardiovasc. Dis., 11:488, 1969; with permission.)*

ward Na^+ currents elicited when some Na^+ channels remain inactivated can cause regenerative depolarization and thus give rise to action potentials. However, the rate and extent of the depolarization and, hence, the conduction velocity of these action potentials are all greatly reduced (Fig. 3-5) and only return to normal values after full repolarization.[17,18] The time during which a second stimulus can elicit these "graded" action potentials is called the *relative refractory period.* The voltage dependence of the removal of inactivation was studied by Weidmann, who found that the rate of rise of an action potential and the potential level at which that action potential was elicited were related by an S-shaped curve, which is also known as the *membrane responsiveness curve.*

The small rate of rise of action potentials initiated during the relative refractory period causes them to propagate slowly, and such action potentials may form the basis of conduction abnormalities such as conduction delay, decrement, and block and may even cause reentrant excitation. These phenomena will be discussed later in this chapter.

In normal cardiac cells, the inward sodium current responsible for the fast upstroke of the action potential is followed by a second inward current that is smaller and slower than the sodium current and that is probably carried mainly by calcium ions.[19,20] This current is generally referred to as *slow inward current* (although it is slow only in comparison to the fast sodium current—other important current changes such as those occurring during repolarization are probably still slower), and it flows through a channel exhibiting time- and voltage-dependent conductance characteristics that has been called the *slow channel* (see Fig. 3-3).[21] The threshold for activation of this conductance (*i.e.*, for the activation gates [d] to begin opening) is thought to be around −30 to −40 mV compared with −60 to −70 mV for the sodium conductance.[20] The regenerative depolarization caused by the fast Na^+ current normally activates the slow inward current conductance, and current flows in both channels during the latter part of the action potential upstroke. The Ca^{++} current is much smaller than the peak fast Na^+ current, however, and so it contributes very little to the action potential until the fast Na^+ current becomes largely inactivated, that is, after the initial rapid upstroke. Since the slow inward current inactivates only slowly, it contributes mainly to the plateau of the action potential. Thus the plateau is shifted in a depolarizing direction when the electrochemical potential gradient for Ca^{++} is enhanced by raising the external Ca^{++} concentration, $[Ca^{++}]_o$, and lowering $[Ca^{++}]_o$ produces a shift in the opposite direction.[22,23] In some cases, however, a contribution of the Ca^{++} current to the rising phase of the action potential can be observed. For example, the upstrokes of action potentials in fibers of the frog ventricle sometimes show an inflection near 0 mV, at which point the initial rapid depolarization gives way to a slower depolarization that continues to the peak of the action potential overshoot. Both the rate of the slower depolarization and the extent of the overshoot have been shown to increase as $[Ca^{++}]_o$ is raised.[23,24]

In addition to the different dependence of these two conductances on membrane potential and time, they are pharmacologically quite distinct. Thus current through the fast Na^+ channel is reduced by tetrodotoxin (TTX),[25] whereas the slow Ca^{++} current is unaffected by TTX[20] but is enhanced by catecholamines[26] and reduced by manganese ions[27] and by the drugs verapamil and D600.[28] It seems likely, at least in the frog heart, that much of the calcium needed to activate the contractile proteins during each heartbeat enters the cell during the action potential through the slow inward current channel. In mammalian cardiac cells, an additional source of Ca^{++} is available in the stores of the sarcoplasmic reticulum.

The Repolarization Phases of the Cardiac Action Potential

Action potentials recorded in Purkinje fibers and in some ventricular muscle fibers show a brief, rapid phase of repolarization (phase 1) immediately following the action potential upstroke (see Fig. 3-1). This phase temporarily returns the membrane potential to near 0 mV, from which level the plateau phase of the action potential arises, and a well-defined notch is sometimes seen between these two phases. The rapid repolarization has been shown (in Purkinje fibers) to result from a transient surge of outward current.[30] This outward current is activated by the depolarization to positive potential levels during the upstroke of the action potential and is then inactivated both by a time-dependent process and by the resulting repolarization. Although it was originally thought that this outward current was carried largely by chloride ions, it now seems more likely that it is carried largely by potassium ions and that only a small component is carried by chloride ions.[29]

During the plateau phase of the action potential, which may last for hundreds of milliseconds, the rate of membrane repolarization is much slower, since the net outward membrane current is small, the inward currents remaining as a result of incomplete inactivation of Na^+ and Ca^{++} channels being approximately balanced by outwardly directed membrane currents.[30,31] At least one of these currents is likely to be a potassium current flowing through a gated, time- and voltage-dependent conductance. Activation of this conductance takes place only slowly at plateau levels of membrane potential. Other small contributions to outward (repolarizing) membrane current at this potential level are expected to be made by inward movements of chloride ions and by the activity of the Na–K exchange pump, which generates a net outward current of Na^+.[39] As the net membrane current at the plateau potential, that is, the algebraic sum of all outward and inward current components, becomes more outward, the membrane potential shifts more rapidly in a negative direction and the final rapid phase of action potential repolarization takes place. This final repolarization, like the initial fast depolarization, is regenerative, but unlike the upstroke, it probably involves conductance changes that are predominantly voltage dependent and not time dependent; its time course, therefore, reflects the time taken for the outward current to charge the membrane capacitance.[34]

Spontaneous Diastolic Depolarization and Automaticity

The membrane potential of normal working atrial and ventricular muscle cells remains steady at its resting level throughout diastole (see Fig. 3-1): if these cells are not excited by a propagating impulse, then the resting potential is maintained. In other cardiac fibers, such as specialized atrial fibers or Purkinje fibers of the ventricular conducting system, the membrane potential is not steady during diastole but declines. If such a fiber is not excited by propagating impulses before the membrane potential reaches threshold level, a spontaneous action potential may arise in that cell (Fig. 3-6). The decline of membrane potential during diastole is called *spontaneous, diastolic,* or *phase 4, depolarization,* and by initiating action potentials, this mechanism forms the basis of automaticity. Automaticity is a normal property of cells in the sinus node, in the muscle of the mitral and tricuspid valves, in some parts of the atrium, in the distal part of the AV node, and in the His-Purkinje system. In the normal heart, the rate of impulse initiation due to automaticity of cells in the sinus node is sufficiently high that these propagated impulses excite other potentially automatic cells before they spontaneously depolarize to threshold potential. In this way, the potential automaticity of other cells is normally suppressed, although it may be revealed under a number of physiologic and pathologic conditions, as discussed later.

Spontaneous diastolic depolarization results from a gradual shift in the balance between inward and outward components of membrane current in favor of net inward (depolarizing) currents. This pacemaker current shows both time- and voltage-dependent gating properties when investigated with the voltage-clamp technique in Purkinje fibers[34–37] and in nodal pacemakers.[38] Initial studies of the potential levels at which these pacemaker current changes reversed their direction strongly suggested that an outward pacemaker current, carried by K^+, gradually declined and so allowed inwardly di-

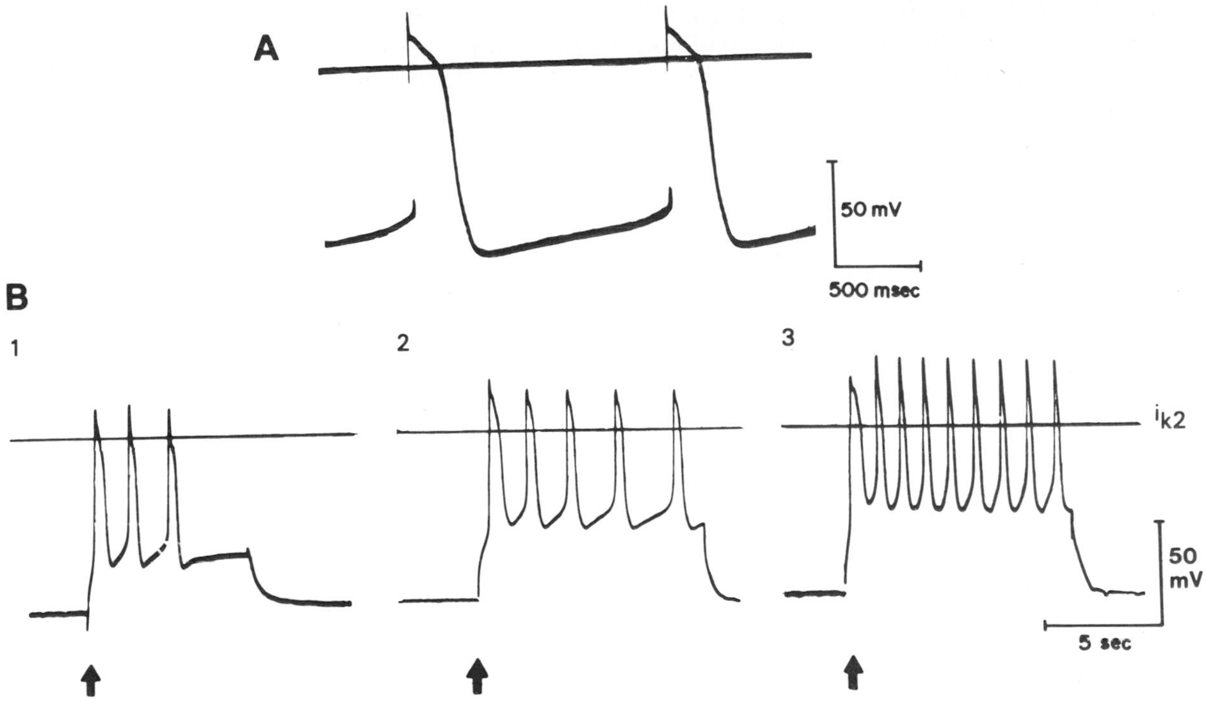

Figure 3-6. *Spontaneous diastolic depolarization and automaticity in canine Purkinje fibers. Panel A shows automatic firing of a Purkinje fiber with a maximum diastolic potential of −85 mV. The diastolic depolarization results from the decay of the i_{K_2}, or pacemaker, current, as discussed in the text. Panel B shows the automaticity that can occur when membrane potential is decreased. This record was obtained from a Purkinje fiber superfused with a Na^+-free solution, but similar activity is seen in a normal, Na^+-containing Tyrode's solution. In B_1, when the fiber is depolarized (at the arrow) from a resting potential of −60 mV to −45 mV by injecting a long-lasting current pulse through a microelectrode, three nondriven action potentials occur. In B_2, a larger amplitude current pulse reduces the membrane potential to −40 mV, resulting in sustained rhythmic activity. In B_3, a still larger current pulse reduces the membrane potential to −30 mV, and sustained rhythmic activity then occurs at a higher rate. Such rhythmic activity occurring at membrane potentials less negative then −60 mV probably depends on different pacemaker currents than the rhythmic activity shown in A. (Wit, A. L., and Friedman, P. F.: Basis for ventricular arrhythmias accompanying myocardial infarction. Arch. Intern. Med., 135:459, 1975; with permission.)*

rected background current to depolarize the cell membrane.[34–36] More recent experiments, however, are interpreted as suggesting that the normal pacemaker current is an inward current, carried predominantly by Na^+, that gradually increases with time, thereby causing the gradual diastolic depolarization.[37,38] When the depolarization reaches threshold potential, an impulse is initiated and the pacemaker conductance is then switched off by the depolarization, only to be reactivated after repolarization of the action potential. Clearly, the pacemaker rate is determined by the time taken for diastolic depolarization to carry the membrane potential to threshold, so that changes in either the threshold potential or the rate of diastolic depolarization, such as that caused by epinephrine in Purkinje fibers, can alter the rate of automaticity.

Delayed Afterdepolarizations and Triggered Sustained Rhythmic Activity

In addition to automaticity, there is another mechanism by which impulses may be rhythmically initiated in normal cardiac cells. The mechanism of impulse initiation depends on delayed afterdepolarizations, and the resulting nondriven rhythmic impulses are called *triggered action potentials*.[20,39] As described above, automatic activity is characterized by the spontaneous initiation of each impulse. Thus, if an automatic fiber is not excited by a propagated impulse, it does not remain quiescent but undergoes spontaneous diastolic depolarization until an action potential is initiated. This accords with the use of the adjective "automatic," which is defined as "having the power of self-motion." In contrast to this, if a triggerable fiber is not excited by a propagated impulse, it will remain quiescent. Since a triggered impulse is one that arises after, and as a result of, another impulse, triggered activity cannot occur until the fiber is excited at least once by a propagating impulse. Triggered activity is a form of rhythmic activity in which each impulse arises as a result of the preceding impulse, except, of course, in the case of the first triggering action potential, which must be driven.

Triggered impulses arise from delayed afterdepolarizations that are large enough to bring the membrane potential to threshold. Delayed afterdepolarizations are transient depolarizations that occur after termination of an action potential but that arise as a result of that action potential. Delayed afterdepolarizations have been recorded in atrial fibers of the mitral valve[40] and in fibers of the coronary sinus[41] and atrial pectinate muscles[42] of normal hearts. As shown in Figure 3-7, delayed afterdepolarizations are often preceded by an afterhyperpolarization; following the action potential the membrane potential transiently becomes more negative than it was just before the action potential. Following the decay of this afterhyperpolarization, the membrane potential transiently becomes more positive than it was just before the action potential. The transient nature of this afterdepolarization clearly distinguishes it from normal spontaneous diastolic (pacemaker) depolarization, during which the membrane potential declines monotonically until the next action potential occurs.

Delayed afterdepolarizations may be subthreshold, but under certain conditions they may exceed threshold potential; when this occurs a nondriven action potential arises from the afterdepolarization. In the atrial fibers mentioned above, catecholamines increase the amplitude of afterdepolarizations, causing them to reach threshold potential.[40,41] The amplitude of subthreshold afterdepolarizations is also highly sensitive to the rate at which action potentials are elicited.[39,42] An increase in drive rate is accompanied by an increase in the amplitude of afterdepolarizations (Fig. 3-8), and, conversely, a reduction in the rate of stimulation leads to a decline in afterdepolarization amplitude. In addition, when a premature action potential is elicited during stimulation at a regular rate, the afterdepolarization following the premature action potential is larger than that following the regular action potential. Furthermore, the amplitude of that premature afterdepolarization increases as the premature action potential is elicited earlier during the basic cycle. At a sufficiently high rate of regular stimulation or following a sufficiently early premature stimulus, afterdepolarizations may reach threshold and initiate nondriven action potentials. The first nondriven impulse arises after an interval shorter than the basic cycle length because the afterdepolarization from which it arises occurs soon after repolarization of the preceding action potential. Therefore, that nondriven impulse gives rise to another afterdepolarization that also reaches threshold, causing a second nondriven impulse (Fig. 3-8). The latter impulse gives rise to the afterdepolarization that initiates a third nondriven impulse and so on for the duration of the triggered activity. The triggered activity may eventually terminate spontaneously, and when it does so the last nondriven impulse is usually followed by one or more subthreshold afterdepolarizations.

The ionic basis of the currents underlying the appearance of afterdepolarizations and the mechanism by which afterdepolarization amplitude is altered by changes in stimulus cycle length are not known. The amplitude of afterdepolarizations can be reduced by drugs that are known to reduce current flowing through the slow inward (Na^+/Ca^{++}) channel. These drugs can also prevent the appearance of triggered activity.[39-41] It is believed, however, that the slow inward current is not involved directly in the initiation of afterdepolarizations, but that calcium ions entering the cell through this and possibly other routes give rise in some other way to the delayed inward current that causes afterdepolarizations.[43]

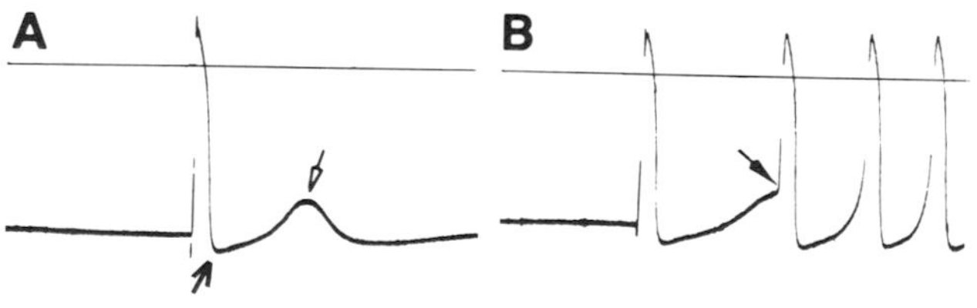

Figure 3-7. *Afterdepolarizations and triggered activity in an atrial fiber in the canine coronary sinus. In A, the fiber is stimulated once and a single action potential is elicited; that action potential is followed by an afterhyperpolarization (solid arrow) and then a delayed afterdepolarization (open arrow). B shows recordings from a different cell; the first action potential (at the left) is elicited by a stimulus, but the delayed afterdepolarization (black arrow) that follows it reaches threshold potential and gives rise to a nondriven action potential. This first nondriven action potential is then followed by more nondriven action potentials; the nondriven impulses are "triggered" impulses, and they constitute what is called* "triggered activity."

The Resting and Action Potentials of Normal Sinus and Atrioventricular Node Cells

The electrical activity of cells in the sinus and AV nodes is quite different from that of cells in the ventricular specialized conducting system and in the working myocardium of the atria and ventricles, which has been dis-

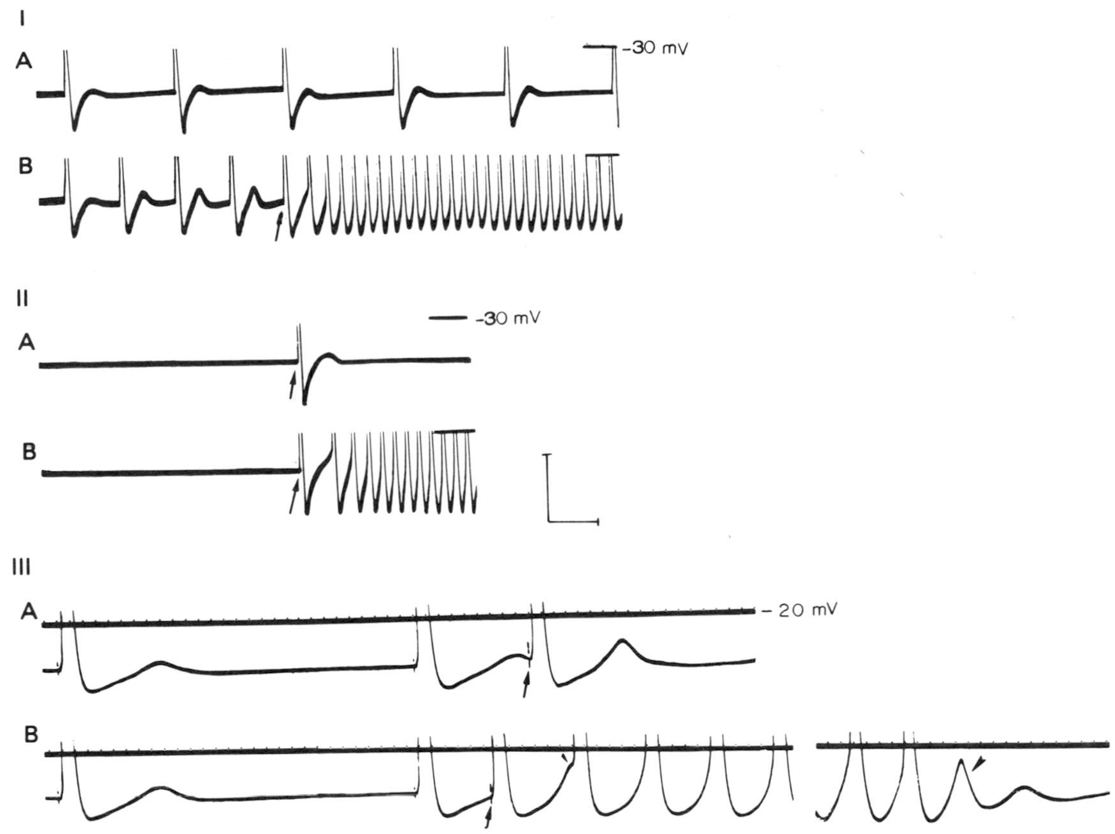

Figure 3-8. *Induction of triggered activity in an atrial fiber in the simian mitral valve. In each panel only the lower parts of the action potentials are shown. Horizontal lines in panels I and II are drawn at −30 mV; the top trace in III is at −20 mV. Panels IA and IB show triggered activity initiated as a result of decreasing the basic stimulus cycle length. In IA, stimulus cycle length was 3400 msec, and a subthreshold delayed afterdepolarization follows each action potential. At the start of IB, the stimulus cycle length was reduced to 1750 msec, and a progressive increase is seen in the amplitude of the afterdepolarization that follows each of the first four driven action potentials. The last driven action potential (arrow) is followed by a nondriven action potential and then by sustained rhythmic activity at a rate higher than the drive rate. Panels IIA and IIB show triggering caused by a single driven impulse. In IIA, after a period of quiescence, a single, stimulated action potential (arrow) is followed by a subthreshold afterdepolarization. In IIB, under slightly different conditions, a single, stimulated action potential (arrow) is followed by sustained rhythmic activity. Panels IIIA and IIIB show how triggered activity may be induced by premature stimulation. In IIIA, when the premature impulse (arrow) was elicited during the repolarization phase of the afterdepolarization, the amplitude of the subsequent afterdepolarization was increased. In IIIB, the premature impulse (large arrow) was followed by an afterdepolarization that just reached threshold (small arrow) and initiated a train of triggered impulses. (Wit, A. L., and Cranefield, P. F.: Triggered activity in cardiac muscle fibers of the simian mitral valve. Circ. Res., 38:85, 1975; by permission of the American Heart Association, Inc.)*

cussed above. By virtue of their unusual electrophysiologic characteristics, nodal cells are often involved in the initiation and maintenance of arrhythmias. Because of the important differences between nodal and other cardiac cells, it is convenient to discuss the normal electrical characteristics of the nodes separately.

The Resting Potential

Cells of the sinus node are usually continuously active and rarely at rest so that, strictly speaking, the term *resting potential* should not be used. However, the maximum diastolic potential (the most negative level of the membrane potential immediately following action potential repolarization) is easily measured and is much less negative (by about 20 mV) than the maximum diastolic potential of Purkinje fibers or atrial or ventricular fibers (Fig. 3-9). The maximum diastolic potential of AV nodal cells is similar to that of sinus nodal cells. The measured levels of intracellular K^+ concentration (and thus the level of E_K) in sinus nodal cells appear to be similar to those of cardiac cells with much higher resting potentials.[44] It is likely, therefore, that the lower membrane potential of sinus and AV nodal cells results from a higher ratio of the Na^+ to the K^+ permeability coefficient (P_{Na}/P_K) of the membrane of these cells in comparison with that of atrial, ventricular, and Purkinje cells. It is not yet clear how much the larger ratio P_{Na}/P_K of nodal cells reflects a lower P_K, as opposed to a higher P_{Na}, than exists in the other cardiac cells. Further experiments should indicate, however, whether nodal cells have an unusually high resting permeability to Na^+ or an unusually low permeability to K^+

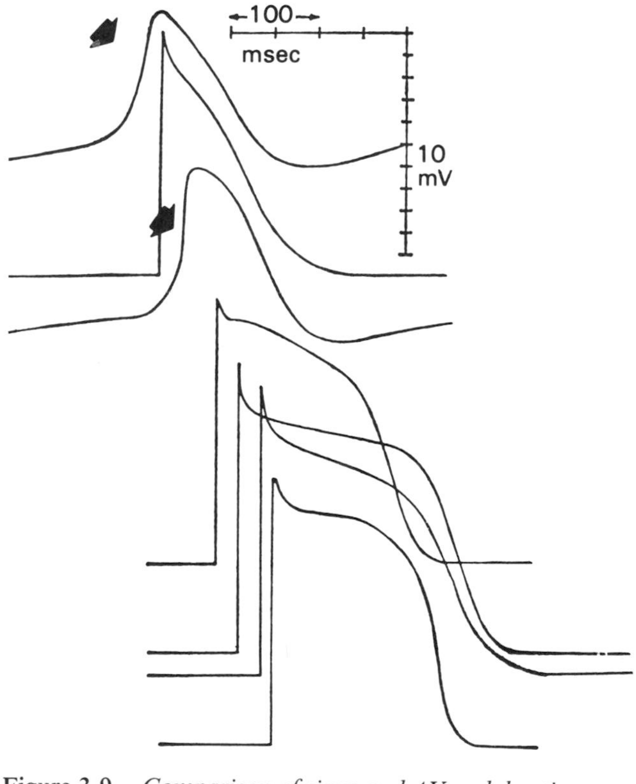

Figure 3-9. *Comparison of sinus and AV nodal action potentials (indicated by arrows) with action potentials of working myocardium and Purkinje fibers. Drawings of action potentials recorded from the following sites, starting at the top: sinoatrial node, atrium, atrioventricular node, bundle of His, Purkinje fiber in a false tendon, terminal Purkinje fiber, and ventricular muscle fiber. Note that the upstroke velocity and amplitude of sinus and AV nodal action potentials are both smaller than those of the action potentials of the other cells. (Hoffman, B. F., and Cranefield, P. F.: Electrophysiology of the Heart. New York, McGraw-Hill, 1960)*

The Depolarization and Repolarization Phases of the Action Potential

Sinus and AV nodal cells exhibit a much lower rate of phase 0 depolarization (1–20 V/sec) than normal Purkinje or working myocardial cells (Fig. 3-9). The amplitude of the action potentials is also quite small (60 to 80 mV), and in some fibers the peak of the action potential might not exceed 0 mV.[3] The slower upstroke and the lower amplitude of the action potential of nodal cells both reflect the much smaller inward current underlying the phase 0 depolarization of these cells in comparison with that of other cardiac cells. Present evidence strongly suggests that this smaller inward current of sinus and AV nodal cells flows not through the fast Na^+ channel but through the slow inward channel and is carried by calcium and sodium ions.[45-47] Such action potentials with upstrokes dependent on slow inward current are often called *slow responses* to distinguish them from the more usual *fast response* action potentials in which the upstroke depends on the fast Na^+ current.[20] Because of the small net inward current and the slow phase 0 depolarization, the slow response action potentials conduct only slowly (0.01 to 0.1 m/sec) through the nodes, and it is this slow conduction that, under certain conditions, can cause arrhythmias to arise in the nodes. As already described, the slow inward current channel has quite different time- and voltage-dependent properties than the fast sodium channel. The slow inward current turns on and also turns off, or inactivates, much more slowly than the fast sodium current. Following the upstroke of the nodal action potential, therefore, the slow inward current inactivates only slowly and contributes to the membrane depolarization throughout the action potential plateau. Activation of a time- and voltage-dependent outward K^+ current coupled with inactivation of the slow inward current probably causes repolarization of nodal cells as described above for termination of the action potential of other cardiac fibers.

The slow inward channel conductance is also much slower to reactivate following membrane repolarization than the fast Na^+ channel conductance.[20,21] In contrast to the other cardiac cells, nodal cells do not respond to premature stimuli applied during the terminal repolarization phase by giving action potentials. In fact, sufficient inactivation of the slow inward conductance may persist even after full repolarization for the cells still to be absolutely refractory to applied stimuli.[48] Reactivation then occurs gradually throughout diastole; premature impulses elicited soon after full repolarization have slower upstrokes and lower amplitudes than normal and conduct more slowly. Premature impulses initiated later in diastole have correspondingly faster upstrokes and higher amplitudes and, therefore, conduct more rapidly.[49] This behavior reflects the long time course for reactivation of the slow channel. The resulting long refractory period of the nodes and the markedly slowed conduction through them of premature impulses can be an important factor in the initiation of some arrhythmias.

Automaticity

Sinus node cells are usually automatic, each action potential apparently being initiated as a result of spontaneous diastolic depolarization, and AV nodal cells can also fire automatically, especially when disconnected from surrounding atrial myocardium.[50] It therefore appears that electrotonic interaction between atrium and node suppresses automaticity through atrio–nodal connections. Automaticity of sinus node cells might not be due to the same pacemaker current as described above for Purkinje fibers. The gating variable of the membrane conductance responsible for normal Purkinje fiber automaticity changes only between membrane potential levels of −90 and −60 mV.[36] Such conductance changes seem unlikely to provide an explanation of spontaneous diastolic depolarization of sinus node cells, since the maximum diastolic potential in these cells is usually less negative than −60 mV. However, available evidence suggests that the pacemaker current in the sinus node is at least partly carried by K^+,[38] and the decay of this outward current against a steady background inward current results in gradual membrane depolarization. In addition, it appears that an inward current that can be activated by hyperpolarization and that is called, i_f, plays an important role.[38]

The Effects of Cardiac Disease on the Resting and Action Potential of Cardiac Fibers

Cardiac arrhythmias and conduction disturbances can occur as a result of alterations in the electrical properties of cardiac fibers due to disease, and recent investigations have been aimed at characterizing some of these changes. Microelectrodes have been used to record electrical activity of cells in pieces of myocardium isolated from diseased human and experimental animal hearts. Results from such studies can often be correlated with other data obtained in studies on normal myocardial tissue exposed to an altered extracellular environment in order to mimic conditions existing during certain cardiac diseases.

The Resting Potential

It appears that many diseases that affect the heart, causing arrhythmias, tend to depolarize the membrane of cardiac cells. At the time of writing this chapter, membrane potentials have been recorded in atrial cells from hearts with rheumatic and congenital disease[51] and with cardiomyopathy[52] and from cells in both ventricular muscle and ventricular conducting fibers in areas of ischemia and infarction.[53–56] In each instance, resting membrane potentials were found to be less negative than those of cells from similar regions of normal hearts (Fig. 3-10).

The reasons for the decline in resting potential in each of these cases are not completely understood, but several factors might contribute. These are best considered in terms of the Goldman and Hodgkin and Katz equation that, as we have already shown, approximates well the resting potentials of Purkinje fibers exposed to a wide range of extracellular K^+ concentrations:

$$V_r = \frac{RT}{F} \ln \frac{[K^+]_o + (P_{Na}/P_K)[Na^+]_o}{[K^+]_i + (P_{Na}/P_K)[Na^+]_i}$$

Remembering that typical values for the ion concentrations and permeability ratio in this equation are roughly $[K^+]_o = 4$ mM; $[K^+]_i = 150$ mM; $[Na^+]_o = 150$ mM; $[Na^+]_i = 10$ mM; and $P_{Na}/P_K = 1/100$, it can be seen that, in the absence of large temperature changes, there are four separate ways in which the resting potential, V_r, might readily be made less negative. These are as follows: (1) the extracellular K^+ concentration, $[K^+]_o$, might be increased; (2) the intracellular K^+ concentration, $[K^+]_i$, might be decreased; and the ratio P_{Na}/P_K might be increased following either (3) an increase in membrane Na^+ permeability, P_{Na}, or (4) a decrease in membrane K^+ permeability, P_K. Any one of these changes would by itself cause the resting potential to decline, but of course more than one of them might occur in diseased cells. For example, any pathologic condition that results in impaired activity of the sodium pump would be expected to lead to depolarization of the affected cells, probably as a result of both an increase in $[K^+]_o$ and a decrease in $[K^+]_i$. The normal loss of cellular K^+ and gain of Na^+ that accompanies electrical activity (and that occurs, to a smaller extent, even at rest) is therefore not easily reversed, as it usually is, by the sodium pump. In other words, there is a continuous net loss of K^+ from the cells (the cellular K^+ effectively being replaced by Na^+), and $[K^+]_i$ gradually declines. Since diffusion of ions from the extracellular spaces is somewhat restricted, and therefore slow, the potassium ions lost by the cells tend to accumulate in these spaces, causing $[K^+]_o$ to rise. As noted above, both the fall in $[K^+]_i$ and the rise in $[K^+]_o$ may be expected to contribute to the decline in resting membrane potential.

Just as changes in both $[K^+]_o$ and $[K^+]_i$ may simultaneously contribute to a fall in resting potential, it is likely that complementary changes in both P_{Na} and P_K also combine to cause membrane depolarization in the following way. Suppose that a certain pathologic condition

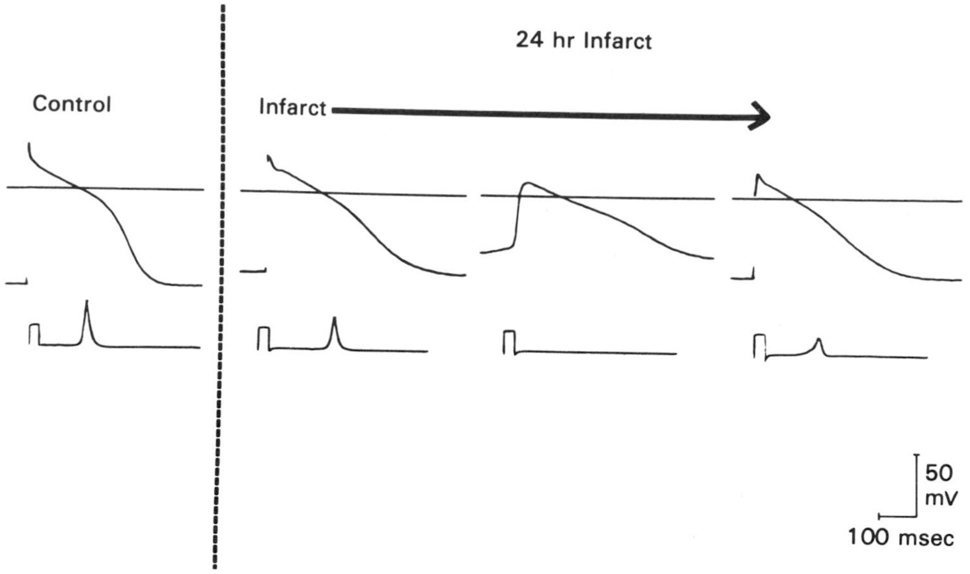

Figure 3-10. *Changes in the action potentials recorded from Purkinje fibers as a result of infarction in the canine heart. The bottom trace in each panel (recorded with a faster sweep) shows the differentiated upstroke of the action potential preceded by a differentiated calibration signal with a 200 V/sec slope of depolarization; the differentiated calibration pulse appears as a square wave. The left (control) panel shows the action potential recorded from a Purkinje fiber in a noninfarcted region; it has a normal maximum diastolic, or resting, potential and a rapid upstroke. The right panel shows action potentials recorded from three different Purkinje fibers on the endocardial surface of the infarct. Note that maximum diastolic potential, action potential amplitude, and upstroke velocity ($\dot{V}_{max}$) were all diminished in the infarct as compared to the control region. Depression of the resting potential and action potential in the middle infarct panel is particularly severe. (Friedman, P. L., Stewart, J. R., Fenoglio, J. J., Jr., and Wit, A. L.: Survival of subendocardial Purkinje fibers after extensive infarction in dogs: In vitro and in vivo correlations. Circ. Res., 33:597, 1973; by permission of the American Heart Association, Inc.)*

were associated with an increase in the "leakiness" of cell membranes to Na ions (in other words, P_{Na} is increased). In this case the ratio P_{Na}/P_K would be increased and, from the above equation, the resting potential would be reduced. Since this depolarization might occur in the absence of any significant change in $[K^+]_o$ or $[K^+]_i$, the K^+ equilibrium potential would remain unchanged. However, the outward driving force on K^+, given by $(V_m - E_K)$, is now greater than normal, and as a result of inward rectification, the K^+ conductance and, therefore, the K^+ permeability coefficient, P_K, would be smaller than normal. The steady membrane depolarization under these conditions would indeed be associated with an enhanced ratio, P_{Na}/P_K, but both an increase in P_{Na} and a decrease in P_K contribute to this change.

If, on the other hand, some cardiac disease were to lead specifically to a reduction in P_K (as a result of alterations in the chemical composition of the membrane due to abnormal protein or lipid metabolism, for example) the ratio P_{Na}/P_K would still increase and depolarization occur, while P_{Na} remained unchanged. It should be stressed that such a specific decline in P_K has not yet been demonstrated in diseased cardiac cells, although a similar effect may be artificially produced in isolated tissue preparations by including millimolar concentrations of cesium ions in the bathing solution.[57] Of course a large, maintained increase in the leakiness of cell membranes to Na^+ might eventually lead to changes in the cation distributions across the membrane if the sodium pump were unable to keep pace with the resulting increased fluxes of Na^+ and K^+. An initial depolarization would occur in response to the relative increase in sodium permeability, as described above, but then a more gradual, secondary depolarization might occur, reflecting a fall in intracellular K^+ concentration. This is because K^+ would leave the cells as Na^+ entered in order to preserve electroneutrality. Although chloride ion permeability is generally thought to be small in cardiac cells, some chloride ions may be expected to enter the cells along with Na^+, together with some water; the cells would therefore swell slightly, leading to a corresponding further fall in $[K^+]_i$. Since the rate of sodium pump activity is predominantly determined by the level of $[Na^+]_i$, pump activity would be increased in these leaky cells with raised $[Na^+]_i$. If the passive movements of Na^+ and K^+ were large, however, or if pump activity were impaired in some way substantial changes in the levels of $[Na^+]_i$ and $[K^+]_i$ would still occur despite this pump activation by internal Na^+.

Phase 0 Depolarization

Under most pathologic conditions investigated, the upstroke of the action potential (phase 0) of Purkinje fibers or atrial or ventricular myocardial cells is slowed and reduced in amplitude.[51-56,58] These changes are probably largely due to the reduced membrane potentials of the diseased cells, although similar changes could also arise as a result of specific disease-related alterations in the underlying conductance mechanisms in the absence of any resting potential changes. There is, as yet, little detailed information about the specific primary effects of diseases on the conductance mechanisms underlying the inward current that causes the action potential upstroke.

We have already described how the fast Na^+ conductance inactivates during prolonged membrane depolarization (after the upstroke of the action potential) and how full membrane repolarization to large negative potential levels (*e.g.*, the repolarization of the action potential) is necessary to remove this inactivation completely. Incomplete membrane repolarization leads to only partial removal of inactivation in the steady state. Thus, following complete activation of the Na^+ conductance, a steady hyperpolarization to about −100 mV suffices to remove inactivation fully, leaving all Na^+ channels available for reactivation by a subsequent depolarizing stimulus, whereas steady repolarization to between −60 and −70 mV would leave about 50% of the sodium channels inactivated and, therefore, unavailable for reactivation by a depolarizing stimulus. At a potential level of −50 mV practically all the sodium channels remain inactivated and so are unavailable for immediate reactivation (see Fig. 3-3).

Thus in cardiac cells depolarized as a result of disease, only a fraction of the total population of fast Na^+ channels may be available to carry inward current. In this case the magnitude of the net inward current during phase 0 of the action potential would be reduced, and, consequently, both the speed and amplitude of the upstroke would be diminished (see Fig. 3-10). Such action potentials, with upstrokes dependent on inward current flowing through partially inactivated Na^+ conductance, are sometimes referred to as *depressed fast responses*[16] to distinguish them from *slow responses,*[20] which also have slow upstrokes but which depend on inward current flowing in quite different, pharmacologically distinct, membrane channels (see above). Because of their slow upstrokes and diminished amplitudes the conduction velocity of depressed fast responses is much reduced. For example, the conduction velocity of Purkinje fiber action potentials may be reduced from 2 to 4 m/sec to less than 0.5 m/sec because of steady state Na^+ channel inactivation resulting from membrane depolarization. Further depolarization and inactivation of the Na^+ channel may render the fiber inexcitable so that it may become a site of conduction block. However, although the fast Na^+ conductance may be completely inactivated near −50 mV, the slow inward conductance (Na^+/Ca^{++} channel) is still available for activation below this potential.[20,21] Under these conditions, therefore, a strong depolarizing stimulus can still elicit a slow inward current. Whether this normally weak, slow inward current gives rise to the regenerative depolarization characteristic of a propagated slow response action potential depends on the relative magnitude of the membrane K^+ conductance. As mentioned in our discussion of the resting potential, membrane depolarization caused by a small increase in Na^+ permeability, for instance, would be expected to result in a reduction in K^+ conductance because of the presence of inward-going rectification. Under these conditions, the slow inward current may suffice to initiate a slow response action potential (see Fig. 3-3). On the other hand, membrane depolarization resulting from an increase in $[K^+]_o$ is associated with an increase in K^+ conductance, so that in this case the same weak, slow inward current may give rise to only a negligibly small depolarization. However, if the slow inward current is enhanced, as for example, in the presence of catecholamines, slow response action potentials can also be elicited when $[K^+]_o$ is elevated.[59] Because of their slow upstrokes the conduction velocity of slow response action potentials is low. The conduction velocity of Purkinje fiber action potentials may thus be reduced to less than 0.1 m/sec as a result of severe membrane depolarization.[20]

When phase 0 depolarization is slowed to a critical degree, unidirectional conduction block may occur.[1] In bundles of atrial, ventricular, or Purkinje fibers, stimulated at either end to elicit normal action potentials, the impulse conducts at almost equal velocities in either direction along the bundle. As the upstroke velocity and amplitude of the action potential decrease, conduction velocity is slowed in both directions. At a critical degree of depression of the action potential upstroke velocity, conduction may fail in one direction but proceed slowly in the other direction (Fig. 3-11). The critical degree of depression varies in different regions of the heart and depends partly on the geometry of the cardiac syncytium. Further depression of the action potential upstroke and amplitude usually results in conduction block in both directions. Slow conduction or unidirectional conduction block can occur in bundles of fibers showing

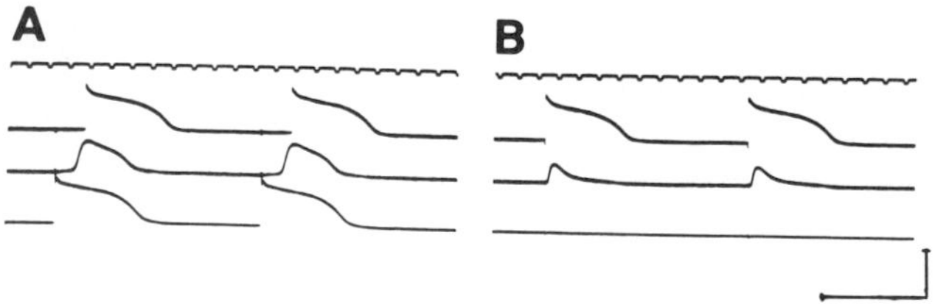

Figure 3-11. *Unidirectional conduction block in a bundle of canine Purkinje fibers. The top line shows time marks at 100-msec intervals. The three traces beneath show action potentials recorded from three different cells along the length of a Purkinje fiber bundle. The action potentials on the upper trace were recorded from the near end of the bundle, those on the middle trace were recorded from the center, and those on the bottom trace were recorded from the far end of the bundle. The cells in the center segment of the bundle were depolarized by perfusion with high $[K^+]_o$ solution, and the action potentials recorded there have slow upstrokes and low amplitudes. Panel A shows records obtained by stimulating the bundle at the far end. The impulse was first recorded in the cell at the far end of the bundle (bottom trace), and then it conducted through the center segment (middle trace) to finally excite the cells at the near end of the bundle (top trace). Panel B shows records obtained when the near end of the bundle was stimulated instead. The cell monitored by the top trace was excited, since this was near the region of stimulation, but conduction block occurred in the depressed area (middle trace) and so the far end of the bundle (bottom trace) was not activated. (Cranefield, P. F., Wit, A. L., and Hoffman, B. F.: The genesis of cardiac arrhythmias. Circulation, 47:190, 1973; by permission of the American Heart Association, Inc.)*

either depressed fast response or slow response action potentials.

Since it is unlikely that there will be a uniform reduction in membrane potential in diseased areas of the heart, it seems reasonable to expect varying degrees of Na^+ channel inactivation in these areas, ranging from very little inactivation (impulses conducted rapidly in the form of fast response action potentials), through moderate inactivation (impulses conducted relatively slowly as depressed fast responses), to full inactivation (impulses, if any, conducted very slowly as slow response action potentials).

Repolarization and Refractoriness

As described in the section on normal action potentials, the relative refractory period of normal Purkinje or atrial or ventricular myocardial cells (with maximum diastolic potentials near −90 mV) lasts until action potential repolarization is complete. Premature action potentials elicited during this period have reduced rates of rise and reduced amplitudes due to persisting, partial inactivation of the Na^+ conductance. This inactivation is removed within a few milliseconds after repolarization to about −90 mV, and then action potential upstrokes regain their normal speed and amplitude. However, the rate of removal of Na^+ current inactivation (and, therefore, the rate of recovery of the maximum rate of depolarization) depends strongly on the steady level of membrane potential: recovery occurs rapidly (within 20 msec) at −90 mV but takes longer (more than 100 msec) at −60 mV.[60] In cardiac cells depolarized by disease, therefore, recovery of the action potential upstroke may be prolonged. Since the upstrokes of action potentials in these cells are already slowed as a result of the steady membrane depolarization, premature action potentials elicited during the prolonged relative refractory period will have even slower upstrokes and correspondingly lower conduction velocities. If the cells are so depolarized that the Na^+ conductance remains fully inactivated and only slow response action potentials can be initiated, then the relative refractory period will still extend into diastole because removal of inactivation of the slow inward current also occurs very slowly. In this case the absolute refractory period may last until action potential repolarization is complete, and full recovery of the upstroke of a premature impulse may not be achieved for hundreds of milliseconds after that time. The greatly slowed conduction of premature impulses in cardiac fibers with low membrane potentials can lead to reentry, and the premature impulses that cause reentry in these fibers may arise long after complete repolarization.

Large alterations in the refractory periods can also be brought about by changes in action potential duration in cells with large negative resting potentials, since, in this case, removal of inactivation is complete soon after action potential repolarization. A shortening of the action potential in these cells, such as that resulting from an increase in stimulation rate, is therefore accompanied by a corresponding shortening of the effective and relative refractory periods.[3] In cells with very low resting potentials, on the other hand, removal of inactivation may occur so slowly that the relative refractory period is practically independent of action potential duration.

Several examples of changes in action potential duration caused by cardiac disease are the following. The action potential of ventricular muscle cells shortens soon after the onset of ischemia, before the resting potential declines significantly.[55,61,62] The effective and relative refractory periods of such ischemic cells are decreased accordingly. In areas that are chronically ischemic, action potential duration of ventricular muscle and Purkinje fibers may be markedly prolonged,[53,54,63] and therefore the relative and effective refractory periods of these cells are increased. Vagal stimulation causes atrial action potential duration and refractory periods to decrease.[64] Such changes in action potential duration and refractoriness can markedly alter conduction properties and thereby cause arrhythmias (see below).

Abnormal Automaticity and Triggered Activity

Previously, we discussed the automaticity that is a normal property of certain types of cardiac fibers. Working atrial and ventricular myocardial cells do not normally develop spontaneous diastolic depolarization and do not initiate spontaneous impulses. However, when the membrane potential of atrial or ventricular fibers is experimentally reduced to less than about −60 mV, "spontaneous" diastolic depolarization and automatic impulse initiation may occur in these cells.[65–67] The "spontaneously" occurring action potentials are slow responses. The decrease in membrane potential that may lead to this abnormal automaticity, however, might also be caused by disease (Fig. 3-12). Automaticity may occur also in Purkinje fibers when the membrane is depolarized to less than −60 mV (see Fig. 3-6).[68] As discussed before, in order for propagated action potentials to occur at these low membrane potentials in atrial, ventricular, or Purkinje fibers, membrane K^+ conductance must be low. In cells depolarized by an increase in $[K^+]_o$, such automaticity is usually not seen because the membrane K^+ conductance is also increased under these conditions.

The ionic currents underlying the automaticity at low membrane potentials have not yet been elucidated, but it is unlikely that the pacemaker current described above for normal Purkinje fibers is involved, because the gating variable for this channel does not change at membrane potentials less negative than about −60 mV.

Delayed afterdepolarizations may follow the action potentials of working atrial fibers[52,69] and of Purkinje fibers[70] when the membrane potential is reduced by cardiac disease. The amplitude of these afterdepolarizations increases when the dominant rhythm becomes faster or after a premature impulse, and triggered activity may occur in such cells if the afterdepolarizations reach threshold potential. The mechanism by which afterdepolarizations arise in diseased cardiac cells is not yet clear but is probably related to an increase in intracellular Ca.

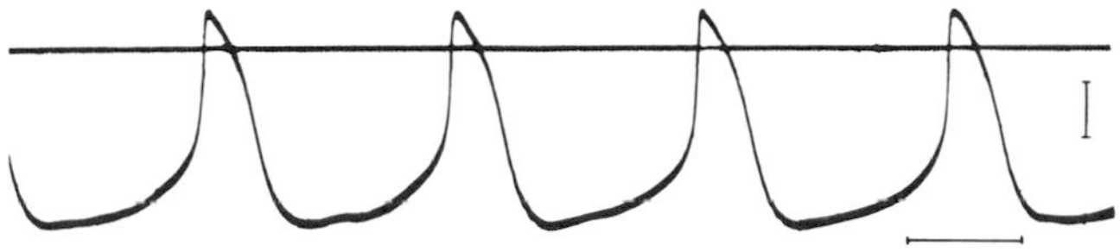

Figure 3-12. *Abnormal automaticity recorded from a left atrial fiber in an isolated preparation obtained from a failed canine heart. The left atrium was markedly dilated, and resting potentials of the atrial cells were generally very low. The automaticity in this cell may have been initiated as a result of the fall in resting membrane potential. (Vertical calibration = 15 mV; horizontal calibration = 300 msec)*

The Genesis of Cardiac Arrhythmias

In this section we will describe how the site of origin of the dominant pacemaker may shift from the sinus node to an ectopic site, thereby causing ectopic beats and tachycardia. This change in the locus of impulse initiation is often a consequence of the alterations in electrical activity of cardiac cells that accompany disease. Although arrhythmias may also occur in clinically normal hearts, these arrhythmias might be initiated by similar alterations in cellular electrophysiology that occur in only a limited region of the heart and may, therefore, be too small to be detected by clinical examination.

Arrhythmias Caused by Reentry

In the heart driven by the sinus rhythm, the conducting impulse dies out after sequential activation of the atria and ventricles because it is surrounded by refractory tissue that it has recently excited. The heart then must await a new impulse arising in the sinus node for subsequent activation. The phenomenon of reentry occurs when the propagating impulse does not die out after complete activation of the heart but persists to reexcite the heart after the end of the refractory period.[71] In order for this to happen, the impulse must remain somewhere in the heart while the recently excited cardiac fibers regain excitability so that the impulse can subsequently reenter and reactivate them.

The effective refractory period of cardiac fibers is long, ranging from 150 msec in the atrium to about 300 to 500 msec in the ventricular specialized conducting system.[3] An impulse destined to reenter or reexcite the heart must therefore survive for at least this time if it is to outlast the refractory period. However, it cannot remain stationary while waiting out the refractory period but must continue to travel over a pathway that is functionally isolated from the rest of the heart. Such a conduction pathway must provide a return route to the regions previously excited and must be sufficiently long to permit propagation of the impulse during the entire refractory period. The cardiac impulse normally conducts at a velocity of 0.5 to 5 m/sec in cardiac fibers other than those in the sinus and atrioventricular nodes. If it traveled at these speeds for the duration of the refractory period, it would have to travel in a pathway between 7.5 cm and 2.5 m long. Cranefield and Hoffman have stated "that so long a path, however circuitous, could exist in functional isolation from the rest of the heart has never seemed likely."[72]

Of course, travel at a normal velocity is not the only way in which the impulse, destined to reenter, might persist during the refractory period: a reduction of the conduction velocity obviates the need for such a long conduction pathway. For example, if conduction is slowed to 0.02 m/sec, the impulse would travel only 6 mm during a refractory period of 300 msec.[72] In the previous section we have described how cardiac disease can give rise to such slow impulse conduction, and pathways of this length are readily available in the heart.

Alterations in the duration of the refractory period also may facilitate reentry. For example, a shortening of the effective refractory period, which usually occurs when repolarization of the action potential is accelerated, reduces the time during which the impulse must conduct through the functionally isolated pathway while awaiting the recovery of excitability of the rest of the heart.

Reentry Caused by Slow Conduction and Unidirectional Conduction Block in Cardiac Fibers With Low Resting Potentials and Low Upstroke Velocities

The occurrence of reentry depends on the presence of slow conduction and unidirectional conduction block. The basic principles that enable reentry to occur are illustrated in Fig. 3-13, which reproduces in modified form a figure published by Mines in 1914.[71] His data was obtained from isolated rings of cardiac tissue. Similar studies that also contributed to the modern concepts on reentrant excitation were performed by Mayer[73] in rings of jellyfish subumbrella tissue. Figure 3-13 shows that if a ring of excitable tissue is stimulated at one point, two waves of excitation start at this point and progress in opposite directions around the ring, with only one excitation of the ring occurring, since the waves collide and die out. However, by temporarily applying pressure near the site of stimulation, an excitation wave can be induced to progress in only one direction around the ring, the area of compression preventing the conduction of a wave in the other direction. The wave conducting in one direction returns to its point of origin (by which time pressure is no longer being applied to the ring) and then conducts around the ring again. The impulse is able to conduct around the ring an indefinite number of times because each time it returns to its point of origin, that part of the ring has recovered excitability.[71,73]

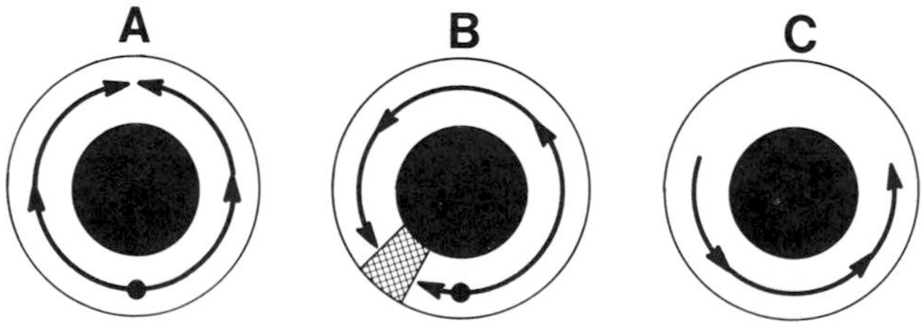

Figure 3-13. *Schematic representation of reentry in a ring of excitable tissue as described by Mayer and by Mines. In A, the ring was stimulated in the area indicated by the black dot, and impulses propagated away from the point of stimulation, in both directions, and collided; no reentry occurred. In B, the cross-hatched area was compressed while the ring was stimulated, again at the black dot. The impulse propagated around the ring in only one direction, having been blocked in the other direction by the area of compression; immediately after stimulation the compression was relieved. In C, the unidirectionally circulating impulse is shown returning to its point of origin and then continuing around the loop.*

Reentry can occur in a similar manner in loops composed of bundles of cardiac fibers, whether they be atrial, ventricular, or Purkinje fibers. For example, the anatomy of the ventricular specialized conducting system provides conduction pathways that are functionally suitable for reentry. Bundles of interconnecting Purkinje fibers are surrounded by connective tissue that separates them from the ventricular myocardium. In peripheral regions of the conducting system such Purkinje fiber bundles often arborize into many branches; where these branches make contact with ventricular muscle, anatomic loops composed of the Purkinje fiber bundles and the muscle are often formed (Fig. 3-14). Loops composed entirely of Purkinje fiber bundles are also known to exist in the peripheral ventricular conducting system.

Purkinje fibers normally have fast response action potentials that conduct rapidly at a velocity of 1 to 4 m/sec. Under normal circumstances the rapidly conducting impulse of sinus origin will invade all Purkinje fiber bundles of a distal loop and conduct into ventricular muscle, where impulses collide and die out because they are surrounded by refractory tissue (Fig. 3-15). For reentry to occur in the distal ventricular specialized conducting system, conduction must be slowed and a strategically located region of unidirectional block must be present. Slow conduction may occur when the loop of fibers is in a diseased region of the heart. In this case both the rate of phase 0 depolarization and the overshoot of the action potential of the Purkinje fibers in the loop may be reduced, possibly because of a decrease in resting potential. Depression of the resting potential and action potential upstroke is rarely uniform in regions of disease, and in areas where the action potential is severely depressed unidirectional block may occur.

The mechanism by which slowed conduction and unidirectional block can result in reentry is illustrated in the left panel of Figure 3-14.[74,75] In the distal loop, composed of Purkinje fiber bundles and ventricular muscle, an area of unidirectional conduction block is located

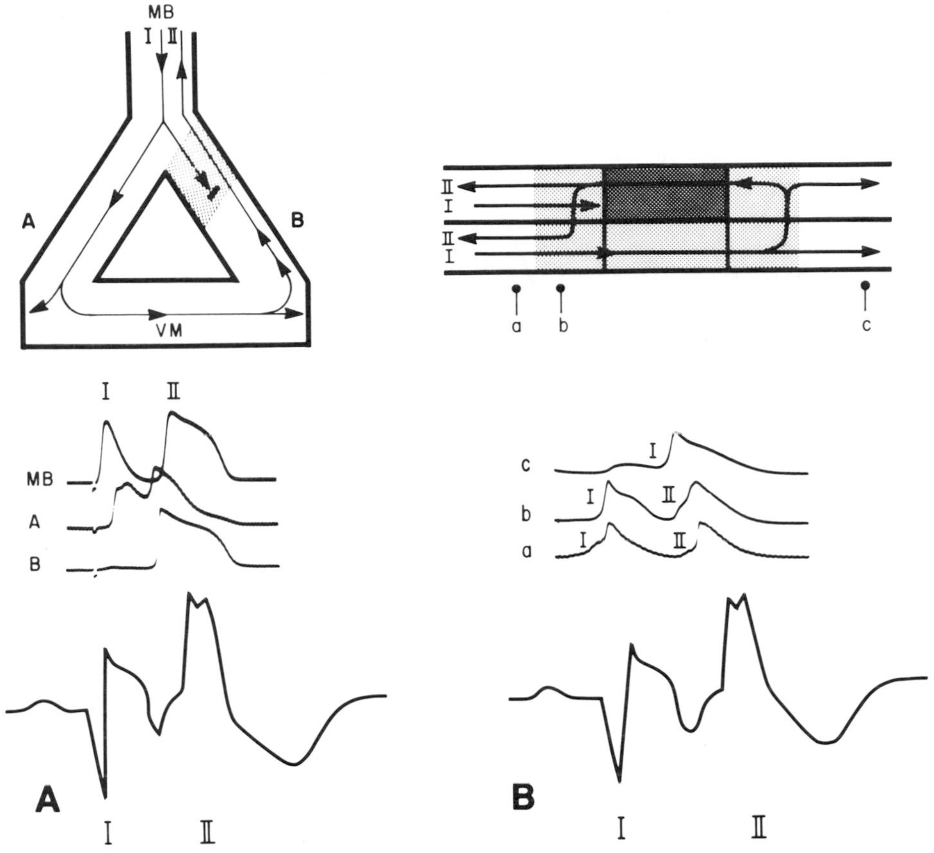

Figure 3-14. *Possible mechanisms for reentry resulting from slow conduction and unidirectional conduction block. The left panel shows a main bundle of Purkinje fibers (MB), which divides into two branches (A and B) before terminating on ventricular muscle (VM). A severely depressed area in which unidirectional conductional block, in the antegrade direction, occurs is located in branch B (shaded area). Conduction is slow throughout the rest of the loop because the Purkinje fibers have low resting potentials; their action potentials, consequently, have slow upstrokes. The arrows indicate the sequence of activation of the loop by the conducting impulse: the arrow labeled I represents an impulse of sinus origin entering the loop; the arrow labeled II is the reentering impulse leaving the loop. Details of the mechanism by which reentry occurs are given in the text. Action potentials recorded from MB and branches A and B are shown below, together with an example of how the electrocardiogram might appear. Action potential I in the MB trace was recorded as the impulse entered the loop. The action potentials in A and B were recorded as the impulse conducted around the loop. The action potential II in the MB trace occurred when the impulse reexcited the main bundle. Impulse I would cause ventricular depolarization I on the electrocardiogram and impulse II would cause a ventricular extrasystole (ventricular depolarization II). The right panel shows, at the top, how reentry can occur even in a single bundle of muscle or Purkinje fibers. The diagram depicts two adjacent fibers in a bundle; the entire shaded area is depressed, but depression in the darker area of the upper fiber is so severe that unidirectional conduction block occurs there. The arrows indicate the sequence of activation in the bundle; arrows labeled I show the impulse entering the bundle, and the arrows labeled II show the reentrant impulse returning to reexcite the left end of the bundle (see text). Action potentials recorded from sites a, b, and c in the lower fiber are shown below: action potentials labeled I were recorded as the impulse conducted from left to right, and action potentials labeled II were recorded as the impulse returned to its origin. The bottom trace shows how such events would appear on the electrocardiogram. (Wit, A. L., and Bigger, J. T.: Possible electrophysiological mechanisms for lethal arrhythmias accompanying myocardial ischemia and infarction. Circulation [Suppl.] 51 and 52, III–96, 1975; by permission of the American Heart Association, Inc.)*

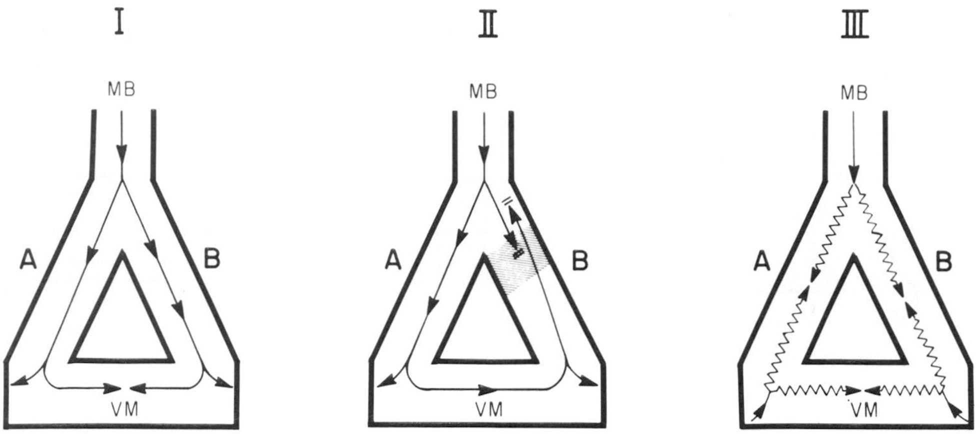

Figure 3-15. *Schematic representation of a bundle of Purkinje fibers (MB) in the distal ventricular conducting system, which divides into two branches (A and B) before making contact with ventricular muscle (VM) to form a loop. Panel I shows the sequence of activation under normal conditions; the impulse of sinus origin invades the main bundle (MB) leading to the loop and conducts through both branches A and B into ventricular muscle, where the impulses collide and die out. Panel II shows the sequence of activation in the presence of an area of unidirectional conduction block (shaded area in branch B); conduction is blocked in the antegrade direction (from B to VM) but not in the retrograde direction (from VM to B). Conduction velocity is normal in the rest of the loop, since this is not depressed, and, therefore, the impulse conducts rapidly around the loop, returning to the main bundle (MB) before it has recovered excitability and is then blocked in this refractory tissue. Panel III indicates a possible sequence of activation when conduction is slowed throughout the loop, but no region of unidirectional conduction block is present. Thus the impulse conducts slowly from the main bundle through both branches. However, the ventricular muscle is first activated by impulses conducting rapidly from other regions where conduction is not depressed. Again, there is no excitable return pathway through which reentry can take place. (Wit, A. L., Rosen, M. R., and Hoffman, B. F.: Electrophysiology and pharmacology of cardiac arrhythmias. II. Relationship of normal and abnormal electrical activity of cardiac fibers to the genesis of arrhythmias. B. Reentry. Am. Heart J., 88:664, 1974; with permission.)*

near the origin of branch B; an impulse cannot conduct through this area in the antegrade direction but it can in the retrograde direction. Slow conduction is assumed to occur in the rest of the loop. An impulse of sinus origin conducting into the loop through the main Purkinje fiber bundle blocks near the origin of branch B and can enter only branch A, through which it conducts slowly into the ventricular muscle. This impulse can then invade branch B at its myocardial end. This branch had not been excited initially because of the unidirectional block at its origin, and so the impulse can conduct in the retrograde direction in branch B, through the region of unidirectional block, and then reexcite the main bundle from which it entered the loop (Fig. 3-14).

The reentering impulse will, of course, block if it returns to the main bundle while the fibers in that region are still effectively refractory (Fig. 3-15). Hence, the necessity for slowly conducting action potentials around the loop. The region of unidirectional conduction block is necessary to prevent one part of the loop from being invaded by the antegrade impulse and so provide a return excitable pathway for the reentering impulse.

When the reentrant impulse returns to the main bundle, it may travel throughout the conducting system to reactivate the ventricles, causing a premature ventricular beat. It may also reinvade the bundle of Purkinje fibers through which it originally excited the ventricular muscle (branch A in Fig. 3-14) and once again propagate back through the reentrant pathway. This may result in a continuous circling of the impulse around the loop or "circus movement," much like the circling of the impulse around the ring of tissue observed by Mines and Mayer. In the loop just described, however, the continuous circling would result in repetitive excitation of the ventricles.

If, during normal activation of the heart, conduction in the loop of Purkinje fibers and ventricular muscle is not slowed sufficiently to permit reentry, or if there is not a strategically located site of unidirectional block, reentry might still be induced by premature activation. The basic impulse may spread through the Purkinje bundles and ventricular muscle in any of the ways indicated in Figure 3-15. If these Purkinje fibers are then reactivated prematurely, before they have completely recovered excitability, the premature impulse may be expected to conduct even more slowly than the basic impulse. Premature activation may also result in unidirectional block because of the low safety margin for conduction in partially refractory tissue. Premature activation may therefore lead to reentry of the kind illustrated in Figure 3-14.

Although we have used the peripheral Purkinje system as an example in describing the mechanism for reentry in a loop caused by depressed conduction, reentry may occur by a similar mechanism in other regions of the heart. For instance, rheumatic heart disease in the atrium or infarction of the ventricle can leave discrete areas of inexcitable tissue in addition to depressing the resting potential and action potential upstroke[52,55]: conduction around these areas may then be circular, as described above for the peripheral Purkinje system and schematically illustrated in Figure 3-14.

Gross anatomic loops are not a prerequisite for the occurrence of reentry: reentry caused by slow conduction and unidirectional block can also occur in unbranched bundles of muscle fibers, and the same general principles apply as already discussed for reentry in discrete loops of tissue.[74–76] A mechanism for reentry in an unbranched bundle of Purkinje or muscle fibers, called reflection, is shown in the right panel of Figure 3-14. In these structures individual fibers are arranged predominantly in parallel with lateral connections in some regions. An example of nonuniform reduction of membrane potential as a result of disease in such an unbranched structure is depicted in the top part of the diagram. Cells in the mid-region of the upper fiber are assumed to have lower resting potentials than those in the lower fiber, so that unidirectional conduction block occurs in the upper fiber while slow conduction occurs in the lower one. An impulse propagating through this unbranched bundle will therefore be blocked near the mid-region of the upper fiber but will conduct slowly along the lower fiber. Once past the mid-region, the impulse may then travel laterally into the upper fiber and conduct in both antegrade and retrograde directions (see Fig. 3-14). In this way the impulse can reenter and reexcite the unbranched structure in the retrograde direction and thereby reexcite other parts of the heart.

Recently, another mechanism that may cause reflection has been described.[77] Slow conduction does not occur along the entire bundle because of depressed transmembrane potentials, as illustrated in Figure 3-14B. Instead, there is delayed activation of part of the bundle, resulting from electrotonic excitation of a region distal to an inexcitable segment. The inexcitable segment may be caused by a depressed resting potential and subsequent inactivation of the Na channels. The reader is referred to the original article for further details.[77]

Reentry Caused by Dispersion of Refractoriness

Reentry can also occur in the absence of disease-induced steady-state reduction in resting membrane potential and depression of phase 0 depolarization. However, the two essential conditions for the occurrence of reentry remain slow conduction and unidirectional conduction block. Both these conditions may be met in healthy cardiac fibers when premature impulses are elicited within the relative refractory period, particularly if the refractory periods of adjacent groups of cardiac fibers differ markedly. The differences in refractory periods of adjacent groups of fibers can also be accentuated by cardiac disease. The following are some examples of reentry caused by such dispersion of refractoriness.

The refractory periods of cells in the normal AV node vary considerably. Cells at the atrial end of the node (AN region) appear to comprise at least two populations, each with a different refractory period (Fig. 3-16).[78] Under appropriate conditions, this difference in refractoriness of cells in the upper nodal region may lead to the formation of a functional reentrant pathway.[78] Normally, the sinus impulse reaches the AV node long after both groups of cells recover excitability and so conducts through all these fibers to the His bundle. Similarly, a premature atrial impulse occurring late enough in the basic cycle length usually propagates through all the fibers in the AV node. However, the disparity in refractoriness of upper nodal fibers becomes significant in determining conduction patterns of frequent irregular impulses or early premature impulses. Early premature atrial impulses conducting into the node may encounter a region of unidirectional block where the refractory periods of the cells are the longest but may still conduct slowly through upper nodal fibers, which have somewhat shorter effective refractory periods (Fig. 3-16). If conduction of the early premature impulses through these fibers is slow enough, the impulse may enter the region of unidirectional block in a retrograde direction after fibers in this region have recovered excitability and then return to reexcite the atrium as a reentrant impulse or return extrasystole (Fig. 3-16). The "antegrade" conduction pathway, with the shorter refractory period, has been called the *alpha pathway* by Mendez and Moe, while the "retrograde" pathway, with the longer refractory period, has been called the *beta pathway*.[78] Since the

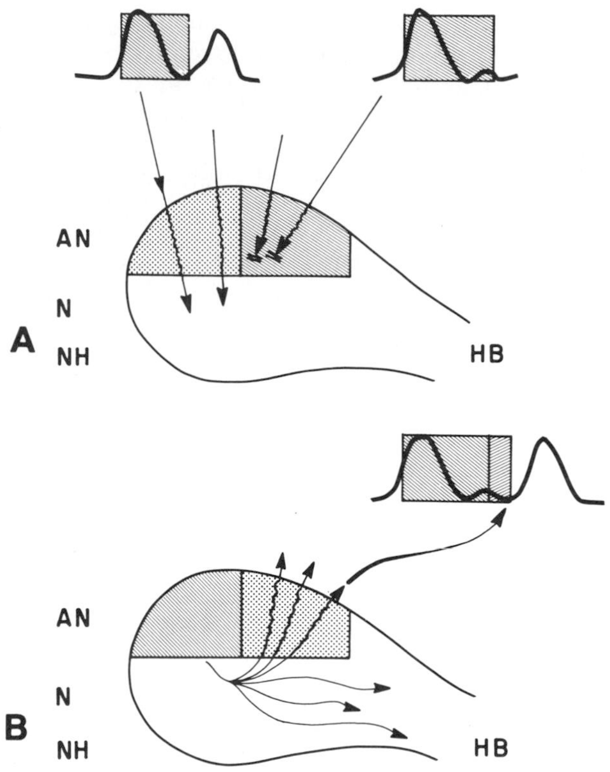

Figure 3-16. *Reentry of an atrial impulse in the AV node. Both A and B show diagrammatic representations of the AV node with the upper (AN), middle (N), and lower (NH) node indicated; HB indicates the His bundle. In A, action potentials recorded from two regions of the upper node are illustrated at the top: the action potential at the left has a shorter refractory period than that shown at the right, as indicated by the shaded area. Therefore, when a premature atrial impulse enters the AV node (arrows), it may be able to propagate through the part of the upper node with the shorter refractory period but blocks in the region with the longer refractory period. This is also depicted in the action potential recordings at the top. Panel B shows a possible continuation of these events: the propagating impulse (indicated by the arrows) can return to excite the area of the node in which antegrade conduction block had occurred and thereby reenter the atrium; action potentials recorded from the return nodal pathway are shown above. The impulse can also conduct into the His bundle. (Wit, A. L., Rosen, M. R., and Hoffman, B. F.: Electrophysiology and pharmacology of cardiac arrhythmias. II. Relationship of normal and abnormal electrical activity of cardiac fibers to the genesis of arrhythmias. B. Reentry. Am. Heart J., 88:799, 1974; with permission.)*

lower region of the AV node is not part of the reentrant pathway,[78] a premature atrial impulse can reenter whether or not that impulse is also conducted in an antegrade direction to activate the His bundle and the ventricles.

The mechanisms described above for single reentry of atrial impulses in the AV node can also result in continuous reentry. If an impulse reenters the atrium when the nodal fibers it previously excited in the antegrade pathway have recovered excitability, the impulse can once again enter the AV node and conduct around the circuit.[79-81] This can become a repetitive process, the atrium being activated each time the impulse conducts around the reentrant loop. This is one of the possible mechanisms for supraventricular tachycardia and is discussed further in Chapter 10.

Differences in refractoriness of adjacent groups of cells can also cause reentry in atrial,[82,83] ventricular,[84] or Purkinje fibers[85,86] with normal electrophysiologic characteristics, although pathologic changes that tend to accentuate local differences in refractoriness will of course facilitate reentry.[87] As in the example given above of reentry in the AV node, a premature impulse is necessary for reentry to occur. Reentry in the atrium resulting from the leading circle mechanism[83] is described in Chapter 6. An illustration of reentry resulting from dispersion of refractoriness in the Purkinje system surviving in a region of myocardial infarction is presented in Figure 3-17. The action potential duration of these fibers is extremely prolonged, as are the relative and effective refractory periods compared to Purkinje fibers in surrounding noninfarcted regions. In addition, the action potential duration of adjacent fibers in the infarct are not homogeneous; action potential duration and refractoriness are prolonged more in some fibers than in others. Marked differences in the effective refractory periods of cells in adjacent regions result in an early premature impulse being blocked in the region with the longest effective refractory period, yet conducting slowly through relatively refractory regions with a shorter effective refractory period (Fig. 3-17*A*). While the impulse conducts slowly through the excitable tissue, the region of block recovers excitability so that the premature impulse eventually excites these regions and then returns to its site of origin as a reentrant impulse. Reentry caused by this mechanism can also be repetitive and give rise to tachycardias.

The premature impulses that are necessarily responsible for the above types of reentry can arise in several ways. These impulses may arise spontaneously in the sinus node, for example, or in an ectopic pacemaker, or they may be elicited by electrical stimulation of the heart.

Slow Conduction and Reentrant Excitation Caused by the Anisotropic Structure of Cardiac Muscle

Cardiac muscle is anisotropic, that is, its anatomic and biophysical properties vary according to the direction in

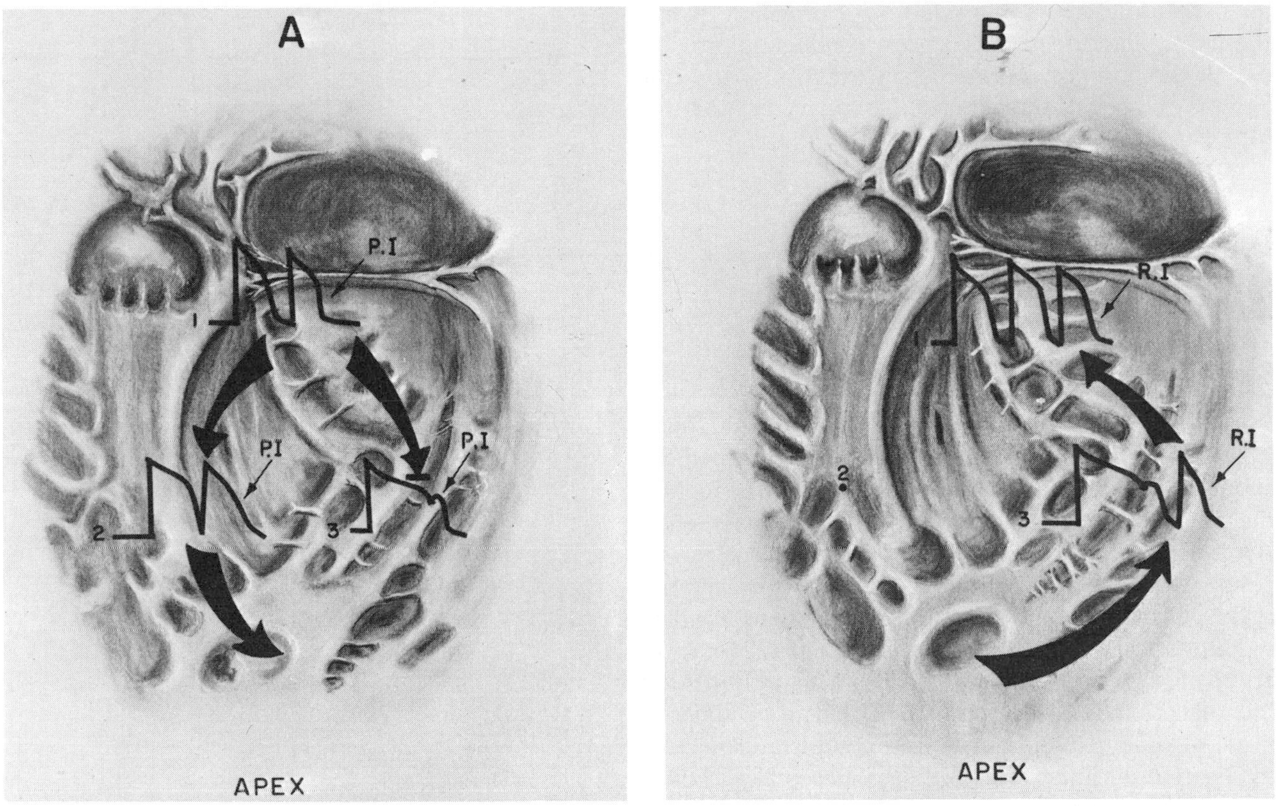

Figure 3-17. *Mechanism for reentry resulting from dispersion of refractoriness in the subendocardial Purkinje fiber network over an area of extensive myocardial infarction. Both A and B show the endocardial surface of the left ventricular anterior papillary muscle (to the left) and the anterior interventricular septum (to the right). The light area in each diagram is the infarcted region, which is covered by a blanket of surviving Purkinje fibers.*[53] *Purkinje fibers in different regions have action potentials with markedly different durations and refractory periods. Action potentials recorded from a subendocardial Purkinje fiber at the border of the infarcted region and normal tissue (site 1) and from subendocardial Purkinje fibers with prolonged repolarization phases (sites 2 and 3),*[53] *surviving in the infarct, are shown in the diagrams. In A, a premature impulse (P.I.) occurs at site 1, at the infarct border, and conducts into the infarcted regions (as indicated by the curved arrows), where action potentials are prolonged; the action potential at site 3 is longer than that at site 2 in the infarct. Consequently, the premature impulse can excite cells at site 2 but conduction blocks at site 3. Panel B shows the continuation of these events: the premature impulse, after conducting through site 2, activates the cells at site 3 as a reentering impulse (R.I.) and then proceeds to its site of origin, site 1, which it also reexcites as a reentrant impulse (R.I.). (Wit, A. L., Rosen, M. R., and Hoffman, B. F.: Electrophysiology and pharmacology of cardiac arrhythmias. II. Relationship of normal and abnormal electrical activity of cardiac fibers to the genesis of arrhythmias. B. Reentry. Am. Heart J., 88:799, 1974; with permission.)*

the cardiac syncytium in which they are measured.[88] These anisotropic properties might sometimes cause reentry by affecting conduction of the cardiac impulse.[89,90] Impulse conduction velocity in a direction that is perpendicular to the long axis of orientation of atrial or ventricular fibers is much slower than parallel to the long axis. Very slow conduction occurs even though resting potentials and action-potential upstrokes are normal. The slow conduction is caused by an effective axial resistivity (resistance to current flow in the direction of propagation), which is much higher in the direction perpendicular to fiber orientation than parallel to fiber orientation.[88-90] This higher axial resistivity results in part from fewer and shorter intercalated disks connecting myocardial fibers in a side-to-side direction than in the end-to-end direction. The slow conduction provides one of the components necessary for reentry to occur and may be one of the factors enabling reentry to occur in normal atrial or ventricular muscle.

Arrhythmias Caused by Automaticity and Triggered Activity

Sinus Node Domination of Subsidiary Pacemakers

Cells in many regions of the normal heart are capable of spontaneous impulse initiation. These regions include the sinus node, atrial specialized fibers, coronary sinus, AV junction and valves, and the ventricular specialized conducting system. In the diseased heart, however, impulse initiation can occur almost anywhere, even in working atrial and ventricular muscle. The cell (or small group of cells) that become the pacemaker of the heart is the cell that first depolarizes to threshold and initiates an impulse, provided that the impulse conducts throughout the heart and excites other potential pacemakers before they can spontaneously depolarize to threshold. The site of impulse initiation is known as the *dominant pacemaker.* Other regions that are capable of pacemaking but that are being driven by the dominant pacemaker are called *subsidiary* or *latent pacemakers.*

The intrinsic rate at which a pacemaker cell initiates impulses is determined by the interplay of three factors: (1) the level of the maximum diastolic potential, (2) the level of the threshold potential, and (3) the steepness of phase 4 depolarization. A change in any one of these factors will alter the time taken for phase 4 depolarization to carry the membrane potential from the maximum diastolic level to the threshold level (Fig. 3-18) and, therefore, alter the rate of impulse initiation. For example, if maximum diastolic potential increases (becomes more negative), spontaneous depolarization to threshold potential will take longer and the rate of impulse initiation will fall (Fig. 3-18). Conversely, a decrease in maximum diastolic potential will increase the rate of impulse initiation. Similarly, changes in threshold potential level or changes in the slope of phase 4 depolarization will alter the rate of impulse initiation. In the normal heart, cells in the sinus node are the quickest to depolarize to threshold, and so the intrinsic rate of the sinus node is faster than that of other cells. Therefore, the sinus node is usually the dominant pacemaker.

If sinus node activity is suddenly stopped, impulse initiation by some subsidiary pacemaker does not occur immediately but usually follows a long period of quiescence. The initial rate of impulse initiation by the subsidiary pacemaker is then quite slow and only gradually speeds up to a steady rate, which is still lower than the original sinus rate.[91] The quiescent period that follows abolition of the sinus rhythm reflects the wearing off of an inhibitory influence exerted on subsidiary pacemakers by the dominant pacemaker. This type of inhibition ensures that the sinus node usually functions as the only pacemaker in the normal heart and is called *overdrive suppression.*

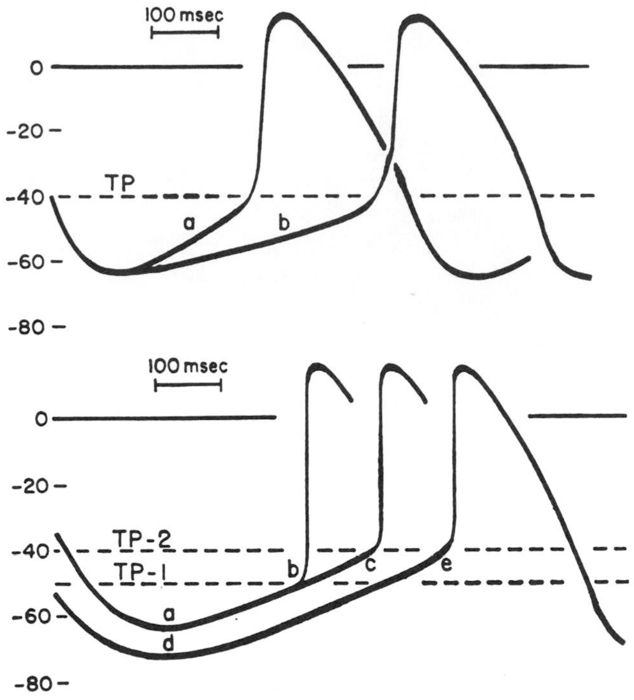

Figure 3-18. *Diagram illustrating the principal mechanisms underlying changes in the frequency of discharge of a pacemaker fiber. The upper diagram shows a reduction in rate caused by a decrease in the slope of diastolic, or pacemaker, depolarization, from a to b, and thus an increase in the time required for the membrane potential to decline to the threshold potential level (TP). The lower diagram shows the reduction in rate associated with a shift in the level of the threshold potential from TP-1 to TP-2 and a corresponding increase in cycle length (b to c); also illustrated is a further reduction in rate due to an increase in the maximum diastolic potential level (compare a to c with d to e). (Hoffman, B. F., and Cranefield, P. F.: Electrophysiology of the Heart. New York, McGraw-Hill, 1960; with permission.)*

Overdrive suppression results from driving a pacemaker cell faster than its intrinsic spontaneous rate and is mediated by enhanced activity of the Na-K exchange pump. Since sodium ions enter the cell during each action potential, the higher the rate of stimulation, the greater will be the amount of Na^+ entering the cell over a given time. The rate of activity of the sodium pump is largely determined by the level of intracellular sodium concentration, so that pump activity is enhanced during high rates of stimulation.[92] As already discussed, the Na–K exchange pump usually moves more Na^+ outward than K^+ inward, thereby effectively generating a net outward (hyperpolarizing) current of Na^+. When subsidiary pacemaker cells are driven faster than their intrinsic rate, this hyperpolarizing pump current further suppresses spontaneous impulse initiation in these cells. Following cessation of activity by the dominant pacemaker, this suppression of subsidiary pacemakers is responsible for the period of quiescence that lasts until the intracellular Na^+ concentration, and hence the pump current, becomes small enough to allow subsidiary pacemaking cells to depolarize to threshold and so initiate the next impulse. It seems likely that the dominant pacemaker subordinates other potential pacemakers by the mechanism of overdrive suppression, whether pacemaking in these other cells depends on normal automaticity or on triggered activity, since the amplitude of the afterdepolarizations from which triggered impulses arise is also expected to be reduced by enhanced pump current. However, an important distinction may be made between the effects of the dominant sinus pacemaker on abnormal automaticity (automaticity at low membrane potentials) and normal automaticity. Unlike normal automaticity, abnormal automaticity may not be overdrive suppressed.[93] Therefore, if sinus node activity is suddenly stopped, impulse initiation by subsidiary pacemakers with abnormal automaticity might occur immediately.

Mechanisms for a Shift in the Pacemaker

A shift in the site of impulse initiation (the pacemaker) to a region other than the sinus can result either from failure of the sinus impulse to activate the heart or from enhancement of impulse initiation in a subsidiary pacemaker. The rate of impulse initiation by the sinus node may be slowed, or impulse initiation may be inhibited altogether by either the autonomic nervous system[94] or by sinus node disease.[95] A decrease in sympathetic activity or an increase in vagal (parasympathetic) activity suppresses sinus node automaticity; sinus node disease may lead to degeneration of sinus node cells. Alternatively, impulse conduction from the sinus node to the atrium might be impaired in some way. Under any of these conditions there may be escape of a subsidiary pacemaker. Removal of overdrive suppression resulting from a decrease in, or abolition of, sinus rate enables spontaneous diastolic depolarization in a latent pacemaker to proceed to threshold and initiate impulses. Such escape rhythms normally arise in the AV junction (AV node or His bundle) because cells in this region have faster intrinsic rates than other ectopic sites. Sometimes, however, pathologic processes that suppress impulse initiation in the sinus node also suppress it in the AV junction,[95] and then the site of ectopic impulse initiation usually resides at some other site in the atria or ventricular conducting system. The mechanism for spontaneous diastolic depolarization underlying the ectopic rhythm may be the normal pacemaker current that occurs at high levels of membrane potential in normal Purkinje fibers, or it may be a pacemaker current occurring at lower levels of membrane potential in the AV valves or AV node.

Many factors can enhance subsidiary pacemaker activity and cause impulse initiation to shift to ectopic sites, even when sinus node function is normal. For example, norepinephrine released from sympathetic nerves increases the slope of spontaneous diastolic depolarization of most ectopic pacemaker cells, enabling the membrane potential to reach threshold level in these cells before they are activated by an impulse conducting from the sinus node.[96] The norepinephrine may be released locally at discrete ectopic sites, thereby causing a shift of the pacemaker.[97,98] This effect of the catecholamine may result from its known action on the normal pacemaker current in Purkinje fibers[99] or an action on pacemaker currents occurring at lower levels of membrane potential. Norepinephrine is also known to increase the amplitude of delayed afterdepolarizations in mitral valve and coronary sinus fibers,[40,41] and if the afterdepolarizations reach threshold then triggered activity might be initiated at a higher rate than the sinus rate. Cardiac disease can also lead to subsidiary pacemaker activity; thus, a reduction in membrane potential can result in automatic activity in atrial, ventricular, and Purkinje fibers, as already described. This type of spontaneous activity often occurs at higher rates than the sinus rate, and hence impulse initiation may shift to a diseased area of the heart. As mentioned above, the automaticity caused by a reduction in membrane potential is probably not suppressed by overdrive from the sinus node.

References

1. Cranefield, P. F., Wit, A. L., and Hoffman, B. F.: The genesis of cardiac arrhythmias. Circulation, 47:190, 1973.
2. Hoffman, B. F., and Cranefield, P. F.: Physiologic basis of cardiac arrhythmias. Am. J. Med., 37:670, 1964.
3. Hoffman, B. F., and Cranefield, P. F.: Electrophysiology of the Heart. New York, McGraw-Hill, 1960.
4. Hodgkin, A. L.: Ionic movements and electrical activity in giant nerve fibers. Proc R. Soc. Biol. (Lond.), 148:1, 1957.
5. Weidmann, S.: Elektrophysiologie der herzmuskelfaser. Bern, Medizinischer Verlag Hans Huber, 1956.
6. Draper, M. H., and Weidmann, S.: Cardiac resting and action potentials recorded with an intracellular electrode. J. Physiol., 115:74, 1951.
7. Miura, D. S., Hoffman, B. F., and Rosen, M. R.: The effect of extracellular potassium on the intracellular potassium ion activity and transmembrane potentials of beating canine cardiac Purkinje fibers. J. Gen. Physiol., 69:463, 1977.

8. Ellis, D.: The effects of external cations and ouabain on the intracellular sodium activity of sheep heart Purkinje fibers. J. Physiol (Lond.), 273, 211, 1977.
9. Thomas, R. C.: Electrogenic sodium pump in nerve and muscle cells. Physiol. Rev., 52:563, 1972.
10. Adrian, R. H.: Potassium chloride movement and the membrane potential of frog muscle. J. Physiol., 151:154, 1960.
11. Gadsby, D. C., and Cranefield, P. F.: Two levels of resting potential in cardiac Purkinje fibers. J. Gen Physiol., 70:725, 1977.
12. Goldman, D. E.: Potential, impedance and rectification in membranes. J. Gen. Physiol., 27:27, 1943.
13. Hodgkin, A. L., and Katz, B.: The effect of sodium ions on the electrical activity of the giant axon of the squid. J. Physiol., 108:37, 1949.
14. Hodgkin, A. L., and Huxley, A. F.: A quantitative description of membrane currents and its application to conduction and excitation in nerve. J. Physiol., 117:500, 1952.
15. Dudel, J.: Excitation process in heart cells. In De Mello, W. C. (ed.): Electrical phenomena in the heart. New York, Academic Press, 1972.
16. Wit, A. L., Rosen, M. R., and Hoffman, B. F.: Electrophysiology and pharmacology of cardiac arrhythmias. II. Relation of normal and abnormal electrical activity of cardiac fibers to the genesis of arrhythmias. Am. Heart J., 88:515, 1974.
17. Weidmann, S.: The effect of the cardiac membrane potential on the rapid availability of the sodium carrying system. J. Physiol (Lond.), 127:213, 1955a.
18. Van Dam, R. T., Moore, E. N., and Hoffman, B. F.: Initiation and conduction of impulses in partially depolarized cardiac fibers. Am J. Physiol., 204:1133, 1963.
19. Reuter, H.: The dependence of slow inward current in Purkinje fibers on the extracellular calcium concentration. J. Physiol. (Lond.), 192:479, 1967.
20. Cranefield, P. F.: The Conduction of the Cardiac Impulse. Mt. Kisco, NY, Futura, 1975.
21. Reuter, H.: Divalent cations as charge carriers in excitable membranes. In Butler, J. A. V., and Noble, D. (eds.): Progress in Biophysics and Molecular Biology 26, p. 3. New York, Pergamon Press, 1973.
22. Kass, R. S., and Tsien, R. W.: Control of action potential duration by calcium ions in Purkinje fibers. J. Gen. Physiol., 67:599, 1976.
23. Niedergerke, R., and Orkand, R. K.: The dual effect of calcium on the action potential of the frog's heart. J. Physiol. (Lond.), 184:291, 1966.
24. Niedergerke, R., and Orkand, R. K.: The dependence of the action potential of the frog's heart on the external and intracellular sodium concentration. J. Physiol. (Lond.), 184:312, 1966.
25. Kao, C. Y.: Tetrodotoxin, saxitoxin and their significance in the study of excitation phenomena. Pharmacol Rev., 18:998, 1966.
26. Vassort, G., Rougier, O., Garnier, D., et al.: Effects of adrenaline on membrane inward currents during the cardiac action potential. Pfluegers Arch. 309:70, 1969.
27. Hagiwara, S., and Nakajima, S.: Differences in Na and Ca spikes as examined by application of tetrodotoxin, procaine and manganese ions. J. Gen. Physiol., 49:793, 1966.
28. Kolhardt, M., Bauer, B., Krause, H., and Fleckenstein, A.: Differentiation of the transmembrane Na and Ca channels in mammalian cardiac fibers by the use of specific inhibitors. Pfluegers Arch. 335:309, 1972.
29. Kenyon, J. L., and Gibbons, W. R.: Effects of low-chloride solutions on action potentials of sheep cardiac Purkinje fibers. J. Gen. Physiol., 70:635, 1977.
30. Trautwein, W.: Membrane currents in cardiac muscle fibers. Physiol. Rev., 53:793, 1973.
31. Noble, D., and Tsien, R. W.: Outward membrane currents activated in the plateau range of potentials in cardiac Purkinje fibers. J. Physiol. (Lond.), 200:205, 1969a.
32. Isenberg, G., and Trautwein, W.: The effect of dihydro-ouabain and lithium-ions on the outward current in cardiac Purkinje fibers; evidence for electrogenicity of active transport. Pfluegers Arch., 35:41, 1974.
33. Isenberg, G., and Trautwein, W.: Outward current and electrogenic sodium pump in Purkinje fibers. In Fleckenstein, A., and Dhalla, N. S. (eds.): Recent Advances in Studies on Cardiac Structure and Metabolism, vol. 5, pp. 43–49. Baltimore, University Park Press, 1975.
34. Vassalle, M.: Analysis of cardiac pacemaker potential using a "voltage clamp" technique. Am. J. Physiol. 210:1335, 1966.
35. Vassalle, M.: Cardiac pacemaker potentials at different extracellular and intracellular K concentrations. Am. J. Physiol. 208:770, 1965.
36. Noble, D., and Tsien, R. W.: The kinetics and rectifier properties of the slow potassium current in cardiac Purkinje fibers. J. Physiol. (Lond), 195:185, 1968.
37. DiFrancesco, D.: A new interpretation of the pace-maker current in Purkinje fibers. J. Physiol. (Lond), 314:359–376, 1981.
38. DiFrancesco, D., and Ojeda, C.: Properties of the current i_f in the sino–atrial node of the rabbit compared with those of the current i_{K_2} in Purkinje fibres. J. Physiol. (Lond), 308:353–367, 1980.
39. Cranefield, P. F.: Action potentials, afterpotentials and arrhythmias. Circ. Res. 41:415, 1977.
40. Wit, A. L., and Cranefield, P. F.: Triggered activity in cardiac muscle fibers of the simian mitral valve. Circ. Res. 38:85, 1976.
41. Wit, A. L., and Cranefield, P. F.: Triggered and automatic activity in the canine coronary sinus. Circ. Res. 41:435, 1977.
42. Saito, T., Otoguro, M., and Matsubara, T.: Electrophysiological studies on the mechanism of electrically induced sustained rhythmic activity in the rabbit right atrium. Circ. Res. 42:199, 1978.
43. Weingart, R., Kass, R. S., and Tsien, R. W.: Role of calcium and sodium ions in the transient inward current induced by strophanthidin in cardiac Purkinje fibers. Biophys J., 17:3A, 1977.
44. Grant, A. O., and Strauss, H. C.: Intracellular potassium activity in rabbit sinoatrial node. Evaluation during spontaneous activity and arrest. Circ. Res. 51:271, 1982.
45. Paes de Carvalho, A., Hoffman, B. F., and de Paula Carvalho, M.: Two components of the cardiac action potential. I. Voltage time course and the effect of acetylcholine on atrial and nodal cells of the rabbit heart. J. Gen. Physiol. 54:607, 1969.
46. Zipes, D. P., and Mendez, C.: Action of manganese ions and tetrodotoxin on atrioventricular nodal transmembrane potentials in isolated rabbit hearts. Circ. Res. 32:447, 1973.
47. Wit, A. L., and Cranefield, P. F.: Effect of verapamil on the sinoatrial and atrioventricular nodes of the rabbit and the mechanism by which it arrests reentrant atrioventricular nodal tachycardia. Circ. Res. 35:413, 1974.
48. Merideth, J., Mendez, C., Mueller, W. J., and Moe, G. K.: Electrical excitability of atrioventricular nodal cells. Circ. Res. 23:69, 1968.
49. Mendez, C., and Moe, G. K.: Some characteristics of transmembrane potentials of AV nodal cells during propagation of premature beats. Circ. Res. 19:993, 1966.
50. Kokubun, S., Nishimura, M., Noma, A., and Irisawa, A.: The spontaneous action potential of rabbit atrioventricular nodal cells. Jpn. J. Physiol. 30:529, 1980.
51. Hordof, A. J., Edie, R., Malm, J. R., et al.: Electrophysiologic properties and response to pharmacologic agents of fibers from diseased human atria. Circulation, 54:774, 1976.
52. Boyden, P. A., Tilley, L. P., Albala, A., et al.: Mechanisms for atrial arrhythmias associated with cardiomyopathy: A study of feline

hearts with primary myocardial disease. Circulation, 69:1036, 1984.
53. Friedman, P. L., Stewart, J. R., Fenoglio, J. J., Jr., and Wit, A. L.: Survival of subendocardial Purkinje fibers after extensive myocardial infarction in dogs: In vitro and in vivo correlations. Circ. Res. 33:597, 1973.
54. Lazzara, R., El-Sherif, N., and Scherlag, B. J.: Early and late effects of coronary artery occlusion on canine Purkinje fibers. Circ. Res. 35: 391, 1974.
55. Downar, E., Janse, M. J., and Durrer, D.: The effect of acute coronary artery occlusion on subepicardial transmembrane potentials in the intact Porcine heart. Circulation, 56:217, 1977.
56. Lazzara, R., El-Sherif, N., Befeler, B., and Scherlag, B. J.: Lidocaine action on depressed cardiac cells. Circulation 52:II-85, 1975.
57. Isenberg, G.: Cardiac Purkinje fibers: Cesium as a tool to block inward rectifying potassium currents. Pfluegers Arch., 365:99, 1976.
58. Lazzara, R., El-Sherif, N., and Scherlag, B. J.: Disorders of cellular electrophysiology produced by ischemia of the canine His bundle. Circ. Res., 36:444, 1975.
59. Carmeliet, E., and Vereecke, J.: Adrenaline and the plateau phase of the cardiac action potential. Importance of Ca^{++}, Na^{+}, and K^{+} conductance. Pfluegers Arch., 313:300, 1969.
60. Gettes, L. S., and Reuter, H.: Slow recovery from inactivation of inward currents in mammalian myocardial fibers. J. Physiol. (Lond.), 240:703, 1974.
61. MacLeod, D. P., and Prasad, K.: Influence of glucose on the transmembrane action potential of papillary muscle. J. Gen. Physsiol., 53:792, 1969.
62. Han, J.: Ventricular ectopic activity in myocardial infarction. In Han, J. (ed.): Cardiac Arrhythmias, p. 171. *A symposium edited by J. Han,* Springfield, Ill., Charles C Thomas, 1972.
63. Lazzara, R., El-Sherif, N., and Scherlag, B. J.: Electrophysiological properties of canine Purkinje cells in one-day-old myocardial infarction. Circ. Res., 33:722, 1973.
64. Alessi, R., Nusynowitz, M., Abildskov, J. A., and Moe, G. K.: Nonuniform distribution of vagal effects on the atrial refractory period. Am. J. Physiol., 194:406–410, 1968.
65. Katzung, B.: Effects of extracellular calcium and sodium on depolarization-induced automaticity in guinea pig papillary muscle. Circ. Res., 37:118, 1975.
66. Brown, H. F., and Noble, S. J.: Membrane currents underlying delayed rectification and pacemaker activity in frog atrial muscle. J. Physiol. (Lond.), 204:717, 1969.
67. Imanishi, S., and Surawicz, B.: Automatic activity in depolarized guinea pig ventricular myocardium: Characteristics and mechanisms. Circ. Res., 39:751, 1976.
68. Imanishi, S.: Calcium-sensitive discharges in canine Purkinje fibers. Jpn. J. Physiol., 21:443, 1971.
69. Mary-Rabine, L., Hordof, A. J., Daniels, P., Jr., et al.: Mechanisms for impulse initiation in isolated human atrial fibers. Circ. Res., 47:267, 1980.
70. El-Sherif, N., Gough, W. B., Zeiler, R. H., and Mehra R.: Triggered ventricular rhythms in 1-day-old myocardial infarction in the dog. Circ. Res., 52:566, 1983.
71. Mines, G.R.: On circulating excitations in heart muscle and their possible relations to tachycardia and fibrillation. Trans. R. Soc. Can. (Ser 3 Sec. 4), 8:43, 1914.
72. Cranefield, P. F., and Hoffman, B. F.: Reentry: Slow conduction, summation and inhibition. Circulation, 44:309, 1971.
73. Mayer, A. G.: Rhythmical pulsation in scyphomedusae II. Papers from the Tortugar Laboratory of the Carnegie Institute of Washington 1:113. Carnegie Institution of Washington Publication No. 102, part VII, 1908.
74. Schmitt, F. O., and Erlanger, J.: Directional differences in the conduction of the impulse through heart muscle and their possible relation to extrasystolic and fibrillary contractions. Am. J. Physiol., 87:326, 1928–1929.
75. Wit, A. L., Cranefield, P. F., and Hoffman, B. F.: Slow conduction and reentry in the ventricular conducting system. II. Single and sustained circus movement in networks of canine and bovine Purkinje fibers. Circ. Res., 30:11, 1972.
76. Wit, A. L., Hoffman, B. F., and Cranefield, P. F.: Slow conduction and reentry in the ventricular conducting system. I. Return extrasystole in canine Purkinje fibers. Circ. Res., 30:1, 1972.
77. Antzelevitch, C., Jalife, J., and Moe, G. K.: Characteristics of reflection as a mechanism of reentrant arrhythmias and its relationship to parasystole. Circulation, 61:182, 1980.
78. Mendez, C., and Moe, G. K.: Demonstration of a dual A-V nodal conduction system in the isolated rabbit heart. Circ. Res., 29:378, 1966.
79. Wit, A. L., Goldreyer, B. N., and Damato, A. N.: An in vitro model of paroxysmal supraventricular tachycardia. Circulation, 43:862, 1971.
80. Janse, M. J., van Capelle, F. J. L., Freud, G. E., and Durrer, D.: Circus movement within the AV node. Circ. Res., 28:403, 1971.
81. Coumel, P.: Mechanism of supraventricular tachycardia. In Narula, O. S. (ed.): His bundle Electrocardiography and Clinical Electrophysiology. Philadelphia, F. A. Davis, 1975.
82. Moe, G. K.: On the multiple wavelet hypothesis of atrial fibrillation. Arch. Int. Pharmacodyn., 140:183, 1962.
83. Allessie, M. A., Bonke, F. I. M., and Schopman, F. J. G.: Circus movement in rabbit atrial muscle as a mechanism of tachycardia. III. The "leading circle" concept: A new model of circus movement in cardiac tissue without the involvement of an anatomical obstacle. Circ. Res., 41:9, 1977.
84. Moe, G. K.: Evidence for reentry as a mechanism for cardiac arrhythmias. Rev. Physiol. Biochem. Pharmacol., 72:56, 1975.
85. Sasyniuk, B. I., and Mendez, C.: A mechanism for reentry in canine ventricular tissue. Circ. Res., 28:3, 1973.
86. Myerburg, R. J., Stewart, J. W., and Hoffman, B. F.: Electrophysiological properties of the canine peripheral AV conducting system. Circ. Res., 26:361, 1970.
87. Friedman, P. L., Stewart, J. R., and Wit, A. L.: Spontaneous and induced cardiac arrhythmias in subendocardial Purkinje fibers surviving extensive myocardial infarction in dogs. Circ. Res., 22:612, 1973.
88. Clerc L.: Directional differences of impulse spread in trabecular muscle from mammalian heart. J. Physiol. (Lond.), 255:355, 1976.
89. Spach, M., Miller, W. T., Geselowitz, D. B., et al.: The discontinuous nature of propagation in normal canine cardiac muscle: Evidence for recurrent discontinuities of intracellular resistance that effect the membrane currents. Circ. Res., 48:39, 1981.
90. Spach, M., Miller, W. T., Dolber, P. C., et al.: The functional role of structural complexities in the propagation of depolarization in the atrium of the dog: Cardiac conduction disturbances due to discontinuities of effective axial resistivity. Circ. Res., 50:175, 1982.
91. Vassalle, M.: The relationship among cardiac pacemakers: Overdrive suppression. Circ. Res., 41:269, 1977.
92. Vassalle, M.: Electrogenic suppression of automaticity in sheep and dog Purkinje fibers. Circ. Res., 27:361, 1970.
93. Dangman, K. H., and Hoffman, B. F.: Studies on overdrive stimulation of canine cardiac Purkinje fibers: Maximum diastolic potential as a determinant of the response. J. Am. Coll. Cardiol. 2:1183, 1983.
94. Trautwein, W., Kuffler, S. W., and Edwards, C.: Changes in membrane characteristics of heart muscle during inhibition. J. Gen. Physiol., 40:135, 1956.

95. Ferrer, M. I.: The Sick Sinus Syndrome. Mt. Kisco, N.Y., Futura, 1974.
96. Wit, A. L., Hoffman, B. F., and Rosen, M. R.: Electrophysiology and pharmacology of cardiac arrhythmias. IX. Cardiac electrophysiologic effects of beta adrenergic receptor stimulation and blockade. Am. Heart J., 90:521, 1975.
97. Armour, J. A., Hageman, G. R., and Randall, W. C.: Arrhythmias induced by local cardiac nerve stimulation. Am. J. Physiol., 223:1068, 1972.
98. Geesbreght, J. M., and Randall, W. C.: Area localization of shifting cardiac pacemakers during sympathetic stimulation. Am. J. Physiol., 220:1522, 1971.
99. Tsien, R. W.: Effect of epinephrine on the pacemaker potassium current of cardiac Purkinje fibers. J. Gen. Physiol., 64:293, 1974.

4

The Interrelationship of Electrolyte Abnormalities and Arrhythmias

Borys Surawicz

The electrical activity in the excitable tissues is accompanied by changes in membrane permeability and transmembrane fluxes of ions. Some background knowledge of these phenomena is required to study the material presented in this chapter, and for this the reader is referred to excellent textbooks, review articles,[1,2] and Chapter 3 in this book. The following discussion of the electrophysiologic theory is limited to the phenomena that are directly related to the clinical observations described in this chapter. Therefore, the experimental background is confined almost exclusively to the ranges of electrolyte concentrations encountered in clinical practice. In the following discussion, the largest portion of the text is allotted to potassium, because the role of this ion in arrhythmias appears to be more important and better known than the role played by other ions.

Hyperkalemia

Electrophysiologic Mechanism

1. Resting membrane potential (RMP), or maximal diastolic potential (MDP),* decreases (*i.e.,* becomes less negative) with increasing extracellular potassium concentration. Within the range of plasma potassium concentrations encountered *in vivo,* intracellular potassium concentration stays within narrow limits and therefore is not expected to play a major role in the determination of RMP or MDP values. This allows us to consider the changes in extracellular plasma potassium concentration as the principal factor in the determination of RMP or MDP.[3] Depolarization due to increased extracellular potassium concentration brings the membrane potential to an approximate value expected from the Nernst equation for a membrane freely permeable to K^+. This means that at plasma potassium concentrations higher than normal the membrane acts like a potassium electrode. The value of RMP in the ventricular myocardium is about −84 mV at $K_o = 5.4$, about −67 mV at $K_o = 10.0$ mM/liter, and about −60 mV at $K_o = 16.2$ mM/liter. At less negative levels of RMP, the fibers are usually

This study was supported in part by the Herman C. Krannert Fund; by Grants HL-06308 and HL-07182 from the National Heart, Lung, and Blood Institute of the National Institutes of Health; by the American Heart Association, Indiana Affiliate; and by the Veterans Administration.

* Refers to myocardial fibers of the atria or the ventricles and to the Purkinje fibers.

no longer excitable, at least in response to stimuli of ordinary strength.

2. Repolarization becomes more rapid because increased K_o increases membrane permeability to potassium and shortens the duration of the action potential. In the ventricular myocardial fibers, this shortening is due predominantly to a more rapid slope of phase 3.
3. Diastolic depolarization in Purkinje fibers is attributed to increasing membrane permeability to Na^+ and, perhaps, to decreasing membrane permeability to K^+. Hyperkalemia, which increases membrane permeability to potassium, decreases the slope of phase 4 (diastolic depolarization) and thereby decreases or suppresses automaticity.
4. Threshold potential decreases (becomes less negative) with increasing depolarization (less negative RMP or MDP). However, hyperkalemia usually causes a greater shift of the RMP in the depolarizing direction than the shift of the threshold potential. This may cause a decrease in the "distance" (difference) between the RMP and the threshold potential. Therefore, an increase in K_o does not always decrease conduction velocity or the rate of the pacemaker fibers. On the contrary, as will be described later, moderate increase in K_o may improve conduction without changing the rate of pacemakers.
5. Biphasic effect of increased K_o on conduction and excitability results from the dependence of conduction and excitability on both the absolute level of RMP and the difference between RMP and threshold potential. When K_o increases gradually, the conduction at first becomes more rapid and the excitability threshold decreases because of the decreased difference between RMP and threshold potential. Afterward, the conduction becomes slower and the threshold of excitability increases due to the absolute decrease in the level of RMP.[4] Increase in K_o may have the same biphasic effect on the rate of firing of the Purkinje fibers, first an increase and then a decrease and arrest.
6. Differences in sensitivity to potassium among different types of cardiac fibers are quite prominent.[5] Thus, the depression of excitability and conduction in atrial myocardial fibers takes place at lower K_o than in other types of myocardial fibers. In isolated preparations the sinus node and the His bundle are more "resistant" to the increased K_o than the ventricular myocardium, which in turn is more "resistant" to high potassium concentration than is the atrial myocardium.
7. "Injury currents" may result from differences in potassium concentration in different parts of the myocardium.
8. Increased potassium concentration tends to decrease the dispersion of refractoriness because it shortens action potential duration at all heart rates and decreases the rate-dependent differences in action potential duration in both ventricular muscle and Purkinje fibers. It also decreases the difference between the duration of action potentials in Purkinje and ventricular fibers at all heart rates.[6] The decrease in dispersion of refractoriness in the myocardium caused by these factors predominantly affects the nonpremature complexes. However, a very marked shortening of the action potential in the early premature complexes can contribute to an increase in dispersion.
9. Moderate hyperkalemia abolishes supernormal conduction and excitability. This effect has been observed both *in vitro* and *in vivo* in the Purkinje fibers and bundle branches.[7] A similar phenomenon in the ventricular myocardium can suppress the dip in the excitability curve.[8]
10. The negative inotropic effect of hyperkalemia, which may play an indirect role in the genesis of arrhythmias, appears to be more pronounced in the failing heart than in the normal heart.[9] In animal experiments the depression of contractility by potassium is associated with myocardial K^+ uptake and is related to the rate of K_o rise rather than to the absolute K_o value.[10]

Electrocardiographic Manifestations

When the plasma potassium concentration exceeds approximately 5.5 mEq/liter, the T waves become tall and peaked, and when the plasma potassium concentration exceeds 6.5 mEq/liter, QRS changes are usually present. The diagnosis of hyperkalemia cannot be made with certainty on the basis of T wave changes alone. In one study, the characteristic tall, steep, narrow, and pointed T waves were present in only 22% of patients with hyperkalemia, while in the remainder the tall T wave could not be distinguished from similar T waves of other etiology. The differential diagnosis may be helped by the measurement of the QTc interval. When the tall, peaked T wave is the only electrocardiographic abnormality produced by hyperkalemia, and the duration of the QRS complex and the ST segment is normal, the QTc interval is normal or shortened, whereas in other conditions associated with tall T waves, the QTc interval is nearly always prolonged.[11] The U waves in patients with hyperkalemia are usually low or absent.[11]

A correct electrocardiographic diagnosis of hyperkalemia can usually be made when plasma potassium concentrations exceed 6.7 mEq/liter. The uniformly wide QRS complex due to hyperkalemia differs from the electrocardiographic pattern of bundle branch block or preexcitation because widening affects both the initial and the terminal portions of the QRS complex. The wide S wave in the left precordial leads helps to differentiate a pattern of hyperkalemia from a typical left bundle branch block and the wide initial portion from a right bundle branch block. However, the wide QRS complex in patients with hyperkalemia may resemble the typical pattern of left bundle branch block. Not infrequently the QRS axis shifts superiorly and sometimes inferiorly. This suggests a nonuniform delay of conduction in the major divisions of left bundle branch. As may be expected, slow intraventricular conduction is associated with prolongation of the HV interval, and this prolongation parallels the increase in QRS duration.[12] QRS duration increases progressively with an increasing plasma potassium concentration, and there is a rough correlation between the duration of the QRS complex and plasma potassium concentration.

The pattern of advanced hyperkalemia is nearly identical to that recorded in dying hearts. Sometimes in patients with advanced hyperkalemia the ST segment deviates appreciably from the baseline and simulates the "acute injury" pattern, which resembles the pattern of acute myocardial ischemia. Such ST deviation disappears rapidly when the pattern of hyperkalemia regresses during treatment with hemodialysis.[13] The "injury current" responsible for the ST segment deviation is probably caused by nonhomogeneous depolarization in different portions of the myocardium. Deviation of the ST segment or a monophasic pattern can be readily produced by topical application of potassium on the ventricular surface or an intracoronary KC1 injection.[10]

When the plasma potassium concentration exceeds 7 mEq/liter, the P wave amplitude usually decreases and the duration of the P wave increases because of the slower conduction in the atria. The PR interval is frequently prolonged, but most of the prolongation tends to be due to an increase in P wave duration. When the plasma potassium concentration exceeds 8.8 mEq/liter, the P wave frequently becomes invisible. In the presence of a wide QRS complex, a low or absent P wave helps to differentiate the pattern of hyperkalemia from intraventricular conduction disturbance of other origin. A regular rhythm in the absence of P waves has been attributed to sinoventricular conduction in the presence of sinoatrial block.[14] This concept is supported by recent experiments in dogs,[15] which showed that even when the P wave disappeared during hyperkalemia, the electrical activity was recorded from the sinoatrial node and crista terminalis, and each QRS complex was preceded by a His bundle electrogram (Fig. 4-1). A regular rhythm in the absence of P waves can be caused by a displacement of the pacemaker into the AV junction or the Purkinje fibers, but precise localization of the pacemaker in patients with absent P waves is usually not possible. When the plasma potassium concentration exceeds about 10 mEq/liter, the ventricular rhythm may become irregular due to the simultaneous activity of several escape pacemakers in the depressed myocardium. The combination

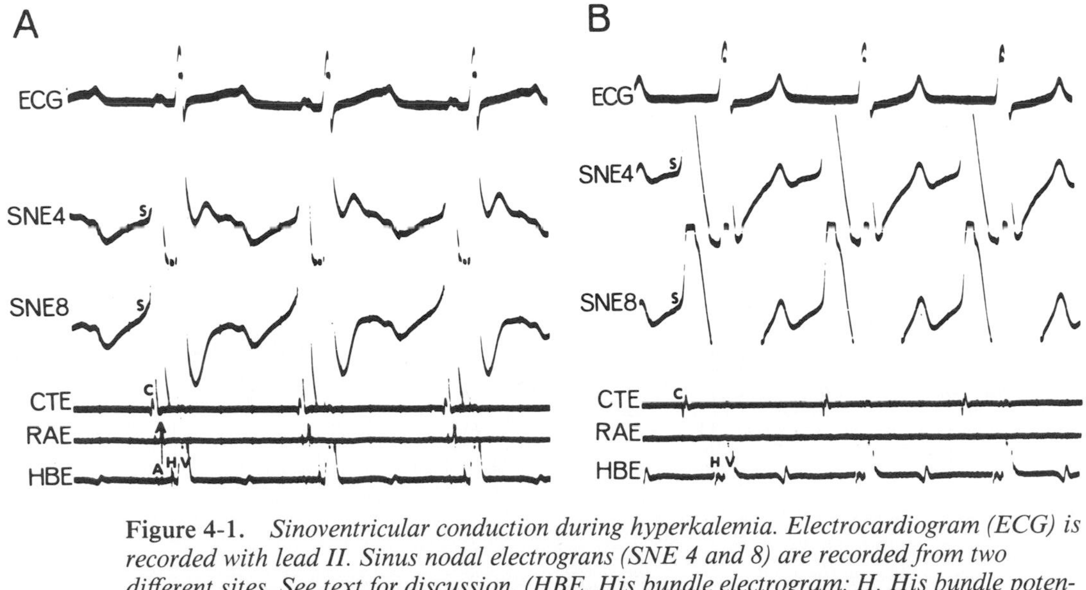

Figure 4-1. *Sinoventricular conduction during hyperkalemia. Electrocardiogram (ECG) is recorded with lead II. Sinus nodal electrograns (SNE 4 and 8) are recorded from two different sites. See text for discussion. (HBE, His bundle electrogram; H, His bundle potential; CTE, crista terminalis potential; RAE, right atrial appendage) (Hariman, R. J., and Chen, C. M.: Effects of hyperkalemia on sinus nodal function in dog: Sino-ventricular conduction. Cardiovasc. Res., 17:509, 1983)*

of an irregular rhythm and an absent P wave may simulate atrial fibrillation.

An increase in the plasma potassium concentration above 12 to 14 mEq/liter causes ventricular asystole or ventricular fibrillation. The latter may be preceded by an acceleration of the ventricular rate.[16] Ventricular fibrillation probably results from reentry, which is facilitated by the slow intraventricular conduction and the short duration of the ventricular action potential. Experiments in dogs have shown that advanced intraventricular conduction disturbances may be associated with a change or even a reversal of the activation sequence (*i.e.*, the epicardial excitation occurring before the endocardial excitation).[12]

The electrocardiographic pattern of hyperkalemia can be made more normal by increasing the concentration of plasma calcium and sodium[17] and more abnormal by decreasing the concentration of plasma calcium and, possibly, sodium.

The understanding of the above-described electrocardiographic changes produced by hyperkalemia may be facilitated by correlating these changes with the concomittant changes in the atrial and ventricular action potential, as shown in the diagram in Figure 4-2, which is based on experimental work in isolated perfused rabbit hearts. Except for the difference in the QRS and the QT durations, the normal electrocardiogram and various electrolyte imbalance patterns in the rabbit are almost identical with those in humans.[18] Figure 4-2 shows that the duration of action potential in the atrial fibers is shorter than in the ventricular fibers. We assume that the sum of all depolarizations and repolarizations of the atrial fibers is responsible for the origin of the P wave and the Ta wave and that of the ventricular fibers is responsible for the origin of the QRS complex, ST segment, and T wave. The duration of phase 0 is only approximately a few milliseconds, but the time required to depolarize all fibers is represented by the duration of the QRS complex. The duration of phase 2 corresponds approximately to the duration of the ST segment, and the duration of phase 3 corresponds to the duration of the T wave. The end of the T wave corresponds approximately to the termination of ventricular action potentials on the ventricular surface. The slope of phase 3 is usually similar to the slope of the terminal portion of the T wave. The end of the T wave coincides approximately with the end of the ventricular ejection, and the U wave is usually inscribed during relaxation. Figure 4-2B shows the effect on repolarization, which is responsible for the narrow and peaked T wave when the potassium concentration is increased to 6 mEq/liter. At this concentration, the effects of slight lowering of RMP are still not evident. Figure 4-2C to E demonstrates that a progressive increase in potassium concentration produces a progres-

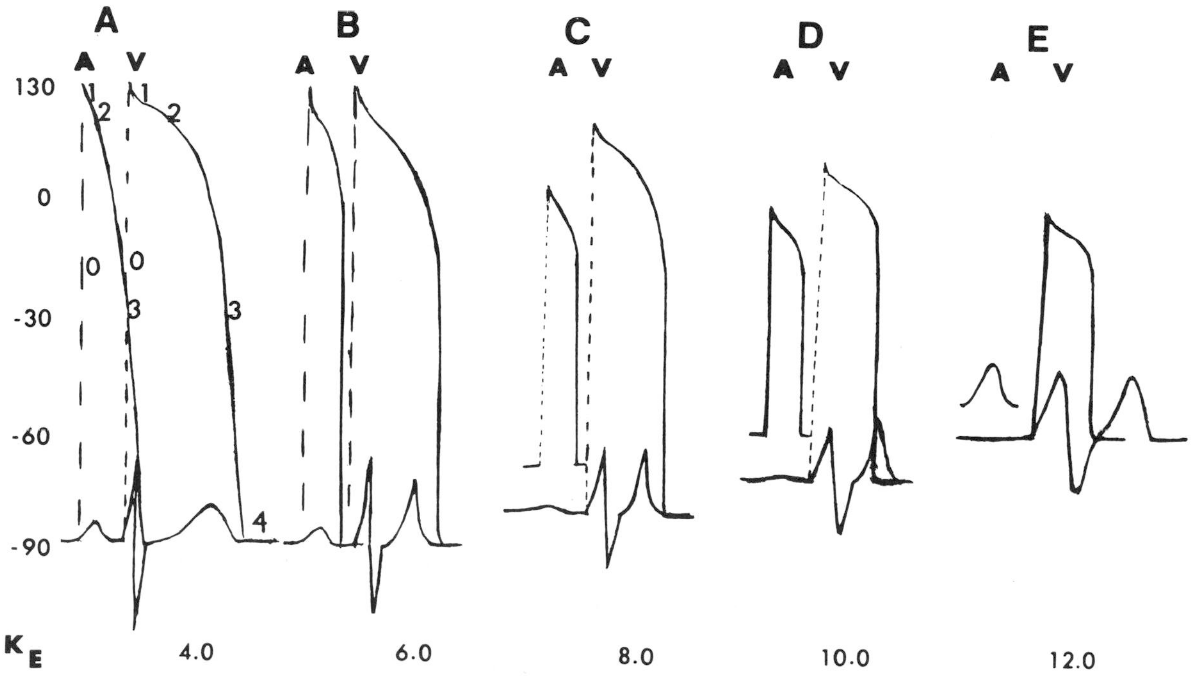

Figure 4-2. *Diagram of an atrial (A) and ventricular (V) action potential superimposed on the electrocardiogram. The numbers on the left designate the transmembrane potential in millivolts, and the numbers at the bottom, $[K]_o$ in mEq/liter. (Surawicz, B.: Relation between electrocardiogram and electrolytes. Am. Heart J., 73:814, 1967)*

sive decrease in RMP, which decreases the upstroke velocity of the action potential. This in turn slows the intra-atrial and intraventricular conduction and thereby increases the duration of the P wave and the QRS complex, respectively.[19] At the potassium concentration of 12 mEq/liter, ventricular depolarization is very slow, portions of the ventricular myocardium undergo repolarization before depolarization is completed, and the determination of the end of the QRS complex may be difficult to impossible (Figure 4-2E). Figure 2C and D shows that the depolarization of the atrial fibers is more pronounced than that of the ventricular fiber. In Figure 4-2C, the P wave is wide and of low amplitude; in Figure 4-2D, the P wave is barely discernible. In Figure 4-2E, the P wave is absent because the low amplitude impulse does not reach the threshold and does not produce a propagated response.[20] The disappearance of the P wave at the time when the ventricular complex is still well defined indicates that excitability of the atrial fibers is abolished at a lower potassium concentration than is the excitability of the ventricular fibers.

Antiarrhythmic Effects of Potassium

Patients with moderate hyperkalemia (*i.e.*, potassium concentrations from 5.5 to 7.5 mEq/liter) rarely have ectopic beats. Disturbances of AV conduction are also uncommon at this stage of hyperkalemia. The antiarrhythmic effects of increased potassium concentration may be due to one of the following mechanisms: (1) depression of automaticity of ectopic pacemakers caused by slowed diastolic depolarization; (2) termination of reentry due to improved conduction (*i.e.*, dissipation of unidirectional block); (3) termination of reentry due to impaired conduction (*i.e.*, change from a unidirectional to a bidirectional block); (4) decreased dispersion of refractoriness within the myocardium and between Purkinje fibers and ventricular myocardium; and (5) abolition of supernormal conduction and excitability. Of all the above effects, the first is probably of greatest clinical interest, at least after a slight to moderate increase in plasma potassium concentration.

The effect of potassium administration on cardiac rhythm and conduction depends on the integrity of the myocardium, the initial plasma potassium concentration, the amount of administered potassium, and the change or the rate of change of plasma potassium concentration. In our study, intravenous administration of potassium suppressed supraventricular and ventricular ectopic beats, with the exception of atrial fibrillation and flutter, in about 80% of patients[21]; the incidence of suppression was not influenced by the presence or absence of heart disease and treatment with digitalis.[21] The margin between the therapeutic and the toxic dose of potassium was rather narrow,[21] and the antiarrhythmic effect usually occurred when the plasma potassium concentration increased by 0.5 to 1 mEq/liter to a level of 5 to 6.5 mEq/liter. Such an increase of plasma potassium concentration usually had no effect on sinus rate.

The therapeutic effect of potassium administration is usually transient, and therapy must be monitored by a physician thoroughly familiar with the effect of potassium on the electrocardiogram. Observations of the T wave and the P wave are very helpful because peaking of the T wave or a marked decrease of P wave amplitude will usually precede the appearance of serious effects of increased potassium concentration on the QRS duration and atrioventricular conduction. However, in certain patients with impaired atrioventricular conduction, administration of potassium at a safe rate produces a high degree of atrioventricular block before the T wave configuration is appreciably altered.[21] This is more likely to occur in patients treated with digitalis because of the synergistic action of potassium and digitalis on the AV conduction.[22]

It should also be remembered that administration of potassium salts with glucose at a slow rate may precipitate serious arrhythmias in patients with hypokalemia, severe potassium depletion, or digitalis toxicity.[23] In these patients, potassium is apparently avidly taken up by the cells, and when it is administered slowly, plasma potassium concentration decreases, which may precipitate ectopic complexes and ventricular tachycardia or fibrillation.[23]

The therapeutic antiarrhythmic dose of potassium is not readily predictable. Frequently, only a few milliequivalents of potassium are required to suppress ectopic complexes. Should an undesirable arrhythmia reappear, potassium is again administered until the arrhythmia is suppressed. Some of the failures of treatment of arrhythmia with potassium are due to the continuation of potassium administration after the suppression of arrhythmia. In treating arrhythmia, potassium should be administered intermittently, particularly in patients with digitalis-induced ectopic tachycardias, when potassium excretion may be impaired by low cardiac output or hypotension. In these patients, small amounts of potassium may suppress the arrhythmia, but the suppression probably depends more on the transient rate of increase in potassium concentration than on the absolute plasma potassium concentration. Therefore, as long as excessive amounts of digitalis remain in the body, arrhythmia can recur even when the plasma potassium concentration is higher than normal. When potassium administration is continued during an arrhythmia-free interval, hyperkalemia may be produced, precluding further use of potassium if the arrhythmia recurs.

The effect of potassium on arrhythmias is nonspecific. Potassium is equally effective in abolishing ectopic complexes in patients with low and normal plasma potassium concentrations and in patients receiving and not receiving digitalis. However, potassium is most frequently used for the treatment of patients with ectopic complexes and AV conduction disturbances precipitated by hypokalemia and those with ectopic supraventricular tachycardias with 1 : 1 or 2 : 1 conduction and ventricular tachycardia induced by digitalis. The latter are frequently precipitated by hypokalemia and possibly also by potassium depletion without hypokalemia. In these patients, correction of hypokalemia and potassium deficiency restores more normal digitalis tolerance and prevents the recurrence of life-threatening arrhythmias. When the ectopic rhythms and complexes are not due to hypokalemia or digitalis toxicity, the duration of the nonspecific antiarrhythmic potassium effect may be short and the arrhythmias may recur as soon as the treatment is discontinued and potassium concentration returns to control value. Even in patients without hypokalemia or digitalis toxicity, the use of potassium may sometimes be desirable because it causes no hypotensive effect. Potassium is very effective in the treatment of patients with ectopic complexes and rapid ectopic rhythms after open-heart operations. Even when these patients have no hypokalemia before operation, their total body potassium is frequently low. After the operation, hypokalemia may appear because of hemodilution, use of glucose, and large potassium losses in the urine. Since many candidates for open-heart operations receive digitalis, the incidence of postoperative arrhythmias is high. These arrhythmias can often be effectively suppressed by single or repeated administrations of 2 to 5 mEq of potassium intravenously. The antiarrhythmic effect of potassium usually occurs in the absence of significant change in sinus rate, probably because the SA node is less sensitive to potassium than are the Purkinje fibers[24] (see below).

Administration of potassium may occasionally abruptly terminate an ectopic supraventricular or ventricular tachycardia,[25] but more commonly the rate of the ectopic rhythms decreases gradually (Fig. 4-3). Atrial flutter and fibrillation usually do not revert to sinus rhythm after potassium administration, probably because the doses used in the therapy of arrhythmia do not achieve the appropriate potassium concentrations. Clinical and laboratory observations suggest that the defibrillation of the atria can be expected when the plasma potassium concentration exceeds 7 mEq/liter. Spontaneous atrial defibrillation in patients with chronic fibrillation has been reported in patients with severe hyperkalemia.[5,21] The defibrillatory effect of potassium in the ventricles has been known since the beginning of this century. It may be worthwhile to remember that in an emergency, when a defibrillator is not available, the ventricles can be defibrillated using concentrated potassium solution intravenously.[5]

Effects of Potassium on the SA Node and the AV Node

The SA node and the AV node require separate consideration because the automaticity, conduction, and refractoriness in these tissues depend considerably on the membrane current carried predominantly by current passing through a so-called slow channel (see below). This dependence on "calcium current" may be, in part, responsible for the apparent decreased sensitivity of these fibers to hyperkalemia.[26] During regional perfusion of the SA node in the dog, the electrical activity of the SA node persisted when the K_o concentration increased to 21.6 mM/liter but was suppressed at lower K_o concentration when sympathetic influences were eliminated or calcium concentration was decreased.[26] In the cat or the rabbit, high K_o concentrations caused a shift of pacemaker within the perfused SA node, usually from above downward but sometimes from below upward. Such a shift of the pacemaker within the SA node could be recognized in the electrocardiogram only by recording electrocardiograms from the SA node and its vicinity.

High potassium concentration depresses the conduction in the AV node less than in the Purkinje fibers and in the ventricles. Moderate hyperkalemia (*i.e.*, increase of plasma K concentration to 5 to 6.5 mEq) may shorten the PR interval or even abolish second or third degree AV block,[21] probably because optimal AV conduction occurs at potassium concentrations that are near or slightly above the upper limits of normal potassium concentration. However, there are marked individual variations that depend both on the structural integrity of the AV node and on physiologic factors, such as a complex interplay between potassium and acetylcholine.[27] Thus, in some patients the AV block increased after a small increase in potassium concentration.[21] It should be added that most clinical studies of the effect of potassium on atrioventricular conduction were performed before the widespread use of His bundle electrocardiography and therefore do not establish whether the reported impairment of atrioventicular conduction after potassium administration was due to the effect of potassium on the AV node *per se* or on the infranodal portions of the atrioventricular conduction system.[28]

Biphasic Effects of Potassium on Excitability and Intraventricular Conduction

In dogs, the ventricular threshold of excitability decreases when the plasma potassium concentration is moderately elevated[8] but increases sharply when plasma potassium concentration exceeds about 7 to 9 mEq/liter. In humans, gradual increase in the plasma potassium concentration failed to reproduce the expected initial

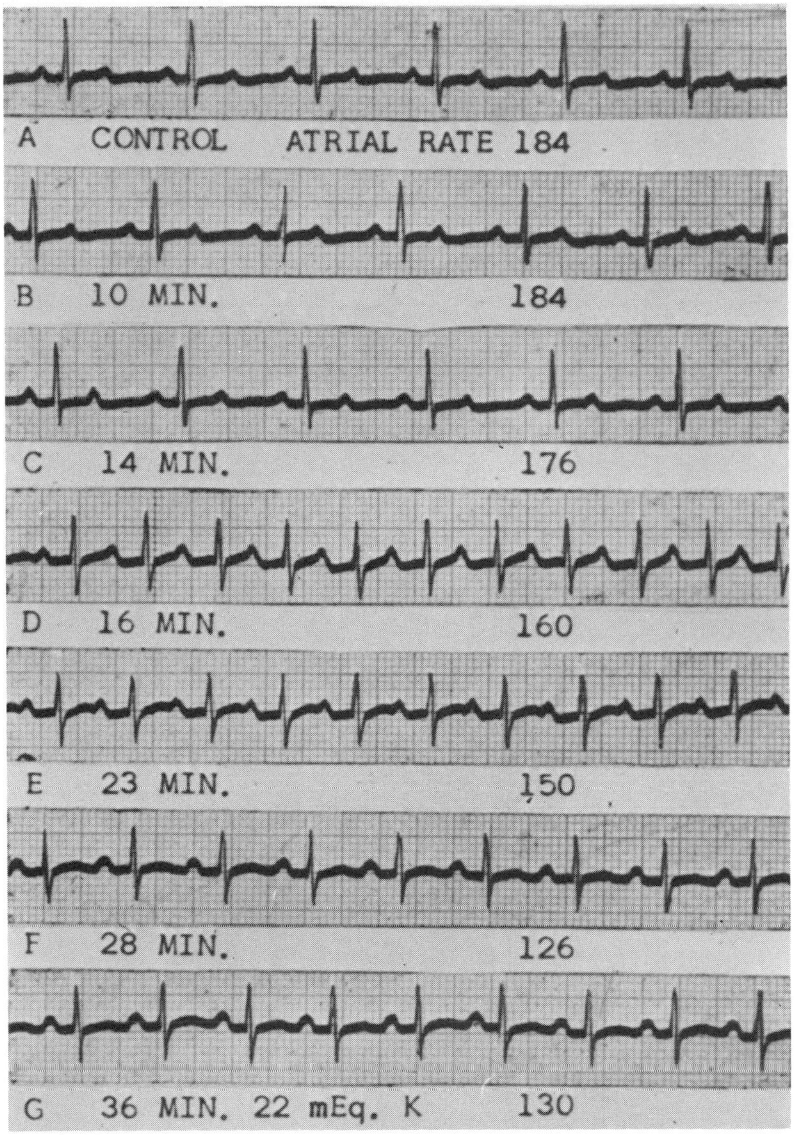

Figure 4-3. *Effect of intravenous KCl administration on the rate of an ectopic atrial pacemaker. Note the gradual decrease of atrial rate. In strips A, B, and C, the atrioventricular conduction is 2:1; in the remaining strips it is 1:1. (Surawicz, B.: Antiarrhythmic properties of potassium salts. In Brest, A. N., and Moyer, J. H. [eds.]: Cardiovascular Drug Therapy. New York, Grune & Stratton, 1964)*

decrease in the excitability threshold, which increased when the plasma potassium concentration had exceeded about 7 mEq/liter[29] (Fig. 4-4). However, certain clinical observations suggest that a slight increase in potassium concentration may increase the excitability threshold. Thus, occasionally a normal response to pacemaker stimulation could be restored by the administration of potassium, possibly due to lowering of the excitability threshold.[30] It should be added that the measurement of the excitability threshold in patients with pacemakers does not differentiate between a lack of response to stimulation and the lack of propagation of local response. However, this is probably of little practical significance, since potassium appears to affect both the excitability threshold and the conduction velocity in the same manner. The lowest excitability threshold and the most rapid intraventricular conduction in humans probably occurs when the plasma potassium concentration is close to 6 mEq/liter. Both lower and higher potassium concentrations are expected to slow the conduction and increase the excitability threshold. Therefore, within normal ranges of K_o, potassium administration may increase the intraventricular conduction velocity.[20,31] It has been shown that during rapid administration of potassium intravenously, the duration of the QRS interval first decreased and then increased.[31] An initial decrease in QRS duration was also observed during intracoronary infusions of potassium salts.[10]

Arrhythmogenic Effects of High K_o

Progressive slowing of conduction and decrease in excitability terminate in cardiac arrest when potassium depolarizes ventricular fibers to a critical level at which these

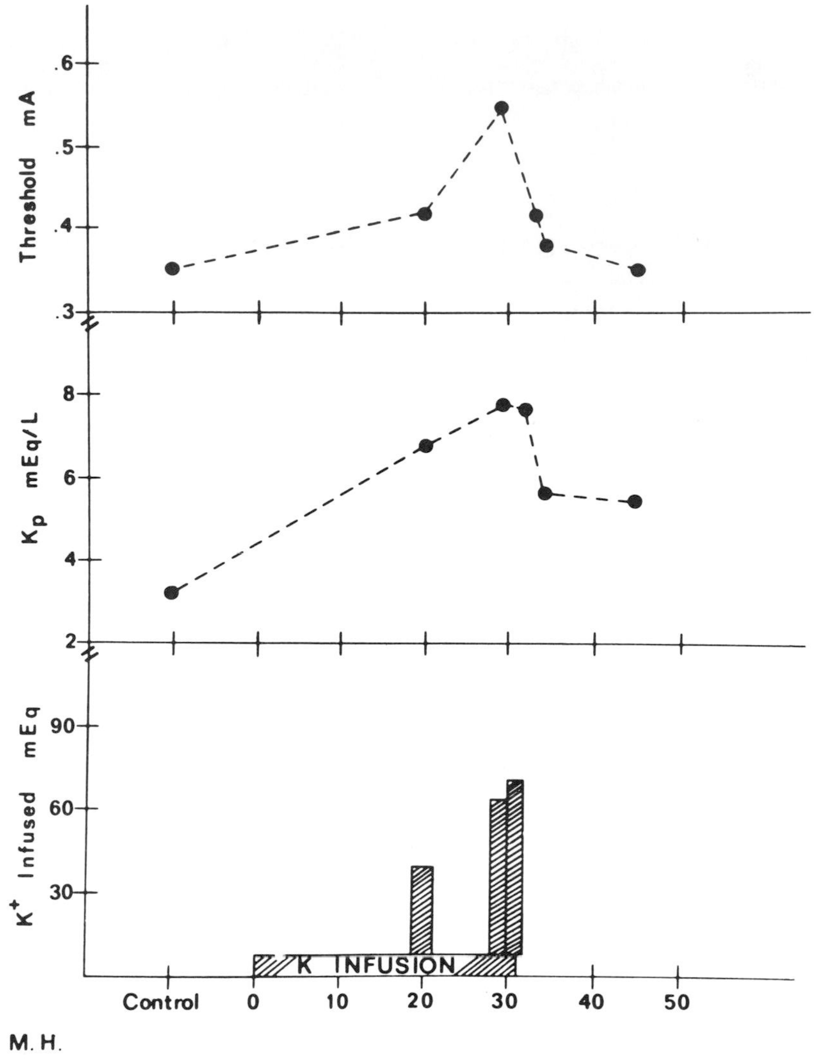

Figure 4-4. *Changes in diastolic threshold and plasma potassium concentration (K_p) during the infusion of KCl. Time in minutes is given along the horizontal axis. See text for details. (Gettes, L. S., Shabetai, R., Downs, T. A., and Surawicz, B.: Effect of changes in potassium and calcium concentrations on diastolic threshold and strength-interval relationship of the human heart. Ann. N.Y. Acad. Sci., 167:693, 1969)*

fibers become nonexcitable, but a more common terminal event produced by hyperkalemia is ventricular fibrillation. Ventricular fibrillation caused by hyperkalemia is most likely due to reentry precipitated by both slow conduction and short refractory period. The greatest shortening of action potential (*i.e.*, refractory period) may be expected in the early premature complexes, an effect attributed to the repolarizing action of membrane currents carried by potassium.[32,33]

Lethal hyperkalemia in humans is predominantly due to uremia and occasionally to an accidental error in the amount of potassium administered intravenously (*e.g.*, therapy with massive doses of potassium salts of penicillin). Also, large doses of orally administered potassium can be lethal in certain patients with low cardiac output or impaired renal function.

Effects of intravenously administered potassium depend on the rate of administration rather than an absolute amount of administered potassium. Large amounts of potassium can be administered at a slow rate, which allows the potassium to be excreted through the kidneys or transferred into the cells. However, at rapid rates of administration even small amounts of potassium can be lethal. Thus, in a dog, rapid intravenous administration of 2 to 4 mEq of KC1 produced ventricular fibrillation.[16] Figure 4-5 shows that such ventricular fibrillation may be initiated by a single ectopic complex and that it may not be preceded by any of the usual manifestations of potassium toxicity such as wide QRS complex, prolonged PR interval, or bradycardia. Similar effects, but after smaller doses of administered potassium, occur during administration of potassium salts directly into coronary arteries. In dogs, ventricular fibrillation occurred when potassium was administered at a rate of 1.6 μEq/kg/sec into the left anterior descending artery or at a rate of 0.8 μEq/kg/sec into the right coronary artery.[10] The total amounts of potassium that caused ventricular fibrillation in these experiments were within the range of 0.25 to 0.5 mEq. Electrophysiologic studies in dogs have shown that ventricular fibrillation induced by regional

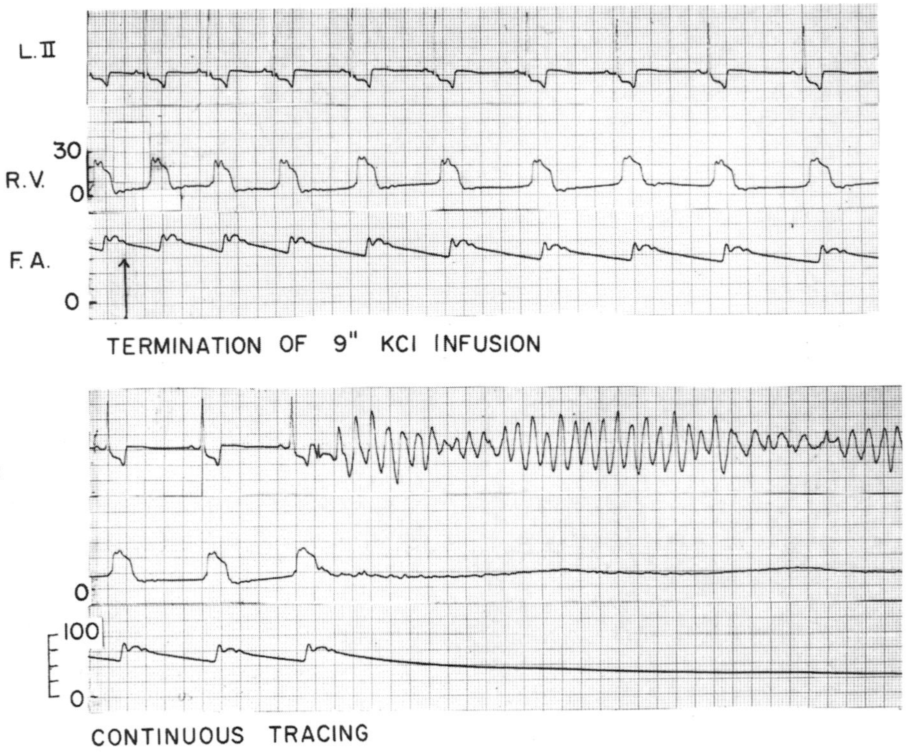

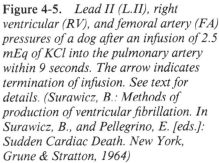

Figure 4-5. *Lead II (L.II), right ventricular (RV), and femoral artery (FA) pressures of a dog after an infusion of 2.5 mEq of KCl into the pulmonary artery within 9 seconds. The arrow indicates termination of infusion. See text for details. (Surawicz, B.: Methods of production of ventricular fibrillation. In Surawicz, B., and Pellegrino, E. [eds.]: Sudden Cardiac Death. New York, Grune & Stratton, 1964)*

hyperkalemia is preceded by the appearance of injury current,[10] increased duration of the vulnerable period, and reversal of the normal endocardial to epicardial sequence of excitation.[12] The latter observation suggested that the origin of the ventricular ectopic activity was within the myocardium rather than the conducting system.[12]

Role of Increased Potassium Concentration in Myocardial Ischemia

Animal experiments have suggested that sudden death after myocardial infarction may be due to ventricular fibrillation induced by liberation of potassium from the ischemic myocardium.[34] Harris has demonstrated that the onset of arrhythmias in dogs with coronary occlusion coincided with an increase in potassium concentration in a coronary vein draining the infarcted area.[34] In humans, loss of potassium during myocardial ischemia can be induced by pacing. The mechanism of this potassium loss is still poorly understood. Studies of Shine and co-workers in rabbit myocardium showed that the potassium loss during the first 30 to 45 minutes of total ischemia could not be explained by the impairment of sodium-potassium ATPase activity ("pump").[35] Therefore, the more likely cause of transient ischemic injury and potassium loss is an increased cell membrane permeability.[36]

The recent development of the K^+-sensitive electrode enabled several groups of investigators in this country[37] and abroad[38] to measure directly potassium concentration changes in the interstitial fluid in the area of acute myocardial ischemia. These studies have demonstrated close correlation between the rise in extracellular potassium concentration and the development of current of injury, shortening of refractory period, slowing of conduction, ventricular fibrillation (Fig. 4-6), and depression of contractility immediately after coronary ligation in dogs and pigs.[37,38] These observations strongly support the "potassium theory" of ventricular arrhythmias during acute myocardial ischemia but do not exclude the possible role of additional factors.

Effects Peculiar to Nonsteady State During Rapid Changes of Potassium Concentration

Rapid changes in extracellular potassium concentration can produce electrophysiologic effects that differ from those occurring at the corresponding K_o concentrations during steady state. An example of such phenomenon is the "paradoxic" Zwaardemaker-Libbrecht effect, which consists of a transient arrest of pacemaker fibers, shortening of action potential duration, and hyperpolarization following change from low to normal or high extracellular potassium concentration. This phenomenon was studied in perfused rabbit hearts,[18,20] isolated Purkinje fibers,[6,39] and anesthetized potassium-depleted dogs[31] and was attributed to sudden increase in potas-

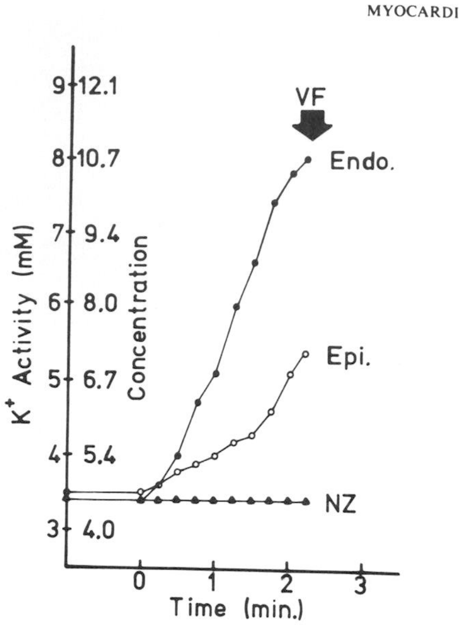

Figure 4-6. *Changes in subendocardial (Endo) and subepicardial (Epi) extracellular K^+ activity (a_{K+}) recorded in the center of the ischemic zone by two double barrel K^+ electrodes fused together with their tips positioned 8 mm apart. (NZ, nonischemic zone; VF, ventricular fibrillation) (Hill, J. L., and Gettes, L. S.: Effect of coronary artery occlusion on local myocardial extracellular K^+ activity in swine. Circulation, 61:768, 1980; by permission of the American Heart Association, Inc.)*

sium permeability and increased activity of the sodium pump.[6,39] The clinical significance of the Zwaardemaker-Libbrecht effect is probably limited to an occasional episode of bradycardia or AV block during administration of potassium at a rapid rate in patients with severe hypokalemia and potassium depletion.[11]

Other examples of the "paradoxic" effect of potassium during the nonsteady state are the decrease in QRS duration observed during the rapid administration of potassium in dogs[31] and the negative inotropic effect of potassium dependent on the rate of potassium administration rather than on the absolute value of extracellular potassium concentration.[10]

Hypokalemia

Electrophysiologic Mechanisms

The RMP or MDP* of cardiac fibers increases (*i.e.,* becomes more negative) with decreasing extracellular potassium concentration. However, this increase (*i.e.,* the hyperpolarization) is not as large as might be expected from the calculation based on the Nernst equation for a membrane freely permeable to K^+. The hyperpolarization can be demonstrated in all types of cardiac fibers, but its time course is different in myocardial and pacemaker (*e.g.,* Purkinje) fibers.[6,40] In the nonpacemaker fibers, perfusion with low potassium solution (*i.e.,* 0.54 mM/liter) produces long-lasting hyperpolarization, but in the Purkinje fibers the hyperpolarization is brief and transient and is rapidly succeeded by progressive depolarization due to marked increase in the slope of diastolic depolarization. This is followed by the appearance of spontaneous automatic activity, during which MDP becomes progressively less negative until the fiber becomes nonexcitable.

Repolarization

With decreasing K_o concentration, repolarization becomes slower and action potential duration increases.[18] The latter effect is associated with a progressively steeper slope of phase 2 and a less steep slope of phase 3 that causes a prolonged "tail" of the action potential (AP). The repolarization slope not only becomes slower but also changes progressively from convex to concave. When repolarization is prolonged, there is a longer interval during which the difference between the diastolic potential and the threshold potential is small. This means that the period of increased excitability is prolonged and the appearance of ectopic complexes is facilitated.[18,19] Hypokalemia prolongs the "tail" of the AP in the conducting system more than in the ventricles, so that the period of incomplete repolarization is longer in the Purkinje fibers than in the ventricular fibers.

Diastolic Depolarization

Hypokalemia increases diastolic depolarization in the Purkinje fibers[6,24,40] and therefore promotes automatic activity in quiescent Purkinje fibers. When such fibers are depolarized from a level of membrane potential that is less negative than the maximal diastolic potential, the upstroke velocity of the action potential and the conduction velocity decrease. Increased automaticity of Purkinje fibers may cause ventricular ectopic complexes and rhythms. Automaticity can appear even in ventricular myocardial (nonpacemaker) fibers when the repolarization of these fibers becomes slow, and the threshold potential is reached before the repolarization is completed.[19] This type of automaticity may be triggered by repetitive stimulation.[41]

Other Effects

Gettes and Surawicz have shown that hypokalemia increases the difference between the action potential duration of the Purkinje and ventricular fibers.[6] Initially, prolonged duration of the action potential was associated with prolonged refractoriness,[6] but the subse-

* Refers to myocardial fibers of the atria or the ventricles and to the Purkinje fibers.

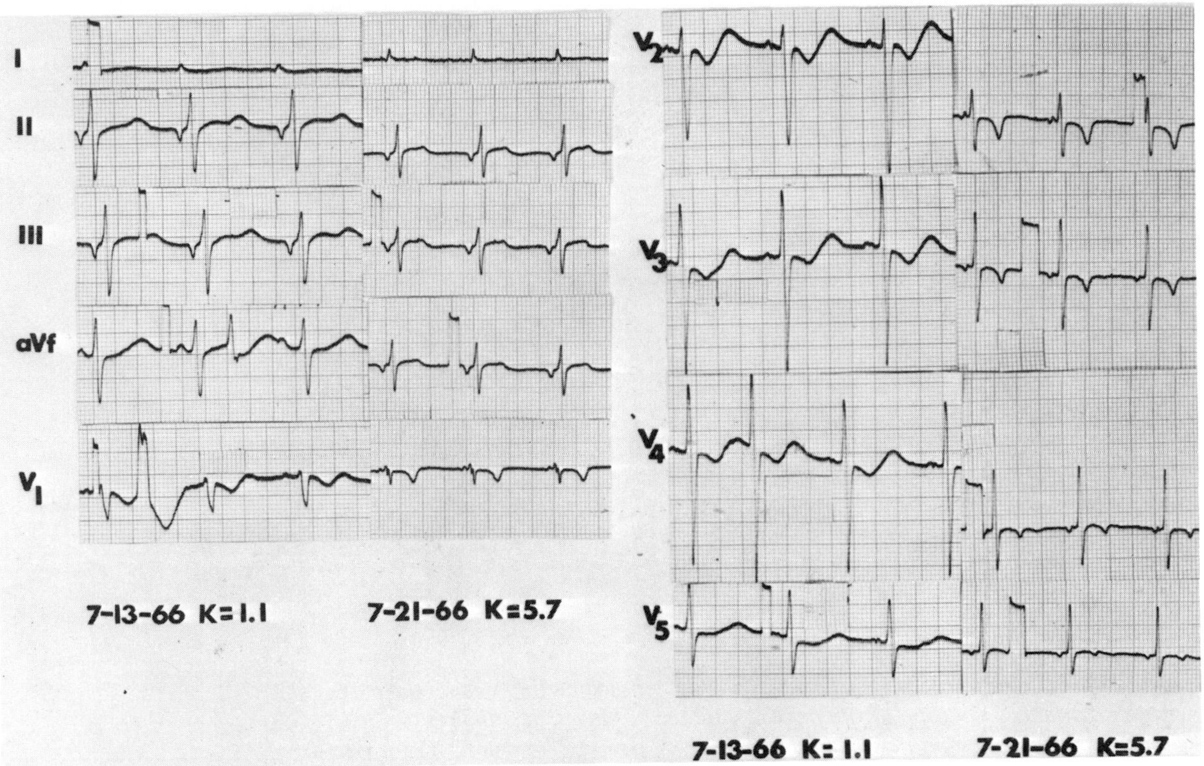

Figure 4-7. *Electrocardiograms of a woman aged 65 years with chronic pyelonephritis and vomiting before and after treatment with potassium salts. Note the typical pattern of hypokalemia on July 13, 1966, and the short coupling interval of the ventricular ectopic beats in leads aVF and V_1. Plasma K concentration is in mEq/liter. (Surawicz, B.: Relation between electrocardiogram and electrolytes. Am. Heart J., 73:814, 1967)*

quent shortening of phase 2 and the slow rate of phase 3 repolarization allowed the fiber to reach the threshold potential earlier than in the presence of normal potassium concentration and thus resulted in a shortened refractory period. Clinical observations also suggest that hypokalemia shortens the effective refractory period because atrial and ventricular premature complexes in patients with hypokalemia frequently appear after a short coupling interval (Fig. 4-7).

Hypokalemia frequently slows conduction because the depolarization begins in incompletely repolarized fibers and probably also because there is an increased difference between the resting membrane potential and the threshold potential.[19]

Electrocardiograms

The understanding of the electrocardiographic changes due to hypokalemia may be facilitated by correlating these changes with the concomitant changes in the ventricular action potential, as shown in the diagram in Figure 4-8. It can be seen that progressive changes in repolarization are reflected in the electrocardiogram as a progressive depression of the ST segment, a decrease in the T wave amplitude, and an increase in the U wave amplitude in the standard limb and precordial leads. As long as the T wave and the U wave are separated by a notch, the duration of the QT interval is unchanged. In more advanced stages of hypokalemia, the T wave and U wave are fused, and an accurate measurement of the QT interval is not possible.[11] Since the duration of mechanical systole does not change in hypokalemia, one can best describe the pattern of hypokalemia as a gradual shift of the major repolarization wave from systole into diastole. In Figure 4-8A, the amplitude of the repolarization wave inscribed during systole (T) is appreciably greater than the amplitude of the repolarization wave inscribed during diastole (U). In Figure 4-8B, both waves are of equal amplitude, whereas in C and D the amplitude of the repolarization wave inscribed during diastole is greater than that inscribed during systole. The latter two types of electrocardiographic pattern of hypokalemia are most frequently encountered when the plasma concentration is less than 2.7 mEq/liter.[11,42]

When hypokalemia is advanced, the amplitude and duration of the QRS interval are increased. The QRS complex is widened diffusely but in adults seldom by more than 0.02 second. In children, the QRS widening

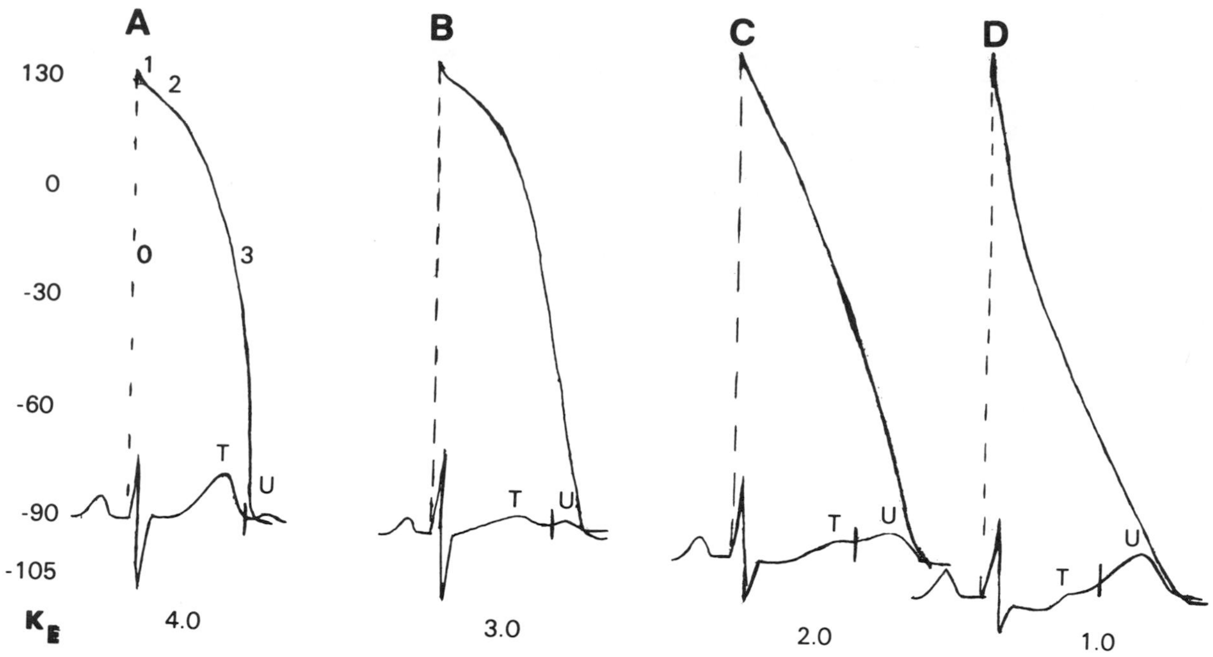

Figure 4-8. *Diagram of the ventricular action potential superimposed on the ECG for extracellular potassium concentrations (K_E) 4 to 1 mEq/liter. The numbers on the left designate the transmembrane potential in millivolts. See text for details. (Surawicz, B.: Relation between electrocardiogram and electrolytes. Am. Heart J., 73:814, 1967)*

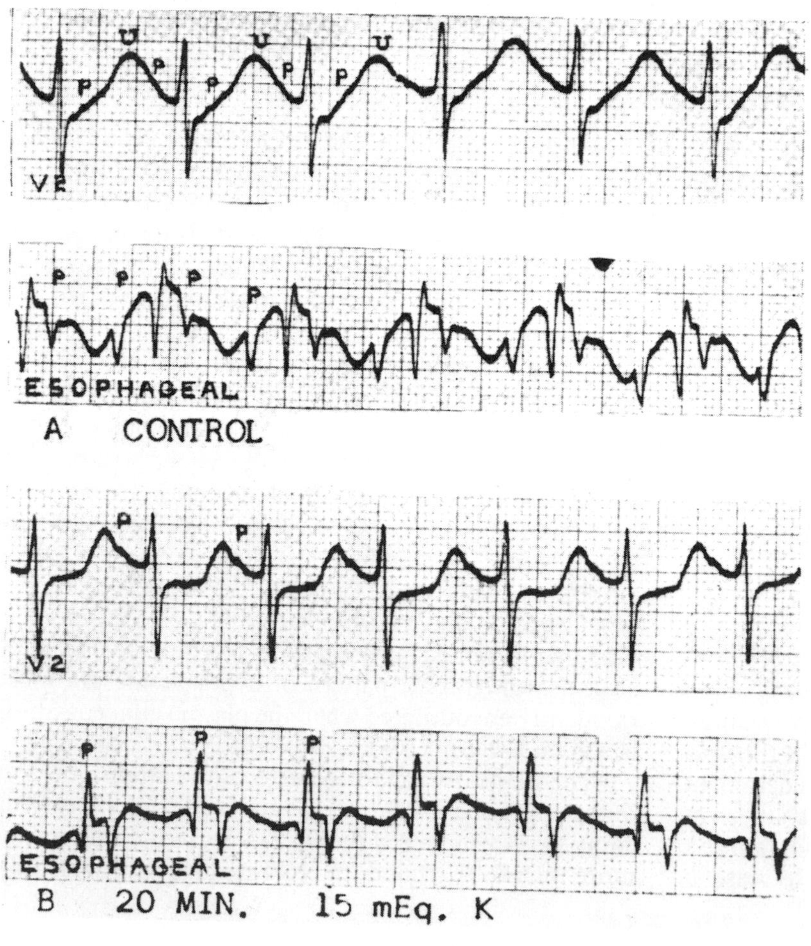

Figure 4-9. *Electrocardiogram of a woman aged 34 years with vomiting and plasma potassium concentration of 1 mEq/liter. The upper strip shows hypokalemia pattern and indistinct P waves in lead V_2. The P waves and the 2:1 AV block are clearly seen in the esophageal lead. Following intravenous administration of 15 mEq of potassium (lower two strips), ectopic atrial tachycardia and 2:1 block are no longer present. (Bettinger, J. C., Surawicz, B., Bryfogle, J. W. et al.: The effect of intravenous administration of potassium chloride on ectopic rhythms, ectopic beats and disturbances in AV conduction. Am. J. Med., 21:521, 1956)*

may be more pronounced. The increased duration of the QRS is the result of widening without change in the shape, which suggests that this is caused by slower intraventricular conduction without changes in the sequence of depolarization. As discussed earlier, the slowing of intraventricular conduction in hypokalemia may be due to hyperpolarization of ventricular fibers or to a slower propagation in the incompletely repolarized Purkinje and ventricular fibers.

The amplitude and duration of the P wave in hypokalemia is usually increased, and the PR interval is frequently slightly or moderately prolonged.

Arrhythmogenic Effects

Hypokalemia precipitates ectopic complexes and rhythms due to increased automaticity and facilitation of reentry. The latter can be caused by slow conduction during the prolonged relative refractory period, increased dispersion of refractoriness,[6] and decreased threshold of excitability. Perfusion of isolated rabbit hearts with potassium-deficient solutions produced intraventricular conduction disturbances and AV block as well as supraventricular and ventricular ectopic complexes.[18,19] In humans, hypokalemia promotes the appearance of supraventricular and ventricular ectopic complexes. In one study of 81 patients not treated with digitalis and who had a plasma potassium concentration 3.2 mEq/liter or less, ventricular ectopic complexes occurred in 28%, supraventricular ectopic complexes in 22%, and AV conduction disturbances in 12%.[42] Ectopic complexes occurred three times and AV conduction two times more frequently than in the control hospital population.[42]

Arrhythmias appearing in patients with severe hypokalemia are of the same type as in patients with digitalis toxicity, that is, nonparoxysmal atrial tachycardia with block (Fig. 4-9) and various types of AV dissociation. These arrhythmias are attributed to a combination of increased automaticity of ectopic pacemakers and at least some degree of AV conduction disturbance. Like digitalis, hypokalemia increases sensitivity to vagal stimulation.

Perfusion of isolated hearts with potassium-deficient solutions produces ventricular fibrillation.[18] This may be due to a combination of increased ventricular automaticity, slow conduction, short effective refractory period, and prolonged relative refractory period. In patients with severe hypokalemia, serious ventricular tachyarrhythmias, including ventricular tachycardia and fibrillation, have been reported in the absence of heart disease or digitalis therapy (Fig. 4-10).[23,42,44,45] A pattern of ventricular tachycardia called *torsade de pointe* has been recorded in some of these patients.[45] Hypokalemia is frequently present in patients with acute myocardial infarction[46-51] as is seen after resuscitation from out-of-hospital ventricular fibrillation,[52] possibly due to previous treatment with thiazide diuretics[46,48,52]

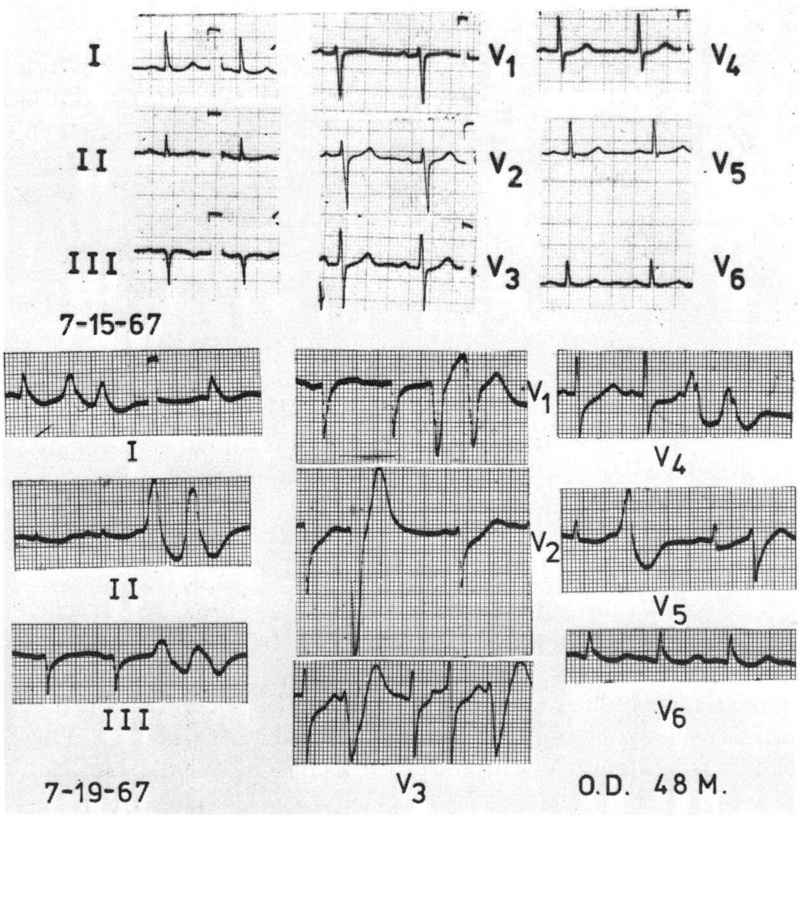

Figure 4-10. *Electrocardiographic pattern of hypokalemia with ventricular ectopic beats during treatment of diabetic ketoacidosis (7-19-67) in a patient with normal electrocardiogram before the episode of ketoacidosis (7-15-67). (Surawicz, B., and Mangiardi, M. L.: Electrocardiogram in endocrine and metabolic disorders. In Rios, J. (ed.): Clinical Electrocardiographic Correlations. Cardiovascular Clinics 8/3. Philadelphia, F. A. Davis, 1977)*

or administration of sodium bicarbonate during resuscitation.[52] In addition, hypokalemia may be precipitated by intense sympathetic stimulation, which shifts potassium into the skeletal muscle and the liver,[53] an effect attributed to beta$_2$-receptor stimulation by the circulating epinephrine.[54] The presence of hypokalemia in patients with acute myocardial infarction increases the incidence of serious ventricular arrhythmias.[46–51]

Modification of Potassium Effects by Other Electrolytes

In patients with hyperkalemia, calcium concentration may be the important factor determining the severity of atrioventricular and intraventricular conduction disturbance and vulnerability to ventricular fibrillation. Hypocalcemia frequently accompanies hyperkalemia in patients with renal insufficiency. It may be expected to aggravate the atrioventricular and intraventricular conduction disturbances and facilitate the appearance of ventricular fibrillation.

In some patients with renal insufficiency and hyperkalemia, hypercalcemia may also be present because of secondary hyperparathyroidism or overzealous therapy with calcium. Hypercalcemia may be expected to counteract the effect of hyperkalemia on the atrioventricular and intraventricular conduction disturbances and to prevent ventricular fibrillation.

Arrhythmias have been frequently reported during dialysis in both patients treated and patients not treated with digitalis. However, the effect of dialysis on the relationship between arrhythmias and electrolyte disturbances is difficult to evaluate because the dialysis aims at correcting several electrolyte disorders simultaneously.

Abnormal sodium and magnesium concentrations may also modify the electrocardiographic pattern of hyperkalemia. Hypernatremia may be expected to counteract, and hyponatremia to augment, the effects of increased potassium concentration on atrioventricular and intraventricular conduction disturbances. Hypermagnesemia could also possibly augment the effect of hyperkalemia on conduction disturbances. In hypokalemic patients with hypocalcemia, arrhythmias were as common as in those without hypocalcemia.[42] Similarly, the incidence of arrhythmias was the same in hypokalemic patients with and without acidosis.[42]

Other Ions

Electrophysiologic Mechanisms

Only extremely high or low concentrations of calcium produce electrophysiologic abnormalities that are of clinical importance. Within the range of concentrations compatible with life, calcium has relatively little effect on the resting membrane potential. Low calcium prolongs, and high calcium shortens, the phase 2 of the action potential, the total action potential duration, and the duration of the effective refractory period.[55] The effects appear to be secondary to changes in potassium currents due, in part, to changes in the intracellular calcium concentration and in part to the changes in the plateau amplitude of the action potential.[56] The changes also depend on the heart rate and magnesium concentration.[55,57] Low calcium depresses contractility, lowers the excitability threshold, and slightly decreases the rate of diastolic depolarization in Purkinje fibers. High calcium has a positive inotropic effect, increases the excitability threshold, and slightly increases the rate of diastolic depolarization in Purkinje fibers. Calcium plays an important role in the conduction of impulses dependent on the flow of ions through the so-called slow channel. These effects will be discussed later.

High sodium concentration increases and low sodium concentration decreases the upstroke velocity of the action potential. Increased sodium concentration counteracts many effects of hyperkalemia by increasing the rate of depolarization. High sodium prolongs the duration of the action potential, but the clinical significance of this is uncertain.

Magnesium concentrations within the range encountered in clinical situations have no important effect on the action potential, at least at normal potassium and calcium concentrations.[57] At low calcium concentration, low magnesium concentration exaggerates the effect of low calcium and high magnesium concentration corrects the effect of low calcium.[55,57] This suggests some limited competition between calcium and magnesium at the cell membrane. Also, high potassium concentration can modify the electrophysiologic effects of high magnesium concentration.

Effects on Electrocardiogram and Cardiac Arrhythmias

In patients with hypercalcemia, the ST segment is short or absent and the duration of the QTc interval is decreased.[11] Experimental hypercalcemia increases the duration of the PR interval and QRS complex and produces ectopic complexes and ventricular fibrillation. In dogs, hypercalcemia decreased the sinus rate and prolonged the AH interval during atrial pacing, but these effects occurred when plasma calcium concentrations reached levels of 10.5 and 9.6 mEq/liter, respectively.[58] In patients with severe hypercalcemia, QRS and PR intervals are frequently prolonged, and second or third degree AV block is occasionally present.[59]

There is no firm evidence that the incidence of ectopic beats in patients with hypercalcemia is increased. However, it has been postulated that sudden death of patients during hyperparathyroid crisis and other conditions associated with severe hypercalcemia may be caused by ventricular fibrillation.[59] In one case, the sudden postoperative death of a patient with a plasma calcium concentration of 18 mEq/liter was attributed to arrhythmia.

In patients with hypocalcemia, the ST segment and the QTc interval are prolonged. The duration of the ST segment is inversely related to plasma calcium concentration.[11] Prolongation of the QTc interval is associated with increased duration of the ventricular refractory period. This effect *per se,* in the absence of concomitant increase in dispersion of refractoriness or changes in conduction, may be expected to produce an antiarrhythmic action. Moderate hypocalcemia induced by administration of Na_2EDTA suppressed supraventricular and ventricular ectopic complexes in about 50% of patients.[60] Ectopic complexes suppressed by hypocalcemia reappeared after calcium administration.[60]

The effects of high or low sodium on the electrocardiogram, cardiac rhythm, and conduction are probably negligible within limits of plasma sodium concentration compatible with life. However, in patients with intraventricular conduction disturbances caused by hyperkalemia, hypernatremia shortens, and hyponatremia prolongs, the duration of the QRS complex.

Although both hypomagnesemia and hypermagnesemia may be expected to produce some effects on refractoriness and conduction, there are no recognizable specific electrocardiographic patterns caused by these disturbances.[11] Hypermagnesemia depresses atrioventricular and intraventricular conduction. In the animal experiments, the depression of atrioventricular conduction may occur when the magnesium concentration reaches 3 to 5 mM/liter.[57] The latter concentrations are considerably higher than those that cause respiratory arrest. Intravenous administration of magnesium salts may suppress cardiac arrhythmias in both patients receiving and not receiving digitalis.[61] Serious ventricular arrhythmias ascribed to hypomagnesemia have been reported in a variety of clinical settings, usually in association with hypokalemia and other electrolyte disturbances. The independent role of hypomagnesemia in the genesis of arrhythmias is difficult to establish. Abolishing arrhythmia by magnesium administration is not proof that arrhythmia was caused by magnesium deficiency, because magnesium has an inherent antiarrhythmic effect. Moreover, there is no conclusive evidence of arrhythmias in animals with experimental magnesium deficiency.

Acidosis and alkalosis are usually associated with altered concentration of potassium and ionized calcium. Whether the modifications of extracellular *p*H *per se* cause specific electrocardiographic changes is difficult to determine.

Interaction of Electrolytes With Digitalis and Antiarrhythmic Drugs

The action of all cardioactive and antiarrhythmic drugs produces various changes in membrane permeability to ions and is influenced by altered intracellular and extracellular ionic concentrations. A detailed review of this subject is beyond the scope of this chapter, but some of the more important clinical interactions will be mentioned.

Digitalis

Increased extracellular potassium concentration inhibits glycoside binding to (Na^+ K^+) ATPase, decreases the inotropic effect of digitalis, and suppresses digitalis-induced ectopic rhythms.[62–64] Accordingly, hyperkalemic animals and humans can tolerate large doses of digitalis without developing ectopic activity.[65] Conversely, hypokalemia increases glycoside binding to (Na^+, K^+) ATPase, decreases rate of digoxin elimination,[66] and potentiates toxic effects of digitalis. In hypokalemic animals, ectopic complexes and rhythms may appear after administration of unusually small doses of glycosides. In patients treated with digitalis, arrhythmias may be precipitated by carbohydrate administration, by removal of potassium by dialysis,[67] and, most frequently, by treatment with diuretic drugs.

The effect of interaction of potassium and digitalis on atrioventricular conduction reflects the complex effects of potassium on atrioventricular conduction, which may be depressed by both low and high potassium concentration. Moderate hyperkalemia may improve atrioventricular conduction in patients with digitalis-induced atrioventricular block,[21] but an opposite effect can occur due to a synergistic depressive effect of hyperkalemia on the atrioventricular conduction, as reported both in dogs and humans.[68] Therefore, the net effects of hyperkalemia on the atrioventricular conduction changes induced by digitalis are not predictable in individual cases. Moreover, these effects depend not only on the absolute plasma potassium concentration, but also on the rate of potassium administration and the structural integrity of the AV junction. Personal experience suggests that a combination of hyperkalemia and digitalis causes serious atrioventricular conduction disturbances only in patients with preexisting first degree AV block. In patients without preexisting AV block, the rate of the escape pacemakers is either normal or rapid. Figure 4-11 shows an electrocardiogram of a patient with atrial fibrillation and renal insufficiency treated with a maintenance dose of 0.5 mg of digoxin daily. In this patient, the rhythm and the rate are the same when plasma potassium concentration is (A) 8.4, (B) 6.7, and (C) 4.4 mEq/liter.

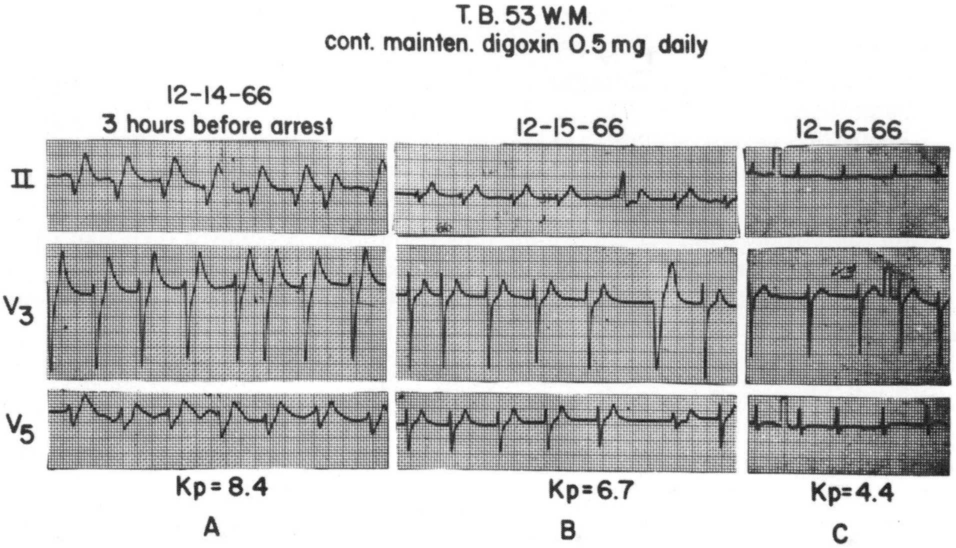

Figure 4-11. *Electrocardiogram of a patient aged 53 years with atrial fibrillation treated with a maintenance dose of digoxin, 0.5 mg daily. Note pattern of hypokalemia 3 hours before "cardiac arrest" (A) and after treatment with sodium lactate, glucose, and insulin (B and C). Ventricular rate is about 95/min in all three tracings. See text for details. (Surawicz, B.: Arrhythmias and electrolyte disturbances. Bull. N.Y. Acad. Med., 43:1160, 1967)*

Hypokalemia may augment the digitalis-induced depression of atrioventricular conduction. The most characteristic arrhythmias are nonparoxysmal supraventricular tachycardia with block and AV junctional tachycardia either during sinus rhythm (AV dissociation) or during atrial fibrillation. These types of arrhythmia are caused by a combination of increased ectopic pacemaker activity and depression at the atrioventricular conduction. Both hypokalemia and digitalis shorten the effective refractory period of the ventricles and the coupling interval of the ventricular ectopic complexes. Slow propagation of the early premature ectopic impulses may result in reentry and cause ventricular fibrillation (Fig. 4-12). The synergistic effect of hypokalemia and digitalis on automaticity of ectopic pacemakers and atrioventricular conduction explains the low digitalis tolerance of patients with hypokalemia. In these patients, nonparoxysmal atrial tachycardia with block or atrioventricular dissociation with AV junctional tachycardia may appear after the administration of 0.75 to 2 mg of digoxin.

Digitalis and hypercalcemia have similar effects on the automaticity of ectopic pacemakers. At the same time, both increase the threshold of excitability and shorten the effective refractory period in the ventricles. Recent studies also show that increased calcium concentration increases the transient diastolic depolarization induced by glycosides. Although observations *in vitro* suggest that hypercalcemia may be expected to increase ectopic activity in patients treated with digitalis, there is no convincing clinical or experimental support of this hypothesis. The clinical examples of an alleged synergism between hypercalcemia and digitalis date back about 40 to 50 years[60]; more recent information on this subject is lacking. In experimental animals treated with digitalis and calcium, hypercalcemia produced ectopic rhythms only when the animals had received more than 95% of the toxic dose of ouabain. Animals that received 90% of the toxic glycoside dose had no arrhythmia when their plasma concentration was 46.2 mg/100 ml. This confirmed data from an earlier study in dogs, which failed to show important synergistic or additive effects of calcium and digitalis on cardiac rhythm and conduction.

Hypocalcemia induced by administration of Na_2EDTA or citrate salts is believed to suppress ectopic complexes induced by digitalis. However, personal experience suggests that Na_2EDTA is equally effective in suppressing ectopic complexes and rhythms in both patients receiving and those not receiving digitalis.[60]

Hypomagnesemia decreases the dose of digitalis required to induce ectopic rhythms in both experimental animals and in humans.[69,70] Intravenous administration of magnesium salts suppresses ectopic complexes in patients treated with digitalis, but the same effect can occur in patients not receiving digitalis.[61]

Antiarrhythmic Drugs

In animal experiments, hyperkalemia and quinidine exert synergistic effects on the rate of rise of cardiac

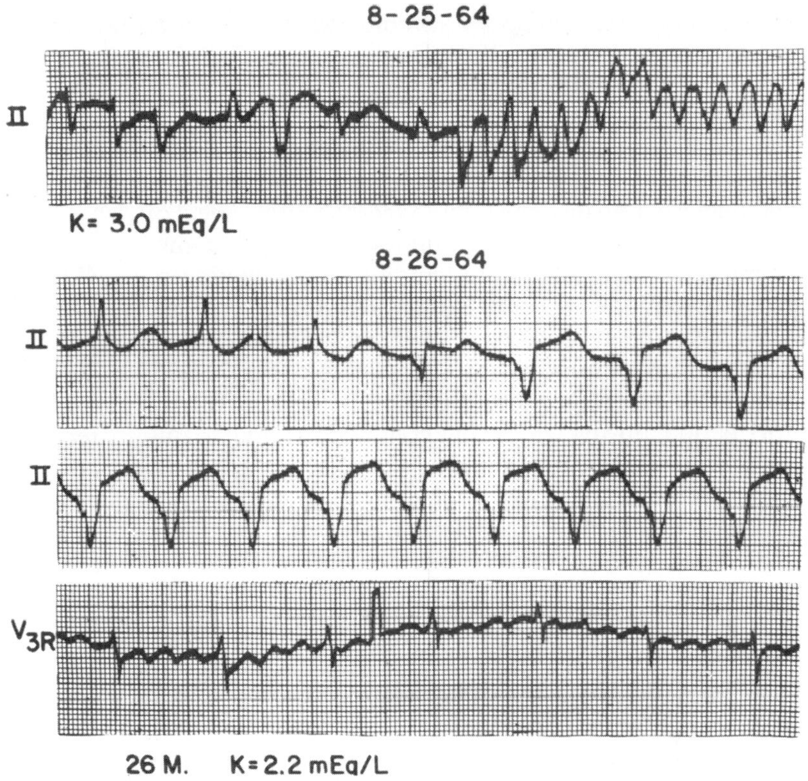

Figure 4-12. *Electrocardiogram of a patient aged 26 years with rheumatic heart disease treated with a maintenance dose of 0.25-mg digoxin daily. On Aug. 25, 1964, ventricular fibrillation begins after a ventricular premature beat with a short coupling interval. On the following day (8-26-64), the electrocardiographic pattern of hypokalemia and regular rhythm is attributed to an ectopic escape pacemaker. (Davidson, S., and Surawicz, B.: Ectopic beats and atrioventricular conduction disturbances in patients with hypopotassemia. Arch. Intern. Med., 120:280, 1967)*

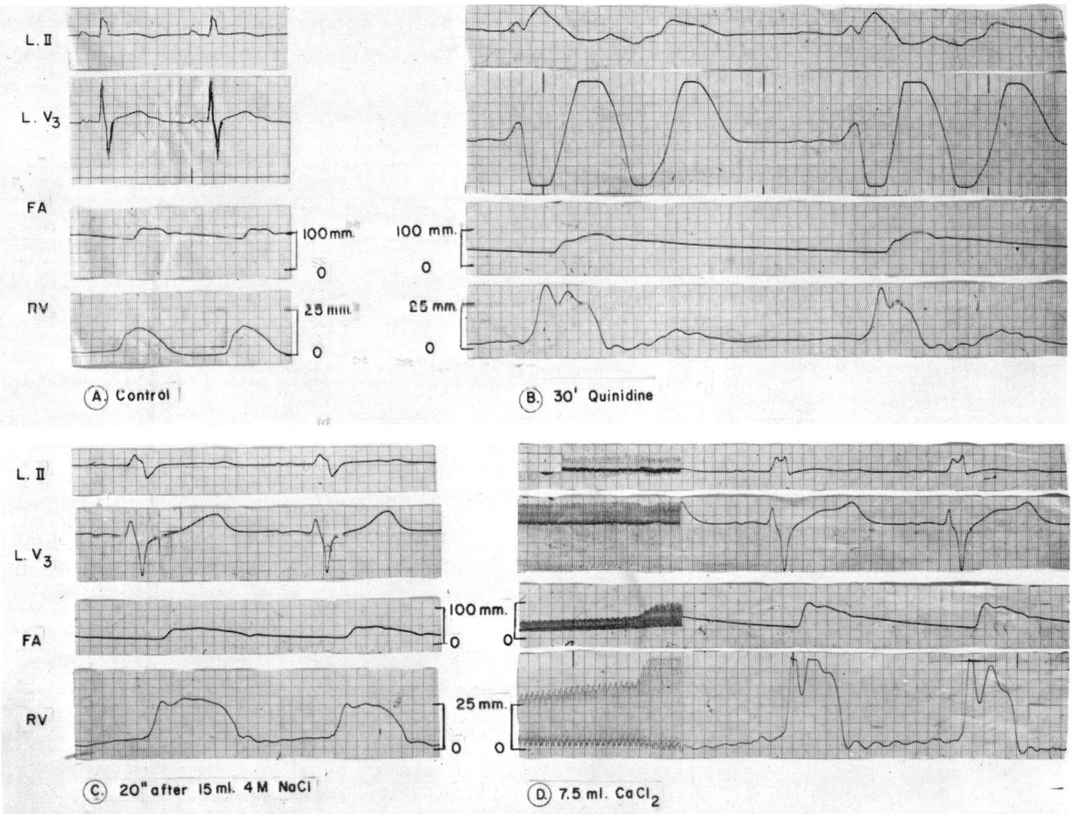

Figure 4-13. *Leads II (L.II) and V_3 (L.V_3) electrocardiograms and femoral artery (FA) and right ventricular (RV) pressure of a 20-kg dog before (A) and after (B) 30 minutes of intravenous administration of quinidine gluconate solution. Note that the very wide QRS complex in B becomes more narrow after administration of 15 ml of 4 molar NaCl solution in C. Note further the increase in pressure after administration of calcium chloride (D). (Surawicz, B.: Relation between electrocardiogram and electrolytes. Am. Heart J., 73:814, 1967)*

action potential and conduction velocity. Therefore, hyperkalemia augments quinidine toxicity. However, the effects of hypokalemia are less predictable: at slower heart rates, hypokalemia improved quinidine-depressed conduction, possibly due to the hyperpolarizing effect of low potassium. At more rapid rates, hypokalemia augmented the toxic effects of quinidine on conduction in isolated rabbit hearts and anesthetized dogs,[19] presumably due to greater prolongation of repolarization by low potassium and quinidine together than by either alone.[19] This in turn increased the duration of the relative refractory period, during which slow conduction is due to impulse propagation in incompletely repolarized fibers. In addition, quinidine administration can produce hypokalemia, which may possibly contribute to quinidine toxicity. Also, quinine, which causes the same electrophysiologic effects as quinidine, can induce serious ventricular arrhythmias associated with drug-induced hypokalemia.

Other antiarrhythmic drugs that increase the action potential duration have similar interactions with potassium, particularly in the presence of hypokalemia, when the drug-induced prolongation of QT appears to facilitate the occurrence of ventricular arrhythmia, especially torsades de pointes.[71,72] Class I antiarrhythmic drugs exaggerate the slowing of conduction induced by hyperkalemia,[73] and the effects of these drugs on conduction is influenced by potassium concentration. For instance, therapeutic concentrations of lidocaine have little effect on rate of depolarization when extracellular potassium concentration is less than 4.5 mM,[74] but may be expected to cause a decrease in the rate of depolarization when potassium concentration is elevated in depolarized, infarcted myocardium.[75]

Toxic effects of quinidine on atrioventricular and intraventricular conduction in dogs are reversed by administration of sodium lactate or NaCl. Figure 4-13 shows the effect of the administration of NaCl on the electrocardiogram of a dog with quinidine-induced intraventricular conduction disturbance. The improvement in conduction is probably due to the increase of the rate of rise of the action potential by sodium. This effect of sodium is not specific for quinidine because it is also present when conduction is depressed by potassium and certain drugs. Administration of calcium aggravates conduction disturbances produced by quinidine.

Arrhythmias Related to Slow Channel–Dependent Conduction and Automaticity

The recent discovery of an inward ionic membrane current flowing through a so-called slow channel has been of great theoretic and practical importance.[76] This current, carried predominantly by calcium and, to some extent, by sodium ions, plays a major role in the depolarization of the fibers in the SA and AV nodes. In addition, this current is capable of depolarizing all types of cardiac fibers when the rapid inward sodium current is inactivated at membrane potentials that are less negative than about −55 mV. The slow channel–dependent depolarization can maintain impulse propagation at a very slow rate and thus contribute to unidirectional or bidirectional block and reentry. Automatic activity can also develop in the myocardium depolarized to the level of membrane potential at which rapid inward sodium current is inactivated (Fig. 4-14).[77,78] Also, digitalis glycosides can induce transient diastolic depolarizations dependent on the membrane current flowing through the slow channel.[76]

Although a detailed discussion of the slow inward current is beyond the scope of this chapter, it is important to remember that the clinical significance of possible arrhythmias dependent on this current has not been conclusively established.

The slow inward current will be decreased by low and increased by high extracellular calcium concentration. The role of potassium in slow channel–dependent impulse propagation appears to be complex. Thus, high extracellular potassium concentration may contribute to depolarization and inactivation of rapid inward sodium current and thereby create conditions that would favor slow channel–dependent activity. On the other hand, high potassium concentration *per se* depresses the

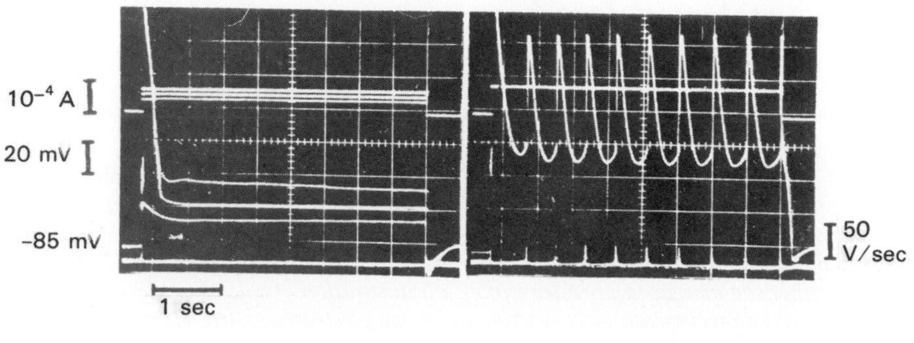

Figure 4-14. *Transmembrane action potentials of guinea pig papillary muscle during application of depolarizing current pulses (upper trace). On the left are subthreshold depolarization and single action potentials. On the right, depolarization to about −35 mV causes rhythmic automatic activity. (Unpublished data, S Imanishi and B. Surawicz)*

slow channel–dependent automaticity. Conversely, low extracellular potassium concentration may be expected to enhance slow channel–dependent automaticity. The possible role of other ions on the slow channel–dependent impulse propagation appears to be negligible, at least within the limits of concentrations encountered *in vivo*.

References

1. Hoffman, B. F., and Cranefield, P. F.: Electrophysiology of the Heart. New York, McGraw-Hill, 1960.
2. Noble, D.: The Initiation of the Heartbeat. Oxford, Clarendon Press, 1975.
3. Fozzard, H. A., and Sheu, S. S.: The resting potential in heart muscle. Adv. Myocardiol., 3:125, 1982.
4. Dominguez, G., and Fozzard, H. A.: Influence of extracellular K^+ concentration on cable properties and excitability of sheep cardiac Purkinje fibers. Circ. Res., 26:565, 1970.
5. Surawicz, B.: Role of electrolytes in etiology and management of cardiac arrhythmias. Prog. Cardiovasc. Dis., 8:364, 1966.
6. Gettes, L., and Surawicz, B.: Effects of low and high concentrations of potassium on the simultaneously recorded Purkinje and ventricular action potentials of the perfused pig moderator band. Circ. Res., 23,717, 1968.
7. Spear, J. F., and Moore, E. N.: Effect of potassium on supernormal conduction in the bundle branch Purkinje system of the dog. Am. J. Cardiol., 40:923, 1977.
8. Lyons, C. J., Burgess, M. J., and Abildskov, J. A.: Effects of acute hyperkalemia on cardiac excitability. Am. Heart J., 94:755, 1977.
9. Kaseno, K., Sugimoto, T., Hirazawa, K., et al.: The effects of hyperpotassemia on cardiac performance. Cardiovasc. Res., 9:212, 1975.
10. Logic, J. R., Krotkiewski, A., Koppius, A., and Surawicz, B.: Negative inotropic effects of K^+: Its modification by Ca^{++} and acetylstrophanthidin in dogs. Am. J. Physiol., 215:14, 1968.
11. Surawicz, B.: Relation between electrocardiogram and electrolytes. Am. Heart J., 73:814, 1967.
12. Ettinger, P. O., Regan, T. J., and Oldewurtel, H. A.: Hyperkalemia, cardiac conduction and the electrocardiogram: A review. Am. Heart J., 88:360, 1974.
13. Levine, H. D., Wanzer, S. H., and Merrill, J. P.: Dialyzable currents of injury in potassium intoxication resembling acute myocardial infarction or pericarditis. Circulation, 13:29, 1956.
14. DeMello, W. C., and Hoffman, B. F.: Potassium ions and electrical activity of specialized cardiac fibers. Am. J. Physiol., 199:1125, 1960.
15. Hariman, R. J., and Chen, Chai-M.: Effects of hyperkalemia on sinus nodal function in dog: Sino-ventricular conduction. Cardiovasc. Res., 17:509, 1983.
16. Surawicz, B.: Methods of production of ventricular fibrillation. In Surawicz, B., and Pellegrino, E. (eds.): Sudden Cardiac Death, p 64. New York, Grune & Stratton, 1964.
17. Garcia-Palmieri, M. R.: Reversal of hyperkalemic cardiotoxicity with hypertonic saline. Am. Heart J., 64:483, 1962.
18. Surawicz, B., Lepeschkin, E., Herrlich, H. C., and Hoffman, B. F.: Effect of potassium and calcium deficiency on the monophasic action potential, electrocardiogram and contractility of isolated rabbit hearts. Am. J. Physiol., 196:1302, 1959.
19. Gettes, L. S., Surawicz, B., and Shiue, J. C.: Effect of high K, low K, and quinidine on QRS duration and ventricular action potential. Am. J. Physiol., 203:1135, 1962.
20. Surawicz, B., and Gettes, L. S.: Two mechanisms of cardiac arrest produced by potassium. Circ. Res., 12:415, 1963.
21. Bettinger, J. C., Surawicz, B., Bryfogle, J. W., et al.: The effect of intravenous administration of potassium chloride on ectopic rhythms, ectopic beats and disturbances in A-V conduction. Am. J. Med., 21:521, 1956.
22. Fisch, C., Martz, B. L., and Priebe, F. H.: Enhancement of potassium induced atrioventricular block by doses of digitalis drugs. J. Clin. Invest., 39:1885, 1960.
23. Kunin, A. S., Surawicz, B., and Sims, E. A. H.: Decrease in serum potassium concentration and appearance of cardiac arrhythmias during infusion of potassium with glucose in potassium-depleted patients. N. Engl. J. Med., 266:228, 1962.
24. Vassalle, M.: Cardiac pacemaker potentials at different extra and intracellular K concentrations. Am. J. Physiol., 208:770, 1965.
25. Surawicz, B.: Arrhythmias and electrolyte disturbances. Bull. N.Y. Acad. Med., 43:1160, 1967.
26. Vassalle, M., Greineder, J. K., and Stuckey, J. H.: Role of the sympathetic nervous system in the sinus node resistance to high potassium. Circ. Res., 32:348, 1973.
27. Feigenbaum, H., Wunsch, C., and Fisch, C.: Effect of intracoronary infusion of potassium on the vagal action on A-V transmission. J. Clin. Invest., 44:339, 1965.
28. Cohen, H. C., Gozo, E. G., Jr., and Pick, A.: The nature and types of arrhythmias in acute experimental hyperkalemia in the intact dog. Am. Heart J., 86:777, 1971.
29. Gettes, L. S., Shabetai, R., Downs, T. A., and Surawicz, B.: Effect of changes in potassium and calcium concentrations on diastolic threshold and strength-interval relationship of the human heart. Ann. N.Y. Acad. Sci., 167:693, 1969.
30. Walker, W. J., Elkins, J. T., and Wood, L. W.: Effect of potassium in restoring myocardial response to a subthreshold cardiac pacemaker. N. Engl. J. Med., 271:597, 1964.
31. Surawicz, B., Chlebus, H., and Mazzoleni, A.: Hemodynamic and electrocardiographic effects of hyperpotassemia. Differences in responses to slow and rapid increases in concentration of plasma K. Am. Heart J., 73:647, 1967.
32. Gettes, L. S., Morehouse, N., and Surawicz, B.: Effect of premature depolarization on the duration of action potentials in Purkinje and ventricular fibers of the moderator band of the pig heart. Circ. Res., 30:55, 1972.
33. Hauswirth, O., Noble, D., and Tsien, R. W.: The dependence of plateau currents in cardiac Purkinje fibers on the interval between action potentials. J. Physiol. (Lond.), 222:211, 1972.
34. Harris, A. S., Bisteni, A., Russell, R. A., et al.: Excitatory factors in ventricular tachycardia resulting from myocardial ischemia: Potassium a major excitant. Science, 119:797, 1954.
35. Shine, K. I., Douglas, A. M., and Ricchiuti, N.: K exchange during myocardial ischemia (abstr.). Am. J. Physiol., 564, 1977.
36. Ganote, C. E., Jennings, R. B., Hill, M. L., and Grochowski, E. C.: Experimental myocardial ischemia injury. II. Effect of in vivo ischemia on dog heart slice function in vitro. J. Mol. Cell. Cardiol., 8:189, 1976.
37. Hill, J. L., and Gettes, L. S.: Effect of coronary artery occlusion on local myocardial extracellular K^+ activity in swine. Circulation, 61:768, 1980.
38. Franz, C., Bös., L., Hirche, H., and Schramm, M. P.: Extracellular K^+ activity and ventricular fibrillation during myocardial ischemia in pigs. Pfluegers Arch. (Suppl.), 373:R17, 1978.
39. Ito, S., and Surawicz, B.: Transient "paradoxical" effects of increasing extracellular K^+ concentration on transmembrane potential in canine cardiac Purkinje fibers. Circ. Res., 41:799, 1977.
40. Christé G.: Effects of low $[K^+]_o$ on the electrical activity of human cardiac ventricular and Purkinje cells. Cardiovasc. Res., 17:243, 1982.

41. Hiraoka, M., and Kawano, S.: Triggered tachycardia of guinea pig papillary muscle in the low K^+ solution. In Ueda, H., Murao, S., Yamada, K., et al. (eds.): Recent Advances in Electrocardiology, p 69. Jap. Heart J., 23:1982, Suppl. J.
42. Davidson, S., and Surawicz, B.: Ectopic beats and atrioventricular conduction disturbances in patients with hypopotassemia. Arch. Intern. Med., 120:280, 1967.
43. Surawicz, B., Braun, A. H., Crum, W. B., et al.: Quantitative analysis of the electrocardiographic pattern of hypopotassemia. Circulation, 16:750, 1957.
44. Redleaf, P. D., and Lerner, I. J.: Thiazide-induced hypokalemia with associated major ventricular arrhythmia. J.A.M.A., 206:1302, 1968.
45. Salvador, M., Thomas, C., Mazenq, M., et al.: Troubles du rhythme directment induits ou favorises par les depletions potassiques. Arch. Mal. Coeur, 63:230, 1970.
46. Beck, O. A., and Hochrein, H.: Initial serum potassium level in relation to cardiac arrhythmias in acute myocardial infarction. Z. Kardiol., 66:187, 1977.
47. Duke, M.: Thiazide-induced hypokalemia: Association with acute myocardial infarction and ventricular fibrillation. J.A.M.A., 239:43, 1978.
48. Hulting, J.: In-hospital ventricular fibrillation and its relation to serum potassium. Acta Med. Scand. (Suppl.), 647:109, 1981.
49. Nordrehaug, J. E.: Malignant arrhythmias in relation to serum potassium values in patients with an acute myocardial infarction. Acta Med. Scand. (Suppl.), 647:101, 1981.
50. Reuben, S. R., and Thomas, R. D.: The relationship between serum potassium and cardiac arrhythmias following cardiac infarction in patients aged over 65 years. Curr. Med. Res. Opin. (Suppl. 1), 7:79, 1982.
51. Solomon, R. J., and Cole, A. G.: Importance of potassium in patients with acute myocardial infarction. Acta Med. Scand. (Suppl.), 647:87, 1981.
52. Thompson, R. G., and Cobb, L. A.: Hypokalemia after resuscitation from out-of-hospital ventricular fibrillation. J.A.M.A., 248:2860, 1982.
53. Vick, R. L., Todd, E. P., and Luedke, D. W.: Epinephrine-induced hypokalemia: Relation to liver and skeletal muscle. J. Pharmacol. Exp. Ther., 181:139, 1972.
54. Brown, M. J., Brown, D. C., and Murphy, M. B.: Hypokalemia from $beta_2$-receptor stimulation by circulating epinephrine. N. Engl. J. Med., 309:1414, 1983.
55. Hoffman, B. F., and Suckling, E. E.: Effect of several cations on transmembrane potentials of cardiac muscle. Am. J. Physiol., 186:317, 1956.
56. Munakata, K., Dominic, J. A., and Surawicz, B.: Variable effects of isoproterenol on action potential duration in guinea pig papillary muscle: differences between nonsteady and steady—role of extracellular calcium concentration. J. Pharmacol. Exp. Ther., 221:806, 1982.
57. Surawicz, B., Lepeschkin, E., and Herrlich, H. C.: Low and high magnesium concentrations at various calcium levels. Effect on the monophasic action potential, electrocardiogram and contractility of isolated rabbit hearts. Circ. Res., 9:811, 1961.
58. Hariman, J., Mangiardi, L. M., McAllister, R. G., et al.: Reversal of the cardiovascular effects of verapamil by calcium and sodium: Differences between the electrophysiological and the hemodynamic response. Circulation, 59:797, 1979.
59. Voss, D. M., and Drake, E. H.: Cardiac manifestations of hyperparathyroidism, with presentation of a previously unreported arrhythmia. Am. Heart J., 73:235, 1967.
60. Surawicz, B.: Use of the chelating agent, EDTA, in digitalis intoxication and cardiac arrhythmias. Prog. Cardiovasc. Dis., 2:432, 1959–1960.
61. Szekely, P.: The action of magnesium on the heart. Br. Heart J., 8:116, 1946–1947.
62. Lown, B., and Levine, H. D.: Atrial Arrhythmias, Digitalis, and Potassium. New York, Lansberger, 1958.
63. Vassale, M., and Greenspan, K.: Effects of potassium on ouabain-induced arrhythmias. Am. J. Cardiol., 12:692, 1963.
64. Fisch, C., Knoebel, S. B., Feigenbaum, H., and Greenspan, K.: Potassium and the monophasic action potential, ECG, conduction and arrhythmias. Prog. Cardiovasc. Dis., 8:387, 1966.
65. Williams, J. F., Klocke, F. J., and Braunwald, E.: Studies on digitalis. XIII. A comparison of the effects of potassium on the inotropic and arrhythmic producing actions of ouabain. J. Clin. Invest., 45:346, 1966.
66. Steiness, E.: Diuretics, digitalis, and arrhythmias. Acta Med. Scand. (Suppl.), 647:75, 1981.
67. Lown, B., and Levine, S. A.: Current concepts in digitalis therapy. N. Engl. J. Med., 25:771, 1954.
68. Fisch, C., Greenspan, K., Knoebel, S. B., and Feigenbaum, H.: Effect of digitalis on conduction of the heart. Prog. Cardiovasc. Dis., 6:343, 1964.
69. Sellers, R. H., Cangrario, J., Kim, K. E., et al.: Digitalis toxicity and hypomagnesemia. Am. Heart J., 79:57, 1970.
70. Beller, J. A., Hood, W. D., Jr., Smith, T. W., et al.: Correlation of serum magnesium levels and cardiac digitalis intoxication. Am. J. Cardiol., 33:225, 1974.
71. McKibbin, J. K., Pocock, W. A., Barlow, J. B., et al.: Sotalol, hypokalemia, syncope, and torsade de pointes. Br. Heart J., 51:157, 1984.
72. Santinelli, V., Chiariello, M., Santinelli, C., and Condorelli, M.: Ventricular tachyarrhythmias complicating amiodarone therapy in the presence of hypokalemia. Am. J. Cardiol., 53:1462, 1984.
73. Surawicz, B.: Pharmacologic treatment of cardiac arrhythmias: 25 years of progress. J. Am. Coll. Cardiol., 1:365, 1983.
74. Singh, B. N., Vaughan Williams, E. M.: Effect of altering potassium concentration on the action of lidocaine and diphenylthydantoin on rabbit atrial and ventricular muscle. Circ. Res., 29:286, 1971.
75. Saito, S., Chen, C. M., Buchanan, J., Jr., et al.: Steady state and time-dependent slowing of conduction in canine hearts. Effects of potassium and lidocaine. Circ. Res., 42:246, 1978.
76. Cranefield, P. I.: The Conduction and the Cardiac Impulse. Mount Kisco, N.Y., Futura, 1975.
77. Katzung, B. G.: Effects of extracellular calcium and sodium on depolarization-induced automaticity in guinea pig papillary muscle. Circ. Res., 37:118, 1975.
78. Imanishi, S., and Surawicz, B.: Automatic activity in depolarized guinea pig ventricular myocardium. Characteristics and mechanism. Circ. Res., 39:751, 1976.

5

Invasive Cardiac Electrophysiologic Testing

Thomas F. Ross and William J. Mandel

Indications

Invasive electrophysiologic study of the heart has been available for clinical use since the late 1960s, when the procedure for reproducible recording of His bundle electrograms was described. The technique has since been expanded to include the use of multiple intracardiac recording electrodes with programmed electrical stimulation. It is currently being used as a diagnostic, therapeutic, and prognostic tool in a variety of clinical situations. Despite this, controversy still exists about its clinical use. Clinical use is an important issue because what began as a sophisticated research tool in select universities is now available in many local medical centers.

Given the financial constraints in present-day medicine, the clinical use of such a technique must include consideration not only of risk-benefit ratio but also of cost-effectiveness. Establishing an electrophysiology laboratory can require more than $100,000.[1] The procedures are time consuming and can present major scheduling problems if performed in a laboratory that also does standard cardiac catheterizations. Catheter insertion times range from 30 to 60 minutes, and programmed stimulation adds an additional 120 to 210 minutes. In-depth analysis of tracings may require 2 to 5 additional hours. Several personnel are needed to perform each study; two technicians and two physicians are present in our laboratory. The cost to the patient is considerable. The basic laboratory charge is approximately $1000, with additional fees for more lengthy procedures requiring extra catheters, drugs, and equipment. Including the cost of 1 to 2 days of hospitalization and the physician's fee, the total charge to the patient can be greater than $3,000. The use of such a costly and time-consuming procedure must therefore be carefully reviewed.

Electrophysiologic studies have become a basic research tool to investigate mechanisms of arrhythmias and conduction disorders. Extrapolation of these findings to prospective clinical situations has resulted in considerable controversy and confusion.[2–5] Current and future clinical uses of electrophysiologic studies involve three areas: diagnostic testing, therapeutic uses (medical and surgical therapy), and prognosis.

Diagnostic Uses

The necessity for electrophysiologic testing in diagnosing arrhythmias and conduction disorders depends not only on the nature of the rhythm disturbance but also on its clinical consequences. A patient with asymptomatic arrhythmia may warrant no therapy or simply an empiric trial of medication rather than a costly invasive evaluation of etiology. On the other hand, a person with recurrent syncope may benefit considerably from invasive investigation of possible arrhythmic causes and appropriately tailored therapy. A variety of neurologic, cardiac, pulmonary, and constitutional symptoms can be caused by rhythm disturbances. Poor cardiac reserve, secondary to associated cardiovascular and pulmonary disorders, can worsen any clinical manifestation. Supraventricular tachycardia in a young, otherwise healthy person may produce little or no symptoms. The same arrhythmia in a person with coronary artery disease can precipitate angina, infarction, or congestive heart failure.

Before invasive diagnostic studies are begun, a careful review of the results of noninvasive electrophysiologic tests is needed. These range from static resting 12-lead electrocardiograms to dynamic studies such as ambulatory Holter monitoring or exercise stress tests. Additional noninvasive tests may be forthcoming. Delayed low amplitude signals after the end of the QRS complex on the surface electrocardiogram are a marker for ventricular tachycardia in certain subsets of patients.[6] In many cases, these studies will obviate the need for further costly diagnostic testing.

Bradyarrhythmias

Sick sinus syndrome is the term applied to disorders of sinus node function that result in clinical bradyarrhythmias. These have generally been considered in three groups: (1) sinus bradycardia (less than 60 beats/min), (2) sinus arrest with junctional or ventricular escape rhythms, and (3) bradycardia-tachycardia syndrome. Most patients with these disorders are easily diagnosed by standard electrocardiograms or ambulatory monitoring.

Asymptomatic patients require no treatment, and invasive diagnostic studies will add little to their management.[7] If symptoms clearly related to sinus node dysfunction are present, a pacemaker is required. In this setting, electrophysiologic studies can provide information on the presence or absence of associated conduction defects that may influence the type of pacemaker (atrial, ventricular, or AV sequential) used. More than 50% of patients with sinus bradycardia or symptomatic sinus node disease have associated atrioventricular conduction abnormalities.[8,9]

Many patients present with symptoms such as syncope or fatigue and have undergone noninvasive studies that reveal no abnormalities or mild sinus bradycardia. Sinus bradycardia has been shown to occur in young and elderly persons without apparent cardiac abnormalities.[10,11] It may also result from autonomic dysfunction with excessive vagal tone rather than from intrinsic sinus node abnormality.[12] In these settings, electrophysiologic studies help establish the presence of sinus node dysfunction and examine the relationship between symptoms and the rhythm disturbance. An approach to the use of invasive testing in patients with bradyarrythmias is summarized in Table 5-1.

Conduction Disorders

Major goals in evaluating patients with atrioventricular conduction disorders include determining the site of block, establishing the relationship between the conduction abnormality and symptoms, and evaluating the likelihood of progression to high grades of atrioventricular block with attendant morbidity and mortality. Given this information, appropriate decisions regarding pacemaker therapy can then be made. In most situations this is accomplished without invasive electrophysiologic investigation (Table 5-2).

Although lesions throughout the conduction system may cause first degree AV block, the most common site of delay is in the AV node. The rate of progression to

Table 5-1. Indications for Electrophysiologic Studies: Bradyarrhythmias

	Indication for Electrophysiologic Study	
Surface ECG	*Symptoms*	*No Symptoms*
Sinus bradycardia	Possible	No
"Sick sinus syndrome"	Pacemaker (No electrophysiologic study)*	No

* Electrophysiologic study may be indicated to diagnose associated conduction abnormalities or aid in choice of pacemaker (see text).

Table 5-2. Indications for Electrophysiologic Studies: AV Conduction Abnormalities

		Indication for Electrophysiologic Study	
Surface ECG	Site of Block*	*Symptoms*	*No Symptoms*
First Degree AV	AVN >> HPS	Rare	No
Second Degree AV			
Type I—normal QRS	AVN >>>> HPS	Pacemaker (no electrophysiologic)†	No
Type I—wide QRS	AVN > HPS	Pacemaker (no electrophysiologic)†	Yes
Type II—normal QRS	HPS > AVN	Pacemaker (no electrophysiologic)†	Yes
Type II—wide QRS	HPS >>>> AVN	Pacemaker (no electrophysiologic)†	Yes‡
2:1 Normal QRS	HPS = AVN	Pacemaker (no electrophysiologic)†	Yes
2:1 Wide QRS	HPS >> AVN	Pacemaker (no electrophysiologic)†	Yes‡
Complete Heart Block			
Normal QRS	HPS = AVN	Pacemaker (no electrophysiologic)†	Yes
Wide QRS	HPS >> AVN	Pacemaker (no electrophysiologic)†	Yes‡

* (After Zipes, D. P.: Second degree atrioventricular block. Circulation, 60:465–472, 1979).
† Electrophysiologic study may be indicated to aid in choice of pacemaker.
‡ Pacemaker without electrophysiologic study is also an option.

high-grade block in asymptomatic persons is extremely low, and evaluation or therapy is not needed. Symptomatic persons with first degree AV block warrant electrophysiologic studies only if the symptoms are recurring or disabling, such as syncope, or if they occur in the setting of other arrhythmias and conduction disorders that warrant such studies in their own right.

Chronic second degree heart block, localized to the AV node, has a benign prognosis in persons without organic heart disease. In the setting of cardiac pathology, however, the prognosis is poor, with 27% of patients requiring pacemakers for symptoms and 47% mortality over $3\frac{1}{2}$ years.[15] Lesions within the bundle of His that result in second degree AV block usually occur in the setting of organic heart disease and result in congestive heart failure, fatigue, dizziness, or syncope.[16,17] In these studies, 86% of persons required pacemakers for symptoms, with 36% mortality over 20 months. Too few asymptomatic persons with second degree intra-Hisian block have been followed to draw conclusions regarding the need for pacemaker therapy. Second degree AV block due to infra-Hisian lesions usually requires pacemaker therapy for symptoms; such patients have a high rate of progression to complete heart block with excessive mortality.[18] Asymptomatic persons with infra-Hisian second degree block are at high risk for syncope and sudden death and are candidates for prophylactic pacemakers.[19]

As described above, the site of block, presence of underlying heart disease, and presence or absence of symptoms are key factors in the morbidity and mortality associated with second degree heart block. The site of block can usually be inferred from surface electrocardiograms in conjunction with provocative maneuvers such as carotid sinus massage and the administration of atropine.[20,21] Symptomatic persons usually require pacemakers unless a reversible etiology is found. In this setting, invasive studies are not needed. If the site of block is uncertain from surface electrocardiograms in asymptomatic persons, an electrophysiologic study can be of value to identify high-risk subgroups (patients with intra-Hisian or infra-Hisian block. Table 5-2 summarizes the indications for invasive electrophysiologic testing in patients with second degree AV block based on their surface electrocardiograms and presence or absence of symptoms.

An additional setting in which electrophysiologic testing is of diagnostic value is in persons with second degree heart block and junctional premature beats. Pseudo-AV block has been reported to occur in patients with frequent, nonpropagated, junctional extrasystoles due to their concealed conduction within the AV node.[22] His bundle studies are required to document this phenomenon.

As with other types of atrioventricular conduction disorders, the lesions producing complete heart block can occur at any level of the conduction system. In 70% to 80% of patients this is within or below the bundle of His.[23] This is usually accompanied by an unstable, wide QRS escape rhythm and bradycardia-related symptoms. In these and other forms of symptomatic complete heart block, pacemaker therapy is required and electrophysiologic studies are not needed. Invasive studies may be used in this setting, however, to determine the optimal pacing mode (ventricular or AV synchronous). Asymptomatic persons with complete heart block are more likely to have lesions involving the AV node or within the His bundle. For these patients, electrophysiologic studies are useful to delineate the site of block and assess the stability of escape pacemakers.[24] This permits a rational approach to the use of prophylactic pacemakers.

The long-term mortality of patients with asymptomatic intraventricular conduction abnormalities (right bundle branch block, left bundle branch block, left anterior fascicular block, left posterior fascicular block) has been reported as high as 50% in those with newly acquired left bundle branch block, or no greater than matched controls in persons with right bundle branch block.[25,26] These discrepancies are most likely explained by differences in the population studied. Morbidity and mortality in these groups reflect the severity of underlying cardiac pathology, with few people progressing to high-grade block. Prospective studies of patients with chronic bundle branch block revealed progression to complete heart block at only 1% to 2% per year. Sudden death was observed in 3% to 5% per year, but most of these were due to tachyarrhythmias and myocardial infarction rather than to bradyarrhythmias.[27,28]

Because prophylactic pacing may benefit some of these persons, attempts have been made to identify high-risk groups. Analysis of surface electrocardiograms and categorization of patients with a combination of conduction defects (such as bifascicular and trifascicular block) does not improve diagnostic sensitivity and specificity. Several prospective studies have used invasive electrophysiologic studies to categorize persons on the basis of their HV interval.[27-29] Although different populations were examined, 31% to 63% had a normal HV interval (less than or equal to 55 msec) and 37% to 69% had a prolonged HV interval. The average annual rate of progression to high-grade block was 0.15% to 1.3% in the former group and 1.2% to 2.4% in the latter. The sensitivity of a prolonged HV interval in these studies was similar at 80%, but the specificity varied from 32% to 64%, with a positive predictive value of only 5% to 7%. One study suggested the longer the abnormal HV interval, the higher the risk; an HV interval of greater than or equal to 70 msec was associated with 4% annual progression and an HV interval greater than or equal to 100 msec with 8% annual progression. Unfortunately, few patients had such prolonged conduction times, 37% and 5%, respectively. Incremental atrial pacing has been performed to enhance the sensitivity and specificity of electrophysiologic studies by stressing the conduction system to reveal occult abnormalities. In patients with intact AV nodal conduction, those who developed infranodal block during pacing progressed to second or third degree AV block at a rate of 14% per year. Only 3% of all patients studied had this finding, but pacing predicted 60% of all episodes of high-grade block.[30] Using this approach, diagnostic sensitivity is 60%; specificity, 98%; and positive predictive value, 43%.

The poor predictive value of such electrophysiologic testing in asymptomatic persons reflects the slow progression of conduction system disease. Also, serial electrophysiologic studies have shown that AV nodal and infranodal conduction disease progress independently. As many as 50% of cases of high-grade heart block, which develop in persons with bifascicular block, occur in the AV node rather than in the infranodal tissues.[31,32]

Neurologic and cardiac symptoms in patients with intraventricular conduction disturbances may be a manifestation of intermittent high-grade block. Evaluation of such patients should include a complete neurologic and medical work-up with extended ambulatory electrocardiographic monitoring. Electrophysiologic testing may provide additional diagnostic information. Through this technique, heart block was thought to be the cause of transient neurologic symptoms in 17% to 47% of persons with bifascicular block.[33-35] Patients with prolonged HV intervals ($>$60 msec in one study and $\geqq$80 msec in another study), or infra-Hisian block during incremental atrial pacing, appear to benefit most from permanent pacing.

Despite these findings, several points should be emphasized: (1) arrhythmias other than high-grade block are the cause of symptoms in more than 50% of patients with bifascicular block, (2) progression to complete AV block can occur despite a normal HV interval, presumably due to AV nodal block, and (3) long-term mortality may not be improved by prophylactic pacing. Table 5-3 summarizes the use of electrophysiologic testing in patients with bundle branch and fascicular blocks.

Conduction abnormalities have been reported in 15% of patients with acute myocardial infarction. Although morbidity and mortality in this group are primarily due to associated pump failure, an increased incidence of progression to high-grade AV block exists as well. There

Table 5-3. Indications for Electrophysiologic Studies: Intraventricular Conduction Abnormalities

Surface ECG		Indication for Electrophysiologic Study: Symptoms	No Symptoms
RBBB, LAFB, LPFB		Rare	No
LBBB			
RBBB + LAFB	Bifascicular Block	Possible	No
RBBB + LPFB			

is considerable controversy about the selection of patients with conduction abnormalities for temporary and permanent pacemakers. Current approaches use infarct location and surface electrocardiogram categorization of conduction abnormalities.[36] Several studies have investigated the use of His bundle recordings to further identify high-risk subgroups. Lie and colleagues found that an HV interval of greater than 60 msec predicted a high rate of progression to complete AV block and death in patients with bundle branch block complicating anteroseptal infarction.[37] Subsequent investigators, however, have failed to demonstrate the prognostic value of a prolonged HV interval in the postinfarct patient.[38,39]

Tachyarrhythmias

Diagnostic electrophysiologic studies are performed in persons with tachyarrhythmias for two major purposes: (1) to guide therapy of documented arrhythmias by determining underlying electrophysiologic mechanisms, and (2) to evaluate the etiology of wide QRS complex tachycardias.

Supraventricular Tachycardia

Examination of the surface electrocardiograms during supraventricular tachycardia may provide clues to underlying electrophysiologic mechanisms.[40] This is often adequate information on which to base empiric drug therapy in patients with infrequent episodes or minimal symptoms. Several groups of patients, however, warrant more invasive diagnostic testing. Persons in whom the occurrence of tachycardia results in disabling or life-threatening symptoms such as hypotension, syncope, or pulmonary edema require rapid diagnosis of the type of tachycardia and appropriate, effective drug therapy. Similarly, patients with recurrent supraventricular tachycardias refractory to conventional antiarrhythmic therapy need electrophysiologic testing on which to base other therapeutic options, among them investigational drugs, antitachycardia pacemakers, and ablation of accessory atrioventricular connections.

Another group that may benefit from electrophysiologic therapy is patients with ventricular preexcitation. Paroxysmal supraventricular tachycardia in these persons can usually be approached as described above, with invasive studies limited to patients with severe symptoms or refractory arrhythmias. Despite the presence of ventricular preexcitation on the surface electrocardiogram, symptoms in these patients may be due to arrhythmias other than those using the accessory pathway. Electrophysiologic testing may be the only way to diagnose such problems.[41] Atrial fibrillation occurs in 20% of patients with Wolff-Parkinson-White syndrome. If the anterograde refractory period of the bypass tract is short, conduction can result in a rapid ventricular response. In addition to severe symptoms, this rhythm can degenerate into ventricular fibrillation.[42] Electrophysiologic studies are necessary in this setting to guide medical or surgical intervention.[43]

Controversy exists on the management of asymptomatic persons with evidence of ventricular preexcitation on their resting electrocardiogram. Although most such persons have a good prognosis, atrial fibrillation with rapid ventricular responses and ventricular fibrillation have been reported.[42] The induction of anterograde block in the accessory pathway with normalization of the QRS complex during exercise or after the administration of procainamide has been used to identify persons thought to be at low risk.[44,45] Whether electrophysiologic testing should be performed in persons who do not respond to such provocative manuevers remains to be determined.

Wide QRS Complex Tachycardias

Differentiation between a supraventricular rhythm with aberrant conduction and a ventricular rhythm in patients with wide QRS complex tachycardias has important therapeutic implications. Traditional approaches have used clinical and electrocardiographic findings.[46] In many cases, however, these criteria are inadequate to make such a distinction. Electrophysiologic testing can provide valuable information in this setting. The rationale for such testing is based on the finding that most supraventricular and ventricular tachycardias are reentrant arrhythmias and, as such, can be reproducibly initiated and terminated by atrial or ventricular stimulation.[47,48] Findings that differentiate supraventricular tachycardia from ventricular tachycardia include (1) the temporal relationship between the atrial, His bundle, and ventricular depolarizations, (2) the atrial activation sequence, (3) the mode of initiation of tachycardia, and (4) the response of the arrhythmia to atrial and ventricular stimuli.

Sudden Cardiac Death and Ventricular Tachyarrhythmias

The use of electrophysiologic testing in the management of survivors of sudden cardiac death has been controversial. Prognosis after survival of cardiac arrest appears poor, with reported mortalities of 24% to 30% at 1 year, 34% to 40% at 2 years, and 51% to 60% at 4 years.[49,50] The cause of death is usually a recurrence of the original arrhythmia. There is considerable variability in the rhythm first recorded in this setting.[51-56] Bradyarrhythmias or asystole occur in 0% to 31%, ventricular tachycardia in 0% to 38%, and ventricular fibrillation in 58% to 87% of patients. This range is in part explained by different patient populations. Also, the first recorded rhythm may not be identical to that which initiated the event. The degeneration of ventricular tachycardia into ventricular fibrillation or asystole has been reported.[57,58]

Empiric antiarrhythmic therapy has had no major impact on these statistics. Sudden death occurred in 50% of patients treated empirically with either quinidine or procainamide.[59] Improved survival has been reported, however, if persons with documented tachyarrhythmias are treated with drugs chosen on the basis of their ability to suppress certain forms of complex ventricular ectopy during both extended ambulatory monitoring and exercise stress testing.[60] Criticism of this technique has been based on the poor relationship between such ectopy and ventricular tachyarrhythmias and the prolonged hospitalization necessary to choose an appropriate drug regimen.[61] Improved survival has also been reported with empiric therapy using amiodarone.[62] In this study, the recurrence of sudden death was only 7% after 12 months. Empiric use of drugs is limited by a lack of parameters with which to judge therapeutic efficacy. Sustained ventricular tachyarrhythmias are infrequent, random events. To use the arrhythmia itself as an endpoint can require many months, and failure may be fatal. These are major limitations given recent data that suggest that any single drug will be effective in only one third of patients and may worsen the arrhythmia in 16%.[63,64]

Electrophysiologic testing has been used during the past several years as an adjunct to the diagnosis and

Table 5-4. Diagnostic Value of Electrophysiologic Studies in Patients With Ventricular Tachyarrhythmias

Study (Reference)	Sensitivity (%)	Specificity (%)	Positive Predictive Value (%)	Negative Predictive Value (%)
Underlying Arrhythmia: Sudden Death (Ventricular Tachycardia + Ventricular Fibrillation)				
Ruskin[53]	81			
Myerburg[52]	29			
Josephson[54]	60			
Ruskin[65]	75			
Mason[73]	89			
Morady[55]	76			
Benditt[66]	88			
Roy[74]	61			
Underlying Arrhythmia: Ventricular Tachycardia				
Ruskin[53]	100			
Myerburg[52]	83			
Josephson[54]	85			
Vandepol[67]	84	99	96	97
Fisher[71]	85	95	94	87
Naccarelli[68]	51			
Livelli[69]	65	98	97	75
Morady[61]	83			
Benditt[66]	100			
Mann[70]	83	88	85	87
Underlying Arrhythmia: Ventricular Fibrillation				
Ruskin[53]	74			
Myerburg[52]	0			
Josephson[54]	43			
Kehoe[72]	64			
Morady[55]	77			
Benditt[66]	86			

Table 5-5. Diagnostic Value of the Number of Ventricular Extra Stimuli in Electrophysiologic Studies in Patients with Ventricular Tachyarrhythmias

Study (Reference)	Arrhythmia	Number of Extra Stimuli	Sensitivity (%)	Specificity (%)	Positive Predictive Value (%)	Negative Predictive Value (%)
Morady[55]	Ventricular tachycardia + ventricular fibrillation	1	2			
		2	26			
		3	67			
Benditt[66]	Ventricular tachycardia + ventricular fibrillation	1	6			
		2	44			
		3	79			
Fisher[71]	Ventricular tachycardia	1	15	100	100	56
		2	42	98	98	49
		3	82	86	94	65
Mann[70]	Ventricular tachycardia	1	17	99	90	60
		2	45	96	89	69
		3	68	90	84	78
		4	83	88	85	87
Brugada[75]	None	4		60		

therapy of persons with sudden death and recurrent ventricular tachyarrhythmias. The purpose of the study is to induce reproducibly the patient's ventricular arrhythmia and judge therapeutic efficacy by the inability to induce the same arrhythmia after appropriate therapy. The rationale for this approach is based on two points: (1) electrophysiologic study is a diagnostic test with suitable sensitivity and specificity, and (2) medical or surgical therapy, based on test results, is superior to conventional empiric drug therapy. Determination of sensitivity and specificity has been hampered by different stimulation protocols used by various investigators, including (1) stimulus intensity (current amplitude and pulse width), (2) rates of pacing, (3) number of extra stimuli (one to four), (4) number of sites stimulated (right ventricle and left ventricle), (5) stimulation during provocative drug infusions (isoproterenol), and (6) definition of a positive response (sustained ventricular tachycardia versus nonsustained ventricular tachycardia versus repetitive ventricular response). In addition, patients with different arrhythmias (ventricular tachycardia versus ventricular fibrillation) and drug histories have been compared.

Tables 5-4 to 5-6 list the sensitivity, specificity, and predictive values of a variety of stimulation protocols. The more aggressive the induction (*i.e.*, multiple ventricular sites with an isoproterenol infusion and multiple extra stimuli, the greater the sensitivity but the lower the specificity). Our current procedure includes burst ventricular pacing and insertion of one to three extra stimuli during ventricular pacing at multiple-paced cycle lengths and multiple locations within the right ventricle. In patients with documented sustained ventricular tachycardia, the sensitivity and specificity of this protocol are approximately 85%. If ventricular fibrillation is the underlying rhythm, the sensitivity is decreased by 10% to 25%.

Table 5-7 describes the rate of recurrence of sudden death or arrhythmia in patients whose therapy was guided by electropharmacologic testing. Early reports suggested that the inability to induce a tachyarrhythmia was a good prognostic sign. Recent reports, however, describe a 35% recurrence at 18 months, similar to that of conventional therapy. Patients with inducible tachycardias that are suppressible with drugs or surgery have a much lower recurrence (0% to 33 % at 14 to 22 months) than do those patients whose arrhythmias are not suppressible (9% to 91%).

Electrophysiologic testing in the diagnosis and treatment of patients with sudden death and ventricular tachyarrhythmias has several limitations and uncertainties. The ideal stimulation protocol has yet to be determined. There is debate about the definition of a positive response. Is nonsustained (less than 30 seconds) polymorphic ventricular tachycardia an abnormal response with the more recent aggressive stimulation protocols? Electropharmacologic testing may not predict the clinical response of certain drugs, such as amiodarone. What is the role of invasive testing in patients with nonsustained ventricular tachycardia and torsade de pointes? Despite these limitations, electrophysiologic testing appears superior to conventional, empiric antiarrhythmic therapy. It identifies persons at high risk for recurrence and permits a more rational approach to drug therapy. In patients requiring cardiac electrosurgery or implantable antitachycardia devices it is essential.

Table 5-6. Stimulation Protocols Used in Electrophysiologic Studies in Patients with Ventricular Tachyarrhythmias

Study (Reference)	Number of Patients	Maximum No. Extra Stimuli	Sites Stimulated: *Right Ventricle (Multiple)*	Sites Stimulated: *Left Ventricle*	Isoproterenol	Burst Pacing	Definition of Minimum Positive Response
Ruskin[53]	31	2	N	N	Y	Y	three repetitive beats
Myerburg[52]	17	1	Y	N	N	Y	sustained ventricular tachycardia
Josephson[54]	50	2	N	Y	N	Y	nonsustained ventricular tachycardia
Vandepol[67]	529	2	Y	Y	N	Y	three repetitive beats
Fisher[71]	203	3	?	?	?	?	?
Ruskin[65]	82	?	?	?	?	?	three repetitive beats
Naccarelli[68]	83	2	Y	Y	N	Y	nonsustained ventricular tachycardia
Livelli[69]	100	2	Y	N	N	Y	three repetitive beats
Kehoe[72]	44	?	?	?	?	?	sustained ventricular tachycardia
Mason[73]	186	3	?	?	?	?	nonsustained ventricular tachycardia
Morady[55]	42	3	N	Y	Y	Y	six repetitive beats
Benditt[66]	34	3	N	N	N	Y	six repetitive beats
Roy[74]	119	3	Y	Y	Y	Y	sustained ventricular tachycardia (>30 sec)
Mann[70]	121	4	Y	N	N	Y	six repetitive beats

Y = Yes. N = No.

Evaluation of Symptoms

Despite extensive cardiac and neurologic evaluation, including ambulatory Holter monitoring, the etiology of transient neurologic and cardiovascular symptoms is often unclear.[79] In this setting, electrophysiologic testing may reveal the presence of arrhythmias or conduction abnormalities. Perhaps the most widely investigated symptom is syncope.[33,80–82] Prospective studies of unexplained syncope have demonstrated possible electro-

Table 5-7. Rate of Recurrence of Sudden Death or Ventricular Tachyarrhythmias Based on Therapy Guided by Electrophysiologic Testing

Study (Reference)	No. of Patients	Months of Follow-up	Inducible Arrhythmia: *Suppressed by RX* (%) Frequency	Inducible Arrhythmia: *Suppressed by RX* (%) Recurrence	Inducible Arrhythmia: *Nonsuppressed by RX* (%) Frequency	Inducible Arrhythmia: *Nonsuppressed by RX* (%) Recurrence	Noninducible Arrhythmia (%) Recurrence
Ruskin[53]	31	15	76	0	24	50	0
Mason[76]	51	18	67	32	33	89	
Kehoe[72]	44	14	64	0	36	78	0
Ruskin[65]	61	18	77	5	23	16	0
Horowitz[77]	111	18	59	6	41	91	
Morady[55]	45	22	26	33	74	9*	0
Schoenfeld[78]	72	16					11
Benditt[66]	34	18	62	5	15	40	38
Roy[74]	119	18	60	15	40	19*	32

* Some patients were treated with Amiodarone.

Table 5-8. Electrophysiologic Effects of Drugs

				Sinus Node			Atrium	AV Node				His-Purkinje		Ventricle	Accessory Pathway
Class	Drug	*QRS*	*QTc*	*SCL*	*SNRT*	*SACT*	*A-ERP*	*Threshold*	*AH*	*AV-ERP*	*AV-FRP*	*HV*	*HP-ERP*	*V-ERP*	*ERP*
I	Quinidine	+	+	0–	V	0+	+	+	V	V	0	0+	0+	+	+
	Procainamide	+	+	0–	0+	0+	+	+	0+	0–	0	0+	0+	+	+
	Disopyramide	+	+	0–	V	V	+	+	V	V	0	0+	0+	+	+
	Lidocaine	0	0+	0	0	0	0	0	0–	0–	0–	0	0–	0–	V
	Diphenylhydantoin	0	0–	–	0	0+	0	0–	0–	0–	0–	0	–	–	V
	Aprindine	+	0+	+			+	–	+	+	+	+	+	+	+
	Mexiletine	0	0	0–	0–		0	–	0+	0+	0+	0+	0+	0	+
	Tocainide	0	0–	0+		0	0–	0	0+	0–	0–	0	0–	0–	+
	Encainide	+	0+	0			0+	–	0+	0+	+	+	+	0+	+
	Flecainide	0+	0	0	+		0	0	+	0	0	+		0+	+
	Ajmaline						+	0+	0+	±	+	+	+	+	+
II	Propranolol	0	0–	+	+	+	0	–	0+	0+	+	0	0	0–	0
III	Bretylium	0	0+	0+	0		0–	0	0	V	–	0	–	–	
	Amiodarone	0	+	+	0	0	+	–	+	+	+	0+	+	+	+
IV	Verapamil	0	0	0+	0+	0	0	–	+	+	+	0	0	0	V
Other	Digoxin	0	–	0–			0–	–	+	+	+	0	0	–	0–
	Atropine			–	–	–	0	+	–	–	0–	0	0	0	0
	Isoproterenol			–	–	–	0–	+	–	–	–	0	0	0–	–

+ = Increase. – = Decrease. 0 = No significant change. V = Variable (reports of increases, decreases, and no significant change).

physiologic causes in 12% to 68% of patients. Factors that explain this variation include (1) different populations with respect to prevalence of underlying heart disease, (2) variable stimulation protocols, and (3) different definitions of significant electrophysiologic abnormalities and arrhythmias. Electrophysiologic testing has its highest diagnostic yield in patients with syncope and clinical evidence of organic heart disease. The importance of identifying the cause of syncope is emphasized by a recent study that demonstrated a 24% incidence of sudden death in patients with a cardiovascular etiology as compared with 4% in patients with a noncardiovascular cause.[79] In addition, if drug or pacemaker therapy is directed by the result of such testing, syncope rarely recurs. The evaluation of other possible arrhythmic-related symptoms such as palpatations or dizziness should include electrophysiologic testing only if noninvasive investigation has been unrevealing and symptoms are recurrent and disabling.

Electropharmacologic Testing

Antiarrhythmic drugs have different effects on the various electrophysiologic parameters of the heart (Table 5-8). Attempts have been made to use such effects on cardiac conduction, refractoriness, and automaticity to enhance the diagnostic sensitivity and specificity of electrophysiologic testing. The use of procainamide and Ajmaline to screen asymptomatic persons with Wolff-Parkinson-White syndrome is one such example.[45] The normalization of the QRS complex after administration of these agents suggests a long anterograde refractory period in the bypass tract. This correlates well with a slow ventricular response to spontaneous or induced atrial fibrillation and suggests a good prognosis in these patients.

Procainamide has been used in patients with bundle branch block during electrophysiologic testing in an attempt to provoke infra-Hisian block and thus identify persons at high risk for spontaneous AV block.[83,84] The results of these studies suggest only a limited role for this agent. Electrophysiologic testing may be of value to screen patients with sinus node dysfunction or conduction abnormalities before beginning antiarrhythmic therapy that may exacerbate these disorders. Measurements of electrophysiologic parameters after administration of drugs may identify patients at high risk to encounter worsening of bradyarrhythmias or conduction abnormalities during chronic use.[85] Studies have not been performed, however, to compare the benefit of electrophysiologic testing with drug administration compared to cautious empiric therapy with ambulatory monitoring.

Therapeutic Uses

Medical Therapy

Much of the rationale in using electropharmacologic testing in the treatment of tachyarrhythmias has been previously discussed. Major limitations in conventional empiric drug therapy include (1) the random nature of spontaneous tachycardias, (2) the lack of noninvasive parameters with which to guide therapeutic efficacy, (3) major morbidity and mortality associated with tachyarrhythmias, and (4) inadequate knowledge of the electrophysiologic mechanism of many arrythmias. The clinical use of electropharmacologic testing is based on its ability to induce the patient's underlying tachycardia. This then provides a reliable tool with which to judge drug efficacy rapidly. The ability of a drug to prevent the induction of a tachycardia has been shown to correlate with long-term efficacy in patients with a ventricular tachyarrhythmia. Similar findings using electropharmacologic therapy have been reported in patients with paroxysmal supraventricular tachycardia.[86,87]

Pacemaker Use

The decision to insert a permanent pacemaker for symptomatic bradyarrhythmias and conduction disorders can usually be made without invasive testing. Although most patients continue to receive single-chamber (VVI) models, during the past several years a wide array of dual-chamber pacemakers (DVI and DDD) have been introduced. Cost and technical complexity of the latter have limited their use despite evidence supporting the physiologic benefit of maintaining atrioventricular synchrony.[88] Hemodynamic assessment during ventricular or atrioventricular synchronous pacing provides a method to evaluate patients in whom the decision between implanting single and dual chamber models is difficult to make. Patients with existing VVI pacemakers who experience fatigue, exercise intolerance, symptomatic worsening of underlying cardiac disorders, and pacemaker syndrome may also be evaluated to assess the potential benefit of conversion to a dual-chamber system. Table 5-9 shows the results of such a study in a man with AV block and exercise intolerance. Ventricular pacing would have resulted in only modest increments in cardiac output with the additional burden of mitral regurgitation. Synchronized AV pacing, however, increased cardiac output without significant mitral regurgitation.

Pacing techniques learned in the electrophysiology laboratory have been expanded and are now applied in the treatment of patients with tachycardias.[89,90] Underdrive pacing, overdrive pacing, and the insertion of one or more extra stimuli have been used to terminate a wide array of reentrant tachyarrhythmias in the acute care setting.

Successful termination of atrial flutter by rapid atrial pacing has been reported in 75% of cases.[91] Rapid ventricular pacing and ventricular extra stimuli can terminate ventricular tachyarrhythmias in up to 79% of cases.[92] Currently under investigation are a wide variety of permanently implanted pacemakers with programmable features to terminate tachyarrhythmias.[93] Early models required patient activation, but recent technologic advances permit automatic sensing of the tachycardia and initiation of a preprogrammed termination sequence. These pacemakers are currently restricted to patients who are not candidates for or do not improve with conventional therapeutic approaches. In addition, extensive preimplant electrophysiologic testing is required to determine suitability for this mode of therapy and the most effective pacing termination sequence for the tachycardia. Another use of electrical stimulation in the treatment of patients with tachycardias has been the development of implantable automatic defibrillators. Early reports suggest a 52% decrease in mortality in patients using this device.[94]

Surgical Therapy

Despite the use of conventional or investigational antiarrhythmic drugs and implantable antitachycardia pacemakers, a number of patients continue to have disabling or life-threatening tachycardias. Electrophysiologic-guided surgical techniques have been developed to aid these persons.

Atrioventricular electrical connections include the normal AV node–His Purkinje system and accessory pathways. These connections may be a vital link in the reentrant pathway of a supraventricular arrhythmia such as orthodromic reciprocating tachycardia, or they may act as passive conduits for rapid atrial impulses such as in atrial flutter. Mechanical disruption of these connections will either terminate the arrhythmia in the former or block conduction to the ventricle in the latter.

Table 5-9. Hemodynamic Effects of Ventricular and AV Sequential Pacing

Pacing Rate	Pacing Mode	PA (mm)	PCW (mm)	CI (1/min/m)	SVI (1/min/m)	Comments
50		25/12	11	2.3	46	Baseline 2:1 AV block
70	Ventricular	28/15	15	2.69	38	6-mm ventricular waves
90	Ventricular	30/16	17	3.08	34	10-mm ventricular waves
110	Ventricular	34/18	19	2.74	25	16-mm ventricular waves
70	AV sequential	25/12	12	3.23	46	
90	AV sequential	26/13	12	3.72	41	4-mm ventricular waves
110	AV sequential	28/14	13	4.07	37	6-mm ventricular waves

If additional atrioventricular connections are not present, the ventricular rate subsequently becomes dependent on a junctional or ventricular escape focus or an implanted pacemaker. Intraoperative electrophysiologic studies are required to map the location of these pathways. Endocardial mapping with cryosurgical ablation of the AV node–His bundle has been successful in producing AV block in 17 of 22 patients with disabling supraventricular tachycardia.[95] Epicardial mapping has been used to locate accessory atrioventricular pathways. Surgical excision, based on mapping, was successful in ablating 80% of pathways in a recent report of patients with the Wolff-Parkinson-White syndrome.[96] Surgical mortality in both these studies was 0%.

Sustained ventricular tachyarrhythmias usually occur in the setting of severe coronary artery disease, often with prior infarction and aneurysm formation. Coronary artery revascularization and aneurysmectomy have been used to treat recurrent ventricular tachycardia in these patients. Early reports suggested short-term survivals as high as 87% with these techniques.[97] Recent studies have questioned these statistics and have reported arrhythmia recurrence rates of 50%.[97,98] Electrophysiologic studies have been performed, both preoperatively and postoperatively, on patients undergoing coronary revascularization for ventricular tachyarrhythmias; 40% had either spontaneously occurring or inducible ventricular tachycardia postoperatively.[99]

New electrophysiologic techniques can, by endocardial or epicardial mapping, localize early sites of ventricular activation during ventricular tachycardia. These areas are usually on the endocardial border zone of a myocardial scar and, when excised by a variety of surgical techniques, terminate the tachycardia and prevent its reinduction. With these procedures, the recurrence of tachyarrhythmias has been reported to be less than 30%.[98–100] These encouraging results suggest that electrophysiologically guided surgery is superior to conventional revascularization and aneurysmectomy in the treatment of patients with intractible ventricular tachyarrhythmias. Similar techniques have also been successfully used in patients with tachycardias unrelated to ischemic heart disease.[101]

Catheter Ablation

Despite the low mortality reported with surgical ablation of the AV node and accessory AV pathways, alternative techniques have been sought to avoid the cost and potential morbidity of an open-chest procedure. One such technique is catheter ablation. In this technique, a conventional pacing catheter is positioned through endocardial electrophysiologic mapping adjacent to the structure of interest and a synchronized direct current shock is delivered. Several groups have reported successful ablation of the AV node–His Purkinje region in patients with refractory supraventricular tachycardia.[102,103] Similar success has been reported in patients with accessory AV pathways, junctional ectopic arrhythmias, and focal ventricular tachycardias.[104–106]

Prognosis

Attempts have been made to use the data obtained during invasive electrophysiologic studies as markers for subsequent morbidity and mortality. This was initially done in patients with conduction disorders to identify those at high risk for complete heart block. As previously discussed, the tests have inadequate specificity in most such patients. Attempts to enhance the specificity by provocative drug administration in conjunction with electrophysiologic testing have also met with limited success in patients with conduction abnormalities and sinus node disorders.[83–85]

Numerous studies support the prognostic value of electrophysiologic testing in survivors of sudden cardiac death.[53,55,65,72,76–78] Noninducibility of ventricular tachyarrhythmias predicts a low rate of recurrence over subsequent months. Similarly, the inability to suppress medically or surgically an induced tachycardia is associated with recurrence rates as high as 90%. Two recent studies have questioned these findings.[66,74] Major limitations in comparing the results of these studies are the use of markedly different stimulation protocols and different definitions of a positive response. Using regression analysis, Swerdlow and associates were able to demonstrate that response to therapy during electrophysiologic study was an independent predictor of survival in patients with ventricular tachyarrhythmias.[107]

Electrophysiologic testing has recently been used in survivors of myocardial infarction to predict groups at high risk for sudden death.[108–110] Although such testing appears to have prognostic value, less invasive and costly techniques, such as determination of left ventricular ejection fraction, appear equally if not more valuable. Other areas in which investigation of the clinical use of electrophysiologic testing has begun include patients with stable coronary artery disease and nonsustained ventricular tachycardia.[111,112]

Methodology

Early electrophysiologic studies consisted of recording intracavitary electrical activity during spontaneous rhythms with conventional pacemaker electrodes. Current methodology uses electrodes in several intracardiac positions for simultaneous pacing and recording. An array of electrophysiologic parameters are then measured during both spontaneous and paced rhythms.

With programmed stimulation, a variety of arrhythmias can be induced and their electrical substrate defined through mapping techniques. Modalities for the treatment and prophylaxis of patients with such arrhythmias can also be evaluated. Each electrophysiologic study must be tailored to the individual patient to minimize time, cost, and morbidity. To provide such services, an investigator must be fully trained in all aspects of electrophysiology and have available a well-equipped catheterization laboratory.

Equipment

A fully equipped catheterization laboratory is a prerequisite. It must be adapted for electrophysiologic testing through the addition of special catheters, amplifiers, recording devices, and stimulators. Intracavitary electrical activity is best recorded from platinum ring electrodes incorporated into woven Dacron catheters. This form of construction allows good torque control, yet sufficient pliability exists to bend and loop the catheter within the vascular system for accurate positioning. The choice of catheter size is generally based on vessel size. No. 6 French catheters are routinely used in adults. Smaller sizes have better pliability but less torque control. Large catheters often have more electrodes or are lumenal; these have greater torque control but are stiffer and may increase the risk of vascular perforation. Intracardiac electrical activity is usually recorded in a bipolar fashion to evaluate local events. This requires at least two ring electrodes per catheter. Commercially available catheters have two (bipolar), three (tripolar), four (quadrapolar), or six (hexapolar) electrodes positioned 0.5, 1, or 2.5 cm apart. Closely positioned electrodes permit electrical activity to be recorded from small areas of endocardium. Accurate mapping studies require interelectrode distances of 1 cm or less.

Selection of an electrode catheter is based on its use in the individual patient. Bipolar catheters with an interelectrode distance of 1 cm are used for intracavitary recordings. If simultaneous pacing (two electrodes) and recording (two electrodes) are desired, a quadripolar catheter is necessary. His bundle potentials can usually be recorded from a bipolar catheter. Continuous His recording is sometimes not possible, however, because of an unstable catheter position. In that case, a tripolar or quadripolar catheter may allow a more stable position with a His potential recorded from one of the possible combinations of electrodes. Uniquely designed catheters are used in some clinical situations. For coronary sinus studies, we use a preshaped no. 7 French lumenal hexapolar catheter. Preshaping the catheter facilitates its introduction into the coronary sinus (Figs. 5-1 and 5-2).

Once positioned, electrode catheters are connected to appropriate amplifiers and recorders. Connecting cables should be shielded to minimize extraneous electrical noise. Sources of such 60-cycle interference include fluoroscopy equipment, overhead lights, and recording devices themselves. Cables must be kept as short as possible to reduce wave form distortion, while leakage currents are minimized to prevent induction of undesired arrhythmias. Before being permanently recorded, intracavitary electrical signals are amplified and filtered. Atrial and ventricular electrograms have an amplitude greater than 1 mV. His bundle potentials are smaller, and adequate visualization requires a sensitivity of 0.1 to 0.2 mV. Intracavitary electrograms are recorded primarily to time local cardiac electrical events. This requires reproduction of the local depolarizing wave front, a medium-frequency event. Examination of waveform morphology is less important. Conventional surface electrocardiographic records require an accurate reproduction of waveform morphology. ST segments, and repolarization phenomena such as T waves, are low-frequency events, and thus diagnostic electrocardiogram amplifiers use a 0.5- to 100-Hz frequency response. To eliminate these repolarization phenomena and other low-frequency events, respiration, body movement, tremor, and electrical interference special filters have been incorporated into intracardiac–His bundle amplifiers. Extremely high frequencies are excluded as well. Most commercial amplifiers use a frequency response of 40 to 500 Hz.

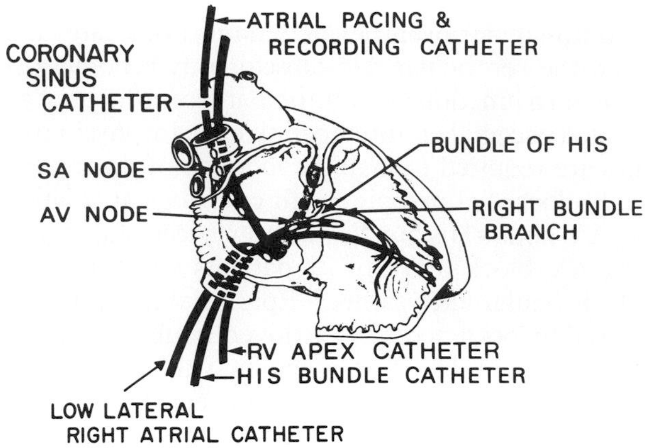

Figure 5-1. *Diagnostic representation of catheter placement for electrophysiologic investigations. Two catheters (atrial pacing, coronary sinus) are shown as they would be introduced from an arm, interval jugular, or subclavian entry site. They also may be introduced from the femoral venous route. The coronary sinus catheter should have multiple poles (see Fig. 5-2). The low atrial catheter may be of the mapping type (see Fig. 5-3). The atrial pacing catheter, when inserted from the femoral route, is usually positioned in the right atrial appendage. The His bundle catheter may also have four poles to allow recording of low atrial or right ventricular inflow electrograms.*

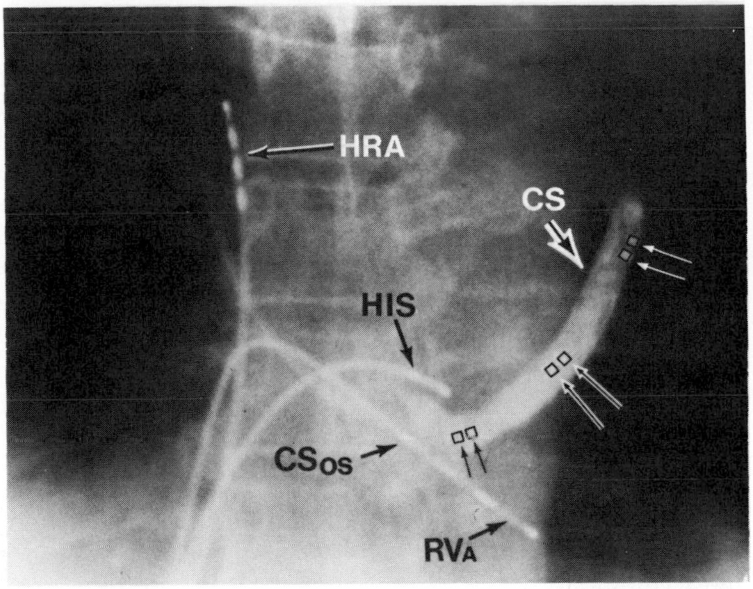

Figure 5-2. *Still frame from angiographic film during contrast injection from °A coronary sinus catheter. This no. 7 French catheter has three bipolar electrode pairs to record distal mid- and proximal coronary sinus electrograms. The coronary sinus and its atrium are easily identified. The catheter was introduced from a left medial antecubital vein via cutdown. Additional catheters, inserted via the femoral route are positioned in the high right atrium (HRA), His bundle (His), and right ventricular apex (RVa) regions.*

After the electrical signal has been amplified and filtered, it is visualized on an oscilloscope and recorded on hard copy. This permanent record can be made during the initial study or later if signals have been stored on a tape or disk recorder. Various available devices use ink jet, ultraviolet light, heat, or photographic techniques to produce a permanent record. Although considerable differences in cost and ease of use exist, all devices must be capable of frequency responses greater than 500 Hz at paper speeds of 100 to 200 mm/sec. High speeds are necessary to permit accurate measurement of closely timed electrical events with a resolution of 5 to 10 msec. The recording system must have multiple channels to permit simultaneous visualization of surface and intracardiac electrical events. Ideally, three surface leads, I, aV_F, and V_1, should be used for accurate analysis of P wave or QRS morphology. Most electrophysiologic studies require two or three intracardiac channels, but additional channels may be needed in some clinical situations. One to two channels should also be available for hemodynamic measurements. If not already integrated into the system, a channel should be available to provide time markers. In complex studies, a marker channel to identify electrical stimuli is also useful. An eight-channel oscilloscope and recorder is usually satisfactory to meet these needs.

The system described above is adequate to evaluate electrical events present during spontaneous rhythms. The introduction of programmed stimulation techniques has expanded the use of these systems. Conventional external pacing devices permit simple incremental pacing, which is sufficient to evaluate sinus node recovery time and AV Wenckebach threshold. Sophisticated electrophysiologic testing, including the induction and termination of arrhythmias, requires a more versatile stimulator. Several models are currently available. Important features include (1) incremental pacing from less than 60 beats/min to greater than 500 beats/min, (2) multiple channels for dual chamber pacing, (3) a variable, constant current source to regulate current output at different pacing thresholds, (4) at least three programmable extra stimuli, and (5) the ability to sense intracardiac electrocardiograms and synchronize stimulation to these events. In addition to shielding connecting cables, all equipment must be well grounded and inspected for leakage currents. These should be less than 10 μamps to minimize accidental induction of potentially lethal cardiac arrhythmias. A defibrillator, which can be synchronized off intracardiac or surface leads, is also needed.

Catheterization Technique

Patients are prepared for electrophysiologic testing just as for conventional diagnostic cardiac catheterization. Food and liquids are withheld for 6 hours before study. Essential medications can be continued, but drugs with antiarrhythmic properties should be stopped for at least five half-lives. In some situations, it may be clinically important to continue antiarrhythmic agents. An example would be a patient being tested for ventricular arrhythmias who is taking therapeutic doses of digoxin to control the ventricular response in atrial fibrillation. In this situation, digoxin should be continued to prevent an acceleration in ventricular rate, but its electrophysiologic effects should be carefully considered. Diazepam can be used if a sedative is required, since it has no major direct electrophysiologic effects.[113] This and similar agents, however, may have indirect electrophysiologic effects because they affect the central nervous system. Lidocaine is used for local anesthesia during catheter insertion. It is preferable to use a 1% solution and limit the total dose to less than 2.5 mg/kg body weight (0.25 ml/kg of 1% solution, or 17.5 ml for a 70-kg person). Larger subcutaneous doses have been shown to result in therapeutic blood concentrations of lidocaine.[114]

Most electrode catheters are positioned in the right heart and thus require access to the venous system. The modified percutaneous Seldinger technique is preferred because of the ease and speed of access, simplicity of catheter exchange and removal, and ability to reuse the vein for subsequent studies. A large vein, as in the femoral area, will accommodate two or more no. 6 French catheters. Direct venous exposure through a cutdown is occasionally used in the upper extremities when a percutaneous procedure is not possible or a special large catheter must be introduced into a small vein. Venous access can be obtained from the femoral, antecubital, subclavian, and internal jugular veins. The femoral veins are most commonly used. Upper extremity veins are of value when additional catheters are needed or the femoral veins cannot be safely cannulated. Use of antecubital veins may facilitate catheterization of the coronary sinus and are often used when a catheter is left in position on completion of the study. Subclavian and jugular veins have been used but may lead to a higher incidence of complications, particularly pneumothorax.[115] Catheters are ultimately positioned in their appropriate intracardiac locations through fluoroscopic visualization. This can be confirmed by recording intracavitary electrograms, using lumenal catheters, examining pressure waveforms, and injecting dye. The choice of catheter location and technical features for accurately positioning each catheter are described below and in Table 5-10. Although the risk of thromboembolic complications is low, 2500 to 5000 U of heparin is routinely administered in procedures lasting longer than 2 hours or when a catheter is introduced into the arterial circulation.

Table 5-10. Common Electrode Catheter Locations in Electrophysiologic Studies

	Type of Study	
Location	*Recording*	*Pacing*
Right atrium	Sinus node SVT Mapping	Sinus node SVT AV conduction
Left atrium	SVT Mapping	SVT
His bundle catheter	AV conduction VA conduction SVT VT	Confirm catheter position
Right ventricle	SVT VT Mapping	SVT VT VA conduction
Left ventricle	VT Mapping	VT
Coronary sinus	As per left atrium and left ventricle	As per left atrium and left ventricle

SVT, supraventricular tachycardias (includes evaluation of bypass tracts); VT, ventricular tachyarrhythmias; AV conduction, anterograde conduction through the AV node–His-Purkinje system; VA conduction, retrograde conduction through the AV node–His-Purkinje system.

Catheter Placement

Right Atrium

Electrode catheters can be positioned in the right atrium from a variety of access sites, although stable recording and pacing may be difficult to maintain because of poor endocardial contact. The atrial appendage provides a stable catheter position and is easily approached from the femoral vein. J-tipped temporary pacing catheters now facilitate entry into the appendage from upper extremity veins.[116] Patients who have undergone open heart surgery with cardiopulmonary bypass have had their atrial appendages ligated. A remnant stump is often present, which may allow a stable catheter position. Another commonly used location is the high posterolateral wall near the origin of the superior vena cava. This location also facilitates direct recordings of sinus node activity.[117] Accurate positioning of catheters is important when atrial mapping is performed. In addition to the high right atrium and atrial appendage, other commonly used right atrium sites include the low right atrium at the junction of the inferior vena cava, the os of the coronary sinus, and the AV junction near the tricuspid valve[118] (see Figs. 5-1 and 5-2). The latter is best recorded in conjunction with His bundle studies. (Mapping of the tricuspid ring is facilitated with the use of a bipolar catheter with a steerable tip [Fig. 5-3].) Common clinical uses for right atrial catheters are listed in Table 5-10.

Left Atrium

Direct placement of an electrode catheter in the left atrium is rarely required. Most atrial electrical studies can be performed from the right atrium. Additional sites are needed, however, in evaluating patients with supraventricular tachyarrhythmias and accessory atrioventricular connections. Although the left atrium can be entered directly through a patent foramen ovale or transseptal puncture or retrogradely across the mitral valve, indirect approaches are preferred. Catheters positioned in the coronary sinus, main pulmonary artery, and esophagus have been used for left atrial recording and pacing. The coronary sinus location allows catheter stability with both recording and pacing capabilities. The main pulmonary artery is useful for recording electrical

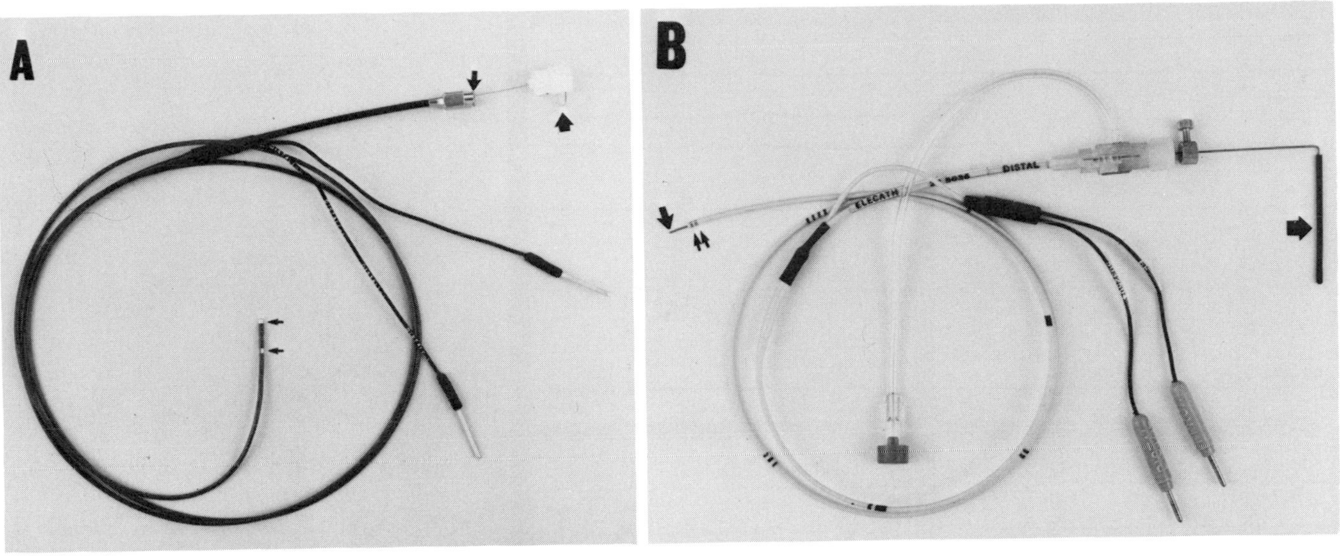

Figure 5-3. *Two types of mapping catheters for use in recording bipolar electrograms from multiple sites. The tips of these catheters can be manipulated with the use of a stiff guide wire, which is inserted and positioned according to the position of its distal "handle." The catheter in A has no lumen, whereas the catheter in B has both a lumen and a side arm for flushing. These catheters are most useful for mapping the tricuspid ring in patients with WPW syndrome, but they are also useful for mapping the right atrium and possibly the left ventricle.*

signals when other techniques are not possible, but left atrial pacing from this site is not practical. Esophageal leads have been used for both recording and pacing. Recent reports, however, suggest that the electrogram recorded from this position reflects paraseptal atrial depolarization rather than true left atrial activation.

His Bundle Electrograms

His bundle recordings are used in most electrophysiologic studies. They are necessary to evaluate anterograde and retrograde AV conduction, supraventricular arrhythmias, and the etiology of wide QRS tachycardias. During ventricular tachycardia studies they are used to confirm a ventricular origin. His bundle pacing has been used to confirm proper catheter position but has limited clinical value. The His bundle recording is best obtained from a bipolar catheter inserted through a femoral vein. It is advanced into the right ventricle and then withdrawn using clockwise torque with final positioning near the septal leaflet of the tricuspid valve (see Fig. 5-1). The endocardial electrogram is recorded during catheter positioning. With the catheter in the right ventricle, a large ventricular electrogram with little or no atrial activity is recorded. As the catheter is withdrawn, the ventricular electrogram becomes smaller as the atrial signal increases. His bundle activity is a biphasic or triphasic signal located between the atrial and ventricular electrograms. The ideal His bundle recording is that recorded with the largest atrial potential, representing proximal His activity in the membranous atrial septum (Fig. 5-4). This is often found with approximately equal atrial and ventricular electrograms. It is extremely important to scan the entire His bundle area (Fig. 5-4). The normal His bundle potential has a duration of 15 to 20 msec, with an HV interval of 35 to 55 msec. Intra-Hisian abnormalities with a split or widened His potential may be missed unless the entire area is adequately explored and recorded.[121] An HV interval less than 30 msec may reflect recording of a right bundle branch potential rather than true His bundle activity. If a stable His bundle recording is not achieved despite repeated attempts at positioning, a tripolar or quadrapolar catheter can be used. This catheter is positioned in a similar fashion with recordings made between various pairs of electrodes. Using this technique, an adequate His bundle can be recorded in over 90% of patients. Procedures for obtaining His bundle studies using upper extremity or retrograde arterial approaches have been described but are technically more difficult and are rarely necessary.

Right Ventricle

Electrode catheters are positioned in the right ventricle to evaluate retrograde ventriculoatrial conduction, supraventricular tachycardia, and ventricular tachycardia. The right ventricular apex is the most widely used position and can easily be approached from both upper and lower extremity veins (see Fig. 5-1). Additional sites, such as the inflow and outflow tracts, may be needed for

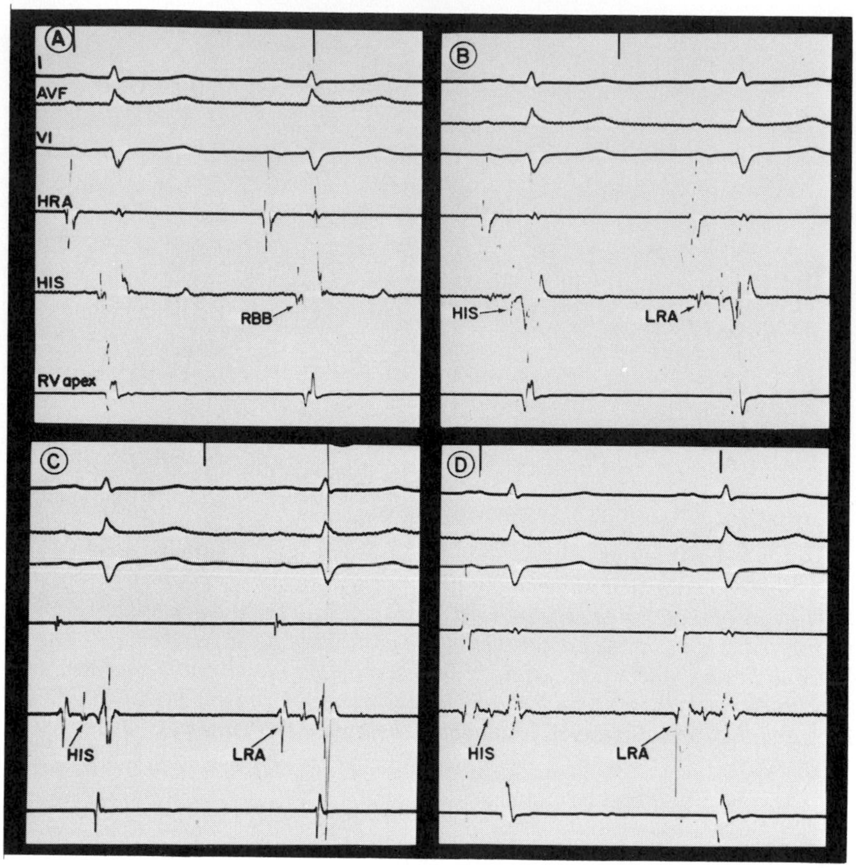

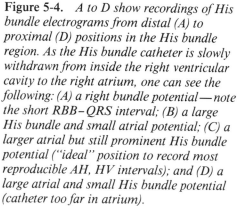

Figure 5-4. *A to D show recordings of His bundle electrograms from distal (A) to proximal (D) positions in the His bundle region. As the His bundle catheter is slowly withdrawn from inside the right ventricular cavity to the right atrium, one can see the following: (A) a right bundle potential—note the short RBB–QRS interval; (B) a large His bundle and small atrial potential; (C) a larger atrial but still prominent His bundle potential ("ideal" position to record most reproducible AH, HV intervals); and (D) a large atrial and small His bundle potential (catheter too far in atrium).*

pacing and mapping in the investigation of ventricular tachycardia.

Left Ventricle

Left ventricular pacing may be required to initiate ventricular tachyarrhythmias if they cannot be induced by conventional right ventricle pacing. Detailed mapping of these arrhythmias also requires access to the left ventricle. Left ventricle pacing and electrogram recording may rarely be needed in evaluating patients with supraventricular tachycardia. Retrograde arterial catheterization is the most widely used technique and allows access to multiple left ventricular sites, including aneurysms.

Coronary Sinus

The coronary sinus is a venous structure that lies in the posterior AV groove. An electrode catheter in this location allows indirect electrogram recording and pacing of both the left atrium and ventricle, which is useful for many clinical situations in which electrophysiologic evaluation of these chambers is needed. Coronary sinus pacing and recording is used to locate accessory AV connections in patients with supraventricular arrhythmias. Direct left atrium catheters are rarely needed if stable coronary sinus pacing and recording is achieved. The coronary sinus is also adjacent to the posterobasal portion of the left ventricle, and ventricular pacing can be achieved in 50% to 75% of patients. If stable left ventricular pacing cannot be achieved, or if detailed ventricular mapping is required, retrograde arterial catheterization is necessary.

Because of the anatomic arrangement of the os of the coronary sinus, it is best cannulated with a catheter inserted from the left arm. We use a preshaped no. 7 French hexapolar lumenal catheter (see Figs. 5-1 and 5-2). Continuous recording of a pressure waveform from a catheter tip during insertion facilitates its placement. Inadvertent advancement of the catheter into the right ventricle rather than the coronary sinus is immediately recognized by a change from a venous to a ventricular waveform. Proper catheter position can be confirmed by several methods. Fluoroscopic location is of value but may be misleading if the coronary sinus is short or the catheter cannot be fully advanced. A lumenal catheter permits analysis of the pressure waveform recorded at the distal tip and injection of renograffin dye to opacify the coronary sinus. Further confirmation is provided by recording left atrial and left ventricular electrograms or by the appearance of a left atrial or left ventricular rhythm during coronary sinus pacing.

Table 5-11. Complications From Electrophysiologic Studies

Complication	Percentage of Patients
Hemmorrhage	<1
Phlebitis/thromboembolism	0.2–2.2
Infection	0.6–1.7
Arrhythmias	
Requiring cardioversion	17
Unsuccessful cardioversion	0
Myocardial infarction or CVA	0
Mortality	0

Complications

Despite the use of multiple intracardiac catheters and lengthy studies, the incidence of complications in electrophysiologic studies is similar to conventional diagnostic catheterizations[115,122] (Table 5-11). The use of multiple catheters increases the risk of significant bleeding. Careful attention to venous and arterial access sites immediately after catheter removal and minimal patient movement for several hours lower the risk of hemorrhage. A low rate of phlebitis and thromboembolic phenomena can be achieved by careful catheterization technique by experienced physicians. Systemic heparin is used for procedures lasting longer than 2 hours or when a catheter is introduced into the arterial circulation. Infection is minimized by proper sterile technique. Antibiotics are not routinely used. In a subclavian or internal jugular approach, care must be taken to avoid pneumothorax.

Arrhythmias are often initiated during electrophysiologic testing and can occur in patients without known clinical arrhythmias. These are usually self-terminating or nonsustained atrial or ventricular tachyarrhythmias. Hemodynamic stability is determined by the rate of the tachycardia, its duration, and the patient's underlying cardiovascular status. Hemodynamically unstable rhythms must be quickly terminated with programmed stimulation techniques or, if this is unsuccessful, electrical cardioversion. The success rate of cardioversion approaches 100% because of the controlled setting and termination of arrhythmias before irreversible metabolic derangements arise. (A significant advance in cardioversion and defibrillation has occurred with the use of adhesive electrode patches connected directly to the defibrillator [Fig. 5-5].) Extreme caution must be exercised, however, in testing patients with unstable clinical conditions. Electrophysiologic studies should be deferred in such patients until they have been stabilized, especially those with severe left ventricular dysfunction. If patients are chosen carefully, and the above precautions are taken, the mortality from electrophysiologic testing, even in patients with malignant ventricular arrhythmias, should approach 0%.

Conduction Intervals and Refractory Periods

Electrical activity is conducted through the heart through a series of specialized tissues with different electrophysiologic characteristics. Measureable parameters have been devised to assess these characteristics and distinguish normal from pathologic conditions. The two most commonly used are *conduction intervals* and *re-*

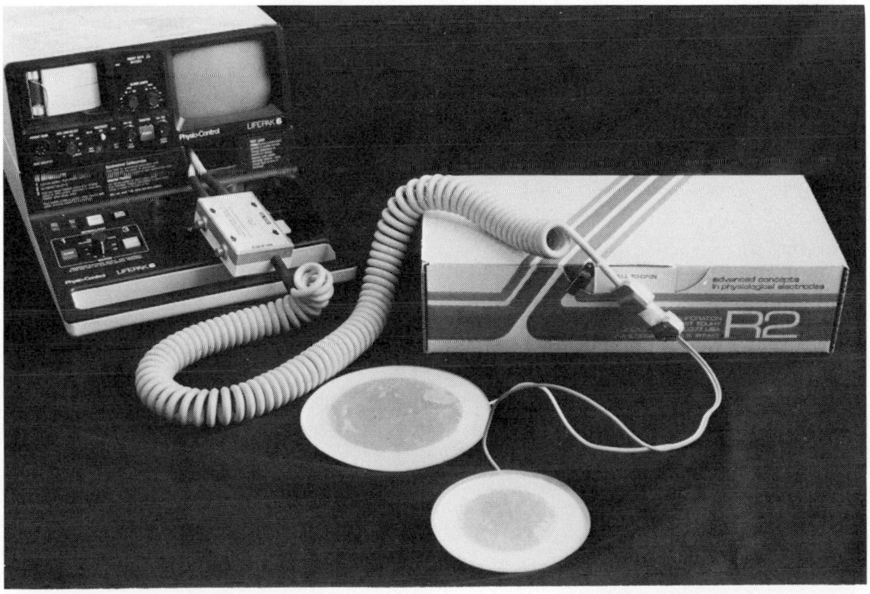

Figure 5-5. *A commercially available defibrillator pad system, which allows a "hands-off" operation in the case of rapid application of D/C transthoracic shock(s).*

fractory periods. The former refers to the time taken for a single spontaneous or paced electrical impulse to traverse one or more portions of the cardiac conduction system. The latter assesses the ability of a tissue to conduct two sequential electrical impulses.

Table 5-12. Normal Conduction Intervals

Study (Reference)	PA	AH	H	HV
Castellanos[123]	20–50	50–120		25–55
Gallagher[124]	24–45	60–140	10–15	30–55
Josephson[125]		60–125	10–25	35–55
Narula[126]	25–60	50–120	25	35–45
Rosen[127]	9–45	54–130		31–55
Ross and Mandel	20–45	60–125		35–55

Conduction Intervals

A conduction interval is merely a measurement of the time it takes for electrical activity to spread through the portion of the heart under study. Surface electrocardiograms have crudely examined atrial, AV, and ventricular conduction through P, PR, and QRS durations. The use of multiple electrodes and recordings made at high paper speeds (≥ 100 mm/sec) permits accurate measurement of a variety of intracardiac conduction times. The most commonly used intervals are as follows:

PA — measure of intra-atrial conduction. The interval from onset of the P wave on surface leads to onset of low atrial activity in the His bundle recording.

AH — measure of low atrial and AV node conduction. The interval from onset of low atrial activity to onset of His potential; both are measured in the His bundle recording.

His potential — measure of conduction through the

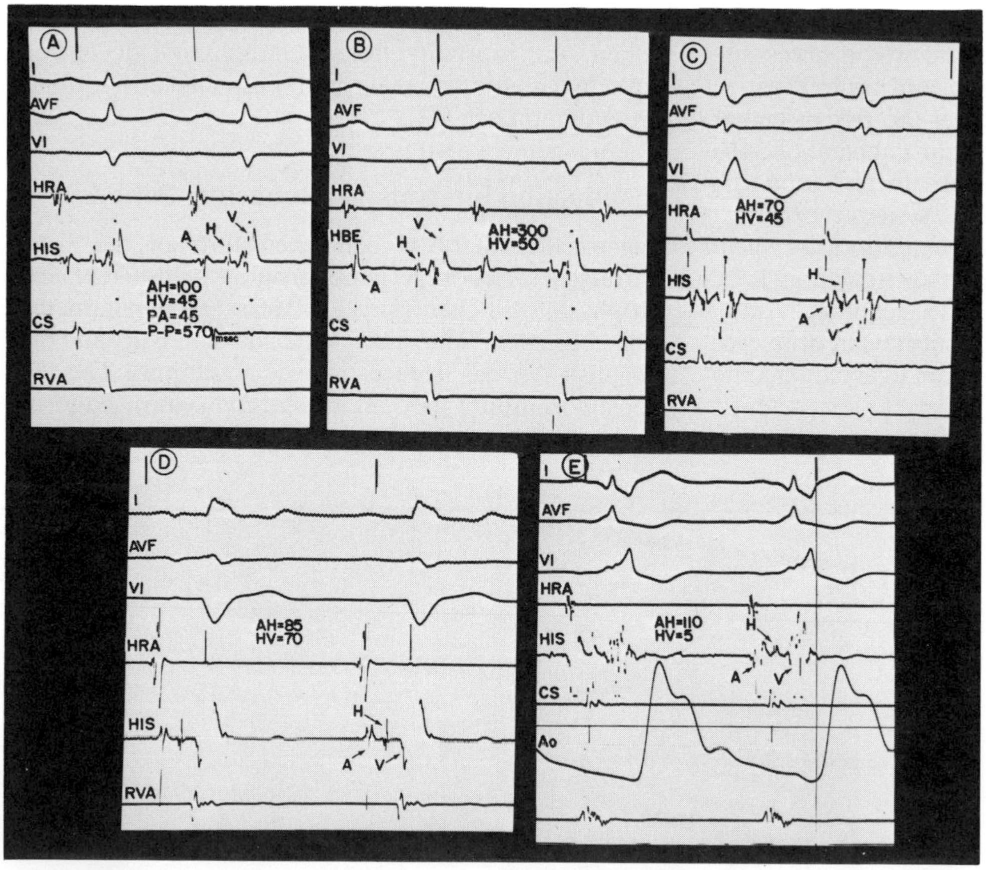

Figure 5-6. *A to E show recordings of three surface ECG leads (I, Avf, V_1) and electrogram recordings from the high right atrium (HRA), His bundle region (His), coronary sinus (CS), and right ventricular apex (RVA). AH and HV intervals are listed for all panels. In A the AH, HV, and PA intervals are all normal. In B there is a marked prolongation of the AH interval. In C, in a patient with RBBB, the AH and HV intervals are also normal. However, in D, in a patient with LBBB, the HV is prolonged (70 msec). Finally, E shows data from a patient with ventricular preexcitation (WPW syndrome). Note the normal AH interval but the very short HV (QRS) interval of only 5 msec.*

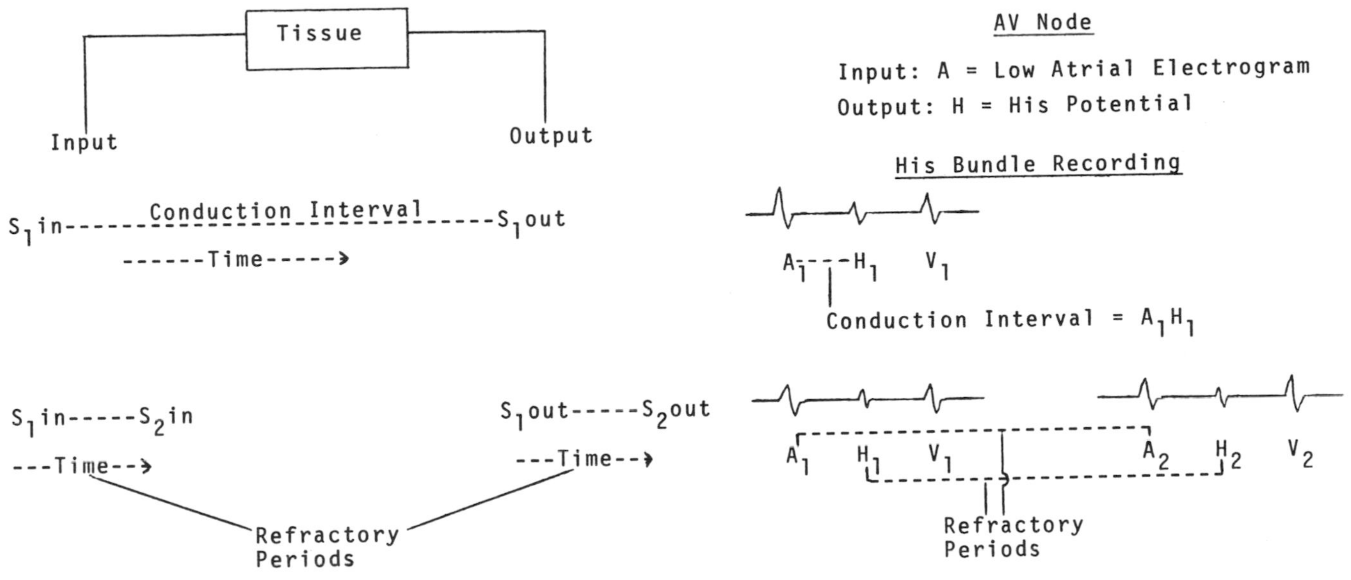

Refractory Period*	Definition*	AV Node*
Relative	$(S_1S_2)out > (S_1S_2)in$	$H_1H_2 > A_1A_2$
Effective	No S_2 out	No H_2
Functional	Shortest $(S_1S_2)out$	Shortest H_1H_2

S_1 = First Impulse
S_2 = Second Impulse
* = See text for details

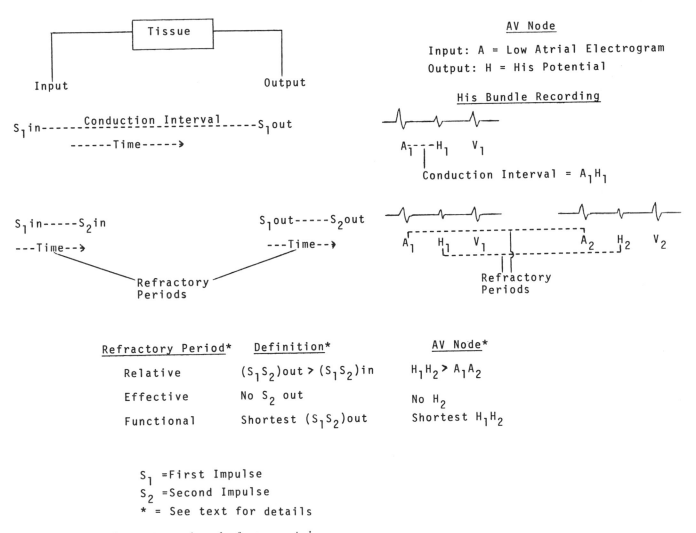

Figure 5-7. *Conduction intervals and refractory periods.*

His bundle. The interval from onset to conclusion of the His potential in the His bundle recording.

HV—measure of His-Purkinje conduction. The interval from onset of His potential in the His bundle recording to the earliest onset of ventricular activation in any intracardiac or surface leads.

Reported normal values are listed in Table 5-12. The variation noted reflects different populations, number of persons studied, catheter positions, criteria for measurements, and statistical methods used. Our normal range reflects the techniques and measurements described above as applied to 243 patients between 1981 and 1983. This represents 85% of all electrophysiologic studies performed during that period. Fifty-three patients were excluded because they were taking medications that might have affected electrophysiologic parameters; thus 190 patients were available for comparison. To define the normal population for each parameter, patients with a clinical or electrophysiologic diagnosis that might significantly affect the measured variable were excluded. As an example, all patients referred for testing for AV block would be excluded from the determination of the normal range of AH and HV intervals. For each group, the 10th through 90th percentile of measured values was used as the normal range.

Determination of these intervals requires a His bundle catheter and one or more surface leads (Figs. 5-1, 5-4, and 5-6). Abnormal autonomic tone or cardiac drugs (Table 5-8) may markedly alter these intervals. Although measurements are usually made in spontaneous sinus rhythm, their response to incremental pacing can be of clinical value. As with other cardiac structures, a stress applied to the conduction system, such as pacing, may unmask otherwise occult disorders. An abrupt increase in the HV interval during slow atrial pacing can indicate His–Purkinje system dysfunction. Quantitative analysis of the effect of pacing is limited for several reasons. Pacing from different sites can result in varying intervals because of altered atrial activation and entry into the

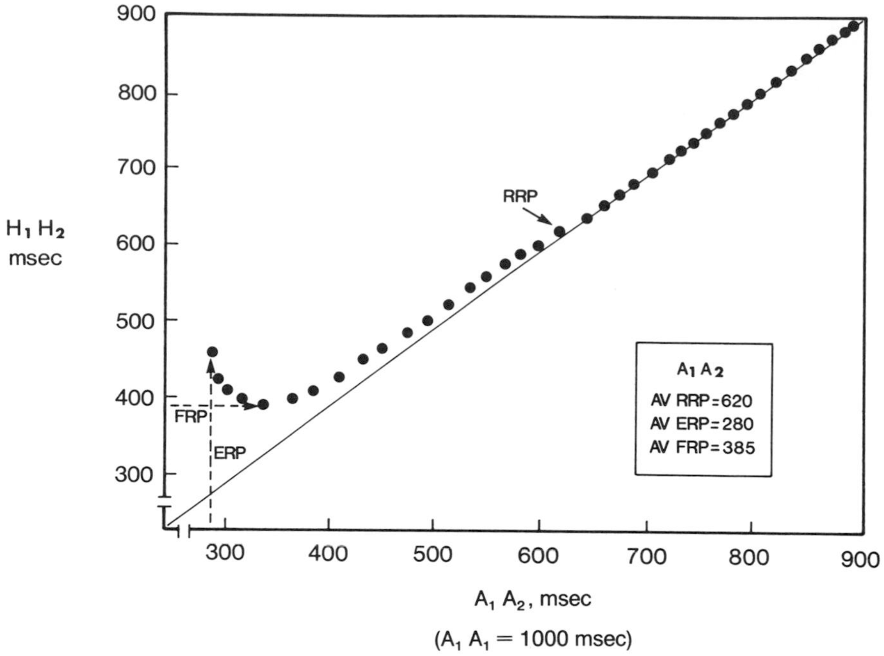

Figure 5-8. *Graph of test stimulus intervals (S_1S_2) on the horizontal axis versus response intervals (H_1H_2) obtained from the His bundle recordings to determine the AV nodal refractory periods. The relative refractory period (RRP) of the AV node begins when there is deviation off the line of identity. The functional refractory period of the AV node (FRF) is the shortest H_1H_2 interval observed. The effective refractory period of the AV node (ERP) is the shortest A_1A_2 interval that conducts to the His bundle.*

conduction system. Rapid pacing may cause catheter artifact and movement, making accurate measurements difficult. Finally, faster heart rates can produce hemodynamic changes that alter autonomic tone and thus indirectly influence conduction intervals.

Refractory Periods

Refractory periods evaluate the capacity of tissues to conduct two sequential impulses. The second impulse is a paced beat; the first can be spontaneous or paced. Refractory periods do not directly measure conduction time. This difference is illustrated in Figure 5-7. It describes a portion of the conduction system with the AV node used as an example. Electrical activity is recorded from electrodes positioned near the input and output of this system. For the AV node, both input (low atrial electrogram) and output (His bundle potential) are measured from the same electrode. For other tissues, separate electrodes may be needed. The conduction interval is the absolute time taken for a single impulse (S_1) to travel through the tissue—in the case of the AV node, the AH interval (A_1H_1).

Refractory periods analyze the difference in conduction between two consecutive impulses, S_1 (spontaneous or paced) and S_2 (paced). They describe not absolute conduction time, but rather the delay between impulses as they exit a tissue compared with the delay at their input. The more closely coupled the two impulses, the more likely the second will encounter refractoriness and delay during its conduction. Refractoriness results in a longer S_1 S_2 interval measured at output than that measured at input. For the AV node, the exit delay (H_1H_2) is compared with the input coupling interval (A_1A_2). If refractoriness is absent, there is no difference in conduction between the two impulses, and A_1A_2 equals H_1H_2. This is usually observed at relatively long coupling intervals between S_1 and S_2. As the second impulse becomes more premature, it will encounter refractoriness and consequently take longer to conduct through the AV node. Thus H_1H_2 becomes longer than A_1A_2, or, put in another way, the AH conduction interval of S_2 becomes longer than that of S_1. The longest coupling interval (A_1A_2) at which this occurs is the relative refractory period of the tissue. This can be illustrated by a graph of the coupling interval at the input versus the output (Fig. 5-7*A*). The coupling interval measured at the output of the AV node (H_1H_2) will be influenced by the degree of prematurity (shortening H_1H_2 because A_1A_2 is less) and the amount of refractoriness encountered (lengthening H_1H_2 because of delayed conduction with increasing A_2H_2). As shown in Figure 5-8, with more premature impulses, the H_1H_2 interval continues to decrease but

Table 5-13. Measurements Necessary to Determine Refractory Periods

Anterograde Conduction		
Structure	*Input*	*Output*
Atrium	S_1S_2	A_1A_2
AV node	A_1A_2	H_1H_2
H-P system	H_1H_2	V_1V_2
Entire conduction system	S_1S_2	V_1V_2
Retrograde Conduction		
Structure	*Input*	*Output*
Ventricle	S_1S_2	V_1V_2
H-P system	V_1V_2	H_1H_2*
AV node	H_1H_2*	A_1A_2
Entire conduction system	S_1S_2	A_1A_2

* Retrograde His potential. S, stimulus artifact; A, atrial electrogram; H, His bundle potential; V, ventricular electrogram; 1, first impulse; 2, second impulse.

more slowly because of increasing refractoriness. A point is often reached at which the increment in conduction delay is greater than the decrement in prematurity, and the H_1H_2 interval actually becomes longer than it was for less premature impulses. This represents the ascending limb of the refractory period curve. Eventually a point comes at which complete refractoriness exists. The second impulse is then blocked within the AV node, and no output (H_2) is recorded. The effective refractory period (ERP) is the longest coupling interval (A_1A_2) at which there is *no* conduction. Examination of the curve shows that there is a minimum output interval (H_1H_2) over the entire range of conducted premature impulses; this represents the functional refractory period (FRP).

Refractory periods have been determined for a variety of tissues in both an anterograde and retrograde direction. The input and output signals necessary to access these are listed in Table 5-13. Table 5-14 shows reported normal ranges for commonly measured refractory periods. In addition to different absolute refractory periods, various cardiac tissues demonstrate different refractory period curves. The AV node often has a prominent ascending curve, and its FRP is significantly greater than its ERP. Atrial and ventricular refractory period curves usually lie close to the line of identity, with their FRP often being only 10 to 30 msec greater than their ERP.

Note that the FRP and ERP are defined as coupling intervals measured at the input of the system, at which point critical conduction changes occur, whereas the FRP is defined as an interval measured at the output. Thus to characterize fully the refractory periods of a tissue, one must be able to measure electrical events on each side. This can be difficult in many situations. AV node refractory periods are measured based on differences between A_1A_2 and H_1H_2, but this requires no limitation in atrial refractoriness during the insertion of premature stimuli. If the atrial FRP is greater than the AV node ERP, the latter can never be accurately determined because refractoriness in the atrium limits the degree of prematurity of input into the AV node; this occurs in 36% of patients. It is often difficult to assess retrograde conduction in the His–Purkinje system because of the inability to record a retrograde His bundle potential in many cases. Refractoriness can be influenced by many factors. Drugs and changes in autonomic tone can have considerable impact on measured values (see Table 5-8). In addition, the basic heart rate at which a refractory period is measured also has an impact. Refractory periods of the atrium, His–Purkinje system, and ventricle shorten with faster heart rates, whereas those of the AV node lengthen.

Principles of Arrhythmia Induction and Termination

Recent research supports the concept that several electrophysiologic mechanisms can cause arrhythmias, including enhanced automaticity, delayed after potentials, triggered automaticity, and reentry.[131] The latter is thought responsible for more than 90% of supraventricular and ventricular tachyarrhythmias. Current electro-

Table 5-14. Normal Refractory Periods

Study (Reference)	ERP Atrium	FRP Atrium	ERP AVN	FRP AVN	ERP HPS	ERP V
Akhtar[128]	230–330		280–430	320–680	340–430	190–290
Denes[129]	150–360	190–390	250–365	350–495		
Josephson[125]	170–300		230–425	330–525	330–450	170–290
Schuilenburg[130]			230–390	330–500		
Ross and Mandel	200–300	235–340	260–430*	355–550		205–270

* AV node ERP limited by atrial FRP in 36% of patients. AVN, AN node; HPS, His–Purkinje system; V, ventricle.

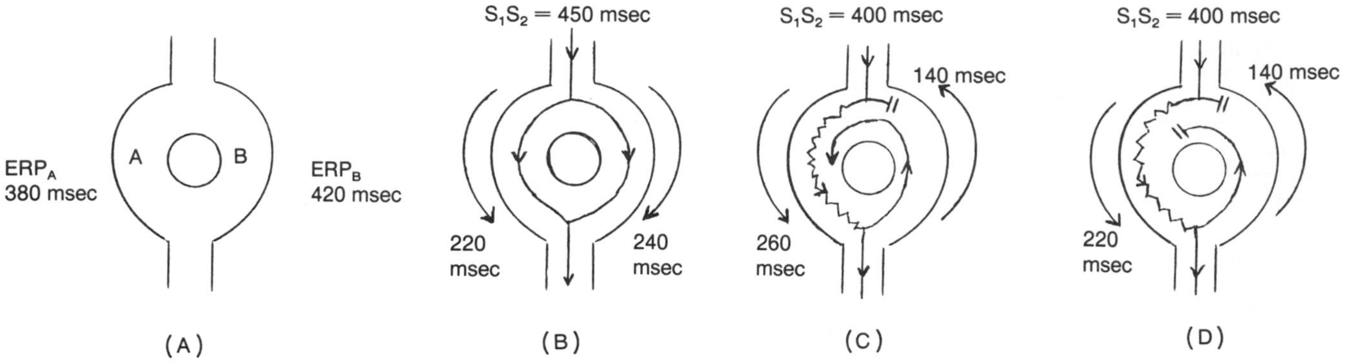

Figure 5-9. *Schematic of AV nodal activity in a patient with dual AV nodal pathways. See text for discussion.*

physiologic techniques are most suitable for initiating and terminating triggered and reentrant arrhythmias. Automatic arrhythmias are diagnosed by their inability to be initiated or terminated by electrophysiologic techniques and the characteristic common to most automatic foci, overdrive suppression. Reentrant arrhythmias are initiated and terminated by incremental pacing and extra stimulus techniques. Under pathologic conditions, tissues or portions thereof may exhibit variable refractoriness. In this setting, these electrophysiologic techniques alter conduction and cause unidirectional block, which is critical to the initiation of reentrant events.

Figure 5-9 illustrates these principles in more detail. An area of the conduction system is illustrated that has two limbs with different refractoriness. These limbs join proximally and distally and have the capacity, as do most cardiac tissues, for anterograde and retrograde conduction. Conduction times through each pathway are listed when appropriate. Dispersion of refractoriness is illustrated by the longer anterograde ERP of pathway B. As shown in Panel B, if two sequential impulses are introduced with a coupling interval of 450 msec, both are conducted in a normal anterograde fashion through each limb. Conduction is intact, although conduction times may vary through each portion. In Panel C, two impulses are introduced with a coupling interval of 400 msec. This is close to the effective refractory period of A; thus conduction may slow but remains intact. Anterograde conduction through B is blocked, however, because the coupling interval is shorter than the ERP of that path. Because of slowed conduction through A, as the impulse reaches its distal connection with pathway B it finds the latter no longer refractory and capable of conducting in a retrograde direction. The transit time around the reentrant circuit is 400 msec, which allows time for pathway A to recover from its refractoriness and conduct another anterograde cycle. The resulting tachycardia will have a cycle length of 400 msec, equivalent to a rate of 150 beats/min. The arrhythmia can be terminated by the introduction of one or more critically timed impulses into the circuit, which induce additional unidirectional or bidirectional blocks and stop the reentrant wave front.

This example uses a single extra stimulus to initiate the arrhythmia. In some cases, the critical degree of refractoriness cannot be reached and a second or third extra stimulus is needed. Multiple extra stimuli allow refractoriness to be "peeled back." Refractory periods vary with different physiologic conditions, including the rate at which a tissue is being paced and the coupling interval of previously introduced extra stimuli. Using Figure 5-9*D* as an example, let us examine the effect of inserting a single extra stimulus, S_2, with a coupling interval of 400 msec but without the marked delay in conduction through limb A. Let us assume that this conduction time is only 220 msec. Unidirectional anterograde block will still occur in limb B. If retrograde conduction occurs through limb B, the transit time of the reentrant cycle would be 360 msec, rather than the 400 msec noted in Panel C. Such a rapid circuit time would result in anterograde block in pathway A after the first circuit because its anterograde refractory period is only 380 msec. A second or third extra stimulus is used to peel back this refractory period. The first extra stimulus (S_2) is introduced just beyond its effective refractory period—in this case, at approximately 390 msec, permitting conduction. A second extra stimulus (S_3) is then introduced with progressively closer and closer coupling intervals. Using this procedure, the effective refractory period of S_3 will be less than S_2 and so on, if a third extra stimulus (S_4) is introduced.

The use of multiple extra stimuli to peel back refractoriness in pathway A may also alter the refractory period in B. Initiation of reentrant arrhythmias requires a critical interplay of refractory periods, delayed conduction, and unidirectional block. By shortening refractory periods with multiple extra stimuli, dispersion in refractoriness will more likely be uncovered, thus fostering the critical electrical milieu for reentry. Incremental pacing serves the same purpose by introducing multiple impulses until a critical degree of conduction delay and unidirectional block occurs. Pacing at faster rates allow refractoriness to be peeled back in a fashion similar to the introduction of multiple extra stimuli. Given this understanding of the principles underlying conduction intervals, refractory periods, and the initiation of arrhythmias, the techniques of incremental pacing and insertion of extra stimuli can be applied to the conduction system in a systematic fashion.

Measurements in Spontaneous Rhythm

Before initiating pacing, the clinician must measure various conduction intervals during normal sinus rhythm. These include the PA, AH, His potential, HV, QRS, and QT intervals (see Fig. 5-6). These measurements are compared to reported normal values and interpreted in light of the surface electrocardiogram. In most patients with arrhythmias and conduction disorders, the abnormality is rarely present in the resting state and must be unmasked by pacing techniques. In some situations, however, the arrhythmia may occur spontaneously. The analysis of conduction intervals and the order of atrial and ventricular activation during these spontaneous events is extremely valuable, particularly if the arrhythmia cannot be initiated by standard electrophysiologic techniques.

Atrial Pacing Studies

Incremental pacing and the insertion of extra stimuli in the right atrium are used to assess sinus node, AV node, and atrial function in addition to initiating and terminating tachyarrhythmias.

Sinus Node Function

A detailed analysis of techniques used to assess sinus node function is provided elsewhere in this text. The most commonly used procedure is overdrive suppression to determine sinus node recovery time (SNRT).[132] Pacing in the high right atrium is initiated and maintained for more than 30 seconds and then abruptly terminated. The interval from the last paced complex to the onset of the first sinus beat, as measured from high right atrium electrograms, is the sinus node recovery time (Fig. 5-10). This interval is often corrected for the underlying sinus rate by subtracting the sinus cycle length ($SNRT_c$). This manuever is performed over a wide range of paced rates, and the maximum sinus node recovery time is defined as the longest recovery time recorded. The normal range for maximum $SNRT_c$ in our laboratory is 180 to 500 msec. We commonly measure this parameter at the following rates: 100, 110, 120, 130, 150, and 170 beats/min. The SNRT lengthens as the paced rate is increased up to heart rates of 120 to 150, after which it frequently shortens. The cause of this paradoxic shortening at high paced rates is unknown, but contributing factors include changes in autonomic tone, neuro-

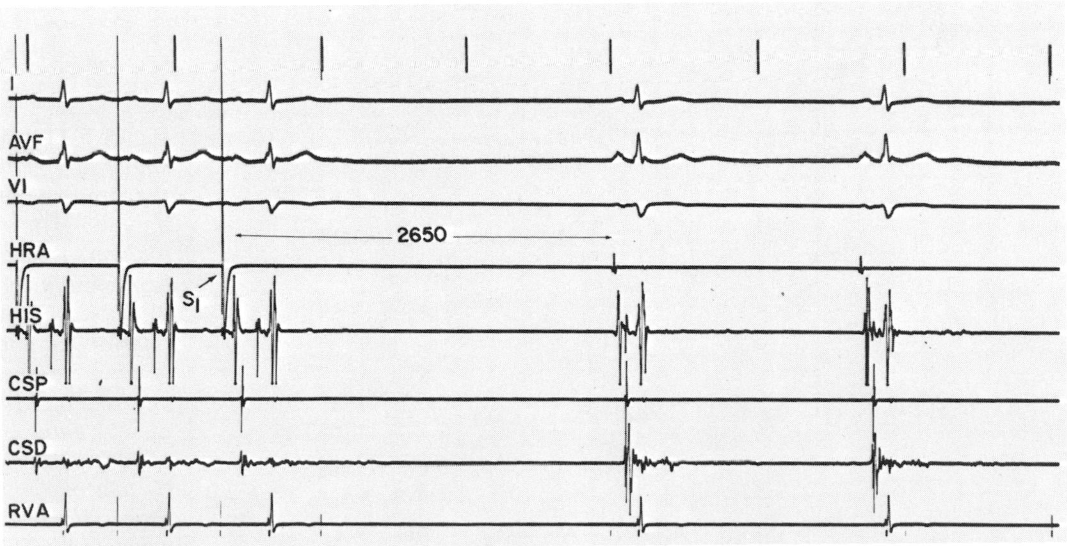

Figure 5-10. *Abnormal sinus node recovery time three surface ECG (I, avf, V_1) recordings, as well as electrogram recordings from the high right atrium (HRA), His bundle region (His), proximal (CSP), and distal (CSD) coronary sinus, and the right ventricular apex (RVA) are displayed. The first three complexes are obtained during atrial pacing, which is discontinued abruptly after the third QRS (S_1), the first complex seen following termination of pacing occurs 2650 msec later. See text.*

transmitter levels, hemodynamics, or variable entrance block of paced beats into the sinus node. In addition to the SNRT, cycle lengths of the subsequent 8 to 10 beats after termination of overdrive pacing are examined. During this period the cycle length gradually returns to that of the underlying sinus rate. Prolonged secondary pauses may indicate sinus node dysfunction despite a normal SNRT.

Another widely measured parameter is sinoatrial conduction time (SACT). This is an estimate of conduction time into and out of the sinus node. Three techniques are currently in clinical use. The first involves an analysis of the response of the sinus node to premature atrial extra stimuli.[133] After eight to ten sinus beats (A_1), a premature atrial extra stimulus (A_2) is introduced. The return interval (A_2A_3) is compared to the coupling interval of the premature impulse (A_1A_2), where A_1 represents the last sinus beat, A_2 the premature atrial extra stimulus, and A_3 the first sinus return beat. Measurements are made from a high right atrial electrode catheter, and impulses are introduced throughout diastole at 10- to 20-msec decrements. To facilitate analysis, these cycle lengths are normalized by dividing by the spontaneous sinus cycle length (A_1A_1). Figure 5-11 is a graph of the normalized premature cycle ($A_1A_2 \div A_1A_1$) plotted against the normalized return cycle ($A_2A_3 \div A_1A_1$). Figure 5-12 illustrates various zones encountered as the atrial extra stimulus is scanned through diastole. In late diastole, there is a period of compensation where premature atrial impulses are followed by a full compensatory

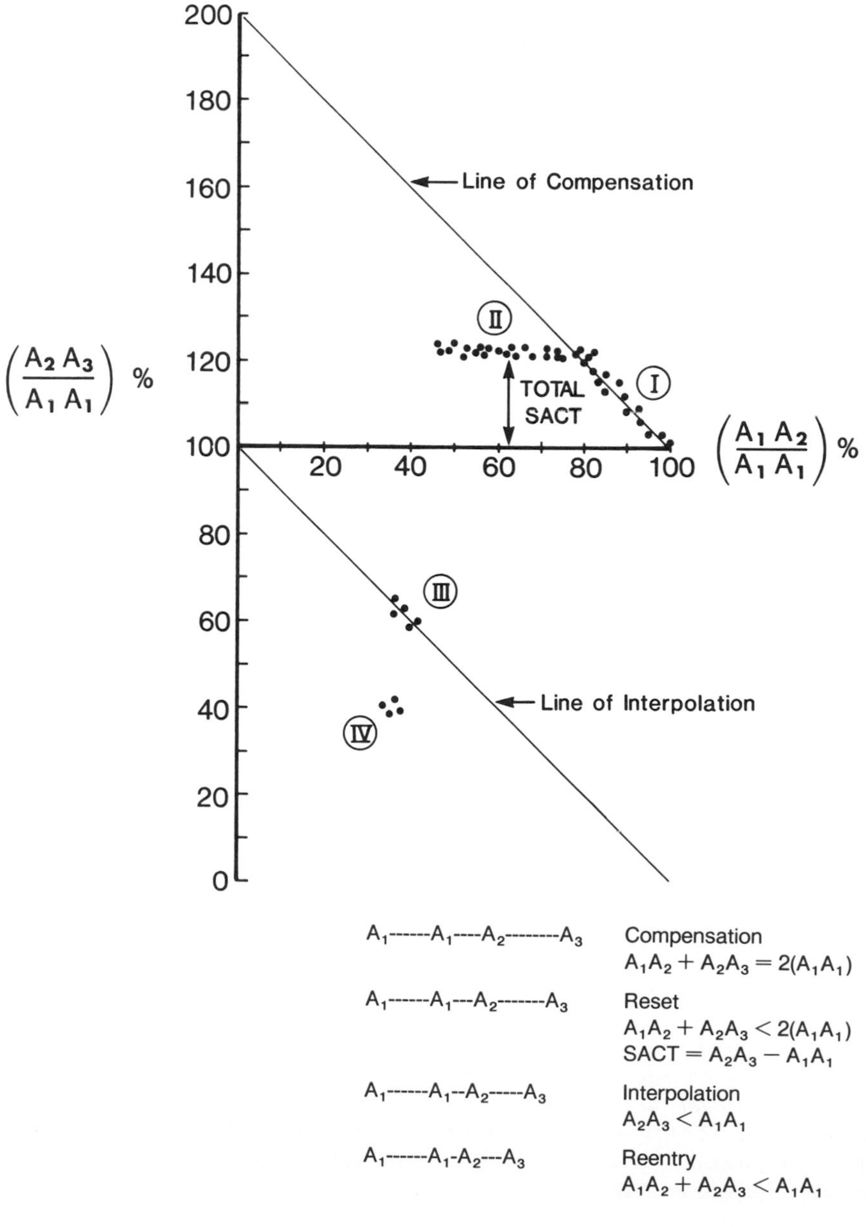

Figure 5-11. *Method of determination of sinoatrial conduction time (SACT) using the Strauss technique. The ventrical axis is the ratio of the A_2A_3 interval (return cycle) to the A_1A_1 interval (sinus cycle length) expressed in percentage from 0 to 200%. The horizontal axis is the ratio of the A_1A_2 interval (test interval) to the A_1A_1 interval (sinus cycle length) expressed in percentage from 0 to 100%. The diagonal lines identify a line of compensation and a line of interpolation. Four zones are identified: (I) zone of compensation, (II) zone of reset, (III) zone of interpolation, and (IV) zone of reset. The total SACT is measured in the zone of reset (II) at the area identified with the line with two arrowheads. See text for discussion. A_1A_1 = sinus cycle length; A_1A_2 = coupling interval of premature atrial extrastimulus; A_2A_3 = cycle length of return sinus impulse.*

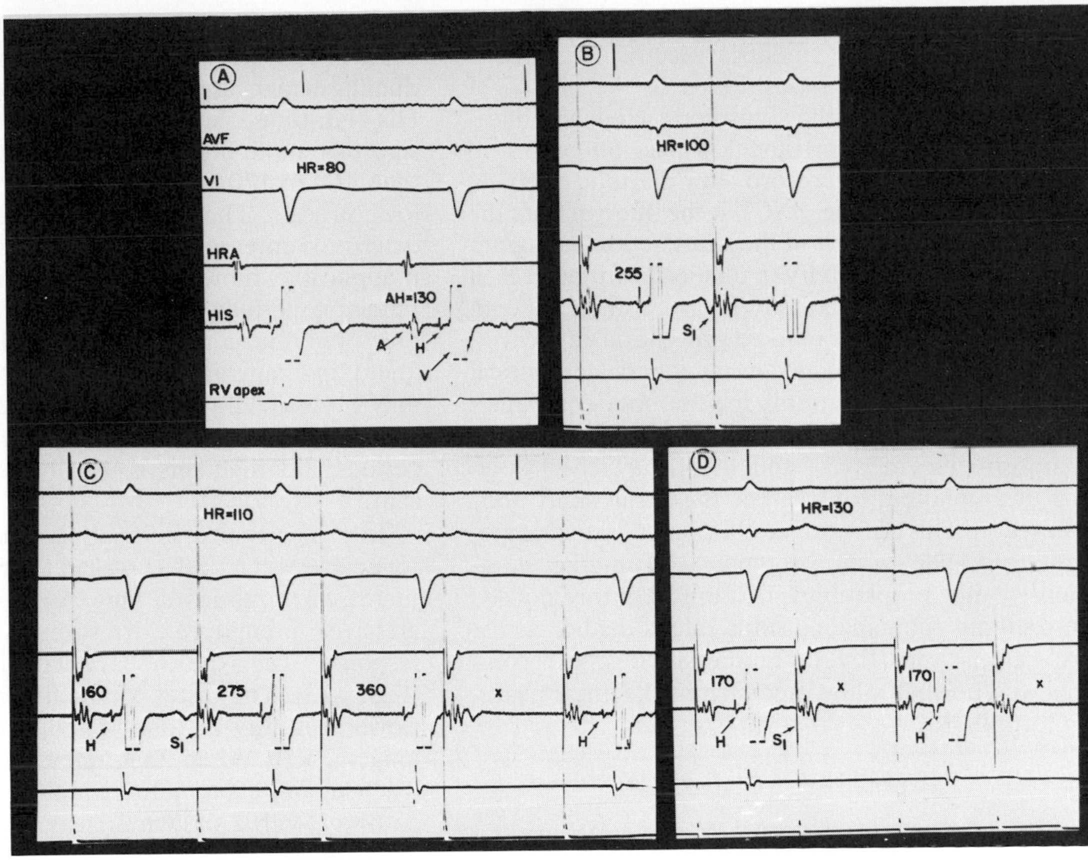

Figure 5-12. *AV Nodal Wenckebach. Three surface ECG leads (I, AVF, V_1) as well as intracardiac electrograms recorded from the high right atrium (HRA), His bundle region (His), and right ventricular apex (RV apex) are shown. In A (sinus rhythm) the AH interval is prolonged (130 msec); atrial pacing is then performed (S_1), and at a heart rate of 100/min (B), the AH interval is markedly prolonged (255 msec). In C, as the pacing rate was increased to 110/min, 4:3 AV nodal Wenckebach occurs; there is no His bundle spike or QRS after the fourth paced p wave. Progressive AH interval prolongation occurred (160, 275, and 360 msec) prior to the blocked p wave. In D, as the paced rate is increased further (130/min), 2:1 AV conduction occurs with block occurring at the AV mode; no His spike is seen following the nonconducted p wave.*

pause, $A_1A_2 + A_2A_3 = 2$ times A_1A_1. Through mid-diastole, a plateau is noticed in Figure 5-11. This represents a reset zone in which the premature extra stimulus has reset the sinus node pacemaker without changing its underlying cycle length; A_1A_3 is less than two times A_1A_1. Since sinus node automaticity is unchanged, in the return cycle $A_2A_3 = A_1A_1 + \text{SACT}$, the latter being the conduction time into and out of the sinus node to the recording electrode. During early diastole, premature atrial extra stimuli may result in interpolation, so that A_2A_3 is less than A_1A_1, or in reentry, so that $A_1A_2 + A_2A_3$ is less than A_1A_1.

Sinoatrial conduction time is an estimate of perinodal conduction time. Using the premature atrial extra stimulus technique, the total conduction time into and out of the sinus node is measured. A wide range of normal values has been reported; 100 to 250 msec represents the normal values as determined by our laboratory. Variables that may influence this measurement include location of the HRA pacing and recording electrode, atrial conduction abnormalities, sinus arrhythmia, and the possibility that the premature atrial impulse may suppress the sinus node and alter its automaticity.

An alternative approach to measuring SACT has been developed by Narula.[134] In this technique, the atrium is paced for eight beats, 10 beats/min faster than the underlying sinus rate. The interval from the last paced beat to the first return sinus beat, recorded in the HRA, is measured. The SACT is this interval minus the mean sinus cycle length. This is analogous to measurement of sinus node recovery time, but pacing at this rate is felt not to suppress sinus node automaticity. This method is easier and faster than the atrial extra stimulus technique and also overcomes the limitations of sinus arrhythmia.

The most recent technique developed to measure SACT uses direct recording of sinoatrial electrical activity.[135] An electrode catheter is positioned in the high right atrium in proximity to the sinus node. High amplification (50 to 100 mV/cm) and low-pass filters (0.1 to 20 Hz) are employed to record slow diastolic electrical activity of the sinus node. SACT is the interval from the beginning of the upstroke of the sinus node electrogram to the onset of atrial activity in that lead. Although each of these techniques purports to measure sinoatrial conduction time, given their marked procedural differences, it is unlikely that they examine identical electrical events. This in part accounts for the poor correlation between methods in certain clinical situations.[136]

Abnormalities in SNRT and SACT may reflect variations in autonomic tone rather than true sinus node dysfunction. This effect can be eliminated through autonomic blockade with atropine, 0.04 mg/kg intravenously, and propranolol, 0.2 mg/kg intravenously. The resultant spontaneous sinus rate is defined as the intrinsic heart rate (IHR). The measured value is compared with normal values predicted by the linear regression formula[137]:

$$IHR_p = 118.1 - (0.57 \times \text{age})$$

The 95% confidence limit is plus or minus 14% for people under 45 years of age and plus or minus 18% for people over 45 years of age. An abnormal SNRT or SACT with a normal IHR suggests abnormal autonomic activity, whereas an abnormal IHR indicates intrinsic sinus node dysfunction. To assess sinus node function, we currently measure maximum $SNRT_c$ and one or more measurements of SACT in all patients undergoing electrophysiologic testing. If there are significant abnormalities in these results, or if the patient is being tested primarily for sinus node dysfunction, autonomic blockade with termination of intrinsic heart rate is performed.

AV Node–His-Purkinje Function

The same electrophysiologic techniques, incremental atrial pacing and the insertion of premature atrial extra stimuli, are used to assess sinus node and AV node function. During incremental atrial pacing, AH interval prolongation occurs with faster rates due to encroachment on the relative refractory period of the AV node. At a critical rate long-cycle AV node–Wenckebach occurs (Fig. 5-12). This is confirmed by incremental lengthening of the AH interval with the dropped ventricular complex showing paced atrial activity but no His bundle activity. The rate at which AV node–Wenckebach occurs varies because of differing refractory periods and autonomic nervous system activity. The normal range in our laboratory is 120 to 200 beats/min. Although the usual response to incremental atrial pacing is block within the AV node, infra-Hisian block can occur in some healthy persons. If the AV node is capable of conducting at high rates, the refractory periods of the normal His–Purkinje system can be encroached on. Infra-Hisian or bundle branch block occurring at rates of less than 160 to 170 beats/min usually represents a pathologic process. The extra stimulus technique is used to determine anterograde AV node refractory periods and, if applicable, bundle branch and His–Purkinje system refractory periods. In our laboratory, these are routinely measured during pacing at 100 to 110 beats/min. Frequent spontaneous extrasystoles or other arrhythmias may necessitate a faster basic drive rate. A change in cycle length, however, can affect the measured refractory periods, although this is usually not clinically significant.[138]

In some persons, an analysis of the AV node refractory curve will reveal a break in the curve with a marked increase in conduction time (A_2H_2 or H_1H_2) with progressively premature extra stimuli. This discontinuous response reflects the presence of dual AV node pathways (Fig. 5-13). The faster conducting pathway masks the slower pathway at long coupling intervals but has a longer ERP. When that refractory period has been reached, more premature impulses unmask the slow pathway, with a sudden increase in the A_2H_2 interval. This abnormality is present in approximately 75% of patients with clinical AV node reentrant tachycardia, but it is also seen in persons without a history of clinical arrhythmias.

Atrial Function

Techniques similar to those described above are used to evaluate atrial function. The clinical significance of such findings is not as well understood as for the AV node and His–Purkinje system. The PA interval is used to measure intra-atrial conduction but has many limitations. It represents the conduction interval from the onset of P wave activity on the surface electrocardiogram to the onset of low right atrial activity in the His bundle electrogram. As such, it is a crude index of right atrial activation. In many cases, endocardial atrial activity, as measured by other atrial electrograms, will often precede the onset of surface P wave activity. A more extensive analysis of atrial conduction requires mapping techniques.

With stimulation currents of two to three times diastolic threshold, incremental atrial pacing should result in 1 : 1 capture to rates greater than 250 beats/min. Loss of capture before this point is usually due to unstable catheter position and can be corrected by increasing current intensity or repositioning the pacing catheter. Atrial pacing at rates greater than 250 beats per minute may induce atrial fibrillation or flutter in normal persons (Fig. 5-14). These arrhythmias usually terminate spontaneously in a few seconds or minutes. Atrial refractory

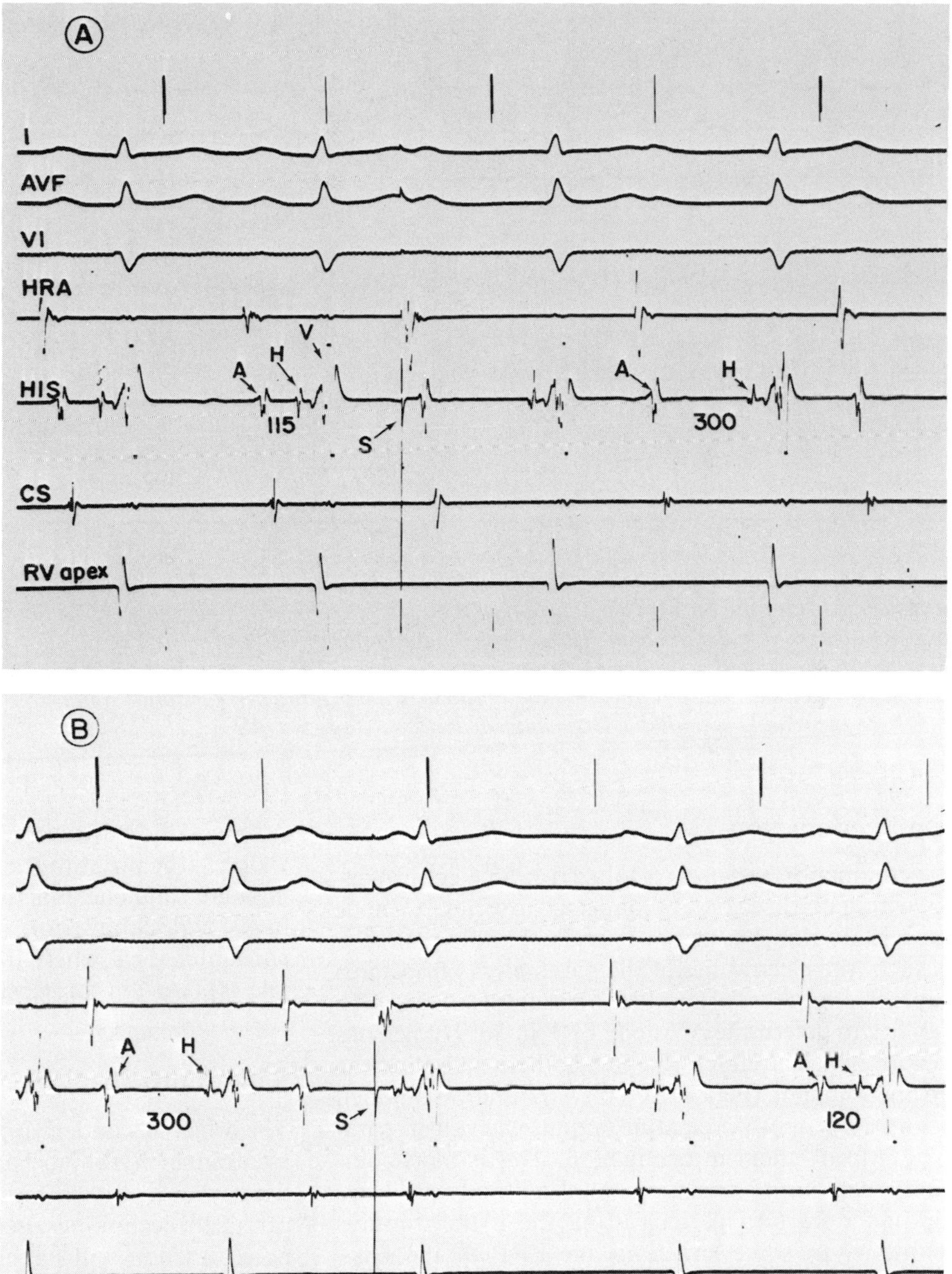

Figure 5-13. *Dual AV nodal pathways. In A two sinus complexes precede an electrically stimulated atrial premature complex (S_1). The AH intervals before the APC were 115 msec, but the AH interval in the sinus complex following the APC is 300 msec. In B a second APC is induced, and the previously prolonged AH interval (300 msec) is now followed by sinus complexes with an AH interval of 120 msec. See text for discussion.*

periods are measured with the extra stimulus technique. Caution must be used during atrial pacing in persons with a clinical history of atrial fibrillation and flutter. Rapid atrial pacing (greater than 200 beats/minute) or the insertion of premature atrial extra stimuli close to the atrial ERP may induce sustained atrial fibrillation or flutter. This may preclude further analysis of sinus node, atrial and AV node function unless the arrhythmia can be terminated. Electrical cardioversion may be required to terminate atrial fibrillation in this setting.

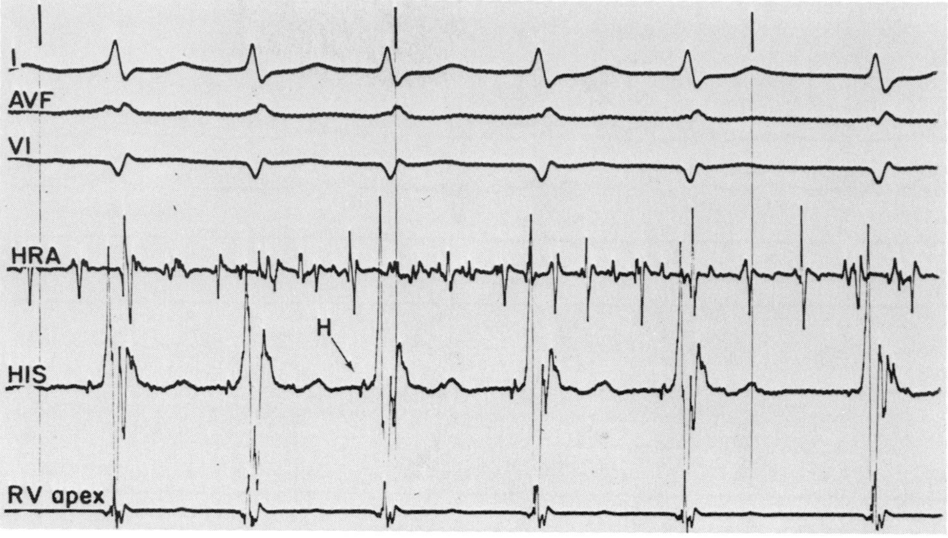

Figure 5-14. *Atrial fibrillation. Three surface ECG leads (I, AVF, V_1) are recorded with intracardiac leads from the high right atrium (HRA), His bundle (HIS), and right ventricular apex (RV apex). Note the irregular RR intervals on the surface ECG leads. The HRA recording shows a rapid, irregular pattern of atrial discharge. The His recording is obtained with the catheter introduced further into the ventricle to lower atrial depolarization amplitude. Note the readily identifiable His bundle deflection with each QRS.*

Gap Phenomenon

The conduction system is organized as an electrical circuit with specialized tissues connected in series, AV node and His–Purkinje system, or parallel bundle branches. As such, the electrophysiologic parameters of one area may influence those of another. An example of this is the inability to determine AV node ERP in 36% of persons because of atrial refractoriness. Another example is the gap phenomenon (Fig. 5-15). This is a situation in which progressively more premature impulses result in paradoxic improvement in conduction. This is most commonly seen during measurement of AV node and His–Purkinje refractory periods using the extra stimulus technique. In some situations the ERP of the His–Purkinje system or bundle branches is reached while the AV node is still capable of conduction. At this point, either infra-Hisian or bundle branch block occurs. As progressively more premature impulses are delivered, the infra-Hisian or bundle branch block is noted to resolve, an apparent paradox. This is explained by the gap phenomenon. Premature extra stimuli are being introduced into the high right atrium and must traverse the atrium and AV node before reaching the input to the His–Purkinje system. These impulses are thus subject to conduction delays at several sites. In the example noted above, more premature atrial impulses can encounter the ascending limb of the AV node refractory period curve, producing marked AV node delay and allowing the His–Purkinje system to recover from refractoriness. Although the extra stimulus is more premature (A_1A_2 is shorter), the input to the His–Purkinje system (H_1H_2) or bundle branches is actually longer because of the delay in AV node conduction. This same phenomenon can be encountered elsewhere in the conduction system and is one explanation for accelerated conduction.

Supraventricular Arrhythmias

The principles underlying initiation and termination of reentrant arrhythmias have been discussed. In most patients with a clinical history of supraventricular tachycardia, the techniques used to assess sinus, atrial, and AV node function will be sufficient. These include incremental atrial pacing to a rate of 200 to 250 beats/min and scanning diastole by 10- to 20-msec decrements with premature atrial extra stimuli. In some situations, more rapid pacing rates or multiple extra stimuli are needed. Certain supraventricular tachyarrhythmias require critical alterations in autonomic tone for initiation. Intravenous atropine, 0.5 to 2 mg, or isoproterenol, sufficient to produce a resting sinus rate of 110 to 120 beats/min, can be used in conjunction with pacing techniques if the latter alone fail to initiate the tachycardia. These aggressive techniques are capable of inducing transient atrial arrhythmias in some healthy persons, however. Arrhythmias are terminated by similar techniques—bursts (10 to 20 beats) of more rapid atrial pacing or the introduction of progressively more premature extra stimuli. He-

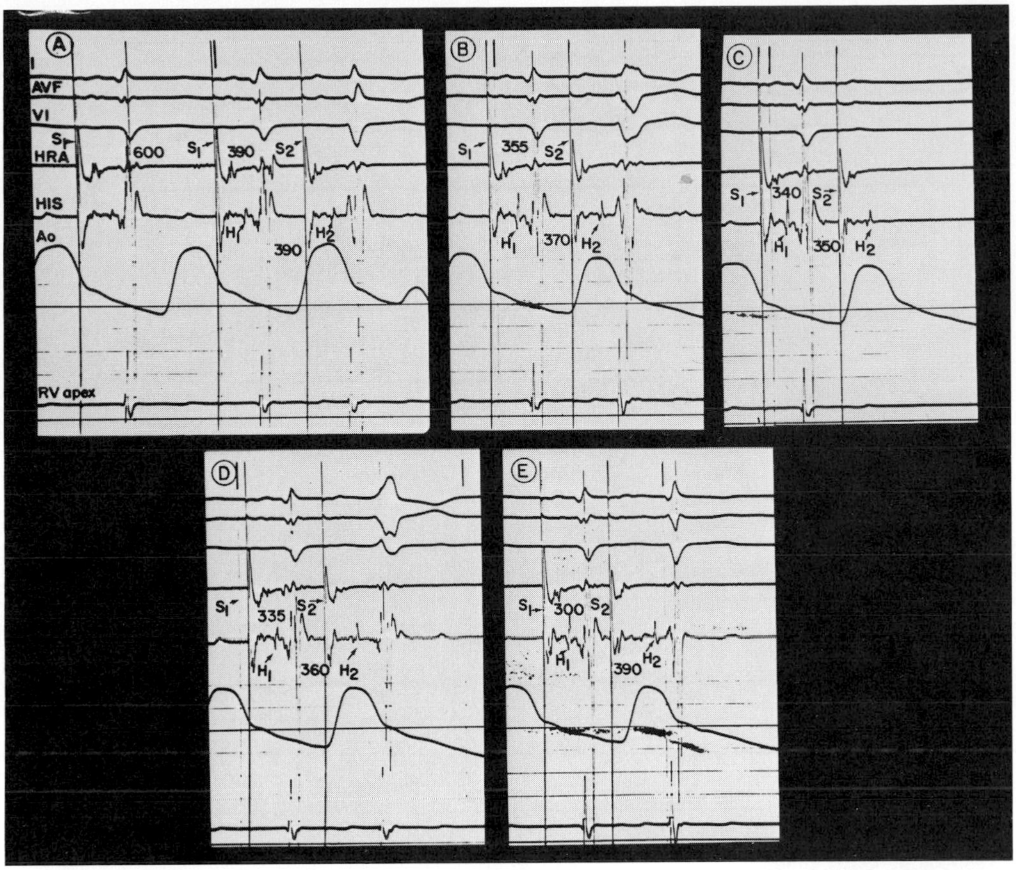

Figure 5-15. *Gap phenomenon panels A to E show three surface ECG leads (I, AVF, V_1), as well as intracardiac electrograms recorded from the high right atrium (HRA), His bundle (His), and right ventricular apex (RV apex). An intra-arterial pulse tracing is also shown (A_o). In A the last two of a train of eight basic drives (S_1) are shown, and then a test pulse (S_2) is delivered. The basic drive cycle length is 600 msec (100/min). The S_1S_2 test interval is 390 msec, and the H_1H_2 response interval is also 390 msec. The resultant QRS demonstrates slight aberration, and the H_2V_2 intervals are prolonged. B to E show further sequences during the stimulation run as the S_1S_2 interval is shortened. In B the test interval was shortened to 355 msec. The H_1H_2 interval is greater than the S_1S_2 interval, and the QRS is grossly aberrant. In C the test interval was shortened to 340 msec, the H_1H_2 was 350 msec, but block occurred below the His. In D the test interval was reduced to 335 msec, and conduction resumed with an aberrant QRS similar to that in B but with a longer HV interval. In E the test interval was shortened to 300 msec. Conduction persisted, but aberration was lessened significantly as the S_2H_2 interval was markedly prolonged (390 msec).*

modynamically unstable arrhythmias require immediate termination with synchronized cardioversion.

These techniques are used to initiate a variety of supraventricular tachycardias, including atrial fibrillation, atrial flutter, sinus node reentry, atrial reentry, AV node reentry, and tachycardias using accessory AV connections with orthodromic or antidromic conduction (Figs. 5-16 and 5-17). These are easily distinguished by their rate, P wave and atrial endocardial electrogram morphology, and atrial activation sequence (Table 5-15).

In some cases, however, more sophisticated electrophysiologic techniques are needed to define the underlying abnormality. These are beyond the scope of this discussion but include analysis of response of the tachycardia to bundle branch block, atrial or ventricular pacing, and premature atrial or ventricular extra stimuli. In rare patients, atrial pacing studies may induce ventricular tachycardia. This occurs in patients capable of 1 : 1 AV conduction at rapid pacing rates. The effect is probably similar to direct ventricular pacing techniques used to induce ventricular tachyarrhythmias. Ventricular tachycardia must therefore be included in the differential diagnoses of wide QRS tachycardias induced during atrial stimulation (see Table 5-15).

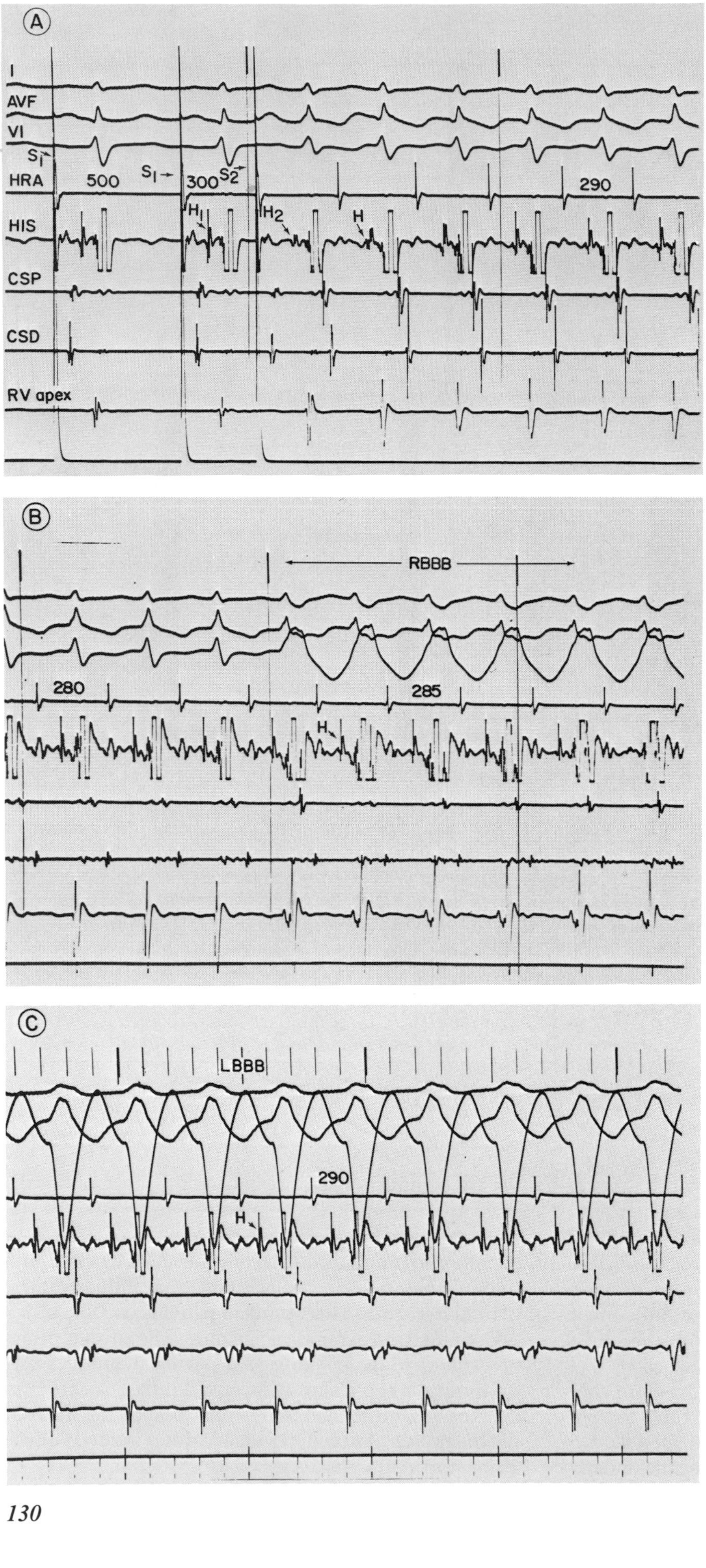

Figure 5-16. *Supraventricular tachycardia. In A three surface ECG leads (I, AVF, V_1) are recorded, along with intracardiac electrograms from the high right atrium (HRA), His bundle (HIS), and the proximal (CSP) and distal (CSD) coronary sinuses, as well as the right ventricular apex (RV apex). The basic drive (S_1S_1) is 500 msec (120/min). An atrial premature complex is initiated with a test interval (S_1S_2) of 300 msec. Supraventricular tachycardia occurs with a cycle length of 290 msec. Review of the activation sequence identifies that proximal coronary sinus electrogram precedes all other atrial electrograms, indicating a left paraseptal bypass tract operating in the retrograde direction. In B spontaneous RBBB occurs with no significant change in tachycardia cycle length or HA or AH intervals. In C spontaneous LBBB occurs, and again no significant change in the tachycardia cycle length is observed. See text for discussion.*

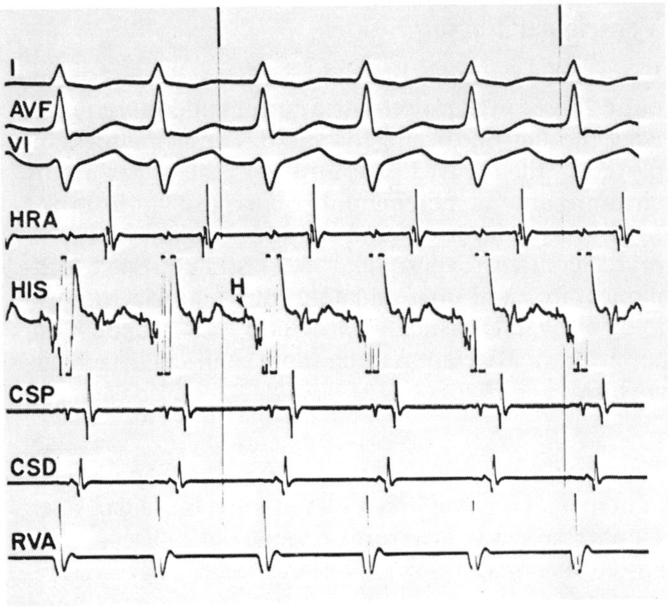

Figure 5-17. *Supraventricular tachycardia. The format is similar to that of Figure 5-16. Recordings obtained in a patient with a left lateral bypass tract are shown. Note, in contrast to Figure 5-16, that the* distal coronary sinus *electrogram occurs first, with atrial activation proceeding in a stepwise fashion from proximal CS, atrial septum (His) to HRA.*

Table 5-15. Common Arrhythmias Induced by Programmed Stimulation

Arrhythmia	Atrial Rate	P Wave Morphology	Atrial Electrogram	P Wave and QRS Relationship	Atrial Activation Sequence	His Potential	Dual AV Node Pathways (%)	Effect of BBB on Cycle Lengths	Atrial Participation Required	Atrial Activation Sequence During V Pacing	AV Node H-P System Required	Atrial Advancement by PVC
Sinus node reentry	80–150	Similar to sinus	Discrete	P > QRS	Similar to sinus	Yes	<10	None	Yes	Retrograde	No	No
Atrial reentry	150–200	Variable	Discrete	P > QRS	Variable	Yes	<10	None	Yes	Retrograde	No	No
AV node reentry	150–250	Variable	Discrete	Variable	Retrograde	Yes	>75	None	No	Retrograde	Yes	No
Reentry with bypass tracts												
Orthodromic	150–250	Variable	Discrete	QRS > P	Variable	Yes	<10	↑ if BBB ipsilateral to bypass tract	Yes (in part)	Same as in SVT	Yes	Yes
Antidromic	150–250	Variable	Discrete	P > QRS	Retrograde	Rare (Retrograde)	<10	—	Yes (in part)	Variable	Yes	Yes
Atrial fibrillation	400–650	Absent	Fibrillatory waves	—	Disorganized	Yes	<10	None	Yes	—	No	No
Atrial flutter	230–450	Flutter waves	Discrete	Variable	Variable	Yes	<10	None	Yes	—	No	No
Ventricular tachycardia	AV dissociation	→Sinus	Discrete	Variable	Sinus	No	<10	—	No	Sinus	No	No
	Retrograde VA conduction	→Variable	Discrete	QRS > P	Retrograde	No	<10	—	No	Retrograde	No	Variable

V, ventricular, BBB, bundle branch block.

Ventricular Pacing Studies

Ventricular pacing is typically performed using an impulse 2 msec in duration with a current intensity equal to twice the diastolic pacing threshold. The techniques employed in the ventricle are similar to those used in the atrium, namely, incremental pacing, usually from the right ventricular apex, and the introduction of one or more premature ventricular extra stimuli. Such techniques are used to evaluate ventricular electrophysiologic characteristics, retrograde VA conduction, supraventricular tachycardia, and ventricular tachyarrhythmias.

Ventricular Function and VA Conduction

Incremental pacing from the right ventricular apex should result in 1 : 1 capture up to rates of 200 beats/min. Faster rates may result in variable ventricular capture. Ventricular refractory periods are derived by scanning diastole with single ventricular extra stimuli. This is usually performed during ventricular pacing at 100 to 120 beats/min for eight beats. This allows sufficient time for the influence of the pacing rate to stabilize. As with atrial muscle, the refractory period curve usually lies close to the line of identity, with minimal conduction delay and a short ascending limb.

Retrograde VA conduction is present in 50% of healthy persons. Conduction can be evaluated in a manner analogous to anterograde AV conduction. With incremental ventricular pacing there will be gradual prolongation in retrograde conduction through the His–Purkinje system and AV node (Fig. 5-18). This is documented by an increase in the VA conduction interval. The VA interval is measured as the time between onset of ventricular activity, usually measured by the right ventricular apex electrogram, and onset of earliest retrograde atrial activity, usually measured in the His-bundle recording. Retrograde VA block occurs at a critical rate, usually with Wenckebach periodicity. The level of retrograde block (His–Purkinje versus AV node) is

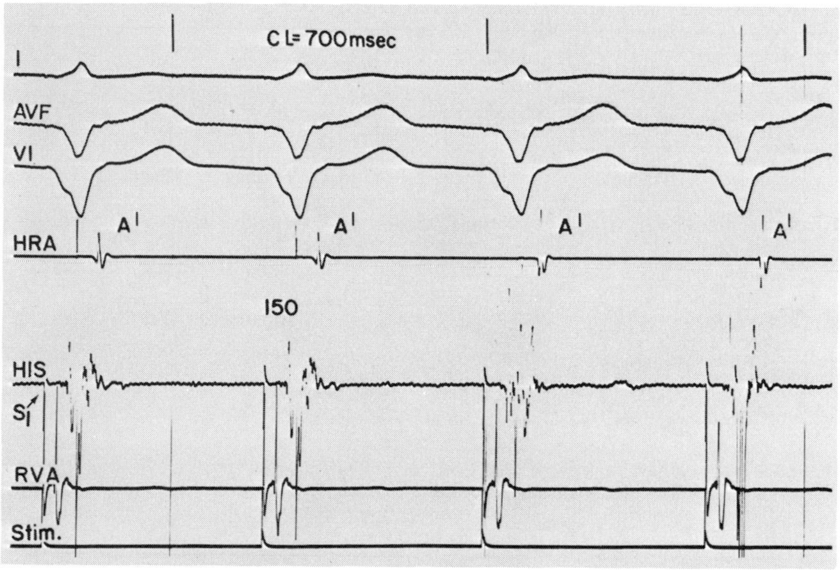

A

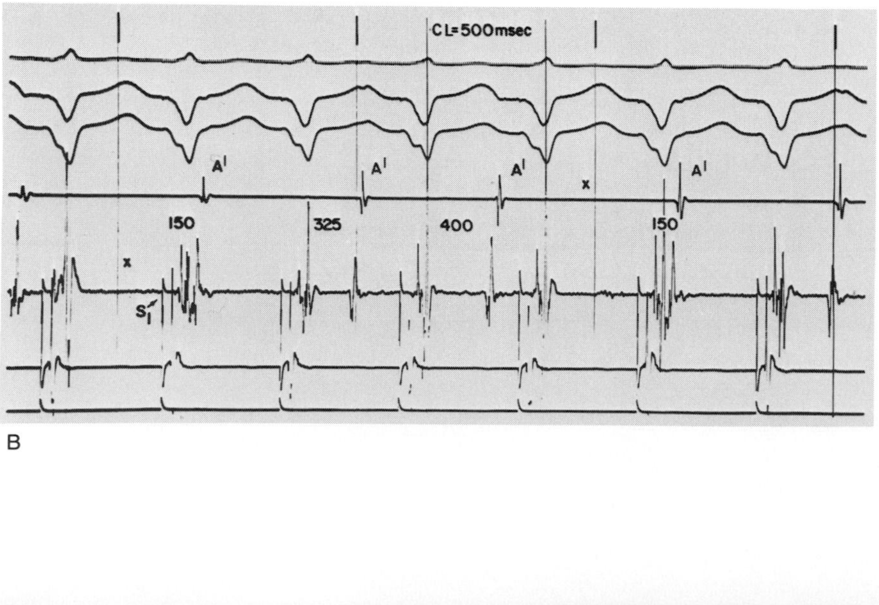

B

Figure 5-18. *VA Wenckebach. In A the ventricle is being paced at a cycle length of 700 msec (85 t/m). One-to-one VA conduction is present, with a VA interval of 150 msec. Stim. represents a display of the stimulus artifact only. The remainder of A is similar to previous figures. In B the ventricular cycle length has been shortened to 500 msec (120 b/min). Note the 4:3 retrograde Wenckebach period with progressive VA delay (150, 325, and 400 msec) until VA block occurs.*

difficult to determine because a retrograde His potential is visualized in only 10% of persons. With intact VA conduction, we have found retrograde conduction to be better than anterograde conduction in 27% of persons, the same in 20%, and worse in 53%. Retrograde VA refractory periods are determined with the extra stimulus technique. As with incremental ventricular pacing, the level of block may be difficult to determine because of an inability to visualize a retrograde His potential. Indirect methods suggest the site of block is the AV node in 90% of patients.[139] Retrograde VA gap phenomena may be seen during the insertion of premature ventricular extra stimuli. This usually occurs when the effective refractory period of the AV node is reached, resulting in retrograde VA block. More premature ventricular extra stimuli paradoxically restore VA conduction by inducing delay in the His–Purkinje system sufficient to allow recovery of AV node conduction.

It is important to examine the sequence of retrograde atrial activation during ventricular pacing. In normal persons, the earliest activity should appear in the low atrial septum, best visualized from the atrial electrogram in the His bundle recording. Early electrical activity in other portions of the atrium suggests the presence of an accessory atrioventricular connection. The order of retrograde atrial activation during ventricular pacing should be compared with atrial activation during supraventricular tachycardia to understand better the mechanism of the arrhythmia (see Table 5-15).

Supraventricular Arrhythmias

Incremental pacing and the extra stimulus technique are used to evaluate supraventricular tachycardias. If the ventricle is part of the reentrant circuit, these techniques may directly initiate and terminate the arrhythmia. Ventricular pacing can initiate supraventricular tachycardia even when the ventricle does not participate in the arrhythmia. If retrograde conduction is intact, ventricular impulses can reach critical portions of the tachycardia circuit, such as the atrium or AV node. The response of an arrhythmia to burst ventricular pacing and premature ventricular extra stimuli is also of diagnostic value (see Table 5-15).

Ventricular Arrhythmias

Ventricular pacing is most widely used during electrophysiologic studies to evaluate patients with sudden death and recurrent ventricular tachycardia. The sensitivity, specificity, and predictive value of numerous ventricular pacing protocols has been discussed. Our current protocol includes incremental ventricular pacing from 100 to 250 beats/min for bursts of 5 to 10 seconds at twice diastolic threshold from the right ventricular apex. This is followed by pacing for eight beats at 100 to 120 beats/min with the sequential insertion of single, double, and triple ventricular extra stimuli carried down to the point of refractoriness (Fig. 5-19). If this fails to induce sustained ventricular tachycardia, the extra stimulus technique is repeated, initially with a higher basic drive rate of 150 beats/min and subsequently with a high pacing rate and increased current strength (five times diastolic threshold). These changes peel back ventricular refractoriness and facilitate initiation of tachyarrhythmias. If this is unsuccessful, the latter pacing sequence is repeated in at least one another location within the right ventricle, usually the outflow tract. These techniques have a sensitivity and specificity of approximately 85% to 90%. In certain clinical situations, additional stimulation is performed during an isoproterenol infusion or from the left ventricle. The latter procedures are not routinely used, despite an increase in sensitivity, for several reasons: (1) their use may decrease specificity and increase morbitity, (2) most patients with ventricular arrhythmias have underlying coronary artery disease, and (3) an isoproterenol infusion can result in worsening angina or myocardial infarction. These techniques also limit the ease of serial drug testing. Evaluation of proper pharmacologic therapy requires serial stimulation using the same procedures as those required to initiate the arrhythmia in the drug-free state. A right ventricular pacing catheter can be safely left in place for 7 to 10 days with serial studies performed at bedside. If left ventricular stimulation is required, multiple left ventricular catheterizations may be necessary. Serial antiarrhythmic drug studies during an isoproterenol infusion may be difficult to interpret because of drug interactions.

The ability to quickly and safely terminate sustained ventricular arrhythmias is critical. The hemodynamic response to such arrhythmias depends on their rate and the severity of underlying cardiac disorders. Left ventricular function is a critical factor. Most patients with good left ventricular function will tolerate tachycardias with rates up to 200 beats/min without hemodynamic deterioration. Ventricular mapping studies and response to drug infusions can be examined in clinically stable patients. Hemodynamic compromise, either initially or after several minutes, requires prompt intervention. The electrophysiologic mechanisms underlying the termination of reentrant arrhythmias with pacing techniques have been discussed. Programmed stimulation techniques are successful in terminating ventricular tachycardia in up to 80% of patients. The remainder require cardioversion.[92] The insertion of one to three extra stimuli results in termination in 27% to 63% of attempts. Burst pacing is successful in 76% of trials. Acceleration of the tachycardia occurs in 20%. The rate of the tachycardia is critical to successful termination by pacing techniques. Programmed extra stimuli are successful in only 15% when the tachycardia is faster than 200 beats/min. Burst ventricular pacing is successful in 49% at similar

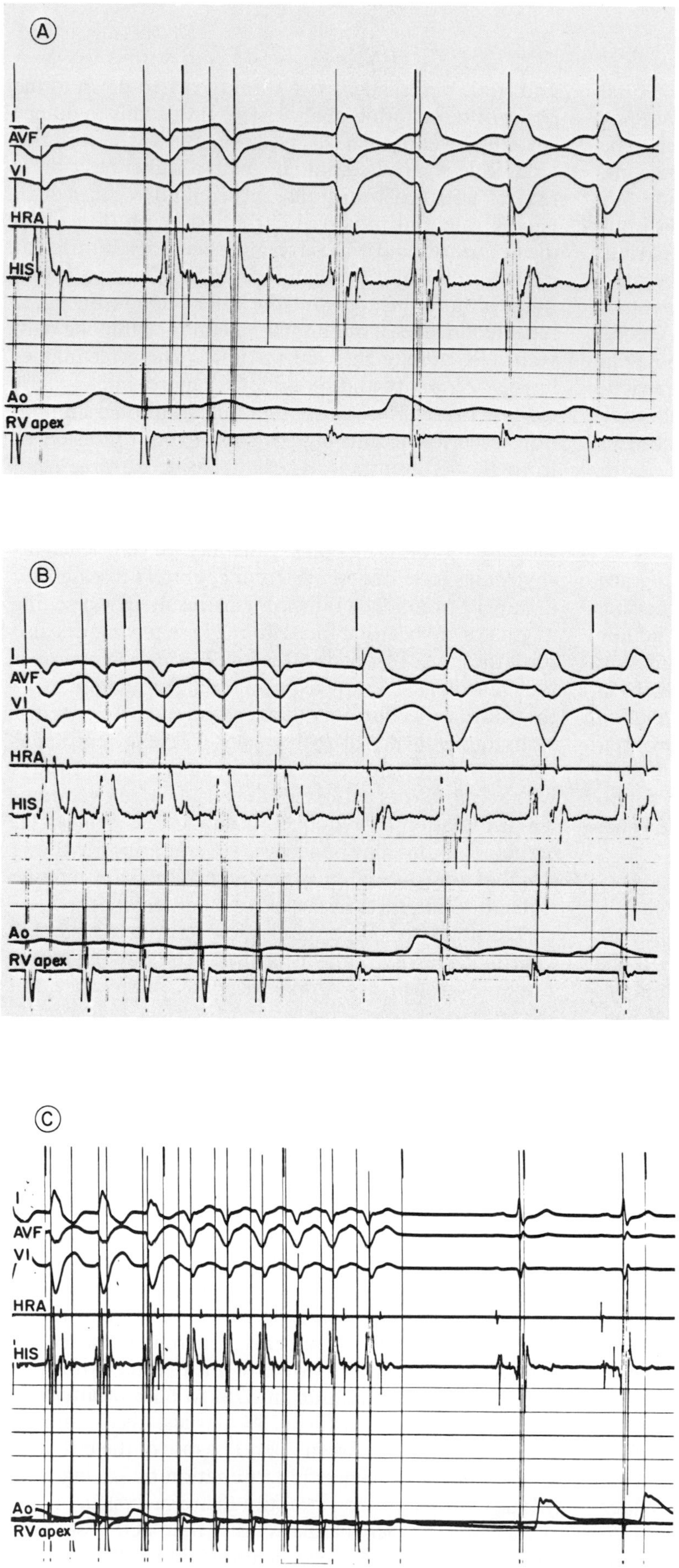

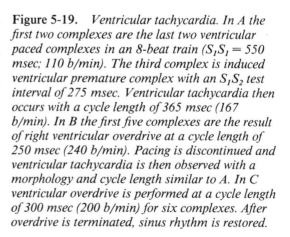

Figure 5-19. *Ventricular tachycardia. In A the first two complexes are the last two ventricular paced complexes in an 8-beat train (S_1S_1 = 550 msec; 110 b/min). The third complex is induced ventricular premature complex with an S_1S_2 test interval of 275 msec. Ventricular tachycardia then occurs with a cycle length of 365 msec (167 b/min). In B the first five complexes are the result of right ventricular overdrive at a cycle length of 250 msec (240 b/min). Pacing is discontinued and ventricular tachycardia is then observed with a morphology and cycle length similar to A. In C ventricular overdrive is performed at a cycle length of 300 msec (200 b/min) for six complexes. After overdrive is terminated, sinus rhythm is restored.*

tachycardia rates. Other techniques, such as ultrarapid stimulation or rapid pacing plus extra stimuli, have been reported to terminate ventricular tachycardia.[140,141] These methods, however, require further investigation.

When a hemodynamically unstable rhythm causes loss of consciousness, direct current cardioversion is immediately performed, with 200 watt-sec used initially, followed by higher energies if additional countershocks are necessary. If the rhythm is hemodynamically stable, burst ventricular pacing for 10 to 15 beats is attempted at a rate 10 to 20 beats/min faster than the tachycardia. If this is unsuccessful or acceleration occurs and the patient remains clinically stable, faster overdrive rates or premature extra stimuli are used.

Coronary Sinus Pacing Studies

The coronary sinus provides an additional site for electrogram recording and pacing in evaluating supraventricular and ventricular arrhythmias. Because of its location, it allows indirect electrical access to the left atrium and ventricle. The pacing techniques used are identical to those described elsewhere, namely, incremental pacing and insertion of one or more extra stimuli. Greater current intensity may be needed to achieve stable left atrial or left ventricular pacing from the coronary sinus than with direct electrical contact against the endocardium.

Coronary sinus studies are important in patients with supraventricular tachycardia using accessory AV connections because most of these tracts are left sided. If anterograde conduction is present (Wolff-Parkinson-White syndrome), the location of the bypass tract can be located by comparing the stimulus-to-delta wave interval and degree of ventricular preexcitation at different paced sites with similar rates. Proximity of the pacing site to the origin of the accessory tract will shorten the stimulus-to-delta interval and increase the degree of preexcitation. The tract is likely to be in the left free wall when this occurs during distal coronary sinus pacing. A paraseptal tract should be suspected when maximal preexcitation occurs with proximal coronary sinus or low atrial septum pacing. Coronary sinus stimulation can initiate supraventricular tachycardia, but this does not happen from other atrial sites. Critical tachycardia zones may be encountered because of proximity to bypass tracts and altered atrial activation or conduction.

Indirect left ventricular stimulation through coronary sinus pacing can be used to initiate and terminate ventricular tachycardias that were unprovokable from right ventricular sites. Direct left ventricle stimulation has been reported necessary for induction in 11% of patients with recurrent ventricular tachycardia.[142] Indirect left ventricle pacing may decrease morbidity associated with retrograde left ventricle catheterization. Left ventricular stimulation has also been reported to enhance the evaluation of drug efficacy in patients with ventricular arrhythmias.[143] Since such testing takes place over several days, a coronary sinus catheter can be left in place for repeated use rather than performing multiple retrograde left ventricle catheterizations.

Drug Testing

Drugs are used in conjunction with electrophysiologic studies to enhance the sensitivity and specificity of diagnostic testing and to treat a variety of arrhythmias. Atropine and propranolol are used to produce autonomic blockade in evaluating patients for sick sinus syndrome. Similar agents may facilitate the initiation of tachyarrhythmias where standard programmed stimulation techniques have been unsuccessful. Because of their electrophysiologic effects, atropine, 0.01 to 0.04 mg/kg, and isoproterenol, 0.5 to 10.0 μg/min, enhance the initiation of a variety of supraventricular arrhythmias. Isoproterenol in comparable doses is used to facilitate the initiation of ventricular tachycardia.

Antiarrhythmic agents can be tested for their ability to terminate or prevent the initiation of tachyarrhythmias. Most electropharmacologic testing is performed for the latter purpose. Once it has been demonstrated that programmed stimulation can reproducibly initiate a tachyarrhythmia, a series of drugs are administered and repeat stimulation studies are performed. Dose is adjusted to achieve therapeutic serum levels if available. That drug that best prevents the induction of the same tachycardia is subsequently used for long-term therapy. During the initial electrophysiologic study, pharmacologic testing is usually performed with an intravenous preparation. If this is successful, the patient is given an oral form and repeat testing is performed in several days. If the initial drug is unsuccessful, another type of agent is then tested. It is important to allow a suitable length of time ($\geq$ five drug half-lives) for steady-state levels to be achieved.

The choice of drugs is dictated by the nature of the arrhythmia, side-effects, left ventricular function, and any potential drug-drug or drug-disease interactions. For supraventricular tachycardia, we test the effectiveness of a type I agent (quinidine, procainamide, or disopyramide) alone and in combination with a different type of drug (propranolol, digoxin, or verapamil). If these are unsuccessful, an experimental agent may be considered.

Considerable controversy exists regarding the choice of drugs to treat ventricular tachyarrhythmias. During the initial electrophysiologic study, an intravenous preparation of a type I agent is usually tested, such as procainamide, 15 mg/kg, or quinidine, 10 mg/kg. If the arrhythmia is noninducible, repeat testing is performed after a steady-state level has been achieved on an oral regimen. It has been suggested that a negative response to a type I agent predicts a poor response to other conventional drugs and that further therapy should involve experimental agents, surgery, or antitachycardia pacemakers.[63] Any single agent has an efficacy less than 33%.[55,63,73] The testing of other conventional drugs improves this response by 10%. Given the low rate of initial response, however, the testing of multiple drugs improves the overall response rate by 25% to 30%. The testing of combinations of drugs does not improve therapeutic efficacy.[144,145] Our current approach is to test a minimum of two conventional antiarrhythmic drugs before using investigational agents. Experimental drugs are tested in a similar fashion, with the exception of amiodarone. There is a poor correlation between the results of electropharmacologic testing and clinical response with this agent.[146]

Mapping Studies

Mapping studies are performed to localize electrophysiologic areas for surgical or catheter ablation. Preliminary mapping is done in the catheterization laboratory, with more detailed studies at the time of surgery. In the evaluation of supraventricular tachycardia, mapping is most often performed to localize accessory AV connections. If the pathway shows evidence of anterograde conduction (Wolff-Parkinson-White syndrome), it can be localized by two methods: (1) evaluation of the stimulus-to-delta wave interval and degree of preexcitation during atrial pacing at different sites, and (2) ventricular mapping during atrial pacing. The former is used to locate the bypass tract in the catheterization laboratory; the latter technique is used at surgery. Ventricular mapping can be performed in the catheterization laboratory but requires positioning catheters at multiple points around the AV valve rings in both the right and left ventricles. This is technically difficult because of supporting valvular structures. Intraoperative studies are performed with epicardial rather than endocardial mapping because of the location of most accessory AV connections. A hand-held mapping electrode is moved around the valve rings along the ventricular aspect of the AV groove during atrial pacing. The timing of the ventricular electrogram is compared to that of right and left ventricle reference epicardial electrograms and multiple surface leads. The site of earliest ventricular activity identifies the bypass tract. Mapping must be performed when there is manifest preexcitation on the surface electrocardiogram. If pacing is performed at a rate that results in anterograde block in the bypass tract, conduction to the ventricle will be solely through the AV node.

If retrograde conduction is present, atrial mapping is performed during ventricular pacing. In the catheterization laboratory, the right atrium is mapped through a standard electrode catheter and the left atrium is indirectly mapped through a coronary sinus catheter. The sequence and timing of retrograde atrial activation is compared to reference atrial electrograms from the high right atrium and low septal atrium, the latter from the His bundle electrogram recording. It is important to confirm that retrograde atrial activation is indeed through an accessory AV connection rather than the normal His-Purkinje–AV node pathway. In the latter, the earliest site of retrograde atrial activity will appear in the His bundle recording. Paraseptal bypass tracts may be difficult to distinguish from normal retrograde conduction. Intraoperative retrograde mapping is performed in a similar fashion during ventricular pacing, except the atrial epicardial surface around the AV groove, rather than the endocardial surface, is mapped.

Recent studies suggest that electrophysiologically guided resection of myocardial scar will markedly decrease the recurrence of ventricular tachyarrhythmias.[98–100] These areas are usually on the endocardial border zone of a myocardial scar, often a ventricular aneurysm. Preliminary mapping can be performed in the catheterization laboratory in some patients, with more detailed mapping at surgery.[147,148]

Only those patients with hemodynamically stable tachycardias can be mapped in the catheterization laboratory; 30% to 50% will have tachycardias that are too rapid. Administration of an antiarrhythmic drug may sufficiently slow the tachycardias to permit mapping yet not alter the site of origin. The timing and morphology of ventricular electrograms from a mapping catheter are compared with those of multiple surface leads and a reference endocardial catheter, usually at the right ventricular apex. The earliest recorded presystolic ventricular electrogram, whether discrete or fragmented, locates the site of the tachycardia. In some patients, holodiastolic fragmented activity is recorded. This is thought to represent electrical activity within the reentrant circuit. All catheter positions are confirmed by fluoroscopy in multiple planes. In patients whose ventricular tachycardia has multiple morphologies, an attempt should be made to map each form.

More detailed mapping is performed in the operating room on full cardiopulmonary bypass at a temperature of 37° to 38°C. Endocardial mapping is performed with a ring or hand-held electrode, with an interelectrode distance of 1 to 2 mm, through a ventriculotomy through an area of myocardial scar. If an aneurysm is present, it is first resected and mapping is started at the border zone. The tachycardia is induced through a previously paced right ventricle pacing catheter, and mapping is performed under direct vision in a radial fashion around the ventriculotomy in successive circles 1 cm apart. Ventricular electrograms are compared with the right and left ventricle reference electrograms, recorded from plunge

Table 5-16. Electrophysiologic Pacing Protocols

Sinus Node Studies

Catheters
1. HRA (pacing and recording)

Procedures
1. Incremental atrial pacing (to rates greater than 150 beats/min)
2. Atrial extra stimulus technique (single)
3. Autonomic blockade (atropine and propranolol)

Conduction System Studies

Catheters
1. HRA (pacing)
2. HBE (recording)
3. RV (pacing)

Procedures
1. Baseline conduction intervals
2. Anterograde conduction
   a. Incremental atrial pacing (to development of AV block)
   b. Atrial extra stimulus technique (single)
3. Retrograde conduction
   a. Incremental ventricular pacing (to development of VA block)
   b. Ventricular extra stimulus technique (single)
4. Atropine (repeat 1, 2, and 3)

Supraventricular Tachycardia

Catheters
1. HRA (pacing and recording)
2. HBE (recording)
3. RV (pacing and recording)
4. CS (pacing and recording)

Procedures
1. Baseline conduction intervals
2. Atrial pacing (possible multiple sites)
   a. Incremental pacing (to rates greater than 200 beats/min)
   b. Extra stimulus technique (single; possible double and triple)
3. Coronary sinus pacing (possible multiple sites)
   a. Incremental pacing (to rates greater than 200 beats/min)
   b. Extra stimulus technique (single; possible double and triple)
4. Ventricular pacing
   a. Incremental pacing (to rates greater than 200 beats/min)
   b. Extra stimulus technique (single; possible double and triple)
5. During tachycardia (repeat 1, 2, 3 and 4)
6. Drug studies

Ventricular Tachycardia

Catheters
1. RV (pacing and recording)
2. HBE (recording)
3. CS or LV (possible; pacing and recording)

Procedures
1. Baseline conduction intervals
2. RV pacing
   a. From apex at two times diastolic threshold
      i. Incremental pacing (to 250 beats/min)
      ii. Extra stimulus technique (single, double, and triple; paced rate of 110 and 150 beats/min)
   b. From apex at five times diastolic threshold
      i. Extra stimulus technique (single, double and triple; paced rate of 150 beats/min)
   c. From outflow tract at five times diastolic threshold
      i. Extra stimulus technique (single, double and triple; paced rate of 150 beats/min)
3. LV (direct or from CS)
   a. Two times diastolic threshold
      i. Extra stimulus technique (single, double and triple; paced rate of 150 beats/min)
4. Isoproterenol (repeat 2b, 2c, and 3)

continued

Table 5-16. Electrophysiologic Pacing Protocols (Continued)

Ventricular Tachycardia

5. During tachycardia (hemodynamically stable)
   a. Mapping of LV and RV
   b. Termination
      i. Burst overdrive pacing
      ii. Extra stimulus technique (single, double and triple)
6. Drug studies

electrodes inserted at the time of surgery, and multiple surface leads. Similar criteria are used for locating the site of origin as in the catheterization laboratory. Areas of origin are subsequently resected, and an attempt is made to reinduce the tachycardia. If inducible, mapping and resection are repeated.

Several limitations exist with these techniques. Programmed stimulation is successful in initiating ventricular tachycardia during surgery in only 80% of patients, despite preoperative induction in the catheterization laboratory. Limiting factors include cardiac temperature, presence of antiarrhythmic drugs, electrolyte imbalance, and anesthetic agents. Temperature is an important variable. Ventricular tachycardia can rarely be induced when the patient is hypothermic. Intraoperative studies should thus be performed with a cardiac temperature of 37° to 38°C. All antiarrhythmic drugs should be stopped at least four to five half-lives before surgery. Mapping requires a stable, sustained monomorphic arrhythmia. Nonsustained ventricular tachycardia can be mapped if the morphology is constant but requires repeated induction. Rapid, polymorphic tachycardias can rarely be accurately mapped. Because of these limitations, an attempt has been made to perform intraoperative mapping during normal sinus rhythm.[149] With this technique, endocardial areas showing fragmented electrical activity are resected. Further investigation is needed to confirm this approach.

Conclusion

Invasive electrophysiologic testing is a valuable diagnostic and therapeutic tool. A variety of pacing and recording techniques are available to examine the cardiac electrical system. Each study must be tailored to the individual patient's clinical needs. Table 5-16 summarizes our approach to the evaluation of the more common electrophysiologic disorders. These are often combined to assess multiple areas of the electrical system with the same technique (*e.g.,* evaluation of sinus and AV node function and initiation of supraventricular tachycardia with atrial pacing studies). In the hands of an experienced electrophysiologist, these techniques can be applied with minimal morbidity and facilitate the diagnosis and therapy of complex clinical situations.

References

1. Ross, D. L., Farre, J., Bar, F. W., et al.: Comprehensive clinical electrophysiologic studies in the investigation of documented tachycardias; time, staff, problems and costs. Circulation, 61:1010–1016, 1980.
2. Dreifus, L. S.: Clinical judgement is sufficient for the management of conduction defects. Cardiovasc. Clin., 8:195–201, 1977.
3. Wu, D., Rosen, K. M.: Clinical judgment is not sufficient for the management of conduction defects. (Indications for diagnostic electrophysiologic studies.) Cardiovasc. Clin., 8:203–216, 1977.
4. Weiner, I.: Current applications of clinical electrophysiologic study in the diagnosis and treatment of cardiac arrhythmias. Am. J. Cardiol., 49:1287–1292, 1982.
5. Scheinman, M. M., and Morady, F.: Invasive cardiac electrophysiologic testing: The current state of the art. Circulation, 67:1169–1173, 1983.
6. Simson, M. B.: Use of signals in the terminal QRS complex to identify patients with ventricular tachycardia after myocardial infarction. Circulation, 64:235–242, 1981.
7. Shaw, D. B., Holman, R. R., and Gowers, J. I.: Survival in sinoatrial disorder. Br. Med. J., 1:139–141, 1980.
8. Narula, O. S.: Atrioventricular conduction defects in patients with sinus bradycardia. Circulation, 44:1096–1110, 1974.
9. Rosen, K. M., Loeb, H. S., Sinno, M. Z., et al.: Cardiac conduction in patients with symptomatic sinus node disease. Circulation, 43:836–844, 1971.
10. Brodsky, M., Wu, D., Denes, P., et al.: Arrhythmias documented by 24-hour continuous electrocardiographic monitoring in 50 male medical students without apparent heart disease. Am. J. Cardiol., 39:390–395, 1977.
11. Agruss, N. S., Rosin, E. Y., Adolph, R. J., and Fowler, N. O.: Significance of chronic sinus bradycardia in elderly people. Circulation, 46:924–930, 1972.
12. Thormann, J., Schwarz, F., Ensslen, R., and Sesto, M.: Vagal tone, significance of electrophysiologic findings and clinical course in symptomatic sinus node dysfunction. Am. Heart J., 95:725–731, 1978.
13. Gann, D., Tolentino, A., and Samet, P.: Electrophysiologic evaluation of elderly patients with sinus bradycardia. Ann. Intern. Med., 90:24–29, 1979.
14. Reiffel, J. A., Bigger, J. T., Cramer, M., and Reid, D. S.: Ability of Holter electrocardiographic recording and atrial stimulation to detect sinus nodal dysfunction in symptomatic and asymptomatic patients with sinus bradycardia. Am. J. Cardiol., 40:189–194, 1977.

15. Strasberg, B., Amat-Y-Leon, F., Dhingra, R. C., et al.: Natural history of chronic second degree atrioventricular nodal block. Circulation, 63:1043–1049, 1981.
16. Amat-Y-Leon, F., Dhingra, R., Denes, P., et al.: The clinical spectrum of chronic HIS bundle block. Chest, 70:747–754, 1976.
17. Gupta, P. K., Lichstein, E., and Chadda, K. D.: Chronic HIS bundle block: Clinical, electrocardiographic, electrophysiological and follow-up studies on 16 patients. Br. Heart J., 38:1343–1349, 1976.
18. Ranganathan, N., Dhurandes, R., Phillips, J. H., and Wigle, E. D.: HIS bundle electrogram in bundle-branch block. Circulation, 45:282–294, 1972.
19. Dhingra, R. C., Denes, P., Wu, D., et al.: The significance of second degree atrioventricular block and bundle branch block: Observations regarding site and type of block. Circulation, 49:638–645, 1974.
20. Zipes, D. P.: Second degree atrioventricular block. Circulation, 60:465–472, 1979.
21. Mangiardi, L. M., Bonamini, R., Conte, M., et al.: Bedside evaluation of atrioventricular block with narrow QRS complexes: Usefulness of carotid sinus massage and atropine administration. Am. J. Cardiol. 49:1136–1145, 1982.
22. Rosen, K. M., Rahimtoola, S. H., and Gunnar, R. M.: Pseudo AV block secondary to premature non-propagated HIS bundle depolarizations: Documentation by HIS bundle electrocardiography. Circulation, 42:367–373, 1970.
23. Narula, O. S., Scherlag, B. J., Javier, R. P., et al.: Analysis of the AV conduction defect in complete heart block utilizing HIS bundle electrograms. Circulation, 41:437–448, 1970.
24. Narula, O. S., and Narula, J. T.: Junctional pacemakers in man: Response to overdrive suppression with and without parasympathetic blockade. Circulation, 57:880–889, 1978.
25. Schneider, J. F., Thomas, H. E., Sorlie, P., et al.: Comparative features of newly acquired left and right bundle branch block in the general population: The Framingham study. Am. J. Cardiol., 47:931–940, 1981.
26. Fleg, J. L., Das, D. H., and Lakatta, E. G.: Right bundle branch block: Long term prognosis in apparently healthy men. J. Am. Coll. Cardiol., 1:887–892, 1983.
27. McAnulty, J. H., Rahimtoola, S. H., Murphy, E., et al.: Natural history of "high risk" bundle branch block. N. Engl. J. Med., 307:137–143, 1982.
28. Scheinman, M. M., Peters, R. W., Sauve, M. J., et al.: Value of the H-Q interval in patients with bundle branch block and the role of prophylactic permanent pacing. Am. J. Cardiol., 50:1316–1322, 1982.
29. Rosen, K. M., Dhingra, R. C., and Wyndham, C. R.: Significance of H-V interval in 515 patients with chronic bifascicular block (abstr). Am. J. Cardiol., 45:405, 1980.
30. Dhingra, R. C., Wyndham, C., Baurnfeind, R., et al.: Significance of block distal to the HIS bundle induced by atrial pacing in patients with chronic bifascicular block. Circulation, 60:1455–1464, 1979.
31. Dhingra, R. C., Wyndham, C., Amat-Y-Leon, F., et al.: Incidence and site of atrioventricular block in patients with chronic bifascicular block. Circulation, 59:238–246, 1979.
32. Peters, R. W., Scheinman, M. M., Dhingra, R., et al.: Serial electrophysiologic studies in patients with chronic bundle branch block. Circulation, 65:1480–1485, 1982.
33. Dhingra, R. C., Denes, P., Wu, D., et al.: Syncope in patients with chronic bifascicular block: Significance, causative mechanisms, and clinical implications. Ann. Intern. Med., 81:302–306, 1974.
34. Scheinman, M., Weiss, A., and Kunkel, F.: His bundle recordings in patients with bundle branch block and transient neurologic symptoms. Circulation, 48:322–330, 1973.
35. Altschuler, H., Fisher, J. D., and Furman, S.: Significance of isolated H-V interval prolongation in symptomatic patients without documented heart block. Am. Heart J., 97:19–26, 1979.
36. DeGuzman, M., and Rahimtoola, S. H.: What is the role of pacemakers in patients with coronary artery disease and conduction abnormalities. Cardiovasc. Clin., 13:191–207, 1983.
37. Lie, K. I., Wellens, H. J., Schuilenberg, R. M., et al.: Factors influencing prognosis of bundle branch block complicating acute antero-septal infarction. Circulation, 50:935–941, 1974.
38. Harper, R., Hunt, D., Vohra, J., et al.: His bundle electrogram in patients with acute myocardial infarction complicated by atrioventricular or intraventricular conduction disturbances. Br. Heart J., 37:705–710, 1974.
39. Gould, L., Reddy, C. V., Kim, S. G., and Oh, K. C.: His bundle electrogram in patients with acute myocardial infarction. PACE, 2:428–434, 1979.
40. Wu, D., Denes, P., Amat-Y-Leon, F., et al.: Clinical, electrocardiographic and electrophysiologic observations in patients with paroxysmal supraventricular tachycardia. Am. J. Cardiol., 41:1045–1051, 1978.
41. Lloyd, E. A., Hauer, R. N., Zipes, D. P., et al.: Syncope and ventricular tachycardia in patients with ventricular pre-excitation. Am. J. Cardiol., 52:79–82, 1983.
42. Klein, G. J., Bashare, T. M., Sellers, T. D., et al.: Ventricular fibrillation in the Wolff-Parkinson-White syndrome. N. Engl. J. Med., 301:1080–1085, 1979.
43. Morady, F., Sledge, C., Shen, E., et al.: Electrophysiologic testing in the management of patients with the Wolff-Parkinson-White syndrome and atrial fibrillation. Am. J. Cardiol., 51:1623–1628, 1983.
44. Strasberg, B., Ashley, W. W., Wyndham, C. R., et al.: Treadmill exercise testing in the Wolff-Parkinson-White syndrome. Am. J. Cardiol., 45:742–748, 1980.
45. Wellens, H. J., Braat, S., Brugada, P., et al.: Use of procainamide in patients with the Wolff-Parkinson-White syndrome to disclose a short refractory period of the accessory pathway. Am. J. Cardiol., 50:1087–1089, 1982.
46. Wellens, H. J., Bar, F. W., and Lie, K. I.: The value of the electrocardiogram in the differential diagnosis of a tachycardia with a widened QRS complex. Am. J. Med., 64:27–33, 1978.
47. Josephson, M. E.: Paroxysmal supraventricular tachycardia: An electrophysiologic approach. Am. J. Cardiol., 41:1123–1126, 1978.
48. Kastor, J. A., Horowitz, L. N., Harken, A. H., and Josephson, M. E.: Clinical electrophysiology of ventricular tachycardia. N. Engl. J. Med., 304:1004–1018, 1981.
49. Cobb, L. A., Baum, R. S., Alvarez, H., and Schaffer, W. A.: Resuscitation from out-of-hospital ventricular fibrillation: 4 years of follow-up. Circulation, (Suppl.) 52:III:223–228, 1975.
50. Eisenberg, M. S., Hallstrom, A., and Bergner, L.: Long term survival after out-of-hospital cardiac arrest. N. Engl. J. Med., 22:1340–1343, 1982.
51. Iseri, L. T., Humphrey, S. B., and Siner, E. J.: Prehospital bradyasystolic cardiac arrest. Ann. Intern. Med., 88:741–745, 1978.
52. Myerburg, R. J., Conde, C. A., Sung, R. J., et al.: Clinical, electrophysiologic and hemodynamic profile of patients resuscitated from prehospital cardiac arrest. Am. J. Med., 68:568–576, 1980.
53. Ruskin, J. N., DiMarco, J. P., and Garan, H.: Out-of-hospital cardiac arrest: Electrophysiologic observations and selection of long term antiarrhythmic therapy. N. Engl. J. Med., 303:607–613, 1980.
54. Josephson, M. E., Horowitz, L. N., Spielman, S. R., and Greenspan, A. M.: Electrophysiologic and hemodynamic studies in patients resuscitated from cardiac arrest. Am. J. Cardiol., 46:948–955, 1980.
55. Morady, F., Scheinman, M. M., Hess, D. S., et al.: Electrophysio-

logic testing in the management of survivors of out-of-hospital cardiac arrest. Am. J. Cardiol. 51:85–89, 1983.
56. Longstreth, W. T., Inui, T. S., Cobb, L., and Copass, M. K.: Neurologic recovery after out-of-hospital cardiac arrest. Ann. Intern. Med., 98:588–592, 1983.
57. Panidis, I. P., and Morganroth, J.: Sudden death in hospitalized patients: Cardiac rhythm disturbances detected by ambulatory electrocardiographic monitoring. J. Am. Coll. Cardiol. 2:798–805, 1983.
58. Pratt, C. M., Francis, M. J., Luck, J. C., et al.: Analysis of ambulatory electrocardiograms in 15 patients during spontaneous ventricular fibrillation with special reference to preceding arrhythmic events. J. Am. Coll. Cardiol., 2:789–797, 1983.
59. Myerburg, R. J., Conde, C., Sheps, D. S., et al.: Antiarrhythmic drug therapy in survivors of prehospital cardiac arrest: Comparison of effects on chronic ventricular arrhythmias and recurrent cardiac arrest. Circulation, 59:855–863, 1979.
60. Graboys, T. B., Lown, B., Podrid, P. J., and DeSilva, R.: Long-term survival of patients with malignant ventricular arrhythmia treated with antiarrhythmic drugs. Am. J. Cardiol. 50:437–443, 1982.
61. Winkle, R.: Measuring antiarrhythmic drug efficacy by suppression of asymptomatic ventricular arrhythmias. Ann. Intern. Med., 91:480–482, 1979.
62. Peter, T., Hamer, A., Weiss, D., and Mandel, W.: Sudden death survivors: Experience with long-term empiric therapy with Amiodarone (abstr). Circulation, (Suppl. IV), 64:36, 1981.
63. Waxman, H. L., Buxton, A. E., Sadowski, L. M., and Josephson, M. E.: The response to Procainamide during electrophysiologic study for sustained ventricular tachyarrhythmias predicts the response to other medications. Circulation, 67:30–37, 1983.
64. Velebit, V., Podrid, P., Lown, B., et al.: Aggravation and provocation of ventricular arrhythmias by antiarrhythmic drugs. Circulation, 65:886–894, 1982.
65. Ruskin, J. N., Garan, H., Dimarco, J. P., and Kelly, E.: Electrophysiologic testing in survivors of prehospital cardiac arrest (abstr). Am. J. Cardiol., 49:958, 1982.
66. Benditt, D. G., Benson, D. W., Klein, G. J., et al.: Prevention of recurrent sudden cardiac arrest: Role of provocative electropharmacologic testing. J. Am. Coll. Cardiol., 2:418–425, 1983.
67. Vandepol, C. J., Farshidi, A., Spielman, S. R., et al.: Incidence and clinical significance of induced ventricular tachycardia. Am. J. Cardiol., 45:725–731, 1980.
68. Naccarelli, G. V., Prystowksy, E. N., Jackman, W. M., et al.: Role of electrophysiologic testing in managing patients who have ventricular tachycardia unrelated to coronary artery disease. Am. J. Cardiol., 50:165–171, 1982.
69. Livelli, F. D., Bigger, J. T., Reiffel, J. A., et al.: Response to programmed ventricular stimulation: Sensitivity, specificity, and relation to heart disease. Am. J. Cardiol., 50:452–458, 1982.
70. Mann, D. E., Luch, J. C., Griffin, J. C., et al.: Induction of clinical ventricular tachycardia using programmed stimulation: Value of third and fourth extrastimuli. Am. J. Cardiol., 52:501–506, 1983.
71. Fisher, J. D.: Role of electrophysiologic testing in the diagnosis and treatment of patients with known and suspected bradycardias and tachycardias. Prog. Cardiovasc. Dis., 24:25–90, 1981.
72. Kehoe, R. F., Moran, J. M., Zheutin, T., and Lesch, M.: Electrophysiological study to direct therapy in survivors of pre-hospital ventricular fibrillation (abstr.). Am. J. Cardiol., 49:928, 1982.
73. Mason, J. W., Swerdlow, C. D., Winkle, R. A., et al.: Programmed ventricular stimulation in predicting vulnerability to ventricular arrhythmias and their response to antiarrhythmic therapy. Am. Heart J., 103:633–638, 1982.
74. Roy, D., Waxman, H. L., Kienzle, M. G., et al.: Clinical characteristics and long-term follow-up in 119 survivors of cardiac arrest: Relation to inducibility at electrophysiologic testing. Am. J. Cardiol., 52:969–974, 1983.
75. Brugada, P., Adbollah, H., Heddle, B., Wellens, H. J.: Results of a ventricular stimulation protocol using a maximum of 4 premature stimuli in patients without documented or suspected ventricular arrhythmias. Am. J. Cardiol., 52:1214–1218, 1983.
76. Mason, J. W., and Winkle, R. A.: Accuracy of the ventricular tachycardia-induction study for predicting long-term efficacy and inefficacy of antiarrhythmic drugs. N. Engl. J. Med., 303:1073–1077, 1980.
77. Horowitz, L. N., Spielman, S. R., Greenspan, A. M., and Josephson, M. E.: Role of programmed stimulation in assessing vulnerability to ventricular arrhythmias. Am. Heart J., 103:604–610, 1982.
78. Schoenfeld, M. H., McGovern, B., Garan, H., et al.: Long-term follow-up of patients with ventricular tachycardia or fibrillation with no inducible arrhythmia during programmed cardiac stimulation (abstr.). J. Am. Coll. Cardiol., 1:606, 1983.
79. Kapoor, W. N., Karpf, M., Wieand, S., et al.: A prospective evaluation and follow-up of patients with syncope. N. Engl. J. Med., 309:197–204, 1983.
80. DiMarco, J. P., Garan, H., Harthorne, J. W., and Ruskin, J. N.: Intracardiac electrophysiologic techniques in recurrent syncope of unknown cause. Ann. Intern. Med., 95:542–548, 1981.
81. Gulamhusein, S., Nacarelli, G. V., Ko, P. T., et al.: Value and limitations of clinical electrophysiologic study in assessment of patients with unexplained syncope. Am. J. Med., 73:700–705, 1982.
82. Hess, D. S., Morady, F., and Scheinman, M. M.: Electrophysiologic testing in the evaluation of patients with syncope of undetermined origin. Am. J. Cardiol., 50:1309–1315, 1982.
83. Tonkin, A. M., Heddle, W. F., and Tornos, P.: Intermittent atrioventricular block: Procainamide administration as a provocative test. Aust. N.Z. J. Med., 8:594–602, 1978.
84. Zaher, C., Hamer, A., Peter, T., and Mandel, W.: The use of intravenous procainamide to evaluate the potential etiology of syncope in patients with bundle branch block. PACE, 6:A-104, 1983.
85. LaBarre, A., Strauss, H. C., Scheinman, M. M., et al.: Electrophysiologic effects of disopyramide phosphate on sinus node function in patients with sinus node dysfunction. Circulation, 59:226–235, 1979.
86. Wu, D., Amat-Y-Leon, F., Simpson, R. J., et al.: Electrophysiological studies with multiple drugs in patients with atrioventricular re-entrant tachycardias utilizing an extranodal pathway. Circulation, 56:727–736, 1977.
87. Bauernfiend, R. A., Wyndham, C. R., Dhingra, R. C., et al.: Serial electrophysiologic testing of multiple drugs in patients with atrioventricular nodal re-entrant paroxysmal tachycardia. Circulation, 62:1341–1349, 1980.
88. Kruse, I., Arnman, K., Conradson, T. B., and Rydén, L.: A comparison of the acute and long-term hemodynamic effects of ventricular inhibited and atrial synchronous ventricular inhibited pacing. Circulation, 65:846–855, 1982.
89. Weiner, I.: Pacing techniques in the treatment of tachycardias. Ann. Intern. Med., 93:326–329, 1980.
90. Kowey, P. R., and Engel, T. R.: Overdrive pacing for ventricular tachyarrhythmias: A reassessment. Ann. Intern. Med., 99:651–656, 1983.
91. Wells, J. L., MacLean, W. A., James, T. N., and Waldo, A. L.: Characterization of atrial flutter: Studies in man after open heart surgery using fixed atrial electrodes. Circulation, 60:665–673, 1979.
92. Roy, D., Waxman, H. L., Buxton, A. E., et al.: Termination of ventricular tachycardia: Role of tachycardia cycle length. Am. J. Cardiol., 50:1346–1350, 1982.

93. Fisher, J. D., Kim, S. G., Furman, S., and Matos, J.: Role of implantable pacemakers in control of recurrent ventricular tachycardia. Am. J. Cardiol., 49:194–206, 1982.
94. Mirowski, M., Reid, P. R., Winkle, R. A., et al.: Mortality in patients with implanted automatic defibrillators. Ann. Intern. Med., 98:585–588, 1983.
95. Klein, G. J., Sealy, W. C., Pritchett, E. L., et al.: Cryosurgical ablation of the atrioventricular node—His bundle: Long term follow-up and properties of the junctional pacemaker. Circulation, 61:8–15, 1980.
96. Holmes, D. R., Osborn, M. J., Gersh, B., et al.: The Wolff-Parkinson-White syndrome: A surgical approach. Mayo. Clin. Proc., 57:345–350, 1982.
97. Mason, J. W., Stinson, E. B., Winkle, R. A., et al.: Relative efficacy of blind left ventricular aneurysm resection for the treatment of recurrent ventricular tachycardia. Am. J. Cardiol., 49:241–249, 1982.
98. Mason, J. W., Stinson, E. B., Winkle, R. A., et al.: Surgery for ventricular tachycardia: Efficacy of left ventricular aneurysm resection compared with operation guided by electrical activation mapping. Circulation, 65:1148–1155, 1982.
99. Garan, H., Ruskin, J. N., DiMarco, J. P., et al.: Electrophysiologic studies before and after myocardial revascularization in patients with life-threatening ventricular arrhythmias. Am. J. Cardiol., 51:519–524, 1983.
100. Josephson, M. E., Harken, A. H., Horowitz, L. N.: Long-term results of endocardial resection for sustained ventricular tachycardia in coronary disease patients. Am. Heart J., 104:51–57, 1982.
101. Fontaine, G., Guirandon, G., Frank, R., et al.: Surgical management of ventricular tachycardia unrelated to myocardial ischemia or infarction. Am. J. Cardiol., 49:397–410, 1982.
102. Gallagher, J. J., Svenson, R. H., Kasell, J. H., et al.: Catheter technique for closed-chest ablation of the atrioventricular conduction system. N. Engl. J. Med., 306:194–200, 1982.
103. Wood, D. L., Hammill, S. C., Holmes, D. R., et al.: Catheter ablation of the atrioventricular conduction system in patients with supraventricular tachycardia. Mayo Clin. Proc., 58:791–796, 1983.
104. Weber, H., and Schmitz, L.: Catheter technique for closed-chest ablation of an accessory atrioventricular pathway. N. Engl. J. Med., 308:653–654, 1983.
105. Gillette, P. C., Garson, A., and Porter, C. J.: Junctional automatic ectopic tachycardia: New proposed treatment by transcatheter His bundle ablation. Am. Heart J., 106:619–623, 1983.
106. Hartler, G. O.: Electrode catheter ablation of refractory focal ventricular tachycardia. J. Am. Coll. Cardiol., 2:1107–1113, 1983.
107. Swerdlow, C. D., Winkle, R. A., and Mason, J. W.: Determinants of survival in patients with ventricular tachyarrhythmias. N. Engl. J. Med., 308:1436–1442, 1983.
108. Hamer, A., Vohra, J., Hunt, D., and Sloman, G.: Prediction of sudden death by electrophysiologic studies in high risk patients surviving acute myocardial infarction. Am. J. Cardiol., 50:223–229, 1982.
109. Richards, D. A., Cody, D. V., Denniss, A. R., et al.: Ventricular electrical instability: A predictor of death after myocardial infarction. Am. J. Cardiol., 51:75–80, 1983.
110. Marchlinski, F. E., Buxton, A. E., Waxman, H. L., and Josephson, M. E.: Indentifying patients at risk of sudden death after myocardial infarction: Value of the response to programmed stimulation, degree of ventricular ectopic activity and severity of left ventricular dysfunction. Am. J. Cardiol., 52:1190–1196, 1983.
111. Kowey, P. R., Folland, E. D., Parisi, A. F., and Lown, B.: Programmed electrical stimulation of the heart in coronary artery disease. Am. J. Cardiol., 51:531–536, 1983.
112. Buxton, A. E., Waxman, H. L., Marchlinski, F. E., and Josephson, M. E.: Electrophysiologic studies in nonsustained ventricular tachycardia: relation to underlying heart disease. Am. J. Cardiol., 52:985–991, 1983.
113. Ruskin, J. N., Caracta, A. R., Batsford, W. P., et al.: Electrophysiologic effects of diazepam in man. Clin. Res., 22:302A, 1974.
114. Nattel, S., Rinkenberger, R. L., Lehrman, L. L., and Zipes, D. P.: Therapeutic blood lidocaine concentrations after local anesthesia for cardiac electrophysiologic studies. N. Engl. J. Med., 301:418–420, 1979.
115. Dimarco, J. P., Garan, H., and Ruskin, J. N.: Complications in patients undergoing cardiac electrophysiologic procedures. Ann. Intern. Med., 97:490–493, 1982.
116. Littleford, P. O., Curry, R. C., Schwartz, K. M., and Pepine, C. J.: Clinical evaluation of a new temporary atrial pacing catheter: Results in 100 patients. Am. Heart J., 107:237–240, 1984.
117. Reiffel, J. A., Gang, E., Gliklich, J. et al.: The human sinus node electrogram: A transvenous catheter technique and a comparison of directly measured and indirectly estimated sinoatrial conduction time in adults. Circulation, 62:1324–1334, 1980.
118. Josephson, M. E., Scharf, D. L., Kastor, J. A., Kitchen, J. G.: Atrial endocardial activation in man. Am. J. Cardiol., 39:972–981, 1977.
119. Breithardt, G., and Seipel, L.: Recording of left atrial potentials from pulmonary artery in man. Br. Heart J., 43:689–694, 1980.
120. Prystowsky, E. N., Pritchett, E. L., and Gallagher, J. J.: Origin of the atrial electrogram recorded from the esophagus. Circulation, 61:1017–1023, 1980.
121. Guimond, C., and Puech, P.: Intra-His bundle blocks (102 cases). Eur. J. Cardiol., 4:481–493, 1976.
122. Josephson, M. E., Seides, S. F.: Clinical cardiac electrophysiology; techniques and interpretations, pp. 18–20. Philadelphia, Lea & Febiger, 1979.
123. Castellanos, A., Castillo, C., and Agha, A.: Contribution of His bundle recording to the understanding of clinical arrhythmias. Am. J. Cardiol., 28:499–508, 1971.
124. Gallagher, J. J., and Damato, A. N.: Techniques of recording His bundle activity in man. In Grossman W (ed.): Cardiac Catheterization and Angiography, pp. 283–301. Philadelphia, Lea & Febiger, 1980.
125. Josephson, M. E., and Seides, S. F.: Clinical cardiac electrophysiology: Techniques and interpretations, pp. 23–59. Philadelphia, Lea & Febiger, 1979.
126. Narula, O. S., Scherlag, B. J., Samet, P., and Javier, R. P.: Atrioventricular block: Localization and classification by His bundle recordings. Am. J. Med., 50:146–165, 1971.
127. Rosen, K. M.: Evaluation of cardiac conduction in the cardiac catheterization laboratory. Am. J. Cardiol., 30:701–703, 1972.
128. Akhtar, M., Damato, A. N., Batsford, W. P., et al.: A comparative analysis of antegrade and retrograde conduction patterns in man. Circulation, 52:766–778, 1975.
129. Denes, P., Wu, D., Dhingra, R., et al.: The effects of cycle length on cardiac refractory periods in man. Circulation, 49:32–41, 1974.
130. Schuilenberg, R. M., and Durrer, D.: Conduction disturbances within the His bundle. Circulation, 45:612–628, 1972.
131. Hoffman, B. F., and Rosen, M. R.: Cellular mechanisms for cardiac arrhythmias. Circ. Res., 49:1–15, 1981.
132. Mandel, W. J., Hayakawa, H., Danzig, R., and Marcus, H. S.: Evaluation of sinoatrial node function in man by overdrive suppression. Circulation, 44:59–66, 1971.
133. Strauss, H. C., Saroff, A. L., Bigger, J. T., and Giardina, E. G.:

Premature atrial stimulation as a key to the understanding of sinoatrial conduction in man. Circulation, 47:86–93, 1973.

134. Narula, O. S., Shanto, N., Vasquez, M., et al.: A new method for measurement of sinoatrial conduction time in man. Circulation, 58:706–714, 1978.

135. Hariman, R. J., Krongrad, E., Boxer, R. A., et al.: Method for recording electrical activity of the sinoatrial node and automatic atrial foci during cardiac catheterization in human subjects. Am. J. Cardiol., 45:775–781, 1980.

136. Juillard, A., Guillerm, F., Chuong, H. V., et al.: Sinus node electrogram recording in 59 patients: Comparison with simultaneous estimation of sinoatrial conduction using premature atrial stimulation. Br. Heart J., 50:75–84, 1983.

137. Jose, A. D., and Collison, D.: The normal range and determinants of the intrinsic heart rate in man. Cardiovasc. Res., 4:160–168, 1970.

138. Denes, P., Wu, D., Dhingra, R., et al.: The effects of cycle length on cardiac refractory periods in man. Circulation, 49:32–41, 1974.

139. Josephson, M. E., and Seides, S. F.: Clinical cardiac electrophysiology: Techniques and interpretations, pp. 39–40. Philadelphia, Lea & Febiger, 1979.

140. Fisher, J. D., Ostrow, E., Kim, S. G., and Matos, J. A.: Ultrarapid single-capture train stimulation for termination of ventricular tachycardia. Am. J. Cardiol., 51:1334–1338, 1983.

141. Gardner, M. J., Waxman, H. L., Buxton, A. E., et al.: Termination of ventricular tachycardia: Evaluation of a new pacing method. Am. J. Cardiol., 50:1338–1345, 1982.

142. Robertson, J. F., Cain, M. E., Horowitz, L. N., et al.: Anatomic and electrophysiologic correlates of ventricular tachycardia requiring left ventricular stimulation. Am. J. Cardiol., 48:263–268, 1981.

143. Morady, F., Hess, D., Scheinman, M. M.: Electrophysiologic drug testing in patients with malignant ventricular arrhythmias: Importance of stimulation at more than one ventricular site. Am. J. Cardiol. 50:1055–1060, 1982.

144. Ross, D. L., Sze, D. Y., Keffe, D. L., et al.: Antiarrhythmic drug combinations in the treatment of ventricular tachycardia. Circulation, 66:1205–1210, 1982.

145. Duffy, C. E., Swiryn, S., Bauernfeind, R. A., et al.: Inducible sustained ventricular tachycardia refractory to individual class I drugs: Effect of adding a second class I drug. Am. Heart J., 106:450–458, 1983.

146. Hammer, A. W., Finerman, W. B., Peter, T., and Mandel, W. J.: Disparity between the clinical and electrophysiologic effects of amiodarone in the treatment of recurrent ventricular tachyarrhythmias. Am. Heart J., 102:992–1000, 1981.

147. Josephson, M. E., Horowitz, L. N., Farshidi, A., et al.: Recurrent sustained ventricular tachycardia. II. Endocardial mapping. Circulation, 57:440–447, 1978.

148. Josephson, M. E., Horowitz, L. N., Spielman, S. R., et al.: Comparison of endocardial catheter mapping with intraoperative mapping of ventricular tachycardia. Circulation, 61:395–404, 1980.

149. Weiner, I., Mindich, B., and Pitchon, R.: Fragmented endocardial electrical activity in patients with ventricular tachycardia: A new guide to surgical therapy. Am. Heart J., 107:86–90, 1984.

6

Disorders of Sinus Function

Jay L. Jordan and William J. Mandel

The sinus node is a highly organized cluster of specialized cells located in the area of the junction between the superior vena cava and right atrium.[1] Crescent shaped, it varies in length from 9 to 15 mm and has a central body (5 mm wide and 1.5 to 2 mm thick) and tapering ends. Its anatomic, microscopic, and ultrastructural features have already been described in Chapter 2 of this book (Anderson and Becker). However, an important ultrastructural characteristic of the sinus node includes a sarcolemma composed of a trilaminar unit plasma membrane surrounded by an external glycoprotein coat. The glycoprotein coat may concentrate and bind cations to its surface, thereby in part determining the local ionic environment of the sinus node independent of the actual concentration of cations in the surrounding media.[2–8] This property of the glycoprotein coat could confound the interpretation of voltage-clamp studies designed to identify the ionic currents involved in sinoatrial electrogenesis.

Recently, a perinodal zone of unique cell type surrounding the sinus node of the rabbit has been identified. These perinodal fibers have electrophysiologic characteristics distinct from the sinus node and normal atrial tissue and may represent a buffer zone through which electrical activity must pass on its way out of or into the sinus node. Although the presence of an anatomically distinct perinodal zone and specialized pathways of conduction between the sinus node and atrium have not been demonstrated in humans, there is considerable indirect evidence supporting their functional existence. In view of the failure by some investigators to trace discrete or continuous anatomic tracts of Purkinje-like cells between the sinus and AV nodes, it has been suggested that the spatial orientation of atrial myocardial fibers facilitates preferential routes of conduction.

The vascular supply to the mammalian sinus node region comes from a central artery that does not appear to terminate in the sinus node. A rich supply of collateral vessels, densest centrally and sparser peripherally, is a constant feature. Although some animals, particularly the dog, occasionally have more than one sinus node artery or have a single vessel with multiple origins, this is not the case in humans, in whom a single sinus node artery originates from the proximal 2 to 3 cm of the right coronary artery in 55% and from the proximal 1 cm of the left circumflex artery in 45%.

Sinoatrial Node Electrogenesis

The phenomenon of spontaneous phase 4 depolarization is the electrophysiologic characteristic that distinguishes pacemaker cells from all other cells in the body. Emergence of the sinus node as the dominant cardiac pacemaker is due to two basic electrophysiologic properties of the sinus node pacemaker cells: (1) the low level of the resting or maximum diastolic membrane potential (−60 mV) and (2) the rapid rate of rise of phase 4 diastolic depolarization. Characterization of the ionic events that give rise to spontaneous diastolic depolarization in the sinus node has been hampered because only recently has a technique been developed permitting performance of voltage-clamp experiments in the sinus node.[9] From extensive microelectrode studies, however, the following changes in membrane properties, either singly or in combination, have been proposed as possible mechanisms responsible for phase 4 depolarization: (1) decreased outward permeability to potassium, (2) increased inward permeability to sodium, (3) reduced sodium pump activity, and (4) increased inward permeability to calcium.

Although the most accepted explanation for the initiation of spontaneous pacemaker depolarization is a voltage greater than the time-dependent decay in outward potassium current, several facts mitigate against applying this theory to the sinus node. First, the potential range over which phase 4 depolarization occurs in sinus node cells is in a voltage range in which the pacemaker current is fully activated in pacemaker cells proved to be dependent on decay of outward potassium current (*i.e.*, Purkinje fibers).[10-12] Second, the slope of phase 4 depolarization in sinus node cells is relatively resistant to the depressant effect of an increase in external potassium concentration when compared to Purkinje fibers.[13]

There is now sufficient evidence suggesting that the passive sodium current plays at most a very minimal role in initiating the sinus node impulse. Specifically, changes in the extracellular concentration of sodium have little effect on the slope of phase 4 depolarization.[14] Likewise, active sodium transport appears to contribute little to generating the sinus node impulse; neither tetrodotoxin nor lithium substitution, both of which make the electrogenic sodium pump inoperative, significantly affects the slope of phase 4 depolarization.[15-17]

Our understanding of the mechanisms of the generation of the sinus node impulse has recently been expanded by recognizing the importance of the slow channel.[18,19] Both sodium and calcium have been implicated as the ionic elements participating in a slow inward current that follows closely behind an initial fast inward current in both the sinus and atrioventricular nodes. Although the threshold of activation for the slow current (−30 to −40 mV) is positive to the voltage range over which pacemaking largely occurs, microelectrode studies suggest that the slow current may play a significant role in generating the sinus node impulse. Specifically, slow channel inhibitors such as D-600, Mg^{++}, and verapamil depress sinus node phase 4 depolarization.[20-24] It has been suggested that sluggish inactivation occurs of the slow current that had been activated during the plateau of the previous action potential, thus accounting for its persistence at the level of the sinus node maximum diastolic membrane potential.[25]

Theories and mathematic models that have been proposed to explain the extreme complexity of the relationship between the various ions participating in the generation of slow diastolic depolarization in the sinus node pacemaker cell now must contend with recent observations regarding the role of anion currents. An inward chloride ionic current does seem to participate in slow diastolic depolarization in the sinus node.[26-28] Anion permeability of the sinus node is much greater than that of Purkinje cells. Substitution of anions in the extracellar environment that are more permeant than chloride (*e.g.*, bromide) results in faster rates of spontaneous diastolic depolarization of the isolated sinus node cell. Substitution of anions that are less permeant than chloride (*e.g.*, methyl sulfate), results in slower rates of spontaneous diastolic depolarization. Although it remains unclear how chloride contributes to phase 4 depolarization at any given moment, it is likely that chloride contributes only a part of the current responsible for slow diastolic depolarization in the sinus node cell.

Voltage-clamp studies have determined that part of the difficulty in identifying the precise ionic currents involved in generating diastolic depolarization in the sinus node is that cells in different parts of the node have different electrophysiologic characteristics with participation of different ions. The "dominant pacemaker site" probably lies in the center of the node, where a group of approximately 5000 cells, with identical synchronous activity, show maximum diastolic potentials of about −50mV and have short times halfway between maximum diastolic potential and peak action potential. For technical reasons, most voltage-clamp studies performed thus far have been in the periphery of the sinus node near the crista terminalis, where the most negative maximum diastolic potential seen is between −70 mV and −75 mV. Central cells appear to be slow channel dependent, while peripheral cells are less dependent on the slow channel alone.

The rate of spontaneous depolarization of a pacemaker cell is determined by the level of maximum diastolic potential, the rate or slope of phase 4 depolarization, the level of the threshold potential, the rate of rise and amplitude of phase 0, and duration of the action

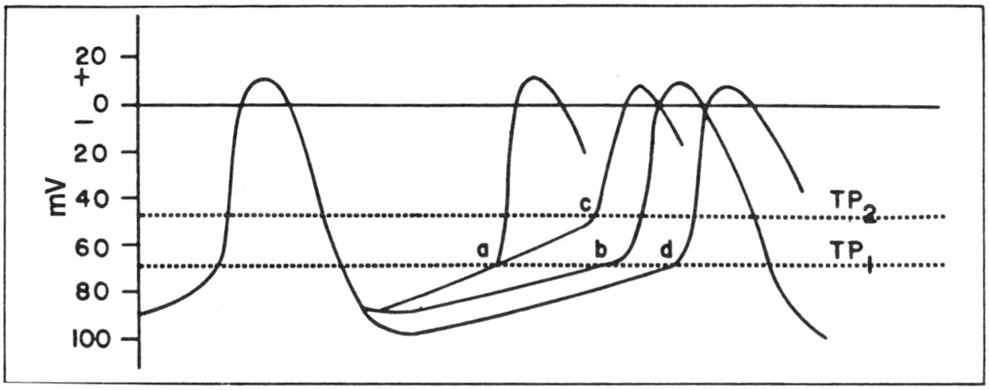

Figure 6-1. *A typical sinus node action potential is seen on this graph. An indication of action potential voltage in millivolts is shown on the vertical axis. Points a and b identify different frequencies of sinus node depolarization dependent on the slope of phase 4 depolarization. In action potentials b and d, with equal slopes of phase 4 depolarization, maximum diastolic potential in b is greater (more negative than in d); therefore, the rate of discharge of the sinus node pacemaker in d is slower than in b. Another feature that will alter the rate of discharge of the sinus node is the threshold potential. At points a, b, and d, the threshold potential is approximately −70 mV; at point c, the threshold potential is approximately −48 mV. This upward shift in the threshold potential (*i.e., *to less negative) results in a slowing in the rate of discharge when points a and c are compared.*

potential (Fig. 6-1). Thus, slowing of the rate of spontaneous sinus node discharge may be due to an increased maximum diastolic potential, a reduced slope of diastolic depolarization, a threshold potential less negative than normal, a reduced slope and amplitude of phase 0, or a prolonged duration of the action potential.

As with phase 4 depolarization, the determinants of the other characteristics of the sinus node action potential are voltage- or time dependent fluctuations in membrane permeability to various ions. Phase 0 appears to depend on both the activation of a fast sodium channel and a second slow channel, the dominant current being determined by the level of the takeoff potential.[29–32] Maintenance of the resting membrane potential probably depends on the electrogenic sodium pump and changes in potassium flux,[17,33–35] although the precise mechanisms involved remain uncertain. The duration of the action potential probably depends on characteristics of slow channel currents as well as potassium conductance.

An apparent slowing of sinus node automaticity, manifesting itself electrocardiographically in a manner indistinguishable from abnormalities of sinus node pacemaker function, may result from slowing of conduction through the sinoatrial junction. Depression of sinoatrial conduction by verapamil in isolated rabbit sinus node preparations suggests that the slow channel plays a significant role in determining the conduction properties of the perinodal zone.[36]

Extrinsic Factors Modifying the Intrinsic Electrophysiologic Characteristics of the Sinus Node

The Role of the Autonomic Nervous System

The mechanisms of initiating spontaneous phase 4 depolarization and the determinants of the rate of spontaneous depolarization are intrinsic properties of the pacemaker cell. Similarly, sinoatrial conduction time is a function of the intrinsic electrophysiologic properties of the sinoatrial junction. However, the characteristics of these intrinsic properties can be modified by parasympathetic and sympathetic influences.

Vagal stimulation or acetylcholine slows the sinus rate and intranodal conduction velocity and lengthens the effective and relative refractory period of the sinus node.[37] Corresponding changes in the sinus node action potential include increased negativity of the maximum diastolic potential and reduced slope of phase 4 diastolic depolarization.[38,39] Considerable evidence suggests that these effects are mediated in part by increased conductance of potassium.[40–45] Parasympathetic effects on sodium conductance are minimal,[17] while effects on the slow channel, independent of an increased maximum diastolic potential, are less clear.[46,47] Furthermore, sinoatrial conduction time is prolonged by parasympathetic stimuli.[48]

In contrast, sympathetic stimulation or catecholamine infusion increases the spontaneous sinus node discharge rate, primarily because the rate of phase 4 depolarization is increased.[37,49] This change in phase 4 slope presumably relates to a decrease in time-dependent potassium conductance.[50] However, sympathetic simulation also increases calcium conductance at all levels of maximum diastolic potential, probably through a nonspecific effect on adenyl cyclase induction.[51,52] Sinoatrial conduction time is shortened by sympathetic stimulation.

During simultaneous stimulation of the sympathetic and parasympathetic systems, deceleration of sinus rate to cholinergic stimulation predominates over the acceleratory effects of sympathetic stimulation. In an elegant series of experiments, MacKary and co-workers[53] determined that when acetylcholine is added to a sinus node preparation, either alone or in combination with epinephrine, pacemaker shift occurs from the superior part of the sinus node to the inferior portion. Pacemaker cells in the inferior portion demonstrate deceleration due to acetylcholine, which is enhanced in the presence of epinephrine. Thus, functional inhomogeneity of the sinus node would seem to explain, in part, the predominance of the effect of cholinergic stimulation over that of sympathetic stimulation.

The Role of the Endocrine System

Although less extensively investigated than the interaction between intrinsic sinus node function and the autonomic nervous system, humoral factors also modify the electrophysiologic characteristics of the sinus node. This modification appears to be independent of any interaction with the autonomic nervous system. For example, sinus node cells isolated from the hearts of thyrotoxic rabbits have an increased rate of diastolic depolarization and a decreased action potential duration. In contrast, sinus node cells isolated from hypothyroid rabbits have a decreased rate of diastolic depolarization and an increased action potential duration.[54]

The Role of the Sinus Node Artery

The sinus node artery is larger than anticipated from knowledge of the extent of the area that it supplies. This disproportionately large size is considered by James to be of physiologic importance.[55,56] Based on predictable responses of the sinus rate to stretch[57,58] and the special arrangement of the sinus node cells around the sinus node artery, James suggests that the distention and collapse of this vessel play an important role in regulating sinus rate. Collapse of the artery results in an increase in tension on pacemaker cells because of the relationship between the cells and the artery through the attachment of collagen to both the nodal cells and the arterial wall. Collapse of the artery thereby increases sinus rate. Distention of the artery has the opposite effect, leading to relaxation of the nodal cells and slowing of the heart rate. The precise intrinsic electrophysiologic properties of the sinus node that are modified by stretch and, therefore, by sinus node artery perfusion pressure have not yet been clearly defined.

Other Extrinsic Factors

Hypothermia depresses sinus automaticity by increasing the negativity of the maximum diastolic membrane potential, an effect mediated through inhibition of the sodium pump, resulting in accumulation of intracellular sodium. Hypothermia also reverses the acceleratory effect of increased extracellular calcium concentration and, therefore, may retard conductance through the slow channel.[59,60] Conversely, hyperthermia in the isolated preparation and fever in humans increase sinus rate.[59] Drugs that interfere with oxidative metabolism (*e.g.*, cyanide, phenobarbital) depress intrinsic sinus node automaticity, whereas aspirin enhances automaticity.

Sinus Node Dysfunction

Definition

The sick sinus syndrome is a descriptive term coined by Lown[61] and popularized by Ferrer[62] to refer to a constellation of signs, symptoms, and electrocardiographic criteria defining sinus node dysfunction in a clinical setting. The syndrome is characterized by syncope or other manifestations of cerebral dysfunction in association with sinus bradycardia, sinus arrest, sinoatrial block, alternating bradyarrhythmias and tachyarrhythmias, or carotid hypersensitivity. However, clinical signs and symptoms result from failure of escape pacemaker function, not from sinus node malfunction *per se*. Thus, the sick sinus syndrome may represent a generalized disorder of the conduction system of the heart, sinus node dysfunction being only one aspect.

Incidence

The incidence of sinus node dysfunction in the general population is unknown. Limited information suggests that in cardiac patients the incidence of sinus node dysfunction is approximately 3 in 5000.[63] Between 6.3% and 24% of all patients with permanent pacemakers followed in pacemaker clinics worldwide have evidence of sinus node disease.[64–70] With increasing clinical awareness of the sick sinus syndrome and more liberal criteria for pacemaker insertion in general, in recent years abnormalities of sinus node function may have been the primary indication for permanent pacing in as many as 50%

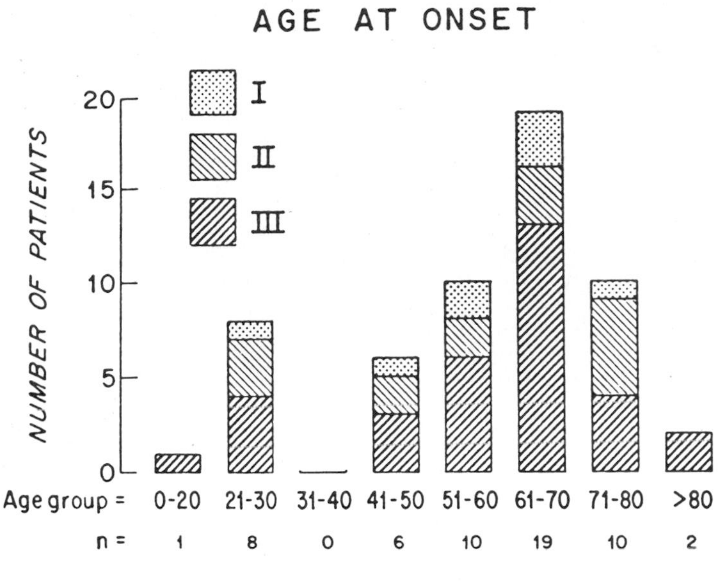

Figure 6-2. *This figure demonstrates the age of onset of sinus node dysfunction in a group of sinus node dysfunction patients. Note the bimodal distribution of the patient population, with the vast majority being over 50 years of age. However, there is a small subgroup of patients who are below the age of 30. (Rubenstein, J. J., et al.: Clinical spectrum of the sick sinus syndrome. Circulation, 46:5, 1972; by permission of the American Heart Association, Inc.)*

of permanently paced patients. Men and women appear to be equally affected by disturbances of sinus node function.[71] In terms of age, there seems to be a bimodal distribution of incidence of sinus node dysfunction, with peaks occurring in the third and fourth decades of life and again in the seventh (Fig. 6-2). The majority of patients in the older age group have coexisting hypertensive heart disease or coronary artery disease,[71-73] although many exceptions to this association have been cited.

Etiology

Many etiologic factors have been implicated in the development of abnormalities of sinus node function.[74-78] The most frequent anatomic findings in patients with sick sinus are coronary atherosclerosis, atrial amyloidosis, and diffuse fibrosis. Although sinus node dysfunction is characteristically thought of as a disease of the aged, the precise anatomic concomitants of the aging process responsible for sinus node dysfunction in the elderly have not been elucidated. The syndrome has also been described in association with other infiltrative disorders, collagen vascular disease, infectious processes including diphtheria, rheumatic fever, and viral myocarditis, as a familial pattern, and in pericardial disease. Drug-induced abnormalities of sinus node function have been recognized with increasing frequency. However, perhaps the most common form of the sick sinus syndrome is the idiopathic variety.

Special consideration should be given to sinus node dysfunction in the setting of acute myocardial infarction. Sinus bradycardia is a common clinical manifestation of acute inferior and lateral myocardial infarction, and even sinus arrest occasionally has been reported.[79-81] Whether these manifestations of sinus node dysfunction are the consequence of ischemia to the sinus node *per se* or reflect local autonomic neural effects or edematous changes in surrounding tissue is speculative.[82,83] Although the majority of patients demonstrate only transient depression of sinus node function during the acute stage of the infarct, a small number will develop evidence of permanent sinus node dysfunction. Unfortunately, no long-term follow-up study of a large population of these patients has been reported to allow a statement on the incidence of permanent sinus node dysfunction following an acute myocardial infarction. Experimental occlusion of the sinus node artery in dogs has resulted in variable degrees of sinus node dysfunction, ranging from profound slowing to no response whatsoever.[84-86] The variability in response has been attributed to differences in extent of collaterals and the occasional multiplicity of sinus node arteries in canine hearts.[87,88]

Electrocardiographic Manifestations of Sinus Node Dysfunction

Regular sinus rhythm is the normal rhythm of the heart. The normal rate of impulse formation by the sinus node in the adult is conventionally accepted as 60 to 100 beats/min. Sinus rhythm has a frontal-plane P vector oriented to the left and inferior generally between $+30°$ and $+60°$ (Fig. 6-3). A regular sinus rhythm with a rate over 100 defines sinus tachycardia. Sinus tachycardia rarely exceeds 160 beats/min in the adult; however, in the young adult, the normal sinus node is probably capable of discharging at rates over 180 beats/min under the influence of maximum physiologic or pharmacologic stimulation. The maximum rate at which the sinoatrial junction is normally able to conduct sinus impulses is unknown. A regular sinus rhythm with a rate less than 60 beats/min defines sinus bradycardia, perhaps the commonest electrocardiographic manifestation of sinus node dysfunction.

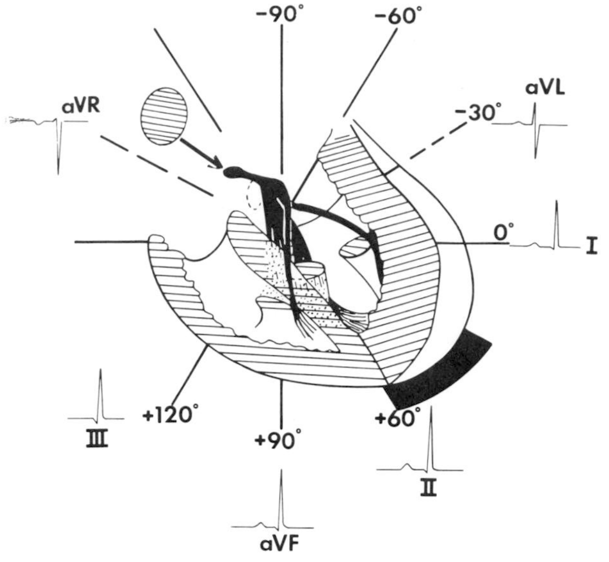

Figure 6-3. *This diagram illustrates the normal P wave activation. Note that the normal P wave vector is between +30° and +60° in the frontal plane, leading to an isoelectric P wave in lead III and a negative P wave in lead aVR.*

Sinus Arrhythmia

In sinus arrhythmia, the pacemaker is the sinus node but the rhythm is irregular. The definition of sinus arrhythmia has not been standardized; some authorities consider sinus arrhythmia to be present when the difference between the shortest P-P interval and the longest P-P interval is greater than 120 msec.[89] Other criteria defining sinus arrhythmia include variations in sinus cycle length of 10% or more[90] and variations in P-P intervals of 160 msec or greater.[91]

Sinus rate varies normally with the phases of respiration, increasing with inspiration and slowing with expiration. Sinus arrhythmia bearing no relationship to respiration probably has little clinical significance; rarely is this rhythm a forerunner of atrial dysrhythmias. It is not possible to distinguish irregularity of sinus impulse formation from variable conduction velocities through the sinoatrial junction on the surface electrocardiogram.

Variations in ventricular rate are often accompanied by parallel variations in sinus rate. This arrhythmia is termed *ventriculophasic arrhythmia* and may relate to variations in coronary flow, carotid flow, or alterations in autonomic tone (Fig. 6-4).

Sinus Arrest

Alternatively designated *sinus pause* or *atrial standstill,* sinus arrest denotes a cessation of sinus node impulse formation. Criteria for minimum duration of a pause that would qualify it as an arrest of sinus activity have not been established. Characteristically, the pause is not an exact multiple of the normal P-P interval.

Typically, the period of sinus arrest in patients with sick sinus is terminated by a sinus beat (Fig. 6-5). Escape pacemakers often fail to assume dominance of the cardiac rhythm despite markedly prolonged durations of sinus arrest. When subsidiary pacemakers are capable of escaping, the pause may be terminated by either AV junctional (see Fig. 5-5) or ventricular automatic foci.

Sinoatrial Exit Block

Sinoatrial exit block is that which denotes failure of the sinus node impulse to conduct normally to the atrium. The site of block may be within the sinus node itself or within the sinoatrial junction. Furthermore, spontaneous sinus node impulse formation may be normal or abnormal.

First degree sinoatrial block describes an abnormal prolongation of the sinoatrial conduction time. Nonetheless, in this situation, each spontaneously generated nodal impulse does arrive at the atrium, albeit the arrival is delayed. First degree sinoatrial block cannot be recognized on the surface electrocardiogram. Its recognition

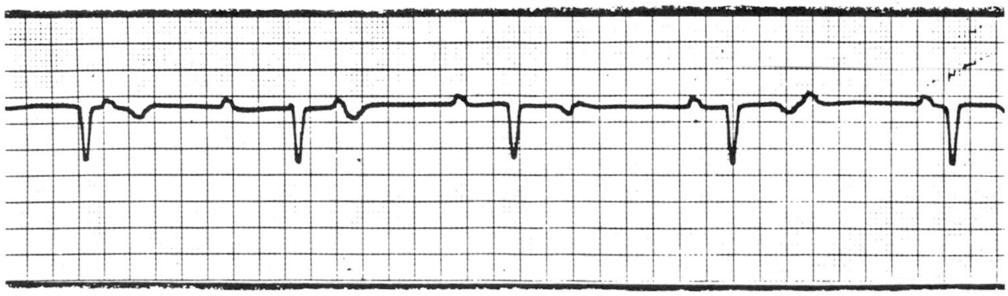

Figure 6-4. *This rhythm strip was obtained from a patient with advanced AV block and a junctional escape pacemaker. When one plots the P-P interval encompassing a QRS and compares this to the P-P interval in cycles without a QRS, one notices that the cycle encompassing the QRS has a shorter P-P interval. This is characteristic of ventriculophasic sinus arrhythmia.*

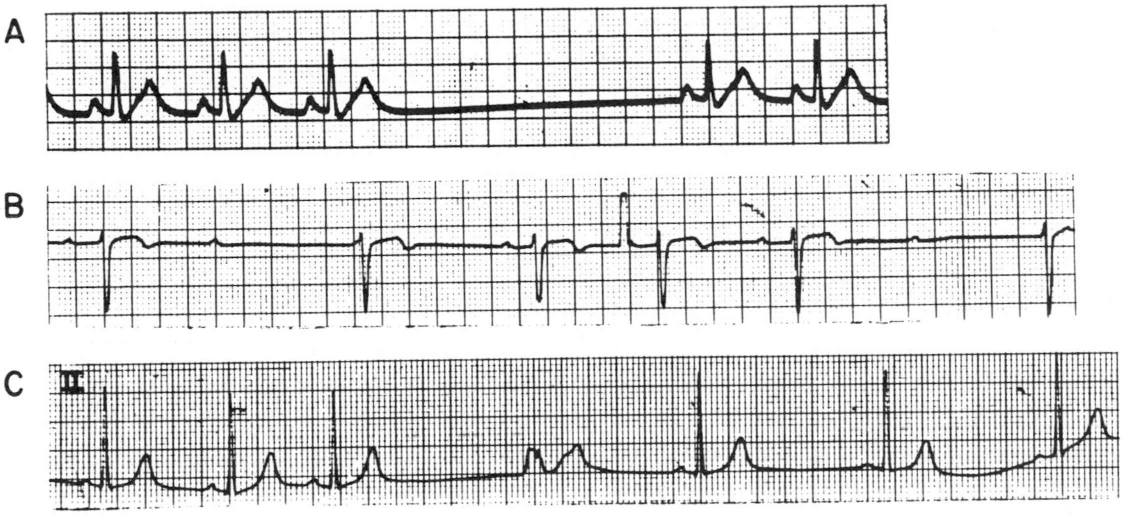

Figure 6-5. *In A, an episode of sinus arrest occurs in which the P-P cycle of the long pause is not a multiple of basic sinus cycle length. There is no escape complex present. In B, during an episode of AV block probably of the Wenckebach type, junctional escape complexes are noted. In C, during a sinus arrhythmia, a ventricular escape complex is noted.*

by the technique of programmed premature atrial stimulation will be described in detail later in this chapter.

Second degree sinoatrial block is characterized by periodic failure of the sinus node impulse to conduct to the atrium, which is manifested as periodic absence of a P wave on the surface electrocardiogram. Sinoatrial Wenckebach periodicity results from progressive delay of sinoatrial conduction in the face of regular sinus node pacemaker activity. Electrocardiographically, this phenomenon is manifested as a progressive shortening of the P-P interval preceding the dropped P wave (Fig. 6-6).

Advanced second degree sinoatrial block occurs when there is a regular interruption of anterograde sinoatrial conduction not preceded by progressive prolongation of sinoatrial conduction. Absence of a P wave on the surface electrocardiogram associated with second degree sinoatrial block can be distinguished from that observed with sinus arrest; characteristically, the pause between P waves in the former circumstance is an exact multiple of the normal P-P interval (Fig. 6-7).

Third degree or complete sinoatrial block cannot be distinguished from prolonged sinus arrest on the surface electrocardiogram. P waves are absent in both circumstances. Irrespective of the etiology, advanced SA block or profound SA arrest invariably is associated with significant clinical symptoms.

The Bradycardia-Tachycardia Syndrome

A frequent electrocardiographic manifestation of sinus node dysfunction is a pattern of slow sinus or subsidiary rhythms alternating with tachyarrhythmias, typically supraventricular in origin (Fig. 6-8). In keeping with the high incidence of atrial disease in patients with the sick

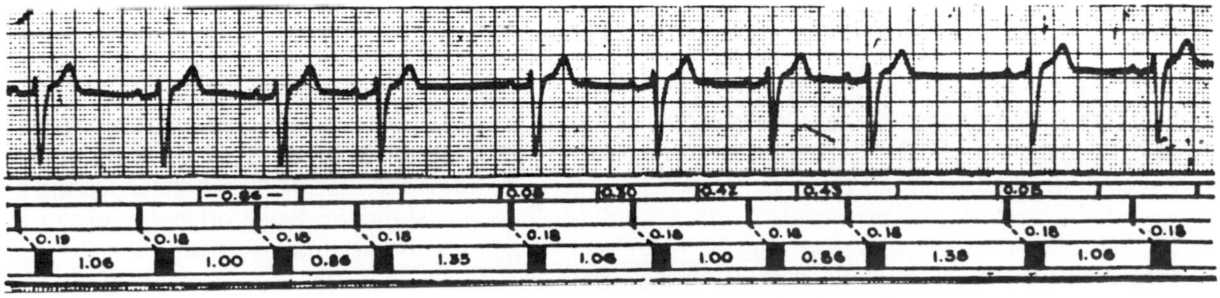

Figure 6-6. *This electrocardiogram rhythm strip demonstrates repetitive group beating with fixed PR relationships but abbreviated R-R relationships followed by a pause. The laddergram below the tracing identifies that SA Wenckebach phenomenon occurs due to progressive delay at the SA junction. (Greenwood, R. J., Finkelstein, D., and Monheit, R.: Sinoatrial heart block with Wenckebach phenomenon. Am. J. Cardiol., 8:141, 1961)*

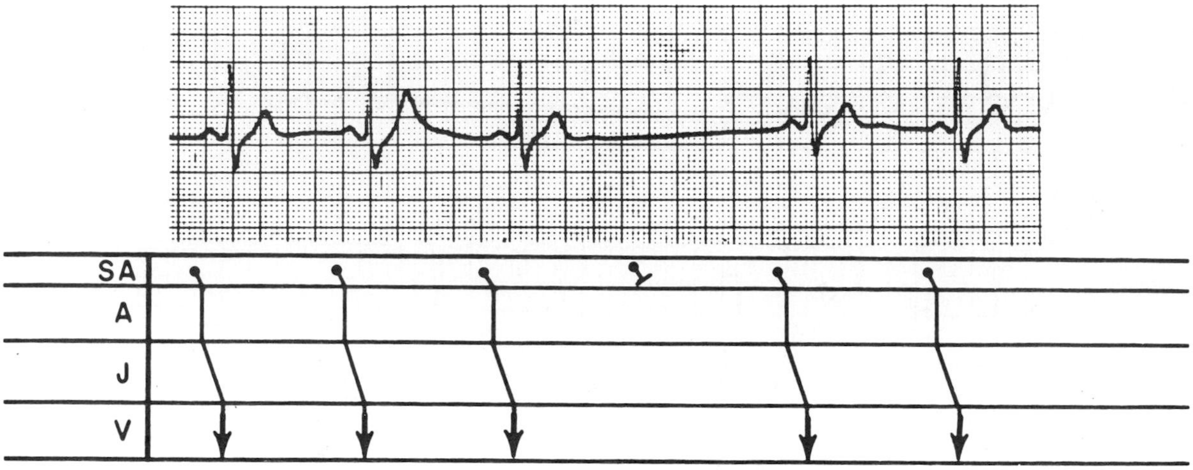

Figure 6-7. *This rhythm strip and its accompanying laddergram identify the etiology of the pause seen on the rhythm strip. The P-P interval encompassing the pause is twice the normal sinus cycle length, identifying that paroxysmal second degree SA block occurs with delay at the SA junction.*

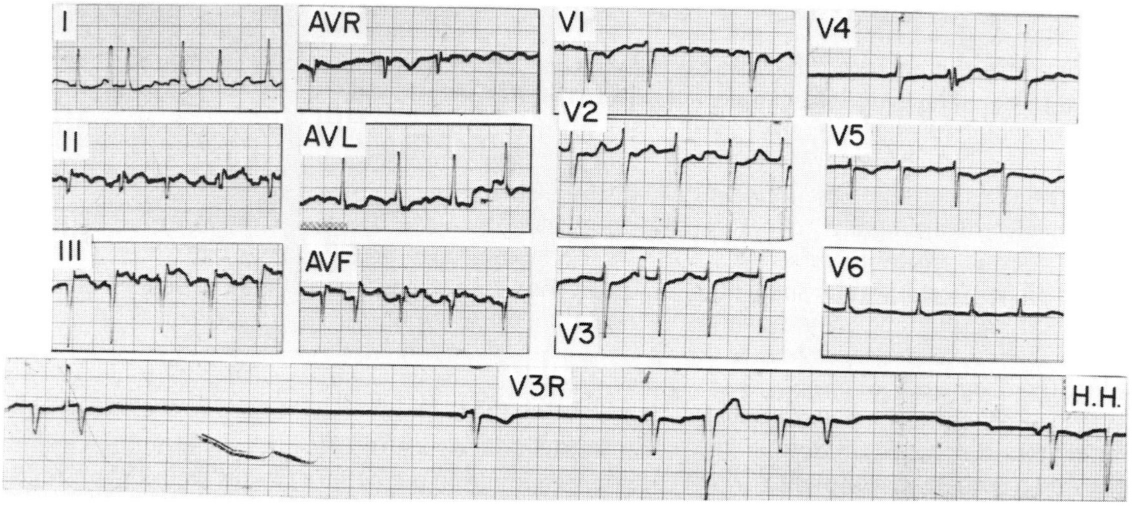

Figure 6-8. *This standard electrocardiogram was obtained from a patient with a history of palpitations and dizziness. The 12-lead electrocardiogram identifies the presence of atrial fibrillation with a moderately rapid ventricular rate. During the rhythm strip (V3R), atrial fibrillation terminates spontaneously with a very pronounced pause followed by a sinus escape complex. This tracing is typical for episodes of bradycardia-tachycardia.*

sinus syndrome, atrial fibrillation is probably the supraventricular tachycardia most frequently observed in this setting. However, atrial flutter, accelerated AV junctional rhythms, and reentrant AV junctional tachycardias are also observed. Although less frequently encountered, ventricular tachycardia also may be witnessed. Indeed, it is surprising that ventricular tachycardia is not a more common concomitant of sinus node dysfunction, since slow supraventricular rhythms could theoretically predispose to ventricular dysrhythmias.[92,93]

Abrupt spontaneous termination of a tachycardia episode is often accompanied by exaggerated suppression of sinus and subsidiary pacemaker activity in patients with the sick sinus syndrome. Electrocardiogram abnormalities and central nervous system symptoms may become manifest only during this posttachycardia period, sinus node dysfunction being otherwise occult in many patients with sick sinus syndrome.

Sinus Node Reentry

A supraventricular tachyarrhythmia unique to patients with sick sinus is sinus node reentry tachycardia. Although some evidence suggests that sinus node reentry is

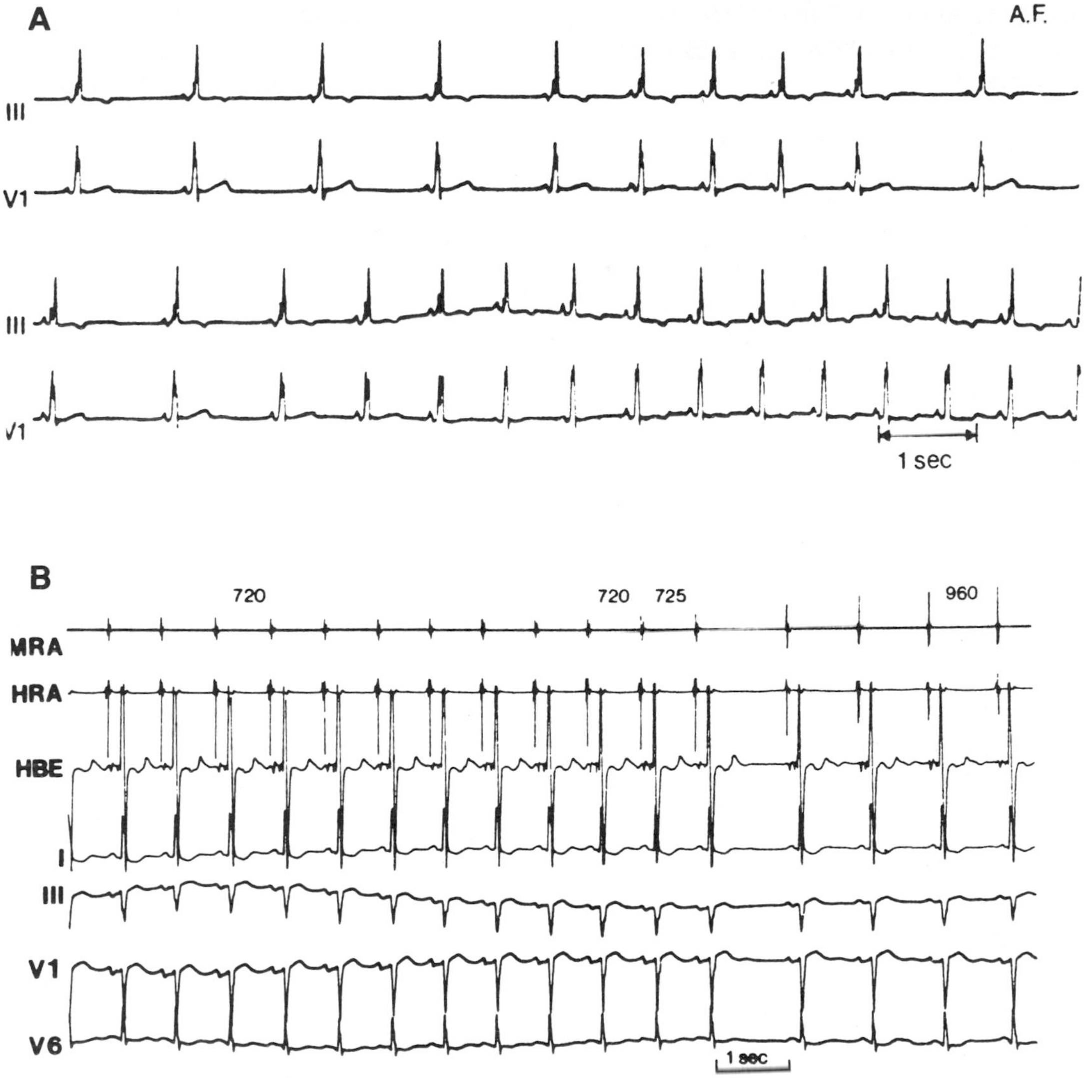

Figure 6-9. *(A) In the upper panel, sinus rhythm is interrupted by a short burst of accelerated sinus rate. In the lower panel, a more sustained episode of sinus rhythm acceleration is noted. (B) In these tracings, from a different patient, termination of an episode of "sinus" tachycardia is seen, with the prompt restoration of sinus rhythm at a rate of approximately 65 per minute. Note the lack of change in P wave morphology in the various surface electrocardiographic leads during the burst of more rapid "sinus" rhythm. The episodes in both A and B are typical of paroxysmal sinus node reentry. (Curry, P. V. L., and Krinkler, D. M.: Paroxysmal reciprocating sinus tachycardia.* In *Kulbertus, H. E. [ed.]: Re-entrant Arrhythmias: Mechanisms and Treatment, p. 39. Baltimore, University Park Press, 1976)*

a genuine phenomenon, certain investigators continue to doubt that the sinus node itself is involved in a tachycardia circuit.[94-100] Nonetheless, to qualify as a sinus node reentrant tachycardia, a supraventricular rhythm must meet certain criteria. It is usually initiated by premature atrial depolarizations occurring early in diastole; P waves during the tachyarrhythmia must have the same shape as P waves during normal sinus rhythm; the rate of the tachyarrhythmia is characteristically slow (100 to 120 beats/min); and the duration of the arrhythmia is often brief (several beats) (Fig. 6-9).[101,102] Additional comments on the mechanism of sinus node reentry will be made in the section dealing with sinus node responses to premature atrial stimuli.

Mechanisms of Sinus Node Dysfunction in the Sick Sinus Syndrome

A proper evaluation of sinus node function must take into account that its normal function depends on a delicately balanced interaction between intact intrinsic electrophysiologic properties of pacemaker automaticity and sinoatrial conduction and factors extrinsic to the sinoatrial region. Thus, not only must the integrity of intrinsic electrophysiologic determinants of sinoatrial function be tested, but the integrity of the autonomic nervous system, the endocrine system, and the sinus node blood supply must also be evaluated. These extrinsic elements exert profound modifying influences on intrinsic electrophysiologic mechanisms of the sinus node and perinodal structures; dysfunction at any one of these sites may become clinically manifest as the sick sinus syndrome. Furthermore, although each component of this complex network of factors, on which normal sinus function depends, may be intact, the interaction between them may be abnormal. Possible disturbances of reflex feedback mechanisms should therefore be considered and explored.

Clinical Evaluation of Sinus Node Function

The sick sinus syndrome must be included in the differential diagnosis of the patient giving a clinical history of palpitations, vague neurologic complaints of intermittent dizziness and lightheadedness, or alarming symptoms related to hypotension and reduced cardiac output (*e.g.,* syncope). However, the intermittency of symptoms and electrocardiographic features so characteristic of the syndrome may frustrate efforts to document a cause-and-effect relationship between clinical presentation and electrophysiologic events. Sophisticated electrophysiologic studies should be reserved for those patients in whom the diagnosis of sinus node dysfunction is in question. Furthermore, the diagnostic situation in which the studies are performed should be optimized to enhance the probability that symptoms and electrocardiographic abnormalities will occur at that time.

Electrocardiogram Monitoring

Exercise Testing

Exercise testing assesses the ability of the sinus node to accelerate in an appropriate fashion to internal physiologic chronotropic stimuli. Although a patient may have no evidence of sinus node dysfunction on the resting electrocardiogram, abnormal sinus node responses to stress may be uncovered by treadmill testing. Established norms for sinus node rate response for standard stress testing protocols for age and sex are available.[103,104]

Although some investigators have found that mean oxygen consumption at maximum stress was significantly lower for patients with sick sinus compared with predicted maximum oxygen consumption for controls,[105] recent reports indicate that maximum oxygen consumption may not differ between the two groups. Thus, in the absence of myocardial disease, for any given oxygen consumption, patients with sick sinus will have slower heart rate responses than healthy patients.

Exercise testing could potentially allow distinction between patients with sick sinus and other groups of patients with slow resting or exercise heart rates.[106] For example, age-matched "healthy" patients with autonomic chronotropic incompetence secondary to myocardial disease will have lower oxygen consumption for any given heart rate during exercise because of the inability to increase cardiac output by increasing stroke volume. Also, these patients usually will not be able to reach as high a peak oxygen consumption as patients with sick sinus with normal myocardial function.[106,107]

In contrast to patients with sick sinus, otherwise normal individuals with sinus node dysfunction primarily as a consequence of heightened vagal tone would be expected to have normal heart rate responses to exercise.[108] Specifically, exercise is vagolytic, eliminating parasympathetic influences on sinus node function in all groups of patients. This explains the lack of effect on the maximum heart rate achieved during exercise by atropine administration.

Finally, patients with sick sinus can be distinguished from physically well-trained persons during exercise although both groups seem to have similar heart rates at similar levels of oxygen consumption. However, the physically well-conditioned individual will be able to ultimately achieve a greater peak oxygen uptake and therefore a greater maximum heart rate response.

As attractive as exercise testing may appear for distinguishing patients with sick sinus from other groups of individuals with slow heart rates, the sensitivity of the method is less than perfect. Some patients with sick sinus will demonstrate normal heart rate responses to exercise.

Holter Monitoring

Ambulatory monitoring with a Holter device is possibly a more useful physiologic technique than exercise testing for assessing sinus node function if performed during normal daily activities[109] (see Chap. 18). The intermittent occurrence of both bradyarrhythmias and tachyarrhythmias in patients with the sick sinus syndrome frequently is missed on a routine resting electrocardiogram.

Furthermore, ambulatory monitoring can be virtually diagnostic of many cases of the sick sinus syndrome if the simultaneous occurrence of symptoms and sinus dysrhythmia is documented. More recent technical advances have enabled a patient to carry a device to be used only when symptoms occur, transmitting an electrocardiogram to a central station by telephone or recording the electrocardiogram on a portable recorder. "Intelligent recorders" are being developed that attempt to record the electrocardiogram only when abnormalities of rate or rhythm occur.

Testing the Sinus Node—Autonomic Nervous System Axis

Tests of Sinus Node Responsiveness to Autonomic Activity

The signs, symptoms, and electrocardiogram features of the sick sinus syndrome may be secondary to sinus node overresponsiveness or underresponsiveness to appropriate autonomic activity. Arguss and co-workers[108] have demonstrated that the well-established phenomenon of slowing of the sinus rate with age may be, in part, secondary to increased parasympathetic tone in many elderly individuals. Other investigators have shown that in some patients sinoatrial block may be mediated by abnormal autonomic tone.[110,111] Furthermore, it has been demonstrated that sinus arrhythmia is often produced primarily by periodic alterations in parasympathetic efferent cardiac activity.[112] Finally, patients with myocardial dysfunction have been shown to have profound abnormalities of parasympathetic and sympathetic control of heart rate.[113–116]

The importance of the autonomic nervous system to intrinsic sinus node function has led some investigators to recommend that heart rate response to sympathomimetic (isoproterenol), sympatholytic (propranolol), vagotonic (bethanechol or edrophonium), and vagolytic (atropine) drugs be employed routinely in the clinical evaluation of patients with the sick sinus syndrome.[117] Unfortunately, no standardized or systematic protocols have been described for administration of these agents to evaluate heart rate response. Furthermore, before abnormalities of heart rate response to these agents can be quantified, dose-response curves in healthy subjects must be described for comparative purposes. In general, it might be anticipated that patients with intrinsic sinus node dysfunction may exhibit all, some, or various combinations of the following abnormal responses: (1) a blunted heart rate acceleration with isoproterenol administration, suggesting sinus node unresponsiveness to appropriate beta-adrenergic stimulation; (2) a blunted acceleration response to atropine, suggesting that sinus node dysfunction is not due to oversensitivity to parasympathetic tone; (3) an exaggerated response to atropine, indicating that oversensitivity to parasympathetic tone or increased parasympathetic tone are etiologic factors; and (4) an exaggerated slowing response to bethanechol or edrophonium, indicating oversensitivity to parasympathetic stimulation.

Testing the Integrity of the Autonomic Nervous System

Having excluded the possibility that the sinus node responds inappropriately to changes in the autonomic environment with the above pharmacologic tests, it is then necessary to verify that the autonomic nervous system is itself intact. A characteristic clinical presentation of patients with the sick sinus syndrome may result from primary dysfunction of the autonomic nervous system. To test this possibility, autonomic activity should be provoked mechanically or pharmacologically. Carotid massage, the Valsalva maneuver, or phenylephrine-induced hypertension should normally produce slowing of the heart rate by reflex responses of the autonomic nervous system.[114–118] In contrast, lowering the blood pressure by titrated nitroprusside infusion should normally result in a reflex increase in heart rate.[118–122] In addition, heart rate changes induced by rapid positional changes should also be studied. Regrettably, blood pressure–heart rate response curves are not available for healthy subjects.

With the combined results of studies designed to test the integrity of sinus node response to direct autonomic stimulation and inhibition and studies testing the integrity of the autonomic nervous system, the status of autonomic regulation of sinus node function can be completely characterized. Recently, Dighton[123] suggested that persons with symptomatic sinus bradycardia are more likely to have an abnormal sinus rate response to autonomic stimulation and inhibition than are asymptomatic patients.

Intrinsic Heart Rate Determination

The intrinsic heart rate (IHR) is defined as the rate of spontaneous sinus node depolarization independent of the effects of the autonomic nervous system. The significance of the IHR is that its value theoretically depends only on intrinsic electrophysiologic mechanisms of sinus node automaticity. Complete autonomic blockade can be achieved with a modification of the protocol of Jose.[124–130] Propranolol, 0.2 mg/kg, is administered intravenously at a rate of 1 mg/min to obtain a dose-response curve of heart rate response to beta blockade. Ten minutes after, atropine sulfate, 0.04 mg/kg, is administered intravenously over 2 minutes. The resultant sinus rate is the observed IHR (IHRo). The dose of propranolol used abolishes the positive beta-adrenergic effects of large doses of isoproterenol for approximately 20 minutes. After atropine has been administered, the intrinsic heart rate remains stable for approximately 30 minutes.[124] Therefore, within the physiologic range, functional autonomic blockade appears to be complete.

With the technique of intrinsic heart rate determination, patients with sick sinus syndrome with intrinsic sinus node dysfunction can be distinguished from patients with disturbed autonomic regulation of sinus node function. Since the observed intrinsic heart rate theoretically depends only on intrinsic electrophysiologic properties of sinus node automaticity, an abnormal IHRo reflects an abnormality of one or more of these intrinsic properties. In contrast, when the heart rate is normal after autonomic blockade, it follows that disturbed autonomic regulation is most likely the underlying mechanism responsible for the manifestations of sinus node dysfunction.

Normal values for intrinsic heart rate can be determined using the linear regression equation derived by Jose, relating predicted IHR (IHRp) to age[124]:

$$\text{IHRp} = 118.1 - (0.57 \times \text{age})$$

For young individuals (under 45 years), the 95% confidence limit of IHRp is ± 14%; for older individuals (over 45 years), the 95% confidence limit of IHRp is ± 18%. An IHRo falling within two standard deviations (SD) of the predicted IHR is considered indicative of normal sinus node function. Conversely, an IHRo falling below and outside the 95% confidence limit of IHRp is considered to be compatible with abnormal intrinsic sinus node function.

A comparative measure of intrinsic sinus node function has also been derived.[125] The ratio of observed IHR to the lowest it could be and still be normal (*i.e.*, IHRo/IHRp − 2 SD) represents a quantitative measure of the integrity of intrinsic sinus node function. By this method a ratio of 1 or greater indicates normal sinus node function.

Autonomic influences on intrinsic electrophysiologic properties of the sinus node vary from moment to moment depending on a host of internal and external stimuli and inhibitors. Moreover, autonomic influences can either mask or exaggerate abnormalities of intrinsic electrophysiologic properties, contributing to the evanescent quality of electrocardiographic features of the sick sinus syndrome. On the other hand, the intrinsic heart rate has been shown to be stable on repeated determinations over extended periods.

The magnitude and direction of autonomic tone at any point can be semiquantitated in humans by using the technique of IHR determination. The percentage of a person's resting heart rate (RHR) attributable to negative or positive autonomic chronotropic influences on intrinsic electrophysiologic mechanisms of sinus node automaticity can be determined by the following formula[125]:

$$(\text{RHR}/\text{IHR} - 1.00) \times 100$$

If a person's RHR is less than his or her IHR, the resultant value will be negative, indicating that net negative autonomic chronotropy is present. When the RHR is greater than the IHR, net positive autonomic chronotropy is present and the value will be positive.

Atrial Overdrive

In 1884, Gaskell reported that termination of rapid cardiac rhythms in the turtle heart resulted in a delay of return of spontaneous pacemaker activity.[126] Subsequent clinical reports emphasized this phenomenon in ventricular pacemakers.[127–129] Using these clinical observations, Lange[130] systematically studied overdrive suppression of the sinus node in the laboratory. With the use of transvenous pacing catheters, overdrive suppression evolved into a means of evaluating sinus node function in humans.[131]

Until recently, "suppression" of sinus node pacemaker automaticity by intra-atrial overdrive pacing was considered a phenomenon that could be of value in unmasking occult sinus node dysfunction in many patients with the sick sinus syndrome.[132–134] However, recent observations suggest that this phenomenon may provide a key to understanding fundamental electrophysiologic properties of pacemaker automaticity itself.

Transient arrest of spontaneous sinus node activity follows cessation of overdrive atrial pacing as an apparent physiologic event. In general, patients with sinus node dysfunction demonstrate longer periods of sinus arrest than do healthy subjects (Fig. 6-10). The mechanism(s) by which overdrive pacing suppresses pacemaker automaticity has been the subject of much speculation. Two general hypotheses have received serious consideration in the clinical and experimental laboratory: (1) suppression is mediated by the release of autonomic neurotransmitters and (2) overdrive pacing directly disrupts intrinsic mechanisms of pacemaker automaticity.[130,135,136]

Atrial overdrive pacing does result in a release of autonomic neurotransmitters from storage sites within myocardial tissue and nerve endings.[38,137] Assuming that there is a net release of a negative chronotropic neurotransmitter, presumably acetylcholine, suppression of sinus node automaticity may indeed be mediated by this neurohumoral agent. Vagal stimulation or acetylcholine administration does in fact prolong sinus node recovery.[13]

That catecholamine release also plays a role in postoverdrive electrophysiologic events is suggested by the observation that the often-seen postoverdrive accelera-

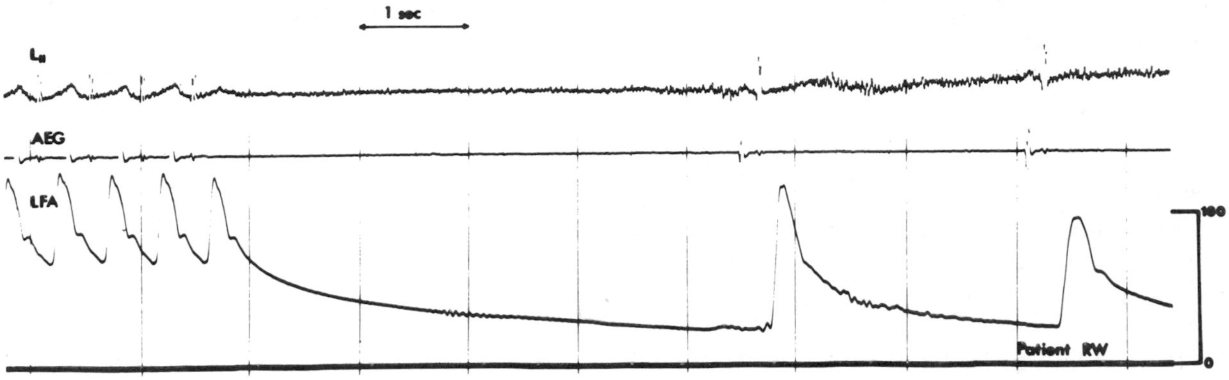

Figure 6-10. *A typical example of marked suppression of sinus function following overdrive pacing. The tracings are, from above downward, lead II electrocardiogram, a high right atrial electrocardiogram, and left femoral artery blood pressure. Right atrial overdrive pacing at a rate of 130/min was abruptly turned off, resulting in a pause of approximately 5 seconds terminated by a sinus complex.*

tion of sinus rate can be abolished by reserpine or propranolol pretreatment.[136] Moreover, isoproterenol infusion results in a predictable shortening of the sinus node recovery time.[13]

That release of autonomic neurotransmitters is not the only mechanism by which overdrive atrial pacing suppresses sinus node pacemaker automaticity is suggested by clinical and experimental observations. First, since the sinus node recovery time is longer than the spontaneous sinus cycle length even after complete autonomic blockade, it seems reasonable that overdrive pacing may directly disrupt intrinsic electrophysiologic determinants of sinus node automaticity.[130] Second, some patients with the sick sinus syndrome exhibit longer corrected sinus node recovery times (SNRTC; see below) than healthy subjects after autonomic blockade, suggesting that overdrive pacing may actually exaggerate abnormalities of these intrinsic properties.[130] Third, some individuals have net release of a positive chronotropic neurotransmitter in the face of overdrive suppression (see below), leading to the conclusion that a direct effect on intrinsic electrophysiologic properties may be the primary mechanism of suppression.[130]

Recent observations in the microelectrode laboratory on the relationship between rate of overdrive pacing and SNRT have significantly advanced our understanding of the mechanisms and determinants of sinus node recovery time.[138,139]

1. Using small sinus node preparations and pacing at a closer proximity to the pacemaker cell (<5 mm) minimizes acetylcholine release and unmasks the direct disruptive effects of overdrive pacing on pacemaker automaticity. These effects on the sinus pacemaker action potential are directly proportional to the rate of penetration of paced beats and are not reversed by atropine.

2. The extent of sinus node pacemaker suppression is directly related to the number of paced beats actually penetrating it per unit of time. Paced beats that fail to penetrate the sinus node do not suppress pacemaker automaticity to the same extent as do paced beats penetrating the sinus pacemaker.

3. The observation that overdrive pacing directly hypopolarizes the sinus node pacemaker cell eliminates activation of the electrogenic sodium pump as a mechanism of pacemaker suppression in the sinus node.

4. Sinus node recovery time cannot be interpreted only in terms of overdrive suppression of sinus node automaticity but is the result of a complex interaction between conduction and impulse formation in the sinoatrial region. The faster the rate of overdrive pacing, the slower is retrograde sinoatrial conduction because of progressive impingement on the relative refractory period of the perinodal zone. The faster the rate of overdrive pacing, the slower is antegrade sinoatrial conduction because of decreased amplitude of the sinus node pacemaker action potential.

5. The mechanism by which overdrive pacing reduces the amplitude of the pacemaker action potential may be prevention of completion of phase 3 when pacing rates are rapid.

To date, abnormalities of only one potential intrinsic mechanism of sinus node automaticity have been studied with the object of uncovering the mechanism of suppression by overdrive pacing. When isolated rabbit sinus node preparations are perfused with the slow channel inhibitor verapamil, 1×10^{-7}M, the corrected sinus node recovery time is prolonged.[140] This finding is reproducible even when the influence of released autonomic neurotransmitters is blocked with atropine and propranolol added to the perfusate.[141] It is therefore reasonable to assume that some patients with sick sinus syndrome demonstrating abnormal prolongation of the sinus node recovery time may have intrinsic slow channel abnormalities. An exaggeration of Na^+, K^+, and anion current abnormalities by atrial pacing has not yet been investigated.

Another mechanism that has been considered as a possible etiology of overdrive suppression is the transient induction of ischemia of the sinus node by rapid atrial pacing. Against this hypothesis is the clinical finding that sinus node recovery time is not prolonged in patients with chronic or acute ischemia of the SA node.[142,143] The possibility that *p*H changes induced by rapid pacing may contribute to ionic current alterations and therefore to abnormal pacemaker suppression has not been specifically investigated. However, sinus node automaticity is certainly influenced by acid-base imbalances.[144]

Intracardiac pacing is performed in the cardiac catheterization laboratory with patients in the fasting state. All cardiac drugs and medications known to interfere with sinus node or autonomic neural function should be withdrawn for at least 48 hours or two half-lives before the study. Mild sedation is achieved with Seconal, 100 mg orally, given 30 minutes before the procedure. After local anesthesia has been achieved, a quadripolar pacing catheter is positioned at the high right atrium. Multiple electrocardiographic leads as well as an intra-atrial electrogram are monitored on a photographic oscillographic recorder. Atrial pacing is performed at a milliamperage two times the diastolic threshold. An initial intra-atrial pacing rate of approximately 20 beats/min faster than the patient's resting heart rate is chosen, with increments of 20 beats/min in succeeding pacing trials, up to a rate of 170 beats/min. Pacing is continued for 30, 60, and 180 seconds at each pacing rate and abruptly terminated; 60 seconds is allowed to elapse between each pacing trial. The SNRT is measured in milliseconds as the time elapsing from the last paced P wave to the first spontaneous depolarization on the intra-atrial electrogram. The shape of the P wave is noted to confirm that the complex ending the sinus pause is indeed sinoatrial in origin.

To control for differences in spontaneous sinus rate between patients and for the influence that it would naturally have on the apparent time it would take the sinus node to recover its automaticity, the sinus node recovery time may be corrected for the spontaneous sinus cycle length (SCL); thus, SNRTC = SNRT − SCL. Benditt and associates[145] expressed SNRT as a ratio of SCL. Accordingly, SNRT/SCL $\leq$ 1.61 was used as the normal value for patients with sinus cycle lengths less than 800 msec. For patients with sinus cycle lengths greater than 800 msec, SNRT/SCL $\leq$ 1.83 was considered normal.

Reported SNRT values for normal subjects include 1400 msec,[146] 1040 ± 56 msec (M ± SEM),[131] and 958 ± 149 msec.[147] Reported normal SNRTC values range from <450 msec[148] to <525 msec.[133]

In humans and animals, SNRT increases slightly as the pacing rate increases. However, at rapid rates (> 130 beats/min) SNRT decreases somewhat.[131] In patients with sick sinus syndrome, maximum SNRT often occurs at rates slower than the pacing rate at which $SNRT_{max}$ occurs in normal subjects.[149,151] It has been suggested that the pacing cycle length at which the longest postpacing pause occurs ("peak paced cycle length," or "PCL_p") be considered when interpreting the meaning of any particular SNRT value. Reiffel and colleagues[152] found that PCL_p was equal to or less than 600 msec in normal subjects and tended to prolong in patients with sick sinus syndrome. The authors invoked the explanation that a prolonged PCL_p is a manifestation of disturbed atriosinus conduction during pacing and a prolonged perinodal refractory period.[153] Furthermore, they suggested that rate-dependent retrograde sinoatrial block[153] during atrial pacing could result in spuriously short SNRT values in patients with sick sinus because of failure of each paced beat to reach and depolarize sinus node pacemaker cells. Therefore, a patient with a normal SNRT but a long PCL_p may actually have a disorder of sinus node pacemaker function that escapes detection through overdrive atrial pacing if an abnormally prolonged PCL_p is not recognized. In microelectrode studies, Kerr and colleagues[154] have confirmed that the PCL_p is determined by the refractory period of the perinodal zone and the occurrence of retrograde sinoatrial block.

In contrast to the sinus node pacemaker, subsidiary pacemakers demonstrate significant proportional increases in recovery time with increasing pacing rates (Fig. 6-11).[155] Of more importance clinically, subsidiary pacemakers have more sustained periods of suppression than the sinus node following overdrive.

Most normal subjects demonstrate little correlation between duration of pacing and SNRT (Fig. 6-12).[155] The correlation in patients with sick sinus is variable. Subsidiary pacemakers generally show a positive correlation between pacing duration and recovery time (see Fig. 6-11)[155]; this finding may reflect different mechanisms mediating overdrive suppression in different pacemaker sites.

The proximity of the pacing catheter to the intrinsic pacemaker being studied appears to be an important determinant of the magnitude of that pacemaker's overdrive suppression. Ventricular pacing results in less depression of AV junctional pacemakers than does atrial pacing and even less suppression of the sinus node.[130] On the other hand, suppression of Purkinje fiber automaticity is best achieved by ventricular pacing.[13] Within the atrium itself, it has been demonstrated in experimental preparations that a premature impulse results in a longer return cycle if delivered in the region of the coronary sinus or crista terminalis than in the intra-atrial septum.[156] By convention, in the clinical laboratory atrial pacing is performed in the high right atrium. Variations

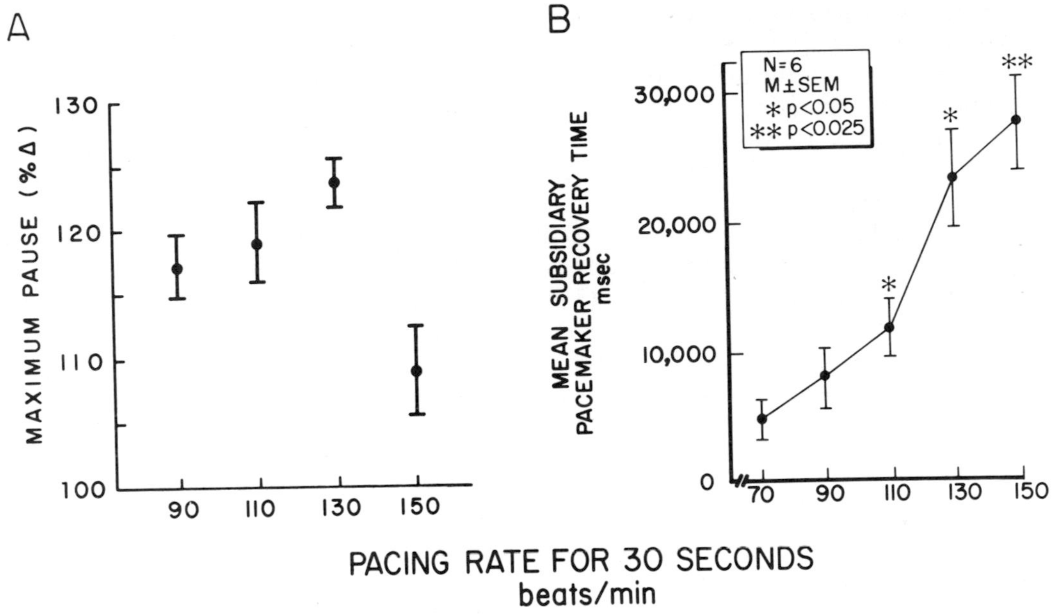

Figure 6-11. *The influence of pacing rate on sinus node recovery time. In both A and B, the horizontal axis indicates the pacing rate used for 30 seconds of overdrive. The vertical axis demonstrates the maximum sinus node recovery time in milliseconds. In A, using data obtained from normal patients, a peak in sinus node recovery time is observed at a rate of 130/min. In contrast, in B, data obtained from animal investigations show that in subsidiary pacemakers (*i.e., *junctional escape pacemakers) overdrive suppression is much more pronounced and has a linear relationship with the frequency of overdrive used.*

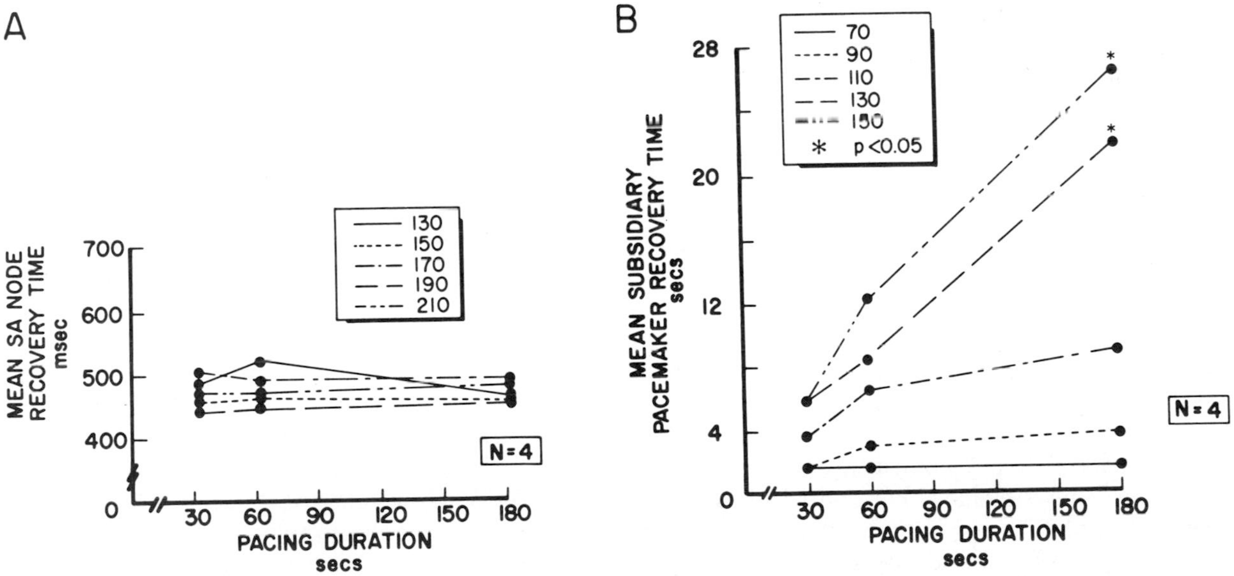

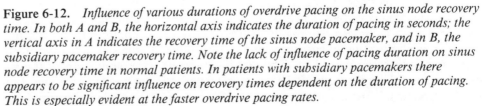

Figure 6-12. *Influence of various durations of overdrive pacing on the sinus node recovery time. In both A and B, the horizontal axis indicates the duration of pacing in seconds; the vertical axis in A indicates the recovery time of the sinus node pacemaker, and in B, the subsidiary pacemaker recovery time. Note the lack of influence of pacing duration on sinus node recovery time in normal patients. In patients with subsidiary pacemakers there appears to be significant influence on recovery times dependent on the duration of pacing. This is especially evident at the faster overdrive pacing rates.*

in pacing amperage cause no significant change in SNRT or SNRTC.[131]

In normal subjects the uncorrected sinus node recovery time prolongs in a linear fashion with longer resting sinus cycle lengths. However, at abnormally slow heart rates the recovery time generally becomes disproportionately prolonged.[131]

It has been shown that the sinus node recovery time in children and in elderly normal subjects is not significantly different from mean values found in the general population.[158,159] The pacing rate at which there is a sudden decrease in SNRT seems to be slower in the elderly, suggesting that sinoatrial entrance block occurs at a slower rate.[149] This phenomenon may represent differential aging of the perinodal zone.

Generally, patients with sick sinus with documented sinus arrest of marked duration (5 seconds or longer) and central nervous system symptoms have relatively longer SNRTC than asymptomatic patients with sinus arrest of lesser magnitude. However, dramatic exceptions to this rule demonstrate that there is probably no direct linear relationship between magnitude of sinus bradycardia or sinus arrest and the duration of SNRTC in patients with the sick sinus syndrome.

Patients with congestive heart failure, independent of etiology, have diminished sinus rate responses to variations in autonomic tone[113–116] as well as significantly slower intrinsic heart rates.[159] Jose[159] suggested that in congestive heart failure the same biochemical abnormality exists in both myocardial and pacemaker cells. However, the relationship between sinus node recovery time and the presence of heart failure has not been specifically investigated.

Atherosclerotic disease of the sinus node artery is not associated with abnormalities of sinus node recovery time.[160] In addition, mild to moderate hypertension in the absence of cardiomegaly or heart failure does not influence sinus node response to overdrive pacing.[125]

Despite the theoretical potential for marked variations in autonomic tone, SNRT and SNRTC have been shown to be remarkably reproducible whether pacing is performed on consecutive days or at an interval of many months.[133,149]

In some instances, sinoatrial conduction time (SACT) appears to be a clinically more sensitive indicator of electrophysiologic abnormalities of the sinoatrial region than SNRT (*e.g.*, in the setting of atherosclerotic involvement of the sinus node artery).[149] Even patients with gross manifestations of the sick sinus syndrome may have an abnormal SACT in association with a normal SNRT.[134,161,162] The comparative insensitivity of SNRT may be a consequence of sinoatrial entrance block in the diseased perinodal zone and inconsistent penetration of the sinus node.[153] The occasional finding of a paradoxical effect of atropine on SNRT (*i.e.*, increased prolongation) may thus be accounted for on the basis of improved retrograde conduction of paced beats into the SA node.[163,164]

That a disparity of sinus node recovery time and sinoatrial conduction time may be artifactual is suggested by observations in isolated tissue preparations in which the calcium current is abnormal. In these preparations, SNRT and SACT abnormalities invariably parallel one another.[141,165] Of course, the relative magnitude of abnormalities of SNRT and SACT may depend on the mechanisms of sinoatrial dysfunction operative in any given patient with the sick sinus syndrome, the calcium current being equally important to both automaticity and sinoatrial conduction.

Limited information suggests that sick sinus patients with abnormalities of AV nodal or intraventicular conduction may have a greater incidence of abnormal SNRT than patients without distal conduction abnormalities.[146]

Recently, the value of the sinus node recovery time as a diagnostic tool in the sick sinus syndrome has been questioned. Specifically, not all patients with sick sinus demonstrate abnormal prolongation of the sinus node recovery time.[166] However, to expect the sinus node recovery time to be prolonged in all patients with the sick sinus syndrome presupposes that the technique of intraatrial overdrive pacing tests an underlying pathophysiologic mechanism that is common to all cases. Based on our knowledge of the large number of potential determinants of sinus node automaticity and overdrive suppression, it is unlikely that the sick sinus syndrome is a homogeneous entity in terms of pathophysiologic mechanisms.

Normal sinus node function depends on a complex and delicately balanced interaction among intrinsic sinus node electrophysiologic properties, sinoatrial conduction properties, and factors extrinsic to the sinoatrial region. Among the extrinsic factors capable of exerting modifying influences on intrinsic sinus node function, the role of the autonomic nervous system is perhaps the most important. However, persons differ in extent and direction of net autonomic tone and perhaps also in end-organ sensitivity to similar levels of autonomic tone. It is also reasonable to assume that individuals differ in the relative and absolute amounts of epinephrine and acetylcholine released during intra-atrial pacing. Considering that abnormalities of different intrinsic electrophysiologic properties of sinus node automaticity may be differentially influenced directly by overdrive pacing and that pacing takes place at different levels of autonomic activity, it is not surprising that all patients with the sick sinus syndrome do not demonstrate abnormal prolongation of the sinus node recovery time. In fact, Chadda and co-workers[167] have suggested that the finding of an abnormal corrected sinus node recovery time should be evaluated in terms of the role that autonomic tone plays in its value before concluding that sinus node dysfunction *per se* caused the abnormality.

Based on observations that many patients with sick sinus have blunted sinus rate acceleration to the administration of atropine and that atropine shortens the sinus node recovery time in normal subjects, this drug has been employed to distinguish patients with sick sinus with intrinsic sinus node disease from those with abnormally exaggerated parasympathetic influences.[157] The effects of atropine on the sinus node recovery time vary in patients with sick sinus, shortening it in some, having no effect in others, and paradoxically prolonging it in a small number.[163,164,168] These different results may represent differences in residual parasympathetic tone, which must be accounted for before comparing the effect of parasympathetic blockade on sinus node recovery time in different persons. Differences in resting sympathetic tone, now unopposed in the postatropine state, also must be taken into account. All atttempts to determine absolute normal values for SNRT in the postatropine state may be thwarted because of the problems encountered in quantifying sympathetic and residual parasympathetic tone.

The problems associated with determining normal values for postpropranolol SNRT are similar to those discussed for atropine. Standards for completeness of sympathetic blockade must be established. Differences in unopposed parasympathetic tone must be taken into account.

Most of the disadvantages of separate atropine and propranolol administration can be overcome by the simultaneous administration of these drugs and determination of intrinsic heart rate at the time of atrial overdrive pacing. With the doses of atropine and propranolol employed with IHRo determination (see above), sinus node recovery time can be automatically adjusted for the role that autonomic influences might play in its value. Alternatively, control sinus node recovery time can be adjusted mathematically for the role of autonomic influences:[125]

$$\text{Adjusted SNRTC} = \text{SNRTC} + \text{SNRTC} \times (\text{RHR}/\text{IHR} - 1.00)$$

In our unit, observed IHRs have been determined in 17 patients with symptomatic sinus bradycardia; 10 patients had normal IHRo. Six of these patients had normal control SNRTC (>450 msec), and four had abnormal control SNRTc. Seven patients had abnormal IHRo, and all seven patients had abnormal control SNRTC. When overdrive pacing was performed following autonomic blockade, all ten patients with normal IHRo had normal adjusted SNRTC, while all seven patients with abnormal IHRo continued to demonstrate abnormal corrected sinus node recovery times (Fig. 6-13). From these findings we concluded that (1) the sick sinus syndrome is clearly not a homogeneous entity in terms of pathophysiologic mechanisms, (2) patients with sick sinus demonstrating normal sinus node recovery times corrected for the magnitude and direction of autonomic chronotropy consistently have normal intrinsic heart rates and, therefore, abnormalities of autonomic regulation of sinus node function, and (3) patients with sick sinus demonstrating abnormal adjusted sinus node recovery times consistently have abnormal intrinsic heart rates and, therefore, abnormalities of intrinsic sinus node function.

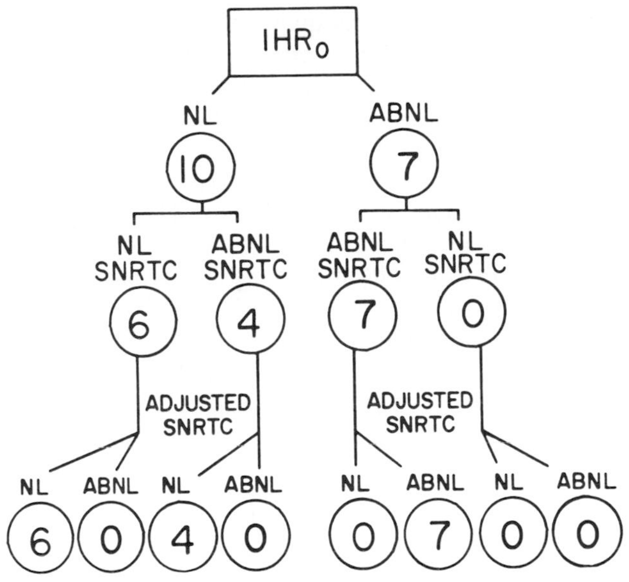

Figure 6-13. *Use of the intrinsic heart rate to separate normal and abnormal sinus node recovery times based on intrinsic or extrinsic sinus node dysfunction. The flow diagram demonstrates that patients with normal intrinsic heart rates who have abnormal sinus node recovery times corrected for basic sinus cycle length will have corrected normal values if their SNRTC is adjusted for the degree of positive or negative chronotropic activity. The latter is based on differences between the observed intrinsic heart rate and the basal heart rate. (NL, normal; ABNL, abnormal; IHR$_O$, observed intrinsic heart rate; SNRTC, corrected sinus node recovery time)*

Subsequent investigators have demonstrated occasional exceptions to these results. However, most agree that the technique does improve the sensitivity and specificity of the sinus node recovery time as well as clarify mechanisms of sinus node dysfunction in patients with the sick sinus syndrome.

Exceptions to our findings include the occasional patient with normal intrinsic heart rate showing abnormal SNRTC after but not before autonomic blockade. This exception emphasizes the fact that unlike IHR, sinus node recovery time is not a function of sinus node automaticity alone. The consequences of atrial overdrive pacing also depend on properties of sinoatrial conduction. Thus, when the effects of cholinergic blockade outweigh the effects of beta-adrenergic blockade in the sinoatrial junction, the net effect is facilitation of retrograde sinoatrial conduction and more consistent penetration into the sinus node by the paced beats. This differential effect of autonomic blockade on the sinus node and sinoatrial junction cannot be anticipated on the basis of IHR alone.

The rare patient with an abnormal intrinsic heart rate but a normal SNRTC both before and after autonomic blockade has been described. In the absence of abnormal retrograde sinoatrial conduction preventing consistent penetration of paced beats into the sinus node, no adequate explanation has yet been offered to account for this phenomenon.

Recently, Mason[168] has reported results of overdrive atrial pacing in denervated transplanted human hearts. Sinus rate was significantly faster in denervated donor hearts than in remnant atrial and control subsets. No significant difference was found between donor SNRTC (300 ± 117 msec) and recipient SNRTC (291 ± 171 msec) or control SNRTC (273 ± 171). Of clinical importance is that these values compare favorably with SNRTC after pharmacologic blockade in patients with normal intrinsic heart rates (287 ± 114 msec).[172] The most dramatic finding was that $SNRT_{max}$ resulted from shorter overdrive cycle lengths in the donor hearts (359 ± 46 msec) than in recipient hearts (491 ± 111 msec) ($P < 0.005$) or in control hearts (499 ± 82 msec) ($P < 0.005$). This latter finding suggests that the sinoatrial junction is particularly sensitive to negative dromotropic effects of resting autonomic tone. Thus, elimination of resting autonomic tone resulted in shortening the retrograde sinoatrial refractory period, allowing more rapidly delivered paced beats to conduct into the sinus node.

After autonomic blockade has been achieved, the acute administration of ouabain, 0.1 mg/kg intravenously, may rarely produce marked prolongation of the sinus node recovery time. This phenomenon has only been observed in patients with sick sinus with abnormal intrinsic heart rates. The mechanism of action is not certain; however, this finding may further improve the sensitivity of SNRTC.

There does not appear to be a correlation between the duration of overdrive pacing and the magnitude of SNRTC in patients with normal intrinsic heart rates.[169] However, preliminary observations suggest that patients with abnormal intrinsic heart rates may show progressively longer recovery times with longer durations of pacing.[169] Recognizing this phenomenon as an abnormal response to overdrive pacing could potentially increase the sensitivity of the technique.

In the healthy subject, the sinus cycles following the first recovery sinus beat are either shorter (secondary acceleration) or initially longer than the basic sinus cycle with gradual but progressive return to the basic sinus cycle length. In some patients with sick sinus the P-P interval immediately following cessation of pacing is not the longest, or even abnormally prolonged, but is followed by longer P-P intervals (Fig. 6-14). This secondary suppression may persist for 10 to 20 beats or more. Instances of secondary suppression have been reported in patients with sick sinus but less frequently in healthy

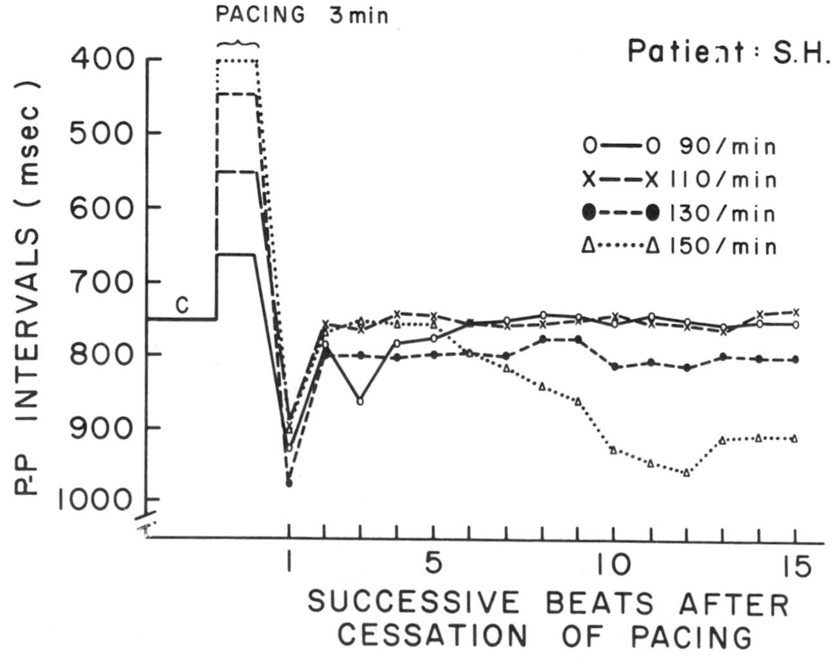

Figure 6-14. *The influence of overdrive pacing at different rates on the sinus cycle length following termination of pacing. After overdrive pacing at rates of 90, 110, and 130 beats/min, sinus cycle length promptly returns to control values. However, following overdrive pacing at a rate of 150/min, initial overdrive suppression is followed, after approximately 10 beats, by subsequent additional suppression (*i.e., *secondary suppression).*

subjects. Recently, Desai and colleagues[170] reported that in the preautonomic blockade state the incidence of secondary pauses was significantly higher in patients with abnormal intrinsic heart rates than in those with normal intrinsic heart rates (5 of 8 versus 2 of 13) ($P<0.05$). Moreover, after autonomic blockade, secondary pauses in patients with abnormal intrinsic heart rates persisted or increased, while secondary pauses in patients with normal intrinsic heart rates tended to disappear. Similarly, Mason[168] reported that secondary pauses seen in 78% of recipient atria and in 45% of control atria were virtually absent in denervated donor hearts (6%). These observations suggest that careful examination of the phenomenon of secondary pauses, especially after autonomic block, increases the sensitivity and specificity of overdrive atrial pacing in the diagnosis of the patient with sick sinus syndrome.

Premature Atrial Stimulation

Analysis of sinus node responses to premature atrial depolarizations has revealed important electrophysiologic features of normal and abnormal sinus node function and sinoatrial conduction.[172-175] With methods similar to those described in the section on sinus node recovery times, premature atrial stimuli are introduced in late diastole during spontaneous sinus rhythm after every eighth beat at progressively decreasing coupling intervals (in 10-msec increments). In this fashion, the sinus cycle length is scanned until atrial capture is lost.

Four types of sinus node responses to atrial premature depolarizations, depending on the timing of the APD in the sinus cycle (A_1-A_1) and whether the APD retrogradely penetrates the sinus node, have been identified: (1) compensation resulting from a late diastolic extra stimulus that fails to depolarize the sinus node because of collision with the normal sinus depolarization; (2) reset, produced by premature depolarization of the sinus node by the extra stimulus resulting in A_2-A_3 interval of shorter duration than a compensatory pause; (3) interpolation, produced by failure of the extra stimulus to enter the sinus node, but not barring conduction to the atrium of the next sinus impulse; and (4) reentry resulting from reflection of the premature complex, producing an early "sinus" depolarization (Fig. 6-15).

Identification of a perinodal zone of tissue in the right atrium of the rabbit by Strauss and Bigger[176] has contributed significantly to our understanding of the above events. The perinodal cells have electrophysiologic characteristics distinct from atrial muscle and sinus node cells and may represent a potential conduction barrier.

The fibers of the sinoatrial node and perinodal zone share some electrophysiologic properties with AV junctional tissue. Specifically, the depolarization velocity of the action potential of an APD progressively slows as the extrasystole is delivered earlier in diastole, exhibiting decremental conduction.[177] Moreover, an APD may be completely blocked in the retrograde direction within the perinodal zone or within the sinoatrial node if it encounters these tissues in the absolute refractory period of excitability.[153,173-175]

The phenomenon of the compensatory pause seen when APDs are introduced late in the sinus cycle may be attributed to the electrophysiologic properties of the perinodal zone because the APD does not penetrate or disturb the sinus node and the subsequent sinus beat occurs on time. If the perinodal zone is abnormal, as might be the case in patients with the sick sinus syndrome, the zone of compensation may be expected to occupy a greater percentage of the sinus cycle than in patients with normal perinodal tissue. Thus, even earlier APDs would encounter the exiting sinus beat in the perinodal zone. These events form the electrophysiologic basis of first degree sinoatrial block, a manifestation of the sick sinus syndrome (Fig. 6-16).[178,179]

During a portion of the zone of sinus node reset, the postextrasystolic pause (A_2-A_3) lengthens progressively as the premature beat is elicited earlier in the midportion of the atrial cycle. Three mechanisms of this lengthening have been proposed: (1) a progressive slowing of the conduction velocity of the premature impulse, (2) a temporary depression of rhythmicity of sinus node pacemaker cells,[172,174,175,180] and (3) intra-SA nodal pacemaker shifts.[15] In patients with abnormalities of sinoatrial conduction, the zone of reset theoretically occupies less of the sinus cycle than in healthy subjects.[161]

Early APDs encounter a perinodal zone that remains effectively refractory in the wake of the preceding sinus impulse, are blocked from entering the sinus node, and fail to reset it. The next spontaneous impulse occurs on schedule, traverses a perinodal zone that has recovered from refractoriness, enters the atrium on schedule, and results in interpolation of the APD. The zone of interpolation has been examined in close detail in the microelectrode laboratory.[181] Progressively earlier premature beats are actually blocked at progressively greater distances from the node. Therefore, the sinoatrial junction provides a progressive gradation of refractoriness rather than a discrete barrier. Furthermore, APDs occurring later in the zone of interpolation may actually penetrate the sinus node. However, their amplitude is so low that they cannot reset the node. Rather, these earlier APDs appear to reduce the maximum diastolic potential, impose a phase delay in attaining maximum diastolic potential, and perturb the terminal part of phase 3 or the early part of phase 4 of the transmembrane action potential, or both, delaying the appearance of the spontaneous recovery beat, resulting in incomplete interpolation.

Very early APDs may find a portion of the perinodal zone and sinus node recovered sufficiently from the pre-

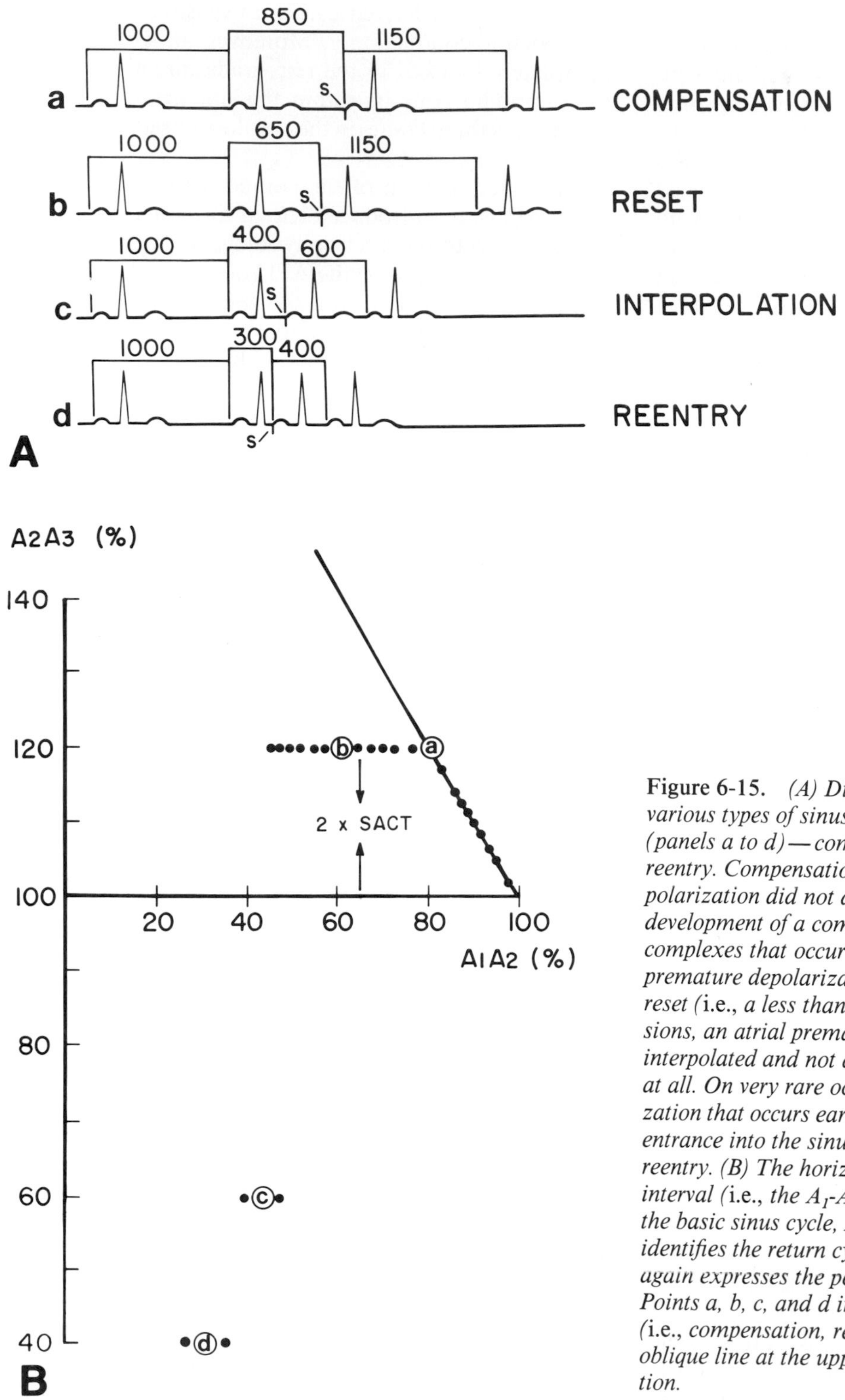

Figure 6-15. *(A) Diagrammatic representation of the various types of sinus node response to atrial extra stimuli (panels a to d)—compensation, reset, interpolation, and reentry. Compensation implies that the atrial premature depolarization did not depolarize the sinus node, leading to the development of a compensatory pause. Atrial premature complexes that occur earlier in the sinus cycle lead to the premature depolarization of the sinus node with subsequent reset (*i.e., *a less than compensatory pause). On rare occasions, an atrial premature depolarization can in fact be interpolated and not disturb the manifest sinus cycle length at all. On very rare occasions, an atrial premature depolarization that occurs early in the diastole can lead to delayed entrance into the sinus node region, followed by sinus node reentry. (B) The horizontal axis identifies the test coupling interval (*i.e., *the A_1-A_2 interval expressed as a percentage of the basic sinus cycle, A_1-A_1 interval). The vertical axis identifies the return cycle length (*i.e., *The A_2-A_3 interval again expresses the percentage of basic sinus cycle length). Points a, b, c, and d in B refer to the similar points seen in A (*i.e., *compensation, reset, interpolation, and reentry). The oblique line at the upper right identifies the line of compensation.*

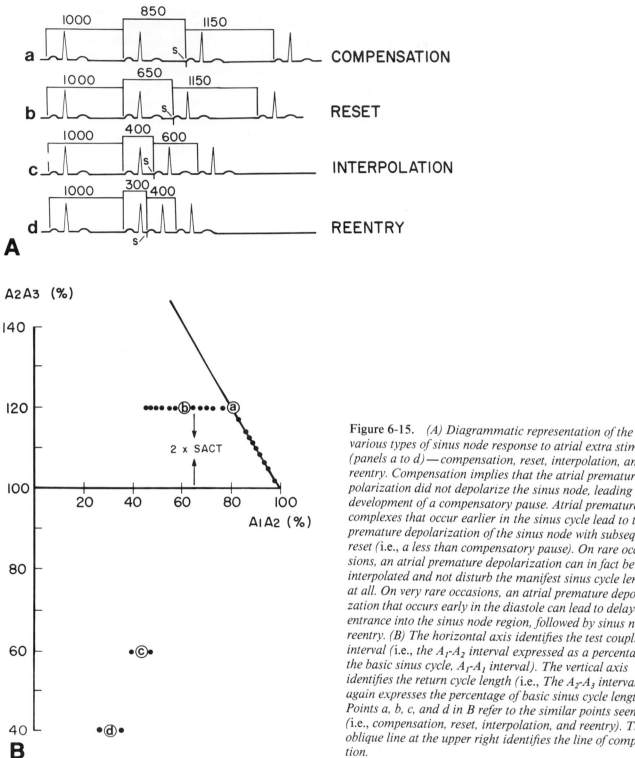

vious spontaneous sinus beat to enter these tissues. However, retrograde conduction would be markedly slowed, allowing other portions of the sinus node and perinodal zone to recover excitability. Such an electrophysiologic circumstance would allow for sinus node reentry. Theoretically, abnormalities of the sinoatrial region should increase the probability of sinus node reentry and the occurrence of atrial arrhythmias.[94,95,182,183] These events may be the underlying electrophysiologic basis for the observed increased frequency of occurrence of supraventricular tachyarrhythmias in patients with the sick sinus syndrome.

In summary, patients with sick sinus with electrophysiologic abnormalities of the sinoatrial junction

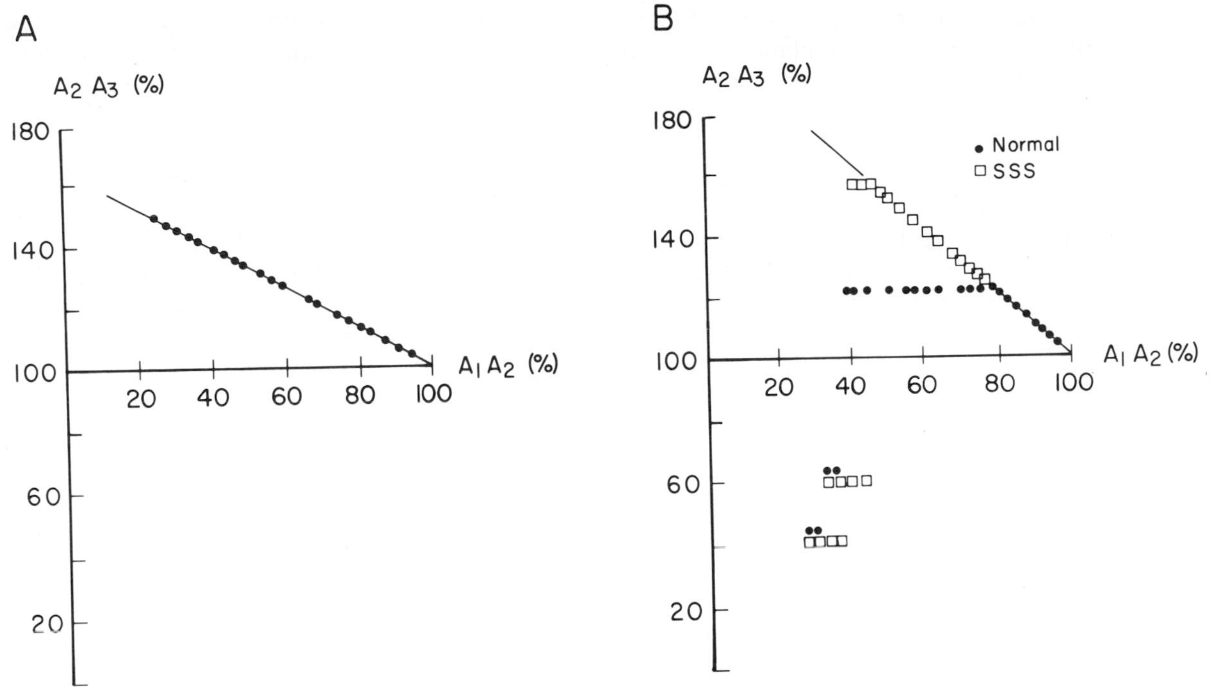

Figure 6-16. *Diagrammatic representation of plots of the A_1-A_2/A_2-A_3 relationships that might be expected in normal patients (B,* solid circles*) and in patients with sinus node dysfunction (*solid circles, *A, and* open squares, *B). In A, all points fall on the line of identity, indicating inability of even early atrial premature depolarizations to enter the sinus node and reset it. This is an example of first degree SA block. In B, patients with sinus node dysfunction may be expected to have prolongation of the compensatory zone, a decrease in the reset zone, and an increase in the interpolation and reentry zone.*

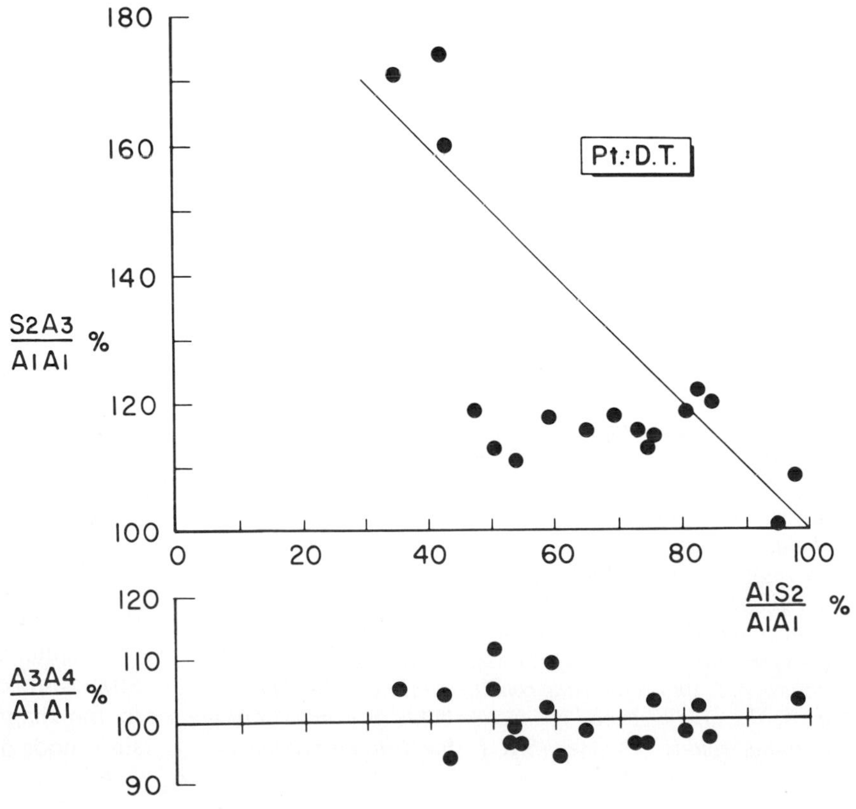

Figure 6-17. *Plot of the A_1-S_2 test interval versus the S_2-A_3 response intervals. The plot at the lower portion of the panel identifies subsequent A_3-A_4 intervals plotted against control A_1-A_1. Note that in the upper portion of this graph a compensatory zone and a reset zone are followed by a second zone of compensation, which occurs with very early atrial premature complexes.*

might be expected to demonstrate the following responses to premature atrial stimulation: (1) a prolonged zone of compensation, (2) a shortened zone of sinus node reset, (3) a prolonged zone of interpolation, and (4) a prolonged zone of sinus node reentry (see Fig. 6-16).

Recently, a fifth type of sinus node response to atrial premature depolarizations has been described, a second compensatory pause following very early APDs (Fig. 6-17).[184] Collision between early APDs and the next sinus beat cannot be merely a consequence of fortuitous timing, as in the case with late APDs. The marked prematurity of early APDs should allow more than sufficient time for retrograde SA conduction before the next sinus discharge. Thus, conduction of these APDs must be significantly slowed in the sinoatrial junction. In short, early APDs followed by a compensatory sinus pause have encountered the relative refractory period of the sinoatrial junction, where decremental conduction becomes electrocardiographically manifest.

In 1962, Langendorf and co-workers[185] deduced some of the functional characteristics of conduction between the sinoatrial node and the atrium from an analysis of the surface electrocardiogram in a patient with atrial parasystole. Based on their clinical observations and the experimental observations of Bonke and co-workers,[173] Strauss and co-workers[175] described how to assess sinoatrial conduction time using programmed atrial stimulation. The calculation of SACT assumes that the difference between the mean return cycle length (A_2-A_3) in the zone of sinus node reset and the spontaneous cycle length (A_1-A_1) is equal to the time required for the APD to retrogradely conduct through the perinodal zone plus the time required for the reset sinus impulse to traverse the perinodal zone anterogradely and enter the atrium (Fig. 6-18). An abnormally prolonged SACT is compatible with first degree sinoatrial block, a characteristic of some patients with the sick sinus syndrome.[134,176,186–189]

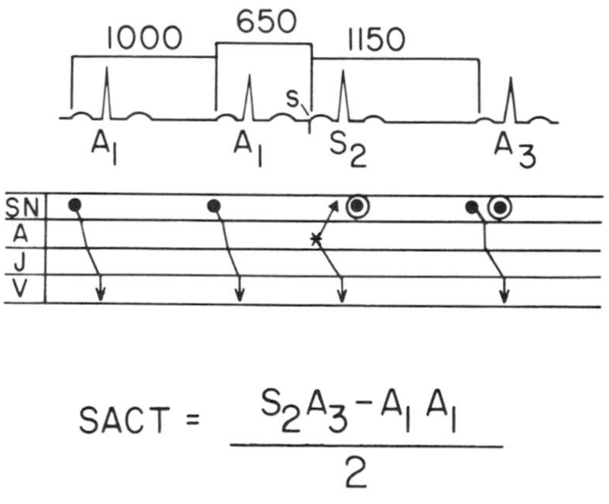

Figure 6-18. *Diagrammatic explanation of the method of calculating sinoatrial conduction time. The electrocardiographic strip identifies the events seen before and after an atrial premature complex. In the laddergram, the asterisk identifies the atrial premature depolarization that prematurely excites the sinus node* (arrowhead); *the double circles identify where the anticipated sinus node depolarization should normally have been; and the last solid circle identifies the reset sinus node discharge point. In the lowest portion of the diagram, SACT is calculated by subtracting the basal A_1-A_1 interval (1000 msec) from the observed recovery time S_2-A_3 interval (1150 msec). The total SACT, that is, the anterograde and retrograde conduction times, would be 150 msec; the unidirectional conduction time, as expressed in the formula, would be 75 msec. (SACT, sinoatrial conduction time)*

However, this method requires certain assumptions: (1) all APDs resulting in a postextrasystolic pause that is less than compensatory must reset the sinus node, (2) APDs must not depress sinus node automaticity, an event that would cause an overestimation of SACT, (3) anterograde and retrograde conduction must be equally influenced by an APD, (4) SACT must be independent of variations in spontaneous sinus rate, a phenomenon common to many patients with sinus node dysfunction, and (5) the velocity of retrograde sinoatrial conduction must be independent of the site of atrial stimulation.

In isolated tissue, Miller and Strauss[190] demonstrated that the transition between compensatory and less than compensatory postextrasystolic pauses included APDs that did not penetrate and reset the sinus node. Shortening of the sinus node return cycle in these cases was due to a shortening of the sinus node action potential by electronic interaction between sinus node and adjacent cells during repolarization. This artifactual shortening of the return cycle resulted in underestimation of the actual sinoatrial conduction time. Furthermore, APDs delivered in the middle of the sinus cycle in animal hearts may depress sinus node automaticity and cause pacemaker shifts.[172] However, differences of opinion do exist concerning the magnitude of the influence of depressed pacemaker automaticity on estimated SACT in humans.[191]

Miller and Strauss[190] noted that measured anterograde and retrograde conduction times are not equal, retrograde conduction usually being faster than anterograde conduction. In addition, SACT appears to vary as a function of the spontaneous sinus cycle length,[192,193] at slower heart rates estimated SACT being shorter than at faster heart rates.

Finally, Yamaguchi and Mandel[156] have recently demonstrated that the speed of retrograde conduction of an APD does depend on the site of atrial stimulation (Table 6-1). This observation may relate to the existence of specialized functional pathways of conduction between the sinus node and the atrium.[194]

Despite these inherent problems, the method of Strauss and co-workers[175] has proved a valuable addition to the diagnostic modalities available for evaluating sinus node dysfunction. Differentiation between abnor-

Table 6-1. Sinoatrial Conduction Times and Transition Points During Crista Terminalis, Coronary Sinus, and Atrial Septal Stimulation

	Crista Terminalis	Coronary Sinus	Atrial Septum
Retrograde conduction time (msec)	19.7 ± 1.1	18.6 ± 1.6	15.7 ± 1.0 ‡
Anterograde conduction time (msec)	32.5 ± 2.6 ΔΔΔ	33.5 ± 2.6 ΔΔΔ	34.7 ± 2.8 ΔΔΔ*
Total measured conduction time (msec)	52.2 ± 3.3	52.1 ± 4.1	50.4 ± 3.0
Estimated conduction time (msec)	57.8 ± 6.3	66.4 ± 10.7	43.6 ± 4.8 †
Transition point (%)	83.6 ± 1.2	83.0 ± 11.9	88.7 ± 0.9 ‡

Key: Values are: mean ± SEM; N = 18; * = significantly different from crista terminalis stimulation; Δ = significantly different from retrograde conduction time. (SEM, standard error of the mean)

Δ* $P < 0.05$
ΔΔ† $P < 0.01$
ΔΔΔ‡ $P < 0.005$

malities of sinus node generator function and impulse conduction is now potentially possible.

Reported ranges of normal values for calculated sinoatrial conduction time in patients without apparent sinus node dysfunction include 56 ± 22 msec[162]; 70 ± 30 msec[161]; 84.5 ± 26 msec[180]; 92 ± 60 msec[195]; 82 ± 19.2 msec[191]; and 88 ± 7 msec.[149] However, many of these patients had evidence of organic heart disease—some with abnormalities of the distal conduction system, many with ischemic heart disease, and others with valvular abnormalities. Jordan and co-workers[160] reported that patients with atherosclerotic involvement of the sinus node artery and no clinical or electrocardiographic evidence of sinus node dysfunction have significantly longer (although "normal") SACT values than do patients with coronary artery disease without such lesions. Similar differences in SACT may eventually be found in patients without apparent sinus node dysfunction dependent on other underlying pathologic processes. The important point is that sinoatrial disease progression to overt clinical and electrocardiographic manifestations may be a dynamic but gradual process.

Furthermore, as sinus node recovery time may be influenced by differences in autonomic tone, so may SACT be modified by changes in autonomic activity. Bonke and co-workers[172] and Klein and co-workers[174] could demonstrate no effect of atropine on sinoatrial conduction. Miller and Strauss[190] found that shortening of the sinus node action potential by APDs was not affected by atropine or propranolol. However, in 17 normal human subjects, Dhingra and co-workers[196] reported a significant shortening of calculated SACT following 1 to 2 mg of atropine (from 103 ± 5.7 msec to 58 ± 3.9 msec) as well as a shortening of the zone of compensation.

That SACT is shortened in humans by the administration of atropine independent of any change in heart rate is suggested by the observation that the return cycle following an APD shortened more than did the sinus cycle length.[196] In keeping with a hypothesis that atropine facilitates perinodal conduction, this drug has been shown to eliminate interpolation and echo responses in some persons.[196] Techniques for lengthening the perinodal refractory period, such as pacing the atrium at a rate faster than the sinus rate, have been shown to increase the number of normal subjects with zones of interpolation and reentry.[195]

The effect of atropine on SACT in patients with sinus node dysfunction is variable. Some patients with sick sinus have marked shortening of SACT after receiving atropine while others have only minimal shortening.[196,197] As a group, Dhingra and co-workers[198] found that mean preatropine and postatropine SACTs in 21 patients with sick sinus did not differ significantly than previously reported mean postatropine SACTs in 17 patients without evidence of sinus node dysfunction.[196] Individual sick sinus patients who do show significant shortening of SACT after atropine administration may have lower levels of resting parasympathetic activity and therefore less residual parasympathetic tone following similar doses of atropine. Alternatively, these patients may have greater resting sympathetic activity than patients failing to demonstrate SACT shortening. Finally, these patients may have no abnormalities of intrinsic electrophysiologic properties of sinoatrial conduction, their sinus node dysfunction being primarily a manifestation of abnormal autonomic control of sinoatrial conduction.

Dhingra and co-workers[198] did not find an overall shortening of the zone of compensation following atropine or a lengthening of the zone of sinus reset in patients with sick sinus. Similarly, interpolation and echo responses were unaffected by atropine in these patients.

Strauss and co-workers[199] found that propranolol, 1 mg/kg, significantly lengthened SACT in patients with sick sinus. However, effects on sinus node automaticity may have contributed to this finding.

As a group, in the control state, patients with sick sinus and abnormal intrinsic heart rates have significantly longer SACT than patients with sick sinus and normal intrinsic heart rates. Also, patients with sick sinus and normal intrinsic heart rates do have significantly greater decreases in SACT than do patients with abnormal intrinsic heart rates after autonomic blockade. However, individual patients do not neatly separate in terms of normal and abnormal SACT on the basis of normal versus abnormal intrinsic heart rates either in the control state or after complete pharmacologic autonomic blockade. That is, many patients with sick sinus and normal intrinsic heart rates have abnormal SACT; many patients with sick sinus and abnormal intrinsic heart rates have normal SACT. Thus, autonomic blockade appears to be a better discriminator of intrinsic sinus node pacemaker dysfunction than of intrinsic sinoatrial conduction abnormalities. However, this judgment may be too hasty. To assess sinoatrial conduction on the basis of sinus node automaticity (*i.e.*, IHR) may not be appropriate. To declare intrinsic sinoatrial conduction abnormal, comparison between known or predicted normal intrinsic SACT values and not normal intrinsic heart rates would be necessary. Thus, the laborious effort of Jose to establish norms for IHR in different age groups would have to be repeated to establish norms for intrinsic SACT. To date, normal intrinsic SACT values have not been established.

The incidence of abnormal prolongation of calculated SACT in 418 patients without evidence of sinus node dysfunction was found to be 2% by Dhingra and co-workers.[188] However, these investigators used a SACT of 152 msec as their criterion for abnormal, a figure considerably greater than other investogators have used. Therefore, their number of "false-positive" results may be spuriously low. This high cut-off value for normal subjects may also explain the low incidence of abnormal SACT found in patients suspected of having sinus node dysfunction (29% of 52 patients). Breithardt and co-workers[189] reported that 45% of 41 patients with various manifestations of sinus dysfunction had prolonged SACT when 120 msec was used as the upper limit of normal. Using a normal value of 215 msec for total anterograde plus retrograde conduction, Strauss and co-workers[134] reported that 38% of 16 patients with sinus node dysfunction demonstrated an abnormally long total SACT.

Recently, Breithardt and co-workers[189] attempted to correlate prolongation of SACT and SNRT with specific electrocardiographic abnormalities in patients with sick

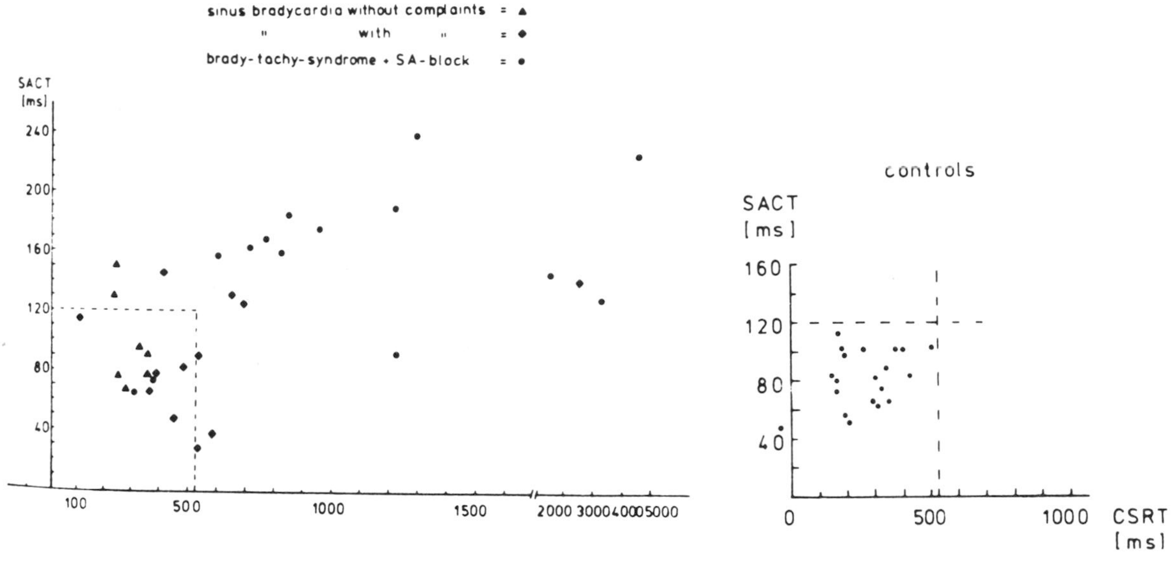

Figure 6-19. *In this figure, the corrected sinus node recovery time is plotted on the horizontal axis and the sinoatrial conduction time is plotted on the vertical axis.*

In the right-hand graph, data on control patients without clinical evidence of sinus node dysfunction are plotted. Note that in all patients, corrected sinus node recovery times and sinoatrial conduction times fall within the normal zone. The left-hand graph shows data for patients with sinus bradycardia but no significant complaints (triangles) *and sinus bradycardia with cardiovascular complaints* (diamonds), *as well as data for patients with bradycardia-tachycardia syndrome with SA block* (circles). *Note that the most abnormal data points for both sinoatrial conduction and sinus node recovery times occur with patients with bradycardia-tachycardia syndrome with SA block. The majority of patients with sinus bradycardia but no central nervous system symptomatology fall within the normal zone. (Breithardt, G., Seipel, L., and Loogan, F.: Sinus node recovery time and calculated sinoatrial conduction time in normal subjects and patients with sinus node dysfunction. Circulation, 56:43, 1977; by permission of the American Heart Association, Inc.)*

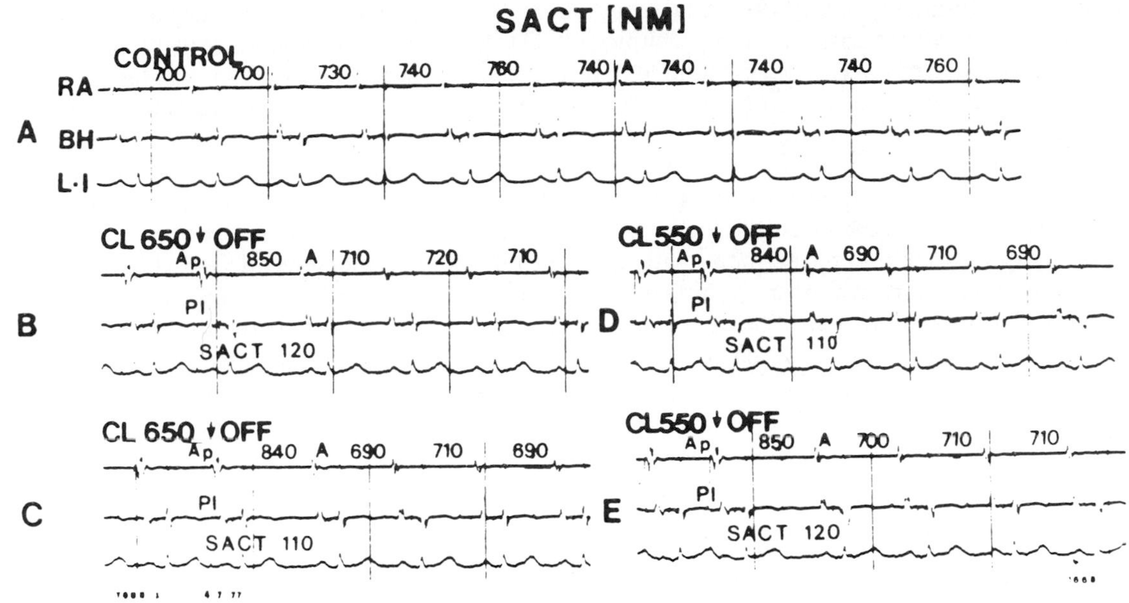

Figure 6-20. *This figure shows the method used to calculate the sinoatrial conduction time using the new method of Narula. In A to E, recordings are shown in the control state and following overdrive pacing at a cycle length of 650 and a cycle length of 550. Note the similarity of sinoatrial conduction times measured following the last paced beats to the onset of the next spontaneous sinus complex. (Narula, O. S., Narashimhan, S., Vasquez, M., et al.: A new method for measurement of sinoatrial conduction time. Circulation, 58:706, 1978; by permission of the American Heart Association, Inc.)*

sinus. Patients with asymptomatic sinus bradycardia did not have significantly longer SNRTC or SACT values than control subjects, whereas patients with symptoms did. Patients with the bradycardia-tachycardia syndrome or episodic sinoatrial block or both demonstrated significantly longer SNRT values than control subjects, although SACT in the bradycardia-tachycardia group did not differ from that of the control patients. SNRT was found to be a somewhat more sensitive measure than SACT, showing fewer false-negative results in patients with sinus node dysfunction (Fig. 6-19). Nonetheless, SACT determination proved to be a better method of distinguishing patients with sick sinus from healthy subjects than had previously been reported.[133]

Continuous Pacing Method for Determining Sinoatrial Conduction Time

Limitations of the atrial premature stimulus technique for determining the sinoatrial conduction time have been reviewed. In order to circumvent sinus node suppression, pacemaker shift, and other variables, Narula described a new method for determining sinoatrial conduction time using overdrive atrial pacing.[200] The atrium is paced 10 beats/min faster than the basic sinus rate for eight beats. The interval in milliseconds from the last paced beat to the first return sinus beat on the intra-atrial electrogram is taken as the total time of retrograde and anterograde sinoatrial conduction (Fig. 6-20). Clinically, at this pacing rate, the sinus node pacemaker does not appear to be suppressed and there is no suggestion of pacemaker shift when postreturn cycles (A_3-A_4, A_4-A_5, and so on) are examined. The measure appears to be reproducible. The advantages of the methods are that complex equipment (*i.e.*, programmed stimulator) and laborious calculations required for sinoatrial conduction time determination with the premature atrial stimulation technique are unnecessary.

The validity of sinoatrial conduction time as estimated by the constant atrial pacing technique has been examined in the microelectrode laboratory.[201] Many of the same difficulties encountered in the premature atrial stimulus technique exist in the constant atrial pacing method. Shortening of sinus node action potential, depression of automacity, and shifts in the primary pacemaker contributed to errors in both techniques. Estimation of SACT by the constant atrial pacing method was further complicated by failure of sinus node capture, especially at slow pacing rates ($\leq$ 5 beats/min faster than the basic sinus rate). Total SACT 5, 10, and 15 beats/min faster than the resting heart rate were 76 $\pm$ 10, 86 $\pm$ 10, and 96 $\pm$ 10 msec; correlation coefficients with measured SACT were 0.7, 0.54, and 0.4, respectively. Estimates of SACT by constant atrial stimulation compared well with estimates by premature atrial stimulation. The mean ± SEM were similar for both techniques. SACTs overestimated by constant pacing tended to be overestimated by premature atrial stimulation. The correlation coefficient for the two methods was 0.85. When the two estimates were compared with measured SACTs, the determinations were not significantly different from each other ($P \geq 0.9$), and both were subject to a mean error of approximately 30%. Pretreatment with atropine and propranolol did not prevent shortening of the sinus node action potential duration. The antegrade conduction time preceding the train of paced beats was 30 msec and 10 msec for the first return sinus beat, possibly reflecting a shift in the pacemaker site toward the crista terminalis and leading to an underestimation of SACT; antegrade conduction time usually returned to its prepacing value in five to ten cycles.

Clinically, Kang and colleagues[202] found that the two methods correlated very well (r = .80) during control and after autonomic blockade (r = .85). In addition, the directional changes in SACT after autonomic blockade were always similar. For each method, 8 of 12 patients with sick sinus demonstrated shortening of SACT and 4 of 12 demonstrated lengthening of SACT following autonomic blockade. The investigators suggested that prolongation of SACT after autonomic blockade is an abnormal response in patients in whom sinus node suppression cannot be demonstrated by examining postpacing or post–extra stimulus cycle lengths. They proposed that an increase in SACT may be related to intrinsic abnormalities of sinoatrial conduction previously masked by sympathetic activity.

Breithardt and Seipel[203] reported a poor correlation between SACTs by the constant atrial stimulation method and the premature atrial stimulation method (r = .45). The investigators suggested that the poor correlation resulted from greater depression of sinus node automaticity by the premature atrial stimulus technique. However, Grant and associates[201] believe that the disparity was more likely related to failure of penetration and reset of the sinus node during pacing at slow pacing rates, an effect that disappeared when pacing rates were increased by as little as 3 beats/min (see above).

Sinus Node Extracellular Potential Recordings

Recently, developments in electrophysiologic techniques have permitted the recording of the sinus node action potential from the endocardial and epicardial surfaces of the intact heart.[204–207] With unipolar recordings through Ag-AgCl electrodes (0.5 mm in diameter), covered to the tip with polyethylene, directly coupled to a preamplifier and positioned 0.2 to 0.5 mm above the sinus node, identification of pacemaker action potentials from the epicardial surface has been substantiated by simultaneous transmembrane recordings in isolated rabbit hearts.[204] A similar technique that obtains both unipolar and bipolar recordings has permitted extracellular action potentials to be recorded from the epicardial surface in humans during open-heart surgery (Fig. 6-21).[205] Hariman and colleagues[208] found that sinoatrial conduction times were 32.4 ± 2.8 msec, at sinus cycle lengths 587.6 ± 35.6 msec for the bipolar method and 38.2 ± 3.2 msec at sinus cycle lengths of 712.2 ± 50.7 msec for the unipolar method.

Finally, a transvenous catheter technique has been developed to record endocardial surface sinoatrial pacemaker potentials in the intact canine heart[206] and, more recently, humans.[209–211] Gomes and co-workers[212] have reported that when the catheter was looped in the right atrium and advanced to the junction of the superior vena cava and right atrium so that the distal poles of the catheter were in direct contact with the right atrial endocardium underlying the area of the sinoatrial node, stable sinoatrial electrograms could be obtained in 18 of 21 (86%) patients. The method was reported superior to the technique of Reiffel and colleagues,[210] in which the catheter tip was only in close proximity to the right atrial endocardium. The former technique minimized baseline drift of the sinoatrial electrogram. Patients with sick sinus syndrome consistently had longer directly measured SACT (1.35 ± 30 msec) than did patients without sick sinus syndrome (87 ± 12 msec), measurements in agreement with those found by Reiffel and co-workers. The discrepancy between SACT recorded from the endocardial surface and SACT recorded from the epicardial surface by Hariman and colleagues[208] was not explained. There was good correlation between direct and indirect SACTs estimated by Narula's pacing method (r = .843, N = 28) and by the premature stimulation method (r = .778, N = 18). The direct method, $SACT_d$, appears superior to the indirect methods, $SATC_i$, for measuring SACT in patients in whom no zone of reset can be obtained and in patients in whom frequent atrial premature complexes are present.

Based on their findings that $SACT_i$ often overestimates $SACT_d$, Reiffel and colleagues[210] have suggested that when $SACT_i$ is normal, $SACT_d$ will be normal; however, if $SACT_i$ is prolonged, $SACT_d$ may be normal. On the other hand, and unexpectedly, Gomes and colleagues found that $SACT_i$ often underestimates $SACT_d$. The discrepancy between these results is disturbing and requires explanation, although it may relate to differences in methodology (see above).

Although these techniques await further confirmation by other investigators and a wider variety of applications, such developments represent major advances in electrophysiologic methodology. The surface electrocardiogram and intracavitary recordings often grossly mis-

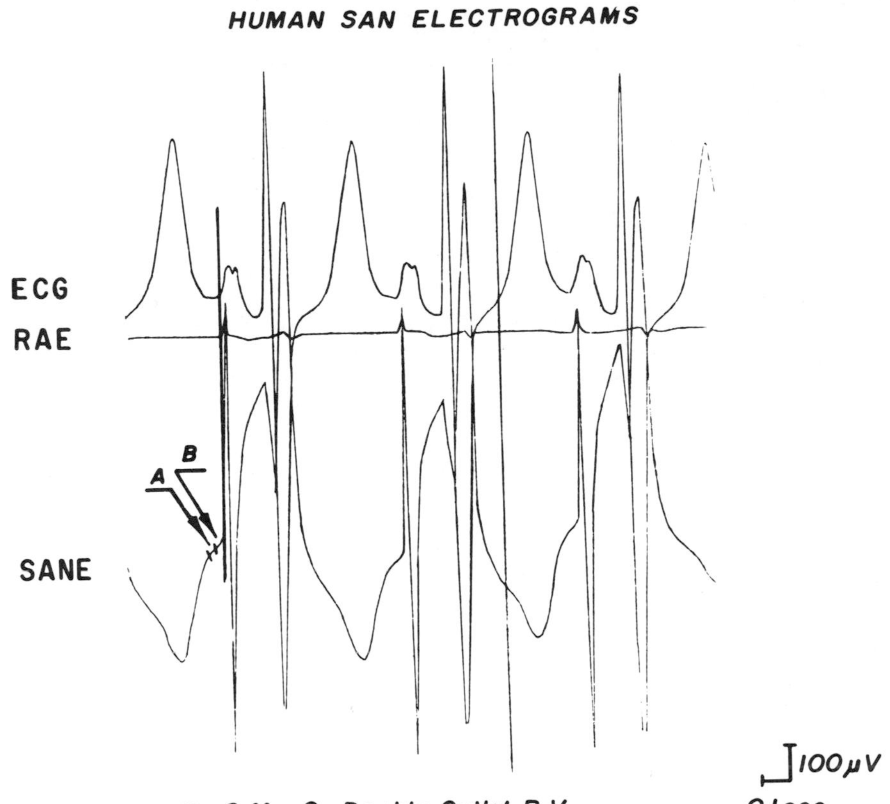

Figure 6-21. *Extracellular recordings obtained from human sinus node at the time of open-heart surgery.* From above downward: *surface electrocardiogram, right atrial electrogram, and a sinoatrial node electrogram. Note the appearance of pre P wave electrical activity in the sinoatrial node electrogram. (Courtesy Robert Harriman, M.D.)*

represent underlying electrophysiologic events in the sinus node and sinoatrial junction in the setting of overdrive pacing and premature atrial stimulation. Applying these new methods of recording surface electrical potentials from the sinoatrial region in humans may provide new insights into the mechanisms of function and dysfunction in the human sinus node.

To date, the most controversial application of sinoatrial electrogram recordings in humans comes from a report by Asseman and colleagues.[213] These investigators studied eight patients with sick sinus with SNRT greater than 1500 msec. In six patients, sinus node electrograms, appearing at a rate similar to the basic sinus rate, persisted during the postpacing pause. The authors concluded that the pause following cessation of atrial overdrive is often caused by overdrive-induced sinoatrial block rather than by sinus node pacemaker suppression in patients with sick sinus. This surprising conclusion is in direct conflict with findings in microelectrode studies that clearly demonstrate suppression of sinus node pacemaker activity by atrial overdrive pacing in both the normal sinus node[214] and in the sinus node made abnormal by the addition of verapamil to the preparation.[141] Moreover, microelectrode studies that do confirm alteration in sinoatrial conduction following overdrive pacing (as a consequence of decreased sinus pacemaker action potential amplitude) also show slowing of pacemaker rate.[215,216] Curiously, Asseman and colleagues reported that overdrive pacing resulted in no sinus rate suppression, despite obvious changes in action potential characteristics. Despite these inconsistencies, the findings of Asseman's group are provocative and demand an explanation, especially in recognition of the complex interaction between conduction and impulse formation that determines sinus node recovery time.

More in keeping with microelectrode findings is the recent report of Gomes and co-workers.[217] Direct sinus node recordings in humans revealed that $SNRT_i$ reflects both sinus node automaticity and sinoatrial conduction. In all 16 patients, overdrive atrial pacing appeared to result in marked prolongation of $SACT_d$ for the first postpacing beat, which was longer in patients with sick sinus than in healthy subjects. Postpacing $SACT_d$ prolongation persisted for 3.6 ± 0.96 beats. Sinus node suppression was seen in 56% of patients, sinus node acceleration was noted in 26%, and no appreciable change in sinus node automaticity was observed in 19%. Insensitive to the contribution of increased SACT to sinus node recovery after overdrive pacing, $SNRT_i$ consistently overestimated $SNRT_d$.

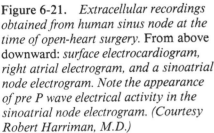

Direct sinoatrial electrogram recordings have exposed the importance of the role of alterations in sinoatrial conduction in other bradycardic situations pre-

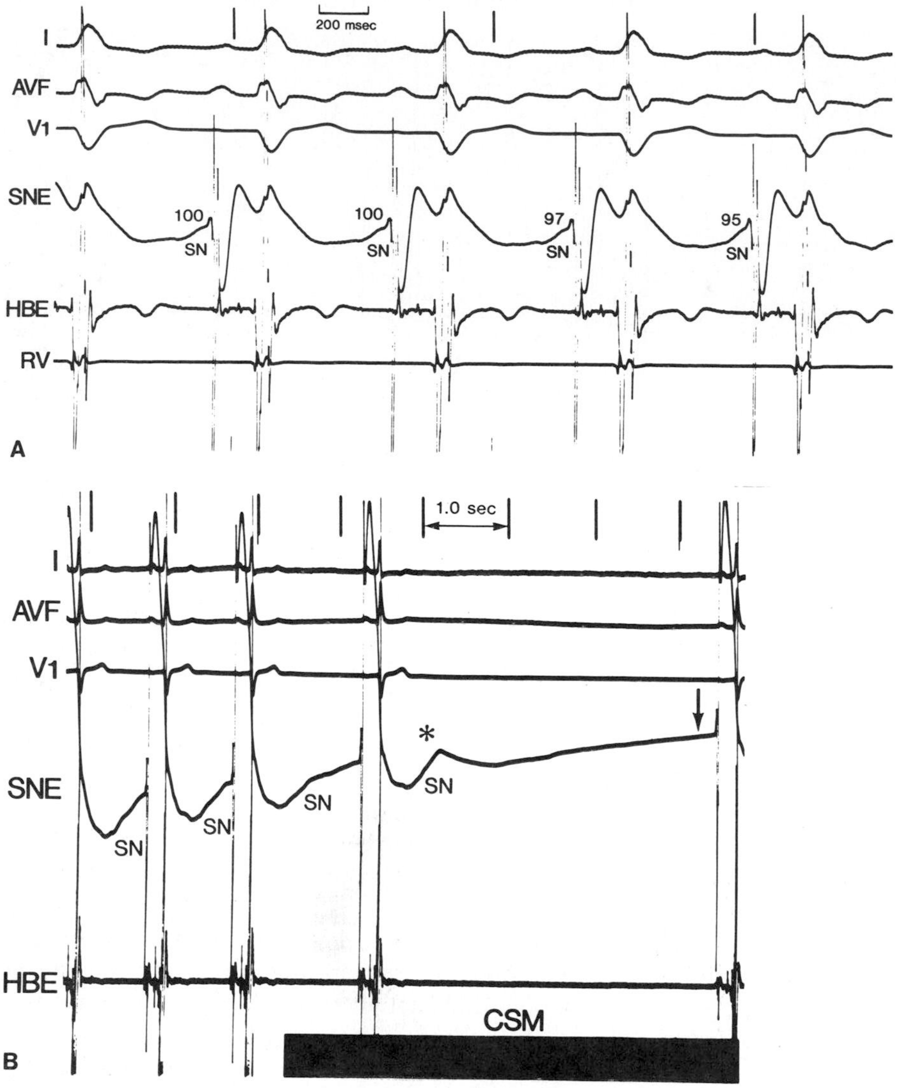

Figure 6-22. *(A) The sinus node electrogram. Surface electrocardiogram leads I, aVF and V_1 are displayed along with intracavitary electrocardiograms from the region of the sinus node, His bundle, and right ventricle. Sinus node potentials are the positive-going, low-frequency deflections preceding each atrial depolarization. The directly measured sinoatrial conduction times are labeled above each SN deflection. (SNE, sinus node; HBE, His bundle; RV, right ventricle; SN, sinus node potentials) (B) Carotid sinus massage in a patient with the hypersensitive carotid sinus syndrome. Surface and intracardiac electrocardiograms are labeled as in A. The onset of carotid sinus massage is followed by profound prolongation in the SN deflection, signifying probable prolongation in the sinoatrial conduction time. Sinoatrial block is then illustrated, since a sinus node impulse is shown to occur* without *subsequent atrial depolarization (asterisk). Sinus node quiescence is then recorded until the inscription of the next atrial impulse, which is not preceded by a SN potential (arrow). The absence of a SN potential suggests a shifting of the primary pacemaker focus out of the sinus node or to another region without the sinus node. (CSM, cardiac sinus massage)*

viously ascribed to depression of sinus node automaticity alone. Using this recording technique, Gang and colleagues[218] have shown that sinoatrial block is an important component of the asystolic pause that occurs in patients with the cardioinhibitory form of the hypersensitive carotid sinus syndrome (Fig. 6-22).

Carotid sinus hypersensitivity may be manifested in two ways, apparently independent of each other.[219,220] The cardioinhibitory type is expressed as an apparent slowing of the heart rate with mechanical stimulation of the carotid sinus and is inhibited by atropine. The less common vasodepressor type is accompanied by vasodilation and hypotension and is often inhibited by epinephrine. The cardioinhibitory type appears to be mediated by the parasympathetic nervous system and is most commonly found in elderly men with coronary atherosclerosis and hypertensive heart disease.[221–223] The precise mechanism of the cardioinhibitory type is not known, although four possibilities have been proposed: (1) a high level of resting vagal tone, (2) excessive release of acetylcholine, (3) inadequate cholinesterase activity, and (4) hyperresponsiveness to acetylcholine. If the latter mechanism is the predominant one, carotid hypersensitivity is properly part of the sick sinus syndrome. The majority of patients with carotid hypersensitivity have normal SNRT and SACT.[220,224–226]

The Effects of Drugs on Normal and Abnormal Sinus Node Function

Sinus node response to any particular pharmacologic agent can be extremely variable and may even appear to be almost idiosyncratic. In any given person, a specific drug may have negligible, profound stimulatory, or marked inhibitory effects on sinus node automaticity or sinoatrial conduction. Moreover, the electrophysiologic effects of many antiarrhythmic agents as observed in isolated tissue preparations often do not correspond to the clinical response witnessed in humans. Furthermore, the effect of a drug on sinus node function may differ significantly when it is given as an acute single intravenous dose or a chronic oral administration. These apparent inconsistencies can be explained when several facts are considered: (1) the effects of a drug on sinus node function may be mediated by indirect (interaction with the autonomic and central nervous systems) as well as direct mechanisms of action, (2) the sinus node response to a specific cardiac drug may differ in the setting of abnormal intrinsic sinoatrial function than when no intrinsic sinus node abnormalities are present, (3) in sinoatrial dysfunction, the clinical response to a pharmacologic agent may be determined by the specific electrophysiologic property that is abnormal as well as the magnitude of the abnormality, (4) drugs may have differential effects on properties of sinus node automaticity and sinoatrial conduction, and (5) the electrophysiologic assumptions on which the technique of premature atrial stimulation are based may be invalid in the sinus node and sinoatrial junction made abnormal by cardioactive drugs.

Established Antiarrhythmic Agents

Digitalis

Digitalis preparations slow sinus rate by slowing the rate of rise of phase 4 of the sinus node action potential. Changes in action potential amplitude and threshold potential have also been reported.[227] Most studies indicate that an interaction with the autonomic nervous system is probably the primary mechanism of action of digitalis on sinus node function.[228–232] However, negative chronotropic responses have also been demonstrated in denervated human hearts[223] and in humans after complete pharmacologic blockade. Gomes and colleagues[234] found that ouabain, 0.01 mg/kg administered intravenously after pharmacologic autonomic blockade, significantly lengthened sinus node recovery time in patients with normal and abnormal intrinsic heart rates. On the other hand, ouabain had no significant effect on sinoatrial conduction time as determined by the continous pacing method after autonomic blockade. Recent reports have described a positive chronotropic response to digitalis preparations in animals[235–237] that may have been due to release of endogenous catecholamines[236] or an increase in preganglionic sympathetic tone.[237]

In healthy subjects, digitalis generally has little effect on sinus rate, sinus node recovery time, or sinoatrial conduction. However, Dhingra and co-workers[238] reported that digitalis shortened sinus node recovery time, and several clinical studies have indicated that digitalis lengthened estimated sinoatrial conduction time.[239,240] This latter finding might suggest that shortening of sinus node recovery time is artifactual, since fewer paced beats would be expected to penetrate the sinus node in the presence of digitalis. However, microelectrode studies in isolated rabbit atria demonstrate that ouabain produces almost no change in refractoriness of perinodal fibers in the retrograde direction (Fig. 6-23).* Furthermore, the premature atrial stimulus technique overestimates sinoatrial conduction time in the presence of ouabain because depression of sinus node automaticity is depressed by the APD (Fig. 6-24).*

The effect of digitalis on sinoatrial function has recently been examined by Harriman and Hoffman,[241] using sinoatrial electrogram recordings in instrumented dogs. These investigators found that ouabain caused beat-to-beat variation in sinus cycles, abnormalities of sinoatrial conduction, and pacemaker shifts. The effects could be abolished by atropine. Ouabain-induced failure of sinoatrial conduction appeared to result by one of two mechanisms. First, failure of sinoatrial conduction can occur if the amplitude of the sinus pacemaker potential is reduced so that it is unable to excite the surrounding tissue. Second, sinoatrial conduction can fail if the effects of ouabain are more intense on the fibers of the sinoatrial junction than on the sinus node pacemaker, resulting in sinoatrial block. Both mechanisms of failure of sinoatrial conduction have also been described in response to vagal stimulation. Because acetylcholine re-

* Yamaguchi, I., Jordan, J. L., and Mandel, W. J.: Antiarrhythmic drug effects on sinus node function during early premature stimulation. Personal communication.

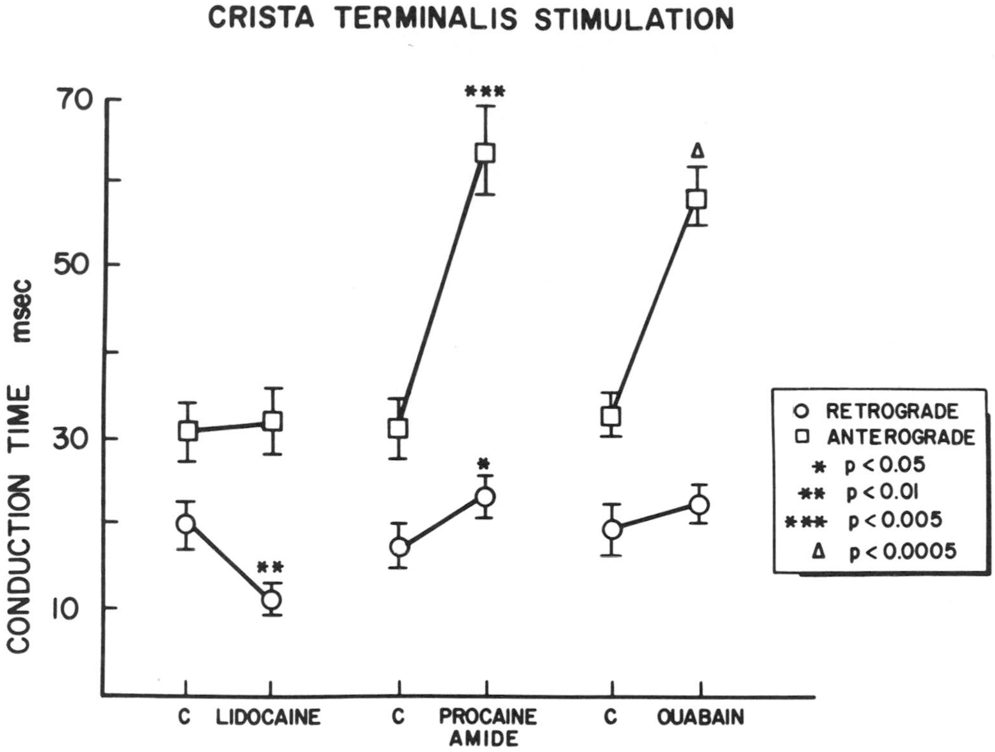

Figure 6-23. *The effect of various antiarrhythmic drugs on anterograde and retrograde sinoatrial conduction time in isolated cardiac tissue. Note that with lidocaine, retrograde conduction time is significantly shortened, whereas with procainamide and ouabain, retrograde and, to a greater extent, anterograde conduction times are significantly prolonged.*

duced sinoatrial conduction time but not pacemaker action potential amplitude, the authors suggested that the effects of ouabain result from different densities of vagal fibers in different areas of the sinoatrial region rather than from differing sensitivities of pacemaker cells and perinodal cells to the drug.

Numerous investigators have cautioned against administering digitalis to patients with sick sinus syndrome.[242-244] However, adverse effects on sinus node function in patients with this syndrome vary, and exaggerated responses cannot be predicted in any given patient.[243,244]

Quinidine

In humans, the usual effect of quinidine is acceleration of sinus rate, believed to be mediated by an interaction with the autonomic nervous system.[245,246] Infrequent negative chronotropic effects on sinus node function do not appear to be related to beta-adrenergic blocking properties of the drug.[247] Mason and co-workers[248] administered quinidine gluconate intravenously to cardiac allograft recipients (mean plasma level 4.3 μg/liter) 8 to 20 months after transplantation. The sinus cycle length increased in all transplanted hearts but decreased in the innervated atrial remnant. The investigators concluded that direct membrane effects of quinidine slow the rate of depolarization of the sinus node while enhancement of sinus node in humans is neurally mediated. In persons without sinus node disease, quinidine-induced abnormalities of sinoatrial dysfunction are probably clinically rare.[249-251] No information is available on the incidence of adverse effects of quinidine in patients with sick sinus.

Procainamide

Consistent with microelectrode observations that procainamide has no significant effect on the characteristics of the spontaneous sinus node action potential,[227] clinical reports of its adverse effects on sinus node function are infrequent. Procainamide does prolong sinoatrial conduction time in isolated tissue preparations, primarily by prolonging anterograde conduction (see Fig. 6-23).[227]

Clinically, Josephson and co-workers[252] observed an increase in sinus rate (mean 7%) in response to intravenous procainamide administration. Although not extensively investigated, enhanced automaticity of the sinus pacemaker has been attributed to a vagolytic effect of procainamide. Reflex sympathetic discharge, because of negative ionotropic actions and vasodilatory effects of procainamide, may also play a role in accelerating heart

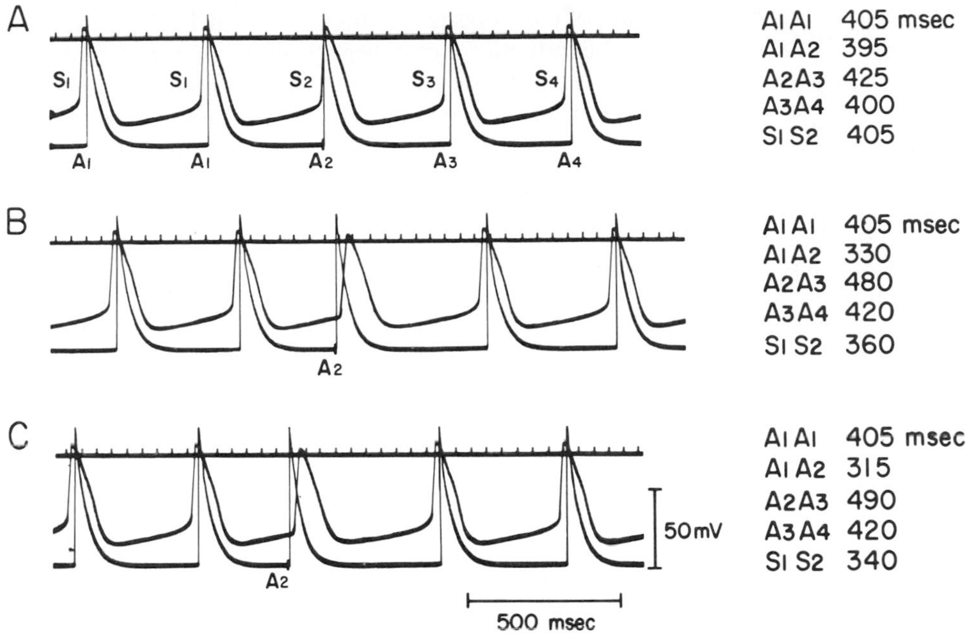

Figure 6-24. *The influence of ouabain on features of indirect sinoatrial conduction time measurements. A to C show the influence of premature atrial depolarizations on sinus node cycle lengths and the indirect measurement of sinoatrial conduction. In A, very late diastolic atrial premature complexes (A_2) do not influence (capture) the sinus node. In B, an earlier A_1-A_2 interval of 330 msec results in sinus node capture, but the test and return cycles are, in fact, compensatory. In C, at an even earlier A_1-A_2 interval, the test and return cycles are now in the zone of reset. The above data indicate that with ouabain the sinus node could be prematurely discharged and reset at a time when the atrial electrograms indicate compensatory response (*i.e., *noncapture). These atrial records result in an apparent upward shift in the point of transition and would therefore lead to false prolongation of the indirectly measured sinoatrial conduction time.*

rate. Goldberg and colleagues[253] reported that procainamide tended to prolong SNRTC by enhancing sinoatrial conduction in patients with sinus node dysfunction. In contrast, procainamide shortened SNRTC in patients without sinus node dysfunction.

Disopyramide

Disopyramide usually (but not invariably) shortens sinus cycle length in healthy persons, presumably by a vagolytic effect.[254] Negative ionotropic effects with reflex sympathetic discharge may also play a role in sinus rate acceleration.[255] In isolated sinoatrial preparations, disopyramide has little effect on sinus node recovery time or sinoatrial conduction regardless of the magnitude of cholinergic tone.[256]

There does appear to be a difference between the effect of disopyramide on normal and abnormal sinus node function. Disopyramide shortens sinus node recovery time in healthy persons[254,257] but significantly prolongs recovery time in patients with sick sinus.[257] LaBarre and co-workers[258] reported that disopyramide slowed the sinus rate in some patients with sick sinus and shortened the estimated sinoatrial conduction time in patients with sinus pauses, SA block, and secondary pauses after overdrive pacing.

Lidocaine

Contrary to microelectrode studies in isolated tissue, which demonstrate lidocaine to have little effect on characteristics of the sinus node action potential,[259] Dhingra and co-workers[260] reported that administration of this drug resulted in a significant decrease in the sinus cycle length in patients with normal and abnormal sinus node function. Positive chronotropic effects of lidocaine on the sinus node in humans may be secondary to the vagolytic properties of the drug.[261]

Dhingra and co-workers[260] reported that lidocaine shortened the mean maximal sinus node recovery time in humans, an effect presumably not artifactual, since lidocaine actually shortens the retrograde absolute refractory period of perinodal fibers* and thus would not

* Yamaguchi, I., Jordan, J. L., and Mandel, W. J.: Antiarrythmic drug effects on sinus node function during early premature stimulation. Personal communication.

be expected to block penetration of paced beats into the sinus node. Estimated sinoatrial conduction times were significantly prolonged in patients with sick sinus but unchanged in patients with normal sinus node function. In contrast, Yamaguchi and co-workers[227] found that measured sinoatrial conduction time significantly shortened in isolated rabbit tissue after lidocaine superfusion (see Fig. 6-23).

Lidocaine has been implicated in the precipitation of exaggeration of abnormalities of sinoatrial function in a number of clinical reports.[262,263] However, at present, adverse effects of lidocaine on sinus node function cannot be reliably predicted.

Mexiletine

Mexiletine is structurally related to lidocaine and has many class IB antidysrhythmic actions. In isolated sinus node tissue, Yamaguchi and co-workers[264] reported that mexiletine slowed the sinus rate only in concentrations exceeding the equivalent of therapeutic plasma levels in humans. In contrast, mexiletine prolonged sinoatrial conduction time at concentrations below the equivalent of toxic plasma levels.

In animals and humans, mexiletine can cause sinus bradycardia.[265,266] However, a slight acceleration in heart rate and decrease in sinus node recovery time have also been observed in some patients. Roos and co-workers[265] reported that three of five patients demonstrating prolongation of sinus node recovery time following mexiletine administration had sick sinus syndrome and in only one patient with sinus node dysfunction did recovery time decrease. These investigators cautioned against using mexiletine in patients with dysfunction of impulse formation.

Tocainide

Tocainide is also structurally related to lidocaine, having class IB effects on the monophasic action potential. Although no reports have appeared to suggest adverse effects on sinus node function, reported experiences with lidocaine and mexiletine warrant caution with the use of tocainide in patients with sick sinus syndrome.

Encainide

Encainide is a class IC antiarrhythmic agent with electrophysiologic properties similar to those of quinidine, except that it does not significantly alter action potential duration. In anesthetized dogs, Samuelsson and Harrison[267] reported a significant reduction in heart rate with intravenous administration of encainide, 2.7 mg/kg. Maximal increase in basic cycle length was reached within 15 to 30 minutes. These results were not confirmed by Sami and colleagues.[268] Furthermore, these investigators found no significant effect of encainide on sinus node recovery time.[269] In humans, neither intravenous nor oral encainide has been shown to significantly affect heart rate or sinus node recovery time.[270]

Flecainide

Flecainide is an antiarrhythmic drug with a predominantly class IC mode of action. In doses of 1 mg/kg given intravenously, Seipel and associates[271] found that it had no significant effect on sinus node function in patients with normal sinus node function. However, at 2 mg/kg, sinus node recovery time increased 37% in these patients, although no effect was observed on spontaneous sinus rate. Vik-Mo and colleagues[272] reported a statistically significant increase in corrected sinus node recovery time in patients with sinus node dysfunction when 1.5 mg/kg of flecainide was administered intravenously. Sinus cycle length and sinoatrial conduction time were not significantly changed. The investigators advised caution in using flecainide in patients with sinus node dysfunction.

Lorcainide

Lorcainide, another antiarrhythmic agent with class IC electrophysiologic properties, was shown in clinical electrophysiologic studies to prolong sinus node recovery time, particularly in patients with sinus node dysfunction.[273–275]

Diphenylhydantoin

Direct membrane effects, an interaction with the autonomic nervous system, and central system effects could all potentially contribute to the electrophysiologic effects of diphenylhydantoin (DPH).[276–278] In humans, heart rate response to DPH may vary. A cardioacceleratory effect may be secondary to an anticholinergic action; in the denervated dog heart, DPH slows the sinus rate.[276] Strauss and co-workers[279] could find no significant effect of DPH on the sinus node action potential in isolated tissue preparations; however, the sinus node that had been depressed by stretch, mechanical trauma, or toxic concentrations of acetylcholine, propranolol, or potassium became markedly more susceptible to toxic concentrations of DPH. Sinoatrial block, however, was not a manifestation of DPH-induced sinoatrial dysfunction in these experimentally depressed preparations.

Examples of sinus node dysfunction in the setting of intravenous DPH administration are well documented but may not be solely the effect of the drug. The solvent for DPH contains propylene glycol, a substance that has been shown to cause marked sinus bradycardia.[280]

Slow Channel Inhibitors

Verapamil

Verapamil is a slow channel blocking agent. It has not yet been established whether it blocks only calcium conductance or the sodium component of the slow channel as well. Verapamil has been demonstrated to affect all aspects of the sinus node action potential, with the possible exception of the maximum diastolic membrane potential. Wit and Cranefield[281] reported that verapamil produced linear dose-related decreases in sinus rate. The negative chronotropic effect of verapamil does not appear to be mediated by interaction with the autonomic nervous system.[282,283] Sinus node recovery time is prolonged after verapamil administration,[284,285] as is sinoatrial conduction time (in the anterograde direction only).[286]

In humans and intact animals, variable effects on heart rate have been demonstrated following intravenous verapamil administration. Most commonly, an increase in sinus rate is observed in the clinical settings following administration of the drug, presumably the result of a reflex autonomic response to hypotension.[287] Verapamil is contraindicated in patients with sick sinus syndrome.

Nifedipine

The effects of nifedipine on SA node transmembrane potentials are identical to the effects of verapamil, although these depressant effects require a much higher concentration of nifedipine.[288] More intense peripheral vasodilatory effects probably result in greater reflex sympathetic activity than is seen with verapamil, usually offsetting the negative chronotropic effects of nifedipine. Nonetheless, nifedipine should be used with caution in patients with sick sinus syndrome.

Diltiazem

Direct negative chronotropic effects of diltiazem are less than verapamil but greater than nifedipine.[289] Extreme caution is advised when using this drug in the setting of sinus node dysfunction.

Newer Antiarrhythmic Agents

Amiodarone

The mechanism of antiarrhythmic action of amiodarone is unknown. The drug appears to have major antimetabolic activity, significantly reducing myocardial oxygen consumption and increasing the ratio of ATP and creatine phosphate to ADP, creatine, and inorganic phosphate.[290]

Amiodarone, 1.5×10^{-5} M, slows spontaneous sinus rate activity. The most significant changes in the sinus node action potential include a depression of phase 4 diastolic depolarization and prolongation of the action potential duration.[291] The negative chronotropic action of amiodarone is enhanced under conditions of low calcium concentration. Autonomic blockade has little or no effect on the negative chronotropic action of amiodarone.[292]

Ajmaline

Ajmaline is a derivative of *Rauwolfia serpentina* and might be expected to depress sinus node function on the basis of catecholamine depletion as well as through direct membrane effects. Obayashi and Mandel[293] observed no significant effect of ajmaline on sinus node automaticity in isolated sinus node preparations at concentrations less than 1×10^{-4} M/liter. In contrast, ajmaline prolonged anterograde sinoatrial conduction. In the intact dog heart, ajmaline slowed sinus rate only at high doses (8 mg/kg); at lower doses (4 mg/kg) an increase in heart rate was observed, perhaps duc to a local (atrial) release of catecholamines.[294]

Aprindine

Aprindine hydrochloride has local anesthetic properties and may also possess significant slow channel blocking properties.[295] Direct membrane effects of the drug cause a dose-dependent slowing of sinus rate.[296] In humans, sinus rate is probably little affected by aprindine; reflex sympathetic activity in response to negative inotropic effects may offset direct membrane-depressant effects.[296]

Propafenone

Propafenone is a new antiarrhythmic agent with complex mechanisms of action, including (1) inhibition of fast sodium current, (2) lidocainelike effects on transmembrane action potentials at low concentrations, (3) beta-sympatholytic actions,[297] and (4) a weakly inhibitory effect on slow calcium inward current at high concentrations.[298] In a dose-dependent fashion, propafenone reduces action potential amplitude, the maximum diastolic potential, and the rate of phase 4 depolarization while prolonging action potential duration.[299] In voltage-clamp studies, Satoh and Hashimoto[299] concluded that the negative chronotropic effects of propafenone are predominantly mediated by decreases in the outward i_k current in the sinus node.

Sotalol

Sotalol is a unique antiarrhythmic agent with both classic beta-adrenergic blocking properties and class III antiarrhythmic effects on the human monophasic action potential.[300] Sotalol slows sinus rate and may precipitate significant exaggeration of sinus node dysfunction in patients with sick sinus syndrome.

Ethmozin

Ethmozin is the first phenothiazine derivative with primarily cardiac antiarrhythmic properties. Its exact modes of action are not known, although voltage-clamp studies in frog atrial muscle suggest that at the very least, ethmozin depresses rapid inward current.[301] Ruffy and colleagues[302] perfused ethmozin directly into the sinus node artery of dogs and found no significant effect on heart rate.

Alinidine

Alinidine, a newly created compound chemically related to clonidine, specifically reduces sinus rate.[303] Miller and Vaughn-Williams[28] have proposed that this compound may represent a fifth class of antiarrhythmic drug. These investigators have published the results of microelectrode studies on isolated sinus node preparations that very strongly suggested that the mechanism by which alinidine decreased the slope of slow diastolic depolarization and increased action potential duration was by restricting inward current through anion-selective channels. Potential antiarrhythmic uses for this drug have not been explored. Because alinidine reduces heart rate without affecting blood pressure, myocardial contractility, or AV conduction, the drug may have important use as an antianginal agent.

Management of Patients with the Sick Sinus Syndrome

The indications for permanent pacing in patients with sick sinus syndrome must be clearly defined.[304-309] The benefits to be realistically expected from pacemaker insertion must be understood by the clinician so that sound judgment, based on well-controlled clinical trials, may prevail. Thus the natural history, complications, morbidity, and mortality of the sick sinus syndrome must be elucidated. Furthermore, electrophysiologic and clinical predictors of the potential for complications must be developed and refined to improve decisions concerning the timing of pacemaker insertion.

Not only is the sick sinus syndrome a heterogeneous entity in underlying pathophysiologic mechanism, but it also occurs in a heterogeneous population having associated cardiovascular diseases. Patients with sick sinus with ischemic heart disease, congestive heart failure, or primary cerebrovascular disease form a higher risk population for sudden death than patients without these associated risk factors.[309-312] Therefore, clinical data concerning the benefits of permanent pacing in terms of reduction in mortality and morbidity should be assessed independently in patients with and without other cardiovascular diseases. In addition, patients with the bradycardia-tachycardia syndrome present therapeutic challenges not encountered in patients with sinus bradycardia, sinus arrest, or sinoatrial block alone.

Provided that central nervous system symptoms have been shown to be unequivocally associated with episodes of sinus node dysfunction and failure of subsidiary pacemakers to escape, artificial pacing has been consistently successful in eliminating cerebral symptoms.[304,309-311] When an adequate cardiac output does not depend on atrial contribution, ventricular pacing has been as successful as atrial or AV sequential pacing in eliminating dizziness or syncope. With severe heart failure, subtle symptoms of fatigue and failing mental acuity may be as much a consequence of diminished stroke volume as an inappropriately slow heart rate. Only prepacing and postpacing hemodynamic studies at a variety of rates will support an assumption that a faster heart rate will increase cerebral perfusion by increasing cardiac output. In patients with myocardial dysfunction, cardiac performance must be assessed in the basal state as well as with atrial and ventricular pacing.

Improvement in symptoms of congestive heart failure, with and without the addition of digitalis, has been reported after pacemaker implantation in some patients with the sick sinus syndrome.[306,309] In an additional group of patients without overt congestive heart failure, patients were noted to achieve improved exercise tolerance following pacemaker insertion.[310]

Since the sick sinus syndrome is probably a diffuse disease of the AV conduction system, His bundle recordings should be performed if atrial pacing is being considered. Frequently, abnormalities of AV nodal and distal pathways of conduction coexist with sinus node dysfunction. If atrial contribution to diastolic ventricular filling is necessary for adequate ventricular performance, sequential AV pacing should be considered in these patients. Although technical problems and malfunctions appear to be more common with these pacemakers, the clinical situation may allow no alternative.

In general, pharmacologic approaches to the management of sinus bradycardia have been disappointing.[305,313-315] However, notable exceptions have been reported, with symptom-free states lasting for 5 years or longer. Atropinelike drugs and sublingual beta-adrenergic drugs have obvious disadvantages. These include short durations of action, intolerable side-effects, irregular and unreliable absorption, and the need for unfaltering patient compliance to a demanding dose schedule. Moreover, these drugs have been shown to worsen or precipitate atrial and ventricular tachyarrhythmias.

Bradyarrhythmias are less well tolerated by patients with significant cerebrovascular disease. In these patients, even short episodes of moderately slow heart rates can be catastrophic. Moreover, a stable sinus bradycardia may have variable central nervous system consequences depending on the relative distribution of blood flow during periods of stress or exercise; blood flow may be diverted to the periphery, "stealing" flow from the cerebral circulation in the absence of compensatory cardioacceleration. Thus, in patients with significant cerebral vascular disease, symptoms may occur even in the absence of gross changes in cardiac rhythm. In addition, cerebral atherosclerosis is a progressive disease, and some patients may have recurrences of central nervous system symptoms after a considerable period of being asymptomatic following artificial pacing. Failure of pacing to improve dizziness or syncopal episodes has been attributed to coexistent severe cerebral vascular disease in most series.[310]

The therapeutic approach to the patient with the bradycardia-tachycardia syndrome is complex and must be individualized. In the absence of central nervous system symptoms, the bradycardia may be observed very closely while antiarrhythmic agents alone are tried in progressive incremental doses. When the tachyarrhythmias are supraventricular, digitalis has been the mainstay of therapy. However, the effect of digitalis on sinus node function in these patients varies, and caution is warranted. Therapy is best started in the hospital while the patient is electrocardiographically monitored. Propranolol and verapamil, documented to be highly effective in supraventricular arrhythmias, probably carry a higher risk of suppressing sinus node function than do digitalis preparations, and the combination of the two drugs is contraindicated in patients with sinus node disease without permanent pacing.

Some investigators have suggested that artificial pacing may not only allow higher doses of antiarrhythmic drugs to be given but also that many patients may have better results with lower doses that failed to control the tachyarrhythmias before pacemaker application.[304,306-307] Certain electrophysiologic principles suggest that a beneficial synergism between atrial or coronary sinus pacing and antiarrhythmic drugs could exist; however, more extensive and well-controlled studies are necessary to prove this. The potential for distal conduction system problems occurring secondary to the use of antiarrhythmic agents alone might be anticipated from the results of His bundle recordings.[309,316-317]

Considerable controversy exists regarding the efficacy of pacing alone for controlling the occurrence of supraventricular tachyarrhythmias in patients with sick sinus syndrome. Rubinstein and others have been unable to limit the frequency of episodes or entirely suppress them without adding antiarrhythmic agents.[305,314,318] Others, however, have met with better success with atrial or coronary sinus pacing alone.[306,319] Some investigators have reported successful prophylaxis with ventricular pacing when retrograde AV conduction is present.[320] At the other extreme, refractoriness to antiarrhythmic agents has continued in a few patients despite permanent pacing.[312] The relative refractoriness to pharmacologic therapy of supraventricular tachyarrhythmias in the bradycardia-tachycardia syndrome compared to other settings has not been specifically investigated. A realistic approach to the control of supraventricular arrhythmias at the present time would be to (1) initiate drug therapy if central nervous system symptomatology permits, (2) proceed with atrial or coronary sinus pacing alone if drugs fail or precipitate symptomatic sinus node dysfunction, and (3) combine antiarrhythmic agents with pacing if pacing alone is ineffectual.

Despite a potential electrophysiologic predisposition for ventricular arrhythmias to occur in the presence of slow heart rates, arrhythmias in patients with the sick sinus syndrome are more often supraventricular.[321-323] When ventricular ectopy or malignant ventricular rhythms do occur, atrial or ventricular pacing may not invariably abolish them without the assistance of antiarrhythmic drugs. However, pacing may facilitate pharmacologic management by shortening the Purkinje fiber refractory period, increasing the threshold for ventricular fibrillation, and minimizing asynchronous recovery of excitability in the ventricles.[321-324]

Prognosis in Patients with the Sick Sinus Syndrome

From the standpoint of mortality and morbidity, the sick sinus syndrome is a discouraging disease entity to treat. The 5-year mortality in these patients is high and does not appear to be significantly influenced by artificial pacing. Skagen and co-workers[311] followed 50 patients with sinoatrial block treated with permanent pacing for 1 to 14 years. They reported survival after 1, 2, 5, and 8 years to be 94%, 85%, 64%, and 48%, respectively. These figures indicate an excess yearly mortality in the first 5 years of 4% to 5% compared with a control population of the same age and sex. Mortality was significantly influenced by the coexistence of cardiovascular and valvular heart disease (Fig. 6-25). Chokski and co-workers[310] reported 1- and 4-year survival rates in 52 permanently paced patients with sick sinus of 85% and 47%, respectively. Krishnaswami and co-workers[312] followed 17 patients with sinus bradycardia or sinus arrest in a pacemaker clinic for a mean duration of 19.4 months and reported a 30% mortality. In 16 patients with alternating bradycardia-tachycardia, these investigators reported a 36% mortality over 16.3 months, half the deaths being secondary to massive cerebral infarction. In a follow-up study of 90 patients for a mean of 23 months after pacemaker implantation, Hartel and Talvensaari[309] reported an annual mortality of 11%. As a group the patients who died did not differ significantly from the survivors with

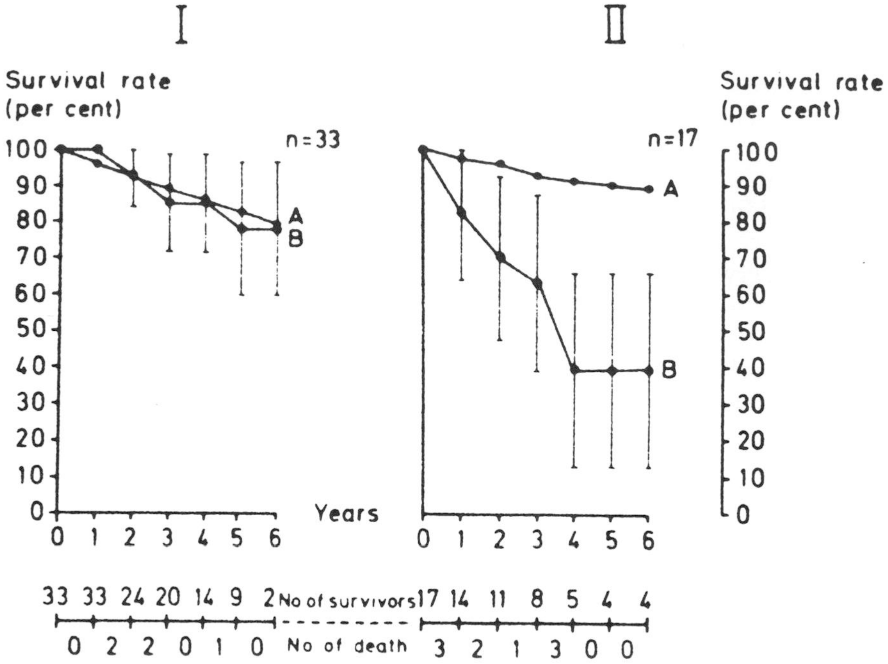

Figure 6-25. *These graphs illustrate survival curves in two groups, one without significant cardiac disease (I) and one with significant cardiac disease (II). All these patients had significant sinus node dysfunction and were treated with permanent cardiac pacing. In each graph, age-matched controls are illustrated by the line marked A, and the index patients are illustrated by the line marked B. Survival rates are shown for group I and group II patients. Note the significant deviation from the expected survival in group II patients without significant underlying disease. (Skagen, K., and Hansen, J. F.: The long-term prognosis for patients with sinoatrial block treated with permanent pacemaker. Acta Med. Scand., 199:13, 1975)*

regard to type of sinus dysfunction, occurrence of tachyarrhythmias, or distal conduction abnormalities.

In all series, death in patients with this syndrome with permanent pacing most frequently results from complications of associated cardiovascular or cerebrovascular disease and not from complications of sinus node and subsidiary pacemaker dysfunction. However, a discouraging fact is that the incidence of embolic events involving the lungs, brain, and peripheral arterial tree remains distressingly high in patients with permanent pacing and the sick sinus syndrome. The frequency of embolic events suggests that the instances of alternating bradyarrhythmias and tachyarrhythmias are more common than appreciated from random electrophysiologic evaluation. Although more extensive use of Holter monitoring to detect cases of inadequate pharmacologic prophylaxis of tachyarrhythmias may reduce the incidence of embolization somewhat, the paroxysmal nature of these arrhythmias would allow many episodes to escape detection. Thus, it has been proposed that all patients exhibiting the bradycardia-tachycardia syndrome be fully anti-coagulated. The benefit-risk argument of chronic anticoagulation has not been resolved, and the issue of anticoagulation in these patients is still controversial. Nevertheless, prevention of life-threatening embolization appears to be the only area in which the physician can potentially favorably influence the high rate of mortality and morbidity in the permanently paced patient with sick sinus syndrome. Thus, a strong case for chronic anticoagulation can be made. However, not all cerebral vascular accidents in these patients are secondary to embolic events. Elderly patients with atherosclerotic cerebral vascular disease may have transient ischemic attacks or frank cerebral infarction if a tachyarrhythmia is associated with a fall in cardiac output. This group of patients will not benefit from anticoagulant therapy and must be distinguished from patients with cerebral embolization.

Finally, the issue of prophylactic permanent pacing in the asymptomatic patient with sick sinus syndrome must be addressed. At present, the natural history of the disease is unknown; furthermore, clinical risk factors for the development of symptoms have not been defined, and no electrophysiologic measure of sinus node function has been demonstrated to have reliable predictive value. Therefore, common practice has been to withhold pacemaker therapy in the asymptomatic patient.

References

1. James, T. N.: Anatomy of the human sinus node. Anat. Rec., 141:109, 1961.
2. Truex, R. C., Smythe, M. Q., and Taylor, M. J.: Reconstruction of the human sinoatrial node. Anat. Rec., 159:371, 1967.
3. James T. N., Scherf, L., and Fine, G.: Comparative ultrastructure of the sinus node in man and dog. Circulation, 34:139, 1966.
4. Howse, N. D., Ferrnas, V. J., and Hibbs, R. G.: A comparative histochemical and electron microscopic study of the surface coatings of cardiac muscle cells. J. Mol. Cell. Cardiol., 1:57, 1970.
5. Kawamura, K., and James, T. N.: Comparative ultrastructure of cellular junctions in working myocardium and the conduction system under normal and pathologic conditions. J. Mol. Cell. Cardiol., 3:31, 1971.
6. DeMello, W. C.: Membrane lipids and cardiac electrogenesis. In DeMello, W. C. (ed.): Electrical Phenomena in the Heart, p. 89. New York, Academic Press, 1972.

7. Langer, G. A., and Frank, J. S.: Lanthanum in heart cell cultures. Effect on localization. J. Cell. Biol., 54:441, 1972.
8. Tranum-Jensen, J.: The fine structure of the atrial and atrioventricular (AV) junctional specialized tissue of the rabbit heart. In Wellen, H. J. J., Lie, K. I., and Janse, M. J. (eds.): The Conduction System of the Heart. Structure, Function and Clinical Implications, p. 55. Leiden, Stenfert Kraese B. V., 1976.
9. Noma, A., and Irisawa, H.: Membrane currents in the rabbit sinoatrial node cell as studied by the double microelectrode method. Pfuegers Arch., 364:45, 1976.
10. Noble, D.: The Initiation of the Heartbeat. Oxford, Clarendon, 1975.
11. Brown, H. F., Clark, A., and Noble, S. J.: Identification of the pacemaker current in frog atrium. J. Physiol., 258:52, 1976.
12. Brown, H. F., Clark, A., and Noble, S. J.: Analysis of pacemaker repolarization currents in frog atrial muscle. J. Physiol., 258:547, 1976.
13. Brooks, C. McC., and Lu, H-H.: The sinoatrial pacemaker of the heart, pp. 109–110. Springfield, Ill., Charles C Thomas, 1972.
14. Hoffman, B. F., and Cranefield, P.: Electrophysiology of the Heart. New York, McGraw-Hill, 1960.
15. West, T. C. L.: Effects of chronotropic influences on subthreshold oscillations in the sinoatrial node. In Pae de Carvalho, A., DeMello, W. C., and Hoffman, B. F. (eds.): Specialized Tissues of the Heart. New York, Elsevier, 1961.
16. Yamagishi, S., and Sano, T.: Effect of tetrodotoxin on the pacemaker action potential of the sinus node. Prac. Jpn. Acad., 42:1194, 1966.
17. Toda, N., and West, T. C.: Interaction of K, Na, and vagal stimulation in the SA node of the rabbit. Am. J. Physiol., 212:426, 1967.
18. Rougier, O., et al.: Existence and role of slow inward current during the frog atrial action potential. Pfluegers Arch., 308:91, 1969.
19. Reuter, H.: Divalent cations as charge carriers in excitable membranes. Prog. Biophys., 26:1, 1973.
20. Kohlhardt, M., Bauer, B., and Krause, H.: Differentiation of the transmembrane Na and Ca channels in mammalian cardiac fibers by the use of specific inhibitors. Pfluegers Arch., 335:309–322, 1972.
21. Wit, A. L., and Cranefield, P.: Effect of verapamil on the sinoatrial and atrioventricular nodes of the rabbit and the mechanism by which it arrests reentrant atrioventricular nodal tachycardia. Circ. Res., 35:413–425, 1974.
22. Zipes, D. P., and Fischer, J. C.: Effects of agents which inhibit the slow channel on sinus node automaticity and atrioventricular conduction in the dog. Circ. Res., 34:184, 1974.
23. Haastert, H. P., and Fleckenstein, A.: Ca-dependence of supraventricular pacemaker activity and its responsiveness to Ca-antagonistic compounds (verapamil, D-600, nifedipine). Arch. Pharmacol., 287 (Suppl. i):R39, 1975.
24. Kolhardt, M., Figulla, H-R, and Tripathi, O.: The slow membrane channel as the predominant mediator of the excitation process of the sinoatrial pacemaker cell. Basic Res. Cardiol., 71:17–26, 1976.
25. Strauss, H. C., Prystowsky, E. N., and Scheinman, M. M.: Sinoatrial and atrial electrogenesis. Prog. Cardiovasc. Dis., 19:385, 1977.
26. DeMello, W. C.: Role of chloride ions in cardiac and pacemaker potentials. Am. J. Physiol. 295:567, 1963.
27. Seyama, I.: Characteristics of the anion channel in the sinoatrial node cell of the rabbit. J. Physiol., 294:447, 1979.
28. Miller, J. S., and Vaughn Williams, E. M.: Pacemaker selectivity: Influence on rabbit atria of ionic environment and of alinidine, a possible anion antagonist. Cardiovasc. Res., 15:335, 1981.
29. Lu, H-H.: The effect of manganese on sinoatrial node pacemaker cells. In Kao, F. F., Koizumi, K., and Vassalle, M. (eds.): Research in Physiology, A Liber Memorials in Honor of C. McC. Brooks, p. 141. Bologna, Gaggi, 1971.
30. Noma, A., and Irisawa, H.: The effect of sodium ion on the initial phase of the sinoatrial action potential in rabbits. Jpn. J. Physiol., 24:617, 1974.
31. Kreiter, D.: Evidence for the existence of a rapid sodium channel in the membrane of rabbit sinoatrial cells. J. Mol. Cell. Cardiol., 7:655, 1975.
32. Noma, A., and Irisawa, H.: Effects of calcium ion on the resting phase of the action potential in rabbit sinoatrial node cells. Jpn. J. Physiol., 25:93, 1976.
33. DeMello, W. C., and Hoffman, B. F.: Potassium ions and electrical activity of specialized cardiac fibers. Am. J. Physiol., 199:1125, 1960.
34. DeMello, W. C.: Some aspects of the interrelationship between ions and electrical activity in specialized tissue of the heart. In Paes de Carvalho, A., DeMello, W. C., and Hoffman, B. F. (eds.): The Specialized Tissue of the Heart, p. 95. New York, Elsevier, 1961.
35. Noma, A., and Irisawa, H.: Effects of Na^+ and K^+ on the resting membrane potential of the rabbit sinoatrial node cell. Jpn. J. Physiol., 25:287, 1975.
36. Jordan, J. L., Yamaguchi, I., and Mandel, W. J.: The effects of verapamil on sinoatrial conduction in isolated tissue. Clin. Res., 26:241, 1977.
37. Hutter, O. F., and Trautwein, W.: Vagal and sympathetic effects on the pacemaker fibers in the sinus venosus of the heart. J. Gen. Physiol., 39:715, 1956.
38. Gaskell, W. H.: The electrical changes in the quiescent cardiac muscle which accompany stimulation of the vagus nerve. J. Physiol., 7:451, 1886.
39. Lu, H-H., Lange, G., and Brooks, C. McC.: Factors controlling pacemaker action in cells of the sinoatrial node. Circ. Res., 42:460, 1965.
40. West, T. C.: Ultramicroelectrode recording from the cardiac pacemaker. J. Pharmacol. Exp. Ther., 115:283, 1955.
41. Harris, E. J., and Hutter, O. F.: The action of acetylcholine on the movements of potassium ions in the sinus venosus of the heart. J. Physiol, 133:58, 1956.
42. Trautwein, W., Kuffler, S. W. L., and Edward, C.: Changes in membrane characteristics of heart muscle during inhibition. J. Gen. Physiol., 40:135, 1956.
43. Trautwein, W., and Dudel, J.: Zum Mechanisms der Membranwirkung des Acetylcholine an der Jerzmuskelfaser. Pfluegers Arch., 266:324, 1958.
44. Vassalle, M.: Electrogenic suppression of automaticity in sheep and dog Purkinje fibers. Circ. Res., 27:361, 1970.
45. Musso, E., and Vassalle, M.: Inhibitory action of acetylcholine on potassium uptake of the sinus node. Cardiovasc. Res., 9:490, 1975.
46. Giles, W., and Tsein, R. W.: Effects of acetylcholine on membrane currents in frog atrial muscle. J. Physiol., 246:64, 1975.
47. Ten Eick, R., Nawrath, H., and McDonald, T. F.: On the mechanism of the negative inotropic effect of acetylcholine. Pfluegers Arch., 361:207, 1976.
48. Brasil, A.: Autonomic sinoatrial block: a new disturbance of the heart mechanism. Arg. Bras. Cardiol., 8:159, 1955.
49. Kassebaum, D. G.: Membrane effects of epinephrine in the heart. In Krays, O., and Kovarikova, A. (eds.): Second International Pharmacologic meeting, vol. 5, Pharmacology of Cardiac Function, pp. 95–100. Oxford, Pergamon Press, 1964.
50. Tsien, R. W. L.: Effects of epinephrine on the pacemaker potassium current of cardiac Purkinje fibers. J. Gen. Physiol., 64:293, 1974.
51. Vassort, G., Rougier, O., and Garmer, D.: Effects of adrenalin on

membrane inward currents during the cardiac action potential. Pfluegers Arch., 309:70, 1969.
52. Watanabe, A. M., and Besch, H. R.: Cyclicadenosine monophosphate modulation of slow calcium influx channels in guinea pig hearts. Circ. Res., 35:316, 1974.
53. Mackary, A. J. C., Hof, T. O., Bkekerwk, et al.: Interaction of adrenaline and acetylcholine on cardiac pacemaker function. Functional inhomogeneity of the rabbit sinus node. J. Pharm. Exp. Therap., 214:417, 1980.
54. Johnson, P. N., Freeberg, A. S., and Marshall, J. M.: Action of thyroid hormone on the transmembrane potentials from sinoatrial node cells and atrial muscle in isolated atria of rabbits. Cardiology, 58:273, 1973.
55. James, T. N., and Nadeau, R. A.: Sinus bradycardia during injections directly into the sinus node artery. Am. J. Physiol., 204:9, 1963.
56. James, T. N.: Pulse and impulse formation in the sinus node. Henry Ford Hosp. Med. J., 15:275, 1967.
57. Brooks, C. McC., et al.: Effects of localized stretch of the sinoatrial node region of the dog heart. Am. J. Physiol., 211:1197, 1966.
58. Lange, G., et al.: Effect of stretch of the isolated cat sinoatrial node. Am. J. Physiol., 211:1192, 1966.
59. Bouman, L. N., and Van der Westen, H. M.: Pacemaker shift in the sinoatrial node induced by a change of temperature. Pfluegers Arch., 318:262, 1970.
60. Bouman, L. N., et al.: Pacemaker shifts in the sinus node: effects of vagal stimulation, temperature and reduction of extra-cellular calcium. In Bonke, F. I. M. (ed.): The Sinus Node: Structure, Function and Clinical Relevance, p. 245. The Hague, Martinus Nijhoff, 1978.
61. Lown, B.: In Dreifus, L., Likoff, W., and Moyer, J. (eds.): Fourteenth Hahnemann Symposium on Mechanisms and Therapy of Cardiac Arrhythmias, p. 185. New York, Grune & Stratton, 1966.
62. Ferrer, M. I.: Sick sinus syndrome in atrial disease. J.A.M.A., 206:645, 1968.
63. Kulbertus, H. E., De Leval-Turren, F., and Demoulin, J. C.: Sinoatrial disease: A report on 13 cases. J. Electrocardiol., 6:303, 1973.
64. Rasmussen, K.: Chronic sinoatrial heart block. Am. Heart J., 81:38, 1971.
65. Conde, C., et al.: Effectiveness of pacemaker treatment in the bradycardia-tachycardia syndrome. Am. J. Cardiol., 32:209, 1973.
66. Sigurd, B., et al.: Adams-Stokes syndrome caused by sinoatrial block. Br. Heart J., 35:1002, 1973.
67. Rokseth, R., and Hatle, L.: Prospective study on the occurrence and management of chronic sinoatrial disease with follow-up. Br. Heart J., 36:582, 1974.
68. Radford, D. J., and Julian, D. G.: Sick sinus syndrome: Expericncc of a cardiac pacemaker clinic. Br. Med. J., 3:155, 1974.
69. Sowton, E., Hendrix, G., and Roy, P.: Ten-year survey of treatment with implanted cardiac pacemaker. Br. Med. J., 3:155, 1974.
70. Hartel, G., and Talvensaari, T.: Treatment of sinoatrial syndrome with permanent cardiac pacing in 90 patients. Acta Med. Scand., 198:341, 1975.
71. Rubenstein, J. J., et al.: Clinical spectrum of the sick sinus syndrome. Circulation, 46:5, 1972.
72. Wan, S. H., Lee, G. S., and Ton, C. S.: The sick sinus syndrome. A study of 15 cases. Br. Heart J., 34:942, 1972.
73. Moss, A. J., and Davis, R. J.: Brady-tachy syndrome Prog. Cardiovasc. Dis., 16:439, 1974.
74. Fraser, G. R., Froggatt, P., and James, T. N.: Congenital deafness associated with electrocardiographic abnormalities, fainting attacks and sudden death: A recessive syndrome. Q. J. Med., 33:361, 1964.
75. Barks, J. B., Bosman, C. K., and Cochrane, J. W. C.: Congenital cardiac arrhythmias. Lancet, 2:531, 1964.
76. Metzger, A. L., Goldberg, A. N., and Hunter, R. L.: Sick sinus node syndrome as the presenting manifestation of reticulum cell sarcoma. Chest, 60:602, 1971.
77. Kaplin, B. M., et al.: Tachycardia-bradycardia syndrome (so-called "sick sinus syndrome"). Pathology, mechanisms and treatment. Am. J. Cardiol., 31:497, 1973.
78. Jordan, J. L., Yamaguchi, I., and Mandel, W. J.: Characteristics of sinoatrial conduction in patients with coronary artery disease. Circulation, 55:569, 1977.
79. Haden, R. F., et al.: The significance of sinus bradycardia in acute myocardial infarction. Dis. Chest, 44:168, 1963.
80. Adgey, A. J. J., et al.: Incidence, significance and management of early bradyarrhythmia complicating acute myocardial infarction. Lancet, 2:1097, 1968.
81. Rokseth, R., and Hattle, L.: Sinus arrest in acute myocardial infarction. Br. Heart. J., 33:639, 1971.
82. Thomas, M., and Goodgate, D.: Effect of atropine on bradycardia and hypotension in acute myocardial infarction. Br. Heart J., 28:409, 1966.
83. Brown, A. M.: Excitation of afferent cardiac sympathetic nerve fibers during myocardial ischemia. J. Physiol., 190:35, 1967.
84. Botti, C., et al.: Effectti imediati della legatura della "arteria del noda del seno" su la funzione ritmica sinusale ne cane. Rass. Fisiof. Cl. Ten., 29:149, 1957.
85. James, T. N., and Reemtsma, K.: The response of sinus node function to ligation of the sinus node artery. Henry Ford Hosp. Med. Bull., 8:129, 1960.
86. Billette, J., et al.: Sinus slowing produced by experimental ischemia of the sinus node in dogs. Am. J. Cardiol., 31:331, 1973.
87. Meck, W. J., Keenan, M., and Theisen, H. J.: Auricular blood supply in the dog. I. General auricular supply with special reference to sino-auricular node. Am. Heart J., 4:591, 1929.
88. Halpern, M. H.: Arterial supply to the nodal tissue in the dog heart. Circulation, 9:547, 1954.
89. Marriott, H. J. L.: Practical Electrocardiography, 5th ed., p. 128. Baltimore, Williams & Wilkins, 1972.
90. Friedman, H. H.: Diagnostic Electrocardiography and Vectorcardiography, p. 432. New York, McGraw-Hill, 1977.
91. Chung, E. K.: Electrocardiography: Practical Applications with Vectorial Principles, p. 167. Hagerstown, Md., Harper & Row, 1974.
92. Han, J., et al.: Incidence of ectopic beats as a function of basic rate in the ventricle. Am. Heart J., 72:632, 1966.
93. Han, J., et al.: Temporal dispersion of recovery of excitability in atrium and ventricle as a function of heart rate. Am. Heart J., 71:481, 1966.
94. Han, J., Malozzi, A. M., and Moe, G. K.: Sinoatrial reciprocation in the isolated rabbit heart. Circ. Res., 22:355, 1968.
95. Paulay, K. L., Varghese, J. P., and Damato, A. N.: Sinus node reentry. An in vivo demonstration in the dog. Circ. Res., 32:455, 1973b.
96. Narula, O. S.: Sinus node reentry. A mechanism for supraventricular tachycardia. Circulation, 50:1114, 1974.
97. Weisfogel, G. M., et al.: Sinus node reentrant tachycardia in man. Am. Heart J., 90:295, 1975.
98. Breithardt, G., and Seipel, L.: Sequence of atrial activation in patients with atrial echo beats. In Bonke, F. I. M. (ed.): The Sinus Node: Structure, Function and Clinical Relevance, pp. 389–408. The Hague, Martinus Nijhoff, 1978.
99. Allessie, M. A., and Bonke, F. I. M.: Re-entry within the sinoatrial node as demonstrated by multiple microelectrode recordings in the isolated rabbit heart. In Bonke, F. I. M. (ed.): The

Sinus Node: Structure, Function and Clinical Relevance, pp. 409–421. The Hague, Martinus Nijhoff, 1978.
100. Damato, A. N.: Clinical evidence for sinus node reentry. In Bonke, F. I. M. (ed.): The Sinus Node: Structure, Function and Clinical Relevance, pp. 379–388. The Hague, Martinus Nijhoff, 1978.
101. Curry, P. V. L., Callowhill, E., and Krikler, D. M.: Paroxysmal re-entry sinus tachycardia. Br. Heart J., 38:311, 1976.
102. Curry, P. V. L., and Krikler, D. M.: Paroxysmal reciprocating sinus tachycardia. In Kulbertus, H. (ed.): Re-entrant Arrhythmias. Mechanisms and Treatment, p. 39. Baltimore, University Park Press, 1977.
103. Balke, B., and Ware, R. W.: An experimental study of physical fitness of Air Force personnel. U.S. Armed Forces Med. J., 10:675, 1959.
104. Goldberg, A. N., Moran, J. F., and Resnekov, L.: Multistage electrocardiographic tests. Am. J. Cardiol., 26:84, 1970.
105. Scheinman, M. M., et al.: The sick sinus and ailing atrium. West. J. Med., 121:473, 1974.
106. Holden, W., McAnulty, J. W., and Rahimotoola, S. N.: Characterization of heart rate response to exercise in the sick sinus syndrome. Br. Heart J., 40:923, 1978.
107. Ellestad, M. H.: Stress Testing: Principles and Practice, p. 38. Philadelphia, F. A. Davis, 1975.
108. Arguss, N. S., et al.: Significance of chronic sinus bradycardia in elderly people. Circulation, 46:924, 1972.
109. Crook, B. R. M., et al.: Tape monitoring of the electrocardiogram in ambulant patients with sinoatrial disease. Br. Heart J., 35:1009, 1973.
110. Brasil, A.: Autonomic sinoatrial block. A new disturbance of the heart mechanism. Arg. Bras. Cardiol., 8:159, 1955.
111. Dighton, D. H.: Sinoatrial block: Autonomic influences and clinical assessment. Br. Heart J., 37:321, 1975.
112. Hamlin, R. L., Smith, C. R., and Smeler, D. L.: Sinus arrhythmia in the dog. Am. J. Physiol., 210:321, 1966.
113. Covell, J. W., Chidsey, C. P., and Braunwald, E.: Reduction of the cardiac responses to postganglionic sympathetic nerve stimulation in patients with cardiac decompensation. Circ. Res., 19:51, 1966.
114. Beiser, G. D., et al.: Impaired heart rate response to sympathetic nerve stimulation in patients with cardiac decompensation. Circulation, 38:VI–40, 1968.
115. Eekberg, D. L., Drabinsky, M., and Braunwald, E.: Defective cardiac parasympathetic control in patients with heart disease. N. Engl. J. Med., 285:877, 1971.
116. Goldstein, R. E., et al.: Impairment of autonomically mediated heart rate control in patients with cardiac dysfunction. Circ. Res., 36:571, 1975.
117. Mandel, W. J., Laks, M. M., and Obayashi, K.: Sinus node function: Evaluation in patients with and without sinus node disease. Arch. Intern. Med., 135:388, 1975.
118. Wang, S. C., and Borison, H. L.: An analysis of the carotid sinus cardiovascular reflex mechanism. Am. J. Physiol., 150:712, 1947.
119. Glick, G., and Braunwald, E.: Relative roles of sympathetic and parasympathetic nervous systems in the reflex control of heart rate. Circ. Res., 16:363, 1965.
120. Robinson, B. F., et al.: Control of heart rate by the autonomic nervous system. Circ. Res., 19:400, 1966.
121. Deuleeschhouwer, G. C., and Heymen, E.: In Kezdi, P. (ed.): Baroreceptors and Hypertension, pp. 187–190. New York, Pergamon Press, 1967.
122. Thomas, M. D., and Kontos, H. A.: Mechanisms of baroreceptor-induced changes in heart rate. Am. J. Physiol., 218:251, 1970.
123. Dighton, D. H.: Sinus bradycardia autonomic influences and clinical assessment. Br. Heart J., 36:791, 1974.
124. Jose, A. D., and Collison, D.: The normal range and determinants of the intrinsic heart rate in man. Cardiovasc. Res., 4:160, 1970.
125. Jordan, J. L., Yamaguchi, I., and Mandel, W. J.: Studies on the mechanism of sinus node dysfunction in the sick sinus syndrome. Circulation, 57:217, 1978.
126. Gaskell, W. H.: On the innervation of the heart with especial reference to the heart of the tortoise. J. Physiol., 4:43, 1884.
127. Cohn, A. E., and Lewis, T.: Auricular fibrillation and complete heart block: a description of a case of Adams-Stokes syndrome including the post-mortem examination. Heart, 4:15, 1912.
128. Parkinson, J., Papp, C., and Evans, W.: The electrocardiogram of the Stokes-Adams attack. Br. Heart J., 3:171, 1941.
129. Pick, A., Langendorf, R., and Katz, L. N.: Depression of cardiac pacemakers by premature impulses. Am. Heart J., 41:49, 1951.
130. Lange, G.: Action of driving stimuli from intrinsic and extrinsic sources on in situ cardiac pacemaker tissues. Circ. Res., 17:449, 1965.
131. Mandel, W. J., et al.: Evaluation of sino-atrial node function in man by overdrive suppression. Circulation, 44:59, 1971.
132. Mandel, W. J., et al.: Assessment of sinus node function in patients with sick sinus syndrome. Circulation, 43:761, 1972.
133. Narula, O. S., Samet, P., and Javier, R. P.: Significance of the sinus node recovery time. Circulation, 45:140, 1972.
134. Strauss, H. C., et.al.: Electrophysiologic evaluation of sinus node function in patients with sinus node dysfunction. Circulation, 53:763, 1976.
135. Vincenzi, F. F., and West, T. C.: Release of autonomic mediators in cardiac tissue by direct subthreshold electrical stimulation. J. Pharmacol. Exp. Ther., 141:185, 1963.
136. Lu, H.-H., Lange, G., and Brooks, C. McC.: Factors controlling pacemaker action in cells of the sinoatrial node. Circ. Res., 17:461, 1965.
137. Furchgott, R. F., DeGubareff, T., and Grossman, A.: Release of autonomic mediators in cardiac tissue by subthreshold stimulation. Science, 129:328, 1959.
138. Kodama, I., Goto, J., Anso, S., et al.: Effects of rapid stimulation on the transmembrane action potentials of rabbit sinus node pacemaker cells. Circ. Res., 46:90, 1980.
139. Steinbeck, G., Haberl, R., and Luderitz, B.: Effects of atrial pacing on atrio-sinus conduction and overdrive suppression in the isolated rabbit sinus node. Circ. Res. 46:859, 1981.
140. Konsai, T.: Electrophysiologic consideration of sick sinus syndrome. Jpn. Circ. J., 40:194, 1976.
141. Jordan, J. L., et al.: Studies on the mechanism of suppression of sinus node pacemaker automaticity by atrial overdrive pacing. Clin. Res., 26:241A, 1978.
142. Engel, T. R., et al.: Appraisal of sinus node artery disease. Circulation, 52:286, 1975.
143. Singer, D., Parameswaran, R., and Goldberg, H.: Sinus and AV nodal dysfunction following myocardial infarction. J. Electrocardiol., 8:281, 1975.
144. Mandel, W. J., and Yamaguchi, I.: The effects of changes in extracellular pH on sinoatrial conduction. Am. J. Cardiol., 39:265, 1977.
145. Benditt, D. C., Strauss, H. C., Scheinman, M. M. et al.: Analysis of secondary pauses following termination of rapid atrial pacing in man. Circulation, 54:436, 1976.
146. Rosen, R. M., et al.: Cardiac conduction in patients with symptomatic sinus node disease. Circulation, 43:836, 1971.
147. Engel, T. R., and Schaal, S. F.: Digitalis in the sick sinus syndrome: the effects of digitalis on sinoatrial automaticity and atrioventricular conduction. Circulation, 48:1201, 1973.
148. Jordan, J. L., Yamaguchi, I., and Mandel, W. J.: The sick sinus syndrome: pathophysiology, significance and treatment. Cardiol. Dig., 12:11, 1977.

149. Kulbertos, H. E., deLeval-Rutten, F., Casters, L.: Sinus node recovery time in elderly. Br. Heart J., 37:420, 1975.
150. Strauss, H. C., Bigger, J. T., Jr., Saroff, A. L., and Giardine, E. G. U.: Electrophysiologic evaluation of sinus node function in patient with sinus node dysfunction. Circulation, 53:763, 1976.
151. Scheinman, M. M., Strauss, H. C., and Abbott, J. A.: Electrophysiologic testing for patients with sinus node dysfunction. J. Electrocardiol., 12:211, 1979.
152. Reiffel, J. A., Gang, E., Bigger, J. T., Jr., et al.: Sinus node recovery time related to paced cycle length in normals and patients with sinoatrial dysfunction. Am. Heart J., 104:746, 1982.
153. Goldreyer, B. N., and Damato, A. N.: Sinoatrial node entrance block. Circulation, 44:789, 1971.
154. Kerr, C. R., Prystowsky, E. N., Browning, D. J., and Strauss, H. C.: Characterization of refractoriness in the sinus node of the rabbit. Circ. Res., 47:742, 1981.
155. Jordan, J., et al.: Comparative effects of overdrive on sinus and subsidiary pacemaker function. Am. Heart J., 93:367, 1977.
156. Yamaguchi, I., and Mandel, W. J.: Alterations in measured and estimated sinus node conduction times: Effects of site stimulation and drug infusion. Arch. Ven. Cardiol., 3:78, 1976.
157. Okimoto, T., et al.: Sinus node recovery time and abnormal post-pacing phase in the aged patients with sick sinus syndrome. Jpn. Heart J., 17:290, 1976.
158. Yabek, S. M., Jarmakani, J. M., and Roberts, N. K.: Sinus node function in children. Factors influencing its evaluation. Circulation, 53:28, 1976.
159. Jose, A. D., and Taylor, R. R.: Autonomic blockade by propranolol and atropine to study myocardial function in man. J. Clin. Invest., 48:2019, 1969.
160. Jordan, J. L., Yamaguchi, E., and Mandel, W. J.: Characteristics of sinoatrial conduction in patients with coronary artery disease. Circulation, 55:569, 1977.
161. Massini, G., Dianda, R., and Grazina, A.: Analysis of sino-atrial conduction in man using premature atrial stimulation. Cardiovasc. Res., 9:498, 1975.
162. Steinbeck, G., and Luderitz, G.: Comparative study of sino-atrial conduction time and sinus node recovery time. Br. Heart J., 37:956, 1975.
163. Bashour, T., et al.: An unusual effect of atropine on overdrive suppression. Circulation, 48:911, 1973.
164. Reiffel, J. P., Bigger, J. T., Jr., and Giardina, E. G. V.: "Paradoxical" prolongation of sinus nodal recovery time after atropine in the sick sinus syndrome. Am. J. Cardiol., 36:98, 1975.
165. Jordan, J. L., et al.: The effects of verapamil on sinoatrial conduction in isolated tissue. Clin. Res., 26:279A, 1978.
166. Gupta, P. K., et al.: Appraisal of sinus nodal recovery time in patients with sick sinus syndrome. Am. J. Cardiol., 34:265, 1974.
167. Chadda, K. D., et al.: Corrected sinus node recovery: Experimental, physiological and pathologic determinants. Circulation, 51:797, 1975.
168. Mason, J. W.: Overdrive suppression in the transplanted heart: Effect of the autonomic nervous system on human sinus node recovery. Circulation, 62:688, 1980.
169. Jordan, J. L., and Mandel, W. J.: Comparative effects of duration of atrial overdrive pacing in patients with and without intrinsic sinus node dysfunction. In preparation.
170. Desai, J. M., Scheinman, M. M., Strauss, H. C., et al.: Electrophysiologic effects of combined autonomic blockade in patients with sinus node disease. Circulation, 63:953, 1981.
171. Delius, W., and Wirtzfeld, A.: Significance of sinus node recovery time in sick sinus syndrome. In Lueritz B. (ed.): Cardiac Pacing, pp. 25–32. Berlin, Springer-Verlag, 1976.
172. Bonke, F. I. M., Bouman, L. N., and VanRisn, H. E.: Change of cardiac rhythm in the rabbit after an atrial premature beat. Circ. Res., 24:533, 1969.
173. Bonke, F. I. M., Bouman, L. N., and Schopman, F. J. G.: Effect of an early atrial premature beat on activity of the sinoatrial rhythm in the rabbit. Circ. Res., 24:704, 1971.
174. Klein, H. O., Singer, D. H., and Hoffman, B. F.: Effects of atrial premature systoles on sinus rhythm in the rabbit. Circ. Res., 32:480, 1973.
175. Strauss, N. C., et al.: Premature atrial stimulation as a key to the understanding of sinoatrial conduction in man. Presentation of data and critical review of the literature. Circulation, 47:86, 1973.
176. Strauss, N. C., and Bigger, J. T., Jr.: Electrophysiological properties of rabbit sinoatrial perinodal fibers. Circ. Res., 31:490, 1972.
177. Pasmooij, J. H., and Bonke, F. I. M.: Influence of stimulus frequency on the depolarization of the action: comparison between atrium and SA node (abstr.). Pfluegers Arch., 318:263, 1970.
178. Rasmussen, K.: Chronic sinoatrial heart block. Am. Heart J., 81:38, 1971.
179. Scherf, D.: The mechanisms of sinoatrial block. Am. J. Cardiol. 23:769, 1969.
180. Engel, T. R., Bond, R. C., and Schaal, S. F.: First degree sinoatrial heart block: Sinoatrial block in the sick sinus syndrome. Am. Heart J., 91:303, 1976.
181. Kerr, C. R., Prytowsky, E. R., Browning, D. J., and Strauss, H. C.: Characterization or refractoriness in the sinus node of the rabbit. Circulation, 47:742, 1980.
182. Childers, R. W., et al.: Sinus node echoes. Am. J. Cardiol., 31:220, 1973.
183. Paritsky, Z., Obayashi, K., and Mandel, W. J.: Atrial tachycardia secondary to sinoatrial node reentry. Chest, 66:526, 1974.
184. Tzivoni, D., Jordan, J. L., Barrett, P., et al.: Two zones of full compensation: An unexpected finding related to alterations in conduction at the sinoatrial junction. Clin. Res., 26:241, 1978.
185. Langendorf, R., et al.: Atrial parasystole with interpolation: Observations on prolonged sinoatrial conduction. Am. Heart J., 63:649, 1962.
186. Scheinman, M. M., et al.: Sinoatrial function and atrial refractoriness in patients with sick sinus syndrome. Circulation, 48:IV-215, 1973.
187. Bigger, J. T.: A simple, rapid method for the diagnosis of first-degree sinoatrial block in man. Am. Heart J., 87:731, 1974.
188. Dhingra, R. C., et al.: Clinical significance of prolonged sinoatrial conduction time. Circulation, 55:8, 1977.
189. Breithardt, G., Seipel, L., and Loogen, F.: Sinus node recovery time and calculated sinoatrial conduction time in normal subjects and patients with sinus node dysfunction. Circulation, 56:43, 1977.
190. Miller, H. C., and Strauss, H. C.: Measurement of sinoatrial conduction time by premature atrial stimulation in the rabbit. Circ. Res., 35:935, 1974.
191. Breithardt, G., and Seipel, L.: The effect of premature atrial depolarization on sinus node automaticity in man. Circulation, 53:920, 1976.
192. Denes, P., Wu, D., and Dhingra, R.: The effects of cycle length on cardiac refractory periods in man. Circulation, 49:32, 1974.
193. Reiffel, J. A., Bigger, J. T., Jr., and Konstam, M. A.: The relationship between sinoatrial conduction time and sinus cycle length during spontaneous sinus arrhythmia in adults. Circulation, 50:924, 1974.
194. Sanot, T., and Yamagishi, S.: Spread of excitation from the sinus node. Circ. Res., 16:423, 1965.
195. Dhingra, R. C., et al.: Sinus nodal responses to atrial extrastimuli in patients without apparent sinus node disease. Am. J. Cardiol., 36:445, 1975.
196. Dhingra, R. C., et al.: Electrophysiologic effects of atropine on human sinus node and atrium. Am. J. Cardiol., 38:429, 1976.
197. Breithardt, G., et al.: The effect of atropine on calculated sino-atrial conduction time in man. Eur. J. Cardiol., 4:49, 1976.

198. Dhingra, R. C., et al.: Electrophysiologic effects of atropine on sinus node and atrium in patients with sinus node dysfunction. Am. J. Cardiol., 38:848, 1976.
199. Strauss, H. C., et al.: Electrophysiologic effects of propranolol on sinus node function in patients with sinus node dysfunction. Circulation, 54:452, 1976.
200. Narula, O. S., Narashimhan, S., Vasquez, M., et al.: A new method for measurement of sinoatrial conduction time. Circulation, 58:706, 1978.
201. Grant, A. O., Kirkorian, G., Benditt, D. G., and Strauss, H. C.: The estimation of sinoatrial conduction time in rabbit heart by the constant atrial pacing technique. Circulation, 60:597, 1979.
202. Kang, P. S., Gomes, J. A. C., Keler, G., and El-Sherif, N.: Role of autonomic regulatory mechanisms in sinoatrial conduction and sinus node automaticity in sick sinus syndrome. Circulation, 64:832, 1981.
203. Breithardt, G., and Seipel, L.: Comparative study of two methods of estimating sinoatrial conduction time in man. Am. J. Cardiol., 42:965, 1978.
204. Cramer, M., et al.: Characteristics of extracellular potentials recorded from the sinoatrial pacemaker of the rabbit. Circ. Res., 41:292, 1977.
205. Hariman, R. J., et al.: A new method for recording of extracellular sinoatrial electrograms during cardiac surgery in man. Am. J. Cardiol., 41:375, 1978.
206. Cramer, M., Hariman, R. J., Boxer, R. A., et al.: Catheter recording of sinoatrial node potentials in the in situ canine heart. Am. J. Cardiol., 41:374, 1978.
207. Cramer, M., Seigal, M., and Hoffman, B. F.: Electrogram of the canine sinus node. Circulation, 54:II-156, 1976.
208. Hariman, R. J., Krongrad, E., Bexer, R. A., et al.: Methods for recording electrograms of the sinoatrial node during cardiac surgery in man. Circulation, 61:1024, 1980.
209. Castillo-Fesnoy, A., Thebaut, J. F., Achard, F., and DeLangenhagen, B.: Identification du potentiel sinusal chez l'homme. Arch. Mol. Coeur, 72:948, 1977.
210. Reiffel, J. A., Gang, E., Glicklich, J., et al.: The human sinus node electrogram: A transvenous catheter technique and a comparison of directly measured and indirectly estimated sinoatrial conduction time in adults. Circulation, 62:1324, 1980.
211. Hariman, R. J., Krongrad, E., Beyer, R. A., et al.: Method for recording electrical activity of the sinoatrial node and automatic atrial foci during cardiac catheterization in human subjects. Am. J. Cardiol., 45:775, 1980.
212. Gomes, J. A. C., Kang, P. S., and El-Sherif, N.: The sinus node electrogram in patients with and without sick sinus syndrome. Techniques and correlation between directly measured and indirectly estimated sinoatrial conduction time. Circulation, 66:864, 1982.
213. Asseman, P., Berzun, B., Desry, D. R., et al.: Persistent sinus nodal electrograms during abnormally prolonged post pacing atrial pauses in sick sinus syndrome in humans: Sinoatrial block vs. overdrive suppression. Circulation, 68:33, 1983.
214. Koniski, T.: Electrophysiological consideration of sick sinus syndrome. Jpn. Circ. J., 40:194, 1976.
215. Kodama, I., Goto, J., Ando, S., et al.: Effects of rapid atrial stimulation on the transmembrane potentials of rabbit sinus node pacemaker cell. Circ. Res., 46:90, 1980.
216. Steinbeck, G., Naberi, R., and Luderitz, B.: Effects of atrial pacing on atriosinus conduction and overdrive suppression in the isolated rabbit sinus node. Circ. Res., 46:859, 1980.
217. Gomes, J. A., Hariman, B. I., and Chowdry, I. A.: New application of direct sinus node recordings in man: Assessment of sinus node recovery time. Circulation, 70:663, 1984.
218. Gang, E. S., Oseran, D. S., Mandel, W. J., and Peter, T.: Sinus node electrogram in patients with the hypersensitive carotid sinus syndrome. J. Am. Coll. Cardiol., in press.
219. Weiss, S., and Baker, J. P.: The cardotid sinus reflex in health and disease; its role in the causation of fainting and convulsions. Medicine, 12:297, 1933.
220. Walter, P. F., Crawley, I. S., and Derney, E. R.: Carotid hypersensitivity and syncope. Am. J. Cardiol., 42:396, 1978.
221. Thomas, J. E.: Hyperactive carotid sinus reflex and carotid sinus syncope. Mayo Clin. Prac., 44:127, 1969.
222. Nathanson, M. H.: Hyperactive cardioinhibitory carotid sinus reflex. Arch. Intern. Med., 77:491, 1946.
223. Sigler, L. H.: The cardioinhibitory carotid sinus reflex. Am. J. Cardiol., 12:175, 1963.
224. Hartzler, G. O., and Maloney, J. D.: Cardioinhibitory carotid sinus hypersensitivity. Arch. Intern. Med., 137:727, 1977.
225. Davies, A. B., Stephens, M. R., and Davies, A. G.: Carotid sinus hypersensitivity in patients presenting with syncope. Br. Heart J., 42:583, 1979.
226. Probst, P., Muhlberger, V., Lederbauer, M., et al.: Electrophysiologic findings in carotid sinus massage. PACE, 6:689, 1983.
227. Yamaguchi, I., Jordan, J. L., and Mandel, W. J.: The effect of antiarrhythmic drugs on estimated and measured sinoatrial conduction. In preparation.
228. Perry, W. L. M., and Reiihert, H.: The action of cardiac glycosides on autonomic ganglia. Br. J. Pharmacol., 9:324, 1954.
229. Mendez, C., Aceves, J., and Mendez, R.: Inhibition of adrenergic cardiac acceleration by cardiac glycosides. J. Pharmacol. Exp. Ther., 81:191, 1961.
230. Nadeau, R. A., and James, T. N.: Antagonistic effects on the sinus node of acetylstrophantidin and adrenergic stimulation. Circ. Res., 13:388, 1963.
231. Ten Eick, R. E., and Hoffman, B. F.: Chronotropic effect of cardiac glyscosides in dogs, cats and rabbits. Circ. Res., 25:305, 1967.
232. Ten Eick, R. E., and Hoffman, B. F.: The effect of digitalis on the excitability of autonomic nerves. J. Pharmacol. Exp. Ther., 109:95, 1969.
233. Goodman, D. J., et al.: Sinus node function in the denervated human heart: Effect of digitalis. Br. Heart J., 37:618, 1975.
234. Gomes, J. A. C., Kang, P. S., and El-Sherif, N.: Effects of digitalis on the human sick sinus node after pharmacologic autonomic blockade. Am. J. Cardiol., 48:783, 1981.
235. Hashimoto, K., Kimura, T., and Kubota, K.: Study of the therapeutic and toxic effects of ouabain by simultaneous observations on the excised and blood-perfused sinoatrial node and papillary muscle preparations and in the heart of dogs. J. Pharmacol. Exp. Ther., 186:463, 1973.
236. Dick, H. L. H., McCawley, E. L., and Fisher, W. A.: Reserpine-digitalis toxicity. Arch. Intern. Med., 109:503, 1962.
237. Gillis, R. A.: Cardiac sympathetic nerve activity: Changes induced by ouabain and propranolol. Science, 166:508, 1969.
238. Dhingra, R. C., et al.: The electrophysiological effects of ouabain on sinus node and atrium in man. J. Clin. Invest., 56:555, 1975.
239. Bond, R. C., Engel, T. R., and Schaal, S. F.: The effect of digitalis on sinoatrial conduction in man. Circulation, 48 (Suppl. IV):147, 1973.
240. Reiffel, J. A., Bigger, J. T., Jr., and Giardina, E. G., Jr.: The effect of digoxin on sinus node automaticity and sinoatrial conduction (SAC) in man (abstr.). J. Clin. Invest., 53:64, 1974.
241. Hariman R. J., Hoffman, B. F.: Effects of ovabain and vagal stimulation on sinus nodal function in conscious dogs. Circ. Res. 51:760, 1982.
242. Rubinstein, J. J., Schulman, C. L., and Yurchak, P. M.: Clinical spectrum of sick sinus syndrome. Circulation, 46:5, 1972.
243. Scherlag, B. J., Abelleira, J. L., and Narula, O. S.: The differential

effects of ouabain on sinus, AV nodal, His bundle and idioventricular rhythmias. Am. Heart J., 81:227, 1971.
244. Engel, T. R., and Schaal, S. F.: Digitalis in the sick sinus syndrome: the effects of digitalis on sinoatrial automaticity and atrioventricular conduction. Circulation, 48:1201, 1973.
245. Wallace, A. G., et al.: Electrophysiological effects of quinidine. Circ. Res., 19:960, 1966.
246. Hoffman, B. F., Rosen, M. R., and Wit, A. L.: Electrophysiology and pharmacology of cardiac arrhythmias. VIII. Cardiac effects of quinidine and procainamide. Am. Heart J., 89:804, 1975.
247. Chiba, S.: Absence of blocking effect of quinidine on response to norepinephrine in the isolated dog atrium. Jpn. Heart J., 17:506, 1976.
248. Mason, J. W., et al.: The electrophysiological effects of quinidine in the transplanted human heart. J. Clin. Invest., 59:481-489, 1977.
249. Josephson, M. E., et al.: The electrophysiological effects of intramuscular quinidine on the atrioventricular conducting system in man. Am. Heart J., 87:55-64, 1974.
250. Cohen, I. S., Jick, H., and Cohen, S. I.: Adverse reactions to quinidinc in hospitalized patients: findings based on data from the Boston collaborative drug surveillance program. Prog. Cardiovasc. Dis., 20:151, 1977.
251. Hirschfield, D. S., et al.: Clinical and electrophysiological effects of intravenous quinidine in man. Br. Heart J., 39:309-316, 1977.
252. Josephson, M. E., et al.: Electrophysiologic properties of procainamide in man. Am. J. Cardiol., 33:596, 1974.
253. Goldberg, D., Reiffel, J. A., Davis, J. C., et al.: Electrophysiologic effects of procainamide on sinus function in patients with and without sinus node disease. Am. Heart J., 103:75-79, 1982.
254. Befeler, B., et al.: Electrophysiologic effects of the antiarrhythmic agent disopyramide phosphate. Am. J. Cardiol., 35:282, 1975.
255. Marrot, P. K., et al.: A study of acute electrophysiological and cardiovascular action of disopyramide in man. Eur. J. Cardiol., 413:303, 1976.
256. Katoh, T., Karagueuzian, H. S., Jordan, J. L., and Mandel, W. J.: The cellular electrophysiologic mechanism of the dual actions of disopyramide on rabbit sinus node function. Circulation, 66:1216, 1982.
257. Seipel, L., and Breithardt, G.: Sinus recovery time after disopyramide phosphate. Am. J. Cardiol., 37:118, 1976.
258. LaBarre, A. B., et al.: Electrophysiologic effects of disopyramide phosphate on sinus node function in patients with sinus node dysfunction. Circulation, 59:226, 1979.
259. Mandel, W. J., and Bigger, J. T.: Electrophysiologic effects of lidocaine on isolated canine and rabbit atrial tissue. J. Pharmacol. Exp. Ther., 185:438, 1973.
260. Dhingra, R. C., et al.: Electrophysiologic effects of lidocaine on sinus node and atrium in patients with and without sinoatrial dysfunction. Circulation, 57:448, 1978.
261. Lieberman, N. A., et al.: The effects of lidocaine on the electrical and mechanical activity of the heart. Am. J. Cardiol., 22:375, 1968.
262. Lippestade, C. T., and Forfang, K.: Production of sinus arrest by lignocaine. Br. Med. J., 1:537, 1971.
263. Parameswaran, R., et al.: Sinus bradycardia due to lidocaine. Clinical electrophysiologic correlations. J. Electrocardiol., 7:75, 1974.
264. Yamaguchi, I., Singh, B. N., and Mandel, W. J.: Electrophysiological actions of mexiletene on isolated rabbit atria and canine ventricular muscle and Purkinje fibers. Cardiovasc. Res., 13:288, 1979.
265. Roos, J. C., Paalman, A. C. A., and Dunning, A. G.: Electrophysiological effects of mexiletene in man. Br. Heart J., 38:1262, 1976.
266. Campbell, R. W. F., et al.: Mexiletine (KO1173) in the management of ventricular dysrhythmias. Lancet, 2:204, 1973.
267. Samuelsson, R. G., and Harrison, D. C.: Electrophysiologic evaluation of encainide with use of monophasic action potential recording. Am. J. Cardiol., 48:871, 1981.
268. Sami, M., Mason, J. W., Al, J. C., and Harrison, D. C.: Canine electrophysiology of encainide, a new antiarrhythmic drug. Am. J. Cardiol., 43:1149-1154, 1979.
269. Sami, M., Mason, J. W., Perbers, F., and Harrison, D. E.: Clinical electrophysiologic effects of encainide, a newly developed antiarrhythmic agent. Am. J. Cardiol., 44:526, 1979.
270. Jackman, W. M., Zipes, D. P., Nacarelli, G. V., et al.: Electrophysiology of oral encainide. Am. J. Cardiol., 49:1270, 1982.
271. Seipel, L., Abendroth, R. R., and Breithardt, G.: Electrophysiological effects of flecainide (R818) in man (abstr). Circulation, 62 (Suppl. III):III-153, 1980.
272. Vik-Mo, H., Ohm, O. J., Lund-Johansen, P.: Electrophysiological effects of flecainide acetate in patients with sinus nodal dysfunction. Am. J. Cardiol., 50:1090, 1982.
273. Ng, C. K., Glottner, M., and Gmeiner, R.: Intracardiac electrophysiological effects of lorcainide in man. Eur. J. Clin. Pharmacol., 15:241, 1979.
274. Bar, F., Farre, J., Ross, D., et al.: Electrophysiological effects of lorcainide, a new antiarrhythmic drug. Observations in patients with and without pre-excitation. Br. Heart J., 45:292, 1981.
275. Manz, M., Steinbeck, G., and Ludentz, B.: Action of lorcainide (RT 15889) on sinoatrial node function and intracardiac conduction. Herz. Kreislauf., 11:192, 1979.
276. Rosati, R. A., et al.: Influence of diphenylhydantoin on electrophysiological properties of the canine heart. Circ. Res., 21:757, 1967.
277. Wit, A. L., Rosen, M. R., and Hoffman, B. F.: Electrophysiology and pharmacology of cardiac arrhythmias. VIII. Cardiac effects of diphenylhydantoin. Am. Heart J., 90:397, 1975.
278. Mercer, E. N., and Osborne, J. A.: Current status of diphenylhydantoin in heart disease. Ann. Intern. Med., 67:1084, 1967.
279. Strauss, H. C., Bigger, J. T., Jr., and Bassett, A. L.: Actions of diphenylhydantoin on the electrical properties of isolated rabbit and canine atria. Circ. Res., 23:463, 1968.
280. Louis, S., Kutt, H., and McDowell, F.: Cardiocirculatory changes caused by intravenous dilantin and its solvents. Am. Heart J., 74:523, 1967.
281. Wit, A. L., and Cravefield, P.: Effects of verapamil on the sinoatrial and atrioventricular nodes of the rabbit and the mechanism by which it arrests atrioventricular nodal tachycardia. Circ. Res., 35:413, 1974.
282. Singh, B. N., and Vaughan-Williams, E. M.: A fourth class of antidysrhythmic action? Effect of verapamil on oubain toxicity and on atrial and ventricular intracellular potentials and on other features of cardiac function. Cardiovasc. Res., 6:109-119, 1972.
283. Zipes, D. P., and Fischer, J. C.: Effects of agents which inhibit the slow channel on sinus node automaticity and atrioventricular conduction in the dog. Circ. Res., 34:184, 1984.
284. Konishi, T.: Electrophysiological consideration of sick sinus syndrome. Jpn. Circ. J., 40:194, 1976
285. Jordan, J. L., Yamaguchi, I., and Mandel, W. J.: Studies on the mechanism of suppression of sinus node automaticity by atrial overdrive pacing. Clin. Res., 26:241, 1978.
286. Jordan, J. L., Yamaguchi, I., and Mandel, W. J.: The effects of verapamil on sinoatrial conduction in isolated tissue. Clin. Res., 26:241, 1978.
287. Singh, B. N., and Roche, A. H. G.: Effects of intravenous verapamil on hemodynamics in patients with heart disease. Am. Heart J., in press.
288. Ning, W., Wit, A. L.: Comparison of the direct effects of nifedipine and verapamil on the electrical activity of the sinoatrial and

atrioventricular nodes of the rabbit heart. Am. Heart J., 106:345, 1983.
289. Henry, P. D.: Comparative pharmacology of calcium antagonists: Nifedipine, verapamil and diltiazem. Am. J. Caridol., 46:1047, 1980.
290. Broekhysen, J., Deltour, G., and Ghislain, M.: Some biochemical effects of amiodarone. Arzneim. Forsch., 19:1850, 1969.
291. Goupil, N., and Lenfant, J.: The effects of amiodarone on the sinus node activity of the rabbit heart. Eur. J. Pharmacol., 39:23, 1976.
292. Gloor, H. O., Urthaler, F., and James, T. N.: Acute effects of amiodarone upon the canine sinus node and atrioventricular junctional region. J. Clin. Invest., 71:1457, 1983.
293. Obayashi, R., and Mandel, W. J.: Electrophysiological effects of ajmaline in isolated cardiac tissue. Cardiovasc. Res., 10:20, 1976.
294. Obayashi, K., Nagasawa, K., Mandel, W. J., et al.: Cardiovascular effects of ajmaline. Am. Heart J., 92:487, 1976.
295. Reiser, J., Freeman, A. R., and Greenspan, K.: Aprindine—a calcium mediated antidysrhythmic. Fed. Proc., 33:476, 1974.
296. Elharrour, V., Foster, P. R., and Zipes, D. P.: Effects of aprindine HCL on cardiac tissue. J. Pharmacol. Exp. Ther., 195:201, 1975.
297. Ledda, E., Mantelli, L., Manzini, S., et al.: Electrophysiological and antiarrhythmic properties of propafenone in isolated cardiac preparations. J. Cardiovasc. Pharmacol., 3:1162, 1981.
298. Kohlhardt, M.: Der Einflus von propafenon auf den transmembranaien Na^+ und Ca^+ strom der Warmbliiter myokard fasermembran. In Hechrein, H., Hapke, H. J., Beck, O. A. (eds.): Fortshritte in der Pharmako Therapie von Herzrhythmusstorungen, pp. 35–38. Stuttgart, Fischer, 1977.
299. Satoh, H., and Hashimoto, K.: Effect of propafenone on the membrane currents of rabbit sinoatrial node cells. Eur. J. Pharmacol., 99:185, 1984.
300. Echt, D. S., Berte, L. E., Clusin, W. T., et al.: Prolongation of the human monophasic action potential by sotalol. Am. J. Cardiol., 51:1082, 1982.
301. Rosenshtraukh, L. V., Yurgavichyus, I. A., Undrovinas, A. I., et al.: Effects of ethmozine on the contractile force, transmembrane action potential, and sodium current in frog auriculat muscle. First US-USSR Symposium of sudden death. Yalta, USSR, Oct. 3–5, 1977.
302. Roffy, R., Rosenshtraukh, L. V., Elharrar, V., and Zipes, D. P.: Electrophysiological effects of ethmozin on canine myocardium. Cardiovasc. Res., 13:354, 1979.
303. Kobinger, W., Lillier, C., and Pichler, L.: N-allyl derivative of clonidine, a substance with specific bradycardia action at a cardiac site. Arch. Pharmacol., 306:255, 1979.
304. Conde, C., Leppo, J., Lipski, J., et al.: Effectiveness of pacemaker treatment in the bradycardia-tachycardia syndrome. Am. J. Cardiol., 32:209, 1973.
305. Sigurd, B., Jensen, G., Melbom, J., et al.: Adams-Stokes syndrome caused by sinoatrial block. Br. Heart J., 35:1002, 1973.
306. Rokseth, R., and Hatle, L.: Prospective study on the occurrence and management of chronic sinoatrial disease, with follow-up. Br. Heart J., 36:582, 1974.
307. Radford, D. J., and Julian, D. G.: Sick sinus syndrome: Experience of a cardiac pacemaker clinic. Br. Med. J., 3:504, 1974.
308. Sowton, E., Hendrix, G., and Roy, P.: Ten-year survey of treatment with implanted cardiac pacemaker. Br. Med. J., 3:155, 1974.
309. Hartel, G., and Talvensaari, T.: Treatment of sinoatrial syndrome with permanent cardiac pacing in 90 patients. Acta Med. Scand., 198:341, 1975.
310. Chokshi, D. S., Mascarenhas, E., Sanet, P., et al.: Treatment of sinoatrial rhythm disturbances with permanent cardiac pacing. Am. J. Cardiol., 32:215, 1973.
311. Skagen, K., and Hansen, J. F.: The long-term prognosis for patients with sinoatrial block treated with permanent pacemaker. Acta Med. Scand., 199:13, 1975.
312. Krishnaswami, K., and Geraci, A. R.: Permanent pacing in disorders of sinus node function. Am. Heart J., 89:579, 1975.
313. Bayley, T. J.: Long-term ventricular pacing in treatment of sinoatrial block. Br. Med. J., 3:456, 1971.
314. Rubenstein, J. J., et al.: Clinical spectrum of the sick sinus syndrome. Circulation, 46:5, 1972.
315. Wan, S. H., Lee, G. S., and Toh, C. C. S.: The sick sinus syndrome. A study of 15 cases. Br. Heart J., 34:942, 1972.
316. Rosen, K., Loeb, H., and Sinno, M. Z.: Cardiac conduction in patients with symptomatic sinus node disease. Circulation, 43:836, 1971.
317. Narula, O.: Atrioventricular conduction defects in patients with sinus bradycardia. Analysis by His bundle recordings. Circulation, 44:1096, 1971.
318. Easley, R. M., and Goldstein, S.: Sinoatrial syncope. Am. J. Med., 50:166, 1971.
319. Zipes, D. P., Wallace, R. G., Sealy, W. C., et al.: Artificial atrial and ventricular pacing in the treatment of arrhythmias. Ann. Intern. Med. 70:885, 1969.
320. Chen, T. O.: Transvenous ventricular pacing in the treatment of paroxysmal atrial tachyarrhythmias alternating with sinus bradycardia and standstill. Am. J. Cardiol., 22:874, 1968.
321. Zoll, P. M., Linenthal, D. J., and Zarsky, L. R. N.: Ventricular fibrillation. Treatment and prevention by external cardiac currents. N. Engl. J. Med., 262:105, 1960.
322. Han, J., Millet D., Chizzonitti, B., et al.: Temporal dispersion of recovery of excitability in atrium and ventricle as a function of heart rate. Am. Heart J., 71:481, 1966.
323. Han, J., De Traglia, J., Millet, D., et al.: Incidence of ectopic beats as a function of basic rate in the ventricle. Am. Heart. J., 72:632, 1966.
324. Sandoe, E., and Flensted Jensen, E.: Adams-Stokes seizures in patients with attacks of both tachy and bradycardia, a therapeutic challenge. Acta Med. Scand., 186:111, 1969.

7

Atrial Arrhythmias: Basic Concepts

Maurits A. Allessie and Felix I. M. Bonke

Several problems are inherent in writing about the concepts of atrial premature beats and tachyarrhythmias. The main difficulty is that despite the extensive and excellent research done in this field, the underlying mechanisms of most human arrhythmias have still not been settled. Therefore, we cannot describe in this chapter the mechanism of each of the different atrial arrhythmias as a circumscript, well-defined scientific fact. Rather, we are forced to present the various theoretical mechanisms for tachyarrhythmias as they are found in experimental studies.

Nevertheless, by comparing experimental data obtained from animal studies with clinical observations, we will try to indicate which of the possible mechanisms seems most likely to be responsible for each of the different arrhythmias encountered in humans.

Classification of Atrial Arrhythmias

Another difficulty caused by the lack of knowledge concerning the underlying mechanisms of atrial arrhythmias is that the clinical classification of supra-ventricular tachyarrhythmias in tachycardia, flutter, and fibrillation is primarily arbitrary; the most important criterion used for this classification is the rate of the arrhythmias. Figure 7-1 shows the different rate scales several authors use to classify atrial tachyarrhythmias. As seems inevitable in medicine when some arbitrary criterion is used, opinions diverge widely on the rate at which a tachycardia should be called *flutter* or when flutter changes into *fibrillation.* In fact, no sharp division exists between the different arrhythmias. As indicated by some authors, there is overlap in rate between tachycardia and flutter and an area of "no man's land" between flutter and fibrillation. Terms such as *impure flutter, flutter-fibrillation,* and *coarse fibrillation* are used to describe the intermediate form between flutter and fibrillation.

The close interrelationship between different atrial arrhythmias is further illustrated by the observation that one arrhythmia may change into another. The transition from atrial flutter into fibrillation, or vice versa, occurring either spontaneously or during the administration of digitalis or quinidine, is well known. All this clarifies that the present classification of atrial arrhythmias does not necessarily mean that each has a different funda-

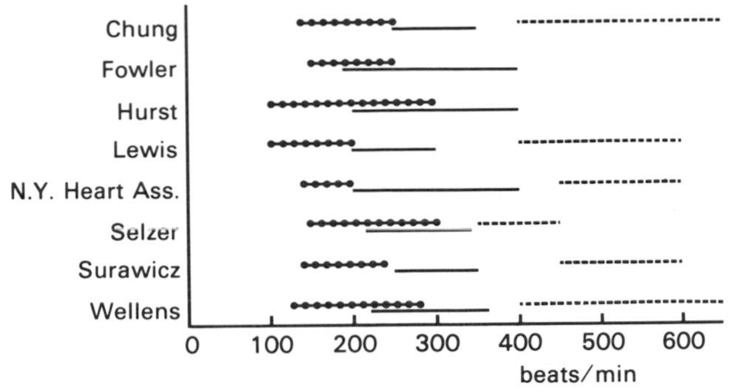

Figure 7-1. *Classification of supraventricular tachyarrhythmia in tachycardia, flutter, and fibrillation, according to the rate of the arrhythmia. A wide variability exists in the criteria used by several authors. There is overlap between the definition of tachycardia and flutter, whereas an undefined area exists between flutter and fibrillation. (•–•–•–•, tachycardia; ———, flutter; ------, fibrillation) (Data from Chung, E. K.: Principles of Cardiac Arrhythmias. Baltimore, Waverly Press, 1977; Fowler, N.: Cardiac Diagnosis. Hagerstown, Md., Harper & Row, 1968; Hurst, J.: The Heart. New York, McGraw-Hill, 1974; Lewis, T.: The Mechanism and Graphic Registration of the Heart Beat. London, Shaw and Sons, 1925; New York Heart Association: Nomenclature and Criteria for Diagnosis of Diseases of the Heart and Great Vessels, 7th ed., 1973; Selsen, A.: Principles of Clinical Cardiology. Philadelphia, W. B. Saunders, 1975; Surawicz, B., et al.: Standardization of terminology and interpretation. Am. J. Cardiol., 41:130–145, 1978; Wellens, H. J. J.: Electrical stimulation of the heart in the study and treatment of tachycardias. Leiden, Stenfert Kroese, 1971)*

mental mechanism. In addition, tachyarrhythmias of about the same rate and of similar clinical appearance may be based on completely different mechanisms. Because of this, another classification based on the underlying mechanisms would be far preferable. However, such classification cannot be made until the various mechanisms underlying atrial arrhythmias are better understood and a set of clinical criteria and diagnostic tests are developed to differentiate the various mechanisms of arrhythmias operative in humans.

Atrial Premature Complexes

A premature atrial complex is an early depolarization that may originate anywhere in the atria outside the sinus node. The propagation of the impulse in the atria from an atrial ectopic focus is usually different from that of the sinus impulse, so that the shape of the resultant P wave is more or less different from the P wave of sinus origin. Depending on the degree of prematurity and whether the pacemaker in the sinus node is reset, an atrial premature complex may be interpolated, followed by a full compensatory pause, or followed by an interval that is only somewhat longer than a normal sinus interval. Furthermore, it may also trigger a bout of rapid repetitive atrial activity.

Atrial Tachycardia

Like atrial premature complexes, atrial tachycardia may originate from anywhere in the atria. There is a rapid and regular succession of P waves of different form compared to the P wave of sinus origin, and an isoelectric segment exists between P waves. Atrial tachycardia frequently occurs in paroxysms, but on rare occasions it may become chronic. It usually has a rate between 140 and 200 beats/min, generally with each atrial impulse conducted to the ventricle (1 : 1 response).

Atrial Flutter

Atrial flutter is characterized by a very rapid, highly regular rhythm of the atria (200 to 350 beats/min). Because of the refractory period in the AV junctional tissue, the ventricular response is usually at half this rate, since a 2 : 1 or greater AV block almost always exists. Atrial activity is represented in the electrocardiogram by regular biphasic oscillations (F waves) of uniform shape. There is no intervening isoelectric segment between the F waves, and the atrial oscillations have a continuous sawtooth type of appearance. Recently atrial flutter has been classified into two different types.[1] Type I, similar to classic or common atrial flutter, has an atrial rate between 240 and 340 beats/min and can be entrained by rapid pacing. Type II flutter, with an atrial rate between 340 and 430 beats/min, cannot be reset or entrained by programmed electrical stimulation. Atrial flutter may occur in paroxysms with spontaneous termination, be a continuous chronic process when not treated, or change into atrial fibrillation. In general, flutter is less stable than fibrillation.

Atrial Fibrillation

During atrial fibrillation, atrial activity is chaotic and uncoordinated. On the electrocardiogram the completely irregular atrial activation is recorded in the form of small waves that constantly vary in amplitude and configuration. It is usually impossible to count accurately the number of atrial responses from the ordinary electrocardiogram, but it has been estimated to vary between 400 and 650 "beats"/min. Not uncommonly, fibrillation is so fine, and activation of the atria so fragmented, that it becomes difficult to distinguish any atrial activity on the electrocardiogram at all. However, local electrograms recorded directly from the surface of the atria under these circumstances still show well-defined, although irregular, electrical activity.[2] The ventricular

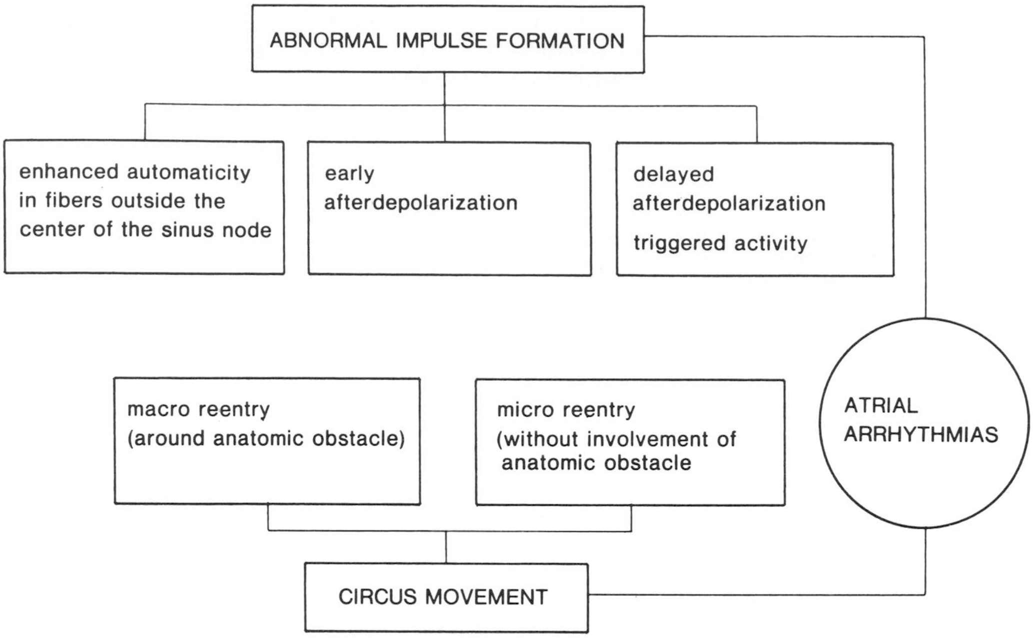

Figure 7-2. *Classification of atrial tachyarrhythmias on the basis of their possible underlying mechanisms.*

rhythm during atrial fibrillation is completely irregular. Atrial fibrillation may occur in a paroxysmal form, or it may become chronic. Generally, paroxysms of atrial fibrillation must be considered a precursor of permanent atrial fibrillation.

Possible Mechanisms of Atrial Tachyarrhythmias

Two groups of fundamentally different mechanisms may be responsible for producing tachyarrhythmias. Group I contains those mechanisms that are based on some form of abnormal impulse formation. Group II is based on a disorder of impulse conduction, leading to circulating excitation or reentry. Figure 7-2 summarizes the different types of abnormal impulse formation and the two types of circus movement that have been recognized in experimental studies.

Abnormal Impulse Formation

Abnormal impulse formation may be defined as the generation of impulses by fibers other than the dominant pacemaker fibers in the center of the sinus node, regardless of whether the abnormal impulse is generated spontaneously or induced by foregoing normal or abnormal activities. According to this definition, abnormal impulse formation is the same as ectopic impulse formation.

However, it is also possible to use a definition based more on the mechanism underlying impulse formation. Normal impulse formation is the occurrence of a spontaneous depolarization before the onset of an action potential, the so-called diastolic depolarization. If depolarization occurs either during repolarization or under special conditions directly after repolarization, the term *abnormal impulse formation* may be used.

Under normal conditions, the fibers in the atrium that show spontaneous depolarization (diastolic depolarization) are located in the sinus node, the region of the AV node, and perhaps around the orifices of the pulmonary veins in the left atrium (these fibers are present in the rabbit but perhaps not in all other species). Furthermore, there are fibers in the vicinity of the coronary sinus (at least in the dog) and in the leaflets of the AV valves that have a relatively low resting potential and develop spontaneous depolarization under certain conditions.

Finally, Hashimoto and Moe[3] have described fibers in the canine right atrium close to the crista terminalis that have some characteristics of Purkinje fibers (*i.e.*, spontaneous depolarization). It is not known whether these fibers are also present in other species.

The spontaneous depolarization in the fibers in the center of the sinus node is normally the fastest, and therefore this depolarization brings these fibers to a discharge before others. Thus, under normal conditions, automaticity of the dominant pacemaker in the center of the sinus node suppresses the subsidiary pacemakers in the atria.

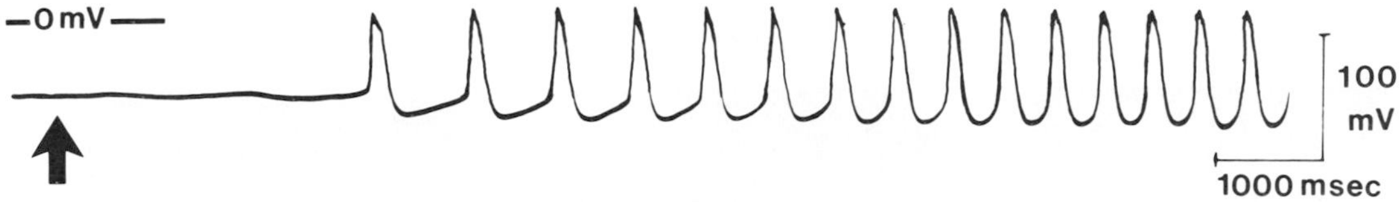

Figure 7-3. *Spontaneous impulse initiation in atrial fibers outside the coronary sinus ostium (dog). Norepinephrine, 10^{-6} g/ml, was added to the tissue bath at the moment indicated by the arrow* (left). *Small oscillations in membrane potential then occurred and led to the first spontaneous impulse; the slope of the diastolic depolarization increased with each subsequent spontaneous impulse by which the rate of the focal discharge increased. (Wit, A. L., and Cranefield, P. F.: Triggered and automatic activity in the canine coronary sinus. Circ. Res., 41:435–445, 1977. By permission of the American Heart Association, Inc.)*

Enhanced Automaticity in Fibers Outside the Center of the Sinus Node

A certain agent can perhaps differentially enhance the spontaneous depolarization in a subsidiary pacemaker without affecting the sinus node or influencing it only to a lesser extent. Thus, for instance, when extracellular potassium concentration is reduced, diastolic depolarization (phase 4 depolarization) may be enhanced in subsidiary pacemaker fibers while fibers within the center of the sinus node remain relatively insensitive. Similarly, although catecholamines enhance diastolic depolarization both in the dominant and subsidiary pacemakers, this effect could be more pronounced on subsidiary pacemakers than on sinus node fibers. Vagal influences may also preferentially suppress the dominant pacemaker so much that subsidiary pacemakers generate either one or a series of spontaneous discharges.

If the normal function of the pacemaker of the sinus node is severely depressed by whatever cause, or if the impulse from the pacemaker does not reach the atrium (sinoatrial block), automaticity in subsidiary pacemaker fibers may generate an impulse or even take over pacemaker function. In an isolated preparation of the coronary sinus region of the canine atrium, Wit and Cranefield[4] were able to induce automaticity by adding catecholamines to the tissue bath and to increase the rate to a range similar to the sinus rate in an isolated canine right atrium preparation (Fig. 7-3).

Early Afterdepolarizations

Depolarization may also occur during repolarization or before repolarization is completed. It is incorrect to call this a phase 4 depolarization, since the depolarization starts from a low level of membrane potential (*e.g.*, −30 mV). Cranefield[5] has used the term *early afterdepolarization.* If such an afterdepolarization is strong enough, it may lead to an action potential with a low amplitude.

Normally, the net ionic current through the cell membrane during repolarization is directed outward. If the outward current is depressed or if the background inward current is enhanced, the net current may become inward; this means that a depolarization of the membrane will occur, and such a depolarization may excite the fiber again. Such decrease of outward (repolarizing) current may occur if the membrane conductance for potassium ions is reduced, as is, for instance, the case if the extracellular potassium concentration is markedly reduced. An increase of background inward current may result from hypoxia, injury, or some drugs.[6] An example

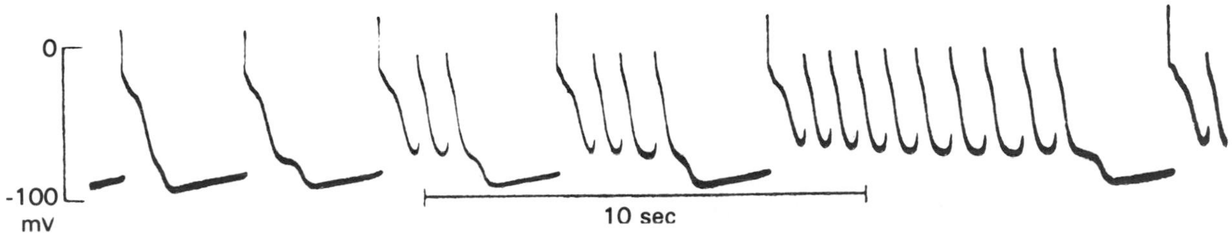

Figure 7-4. *Isolated Purkinje fibers of the dog showing spontaneous activity. Aconitine is added to the tissue bath in a low concentration (10^{-6}–10^{-8} g/ml). This slows the repolarization, and the third action potential is followed by two spontaneous, nondriven impulses. The fourth and fifth action potentials are followed by a series of these impulses. (Schmidt, R. F.: Versuche mit Aconitin zum Problem der spontanen Erregungsbildung im Herzen. Pfluegers Arch., 271:526–536, 1960)*

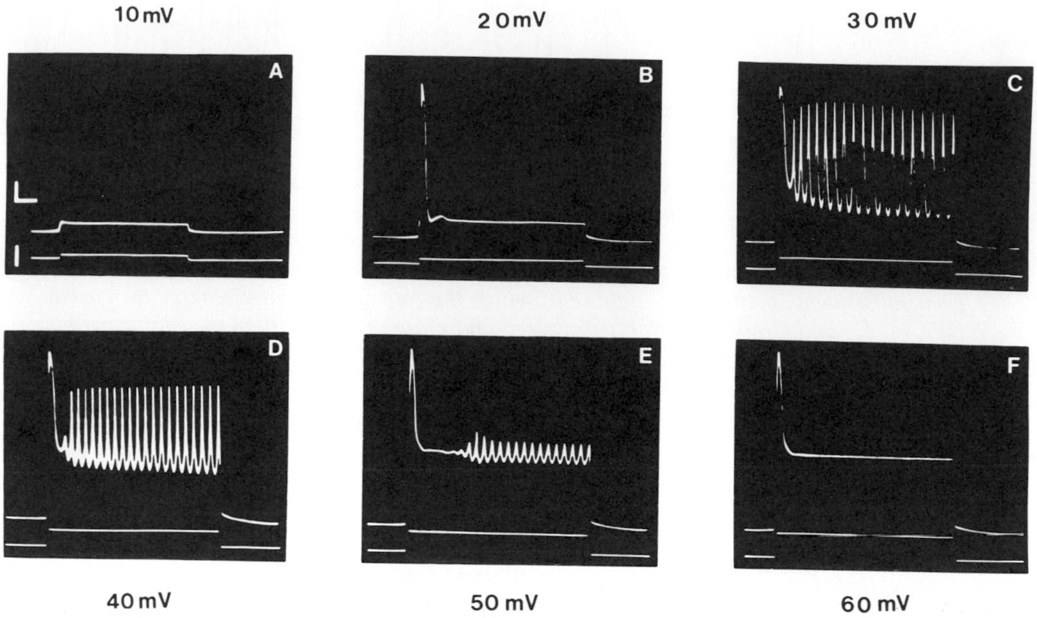

Figure 7-5. *The effect of depolarizing current on frog atrial trabecula. The upper trace in each panel represents the membrane potential; the lower trace, the amount of current that is given to the preparation. In the first panel (A), the current causes a depolarization of 10 mV, whereas a depolarization of 20 mV (in B) causes one single action potential followed by an oscillation. More current causes a stronger depolarization (30 mV in C and 40 mV in D), and sustained rhythmic activity follows the first-induced action potential. If the membrane is depolarized with 50 mV (E), only small oscillations are present, whereas in case of a depolarization with 60 mV (F), a stable membrane potential is reached after the action potential.*

In the first panel (A), calibrations are given, namely, 20 mV and 1 second for the first trace and 5×10^{-7} A for the current trace (second trace). Measurements were made with a double-sucrose-gap technique. (Lenfant, J., Mironneau, J., Aka, J. K.: Activité répétitive de la fibre sino-auriculaire de grenouille: analyse des courants membranaires responsables de l'automatisme cardiaque. J. Physiol. (Paris), 64:5–18, 1972)

of the latter is the demonstration by Scherf[7] that focal application of aconitine to the surface of the canine atrium produced a tachycardia with a rate of 200 to 300 beats/min originating at the site where aconitine was applied. Although this drug has no significance for practical use, it illustrates well the phenomenon of early afterdepolarizations. Matsuda and co-workers[8] have shown that in isolated dog ventricular myocardium, focal application of aconitine prolonged the repolarization and subsequently the occurrence of "spontaneous" or "nondriven" action potentials. This has also been demonstrated by Schmidt,[9] and Figure 7-4 is taken from his publication. Peper and Trautwein[10] were able to demonstrate that aconitine inhibits or postpones the inactivation of the sodium influx system, so that the background inward current is strongly increased during repolarization. If the membrane potential of a group of fibers is brought artificially, for instance through depolarizing current, to a level between −40 and −10 mV, spontaneous action potentials may occur. This is illustrated in Figure 7-5, taken from the work of Lenfant and co-workers[11] using atrial trabecula of the frog. In principle, the same phenomena were demonstrated in ventricular muscle of the guinea pig.[12,13] The same phenomenon may be present in diseased human atrial tissue; if these fibers are brought in a tissue bath they turned out to be depolarized and spontaneously active.[14]

Delayed Afterdepolarizations

An afterdepolarization may also occur after the fiber is repolarized completely or almost completely. If the amplitude of such an afterdepolarization is large enough, a single or a series of nondriven action potentials may arise. Afterdepolarizations of this kind have been recorded in experimental studies in which cardiac tissue was exposed to toxic concentrations of cardiac glycosides; this is true not only in Purkinje and ventricular fibers[15] but also in specialized atrial fibers[3] and diseased human atrial tissue.[16] On the other hand, Saito and co-workers[17] recently described that in isolated rabbit right atrium preparations it was possible under special condi-

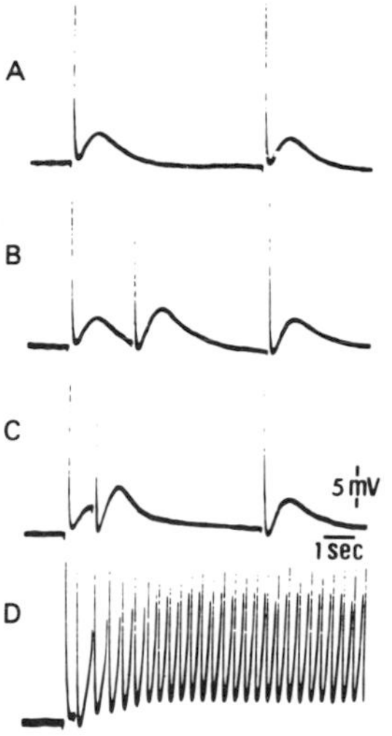

Figure 7-6. *In isolated right atrium of the rabbit, it is sometimes possible to find fibers showing afterpotentials. In this experiment, the preparation was electrically stimulated every 6 seconds. Only the foot of the action potential is shown in this recording (note the calibration). Record A shows the control recording, whereas an extra stimulus was given in the other records: in B with a coupling of 2 seconds; in C, of 1 second; and in D, of 500 msec. In D, the extra response is followed by a series of nondriven impulses. (Saito, T., Otoguro, M., and Matsubara, T.: Electrophysiological studies on the mechanism of electrically induced sustained rhythmic activity in the rabbit right atrium. Circ. Res., 42:199–206, 1978. By permission of the American Heart Association, Inc.)*

tions (no spontaneous activity, $K_o = 2.6$ mM, and with the temperature of the superfusate at 32°C) to induce, by regular drive, delayed afterpotentials and, by an extra stimulus, sustained rhythmic activity. This is illustrated in Figure 7-6. Saito mentioned that some of the spontaneously active preparations became quiescent when the external potassium concentration was raised from 2.6 to 5.2 mM. It is unclear whether this phenomenon is important under normal conditions and in the human heart.

Furthermore, these delayed afterdepolarizations also occur in canine, simian, and human valvular fibers,[18–20] in the canine coronary sinus,[4] and in diseased human atrium.[21] In all these cases the afterdepolarizations only occur in relation to a preceding action potential and never develop spontaneously. Therefore the term *triggered activity* is used in case an afterdepolarization is strong enough to initiate a nondriven action potential (Fig. 7-7).[4] Wit and Cranefield[4] demonstrated that triggered sustained tachycardias are characterized by the fact that during the first 10 to 20 beats there is a progressive decrease of the cycle length (the rate increases; "warming-up" phenomenon). The sustained activity always subsides spontaneously after some seconds to minutes. Preceding termination, the rate slows down and the last nondriven action potential is followed by one or more subthreshold afterdepolarizations. Then in

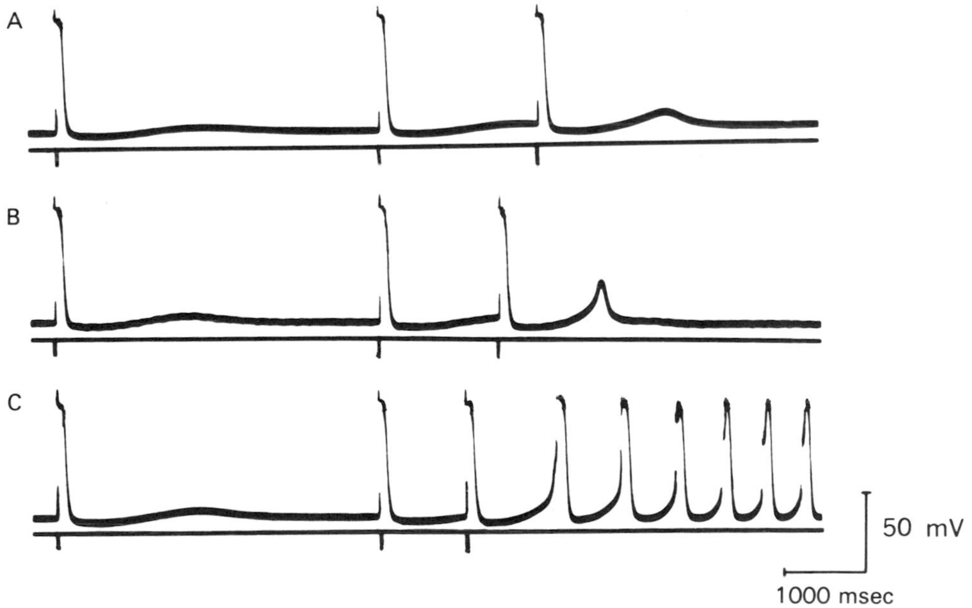

Figure 7-7. *Recording from a canine coronary sinus fiber while norepinephrine (10^{-6} g/ml) was in the tissue bath. Each panel shows the last two impulses of a series of 10 driven beats with an interval of 4000 msec, after which a premature impulse was induced at progressively shorter coupling intervals (A, 2000 msec; B, 1400 msec; and C, 1000 msec). In B, the premature action potential is followed by an afterdepolarization of about 30 mV, whereas in C, sustained rhythmic activity is triggered by the afterdepolarization following the premature action potential. (Wit, A. L., and Cranefield, P. F.: Triggered and automatic activity in the canine coronary sinus. Circ. Res., 41:435–445, 1977. By permission of the American Heart Association, Inc.)*

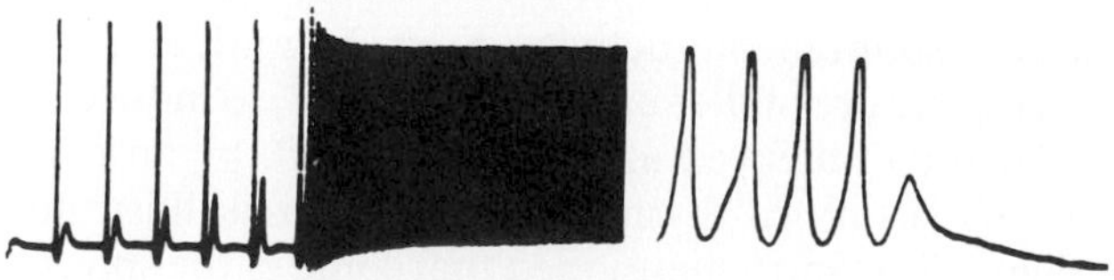

Figure 7-8. *Recording from a canine coronary sinus fiber stimulated with an interval of 4000 msec. The afterdepolarizations progressively increase in amplitude until rapid sustained rhythmic activity is triggered. During this rapid rhythm the membrane potential and the amplitude of the action potentials are decreased. At the right, the end of the rapid rhythm is shown while the paper speed of the recorder is ten times faster than at the left. The last action potential is followed by an afterdepolarization, and then the membrane potential returns to the level present before triggering. The interval at the end of the period of rapid rhythm is about 440 msec in this case. The amplitude of the action potential shown at the left is about 90 mV. Norepinephrine (10^{-6} g/ml) was added to the superfusing fluid. (Wit, A. L., and Cranefield, P. F.: Triggered and automatic activity in the canine coronary sinus. Circ. Res., 41:435–445, 1977. By permission of the American Heart Association, Inc.)*

a few seconds the membrane potential increases to the level present just before triggering (Fig. 7-8).

The mechanism for delayed afterdepolarizations is still unclear. Probably calcium plays an important role, since the amplitude of afterdepolarizations is increased by catecholamines and by an increase of extracellular calcium. On the other hand, the amplitude is lowered by calcium entry blockers (*e.g.*, verapamil). However, sodium is also important, since the amplitude of the afterdepolarizations is reduced by lowering the extracellular sodium concentration, by TTX, and by class I antiarrhythmic drugs. It seems that during the delayed afterdepolarization the transient inward (depolarizing) current is carried by sodium ions, whereas the membrane conductance is modulated by the intracellular calcium concentration.[22]

In Figure 7-9, the three different types of abnormal impulse formation (enhanced automaticity, early afterdepolarization, and delayed afterdepolarization–triggered activity) are summarized schematically.

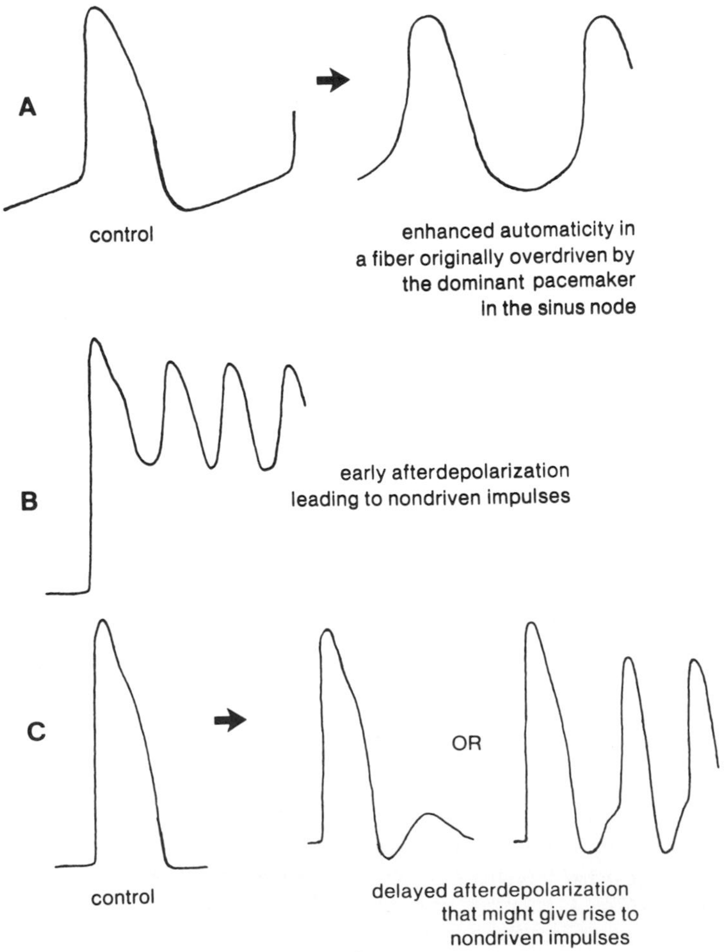

Figure 7-9. *(A) Enhanced automaticity (diastolic depolarization). (B) Early afterdepolarization leading to nondriven impulses. (C) Delayed afterdepolarization that might give rise to nondriven impulses.*

Circus Movement

General Considerations

The concept of the electrical impulse being entrapped in a circus movement somewhere in the heart dates from the end of the 19th century. As an alternative to the earlier proposed possibility of enhanced automaticity, in an article about fibrillar contraction of the heart, McWilliam[23] wrote:

> For apart from the possibility of rapid spontaneous discharges of energy by the muscular fibers, there seems to be another probable cause of continued and rapid movement. The peristaltic contraction travelling along such a structure as that of the ventricular wall must reach adjacent muscle bundles at different points of time, and since these bundles are connected with one another by anastomosing branches the contraction would naturally be propagated from one contracting fiber to another over which the contraction wave had already passed. Hence if the fibers are sufficiently excitable and ready to respond to contraction waves reaching them there would evidently be a more or less rapid series of contractions in each muscular bundle in consequence of the successive contraction waves reaching that bundle from different directions along its fibers of anastomosis with other bundles.

It is a very interesting detail that the first observations about circulating excitation were not done on the heart but on an animal bearing close resemblance to the heart, namely, the jellyfish. In 1906 Mayer,[24] studying the nature of rhythmic pulsation of the jellyfish, found that a strip of paralyzed subumbrella tissue of the jellyfish *Scyphomedusa,* cut in the shape of a ring or closed circuit, will pulsate rhythmically again, provided a contraction wave is initiated in the circuit. The rate of this rhythm, based on a continuous circus movement of the impulse around the ring, was about three to four times as rapid as the normal rhythm of the Medusa originating from its marginal sense organs. The analogy with atrial flutter and sinus rhythm is indeed striking.

It seems questionable whether Mayer himself was aware of the utmost importance of his observations with respect to cardiac arrhythmias. Although he repeated his experiments on ring-shaped strips of turtle ventricle, in which he found the same phenomena as in the rings of the jellyfish, he emphasized:

> It is remarkable that these isolated circuit waves, moving constantly in one direction through a circuit, are not met with in nature. Indeed, the heart, or pulsating Medusa, contains within itself the means to prevent any single pulsation wave from coursing constantly in one direction through the tissues. . . . Such a circuit cannot take possession of the vertebrate heart.

Fortunately two contemporary physiologists immediately understood the fundamental significance of Mayer's observations in respect to cardiac arrhythmias. Independently of each other, Mines[25,26] and Garrey[27] extended Mayer's studies on rings cut from atria, ventricles, or both. These studies resulted in a concept of circulating excitation that has survived 65 years of extensive research on the electrophysiology of the heart. Ever since, this early model of Mines as a basis for tachyarrhythmias has not lost its validity. It still gives a good and complete description of the properties of a rhythm based on the circulation of an excitation wave in a relatively large, anatomically defined circuit. However, more recent investigations have pointed out that in contrast to this classic model of circus movement, many tachyarrhythmias seem to arise from circus movement in a small circuit without involving a gross anatomic obstacle. The behavior of this type of circus movement differs from circus movement around a large anatomically determined circuit. Instead of being determined by the length of the circuit, this circus movement is completely governed by the functional electrophysiologic properties of the tissue composing the circuit. Circus movement tachycardias within the AV and SA nodes are probably the best-known examples of such microreentry,[28–31] but sustained microreentry is also possible in ordinary working myocardium.[32] These recent investigations have led to the description of a second model of circus movement that, in contrast to the classic anatomic model, is based solely on the functional electrophysiologic properties of cardiac muscle.[33] We will first describe these two fundamental models of circulating excitation in the heart, emphasizing the similarities and differences between macroreentry and microreentry.

Circus Movement in an Anatomically Defined Pathway

Figure 7-10 shows the original diagrams drawn by Mines to illustrate the conditions required for initiation of circulating excitation in an anatomically defined circuit. It also shows the electrophysiologic situation during a sustained circus movement of the impulse. Shown in this figure is a series of images of the electrophysiologic state of a ring of cardiac muscle, and the impulse is assumed to travel exclusively in a clockwise direction. The part of the circuit in the absolute refractory period is indicated by black, while the phase of the relative refractory period is represented by dots. The white area in the ring represents the fibers that have completely restored their excitability after the foregoing excitation.

Two prerequisites must be fulfilled to capture the im-

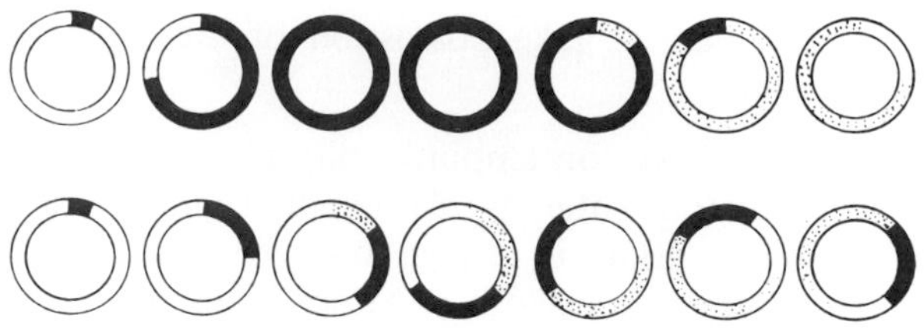

Figure 7-10. *Original diagrams drawn by Mines to illustrate the conditions under which circulating excitation can occur. The absolute refractory period is indicated in black, while the condition of depressed excitability that exists during the relative refractory period is represented by dots. (Mines, G. R.: On dynamic equilibrium in the heart. J. Physiol., 46:349–383, 1913)*

pulse in a continuous circus movement around a ring: (1) the conduction of the impulse must be blocked into one direction around the ring while it continues to propagate into the other direction, and (2) the conduction time of the impulse around the circuit must be long enough to enable each part of the ring to restore its excitability sufficiently to respond to the next impulse.

The first condition of local conduction block can arise under many circumstances, the common cause being some kind of spatial inhomogeneity in the ability to propagate an excitation wave. The second condition is emphasized in Figure 7-10.

Figure 7-10*A* depicts a situation that arises if the rate of propagation is rapid as compared with the length of the circuitous pathway or the duration of the refractory period or both. If the conduction velocity is too rapid, the circuit too small, or the refractory period too long, the impulse will return to its point of origin at a moment when the fibers have not yet recovered their excitability. Consequently, after one circuit around the ring, the excitation will die out and sustained circus movement will be prevented. However, if the dimensions of the circuit are large, if the conduction velocity is low, or if the refractory period is short, the region where the excitation started will have restored its excitability again before the impulse returns to this point of the ring; consequently, the impulse will reenter the ring for a second time (Fig. 7-10*B*). Once started in this way, the impulse may continue to circulate for many revolutions, resulting in a sustained regular rhythm, the rate of which is determined by the conduction time of the activation wave around the circuit.

Figure 7-11 summarizes the properties of such sustained circus movement in a large anatomic circuit. The main characteristics are as follows:

1. The length of the circuit is fixed, being determined by the perimeter of the anatomic structure which forms the inexcitable center of the circuit.
2. The rate of the tachycardia is given by the following equation:

   $$\text{Rate of tachycardia (beats/sec)} = \frac{\text{conduction velocity}}{\text{length of circuit}}$$

   because

   $$\text{Rate} = \frac{1}{\text{revolution time}}$$

   and

   $$\text{Revolution time} = \frac{\text{length of circuit}}{\text{conduction velocity}}$$

Thus, the rate is governed by two parameters, the length of the circuit and the average conduction velocity of the circulating impulse. When the circuit is small or the conduction velocity is high, the resulting rhythm will be fast. On the other hand, when the circuit is large or the impulse conducts slowly in all or part of the circuit, the rate of the arrhythmia will be slow.

CIRCUS MOVEMENT AROUND ANATOMIC OBSTACLE (MINES 1913)

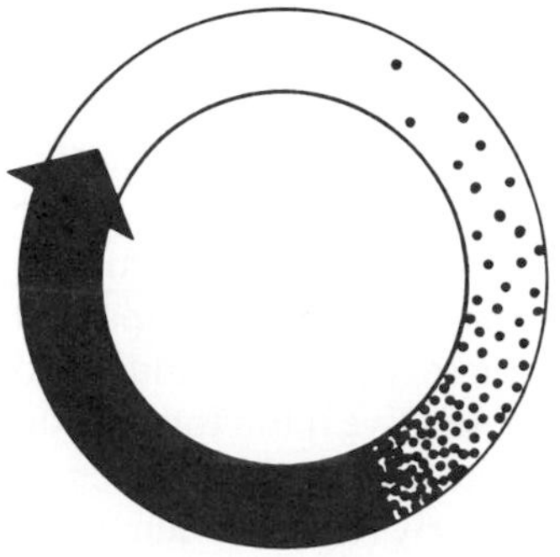

1. Length of circuit is fixed (given by perimeter of obstacle)
2. Rate of reentrant rhythm is proportional to $\frac{\text{conduction velocity}}{\text{length of circuit}}$
3. There is a gap of full excitability in the circuit (white part of the circuit)
4. Shortening of the refractory period does not affect the rate of the circus movement

Figure 7-11. *Properties of circus movement in a gross anatomic circuit.*

3. There exists an excitable gap in the circuit (see white area in Figs. 7-10 and 7-11). When the length of the circuit is longer than the wavelength of the circulating excitation wave, the fibers ahead of the circulating depolarization front have completely restored their excitability. This means that a stimulus, or approaching depolarization wave, of diastolic threshold may already interfere with this circus movement rhythm. This is significant for the behavior of this type of circus movement when confronted with wavefronts of other origin, either occurring spontaneously or induced by electrical stimulation.
4. Note that this type of circus movement is rather insensitive to changes in duration of the effective refractory period in (parts of) the ring. A shortened refractory period will further enlarge the gap of full excitability, whereas a prolonged refractory period will only narrow the excitable gap without affecting the actual rate of the tachycardia. Only after marked prolongation of the refractory period will the excitable gap be closed, and the circulating activation wave will encounter fibers that are still in their relative refractory state. This eventually will lead either to a slowing of conduction of the circulating wavefront and a concomitant slowing of the tachycardia or to termination of the arrhythmia.

Circus Movement Without the Involvement of an Anatomic Obstacle

Over the years, little attention has been paid to circus movement without the involvement of an anatomically preformed pathway. However, the question of whether an anatomic obstacle is involved has important consequences for the properties of a circus movement tachycardia.

Lewis was one of the few who realized that the behavior of circulating waves in the intact heart probably would be much more complicated than in artificial narrow rings of muscle. In his famous monograph *The Mechanism and Graphic Registration of the Heart Beat,*[34] he spends an entire chapter (Chap. XXVIII) on this subject. He gives some early theoretic considerations about the properties of circulating excitation in a simple narrow ring compared with circus movement in a sheet of muscle. Because these early ideas seem to be ignored by many later investigators, and because Lewis predicted a kind of circus movement similar to that described in this chapter, the relevant passage is given below in full.

After having described the properties of circus movement in a narrow ring, Lewis continues:

> We have been dealing, in speaking of circus movement, with a simple and narrow ring of muscle of fixed circumference; such does not exist in the auricle. It is true that there are natural rings of tissue around the mouths of the great vessels and around the auriculo-ventricular orifices, but each of these is more correctly viewed as a circular hole in a flat sheet of muscle. Thus, there is a ring adjoining the orifice; there are also outer rings, greater in circumference, at distances more removed from the orifice. These outer rings provide optional paths for the wave and introduce a new possibility, namely, change in the length of circuit travelled. Suppose that the responsive gap in a ring of tissue immediately surrounding a natural auricular orifice is represented by Figure 310*A* [see Fig. 7-12], and supposing that for some reason the refractory period becomes longer, the gap will close (Fig. 310*B*). This closure will not end the circus movement,

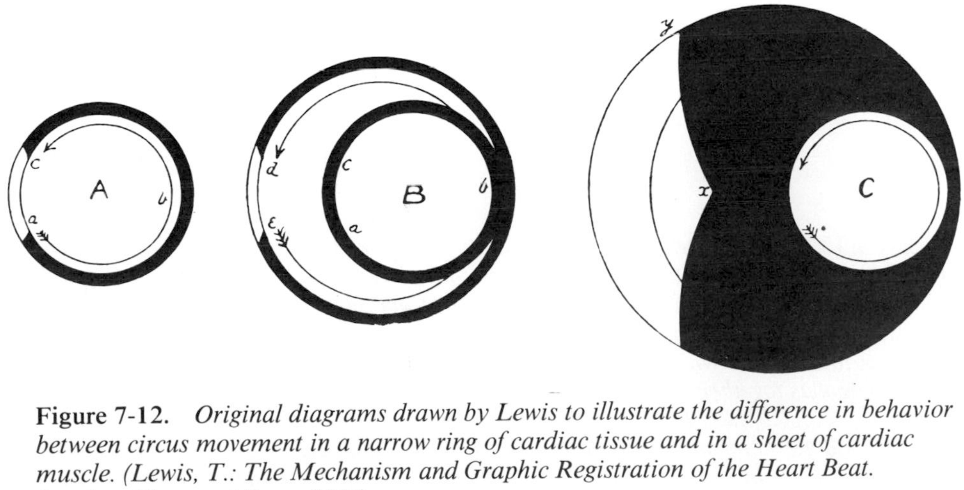

Figure 7-12. *Original diagrams drawn by Lewis to illustrate the difference in behavior between circus movement in a narrow ring of cardiac tissue and in a sheet of cardiac muscle. (Lewis, T.: The Mechanism and Graphic Registration of the Heart Beat. London, Shaw and Sons, 1925)*

providing there are longer paths open to the wave; it can still circulate and will circulate, upon such a new path if the conditions are there suitable (Fig. 310*B*). When a wave circulates around an orifice in a sheet of muscle the size of the gap will be greater if we pass from inner to outer circles of muscle, as is shown in Figure 310*C*. At any given instant the gap is represented by a wedge of tissue, its point (x) lying towards the center and its base (y-z) lying peripherally.

The conditions existing in the circle of muscle in which the gap is shortest, the circle which includes the point of this wedge in the diagram, are those which determine the rate of beating of the muscle sheet as a whole. That is to say, the rate of beating is not controlled by the length of path, providing sufficient optional paths are available, for the length of path is determined by the remaining factors. It is probable, too, that the rate of conduction in these circumstances would not influence the rate of beating, since a change in conduction would at once be balanced by an appropriate change in the length of path followed. It is impossible to visualize the precise paths followed by, and available to, a circulating wave in the auricle, but it would seem from the consideration here set forth that when a circus movement is established and *when shorter or longer paths become available, the length of the refractory period is in sole control of the rate of beating.**

Later studies have demonstrated that the central aperture, still present in the above-cited theoretic considerations, is not essential for the initiation and continuation of circus movement.[32,33,35-39] It has been demonstrated that sustained tachyarrhythmia can be electrically induced in isolated small segments of ordinary atrial muscle. The mechanism of this tachyarrhythmia was extensively studied by the authors.[32,33,39] These studies have led to the description of a second type of circus movement, the *leading circle* concept, which is completely determined by the electrophysiologic properties of cardiac tissue.

In Figures 7-13 and 7-14 the phenomenon of circus movement in the absence of an anatomic obstacle is documented. In isolated pieces of the left atrium of the rabbit (15 × 20 mm), paroxysms of a rapid regular

* Figure numbers given in Lewis's quote refer to illustrations in Lewis's book and not to illustrations in this text, except for Figure 7-12.

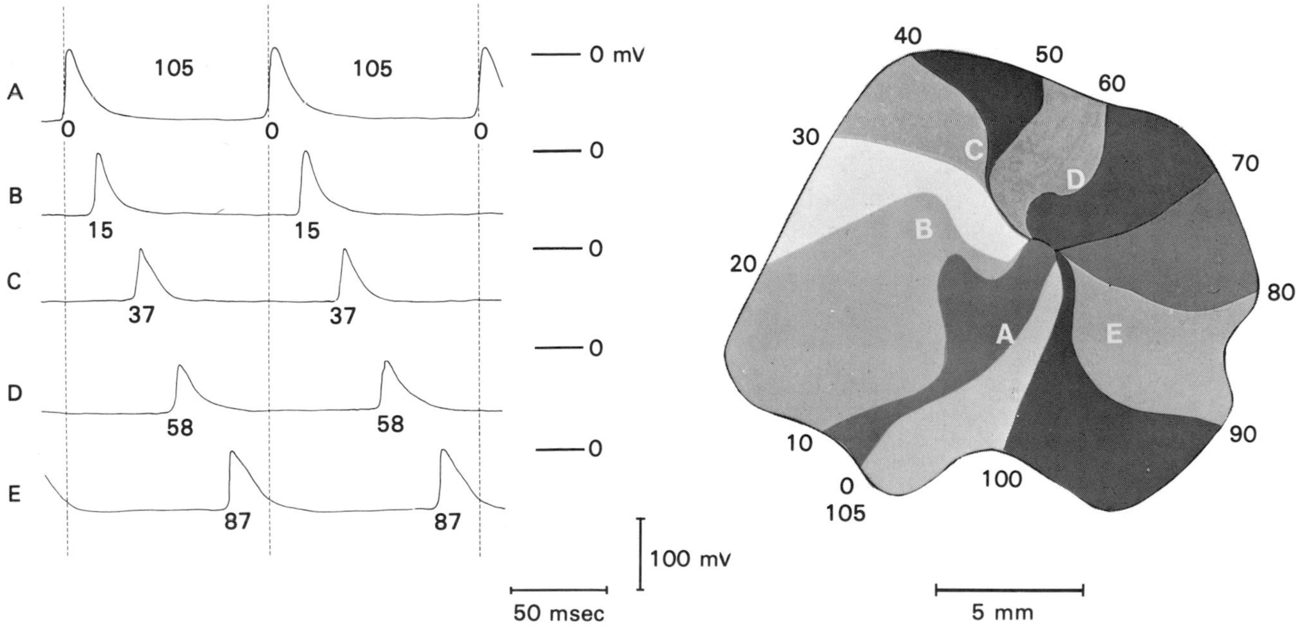

Figure 7-13. *Map of the spread of activation in a piece of isolated left atrial muscle of the rabbit during sustained flutter. The map was constructed from time measurements of the intracellular recordings of 94 different fibers. The impulse was rotating in a clockwise direction with a revolution time of 105 msec. At the left, the transmembrane potentials of 5 fibers (A to E) are shown that lie along the circular pathway. The activation times are given in milliseconds together with the action potentials and the isochronic lines of the map. (Allessie, M. A., Bonke, F. I. M., and Schopman, F. J. G.: Circus movement in rabbit atrial muscle as a mechanism of tachycardia. III. The "leading circle" concept: A new model of circus movement in cardiac tissue without the involvement of an anatomic obstacle. Circ. Res., 41:9–18, 1977. By permission of the American Heart Association, Inc.)*

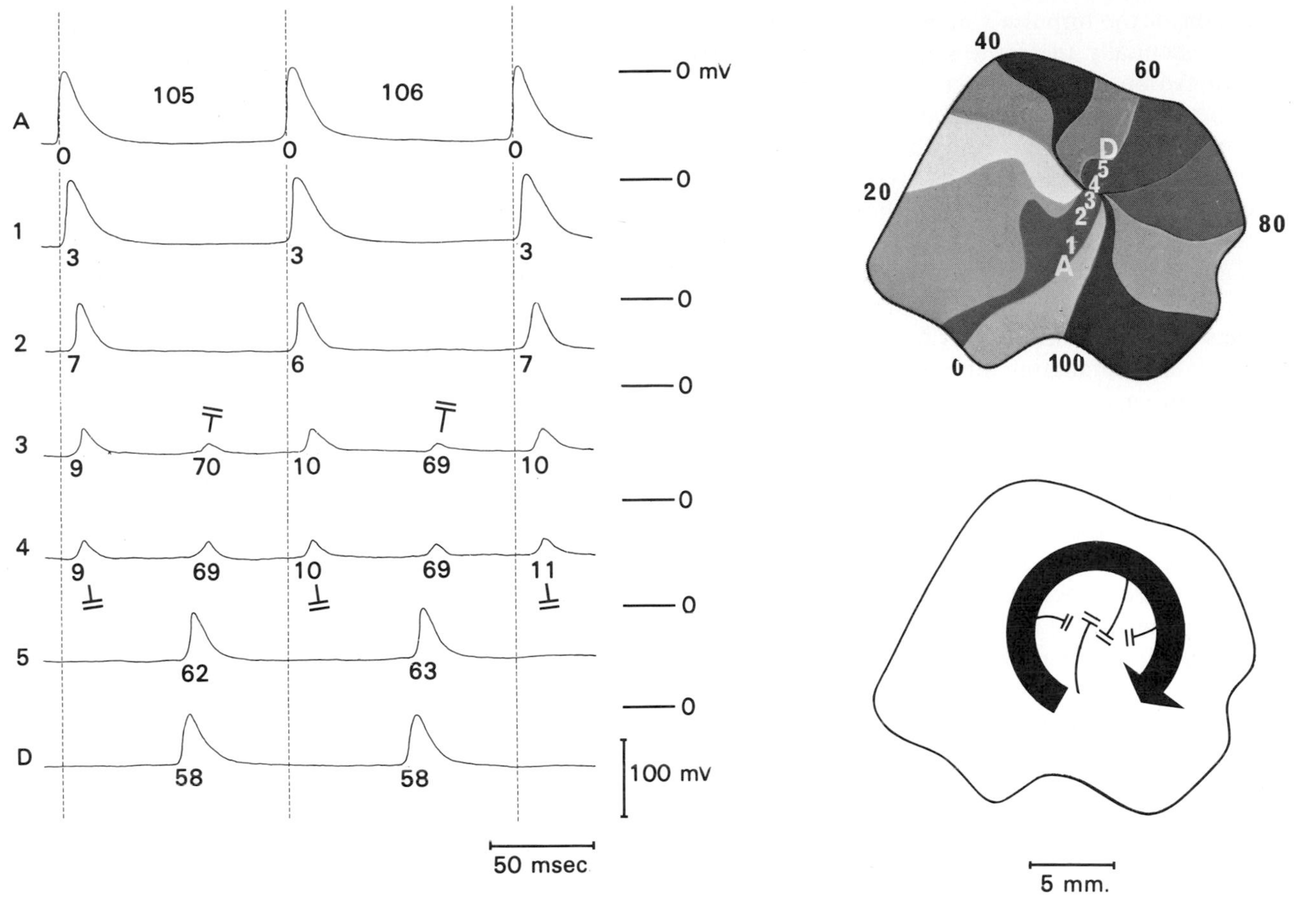

Figure 7-14. *Same experiment as in Figure 7-13. The transmembrane potentials of seven fibers (marked A, D, and 1 to 5) located on a straight line through the center of the circus movement are shown. Fibers A and D are the same as in Figure 7-13. This figure demonstrates that the central area is activated by centripetal wavelets. Note that the fibers in the central point of the circuit (fibers 3 and 4) show double responses of subnormal amplitude. Both responses are unable to propagate beyond the center, thus preventing the impulse from short-circuiting. Below the map the activation pattern is given schematically, showing the "leading circuit" with the converging wavelets in the center. Block is indicated by double bars. (Allessie, M. A., Bonke, F. I. M., and Schopman, F. J. G.: Circus movement in rabbit atrial muscle as a mechanism of tachycardia. III. The "leading circle" concept: A new model of circus movement in cardiac tissue without the involvement of an anatomic obstacle. Circ. Res., 41:9–18, 1977. By permission of the American Heart Association, Inc.)*

rhythm (rate between 400 and 800 beats/min) were produced by the induction of a single premature beat. The spread of the excitation wave in the sheet of atrial myocardium was mapped accurately both during initiation and perpetuation of atrial flutter.

In Figure 7-13 an activation map is given that was reconstructed from more than 100 intracellular recordings during a single period of sustained tachycardia. The map clearly shows a circus movement of the depolarization wave in a clockwise direction with a revolution time of 105 msec (rate 550 beats/min). The dimensions of the circuit are remarkably small. In this case the diameter can be estimated to be about 0.6 cm. Hence the total length of the circular pathway is no more than 2 cm.

Figure 7-14 shows the intracellular recordings of seven fibers located on a straight line through the center of the circuit. The most peripheral fibers lying along the circuit (*A* and *D*) are the same as in Figure 7-13. The fibers in the center are marked by numerals (*1* to *5*). As can be read from the time measurements of these fibers, the central area of the circuit is activated in a centripetal direction. From fiber *A* the impulse excites fibers *1, 2, 3,* and *4,* in that order. When penetrating deeper into the center of the vortex, the centripetal wavelets lose more and more of their "stimulating efficacy" until they are unable to excite the tissue ahead. Going from fiber *1* to *4,* amplitude, rate of rise, and duration of the responses are all gradually decreasing, finally resulting in complete extinction of the impulse somewhere between fibers *4* and *5*. Essentially the same sequence of events takes place at the opposite side of the circuit. There, half a revolution time later, the circulating impulse penetrates the center again, traveling from fiber *D* to fibers *5, 4,* and *3*. Again, the centripetal wavelet is conducted with decrement, resulting in extinction of the impulse between fibers *3* and *2*.

As a result of this course of events, the center of the vortex is continuously invaded by multiple centripetal wavelets that collide in the very center of the circuit. In this way, the circulating impulse is prevented from short-circuiting, whereas the area of converging wavelets serves as a functional "obstacle" for the impulse to turn around. In the diagram beneath the map in Figure 7-14 the sequence of excitation is summarized schematically. It can be described as a "leading" circulating wavefront that activates both the periphery and the center of this circle. It is this leading circuit that determines the rate of beating of the rest of the heart. With more than one circuit available (and a sheet of muscle can be regarded as being composed of numerous circles of different diameter), the circuit with the shortest revolution time will take the lead. In fact, the situation is highly analogous with the competition between pacemakers. There the fibers with the most rapid rate of diastolic depolarization act as the dominant pacemaker, whereas all the other optional pacemakers with a slower intrinsic rate of discharge are under the control of the fastest rhythm.

Usually the circuit with the smallest diameter will also exhibit the shortest revolution time. In the smallest possible circuit, the stimulating efficacy of the circulating wavefront is just enough to excite the tissue ahead, which is still in its relative refractory phase. In other words, on the leading circuit the head of the circulating wave is continuously biting its own tail of refractoriness.

Because of this tight fit, the length of the leading circuit is defined by, and equal to, the "wavelength" of the impulse (*i.e.,* the product of conduction velocity and refractory period). In the center of the leading circuit, dimensions are too small for sustained circus movement. Within this area a circulating impulse would encounter tissue in which excitability had not yet recovered sufficiently, and the conduction velocity of the impulse would be secondarily depressed below some minimal value where successful impulse propagation was no longer possible.

The properties of circus movement without the involvement of an anatomic obstacle are summarized in Figure 7-15. The main characteristics are as follows:

1. The dimensions of the leading circuit are not fixed but are variable, the length of the circuit being equal to the wave length of the impulse. Since the wavelength is given by the product of conduction velocity and functional refractory period, a change in either of these electrophysiologic parameters will result in a shift of the leading circle to another circuit of different dimensions. Again, this situation is highly analogous with the competition between pacemaker fibers. A shift in the pacemaker will occur if the electrophysiologic properties of pacemaker fibers (*e.g.,* phase 4 depolarization) are changed by maneuvers such as stimulation of the vagal nerves.[40] Thus, a shortening of the functional refractory period or a slowing of conduction velocity in the myocardium will result in a narrowing of the leading circuit. On the other hand, when the refractory period is long, or when the conduction velocity is fast, the minimal dimensions for a sustained circus movement will be large.
2. By definition, there is no gap of full excitability within the circuit. This implies that a stimulus, or depolarization of greater than diastolic threshold, is required to influence this type of circus movement.
3. The rate of this reentrant rhythm is inversely related to the refractory period. A shortening of the functional refractory period will enable the impulse to circulate in a smaller circuit with a shorter

CIRCUS MOVEMENT WITHOUT ANATOMIC OBSTACLE (Leading circle model)

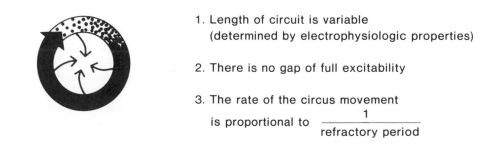

1. Length of circuit is variable (determined by electrophysiologic properties)
2. There is no gap of full excitability
3. The rate of the circus movement is proportional to $\frac{1}{\text{refractory period}}$

Figure 7-15. *Properties of circus movement without an anatomic obstacle being involved.*

revolution time, accelerating the circus rhythm. On the other hand, a prolonged refractory period will force the impulse to find a larger circular pathway, resulting in deceleration of the tachycardia. If such a larger circuit is not available, the circus movement will suddenly terminate.

Note that in contrast to circus movement around an obstacle, the rate of the functionally determined circus movement does *not* depend directly on conduction velocity, since a change in conduction velocity is immediately neutralized by a change in length of the circuitous pathway. However, when a change in conduction velocity is caused by a change in the stimulating efficacy of the impulse, an indirect effect on the rate of circus rhythm may be expected. This can be understood by realizing that a decrease of the stimulating efficacy of the depolarization wave will not only depress conduction velocity but will also prolong the functional refractory period.

Relationship of the Different Basic Mechanisms to Clinical Arrhythmias

Atrial Premature Depolarizations

Many textbooks state that atrial premature beats can occur in persons of all ages and in the absence of heart disease. However, emotional stress, fatigue, or excessive use of alcohol, tobacco, or coffee may be associated with a higher incidence of premature complexes, atrial as well as ventricular. Furthermore, premature complexes are "normal" in ischemia of the myocardium and are often seen following the use of cardiac drugs such as digitalis, quinidine, and procainamide, in which case they may indicate a toxic reaction to these drugs. The incidence of atrial premature contractions and other atrial arrhythmias is greater in distention of the atrium. Furthermore, atrial premature complexes occurring at rest often disappear during exercise. All the above should be kept in mind during the discussion of the possible underlying mechanisms of atrial premature beats.

The normal impulse formation in the sinus node is strongly influenced by the autonomic nervous system. Although vagal as well as sympathetic nerves do influence the atrial myocardium and the AV node, it is not clear whether these structures are always influenced to the same degree as the sinus node. Therefore, the automaticity in one of the subsidiary pacemakers might be fast enough to produce an impulse that activates the rest of the atrium, especially if the sinus node is under vagal influence. This hypothesis agrees with the fact that during exercise, and thus with less vagal influence, atrial premature complexes often disappear. The second possible mechanism of abnormal impulse formation, namely, the occurrence of an early afterdepolarization, is very unlikely to be the cause of atrial premature depolarizations, since it demands unusual circumstances. If such circumstances are present, a series of impulses rather than one single premature complex can be expected.

A premature atrial complex can also be induced or triggered. The studies of Wit and Cranefield[4,19] show sustained triggered activity, but it is also possible to trigger only one single impulse with the appropriate concentration of catecholamines.

Most textbooks mention a reentrant mechanism as the primary cause for atrial premature complexes. If the impulse coming from the sinus node is blocked somewhere in the atrium (the first prerequisite for reentry) and the area of block is relatively large, the area of block may be activated retrogradely, and from this region the atrium may be reentered, creating an atrial premature beat. This may occur more easily if the impulse is conducted very slowly; therefore, if the impulse on its way through the AV node is blocked in one part of the node, conduction may go on through the rest of the node and, because of slow conduction in this tissue, may retrogradely excite the area of block and reenter the atrium. In the literature this is often referred to as *return extrasystole* or *AV nodal echo beat.*

If one atrial premature beat exists, this impulse can set the stage for another reentry either in the atrium or through the AV node or the sinus node. Therefore, a premature impulse coming from the atrium may invade part of the sinus node while the entrance to other parts of the sinus node is blocked. The impulse can then find a way through the slowly conducting tissue of the sinus node and find an exit to the atrium that has meanwhile restored its excitability. The impulse then reenters the atrium. The existence of such a sinus echo has recently been demonstrated by Allessie and Bonke.[31] The same is possible in the AV node, as was demonstrated experimentally by Moe and co-workers[28] and Mendez and Moe[41] and clinically by Schuilenburg and Durrer.[42] In general, a reentrant mechanism is well reconciled with a fixed coupling interval of atrial premature beats.

Atrial Tachycardia

If the impulse generation in the dominant pacemaker in the sinus node is enhanced, for instance because of a high sympathetic activity, sinus tachycardia will occur. If the impulse formation outside the sinus node is enhanced, atrial or nodal tachycardia will be present. This is demonstrated in Figure 7-3. The rate of such atrial tachycardias will increase if catecholamines are administered, whereas it will slow down or even be interrupted by acetylcholine or vagal stimulation (carotid sinus massage).

Sustained rhythmic activity may be induced or triggered by a relatively rapid sinus nodal or atrial rhythm as well as by a premature atrial beat. Triggering will only occur if catecholamines are present and therefore depends on the equilibrium of the autonomic nervous system. Furthermore, the rate of such a tachycardia will diminish or the tachycardia may even be stopped by the administration of acetylcholine and also by a drug such as verapamil. Also, triggered rhythmic activity not only can be started but also can be stopped by a single premature complex.

From a theoretic point of view, the third possible cause of abnormal impulse formation, namely, the occurrence of early afterdepolarizations, may induce a rapid-firing atrial focus. However, under normal conditions this is very unlikely. Theoretically, tachycardias based on this mechanism will be stopped by the administration of acetylcholine (or vagal stimulation) because this will increase membrane conductance for potassium and therefore repolarize the fibers. Thus, acetylcholine will not enable the clinician to distinguish among tachycardias.

The underlying mechanism for supraventricular tachycardia may also be a circus movement of the impulse. However, if the circuit of the circus movement is purely within the atrial myocardium, the length of such a pathway should be between 20 and 26 cm, assuming a mean conduction velocity of the impulse in the atrium during tachycardia of about 60 cm/sec (normally during sinus rhythm this will be between 60 and 100 cm/sec) and a rate of the tachycardia between 140 and 180 beats/min. These long circuits are very unlikely in the atrium. On the other hand, if part of the circuit has properties of slow conduction, the circuit may be considerably smaller, and this will make a circus movement as a cause of atrial tachycardia much more probable. Slow conduction will be present if the sinus node or the AV node is part of the circuit. In these cases the terminology of *sinus nodal reentrant tachycardia* or *AV junctional tachycardia* is used. Both kinds of tachycardia can frequently be slowed down or even converted to sinus rhythm by carotid sinus massage. This agrees with the fact that acetylcholine slows down or even blocks conduction in the SA or AV node.

Tachycardia based on a circus movement can be started or terminated by a single premature beat. Since this is the case for "triggered" sustained rhythmicity as well, it is not a good way to distinguish between these two mechanisms.

Therefore, if a patient has (paroxysmal) supraventricular tachycardia, enhanced automaticity, triggered activity, and circus movement must be considered, and it may be difficult to distinguish among these possible mechanisms.

Atrial Flutter

Atrial flutter has never been satisfactorily defined. Lewis[34] emphasized that a high degree of regularity in both beat-to-beat interval and configuration of the atrial complexes in the electrocardiogram is the most prominent characteristic of atrial flutter. Realizing that the boundaries between atrial tachycardia and atrial flutter are not very sharp and that the rates of the two arrhythmias may overlap, atrial flutter can be defined as any regular atrial rhythm faster than 200 beats/min. This is a rather wide definition, and subdivision of atrial flutter into different types is helpful. On the basis of the polarity of the flutter waves, Lewis[34] distinguished a "common" form of atrial flutter with F waves inverted in leads II, III, and aV_F and upright in lead aV_R and an "uncommon" form with F waves upright in leads II, III, and aV_F and inverted in lead aV_R. No differences in rate have been found between these two types of flutter.[43] Because of the similarity between the F waves during uncommon flutter and P waves during subsequent sinus rhythm, it has been suggested that uncommon flutter arises from the high right atrium. However, many examples of clinical atrial flutter can be found with F waves somewhere intermediate between the two extreme forms representing common and uncommon flutter.

Recently Wells and colleagues[1] distinguished two different types of atrial flutter primarily based on differences in atrial rate. They divided 27 patients developing atrial flutter after open-heart surgery into two groups. Group I consisted of 18 patients with classic (common) atrial flutter with an atrial rate ranging from 240 to 338 beats/min. In group II (nine patients) the atrial rates ranged from 340 to 433 beats/min. Both types of flutter were characterized by a strikingly constant beat-to-beat interval, morphology, polarity, and amplitude of the atrial electrograms. The authors separated atrial flutter into two categories because they observed that rapid atrial pacing from the high right atrium always influenced type I flutter[2] but never influenced type II flutter. Conversion of atrial flutter by rapid pacing or reset of the flutter cycle with a properly timed single stimulus strongly points to the existence of a reentry circuit with an excitable gap.[44–46] Thus the slower examples of atrial flutter (type I) should be based on circus movement including an appreciable excitable gap. On the other hand, failure to interrupt type II flutter by overdrive pacing suggests that the excitable gap is either very small or absent, resulting in effective shielding of the circuit from interference with oncoming activation waves.

There is considerable experimental evidence that circus movement around an anatomic obstacle can cause atrial flutter. This concept was first introduced by Lewis and co-workers[47] on the basis of multiple record-

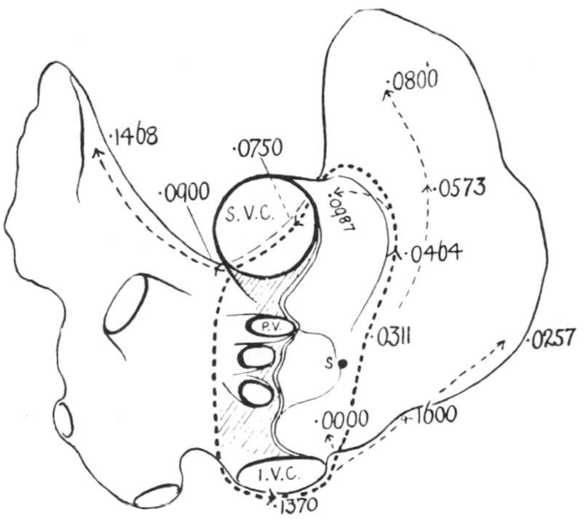

Figure 7-16. *The spread of excitation in the atria of a dog, measured by Lewis and co-workers, during a period of electrically induced atrial flutter. Local activation times are expressed as parts of a second, and the broken lines and arrows indicate the course taken by the excitation wave. Note that recordings were not obtained at the left side of the entrances of the caval veins.* **S** *marks the point that was originally stimulated to induce flutter. (Lewis, T., Feil, H. S., and Stroud, W. D.: Observations upon flutter and fibrillation. II. Nature of auricular flutter. Heart, 7:191–245, 1920)*

ings during long-lasting periods of atrial flutter induced by weak faradic stimulation of the auricle. Figure 7-16 shows the spread of the excitation process during such a period of atrial flutter. A large part of the pathway taken by the activation waves could be identified by this method. During one cycle of the flutter (beat-to-beat interval, 0.16 second), the wave travels from the inferior cava up along the crista terminalis and to the right auricular appendage. It then turns around the orifice of the superior cava and passes along the interatrial band to the left atrium; a little later a new wave appears behind the inferior cava, and the same sequence of activation is repeated. However, as Lewis himself emphasized: "It remains to ascertain if this new wave is a continuation of the old one; if so, than a circus movement is proved."

Unfortunately, direct measurements along the left side of the entrances of the caval veins were not obtained, but on the basis of indirect evidence Lewis decided that "there remains little doubt that we are dealing with a wave moving around the cavae, the movement being continuous and completes once during each auricular cycle."

Later studies show the same conclusion.[48–51] The studies of Kimura and co-workers[49] supplied complementary data on the spread of excitation at the left side of the venae cavae, where Lewis was unable to take records. Figure 7-17 shows the complete map of the pathway of the excitation wave during flutter. The results confirm Lewis's conclusions. The involvement of artificial or pathologic obstacles in atrial flutter was emphasized by Rosenblueth and Garcia Ramos[48] and later by Kimura and co-workers.[49] These authors found that crushing the conducting bridge between the two venae cavae, which converted the two orifices into a single obstacle, markedly facilitated the induction of flutter by rapid stimulation. Further enlargement of the obstacle decreased the rate of flutter. When the lesion was extended to the auriculoventricular groove (*i.e.*, as soon as the obstacle was no longer entirely surrounded by conducting tissue), the flutter suddenly terminated and could no longer be reinitiated. However, more anatomically defined circuits exist in the atria. A list of the possible anatomic circuits

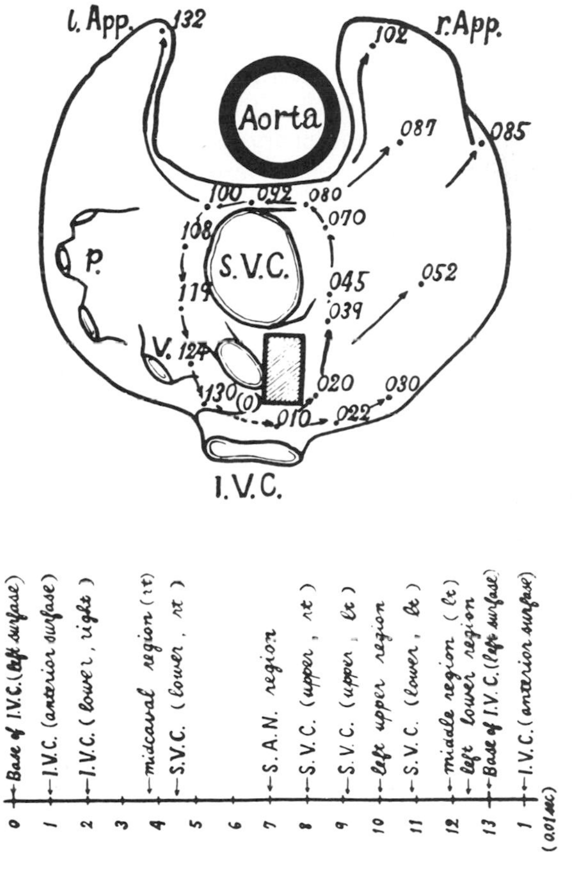

Figure 7-17. *Recordings taken during atrial flutter induced by rapid stimulation of the left appendage. To facilitate the induction of atrial flutter, the conducting bridge between the two venae cavae was crushed. In this study, the left side of the caval veins was also mapped. It is demonstrated that the impulse turns around the superior vena cava and a right pulmonary vein. The revolution time is 0.13 second. A chart is given below the map, showing the time relation of the different recording sites during one cycle of the flutter. (Kimura, E., Kato, K., Murao, S., et al.: Experimental studies on the mechanism of the auricular flutter. Tohoku J. Exp. Med., 60:197–207, 1954)*

in the human atria, together with the estimated length of the pathways, is given below.[52]

1. Circuit around the orifices of all atrial veins (superior vena cava [SVC], inferior vena cava [IVC], left and right pulmonary veins) — 26 cm
2. Around SVC, IVC, and right pulmonary veins — 23 cm
3. Around IVC and right pulmonary veins — 20 cm
4. Around SVC and right pulmonary veins — 18 cm
5. Around SVC and IVC — 18 cm
6. Around right and left pulmonary veins — 17 cm
7. Around SVC and upper right pulmonary veins — 16 cm
8. Around IVC and lower right pulmonary veins — 16 cm
9. Around right pulmonary veins — 12 cm
10. Around left pulmonary veins — 12 cm
11. Around tricuspid orifice — 12 cm
12. Around mitral orifice — 12 cm
13. Around SVC — 9 cm
14. Around IVC — 9 cm
15. Around one pulmonary vein — 3 cm–6 cm

In the above list, pathways course around a combination of cardiac veins. Such long loops do not exist in a normal heart, since the intact muscle bands between the orifices of the veins will short-circuit these loops.

However, when the atria are diseased, for instance by coronary artery disease or mitral stenosis, and the conduction properties in (parts of) the atrial myocardium are lost, large circuits may result, either by a loss of excitability in the muscle bands between two or more veins or by the presence of hypoplastic or fibrotic areas lying as an island in the myocardium or in close opposition to one of the natural openings in the atria.

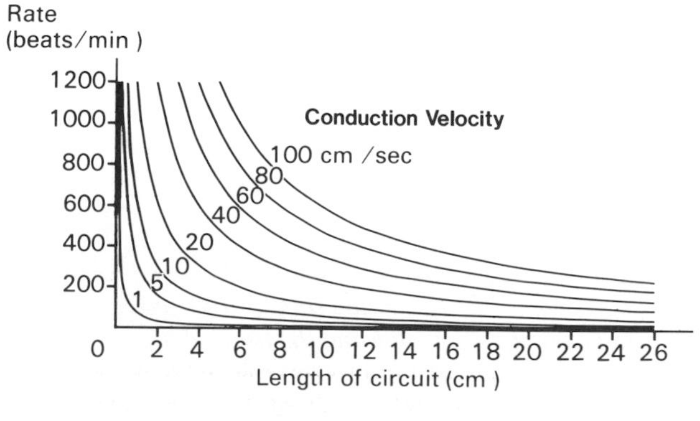

Figure 7-18. *Graph relating the rate of a circus movement to the length of the circuitous pathway at different conduction velocities of the impulse.*

Figure 7-18 shows a graph relating the length of a given circuit to the rate of the related reentrant rhythm as calculated for different conduction velocities. From this graph it can be seen that at the normal conduction velocity in the atrium of 70 cm/sec, to get a tachyarrhythmia that is classified as atrial flutter the length of the circuit must be between 12 and 20 cm. Such long pathways are not available in the normal heart. On the other hand, when the conduction velocity of the impulse in the atrial myocardium is decreased to, for instance, 40 cm/sec, an obstacle with a perimeter of only 9 cm may be adequate to serve as a center for circus movement with a rate of 300 beats/min.

Recently the activation during acetylcholine-induced rapid atrial flutter has been mapped in the isolated canine heart.[53] Figure 7-19 has been taken from this study. In all cases atrial flutter was based on continuous circus movement of the impulse in the atrial myocardium. However, the localization and dimensions of the circuit differed from case to case. In most cases a gross anatomic obstacle was not involved in this type of atrial flutter.

Atrial Fibrillation

The most likely mechanism underlying fibrillation of the atria is the presence of multiple circus movements of the leading circle type. According to this theory, in "coarse" fibrillation the number of circuits will be small and circuit dimension relatively large, whereas in "fine" fibrillation numerous circuits of small dimension may exist. Conditions that facilitate the induction of atrial fibrillation, such as vagal stimulation, rapid pacing, distention of the atria, ischemia, and the presence of conduction disturbances, all cause shortening of the refractory period, lowering of conduction velocity, or both and thus a shortening of the dimension of a leading circuit. If there exists one single circus movement as cause of atrial flutter, shortening of the minimum dimension of that circuit (*e.g.*, by vagal stimulation) creates a situation in which there is room for more than one circuit. As soon as a second or third circuit is established, flutter converts into fibrillation. As the conditions that favored the initiation of multiple small circuits wane, the small circuits may die out one after the other, and fibrillation may convert to flutter again if a single circus movement remains, or, if not, fibrillation will be terminated completely and sinus rhythm will resume. Because of the complexity of the above-described situation, no one has been able to analyze the activation of the atria during fibrillation. However, in a computer simulation, Moe and co-workers[54–56] succeeded in producing fibrillation in a mathematic two-dimensional area or in a closed surface without holes. In this model, multiple circulating wavefronts were shown to occur during fibrillation: "reentry oc-

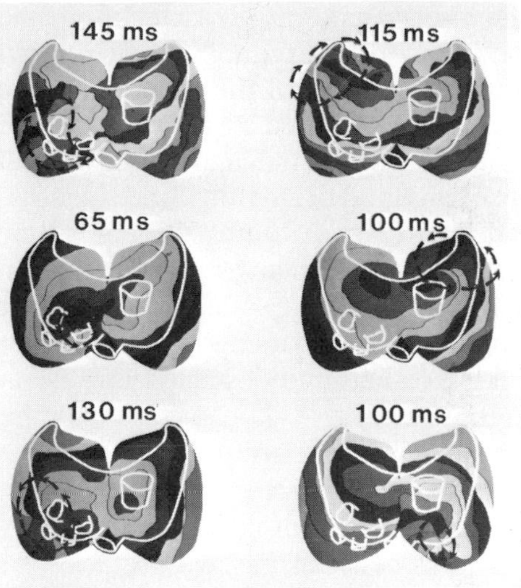

Figure 7-19. *Atrial excitation maps of six different cases of rapid atrial flutter. In all cases atrial flutter was based on intra-atrial reentry. There was marked variation in both the rate of the flutter and the localization of the circuit responsible for the arrhythmia. In the upper left panel the circuit (cycle length = 145 msec) was found in the inferolateral wall of the left atrium. In the upper right panel the impulse circulated around the left atrial appendage with a revolution time of 115 msec. The extremely rapid flutter shown in the middle left panel (cycle length = 65 msec) was based on a circuit in the posterior wall of the left atrium. The episodes of the other three cases of atrial flutter were caused by an intra-atrial circuit located around the right atrial appendage (middle right panel), in the free wall of the left atrium (lower left panel), and in the posterior right atrium (lower right panel), respectively. Estimated circuit size varied between 5 and 10 cm. Each shade of gray represents an isochrone of 10 msec. (Allessie M. A., et al.: Circulation, in press. By permission of the American Heart Association, Inc.)*

curred over numerous loops of varying size and position, wandering over the excitable surface like eddies in a turbulent pool."

If fibrillation is caused by the presence of multiple circulating wavelets, its persistence is a matter of statistical probability. Circus movement without the involvement of an anatomic obstacle is not a very stable phenomenon; as a rule, spontaneous termination occurs after a shorter or longer period.[32] However, if many circuits exist, it is unlikely they will stop at the same time. The crucial factor for induction and termination of fibrillation is the *dimension of the heart relative to the dimension of the smallest possible circuit in the myocardium.* If the heart is large or the dimension of a functionally determined circuit is small, many circuits can exist in the heart and the statistical chance for spontaneous termination of fibrillation is low. On the other hand, if the heart is small or the dimension of the "leading circuit" is large, the heart can accommodate only a limited number of circuits, and in this situation the probability of conversion of fibrillation to sinus rhythm is great. According to this concept, interventions that either decrease the dimension of the heart (diminishing of the atrial distention) or increase the dimension of a functionally determined circuit (drugs that increase refractory period or conduction velocity or both) will decrease the chance for induction of fibrillation and increase the probability of its spontaneous termination.

A Unified Concept of Intra-Atrial Reentry as a Basis for Atrial Flutter and Fibrillation

We postulate that all cases of clinical atrial flutter and fibrillation are based on a reentrant mechanism, since any positive proof for a different mechanism is lacking. The evidence in favor of a focus of some form of rapid automaticity is either exclusively based on experiments performed with aconitine, or, in the case of triggered activity, the rate of abnormal impulse generation is too slow to account for atrial flutter or fibrillation. There is no doubt that topical application of aconitine produces rapid abnormal automaticity in the atrium, precipitating atrial flutter or fibrillation.[7] However, this cannot be regarded as evidence that in clinical flutter a similar mechanism is operative. Triggered activity has been elicited in several parts of the heart under a variety of circumstances.[3–6,18–20] However, the rate of this abnormal rhythm is usually about 140 beats/min and rarely exceeds 200 beats/min. Another argument that speaks against triggered activity as a mechanism for atrial flutter or fibrillation is the observation that delayed afterdepolarizations and sustained triggered activity are inhibited by acetylcholine,[4] whereas in human atrial flutter or fibrillation the rate of the F waves either remains unchanged or is accelerated by vagal stimulation.[57–58] Furthermore, study of the electrophysiologic properties of pieces of diseased atrium taken from patients exhibiting atrial arrhythmias failed to demonstrate the presence of rapid automaticity in diseased atrial myocardium.[14,21]

In considering circus movement in the atria as cause for atrial flutter and fibrillation, many possibilities exist. At one end is circus movement around a large anatomic obstacle; at the other is the possibility of a small functional intramyocardial circuit without an excitable gap, originally identified in isolated pieces of rabbit myocardium[32,33,39] and later confirmed in the canine heart.[53] Between these two extremes a wide variety of intermediate types of reentry of various sizes and with different excitable gaps may exist. The presence of diseased atrial tissue with abnormal electrophysiologic properties may further add to the complexity of intra-atrial circus movement in patients.

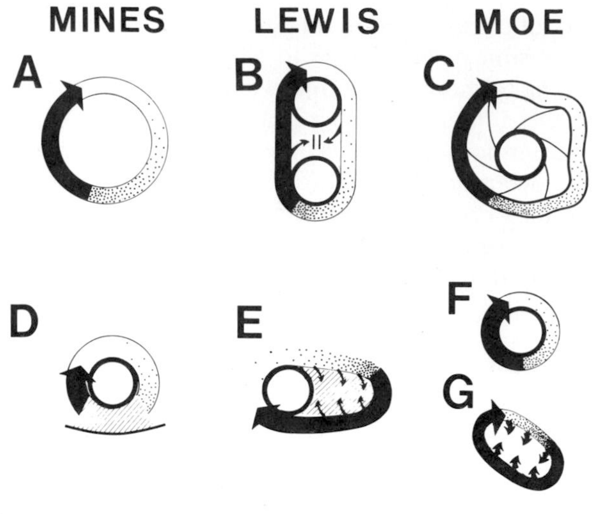

Figure 7-20. *Schematic representation of various possible types of circus movement in the atria. The black arrow represents the crest of a circulating depolarization wave with the area that is in the absolute refractory phase in its wake. The dotted area indicates the tail of relative refractory tissue. In A circus movement around a gross anatomic obstacle as introduced by Mines[25] is given. Essential characteristics of this model are the presence of an excitable gap (white part of the circuit) and the fact that the size and location of the reentrant pathway are anatomically determined. In B circus movement around the orifices of two (or more) veins, as suggested by Lewis[34] to be responsible for atrial flutter, is given. The main difference with the model in A is the presence of a bridge of conductive tissue between the two obstacles through which shortcut of the circuit can take place. Panel C shows the model of circus movement, as recently introduced by Moe and colleagues,[59] in which the impulse is thought to circulate in a loop composed of atrial bundles exhibiting a faster conduction velocity than the atrial tissue within the loop. The types of circus movement diagrammed in D and E are based on a combination of an anatomic obstacle and an adjacent area of diseased atrium exhibiting depressed conduction (hatched area). In F circus movement around a relatively small obstacle has become possible because of alterations in the refractory period and the conduction velocity, resulting in a shortening of the wavelength of the impulse. Panel G depicts circus movement without the involvement of an anatomic obstacle.[33,53] This kind of intra-atrial reentry is completely determined by the electrophysiologic properties of the myocardium. The impulse is circulating around a functional arc of conduction block. The rate of the resulting arrhythmia is the highest of all models of circus movement summarized in this figure. However, its dimension is the smallest, the length of the circular pathway being equal to the length of the excitation wave itself. (Allessie, M. A., et al.: Circulation, 70:123–135, 1985. By permission of the American Heart Association, Inc.)*

Figure 7-20 diagrams various types of intra-atrial circus movement. Panel *A* shows the earliest model of circus movement, introduced by Mines in 1913.[25] It is the simplest model of reentry, in which the impulse continuously encircles a large anatomic obstacle. Implicit to this model is the existence of an excitable gap (white part of the circuit) between the crest of the excitation wave and its tail of refractoriness (dotted area). The presence of such an excitable gap explains the high degree of regularity and stability of this kind of rhythm. Since the studies of Rosenblueth and Garcia Ramos,[48] there is little doubt that by creating a large obstacle in the atria, atrial flutter based on this mechanism can be produced. The problem, however, is that in patients suffering from atrial flutter, such large anatomic obstacles have never actually been demonstrated.

In panel *B* circus movement around two obstacles (*e.g.*, the venae cavae) as popularized by Lewis[34] is given schematically. A functional arc of conduction block is assumed in the isthmus between the two obstacles. As long as the excitable gap remains *shorter* than the circumference of the *smallest* of the two obstacles, short-circuit of the circulating impulse through the interobstacle band is prevented and the flutter rate is determined by the revolution time of the impulse around both obstacles. The behavior of this type of reentry is identical to the model given in panel *A*, with one exception. As soon as the excitable gap gets larger than the perimeter of the smallest obstacle, the impulse can shortcut the circuit. This may result in sudden termination of flutter (an event that occurred so frequently in Lewis's experiments that it almost invariably prevented complete mapping of the excitation of the atria) or, when the impulse continues to circulate around the larger obstacle, cause the flutter to accelerate abruptly. When other parts of the atria cannot follow the higher rate, degeneration into atrial fibrillation will occur.

In another attempt to overcome the problem that natural obstacles in the atria do not seem to be large enough to allow for sustained circus movement, Moe and collaborators[59] modified the early model of Mines by taking into account differences in conduction velocity in the atrium. In Moe's model (panel *C*) the role of rapidly conducting muscle bundles (*e.g.*, the internodal bands and the bundle of Bachmann) is emphasized. The idea is that the internodal pathways forming closed loops may serve as preferential circuits through which flutter waves may circulate. The greater conduction velocity in these muscle bundles would abandon the necessity for a large physical obstacle. For instance, by assuming that the conduction velocity in a loop of internodal bands is twice as rapid as in normal myocardium, the *effective* perimeter of any natural opening present within that loop will be doubled.

In panels *D* and *E* we propose some additional variants of intra-atrial circus movement that may be responsible for common atrial flutter in humans. They are based on a *combination* of a physical obstacle and an adjacent area of diseased tissue. In panel *D* an area of depressed conduction is assumed in the inferior atrium between an internal obstacle (*e.g.,* a pulmonary vein or the inferior vena cava) and the atrioventricular ring. Assume that the circumference of the internal obstacle is 9 cm, and let the shortest possible cycle length of a sustained atrial rhythm be 140 msec at a conduction velocity of 70 cm/sec. If the obstacle is completely surrounded by healthy tissue, circus movement around the obstacle would be impossible because the impulse would complete a full cycle within 130 msec, 10 msec less than the atrial fibers need to restore their excitability. However, if one third of the loop in the isthmus between the internal obstacle and the anulus fibrosis consists of depressed atrial tissue with a conduction velocity of 30 cm/sec, it would take the impulse 190 msec to travel around the orifice. Not only would the rate of such reentrant rhythm be within the range of common atrial flutter, but it would most likely be stable and long lasting because now in the healthy segment of the circuit exists an excitable gap of 50 msec.

In panel *E* a functional arc of conduction block extends to an internal anatomic obstacle. The revolution time in such a circular pathway may be long enough to create an excitable gap in the normal atrial myocardium. Only at the free end of the arc of conduction block is there a tight fit between the crest of the circulating depolarization wave and its tail of refractoriness. This functionally determined turning point is the only unstable part of the circuit. During subsequent cycles the impulse may pivot at slightly different points, resulting in minor variations in size and cycle length of the circuit. However, the localization of the circuit will be fixed and the resulting flutter could last for a long period.

Another way to facilitate intra-atrial reentry is shortening of the wavelength of the impulse. The wavelength is defined as the distance traveled by the impulse during the time equal to the functional refractory period. When this occurs, the size of natural openings in the atria may suffice as central anatomic obstacles for stable circus movement (panel *F*). Conditions that shorten the excitation wave also favor circus movement without involving any physical obstacle. Relatively small arcs of functional conduction block that may arise during atrial premature beats or rapid pacing may then be sufficiently large to permit rapid self-sustained reentry (panel *G*).

When the different types of circus movement are compared with the different atrial tachyarrhythmias, the following concepts are evident:

1. Intra-atrial reentry without the involvement of an anatomic obstacle (panel *G*) generates the fastest possible atrial rhythm. If only one circuit is present and the rest of the atria can follow the high rate in a 1:1 way, rapid atrial flutter will result. The episodes of acetylcholine-induced atrial flutter analyzed in the present studies were based on this type of reentry. Most of the rapid atrial flutters found after cardiac surgery[1] are probably based on this mechanism. In our experiments, rapid atrial flutter was not a very stable arrhythmia. Because of the absence of a clear excitable gap, the chances for conduction block of the circulating impulse, leading to sudden termination of flutter, are rather high. Another reason why this rhythm was not stable for prolonged periods is that because of the extremely high rate, degeneration into atrial fibrillation may easily occur.
2. The same type of intra-atrial circus movement (around a functional arc of conduction block) is the basic element underlying atrial fibrillation. Atrial fibrillation may result from two different mechanisms. One possibility is that a *single* intramyocardial circuit is operative whose circulation rate is so high that it causes conduction disturbances in other parts of the atria. In fact, this kind of fibrillation is more adequately described as *rapid flutter with fibrillatory conduction.* The other type of atrial fibrillation ("true fibrillation") is based on the presence of multiple wandering wavelets.[54]
3. We do not believe that reentry without an anatomic obstacle is responsible for the slower type of atrial flutter. Not only would the rate of this type of reentry be higher than the rate of common atrial flutter, but the absence of an appreciable excitable gap excludes that such rhythm can persist for weeks, months, or even years. Recent evidence shows that an excitable gap of about 15% to 25% of the flutter cycle exists in human atrial flutter.[43–46] The crucial point to be elucidated about the mechanism of classic atrial flutter is which electrophysiologic or structural abnormalities create the appropriate conditions for an excitable gap. Catheter mapping and programmed electrical stimulation during atrial flutter point to an area of slow conduction located somewhere in the inferior atrium. Puech[43] noted an isthmus of slow conduction in the inferior right atrium in the vicinity of the coronary sinus: "la partie occulte de la depolarisation auriculaire droite correspond au front d'onde d'excitation qui occupe le bas fond de l'oreillette entre la partie externe et basse de la paroi anterieure et la septum interauriculaire." Using programmed electrical stimulation, Inoue and colleagues[45] and Disertori and colleagues[46] reported that the degree of reset of the flutter cycle by the application of a single premature stimulus depended on both the site of stimulation and the site of recording. Together with the studies of Leier and associates[60] and Cosio and associates[61] who showed that clinical atrial flutter is associated with depressed atrial conduction, these observations make us believe that common atrial flutter can

best be understood by a special interplay between the anatomy of the atria and the presence of abnormal electrophysiologic properties at some strategic areas (see Fig. 7-20 *D* and *E*).

References

1. Wells, J. L., Maclean W. A. H., James, T. N., and Waldo, A. L.: Characterization of atrial flutter. Studies in man after open heart surgery using fixed atrial electrodes. Circulation, 60:665–673, 1979.
2. Waldo, A. L., Maclean, W. A. H., Karp, R. B., et al.: Entrainment and interruption of atrial flutter with atrial pacing. Studies in man following open heart surgery. Circulation, 56:737–745, 1977.
3. Hashimoto, K., and Moe, G. K.: Transient depolarizations induced by acetylstrophantidin in specialized tissue of dog atrium and ventricle. Circ. Res., 32:618–624, 1973.
4. Wit, A. L., and Cranefield, P. F.: Triggered and automatic activity in the canine coronary sinus. Circ. Res., 41:435–445, 1977.
5. Cranefield, P. F.: The Conduction of the Cardiac Impulse. New York, Futura, 1975.
6. Cranefield, P. F.: Action potentials, afterpotentials and arrhythmias. Circ. Res., 41:415–423, 1977.
7. Scherf, D.: Studies on auricular tachycardia caused by aconitine administration. Proc. Soc. Exp. Biol. Med., 64:233–239, 1947.
8. Matsuda, K., Hoshi, T., and Kameyama, S.: Effects of aconinitine on the cardiac membrane potential of the dog. Jpn. J. Physiol. 9:419–429, 1959.
9. Schmidt, R. F.: Versuch mit Aconitin zum Problem der spontanen Erregungsbildung im Herzen. Pfluegers Arch., 271:526–536, 1960.
10. Peper, K., and Trautwein, W.: The effect of aconitine on the membrane current in cardiac muscle. Pfluegers Arch., 296:328–336, 1967.
11. Lenfant, J., Mironneau, J., and Aka J. K.: Activitẽ rẽpẽtitive de la fibre sino-auriculaire de grenouille: analyse des courants membranaire responsables de l'automatisme cardiaque. J. Physiol. (Paris), 64:5–18, 1972.
12. Imanishi, S., and Surawicz, B.: Automatic activity in depolarized guinea pig ventricular myocardium. Characteristics and mechanisms. Circ. Res., 39:751–759, 1976.
13. Katzung, B. G.: Effects of extracellular calcium and sodium on depolarization-induced automaticity in guinea pig papillary muscle. Circ. Res., 37:118–127, 1975.
14. Hordof, A. J., Edie, R., Malm, J., et al.: Electrophysiologic properties and response to pharmacologic agents of fibers from diseased human atria. Circulation, 54:774–779, 1976.
15. Rosen, M. R., and Reder, R. F.: Does triggered activity have a role in the genesis of cardiac arrhythmias? Ann. Intern. Med. 94:794–801, 1981.
16. Hordof, A. J., Spotnitz, A., Mary-Rabine, L., et al.: The cellular electrophysiologic effects of digitalis on human atrial fibers. Circulation, 57:223–229, 1978.
17. Saito, T., Otoguro, M., and Matsubara, T.: Electrophysiological studies on the mechanisms of electrically induced sustained rhythmic activity in the rabbit right atrium. Circ. Res., 42:199–206, 1978.
18. Wit, A. L., Fenoglio, J. J., Wagner, B. M., and Bassett, A. L.: Electrophysiological properties of cardiac muscle in the anterior mitral valve leaflet and the adjacent atrium in the dog: possible implications for the genesis of atrial dysrhythmias. Circ. Res., 32:731–745, 1973.
19. Wit, A. L., and Cranefield, P. F.: Triggered activity in cardiac muscle fibers of the simian mitral valve. Circ. Res., 38:85–98, 1976.
20. Wit, A. L., Fenoglio, J. J., Hordof, A. J., and Reemtsma, K.: Ultrastructure and transmembrane potentials of cardiac muscle in the human anterior mitral valve leaflet. Circulation, 59:1284–1292, 1979.
21. Mary-Rabine, L., Hordof, A. J., Danilo, P., et al.: Mechanisms for impulse initiation in isolated human atrial fibers. Circ. Res., 47:267–277, 1980.
22. Hoffman, B. F., and Rosen, M. R.: Cellular mechanisms for cardiac arrhythmias. Circ. Res., 49:1–15, 1981.
23. McWilliam, J. A.: Fibrillar contraction of the heart. J. Physiol., 8:296–310, 1887.
24. Mayer, A. G.: Rhythmical Pulsation in Scyphomedusae, Pub. no. 47. Washington, D. C., Carnegie Institution, 1906.
25. Mines, G. R.: On dynamic equilibrium in the heart. J. Physiol., 46:349–383, 1913.
26. Mines, G. R.: On circulating excitations in heart muscles and their possible relation to tachycardia and fibrillation. Trans. R. Soc. Canad. Section IV, 43–53, 1914.
27. Garrey, W. E.: The nature of fibrillary contraction of the heart. Its relation to tissue mass and form. Am. J. Physiol., 33:397–414, 1914.
28. Moe, G. K., Preston, J. B., and Burlington, H.: Physiologic evidence for a dual AV transmission system. Circ. Res., 4:357–375, 1956.
29. Janse, M. J., Van Capelle, F. J. L., Freud, G. E., and Durrer, D.: Circus movement within the AV node as a basis for supraventricular tachycardia as shown by multiple microelectrode recordings in the isolated rabbit heart. Circ. Res., 28:403–414, 1971.
30. Han, J., Malozzi, A. M., and Moe, G. K.: Sinoatrial reciprocation in the isolated rabbit heart. Circ. Res., 44:355–362, 1968.
31. Allessie, M. A., and Bonke, F. I. M.: Direct demonstration of sinus node reentry in the rabbit heart. Circ. Res., 44:557–568, 1979.
32. Allessie, M. A., Bonke, F. I. M., and Schopman, F. J. G.: Circus movement in rabbit atrial muscle as a mechanism of tachycardia. Circ. Res., 33: 54–62, 1973.
33. Allessie, M. A., Bonke, F. I. M., and Schopman, F. J. G.: Circus movement in rabbit atrial muscle as a mechanism of tachycardia. III. The "leading circle" concept: A new model of circus movement in cardiac tissue without the involvement of an anatomic obstacle. Circ. Res., 41:9–18, 1977.
34. Lewis, T.: The Mechanism and Graphic Registration of the Heart Beat. London, Shaw and Sons, 1925.
35. Dawes, G. S., and Vane, J. R.: Repetitive discharges from the isolated atria. J. Physiol., 112:28P, 1951.
36. Dawes, G. S.: Experimental cardiac arrhythmias and quinidine-like drugs. Pharmacol. Rev., 4:43–84, 1952.
37. West, T. C., and Cox, A. R.: Single fiber recording during the production and control of flutter in the isolated atrium of the rabbit. J. Pharmacol. Exp. Ther., 130:303–310, 1960.
38. West, T. C., and Landa, J. F.: Minimal mass required for induction of a sustained arrhythmia in isolated atrial segments. Am. J. Physiol., 202:232–236, 1962.
39. Allessie, M. A., Bonke, F. I. M., and Schopman, F. J. G.: Circus movement in rabbit atrial muscle as a mechanism of tachycardia. II. The role of nonuniform recovery of excitability in the occurrence of unidirectional block as studied with multiple microelectrodes. Circ. Res., 39:168–177, 1976.
40. Bouman, L. N., Gerlings, E. D., Biersteker, P. A., and Bonke, F. I. M.: Pacemakershift in the sinoatrial node during vagal stimulation. Pfluegers Arch., 302:255–267, 1968.
41. Mendez, C., and Moe, G. K.: Demonstration of a dual AV nodal conduction system in isolated rabbit heart. Circ. Res., 19:378–393, 1966.
42. Schuilenburg, R. M., and Durrer, D.: Atrial echo beats in the

human heart elicited by induced atrial premature beats. Circulation, 37:680–692, 1968.
43. Puech, P., Latour, H., and Grolleau, R.: Le flutter et ses limites. Arch. Mal. Coeur, 61:116–144, 1970.
44. Watson, R. M., and Josephson, M. E.: Atrial flutter. I. Electrophysiologic substrates and modes of initiation and termination. Am. J. Cardiol., 45:732–741, 1980.
45. Inoue, H., Matsuo, H., Takayanagi, K., and Murao, S.: Clinical and experimental studies of the effects of atrial extrastimulation and rapid pacing on atrial flutter cycle. Am. J. Cardiol., 48:623–631, 1981.
46. Disertori, M., Inama, G., Vergara, G., et al.: Evidence of a reentry circuit in the common type of atrial flutter in man. Circulation, 67:434–440, 1983.
47. Lewis, T., Feil, H. S., and Stroud, W. D.: Observations upon flutter and fibrillation. II. Nature of auricular flutter. Heart, 7:191–245, 1920.
48. Rosenblueth, A., and Garcia Ramos, J.: Studies on flutter and fibrillation. II. The influence of artificial obstacles on experimental auricular flutter. Am. Heart J., 33:677–684, 1947.
49. Kimura, E., Kato, K., Murao, S., et al.: Experimental studies on the mechanism of the auricular flutter. Tohoku J. Exp. Med. 60:197–207, 1954.
50. Lanari, A., Lambertini, A., and Ravin, A.: Mechanism of experimental atrial flutter. Circ. Res. 4:282–287, 1956.
51. Hayden, W. G., Hurley, E. J., and Rytand, D. A.: The mechanism of canine atrial flutter. Circ. Res., 20:496–505, 1967.
52. McAlpine, W. A.: Heart and Coronary Arteries. Berlin, Springer-Verlag, 1975.
53. Allessie, M. A., Lammers, W. J. E. P., Bonke, F. I. M., and Hollen, J.: Intra-atrial reentry as a mechanism for atrial flutter induced by acetylcholine and rapid pacing in the dog. Circulation, 70:123–135, 1985.
54. Moe, G. K.: On the multiple wavelet hypothesis of atrial fibrillation. Arch. Intern. Pharm. Ther., 140:183–188, 1962.
55. Moe, G. K., Rheinboldt, W. C., and Abildskov, J. A.: A computer model of atrial fibrillation. Am. Heart J., 67:200–220, 1964.
56. Moe, G. K.: In Stacy, R. W., and Waxman, B. D. (eds.): Computers in Biomedical Research, vol. 2. New York, Academic Press, 1965.
57. Lewis, T., Drury, A. N., and Bulger, H. A.: Flutter and fibrillation; the effects of vagal stimulation. Heart, 8:141–169, 1921.
58. Wilson, F. N.: Report of a case of auricular flutter in which vagus stimulation was followed by an increase in the rate of the circus rhythm. Heart, 11:61–66, 1924.
59. Moe, G. K., Pastelin, G., and Mendez, R.: Circus movement excitation of the atria. In Little, R. C. (ed.): Physiology of Atrial Pacemakers and Conductive Tissues, pp. 207–220. New York, Futura, 1980.
60. Leier, C. V., Meacham, J. A., and Schaal, S. F.: Prolonged atrial conduction. A major predisposing factor for the development of atrial flutter. Circulation, 57:213–216, 1978.
61. Cosio, F. G., Palacios, J., Vidal, J., et al.: Electrophysiologic studies in atrial fibrillation. Slow conduction of premature impulses: A possible manifestation of the background for reentry. Am. J. Cardiol., 51:122–130, 1983.

8

Atrial Arrhythmias: Clinical Concepts

Paul V. L. Curry and Mohammad Shenasa

Approximately 60% of all cardiac arrhythmias encountered clinically either arise in or involve the atria.[1] The spectrum of such atrial arrhythmias includes, at one extreme, single atrial extrasystoles of dubious significance and, at the other, chronic irreversible atrial fibrillation. Between these two extremes are atrial tachycardias of varying rate and regularity such as paroxysmal sinus node tachycardia, pure atrial tachycardia, "chaotic" or multifocal atrial tachycardia, and atrial flutter. There are also disorders of intra-atrial and interatrial conduction. Despite such diversity, atrial arrhythmias have much in common, especially in regard to their etiology and management.

Atrial Arrhythmias

Atrial extrasystoles, echo beats, and parasystole
Paroxysmal sinus node tachycardia
Pure atrial tachycardia
Multifocal atrial tachycardia
Atrial flutter
Atrial fibrillation
First, second, and third degree intra-atrial block

Pathophysiology

The many pathologic and functional conditions that can affect the atria, thereby causing atrial arrhythmias, are summarized in Table 8-1. The majority of such pathologic processes affect not only working atrial myocardium,[2] but also the sinus and sometimes the atrioventricular nodes that are also situated within the atria. When this occurs, it does not necessarily give rise to arrhythmias that fairly represent the degree of involvement of each site; indeed, many atrial tachyarrhythmias can arise with sinus node disease alone and in the absence of overt atrial myocardial involvement. In fact, often atrial arrhythmias arise as part of the sick sinus syndrome or the atrial bradycardia-tachycardia syndrome (Fig. 8-1), sometimes before the bradycardia component has developed.[3,4] Hudson,[5] in 1965, suggested that damage to the sinoatrial node was a necessary precursor to the occurrence of atrial arrhythmias. Direct damage to atrial muscle,[6] atrial dilatation,[7] and occlusion of the sinus node artery[8] were also felt to be predominant factors responsible for atrial arrhythmias.

Davies and Pomerance[9] undertook pathologic studies of 100 hearts from patients coming to autopsy who had

We wish to thank the British Heart Foundation for supporting this work.

Table 8-1. Disorders Affecting Sinus Node, Atrium, and AV Node

General Type of Disorder	Specific Disorder or Cause
Acute	
Vascular	Acute myocardial infarction
Inflammatory	Viral myocarditis Rheumatic carditis Collagen disease Bacterial carditis
Trauma	
Surgery	
Distention	Raised atrial pressure
Distortion	From within or externally
Tumor	Infiltration (including leukemia)
Radiation	
Toxic carditis	
Drugs	*e.g.*, Digoxin
Endocrine and metabolic disorder	*e.g.*, Acute electrolyte imbalance
Bronchopulmonary disease (acute)	
Bradycardia with hypervagotonia	
Chronic	
Rheumatic heart disease	
Cardiomyopathy	(Primary or secondary)
Coronary artery disease	
Idiopathic atrial fibrosis	(Sclerodegenerative)
Infiltrations	(Including slow neoplasia, amyloid, hemochromatosis, etc.)
Collagen disease	
Chronic infections	*e.g.*, Tuberculosis, carditis, sacroid, Chagas disease
Congenital	*e.g.*, Atrial septal defect, SA node mat development, etc.
Chronic dilatation or hypertrophy	*e.g.*, Mitral valve disease, hypertension
Bronchopulmonary disease (chronic)	
Endocrine	*e.g.*, Thyroid disease

had atrial fibrillation. Examining specifically both the sinoatrial node and atrial tissue, they found that patients with either recent or rare atrial fibrillation had atrial dilatation but essentially preserved sinus node and atrial myocardium. In contrast, patients with long-term atrial tachyarrhythmias such as atrial fibrillation showed combinations of sinoatrial node artery stenosis and muscle loss within the SA node or main intra-atrial bundles, as well as atrial dilatation. The underlying pathologic conditions found most commonly in this group were chronic rheumatic valvular disease, ischemic heart disease, hypertension, and cor pulmonale. Occasionally, in some aged patients, atrial fibrillation had occurred in association with loss of muscle fibers and increased fibrosis within the SA node, but for which there was no clear underlying pathologic cause and no atrial involvement. Sims[10] reported similar findings.

The precise form of atrial arrhythmia is often independent of the nature of the causative atrial disease and relates more to the extent and location of the disease process within the atria and to prevailing autonomic tone. However, certain arrhythmias are more common with acute atrial disturbance. It is known that atrial fibrillation can even occur in the absence of both atrial and sinus node disease, possibly as a result of sudden changes in autonomic tone.[11] Pharmacologic interventions can have the same effect.[9,12–15] Atrial arrhythmias may "escape" during transient bradycardia or may be precipitated by either physical or emotional stress (Fig. 8-2).[16]

Other conditions within the chest, but remote from the heart, can precipitate atrial arrhythmias (*e.g.*, pleurisy or trauma, chest infection, etc.), possibly through reflex mechanisms. Neuromuscular disorders such as myotonia dystrophica and metabolic disorders such as either thyroid over- or underactivity, diabetes, uremia, and pheochromocytoma can cause atrial arrhythmias.[16] Paroxysmal or acute atrial arrhythmias may also be precipitated by toxic states, hypoxia, alcohol, nicotine, caffeine, digitalis, and adrenergic stimulants.

Sometimes atrial arrhythmias are caused by other tachycardias that either directly (Wolff-Parkinson-White syndrome or intra-AV nodal reentrant tachycardia) involve the atria or secondarily affect atrial electrophysiologic behavior (*e.g.*, rapid ventricular tachycardia). Atrial arrhythmias can even be precipitated by permanent endocardial pacing leads as they course through or impinge on the right atrium. It has also been postulated that certain rapid atrial arrhythmias may arise as a result of conduction of premature ventricular impulses retrogradely up functional bypasses of the atrioventricular node, which then arrive in the atria during their vulnerable period, precipitating the fibrillation process (see Fig. 8-29).

Arrhythmias can arise anywhere within the atria, even within the sinus node.[17] They can then either involve both atria or be isolated to one part of either the left or right atrium while another atrial rhythm prevails elsewhere[18]; recently, however, the simultaneous occurrence of dissimilar atrial rhythms has been requestioned.[19]

The abnormal electrophysiologic mechanisms underlying such arrhythmias include both enhanced focal automaticity and impulse reentry (Fig. 8-3). In the latter

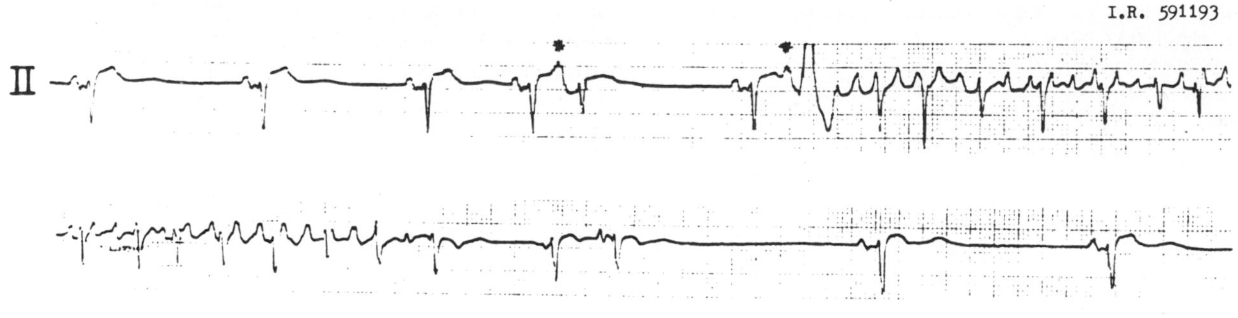

Figure 8-1. *Atypical atrial flutter arising in association with sinoatrial disease. Some of the atrial extrasystoles appear to rise from a site in the atrium in common with that for the tachycardia.*

case, circus movement can occur either within a closed anatomic circuit—perhaps formed by divisive structures such as caval orifices and foramina within the atria—or by the "leading circle" mechanism without necessarily involving fixed anatomic features.[20] A third recently recognized mechanism—"triggered activity"—may underlie some forms of atrial and sinus node tachycardia. Abnormalities of intra-atrial conduction can also occur either alone or in association with atrial tachyarrhythmias.[21] In general, such abnormal electrophysiologic mechanisms arise as a result of atrial disease. This is in marked contrast to the occurrence of reentrant tachycardias at the AV junction in patients who, most often, have otherwise normal hearts.

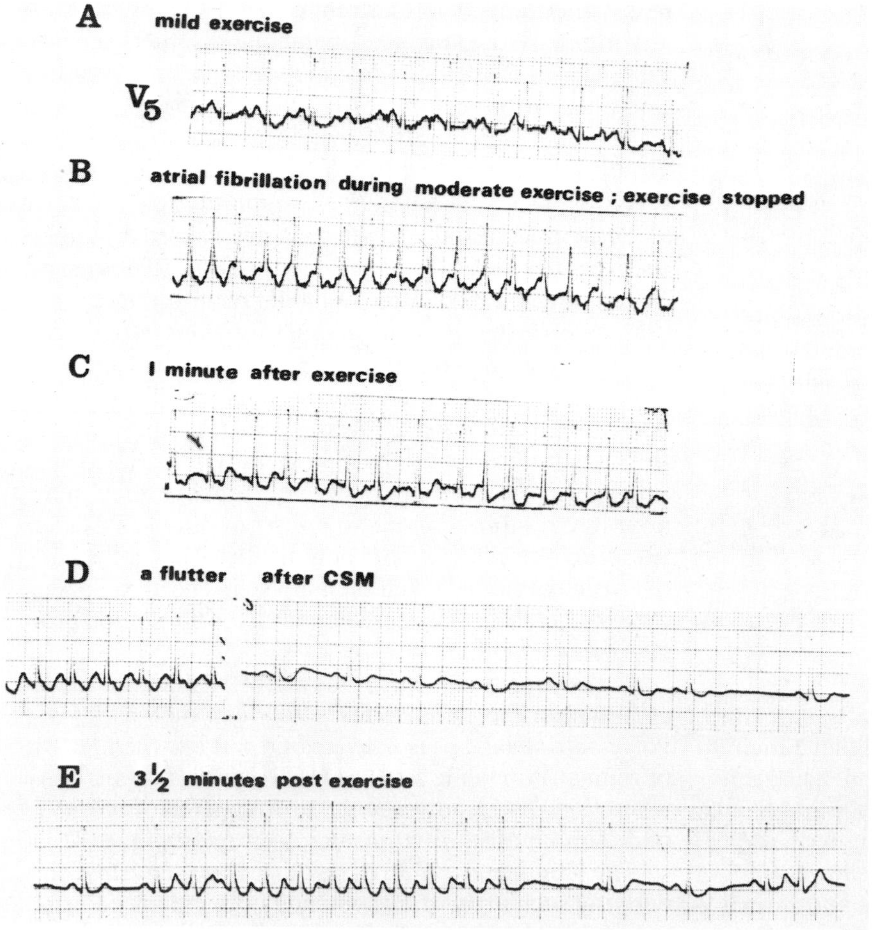

Figure 8-2. *Paroxysmal atrial fibrillation and flutter provoked by exercise.* (CSM, *carotid sinus massage)*

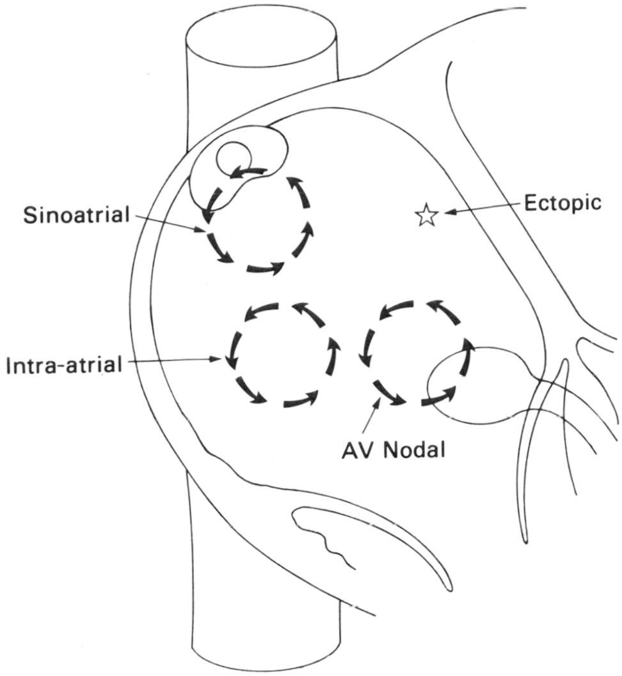

Figure 8-3. *Sites and mechanisms of atrial tachyarrhythmias. Proximity to nodal tissue confers increasing sensitivity to alterations in autonomic nervous tone.*

Atrial Extrasystoles, Echoes, and Parasystole

Neither the incidence nor the significance of these arrhythmias is fully known. Undoubtedly they occur in otherwise normal individuals, whether adults[22] or children.[23] Atrial parasystole is relatively infrequent.[24-26] We have found a 10% incidence of "minor atrial arrhythmias" in normal subjects, compared with a 30% incidence in patients with complete heart block and an 88% incidence in patients with the sick sinus syndrome.[27]

Mostly, the occurrence of atrial arrhythmias goes unnoticed, although long compensatory or "reset" pauses may be detected by the patient as transient dizziness with a characteristic precordial discomfort and a stronger postectopic impulse, especially in hypertensive patients. The effects of exercise, emotion, sudden deep breathing, and vagal tone on such arrhythmias are individual. Responses are inconsistent even in the same patient on differing occasions.[26,28,29] Most often, "atrial transport" is retained and unpleasant canon-wave reflexes avoided.[30]

The electrocardiographic features of such arrhythmias are well known. The P wave configuration of the extra atrial beat, when examined in all twelve conventional surface ECG leads, portrays its approximate site of origin.[31] Atrial parasystole is suspected if there is a constant short interectopic P wave interval and there are atrial fusion beats. However, the clinical value of this diagnostic achievement is less clear unless it is associated, in a particular case, with recurrent atrial tachycardia, flutter, or fibrillation due to the atrial R-on-T phenomenon. Rarely, such foci require ablation because of this phenomenon.

Similarly, atrial echo beats may reflect a latent predisposition to reentrant or junctional tachycardia; sinus node, atrial, and junctional echoes are commonly elicited during intracardiac extra stimulation tests.[32]

Wandering Atrial Pacemaker

Typically, the atrial rate during this arrhythmia is approximately 100 beats per minute or less, and P-P intervals vary at random (Fig. 8-4). The P wave may be hidden if it occurs simultaneously with a junctional beat during a relative bradycardia phase. The ventricular response is usually 1 : 1[33] with the exception of concealed premature impulses that arise at a time when the AV node is refractory.

Investigation, if indicated for such minor atrial ar-

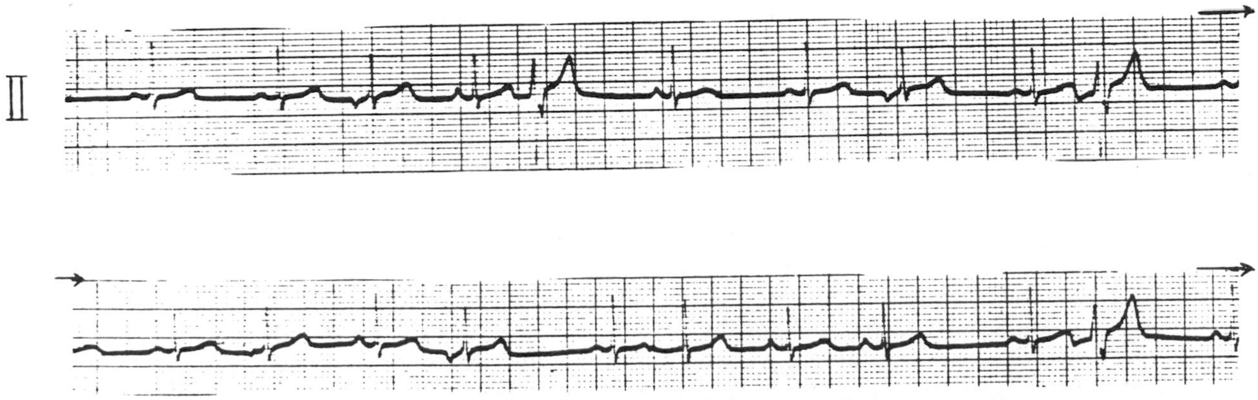

Figure 8-4. *Wandering atrial pacemaker.*

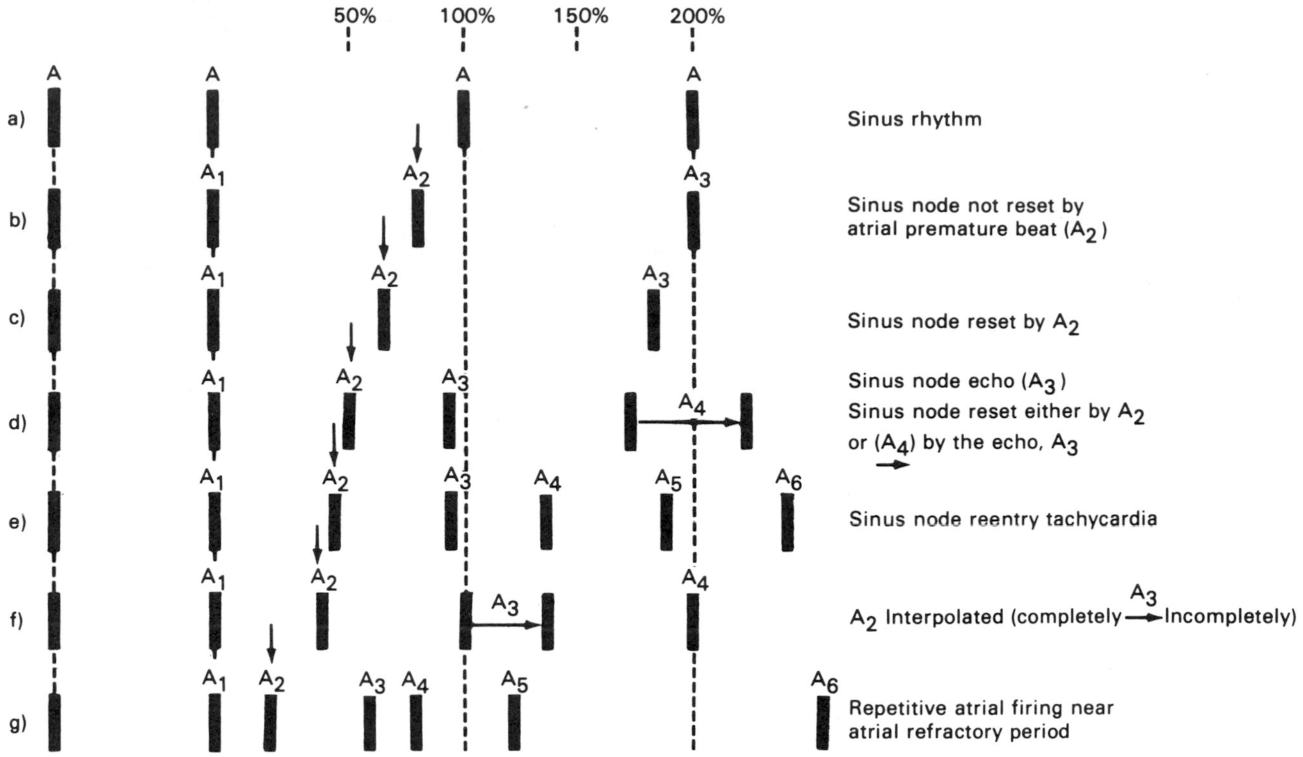

Figure 8-5. *Diagram of responses seen variably with programmed atrial extra stimulation (non-sinus reset; sinus node reset, sinus node or atrial echoes and tachycardias; atrial repetitive firing or local reentry sometimes leading to atrial flutter or fibrillation as the extra stimulus is given more prematurely).*

rhythmias, is with 24-hour continuous ECG recording and, perhaps, monitored stress testing. The occurrence of echoes and extrasystoles during clinical electrophysiologic studies is standard, especially during the functional refractory periods of the different regions comprising the atrium (Fig. 8-5).

Since most patients with such arrhythmias are unaware of their occurrence, treatment is very rarely required. However, the nature and frequency of such arrhythmias should be noted for serial assessment. Occasionally, their occurrence heralds thyroid overactivity before it is otherwise clinically overt.

Paroxysmal Sinus Tachycardia

Paroxysmal apparent sinus tachycardia is a relatively "new" clinical arrhythmia, at least as regards its recognition (Fig. 8-6).[17] Over thirty years ago, Barker, Wilson, and Johnson[34] put forward the concept that one form of paroxysmal supraventricular tachycardia might be due to sustained impulse reentry within the region of the sinoatrial node, a concept reiterated more recently by Wallace and Daggett.[35] During clinical intracardiac studies, the underlying electrophysiologic mechanism behaves as if it were reentrant, that is, such tachycardias can be both initiated and terminated, reproducibly and over a "critical zone" during atrial diastole by a single triggered atrial extra stimulus, although "triggered activity" cannot be excluded. Support for the reentrant hypothesis came from the work of Han, Mallozzi, and Moe,[36] and more recently from that of Allessie and Bonke.[37] However, knowledge of the precise mechanism is of little consequence to therapy in this particular instance.

The incidence of paroxysmal sinus tachycardia is not known, but the number of newly reported cases has grown rapidly since its recognition. We now have observed 25 such cases. Most early examples were seen incidentally during intracardiac studies, but recently cases have been diagnosed electrocardiographically on suspicion of their occurrence. Continuous 24-hour ECG monitoring is especially applicable to the diagnosis and assessment of this arrhythmia.

Most patients with paroxysmal sinus tachycardia have some form of heart disease and over half have other features of sinoatrial disease. However, its occurrence in normal subjects is well described.[38–41] In some patients, the only additional finding is a ventricular preexcitation syndrome.[41,42] Sinus node echo responses have been re-

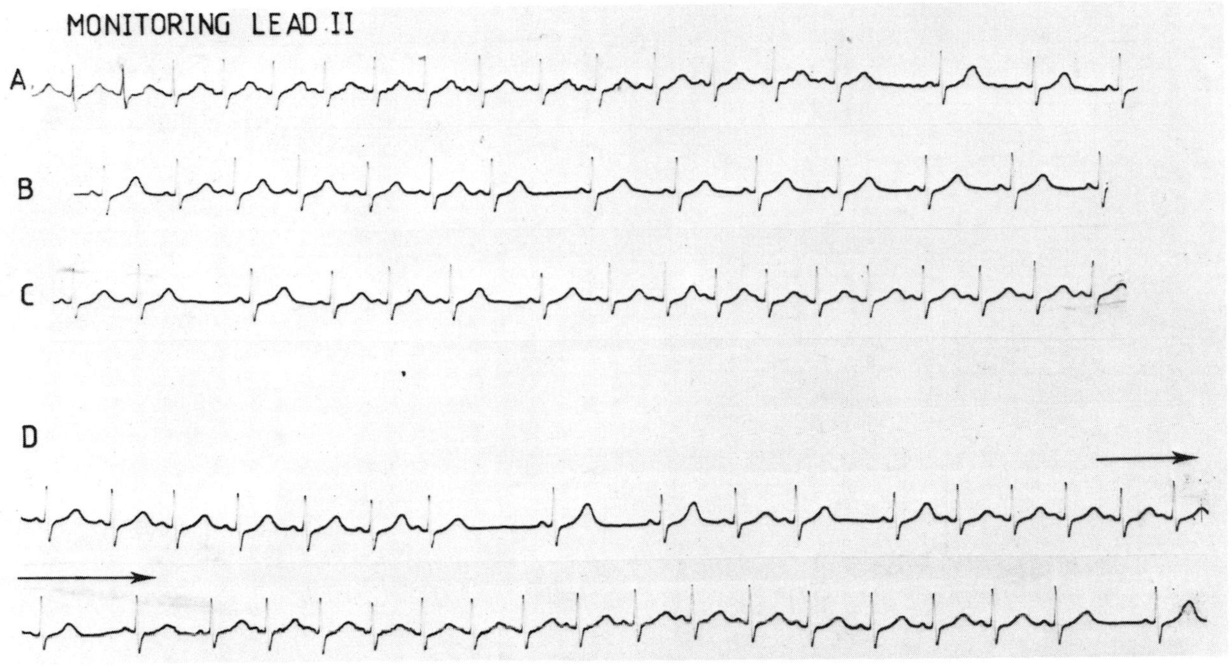

Figure 8-6. *Repetitive paroxysmal sinus tachycardia. The lower two panels (D) are continuous.*

ported as occurring in up to 11% of patients without SA node disease.[43]

Heart rates during paroxysmal sinus tachycardia are slower than those in most other forms of supraventricular tachycardia, usually between 80 and 150 beats per minute, although faster rates have been reported.[39–41] When heart rates during tachycardia are below 90 beats per minute, this is a relative tachycardia occurring in patients with sinus bradycardia. Symptoms are usually mild, and most attacks probably pass unnoticed except when the rate in tachycardia is above 120 beats per minute. Most attacks are short-lived, usually lasting for no more than 10 to 20 beats (Fig. 8-7), but they are repetitive, being characteristically sensitive to changes in autonomic tone, including even those changes associated with normal breathing. This last feature occasionally

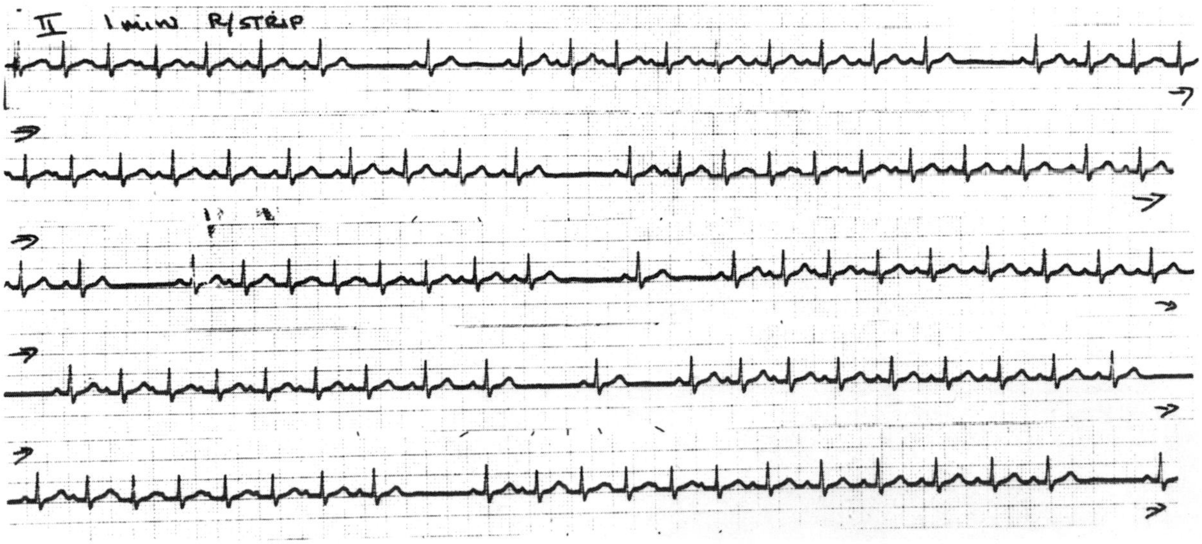

Figure 8-7. *Repetitive paroxysmal sinus tachycardia. Atrial rate-related functional prolongation of the PR interval is seen, a feature that distinguishes this arrhythmia from normal sinus rhythm.*

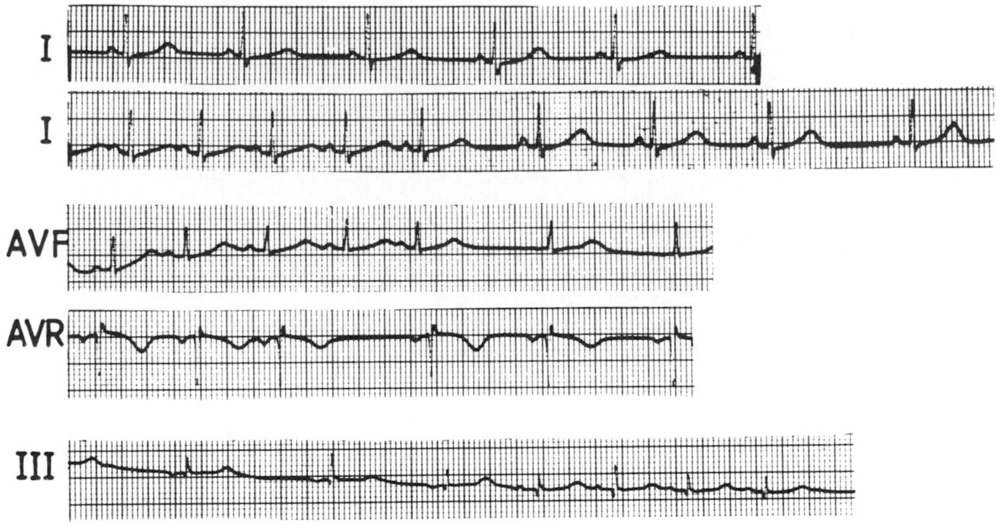

Figure 8-8. *In these ECG strips, paroxysmal sinus tachycardia can be distinguished from sinus arrhythmia by the minor alteration in P wave morphology and the slight lengthening of the PR interval.*

makes distinction from sinus arrhythmia almost impossible (Fig. 8-8). More persistent attacks last for some minutes but rarely longer.

It would be interesting to know how often patients with this arrhythmia are mistakenly diagnosed as suffering from anxiety. Reassurance and tranquilizers have little effect on the occurrence of attacks; however, close questioning reveals that their tachycardias are truly paroxysmal. While most attacks are only a mild nuisance (once recognized and their significance explained), others can cause angina, breathlessness, and syncope—especially in those with associated heart disease and the sick sinus syndrome. The similarity to normal sinus rhythm extends to hemodynamic considerations such as

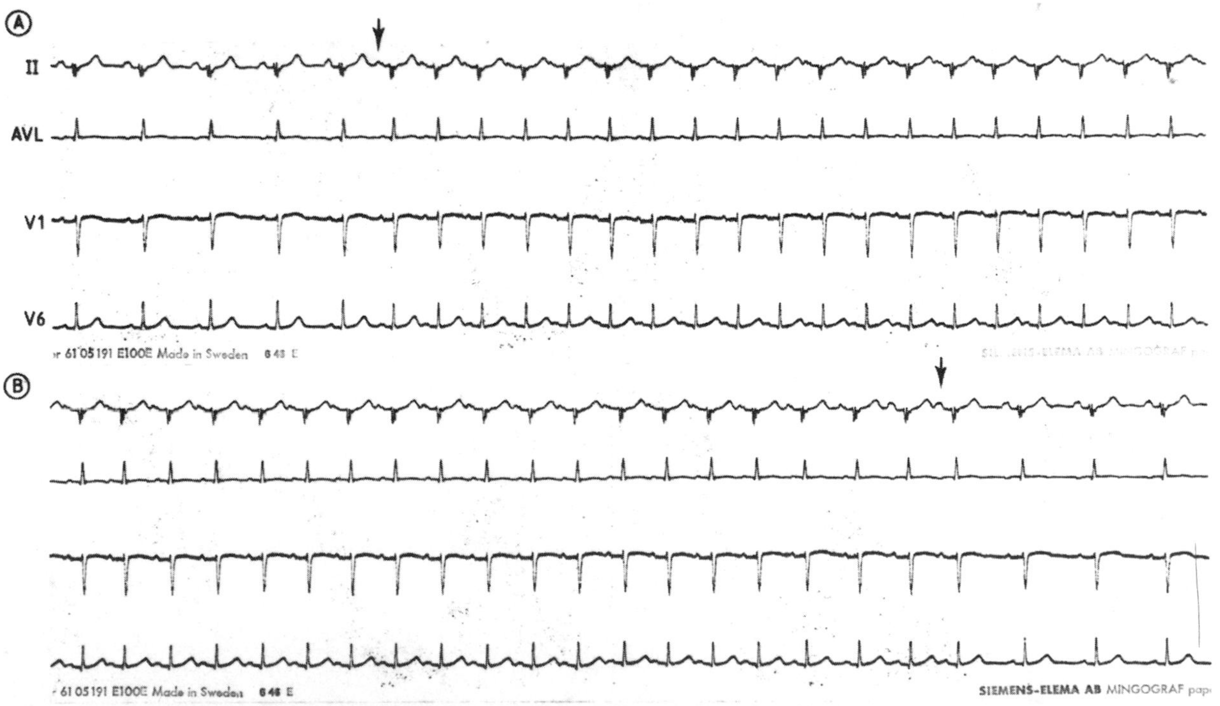

Figure 8-9. *A more sustained example of paroxysmal sinus tachycardia. The arrows simply show the spontaneous onset and termination. Interestingly, the minor aberration in P wave morphology in the tachycardia recovers just before the tachycardia stops, so that the last two P waves are identical to those of the ensuing normal sinus rhythm.*

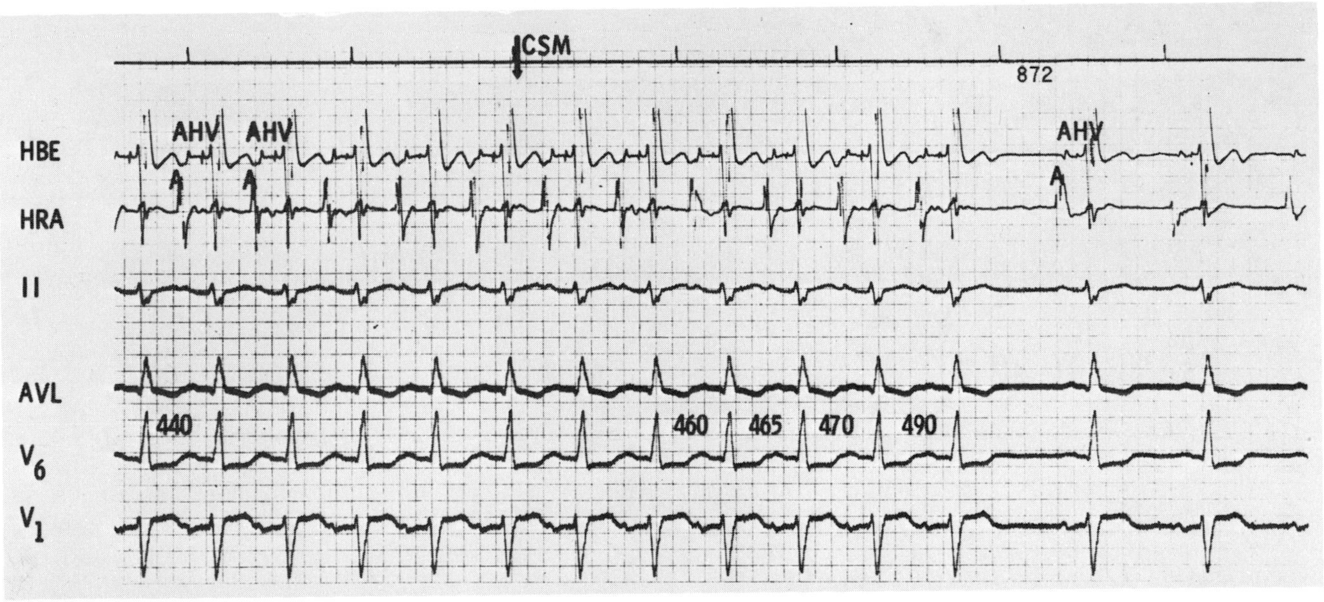

Figure 8-10. *Carotid sinus massage* (CSM) *slows and then stops an attack of paroxysmal sinus node tachycardia.* (HBE, *His bundle electrogram;* HRA, *high right atrial electrogram)*

appropriate atrial systole and "transport"—only the rate is inappropriate.

Electrocardiographic Features

The electrocardiographic features of this arrhythmia are now well described and consist of the sudden onset and termination of a supraventricular tachycardia, the appearances of which suggest a regular (but inappropriate) sinus tachycardia. Although P wave morphology in the tachycardia may be indistinguishable from that in basic sinus rhythm in all twelve leads of the conventional ECG, more often the P waves are similar but not identical. The sequence of atrial activation, however, remains one of high to low, and right to left, even for nonidentical P waves, suggesting an origin for the arrhythmia in the high right atrium. Mostly, attacks arise without antecedent premature spontaneous extrasystoles—a distinction from most other such apparently reentrant supraventricular tachycardias, although their initiation by prior sinus node acceleration is similar to the mechanism of initiation that is sometimes seen with paroxysmal reentry AV tachycardias that have a wide "initiation zone."[44]

As a rule, attacks slow before terminating spontaneously, again without prompting by spontaneously occurring premature extrasystolic activity (Figs. 8-9 and 8-16). Termination can be encouraged by carotid sinus massage or similar maneuvers to which this arrhythmia is supremely sensitive (Fig. 8-10). The paroxysm may terminate with cycle length alteration—a feature that suggests an underlying reentrant mechanism (Fig. 8-11).[45] The post-termination pause resembles that seen after

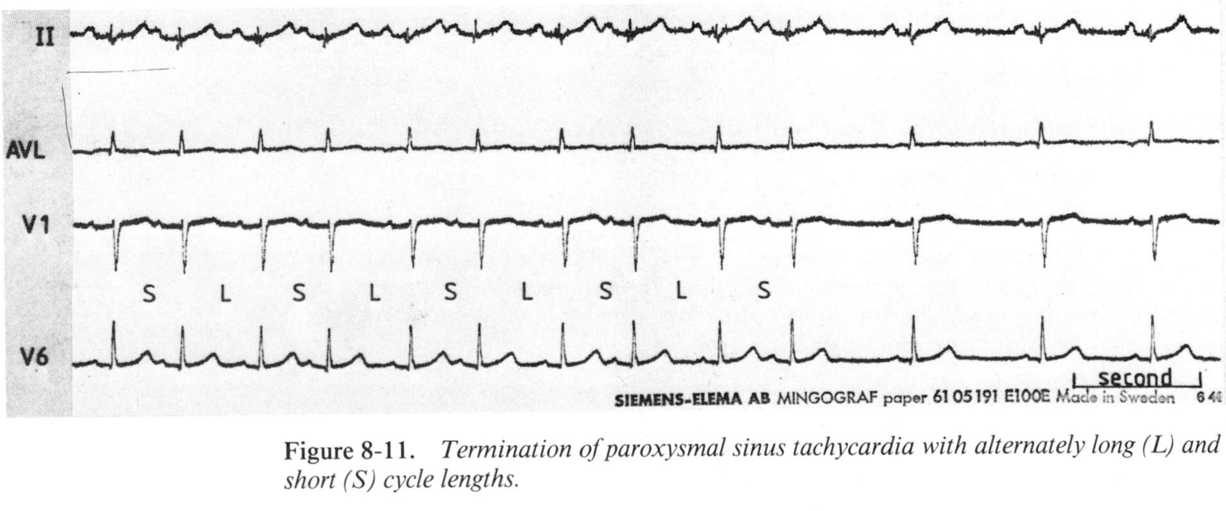

Figure 8-11. *Termination of paroxysmal sinus tachycardia with alternately long (L) and short (S) cycle lengths.*

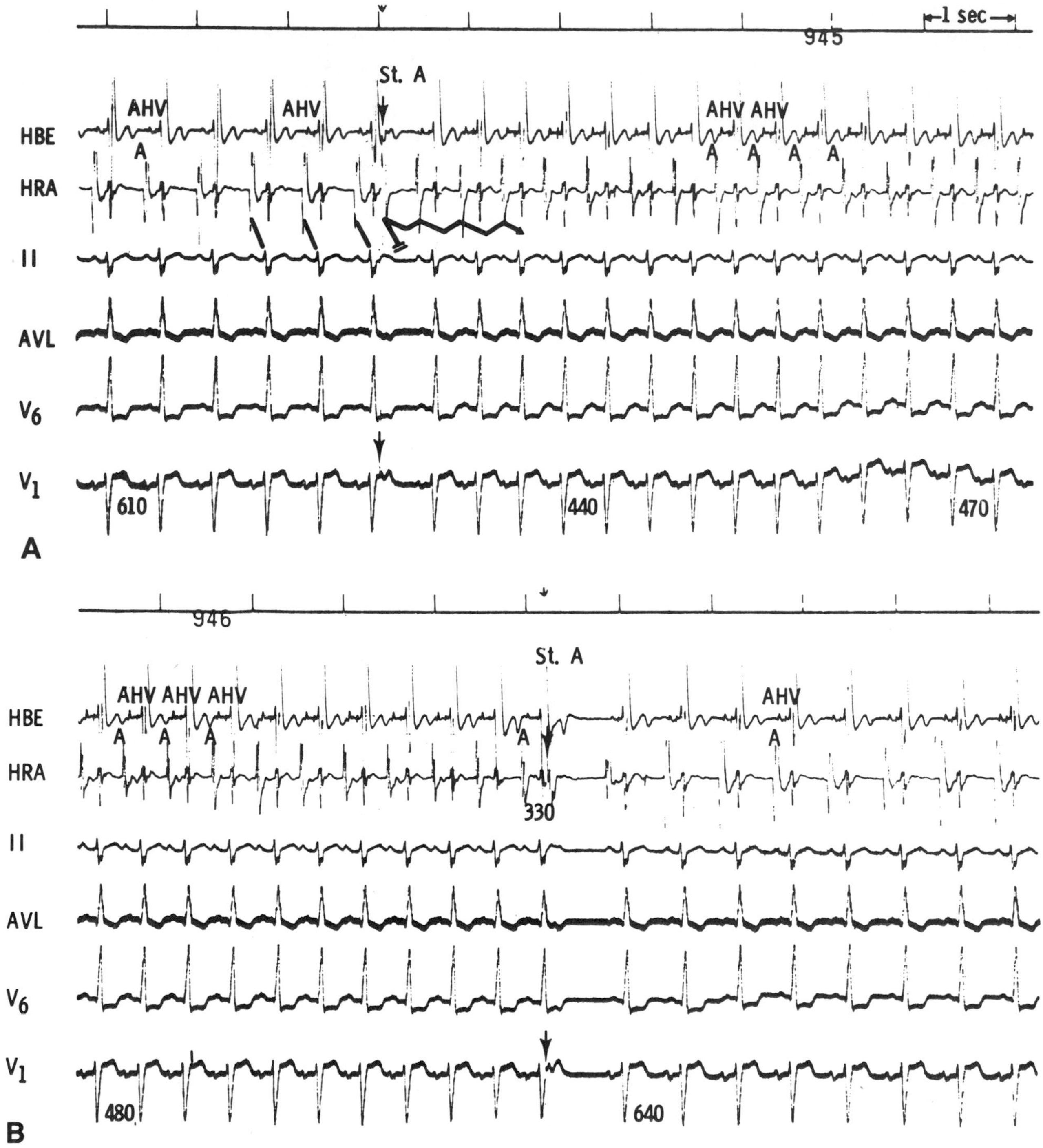

Figure 8-12. *Initiation and termination of paroxysmal sinus tachycardia by programmed atrial extra stimulation. Note that the initiating atrial extra stimulus itself fails to traverse the AV node, thereby excluding this structure from participation in the atrial tachycardia mechanism. (*St. A, *induced premature atrial extra beat)*

moderate overdrive atrial pacing as performed in studies of sinus node recovery, confirming the conflict of interests within the region of the SA node.

Perhaps the most important electrocardiographic sign that distinguishes this arrhythmia from "appropriate" sinus tachycardia is prolongation of the PR interval in accordance with inherent functional properties of reserve-delay within the AV node when this is traversed by impulses other than those of natural sinus rhythm. The degree of prolongation is mild, but so is the stress imposed on the AV node by this relatively slow atrial tachycardia. Figure 8-7 shows this phenomenon most clearly as each new tachycardia arises. By contrast, autonomically mediated sinus tachycardia would show little change or even shortening of the PR interval. Rarely, variable AV conduction occurs at the onset of such tachycardias, with some impulses failing to traverse the AV node (Fig. 8-12). Both functional patterns of disturbed AV conduction are "passive" phenomena and exclude participation of the AV node in the mechanism of the arrhythmia.

Intracardiac Studies of Paroxysmal Sinus Tachycardia

Characteristically, attacks can be both initiated and terminated reproducibly with programmed extra stimulation (Figs. 8-12, 8-13, and 8-14). However, termination by this method requires that the tachycardia is sufficiently sustained before application, a feature that is not always forthcoming although small amounts of atropine are persuasive.[41] Such extra stimuli are most effective when introduced near the sinus node, except when delivered with antecedent paced rhythm, in which case they are equally effective from any site, providing "effective prematurity" is maintained in transit to the SA node. Initiation by ventricular extra stimulation has been observed (Fig. 8-15).

Simultaneous multipoint atrial mapping confirms the direction of atrial activation during paroxysmal sinus tachycardia as being similar to that of natural sinus rhythm, although minor alterations in the configuration of the high right atrial electrograms and of the initial P wave vector are to be expected since the pattern of atrial activation within the immediate vicinity of the SA node must be affected if the circuit partially includes extranodal atrial myocardium. Intra-sinus node aberration and a shifting sinus node pacemaker would have similar effects, however (Fig. 8-14).[44,46]

Incremental atrial pacing also initiates attacks whereas overdrive pacing may suppress them. Spontaneous termination is never long awaited (Fig. 8-16). Direct recording of the sinus node electrogram during sinus rhythm and sinus node reentry may further elucidate the

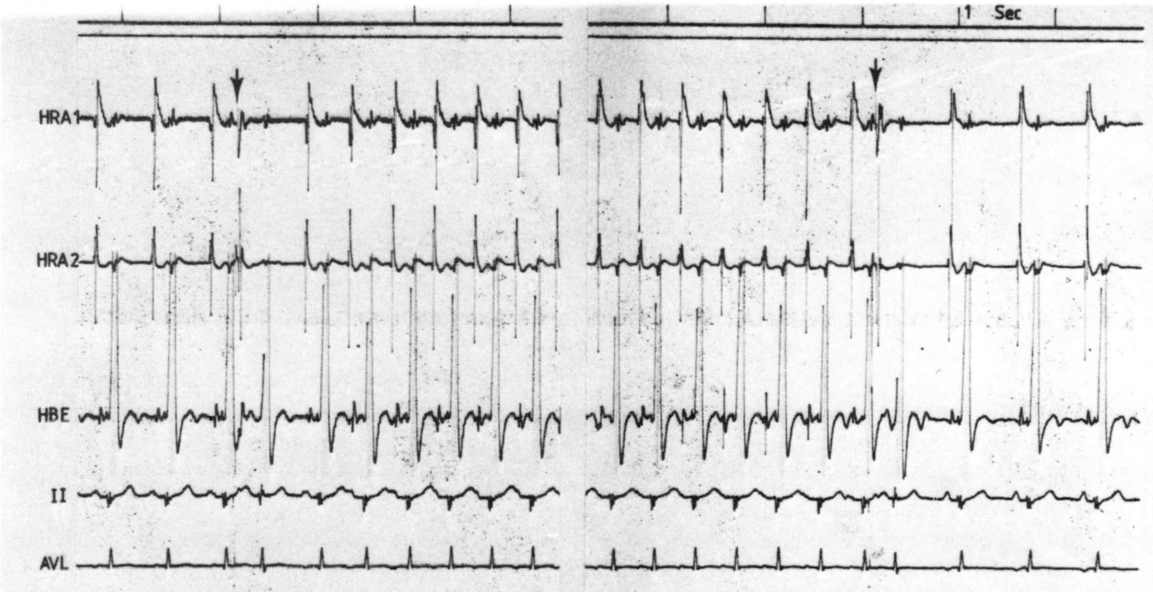

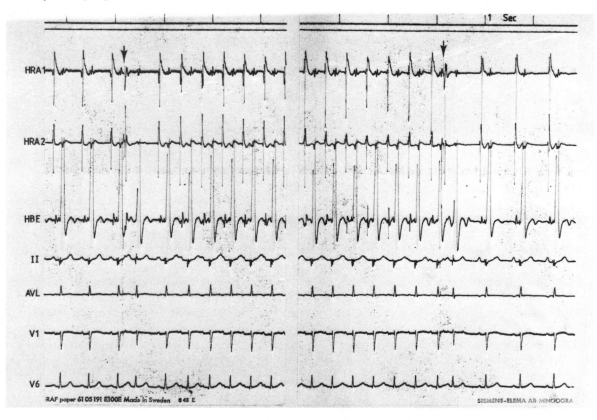

Figure 8-13. *Initiation and termination of paroxysmal sinus tachycardia by programmed extra stimulation.*

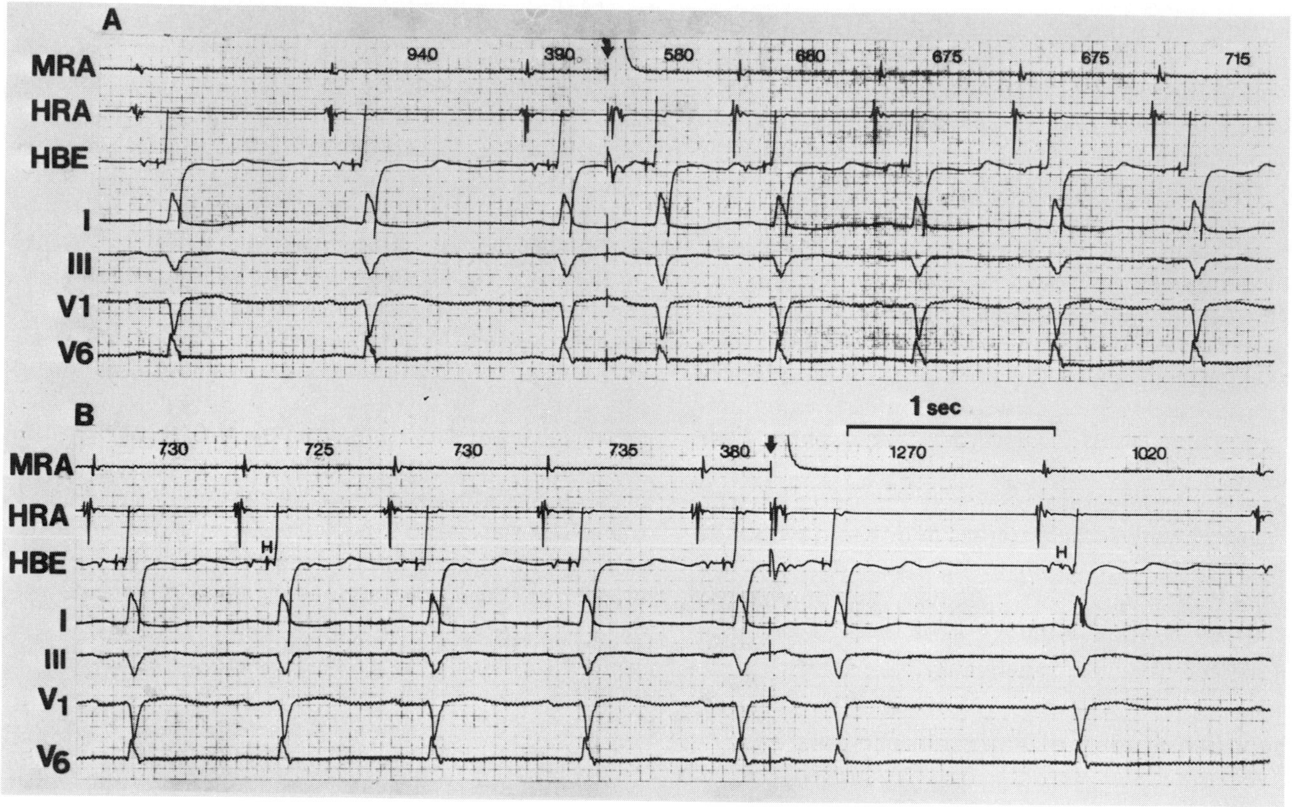

Figure 8-14. *The sequence of atrial activation in the initiated attack of paroxysmal sinus tachycardia is identical to that in normal sinus beats seen before (first three beats,* upper panel*) and after (last two atrial beats,* lower panel*) the tachycardia. The heart rate in tachycardia is only about 85 beats per minute. Sinus node recovery is affected by the preceding tachycardia—not a feature of normal sinus rhythm. Note the subtle change in configuration of the high right atrial electrogram* (HRA) *at the onset of tachycardia.*

mechanisms and electrophysiologic characteristics of this arrhythmia.[47]

Management

Only symptomatic attacks require treatment, which is best achieved with beta blocking drugs (Fig. 8-17, same case as Fig. 8-9), but these can only be used in the absence of other features of sinus node disease. Both digoxin and verapamil have also been effective. Only rarely is this arrhythmia relatively more responsive to the quinidine-like antiarrhythmic drugs. Permanent pacing to either overdrive or interrupt attacks has so far not been required, although pacemaker implantation might conceivably be needed were antiarrhythmic drugs to be necessary for the control of attacks in a patient with associated sinoatrial node disease at risk of sinus arrest.

Most often, reassurance through accurate diagnosis is all the treatment the patient requires of the physician.

Paroxysmal Atrial Tachycardia (Not Involving the Sinus or Atrioventricular Nodes)

Focal and reentrant mechanisms are probably equally important as causative factors in this group of pure atrial arrhythmias that usually arise independently of abnormalities of either the sinus or AV nodes. The acronym "PAT" has previously been widely applied, but it is now clear that true PAT (paroxysmal *atrial* tachycardia) is a comparatively rare, or infrequently recognized, arrhythmia, and PSVT (paroxysmal supraventricular tachycardia) is a better generalization when this is meant.

Most often, the patient with paroxysmal or chronic atrial tachycardia is a child or young adult; alternatively, digoxin toxicity is causative.[48] There are but few reports in the literature that permit exclusion of both paroxysmal sinus tachycardia as well as the permanent form of junctional reentrant tachycardia (Coumel's tachycar-

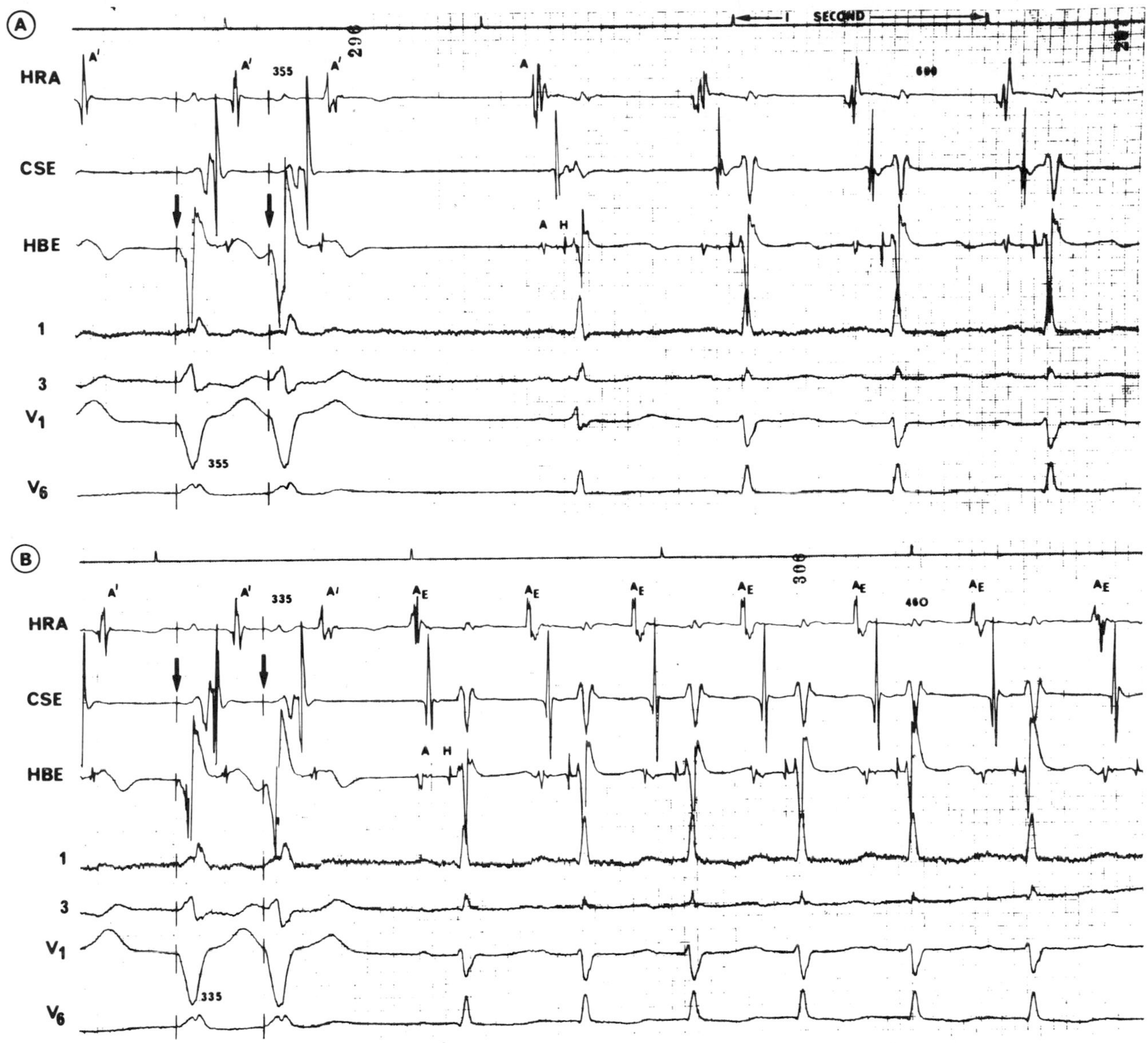

Figure 8-15. *Initiation of paroxysmal sinus tachycardia by ventricular extra stimulation with retrograde conduction to the atria occurring across a left-sided accessory AV pathway that is "latent" in sinus rhythm (*CSE, *left atrial electrogram from electrode in coronary sinus precedes atrial activity on other atrial leads during ventricular pacing). (A) Normal sinus rhythm after ventricular pacing (B) induced sinus tachycardia.*

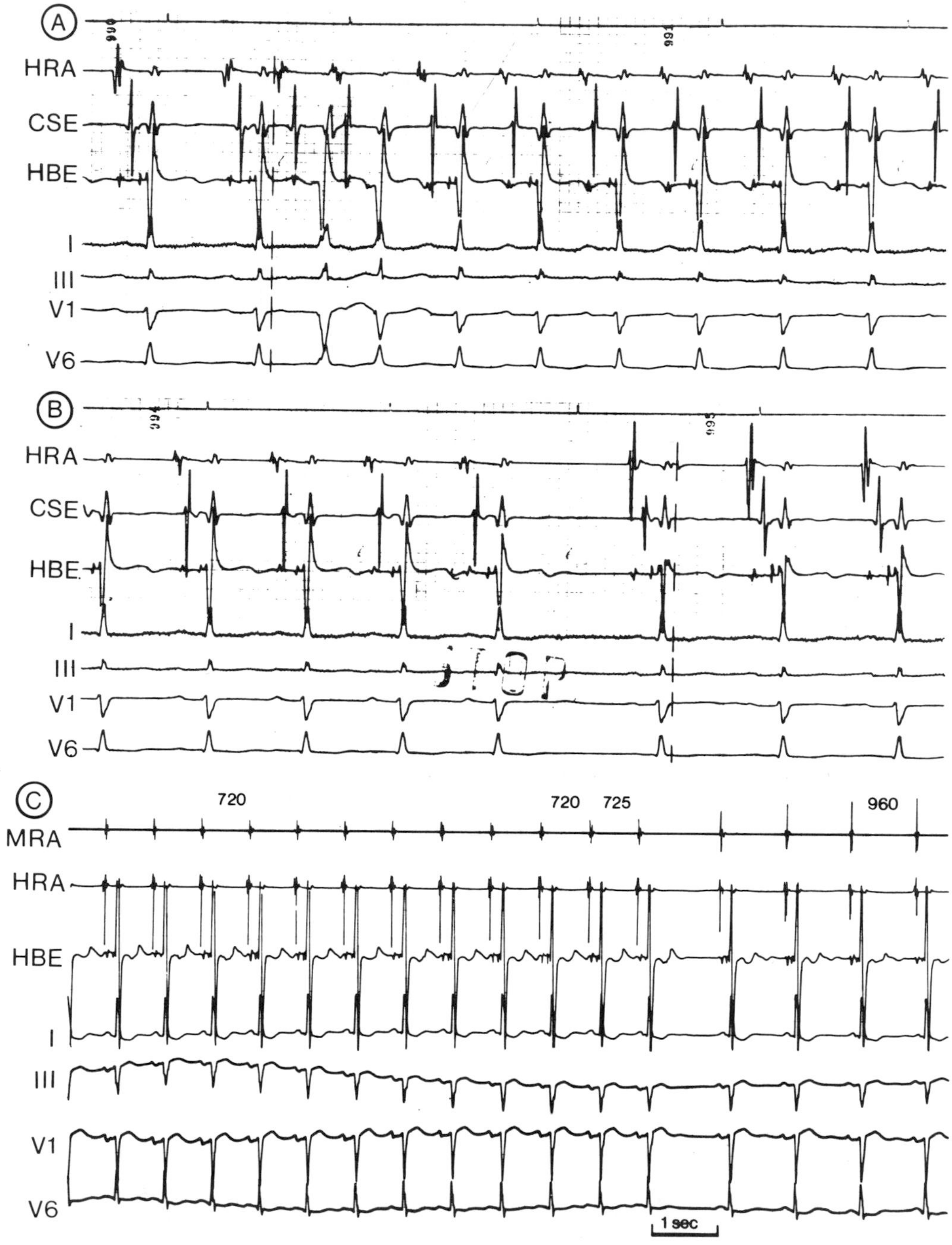

Figure 8-16. *Examples of gradual slowing of paroxysmal sinus tachycardia before spontaneously terminating (A, initiation, and B, termination), and, on the other hand, abrupt termination (C) in different patients.*

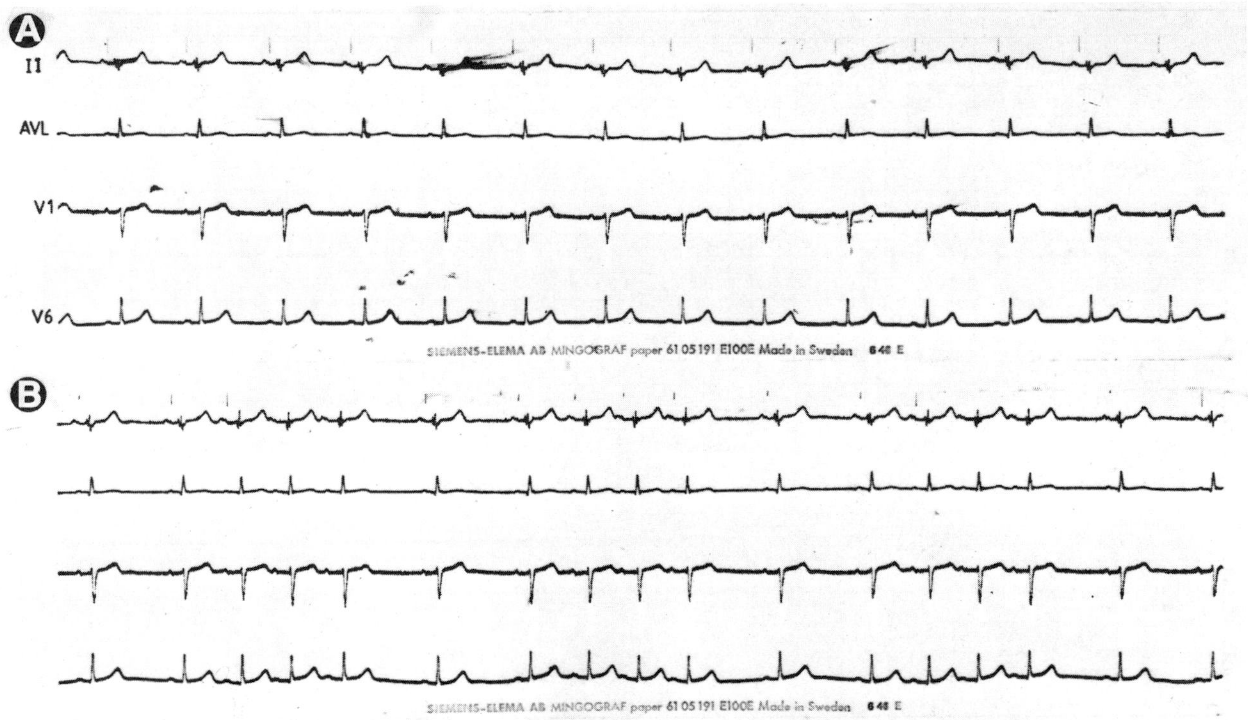

Figure 8-17. *(A) Same case of paroxysmal sinus tachycardia as in Figure 8-9, showing suppression of the tachycardia after practolol (a beta blocking drug), an effect that wears off as time passes (B) although attacks are not so sustained.*

dia), these being the two main differential diagnoses.[49] Any association with sinoatrial disease is tenuous.

The symptoms are those of any regular paroxysmal supraventricular tachycardia whose rate is of the order of 150 to 200 beats per minute. The electrocardiographic features are specific and include eccentric P wave activity that, in more than half the cases, does *not* suggest an origin in the environs of either of the two nodal areas (Fig. 8-18) and obvious functional independence of the properties of the AV node. In fact, the PR interval must be prolonged if the tachycardia arises remote from the AV node. A short PR interval suggests an origin within, or with rapid access to, the AV node.

Initiation usually occurs spontaneously and, in common with paroxysmal sinus tachycardia, without the need for antecedent premature extrasystoles. Sometimes, however, it appears to arise in association with a late-coupled atrial extrasystole, but the P wave configuration in tachycardia remains that of the extrasystole, suggesting either enhanced spontaneous focal activity or wide-zone reentrant tachycardia with "atypical" initiation.[44]

Spontaneous termination and duration of attacks are less predictable than for sinus node tachycardia. Undoubtedly, pure atrial tachycardia is relatively insensitive to the effects of alterations in vagal tone, a feature that is used in differential diagnosis (Table 8-2).

Intracardiac Studies in Patients with Atrial Tachycardia

Attacks start in one of three ways: (1) following premature extra stimulation; (2) spontaneously with late-coupled atrial extrasystoles whose P wave configuration is identical to that seen during tachycardia; and (3) following sinus acceleration (Fig. 8-19). Initiation of attacks with either programmed extra stimulation or incremental pacing is rarely reproducible,[49,50] although we now have experience of five cases with reentrant features (Figs. 8-20 and 8-21). A "warm-up" or acceleration phase often follows an initiation of the tachycardia.[51] Atrial mapping during established attacks of the atrial tachycardia confirms the eccentric, extranodal origin of such arrhythmias. The fact that ventricular extra stimuli during tachycardia fail to capture the atria either exactly, paradoxically prematurely, or with minor distance-related delays excludes participation of an accessory AV pathway in the tachycardia mechanism (this might otherwise explain eccentric atrial activation during attacks).

A macro-reentrant atrial circuit is assumed to be the underlying mechanism of the PAT if certain "capture phenomena" are obtained with triggered *atrial* extra stimuli or if the tachycardia can be terminated with this method from a pacing site that is remote from, and later

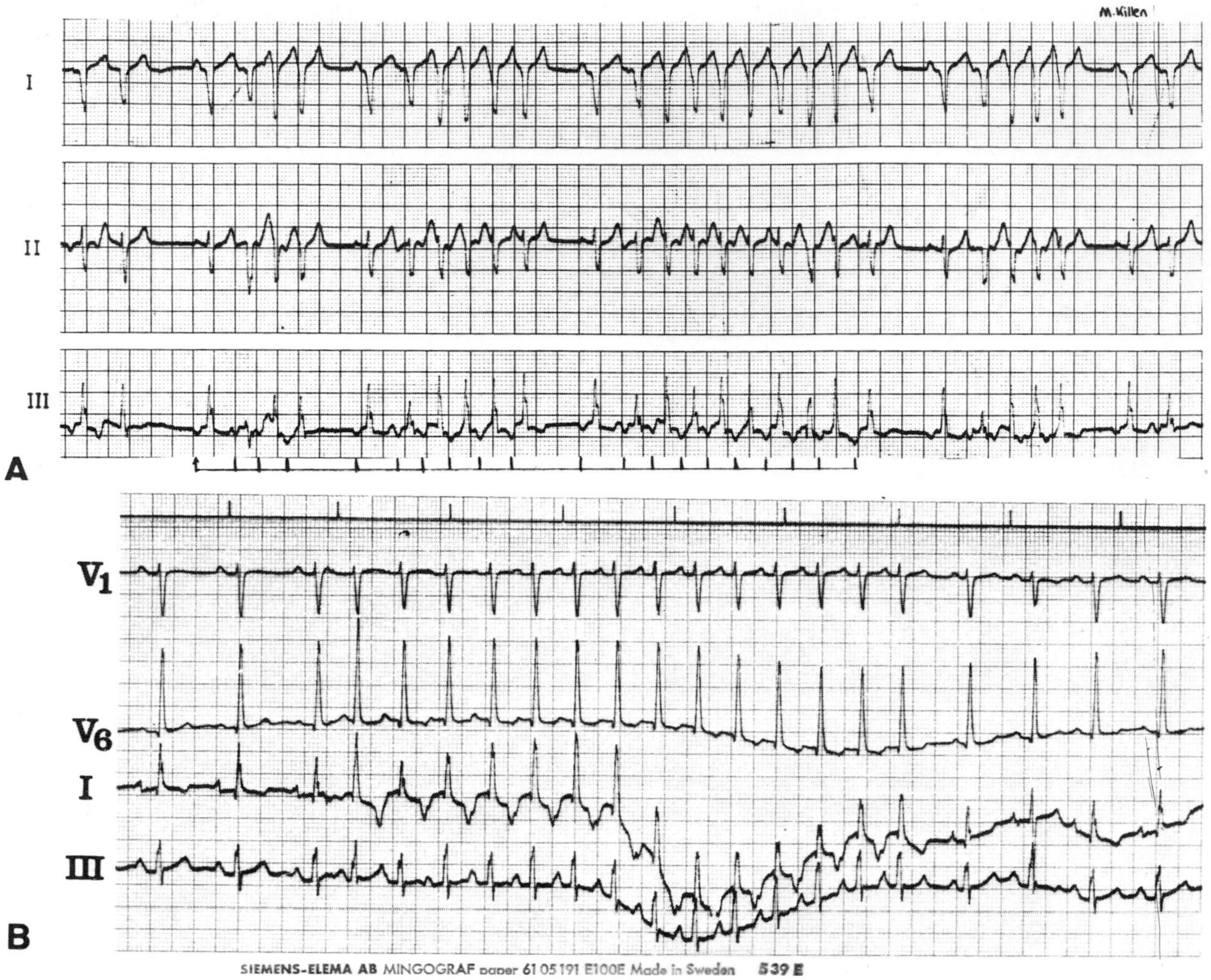

Figure 8-18. *Two different examples of spontaneously occurring paroxysmal atrial tachycardia. Mild ventricular aberration in the upper ECG strips compounds diagnosis, although careful scrutiny of the traces finds the P waves of the tachycardia. The negative P waves in tachycardia in ECG lead I of the lower example suggest that they are arising in the left atrium.*

than, sites of earliest activation during tachycardia. In effect, such impulses gain access to the reentrant circuit through the "back door" and closer to the "weak link" in the circuit where the refractory period is longest (Fig. 8-21). On most occasions, however, persistent attempts with atrial overdrive pacing are required to suppress the tachycardia if it shows features of enhanced focal activity (Fig. 8-22).[40,52]

Management

The most effective treatment is with a combination of digoxin (for ventricular protection) and a quinidine-like drug specifically for the arrhythmia as it arises within the working atrial myocardium. Disopyramide is currently the most useful drug in this latter category. This therapeutic regimen is based on the results of acute pharmacologic studies during intracardiac tests in which it was found that verapamil effectively increased the protection afforded by the AV node against the transmission of rapid atrial impulses (Fig. 8-23), but sometimes had the paradoxical effect of accelerating the atrial rate. It is well known that verapamil may convert atrial flutter to atrial fibrillation, as does carotid sinus massage on occasion, presumably by shortening the refractory period of the atrial myocardium. By contrast, ajmaline (a quinidine-like drug) slowed and finally stopped the tachycardia to restore sinus rhythm (Fig. 8-23). Amiodarone is most effective for such arrhythmias, as is a combination of digoxin and beta blocking drug.[53,54] Drugs such as fle-

Table 8-2. Characteristic Differences Between Paroxysmal Sinus Tachycardia and Paroxysmal Pure Atrial Tachycardia

	High Right Atrial Tachycardia	Other Atrial Tachycardia
Rate (beats/min.)	90–150	150–250
P wave	Similar to sinus rate	Different from sinus rate
Atrial mapping	Similar to sinus rate	Different from sinus rate
Initiation		
S.R. rate change	+++	0
Paced rate change	+++	++
Premature beat	+++ (Effective zone in sinus rate is near sinoatrial node)	++
Duration	Short-lived	Often sustained
Termination		
Spontanteous with slowing	+++	+
Carotid sinus massage	+++	0 or +
Premature beat	+++	+
Drug effects		
Atropine	+++	0
Verapamil	−−−	++ or 0 or −
Beta blocker	−−−	−−
Lanoxin	−−	−
Quinidine-like	−−	−−−
Independence of AV node	+	+
Cycle length Alternation	++	+

Key: + = enhances; − = depresses; 0 = not important feature.

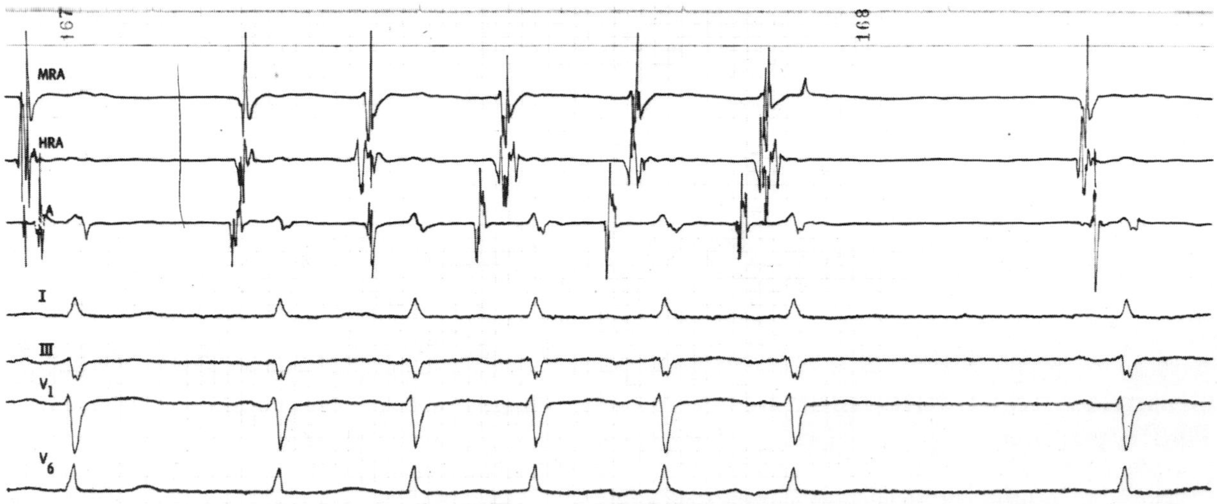

Figure 8-19. *Short-lived spontaneously occurring atrial tachycardia showing "shifting" activation sequence, the left atrium finally winning the atrium on the last three beats (*MRA, *mid right atrium;* HRA, *high right atrium;* LA, *left atrium;* I, II, V_1, *and* V_6, *ECG leads). That the electrodes had not moved is shown by the comparable appearances of the atrial "map" in the two sinus beats that frame the tachycardia.*

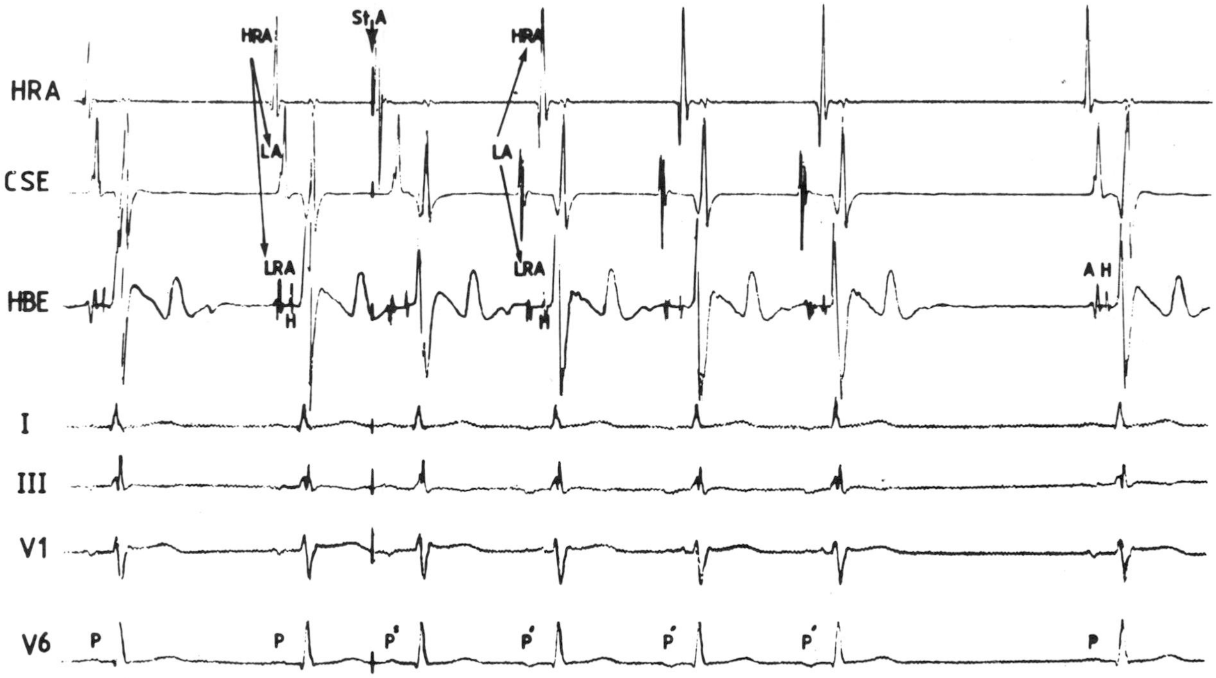

Figure 8-20. *Short run of low-left atrial tachycardia (CSE activity precedes that of other leads), initiated by a right atrial extra stimulus* (StA). *The first two beats and the last beat are normal sinus beats.*

cainide or propafenon may be worth trying, although further experience with these agents is needed to determine their efficacy.

In cases where atrial tachycardia arises in a setting of possible digoxin toxicity, this drug should temporarily be withdrawn pending results of a plasma digoxin assay. Verapamil can be used in the meantime if an alternative is really needed.

Special pacing techniques are rarely needed on a long-term basis.[55] Even more rare is the need to resort to surgery to ablate the refractory focus.[56,57] Transvenous catheter ablation of the ectopic focus has been done successfully.[58] Needless to say, these approaches require further experience and long-term follow-up.

Chaotic and Multifocal Atrial Tachycardia

Chaotic and multifocal atrial tachycardia is a moderately uncommon arrhythmia usually seen with acute disturbances of atrial function or as a transitional atrial tachyarrhythmia in a natural history of atrial disease that culminates in atrial fibrillation.[1,59–62] There appears to be a higher incidence of this arrhythmia in the elderly and in those with chronic pulmonary disease, although it is not known whether the chronic use of medications such as bronchodilators and beta-2 adrenoreceptor stimulants is a causative factor in this latter group.[63] It is an unusual arrhythmia if occurring with suspected digoxin toxicity.[64]

Electrocardiographic Features

The mean atrial rate during multifocal atrial tachycardia often exceeds 100 beats per minute but is rarely greater than 150 (Fig. 8-24). Random variation is seen in the P-P interval, and P wave morphology shows at least three different successive foci.[65] The different P waves occur in random arrangement variously interspersed with periods of more normal atrial activity (sinus rhythm). Most atrial impulses are conducted so that the net hemodynamic and, thereby, symptomatic effects are determined by the atrial arrhythmia more than by the AV node—a subtle distinction from the situation in atrial fibrillation. Most often, the resultant mean ventricular rate is tolerable; indeed, the patient may be unaware of the arrhythmia. Exercise is provocative, as is fever. Often, it is the underlying cardiovascular or respiratory disease that causes more symptoms than this arrhythmia.

Twenty-four hour ECG monitoring is appropriate

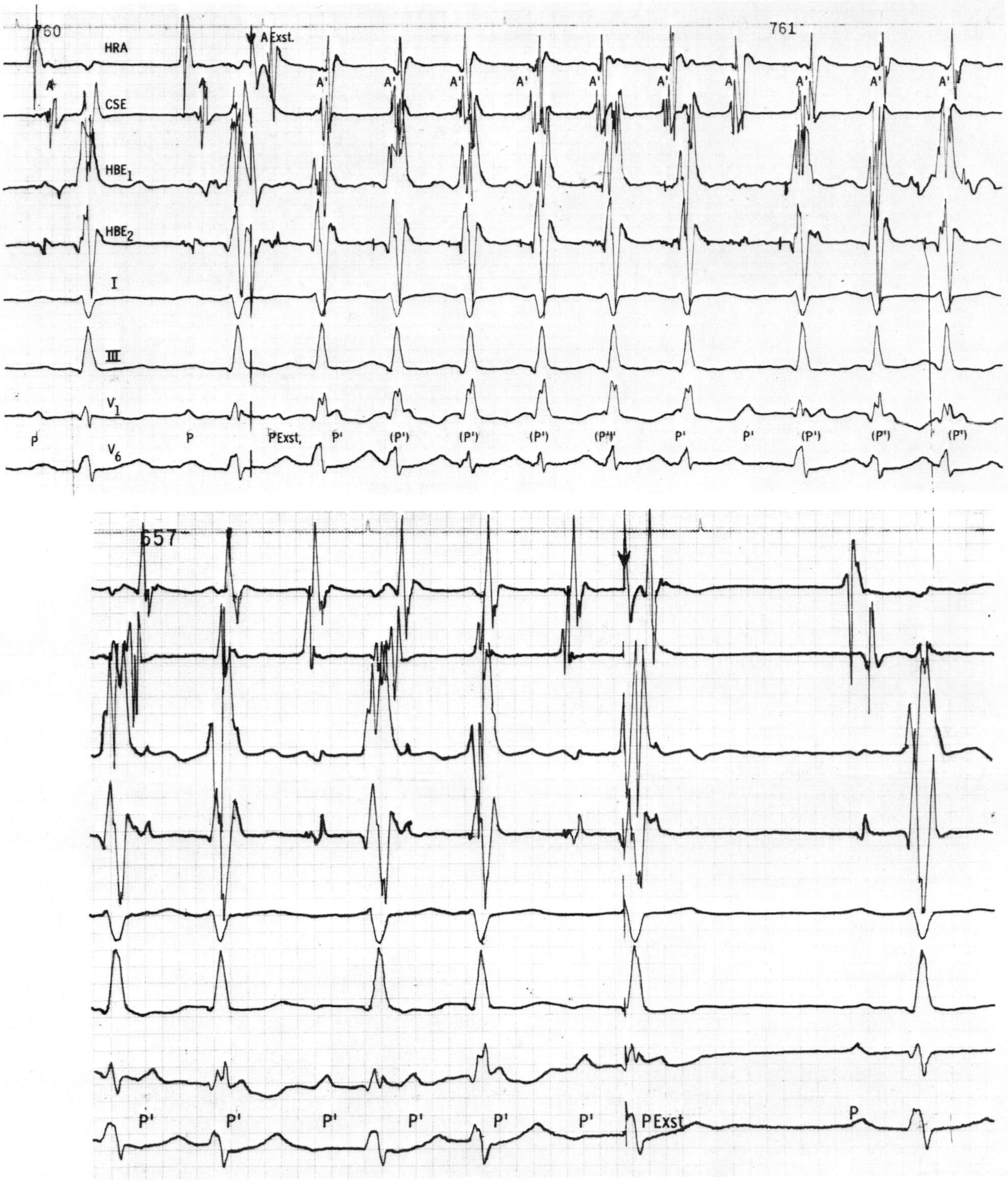

Figure 8-21. *Initiation and termination of a mid atrial paroxysmal tachycardia by programmed extra-atrial stimulation* (P Exst, arrowhead). *Variable* AV *conduction occurs during the attack that excludes participation of the* AV *node in the arrhythmia mechanism.*

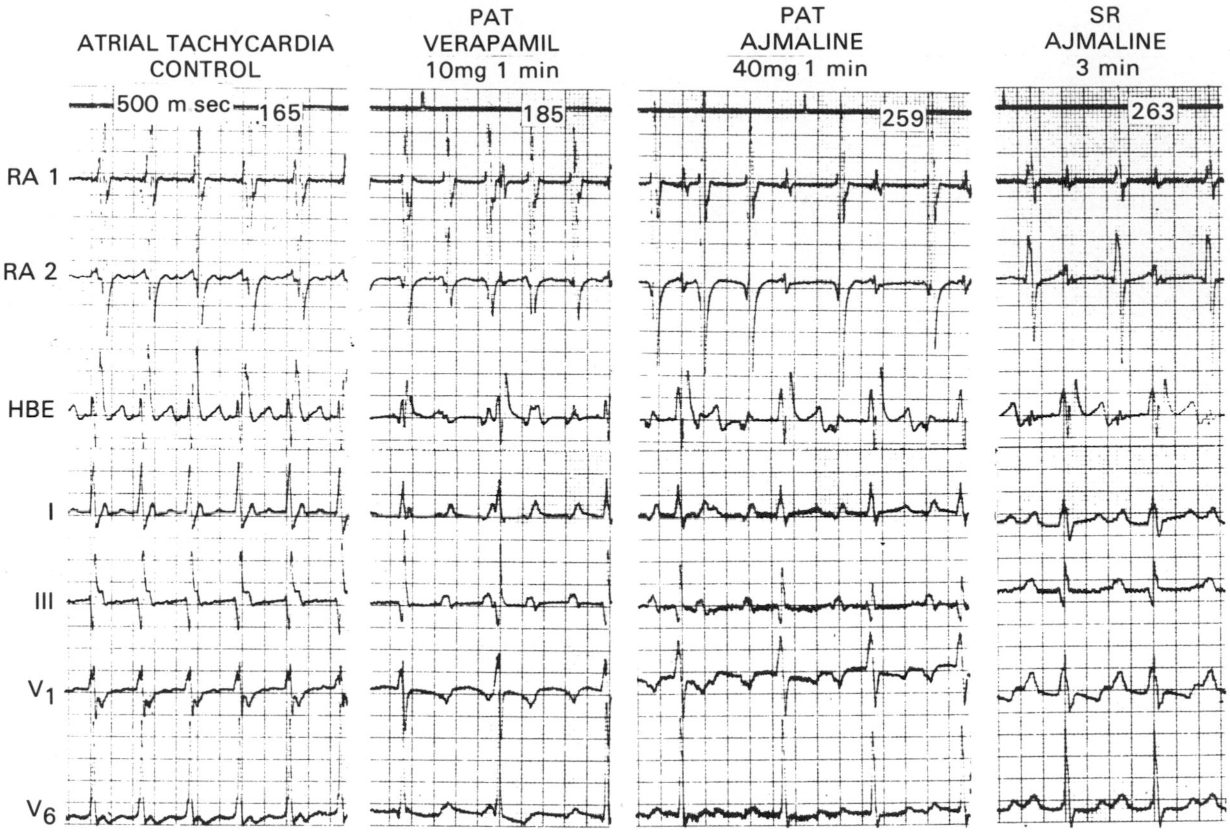

Figure 8-22. *The four panels show the relative sensitivity of paroxysmal "pure" atrial tachycardia (control) to, first, verapamil (this slows the ventricular rate through partial* AV *nodal block, but* increases *the atrial rate) and then to ajmaline, which slows and finally terminates the tachycardia, restoring sinus rhythm* (last panel). *Carotid sinus massage had the same effect as verapamil in this case.*

both for the diagnosis and assessment of this arrhythmia. It is also appropriate for assessing any response to therapy if such is needed. The need for pacing studies is rare.

Management

Treatment is usually primarily directed toward the causative illness, but a combination of digoxin with a quinidine-like drug will tend to control the situation pending spontaneous improvement or progression to chronic atrial fibrillation when the quinidine-like agent can be discontinued. Fortunately, only a tenuous link exists between this arrhythmia and sinoatrial disease, so that further sinus node depression and the need for support pacing are not usually part of management of this disorder. Amiodarone is also effective in the management of this arrhythmia. When this arrhythmia becomes unresponsive to pharmacologic agents or when it is difficult to control the ventricular response during tachycardia, transvenous catheter ablation of the AV node and insertion of a permanent pacemaker may be required to control symptomatic attacks in these patients.[66]

Atrial Flutter

The basic electrophysiologic mechanisms of atrial flutter and its speculative mechanisms are well described in Chapter 6.

Atrial flutter is one of the most common causes of regular supraventricular tachycardia encountered clinically, but unlike the situation that exists with paroxysmal reentrant atrioventricular tachycardia, atrial flutter usually occurs in association with atrial disease. Both atrial distention and intra-atrial delay are predisposing factors.[67] Although still the subject of significant debate, the precise underlying abnormal electrophysiologic mechanism, whether reentrant or focal,[68–70] is of little importance to those involved with the clinical management of such cases. What does remain extremely important, however, is the atrial rate and its regularity and the AV conduction ratio during this arrhythmia since practical management aims to affect these aspects, the priorities being in reverse order.

Most often an acute or transitory arrhythmia, atrial flutter may be chronic, paroxysmal, or repetitive, and

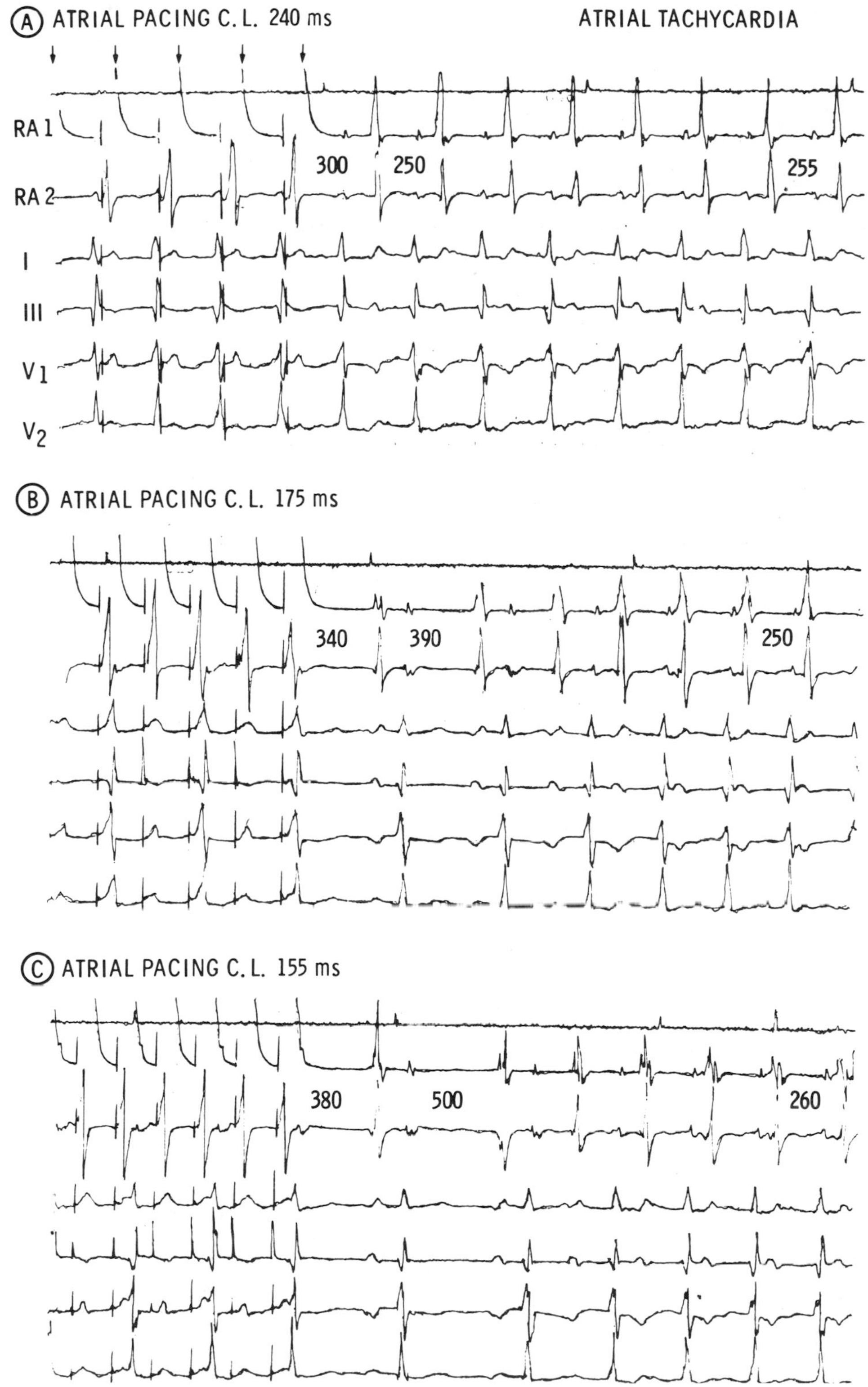

Figure 8-23. *Overdrive atrial pacing at three different rates in an attempt to terminate paroxysmal atrial tachycardia. With higher-paced atrial frequencies, more suppression of the focus is obtained, but it recovers before the sinus node on each occasion. Ajmaline was used successfully to stop the attack.*

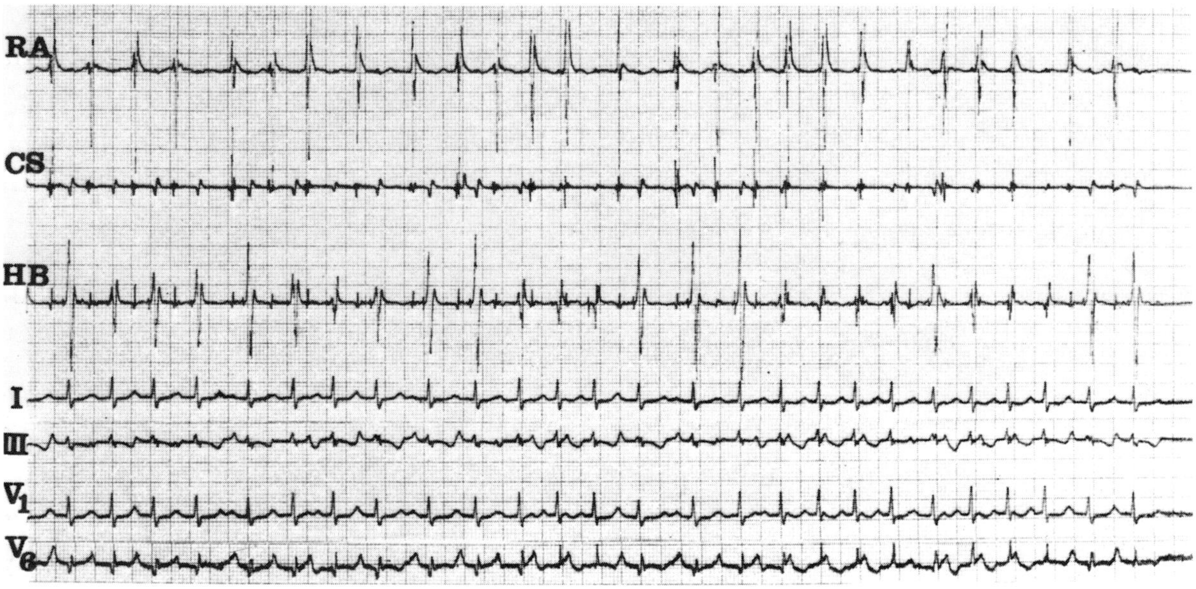

Figure 8-24. *Multifocal atrial tachycardia.*

sometimes without apparent cause (lone atrial flutter). It is a common complication of acute myocardial infarction,[15,71,72] occurs in 14% of those with atrial arrhythmias and the sick sinus syndrome,[27] but is uncommonly seen in children with cardiac disease. It is a common feature after cardiac surgery[73] and during digoxin toxicity.

Characteristically, atrial rates in atrial flutter are on the order of 230 to 450 beats per minute, the ventricular rate and ratio varying in accordance also with the refractory properties of the AV conducting system (Figs. 8-25 and 8-26). One-to-one conduction during atrial flutter produces perhaps one of the most serious arrhythmias known and may occur if AV refractoriness is short as is indeed the case with some patients with either en-

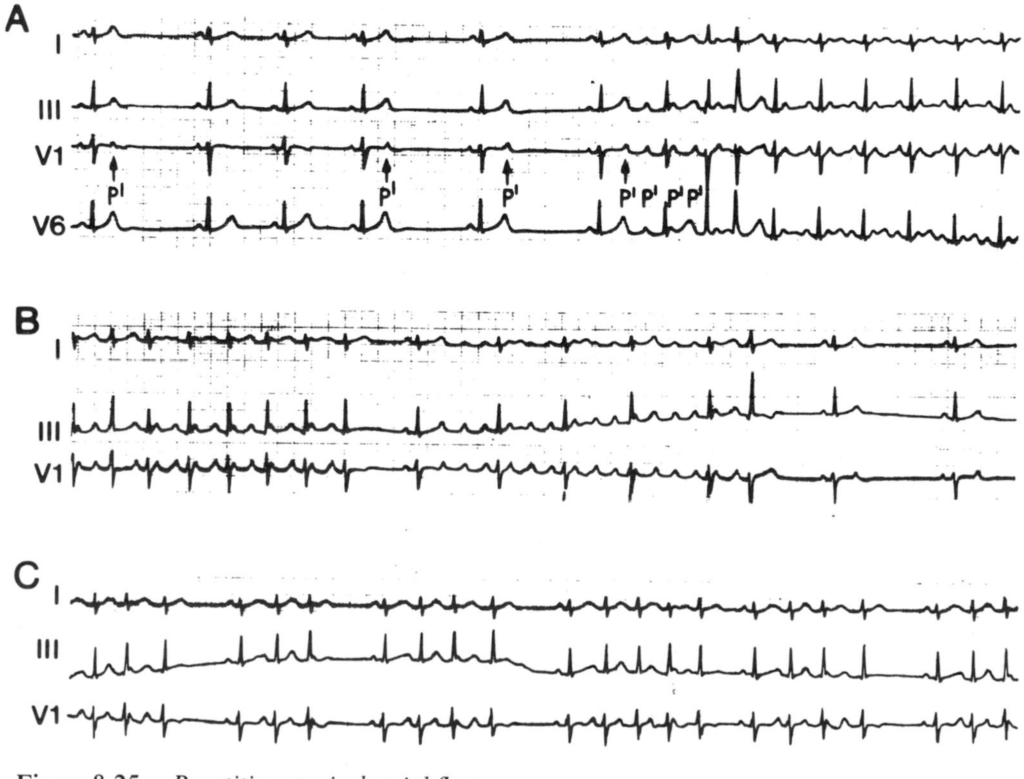

Figure 8-25. *Repetitive atypical atrial flutter.*

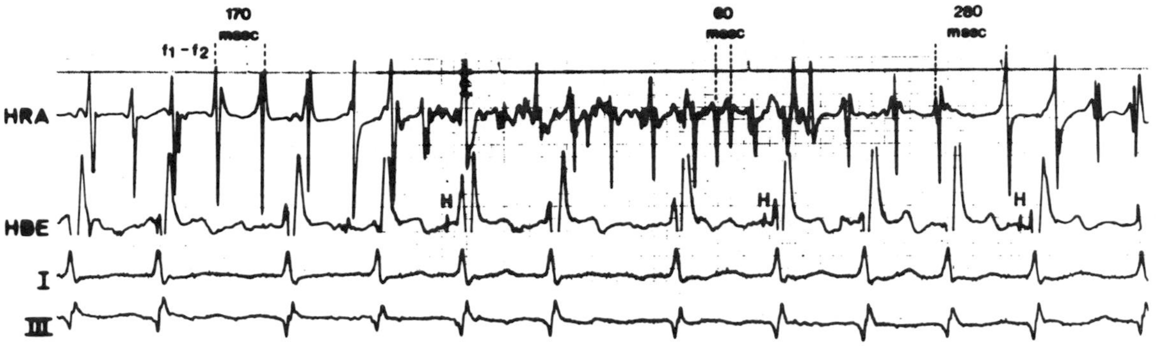

Figure 8-26. *Atrial fibrillation among atrial flutter.*

hanced[74] or anomalous AV conduction. It may also occur if the atrial rate is slowed by a quinidine-like drug while AV conduction capacity remains enhanced. Cardiovascular reflex compensation is insufficient to avoid significant hypotension when ventricular rates exceed 250 beats per minute, even in those with otherwise normal cardiovascular systems.[51] Exercise and emotional stress increase the ventricular rate during atrial flutter, but when the initial AV conduction ratio is only 4 : 1, the patient may be unaware of his arrhythmia. Increased vagal tone has varying effects. It may reduce the ventricular rate through its effects of increasing AV nodal refractoriness, a feature used in diagnosis to reveal underlying characteristic sawtooth atrial flutter waves on the ECG. The atrial flutter frequency, however, may increase with maneuvers that increase vagal tone, sometimes precipitating atrial fibrillation.[11,75,76] Rarely, such maneuvers restore sinus rhythm, but they can precipitate the arrhythmia when applied in sinus rhythm.[11]

The discrete mechanical atrial activity that occurs during atrial flutter, even at rates of 340 beats per minute, many explain the relatively rare occurrence of both atrial thrombi and systemic emboli with this arrhythmia as compared with atrial fibrillation. Tricuspid regurgita-

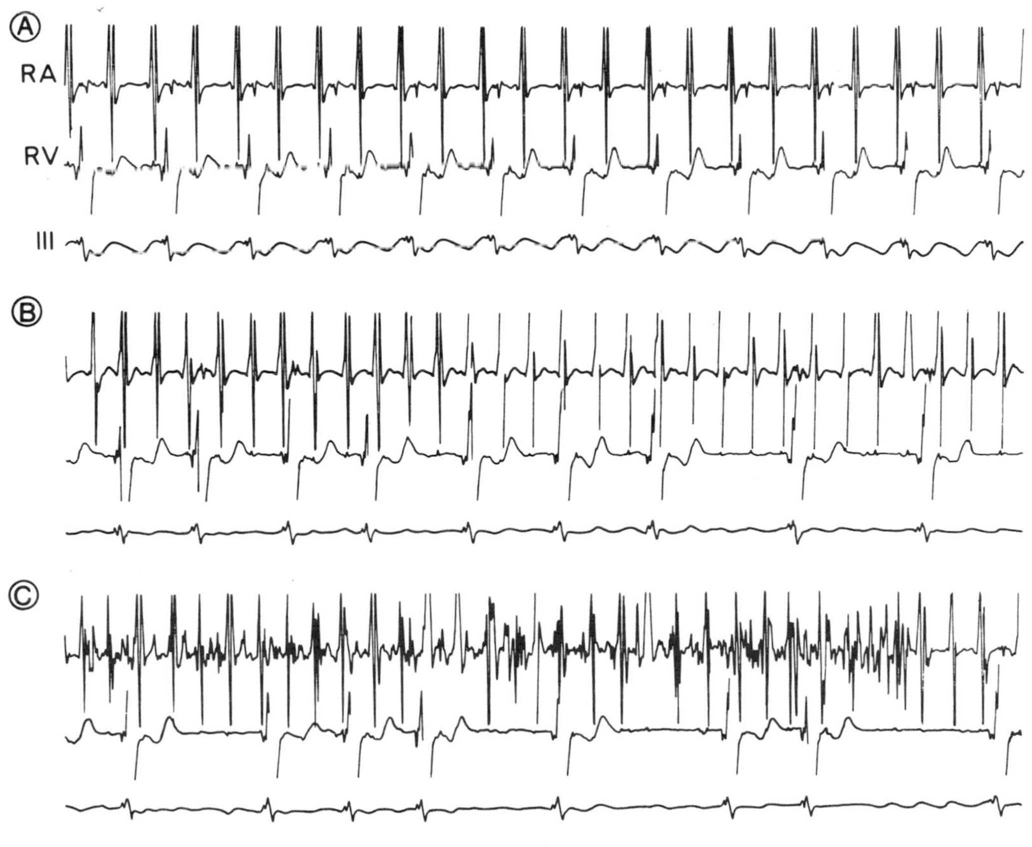

Figure 8-27. *Differing atrial frequencies in atrial flutter (A and B) and in flutter/fibrillation (C) in the same patient.*

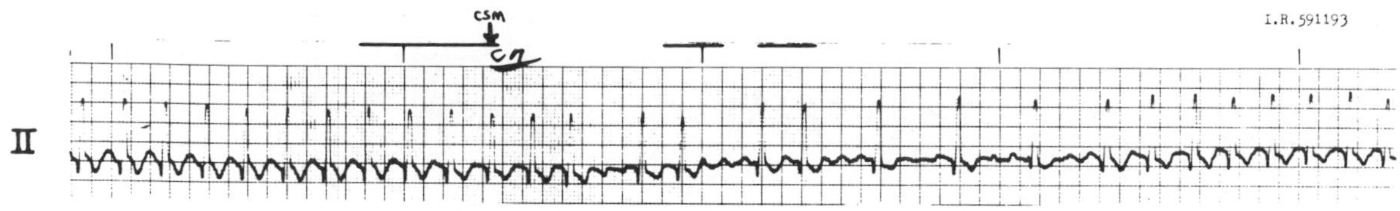

Figure 8-28. *Transient conversion of atrial flutter to atrial fibrillation with carotid sinus massage (CSM).*

tion is rarely seen. Symptoms depend mainly on the rate and regularity of the ventricular response. Restoring sinus rhythm in those with low cardiac output and atrial flutter improves cardiac output by about 38%. Lone atrial flutter, on the other hand, adversely affects only reserve cardiac output for exercise.[77]

During clinical electrophysiologic studies, atrial electrograms show that the flutter frequency varies both in rate and regularity (Fig. 8-27), especially with changing autonomic tone that occurs, for example, with carotid sinus massage (Fig. 8-28). Programmed extra stimulation produces inconsistent effects that only rarely support the concept that such arrhythmias are macro-reentrant in nature (Fig. 8-29). Most often, rapid overdrive pacing is used to terminate the atrial flutter *either* directly, when atrial "entrainment" must be achieved at an appropriate frequency and for an appropriate duration (Fig. 8-30),[78] *or* to induce atrial fibrillation—a more stable arrhythmia that has both a lower mean ventricular rate and a greater potential for spontaneous termination. Several comprehensive studies by Waldo[79,80] described the types and determinants of successful conversion of atrial flutter to sinus rhythm during atrial overdrive pacing. Acute pharmacologic studies give results similar to those described for "pure" atrial tachycardia as regards relative responsiveness of the atrial arrhythmia on the one hand and of the AV node on the other. The main indications for intracardiac pacing studies are (1) therapeutic (overdrive termination) and (2) when this arrhythmia occurs as part of the sick sinus syndrome and when the need both for pacing and antiarrhythmic drugs can be examined safely. Atrial pacing can also be used in patients with overt ventricular or junctional preexcitation who present with syncope, one cause of which could be atrial tachyarrhythmia with rapid rates of 1 : 1 AV conduction across the accessory AV pathway.

Management

Where possible, precipitating factors are removed; otherwise, prophylaxis for attacks of atrial flutter is best obtained with the safe combination of digoxin with disopyramide (or a similar quinidine-like drug). Amiodarone is used for refractory attacks. Permanent pacing will also be required if this arrhythmia occurs as part of the sick sinus syndrome. Quinidine-like drugs should never be given alone, either orally or intravenously, to patients with known 2 : 1 conduction during atrial flutter for fear of inducing a 1 : 1 AV response,[81] but they may be safe for those with low maximum rates of 1 : 1 AV conduction (*i.e.,* less than 130 beats per minute). Attacks of rapid atrial flutter can be treated with verapamil, which readily controls the ventricular rate (at little cost to cardiovascular compensation unless heart failure is overt) and fol-

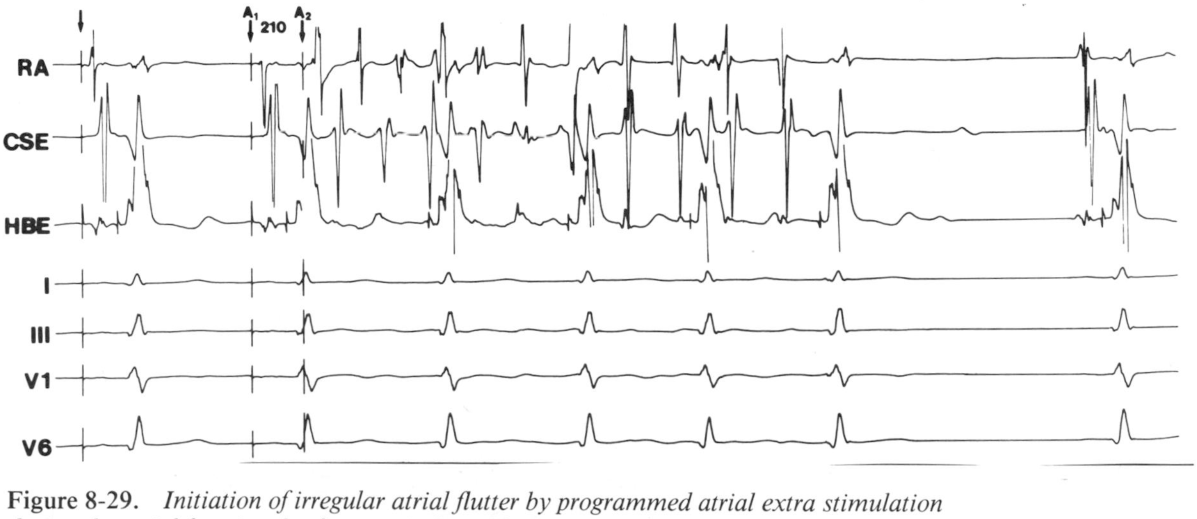

Figure 8-29. *Initiation of irregular atrial flutter by programmed atrial extra stimulation during the atrial functional refractory (vulnerable) period.*

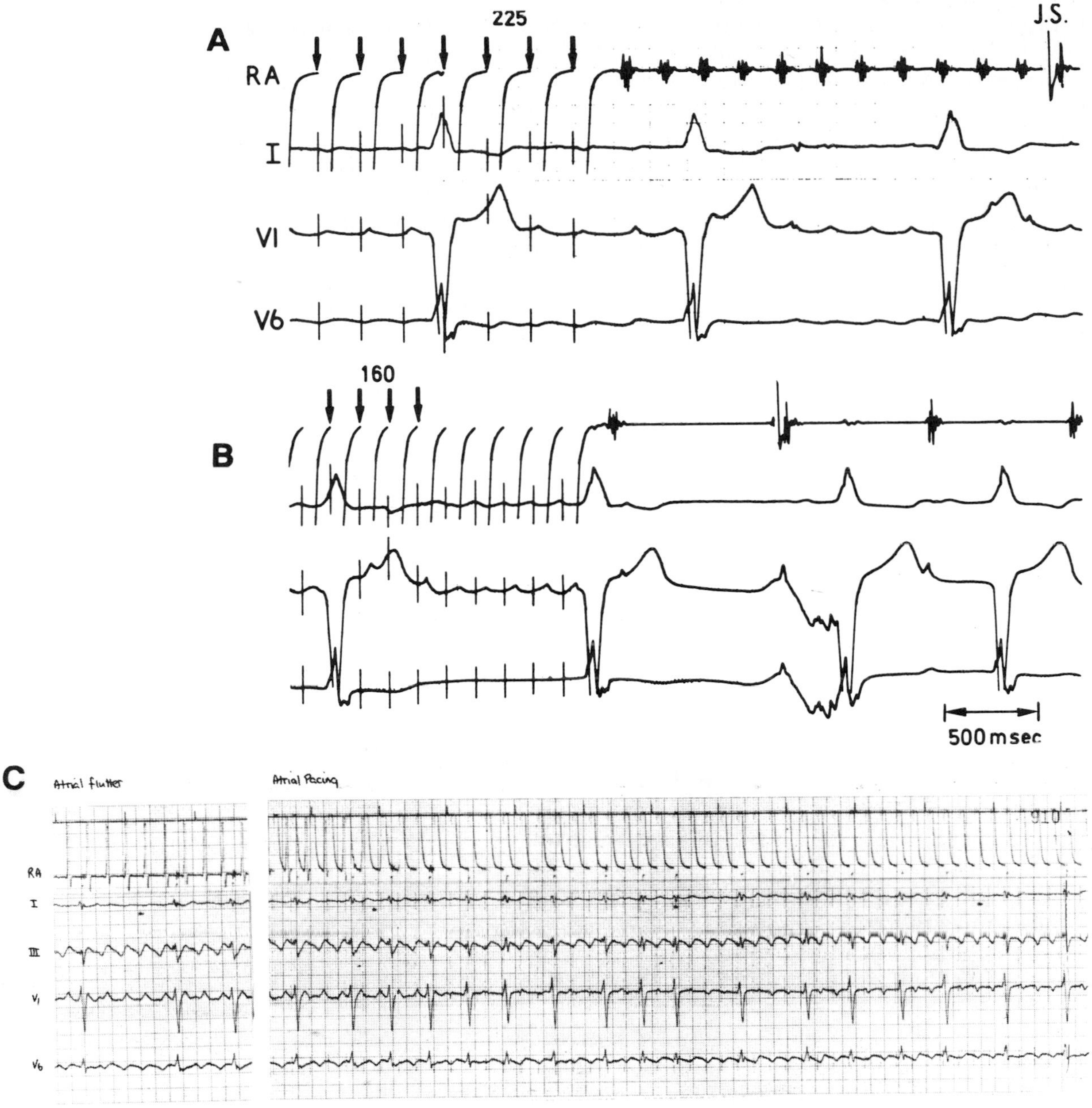

Figure 8-30. *(A) Inadequate, then (B) successful atrial overdrive pacing to terminate atrial flutter. The lowest panel (C) shows that entrainment is best seen when more than one surface ECG lead is recorded during atrial overdrive pacing for atrial flutter.*

lowing which either atrial fibrillation or sinus rhythm can occur.[82] When digoxin has caused the atrial flutter, digoxin should be withdrawn and consideration should be given to the method of overdrive pacing to stop the attack safely.[83] Requirements for successful overdrive pacing have been well reported and consist of (1) ensuring good atrial contact; (2) effective atrial activation (entrainment) best followed electrocardiographically on three leads simultaneously; and (3) diligent atrial pacing that should be gently increased once entrainment is obtained to steady rates that are initially 20, then 40, then 60 beats per minute, and so on, faster than the inherent flutter rate, which should have been recorded and measured before pacing commenced. Most successes are obtained when the initial atrial rhythm is regular. Flutter-fibrillation, on the other hand, is more difficult to capture. Atrial fibrillation is the more likely outcome of overdrive pacing in this latter group (but this is an acceptable outcome!). Skill in this "art" comes only with experience, assisted, of course, by use of the right equipment.[52,70,78,84,85] Temporary epicardial atrial electrodes are extremely useful in this context after heart surgery, both for diagnosis and management (see Chap. 20). Only "synchronized" cardioversion should be used if this alternative is chosen to restore sinus rhythm, and we prefer to use heparin to cover the conversion. We also give long-term oral anticoagulants to those patients with a history either of previous embolism or of associated episodes of atrial fibrillation. Repetitive attacks are also managed this way until consistent control is established (often with amiodarone). Again, in some drug-refractory patients in whom rapid ventricular response produces hemodynamic embarrassment, ablation of the AV node and implantation of a permanent pacemaker remain a suitable therapy.[66]

Atrial Fibrillation

We now appreciate that atrial fibrillation is not an electrophysiologically homogenous process when compared either among different patients or *ad seriatim* in the same patient.[19] Precipitating factors variously include extent of atrial disease (which provides enhanced automaticity, slow intra-atrial conduction, and heterogeneity in refractory properties), autonomic imbalance,[11,12,76] sinus node dysfunction and atrial ischemia,[3,14,16,72,86] and provoked vulnerability.[87]

Resnekov[88] and Abildskov, Millar, and Burgess[89] have recently reviewed the known symptomatic and hemodynamic effects of atrial fibrillation. Atrial fibrillation is now known to occur in 7% to 10% of patients with acute myocardial infarction. Systemic emboli occur in 30% of those with chronic atrial fibrillation, while atrial fibrillation is present in 90% of those with both emboli and mitral stenosis. Kastor[90] has reviewed the management of atrial fibrillation occurring in patients already on digoxin.

Therapeutically, both digoxin and oral anticoagulants remain most appropriate for those with paroxysmal and established atrial fibrillation. Concurrent use of a quinidine-like drug helps reduce the number of attacks in cases of paroxysmal atrial fibrillation and supports the mild prophylactic effect of digoxin in this context.[91] Amiodarone is supremely useful in this capacity.

Serum levels of digoxin do not always relate to therapeutic effect, especially when there is a concurrent pyrexial illness.[92] This is also true for some patients with enhanced AV nodal conduction, when the sensitivity of the AV node may be reduced as regards depression of conduction by digoxin. In both instances, improved control of the ventricular rate can be obtained either temporarily or in the long term with the concurrent use of verapamil.[82] Propafenone and flecainide are both effective against induced atrial fibrillation in the electrophysiology laboratory; however, their long-term effectiveness in chronic atrial fibrillation deserves further investigation.

Management of new cases is either with cardioversion or rapid digitalization. Reversion to sinus rhythm with digoxin is most likely to occur when the initial rate in atrial fibrillation is fast but usually occurs only after 4 to 8 hours. Digitalization is preferred if the precipitating stimulus is likely to last for more than a few hours since recurrence after successful cardioversion is a frequent event. We prefer to review the need for cardioversion "after the storm has died down." In refractory cases with poorly controlled ventricular response, ablation of the AV node is increasingly used.[66]

References

1. Katz, L. N., and Pick, A.: Clinical Electrocardiography. Part I. Arrhythmias With an Atlas of Electrocardiograms. p. 595. Philadelphia, Lea & Febiger, 1956.
2. Legato, M. J., Bull, M. B., and Ferrer, M. I.: Atrial ultrastructure in patients with fixed intra-atrial block. Chest, 65:252, 1974.
3. Kaplan, B. M., Langendorf, R., Lev, M., and Pick, A.: Tachycardia-bradycardia syndrome (so called "sick sinus syndrome"). Pathology, mechanisms and treatment. Am. J. Cardiol., 31:497, 1973.
4. Demoulin, J. C., and Kulbertus, H. E.: Pathological correlates of atrial arrhythmias. *In* Kulbertus, H. E. (ed.): Re-entrant Arrhythmias: Mechanisms and Treatment. p. 99. Lancaster, MTP Press, 1977.
5. Hudson, R. E. B. (ed.): Cardiovascular Pathology. London, Edward Arnold, 1965.
6. James, T. N.: Arrhythmias and conduction disturbances in acute myocardial infarction. Am. Heart J., 64:416, 1962.
7. Laas, E.: Das Arrhythmieherz. Zentrabl. Allg. Pathol., 103:552, 1962.
8. Lippestad, C. T., and Marton, P. F.: Sinus arrest in proximal right coronary artery occlusion. Am. Heart J., 74:551, 1967.
9. Davies, M. J., and Pomerance, A.: Pathology of atrial fibrillation in man. Br. Heart J., 34:520, 1972.
10. Sims, B. A.: Pathogenesis of atrial arrhythmias. Br. Heart J., 34:336, 1972.
11. El-Sherif, N.: Paroxysmal atrial flutter and fibrillation induced by carotid sinus compression and prevention by atropine. Br. Heart J., 34:1024, 1972.
12. Loomis, T. A., Captain, M. C., and Krop, S.: Auricular fibrillation induced and maintained in animals by acetylcholine or vagal stimulation. Circ. Res., 3:390, 1955.
13. Friedberg, C. K., and Donoso, E.: Arrhythmias and conduction disturbances due to digitalis. Prog. Cardiovasc. Dis., 2:408, 1960.
14. Burns, J. H.: The cause of fibrillation. Br. Med. J., 1:1379, 1960.
15. Lindsay, J., and Hurst, J. W.: The clinical features of atrial flutter and their clinical implications. Chest, 66:114, 1974.
16. Hecht, H. H.: Mechanisms, causes and treatment of paroxysmal atrial fibrillation. *In* Sandoe, E., Flensted-Jensen, E., and Olesen, K. H. (eds.): Symposium on Cardiac Arrhythmias. p. 747. Elsinore, Astra, 1970.
17. Narula, O. S.: Sinus node re-entry: mechanism of supraventricular tachycardia (SVT) in man. Circulation, 46(Suppl.2):11, 1972.
18. Chung, E. K.: A reappraisal of atrial dissociation. Am. J. Cardiol., 28:111, 1971.
19. Wells, J. L., et al.: Characterisation of atrial fibrillation in man: studies following open heart surgery. PACE, 1:4, 1978.
20. Allessie, M. A., Bonke, F. I. M., and Schopman, F. J. G.: Circus movement in rabbit atrial muscle as a mechanism of tachycardia. III. The "leading circle" concept: a new model of circus movement

in cardiac tissue without the involvement of an anatomical obstacle. Circ. Res., 41:9, 1977.
21. Warin, J. F., and Fauchier, J. P.: Les troubles de la conduction intra-auriculaire. *In* Peuch, P., and Slama, R. (eds.): Les Troubles du Rythme Cardiaque. p. 95. Paris, Roussel, 1978.
22. Hiss, R. G., and Lamb, L. E.: Electrocardiographic findings in 122,043 individuals. Circulation, 25:947, 1962.
23. Nagira, S.: Arrhythmias in children. Acta Med. Jpn., 16:795, 1975.
24. Chung, K-Y., Walsh, T. J., and Massie, E.: Atrial parasystole. Am. J. Cardiol., 14:255, 1964.
25. Chung, E. K.: Diagnosis and clinical significance of parasystole. *In* Sandoe, E., Flensted-Jensen, E., and Olesen, K. H. (eds.): Symposium on Cardiac Arrhythmias. p. 271. Elsinore, Astra, 1970.
26. Eliakim, M.: Atrial parasystole. Effect of carotid sinus stimulation, Valsalva maneuver, and exercise. Am. J. Cardiol., 16:457, 1965.
27. Shenasa, M., Curry, P. V. L., and Sowton, E.: Comparison of atrial arrhythmias with atrial stimulation threshold and conduction times in patients with sick sinus syndrome. Br. Heart J., 42:237, 1979.
28. Scherf, D., Yildiz, M., and DeArmas, D.: Atrial parasystole. Am. Heart J., 57:507, 1959.
29. Goel, B. G., and Han, J.: Atrial ectopic activity associated with sinus bradycardia. Circulation, 42:853, 1970.
30. Alicandri, C., Fouad, F. M., Terazi, R. C., Castle, L., and Moraut, V.: Three cases of hypotension and syncope with ventricular pacing: possible role of atrial reflexes. Am. J. Cardiol., 42:137, 1978.
31. Maclean, W. A. H., Karp, R. B., Kouchoukos, N. T., James, T. N., and Waldo, A. L.: P waves during ectopic atrial rhythms in man. A study utilizing atrial pacing with fixed electrodes. Circulation, 52:426, 1975.
32. Strauss, H. C., and Geer, M. R.: Sino-atrial node re-entry. *In* Kulbertus, H. E. (ed.): Re-entrant Arrhythmias: Mechanism and Treatment. p. 27. Lancaster, MTP Press, 1977.
33. Marriott, H. J.: Tampa Tracings, p. 77, 1965.
34. Barker, P. S., Wilson, F. N., and Johnson, F. D.: The mechanism of auricular paroxysmal tachycardia. Am. Heart J., 26:435, 1943.
35. Wallace, A. C., and Daggett, W. M.: Re-excitation of the atrium; the echo phenomenon. Am. Heart J., 68:661, 1964.
36. Han, J., Malozzi, A. M., and Moe, G. A.: Sino-atrial reciprocation in the isolated rabbit heart. Circ. Res., 22:355, 1968.
37. Allessie, M. A., and Bonke, F. I. M.: Re-entry within the sinoatrial node as demonstrated by multiple micro-electrode recordings in the isolated rabbit heart. *In* Bonke, F. I. M. (ed.): The Sinus Node: Structure, Function and Clinical Relevance. p. 409. The Hague, Nijhoff, 1978.
38. Pahlajani, D. B., Millar, R. A., and Serrato, M.: Sinus node re-entry and sinus node tachycardia. Am. Heart J., 90:305, 1975.
39. Weisfogel, G. M., et al.: Sinus node re-entrant tachycardia in man. Am. Heart J., 90:295, 1975.
40. Gillette, P. G.: The mechanisms of supraventricular tachycardia in children. Circulation, 54:133, 1976.
41. Curry, P. V. L., Evans, T. R., and Krikler, D. M.: Paroxysmal reciprocating sinus tachycardia. Eur. J. Cardiol., 6:199, 1977.
42. Wu, D., et al.: Demonstration of sustained sinus node and atrial re-entry as a mechanism of paroxysmal supraventricular tachycardia. Circulation, 51:234, 1975.
43. Dhingra, A. C., et al.: Sinus node response to atrial extrastimuli in patients without apparent sinus node disease. Am. J. Cardiol., 36:445, 1975.
44. Krikler, D. M., and Curry, P. V. L.: Atypical initiation of reciprocating tachycardia in the Wolff-Parkinson-White syndrome. *In* Kulbertus, H. E. (ed.): Re-entrant Arrhythmias: Mechanisms and Treatment. Lancaster, MTP Press, 1977.
45. Curry, P. V. L., and Krikler, D.M.: Significance of cycle length alternation during drug treatment of supraventricular tachycardia. Br. Heart J., 38:882, 1976.
46. Breithardt, G., and Seipel, L.: Sequence of atrial activation in patients with atrial echo beats. *In* Bonke, F. I. M. (ed.): The Sinus Node: Structure, Function and Clinical Relevance. p. 389. The Hague, Nijhoff, 1978.
47. Reiffel, J. A., and Bigger, T. J., Jr.: Current status of direct recording of the sinus node electrogram in man. PACE, 6:1143, 1983.
48. Keane, J. F., Plauth, W. H., and Nadas, A. S.: Chronic ectopic tachycardia of infancy and children. Am. Heart J., 84:748, 1972.
49. Scheinman, M. M., Basu, D., and Hollenberg, M.: Electrophysiologic studies in patients with persistent atrial tachycardia. Circulation, 50:266, 1974.
50. Goldreyer, B. N., Gallagher, J. J., and Damato, A. N.: The electrophysiologic demonstration of atrial ectopic tachycardia in man. Am. Heart J., 85:205, 1973.
51. Curry, P. V. L.: The haemodynamic and electrophysiological effects of paroxysmal tachycardia. *In* Narula, O. S. (ed.): Cardiac Arrhythmias: Electrophysiology, Diagnosis and Management. p. 579. Baltimore, Williams & Wilkins, 1979.
52. Pittman, D. E., Makar, J. S., Kooros, K. S., and Joyner, C. R.: Rapid atrial stimulation: successful method of conversion of atrial flutter and atrial tachycardia. Am. J. Cardiol., 32:700, 1973.
53. Gillette, P. G., and Garson, A., Jr.: Electrophysiologic and pharmacologic characteristics of automatic ectopic atrial tachycardia. Circulation, 56:571, 1977.
54. Haines, D. E., Lerman, B. B., Sellers, T. D., Dipparco, J. P.: Intra-atrial reentrant tachycardia: clinical characteristics and response to chronic amiodarone therapy. Circulation, 72(Suppl. III):III–126, 1985.
55. Arbel, E. R., Cohen, H. C., Langendorf, R., and Glick, G.: Successful treatment of drug resistant atrial tachycardia and intractable congestive heart failure with permanent coupled atrial pacing. Am. J. Cardiol., 41:336, 1978.
56. Coumel, Ph., et al.: Repérage et tentative d'exérèse chirurgicale d'un foyer ectopique avriculaire gauche avec tachycardie rebelle: évolution favorable. Ann. Cardiol. Angéiol., 22:189, 1973.
57. Coumel, Ph., and Barold, S. S.: Mechanisms of supraventricular tachycardias. In Narula, O. S. (ed.): His Bundle Electrocardiography and Clinical Electrophysiology. p. 235. Philadelphia, F. A. Davis, 1975.
58. Silka, M. J., Gillette, P. C., Garson, A., Jr., and Zinner, A.: Transvenous catheter ablation of a right atrial automatic ectopic tachycardia. J. Am. Coll. Cardiol., 5:999, 1985.
59. Marriott, H. J.: Diagnosis of cardiac arrhythmias. G. P., 30:96, 1964.
60. Abrams, D. L., and Eaddy, J. A.: Repetitive multifocal paroxysmal atrial tachycardia with second degree AV block type I, and concealed and aberrant conduction. Am. J. Cardiol., 15:871, 1965.
61. Shine, K. I., Kastor, J. A., and Yurchak, P. M.: Multifocal atrial tachycardia. Clinical and electrocardiographic features in 32 patients. N. Engl. J. Med., 279:344, 1968.
62. Lipson, M. J., and Naimi, S.: Multifocal atrial tachycardia (chaotic atrial tachycardia). Circulation, 42:397, 1970.
63. Corazza, L. J., and Pastor, B. H.: Cardiac arrhythmias in chronic cor pulmonale. N. Engl. J. Med., 258:862, 1958.
64. Berlinerblau, R., and Feder, W.: Chaotic atrial rhythm. J. Electrocardiol., 5:135, 1972.
65. Phillips, J., Spano, J., and Burch, G. E.: Chaotic atrial mechanism. Am. Heart J., 78:171, 1969.
66. Gallagher, J. J., Svenson, R. H., Kasell, J. H., et al.: Catheter technique for closed chest ablation of the atrioventricular conduction system: a therapeutic alternative for treatment of refractory supraventricular tachycardia. N. Engl. J. Med., 306:194, 1982.
67. Leier, C. V., Meacham, J. A., and Schaal, S. F.: Prolonged atrial conduction; a major predisposing factor for the development of atrial flutter. Circulation, 57:213, 1978.

68. Hayden, W. G., Hurley, E. J., and Rytand, D. A.: The mechanism of canine atrial flutter. Circ. Res., 20:496, 1967.
69. Lewis, T., Drury, A. N., and Iliescu, C. C.: A demonstration of circus movement in clinical flutter of the auricles. Heart, 8:341, 1921.
70. Guiney, T. E., and Lown, B.: Electrical conversion of atrial flutter to atrial fibrillation; flutter mechanism in man. Br. Heart J., 34:1215, 1972.
71. Cristal, N., Szwarcberg, J., and Gueron, M.: Supraventricular arrhythmias in acute myocardial infarction. Ann. Intern. Med., 82:35, 1975.
72. Liberthson, R. R., Salisbury, K. W., Hutter, A. M., and DeSanctis, R. W.: Atrial tachycardias in acute myocardial infarction. Am. J. Med., 60:956, 1976.
73. Roberts, N. K., and Yabek, S.: Arrhythmias following atrial and ventricular surgery. *In* Roberts, N. K., and Gelband, H. (eds.): Cardiac Arrhythmias in the Neonate, Infant and Child. p. 405. New York, Appleton-Century-Crofts, 1977.
74. Kennelly, B. M., and Lane, G. K.: Electrophysiological studies in four patients with 1 : 1 atrioventricular conduction. Am. Heart J., 96:723, 1978.
75. Allesie, R., Nusynowitz, M., Abildskov, J. A., and Moe, G. K.: Non-uniform distribution of vagal effects on the atrial refractory period. Am. J. Physiol., 194:406, 1958.
76. Anbe, D. T., Rubenfire, M., and Drake, E. H.: Conversion of atrial flutter to atrial fibrillation with carotid sinus pressure. J. Electrocardiol., 2:377, 1969.
77. Ferret, M. I.: Atrial flutter. Chest, 66:111, 1974.
78. Waldo, A. L., Maclean, W. A. H., Karp, R. B., Kouchoukos, N. T., and James, T. N.: Entrainment and interruption of atrial flutter with atrial pacing. Studies in man following open heart surgery. Circulation, 56:737, 1977.
79. Waldo, A. L.: Some observations concerning atrial flutter in man. PACE, 6:1181, 1983.
80. Waldo, A. L., Henthorn, R. W., and Plumb, V. J.: Atrial flutter. Recent observations in man. *In* Josephson, M. E., and Wellens, H. J. J. (eds.): Tachycardias: Mechanisms, diagnosis and treatment. Philadelphia, Lea & Febiger, 1984.
81. Danahy, D. T., and Aronow, W. S.: Lidocaine-induced cardiac rate changes in atrial fibrillation and flutter. Am. Heart J., 95:474, 1978.
82. Schamroth, L., Krikler, D. M., and Garret, G.: Immediate effects of intravenous verapamil in cardiac arrhythmias. Br. Med. J., 1:660, 1972.
83. Das, G., et al.: Atrial pacing for conversion of atrial flutter in digitalized patients. Am. J. Cardiol., 41:308, 1978.
84. Rosen, K. M., Sinno, M. Z., Gunnar, R. M., and Rahimtoola, S. H.: Failure of rapid atrial pacing in the conversion of atrial flutter. Am. J. Cardiol., 29:524, 1972.
85. Preston, T. A.: Atrial pacing to convert atrial flutter. Am. J. Cardiol., 32:737, 1973.
86. Scherf, D.: The mechanism of flutter and fibrillation. Am. Heart J., 71:273, 1966.
87. Paulay, K. L., Varghese, P. J., and Damato, A. N.: Atrial rhythms in response to an early atrial premature depolarization in man. Am. Heart J., 85:323, 1973.
88. Resnekov, L.: Circulatory effects of cardiac dysrhythmias. *In* Dreifus, L. (ed.): Arrhythmias. Cardiovasc. Clin, 2(2):27, 1970.
89. Abildskov, J. A., Millar, K., and Burgess, M. J.: Atrial fibrillation. Am. J. Cardiol., 28:263, 1971.
90. Kastor, J. A.: Digitalis intoxication in patients with atrial fibrillation. Circulation, 47:888, 1973.
91. Hordof, A. J., Spotnitz, A., Mary-Rabin, L., Edie, R. N., and Rosen, M. R.: The cellular electrophysiologic effects of digitalis on human atrial fibers. Circulation, 57:223, 1978.
92. Goldman, S., Probst, P., Selzer, A., and Cohn, K.: Inefficacy of "therapeutic" serum levels of digoxin in controlling the ventricular rate in atrial fibrillation. Am. J. Cardiol., 35:651, 1975.

9

Atrioventricular Junctional Rhythms

R. A. Massumi

Rhythms arising from the atrioventricular junction (AVJ) in the form of single extrasystoles, parasystoles, slow escape rhythms, and nonparoxysmal tachycardias are the best-known varieties of AV junctional rhythms. Other less appreciated arrhythmias include conduction impairments (pseudo-AV block) and reciprocal atrial or ventricular beatings that result from manifest or concealed automatic activity or conduction delay within the AV junctional region. In addition, the bizarre phenomena encountered in patients possessing dual pathways within the AV node, and the "pseudotachycardias" caused by interpolation of junctional beats between sinus beats, make the AV junction the most colorful and versatile of the cardiac regions in terms of rhythm disturbances. The marked versatility of the AVJ owes itself, first, to its central location, situated at the crossroads of the cardiac conduction system, thereby influencing the electrical phenomena as they approach or attempt to pass through the AV junction in either antegrade or retrograde direction and, second, to its ability to produce tachycardias and slower rhythms by both automatic firing and reentry. The responsiveness of the AV node to autonomic influences adds still more nuances to AVJ rhythms.

Deductive analysis of every complex arrhythmia necessitates consideration of the possible interactions between the basic cardiac rhythm and one or more of the AVJ phenomena enumerated above. In this chapter, an attempt is made to demonstrate the multitudinous manifestations of AVJ rhythms and their intriguing ways of interfering with the prevailing cardiac mechanisms.

Difficulties With the Definition of the Term *Atrioventricular Junction*

The term *atrioventricular junction* cannot be defined without taking into consideration both the anatomic and electrophysiologic characteristics as far as they are known. To most authorities, AVJ encompasses the AV node with its three electrophysically distinct regions (AN, N, and NH) and the bundle of His.[1,2] From the standpoint of surface electrocardiography, the common denominator of all the AVJ rhythms is the caudocranial direction of atrial activation, resulting in negative P waves in leads II, III, and aV_F and PR intervals that are shorter than those of the basic sinus beats in the same tracing.[3–6] The same features, however, may also be found in beats originating from the coronary sinus and the lower regions of both right and left atria. It may therefore be necessary to include all these regions under the umbrella of AVJ as has been done by Scherf[2] and suggested by Bellet.[4] This practice may be justified because electrocardiographic differentiation of rhythms originating from the upper regions of the AV node and those arising from the floor of the right and left atria and from the coronary sinus is probably impossible. In the only indisputable example of early left atrial activation occurring in cases of distal coronary sinus pacing, and retrograde left atrial activation during tachycardia in cases of left posterior bypass tracts, P wave polarity is from left to right, giving rise to negative P waves in leads I and V_6 and, frequently but not invariably, negative P waves in leads II, III, and aV_F. How far the pacing catheter must be advanced inside the coronary sinus to obtain clearly negative P waves in leads I and V_6 is not known; moreover, electrical stimulation of the left atrium in the human heart has produced a variety of P waves with diverse morphologies.[7–8] To compound the difficulties in determining the origin of P waves on the basis of their polarity, Moore and colleagues[9] and Waldo and associates[10] have observed P wave positivity in leads II, III, and aV_F following stimulation of the AV nodal region. The lack of uniformity of P wave polarity probably reflects the different modes of spread of the retro-

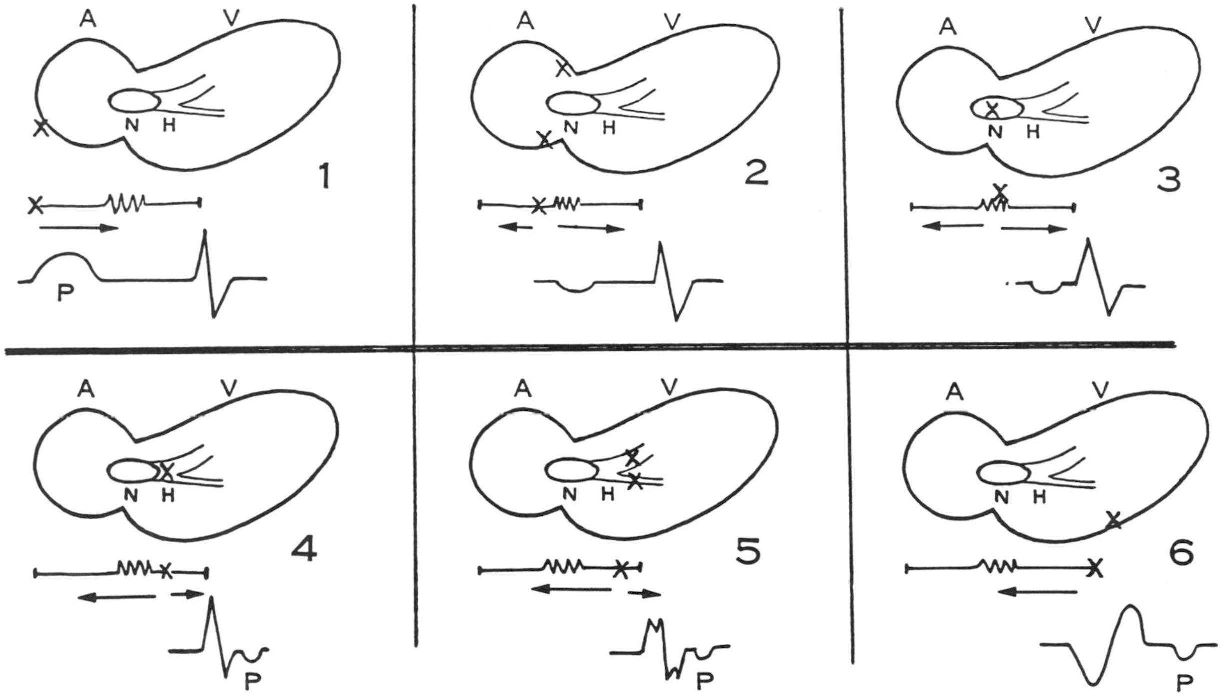

Figure 9-1. *Diagrammatic representations of the atria (A), the ventricles (V), the AV node (N), and the His bundle (H), with variable origins of the P waves (marked by X within the diagrams). The resultant electrocardiograms of lead 2 are schematically drawn beneath the anatomic diagrams. Between the anatomic diagrams and the electrocardiograms, horizontal line drawings depict the origin of the P waves (X) and the direction of spread of the activation process toward the atria and ventricles (arrows). The zigzag portion of the drawing indicates slow conduction through the AV node.*

In 1, the P wave originates within the sinus node and must travel the entire length of the atrium before reaching the AV node; hence, this is the longest PR interval with a positive P wave. In 2, the P wave originates in the lower regions of the atria and depolarizes the atria in a retrograde fashion; the atrial depolarization wave reaches the AV node earlier than in 1. The result is a negative P with a shorter PR interval. In 3, the impulse originates within the AV node and depolarizes the atria and ventricles almost simultaneously. Assuming no significant delay in either direction, the result is a negative P wave with a very short or zero PR interval. In 4, 5, and 6, the origin of the impulse moves distally and originates in the main His bundle (4), bundle branches (5), and ventricular-Purkinje system (6). P waves are retrograde and necessarily occur after the QRS in all these examples. The further from the atria the origin of the P wave, the further or later the retrograde P wave appears after the QRS.

grade impulses within the atria and the possible use of the interatrial septum for its cephalad spread before cascading over both atria caudally. Similarly, rapid spread of a left atrial impulse over Bachmann's bundle may deliver the impulse to the right atrium before it has had time to depolarize the left atrium, thereby giving rise to apparent right atrial P waves. The P wave polarity in lead I has been addressed by Schamroth,[11] who states that the frontal plane axis of the P waves in "idionodal" rhythms is usually −60° to −90°, giving rise to flat or slightly positive P waves in lead I, whereas it is −90° to −110° in reciprocal rhythms using the AV node, thus producing negative P waves in lead I.[12] However, the reason for the different spatial orientations is not discussed.

A beat arising in the AVJ or low atrial regions does not travel the whole extent of the right atrial wall before reaching the His bundle, and its PR interval is necessarily shorter than the PR of a sinus beat in the same person (0.1 to 0.14 second) (Fig. 9-1). Note, however, that a very early AV junctional premature beat may enter the AV node or the bundle of His before the latter has completely recovered conductivity and reach the ventricle with a PR interval that is much longer than 0.1 to 0.14 second. In any case, in a given person, the PR interval of

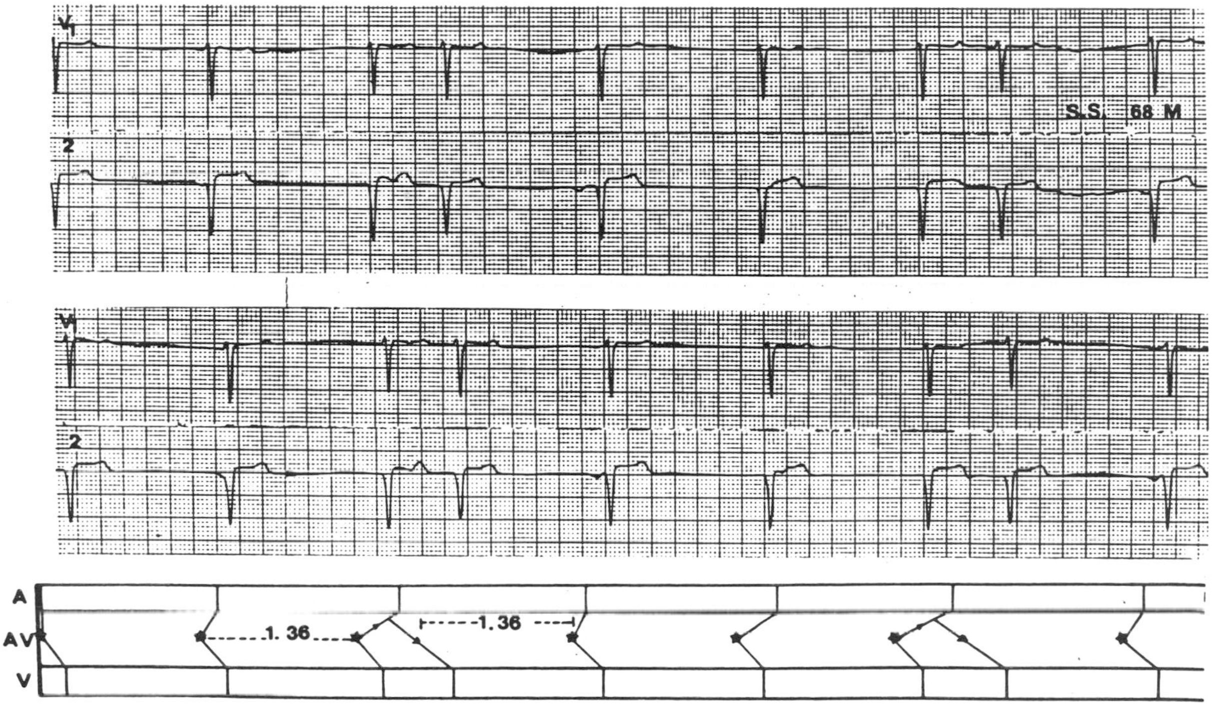

Figure 9-2. *Rhythm strips of simultaneous leads V_1 and V_2, taken on the second day of an acute inferior wall myocardial infarction complicated by sinus node depression, show a slow AVJ rhythm with the rate of 43 beats/min. The P waves are negative in lead 2 and are presumed to be retrograde, originating in the same AVJ focus that drives the ventricles. The tracing could best be analyzed if the pacemaker is assumed to be situated somewhere in the distal AV node, whence impulses conduct to the ventricles without delay but suffer gradual slowing on their way to the atria. Consequently, the retrograde P waves appear increasingly later in relation to the QRS. When the retrograde P wave is so delayed as to appear within the T wave, it can echo back into the ventricle and produce a capture QRS. On its passage through the AV junction, this returning P wave depolarizes the pacemaker focus and resets it, thus delaying the next discharge by exactly the length of the basic AVJ pacemaker cycle (1.36 second). The increasing delay in retrograde propagation of the P wave to the atria must take place within the AV node. The pacemaking focus therefore must be somewhere in the lower regions of the AV node. It cannot be low atrial because all P waves do not occur before the QRS, and it cannot be in the His bundle because the His-Purkinje conduction delay required to place the QRS after the P wave would be outside the range of observed His-Q intervals. In this and all subsequent clinical tracings, intervals are expressed in hundredths of a second and not in milliseconds, because milliseconds cannot possibly be measured in a 25 mm/sec recording. The use of such "pseudo"-precision is probably unwarranted.*

an AVJ or low atrial impulse—provided it is not very premature—is shorter than the PR interval of the sinus beats (see Fig. 9-1).

The terms *upper, middle,* and *lower* nodal rhythms derived from the occurrence of retrograde P waves before, concomitant, and after the QRS, respectively,[1,4] have been abandoned because the temporal relationship between the P and the QRS in an AV nodal beat is more a function of its conduction velocity in antegrade and retrograde directions than its exact anatomic point of origin. Figure 9-2 depicts an AVJ rhythm in which retrograde P waves occur before or after the QRS depending on the conduction time to the atria.

With the electrophysiologic techniques currently available, it is virtually impossible to determine exactly the site of origin of an impulse arising from AVJ–low atrial regions, possibly justifying the expression *AVJ* or *low atrial* in interpreting tracings with abnormal P waves with short PR intervals. The response of a given rhythm to vagal and sympathetic maneuvers may contribute somewhat to delineation of the origin of the rhythm (see below). The difficulties enumerated so far are compounded when one realizes the impossibility of ascertaining the presence of centrally situated, paranodal bypasses capable of rapidly transmitting impulses from atria to ventricles, or vice versa, without having to go through the slowly conducting AV node. The short PR interval thus produced may bring to mind the presence of AVJ beats.

Based on the foregoing discussions and a review of the related literature, it becomes clear that clinical consideration of AVJ rhythms must necessarily be based on few reasonable assumptions:

1. The QRS complexes should be similar to those of sinus beats unless aberrant conduction due to prematurity is present.
2. The areas of greatest automaticity are the perinodal regions of the AV node (coronary sinus, low atrial) and the main His bundle.
3. Impulses arising from the low atrial regions are

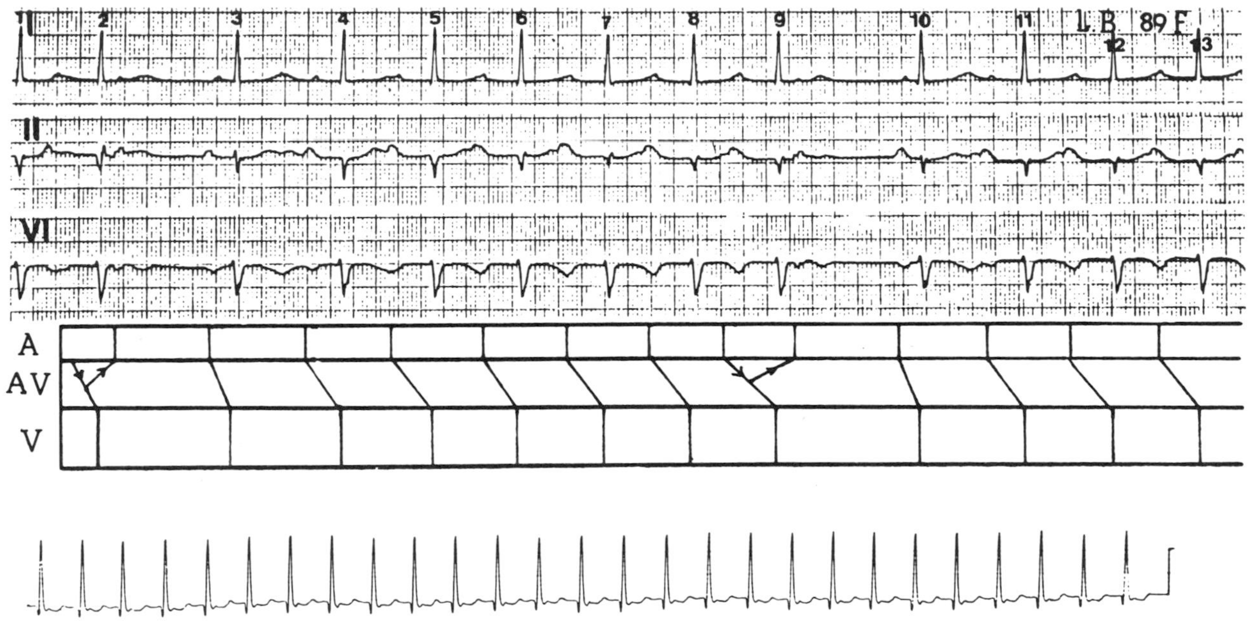

Figure 9-3. *Simultaneously recorded rhythm strips show the Wenckebach type of AV block in this case of acute inferior wall myocardial infarction. The Wenckebach cycles are terminated when echo P waves (negative deflection attached to the end of QRS complexes 2 and 9) follow the longest PR intervals (0.48 second). This phenomenon is not rare and should be looked for whenever the sinus P wave expected to occur in the middle of the pause is absent. Echo P waves may be hidden within the QRS complex and are not always easy to identify. Their presence is suggested by the absence of the expected sinus P wave within the pauses. The combination of long PR–echo is the necessary substrate for AV nodal reentrant tachycardia (shown in the bottom panel). This type of reentrant tachycardia resulting from the Wenckebach type of AV block has been observed in several other cases.*

much more likely to depolarize the atria first and the ventricles last.

4. Beats arising from the His bundle are infinitely more likely to activate ventricles before atria.
5. Impulses originating within the AV node will activate both atria and ventricles almost simultaneously or in quick sequence unless the propagation in one or other direction is impeded.
6. The configuration and polarity of the P waves may be the same regardless of where in the AVJ–low atrial regions the impulses originate.

Lending support to these assumptions are the following observations:

1. Electrical stimulation of the coronary sinus orifice and the low right atrial regions results in retrograde P waves always appearing before the QRS.
2. Pacing of the His bundle always produces QRS complexes before the P wave.
3. AVJ escape beats occurring after pauses in cases of AV nodal–Wenckebach cycles, arising necessarily from the infranodal regions (main His bundle), are characterized invariably by QRS complexes that are not preceded by retrograde P waves.
4. In AVJ echo beats usually occurring after long PR intervals, where the "U turn" occurs in the lower regions of the AV node, the retrograde P always occurs after the QRS complex (Figs. 9-3 to 9-5).
5. In AV nodal reentrant tachycardias, where the antegrade impulse turns around in the lower AV node, activation of the ventricle almost always precedes the retrograde P waves.
6. In slow AVJ escape rhythms emerging because of sinus bradycardia or standstill, and probably originating in the lower regions of the AV node or the upper regions of the His bundle, the QRS complex precedes the retrograde P waves. These AVJ escape rhythms, arising from structures known to

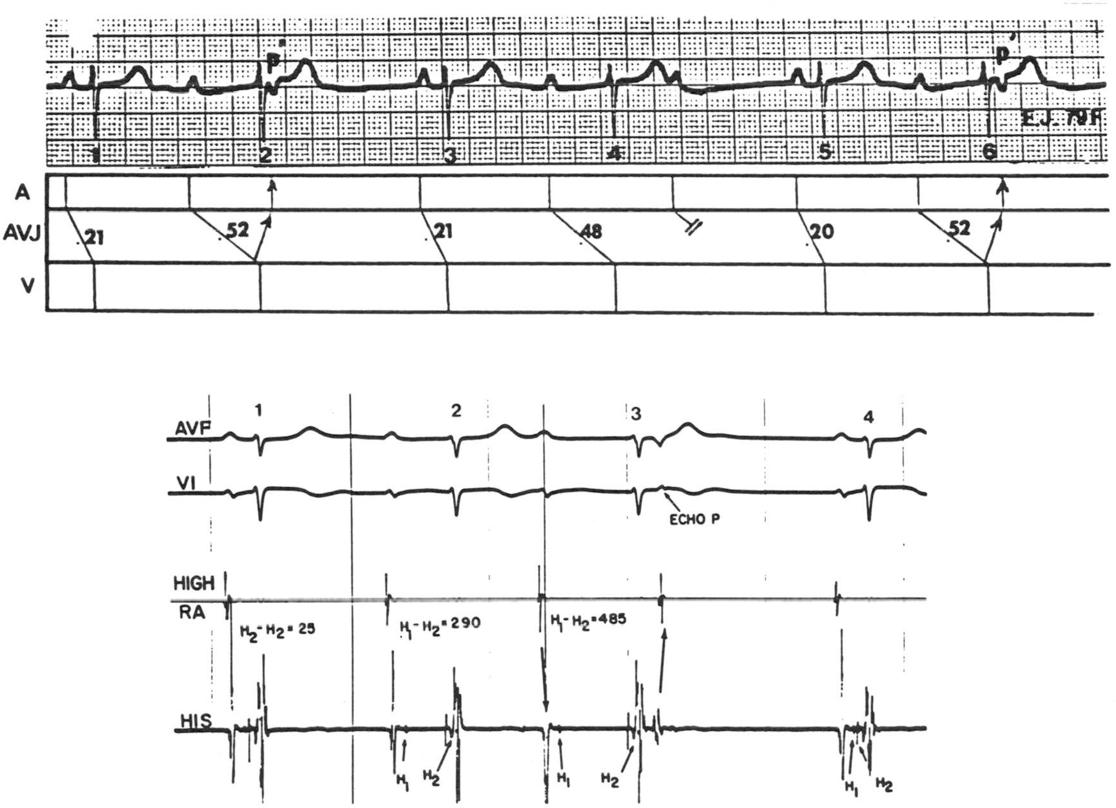

Figure 9-4. *The top panel shows a segment of lead 2 in a case of atypical Wenckebach block with echo P waves marked P′ that are present whenever the PR interval exceeds 0.5 second. The bottom panel shows His bundle recordings and demonstrates two distinct His spikes belonging to the proximal and distal regions of the His bundle, with block situated somewhere between these two sites. In the middle of the panel, an echo P wave occurs when the H_1-H_2 interval reaches 485 msec. Clearly, echo takes place downstream to the distal His bundle, probably just before its bifurcation. Whether the echo P wave uses the His bundle* per se *or an adjacent James fiber cannot be ascertained from this tracing.*

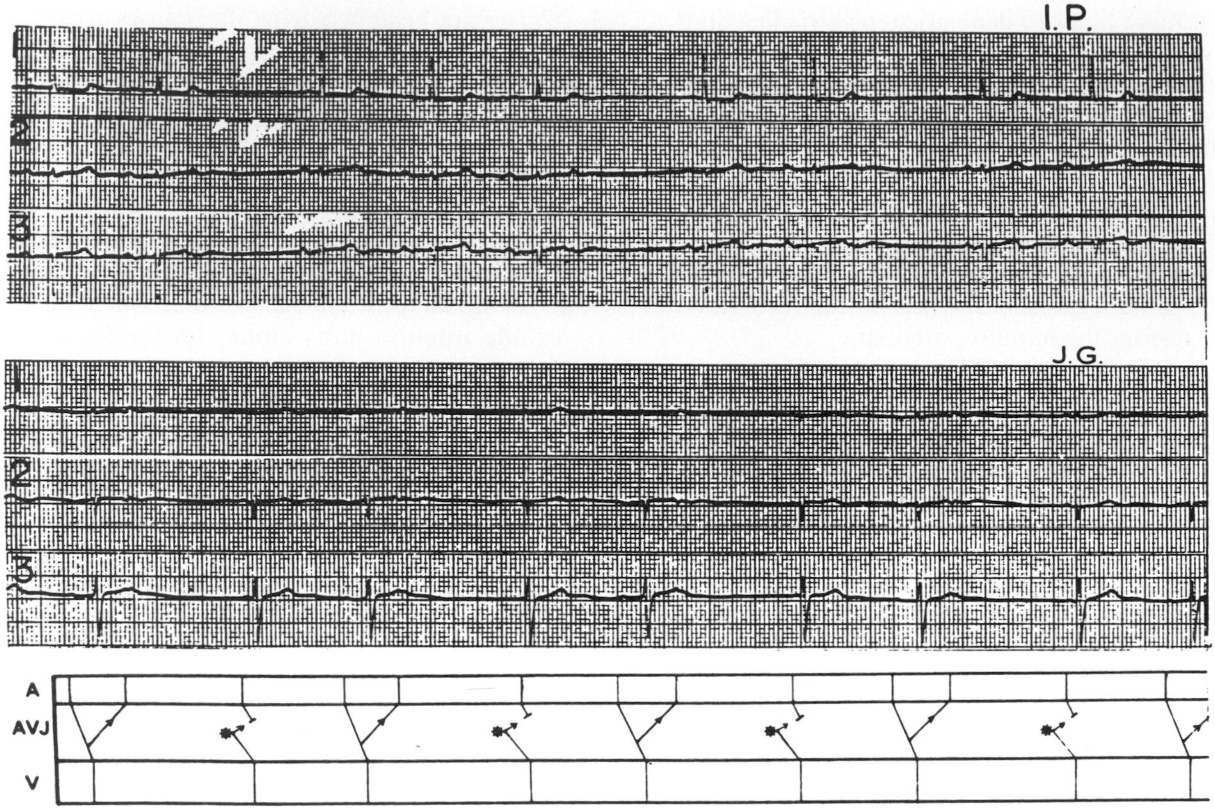

Figure 9-5. *Two cases of echo in Wenckebach cycles characterized by the late appearance of retrograde echo P waves suggesting the use of the slow pathway within the AV node for return to the atria. The contrast with early-appearing retrograde P waves in Figures 9-3 and 9-4 is noteworthy.*

be sensitive to autonomic influences, respond to vagal stimulation and inhibition by slowing and accelerating, respectively (Fig. 9-6).

7. Rhythms marked by retrograde P waves preceding the QRS complex have generally been unresponsive to autonomic influences in the author's experience. This observation is consistent with a low atrial or coronary sinus origin of such rhythms (Fig. 9-7).

These observations provide reason to believe that in AVJ rhythms the sequence of P waves and QRS complexes is probably helpful in determining the origin of the impulses. A beat or rhythm showing the retrograde P wave clearly before the QRS complex is most probably of coronary sinus or low atrial origin, while an aftercoming P wave places the pacemaker in the distal AV node or bundle of His. Between these two extremes lies a large proportion of cases of escape rhythms in which the P waves and QRS complexes occur almost simultaneously or in quick sequence (Fig. 9-8). These rhythms probably arise from the AV node. However, accessory pathway or rapid conduction of a low atrial impulse through the AV node would also place the QRS complex in the proximity of the P wave. Finally, in certain cases several morphologically different P waves at virtually identical rates, with innumerable intermediate forms, occur in the same rhythm strip. It is difficult if not impossible to determine whether the morphologic shifts in the P waves reflect frequent shifts of the atrial pacemaker focus or beat-to-beat variations in the mode of spread of unifocal P waves. The latter explanation appears more tenable.

If the P wave is completely enveloped within the QRS complex, it may be difficult or impossible to determine its spatial orientation unless at least two intra-atrial leads are recorded simultaneously, thus allowing the sequence of atrial activation to be recognized. In a certain percentage of cases, the P waves, because they are wider than the QRS complexes, "hang out" at the beginning or the end of the QRS and may create the erroneous impression of a

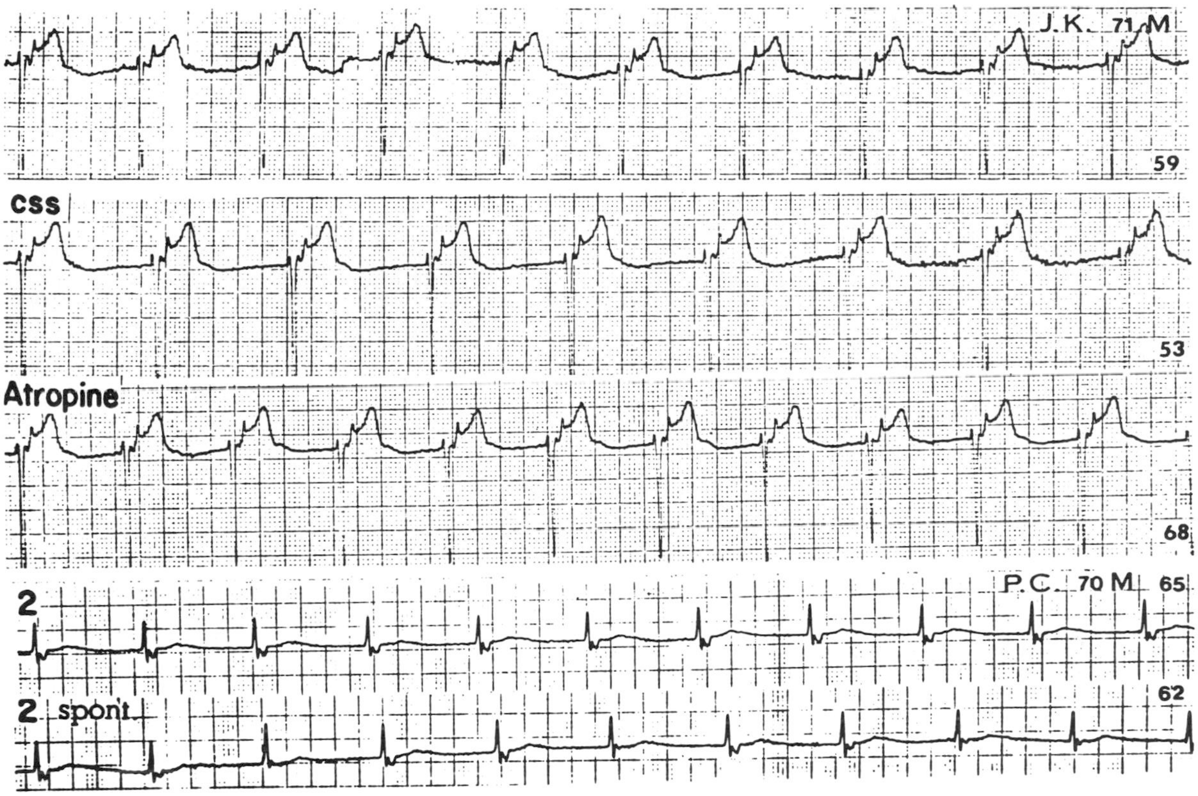

Figure 9-6. *Two cases of AVJ rhythm in which negative P waves persistently occur after the QRS complexes. The most logical location of the pacemaker in such a rhythm is the distal AV node–proximal His bundle. In the top panel, the pacemaking rate slows with carotid sinus stimulation (CSS) and accelerates with atropine, a behavior consistent with the known autonomic responsiveness of the AV node–proximal His bundle. In the bottom panel, spontaneous rate variations related to spontaneous fluctuations of the autonomic tone are noted.*

wide QRS complex (Fig. 9-9). In such tracings, recognition of P wave polarity may be difficult or impossible because it is not recorded on a flat or horizontal baseline. In fact, it may not be easy to determine P wave polarity when any P wave, regardless of its origin, is superimposed on a slanted ST segment or on the T wave (Fig. 9-10).

Clinical Recognition of Atrioventricular Junctional Beats

The most easily recognized AVJ beat is the AVJ escape, which occurs when the dominant sinus rhythm slows or when P waves are blocked. Frequently, the AVJ escape beat occurs shortly after a sinus P wave has been inscribed. Here, the atrial and ventricular activations remain independent even though the P wave may appear to be responsible for the QRS complex. In some cases, the apparent PR interval is so close to the actual AV conduction time as to make it impossible to ascertain whether the QRS complex followed conduction from the atria or was generated from a junctional discharge. Retrograde activation of the atria in a 1 : 1 pattern occurs in over half the cases of AVJ escape rhythm (see Fig. 9-6). The unfavorable position of the P waves after the QRS complexes may cause significant hypotension, necessitating temporary atrial or ventricular or AV pacing. AV junctional escape beats having aberrant QRS complexes were thought to arise eccentrically from the AV node and propagate to the ventricles following an eccentric path within the His bundle. However, Massumi and colleagues were able to demonstrate by His bundle electrography that such beats arose from the fascicles of the left bundle or from the right bundle, thus possessing abnormal QRS complexes.[12] Next in frequency are premature junctional beats occurring either singly or, more frequently, as members of a parasystolic rhythm. AVJ dis-

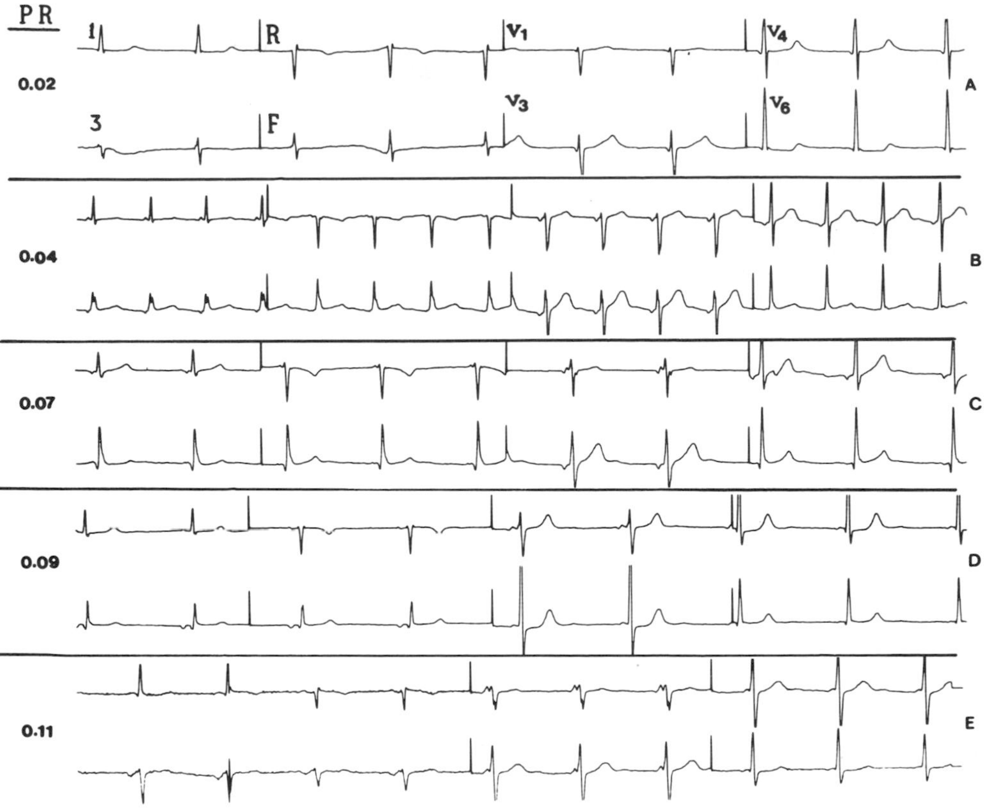

Figure 9-7. *Selected leads (1, 3, aV_R, aV_F, V_1, V_3, V_4, and V_6) in five cases of AVJ–low atrial rhythms in which P waves precede the QRS at PR intervals varying from 0.02 to 0.11 second. The rate was unresponsive to carotid sinus stimulation and atropine in all patients, suggesting an autonomic insensitive focus, probably somewhere in the low atrial–coronary sinus regions. The spatial orientation of the P waves are different in these five patients, reflecting either different pacemaker sites or different patterns of spread. In all patients, P waves are negative in inferior leads and positive in aV_R, indicating a cephalad direction; however, the chest leads differ among the five patients.*

charges resulting from reentry of sinus beats are coupled to the sinus beats at relatively constant intervals and occur in bigeminal and trigeminal modes or in variations thereof, such as concealed bigeminy (Fig. 9-11).

The QRS complexes of AVJ beats are generally similar to those of normally conducted sinus beats unless aberrancy is present. If so, the magnitude of aberrancy is likely to vary depending on the degree of prematurity and the length of the preceding cycle (Fig. 9-12). Monomorphic premature beats with aberrant QRS complexes indicate a fascicular origin. In the presence of atrial fibrillation or flutter or atrial tachycardia, a dissociated, usually regular ventricular rhythm with QRS complexes similar to those of normally conducted beats indicates the operation of an AVJ pacemaker (Figs. 9-13 and 9-14). Frequently, atrial depolarization waves succeed in invading the ventricles in a premature fashion (capture) and give rise to beats mimicking premature atrial beats with or without QRS aberrancy.

A well-recognized AVJ rhythm is one accompanied by AV dissociation in which intrinsic firing rate of the AVJ pacemaker is faster than that of the sinus node (Fig. 9-15). Retrograde conduction to the atria is absent, and the sinus node remains in command of the atria. The relative rapidity of the AVJ pacemaker frequently reflects acute ischemia (acute inferior wall myocardial infarction [Fig. 9-16], anesthesia, or chronic lung disease). However, the most widely appreciated cause is digitalis intoxication (Fig. 9-17), in which a relatively rapid AVJ rhythm (60 to 90 beats/min) is associated with normal sinus rhythm, an atrial tachycardia with block, or atrial fibrillation or flutter.

In the course of His bundle electrography, AVJ beats are recognized by the presence of normal His spikes with

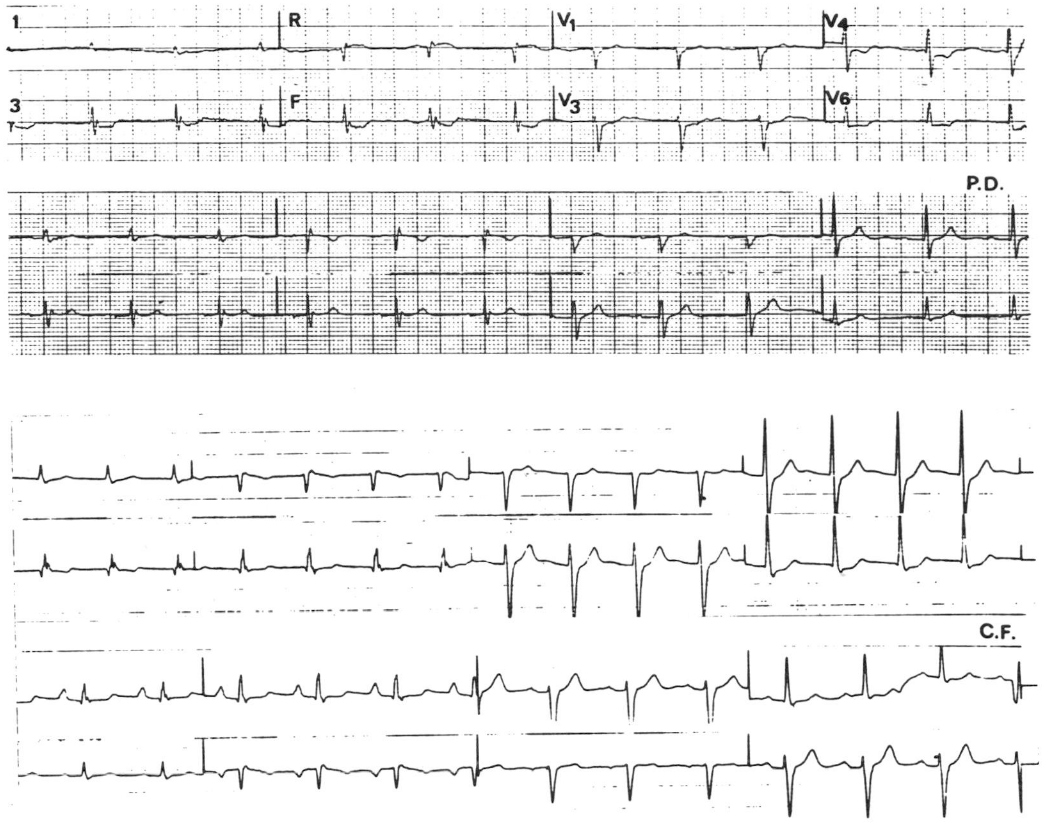

Figure 9-8. *Two cases of AVJ rhythm in which the P wave and the QRS complex are inscribed simultaneously. In both cases, return to normal sinus rhythm is also depicted below the respective tracing. Lead marks are the same as those shown in the top panel. These AVJ rhythms are not likely to arise from the low atrial regions or the coronary sinus because P waves do not precede the QRS complex. They probably do not originate in the main His bundle, since the QRS complex does not precede the P wave. The most likely place for such focus is in the AV node, but the exact location cannot be determined*

normal His-Q intervals, unless slow conduction related to prematurity is present. Note, however, that because of the existing irregularity of the cardiac rhythm, which is often the basis for the emergence of the AVJ beats, the position of the His bundle recording catheter is not stable (variations in atrial filling, forceful A waves, and so on), and His spikes may vary significantly in definition and configuration; they may even disappear intermittently (Fig 9-18).

In the presence of sinus tachycardia, and atrial tachycardia or flutter when 2 : 1 AV conduction is present, the P waves are likely to be superimposed on the T wave or lost within the QRS and become indiscernible, thus suggesting a diagnosis of AVJ tachycardia. The occurrence of premature ventricular beats or slowing of the rate by carotid sinus stimulation may lengthen the cardiac cycle sufficiently to separate the P wave from the T wave and clarify the underlying rhythm (Fig. 9-19). Similar confusion occurs when the P wave is superimposed on the preceding T wave because of very long PR intervals (Fig. 9-20). In cases of AVJ rhythm where visible U waves are present, the latter is frequently mistaken for the P wave, leading to a diagnosis of sinus rhythm with a long PR interval. The clue to the correct identity of the U wave is that its amplitude is highest in leads V_2 and V_3 and quite low in limb leads. P waves, on the contrary, are more prominent in lead V_1 and in limb leads (Fig. 9-21).

Difficult Diagnostic Problems

Tracings with P waves too small to be discernible are found most frequently in very old persons suffering from fibrosis or other destructive processes involving the atrial

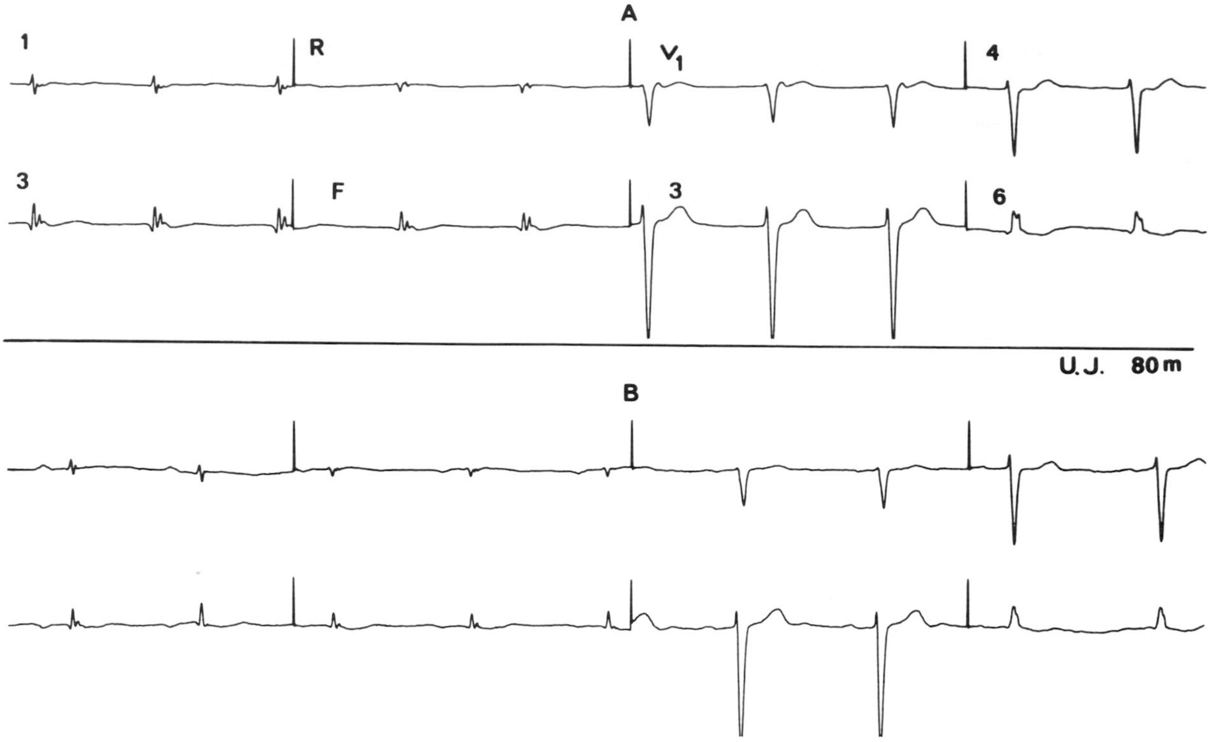

Figure 9-9. *Upper panel shows junctional rhythm in which P waves are attached to the end of the QRS complex, suggesting intraventricular conduction delay with a QRS duration of 0.14 second. During normal sinus rhythm, shown at the bottom, the QRS complexes are no longer attached to the P waves and are only 0.09 second.*

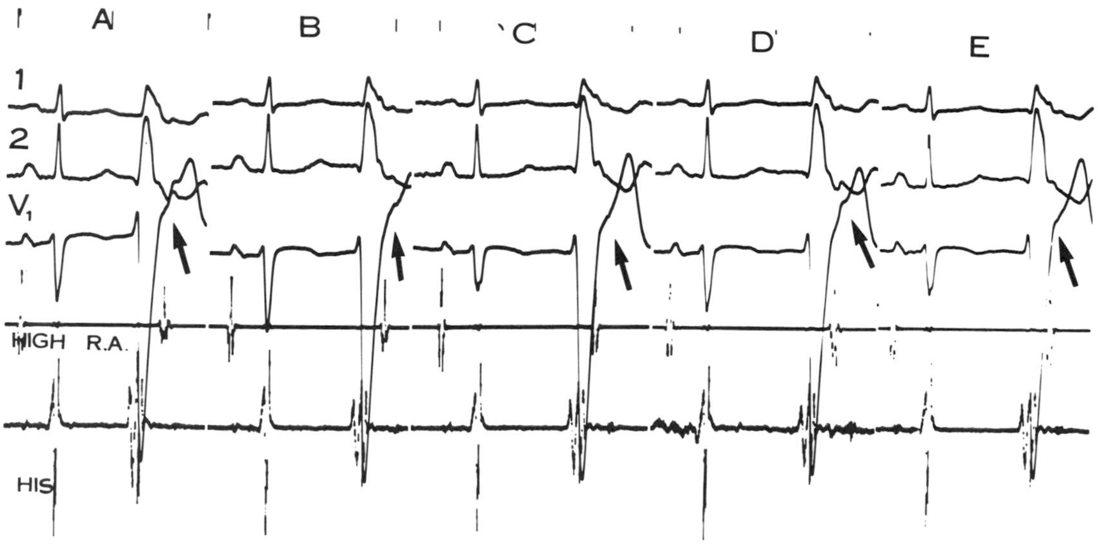

Figure 9-10. *Five panels of leads 1, 2, and V_1 recorded simultaneously with a high right atrial and His bundle electrogram. In each panel (A through E), one sinus beat is followed by a premature ventricular beat. The coupling intervals of the premature ventricular beats vary slightly from panel to panel. Consequently, the sinus P waves following the premature ventricular beats are superimposed on different regions of the ST segments. For this reason, some of the post–premature ventricular beat sinus P waves appear negative in lead 2 (A, B, and D), while others appear positive (C and E).*

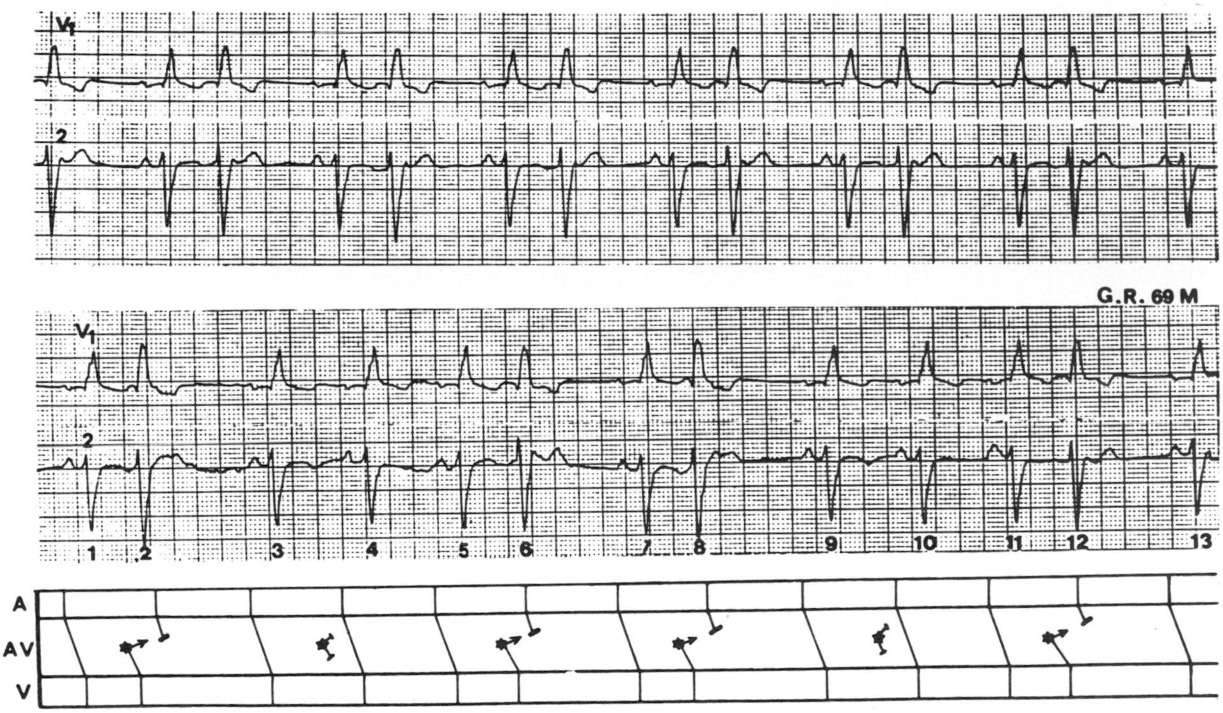

Figure 9-11. *Two rhythm strips of simultaneously recorded leads* V_1 *and* V_2 *show the basic normal sinus rhythm to be interrupted by AVJ premature beats appearing in a bigeminal pattern (top panel) and in the form of concealed bigeminy (bottom panel). The ladder diagram accompanying the bottom panel shows a persistent AVJ bigeminy in which some premature discharges fail to propagate to the ventricles because of exit block (asterisks after beats 3 and 9). The term* concealed bigeminy *is used to describe this phenomenon.*

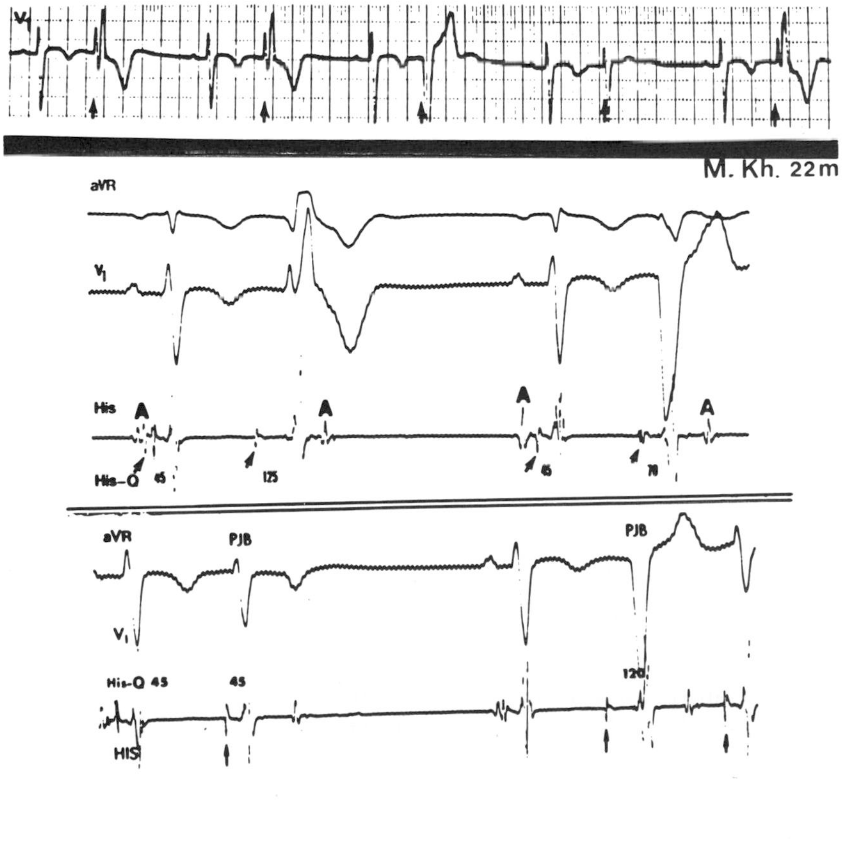

Figure 9-12. *Rhythm strip of* V_1 *shows a basic sinus rhythm and premature beats with greatly variable morphologies appearing in a bigeminal mode. On a His bundle electrogram all the premature beats were preceded by His spikes (beats 2, 4, 6, and 8) with varying His-Q intervals. Conduction of the AVJ impulses from the His bundle to ventricular myocardium met with significant impediment in both bundle branches—hence the shifting of QRS morphology. When both bundles blocked simultaneously, the impulse failed to propagate to the ventricles, and no QRS complex appeared. The effect of the nonpropagated AVJ impulse on AV conduction was striking, ranging from mere prolongation to complete block. The term* pseudo-AV block *is therefore quite appropriate for this phenomenon (see Fig. 9-30).*

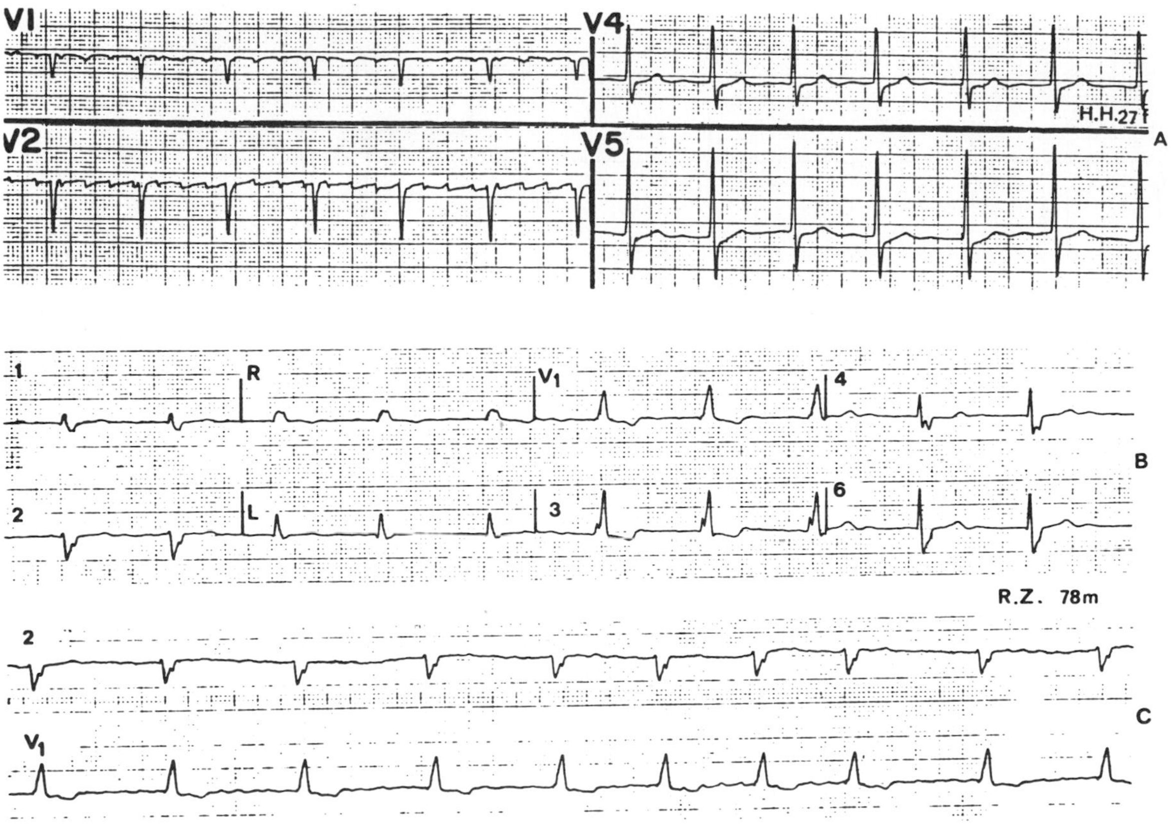

Figure 9-13. *AVJ rhythm in the presence of atrial flutter (top panel) and atrial fibrillation (bottom panel), both resulting from digitalis overdose. In the atrial flutter, P waves are completely dissociated from the QRS complexes, which appear entirely regularly. In the atrial fibrillation, the only feature suggesting the presence of AVJ rhythm is the perfect regularity of the QRS complexes. After the patient was treated for digitalis intoxication, the QRS complexes of the same morphology became irregular (lower portion of the bottom panel).*

myocardium and may mimic junctional rhythms. At times, correct diagnosis can be made only by intra-atrial recordings (Fig. 9-22). In such patients, the atrial myocardium is so severely diseased as to be unable to generate detectable A waves. Another difficult diagnostic dilemma is presented by cases exemplified by Figure 9-23, usually occurring with digitalis overdose. In this instance of nonparoxysmal AVJ tachycardia with exit block and complete AV dissociation, the original diagnosis of sinus tachycardia with Wenckebach periods was refuted because of very long and variable first PR intervals following the pauses. Another especially difficult problem is encountered in persons possessing dual AV nodal pathways. Conduction down the slow pathway occurs with very long PR intervals usually exceeding 0.4 second. This situation places the P waves somewhere within the ST segment or the T wave of the preceding beats (depending on the cycle length), thus mimicking the aftercoming P wave (Fig. 9-24). As pointed out above, recognition of the P wave polarity when it is superimposed on the ST or T wave may be fraught with uncertainty.

Manifestations of Atrioventricular Junctional Rhythms

AVJ rhythms present in one or more of the following patterns:

A AV junctional escape rhythms
B AV junctional extrasystoles (manifest or concealed)
C Nonparoxysmal AV junctional tachycardias (usually relatively slow)
D Isorhythmic AVJ rhythms

(Text continues on p. 252.)

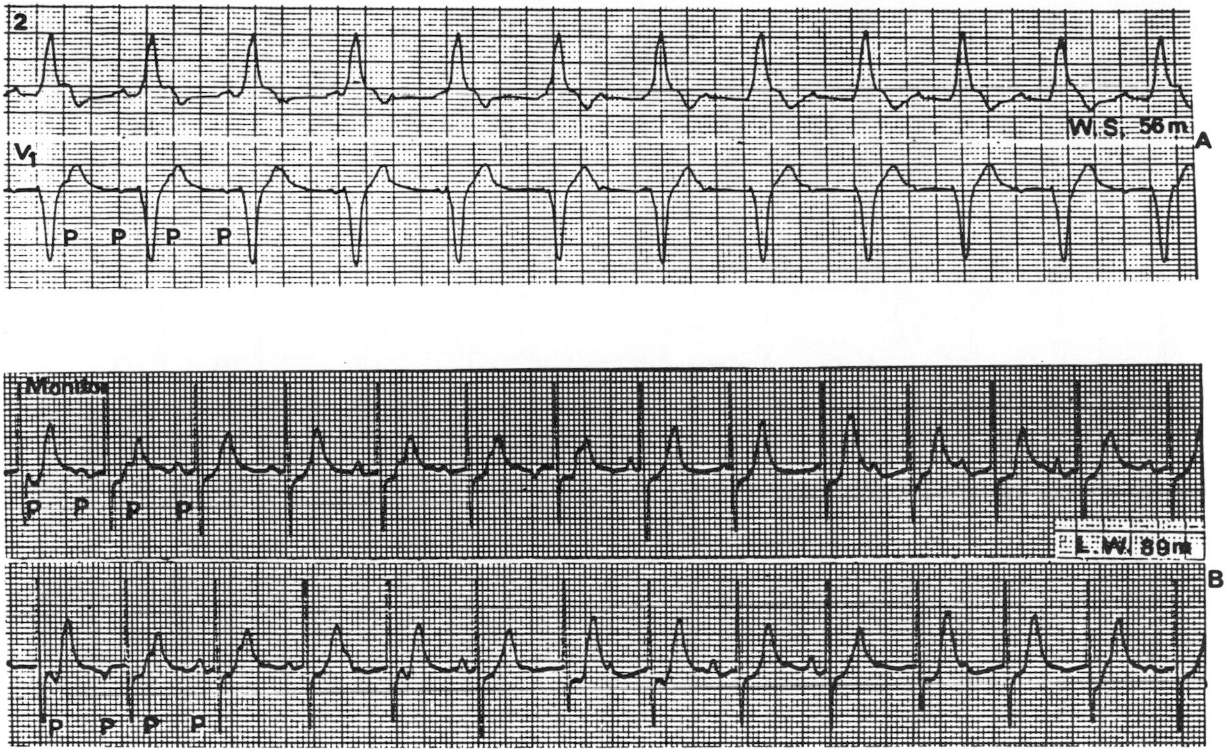

Figure 9-14. *Two examples of AVJ rhythms in the presence of atrial tachycardia due to digitalis intoxication (A) and multifocal atrial tachycardia associated with severe chronic obstructive lung disease in (B). Complete AV dissociation and perfect regularity of the QRS complexes are the reliable diagnostic features.*

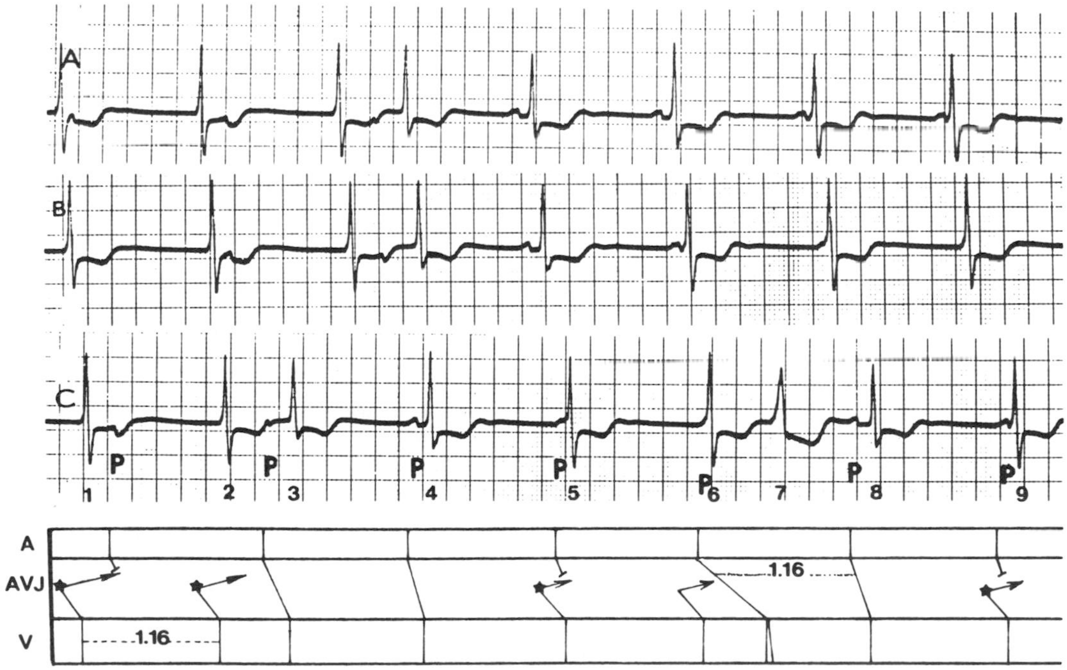

Figure 9-15. *AVJ rhythm of 52 beats/min with AV dissociation. The sinus mechanism is regular at 50 beats/min. Whenever the P waves appear far enough after the QRS complexes, they are successfully conducted to the ventricles, with or without aberrancy (beats 3 and 7). The cycle length of the AVJ rhythm is 1.16 second, as is the return cycle after the AVJ pacemaker has been depolarized by the passing sinus impulse.*

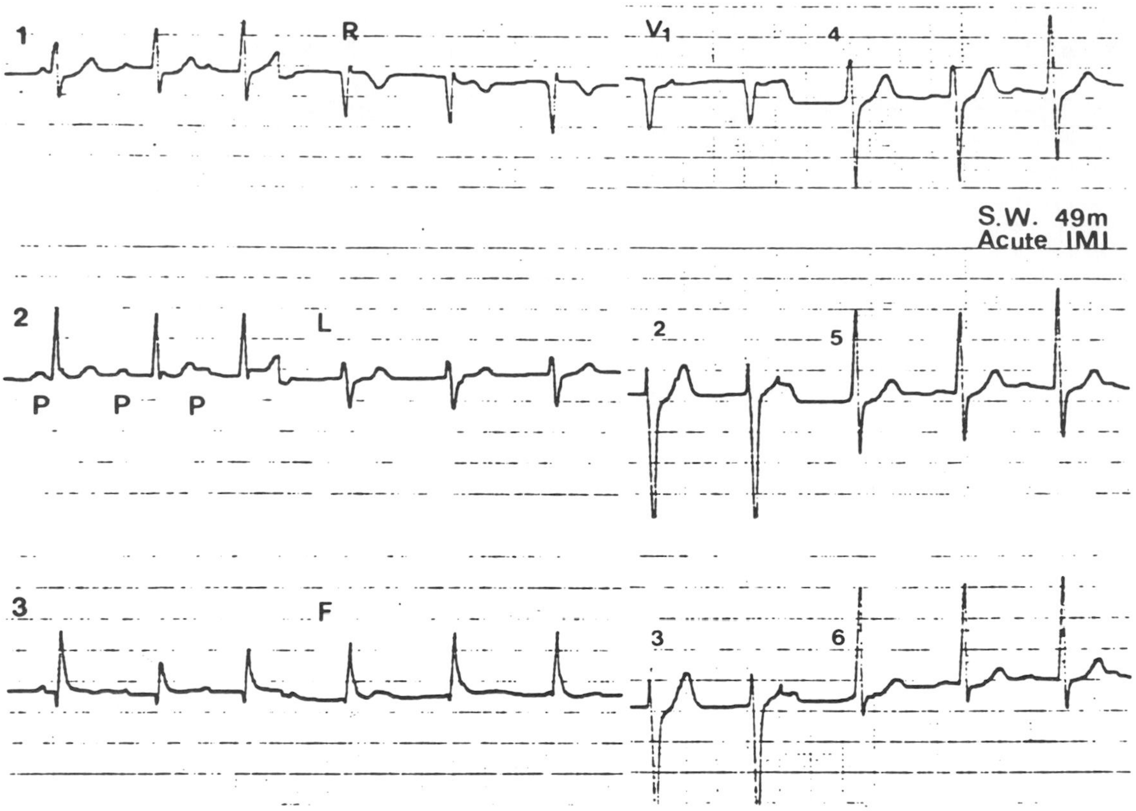

Figure 9-16. *Fast AVJ rhythm in acute inferior wall myocardial infarction (IMI) at 90 beats/min persists despite a sinus rate of 105 beats/min suggesting some degree of coexisting AV block.*

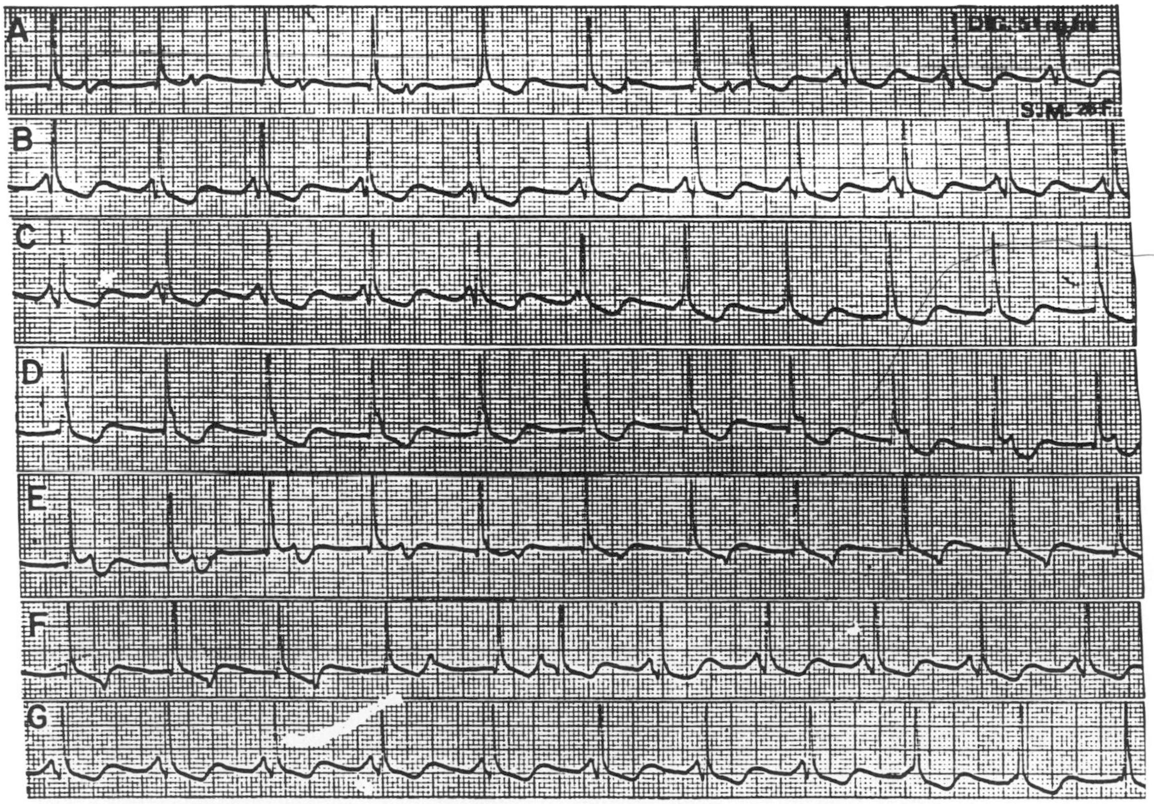

Figure 9-17. *AV dissociation in a case of digitalis intoxication. The sinus and AV junctional rates are very close (isorhythmic), and the two pacemakers, marching in parallel, create an interesting repetitive group beating.*

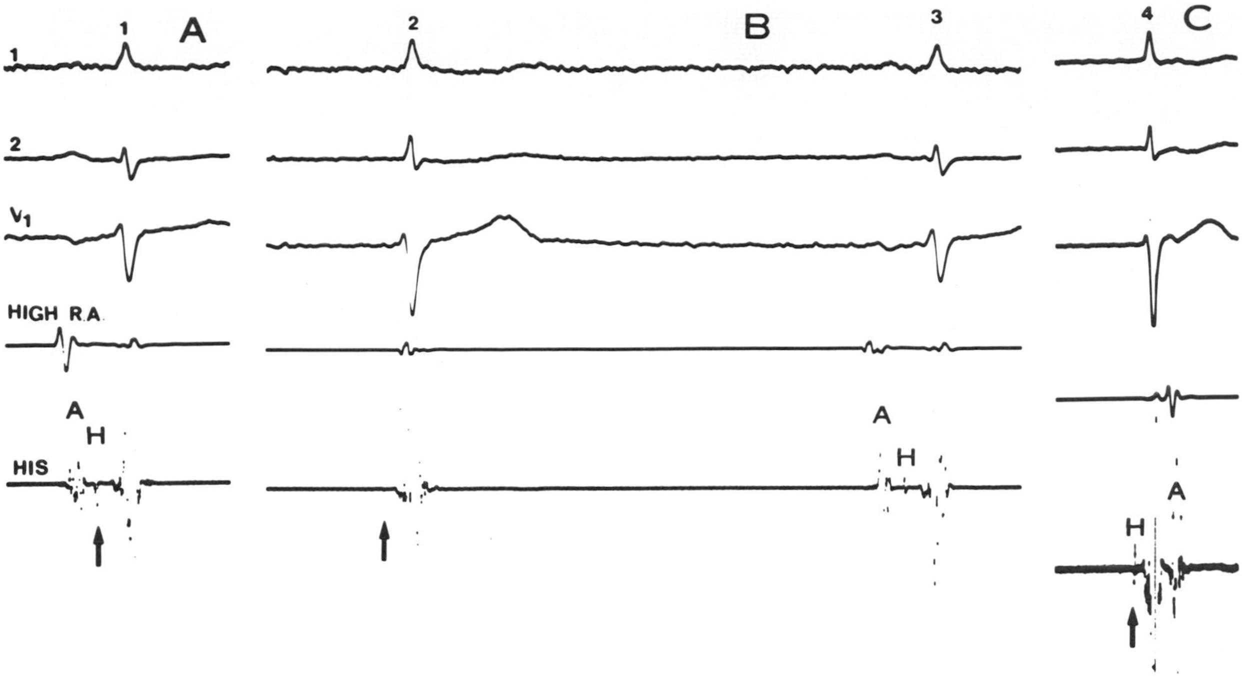

Figure 9-18. *His bundle recordings in a patient with sick sinus syndrome with frequent AVJ escapes. A depicts a normally conducted beat with the His spike clearly seen (arrow). In B an AVJ escape beat is recorded without a visible His spike, while the next sinus beat in the same panel and the next AVJ beat in C both possess sharp His spikes. The absence of the His spike in beat 2 reflects catheter movements caused by the markedly variable degrees of atrial filling because of the underlying variations in cycle lengths.*

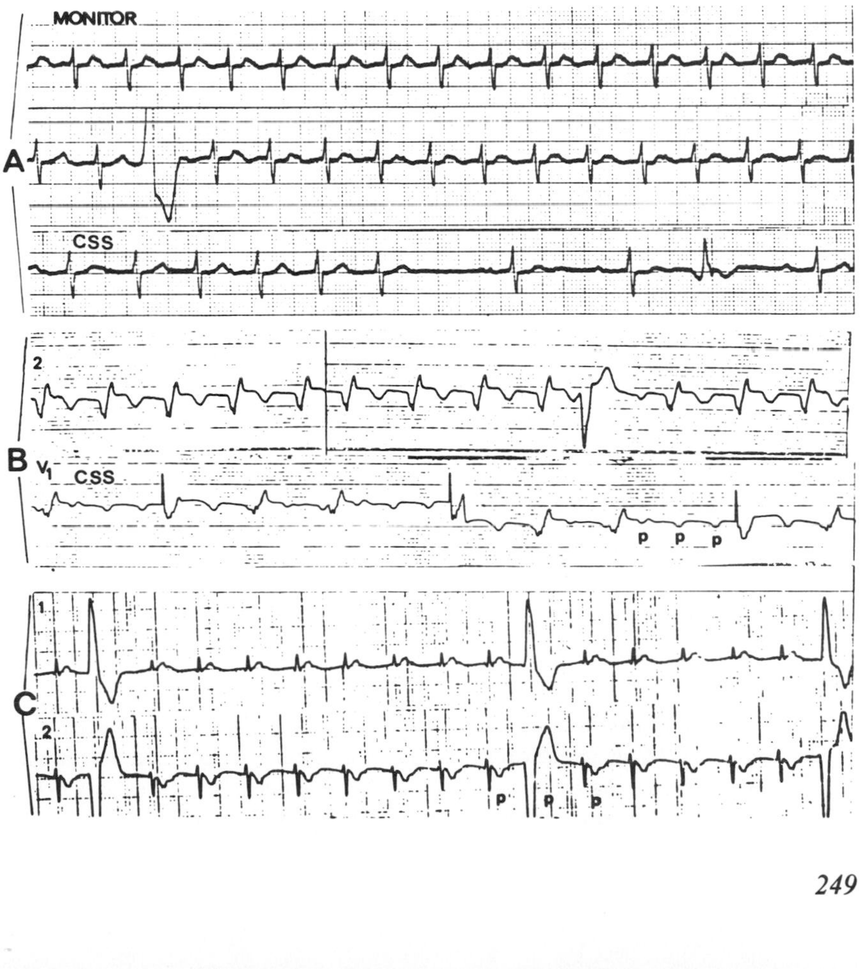

Figure 9-19. *Three cases of superimposition of P and T waves caused by rapid beating, making it difficult to ascertain whether the P wave or the QRS complex comes first. A depicts sinus tachycardia whose true identity was clarified by carotid sinus stimulation (CSS). B shows atrial flutter with 2:1 AV conduction. A premature ventricular beat in lead 2 uncovers negative P waves, thus suggesting an ectopic atrial mechanism. Vagal stimulation (CSS), however, demonstrated the existence of atrial flutter. In C, an AV reentrant tachycardia with negative P waves in the ST segments is clarified during the post–premature ventricular beat pauses.*

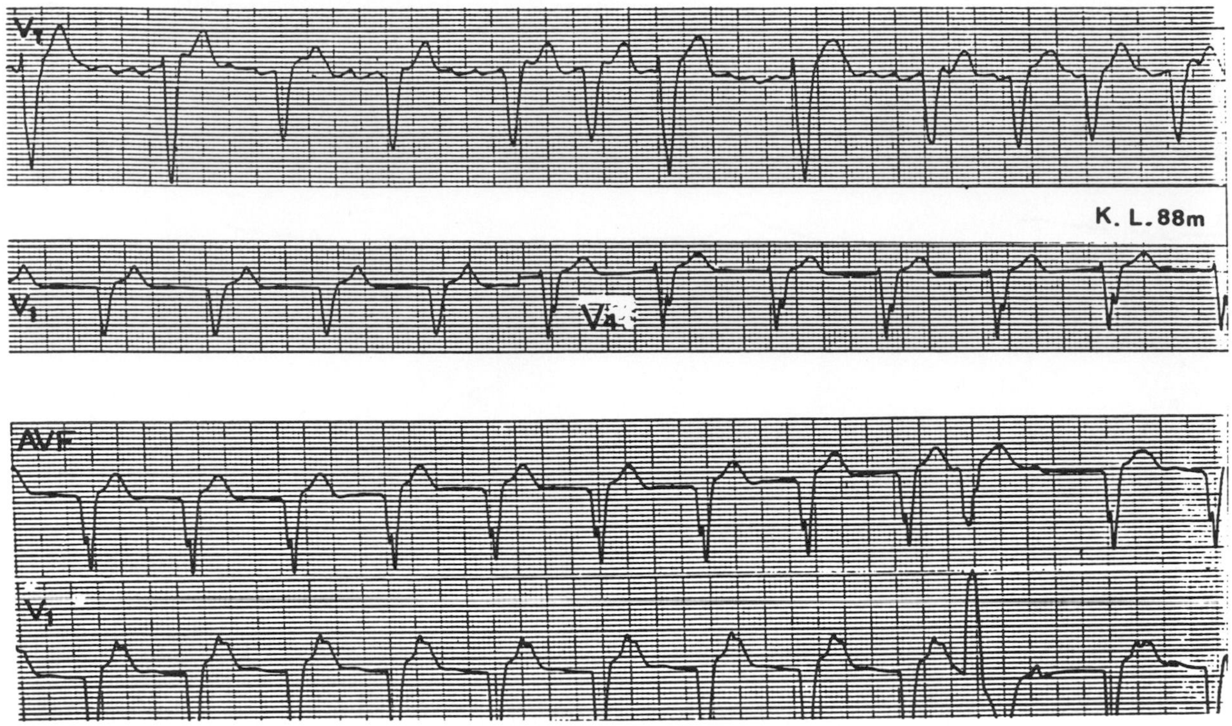

Figure 9-20. *An erroneous diagnosis of AVJ rhythm was made in this patient who was originally in atrial fibrillation (A) and was cardioverted electrically (B). P waves superimposed on apex of the T waves can easily be seen in some leads (C). The relationship between the P wave and the QRS complex, however, could not be determined until a premature ventricular beat occurred (C) and demonstrated the existence of a sinus rhythm with very long PR intervals. Note the normally positive post–premature ventricular beat P wave in lead* aV_F *and the normal positive-negative P wave in lead* V_1*, supporting the sinus origin of the P wave.*

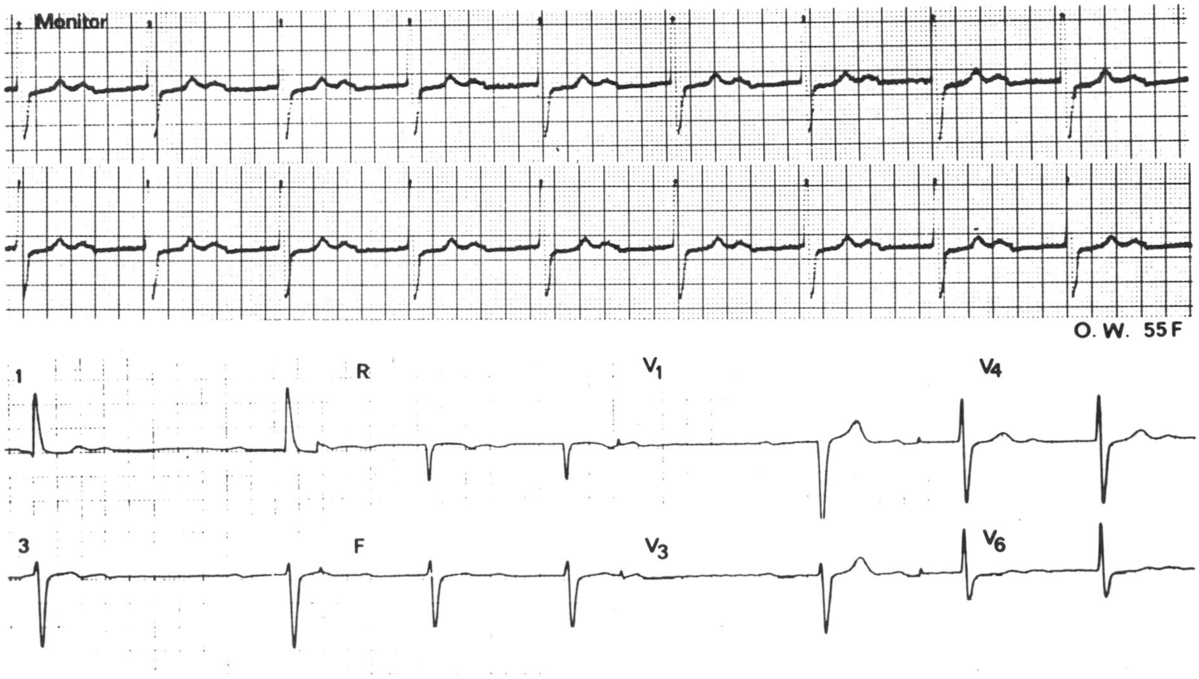

Figure 9-21. *AVJ rhythm with prominent U waves was thought to be present in this case of first degree AV block with PR intervals approaching 0.6 second. The P waves occupied the area of the cycle where U waves are found (top panel). The presence of first degree AV block became substantiated when occasional periods of Wenckebach block appeared between runs of first degree block (bottom panel).*

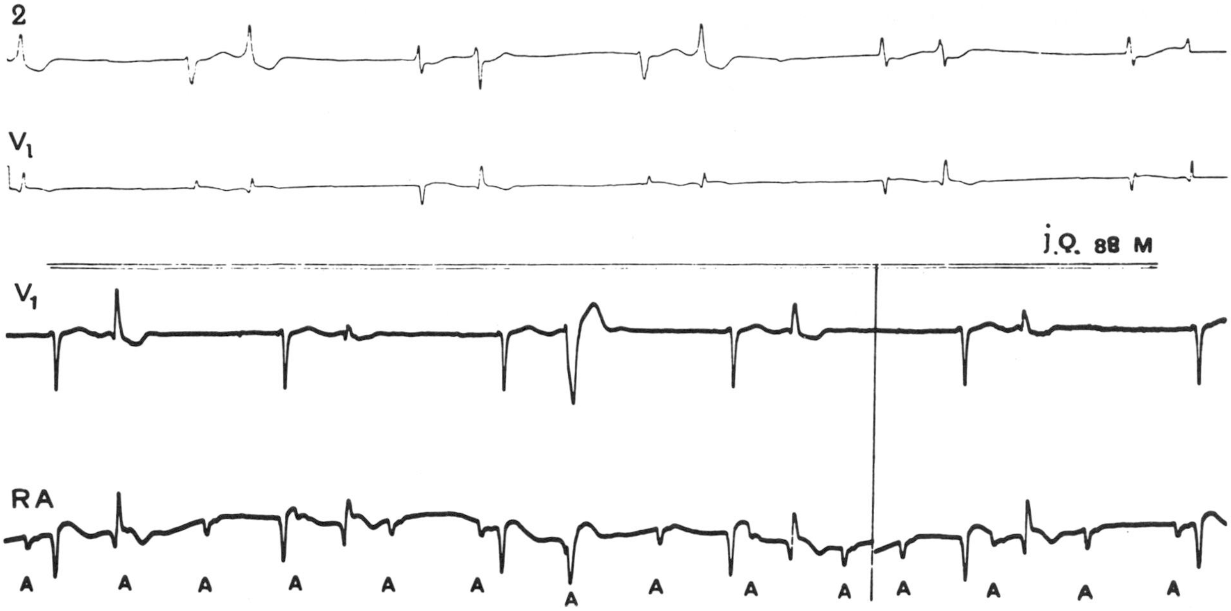

Figure 9-22. *In this case of low-amplitude or invisible P waves, a diagnosis of AVJ escape-bigeminy was entertained until an intra-atrial lead documented the presence of a sinus rhythm together with complete AV block and premature fascicular beats. (A, atrial potentials)*

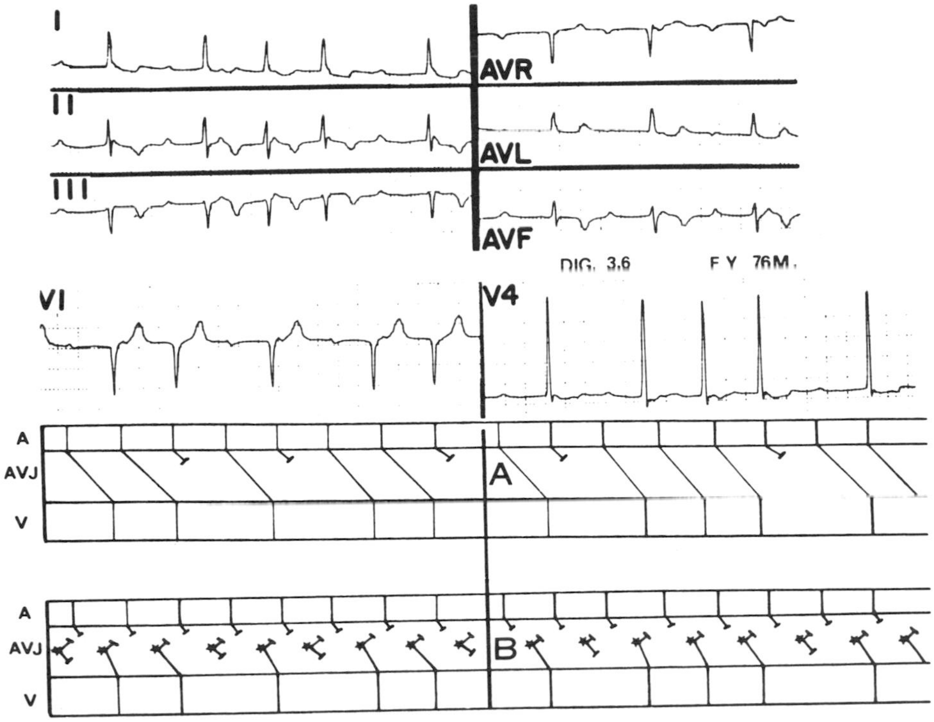

Figure 9-23. *An example of sinus tachycardia with an irregular QRS complex and apparently blocked P waves thought to represent digitalis toxicity (the patient's digoxin blood level was 3.6 ng/ml). The ladder diagram immediately beneath the tracing is based on the above assumption of Wenckebach periodicity. Attention to the length of the pauses and the PR intervals of the first beats after the pauses uncovers some very unusual features, namely, the variable lengths of the pauses and the very long and variable PR intervals of the first beats of the Wenckebach cycles. The ladder diagram at the bottom depicts the existence of an AVJ tachycardia with exit block and complete AV dissociation.*

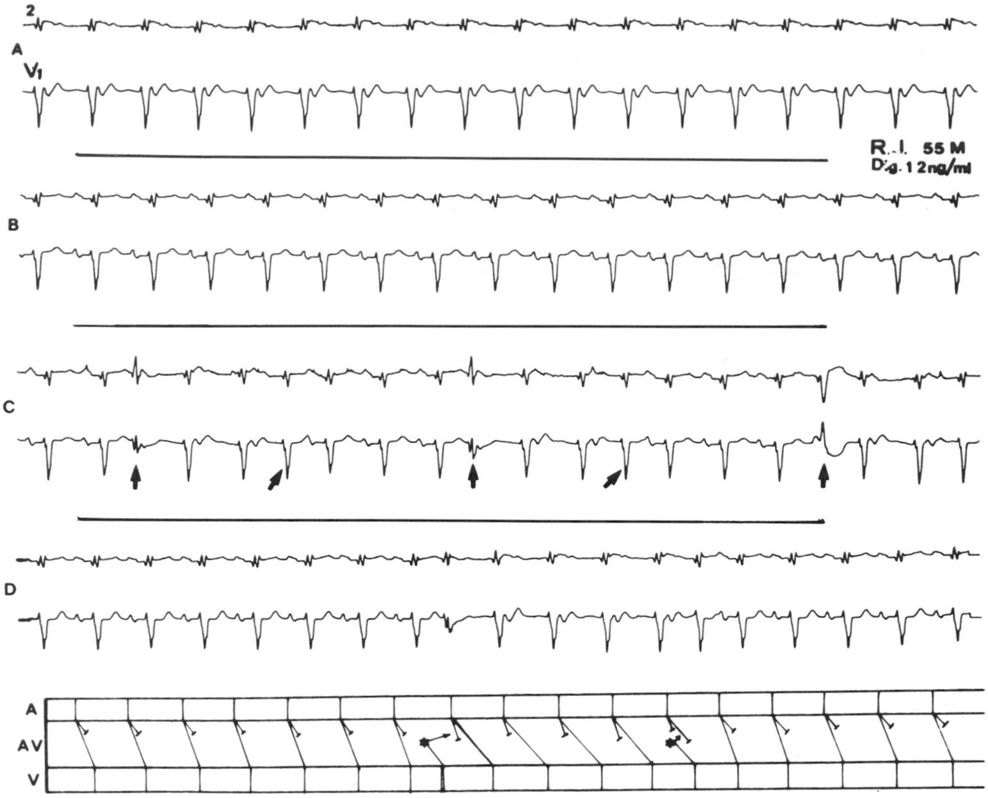

Figure 9-24. *In this man aged 55 years with previous myocardial infarctions, bizarre rhythms occurred during his recovery from the latest inferior wall myocardial infarction. In A, a narrow QRS tachycardia of 104 beats/min, in which P waves of indeterminate polarity appear immediately after the QRS complexes, was thought to be a form of AVJ tachycardia. In B, a sinus rhythm of 101 beats/min with PR intervals of 0.18 second and identical QRS complexes is noted. In C, a shift from NSR to the type of rhythm shown in A occurs after the arrows. The atrial mechanism remained unchanged. The only change was that the PR intervals switched from 0.18 to 0.46 second. Slanted arrows point to junctional extrasystoles conducted normally, while vertical arrows mark junctional extrasystoles conducted aberrantly. D shows another instance of shift from normal to long PR and back to normal PR, caused by premature AVJ extrasystoles. The ladder diagram pertaining to D delineates the effect on AVJ extrasystoles penetrating the functional leg of the dual AV nodal pathways (concealed conduction) and causing block, thereby enabling the same sinus P waves to use the other pathway.*

E Paroxysmal AV junctional tachycardias (usually faster than in C)
F Pseudo-AV block
G "Pseudotachycardia"
H Echo through AVJ
I AV junctional parasystoles (manifest or concealed)
J AV reentrant tachycardias*
K AV nodal reentrant tachycardias*

* These reciprocating tachycardias, which use the AV junction only as a portion of their circus movement pathway, will not be discussed further.

Atrioventricular Junctional Escape Rhythms

The AVJ usually escapes when the cycle length of the dominant rhythm becomes longer than 1.2 second, corresponding to a rate under 50 beats/min. Frequently, the AVJ escape persists for a few beats and then the dominant rhythm returns, either as a result of its basic irregularity or the periodic acceleration of the sinus rate in response to a blood pressure decline that occurs when the optimal PR relationship is lost during the short period of AVJ rhythm. When AVJ rhythm is associated with 1 : 1 retrograde conduction to the atria, the sinus node may be depolarized and kept in check by retrograde P waves and thus not have the opportunity to become the dominant rhythm (see Fig. 9-5). Sinus control will not return until the retrograde conduction fails or the sinus node develops a much faster intrinsic rate. Vagal stimulation during AVJ rhythm with 1 : 1 VA conduction may exert a greater slowing effect on the AVJ pacemaker than on the sinus node, thus enabling the sinus mechanism to become dominant again (Fig. 9-25). Any premature atrial or ventricular depolarization may also disturb the 1 : 1 VA relationship and cause a return to the sinus rhythm.

The slowing of the sinus mechanism, which leads to the emergence of AVJ rhythm, may at the same time bring about premature ventricular beating (PVBs). The resulting post-PVB pause will in turn reactivate the AVJ escape mechanism. This reciprocal relationship will lead to an interesting and self-perpetuating situation known as *escape bigeminy* (Fig. 9-26). This rhythm may be terminated by an acceleration of the sinus mechanism through autonomic maneuvers or by abolition of the PVBs and the disappearance of the post-PVB pauses (see Fig. 9-26). Another interesting variation of AVJ escape rhythms is the so-called escape-capture bigeminy in which each junctional beat is followed by a retrograde or sinus P wave that, in turn, conducts to the ventricles. Frequently, the capture beat is conducted aberrantly because of the operation of so-called long cycle – short cycle sequence.

The intrinsic rate of AVJ escape rhythm is generally slow. However, in patients with acute inferior wall myocardial infarction where ischemia or injury of the AVJ is usually present, the intrinsic rate may be much faster, sometimes over 80 beats/min (see Fig. 9-16). Similarly, fast AVJ escape rhythms are observed in patients with acute myocarditis, chronic obstructive lung disease, and digitalis overdose (see below). In these situations, the AVJ rhythm is ushered in by a gradual or abrupt lengthening of the basic cardiac cycle, and, in this sense, the rhythm must be considered an escape rhythm even though its rate is not slow.

The AVJ escape interval, that is, the interval from the last QRS to the emergence of the first AVJ escape beat, remains constant as long as it is free of autonomic influences and of the effect of concealed conduction of atrial or ventricular depolarizations. Figure 9-27 demonstrates the variations of the escape interval brought about by these interfering mechanisms.

Atrioventricular Junctional Extrasystoles: Manifest and Concealed

Single junctional extrasystoles are far less common than atrial or ventricular extrasystoles and occur most frequently in apparently normal hearts and in young persons. Like all other extrasystoles, they may be interpolated or followed by pauses; they occur in bigeminal, trigeminal, or any other conceivable arithmetic arrangement (see Fig. 9-11). They exert a profound influence on conduction through the AV node, causing marked prolongation or block of the next sinus P wave. In most cases of apparent single extrasystoles, careful study of the long rhythm strips and Holter records show the existence of an actual AV junctional parasystole with infrequent manifest beats (Fig. 9-28). In practice, AVJ extrasystoles should be considered members of a parasystolic rhythm unless proved otherwise.

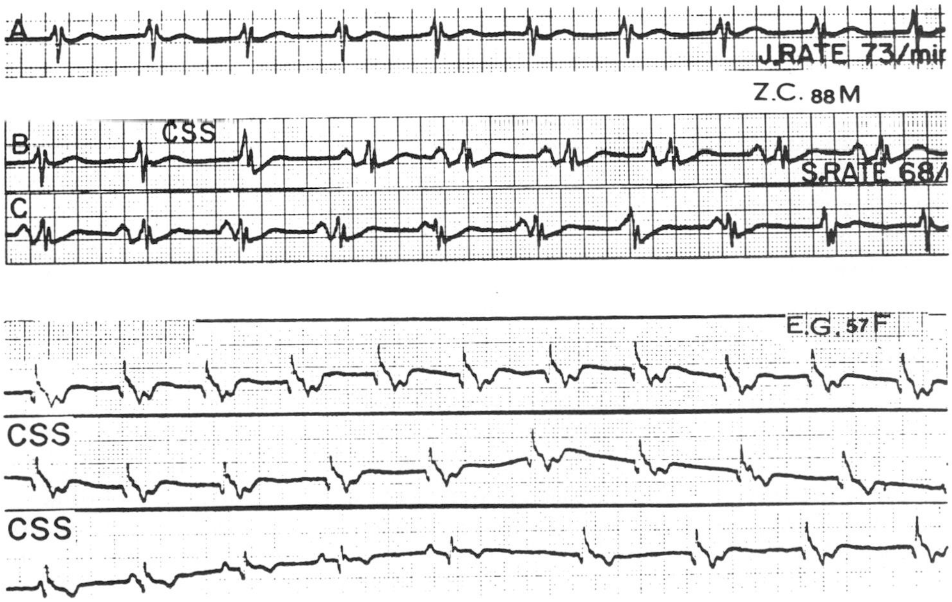

Figure 9-25. *In two cases of AVJ rhythm, with simultaneous activation of both ventricles and atria (top panel) and ventricles before atria (bottom panel), carotid sinus stimulation (CSS) was able to restore normal sinus rhythm by slowing the AVJ pacemaker without simultaneously slowing the sinus node. This behavior is unusual and probably reflects two factors: (1) the inherently sluggish response of the sinus node to vagal stimulation and (2) the presence of an element of sympathetic drive on the sinus node thanks to the fall in blood pressure during the AVJ rhythm with its inappropriate PR relationship.*

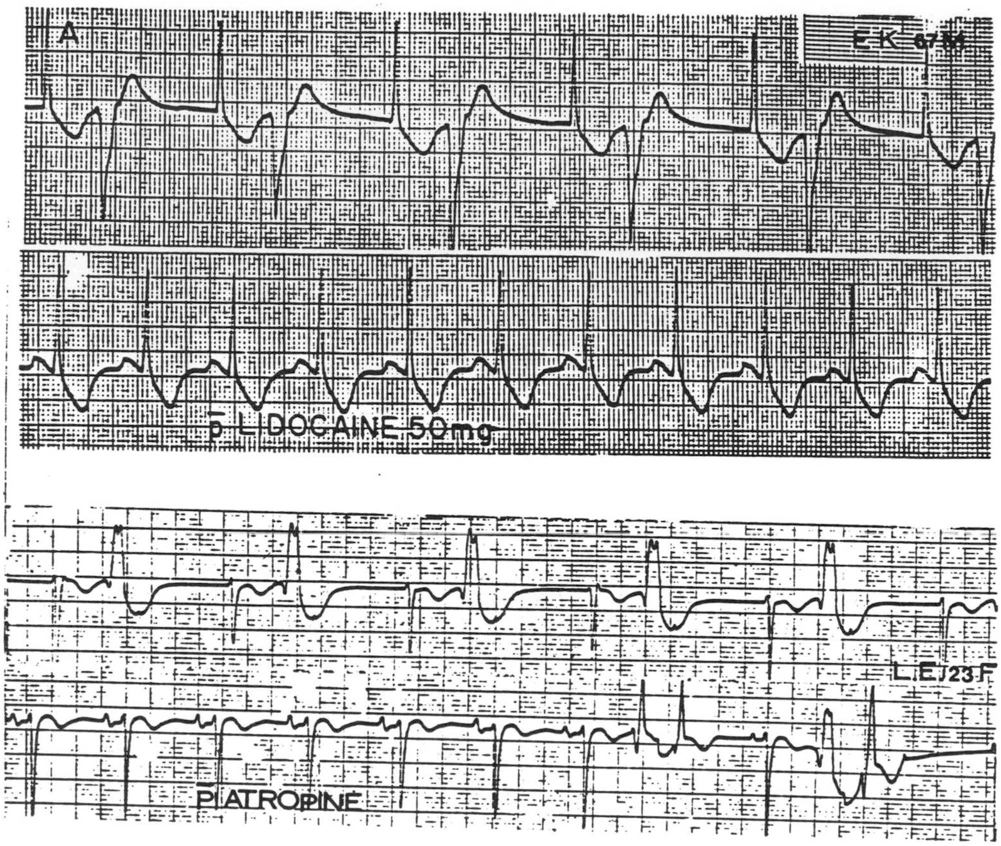

Figure 9-26. *Two cases of AVJ escape-bigeminy are shown in the top panel. Lidocaine administration eliminated the premature ventricular beats and, with them, the post-premature ventricular beat pauses, thereby removing the reason for the emergence of AVJ escapes. In the bottom panel, atropine accelerated the sinus rate and eliminated the AVJ rhythm. At the same time, the premature ventricular beats that followed the long cycles and perpetuated the arrhythmia disappeared. A long post-premature ventricular beat pause at the end of the bottom strip brought back the AJV escape and the escape-bigeminy (rule of bigeminy).*

Nonparoxysmal Atrioventricular Junctional Tachycardias

Nonparoxysmal AV junctional tachycardias (NPJT) are the most common AVJ rhythms and are encountered in a variety of clinical situations including digitalis intoxication, acute inferior wall myocardial infarction, post-operative states, anesthesia, myocarditis, and hypoxia due to any cause. In a sizable number of patients no etiologic agents are apparent. These rhythms appear to result from enhanced automaticity of certain AVJ pacemaker tissue, causing it to discharge at a rate faster than the basic sinus rate (see Fig. 9-16). The range of 70 to 130 beats/min as suggested by Fisch[14] corresponds to Massumi's observations in over 200 such patients. The attribute nonparoxysmal describes the mode of onset and offset of these rhythms, being less abrupt than those of the classic paroxysmal rhythms and ushered in usually by a relative slowing of the dominant sinus rhythm. In this sense, NPJT is identical to AVJ escape rhythms, only with a faster intrinsic rate. It is not rare to observe an AVJ rhythm discharging at the rate of 80 beats/min during the first 24 hours in a patient with an acute inferior wall myocardial infarction when ischemic injury to the junctional tissue is acute, only to slow gradually to rates under 60 beats/min on the second and third days. NPJT may be associated with retrograde conduction to the atria. With 1 : 1 retrograde atrial depolarization, the sinus node may be depolarized with every ascending P wave. Preempted by the retrograde P waves arriving at a relatively fast rate, the sinus node may not find the opportunity of firing, thus allowing the AVJ pacemaker to remain in control of the heart for long periods. The hegemony of the AV junction will be terminated as a result

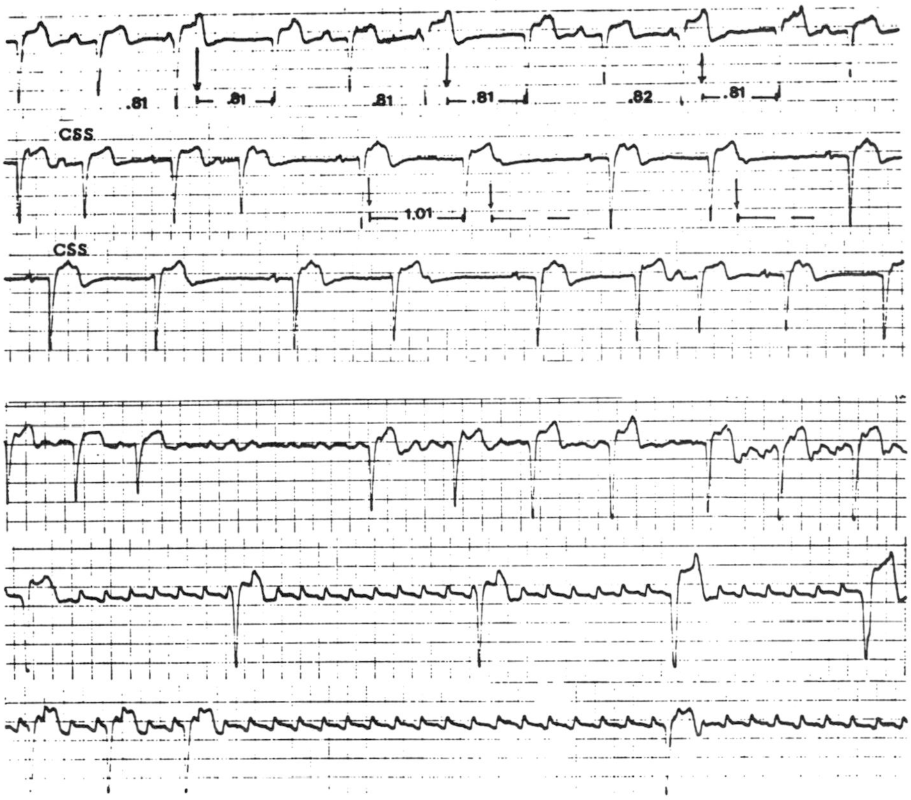

Figure 9-27. *AVJ escape beats occurred frequently in this patient with a sinus rhythm interrupted by premature atrial beats. The AVJ escape interval measured 0.81 second (top strip). In the second and third strips, carotid sinus stimulation (CSS) prolonged the escape interval to over 1 second and then culminated in complete failure of the escape mechanism (see long pauses without AVJ escapes). In strips 4, 5, and 6, atrial fibrillation and flutter caused markedly delayed appearance or even complete inactivation of the AVJ escape focus by concealed penetration and depolarization of the focus.*

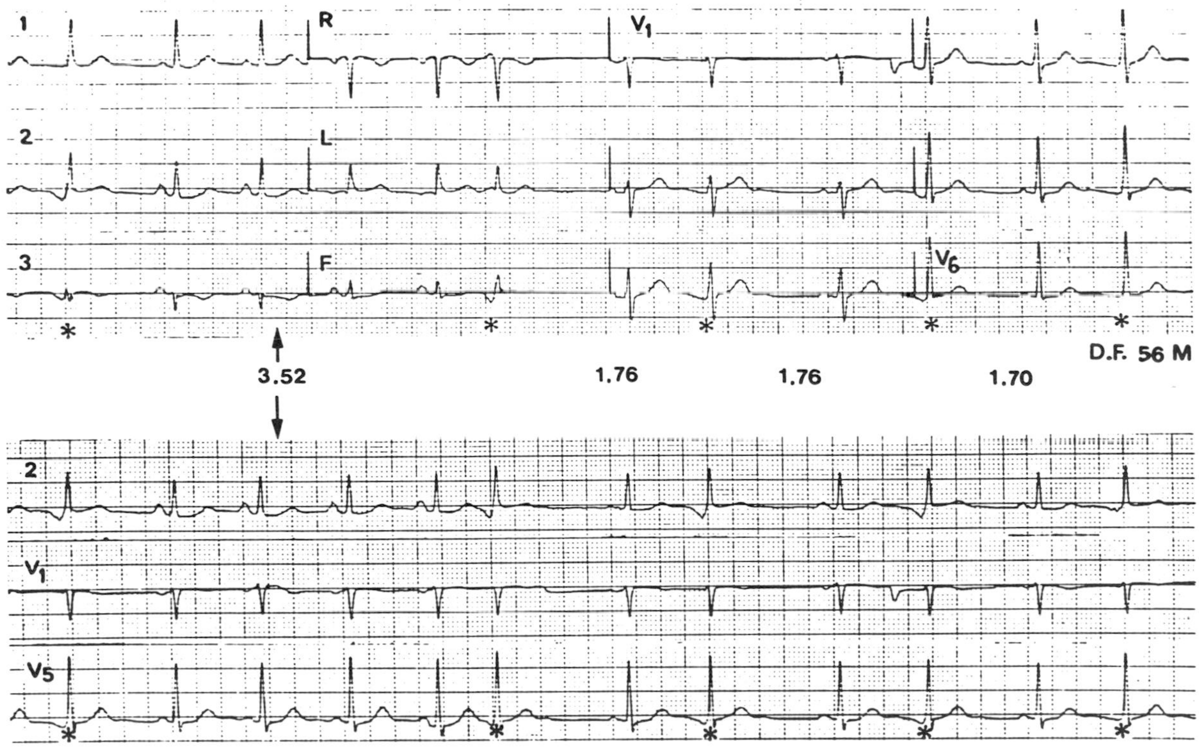

Figure 9-28. *In the 12-lead electrocardiogram in this patient with no documented heart disease, single AVJ extrasystole marked by asterisks was thought to be present. More careful analysis of rhythm strips demonstrated the existence of an AVJ parasystole with an interectopic interval of approximately 1.75 second corresponding to a rate of 34 beats/min.*

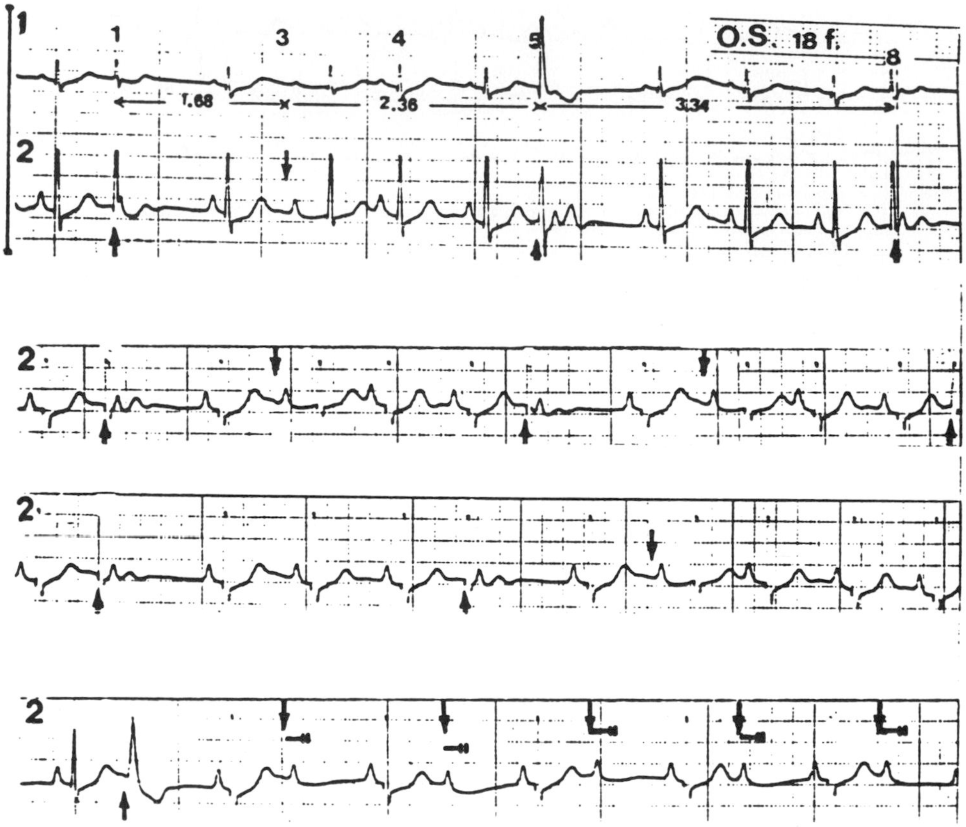

Figure 9-29. *Strips of leads 1 and 2 taken from a girl of 18 years with no heart disease show a basic sinus rhythm interrupted with premature beats having both normal and aberrant QRS complexes (beats 1, 5, and 8). In addition, some PR intervals are inexplicably prolonged (after downward arrows), and some P waves are completely blocked (after downward arrows, bottom strip). Careful attention reveals the existence of a parasystolic rhythm in which some discharges are manifest (upward arrows) but others, situated before the long PR or blocked P waves (downward arrows), remain nonpropagated and serve only to impede conduction through the AV node. The intrinsic rate of the AV junctional parasystolic focus is 71 beats/min. In the bottom strip a pattern of apparent 2:1 AV block has been produced by the occurrence of parasystolic AVJ discharges after every second sinus beat.*

of fatigue and slowing of the automatic focus, or the acceleration of the sinus rate usually caused by a fall in blood pressure during NPJT, or depolarization and resetting of the AVJ tachycardia focus by premature atrial or ventricular beats. Frequently, however, PVBs succeed only in depolarizing the ventricles and rendering them refractory to the next incoming AVJ wave of depolarization, without altering the basic NPJT. Of course, the effect of depolarization of the tachycardia-sustaining tissue by premature beats depends on the basic mechanism of the tachycardia, that is, whether it is due to automatic discharges, reentry, or triggered automaticity.

In the presence of atrial fibrillation, NPJT is recognized by the regularity of the ventricular rhythm. Similarly, in atrial flutter, the regularity of the QRS complexes and the finding of AV dissociation will indicate the presence of NPJT (Fig. 9-13). Intermittent failure of impulses to exit and depolarize the ventricle (exit block) causes unexpected doubling of the RR intervals, thus mimicking advanced AV block (see the discussion on pseudo-AV block). Persistent block of alternate impulses would be indistinguishable from complete AV block. The actual rate of discharge from the AVJ focus may not become apparent until at least two consecutive discharges depolarize the ventricles without being hindered by the exit block. Note that the discharge rate of NPJT may change from time to time and in response to vagal and sympathetic maneuvers such as carotid sinus stimulation and changes of endogenous sympathetic tone.

Paroxysmal Atrioventricular Junction Tachycardia

Excluding the commonly occurring AV nodal reentrant tachycardias (AVNRT), paroxysmal AVJ tachycardias emerging as a result of increased automaticity, be it due to enhanced phase 4 depolarization or triggered (diastolic afterdepolarization), are quite rare. It is not clear how NPJT and PJT can be differentiated clinically unless the onset is recorded. Truly paroxysmal junctional tachycardia with abrupt onset and offset usually proves to be reentrant AVNT. The tachycardia rate tends to be constant in AVNRT, whereas frequent, unprovoked rate changes suggest the existence of an automatically discharging focus.

Perhaps the most useful feature for differentiation between an automatic PJT and AVNRT is that the former is reset by extraneous beats (premature ventricular or supraventricular beats), whereas the latter is either undisturbed or stopped by such interferences.

Pseudo-Atrioventricular Block

Depolarization of the AV junction, caused by whatever impulse is followed by a period of absolute, and then a period of relative, refractoriness during which the passage of other impulses through the AV junction will be blocked or impeded. The impulse causing the delay is most frequently a PVB, and the phenomenon is generally referred to as *concealment.* Impulses arising within the AV junction in the form of premature AVJ beats likewise cause conduction delay or block in the path of sinus beats on their way to the ventricles. Such manifest PJBs are readily recognizable on the electrocardiogram as narrow QRS complexes not preceded by P waves. However, when such AVJ impulses fail to propagate to the ventricles and remain confined to the area of AV junction, no QRS complexes will result but the delay in AV conduction will be exerted nevertheless. On the electrocardiogram such an event will be reflected by unexpected prolongation of the PR interval or complete block of the P waves. This intriguing mechanism was recognized in the 1940s by Langendorf[15] and later documented through His bundle studies by Rosen and colleagues.[16] This phenomenon appears to be quite rare, observed no more than once every 2 years by Massumi in a 1000-bed hospital. Similar to the manifest AVJ extrasystoles, the nonpropagated AVJ extrasystoles causing pseudo-AV block occur in both normal and diseased hearts. In all the six cases studied by Massumi, the nonpropagated and manifest AVJ extrasystoles occurred in a parasystolic mode. In the case reported by Rosen and colleagues,[16] the marked variations in the coupling intervals of the AVJ extrasystoles suggest an AVJ parasystole, although such diagnosis was not discussed by the authors. Figure 9-29 depicts a case of pseudo-AV block.

A more common cause of pseudo-AV block encountered in AVJ rhythm is the type exemplified in Figure 9-23. In this situation of AVJ tachycardia with AV dissociation, the ventricular rate slows unpredictably because of exit block. Retrograde conduction to the atrium exists in about one third of the cases of AVJ rhythm associated with exit block.

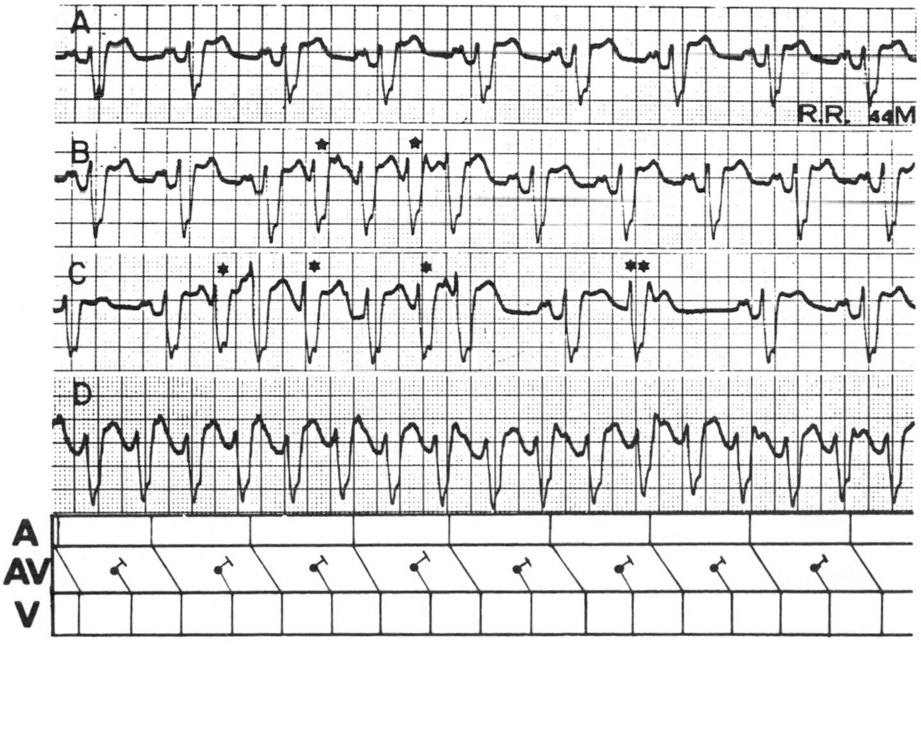

Figure 9-30. *This man of 44 years with known coronary artery disease suffered from recurrent attacks of a wide QRS tachycardia at the rate of 142 beats/min (D). Because of the apparent AV dissociation, a diagnosis of ventricular tachycardia was entertained. The unusual feature, however, was that the QRS complexes during tachycardia were identical with those recorded during sinus rhythm (A to C). The finding of interpolation of some premature beats (asterisks), resulting in doubling of the rate, suggested the mechanism of interpolated premature AVJ extrasystoles causing a pseudotachycardia.*

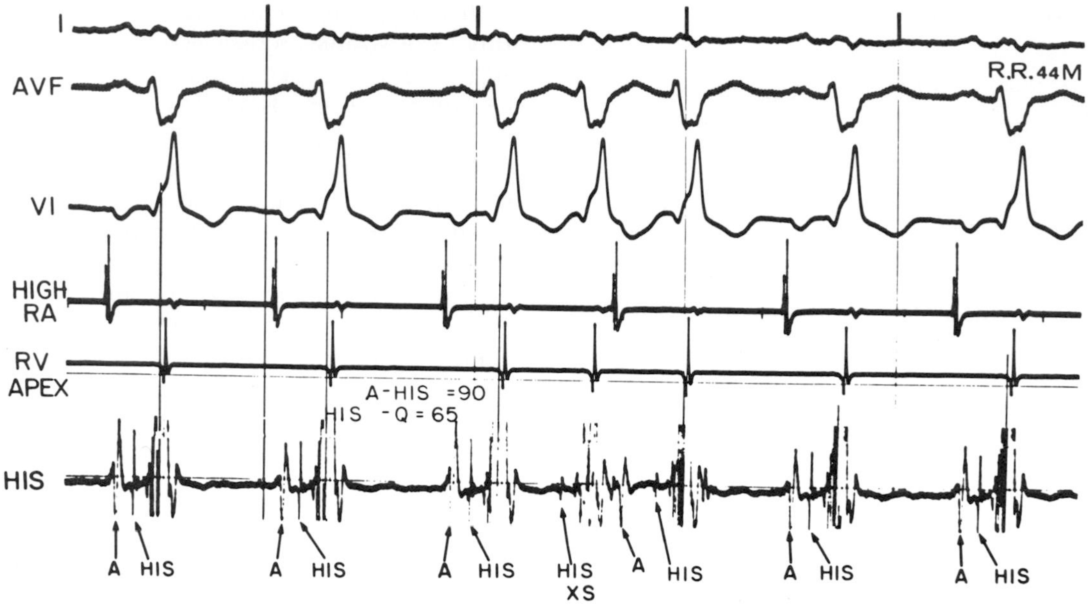

Figure 9-31. *His bundle recordings showing one of the interpolated AVJ extrasystoles possessing a normal His spike with a normal His-Q interval of 65 msec.*

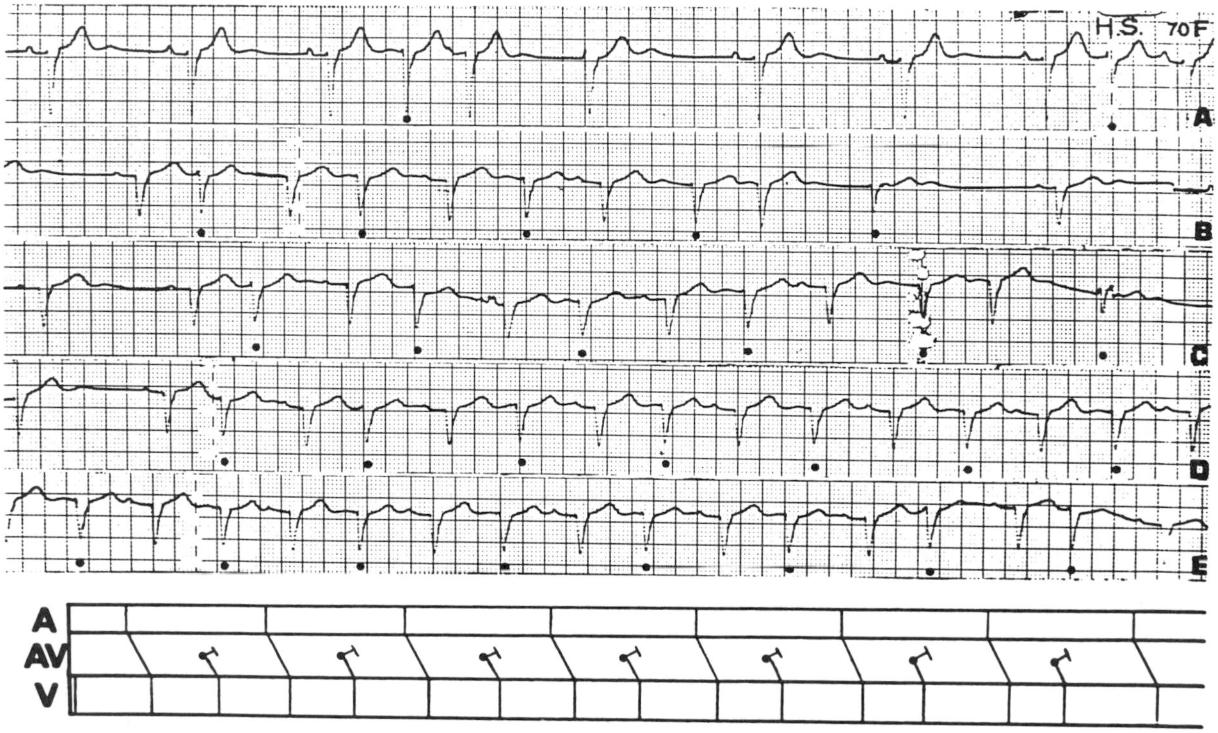

Figure 9-32. *An example of pseudotachycardia in a woman of 70 years complaining of recurrent episodes of rapid heart beating. The Holter monitoring disclosed basic sinus bradycardia with frequent interpolated AVJ extrasystoles (dots) corresponding to an AVJ parasystole discharging 48 beats/min. On several occasions during the 24-hour Holter recording, the sinus rate approximated the rate of AVJ parasystole, allowing the parasystolic discharges to fall between consecutive sinus beats, thereby doubling the effective heart rate (E). The ladder diagram depicts an AVJ parasystole discharging at 48 beats/min with a sinus rate of 47 beats/min.*

Pseudotachycardias

The term *pseudotachycardias* is suggested primarily for the abrupt doubling of the heart rate resulting from interpolation of AVJ extrasystoles between sinus beats. Five cases of this rare arrhythmia have been found in over 6 years of searching electrocardiographic and Holter tracings in a large hospital, and in each case the erroneous diagnosis of paroxysmal supraventricular tachycardia had been entertained.

Treatments usually employed in supraventricular tachycardias (digitalis, class I drugs, calcium channel blockers) had proved completely ineffectual in all five patients. All patients had ischemic heart disease but not digitalis intoxication or any electrolyte abnormalities. Figure 9-30 shows monitor strips taken during normal sinus rhythm (*A*), sinus rhythm with interpolated (asterisk) and noninterpolated (double asterisk) junctional extrasystoles (*B* and *C*), and pseudotachycardia caused by uninterrupted occurrence of interpolated AVJ extrasystoles (*D*). In Figure 9-31 a His bundle recording shows one interpolated AVJ extrasystole in the midst of sinus beats, possessing a normal His spike preceding the ventricular potential. Figure 9-32 depicts another example of pseudotachycardia in a woman of 70 suffering from bouts of fast heartbeats. Here, AVJ discharges occurred in a parasystolic mode, with a discharge rate close to the sinus rate. An even more intriguing mechanism of pseudotachycardia was observed in three patients with sinus tachycardia and dual AV nodal pathways, in whom two families of PR intervals occurred intermittently. A shift from short PR to long PR placed the sinus P waves in the ST segment or the T wave of the preceding beat, thus suggesting an AVJ tachycardia (see Fig. 9-24).

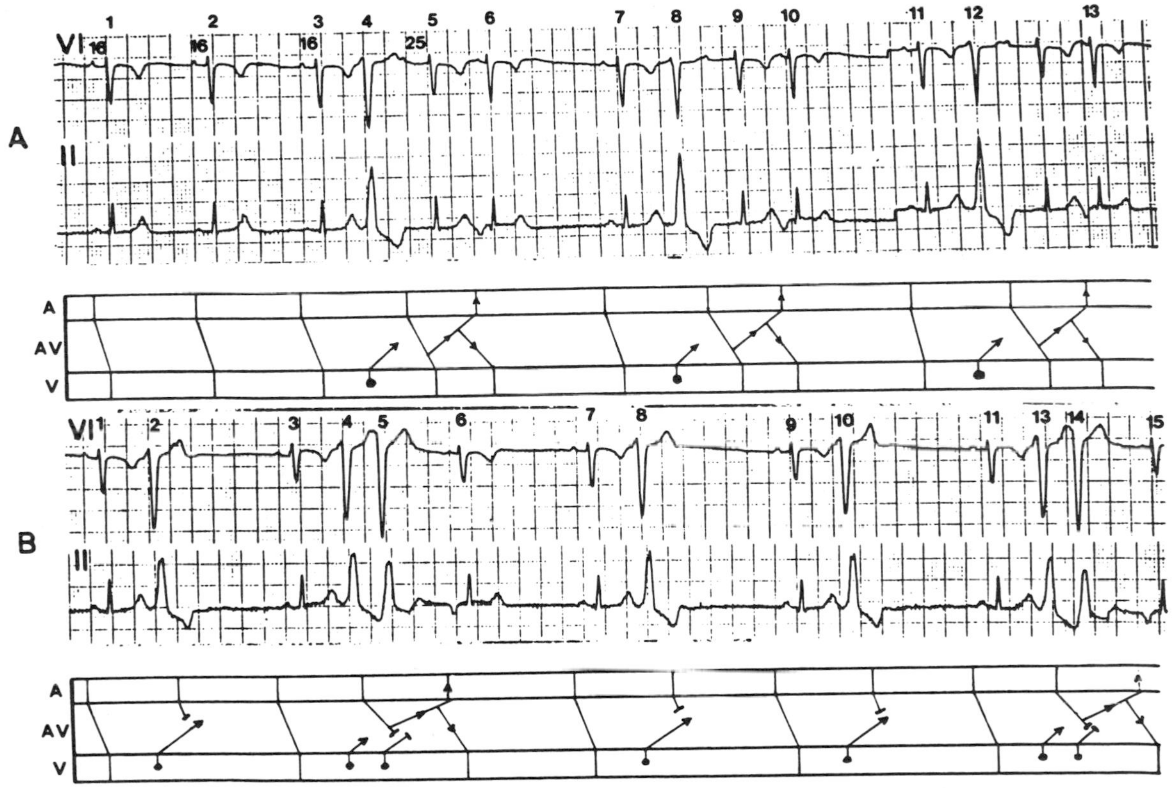

Figure 9-33. *In this woman of 31 years with no detectable heart disease, premature ventricular beats with variable coupling intervals occurred persistently over several years. The concealed conduction of the premature ventricular beats into the AVJ either blocked the next sinus P wave (beats 2, 8, and 10, bottom panel) or prolonged the PR interval (beats 4, 8, and 12, top panel). Following the PR prolongation, the depolarizing impulse passing slowly through the AV node echoed back into the atrium in retrograde fashion, causing a negative P wave (upward arrows in both ladder diagrams). Reciprocation and echo back in the ventricle following the retrograde P waves also occur (QRS 6, 10, and 13 in top panel and 6 and 15 in bottom panel). Perhaps the most remarkable feature of these tracings is the strikingly prolonged retrograde conduction time through the AV junction, placing the retrograde P waves far from the responsible sinus P wave. These far-flung retrograde P waves were originally thought to be AVJ extrasystoles.*

Echo Through the Atrioventricular Junction

In Figures 9-3 to 9-5, examples of an orthograde P wave, conducted slowly through the AVJ and followed by a return to the atrium (echo), were demonstrated. It has been generally assumed that echo occurs through the AV node, where slow conduction, which is the prerequisite for the mechanism of echo, is a common phenomenon.[17] The observation of echo at the distal regions of the main His bundle in a case of intra-Hisian second degree Mobitz type I block (see Fig. 9-4) clearly suggests that echo can also take place in fast-conducting linear structures such as the main His bundle and perhaps the bundle branches. One might reason that a sustained reentrant AVJ tachycardia using the main His bundle may also occur. The majority of echoes occur toward the end of Wenckebach cycles when PR intervals have lengthened to 0.3 second or longer. However, lengthening of the PR interval to the above values for whatever cause may encourage echoing back into the atrium (Fig. 9-33). Echo in the retrograde direction (*i.e.*, an idioventricular impulse ascending through the AV node, making a 180° turn, and reentering the ventricles) also occurs but appears to be rarer than the orthograde echo probably because, most often following a PVB, the AV node has already been penetrated by the orthograde sinus P wave, thus making it impossible for the PVB to penetrate it.

Atrioventricular Junctional Parasystole

As noted in the discussion on pseudo-AV block, extrasystolic discharges from the AVJ frequently occur in a parasystolic mode. This may simply be due to the relative rarity of other forms of AVJ extrasystoles, which tend to be extinguished constantly by the sinus impulses on their way through the AVJ. A measure of entrance block of the type presumed to exist in parasystole may be needed if an AVJ focus is to avoid the extinguishing effect of passing impulses. Many of the patients with AVJ parasystole have had very slow intrinsic rates of 30 beats/min or below, resulting in infrequent manifest beats. Such beats are generally interpreted as AVJ extrasystoles. Correct diagnosis can be made only if long rhythm strips are recorded (see Fig. 9-28).

AVJ parasystoles may remain nonpropagated. Such discharges most frequently go unnoticed or are detected by their slowing effect on AV conduction (pseudo-AV block). An unusual example of AVJ parasystole in which manifest discharges were interpolated between adjacent sinus beats and caused the actual ventricular rate to be doubled (pseudotachycardia) was presented in Figure 9-32.

References

1. Katz, L. N., and Pick, A.: Clinical electrocardiography. I. The arrhythmias. Philadelphia, Lea & Febiger, 1956.
2. Scherf, D., and Cohen J.: The Atrioventricular Node. New York, Grune & Stratton, 1964.
3. Friedberg, C. K.: Disease of the Heart. Philadelphia, W. B. Saunders, 1966.
4. Bellet, S.: Clinical Disorders of the Heart Beat, pp. 419–448. Philadelphia, Lea & Febiger, 1971.
5. Watanabe, Y., and Dreifus, L.: AV junctional rhythms. In Cardiac Arrhythmias: Electrophysiologic Basis for Clinic Interpretation, pp. 98–152. New York, Grune & Stratton, 1977.
6. Bigger, J. T.: In Braunwald, E. (ed.): Heart Disease: A Textbook of Cardiovascular Medicine, pp. 660–664. Philadelphia, W. B. Saunders, 1980.
7. Massumi, R. A., and Tawakkol, A. A.: Direct study of left atrial P waves. Am. J. Cardiol., 20:331, 1967.
8. Massumi, R. A., et al.: Time sequence of right and left atrial depolarization in determining the origin of ectopic P waves. Am. J. Cardiol., 24:28, 1969.
9. Moore, E. N., Jomain, S. L., Stuckey, J. H., et al.: Studies on ectopic atrial rhythms in dogs. Am. J. Cardiol., 19:676, 1967.
10. Waldo, A. L., Vitikainen, K. J., and Hoffman, B. F.: The sequence of retrograde atrial activation in the canine heart: Correlation with positive and negative P waves. Cir. Res., 37:156, 1975.
11. Schamroth, L.: The Disorders of Cardiac Rhythm, p. 305. Oxford, Blackwell Scientific Publishers, 1980.
12. Massumi, R. A., Ertem, G. E., and Vera, Z.: Aberrancy of junctional escape beats: Evidence for origin in the fascicles of the left bundle branch. Am. J. Cardiol., 29:351, 1972.
13. Massumi, R. A., Mason, D. T., Vera, Z., et al.: Fascicular rhythms: Their characteristic morphologic features and protean manifestations. Postgrad. Med., 53:95, 1973.
14. Fisch, C., Sipes, D. P., and McHenry, P. L.: Electrocardiographic manifestations of concealed junctional ectopic impulses. Circulation, 53:217, 1976.
15. Langendorf, R., and Mehlman, J. A.: Blocked (non-conducted) A-V nodal premature systoles imitating first and second degree A-V block. Am. Heart J., 34:500, 1947.
16. Rosen, K. M., Rahimtoola, S. H., and Gunnar, R. M.: Pseudo A-V block secondary to premature nonpropagated His bundle depolarization: Documentation by His bundle electrocardiography. Circulation, 42:367, 1970.
17. Damato, A. N., Varghese, P. J., Lau, S. H., et al.: Manifest and concealed reentry. Circ. Res., 30:283–291, 1972.

10

Paroxysmal Supraventricular Tachycardia

Robert A. Bauernfeind, William J. Welch, and John M. Herre

Paroxysmal supraventricular tachycardia (PSVT) has the following electrocardiographic characteristics: (1) Sudden (paroxysmal) onset and termination, (2) a usually regular rhythm, with only gradual changes in rate, (3) an atrial rate of 100 to 250 beats/min, usually between 140 and 220 beats/min, (4) a ventricular rate that equals the atrial rate or, if AV block exists, is less than the atrial rate, and (5) typically narrow QRS complexes that may be wide when aberrant conduction is present (Fig. 10-1).

Mechanisms

There are presently six well-established types of PSVT.[1–5] Of these, four reflect reentrance: reentrance using an anomalous pathway, AV nodal reentrance, atrial reentrance, and sinus nodal reentrance. Two types appear to reflect automaticity and arise from ectopic foci in the atria or the His bundle.

Reentrance Utilizing an Anomalous Pathway

The conduction system of a patient with Wolff-Parkinson-White (WPW) syndrome (manifest preexcitation) provides an ideal setting for reentrance: There is a proximal common pathway (the atria), a distal common pathway (the ventricles), and two connecting limbs (the AV node and His-Purkinje system and the Kent bundle). During sinus rhythm there is antegrade conduction over both connecting limbs to the ventricles, resulting in fusion QRS complexes (Fig. 10-2). However, a premature atrial beat can find the Kent bundle (anomalous pathway) refractory and conduct antegradely over only the AV node and His-Purkinje system (normal pathway) to the ventricles, resulting in a narrow QRS complex (see Fig. 10-2).[1,6,7] If antegrade conduction delay has been sufficient to enable the anomalous pathway to recover excitability, the wavefront conducts retrogradely over this pathway to the atria.[8,9] If the wavefront then again conducts antegradely over the normal pathway to the ventricles, and retrogradely over the anomalous pathway to the atria, and so on, a circus movement has been initiated (see Fig. 10-2). The same circus movement can be initiated by a premature ventricular beat that blocks retrogradely in the normal pathway but conducts to the atria over the anomalous pathway.[1,6,10]

Reentrance using an anomalous pathway, as de-

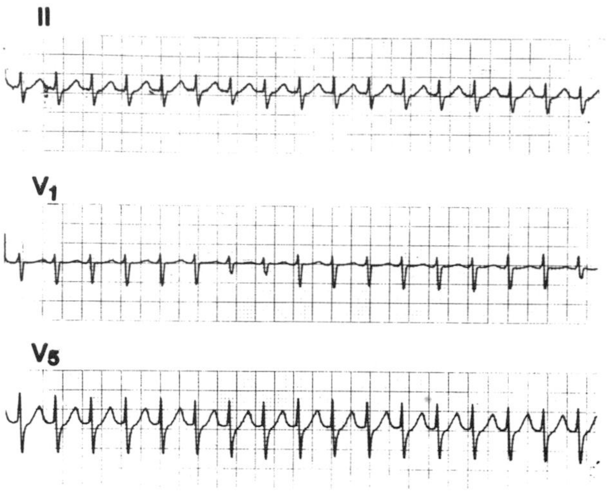

Figure 10-1. *Paroxysmal supraventricular tachycardia.*

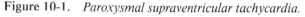

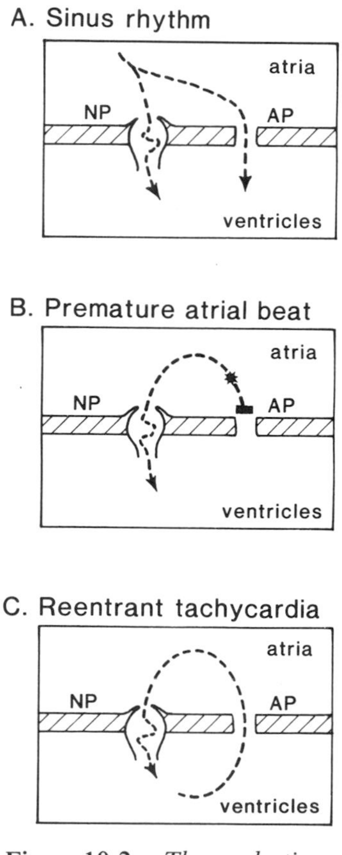

Figure 10-2. *The conduction system in Wolff-Parkinson-White syndrome. (A) Sinus rhythm with antegrade conduction over both pathways. (B) A premature atrial beat (*) blocks in the AP but conducts over the NP to the ventricles. (C) The wavefront then conducts over the AP to the atria and over the NP to the ventricles. Reentrance using an anomalous pathway has been initiated. (NP, normal pathway; AP, anomalous pathway)*

scribed above, occasionally occurs in patients who do not have manifest preexcitation. These patients have "concealed" anomalous pathways, which conduct in only the retrograde direction.[1,2,8,9]

In reentrance using an anomalous pathway, sequential depolarization of the atria and the ventricles exists. Since conduction to the ventricles is over the normal pathway, the QRS complexes are usually narrow, and PSVT is seen on the electrocardiogram.

Atrioventricular Nodal Reentrance

Goldreyer and co-workers suggested that reentrance within the AV node is a common mechanism of PSVT.[11,12] Subsequent studies have shown that the substrate for AV nodal reentrance is provided by functional longitudinal dissociation of the AV node into two pathways (dual AV nodal pathways).[13–18] It is not clear whether this dissociation has an anatomic basis or whether it is a purely physiologic phenomenon.[19,20] Because the two pathways through the AV node are differentiated on the basis of their different conduction times, they are referred to as *fast* and *slow* AV nodal pathways. Most evidence suggests that these pathways join in both the upper (proximal common pathway) and the lower (distal common pathway) part of the node.[21,22]

During sinus rhythm there is antegrade conduction over both the fast and the slow AV nodal pathways. The wavefront conducting over the fast pathway reaches the His bundle first, resulting in a relatively short atrio-His (AH) interval, whereas conduction over the slow pathway is concealed. However, a premature atrial beat can find the fast pathway refractory and conduct antegradely only over the slow pathway, resulting in a relatively long AH interval.[13–18] If antegrade conduction delay has been sufficient to enable the fast pathway to recover excitability, the wavefront conducts retrogradely over this pathway to the proximal common pathway.[11,12] If the wavefront then again conducts antegradely over the slow pathway, and retrogradely over the fast pathway, and so on, a circus movement has been initiated. The same circus movement can be initiated by a premature ventricular beat that blocks in the slow pathway but conducts retrogradely over the fast pathway.

Atrioventricular nodal reentrance occasionally occurs in the opposite direction; that is, the circus movement uses the fast pathway as the antegrade limb and the slow pathway as the retrograde limb.[23,24] This "unusual" variety of AV nodal reentrance can be initiated by a premature atrial beat that blocks in the slow pathway and conducts over the fast pathway or by a premature ventricular beat that blocks in the fast pathway and conducts over the slow pathway.

In most cases of AV nodal reentrance, each depolarization of the proximal common pathway is conducted to the atria and each depolarization of the distal common pathway is conducted to the ventricles. Thus, PSVT is seen on the electrocardiogram.

Sinus Reentrance and Atrial Reentrance

Sinus reentrance is initiated in the following way.[25,26] A premature atrial beat finds one margin of the sinus node refractory (entrance block) but penetrates the node at a different site. If the wavefront traverses the node slowly enough, the atria recover excitability, allowing the wavefront to exit from the node (at the site of original entrance block). If the wavefront conducts back into the node, and then back out to the atria, a circus movement has been initiated. In atrial reentrance, a similar circus movement travels a pathway composed only of atrial tissue.[26] Since sinus and atrial reentrance both occur in structures above the AV node and are frequently difficult to differentiate, they may be considered together as *sinoatrial reentrance.* Sinoatrial reentrance results in tachycardia if P waves are conducted to the ventricles. However, unlike reentrance using an anomalous pathway, AV conduction is not necessary for the continuance of sinoatrial reentrance.[26]

Automatic Ectopic Foci

The types of PSVT discussed to this point have all reflected reentrance and have differed only in the cardiac structures used by their circus movements. However, occasional cases of PSVT reflect spontaneous impulse formation in either the atria or the His bundle.[3,27,28] These tachycardias are not initiated by premature beats but begin spontaneously, with the first beat being identical to the subsequent beats of tachycardia. Automatic ectopic atrial tachycardia and sinoatrial reentrance are *paroxysmal atrial tachycardias* (PAT).

Diagnosis of Paroxysmal Supraventricular Tachycardia Mechanism

Although definitive diagnosis of the mechanism of PSVT usually requires electrophysiologic studies, a tentative diagnosis can frequently be suspected before studies are done. In patients with manifest preexcitation, reentrance using an anomalous pathway is the most common mechanism and should be suspected.[1] In patients without manifest preexcitation, AV nodal reentrance is the most likely diagnosis.[1-5] However, certain clinical features can suggest another diagnosis. For example, if a patient below age 35 years, without apparent heart disease, has PSVT with a rate greater than 200 beats/min, reentrance using an anomalous pathway should be suspected, even if manifest preexcitation is absent.[3] Paroxysmal supraventricular tachycardia that occurs only in an acute clinical setting is frequently automatic ectopic atrial tachycardia.[27] More valuable information, which may yield a specific diagnosis, can frequently be derived from the surface electrocardiogram by examining the onset, the duration, and the termination of PSVT. These electrocardiographic observations are also made during electrophysiologic studies and will be discussed in the context of these studies.

Electrophysiologic Studies

In most cases, a specific type of PSVT can be diagnosed by performing electrophysiologic studies.[1-5] Reentrant tachycardias are differentiated from automatic ectopic tachycardias because they can be initiated and terminated by cardiac pacing.[11,12,27] It is also usually possible to distinguish among reentrance using an anomalous pathway, AV nodal reentrance, and sinoatrial reentrance. In this regard it is useful to consider separately the following portions of the studies: (1) programmed atrial stimulation, (2) programmed ventricular stimulation, (3) observations during paroxysmal tachycardia, and (4) administration of drugs. Each of these portions may yield diagnostic clues regarding the specific type of PSVT. In most cases, clues from two or more parts of the study must be combined to arrive at a diagnosis.

Programmed Atrial Stimulation

Programmed atrial stimulation includes atrial extra stimulus testing and incremental atrial pacing. Extra stimulus testing is continued until atrial refractoriness is encountered, whereas incremental pacing is continued until second degree AV block occurs. Both techniques are performed by stimulating from the high right atrium and, frequently, from a second site such as the coronary sinus. Programmed atrial stimulation, combined with recording of a His bundle electrogram, can yield important information.

Programmed atrial stimulation may reveal ventricular preexcitation that is not apparent during sinus rhythm.[29] Closely coupled atrial beats usually encounter increased AV nodal refractoriness and thus conduct over the normal pathway with increased delay, whereas there is little or no increase in antegrade conduction time over the anomalous pathway. Thus, closely coupled beats can increase the degree of preexcitation, manifested by prolonged QRS complexes and shortened His-ventricular (HV) interval. In rare cases, the ability of an anomalous pathway to conduct antegradely may depend on the direction of input from the atria, and thus ventricular preexcitation may be revealed only when programmed stimulation is performed from the coronary sinus.[29] Demonstration of preexcitation suggests a diagnosis of reentrance using an anomalous pathway.

Programmed atrial stimulation provides information regarding the quality of antegrade normal pathway conduction, which is usually excellent in patients with PSVT. In reentrance using an anomalous pathway, the normal pathway is the antegrade limb and must be capable of repetitive antegrade conduction at short cycle lengths.[30] In AV nodal reentrance, one of the AV nodal pathways (usually the slow pathway) is the antegrade limb and must be capable of repetitive antegrade conduction.[24,31] Although antegrade normal pathway conduction is not required to maintain any of the varieties of atrial tachycardia, these tachycardias are frequently associated with 1 : 1 normal pathway conduction.

Antegrade dual AV nodal pathways are diagnosed when atrial extra stimulus testing reveals discontinuous AV nodal (A_1-A_2, H_1-H_2, and A_1-A_2, A_2-H_2) conduction curves.[13–18] These discontinuous curves are generated when relatively late extra stimuli conduct over the fast pathway (relatively short A_2-H_2 intervals) but slightly earlier extra stimuli block in the fast pathway and conduct over the slow pathway, causing a sudden marked increase in the A_2-H_2 intervals (Fig. 10-3). Discontinuous AV nodal curves can be demonstrated in most patients with the usual variety of AV nodal reentrance. However, in some patients with this variety of tachycardia, discontinuous curves cannot be demonstrated because the effective refractory period of the fast pathway is shorter than the functional refractory period of the atria or because the fast and slow pathways have

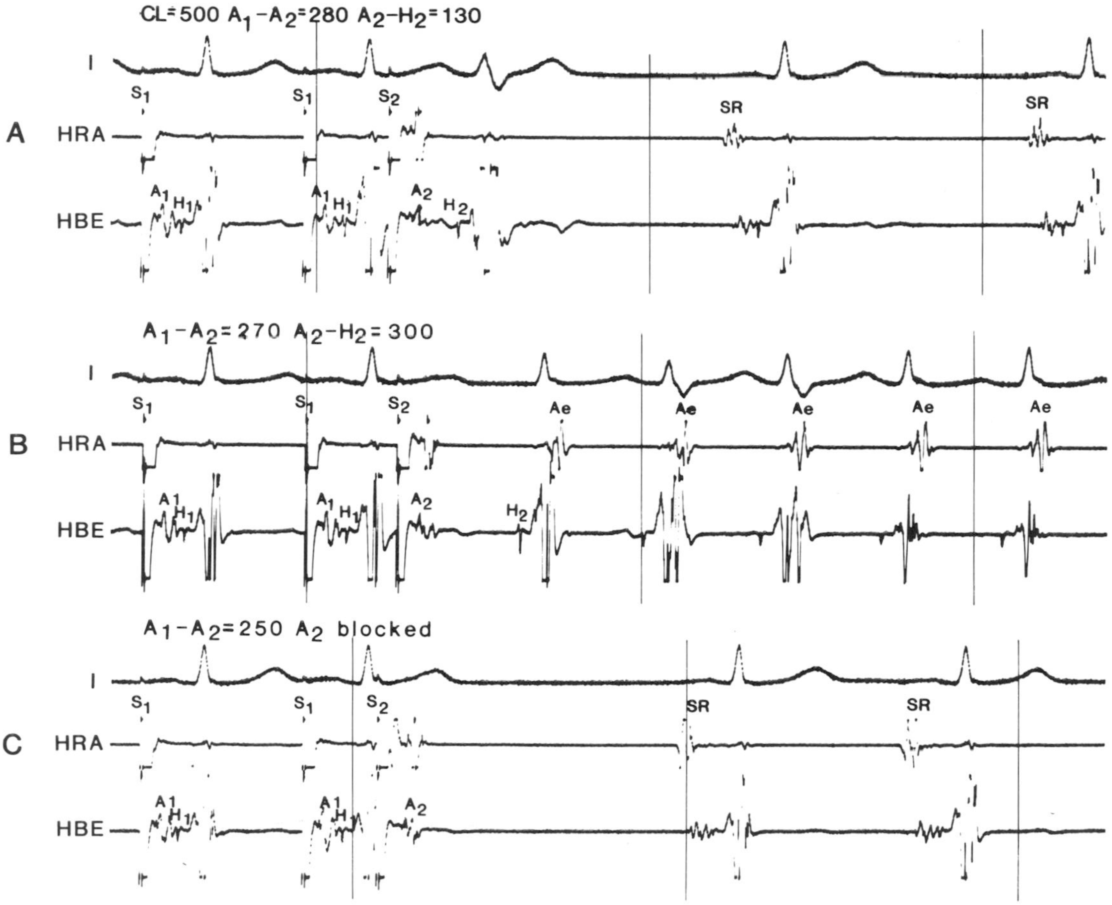

Figure 10-3. *Atrial extra stimulus testing in a patient with antegrade dual AV nodal pathways and AV nodal reentrant tachycardia (usual variety). Shown in each panel are electrocardiographic lead I and high right atrial (HRA) and His bundle (HBE) electrograms. Time lines are at 1-second intervals. (A) A_1-A_2 = 280 msec. A_2 conducts over the fast pathway (A_2-H_2 = 130 msec), and sinus rhythm resumes. (B) A_1-A_2 = 270 msec. A_2 blocks in the fast pathway, conducts over the slow pathway (A_2-H_2 = 300 msec), and induces reentrant tachycardia. (C) A_1-A_2 = 250 msec. A_2 blocks in both the fast and slow pathways, and sinus rhythm resumes. (A_e, atrial echo)*

very similar conduction times.[32-34] Thus, failure to demonstrate discontinuous AV nodal curves does not exclude a diagnosis of AV nodal reentrance. Also, demonstration of discontinuous curves is not specific for a diagnosis of AV nodal reentrance: Discontinuous curves are present in 5% to 10% of patients without AV nodal reentrance, including occasional patients with reentrance using an anomalous pathway or a variety of atrial tachycardia.[32,35-37]

When PSVT is induced during programmed atrial stimulation, it is important to determine whether induction is associated with a specific pattern of AV conduction. Induction of reentrance using an anomalous pathway by an atrial beat requires antegrade block in the anomalous pathway (normalization of the QRS complex in patients with manifest preexcitation) and antegrade conduction to the ventricles over the normal pathway with sufficient delay to allow the anomalous pathway to recover excitability.[1,6-9] The critical delay may be achieved primarily in the AV node (prolonged AH interval) or in the distal conduction system (prolonged HV interval or functional block in the bundle branch ipsilateral to the anomalous pathway).[8,9,38] Induction of the usual variety of AV nodal reentrance by an atrial beat requires antegrade block in the fast pathway and conduction over the slow pathway with sufficient delay (critical AH interval) to allow the fast pathway to recover excitability.[11,12,14-17] Although there is usually conduction to the ventricles, AV nodal reentrance is occasionally induced by atrial beats that block distal to the His bundle or even proximal to the His bundle (presumably in AV nodal tissue distal to the reentrant pathway).[21] Induction of the unusual variety of AV nodal reentrance by an atrial beat requires antegrade block in the slow pathway and conduction over the fast pathway.[39] In antegrade conduction over the fast pathway, antegrade block in the slow pathway is not apparent and can only be inferred. Although induction of sinoatrial reentrance can be achieved by closely coupled atrial beats, the specific characteristics of intra-atrial conduction required for these inductions cannot be established with standard electrophysiologic techniques.[25,26] The presence or absence of AV conduction is irrelevant to induction of sinoatrial reentrance.[26]

The significance of specific patterns of tachycardia induction during programmed atrial stimulation can be summarized as follows. If tachycardia is induced by atrial beats that block proximal to the His bundle, a diagnosis of sinoatrial reentrance should be suspected; this pattern of induction is seen only rarely in patients with AV nodal reentrance and is incompatible with reentrance using an anomalous pathway. This latter diagnosis is also excluded when tachycardia is induced by atrial beats that block distal to the His bundle. In contrast, demonstration that conduction to the His bundle is required for induction of tachycardia excludes a diagnosis of sinoatrial reentrance, and, if conduction to the ventricles is required, AV nodal reentrance can be also excluded, leaving a diagnosis of reentrance using an anomalous pathway. If induction of tachycardia clearly requires achievement of a critical AH interval, a diagnosis of AV nodal reentrance or reentrance using an anomalous pathway is likely, and if induction is facilitated by a prolonged HV interval or functional bundle branch block, the diagnosis is reentrance using an anomalous pathway.

Although the above considerations are frequently useful and, in some cases, can provide a specific diagnosis, their application can be difficult. The information provided by atrial extra stimulus testing is frequently of limited value.[11] Since patients with PSVT usually have excellent antegrade normal pathway conduction, the atrial functional refractory period is frequently longer than the AV nodal effective refractory period. Tachycardia is induced by the most closely coupled atrial extra stimuli, which are conducted with the longest A_2-H_2 and A_2-V_2 intervals. Thus, it is frequently not clear whether induction of tachycardia depends on the presence of short A_1-A_2 intervals (suggesting sinoatrial reentrance), long A_2-H_2 intervals (suggesting AV nodal reentrance), or long A_2-V_2 intervals (suggesting reentrance using an anomalous pathway). Performance of rapid atrial pacing can be useful in this situation.[12] The rate of atrial pacing at which type I second degree blocks occurs in the AV node is determined, and pacing at this rate is repeated, frequently 30 or 40 times. When this is done, the A_1-A_1 interval remains constant but the conduction of the last paced beat varies. Some of these beats will block in the AV node, some will be conducted with short AH and AV intervals, and some will be conducted with long AH and AV intervals. This variability provides an opportunity to determine whether tachycardia can be induced by a blocked atrial beat or whether antegrade conduction (and a critical AH or AV interval) is required.

Programmed Ventricular Stimulation

Programmed ventricular stimulation includes ventricular extra stimulus testing and incremental ventricular pacing. Extra stimulus testing is continued until ventricular refractoriness is encountered, whereas incremental pacing is continued until second degree VA block occurs. It is frequently useful to record electrograms from multiple atrial sites during programmed ventricular stimulation in patients with PSVT.

Programmed ventricular stimulation provides information on the quality of VA conduction, which is usually excellent in patients with PSVT. In reentrance using an anomalous pathway, the anomalous pathway is the retrograde limb and must be capable of repetitive retrograde conduction at short cycle lengths.[30] In AV nodal reentrance, one of the AV nodal pathways (the fast pathway in the usual variety) is the retrograde limb and must be capable of repetitive retrograde conduction.[31] Intact VA conduction is not necessary for atrial tachycardia to occur.[26] Thus, demonstration that VA conduction is absent, or that VA block occurs at a slow ventricular paced rate, suggests a variety of atrial tachycardia.

When VA conduction is excellent, it is important to determine whether conduction occurs over the normal conduction system or over an anomalous pathway. Determination of the sequence of retrograde atrial depolarization can be useful. When the normal pathway is used for retrograde conduction, the earliest atrial electrograms are recorded from the low septal right atrium (His bundle electrogram) or at the os of the coronary sinus.[40] Thus, demonstration that retrograde atrial activation begins at a different site suggests the presence of a retrogradely conducting anomalous pathway.[1,9] Although a normal retrograde sequence suggests that VA conduction is over the normal conduction system, these findings are also compatible with conduction over a septal anomalous pathway.

It is also useful to examine the temporal relationship between retrograde His bundle depolarization and retrograde atrial depolarization. With closely coupled ventricular extra stimuli, the H_2 deflection frequently emerges after V_2.[41] If the V_2-A_2 interval prolongs to a similar degree as the V_2-H_2 interval, the His bundle is probably a part of the pathway used for VA conduction. Conversely, if the V_2-A_2 interval remains relatively constant as the V_2-H_2 interval prolongs, so that the H_2 deflection approaches or even appears later than A_2, then the His bundle cannot be a part of the pathway used for VA conduction and a retrogradely conducting anomalous pathway must be present.[1,42]

Decremental VA conduction, manifested as a progressive increase in VA intervals as the ventricular paced cycle length is decreased, is presumed present when conduction is over the normal A-V conduction system and absent when conduction is over an anomalous pathway. However, in practice, retrograde conduction over the normal conduction system frequently is not decremental, and although retrograde conduction over an anomalous pathway is usually not decremental, exceptions have been noted.[43,44]

Establishing the presence or absence of a retrogradely conducting anomalous pathway is important. If a retrogradely conducting anomalous pathway is present, a diagnosis of reentrance using an anomalous pathway is very likely. On the other hand, the absence of a retrogradely conducting anomalous pathway generally excludes this diagnosis.

Discontinuous V_1-V_2 and V_2-A_2 conduction curves can be relevant to diagnosis of the mechanism of paroxysmal tachycardia. Sometimes one portion (fast or slow) of the curve reflects conduction over an anomalous pathway and the other portion reflects conduction over the normal pathway.[9,10] In this situation, there frequently is a marked change in the sequence of retrograde atrial activation at the point of discontinuity. In other cases, discontinuous V_1-V_2 and V_2-A_2 curves reflect the presence of retrograde dual (fast and slow) AV nodal pathways, which provide the substrate for the unusual variety of AV nodal reentrance.[23,24] It has been recently shown that when retrograde conduction shifts from the fast to the slow pathway, there may be a subtle change in the sequence of atrial activation, with conduction over the slow pathway favoring relatively early activation of the left side of the interatrial septum.[42,45] In other cases, the discontinuous curves merely reflect a shift of VH conduction from the right bundle branch to the left bundle branch, a finding that is not relevant to diagnosis of the mechanism of tachycardia.[46]

It can be useful to analyze the specific events associated with induction of PSVT during programmed ventricular stimulation. Occasional patients with sinoatrial reentrance have excellent VA conduction, which allows critical A_1-A_2 intervals to be achieved during ventricular extra stimulus testing. In this situation, the characteristic pattern at the onset of tachycardia is that A_2 is followed immediately by an atrial echo beat (A_3), which may be conducted to the ventricles.[26] When AV nodal reentrance or reentrance using an anomalous pathway is induced during ventricular extra stimulus testing, the pattern is different: A_2 is immediately followed by a ventricular echo beat (V_3) and only then by an atrial echo beat (A_3). Induction of the unusual variety of AV nodal reentrance by a ventricular beat requires retrograde block in the fast pathway and conduction over the slow pathway with a sufficient delay (critical VA interval) to allow the fast pathway to recover excitability. Therefore, this diagnosis is suggested by demonstration that retrograde dual AV nodal pathways are present and that induction of tachycardia requires achievement of critical (slow pathway) V_2-A_2 intervals. Repetitive performance of rapid ventricular pacing at a rate at which type I second degree VA block occurs is frequently useful in establishing a critical VA interval as a requirement for induction of tachycardia.

It is usually not possible to differentiate between reentrance using an anomalous pathway and the usual variety of AV nodal reentrance by scrutinizing the pattern of induction during programmed ventricular stimulation, because in each of these situations critical events are concealed: Induction of reentrance using an anomalous pathway requires retrograde conduction over the anomalous pathway and also retrograde block in the distal AV node (a concealed event), whereas induction of the usual variety of AV nodal reentrance requires retrograde conduction over the fast pathway and also retrograde block in the distal slow pathway (a concealed event). However, other clues, such as the sequence of retrograde atrial activation at the time of induction, may be useful in differentiating between these two types of tachycardia.[9]

Observations During Paroxysmal Tachycardia

The ability to induce and examine PSVT in the electrophysiology laboratory is crucial in establishing its mechanism. When tachycardia cannot be thus observed, clues such as the presence of a retrogradely conducting anomalous pathway or of antegrade dual AV nodal pathways can suggest, but not establish, a diagnosis. In examining patients with PSVT, it is useful to begin with the relationship between P waves, or atrial electrograms, and QRS complexes (Fig. 10-4). In reentrance using an anomalous pathway, there is an obligatory 1:1 relationship between P waves and QRS complexes. AV nodal reentrance can continue despite the occurrence of block between the reentrant pathway and the atria (apparent VA block) or block between the reentrant pathway and the ventricles (apparent AV block).[20–22,47] In any of the types of atrial tachycardia, antegrade conduction to the ventricles is unnecessary and AV block is common (PAT with block).

The above considerations can be summarized as follows: Continuation of PSVT despite the occurrence of AV block suggests any of the types of atrial tachycardia but is also compatible with either variety of AV nodal reentrance. However, this finding excludes a diagnosis of reentrance using an anomalous pathway. On the other hand, continuation of PSVT despite the occurrence of VA block suggests a diagnosis of AV nodal reentrance (or His bundle tachycardia).

When PSVT is characterized by a 1:1 relationship between P waves and QRS complexes, it is useful to examine the temporal relationship between these events (see Fig. 10-4).[1–5] In reentrance using an anomalous pathway, antegrade conduction over the normal pathway usually takes longer than retrograde conduction over the anomalous pathway. Thus, P waves are usually located in the first half of the RR interval (P after QRS). In the usual variety of AV nodal reentrance, following antegrade conduction over the slow pathway, retrograde conduction over the fast pathway to the atria occurs simultaneously with antegrade conduction over the His-Purkinje system to the ventricles. Thus, P waves tend to occur simultaneously with QRS complexes but may occur slightly before or slightly after. In the unusual variety of AV nodal reentrance, following antegrade conduction over the fast pathway, antegrade conduction over the His-Purkinje system occurs more rapidly than retrograde conduction over the slow pathway, and P waves are usually located in the latter half of the RR interval (P before QRS). In any of the types of atrial tachycardia, the relationship between P waves and QRS complexes is determined by the atrial rate and the PR interval: P waves are usually in front of QRS complexes but may be after QRS complexes if the atrial rate is fast or if there is first degree AV block.

In summary, if during PSVT P waves occur simultaneously (or almost simultaneously) with QRS complexes, the likely diagnosis is the usual variety of AV nodal reentrance. If P waves follow QRS complexes, a diagnosis of reentrance using an anomalous pathway or the usual variety of A-V nodal reentrance is likely. If P waves precede QRS complexes, a diagnosis of atrial tachycardia or the unusual variety of AV nodal reentrance is probable. However, this latter relationship is also seen in occasional patients with reentrance using an

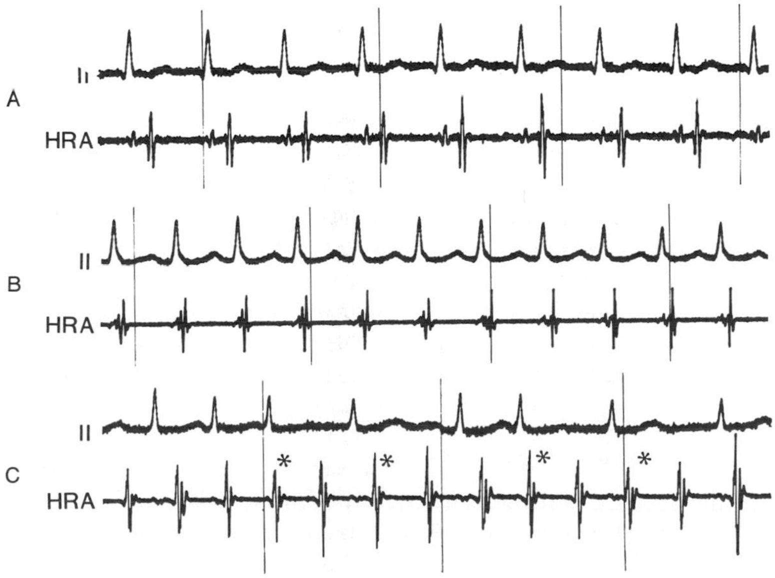

Figure 10-4. *Three types of paroxysmal supraventricular tachycardia. Shown in each panel are electrocardographic lead II and a high right atrial (HRA) electrogram. Time lines are at 1-second intervals. (A) Reentrance using an anomalous pathway. Note the 1:1 relationship between atrial and ventricular depolarizations, with the former occurring in the first half of the RR interval (P after QRS). (B) AV nodal reentrance (usual variety). Note that atrial depolarizations occur simultaneously with QRS complexes. (C) Atrial tachycardia that continues despite the occurrence of AV block (* denotes blocked atrial beats).*

anomalous pathway (when the anomalous pathway conducts slowly).[42]

It is also useful to examine the sequence of atrial activation during PSVT. A normal retrograde sequence (low interatrial septum depolarized first) suggests a diagnosis of AV nodal reentrance but may also occur in reentrance using a septal anomalous pathway or in atrial tachycardia arising low in the interatrial septum.[9] In contrast, an abnormal sequence of retrograde atrial activation suggests a diagnosis of reentrance using an anomalous pathway or atrial tachycardia. The sequence of atrial activation, and P wave morphology, are also used to distinguish sinus nodal reentrance from atrial reentrance.[25,26]

The appearance or disappearance of functional bundle branch block during PSVT may provide observations that are diagnostic of reentrance using an anomalous pathway. In this type of tachycardia, the occurrence of functional block of the bundle branch ipsilateral to the anomalous pathway is associated with an increment of the VA interval.[7,8,48] This increment is less than 25 msec when the anomalous pathway is septal and greater than 35 msec when the anomalous pathway is located in the free wall.[49] Because the increment of the VA interval may be partially compensated for by the antegrade limb (AV node), there may be little (or no) corresponding increment in the cycle length of tachycardia.[48-50] Functional block of the bundle branch contralateral to the anomalous pathway does not affect either the VA interval or the cycle length of tachycardia. In AV nodal reentrance or atrial tachycardia, the occurrence of functional block of either bundle branch does not affect the cycle length of tachycardia.

Performance of ventricular extra stimulus testing during paroxysmal tachycardia can also be useful in diagnosing reentrance using an anomalous pathway. In this type of tachycardia, it may be possible to demonstrate that a ventricular extra stimulus, introduced at a time when the His bundle is being used for antegrade conduction, can reset the atria.[7,8] This finding suggests that an anomalous pathway has been used for retrograde conduction and is probably a part of the reentrant pathway. Inability to reset the atria with ventricular extra stimuli is of little diagnostic value. This is seen not only in AV nodal reentrance and in atrial tachycardia, but also in many cases of reentrance using an anomalous pathway, especially when the rate of tachycardia is fast or the site of ventricular stimulation is distant from the anomalous pathway.

Administration of Drugs

Administration of drugs is frequently of limited value in diagnosing a specific type of PSVT. The expectation that drugs could be useful in determining whether VA conduction occurs over the normal conduction system or an anomalous pathway is seldom fulfilled. Although digitalis, beta-blocking agents, or verapamil usually have little effect on retrograde anomalous pathway refractoriness, they also usually have little effect on retrograde normal pathway refractoriness.[52-56] Although class I antiarrhythmic agents may markedly increase retrograde anomalous pathway refractoriness, they may also markedly increase retrograde normal pathway refractoriness.[56-58]

Administration of digitalis, a beta-blocking agent, or verapamil can occasionally provide useful information by increasing antegrade AV nodal refractoriness. For example, this increased refractoriness may cause early atrial extra stimuli to block in the AV node, thus enabling one to determine whether antegrade conduction to the His bundle is necessary for induction of PSVT. Increased refractoriness may also potentiate the occurrence of AV block during atrial tachycardia. The significance of these observations has been discussed in previous sections of this chapter.

Another situation in which administration of drugs can be useful is when, despite the presence of an anomalous pathway or dual AV nodal pathways, paroxysmal tachycardia cannot be induced because of increased AV nodal refractoriness. In this situation, administration of atropine or isoproterenol may decrease AV nodal refractoriness and thus make it possible to induce tachycardia.[59]

A Strategy

The preceding sections of this chapter have been a catalog of the techniques that can be employed to diagnose the common types of PSVT. However, electrophysiologic studies in a patient with PSVT should not be a gathering of information in a rigidly predetermined order. Rather, these studies should be flexible and aimed at providing the information most relevant to the differential diagnosis at a given time. For example, if the problem is to differentiate between sinoatrial reentrance and AV nodal reentrance, it is most useful to perform repetitive atrial pacing at a rate that causes second-degree block in the AV node. In contrast, this approach is usually of little value in differentiating between AV nodal reentrance and reentrance using an anomalous pathway.

Occasionally the differential diagnosis cannot be narrowed before electrophysiologic studies are done. In this situation, the studies should begin with programmed ventricular stimulation. If VA conduction is absent, a diagnosis of atrial tachycardia is very likely. If VA conduction is present, the presence or absence of a retrogradely conducting anomalous pathway can be determined by noting the sequence of retrograde atrial activation and the temporal relationship between depolarization of the His bundle and depolarization of the atria. If a retrogradely conducting anomalous pathway can be excluded, it is useful to perform rapid atrial pacing to differentiate between sinoatrial reentrance and AV nodal reentrance.

Treatment of Paroxysmal Supraventricular Tachycardia

Paroxysmal supraventricular tachycardia constitutes a broad clinical spectrum. Patients with PSVT vary greatly in frequency of attacks. Furthermore, the severity of symptoms during PSVT varies with the rate of tachycardia, the presence or absence of associated heart disease, and the duration of the attack. Many patients with infrequent or well-tolerated attacks do not need treatment. However, some patients require therapy to achieve one of two goals: to terminate an acute attack of tachycardia or to prevent recurrent attacks.

Termination of an Acute Attack

The rationale for termination of an acute attack of PSVT can be exemplified by the situation in reentrance using an anomalous pathway. The circus movement, and therefore PSVT, continues as long as the circling wavefront finds the reentrant pathway excitable (Fig. 10-5). If the wavefront encounters refractory tissue and blocks, the circus movement is broken and the tachycardia terminates (see Fig. 10-5). In a patient with an acute attack of tachycardia, the goal of therapy is to increase the refractoriness of the antegrade limb (the normal pathway) or the retrograde limb (the anomalous pathway) sufficiently to cause the circling wavefront to block.[30] These considerations are also applicable to the situation in AV nodal reentrance, where the goal of therapy is to increase the refractoriness of the fast or the slow AV nodal pathway.[31]

Several modalities of treatment are available to terminate an acute attack of PSVT. Vagal maneuvers, such as carotid sinus massage or Valsalva, are usually tried first.[60] These maneuvers may increase AV nodal refractoriness sufficiently to terminate the tachycardia. Intravenous drugs can also be used to increase refractoriness in a limb of the reentrant pathway. Verapamil, digitalis, or a beta-blocking agent can increase AV nodal refractoriness, and procainamide can increase retrograde anomalous pathway refractoriness or retrograde fast AV nodal pathway refractoriness (in the usual variety of AV nodal reentrance).[56,61] Intravenous verapamil (5 to 10 mg) is currently the drug of choice, since approximately 90% of attacks of reentrance using an anomalous pathway or AV nodal reentrance can be converted within a few minutes with only rare adverse effects.[54,55] The efficacy of intravenous digitalis, beta-blocking agents, or procainamide in this situation is not known. However, even if effective, these agents usually do not act as quickly as verapamil.

Attacks of PSVT usually reflect reentrance and thus can be terminated by cardiac pacing. If an appropriate pacing site and rate are selected, paced beats can penetrate the reentrant pathway and make it refractory.[6,11] Termination of a single attack of PSVT usually requires insertion of an electrode catheter. However, the development of radiofrequency-triggered pacemakers has made it possible to use a permanent cardiac lead to terminate recurrent attacks of PSVT.[62] This modality of treatment is generally reserved for patients who are refractory to, or intolerant of, the available oral antiarrhythmic drugs. Before a radiofrequency-triggered pacemaker is inserted, electrophysiologic studies are necessary to establish that the tachycardia reflects reentrance and to document that the proposed electrode position will allow paced beats to penetrate the reentrant pathway. Direct-current coun-

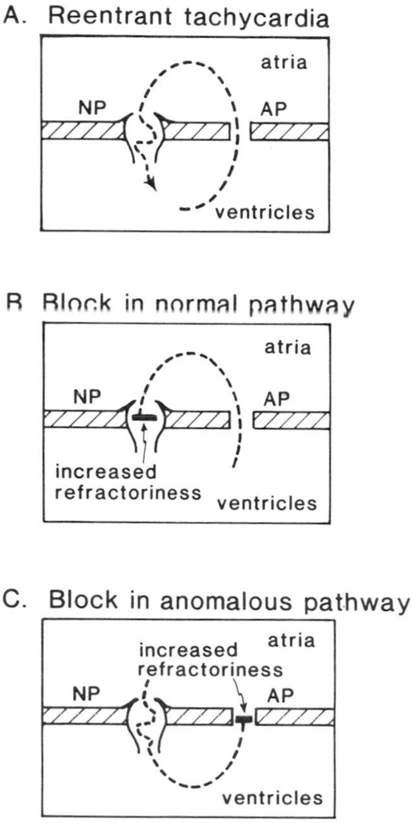

Figure 10-5. *Conduction system in Wolff-Parkinson-White syndrome (see Fig. 10-2). (A) Reentrance using an anomalous pathway. (B) The circus movement blocks in the antegrade limb because of increased AV nodal refractoriness. (C) The circus movement blocks in the retrograde limb because of increased anomalous pathway refractoriness.*

tershock can be used to terminate attacks of PSVT that are very poorly tolerated or refractory to other forms of therapy.

Relatively little is known regarding treatment of the less common varieties of PSVT. Sinoatrial reentrance frequently can be terminated by carotid sinus massage.[26] Automatic ectopic atrial tachycardia is frequently resistant to drugs.[28] However, in this situation administration of verapamil, digitalis, or a beta-blocking agent may increase AV nodal refractoriness sufficiently to control ventricular rate (PAT with block).

Prevention of Recurrent PSVT

Some patients who have recurrent PSVT require therapy to prevent further attacks. In most cases an oral antiarrhythmic drug is administered in an attempt to maintain increased refractoriness in a limb of the reentrant pathway so that a circus movement cannot become established. The drugs currently available for this purpose include digitalis, beta-blocking agents, verapamil, procainamide, quinidine, and disopyramide. Any of these drugs may be effective, and none has emerged as the drug

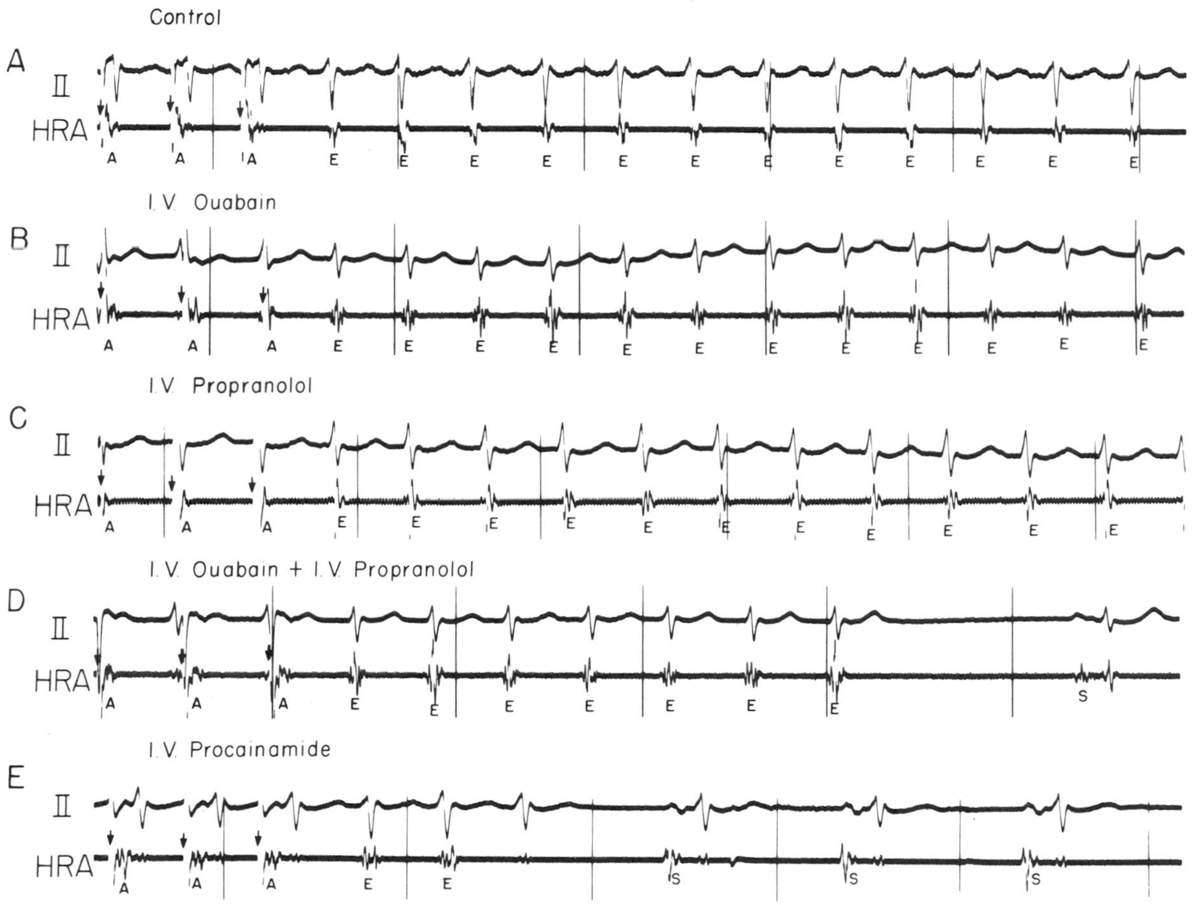

Figure 10-6. *Recordings made during serial electrophysiologic drug studies in a patient with paroxysmal supraventricular tachycardia due to AV nodal reentrance (usual variety). Shown in each panel are electrocardiographic lead II and a high right atrial (HRA) electrogram. Paroxysmal tachycardia was induced by atrial pacing (arrows). Induced tachycardia was sustained in control studies (A), after ouabain administration (B), and after propranolol administration (C). After ouabain plus propranolol were given (D), induced tachycardia was nonsustained because of antegrade block in the slow pathway (the last atrial echo [E] is not followed by a QRS complex). After procainamide was given (E), induced tachycardia was also nonsustained, but in this case because of retrograde block in the fast pathway (the last QRS complex is not associated with an atrial echo). (From Bauernfeind, R. A., Wyndham, C. R., Dhingra, R. C., et al.: Serial electrophysiologic testing of multiple drugs in patients with atrioventricular nodal reentrant paroxysmal tachycardia. Circulation, 62:1341–1349, 1980. By permission of the American Heart Association, Inc.)*

of choice.[56,61] Oral verapamil has not been as frequently effective in prophylaxis of recurrent PSVT as intravenous verapamil has been in termination of acute attacks.[55]

When recurrent PSVT is not associated with severe symptoms, it is reasonable to use the trial and error approach to therapy. Since any of the available antiarrhythmic agents may be effective, the clinician should start with a drug (or drug combination) that is likely to be well tolerated. Thus, digitalis or a beta-blocking agent, alone or in combination, are frequently used in the initial therapeutic trial. If these drugs are not effective in preventing recurrences, one of the class I antiarrhythmic agents can be tried. When this trial and error approach is used, a successful drug regimen is usually delineated within a reasonable time.

Electrophysiologic Drug Studies

The trial and error approach described above is unattractive when recurrent PSVT has been associated with severe symptoms or has been demonstrated to be refractory to several drugs. In these situations, electrophysiologic drug studies can be considered (Fig. 10-6).[56,61,63] A control electrophysiologic study is performed first to delineate the mechanism of the tachycardia and to confirm that the tachycardia can be reliably induced by programmed cardiac stimulation. Following the control study, a hexapolar electrode catheter is positioned so that the distal two poles can be used for pacing the right ventricular apex and the proximal four poles can be used for recording and pacing from the right atrium. Available antiarrhythmic drugs are then administered serially and tested for their ability to prevent reinduction of sustained tachycardia. When a drug prevents reinduction of sustained tachycardia, it is usually possible to delineate the site of action. For example, oral procainamide may prevent reinduction of reentrance using an anomalous pathway by markedly increasing retrograde anomalous pathway refractoriness. This increase in refractoriness can be confirmed by demonstrating that there has been a marked decrease in the maximum ventricular paced rate associated with 1 : 1 VA conduction.

In most cases, electrophysiologic drug studies reveal that one or more of the available antiarrhythmic drugs prevent reinduction of sustained tachycardia. Long-term oral therapy with one of these agents is usually successful in preventing recurrences of sustained PSVT.[56,61] In occasional patients, the studies reveal that none of the available drugs prevents induction of sustained tachycardia. In this situation, surgical therapy or one of the transvenous ablative procedures can be considered.

References

1. Wellens, H. J. J., and Durrer, D.: The role of an accessory atrioventricular pathway in reciprocal tachycardia. Observations in patients with and without the Wolff-Parkinson-White syndrome. Circulation, 52:58–72, 1975.
2. Sung, R. J., Gelband, H., Castellanos, A., et al.: Clinical and electrophysiologic observations in patients with concealed accessory atrioventricular bypass tracts. Am. J. Cardiol., 40:839–847, 1977.
3. Wu, D., Denes, P., Amat-y-Leon, F., et al.: Clinical, electrocardiographic and electrophysiologic observations in patients with paroxysmal supraventricular tachycardia. Am. J. Cardiol., 41:1045–1051, 1978.
4. Farshidi, A., Josephson, M. E., and Horowitz, L. N.: Electrophysiologic characteristics of concealed bypass tracts: Clinical and electrocardiographic correlates. Am. J. Cardiol., 41:1052–1060, 1978.
5. Akhtar, M., Damato, A. N., Ruskin, J. N., et al.: Antegrade and retrograde conduction characteristics in three patterns of paroxysmal atrioventricular junctional reentrant tachycardia. Am. Heart J., 95:22–42, 1978.
6. Durrer, D., Schoo, L., Schuilenburg, R. M., and Wellens, H. J. J.: The role of premature beats in the initiation and the termination of supraventricular tachycardia in the Wolff-Parkinson-White syndrome. Circulation 36:644–662, 1967.
7. Coumel, P., and Attuel, P.: Reciprocating tachycardia in overt and latent preexcitation. Influence of functional bundle branch block on the rate of the tachycardia. Eur. J. Cardiol., 1:423–436, 1974.
8. Neuss, H., Schlepper, M., and Thormann, J.: Analysis of re-entry mechanisms in three patients with concealed Wolff-Parkinson-White syndrome. Circulation, 51:75–81, 1975.
9. Tonkin, A. M., Gallagher, J. J., Svenson, R. H., et al.: Anterograde block in accessory pathways with retrograde conduction in reciprocating tachycardia. Eur. J. Cardiol., 3:143–152, 1975.
10. Wellens, H. J., and Durrer, D.: Patterns of ventriculo-atrial conduction in the Wolff-Parkinson-White syndrome. Circulation, 49:22–31, 1974.
11. Goldreyer, B. N., and Bigger, J. T.: Site of reentry in paroxysmal supraventricular tachycardia in man. Circulation, 43:15–26, 1971.
12. Goldreyer, B. N., and Damato, A. N.: The essential role of atrioventricular conduction delay in the initiation of paroxysmal supraventricular tachycardia. Circulation, 43:679–687, 1971.
13. Rosen, K. M., Mehta, A., and Miller, R. A.: Demonstration of dual atrioventricular pathways in man. Am. J. Cardiol., 33:291–294, 1974.
14. Denes, P., Wu, D., Dhingra, R. C., et al.: Demonstration of dual A-V nodal pathways in patients with paroxysmal supraventricular tachycardia. Circulation, 48:549–555, 1973.
15. Denes, P., Wu, D., and Rosen, K. M.: Demonstration of dual A-V pathways in a patient with Lown-Ganong-Levine syndrome. Chest, 65:343–346, 1974.
16. Touboul, P., Huerta, F., Porte, J., and Delahaye, J. P.: Reciprocal rhythm in patients with normal electrocardiogram: evidence for dual conduction pathways. Am. Heart J., 91:3–10, 1976.
17. Bissett, J. K., de Soyza, N., Kane, J. J., and Murphy, M. L.: Atrioventricular conduction patterns in patients with paroxysmal supraventricular tachycardia. Am. Heart J., 91:287–291, 1976.
18. Bauernfeind, R. A., Ayres, B. F., Wyndham, C. C., et al.: Cycle length in atrioventricular nodal reentrant paroxysmal tachycardia with observations on the Lown-Ganong-Levine syndrome. Am. J. Cardiol., 45:1148–1153, 1980.
19. Bharati, S., Bauernfeind, R., Scheinman, M., et al.: Congenital

abnormalities of the conduction system in two patients with tachyarrhythmias. Circulation, 59:593–606, 1979.
20. Scheinman, M. M., Gonzalez, R., Thomas, A., et al.: Reentry confined to the atrioventricular node: electrophysiologic and anatomic findings. Am. J. Cardiol., 49:1814–1818, 1982.
21. Wellens, H. J. J., Wesdorp, J. C., Duren, D. R., and Lie, K. I.: Second degree block during reciprocal atrioventricular nodal tachycardia. Circulation, 53:595–599, 1976.
22. Josephson, M. E., and Kastor, J. A.: Paroxysmal supraventricular tachycardia. Is the atrium a necessary link? Circulation, 54:430–435, 1976.
23. Wu, D., Denes, P., Amat-y-Leon, F., et al.: An unusual variety of atrioventricular nodal re-entry due to retrograde dual atrioventricular nodal pathways. Circulation, 56:50–59, 1977.
24. Strasberg, B., Swiryn, S., Bauernfeind, R., et al.: Retrograde dual atrioventricular nodal pathways. Am. J. Cardiol., 48:639–646, 1981.
25. Narula, O. S.: Sinus node reentry. A mechanism for supraventricular tachycardia. Circulation, 50:1114–1128, 1974.
26. Wu, D., Amat-y-Leon, F., Denes, P., et al.: Demonstration of sustained sinus and atrial re-entry as a mechanism of paroxysmal supraventricular tachycardia. Circulation, 51:234–243, 1975.
27. Goldreyer, B. N., Gallagher, J. J., and Damato, A. N.: The electrophysiologic demonstration of atrial ectopic tachycardia in man. Am. Heart J., 85:205–215, 1973.
28. Scheinman, M. M., Basu, D., and Hollenberg, M.: Electrophysiologic studies in patients with persistent atrial tachycardia. Circulation, 50:266–273, 1974.
29. Svenson, R. H., Miller, H. C., Gallagher, J. J., and Wallace, A. G.: Electrophysiological evaluation of the Wolff-Parkinson-White syndrome. Problems in assessing antegrade and retrograde conduction over the accessory pathway. Circulation, 52:552–562, 1975.
30. Denes, P., Wu, D., Amat-y-Leon, F., et al.: Determinants of atrioventricular reentrant paroxysmal tachycardia in patients with Wolff-Parkinson-White syndrome. Circulation, 58:415–425, 1978.
31. Denes, P., Wu, D., Amat-y-Leon, F., et al.: The determinants of atrioventricular nodal re-entrance with premature atrial stimulation in patients with dual A-V nodal pathways. Circulation, 56:253–259, 1977.
32. Denes, P., Wu, D., Dhingra, R., et al.: Dual atrioventricular nodal pathways. A common electrophysiological response. Br. Heart J., 37:1069–1076, 1975.
33. Neuss, H., Schlepper, M., and Spies, H. F.: Effects of heart rate and atropine on dual AV conduction. Br. Heart J., 37:1216–1227, 1975.
34. Hess, S. G., Gallastegui, J., and Bauernfeind, R. A.: Failure to demonstrate dual pathways in patients with atrioventricular nodal reentrant tachycardia (abstr.). Circulation, 68:III–11, 1983.
35. Pritchett, E. L. C., Prystowsky, E. N., Benditt, D. G., and Gallagher, J. J.: Dual atrioventricular nodal pathways in patients with Wolff-Parkinson-White syndrome. Br. Heart J., 43:7–13, 1980.
36. Sung, R. J., Styperek, J. L.: Electrophysiologic identification of dual atrioventricular nodal pathway conduction in patients with reciprocating tachycardia using anomalous bypass tracts. Circulation, 60:1464–1476, 1979.
37. Bauernfeind, R. A., Swiryn, S., Strasberg, B., et al.: Analysis of anterograde and retrograde fast pathway properties in patients with dual atrioventricular nodal pathways. Observations regarding the pathophysiology of the Lown-Ganong-Levine syndrome. Am. J. Cardiol., 49:283–290, 1982.
38. Sung, R. J., Castellanos, A., Gelband, H., and Myerburg, R. J.: Mechanism of reciprocating tachycardia initiated during sinus rhythm in concealed Wolff-Parkinson-White syndrome. Circulation, 54:338–344, 1976.
39. Sung, R. J., Styperek, J. L., Myerburg, R. J., and Castellanos, A.: Initiation of two distinct forms of atrioventricular nodal reentrant tachycardia during programmed ventricular stimulation in man. Am. J. Cardiol., 42:404–415, 1978.
40. Amat-y-Leon, F., Dhingra, R. C., Wu, D., et al.: Catheter mapping of retrograde atrial activation. Observations during ventricular pacing and AV nodal re-entrant paroxysmal tachycardia. Br. Heart J., 38:355–362, 1976.
41. Akhtar, M., Damato, A. N., Caracta, A. R., et al.: The gap phenomena during retrograde conduction in man. Circulation, 49:811–817, 1974.
42. Brugada, P., Bar, F. W. H. M., Vanagt, E. J., et al.: Observations in patients showing A-V junctional echoes with a shorter P-R than R-P interval. Am. J. Cardiol., 48:611–622, 1981.
43. Gomes, J. A. C., Dhatt, M. S., Damato, A. N., et al.: Incidence, determinants and significance of fixed retrograde conduction in the region of the atrioventricular node. Evidence for retrograde atrioventricular nodal bypass tracts. Am. J. Cardiol., 44:1089–1098, 1979.
44. Klein, G. J., Prystowsky, E. N., Pritchett, E. L. C., et al.: Atypical patterns of retrograde conduction over accessory atrioventricular pathways in the Wolff-Parkinson-White syndrome. Circulation, 60:1477–1486, 1979.
45. Sung, R. J., Waxman, H. L., Saksena, S., and Juma, Z.: Sequence of retrograde atrial activation in patients with dual atrioventricular nodal pathways. Circulation, 64:1059–1067, 1981.
46. Akhtar, M., Gilbert, C., Wolf, F. G., and Schmidt, D. H.: Reentry within the His-Purkinje system. Elucidation of reentrant circuit using right bundle branch and His bundle recordings. Circulation, 58:295–304, 1978.
47. Bauernfeind, R. A., Wu, D., Denes, P., and Rosen, K. M.: Retrograde block during dual pathway atrioventricular nodal reentrant paroxysmal tachycardia. Am. J. Cardiol., 42:499–505, 1978.
48. Pritchett, E. L. C., Tonkin, A. M., Dugan, F. A., et al.: Ventriculoatrial conduction time during reciprocating tachycardia and intermittent bundle-branch block in Wolff-Parkinson-White syndrome. Br. Heart J., 38:1058–1064, 1976.
49. Kerr, C. R., Gallagher, J. J., and German, L. D.: Changes in ventriculoatrial intervals with bundle branch block aberration during reciprocating tachycardia in patients with accessory atrioventricular pathways. Circulation, 66:196–201, 1982.
50. Bauernfeind, R. A., Strasberg, B., and Rosen, K. M.: Slowing of paroxysmal tachycardia with loss of functional bundle branch block. Br. Heart J., 48:75–77, 1982.
51. Sellers, T. D., Gallagher, J. J., Cope, G. D., et al.: Retrograde atrial preexcitation following premature ventricular beats during reciprocating tachycardia in the Wolff-Parkinson-White syndrome. Eur. J. Cardiol., 4:283–294, 1976.
52. Denes, P., Cummings, J. M., Simpson, R., et al.: Effects of propranolol on anomalous pathway refractoriness and circus movement tachycardias in patients with preexcitation. Am. J. Cardiol., 41:1061–1067, 1978.
53. Dhingra, R. C., Palileo, E. V., Strasberg, B., et al.: Electrophysiologic effects of ouabain in patients with preexcitation and circus movement tachycardia. Am. J. Cardiol., 47:139–144, 1981.
54. Sung, R. J., Elser, B., and McAllister, R. G.: Intravenous verapamil for termination of re-entrant supraventricular tachycardias. Intracardiac studies correlated with plasma verapamil concentrations. Ann. Intern. Med., 93:682–689, 1980.
55. Klein, G. J., Gulamhusein, S., Prystowsky, E. N., et al.: Comparison of the electrophysiologic effects of intravenous and oral verapamil in patients with paroxysmal supraventricular tachycardia. Am. J. Cardiol., 49:117–124, 1982.
56. Bauernfeind, R. A., Wyndham, C. R., Dhingra, R. C., et al.: Serial electrophysiologic testing of multiple drugs in patients with atrio-

ventricular nodal reentrant paroxysmal tachycardia. Circulation, 62:1341–1349, 1980.

57. Wu, D., Denes, P., Bauernfeind, R., et al.: Effects of procainamide on atrioventricular nodal re-entrant paroxysmal tachycardia. Circulation, 57:1171–1179, 1978.
58. Swiryn, S., Bauernfeind, R. A., Wyndham, C. R. C., et al.: Effects of oral disopyramide phosphate on induction of paroxysmal supraventricular tachycardia. Circulation, 64:169–175, 1981.
59. Wu, D., Denes, P., Bauernfeind, R., et al.: Effects of atropine on induction and maintenance of atrioventricular nodal reentrant tachycardia. Circulation, 59:779–788, 1979.
60. Josephson, M. E., Kastor, J. A.: Supraventricular tachycardia: Mechanisms and management. Ann. Intern. Med., 87:346–358, 1977.
61. Wu, D., Amat-y-Leon, F., Simpson, R. J., et al.: Electrophysiologic studies with multiple drugs in patients with atrioventricular re-entrant tachycardias utilizing an extranodal pathway. Circulation, 56:727–736, 1977.
62. Peters, R. W., Shafton, E., Frank, S., et al.: Radiofrequency-triggered pacemakers: Uses and limitations. A long-term study. Ann. Intern. Med., 88:17–22, 1978.
63. Bauernfeind, R. A., Swiryn, S., Petropoulos, A. T., et al.: Concordance and discordance of drug responses in atrioventricular reentrant tachycardia. J. Am. Coll. Cardiol., 2:345–350, 1983.

11

The Wolff-Parkinson-White Syndrome

Hein J. J. Wellens, Jerónimo Farré, and Frits W. H. M. Bär

More than 50 years ago, Wolff, Parkinson, and White described a clinical electrocardiographic entity in a series of 11 healthy young patients consisting of attacks of paroxysmal tachycardia in the presence of an electrocardiogram showing a bundle branch block-like pattern with a short PR interval.[1] Isolated cases showing the same features had been published previously,[2–5] and originally this syndrome was considered to be an electrocardiographic curiosity. Subsequently, however, it became clear that some patients with this condition suffer from incapacitating or even life-threatening arrhythmias.[6] Until recently, the therapeutic approach to the clinical problems of these patients has been more or less empirical.[7] Following the introduction of intracavitary recordings and the technique of programmed stimulation of the heart, mechanisms of arrhythmias and effects of antiarrhythmic drugs can be studied in these patients, allowing a more rational approach to the management of the Wolff-Parkinson-White (WPW) syndrome.[8]

In this chapter we will review present knowledge of the WPW syndrome as derived from recent clinical, electrocardiographic, and electrophysiologic data.

The Anatomic Basis of the Wolff-Parkinson-White Syndrome

Epicardial excitation mapping,[9] electrical stimulation studies,[10] His bundle recordings,[11] intracavitary mapping techniques,[12] and the outcome of surgical interventions[13] have shown that in patients with the WPW syndrome two pathways are present between the atrium and ventricle. Anatomic documentation of the existence of such an accessory atrioventricular connection in these patients is available.[14] Apart from the accessory pathways between the atrium and the ventricle as found in patients with the WPW syndrome, other abnormal connections between the atrium and the specific conduction system and between the specific conduction system and the ventricle have been described.[15] Their electrophysiologic properties, diagnostic features, and clinical significance have been discussed elsewhere.[16]

The Electrocardiogram in Patients With the Wolff-Parkinson-White Syndrome

The typical electrocardiogram of the WPW syndrome (short PR interval with wide QRS complex starting with a delta wave) is the result of fusion of ventricular activation through the normal atrioventricular connection (AV nodal–His-Purkinje axis) and the accessory pathway (AP). In these patients, the pattern of ventricular activation is determined by (1) the location of the AP, (2) the intra-atrial conduction time, (3) the conduction time over the AP, and (4) the atrioventricular conduction time over the normal AV nodal–His-Purkinje pathway.

If, as shown in the left panel of Figure 11-1, the conduction time from the sinus node region to the ventricle over the AP is shorter than that over the normal AV nodal–His axis, ventricular excitation will start earlier than expected (preexcitation).[17] This will result in the following electrocardiographic findings:

1. *Shortening of the PR interval.* If (illustrated in Fig. 11-1, left panel) the total atrioventricular conduction time over the normal AV nodal–His pathway measures 160 msec and the atrioventricular conduction time over the AP measures 95 msec, the actual interval between the beginning of atrial and ventricular activation will measure 95 msec.
2. *Widening of the QRS complex with an initial delta wave.* In most patients, the width of the QRS complex is determined by the degree of ventricular preexcitation. In the example shown in the left panel of Figure 11-1, ventricular excitation starts 65 msec earlier than expected if only the normal AV pathway would have been present ($160 - 95 = 65$ msec), resulting in a wider QRS complex. The initial forces of the QRS complex during preexcited beats represent ventricular activation of the slowly conducting ventricular working myocardium. In the electrocardiogram, this will result in a low-frequency component called the *delta wave.*[18]
3. *Secondary changes in the T wave.* As a result of early asynchronous excitation of a part of the ventricle, the sequence of repolarization will be different, leading to T wave changes. These changes will be related to the area and extent of preexcitation.

In some patients, the contribution of the AP to ventricular activation during sinus rhythm may be minimal, so that PR interval and QRS width are normal. An example of the latter situation is given in the right panel of Figure 11-1. If the atrioventricular conduction time (from the sinus node area) over the AP is not shorter than that over the normal AV nodal–His axis, the PR interval will not be shortened and the QRS will have a normal duration. This can be the result of several factors acting alone or in combination in a given patient:

1. *Location of the AP.* The closer the AP is located to the sinus node, the less time it will take for the impulse to reach the atrial insertion of the AP, resulting in a greater amount of ventricular preexcitation during sinus rhythm. Conversely, in patients with laterally located left-sided APs, contribution to ventricular excitation over the AP may be minimal during sinus rhythm. The importance of distance between the site of supraventricular impulse formation and the accessory pathway on preexcitation is shown in Figures 11-2 to 11-4.
2. *Intra-atrial conduction times.* During sinus rhythm, two intra-atrial conduction times are important: (1) the conduction time from the sinus node to the entrance of the AV node (which corresponds to the interval measured from the beginning of the P wave to the atrial deflection in the His bundle lead or PA interval) and (2) the conduction time from the sinus node to the atrial insertion of the AP. The normal PA interval varies from 30 to 55 msec,[19] but longer values can be observed under pathologic conditions. Left atrial pathology will prolong the time required to reach a left-sided AP. Intra-atrial conduction time can be affected by drugs, resulting in a lesser amount of preexcitation during sinus rhythm in patients with left lateral accessory pathways.
3. *Conduction time over the AP.* The conduction time over the AP depends on the conduction velocity and the length of the AP. Exact figures about conduction velocity in accessory atrioventricular pathways found in the WPW syndrome are not available. Recently, Becker and co-workers[14] reported that the length of the accessory atrioventricular connection in patients with the WPW syndrome varied from 1 to 10 mm. This suggests that with the same conduction velocity of the impulse over the accessory pathway, conduction times over accessory pathways may vary by as much as a factor of 10 from one patient to another.
4. *Conduction time over the AV nodal–His-Purkinje axis.* Some patients with the WPW syndrome have short intranodal conduction times (AH intervals of less than 60 msec).[20] In these patients, especially when a left-sided AP is present, a lesser amount of ventricular preexcitation is observed during sinus rhythm.

In the right panel of Figure 11-1, atrioventricular conduction times through the AP and the AV nodal–His-

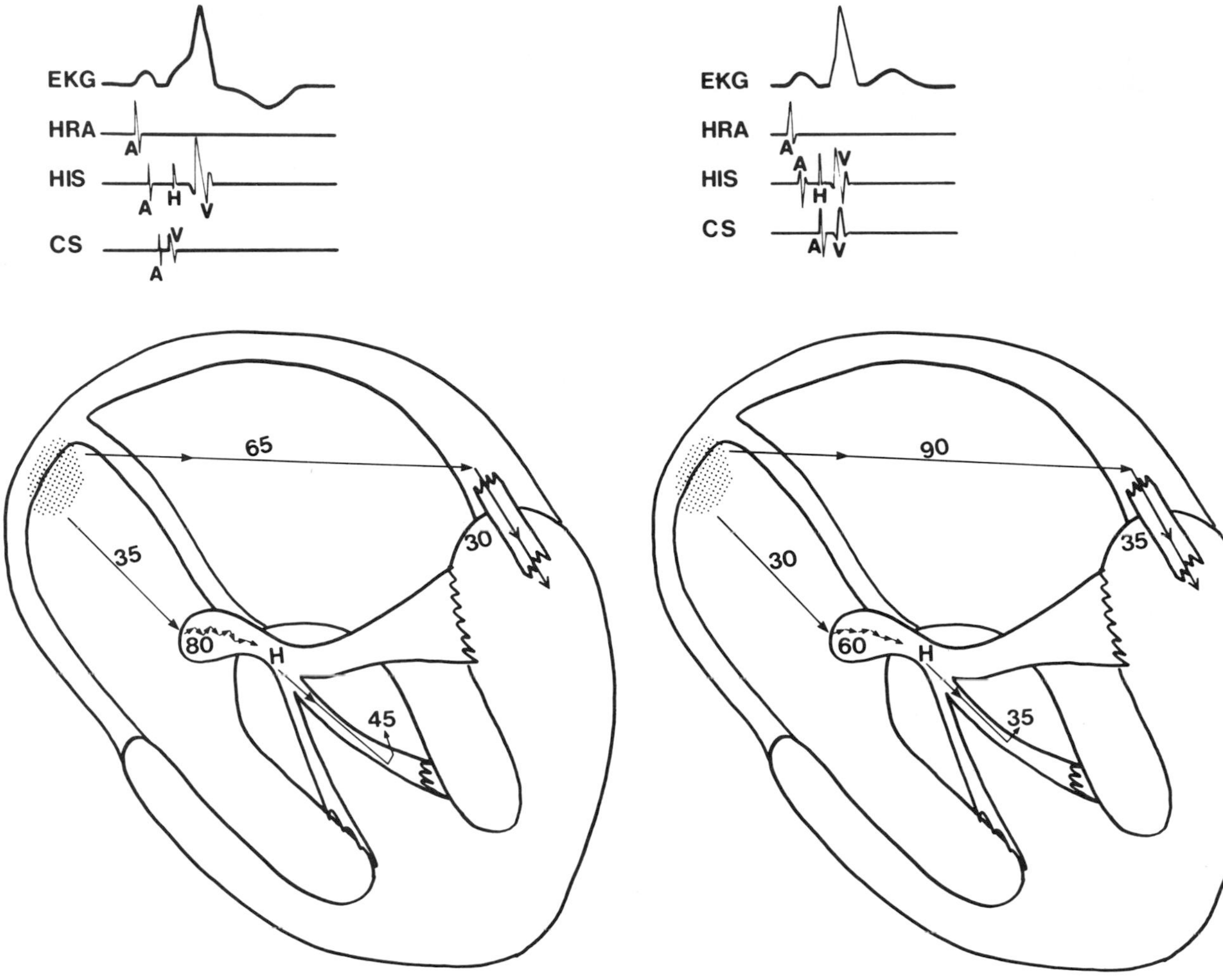

Figure 11-1. *Schematic representation of factors determining the degree of ventricular preexcitation in the Wolff-Parkinson-White patient during sinus rhythm. The corresponding electrocardiogram and intracavitary recordings from the high right atrium (HRA), His bundle region (HIS), and coronary sinus (CS) are shown in the upper part of the figure.* (Left) *The atrioventricular conduction time from the sinus node region over the normal AV pathway measures 160 msec (the time required to travel from the sinus node to the AV node, PA interval, of 35 msec; the transnodal conduction time, AH interval, of 80 msec; and the time needed to travel through the bundle of His and the bundle branches to the ventricular myocardium, HV interval, of 45 msec). The time required to travel from the sinus node to the atrial insertion of the AP measures 65 msec, and the conduction time over the AP measures 30 msec. The total AV conduction time to travel from the sinus node to the ventricle using the AP measures 95 msec. Under these circumstances, the corresponding electrocardiogram will show a P-delta interval of 95 msec and a wide QRS complex with ventricular excitation starting 160 − 95 = 65 msec earlier than expected.* (Right) *In this example, as compared to the left panel, there is (1) a longer conduction time from sinus node to the atrial insertion of the AP, (2) a longer conduction time over the accessory pathway, and (3) a shorter conduction time over the AV node (shorter PA, AH, and HV times). As a result of these differences, the AV conduction times over either the normal or the accessory pathway are identical (both 125 msec). Now the electrocardiogram shows a PR interval of 125 msec and a QRS complex that is not widened.*

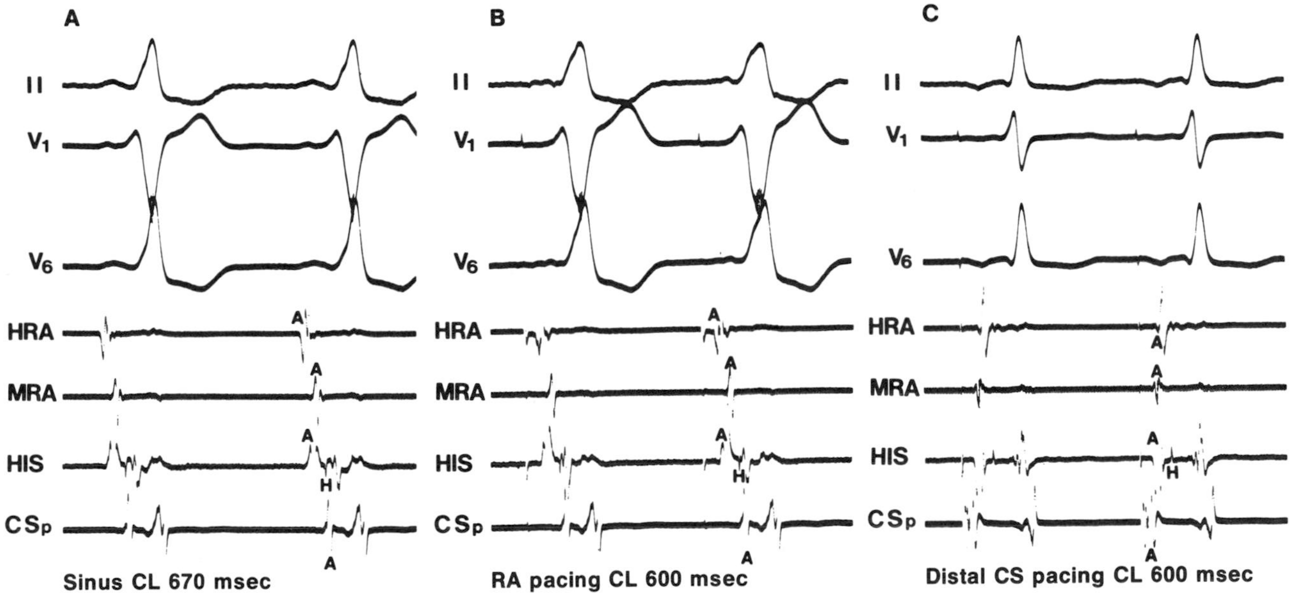

Figure 11-2. *Effect of site of origin of the supraventricular impulse on ventricular excitation and the electrocardiogram in a patient with a right-sided accessory pathway. Leads II, V_1, and V_6 and intracardiac bipolar electrograms from the high right atrium (HRA), mid-right atrium (MRA), His bundle region (HIS), and proximal coronary sinus (CSp) are simultaneously recorded. (A) Recordings obtained during sinus rhythm. (B) Right atrial pacing at a cycle length (CL) of 600 msec, showing enhancement of ventricular preexcitation. (C) Pacing from the distal coronary sinus (CS) at a CL of 600 msec results in disappearance of preexcitation.*

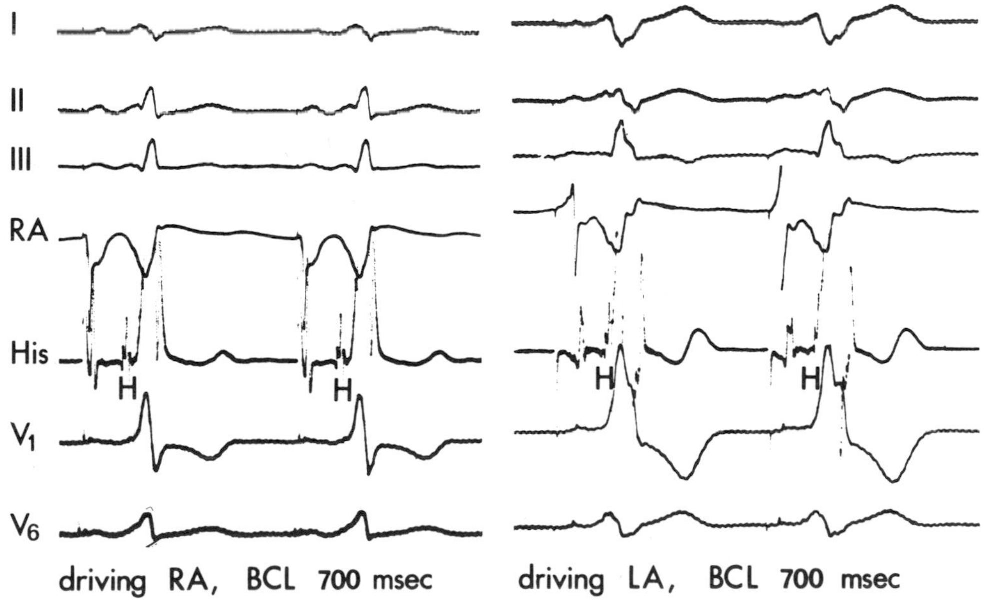

Figure 11-3. (Left) *Right and left atrial stimulation in a patient with a left-sided accessory pathway.* (Right) *Atrial stimulation closer to the accessory pathway results in a greater amount of ventricular preexcitation as compared to atrial pacing at the same rate from the right atrium.*

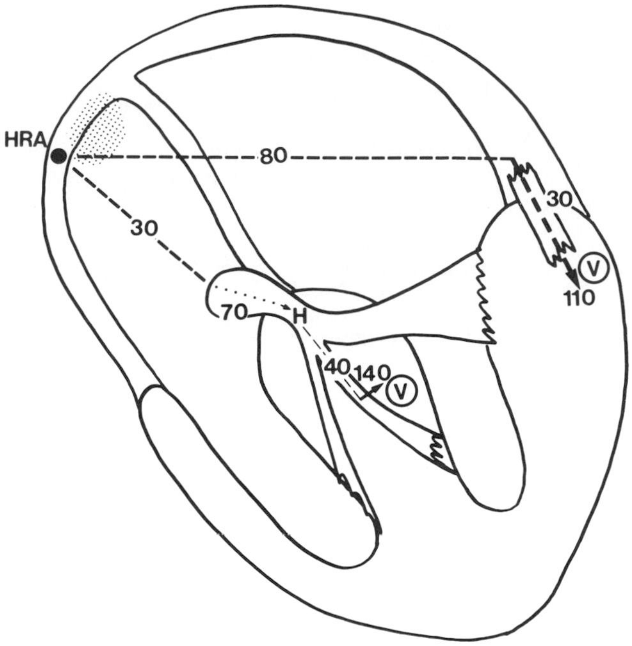

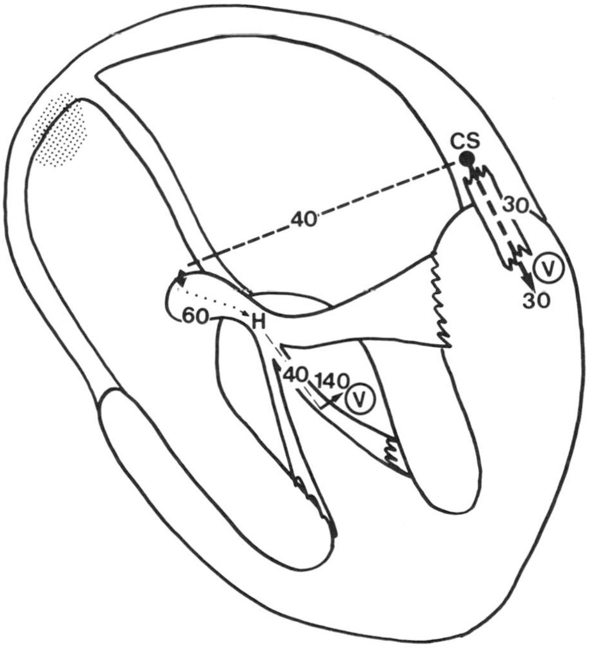

Figure 11-4. *Diagrammatic representation of the relationship between site of atrial stimulation and degree of ventricular preexcitation in patients with the Wolff-Parkinson-White syndrome. A left-sided AP is shown. The upper diagram gives the effects of HRA stimulation. The AV conduction time (from the site of stimulation) over the normal AV nodal–His pathway measures 30 + 70 + 40 = 140 msec, and over the AP, 80 + 30 = 110 msec. In the lower diagram, atrial stimulation is done from the coronary sinus, close to the location of the AP. The AV conduction time through the normal pathway measures 140 msec (the postulated AH is 60, 10 msec shorter as compared to HRA pacing). The AV conduction time through the AP is 30 msec, resulting in a maximal amount of preexcitation.*

Purkinje axis are equal (125 msec). Therefore, the PR interval will be normal (0.125 second) and no QRS widening will be observed. The only abnormalities encountered in such a patient will be in the initial forces of the QRS because the ventricular muscle depolarizing early over the AV nodal–His-Purkinje axis will be excited at the same time as the ventricular myocardium close to the insertion of the AP. This can result in QRS abnormalities, that is, abnormal Q waves, slurring in the ascending limb of the R wave, increased voltage in the R waves, and changes in the axis of the QRS complex. Therefore, QRS abnormalities mimicking myocardial infarction, ventricular hypertrophy, or intraventricular conduction disturbances may be present in the electrocardiogram of these patients. Figure 11-5 shows an example of a patient with mitral valve prolapse and a left-sided AP in whom the electrocardiogram had been erroneously diagnosed as an old posteroinferior myocardial infarction.

Patients in whom the contribution of the AP to ventricular activation is minimal because of the coincidental arrival of the excitation wavefront to the ventricle over both the normal and the accessory pathway should not be diagnosed as having a so-called concealed accessory pathways.[21] Concealed APs are those accessory pathways that only conduct in the retrograde (ventriculoatrial) direction. Anterograde conduction through the

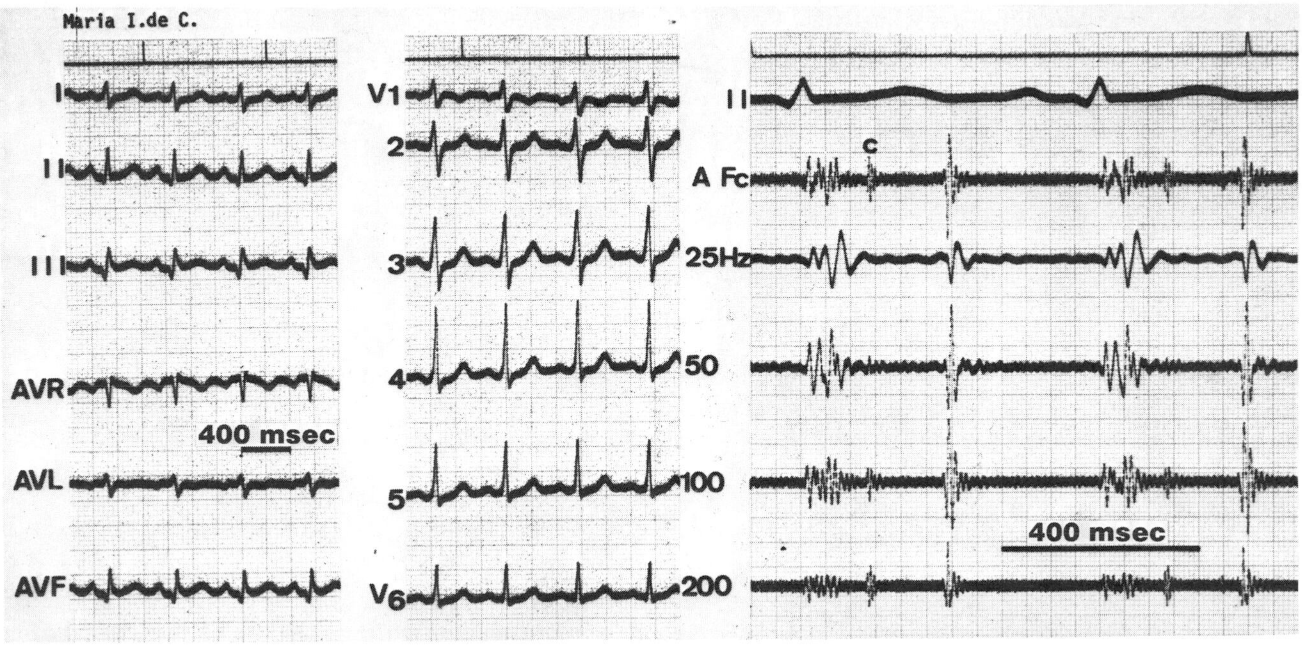

Figure 11-5. *A 12-lead electrocardiogram and phonocardiogram showing a mid-systolic click from a patient with mitral valve prolapse. The electrocardiogram was interpreted as indicative of an old posteroinferior myocardial infarction. The PR interval measured 0.14 second, and the QRS width was 0.08 second. Note that apart from the Q waves in the inferior wall leads and the tall, broad R wave in lead V_1, slurring in the ascending limb of the R wave is present in leads V_4 and V_5. Figure 11-17 belongs to the same patient.*

AP in these patients is absent because the refractory period of the AP in the anterograde direction is longer than the sinus cycle length. The clinical implications of the latter type of AP are discussed elsewhere in this volume.

Incidence of the Wolff-Parkinson-White Syndrome

The true incidence of the WPW syndrome is unknown, the reported figures varying from 0.1 to 3 per 1000 electrocardiograms.[22] The WPW syndrome is undoubtedly underdiagnosed, because many physicians require the presence of the typical electrocardiographic features (short PR interval and wide QRS complex with an initial delta wave) before making the diagnosis. Determination of the real incidence of the syndrome is hampered by (1) the existence of so-called intermittent preexcitation with inconstant atrioventricular conduction over the AP and (2) the presence of left-lateral APs resulting (for reasons given above) in questionable or even normal electrocardiograms.

Table 11-1. Type of Tachycardia Electrocardiographically Documented Prior to the Stimulation Study in a Series of 265 Patients with the Wolff-Parkinson-White Syndrome

Type of Tachycardia*	No. of Patients	%
SVT	162	61
AF	49	18
SVT + AF	29	10

* SVT, supraventricular tachycardia; AF, atrial fibrillation.

Incidence of Tachyarrhythmias in the Wolff-Parkinson-White Syndrome

The incidence of tachyarrhythmias in patients with the WPW syndrome is also unknown. The reported figures vary from 12% to 80%,[7,23] and these figures are obviously affected by patient selection. In our own series of 265 patients with WPW syndrome who had undergone electrophysiologic study, electrocardiographic documentation of either supraventricular tachycardia or atrial fibrillation before the stimulation study was available in 89% of cases (Table 11-1).

Incidence of Wolff-Parkinson-White Syndrome in Patients With Paroxysmal Tachycardia

The WPW abnormality is probably the most important underlying cause of paroxysmal regular supraventricular tachycardia. In a series of 120 consecutive patients admitted to the hospital because of paroxysmal supraventricular tachycardia, an electrocardiogram diagnostic for the WPW syndrome was found during sinus rhythm in 69 patients (57%). This high incidence of WPW syndrome was even more striking on considering the age of the patients. In 45 patients in whom the first attack of paroxysmal tachycardia occurred below the age of 21 years, 33 (73%) had the WPW syndrome on the electrocardiogram recorded during sinus rhythm. In the 75 patients in whom the first attack of tachycardia occurred above the age of 21 years, an electrocardiogram diagnostic for WPW was found in 36 (48%).[24]

Electrocardiographic Classification of the Wolff-Parkinson-White Syndrome

In 1945, Rosenbaum and co-workers[25] proposed a classification of the WPW syndrome according to the QRS configuration in the precordial leads. Type A WPW syndrome showed a predominant R wave in leads V_1, V_2, and Ve, whereas type B showed an S wave as the chief QRS deflection in the right precordial leads.

Durrer and Roos[9] demonstrated by epicardial mapping that type B WPW syndrome was caused by early activation of the lateral aspect of the right ventricle. It was subsequently reported that in patients with type A WPW, early activation of the left ventricle was present.[26]

Extensive studies by the group from Duke University[20] have shown that the accessory atrioventricular pathway responsible for this syndrome can insert not only in the ventricular free wall but also in the interventricular septum. Therefore, Rosenbaum's classification of WPW syndrome into type A and type B oversimplifies the electrocardiographic spectrum of this abnormality. A tentative classification of the location of the accessory pathway based on the initial forces of the QRS complex in both the precordial and extremity leads has been proposed.[27] However, determination of the location of the AP in WPW syndrome from the QRS configuration during sinus rhythm can be extremely difficult. It can only be done confidently during completely preexcited beats (*i.e.,* when ventricular activation is exclusively or mostly over the accessory pathway).[20] As previously mentioned, some patients with WPW syndrome do not show much preexcitation during sinus rhythm, preventing analysis of the initial forces from ventricular excitation through the AP. Other factors hampering localization of the AP are (1) the existence of more than one AP in some patients, (2) the coexistence of congenital or acquired heart disease, (3) the occasional superposition of the terminal part of the P wave on the initial portion of the delta wave, and (4) differences in ventricular activation depending on whether the AP is epicardially or endocardially located.[20]

Associated Cardiovascular Abnormalities

The most frequent forms of associated cardiovascular abnormalities found in patients with the WPW syndrome are listed below. Type B WPW syndrome is found in 5% to 25% of the reported cases of Ebstein's disease.[16] In patients with corrected transposition (L-transposition) of the great arteries, a few cases of WPW syndrome have been reported.[28,29] In those with tricuspid atresia, endocardial fibroelastosis, and double-inlet right ventricle, the WPW syndrome has also been described.[16] Dextrocardia even without cardiac abnormality may also be associated with WPW syndrome.[30] Figure 11-6 illustrates a case of mirror-image dextrocardia without cardiac disease and type B WPW syndrome.

Cardiovascular Abnormalities Associated With Wolff-Parkinson-White Syndrome

- Ebstein's disease
- Corrected transposition (L transposition) of the great arteries
- Tricuspid atresia
- Endocardial fibroelastosis
- Mitral valve prolapse
- Cardiomyopathy
  - Hypertrophic obstructive cardiomyopathy
  - Hypertrophic nonobstructive cardiomyopathy
  - Congestive cardiomyopathy

Association between the WPW syndrome and various forms of cardiomyopathy has been noted.[16,20] Mitral valve proplapse and WPW syndrome (mainly left sided) is another known association (see Fig. 11-5).[20]

Patients with rheumatic and nonrheumatic valve disease, coronary artery disease, and other pathologic conditions affecting the cardiovascular system may have the WPW syndrome as a coincidental feature.

Clinical Manifestations of the Wolff-Parkinson-White Syndrome

The clinical manifestations of the WPW syndrome depend on the physiologic properties of the accessory pathway. The most important problems encountered in these

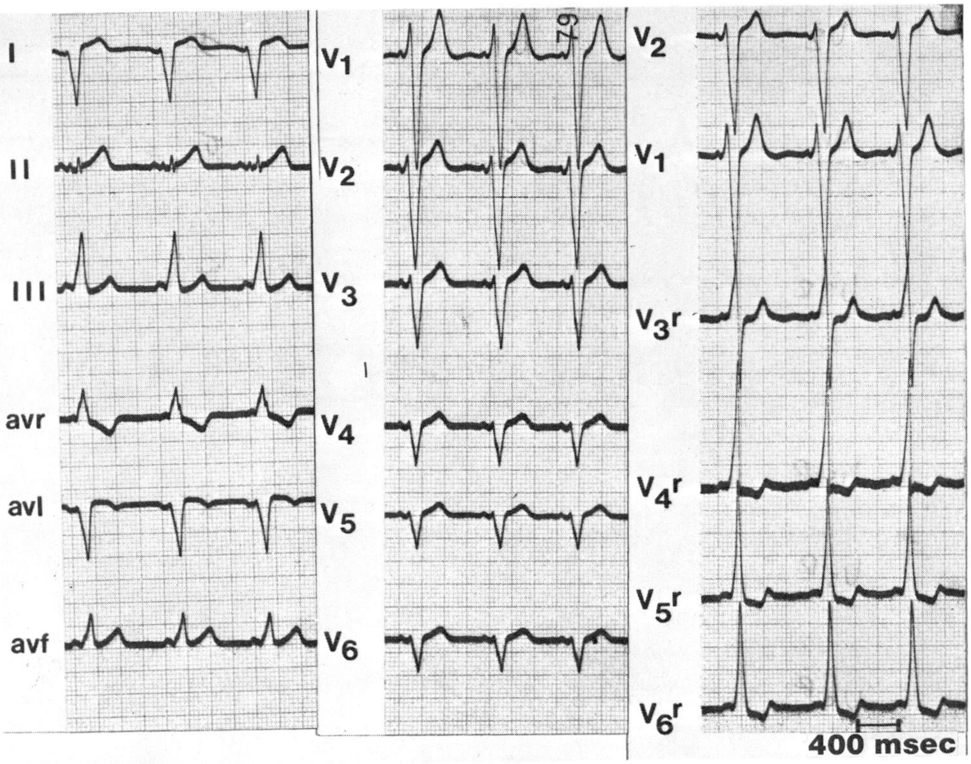

Figure 11-6. *Wolff-Parkinson-White syndrome in a patient with mirror-image dextrocardia. Note the negative P wave in lead I and positive P wave in lead aV_R. The right precordial leads show the accessory pathway located between the anatomic right atrium and right ventricle.*

patients are caused by the development of paroxysmal regular supraventricular tachycardia or atrial fibrillation or both. The occurrence of the latter arrhythmia may even result in sudden death, as discussed below.[6,31–35]

Paroxysmal Tachycardia in the Wolff-Parkinson-White Syndrome

The combination of the technique of programmed electrical stimulaton of the heart with the recording of multiple intracardiac and surface electrocardiographic leads has demonstrated that the most frequent form of paroxysmal tachycardia suffered by patients with WPW syndrome is a circus movement tachycardia (CMT) incorporating the AP in the tachycardia circuit.[20,36] In 69 consecutive patients with WPW syndrome admitted to the hospital with a history of attacks of paroxysmal regular supraventricular tachycardia, during subsequent electrophysiologic investigation it was possible to induce a similar type of tachycardia that proved to be based on an AV junctional reentrant mechanism incorporating the AP.[24]

Circus Movement Tachycardia Incorporating the Accessory Pathway

Circus movement tachycardia incorporating the AP is based on a reentrant circuit that consists of the following structures: (1) AV node, (2) His-Purkinje system, (3) ventricular myocardium, from the terminal Purkinje network to the ventricular end of the AP, (4) the AP itself, and (5) atrial myocardium, from the atrial insertion of the AP to the AV node. This circuit can be used in both directions, resulting in two possible varieties of CMT using the accessory pathway (Table 11-2)[37]:

1. *Type I A CMT.* This is the usual form of CMT in patients with WPW syndrome. Anterograde AV conduction occurs through the normal AV nodal–His pathway, VA conduction, through the AP. Thus, the QRS complex during tachycardia shows either normal intraventricular conduction

Table 11-2. Complaints (Symptoms) During Paroxysmal Circus Movement Tachycardia Incorporating the Accessory Pathway in 69 Patients With Wolff-Parkinson-White Syndrome

Symptom	No. of Patients	%
Palpitations	67	97
Dyspnea	40	57
Anginal pain	39	56
Perspiration	38	55
Fatigue	28	41
Anxiety	20	30
Dizziness	20	30
Polyuria	18	26

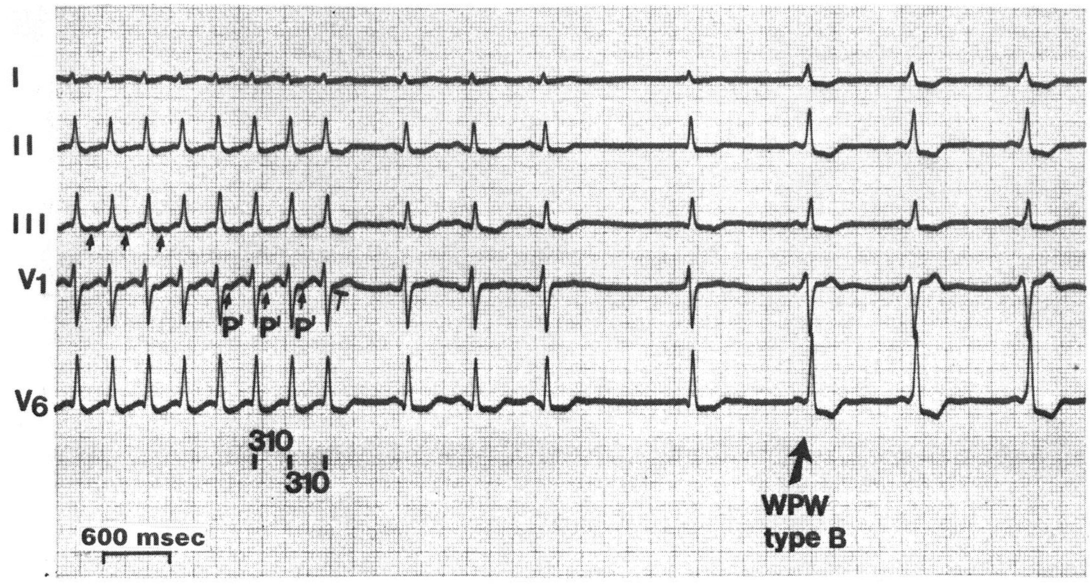

Figure 11-7. *Spontaneous termination of circus movement tachycardia incorporating the AP in the retrograde direction in a patient with right-sided Wolff-Parkinson-White (WPW) syndrome. Note that during tachycardia, the QRS complex indicates anterograde AV conduction over the normal AV nodal–His pathway. Following termination of tachycardia, and after a few beats that do not show preexcitation, right-sided WPW becomes evident during sinus rhythm. Retrograde P waves are identified during tachycardia* (arrows). *This retrograde P wave is not present after the last QRS complex during tachycardia, suggesting that retrograde block in the accessory pathway was the mechanism of spontaneous termination of tachycardia.*

or typical bundle branch block configuration. (Fig. 11-7). Atrial activation during this type of tachycardia starts close to the AP after the ventricular myocardium and the AP have been activated (Fig. 11-8). In some of these patients, the retrograde P wave (P′) can be identified on the electrocardiogram following the QRS complex during tachycardia, the P′R interval usually beng longer than the RP′ intervals (see Figs. 11-7 and 11-8).

2. *Type I B CMT.* Much less frequently, the reversed (antidromic) form of CMT incorporating the AP has been observed in patients with WPW syndrome. During this type of CMT, anterograde AV conduction is through the AP and retrograde VA conduction is through the normal His–AV nodal axis. Therefore, the QRS during tachycardia will show maximal preexcitation (Fig. 11-9). The differential diagnosis of this form of CMT has been recently discussed elsewhere.[38]

Electrophysiologic Requirements for the Development of Circus Movement Tachycardia Incorporating the Accessory Pathway

In 1913, Mines[39] suggested that tachycardia could be the result of an impulse circulating in a circuit consisting of atrium, AV node, ventricle, and an accessory atrioventricular connection. Such a circuit is anatomically present in patients with the WPW syndrome. Essential for the development of a circus movement in this circuit is the creation of unidirectional block in one of the two AV connections, with conduction persisting over the other pathway. The conduction velocity of the impulse should be slow enough to find all parts of the circuit excitable. To use such an anatomic circuit in a reentrant tachycardia, the possibility of VA conduction over at least one of the atrioventricular connections is essential. Patients without VA conduction over the AP can therefore never develop type I A CMT.

The creation of unidirectional block in one of the limbs of the circuit requires differences in duration of the refractory periods of the normal and accessory pathway in AV (anterograde), VA (retrograde), or both directions.[40] Thus, a critically timed premature beat can be blocked in one of the pathways while still being conducted over the other. Figures 11-10 and 11-11 diagrammatically illustrate how the two forms of CMT incorporating the AP can be initiated by an atrial or ventricular premature beat according to the electrophysiologic characteristics of the normal and accessory pathway in both anterograde and retrograde direction. Perpetuation of CMT requires that the time for the impulse to complete the whole circuit (the circulation time) is longer than the duration of the longest refractory period anywhere in the

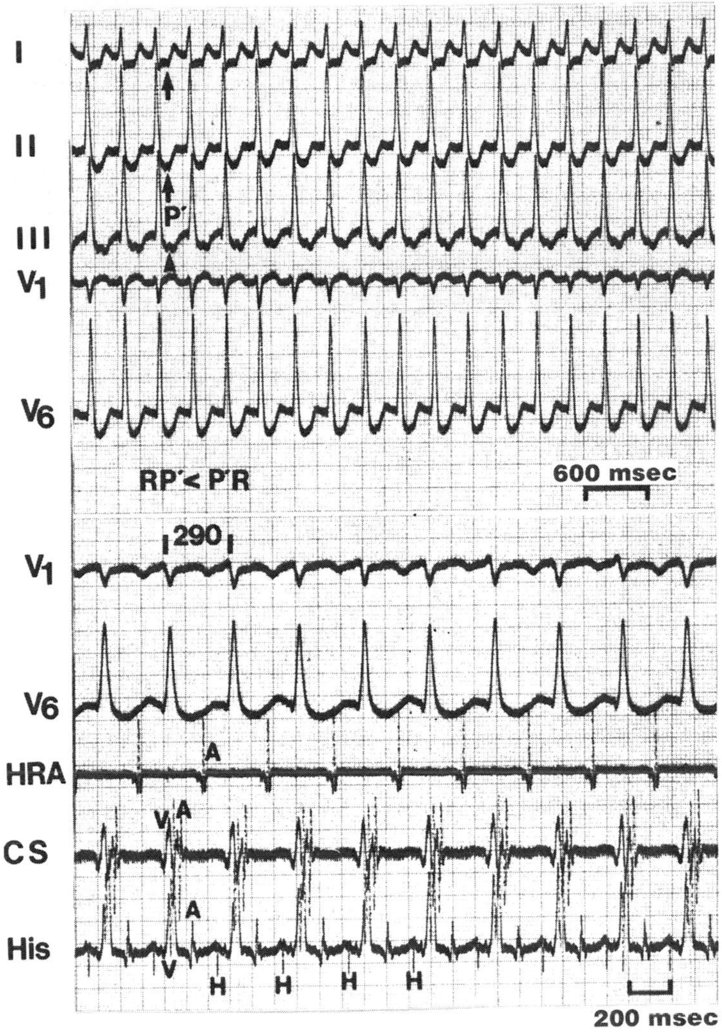

Figure 11-8. *The upper panel shows a 25 mm/sec. electrocardiographic recording of a tachycardia in a patient with a left-sided accessory pathway. QRS complexes during tachycardia show normal intraventricular conduction. A retrograde P wave is identified* (arrows), *the RP′ interval being shorter than the P′R interval. This finding suggests the incorporation of an accessory pathway in retrograde direction during tachycardia. In the lower panel, leads V_1 and V_6 plus intracardiac bipolar electrograms from the high right atrium (HRA), coronary sinus (CS), and His bundle (His) region simultaneously recorded at a paper speed of 50 mm/sec are shown. Note that retrograde atrial activation starts in the CS lead, indicating VA conduction through a left-sided accessory pathway.*

circuit.[40] This explains that circumstances (particularly drugs) promoting slow conduction in any of the components of the circuit can facilitate perpetuation of tachycardia if refractoriness is not prolonged in excess of conduction time.[40]

Symptoms and Signs of Circus Movement Tachycardia in Patients With Wolff-Parkinson-White Syndrome

Wc have recently studied the complaints of 69 consecutive patients with proven CMT incorporating the AP in the retrograde direction (type I A CMT) in the presence of the WPW. As shown in Table 11-2, most of the patients were aware of attacks of rapid heart action starting and stopping abruptly. Anginal pain was not uncommon in the young patient but, when present, was associated wth a high rate during tachycardia (more than 200 beats/min). Polyuria during or after the attack was present in 26% of the patients. Frequently, patients with a longstanding history of paroxysmal tachycardia told us that polyuria tended to disappear gradually over the years.

Other Forms of Paroxysmal Tachycardia in Patients With Wolff-Parkinson-White Syndrome

Table 11-3 shows the types of tachycardias (excluding atrial flutter and atrial fibrillation) induced during the stimulation study in a series of 265 consecutive patients with the WPW syndrome. Except for a few patients in whom atrial tachycardia, AV nodal reentrant tachycardia, or ventricular tachycardia was induced, the great majority had a CMT using the AP initiated during the study. Cases of CMT using two accessory pathways have been observed by others.[41] It is of interest that the reported examples of intranodal reentrant tachycardias in patients with the WPW syndrome showed absence of ventricular preexcitation during tachycardia.[38] Therefore, in patients presenting with a paroxysmal tachycar-

(Text continues on p. 286.)

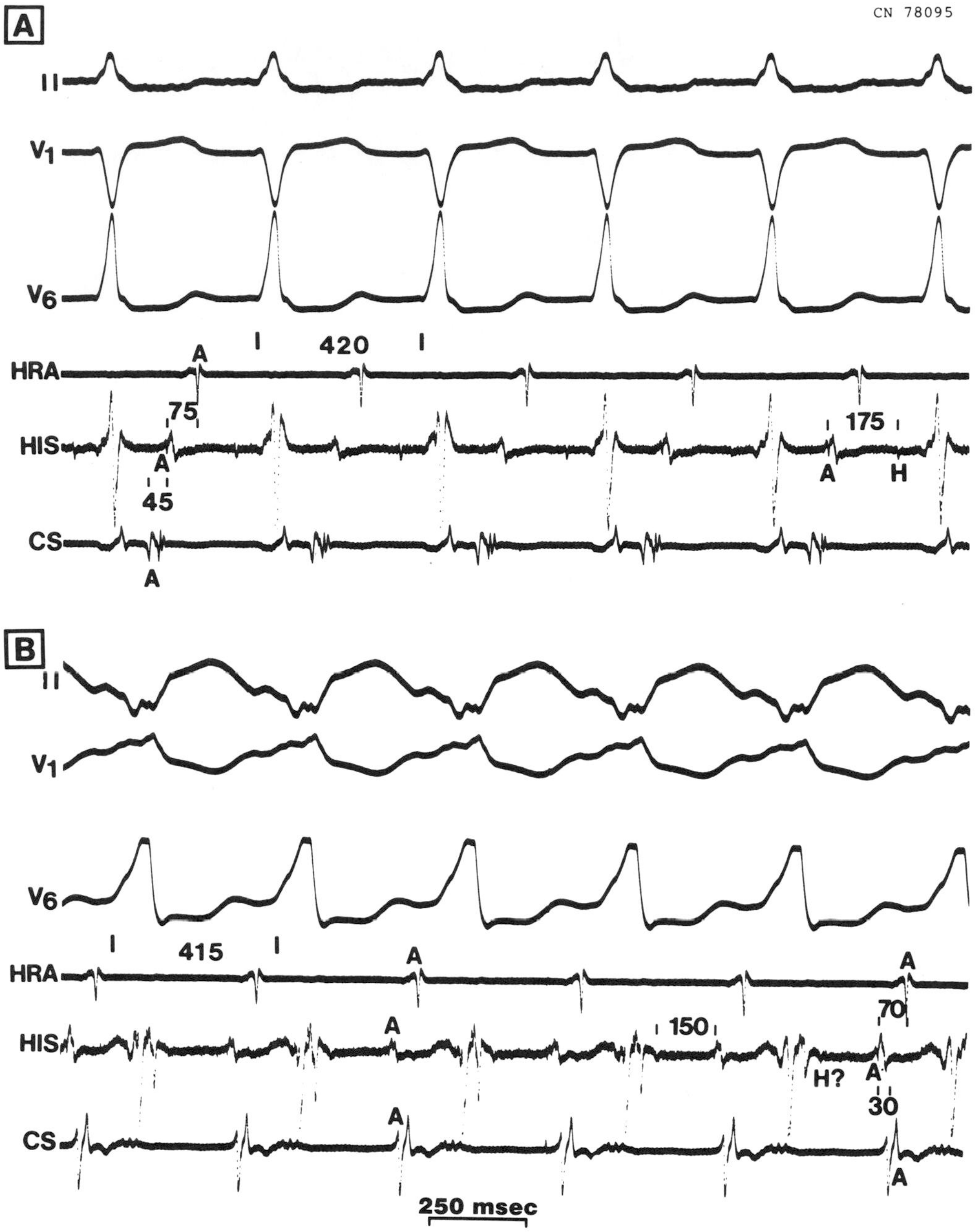

Figure 11-9. *External and intracavitary recordings of both types of CMT incorporating an accessory pathway. Leads II, V_1, and V_6 and bipolar electrograms from high right atrium (HRA), His bundle (HIS), and coronary sinus (CS) region are recorded simultaneously. Both types of tachycardia were induced in the same patient during programmed electrical stimulation of the heart. A shows type I A CMT. Note the narrow QRS indicating normal intraventricular conduction. The RR interval during tachycardia measures 420 msec. The sequence of retrograde atrial activation starts in the coronary sinus lead, indicating VA conduction over a left-sided accessory pathway. As AV conduction occurs by the normal AV pathway, the QRS complex is preceded by a His bundle electrogram. The AH interval during tachycardia is 175 msec. In B, the reversed (antidromic) variety of CMT is illustrated. QRS complexes during tachycardia show maximal preexcitation because of AV conduction over the AP. No His bundle potential precedes the QRS complex. VA conduction is by the normal His–AV nodal pathway, resulting in a different sequence of retrograde atrial activation. The cycle length during tachycardia in 415 msec.*

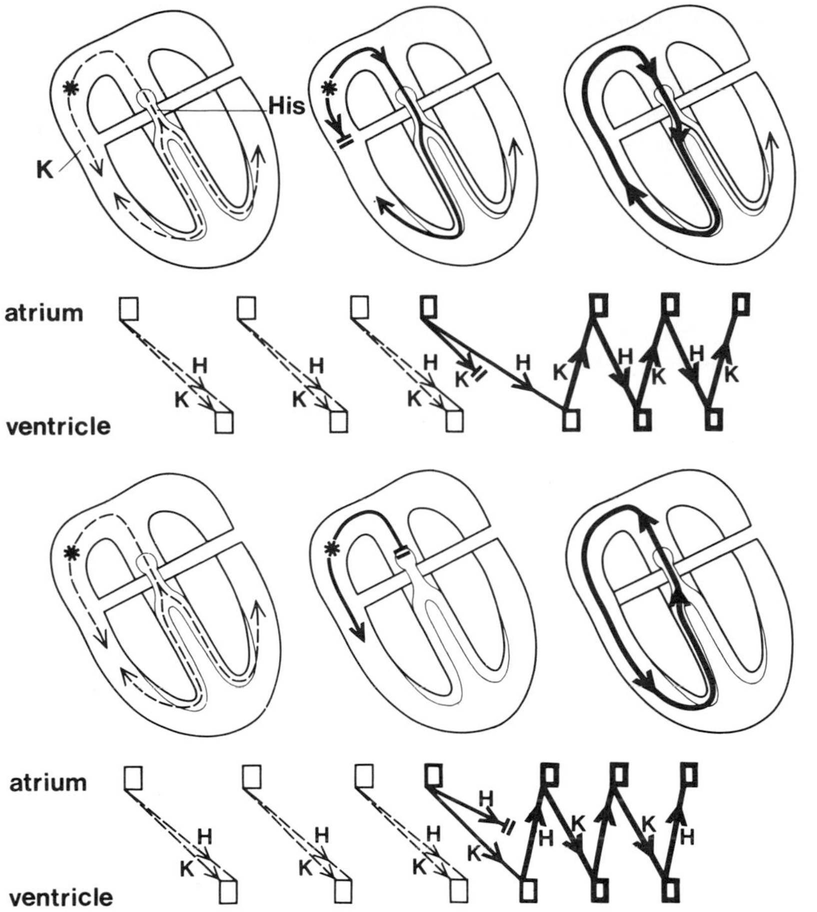

Figure 11-10. *Schematic representation of the modes of initiation of CMT incorporating the AP by an atrial premature beat during atrial pacing. As seen in the upper panel, if the refractory period of the AP is longer than that of the AV nodal–His axis, a precisely timed atrial premature beat is blocked in the AP (K) while still being conducted through the normal pathway (H). Following activation of the ventricle, the impulse is conducted over the AP in the retrograde direction, resulting in an atrial echo beat. If the impulse is conducted to the ventricle through the AV node, a circus movement tachycardia is initiated. The lower panel illustrates the much rarer situation in which the refractory period of the AP is shorter than that of the AV nodal–His pathway and an appropriately timed atrial premature beat is blocked in the normal pathway while still being conducted over the AP to the ventricles. Following activation of the ventricle, this impulse can be conducted in the VA direction over the His–AV nodal pathway, resulting in initiation of the antidromic form of CMT.*

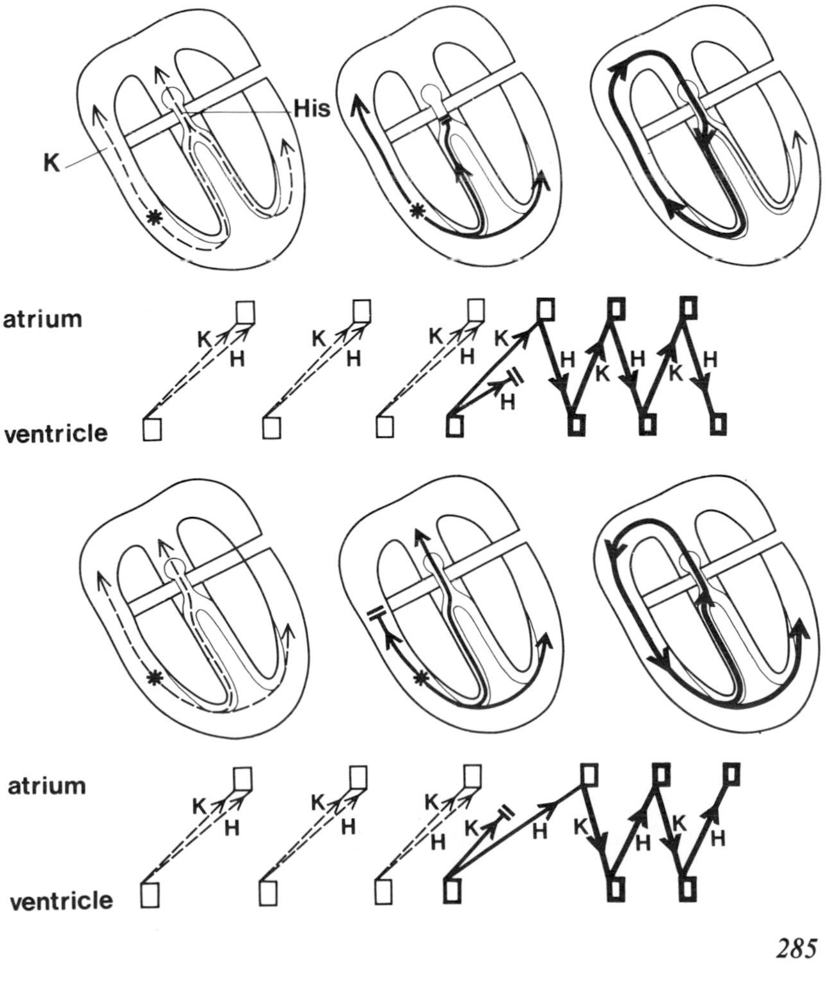

Figure 11-11. *Diagrammatic representation of the modes of initiation of CMT incorporating the AP by a ventricular premature beat during ventricular pacing. In the upper panel, the AP (K) is postulated to have a shorter refractory period than that of the normal AV nodal–His pathway (H). As shown, an appropriately timed ventricular premature beat is blocked in the AV nodal–His pathway while still being conducted over the accessory pathway to the atrium. If this impulse returns to the ventricles over the normal AV nodal–His pathway, a circus movement tachycardia is initiated. The lower panel illustrates the exceptional situation in which an antidromic CMT incorporating the AP is initiated. To have this type of tachycardia initiated, the refractory period of the AP must be longer than that of the AV node. Then an appropriately timed ventricular premature beat can be blocked in the AP while being conducted to the atrium over the His–AV nodal pathway (H). If this impulse on reaching the atrium is conducted back to the ventricles over the AP, an antidromic CMT is initiated.*

Table 11-3. Types of Tachycardia Initiated During Programmed Electrical Stimulation in 265 Patients With the Wolff-Parkinson-White Syndrome

Type of Tachycardia*	No. of Patients	%
Atrial tachycardia	4	1
AVN tachycardia	12	3
CMT incorporating AP	231	90
Ventricular tachycardia	3	1
Undetermined	15	5

* AVN, AV nodal; CMT, circus movement tachycardia; AP, accessory pathway.

dia with a normal QRS configuration (or typical bundle branch block pattern), the differential diagnosis must be made between the common form of CMT incorporating the AP (type I A CMT) and an intranodal reentrant tachycardia.[38] Table 11-4 shows the types of tachycardias possible in patients with WPW syndrome and the differential diagnosis of each variety. Electrophysiologic criteria used to establish the correct diagnosis are discussed elsewhere.[38]

Factors Influencing Clinical Manifestations of Tachycardia in Wolff-Parkinson-White Syndrome

The clinical consequences of paroxysmal tachycardia in patients with WPW syndrome depend on several factors: (1) heart rate during tachycardia (which in CMT depends on conduction velocity of the impulse, size, and functional refractory periods of the components of the circuit), (2) age of the patient (tolerance of the tachycardia tends to decrease with age), (3) presence of associated cardiovascular abnormalities, and (4) number and duration of the attacks of tachycardia.

Atrial Fibrillation in the Wolff-Parkinson-White Syndrome

Atrial fibrillation seems to be frequent in patients with WPW syndrome. As seen in Table 11-1, electrocardiographic documentation of at least one episode of atrial fibrillation was available in 78 of our 265 patients before the stimulation study.

At present, during atrial fibrillation some patients with the WPW syndrome can develop very high, life-

Table 11-4. Possible Types of Paroxysmal Regular Tachycardia in Wolff-Parkinson-White Syndrome and Their Differential Diagnosis*†

	Anterograde Pathway	Retrograde Pathway	Differential Diagnosis
Circus Movement Tachycardias Using AV Junctional Structures			
Type I A CMT	AVN–His pathway	Accessory pathway	Type II CMT
Type I B CMT	Accessory pathway	AVN–His pathway	1. Atrial tachycardia 2. Type II CMT 3. Type III CMT 4. Ventricular tachycardia
Type II CMT (intra-AV nodal)	AVN slow pathway	AVN fast pathway	Type I A CMT
Type III CMT (using two accessory pathways)	Accessory pathway$_1$	Accessory pathway$_2$	1. Type I B CMT 2. Atrial tachycardia 3. Type II CMT 4. Ventricular tachycardia
Atrial Tachycardia			1. Type I B CMT 2. Type II CMT 3. Type III CMT 4. Ventricular tachycardia
Ventricular Tachycardia			1. Type I B CMT 2. Type II CMT 3. Atrial tachycardia

* Criteria used to establish the differential diagnosis of these tachycardias have been discussed elsewhere.[38]
† CMT, Circus movement tachycardia; AVN, AV nodal.

threatening ventricular rates due to exclusive atrioventricular conduction over the AP (Fig. 11-12).[6,31–35] Apart from markedly reducing cardiac output, these rapid ventricular rates may degenerate into ventricular fibrillation.[6,35] It is important to realize that the presenting clinical problem in some patients with the WPW syndrome may be ventricular fibrillation.[35]

Although the ventricular rate during atrial fibrillation in patients with the WPW syndrome depends on several factors,[42] a good correlation has been found between the shortest RR interval showing preexcitation during atrial fibrillation and the effective refractory period of the AP as determined by the single test stimulus technique.[42]

Figure 11-12 shows an example of atrial fibrillation and very high ventricular rate because of exclusive conduction over the AP in a patient with WPW syndrome. Frequently, one can observe that runs of very short RR intervals alternate with groups of RR intervals showing a slower rate. A decrease in refractoriness of both the accessory pathway and ventricular muscle with increasing rates may play an important role in this phenomenon.[42]

The group from Duke University has reported on a series of 16 out of 135 patients with WPW syndrome who presented with ventricular fibrillation.[35] The only important marker for the development of ventricular fibrillation in this series was the occurrence of RR intervals equal to or less than 205 msec during atrial fibrillation. This observation might be of relevance in selecting patients for prophylactic drug treatment (see below).

Note that the degree of ventricular preexcitation observed in the electrocardiogram during sinus rhythm bears no relationship whatsoever to the risk of developing life-threatening ventricular rates during atrial fibrillation. This is illustrated in the electrocardiograms in Figure 11-13 from a patient in whom the AP did not markedly contribute to ventricular excitation during sinus rhythm. As seen in the lower panel, the patient presented with very high ventricular rates due to atrioventricular conduction through the AP during atrial fibrillation (shortest RR interval, 200 msec). In Figure 11-14, which was recorded in the same patient, an atrial premature beat during sinus rhythm is seen to bring out clear-cut ventricular preexcitation for reasons discussed earlier in this chapter. This again stresses the importance of distinguishing patients with little contribution to ventricular excitation through the accessory pathway from

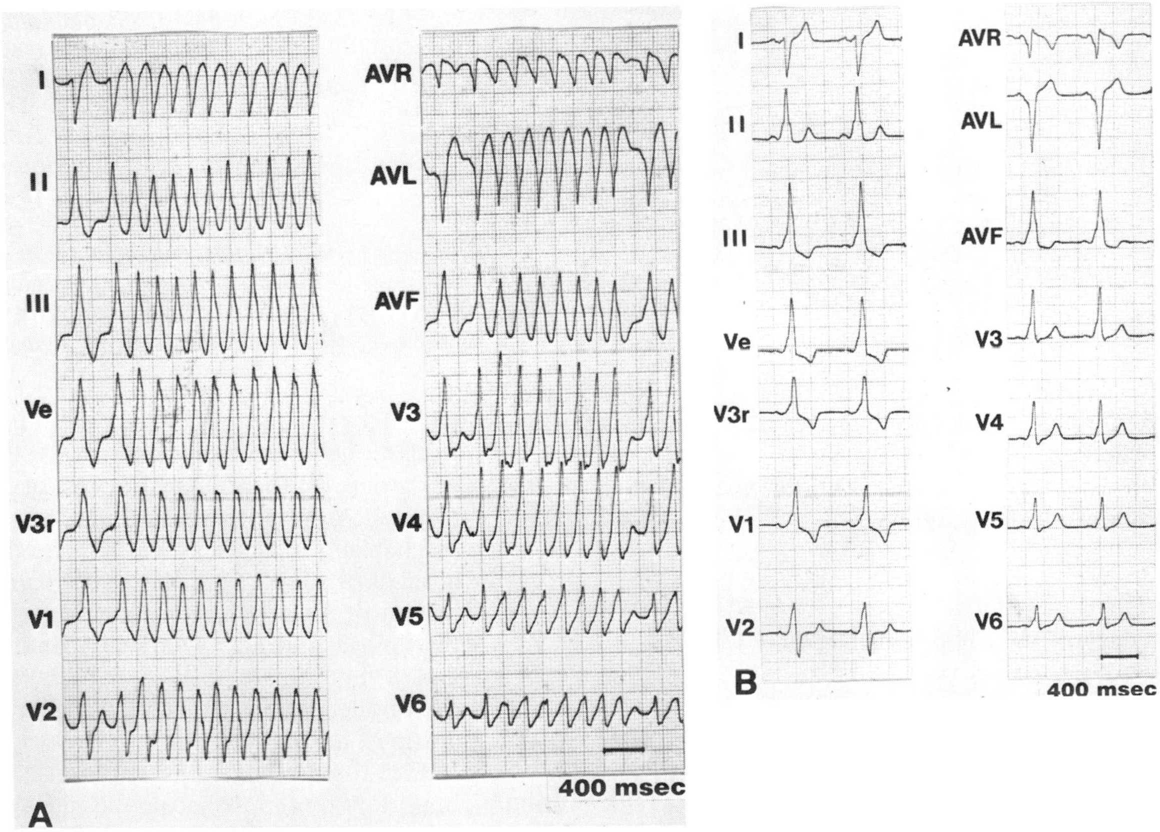

Figure 11-12. *Atrial fibrillation in the presence of an AP with a short refractory period. A shows the typical features of this arrhythmia: (1) irregular RR interval, (2) marked widening of the QRS complex, and (3) a ventricular rate reaching 300 beats/min. B is the electrocardiogram of the same patient during sinus rhythm.*

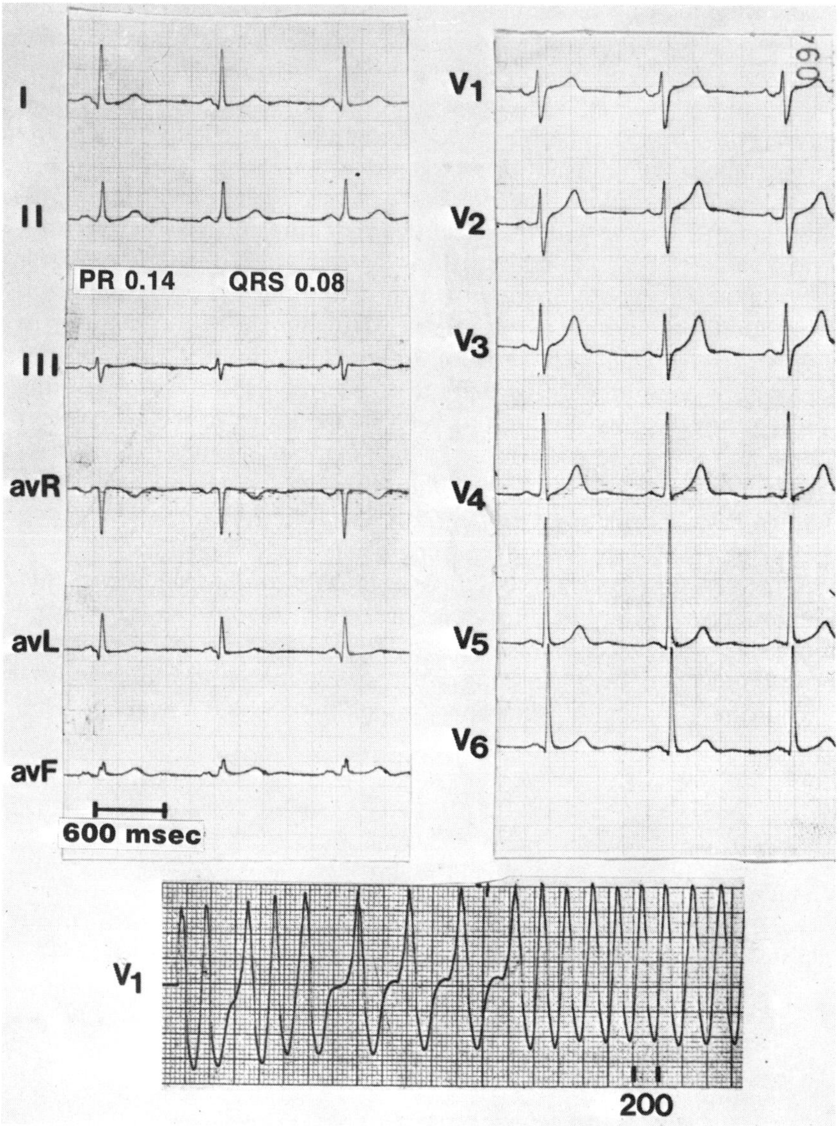

Figure 11-13. *Example of a patient with Wolff-Parkinson-White syndrome with, during sinus rhythm, little contribution to ventricular activation by AV conduction over the accessory pathway. As seen in the upper part of the figure, the PR interval and QRS width were both normal (0.14 and 0.08 second, respectively). The patient was admitted with an attack of atrial fibrillation (with a very high ventricular rate; shortest RR interval, 200 msec) because of conduction from atrium to ventricle over the AP.*

those with the so-called concealed accessory pathways. The latter group of patients are protected against life-threatening ventricular rates if atrial fibrillation develops.

Electrophysiologic Investigations in the Wolff-Parkinson-White Syndrome

Since 1967, many patients with the WPW syndrome have undergone electrophysiologic investigations.[20,36,37] The apparatus used and the protocol followed during these studies have been reviewed recently.[38] The purpose of these studies[38] is (1) to determine the location and number of the accessory pathway(s), (2) to determine the mechanism and pathway of tachycardia, (3) to establish the diagnosis of WPW syndrome in patients with a questionable electrocardiogram, (4) to identify a high-risk group, (5) to evaluate the effect of drugs on the electrophysiologic properties of the heart, especially on mechanisms of tachycardia and ventricular rates during atrial fibrillation, (6) to choose the correct therapy for a patient or for a group of patients with similar electrophysiologic findings, (7) to select candidates for surgery, and (8) to evaluate postoperatively the effect of surgery on conduction over the accessory pathway(s) and mechanism of the tachycardia.

Electrophysiologic investigations have become an important tool in diagnosis and management of the patient with the WPW syndrome. Their value will be commented on during the discussion of our approach to the patient with the WPW syndrome in relation to the problem he or she presents.

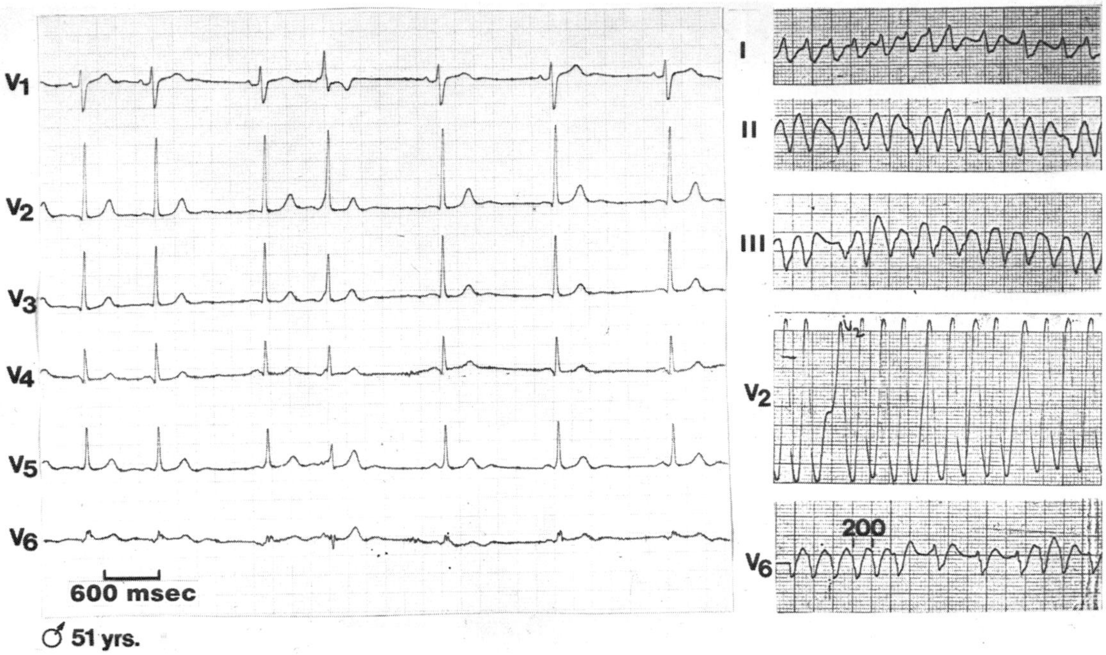

Figure 11-14. *Same patient as in Figure 11-13. A supraventricular premature beat shows clear-cut left-sided preexcitation. On the right part of the figure, several electrocardiographic leads during atrial fibrillation are seen.*

The Diagnostic and Therapeutic Approach to the Patient With Wolff-Parkinson-White Syndrome

A patient with WPW syndrome can be examined by a physician for at least one of the following reasons: (1) a history of palpitations without an electrocardiographically documented tachyarrhythmia, (2) an ongoing attack of palpitations, (3) an electrocardiographic diagnosis of WPW syndrome, and (4) an electrocardiogram with questionable signs of ventricular preexcitation. In the latter two instances, patients are usually referred to the cardiologist following recording of a routine electrocardiogram or because of an electrocardiogram made for evaluation of complaints related to the cardiovascular system. Patients with palpitations are frequently seen for the first time by their general practitioner.

The Patient With Palpitations

Patients Seen After an Attack of Palpitations

The general practitioner tends to misdiagnose complaints of patients suffering from paroxysmal tachycardias when the patient is seen after an attack of tachycardia. In a series of 69 consecutive patients with WPW syndrome admitted to the hospital for evaluation of attacks of paroxysmal supraventricular tachycardia, 39 patients were first seen by their general practitioner following an attack of tachycardia. We found that in only two patients the correct diagnosis was suspected by the general practitioner. In 25 patients, a diagnosis was made of "functional" complaints such as nervousness, fatigue, and so on. Various diagnoses such as "heart murmur" were made in six patients, while six other patients were told that their physician could find no abnormalities at all.[74]

Improvement in diagnosis by the general practitioner can be accomplished by (1) a careful history-taking; (2) the recording of an electrocardiogram (if the WPW electrocardiographic pattern is observed, the patient must be considered as probably suffering from tachyarrhythmias until proved otherwise), (3) instructing the patient to have an electrocardiogram recorded as soon as a tachycardia occurs; and (4) the use of 24-hour electrocardiogram recordings.

As mentioned previously, rapid heart action in patients with WPW syndrome is most frequently the result of either paroxysmal CMT or atrial fibrillation. The presence of accompanying symptoms (see Table 11-2) supports the existence of arrhythmias, either CMT or atrial fibrillation. Abrupt onset and termination of the attack favor the existence of a paroxysmal tachyarrhythmia. Palpitations are regular during CMT and irregular during atrial fibrillation. Patients with WPW paroxysmal CMT have frequently observed that at least some of their attacks could be stopped by vagal maneuvers. Patients with WPW syndrome and atrial fibrillation with a very rapid ventricular rate frequently suffer from dizziness or syncope during the arrhythmia. In patients with palpitations and an electrocardiogram showing the WPW syndrome, the following steps should be taken:

1. A careful history evaluating the frequency and length of the attacks, accompanying symptoms during tachycardia, and physical and psychological tolerance of the attacks, and a physical examination with chest x-ray studies and echocardiogram to assess the presence or absence of concomitant heart disease. The latter may affect tolerance of the attacks of tachycardia and influence therapeutic decisions.
2. The recording of a 24-hour electrocardiogram. This will give information on the nature of the rhythm disturbance when the patient experiences palpitations, and it enables us to confirm the existence of tachyarrhythmias and to determine their type (CMT or atrial fibrillation) and mode of initiation.
3. If the patient's quality of life is affected and the 24-hour electrocardiogram has been negative, a stimulation study should be performed. Inability to induce CMT during the stimulation study makes it very unlikely that the patient suffers from this type of arrhythmia outside the hospital. In a recent study by Denes and co-workers,[43] none of their 22 patients with WPW syndrome in whom CMT could not be induced during the stimulation study had electrocardiographic documentation of paroxysmal supraventricular tachycardia. In this group of patients, 50% were asymptomatic and the other 50% complained of paroxysmal palpitations. Since inability to induce CMT does not exclude atrial fibrillation as a cause of palpitations, we specifically induce this arrhythmia during the stimulation study, asking the patient whether he recognizes the symptoms. Denes and co-workers[43] also reported on 28 patients with WPW syndrome in whom CMT was induced during the stimulation study. Only one of these patients had no symptoms of tachycardia, 19 patients (68%) had electrocardiographic documentation of a similar type of tachycardia outside the cardiac laboratory, and 8 patients (28%) had a history of paroxysmal palpitations without electrocardiographic verifications.

Patients Seen During an Attack of Palpitations

As discussed previously, patients with the WPW syndrome usually suffer from either a CMT incorporating the AP or atrial fibrillation or both.

Paroxysmal Supraventricular Tachycardia. Any patient presenting with a supraventricular tachycardia is first approached by vagal maneuvers (carotid sinus massage, bilateral ocular compression, elevation of the lower extremities, immersion of the face into cold water). If successful, the vagal maneuver terminates the CMT, incorporating the AP by creating block in the AV node (Fig. 11-15).

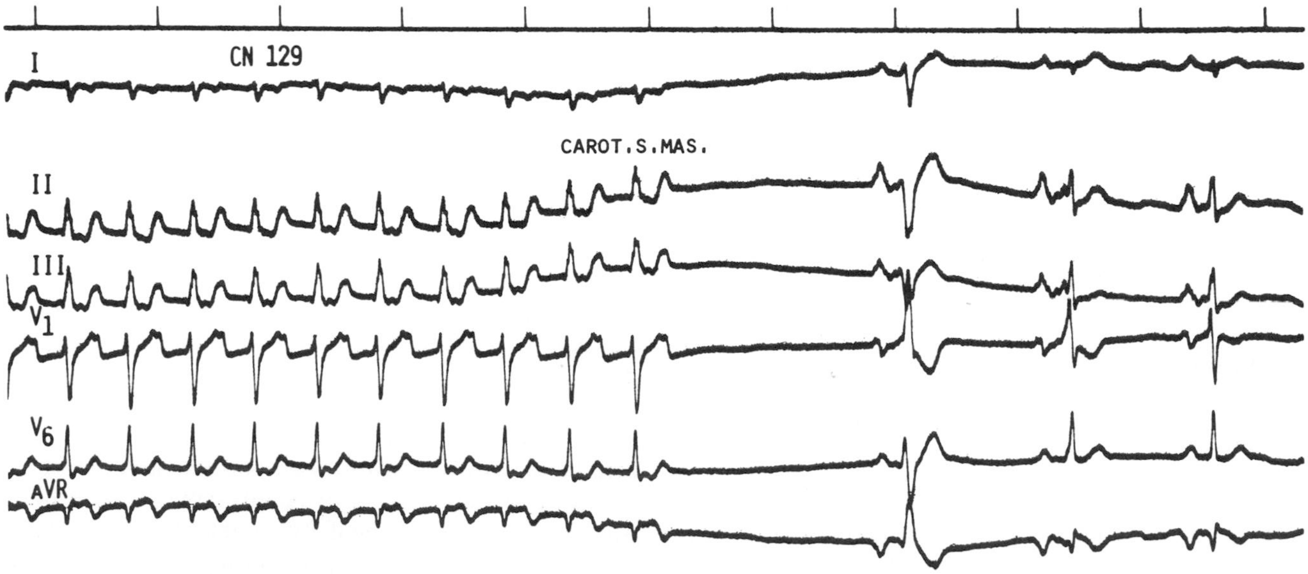

Figure 11-15. *Termination of a CMT incorporating the AP in VA direction by carotid sinus massage. Retrograde P waves are identified following the QRS complex during tachycardia. Note that termination of tachycardia is the result of block in the AV node.*

If vagal maneuvers do not terminate tachycardia, the following information should be obtained: (1) what does the electrocardiogram show during sinus rhythm and (2) was the patient receiving medication, and if so, what has been the success of intravenously and orally given antiarrhythmics in the past. If the patient is known to have WPW syndrome, the supraventricular tachycardia will most likely be a CMT incorporating the AP in the retrograde direction. If no information on the electrocardiogram during sinus rhythm is available, this type of tachycardia is still the most likely one on a statistical basis. In 120 consecutive hospital admissions because of supraventricular tachycardia, we found that during subsequent electrophysiologic evaluation a CMT incorporating an AP in the retrograde direction could be induced in 79 patients (66%), 69 patients having the WPW syndrome and 10 patients having a concealed accessory pathway. In 32 patients (27%), a reentrant tachycardia confined to the AV node was demonstrated. In patients with a tachycardia incorporating an AP, one is often able to identify retrograde P waves (P′) following the QRS, with a P′R interval longer than the RP′ interval (see Fig. 11-8).

As shown in Table 11-5, intravenous verapamil is the first antiarrhythmic drug used in patients with a regular supraventricular tachycardia except if the patient has been receiving a beta-blocking agent.[44] If verapamil is not available, propranolol is given intravenously. Both drugs can terminate CMT, incorporating the AP by creating block in the AV node.[44,45] Digitalis has also been used in the treatment of patients with this arrhythmia. However, because some patients may develop atrial fibrillation during CMT, which is an unpredictable event, digitalis may worsen the situation by abbreviating the refractory period of the AP,[46,47] resulting in higher ventricular rates during atrial fibrillation. Therefore, we do not recommend the use of digitalis in these patients.

If drugs acting on the AV node do not terminate the tachycardia, antiarrhythmic agents known to affect the properties of the accessory pathway should be given intravenously. Ajmaline, procainamide, and disopyramide are used for this purpose.[48–52]

If these methods fail to terminate the tachycardia, or if the patient is tolerating the arrhythmia poorly, electrical methods (direct current cardioversion or pacing) should be employed.[53] Pacing techniques are safer in patients receiving drugs that might endanger direct current cardioversion, that is, digitalis, verapamil, beta-blocking agents, and amiodarone. Electrical stimulation techniques creating block in the tachycardia circuit are preferred in those patients in whom termination of tachycardia is rapidly followed by reinitiation of tachycardia.

Table 11-5. Treatment of Circus Movement Tachycardia in Patients With the Wolff-Parkinson-White Syndrome

Treatment during the Attack of CMT
Vagal maneuvers
Verapamil, 10 mg IV
Propranolol, 5–10 mg IV
Ajmaline, 50 mg IV
Procainamide, up to 10 mg/kg body weight IV
Pacing
DC shock
Prophylaxis of CMT*
Amiodarone
Sotalol
Long-acting quinidine
Long-acting quinidine + propranolol

* Oral drugs are given according to current dose schedules.

Atrial Fibrillation. Patients with high ventricular rates during atrial fibrillation because of AV conduction over an AP, with a short refractory period, deserve special attention. In these patients, mean ventricular rates range from 160 to 300 beats/min. During these high ventricular rates, there usually is not only severe hemodynamic impairment but also the risk of ventricular fibrillation. As a rule, digitalis should be avoided in these patients. During episodes of atrial fibrillation with fast ventricular rates, cardioversion is the treatment of choice. If the patient is receiving drugs that may promote asystole following electrical cardioversion (*e.g.*, verapamil, beta-blocking agents, and probably amiodarone), a temporary pacing lead is positioned in the right ventricle before direct current shock. If the ventricular rate during atrial fibrillation is not excessively high (below 200 beats/min), drugs such as procainamide, ajmaline, disopyramide, and quinidine, which prolong the duration of the refractory period of the accessory pathway, can be given (Table 11-6).

Drug Prophylaxis in Patients With Proven Tachyarrhythmias

Patients with the WPW syndrome should receive prophylactic drug treatment when the arrhythmia is physically and psychologically poorly tolerated. In our experience, of the drugs available in Europe, amiodarone is the most effective drug in the prevention of attacks of paroxysmal tachycardia in patients with WPW syndrome.[54–56] Amiodarone has been shown to act on most of the components of the reentrant circuit in these patients.[55] In the United States, since amiodarone is not available, long-acting quinidine, disopyramide, procainamide, and propranolol, alone or in combination, are used. For reasons

Table 11-6. Treatment of Atrial Fibrillation in Patients With the Wolff-Parkinson-White Syndrome

Treatment During the Attack	
Hemodynamically not tolerated	
	DC shock
Hemodynamically tolerated	
	Procainamide
	Ajmaline
	Disopyramide
Prophylaxis of Atrial Fibrillation	
Amiodarone	
Sotalol	
Long-acting quinidine + propranolol	

already mentioned, digitalis should be avoided whenever possible in patients with the WPW syndrome.

In patients showing life-threatening ventricular rates during atrial fibrillation, prophylactic drug treatment with an antiarrhythmic agent that significantly prolongs the anterograde effective refractory period of the AP is essential. Amiodarone is the most successful drug for these patients because the drug not only reduces the ventricular rate during atrial fibrillation but also prevents the development of the arrhythmia itself.[56,57] Quinidine is an alternative but less effective drug to prevent high ventricular rates during atrial fibrillation. The efficacy of disopyramide as a prophylactic drug under these circumstances has yet to be demonstrated.

Patients with documented atrial fibrillation and high ventricular rates because of a short refractory period of the accessory pathway should be electrophysiologically evaluated to establish the correct choice of antiarrhythmic agent. The necessity of such an evaluation is stressed by our recent observation that the effect of a drug on the duration of the refractory period of the accessory pathway is related to the length of the refractory period of the accessory pathway before drug administration.[58] Preferably, the effect of the orally given drug, selected after the intravenous form has proved to be effective, should be evaluated during a second stimulation study to document that the patient is adequately protected against high ventricular rates during atrial fibrillation. We have recently shown that the duration of the refractory period of the accessory pathway may shorten during sympathetic stimulation.[59] This occurred even in patients receiving amiodarone. We therefore suggest adding a beta-blocking agent to the drug regimen of patients with WPW syndrome who suffer from atrial fibrillation.

The Approach to the Patient With an Electrocardiographic Diagnosis of Wolff-Parkinson-White Syndrome

Patients with an electrocardiographic diagnosis of WPW syndrome should be divided into two groups according to the presence or absence of complaints suggestive of arrhythmias. If a history of palpitations is present, we approach the patients as discussed previously.

As mentioned, the presenting symptom in patients with WPW syndrome can be ventricular fibrillation.[35] Therefore, any patient with an electrocardiogram showing the WPW abnormality should be evaluated to identify the group of patients who seem to be protected against sudden death if atrial fibrillation supervenes.

In patients with WPW syndrome, the development of life-threatening ventricular rates during atrial fibrillation possibly leading to ventricular fibrillation is related to the value of the anterograde effective refractory period of the accessory pathway.[42] We have observed that failure to achieve complete anterograde block in the AP followng the intravenous administration of 50 mg of ajmaline is highly suggestive of an anterograde effective refractory period of the AP with a duration of less than 270 msec.[48] This also holds for procainamide given intravenously in a dosage of 10 mg/kg body weight over a 5-minute period.[60]

Therefore, in patients with the WPW syndrome and no previous complaints of palpitations, a positive ajmaline test (induction of anterograde block over the AP as demonstrated in Figs. 11-16 and 11-17) indicates that the patient has a relatively long duration of the refractory period of the AP and that no further investigations are required. This test should be done in all patients with WPW syndrome independently of their complaints, because the occurrence of paroxysmal supraventricular tachycardias does not give an idea about the duration of the refractory period of the accessory pathway and therefore does not inform about the liability to life-threatening ventricular rates in case atrial fibrillation supervenes.

Patients with WPW syndrome and no previously documented episode of atrial fibrillation, in whom ajmaline or procainamide fails to induce anterograde block over the AP, should be referred to a medical center able to perform an electrophysiologic investigation. During the stimulation study in these patients, the following should be done:

1. The effective refractory period of the AP in the anterograde direction (which requires stimulation close to the atrial end of the AP) should be measured accurately.[38]

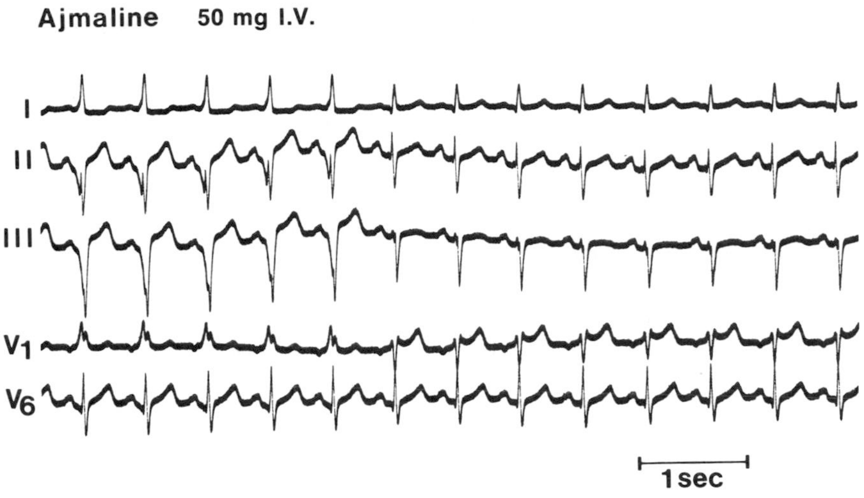

Figure 11-16. *Creation of complete AV block in the accessory pathway by the intravenous administration of 50 mg of ajmaline.*

2. Atrial fibrillation should be induced (by rapid atrial pacing) to evaluate the ventricular rate during the arrhythmia in the controlled and safe environment of the catheterization laboratory. Advice about the treatment of the patient who is asymptomatic and who has atrial fibrillation induced during the stimulation study with RR intervals below 210 msec is extremely difficult at present. This is illustrated by the opinion of the authors of this chapter, one of whom (J.F.) feels that such a patient should receive amiodarone prophylactically because the presenting symptom may be ventricular fibrillation. The two others (H. J. J. W. and F. W. H. M. B.) would like to collect more data about the natural history of the patient with WPW syndrome and a short refractory period of the accessory pathway before prescribing prophylactic drug therapy. In countries where amiodarone is not available, this decision is even more difficult, since the available antiarrhythmic drugs have a high incidence of serious side-effects and the required doses may affect the patient's quality of life.

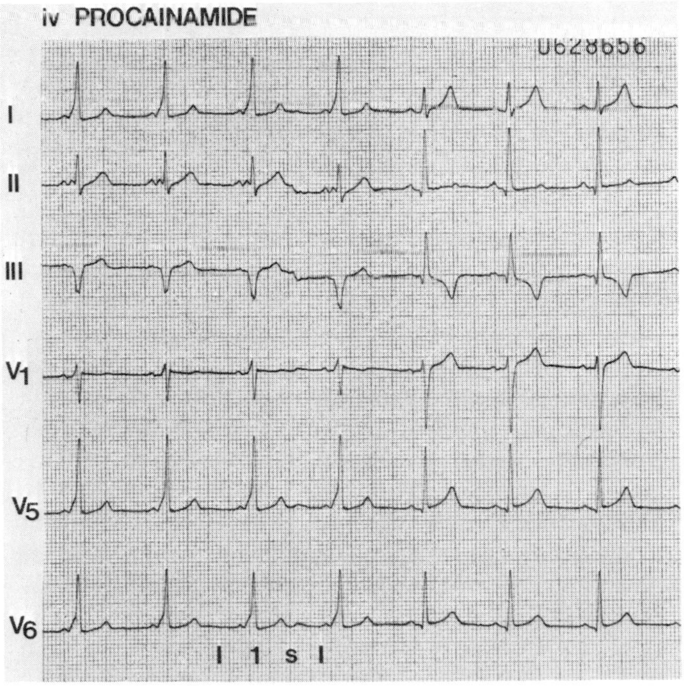

Figure 11-17. *Disappearance of preexcitation in the middle of the figure after the intravenous injection of 300 mg of procainamide.*

The Approach to the Patient With a Questionable Electrocardiogram

In patients with questionable evidence of the WPW syndrome because of little contribution of the AP to ventricular activation during sinus rhythm, resulting in a normal PR interval and normal QRS width, the clinician faces the problem of making the correct diagnosis of preexcitation. In some patients, the diagnosis can be made by the following noninvasive procedures: (1) carotid sinus massage in an attempt to increase AV nodal delay, thereby enhancing ventricular excitation over the accessory pathway, and (2) the intravenous administration of drugs such as ajmaline or procainamide, which by causing block in the AP may cause QRS abnormalities to disappear secondary to preexcitation (see Fig. 11-17). Both tests are only of diagnostic value when positive. The effect of carotid sinus massage on AV nodal conduction depends on many variables, and some patients with WPW syndrome may have a short intra-AV nodal conduction time. The ability to induce block over the AP following the administration of drugs such as ajmaline and procainamide depends on the initial value of the effective refractory period of the accessory pathway.[57]

If both of the aforementioned noninvasive tests are negative, the only way of making the correct diagnosis of WPW syndrome is by (1) atrial pacing at increasing rates or (2) applying atrial test stimuli with increasing prematurity.[38] Both modes of atrial stimulation result in progressive prolongation of the AV nodal conduction time without changing the atrioventricular conduction time over the accessory pathway and will bring out preexcitation.

The Patient With Wolff-Parkinson-White Syndrome and Intractable Tachyarrhythmias

The percentage of patients with WPW syndrome suffering from either paroxysmal supraventricular tachycardia or atrial fibrillation in whom the arrhythmia cannot be controlled is difficult to determine. Many of the patients considered intractable elsewhere and who were referred to us could be adequately controlled by using the drug or combination of drugs found to be active during the stimulation study. Several of these patients were restudied during oral drug administration to establish the effectiveness of the oral drug regimen. Frequent 24-hour recordings are made to document the presence or absence of arrhythmias outside hospital.

The optimal result of prophylactic treatment in patients with WPW syndrome is the complete prevention of attacks of tachycardia. Occasionally one must accept the persistence of attacks of tachycardia that are, however, self-limiting and short. Failure of drug treatment should lead to the following therapeutic interventions. Atrial fibrillation and circus movement tachycardia incorporating the AP will be discussed separately.

Atrial Fibrillation

There are patients who show persisting episodes of atrial fibrillation with high ventricular rates despite an adequate antiarrhythmic drug regimen. The reason for this phenomenon may be that the amount of drug-induced prolongation of the anterograde refractory period of the AP is minimal.[58] As discussed earlier, usually the shorter the anterograde effective refractory period of the AP before drug administration, the less prolongation will result from giving one of the available drugs known to prolong refractoriness in the AP. Also, because the duration of the anterograde refractory period of the accessory pathway is shortened further during sympathetic stimulation,[59] surgical interruption of the AP must be considered in these patients.

Circus Movement Tachycardia Incorporating the Accessory Pathway

Some patients with the WPW syndrome continue to suffer from frequent, incapacitating attacks of paroxysmal CMT even with drug treatment. This can be based on differences in the effect of the drug on electrophysiologic properties of the AP in AV and VA direction.[40]

Drugs that significantly prolong the anterograde refractory period of the AP may have no effect in the retrograde direction.[38,40] If the drug also slows conduction in the tachycardia circuit, both initiation and perpetuation of CMT can be facilitated by administration of such a drug. Other forms of therapy must be considered in these patients, including (1) implantation of a specially designed pacemaker after the stimulation study has demonstrated the feasibility of this approach and (2) surgical interruption of the tachycardia circuit. Preoperative, intraoperative, and postoperative management of these patients has been discussed extensively by the group from Duke University.[20]

References

1. Wolff, J., Parkinson, J., and White, P. D.: Bundle branch block with short P-R interval in healthy young people prone to paroxysmal tachycardia. Am. Heart J., 5:685, 1930.
2. Wilson, F. N.: A case in which the vagus influenced the form of ventricular complex of the electrocardiogram. Arch. Intern. Med., 16:1008, 1915.
3. Wedd, A. M.: Paroxysmal tachycardia. With reference to nomotopic tachycardia and the role of the extrinsic cardiac nerves. Arch. Intern. Med., 27:571, 1921.
4. Bach, F.: Paroxysmal tachycardia of forty-eight years duration and right bundle branch block. Proc. R. Soc. Med., 22:412, 1929.

5. Hamburger, W. W.: Bundle branch block. Four cases of intraventricular blocks showing some interesting and unusual clinical features. Med. Clin. North Am., 13:343, 1929.
6. Dreifus, L. S., Haiat, R., Watanabe, Y., et al.: Ventricular fibrillation, a possible mechanism of sudden death in patients with the Wolff-Parkinson-White syndrome. Circulation, 43:520, 1971.
7. Bellet, S.: Clinical Disorders of the Heart Beat, 3rd ed., p. 506. Philadelphia, Lea & Febiger, 1971.
8. Wellens, H. J. J.: Contribution of cardiac pacing to our understanding of the Wolff-Parkinson-White syndrome. Br. Heart J., 37:231, 1975.
9. Durrer, D., and Roos, J. P.: Epicardial excitation of the ventricles in a patient with Wolff-Parkinson-White syndrome (type B). Circulation, 35:15, 1967.
10. Durrer, D., Schoo, L., Schuilenburg, R. M., and Wellens, H. J. J.: The role of premature beats in the initiation and termination of supraventricular tachycardia in the Wolff-Parkinson-White syndrome. Circulation, 36:644, 1967.
11. Castellanos, A., Jr., Chapunoff, E., Castillo, C. A., et al.: His-bundle electrograms in two cases of WPW (pre-excitation) syndrome. Circulation, 41:399, 1970.
12. Gallagher, J. J., Sealy, W. C., Wallace, A. G., and Kasell, J.: Correlation between catheter electrophysiological studies and findings on mapping of ventricular excitation in the WPW syndrome. In Wellens, H. J. J., Lie, K. I., and Janse, M. J. (eds.): The Conduction System of the Heart, p. 588. Philadelphia, Lea & Febiger, 1976.
13. Sealy, W. C., and Wallace, A. G.: Surgical treatment of the Wolff-Parkinson-White syndrome. J. Thorac. Cardiovasc. Surg., 68:757, 1974.
14. Becker, A. E., Anderson, R. H., Durrer, D., and Wellens, H. J. J.: The anatomical substrates of Wolff-Parkinson-White syndrome. Circulation, 57:870, 1978.
15. Anderson, R. H., Becker, A. E., Brechenmacher, C., et al.: Ventricular pre-excitation. A proposed nomenclature for its substrates. Eur. J. Cardiol., 3:27, 1975.
16. Wellens, H. J. J., Lubbers, J. C., and Losekoot, T. G.: Preexcitation. In Roberts, J., and Gelband, H. (eds.): Cardiac Arrhythmias in Children, p. 231. New York, Appleton-Century-Croft, 1977.
17. Durrer, D., Schuilenburg, R. M., and Wellens, H. J. J.: Preexcitation revised. Am. J. Cardiol., 25:690, 1970.
18. Segers, M., Lequime, J., and Denolin, H.: L'activation ventriculaire précoce de certain coeurs hyperexcitables. Etude de l'onde delta de l'electrocardiogramme. Cardiologia, 8:113, 1944.
19. Puech, P., and Grolleau, R.: L'Activité du Faisceau de His Normale et Pathologique. Paris, Editions Sandoz, 1972.
20. Gallagher, J. J., Pritchett, E. L. C., Sealy, W. C., Kasell, J., and Wallace, A. G.: The preexcitation syndromes. Prog. Cardiovasc. Dis., 20:285, 1978.
21. Coumel, Ph., and Attuel, P.: Reciprocating tachycardia in overt and latent pre-excitation. Eur. J. Cardiol., 1:423, 1974.
22. Chung, K. Y., Walsh, T. J., and Massie, E.: Wolff-Parkinson-White syndrome. Am. Heart J., 69:1, 1965.
23. Averill, K. M., Fosmoe, R. J., and Lamb, L. E.: Electrocardiographic findings in 67,375 asymptomatic subjects. IV Wolff-Parkinson-White syndrome. Am. J. Cardiol., 6:108, 1960.
24. Wellens, H. J. J.: Paroxysmal supraventricular tachycardia. Recognition by the general practitioner. Rev. Lat. Cardiol., 1:51, 1980.
25. Rosenbaum, F. F., Hecht, H. H., Wilson, F. N., and Johnston, F. D.: Potential variations of the thorax and the esophagus in anomalous atrioventricular excitation (Wolff-Parkinson-White syndrome). Am. Heart J., 29:281, 1945.
26. Wallace, A. G., Sealy, W. C., Gallagher, J. J., et al.: Surgical correction of anomalous left ventricular preexcitation: Wolff-Parkinson-White (type A). Circulation, 49:206, 1974.
27. Tonkin, A. M., Wagner, G. S., Gallagher, J. J., and Wallace, A. G.: Initial forces of ventricular depolarization in the Wolff-Parkinson-White syndrome. Circulation, 52:1020, 1975.
28. Schiebler, G. L., Edwards, J. E., and Burchell, H. B.: Congenital corrected transposition of the great vessels. A study of 33 cases. Pediatrics, 27:11, 1960.
29. Ellis, K., Morgan, B. S., Blumenthal, S., and Anderson, D. H.: Congenital corrected transposition of the great vessels. Radiology, 79:35, 1962.
30. Schiebler, G. L., Adams, P., and Anderson, R. C.: The Wolff-Parkinson-White syndrome in infants and children. A review and a report of 28 cases. Pediatrics, 24:585, 1959.
31. Ahlinger, S., Granath, A., and Holmer, S.: Wolff-Parkinson-White syndrom med paroxysmalt atrieflimmer overgaende i ventrikelflimmer. Nord. Med., 70:1336, 1963.
32. Castillo-Fenoy, A., Goupil, A., and Offenstad, G.: Syndrome de Wolff-Parkinson-White et mort subite. Ann. Med. Interne (Paris), 124:871, 1973.
33. Martin-Noel, P., Denis, B., Grunwald, D., and Buisson, M.: Deux cas mortels de syndrome de Wolff-Parkinson-White. Arch. Mal. Coeur, 63:1647, 1970.
34. Touche, M., Jouvet, M., and Touche, S.: Fibrillation ventriculaire au coeurs d'un syndrome de Wolff-Parkinson-White. Réduction par choc électrique externe. Arch. Mal. Coeur, 59:1122, 1966.
35. Bashore, Th.M., Sellers, T. D., Gallagher, J. J., and Wallace, A. G.: Ventricular fibrillation in the Wolff-Parkinson-White syndrome. Circulation, 53:II–187, 1976.
36. Wellens, H. J. J.: The electrophysiological properties of the accessory pathway in the Wolff-Parkinson-White syndrome. In Wellens, H. J. J., Janse, M. J., and Lie, K. I. (eds.): The Conduction System of the Heart, p. 567. Philadelphia, Lea & Febiger, 1976.
37. Wellens, H. J. J.: The Wolff-Parkinson-White and related syndromes. II The value of cardiac pacing in study and treatment. In Krikler, D. M., and Goodwin, J. F. (eds.): Cardiac Arrhythmias, p. 162. Philadelphia, W. B. Saunders, 1975.
38. Wellens, H. J. J., Farré, J., and Bär, F. W.: Stimulation studies in the Wolff-Parkinson-White syndrome. In Narula, O. (ed.): Clinical Electrophysiology. Philadelphia, F. A. Davis, 1979.
39. Mines, G. R.: On dynamic equilibrium in the heart. J. Physiol. 46:23, 1913.
40. Wellens, H. J. J.: Value and limitations of programmed electrical stimulation of the heart in the study and treatment of tachycardias. Circulation, 57:845, 1978.
41. Gallagher, J. J., Sealy, W. C., Kasell, J., and Wallace, A. G.: Multiple accessory pathways in patients with the preexcitation syndrome. Circulation, 54:571, 1976.
42. Wellens, H. J. J., and Durrer, D.: Relation between refractory period of the accessory pathway and ventricular frequency during atrial fibrillation in patients with the Wolff-Parkinson-White syndrome. Am. J. Cardiol., 33:178, 1974.
43. Denes, P., Wu, D., Amat-y-Leon, F., et al.: Determination of atrioventricular reentrant paroxysmal tachycardia in patients with Wolff-Parkinson-White syndrome. Circulation, 58:415, 1978.
44. Krikler, D., and Spurrell, R.: Verapamil in the treatment of paroxysmal supraventricular tachycardia. Postgrad. Med. J., 50:447, 1974.
45. Denes, P., Cummings, J. M., Simpson, R., et al.: Effects of propranolol on anomalous pathway refractoriness and circus movement tachycardias in patients with preexcitation. Am. J. Cardiol., 41:1061.
46. Wellens, H. J. J., and Durrer, D.: Effect of digitalis on atrioventricular conduction and circus movement tachycardia in patients with the Wolff-Parkinson-White syndrome. Circulation, 47:1229, 1973.
47. Sellers, T. D., Bashore, T. M., and Gallagher, J. J.: Digitalis in the pre-excitation syndrome: analysis during atrial fibrillation. Circulation, 56:260, 1977.

48. Wellens, H. J. J., Bär, F. W., Gorgels, A. P., Vanage, E. J.: Use of ajmaline in identifying patients with short refractory period of their accessory pathway in Wolff-Parkinson-White syndrome. Am. J. Cardiol., 45:130, 1980.
49. Wellens, H. J. J., and Durrer, D.: Effect of procaine amide, quinidine and ajmaline on the Wolff-Parkinson-White syndrome. Circulation, 50:114, 1974.
50. Mandel, W. J., Laks, M. M., and Obayashi, K.: The Wolff-Parkinson-White syndrome: pharmacologic effects of procainamide. Am. Heart J., 90:744, 1975.
51. Sellers, T. D., Campbell, R. W. F., Bashore, T. M., and Gallagher, J. J.: Effects of procainamide and quinidine sulfate in the Wolff-Parkinson-White syndrome. Circulation, 55:15, 1977.
52. Spurrell, R. A. J., Thorburn, C. W., Camm, J., et al.: Effects of disopyramide on electrophysiological properties of specialized conduction system in man and on accessory atrioventricular pathway in the Wolff-Parkinson-White syndrome. Br. Heart J., 37:861, 1975.
53. Wellens, H. J. J., Bär, F. W., Gorgels, A. P., and Farré, J.: Electrical management of arrhythmias with emphasis on the tachycardias. Am. J. Cardiol., 41:1025, 1978.
54. Rosenbaum, M. B., Chiale, P. A., Ryba, D., and Elizari, M. V.: Control of tachyarrhythmias associated with Wolff-Parkinson-White syndrome by amiodarone hydrochloride. Am. J. Cardiol., 34:215, 1974.
55. Wellens, H. J. J., Lie, K. I., Bär, F. W., et al.: Effect of amiodarone in the Wolff-Parkinson-White syndrome. Am. J. Cardiol., 38:189, 1976.
56. Wellens, H. J. J., Brugada, P., and Abdollah, H.: Effect of amiodarone in paroxysmal supraventricular tachycardia with or without Wolff-Parkinson-White syndrome. Am. Heart J., 106:876, 1983.
57. Rosenbaum, M. B., Chiale, P. A., Halpern, M. S., et al.: Clinical efficacy of amiodarone as an antiarrhythmic agent. Am. J. Cardiol., 38:934, 1976.
58. Wellens, H. J. J., Bär, F. W., and Gorgels, A. P.: Effect of drugs in WPW syndrome. Importance of initial length of effective refractory period of accessory pathway. Am. J. Cardiol., 41:428, 1978.
59. Wellens, H. J. J., Brugada, P., Roy, D., et al.: Effects of isoproterenol on the antero grade refractory period of the accessory pathway in patients with the Wolff-Parkinson-White syndrome. Am. J. Cardiol., 50:180, 1982.
60. Wellens, H. J. J., Braec, S. H. J. G., Brugada, P., et al.: Use of procainamide in patients with the Wolff-Parkinson-White syndrome to disclose a short refractory period of the accessory pathway. Am. J. Cardiol., 50:921, 1982.

12

Atrioventricular Block: Basic Concepts

Yoshio Watanabe and Leonard S. Dreifus

In recent years, much information has become available concerning the pathology, electrophysiology, anatomy, and clinical significance of disturbances of atrioventricular (AV) conduction. Interest in this subject apparently began in 1827 with a description by Adams[1] of syncope associated with a slow heart rate and with subsequent observations by Stokes[2] in 1846. Wenckebach[3] (1899) and Hay[4] (1906) described AV conduction block and ushered in the era of eponyms and synonyms in the classification of AV conduction disturbances. The issue heated up intensely in 1924 when Mobitz[5] classified AV block according to rather precise criteria. In the following years, numerous clinical and experimental studies appeared in the medical literature.

However, more recent studies indicate that the clinical course and prognosis, as well as the mode of therapy for patients with AV block, depend predominantly on localization of the conduction disturbance within the AV conducting system (e.g., within the AV node or the His-Purkinje system). Hence, it has become increasingly apparent that AV block should be classified by the level of propagation failure rather than by constancy or fluctuations of the PR interval.[6,7]

Moreover, precise determination of the site of conduction block may sometimes be difficult even in those experimental studies using microelectrodes.[8,9] The total AV conduction time contains the following three components: intra-atrial conduction time, intra-AV nodal conduction time, and His-Purkinje (subnodal) conduction time. According to experimental studies using microelectrode techniques, the total AV conduction time in isolated perfused rabbit hearts under normal experimental conditions measures between 90 and 100 msec, of which intra-atrial, intranodal, and His-Purkinje conduction times measure 30, 30 to 35,and 30 msec, respectively.[10,11] Hence, each of these three components roughly corresponds to one third of the total AV interval.

In routine clinical electrocardiograms, these intervals cannot be determined separately, and the AV conduction time is measured from the beginning of the P wave (atrial excitation) to the onset of the QRS complex (ventricular excitation). However, with the use of His bundle electrocardiography, the above three conduction times can be approximately measured (Fig. 12-1). Based on several reports, individual components of the total AV conduction time in the presence of a PR interval between 0.14 and 0.18 second (140 to 180 msec) are as follows: intra-atrial conduction time, 0.04 to 0.05 sec-

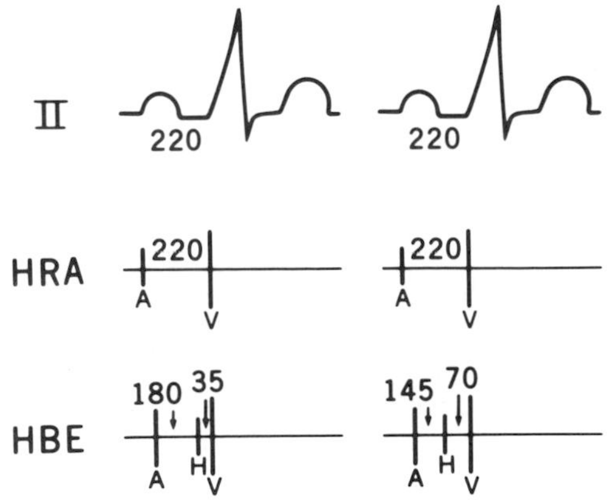

Figure 12-1. *First degree AV block: components of AV interval. The left side of this figure shows conduction delay between the atria and the His bundle. The right side shows subjunctional conduction delay. The duration of the His electrogram is 5 msec.*

ond (40 to 50 msec); intranodal conduction time, 0.05 to 0.07 second (50 to 70 msec); and His-Purkinje conduction time, 0.05 to 0.06 second (50 to 60 msec).[12-14] Thus, the ratio between these three components in human hearts may not be grossly different from that in rabbit hearts. Note that even when the intranodal conduction time and the His-Purkinje conduction time both measure 60 msec, the distance an impulse travels during this time is much shorter for the intranodal conduction. This indicates that the conduction velocity is slowest in the AV node and much higher in the His-Purkinje system. Indeed, the AV node is often said to constitute the weakest point in the entire AV conducting system, although one must be equally aware that AV conduction block does not occur exclusively within the AV nodal tissue.

Classification of Atrioventricular Block

It is customary to divide AV block into first degree, second degree, and third degree (or high grade) according to the severity of conduction disturbance.[15-17] First degree AV block represents a prolongation of the AV conduction time (the PR interval in the electrocardiogram) beyond the normal range. That such prolongation of the AV conduction time may result from a conduction delay within the atria, AV node, or His-Purkinje system or any combinations thereof has been clearly demonstrated in experimental studies[18-20] (see Fig. 12-1) as well as by clinical His bundle electrocardiography.[21] Second degree AV block is diagnosed when some of the impulses originating either in the sinus node or within the atria die out in certain portions of the AV conducting system and fail to reach the ventricles, whereas third degree AV block represents conduction in which impulse transmission from the atria to the ventricles is almost entirely blocked and the ventricles are controlled by a subsidiary pacemaker. Although third degree or high-grade AV block has classically been called *complete AV block,* the former terminology appears to be more adequate, since an occasional occurrence of successful AV conduction in these cases is often observed with continuous electrocardiographic monitoring. Again, note that failure of propagation of impulses in cases with second degree or third degree AV block could occur within the atria, AV node, or in the His-Purkinje system, in both the experimental[8,9] and clinical setting.[22-26]

In addition to the above classification, second degree AV block has been subdivided into two types by the sequence of PR intervals in conducted supraventricular beats. This classification is based on the original observations of Wenckebach[27] and Mobitz[28,29] and can simply be stated as follows: when the AV conduction times in several successive beats are progressively prolonged, culminating in dropping out of one ventricular depolarization, type I is diagnosed; a sudden failure of AV conduction after the maintenance of a constant PR interval is designated type II. It is readily understood that this classification can be applied only when more than two sinus or supraventricular impulses are consecutively conducted the ventricles in the presence of second degree AV block, and the classification is not applicable in third degree AV block.

For clinical purposes, identification of the site of block either within the AV node or in the His-Purkinje system, or above or below the bifurcation of the His bundle, is probably sufficient. This information can now be obtained with the use of His bundle electrocardiography.[12-14,22,26] However, we feel that His bundle electrocardiography should not be used routinely in every patient with AV block because it is an invasive technique. Furthermore, it appears that the level of conduction disturbance can roughly be estimated by studying the QRS duration or the mode of ventricular excitation in the electrocardiogram, at least in the majority of clinical cases.[17,30,31] For instance, if the QRS duration is normal, the site of conduction delay and block is most likely above the bifurcation of the His bundle (either within the AV node or in the main His bundle), whereas abnormally wide QRS complexes suggest the presence of conduction disturbance in bundle branches or fascicles (either alone or in addition to an AV junctional block).

Although the classification of AV transmission disorders has captivated the cardiovascular literature, less attention has been directed to the actual electrophysiologic events responsible for these disorders. Furthermore, it is the site and electrophysiologic behavior of the conduction disorder that offer the most clinical information and prognosis of the patient.[6,7,17,22,23,31-33]

The outline below summarizes the factors controlling AV conduction, and the reader is urged to review the physiology of AV transmission for an in-depth understanding of the nature and mechanisms of AV transmission disorders. Some of the more common electrophysiologic mechanisms of AV block that may have clinical significance will be illustrated.

Factors Controlling Impulse Transmission

I. Primary determinants of conductivity
  A. Physiologic factors
    1. Effectiveness of stimuli produced by depolarization of upstream fibers
    2. Excitability of responding downstream fibers
    3. Temporal fluctuation of 1 or 2
    4. Passive membrane properties and cell-to-cell coupling
  B. Anatomic factors
    1. Fiber diameter
    2. Geometric arrangement of fibers

II. Abnormal conduction phenomena resulting from alterations in the primary determinants of conductivity
  A. Decremental conduction
  B. Inhomogeneous conduction
  C. Conduction delay and block
  D. Unidirectional block
  E. Reentry

III. Abnormal conduction phenomena secondarily affecting conductivity
  A. Conduction delay and block
    1. Effects of conduction delay on the action potential duration (prolongation)
    2. Effects of conduction block on the action potential duration of fibers proximal to thc sitc of propagation failure (shortening)
    3. Effects of conduction block on the action potential duration of fibers distal to the site of propagation failure (prolongation)
    4. Effects of conduction delay or block on excitability of the downstream fibers
    5. Conduction delay or block causing impulse formation in the downstream fibers
  B. Reentry
    1. Collision of reentrant impulse with the more slowly advancing, anterograde wave of excitation resulting in cancellation of both wavefronts
    2. Further disorganization of the excitation front (increased inhomogeneity) in subsequent impulse transmission
    3. Reorganization of the excitation front (decreased inhomogeneity) in subsequent impulse transmission

First Degree Atrioventricular Block

Since the normal range of AV conduction time (PR interval) in an adult is considered to be between 0.12 and 0.21 second, PR intervals longer than 0.22 second will indicate a first degree AV block. These criteria can be applied only in the presence of regular sinus mechanism (or atrial rhythm). If an atrial premature systole is conducted to the ventricles with a PR interval longer than 0.22 second, it is not called a first degree AV block as long as all the other sinus beats show a normal PR interval. Thus, the diagnosis of first degree AV block should not be difficult except in those patients with sinus tachycardia and a markedly prolonged PR interval in which the P waves are superimposed on the T waves of the preceding beats. An example of typical first degree AV block with a PR interval of 0.22 second is shown in Figure 12-1. However, the level of block cannot always be identified.

In clinical cases of simple first degree AV block, no attention is usually paid to the area of conduction delay responsible for the prolonged PR interval. However, when first degree AV block is associated with subjunctional block (*i.e.*, right bundle branch block or a combination of fascicular blocks), His bundle studies may be required to identify those patients at high risk of developing complete heart block because primary conduction delay of the remaining fascicle may be present.

Second Degree Atrioventricular Block With Narrow QRS Complexes

In Figure 12-2, a group of three P-QRS complexes is seen in the middle portion of lead II with progressive prolongation of the PR interval, and a fourth P wave (P4) fails to be conducted to the ventricles, producing a long pause. This pause is terminated by a P wave (P5) that is conducted to the ventricles, again with a shorter PR interval. Since three of the four sinus impulses are transmitted to the ventricles, this is called a *4:3 conduction ratio,* and the sequence is called the *Wenckebach phenomenon.*[15–17,27] Similarly, in lead V_5, six consecutive P waves are conducted to the ventricles, followed by blockage of the seventh P wave (7:6 conduction). Note that the QRS complexes show normal duration, and therefore no intraventricular conduction disturbance is present. It has been said that characteristics of typical Wenckebach phenomenon (type I block) include the following: (1) the PR interval is progressively prolonged in consecutively conducted beats, (2) the RR intervals gradually shorten before a pause (long PP interval), and

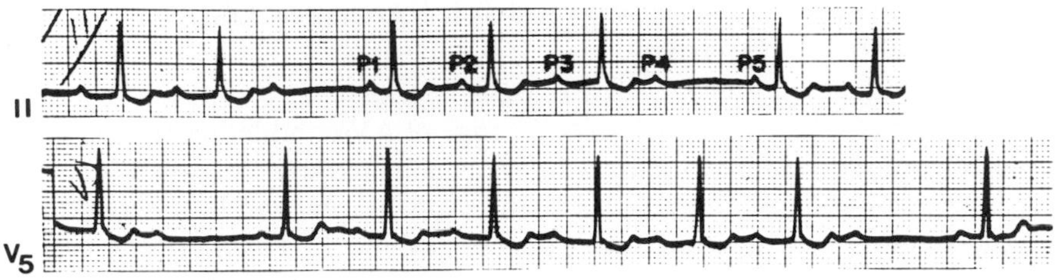

Figure 12-2. *An example of a typical Wenckebach cycle (type I A) with a 4:3 conduction ratio.*

(3) the duration of this pause is shorter than twice the sinus interval (or any RR intervals between two successive conducted beats; see Fig. 12-2).

The mechanism of gradual shortening of the RR cycle in the presence of progressive prolongation of the AV conduction time is shown in Figure 12-3. If the PR interval of two consecutively conducted sinus beats remains constant in the presence of a sinus cycle of 800 msec (0.8 second), the RR interval will also measure 800 msec. In type I block, however, the AV conduction time in the second beat is prolonged compared to that of the first beat. Assume that if the PR interval is prolonged from 180 msec to 300 msec, the RR interval becomes longer than the sinus interval by a difference of 120 msec and attains a value of 920 msec (800 + 120). If the PR interval of the third beat remains at 300 msec, an RR of 800 msec will again be obtained. Since the PR interval is further prolonged, this increment of the PR interval must again be added to the sinus cycle of 800 msec (not to the preceding RR interval of 920 msec). The increment of the PR interval between the second and third conducted beats usually is smaller than that between the first and the second conducted beats and may amount to 60 msec (360 − 300). Therefore, an RR interval of 860 msec (800 + 60) is obtained, which is shorter than the preceding RR interval of 920 msec. Such decreasing increments of AV conduction time would produce a gradual shortening of the ventricular cycle despite the progressive increase in the PR intervals. The reason for the duration of a pause shorter than two sinus cycles will also be readily understood from Figure 12-3. However, note that such a typical sequence of so-called Wenckebach phenomenon is most often noted in the presence of relatively lower conduction ratios such as 4:3 or 5:4 conduction, whereas higher conduction ratios are often associated with more atypical patterns of conduction. Hence, demonstration of a prolongation of the AV interval, at least in any of two consecutive beats, has recently been advocated by certain investigators as a criterion for the Wenckebach periodicity.

Figure 12-4 shows a record of Wenckebach phenomenon obtained in an isolated perfused rabbit heart,[13] in which membrane action potentials from the N (nodal) region of the AV node (N1) and from the proximal portion of the His bundle (N2) were recorded together with an atrial electrogram (*A*) from the sinus nodal region and a ventricular electrogram (*V*) obtained between the right ventricular apex and the left ventricular base. It can be seen from these records and the attached diagram (see Fig. 12-4) that a period of 4:3 conduction is followed by a 3:2 conduction ratio and that in both sequences the AV conduction time is progressively prolonged from 206 msec to 252 msec to 275 msec and from 230 msec to 273 msec. Hence, a typical type I block is present. Furthermore, progressive prolongation of the conduction time from the sinus nodal region to nodal fiber N1 as well as of that between nodal fibers N1 and N2 definitely suggests the presence of intranodal conduction delay. The transmembrane potentials from the N region of the AV node (N1) reveal a gradual decrease in the amplitude and upstroke velocity in successive beats, culminating in an incomplete depolarization (so-called local response) that is associated with failure of propagation to the His bundle (N2) and the ventricles. The reduction in the action potential amplitude as well as the rate of depolarization in fiber N1 may suggest decremental conduction and a decreased efficacy of the excitation wavefront. Although a slight prolongation of the conduction time is

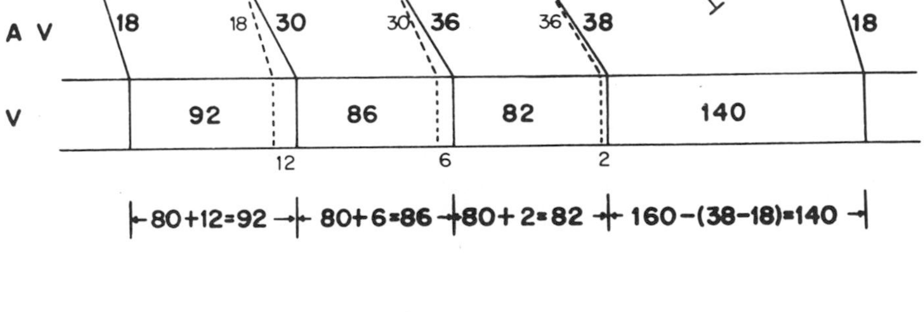

Figure 12-3. *Diagrammatic representation of a typical Wenckebach cycle. Numbers are tenths of a second.*

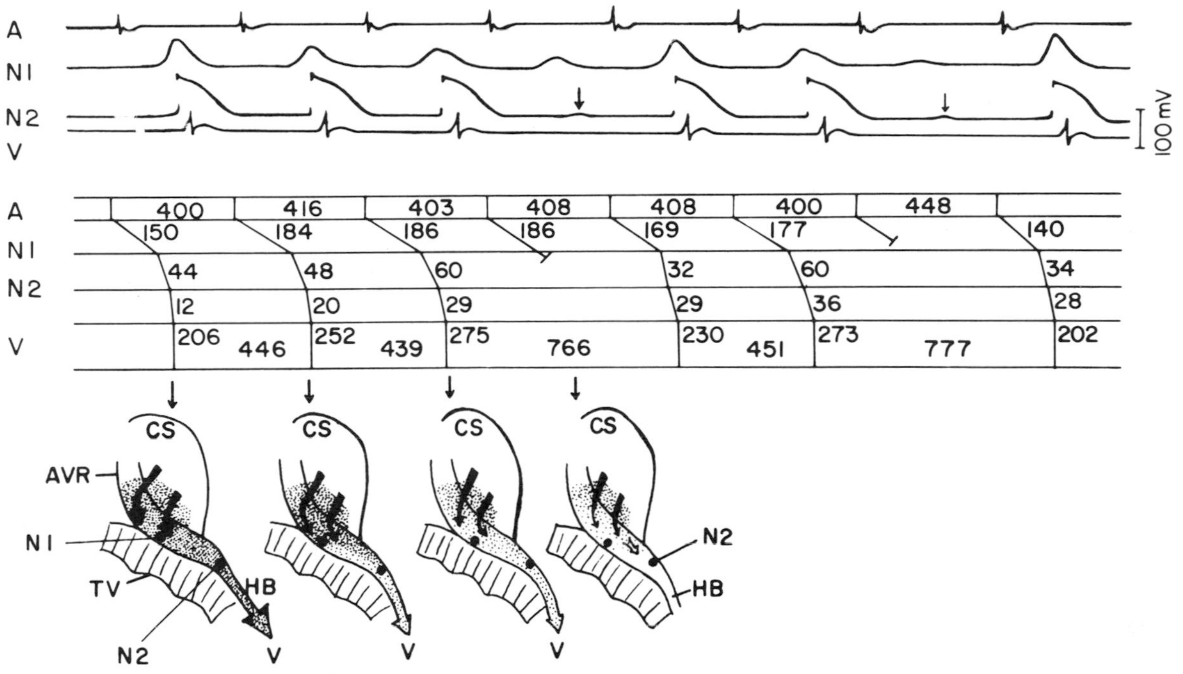

Figure 12-4. *Type I second degree AV block in an isolated perfused rabbit heart. (A, atrial electrogram; N1 and N2, transmembrane potentials from two fibers located in the N region; V, ventricular electrogram; CS, ostium of coronary sinus; AVR, fibrous atrioventricular ring; HB, His bundle)*

also noted below fiber N2 (subnodal), a major conduction delay is definitely localized within the AV node, since other records (not shown in Fig. 12-4) showed a constant conduction time from the sinus node to the atrial muscle fibers adjacent to the AV node.

In certain patients showing atypical Wenckebach phenomenon, especially in the presence of higher conduction ratios such as 7:6 conduction, the RR interval immediately preceding a pause becomes longer than that after the pause because of an increasing increment of PR interval. Identification of a pause, and hence the diagnosis of type I second degree AV block, may be difficult in these instances. It has been shown that, except for those patients with 2:1 conduction, most patients with second degree AV block with narrow QRS complexes show type I or Wenckebach periodicity. Occasionally, exceptions to this rule are noted, as shown in Figure 12-5. In the two strips of lead I shown in this figure, sinus rhythm with slight sinus arrhythmia ranging from 65 to 70 beats/min is present. The bottom record shows a regular 2:1 conduction and cannot be classified as either type I or II. However, in the top record, an initial pause due to 2:1 block is followed by the consecutive appearance of four P waves with associated QRS complexes and

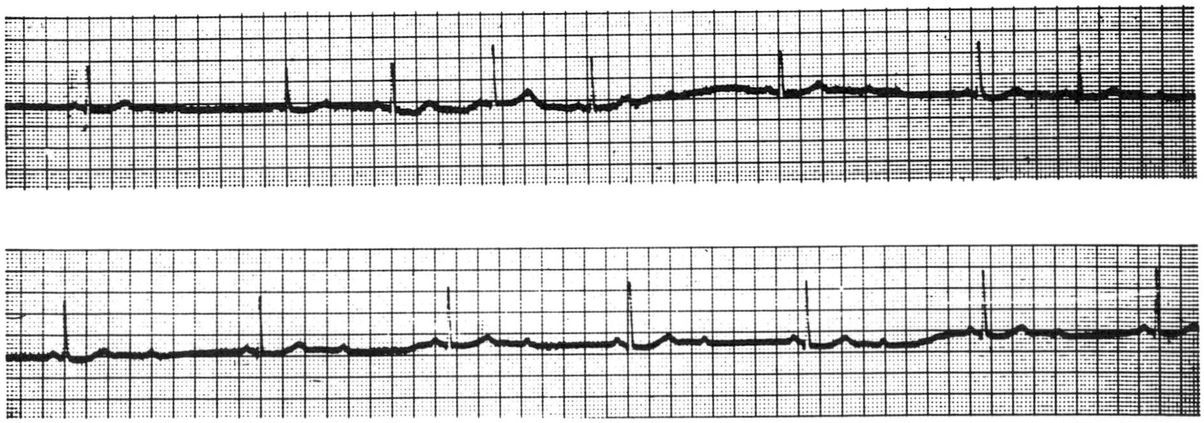

Figure 12-5. *Type II AV block with normal QRS duration.*

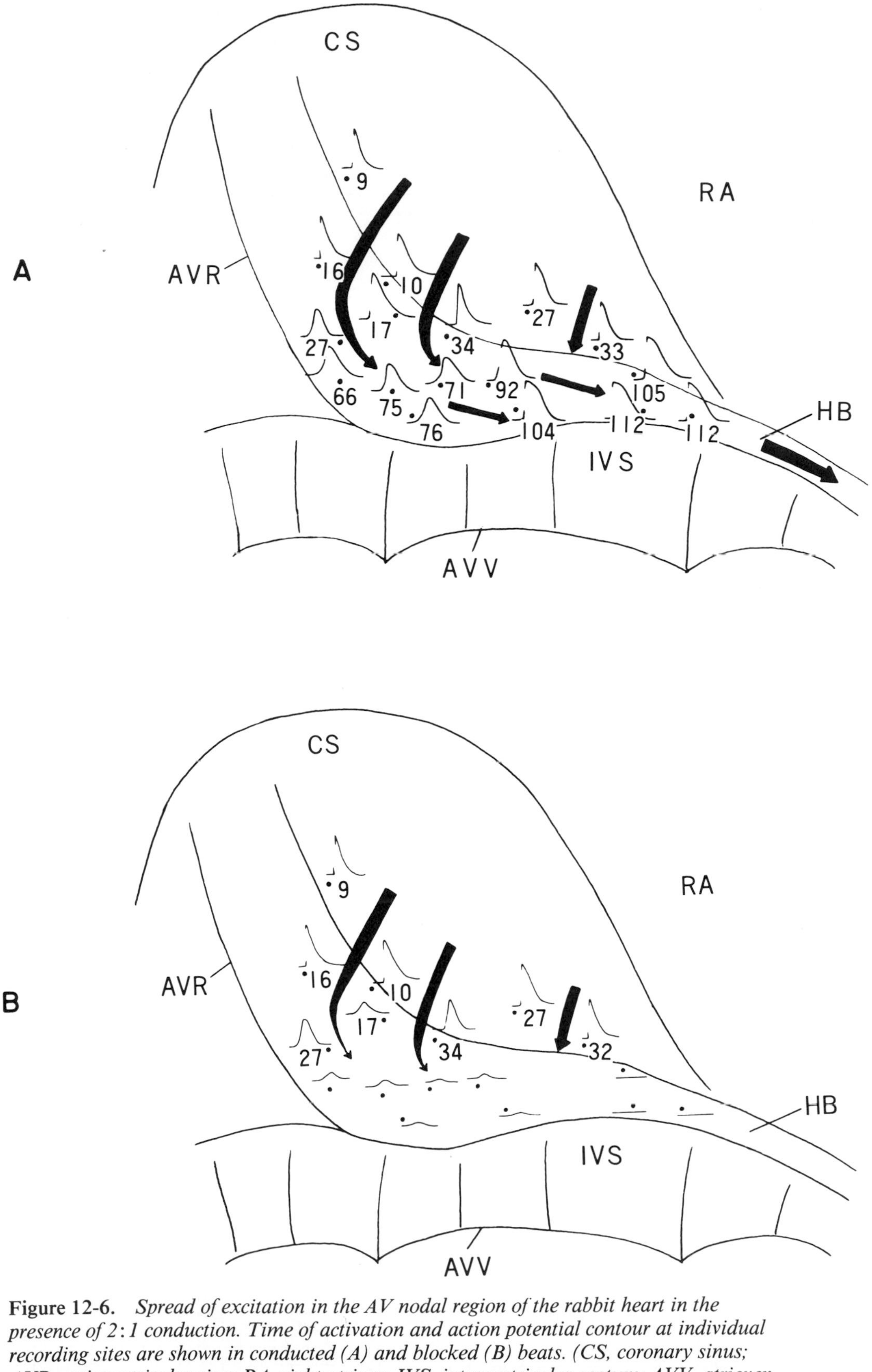

Figure 12-6. *Spread of excitation in the AV nodal region of the rabbit heart in the presence of 2:1 conduction. Time of activation and action potential contour at individual recording sites are shown in conducted (A) and blocked (B) beats. (CS, coronary sinus; AVR, atrioventricular ring; RA, right atrium; IVS, interventricular septum; AVV, atrioventricular valve)*

failure of conduction of the fifth P wave. Hence, a 5:4 conduction ratio is seen. The PR interval in these four beats remains constant at 0.16 second, satisfying the criteria for Mobitz type II AV block. An episode of 3:2 conduction seen toward the end of this strip is also accompanied by a constant AV conduction time. Sudden dropping out of a QRS complex, as seen in this case with a narrow QRS complex, suggests intra-Hisian block.

A question then arises as to the location of the site of propagation failure in these instances. Recordings of His bundle potentials are most likely to provide us with such information. Indeed, His bundle studies carried out in several similar cases suggested a concealed premature depolarization of the His bundle or AV junctional tissue as the cause of this type of block.[37,38] Whether such premature depolarization is caused by automatic impulse formation, concealed reciprocal movement (see Fig. 12-8),[8,34] or local reentry cannot be determined even with His bundle electrocardiography. Nevertheless, blockage of the impulses above the bifurcation of the His bundle appears to be the rule.

Although cases of first and second degree AV block produced by concealed premature discharge of the AV junction have been called pseudo-AV block by Langendorf and others,[37,39] here they will simply be considered as one type of AV conduction block. On the other hand, blockage of atrial impulses within the His bundle (intra-Hisian block) may present a different picture on His bundle electrocardiography. For instance, the His bundle records in certain cases show two His deflections or so-called split His potentials (usually designated as H and H^1). The interval between these two deflections (HH^1 interval) may sometimes vary, and the dropping out of a QRS complex is associated with the disappearance of the H^1 deflection in the presence of a stable AH sequence. In such instances, H and H^1 deflections are thought to be recorded from the portions of the His bundle proximal and distal to the site of depressed conduction, respectively. This type of intra-Hisian block may show either type I or II characteristics of the AV conduction time.

When transmembrane potentials were recorded from numerous fibers of the AV node during a second degree AV block with narrow QRS complexes, varying degrees of reduction in the action potential amplitude and upstroke velocity fibers were usually demonstrated.

Figure 12-6 summarizes the results of such an experiment in the presence of regular 2:1 AV conduction in isolated rabbit hearts. By plotting both the action potential configuration and the conduction time (in milliseconds) from the sinus node for individual recording sites, the spread of AV nodal excitation during conducted beats is shown in Figure 12-6*A* and that during the blocked beat is shown in Figure 12-6*B*. In the blocked beats (see Fig. 12-6*B*), the action potential becomes gradually smaller along the pathway of excitation (as shown by arrows), terminating in small fluctuations in the membrane potential within the NH region. When the action potentials from two fibers (those with activation times of 17 and 27 msec) are compared between parts *A* and *B* of the figure, the N fiber activated at 27 msec maintains a more normal action potential contour than the upstream fiber showing an activation time of 17 msec. This illustrates unequal degrees of decrement of conduction in different portions of the AV node or increased inhomogeneity of conduction.[34] Nevertheless, the occurrence of a major conduction disturbance within the N region of the AV node is evident.[8]

Second Degree Atrioventricular Block With Wide QRS Complexes

Second degree AV block in the presence of intraventricular conduction delay (QRS $\geqq$ 0.12 second) is usually associated with the Mobitz type II variety and appears to offer a more sinister prognosis than AV block with narrow QRS complexes. Hence, it is mandatory that the diagnosis and behavior of this variety of AV block be fully understood.[6,7,9,32,33] A typical example of second degree AV block, type II, is shown in Figure 12-7. In this figure, lead I shows successful transmission of six consec-

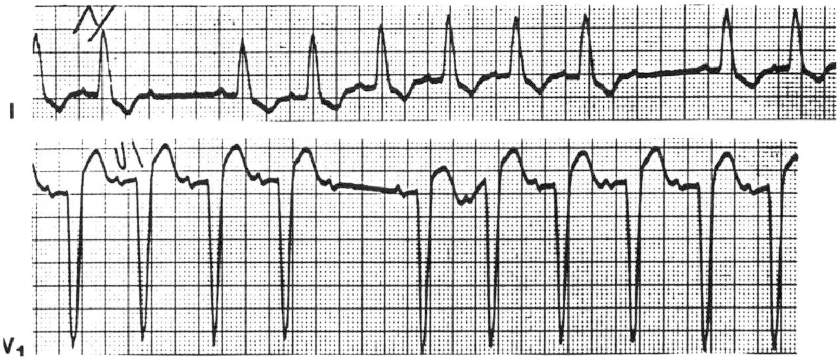

Figure 12-7. *Type II second degree AV block.*

utive sinus impulses, with the seventh P wave not being followed by a QRS complex (7:6 conduction). In this case, the PR interval remains constant in this group of six beats and in those beats occurring after a pause. In other words, a dropped ventricular complex is not preceded by a progressive prolongation of the AV conduction time. This characterizes the classic second degree AV block of Mobitz type II variety, which often is simply called type II block.[15–17,28,29] In this electrocardiogram, the QRS duration is prolonged with the pattern of left bundle branch block.

The presence of intraventricular conduction disturbance as indicated by widened ventricular complexes suggests blockage of these impulses below the bufurcation of the His bundle.

Occasionally, similar type II AV block may be produced by a premature depolarization of the AV junctional tissue that does not appear in clinical electrocardiograms. An experimental record demonstrating this mechanism is shown in Figure 12-8.[8,34] Fibers N1 and N2 in this record were considered to be located within the NH region close to the His bundle, and fiber N1 was slightly upstream to fiber N2. The presence of marked conduction delay below fiber N2 is readily noted by the record as well as the attached diagram (see Fig. 12-8). The first two atrial impulses are successfully conducted to the ventricles, and the action potential configuration in fibers N1 and N2 as well as the conduction time in each subdivision of the AV interval remain constant in these two beats. However, this is followed by a premature depolarization of fibers N1 and N2 occurring almost at the same time as the second ventricular excitation, in which the downstream fiber N2 is depolarized before fiber N1. This indicates retrograde activation of the AV nodal tissue, which does not reach the atria. The third atrial impulse occurring on time produces only a small potential change or a local response in fiber N1 (see Fig. 12-8, *arrow*) and is not transmitted to fiber N2 and the ventricles. Thus, a sudden dropping out of the ventricular complex without a preceding progressive prolongation of the AV conduction time, or typical type II block, was produced by a concealed depolarization of the AV node. The presence of a significant conduction delay below the AV node in this experiment may well suggest the development of a reciprocal movement in the His-Purkinje system. Obviously, similar examples of apparent type II AV block could be produced by a new impulse formation within the AV junction due to automaticity or any other causes, as long as such impulses depolarize only a portion of the AV conducting system and are not conducted to the ventricles. A clinical example of such concealed AV nodal premature systole causing first degree and second degree AV block patterns was reported earlier,[39] and more recent studies using His bundle electrocardiography have reconfirmed these observations.[37,38,40] It is our feeling that many cases of type II AV block without associated intraventricular conduction disturbances (see Fig. 12-7) may result from such concealed ectopic impulse formation in the AV junction. Sudden failure of AV conduction due to concealed His bundle depolarization is shown in Figure 12-8*A*. Spontaneous depolarization or reentry as shown in Figure 12-8 cannot be identified by His bundle electrograms.

Second degree AV block with wide QRS complexes

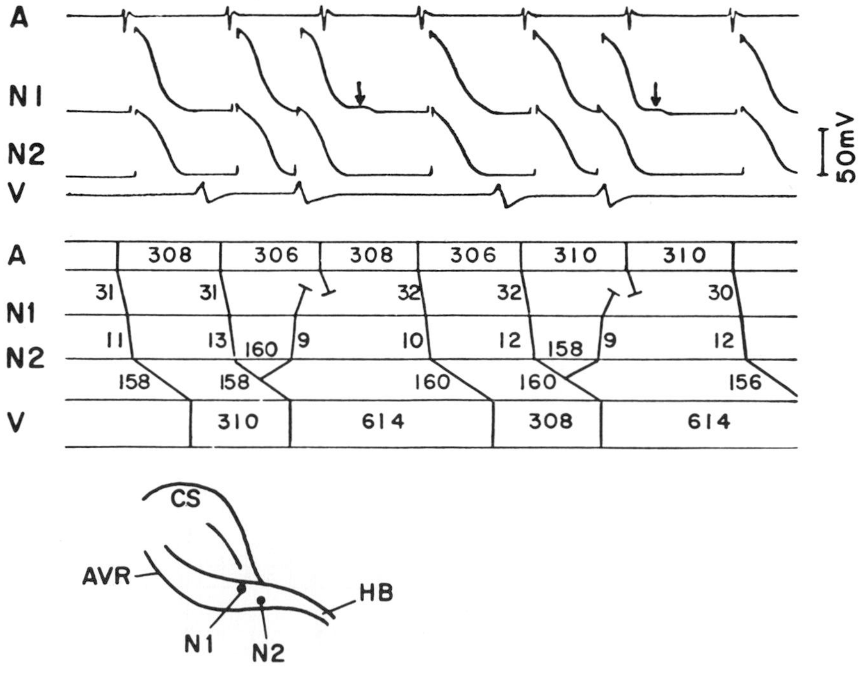

Figure 12-8. *Type II AV block produced by concealed reciprocation with premature discharge of the AV junction. (See Fig. 12-4 for key to abbreviations.)*

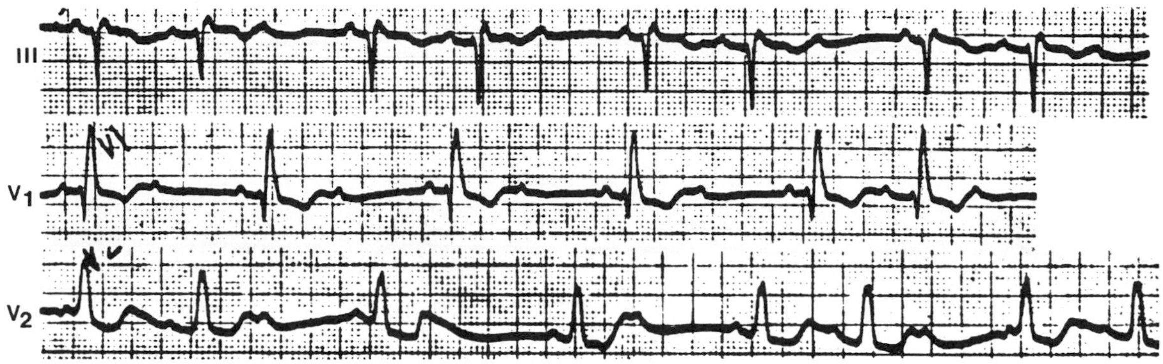

Figure 12-9. *Wenckebach conduction associated with wide QRS complexes.*

may not always be associated with type II block. One such example is shown in Figure 12-9, in which type I block (Wenckebach phenomenon) is associated with wide QRS complexes. Lead III shows persistent 3:2 conduction, with the PR interval of the second conducted beat being significantly prolonged over that of the first beat. Periods of 2:1 block are noted in leads V_1 and V_2 in addition to a similar 3:2 AV response. The QRS duration measures 0.14 second, with a right bundle branch block configuration.

Occasional interruption of typical Wenckebach sequence by an atrial reciprocal beat has often been observed in the presence of second degree AV block. One such example with wide QRS complexes is shown in Figure 12-10. In this tracing, the first three P waves are conducted to the ventricles with a progressive prolongation of the PR interval from 0.28 to 0.34 second, suggesting type I AV block. However, the T wave of the third beat is deformed and the appearance of the following sinus P wave is delayed, indicating superimposition of a premature P wave. In the presence of progressive prolongation of the AV conduction time before the appearance of such early atrial depolarization, reciprocation to the atria is strongly suggested,[41–45] and the activation sequence is interpreted as in the ladder diagram.

Following the return cycle, two consecutive sinus impulses are again successfully transmitted to the ventricles, with increasing PR intervals. This time, however, the third sinus P wave occurring exactly at the expected time is not accompanied by a QRS. Thus, a typical Wenckebach periodicity with a 3:2 conduction ratio is identified. Based on these observations, it is possible to ascribe this 3:2 response to concealed reciprocation of the second sinus impulse, which leaves the AV junction refractory at the time of attempted invasion of the third sinus impulse. Certain investigators appear to emphasize the role of this mechanism in all Wenckebach-type conduction blocks, and concealed reciprocation could actually occur within the AV junction (see Fig. 12-8). The change in the QRS configuration of the sinus beats ter-

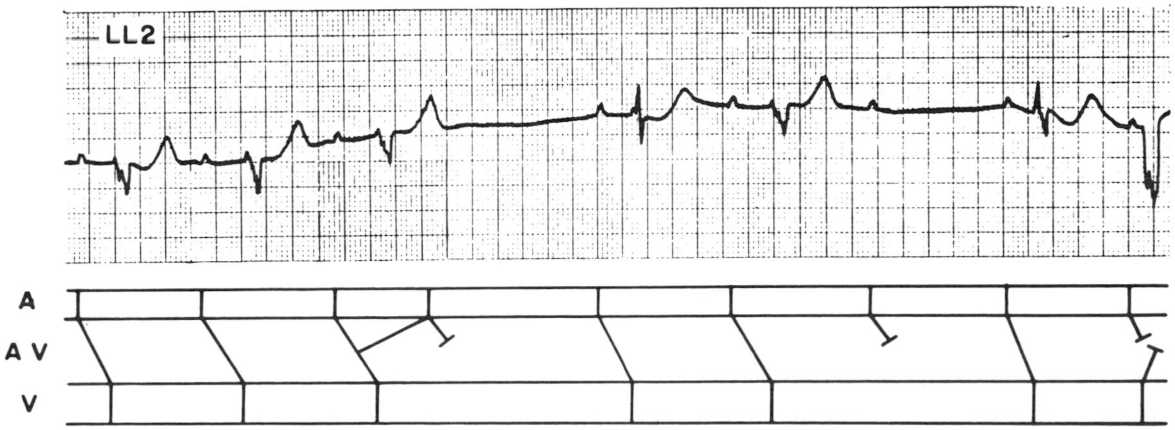

Figure 12-10. *Lead II electrocardiogram, showing interruption of a Wenckebach cycle by an atrial reciprocal complex* (left side), *and second degree block, type I, with 3:2 conduction ratio* (right side).

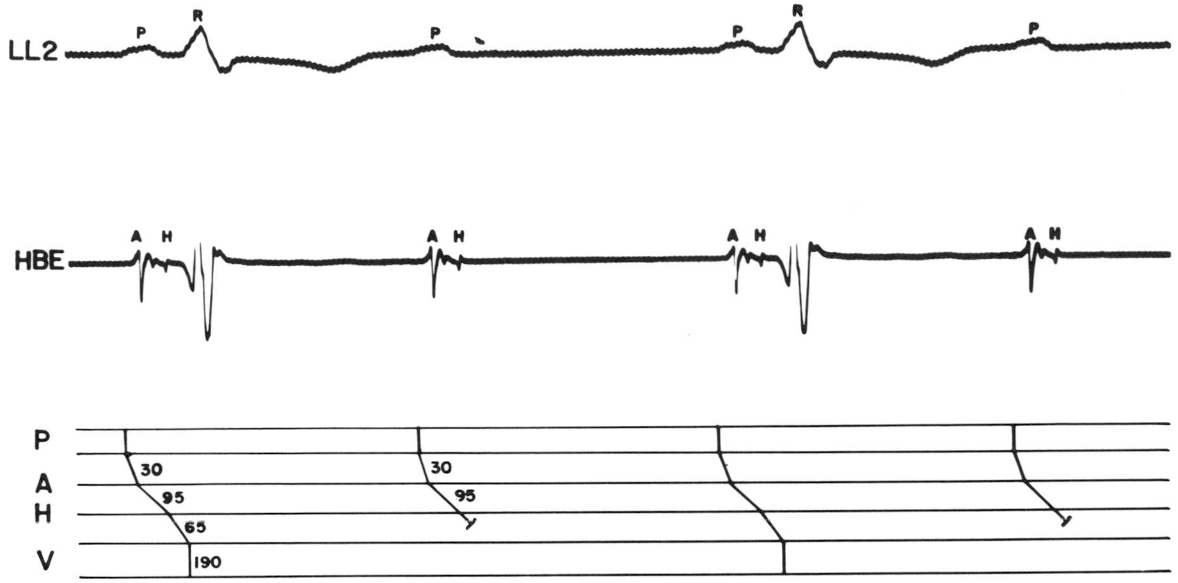

Figure 12-11. *His bundle electrogram in a case of AV block with wide QRS complexes. (P, P wave; A, atria; H, His bundle; V, ventricles)*

minating longer pauses in Figure 12-10 (beats *4* and *6*) may be explained either by a more complete recovery of conductivity in a depressed bundle (or fascicle) or by a conduction delay in other fascicles caused by phase 4 depolarization (so-called phase 4 block) slightly altering the pattern of ventricular excitation. It must also be pointed out that not all cases of premature P waves appearing in the course of a Wenckebach sequence may be attributed to atrial reciprocation, and fortuitous premature impulse formation within the atria may well interrupt the progression of type I AV block.

The Wenckebach phenomenon, or a progressive prolongation of the conduction time followed by blockage of an impulse, can be observed in any portion of myocardial tissue where conductivity is depressed and a state of decremental conduction exists. In other words, this phenomenon is not the property of the AV node alone, and it could be demonstrated even in Purkinje fibers or between contiguous ventricular myocardial fibers.[6,46,47] His bundle recordings in clinical cases also have shown the occurrence of such conduction phenomena below the AV node or in the His-Purkinje system in certain instances.[26] Furthermore, occasional cases are observed in which gradual changes in the QRS contour suggest progressive conduction delay in one of the bundle branches or fascicles, culminating in complete blockage of transmission, although a Wenckebach type of PR prolongation is not usually seen in these instances.[17,48] Thus, at least in the majority of instances, second degree AV block of the type I variety would first suggest a conduction delay within the AV node, as has been shown experimentally.[8] It may be assumed from these considerations that the Wenckebach periodicity suggests a conduction disturbance within the AV node, whereas the right bundle branch block pattern indicates abnormal intraventricular conduction, as in the case shown in Figure 12-9.[30] His bundle electrocardiography obviously would play an important role in the study of similar cases, illustrating its clinical significance. However, when His bundle electrocardiography is not available, assumption of two levels of conduction disorder in these cases will probably be sufficient, as well as safe, in the clinical management of patients with these arrhythmias.[17,30]

A His bundle electrogram obtained in a case of 2:1 conduction with wide QRS complexes is shown in Figure 12-11. Here, every other sinus impulse is conducted to the ventricles with a PR interval of 190 msec, of which the PA interval (from the onset of the P wave to excitation of the lower right atrium recorded on the His bundle electrogram) measures 30 msec, the AH interval measures 95 msec, and the HV interval (from the His deflection to the onset of ventricular depolarization) measures 65 msec. Although this HV interval is prolonged only slightly over normal, the blocked impulses are always accompanied by a His deflection, indicating successful propagation at least to the portion of the His bundle located beneath the recording electrode. Hence, the site of conduction block must be below this portion of the His bundle. Note that the portion of the His bundle that lies closest to the recording electrode cannot be precisely determined. Hence, whether these impulses are blocked below the bifurcation of the His bundle or between the recording site and this bifurcation is difficult to determine, although the presence of wide QRS complexes indicating intraventricular conduction disturbances would probably favor the bundle branch or fascicular level.

More recent studies indicate that two levels of block with so-called concealed conduction are most likely responsible for alternation of the PR interval in the presence of persistent 2 : 1 AV conduction.[9,32] This is shown in Figure 12-12. In this experiment on an isolated perfused rabbit heart, an atrial electrogram from the sinoatrial nodal region (SA), a ventricular electrogram (V), and transmembrane potentials of the NH region of the AV node (NH) were simultaneously recorded. The sinus cycle measures 530 msec, corresponding to a rate of 113 beats/min. In the top record (see Fig. 12-12*A*), every atrial impulse is associated with depolarization of the NH fiber with normal amplitude as well as the upstroke velocity of the action potential, suggesting a 1 : 1 conduction across the N region of the AV node. However, every other NH action potential is not followed by a ventricular excitation, and hence a 2 : 1 conduction block below the AV node or in the His-Purkinje system is indicated. Intraventricular conduction disturbance is evident from the wide and abnormal ventricular electrogram as well as from the marked increase in the subnodal conduction time to 160 msec compared with the normal value of 30 to 35 msec. The conduction time from the sinus node to this distal NH fiber is between 102 and 104 msec. Since a normal intra-atrial conduction time of 35 msec was demonstrated from other records, the intranodal conduction time also was prolonged to 67 to 69 msec. These observations indicate the presence of conduction disturbance both within the AV node and in the His-Purkinje system, although failure of propagation is occurring only in the His-Purkinje system.

In the bottom record (see Fig. 12-12*B*), which was obtained 3 minutes later than the top record (*A*), persistence of 2 : 1 AV block is readily noted from the ventricular electrogram. However, the AV conduction time shows an alternation of long (262 to 264 msec) and short (234 msec) intervals. This also results in alternation of short and long ventricular cycles. The mechanism for such alternation becomes apparent when the action potential record from the NH region is studied. Here it is noted that every fourth sinus impulse fails to depolarize the NH fiber, indicating a 4 : 3 conduction ratio of impulse transmission across the N region of the AV node. This intranodal block shows typical Wenckebach periodicity with progressive prolongation of the SA to NH interval from 104 msec to 116 msec and to 124 msec. Of the three sinus impulses that successfully traversed the AV node, the second one is blocked below the NH region as in Figure 12-12*A*, whereas the first and the third sinus impulses are permitted to reach the ventricles. The AV conduction time in beat 3 is much longer than that in beat 1, which results not only from a prolongation of the intranodal conduction time but also from a prolongation of the His-Purkinje conduction time from 130 msec to 140 msec. Such an increase in the His-Purkinje conduction time can be explained by a partial penetration of

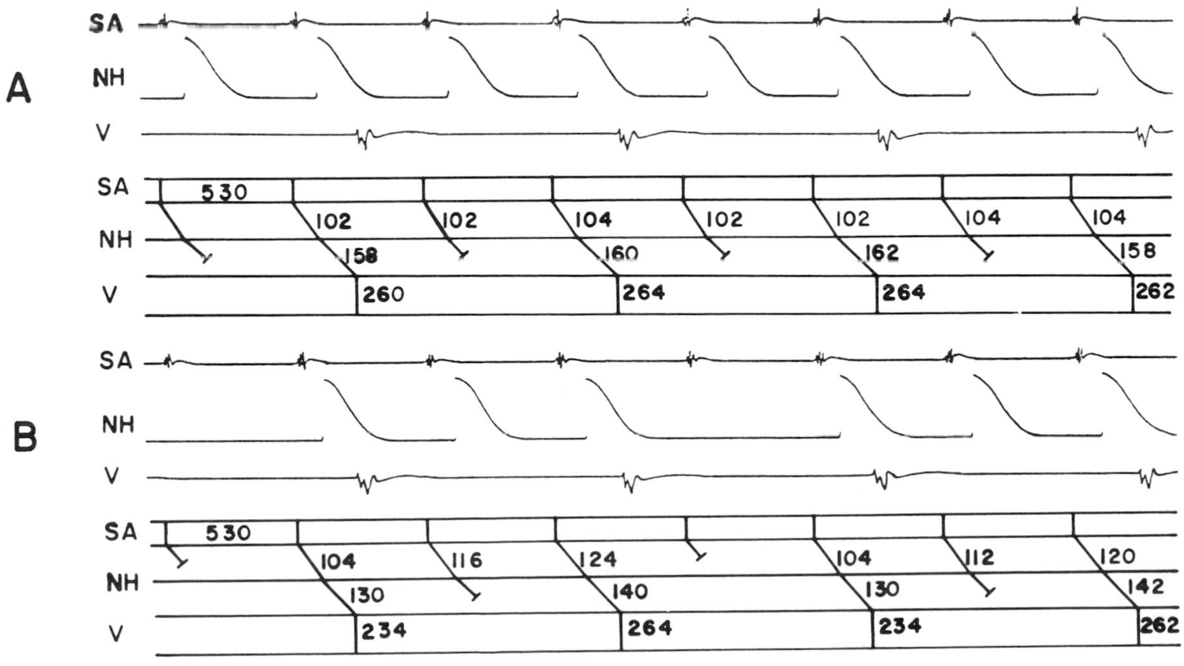

Figure 12-12. *Action potentials recorded from rabbit heart showing 2 : 1 AV block with alternation of long and short AV conduction times.*

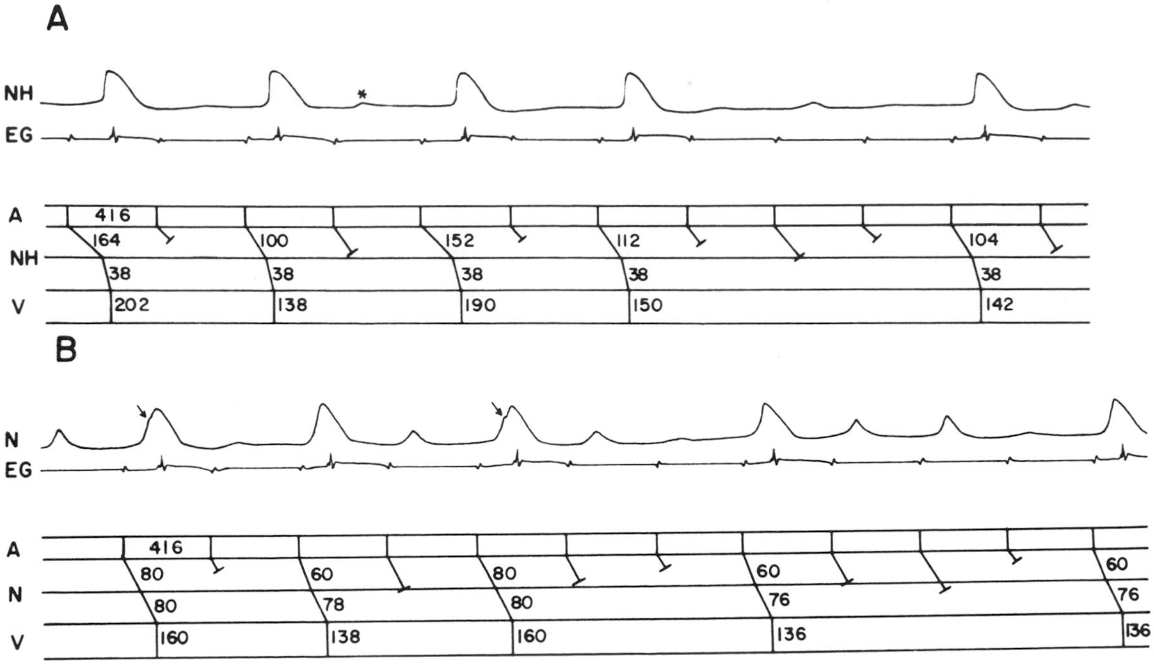

Figure 12-13. *Advanced second degree AV block with fluctuations in the depth of penetration into the AV node.*

the second atrial impulse into the His-Purkinje system, leaving a refractory tissue in its wake. After blockage of the fourth sinus impulse above the NH region of the AV node, both the intranodal and His-Purkinje conduction times are shortened, causing a return of shorter conduction time of 234 msec. Thus, it is evident that in this case 2:1 AV block with alternation of the AV conduction time was caused by the presence of two levels of conduction disturbance and an alternation of subnodal and intranodal block.

Although the longer AV interval seen in Figure 12-12*B* is almost identical to the persistently long AV interval in Figure 12-12*A*, where failure of propagation always occurs below the AV node, the ratio of intranodal and His-Purkinje conduction times is significantly different in these two records. This illustrates that the PR interval in the clinical electrocardiograms is the sum total of intra-atrial, intranodal, and subnodal conduction times, and the role played by these individual components cannot be simply evaluated. Nevertheless, these experimental findings are quite similar to the clinical electrocardiograms, supporting the concept of concealed conduction in explaining its mechanism.[6] It must also be pointed out that a 2 : 1 AV block with alternation of short and long AV conduction times may be seen only in the presence of a 4:3 conduction ratio in the intranodal transmission. When 3:2 conduction is present across the AV node, the ventricular response would show either a 3:2 or a 3:1 conduction ratio (see Fig. 12-15). Type I or type II classification cannot possibly be applied to Figures 12-11 and 12-12. The classification as well as the clinical course will necessarily rest on the lowermost level of block in these electrocardiograms. On the other hand, alternation of short and long PR intervals in the presence of 2 : 1 conduction may be explained by assuming the existence of two functionally (or anatomically) independent conducting fiber groups, a concept termed *dual pathways*.[41–45,49] Indeed, several clinical as well as experimental reports have shown possible roles of dual pathways in AV conduction and intra-atrial or interatrial conduction.[41,42] However, the ultramicroelectrode studies clearly indicate that the conduction patterns seen with so-called dual pathways can be explained by different degrees of inhomogeneous conduction and several levels of conduction delay (see Figs. 12-12 and 12-13).

Advanced Second Degree and Third Degree Atrioventricular Block

The term *advanced second degree AV block* is applied to conditions in which more than two consecutive supraventricular impulses are blocked.[9] Although its differentiation from third degree AV block sometimes becomes difficult in the presence of third degree AV block, most of the ventricular complexes are produced by impulses originating from a subsidiary automatic focus, whereas ventricular excitation in the presence of advanced second degree AV block is predominantly controlled by conducted supraventricular impulses. When one sinus impulse is conducted to the ventricles and this impulse is followed by the blockage of two consecutive impulses, it is called a 3 : 1 conduction, whereas successful transmission of one out of four P waves is termed a 4 : 1 conduction. Several examples of this type of block will be discussed below.

In the experimental records shown in Figure 12-13, transmembrane action potentials from the AV nodal region and an electrocardiogram are reproduced together with analytical diagrams.[9] The initial portion of Figure 12-13*A* shows several periods of 2 : 1 AV conduction in which the AV interval shows alternation of short and long cycles measuring 202 msec, 138 msec, 190 msec, and 150 msec. Failure of propagation always occurs above this NH fiber, and the His-Purkinje or subnodal conduction time remains constant almost within the normal range. Judged from the ventricular complexes in the electrocardiogram, there are no intraventricular conduction disturbances. Thus, it appears that there is only one level of block. However, fluctuations in the size of local responses in this NH fiber suggest that the alternation of the AV conduction time results from different depths of penetration into the AV node by these blocked impulses. For instance, the second and sixth atrial excitation waves (the small diphasic deflections in the electrocardiogram) are followed by hardly any changes in the membrane resting potential of this NH fiber, although the fourth atrial impulse produces a slightly greater potential change (local response), indicating a slightly deeper penetration. This prolongs the AV conduction time of the fifth atrial impulse compared with the other conducted beats, an effect of concealed conduction. A period of 4 : 1 AV response is seen following the period of 2 : 1 conduction, as discussed above. During this 4 : 1 conduction, the second of the three consecutively blocked impulses produces a slightly greater potential change, suggesting a deeper penetration of this particular impulse. A similar phenomenon is commonly seen in the presence of 4 : 1 conduction.

In Figure 12-13*B*, which was recorded 3 minutes after *A*, three periods of 2 : 1 AV conduction are followed by 3 : 1 and 4 : 1 responses. The transmembrane potentials recorded from the N region of the AV node during the periods of 2 : 1 conduction again demonstrate fluctuations in the levels of propagation failure, with resultant alternation of the AV conduction time. When a blocked impulse penetrates deeper into the AV node, the subsequent action potential from this N fiber shows a decreased upstroke velocity, with slurring or notching of phase 0. This finding suggests the presence of either decremental or inhomogeneous conduction. From the sequence of alternating levels of concealment during the periods of 2 : 1 conduction, the sixth atrial impulse is expected to be blocked at a relatively proximal portion of the AV node, but it apparently penetrates again deeper as judged by the amplitude of this local response. Intranodal blockage of the subsequent seventh atrial impulse and the production of a 3 : 1 conduction ratio most likely result from deeper concealment. Thus, in advanced second degree AV block, variations in the depth of penetration appear to be the rule even when failure of propagation always occurs within the AV nodal tissue.

Other mechanisms such as concealed reentry movements could contribute to the development of AV conduction block.[9]

When conditions similar to atrial flutter are produced experimentally by increasing the frequency of atrial stimulation in isolated rabbit hearts, 2 : 1 AV conduction is also commonly seen above certain rapid rates of stimulation. In these instances, every other atrial impulse is blocked within the AV node, although occasional examples similar to those in Figure 12-12 have also been observed.

In third degree or high-grade AV block, ventricular excitation is predominantly controlled by a subsidiary pacemaker and the sinus or atrial impulses are rarely transmitted to the ventricles. It is obvious that the classification of types I and II of second degree AV block cannot be applied to this type of block.

In the example of third degree AV block reproduced in Figure 12-14*A*, there is sinus bradycardia with a moderate sinus arrhythmia. However, the P waves and QRS complexes are independent of each other, with the ventricular rate being constant at 30 beats/min. The QRS duration is within normal limits, measuring 0.07 second, and hence the automatic focus is most likely located above the bifurcation of the His bundle. This suggests a site of block upstream to this subsidiary pacemaker and probably within the AV node.[17,30,33]

In Figure 12-14*B*, fine undulations of the baseline indicate the presence of atrial fibrillation, and the ventricular complexes appear quite regularly at the rate of 40 beats/min. Thus, the presence of a subsidiary pacemaker is diagnosed.[15–17] In order for such an escape mechanism to continue to be active, a high-degree conduction disturbance with blockage of most impulses from the fibrillating atria must be postulated. The normal QRS duration in this instance suggests the site of conduction failure to be within the AV junction and most likely the AV node. With excessive administration of cardiac glycosides, a conduction disturbance due to digitalis should first be suspected as the mechanism of this type of disturbance. On the other hand, when the ventricular cycles in the presence of atrial fibrillation are not exactly regular,

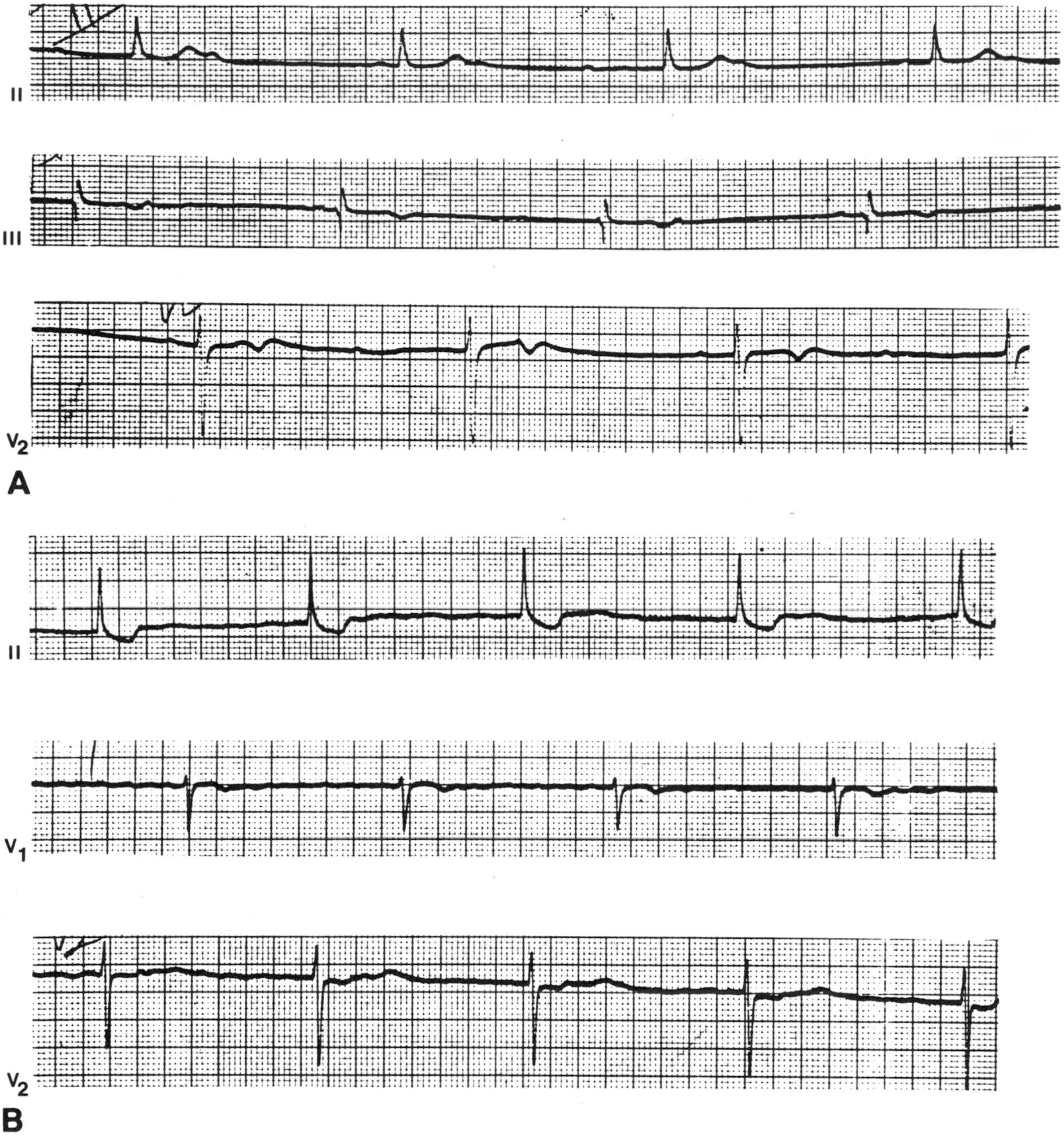

Figure 12-14. *Third degree AV block with narrow QRS complexes in the presence of sinus rhythm (A) and atrial fibrillation (B).*

as in this case, but many RR intervals are identical, frequent occurrence of escape beats because of a possible second degree AV block may be suggested. However, when there are no definite criteria on the percentage of RR intervals that are identical, suggesting escape beats in any long strip, second degree block should be suspected. Hence, the diagnosis in those instances may be more subjective than empirical, in contrast to the cases of third degree AV block as shown in Figure 12-14*B*. Nevertheless, a clinician must be alert to the possibility of digitalis excess in these instances.

Advanced Second Degree and Third Degree Atrioventricular Block, Type B

Advanced second degree and third degree AV block can also be seen in the presence of wide QRS complexes.[33]

The experimental records shown in Figure 12-15 were obtained several minutes after those shown in Figure 12-12. In Figure 12-15, transmembrane potentials from an atrial fiber adjacent to the AV node (A) and from the NH region of the AV node (NH) are shown together with

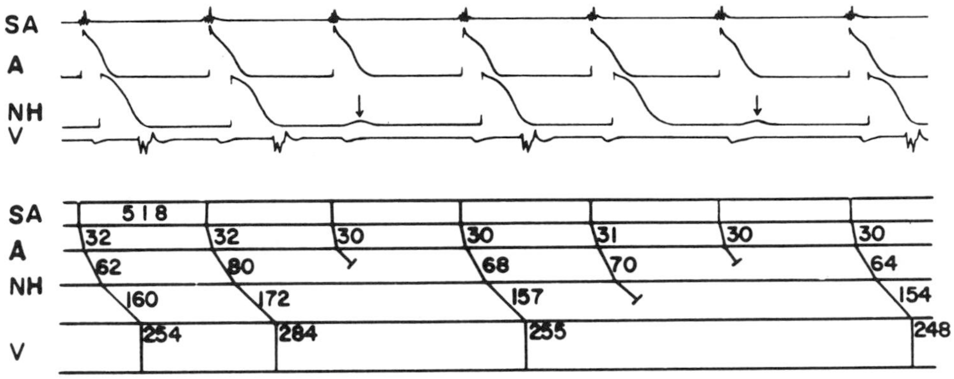

Figure 12-15. *Two levels of block (AV node and His-Purkinje system) causing 3:2 and 3:1 AV conduction ratios in the rabbit heart.*

an electrogram from the sinus node area (SA) and a ventricular electrogram (V). In the initial part of this figure, two consecutive atrial impulses fully depolarize the NH fiber and are conducted to the ventricles, but both the intranodal and His-Purkinje conduction times become prolonged in the second beat. The third atrial impulse causes only incomplete depolarization of the NH fiber (see Fig. 12-15, *arrow*) and fails to propagate to the ventricles. Hence, a 3:2 conduction with Wenckebach periodicity is diagnosed. Subsequently, two atrial impulses again produce normal action potentials in this NH fiber, indicating a successful intra-AV nodal conduction. However, only the first impulse is transmitted to the ventricles, while the second impulse is blocked below the NH region, most likely within the His-Purkinje system. Failure of propagation of the third impulse occurs above this NH fiber as in the initial sequence, thus resulting in a 3:1 response. Note that two such levels of block, one within and the other below the AV node, are associated with an intraventricular conduction disturbance as shown by the widened ventricular complexes and prolonged His-Purkinje conduction time. In contrast to the 4:3 intranodal conduction ratio observed in Figure 12-12, the 3:2 ratio in the record in Figure 12-15 may well suggest further depression of the intranodal conduction. Indeed, a 2:1 intranodal block developed some time after Figure 12-15 was recorded. It is possible that when intraventricular conduction disturbances are sufficiently severe and extensive to cause AV block, the same pathophysiologic mechanisms would often involve the AV nodal region also.

In Figure 12-15 the second of the two atrial impulses successfully traversing the AV node was conducted to the ventricles at one time, but was blocked within the His-Purkinje system at another time, even though a constant conduction ratio of 3:2 is present in the intra-AV nodal conduction. A brief discussion of its mechanism appears in order. First, it is possible that the His-Purkinje conductivity shows temporal fluctuations,[9,32] and thus a slight improvement in conductivity causes a 3:2 response, whereas the lowering of conductivity results in 3:1 conduction (as seen in the right half of Fig. 12-15). On the other hand, blockage of the third atrial impulse within the AV node in the presence of a 3:2 ratio would result in a reduced frequency of excitation in the His-Purkinje system. Therefore, the first conducted beat after such a pause would be associated with a marked prolongation of the action potential duration and the refractory period of these Purkinje fibers. Because of such prolonged refractoriness, the second atrial impulse after the pause may be blocked at the His-Purkinje level, a mechanism often referred to as *phase 3 block.* In this particular record, an action potential duration greater than 500 msec must be postulated in the Purkinje system in order to invoke this latter mechanism. Although this duration appears rather long, such values of action potential duration in the Purkinje fibers have often been observed under various experimental conditions.

Figure 12-16 illustrates a case of third degree AV block with wide QRS complexes as compared to Figure 12-19.[30,33] In the top two strips recorded on June 21 (Fig. 12-16), the sinus P waves as well as several ectopic P waves have no constant time relationship with ventricular excitation, and the QRS complexes appear quite regularly at the rate of 44 beats/min. The wide QRS with a pattern of right bundle branch block indicates the location of the subsidiary pacemaker in or around the left bundle branch system. Third degree AV block is easily diagnosed. The bottom half of Figure 12-16 shows the electrocardiogram recorded 2 days later; a regular ventricular rhythm persists despite the presence of atrial fibrillation as indicated by the undulations in the baseline. The ventricular rate here is slightly faster, at 49 beats/min. That there has been no change in the QRS configuration is seen in leads aV_F and V_1, indicating control of the ventricles by the same subsidiary focus as 2 days previously. The third beat in lead aV_R and the second beat in lead aV_F (the latter is distorted by 1-mV calibration pulse) represent ventricular premature complexes. Since the interval between these premature QRS complexes and the following QRS of the escape rhythm is either equal to (in lead aV_R) or slightly longer than (in

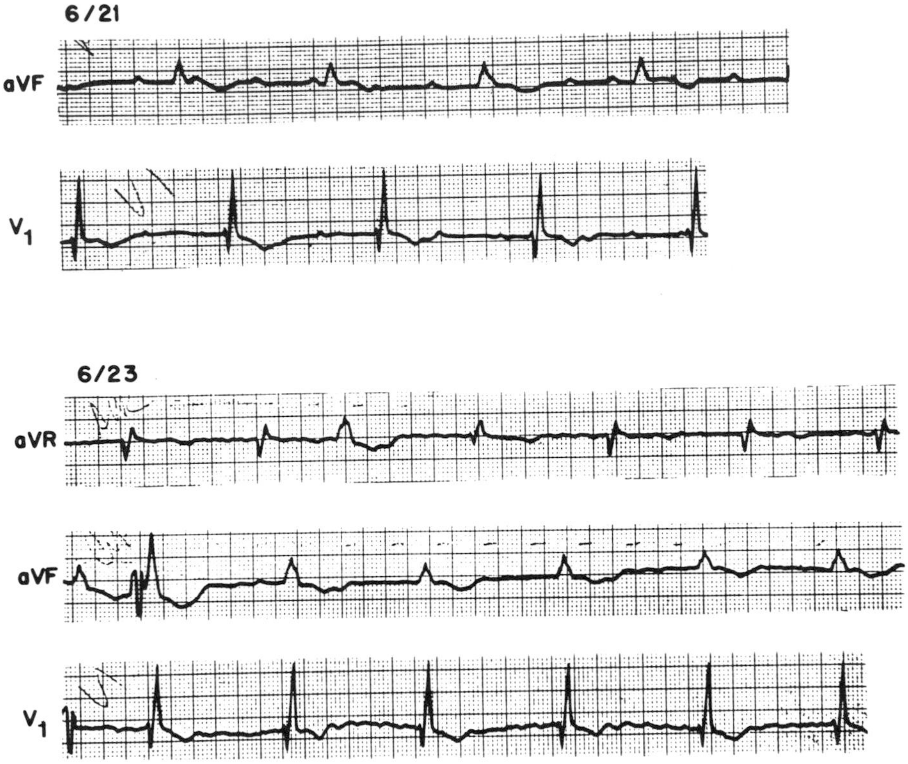

Figure 12-16. *High-grade AV block with escape rhythms originating from the region of the left bundle branch system during both sinus rhythm* (top) *and atrial fibrillation* (bottom).

lead aV_F) other RR intervals, premature discharge of the subsidiary pacemaker by the retrograde conduction of extrasystolic impulses and resetting of its automaticity are suggested. In this instance, the site of propagation failure most likely is below the bifurcation of the His bundle.

However, note that when high grade AV block is observed in the presence of atrial fibrillation, the possibility of intra-AV nodal conduction disturbance in addition to a subjunctional block is much greater compared with the cases of sinus rhythm with high grade AV block. The reason for this is that since the atrial excitation waves during atrial fibrillation are quite irregular and less effective as stimuli to the AV node,[53–56] intranodal block develops more easily than in the presence of a sinus mechanism. Hence, when an electrocardiogram as shown at the bottom of Figure 12-16 is observed alone, especially in the presence of digitalis administration, development of a third degree AV block at the AV nodal level in addition to preexistent bundle branch block must be suspected before a high-grade conduction block within the His-Purkinje system is diagnosed. For this differentiation, comparison of similar electrocardiographic records or a transient withdrawal of digitalis may be of help, but a definitive diagnosis with the use of His bundle electrocardiography may be needed in certain selected cases.

Other Mechanisms Contributing to Atrioventricular Conduction Disorders

Although inhomogeneous conduction and fragmentation in a pathway usually produce conduction delay and block, other conduction phenomena such as unidirectional conduction, summation, and so-called supernormal conduction can be explained by the unusual features seen in the following figures.

With reference to these conduction phenomena, an experimental record from an isolated perfused rabbit heart (Fig. 12-17) is of interest. During the period of 4 : 3 AV conduction seen in the middle portion of this record, the AV conduction time is initially increased from 190 to 210 msec and then again shortened to 197 msec. Such findings contradict the classic type I block (Wenckebach phenomenon), and the paradoxical shortening of the AV interval, instead of a further prolongation, may be interpreted as supernormal conduction. When the action potentials from the N region of the AV node (N) are examined, the first beat of the 4 : 3 conduction shows a normal action potential contour, whereas the second atrial impulse produces a doubly peaked action potential with a markedly decreased rate of depolarization resulting in a prolongation of the conduction time from this N fiber to the ventricles (from 78 to 10 msec). The action potential

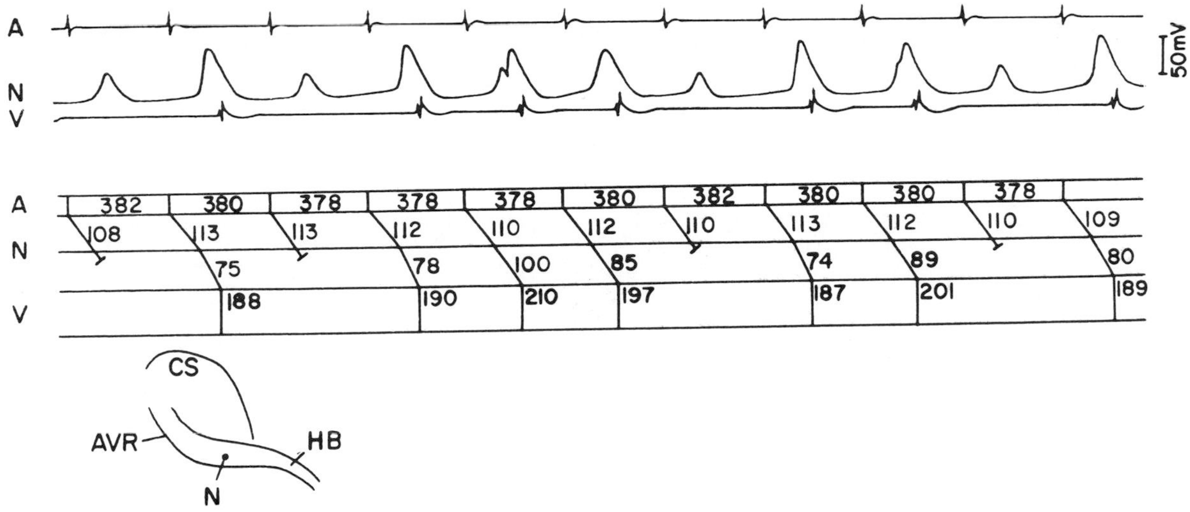

Figure 12-17. *An experimental record of so-called supernormal conduction.*

in the N fiber associated with the third atrial impulse shows a smoother upstroke of phase 0, although the rate of depolarization is not significantly greater, and the conduction time to the ventricles is again shortened to 85 msec. The last (fourth) atrial complex depolarizes the N fiber only incompletely and is not conducted to the ventricles. These findings may be explained by our concept of inhomogeneous conduction as follows: a marked inhomogeneity of intranodal conduction in the second beat resulted in decreased efficacy of its excitation wave, thus delaying conduction below this N region. In contrast, the third beat was somehow associated with a more homogeneous excitation front within the AV node, and its greater efficacy as a stimulus caused a better subnodal conduction. Thus, slight fluctuations of conductivity within the AV junction may well produce this type of supernormal conduction,[9,32,33] although the reason for such fluctuation cannot be readily determined.

Several abnormal conduction phenomena resulting from alterations in the primary determinants of conductivity, as listed on page 299, deserve a brief comment. First, the term *decremental conduction* can be defined as a gradual decrease both in the effectiveness of stimuli and in the magnitude of response along the pathway of conduction in anatomically uniform but functionally depressed tissue.[38,40] From the previous discussion, it will be readily understood that decremental conduction would more easily be produced in the N region of the AV node where the action potentials show inherently slow upstroke and reduced amplitude even under physiologic conditions.[46,57] It is true that the sequential changes in the action potential characteristics from the atrial fiber to the so-called AN region and then to the N region of the AV node may superficially mimic decremental conduction without any depression of conductivity (see Fig. 12-6). However, the changes here probably result from nonuniform anatomic structures and associated differences in their membrane characteristics and hence should not be regarded as decremental conduction.

The second abnormal conduction phenomenon, or what we call *inhomogeneous conduction,*[8,34] is explained as follows: when decremental conduction develops nonuniformly at one portion of the conducting pathway, the wavefront of excitation becomes quite irregular. The overall effectiveness of stimuli is then decreased compared with that in the presence of a smoother excitation front and a synchronous depolarization of neighboring fibers (compare with Fig. 12-4). As a result, conductivity is further depressed, leading to either delay or failure of propagation.[62] It will be easily understood that in a strand of conducting tissue in which fibers run parallel to and in close contact with one another, there would be less chance for inhomogeneous conduction. Contrariwise, when small fibers are rather sparsely distributed or show frequent ramifications and anastomoses to form a complex network as in the AV node, fragmentation of the wavefront is more readily produced.

Several experimental observations supporting this concept include collision of two impulses within the AV node, producing a greater amplitude and upstroke velocity of action potential.[44] It has also been demonstrated that when excitation waves originating from two different portions of the right atrium invade the AV nodal tissue almost simultaneously, transnodal conduction either takes place more rapidly or becomes successful, whereas arrival of only one wavefront or of two grossly asynchronous wavefronts results in much slower conduction or blockage in the node (Fig. 12-18).[9,32,33] Thus,

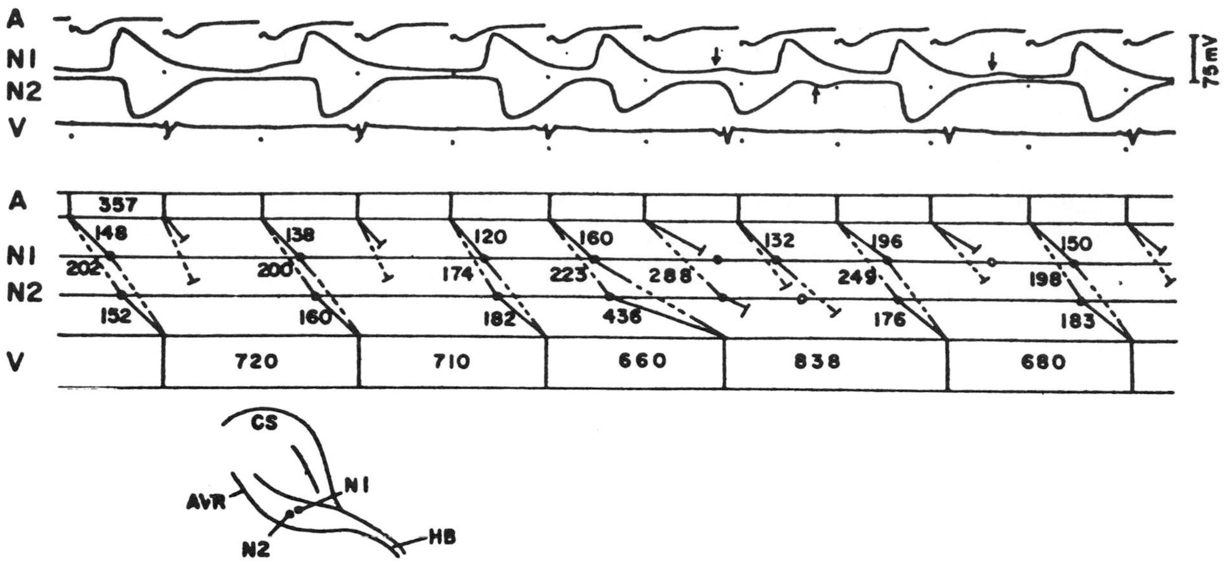

Figure 12-18. *Experimental record illustrating possible role of summation of excitation fronts in successful propagation during second degree AV block in an isolated rabbit heart. (A, atrial electrogram; N1 and N2, transmembrane potentials from two fibers located in the N region; N2 potentials are recorded with reversed polarity; V, ventricular electrogram. Right atrium electrically stimulated at a constant rate.* Schematic map of AV junctional region shown at bottom: *CS, ostium of coronary sinus; AVR, fibrous atrioventricular ring; HB, His bundle.) The Lewis-type diagram at the bottom illustrates sequence of excitation. Although fibers N1 and N2 are located close to each other and almost parallel to the direction of conduction, asynchrony of depolarization is seen between these fibers. Following four atrial beats with a 2:1 AV response, two successive atrial impulses are conducted, the second one showing a reduced action potential amplitude in both fibers and a more prolonged AV interval. The next (seventh) atrial beat produces an action potential in fiber N2 similar in size to that in the preceding conducted beat. However, only a local response* (downward arrow) *is seen in fiber N1, and excitation fails to reach the ventricles. Contrarily, the following (eighth) atrial impulse produces an action potential in fiber N1 but only a local response* (upward arrow) *in fiber N2. Conduction to the ventricles again fails. Finally, the ninth beat is associated with more normal action potentials in both fibers and results in ventricular excitation. Hence, under depressed conduction successful propagation appears to occur when two or more apparently independent wavefronts are simultaneously engaged.*

the significance of inhomogeneous conduction in this tissue must be emphasized. It must further be pointed out that the mode of invasion of impulses into the AV node appears quite important in determining the difficulty or ease of intra-AV nodal conduction.[9,32,34] When inhomogeneity of conduction is markedly increased, failure of propagation may occur in one side of the AV node, while a slow but successful conduction occurs in the other side,[34] a phenomenon called *functional longitudinal dissociation.* Such longitudinal dissociation is said to develop in other cardiac tissues, including the His bundle and bundle branches. Nevertheless, inhomogeneous conduction is considered a parallel (transverse) expression and decremental conduction is considered a series (longitudinal) expression of depressed conductivity.[9,33,34]

A similar concept of dual AV nodal pathways has been advocated by several investigators based on both experimental[19] and clinical electrophysiologic[69] observations, as briefly described earlier. This concept involves the presence of two pathways within the nodal tissue, one having a greater conduction velocity but a longer refractory period and the other having a slower conduction velocity but a shorter refractory period. Hence, a premature atrial impulse can be blocked in the fast pathway because of the longer refractory period and conducted to the ventricles through the slow pathway with a markedly prolonged conduction time.[69] Under appropriate conditions, this slow anterograde conduction allows a successful retrograde conduction to the atria through the slow pathway, engendering a reciprocating AV junctional tachycardia. Such dual pathways

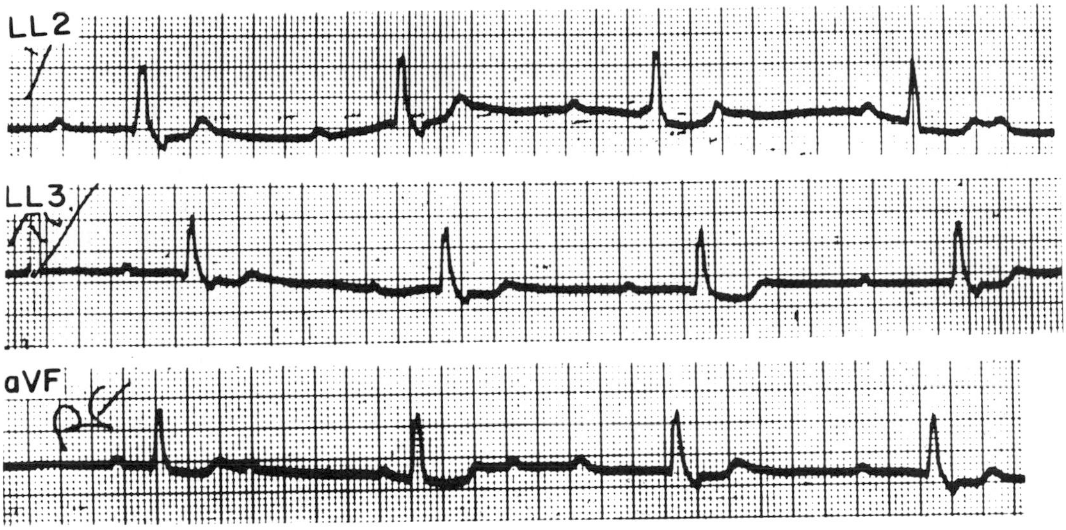

Figure 12-19. *High-grade AV block, type B, with unidirectional retrograde conduction to the atria. (LL2, lead II; LL3, lead III; aVF, lead aV$_F$)*

may then play a more important role in producing tachyarrhythmias rather than in causing AV block. However, more recent studies by Iinuma and associates[44] suggest that the dual AV nodal pathways may simply reflect two atrial inputs to the AV node or the crista terminalis and the interatrial septum. Blockage of an atrial excitation front in one of these two inputs indeed was shown to set up a reentry movement involving the AV node and the perinodal region. With this mechanism, it is also possible that asynchronous engagement of the two inputs can result in a depressed AV nodal conduction, as has been illustrated in Figure 12-18.

Examples of unidirectional conduction are illustrated in Figures 12-19 and 12-20. Other manifestations of AV

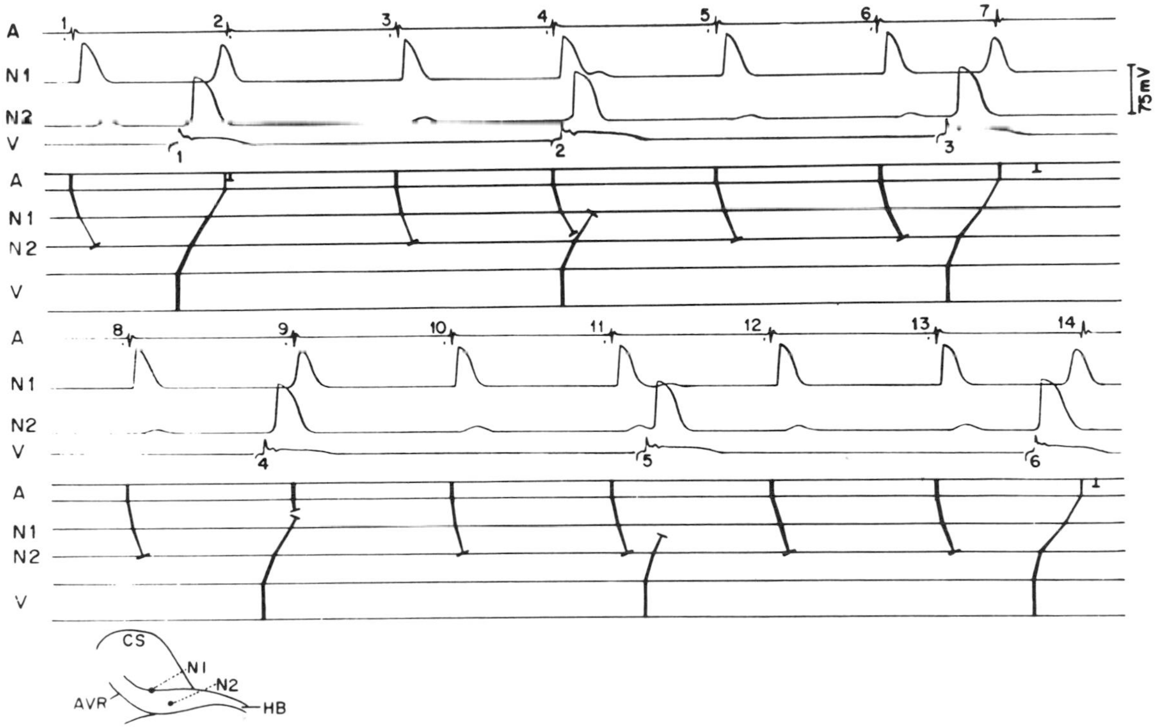

Figure 12-20. *Experimental records showing unidirectional retrograde conduction in an isolated perfused rabbit heart. (See Fig. 12-18 for key to abbreviations.)*

conduction such as unidirectional conduction are shown in Figure 12-19. In this figure, high-grade AV block is easily diagnosed from the regular appearance of ventricular complexes at the rate of 37 beats/min without any fixed relationships with preceding P waves. In lead aV_F, for instance, the first four P waves appear at constant PP intervals showing a rate of 70 beats/min. The fifth P wave appears prematurely and is considered an atrial extrasystole, which also fails to be conducted to the ventricles. Thus, the orthograde (or AV) conduction is always blocked. On the other hand, more than half the ventricular complexes are immediately followed by inverted P waves (beats *1* and *2* in lead II (LL 2); beats *1*, *2*, and *4* in lead III (LL 3); and beats *3* and *4* in lead aV_F), which clearly reset the sinus rhythm and produce the phenomenon of return cycle. Hence, atrial excitation by retrograde (VA) conduction or the presence of unidirectional AV conduction can be diagnosed. A closer examination of the time relationships between the QRS complexes and the P waves reveals that those ventricular complexes terminating relatively short PR intervals (these do not represent AV conduction time, since the P waves are not conducted to the ventricles) are not followed by retrograde conduction. More precisely, retrograde conduction to the atria appears to be permitted when a QRS occurs at least 0.38 second after the attempted invasion of the AV conducting system by the blocked sinus impulses. This indicates that after the refractory period of the AV conducting system caused by concealed orthograde conduction has expired, retrograde impulses may successfully traverse the site of block and reach the atria.

It is noted that in Figure 12-19 the third beat in lead III is not followed by a retrograde P wave even though its interval from the preceding sinus P wave appears to be sufficiently long. This finding can be explained by collision of a retrograde impulse in the AV junctional tissue with attempted forward conduction of an atrial premature systole, which occurred simultaneously with this particular QRS complex. The findings that support this interpretation are as follows: (1) the interval between the third QRS complex and the preceding P wave (0.44 second) is almost identical to the coupling intervals of atrial premature beats seen in other portions of the record (0.44 to 0.46 second) and (2) if an ectopic P wave were hidden in this QRS complex, the interval from this P wave to the following sinus P wave would measure approximately 1.04 second, the same value as other return cycles following retrograde P waves.

One might ask what electrophysiologic mechanisms play a role in producing unidirectional conduction. Some investigators deny the possibility of a retrograde conduction through the site of orthograde block and believe that a mechanical effect of ventricular contraction somehow facilitates impulse formation in the automatic AV junctional fibers above the site of block.[59,60] Another theory states that the electrotonic spread of a retrograde impulse jumps over the site of block and excites the atria.[61] However, we feel that the most likely explanation is different degrees of decrement in forward versus retrograde conduction.[32,33,62] Figure 12-20 shows an experimental record of unidirectional conduction within the AV junctional tissue[62] that is quite similar to the clinical observation in Figure 12-19.

In Figure 12-20, the action potentials from the AN region (N1) and the NH region (N2) of the AV node are recorded together with the atrial (A) and ventricular (V) electrograms. The stimulus artifacts seen in these electrograms clearly indicate that the atria and the ventricles are electrically stimulated at different rates. The action potentials of fiber N1, except for those numbered 2, 7, 9, and 14, always follow the atrial excitation, but they cause only partial depolarization of fiber N2 and fail to be conducted to the ventricles. Thus, high-grade block in a forward direction is present. In contrast, the ventricular impulses always fully depolarize fiber N2 in the NH region. When a N2 action potential occurs immediately after depolarization of fiber N1 due to atrial excitation (ventricular impulses numbered *2* and *5*), it produces local response in fiber N1, and the retrograde conduction does not proceed any further. This suggests that the success or failure of retrograde activation of fiber N1 depends on the excitability or refractoriness in this area. Later appearance of the N2 action potentials with reference to the previous depolarization of fiber N1 (numbers *1*, *3*, *4*, and *6*) is followed by an action potential in N1, which, although showing a slow upstroke velocity, is successfully transmitted to the atria to cause atrial excitation (atrial numbers *2*, *7*, and *14*). When such a retrograde impulse encounters the atrial refractory period (numbered *9*), it is probably blocked between this fiber N1 and the site of the atrial recording electrode. Hence, this is considered an example of unidirectional conduction within the N region of the AV node. It is likely that those clinical cases of high grade AV block[63,64] in which ventricular pacing produces a 1:1 retrograde conduction are associated with similar mechanisms.

On the other hand, a group of clinical phenomena called *supernormal AV conduction* (Figs. 12-21 and 12-22) is still controversial,[15,65–68] with some investigators even denying its presence. Although several different varieties of supernormal AV conduction have been identified, only part of this complex problem will be discussed in this chapter. It must first be pointed out that this term is applied when an unexpected improvement in conduction is noted in the presence of depressed conductivity (either in AV conduction or in conduction in any other portion of the myocardium). For instance, successful conduction when failure of propagation is expected or the occurrence of a shorter conduction time

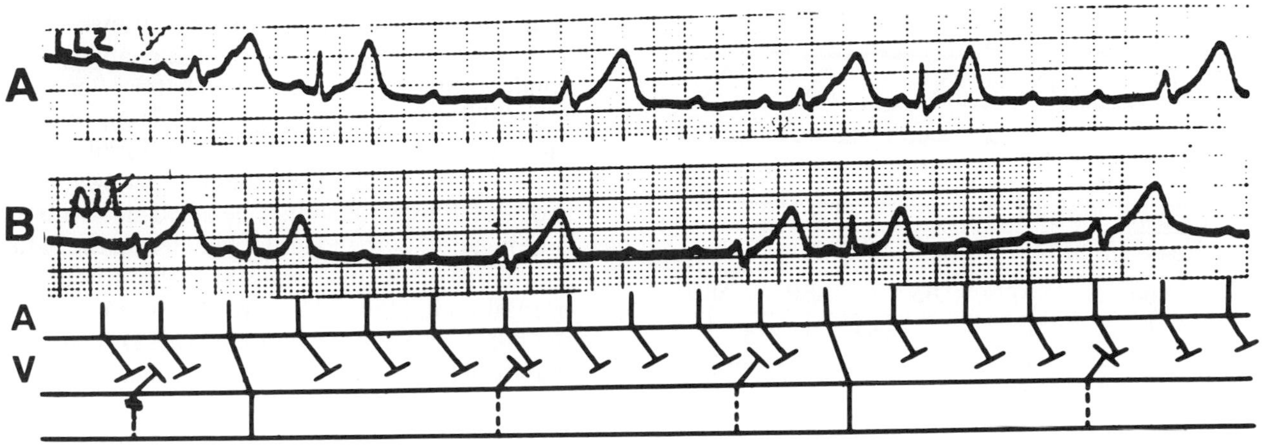

Figure 12-21. *Successful AV conduction of atrial impulses only following the discharge of a subsidiary pacemaker at an appropriate timing. This is considered one type of so-called supernormal conduction.*

when its prolongation is more likely is called supernormal, although it does not represent a condition better than or superior to normal. Possible examples of supernormal conduction are discussed below.

A different type of supernormal conduction is illustrated in Figure 12-21. Since both limb lead II (LL 2) and lead aV_F show identical conduction phenomena, only lead aV_F (with the attached diagram) will be discussed. The P waves appear regularly at the rate of 140 beats/min, suggesting sinus tachycardia as the basic mechanism. The ventricular complexes appear irregularly, showing two different QRS contours. The ones having a wide rS pattern always terminate a long pause measuring 1.50 second without any fixed time relationships with the preceding P waves. Hence, these beats most likely represent either AV junctional or ventricular rhythm caused by a high-grade AV block. On the other hand, beats *2* and *5* with narrow QRS of the R type are preceded by a P wave at an interval of 0.18 second. Exactly the same findings are also noted in lead II, which suggests that these QRS complexes were produced by propagation of atrial impulses. It is further noted that these conducted sinus P waves always show a constant time relationship with the preceding QRS of the escape rhythm. Indeed, the P waves are never conducted to the ventricles unless they appear immediately after the T wave. In order to explain these observations, it has been postulated that invasion of the AV junction by concealed retrograde conduction of the impulses from the subsidiary pacemaker somehow improve the conduction in the forward direction. Since the conducting tissues are ordinarily rendered refractory after their invasion by an impulse and the recovery of excitability is supposed to proceed with time, such improved conductivity immediately after a preceding excitation has been considered a type of supernormal conduction.

With microelectrode techniques, several investigators have explained this phenomenon as follows: a concealed orthograde conduction of atrial impulses into the AV node leaves a long refractory period in this tissue, which prevents transmission of the next impulse. When a retrograde impulse arrives at this area with an appropriate timing (retrograde conduction of the first ventricular impulse in the diagram in Fig. 12-21), it depolarizes the AV nodal tissue rather prematurely, preventing invasion of the second atrial impulse into the region. This earlier depolarization is associated with an earlier termination of the refractory period in the site of conduction block, thus allowing the third sinus impulse to be conducted to the ventricles.[68,70] However, certain criticisms can be presented to challenge this theory, and it is not the only explanation.

One possible mechanism for the above phenomenon is the concept of so-called phase 4 block.[71] When significant diastolic depolarization is present in the His-Purkinje system, causing a decreased membrane potential and resultant depression of conductivity,[72] the propagation of impulses through these fibers becomes more difficult toward later diastole, whereas arrival of an impulse immediately after an action potential, when the membrane potential is the highest, may be associated with improved conduction. Since the QRS complexes of the escape rhythm in Figure 12-21 are wide, suggesting the site of impulse formation (and hence the site of block) to be below the bifurcation of the His bundle, the second theory invoking phase 4 block in the His-Purkinje level may well be the alternative explanation in this case.[73] Another explanation invoking the mechanism of supernormal periods of excitability will not be discussed in detail here but may also be possible.[74]

Finally, there is a phenomenon that has classically been considered as one type of supernormal conduc-

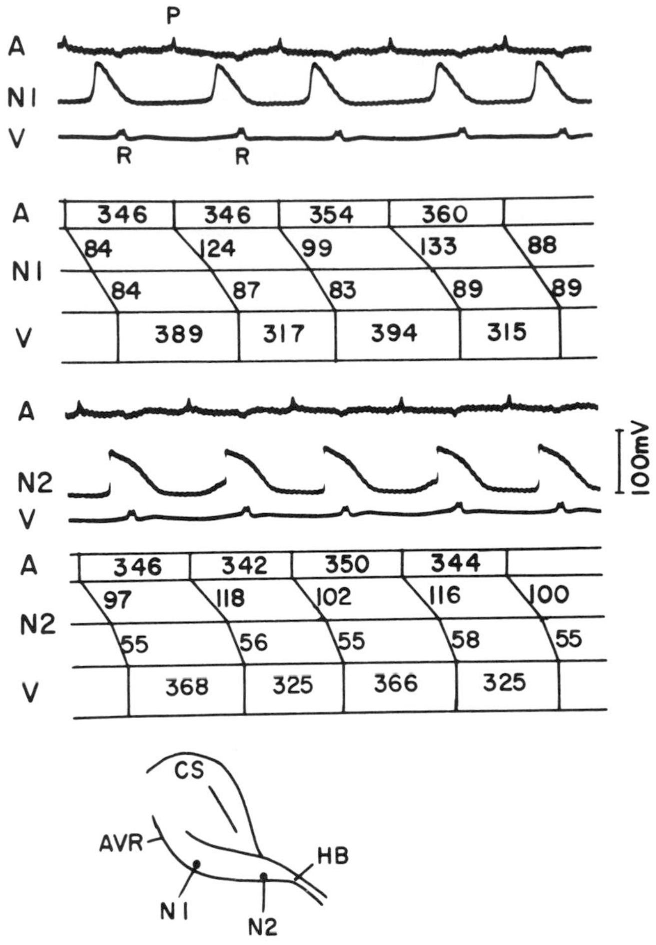

Figure 12-22. *Experimental records showing alternation of short and long AV conduction times in the presence of 1:1 AV response.*

tion,[75] but we feel that this is not the case.[33] This phenomenon is a regular alternation of the PR interval in the presence of 1:1 conduction. In the experimental records shown in Figure 12-22, alternation of long and short AV conduction times is noted in the presence of almost regular sinus rhythm, causing an alternation of the ventricular cycle. In contrast to the several examples of alternating PR intervals in 2:1 AV block (see Figs. 12-12, 12-13, and 12-14), every sinus impulse is transmitted to the ventricles in Figure 12-22. The argument for calling this type of rhythm supernormal conduction has been as follows: the second atrial impulse in the top record of Figure 12-22 (marked P) follows the first ventricular excitation (R) with a relatively long interval (178 msec), and yet its conduction to the ventricles takes a longer time (124 + 87 = 211 msec). On the other hand, the third atrial impulse appears only 135 msec after the second ventricular depolarization R) but is conducted with a shorter AV conduction time (99 + 83 = 182 msec), an apparently paradoxical conduction pattern. In other words, if the AV transmission takes 211 msec when the recovery of excitability of the AV conducting system is considered better after a longer RP interval (the problem involved in this concept is pointed out below), conduction of the next impulse in the presence of poorer recovery of the conducting system after a shorter RP interval should be associated with a further prolongation of the PR interval. Hence, the paradoxical shortening of 182 msec may satisfy the criteria for supernormal conduction. However, a close examination of the attached diagrams (see Fig. 12-22) clearly indicates that the RP interval would have no effect on the recovery of excitability in the AV conducting system. Indeed, the second atrial impulse (P) as well as the third atrial impulse try to invade the AV node with the same cycle length of 346 msec, and not after 178 or 135 msec. The effects of such RP intervals must be taken into consideration only when the ventricles are being controlled by impulses independent from those of the atria, as in the example of Figure 12-21, whereas such values have no meaning when ventricular excitation is caused by supraventricular impulses alone. For this reason, we felt that this phenomenon should not be called a supernormal conduction.[32]

The question then, is how to explain these findings. In this regard, it is noted that the action potentials from fiber N1 in the top record in Figure 12-22 appear to show slight diastolic depolarization, whereas the N2 potential in the bottom record develops a prominent prepotential or step formation when the conduction time is prolonged. These changes suggest that the intra-AV nodal conduction of every other atrial impulse becomes inhomogeneous, and the decreased effectiveness of an irregular excitation front causes depression of conductivity. It may further be postulated that there is functional longitudinal dissociation of the AV junctional tissue in which one fiber group maintains a 1:1 conduction while the other fiber group shows the condition of 2:1 block.[32] Although this latter mechanism may appear similar to the so-called dual AV conducting system,[42,44,45] in which two anatomically separate conduction pathways are often postulated, a functional duality or inhomogeneity is probably sufficient to cause these phenomena. In either case, when the intranodal conduction is delayed, the membrane potential of certain downstream fibers may be decreased due to phase 4 depolarization, which could further delay conduction below the AV node[76] and exaggerate the PR alternation.

Finally, it appears that usually no single electrophysiologic mechanism can explain even the most simple conduction disorders. The site of block and identification of the pathophysiologic mechanism appear essential to clinical management. More detailed experimental studies are probably needed before the final elucidation of the mechanisms causing these complex conduction phenomena.[33]

References

1. Adams, R.: Dublin Hospital Report, 4:353, 1827.
2. Stokes, W.: Dublin Q. J. Med. Sci., 2:73, 1846.
3. Wenckebach, K. F.: Zur Analyse des unregelmassigen Pulses. Z. Klin. Med., 37:475, 1899.
4. Hay, J.: Bradycardia and cardiac arrhythmia produced by depression of certain functions of the heart. Lancet, 1:139, 1906.
5. Mobitz, W.: Über die unvollständige Störung der Erregungsüberleitung zwischen Vorhof und Kammer des menschlichen Herzens. Z. Gesamte Exp. Med., 41:180, 1924.
6. Dreifus, L. S., Watanabe, Y., Haiat, R., and Kimbiris, D.: Atrioventricular block. Am. J. Cardiol., 28:371, 1971.
7. Dreifus, L. S. and Watanabe, Y.: Localization and significance of atrioventricular block. Am. Heart J., 82:435, 1971.
8. Watanabe, Y., and Dreifus, L. S.: Second degree atrioventricular block. Cardiovasc. Res., 1:150, 1967.
9. Watanabe, Y., and Dreifus, L. S.: Levels of concealment in second degree and advanced second degree AV block. Am. Heart J., 84:330, 1972.
10. Watanabe, Y., and Dreifus, L. S.: Sites of impulse formation within the atrioventricular junction of the rabbit. Circ. Res., 22:717, 1968.
11. Watanabe, Y.: Atrioventricular conduction disturbance and electrophysiology. Igaku no Ayumi, 69:339, 1969.
12. Damato, A. N., and Lau, S. H.: Clinical value of the electrogram of the conduction system. Prog. Cardiovasc. Dis., 13:119, 1970.
13. Narula, O. S., Scherlag, B. J., Samet, P., and Javier, R. P.: Atrioventricular block. Localization and classification by His bundle recordings. Am. J. Med., 50:146, 1971.
14. Puech, P., and Grolleau, R.: L'Activite du Faisceau de His Normale et Pathologique. Paris, Editions Sandoz, 1972.
15. Katz, L. N., and Pick, A.: Clinical Electrocardiography. Part I. The Arrhythmias. Philadelphia, Lea & Febiger, 1956.
16. Bellet, S.: Clinical Disorders of the Heart Beat. Philadelphia, Lea & Febiger, 1971.
17. Watanabe, Y.: Cardiac Arrhythmias. Electrophysiologic and Clincal Aspects. Tokyo, Bunkodo, 1973.
18. Watanabe, Y., and Dreifus, L. S.: Electrophysiologic effects of digitalis on A-V transmission. Am. J. Physiol., 211:1461, 1966.
19. Watanabe, Y., and Dreifus, L. S.: Interactions of quinidine and potassium on atrioventricular transmission. Circ. Res., 20:434, 1967.
20. Watanabe, Y., and Dreifus, L. S.: Interactions of lanatoside C and potassium on atrioventricular conduction on rabbits. Circ. Res., 27:931, 1970.
21. Rosen, K. M., Rahimtoola, S. H., Chuquimia, R., et al.: Electrophysiological significance of first degree atrioventricular block with intraventricular conduction disturbance. Circulation, 43:491, 1971.
22. Narula, O. S., Cohen, L. S., Samet, P., et al.: Localization of A-V conduction defects in man by recording of the His bundle electrogram. Am. J. Cardiol., 25:228, 1970.
23. Narula, O. S., Scherlag, B. J., Javier, R. P., et al.: Analysis of the A-V conduction defect in complete heart block utilizing His bundle electrograms. Circulation, 41:437, 1970.
24. Damato, A. N., Lau, S. H., Helfant, R., et al.: A study of heart block in man using His bundle recordings. Circulation, 39:297, 1969.
25. Massumi, R. A., and Ali, N.: Determination of the site of impaired conduction in atrioventricular block. J. Electrocardiol., 3:193, 1970.
26. Narula, O. S., and Samet, P.: Wenckebach and Mobitz type II AV block due to block within the His bundle and bundle branches. Circulation, 41:947, 1970.
27. Wenckebach, K. F.: Zur Analyse des unregelmassigen Pulses. Z. Klin. Med., 37:475, 1889.
28. Mobitz, W.: Über die unvollständige Störung der Erregungsüberleitung zwischen Vorhof und Kammer des menschlichen Herzens. Z. Gesamte Exp. Med., 41:180, 1924.
29. Mobitz, W.: Über den partiellen Herzblock. Z. Klin. Med., 107:449, 1928.
30. Watanabe, Y.: Atrioventricular block. Saishin Igaku, 25:799, 1970 (in Japanese).
31. Haiat, R., Dreifus, L. S., and Watanabe, Y.: Fate of A-V block. An electrocardiographic study. In Han, J. (ed.): Cardiac Arrhythmias. A Symposium. Springfield, Ill., Charles C Thomas, 1972.
32. Watanabe, Y., and Dreifus, L. S.: Factors controlling impulse transmission, with special reference to AV conduction. Am. Heart J., 89:790, 1975.
33. Watanabe, Y., and Dreifus, L. S.: Cardiac Arrhythmias: Electrophysiologic Basis for Clinical Interpretation, pp. 153–217. New York, Grune & Stratton, 1977.
34. Watanabe, Y., and Dreifus, L. S.: Inhomogeneous conduction in the AV node. A model for re-entry. Am. Heart J., 70:505, 1965.
35. Hoffman, B. F., Paes de Carvalho, A., de Mello, W. C., and Cranefield, P. F.: Electrical activity of single fibers of the atrioventricular node. Circ. Res., 7:11, 1959.
36. Damato, A. N., Varghese, P. J., Lau, S. H., et al.: Manifest and concealed reentry: a mechanism of AV nodal Wenckebach phenomenon. Circ. Res., 30:283, 1972.
37. Rosen, K. M., Rahimtoola, S. H., and Gunnar, R. M.: Pseudo A-V block secondary to premature nonpropagated His bundle depolarizations. Documentation by His bundle electrocardiography. Circulation, 42:367, 1970.
38. Lindsay, A. F., and Schamroth, L.: Atrioventricular junctional parasystole with concealed conduction simulating second degree atrioventricular block. Am. J. Cardiol., 31:397, 1973.
39. Langendorf, R., and Mehlman, J. S.: Blocked (nonconducted) AV nodal premature systoles imitating first and second degree AV block. Am. Heart J., 34:500, 1947.
40. Fisch, C., Zipes, D. P., and McHenry, P.: Electrocardiographic manifestations of concealed junctional ectopic impulses. Circulation, 53:217, 1976.
41. Hoffman, B. F., Moore, E. N., Stuckey, J. H., and Cranefield, P. F.: Functional properties of the atrioventricular conduction system. Circ. Res., 13:308, 1963.
42. Wu, D., Denes, P., Dhingra, R., Wyndham, C., and Rosen, K. M.: Determinants of fast and slow pathway conduction in patients with dual atrioventricular nodal pathways. Circ. Res., 36:782, 1975.
43. Noy, Y., and Fleischmann, P.: Electrocardiographic manifestations of dual pathways of retrograde impulse conduction in the human heart. Am. J. Cardiol., 35:293, 1975.
44. Iinuma, H., Dreifus, L. S., Mazgalev, T., et al.: Role of the perinodal region in atrioventricular nodal reentry: Evidence in an isolated rabbit heart preparation. J. Am. Coll. Cardiol., 2:465, 1983.
45. Ogawa, S., and Dreifus, L. S.: Longitudinal dissociation of Bachmann's bundle as a mechanism of paroxysmal supraventricular tachycardia. Am. J. Cardiol., 40:915–922, 1977.
46. Kretz, A., and DaRuos, H. O.: Experimental Luciani-Wenckebach phenomenon in the anterior and posterior divisions of the left bundle branch of the canine heart. Am. Heart J., 84:513, 1972.
47. Wennemark, J. R., and Bandura, J. P.: Microelectrode study of Wenckebach periodicity in canine Purkinje fibers. Am. J. Cardiol., 33:390, 1974.
48. Rosenbaum, M. B., Nau, G. J., Levi, R. J., et al.: Wenckebach periods in the bundle branches. Circulation, 40:79, 1969.
49. Moe, G. K., Preston, J. B., and Burlington, H.: Physiologic evidence for a dual A-V transmission system. Circ. Res., 4:357, 1956.
50. Hoffman, B. F., and Cranefield, P. F.: The Electrophysiology of the Heart. New York, McGraw-Hill, 1960.
51. Moore, E. N., Preston, J. B., and Moe, G. K.: Duration of trans-

membrane potentials and functional refractory periods of canine false tendon and ventricular myocardium. Circ. Res., 17:259, 1965.
52. Watanabe, Y.: Purkinje repolarization as a possible cause of the U wave of the electrocardiogram. Circulation, 51:1030, 1975.
53. Moore, E. N.: Observations on concealed conduction in atrial fibrillation. Circ. Res., 21:201, 1967.
54. Yamada, K., Okajima, M., Hori, K., et al.: On the genesis of the absolute ventricular arrhythmia associated with atrial fibrillation. Circ. Res., 22:707, 1968.
55. Konishi, T., and Matsuyama, G.: Atrial excitation as the input to the AV node: summation in antegrade AV nodal conduction. Jpn. Circ. J. (Suppl.), 40:20, 1976 (in Japanese).
56. de Azevedo, I. M., Watanabe, Y., and Dreifus, L. S.: Form and features of exit heart block. Postgrad. Med., 53:71, 1973.
57. Watanabe, Y.: Recognition of premature systoles originating within the Purkinje system. In Dreifus, L. S., and Likoff, W. (eds.): Cardiac Arrhythmias, p. 379. New York, Grune & Stratton, 1973.
58. Watanabe, Y., Pamintuan, J. C., and Dreifus, L. S.: Role of intraventricular conduction disturbances in ventricular premature systoles. Am. J. Cardiol., 32:188, 1973.
59. Cullis, W. C., and Dixon, W. E.: Excitation and section of the auriculoventricular bundle. J. Physiol., 42:156, 1911.
60. Cohn, A. E., and Fraser, P. R.: The occurrence of auricular contractions in a case of incomplete and complete heart block due to stimuli received from the contracting ventricles. Heart, 5:141, 1913.
61. Scherf, D.: Retrograde conduction in complete heart block. Dis. Chest., 35:320, 1959.
62. Watanabe, Y., and Dreifus, L. S.: Newer concepts in the genesis of cardiac arrhythmias. Am. Heart J., 76:114, 1968.
63. Langendorf, R., Pick, A., Edelist, A., and Katz, L. N.: Experimental demonstration of concealed A-V conduction in the human heart. Circulation, 32:386, 1965.
64. Gubbay, E. R., and Mora, C. A.: Retrograde conduction and isorhythmic dissociation in heart block. Am. Heart J., 68:166, 1964.
65. Mack, I., Langendorf, R., and Katz, L. N.: The supernormal phase of recovery of conduction in the human heart. Am. Heart J., 34:374, 1947.
66. Fisch, C., and Steinmetz, E. F.: Supernormal phase of atrioventricular (A-V) conduction due to potassium. A-V alternans with first degree AV block. Am. Heart J., 62:211, 1961.
67. Pick, A., Langendorf, R., and Katz, L. N.: The supernormal phase of atrioventricular conduction. I. Fundamental mechanisms. Circulation, 26:388, 1962.
68. Moe, G. K., Childers, R. W., and Merideth, J.: An appraisal of "supernormal" A-V conduction. Circulation, 38:5, 1968.
69. Wu, D., Denes, P., Wyndhaums, C.: Demonstration of dual atrioventricular nodal pathways utilizing a ventricular extrastimulus in patients with atrioventricular nodal re-entrant paroxysmal supraventricular tachycardia. Circulation, 52:789, 1975.
70. Moore, E. N., and Spear, J. F.: Experimental studies on the facilitation of A-V conduction by ectopic beats in dogs and rabbits. Circ. Res., 29:29, 1971.
71. Elizari, M. V., Lazzari, J. O., and Rosenbaum, M. B.: Phase 3 and phase 4 intermittent left anterior hemiblock. Report of first case in the literature. Chest, 63:673, 1972.
72. Singer, D. H., Lazzara, R., and Hoffman, B. F.: Interrelationships between automaticity and conduction in Purkinje fibers. Circ. Res., 2:537, 1967.
73. Watanabe, Y.: How to read arrhythmia electrocardiograms. VII. High grade AV block, unidirectional AV conduction and supernormal AV conduction. Clinical All-around, 24:492, 1975 (in Japanese).
74. Spear, J. F., and Moore, E. N.: Supernormal excitability and conduction in the His Purkinje system of the dog. Circ. Res., 35:782, 1974.
75. Ashman, R., and Herrmann, G.: A supernormal phase in conduction and a recovery curve for the human junctional tissue. Am. Heart J., I:594, 1926.
76. Lepeschkin, E.: The electrocardiographic diagnosis of bilateral bundle branch block in relation to heart block. Prog. Cardiovasc. Dis., 6:455, 1964.

13

Clinical Concepts of Spontaneous and Induced Atrioventricular Block

Onkar S. Narula

The term *heart block* was first introduced by Gaskell almost a century ago in 1882.[1,2] In the following two decades, various portions of the specialized atrioventricular conducting system (*i.e.,* AV node, His bundle, and bundle branches) were identified.[3-6] The first electrocardiogram showing experimental and clinical heart block was published by Einthoven in 1906.[7] Numerous histopathologic, experimental, and clinical studies have demonstrated that atrioventricular block may be due to lesions in any portion of the conducting system.[8-15] Although the standard electrocardiogram may indicate AV block or damage to the conduction system, it is limited in identifying the precise site(s) of lesion and the degree of damage to each region. The therapy and prognosis of AV block not only depend on diagnosing AV block, but are also related to the site of lesion in the specialized conducting system. During the early 1970s, the development of His bundle electrocardiography was valuable in enhancing the understanding of normal and abnormal AV impulse transmission.[16] More recently complete AV block has been induced for therapeutic purposes in the management of selected patients with supraventricular tachyarrhythmias. Current investigations are directed toward therapeutic induction of desired degrees of AV delays or AV block through various catheter techniques. Some of these methods appear promising.

Definition of Terms

The PR interval is broken into its three components by the recording of a His bundle electrogram: (1) PA time is an approximation of intra-atrial conduction time and is measured from the high right atrial electrogram or the onset of the P wave on the standard electrocardiogram to the first rapid deflection of the A wave on the bipolar His bundle lead (Fig. 13-1), (2) AH time represents the AV nodal conduction time and is measured from the first rapid deflection of the A wave (in the His bundle lead) to the earliest onset (rapid or slow) of the His bundle (BH) potential, and (3) the HV time represents the conduction time through the His-Purkinje system (HPS) and is measured from the onset of the BH potential to the earliest onset of ventricular activation recorded on either the intracardiac bipolar His bundle lead or any of the multiple surface electrocardiogram leads.[17]

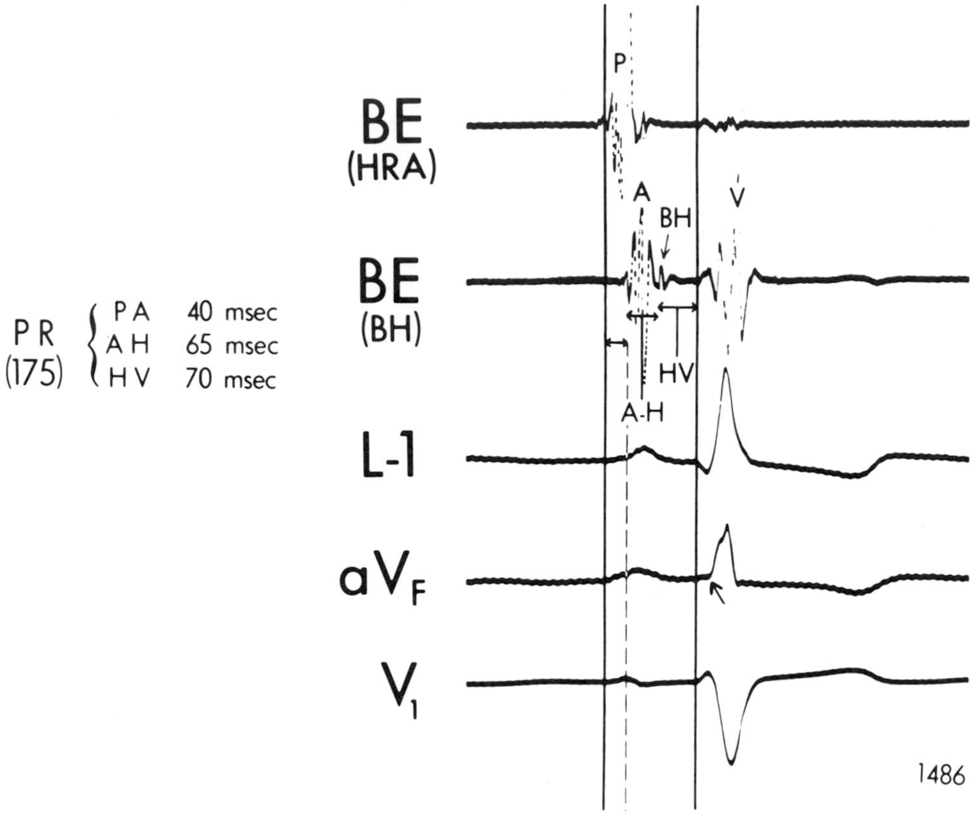

Figure 13-1. *Simultaneous bipolar recordings (BE) from the high right atrium (HRA) and the His bundle (BH) region along with three electrocardiographic leads show the components of the PR interval. The solid vertical lines demarcate the earliest onset of the P wave and the QRS complex. (PA, intra-atrial conduction time; AH, the time interval from the A wave to the BH, representing AV nodal conduction time; HV, the time interval from the BH to the ventricle, V). (Narula, O. S.: Current concepts of A-V block. In Narula, O. S. [ed.]: His Bundle Electrocardiography and Clinical Electrophysiology, p. 139. Philadelphia, F. A. Davis, 1975)*

Normal Atrioventricular Conduction

The normal range and mean, plus or minus standard deviation (SD), for various conduction intervals in our laboratory are as follows: PA, 25 to 45 msec (37 ± 7); AH, 50 to 120 msec (77 ± 16); and HV, 35 to 45 msec (40 ± 3).[18] The His bundle potential duration is 15 to 20 msec. The RBV times are identical and normally range from 20 to 25 msec.[19] The range of conduction values reported by others is essentially similar to ours, except for the difference in the upper limit of normal HV interval, which others consider to be 55 msec.[20–23] The reasons for these differences in the normal values reported by various groups have been previously discussed in detail.[24] The PA and HV intervals are not affected by sympathetic or parasympathetic influences and therefore remain constant from day to day. However, the AH interval is influenced by changes in parasympathetic and sympathetic activity and may vary during the same study.

Normally, the AH interval lengthens with an increase in the atrial pacing rate, whereas the PA and HV intervals remain constant. During atrial pacing, 1 : 1 AV conduction may be noted up to a rate of 150 to 220 beats/min; however, physiologic second degree type I AH block may be manifested at rates of 130 beats/min or greater. Since these observations are based on studies without autonomic blockade, they cannot be applied with certainty to diagnose an abnormal AV node in cases manifesting second degree AH block at rates less than 130 beats/min. In addition, the phenomenon of "AV nodal accommodation" also influences the Wenckebach point, which is related to the size of increment in atrial pacing rate and the duration of pacing between incremental steps.[25] Development of second degree AV block distal to the BH potential with atrial pacing rates less than 150 beats/min is considered abnormal.[24,26]

Spontaneous Atrioventricular Block

First Degree Atrioventricular Block

First degree AV block (PR $\geqq$ 0.21 second) may result from conduction delays in the atrium, AV node, His bundle, or bundle branches (Fig. 13-2).[27] In 79% of our patients with a prolonged PR interval, the conduction delays were localized at more than one site, although the AV node was the dominant site of delay in the majority (83%). Conduction delays at a single site were noted in only 21% of patients (AV node in 11%, atrium in 3%, and HPS in 7%).[28] Patients with a wide QRS complex, especially those with a left bundle branch block, have a very high incidence (50% to 90%) of abnormal HV intervals superimposed on a prolonged AH time.[29–32] Usually with severe intra-atrial delays, the P wave amplitude is markedly diminished, and in some the P waves may be completely absent on the surface electrocardiogram and may fallaciously simulate a junctional rhythm with silent atria.[32] However, a notched and wide P wave does not necessarily indicate an intra-atrial conduction defect, because it may also result from interatrial delays.[32]

In patients with first degree AV block, the response to atrial pacing depends primarily on the site of delay. Patients with intra-atrial (PA) delays usually show 1 : 1 AV conduction at rapid pacing rates. The intra-atrial conduction time may lengthen, and occasionally type I block may be manifested within the atrium.[33] In patients with AV nodal (AH) delays, second degree type I block is usually manifested at slower atrial pacing rates (<130 beats/min). Patients with a prolonged HV time usually exhibit 1 : 1 conduction at rapid pacing rates, and only occasionally is second degree block manifested distal to the His bundle.

Prognosis and therapy are determined not only by the degree of block but also by the site of the block. Patients with intra-atrial conduction defects are usually prone to multiple atrial arrhythmias (*i.e.*, atrial fibrillation, atrial

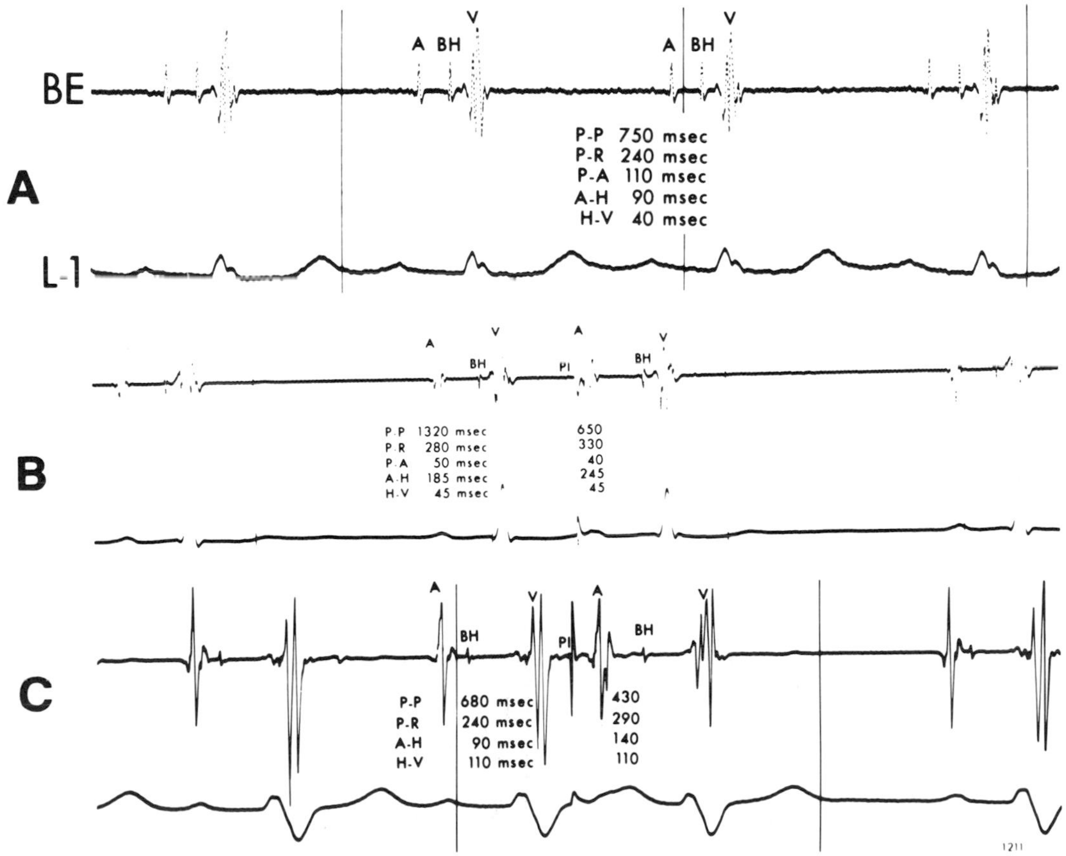

Figure 13-2. *Recordings from three different patients showing first degree AV block due to delays at various sites. The PR interval is prolonged because of (A) intra-atrial conduction delay (PA = 110 msec), in which the AH and HV times are normal; (B) AV nodal delay (AH = 185 msec); and (C) His-Purkinje system delay (HV = 110 msec).*

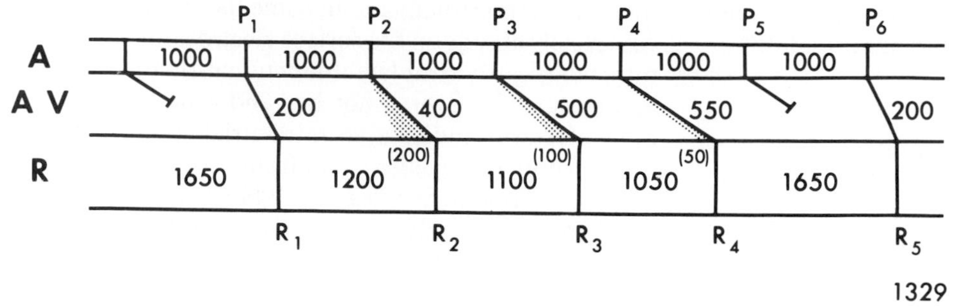

Figure 13-3. *Diagrammatic representation of classic Wenckebach type I AV block. All the intervals are in milliseconds. The shaded area and the numbers in parentheses indicate the amount of the PR interval increment over that of the preceding PR interval (Narula, O. S.: Wenckebach type I and type II atrioventricular block [revisited]. Cardiovasc. Clin., 6[3]:137, 1974)*

flutter, or atrial tachycardia).[34] Conduction delays in the atrium or the AV node are usually stable and slowly progress to higher degrees of AV block. The symptoms of syncope are less likely to be due to intermittent complete heart block if the first degree AV block is localized in the atrium or the AV node. First degree AV block in the HPS usually progresses to Mobitz type II block or complete heart block (CHB) over a relatively shorter period. Therapy with digitalis is not contraindicated in patients with a prolonged PA or HV interval, but the drug should be administered with caution in patients with a prolonged AH time. On the other hand, quinidine or procainamide should be administered with caution in patients with a severely diseased HPS and a prolonged HV interval because these drugs may further lengthen the HV interval. Fortunately, AV block due to antiarrhythmic therapy with quinidine or procainamide is rare.

Second Degree Atrioventricular Block

Second degree AV block is generally divided into two types: Wenckebach I (Mobitz I) and Wenckebach II (Mobitz II).[35,36] High-grade AV block with higher conduction ratios (2:1, 3:1) may be type I or type II.

Wenckebach Type I (Mobitz I) Block

The classic type I block is characterized by a progressive lengthening of the PR interval until a P wave is blocked (Fig. 13-3). The maximum PR increment occurs between the first and second conducted beats of the Wenckebach cycle. The PR interval is usually the longest in the beat preceding the blocked P wave and shortest after the dropped beat. The RR intervals progressively decrease. The pause produced by the nonconducted P wave is equal to the difference between the last PR (before the pause) and the first PR (after the pause) subtracted from twice the PP interval.[37] However, this classic pattern of Wenckebach cycles is seen infrequently (14%).[38,39] During spontaneous type I block, atypical cycles are seen commonly and their frequency increases with conduction ratios greater than 4:3. The atypical cycles are as frequent with lesions in the AV node as in the HPS block.[40] In atypical cycles, various differing patterns of PR intervals may be noted because the PR interval may decrease before the dropped beat or may increase in equal steps; however, the PR interval after the dropped beat is always the shortest (Fig. 13-4). Chronic spontaneous type I block was localized in the AV node in 72% and in the His bundle or the bundle branches in 28%

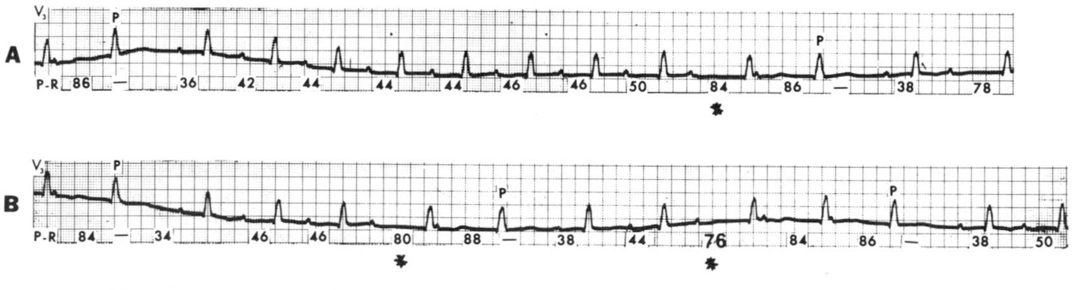

Figure 13-4. *Second degree type I AV block with atypical Wenckebach cycles. The PR interval increases between the first and second conducted beats; however, maximum increment occurs abruptly in the later cycles* (asterisks). *In some of the consecutive beats, the PR interval remains unchanged. All the numbers are given in tenths of a second.*

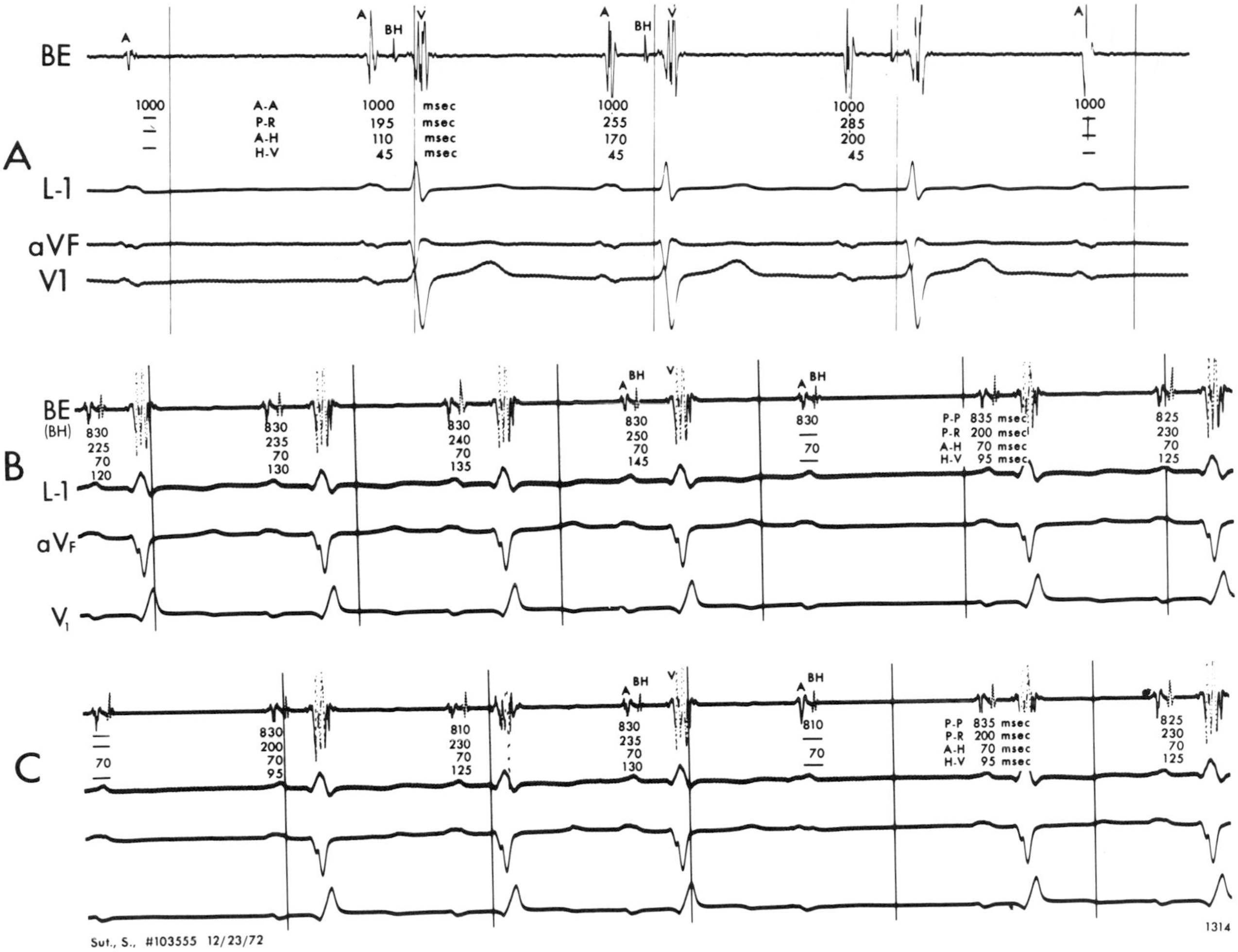

Figure 13-5. *Second degree type I AV block is shown in the AV node and in the His-Purkinje system. (A) The AH time progressively lengthens from 110 to 200 msec before an A wave (fifth) is blocked proximal to the BH (i.e., in the AV node). (B and C) The HV time progressively lengthens until an A wave is blocked distal to the BH deflection. This typical example of type I AV block in the His-Purkinje system also demonstrates that the increments in conduction delay (PR or HV) are minimal. This is in contrast to the larger delays seen in the AV nodal block in A.*

of our patients.[28] Others have reported a similar frequency of block at these sites.[29] In the majority of cases with type I HPS block, the progressive and total increment in the PR interval (or HV) is usually smaller than that seen during AV nodal block (Fig. 13-5). During sinus rhythm, spontaneous type I block has not been documented within the atrium. However, intra-atrial block has been demonstrated during atrial pacing.[33]

Wenckebach periods of alternate beats (AW) have also been reported. These atypical cycles result from simultaneous occurrence of block at two different sites (*i.e.,* His bundle and bundle branches, AV node and the HPS, or atrium and the AV node).[41–43] Wenckebach cycles may also be modified by the occurrence of other phenomena (*i.e.,* supernormal conduction and bradycardia-dependent conduction delays or block). In addition, complete AV dissociation may be simulated by the simultaneous occurrence of second degree block at multiple sites.[44] In rare cases, two consecutive P waves may be blocked in a Wenckebach cycle. Some of these cases may be explained by the occurrence of block at two different sites, whereas in others only a single site of block has been documented.

Electrocardiographic findings of type I second degree AV block and the resultant bradycardia may have different implications depending on the clinical settings. Twenty-four-hour Holter monitor recordings in healthy male medical students, without apparent heart disease, have revealed a 6% incidence of spontaneous occurrences of second degree type I AV block during sleep.[45]

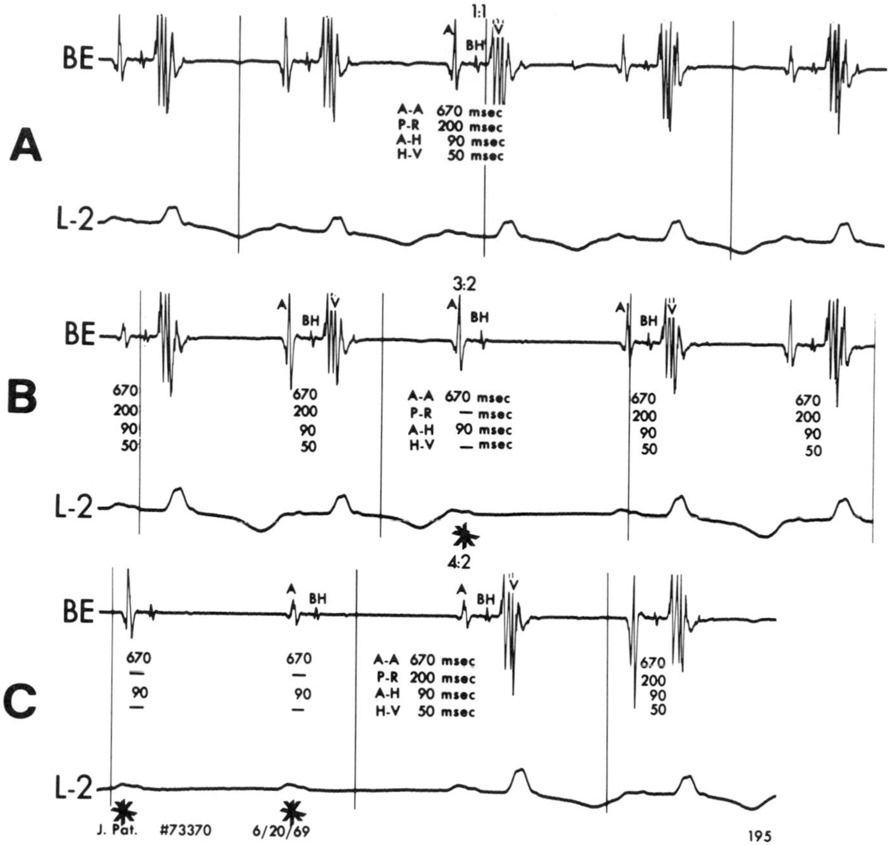

Figure 13-6. *Mobitz type II AV block. His bundle recordings show that the nonconducted P waves* (asterisks) *are blocked distal to the BH deflection. The PR interval remains constant throughout.*

In athletes, a 9% incidence of second degree type I AV block has been reported during periods of complete rest and in the recumbent position. This was considered to be a physiologic phenomenon related to heavy physical training because follow-up observations over 6 years showed no symptoms or progression of block.[46] However, in another study it was suggested that type I block in children should not be considered benign, because during prospective observations 7 of the 16 children progressed to complete heart block, and one experienced dizzy spells.[47]

Wenckebach Type II (Mobitz II) Block

In Mobitz type II second degree AV block, the PR intervals preceding the dropped beats are always constant. This author has previously emphasized that in type II block the PR interval remains constant *throughout* (*i.e.*, even after the dropped beat).[44,48] Although in his original description, Mobitz did not comment on this fact, the Lewis diagram in his paper clearly shows a constant PR interval even after the dropped beat.[36] In cases consistent with the latter criteria, the type II block is limited to the His-Purkinje system (35% in BH and 65% in the distal HPS).[18,29,32,44] Each nonconducted P wave is transmitted through the AV node and is blocked distal to the recorded BH deflection (Fig. 13-6). In the conducted beats, a single or "split" BH potential may be recorded depending on block in the distal or the middle portion of the BH, respectively. In rare cases with block in the uppermost portion of the BH, the A wave may not be followed by a recordable BH deflection and thus may fallaciously simulate AV nodal block.[18,49,50] The PR interval in the conducted beats is usually normal and is less often prolonged.[44] The QRS complex is narrow in over one third of patients (35%) and wide in the others (65%).[28]

Some workers indicate that in type II block the PR interval after the pause may be slightly shorter ($\leqq$20 msec) than that of the remaining conducted beats.[49] Such a modified interpretation or definition of type II block appears unwarranted. Second degree AV block with a shortening of the PR interval, even by 20 msec, should be classified as type I block. A few reports have claimed the demonstration of second degree type II block in the AV node.[51,52] However, a detailed analysis of these reports suggests atypical type I sequences because the PR interval was variable and shortened after the dropped beat. Some cases with type I block and atypical Wenckebach cycles may simulate type II block in the AV node. In these cases, however, the PR interval is always shortened after the dropped beat and long rhythm strips reveal changing PR intervals (Fig. 13-7).

The ability to diagnose the site of block on a standard electrocardiogram is of great clinical value because prognosis and therapy depend on the site of block. It is generally considered that second degree blocks in the HPS often progress to CHB and Adams-Stokes attacks (Fig. 13-8) and require pacemaker implantation. On the other hand, second degree blocks in the AV node have a relatively benign course and do not lead to sudden asystole.[53] The electrocardiographic diagnosis of type II block is always indicative of a HPS lesion, whereas type I block is not predictive of the site of lesion. Cases with type I block require His bundle recordings for the localization of site of lesion. Although minimal increments in the PR interval may suggest block in the HPS, they are not diagnostic. For these reasons, the classification of second degree AV block into types I and II is clinically valuable because it eliminates the need for His bundle recordings in those classified as type II. The clinical importance of this electrocardiographic classification was not accepted by all investigators, but recent data has produced more widespread acceptance.[40,54] In our series, almost one third of patients with chronic second degree AV block fulfilled the strict electrocardiogram definition of type II block, and these cases failed to reveal a shortening of either the PR interval or the HV interval by as much as 5 msec after the dropped beat. In view of these facts, the clinical need for strict adherence to the definition of type II block is self-evident.[48]

2:1 or 3:1 Atrioventricular Block

Cases of 2:1 and 3:1 AV block cannot be classified into type I or type II unless the PR intervals are observed in two consecutively conducted beats during periods of changing conduction ratios (3:2 or 1:1).[53] With a change in conduction ratio, the constancy of the PR interval indicates type II, whereas varying PR intervals are compatible with type I block. A minimal change in conduction delay secondary to a slight alteration in the number of impulses or vagal influences may readily change conduction ratios from 3:2 to 2:1, or vice versa.[32] Irrespective of type I or type II block, an increase in atrial rate, usually by 10 beats/min, changes the conduction ratio from 3:2 to 2:1; however, an increase of 40 to 50 beats/min is required to change the conduction ratios from 2:1 to 3:1. Although a change in AV block from 3:2 to 2:1 may not reflect a progression of the conduction defect, an increase from 2:1 to 3:1 *does* indicate a significant progression. Spontaneous fixed 2:1 block is localized in the AV node in one third of

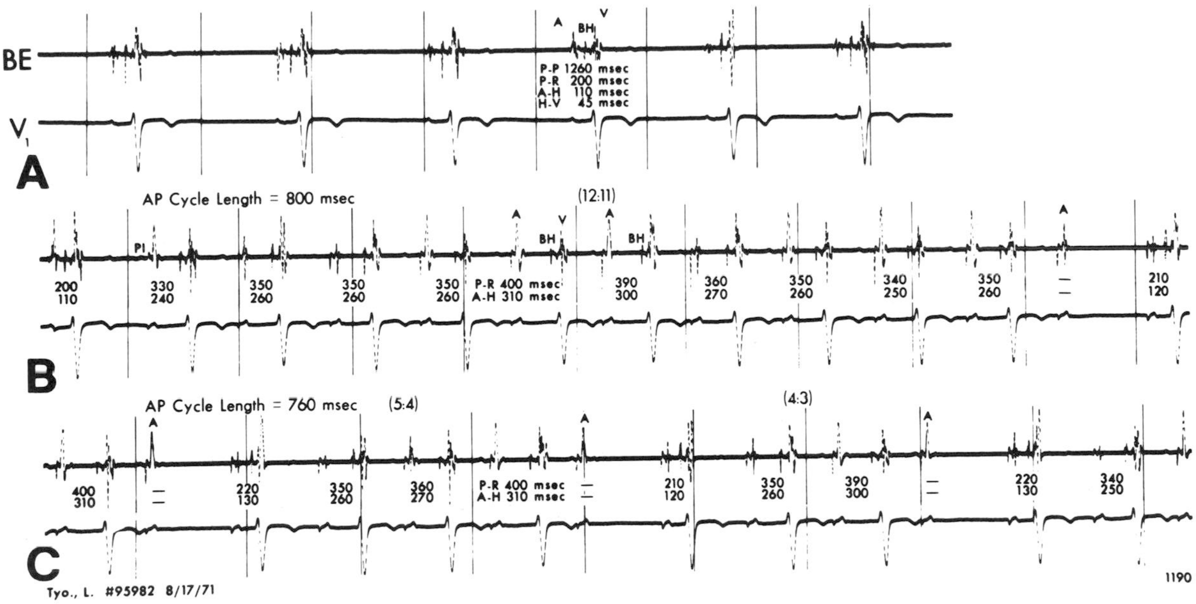

Figure 13-7. *Type I AV block with atypical Wenckebach cycles simulating type II block. (A) Recordings during sinus rhythm show 1:1 AV conduction. (B) Atrial pacing (AP) at a cycle length of 800 msec shows second degree AV block (12:11). The PR and AH intervals in the four consecutive beats immediately preceding the dropped beat do not lengthen and thus fallaciously simulate type II AV block. However, a comparison of the PR intervals in the beats preceding and following the dropped beat shows a marked shortening of the PR interval, diagnostic of type I block. (C) AP at a slightly faster rate (cycle length 760 msec) shows classic Wenckebach cycles, with a progressive prolongation of the PR interval.*

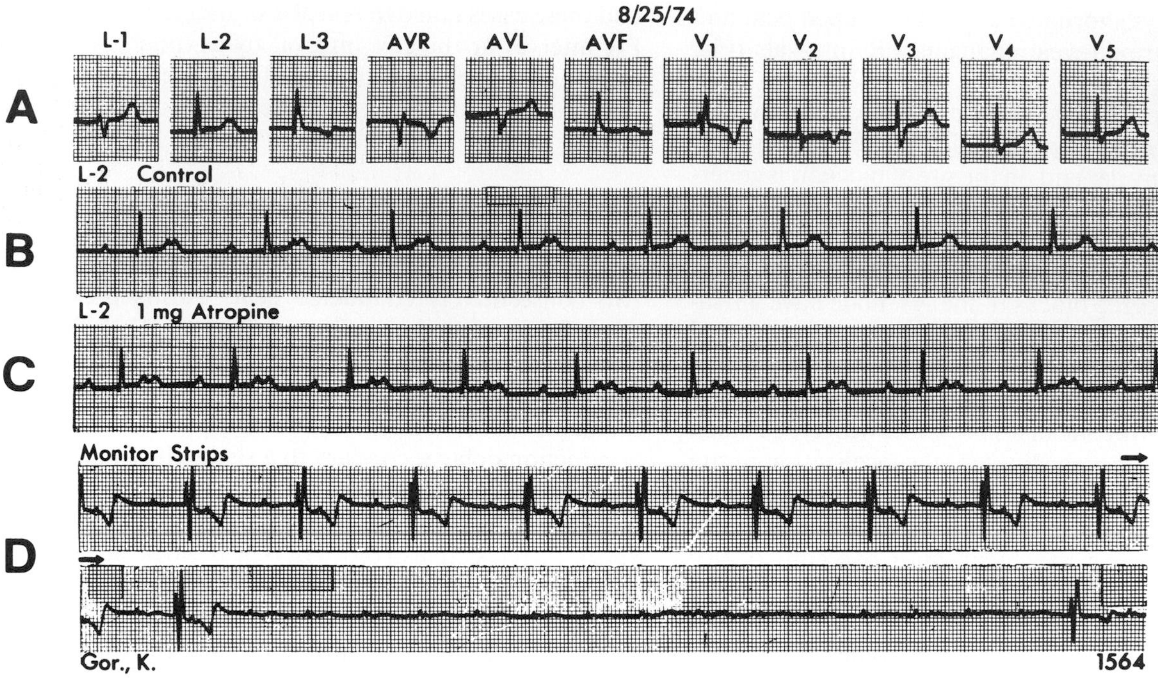

Figure 13-8. *Electrocardiographic recordings from a patient with second degree AV block (2:1) localized in the His-Purkinje system (HPS) show a sudden development of asystole (D). This type of an occurrence is usual in patients with Mobitz type II or HPS block.*

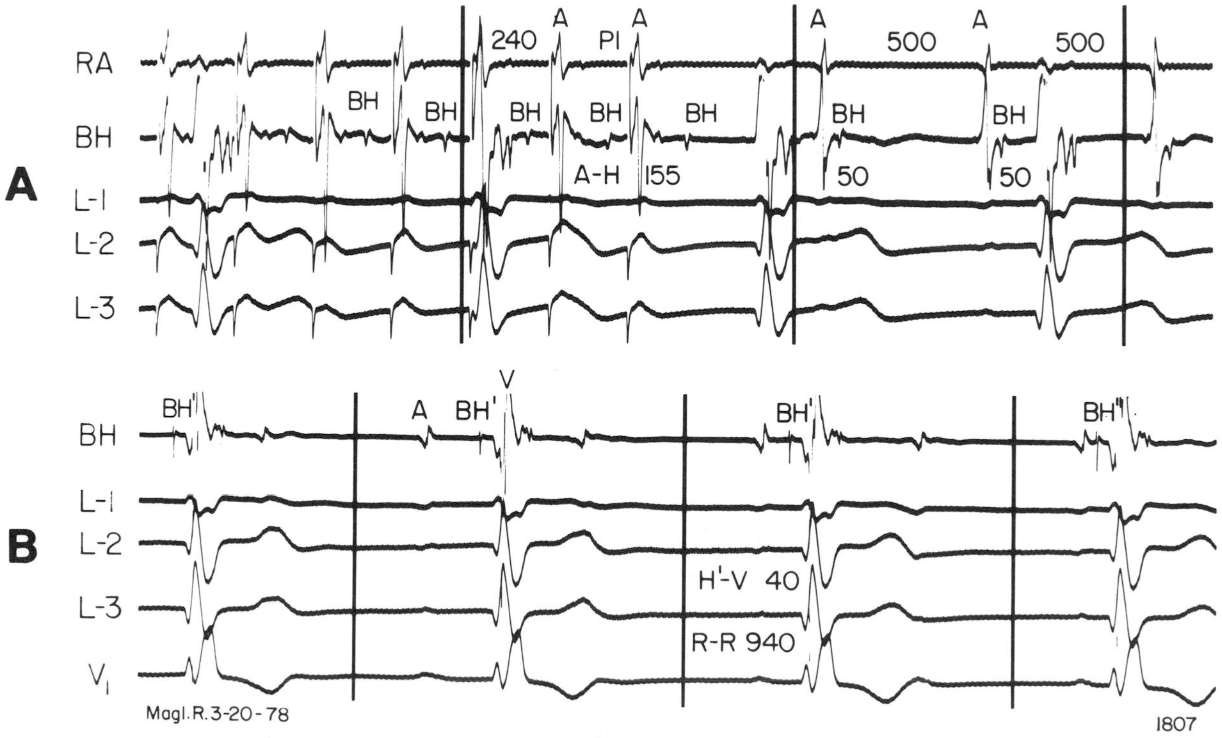

Figure 13-9. *A patient with complete heart block localized within the His bundle. His bundle recordings show "split" BH potentials. (A) Each A wave is blocked distal to a BH deflection (proximal His bundle). (B) Each QRS complex is preceded by a BH′ deflection at an H′V interval of 40 msec. The QRS complex is wide and shows a pattern of right bundle branch block with right axis deviation.*

patients and in the HPS in the other two thirds (17% in BH, 50% in the distal HPS).[28,29] The QRS complex may be narrow or wide.

Carotid massage, if applied with caution, may be clinically useful in suggesting the site of block because the effect of vagal influences is usually limited to the AV node. After carotid massage, the degree of block is likely to increase or decrease depending on the lesion in the AV node or the HPS, respectively. In case of a lesion in the HPS, slowing of the sinus rate with vagal stimulation results in improved AV conduction (1 : 1 or a decrease in block) due to a lesser number of impulses arriving at the abnormal HPS. In rare patients with bradycardia-dependent HPS block, carotid massage may aggravate or aid in the manifestation of second degree AV block and atropine may abolish it.[55,56] In general, however, atropine increases HPS block due to an increase in atrial rate and may improve conduction in AV nodal block. Exercise may also be helpful in differentiating the two types of block. A change in conduction ratios by the above maneuvers may permit classification of 2 : 1 or 3 : 1 block into type I or type II.[32,48]

Complete Heart Block

Complete heart block may be localized at three sites.[27,29,57,58] In different series, the incidence of CHB ranges from 16% to 25% in the AV node, 14% to 20% in the BH, and 56% to 68% in the bundle branches. Complete heart block may occur due to congenital or acquired lesions. All congenital CHBs are not necessarily localized in the AV node, since some have been documented within the BH, especially the middle portion of the BH.[58,62,63] Histologic studies indicate that congenital CHB in otherwise anatomically normal hearts may result from a failure of the atrial myocardium to contact the AV node or may be due to congenital separation of the AV node from the ventricular conducting tissue.[64–66]

The most common cause of CHB is probably bilateral bundle branch block. The block is localized distal to the BH deflection, and the escape rhythm shows a wide QRS complex. Each P wave is followed by a BH deflection. The heart rate may range from 25 to 58 beats/min and does not accelerate with atropine.[32,59] These subsidiary pacemakers are readily suppressed by ventricular stimulation (mechanical or electrical) and are prone to long periods of asystole.

Complete heart block may be localized in any portion of the BH (*i.e.*, proximal, middle, or distal). In cases with middle and distal BH blocks, "split" BH potentials may be documented, and the escape rhythm may either show a narrow or wide QRS complex identical to that seen during intact AV conduction (Fig. 13-9). His bundle recordings may not differentiate a proximal His bundle block from an AV nodal block because in both instances the P waves are not followed by a BH deflection and the QRS complexes are preceded by a BH potential. Following atropine administration, an acceleration in heart rate suggests AV nodal block and a lack of increase suggests a His bundle block.[32,67] However, the latter does not necessarily indicate block in the uppermost portion of the BH because His bundle pacemakers may escape despite a localization of block in the AV node. The heart rate usually ranges from 30 to 50 beats/min and may rarely exceed 70 beats/min, especially in a surgically induced block.[28,29,58] A minimal variation in heart rate over a 24-hour period or from day to day may be noted (Fig. 13-10).[68] Following atropine administration or with ex-

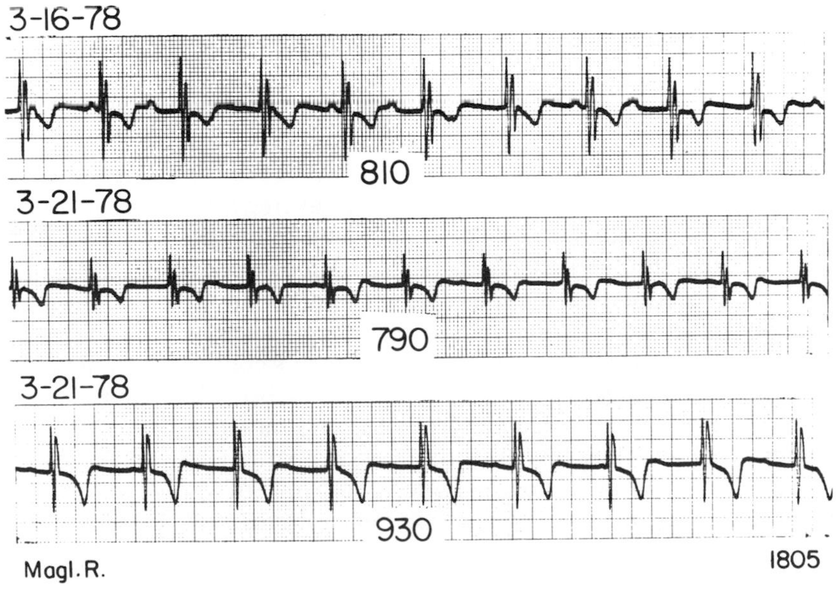

Figure 13-10. *Minor day-to-day fluctuations in the heart rate or cycle length of a subsidiary pacemaker located within the His bundle in a patient with intra-His bundle block (same patient as in Fig. 13-9).*

ercise, the heart rate may remain unchanged or may increase slightly and reach a maximum heart rate of 56 beats/min.[56,59–63,67–69] With carotid stimulation or beta blockade, the heart rate may decrease by 1 or 2 beats/min.[28,56] A majority of these patients have symptoms of snycope or dizziness, and an occasional patient may be asymptomatic.[69] Elderly women are more prone to BH lesions because of degenerative calcific infringement of this region, which occurs three times more often in women than in men.[70,71]

In patients with AV nodal CHB, the P waves are not followed by a BH deflection and the escape QRS complexes may be preceded by a BH deflection (with an HV interval ≧35 msec) if the subsidiary pacemaker originates from the His bundle. The QRS complexes are usually narrow but may be wide in 20% to 50% of patients.[29,32,59] The heart rate usually ranges from 37 to 57 beats/min, and in most (but not all) patients, a significant acceleration in rate is noted following atropine administration or exercise.[27,67,68,72]

Clinically, it has been apparent that symptoms of syncope or dizzincss cannot bc reliably predicted on the basis of electrocardiographic findings. Adams-Stokes attacks have been considered to occur most commonly in those patients with an escape rhythm showing a wide QRS complex, presumably due to complete interruption of both the bundle branches, and less commonly in those patients with escape rhythms showing a narrow QRS complex and an AV nodal block. Following the introduction of His bundlc clectrocardiography, it was suggested that the presence or absence of symptoms may be correlated to the site of block in the HPS (BH or bundle branches) or the AV node, respectively.[32,59,73]

However, subsequent observations suggest that patients with acquired or congenital CHB localized in the AV node (or proximal to the BH deflection) are not a homogeneous group, because in some cases the subsidiary pacemaker is unstable and requires management with an artifical pacemaker (Figs. 13-11 and 13-12).[69] Our recent data suggest that the criteria based on (1) localization of the site of origin, (2) the resting heart rates, and (3) the chronotropic responses to atropine are not sufficicnt for clinical and therapeutic purposes.[69] Despite a significant increase in heart rate following atropine administration (≧72 beats/min), some of the patients with subsidiary pacemakers located proximal to the BH deflection were symptomatic. In addition to the above considerations, the response to overdrive suppression is an important determinant in a patient's clinical course. It was suggested that patients with subsidiary junctional pacemakers may be separated into those patients at risk and those less likely to have syncopal attacks based on electrophysiologic studies consisting of response to overdrive suppression and a measurement of junctional recovery time (JRT) with and without parasympathetic and beta blockade.

The JRT is measured with ventricular pacing at different rates (70 to 150 beats/min). It is the interval between the last paced QRS complex and the first escape QRS complex. The corrected JRT (CJRT) is derived by deducting thc basic control cycle length of the subsidiary rhythm from the JRT. In symptomatic patients with a subsidiary junctional pacemaker, but without documentation of the cause of syncope or dizziness, the diagnosis may be confirmed or rendered less likely by the findings of a CJRT greater or less than 200 msec, with or without atropine, respectively.[69] The measurements of the recovery interval of an escape pacemaker during CHB are of greater value than the mere localization of the site of block in determining the necessity of pacemaker therapy. Contrary to previous clinical views, our recent report documented that an asymptomatic patient with an intra-His bundle block and an escape pacemaker located within the BH is not automatically a candidate for a prophylactic pacemaker insertion (Fig. 13-13).[59,69,73] Note, however, that most of the patients with an intra-His bundle block have unstable escape His bundle rhythms, are symptomatic, and do require an artificial pacemaker (Fig. 13-14).

Atrioventricular Block Triggered by Arrhythmias

All three degrees of AV block may be triggered by an atrial or ventricular arrhythmia. This is generally seen in patients with an abnormal or pathologic conduction system and is rare in those with normal AV conduction. Resetting of the AV node by an atrial or ventricular extrasystole may terminate or induce a sustained PR prolongation.[28] An atrial extrasystole, when conducted with a marked prolongation of the AH (or the PR) interval, may in turn prolong the AH time in the subsequent sinus impulses.[74] The partial compensatory atrial pause may not be long enough to permit complete recovery of the AV node. A sustained prolongation of the PR (AH) interval or induction of second degree AV nodal block following a single extrasystole (atrial or ventricular) is seen only in patients with a prolonged AV nodal refractoriness.

Concealed AV junctional extrasystoles may also simulate first degree or second degree AV block (type I or II) in the absence of true AV block.[18,45,75–78] Concealed His bundle extrasystoles, when conducted in retrograde direction to the atrium, may simulate ectopic atrial extrasystoles.[18,32] In patients with concealed His bundle extrasystoles, the HV time is usually prolonged, and these patients generally exhibit second degree block in the

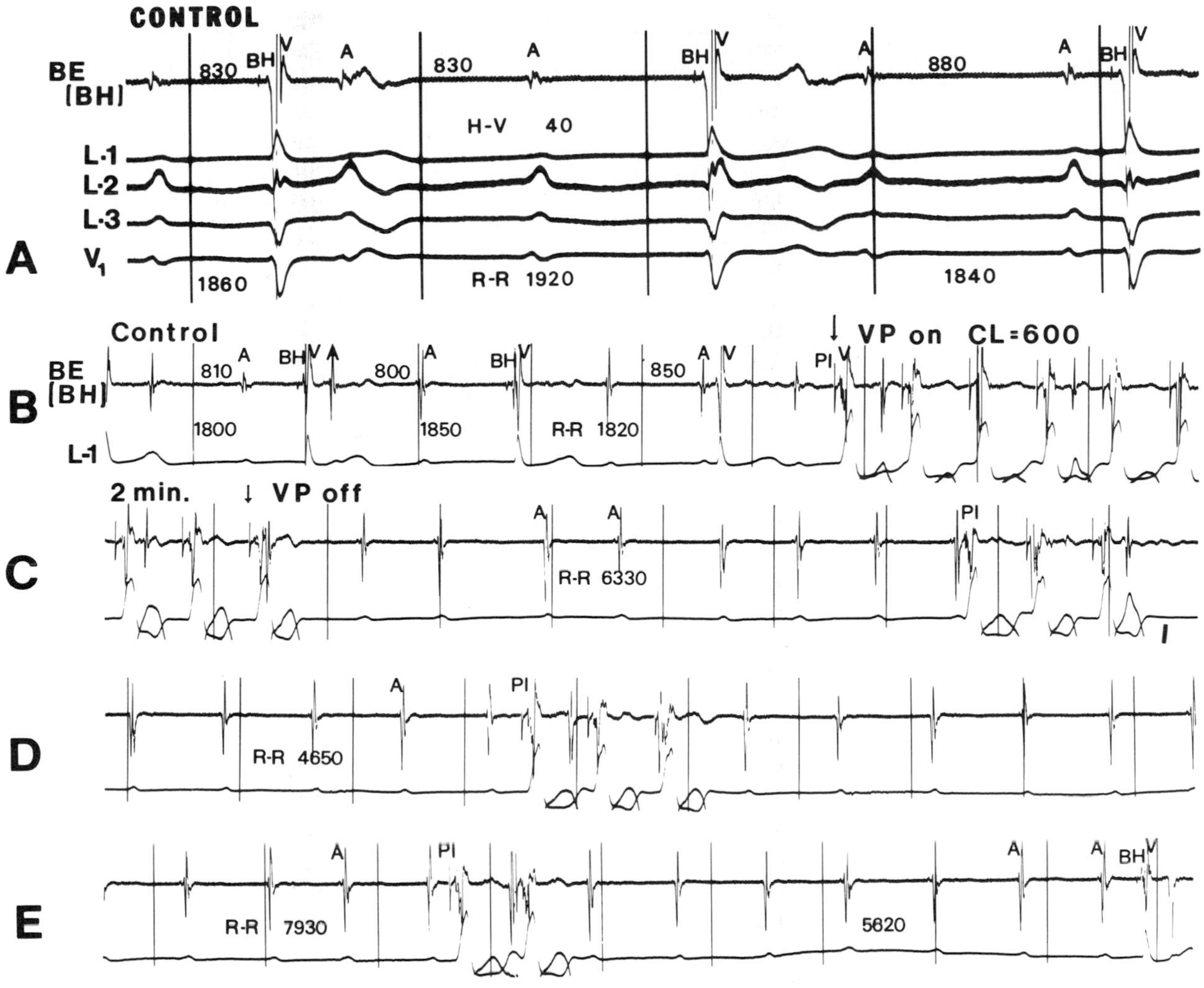

Figure 13-11. *Severely prolonged junctional recovery time in a patient with complete heart block localized in the AV node. (A) Control recordings show that the A waves are not followed by a BH deflection. Each QRS is preceded by a BH potential at an HV interval of 40 msec. (B) Onset of ventricular pacing (VP) at a cycle length (CL) of 600 msec. (C to E) Termination of VP after 2 minutes is followed by a long asystole (6330 msec), indicating a severely prolonged junctional recovery time. The VP was intermittently resumed to prevent Adams-Stokes attacks, and the spontaneous subsidiary pacemaker escapes after 27 seconds (last beat, E). Recordings in panels C to E are continuous. Time lines are at 1-second intervals. (PI, pacing impulse) (Narula, O. S., and Narula, J. T.: Junctional pacemakers in man: Response to overdrive suppression with and without parasympathetic blockade. Circulation, 57:880, 1978. By permission of the American Heart Association, Inc.)*

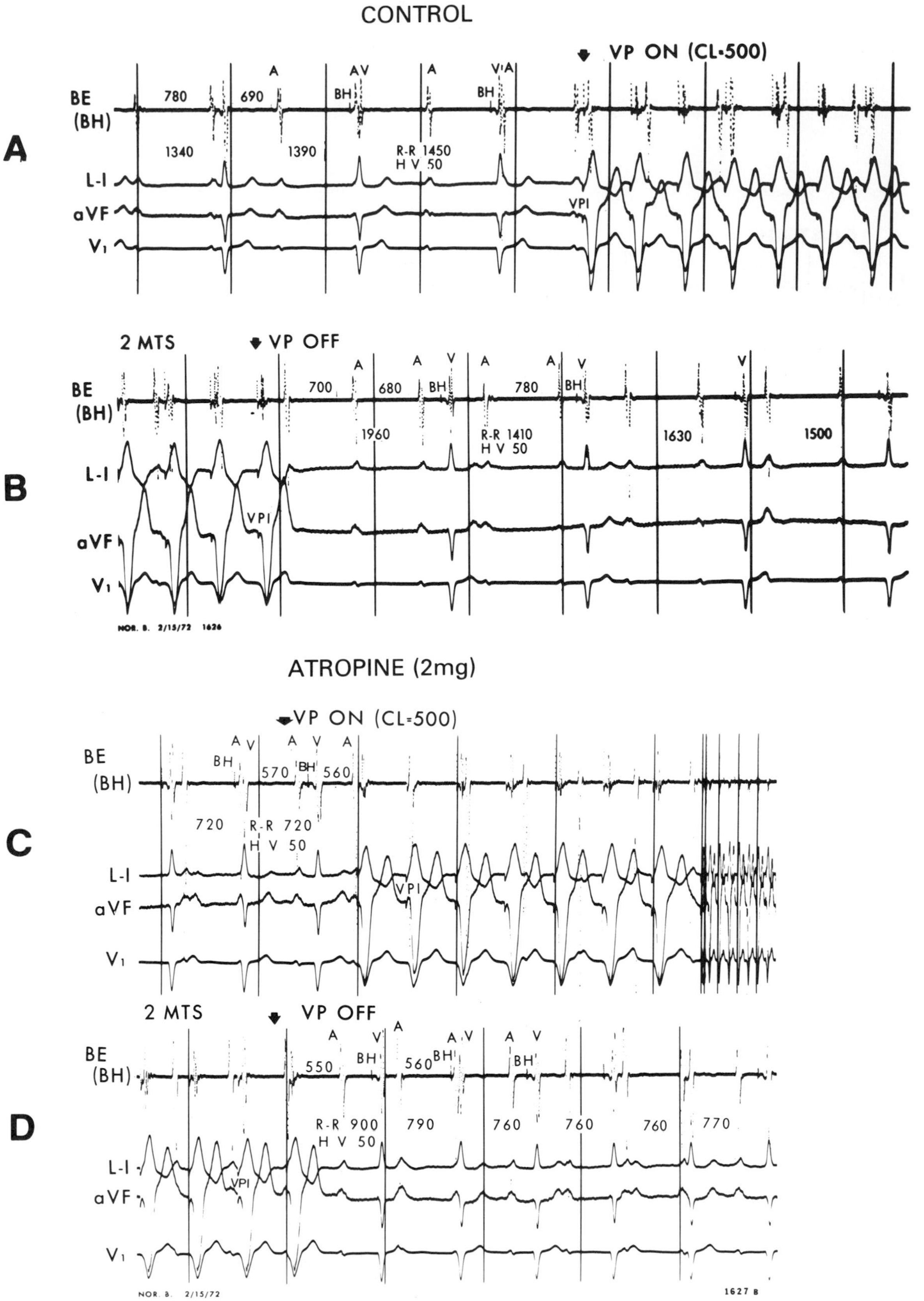

Figure 13-12. *Normalization of junctional recovery time following atropine administration in a patient with complete heart block localized in the AV node. (A and B) Recordings during control, with onset (A) and termination (B) of ventricular pacing (VP). The junctional recovery time is 1960 msec. (C and D) Following atropine administration the heart rate accelerates as the RR interval is shortened from 1450 to 720 msec (A and C). In addition, the junctional recovery time is markedly shortened from 1960 to 900 msec (B and D). (VPI, ventricular pacing impulse) (Narula, O. S., and Narula, J. T.: Junctional pacemakers in man: Response to overdrive suppression with and without parasympathetic blockade. Circulation, 57:880, 1978. By permission of the American Heart Association, Inc.)*

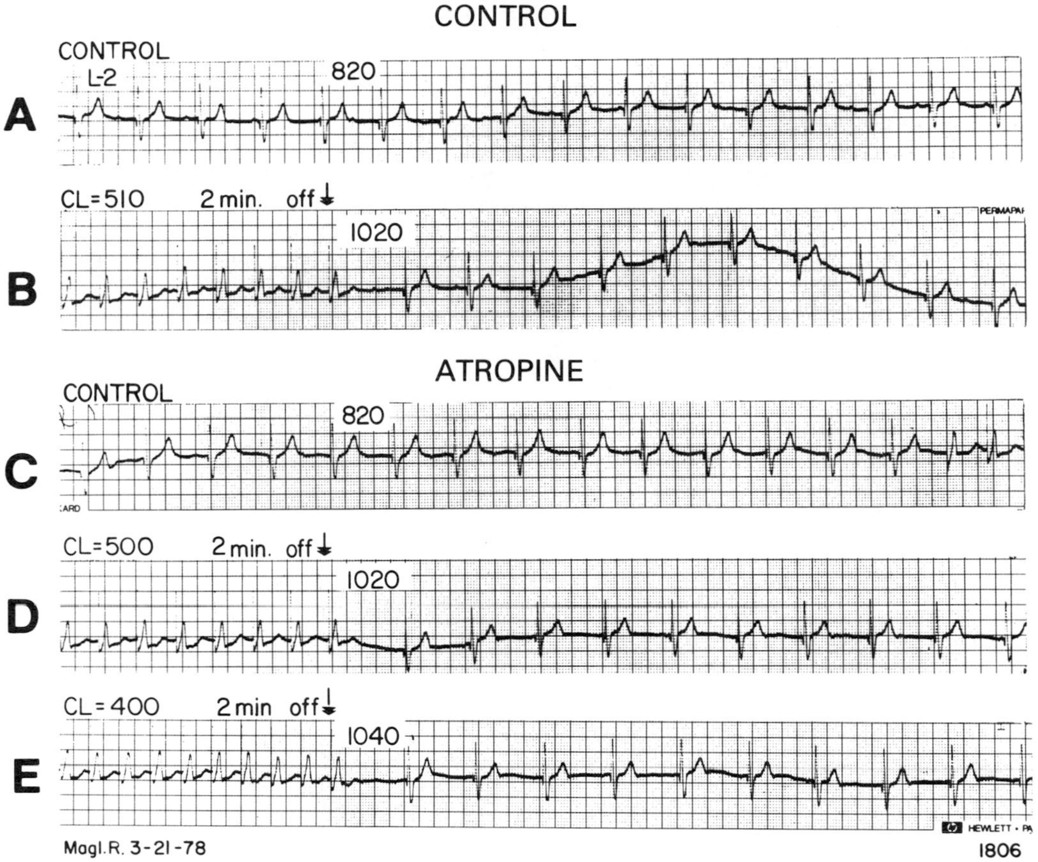

Figure 13-13. *Normal junctional recovery time in a patient with intra-His bundle block and subsidiary pacemaker (same patient as in Fig. 13-9). This patient was not given a permanent pacemaker. (A) During control, the ventricular cycle length (CL) is 820 msec. (B) Control junctional recovery time after VP at a CL of 510 msec is only 1020 msec. (C) Following atropine administration, the ventricular CL remains unchanged (820 msec). (D and E) Following atropine administration, the junctional recovery time is again normal at both the pacing CLS (500 and 400 msec).*

HPS, independent of the extrasystoles, either during sinus rhythm or with atrial pacing (Fig. 13-15).[48,77] The presence of His bundle extrasystoles is in all probability another manifestation of a disease process in the His bundle. Cases with pseudo second degree AV block should not be discounted, because their prognosis may not be benign and may be similar to that of true Mobitz type II block.[32]

Paroxysmal AV block may be triggered following a properly timed premature atrial beat or rapid driving of the heart.[48,79] The block is localized in the HPS, that is, proximal to the BH (upper His bundle), within the BH, or distal to the BH.[48] Paroxysmal AV block is a manifestation of pathologic HPS, as is indicated by a prolonged HV time, or refractory period of the HPS, and by the occurrence of spontaneous Mobitz type II AV block. The underlying mechanism may be related to (1) bradycardia-dependent AV block, which may result from a longer PP or HH interval noted after atrial stimulation,[18,50,55,79,80] (2) supernormal conduction, which is responsible for maintenance of 1:1 AV conduction[18] (atrial stimulation may lead to AV block due to an alteration in the self-perpetuating zone of supernormal conduction), and (3) the "fatigue" phenomenon encountered in the abnormal His-Purkinje system.[25] Thus far, "fatigue" phenomenon has not been seen in the normal conduction system.

Atrioventricular Delays With a Normal Electrocardiogram

The demonstration of a normal PR interval ($\leq$200 msec) and a narrow QRS complex does not exclude sig-

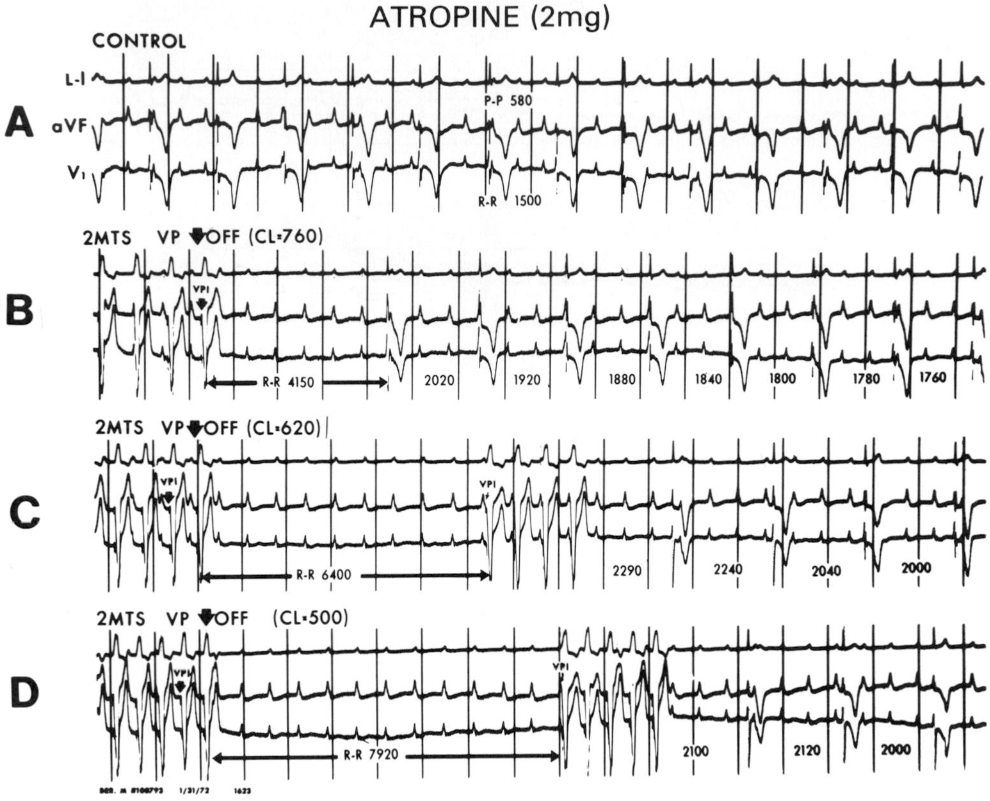

Figure 13-14. *Severely prolonged junctional recovery time in a patient with intra-His bundle complete heart block. The heart rate and the junctional recovery time remained unchanged after atropine administration. The junctional recovery time was directly related to the ventricular pacing (VP) rate and exceeded 7.9 second after VP at 120 beats/min (D).*

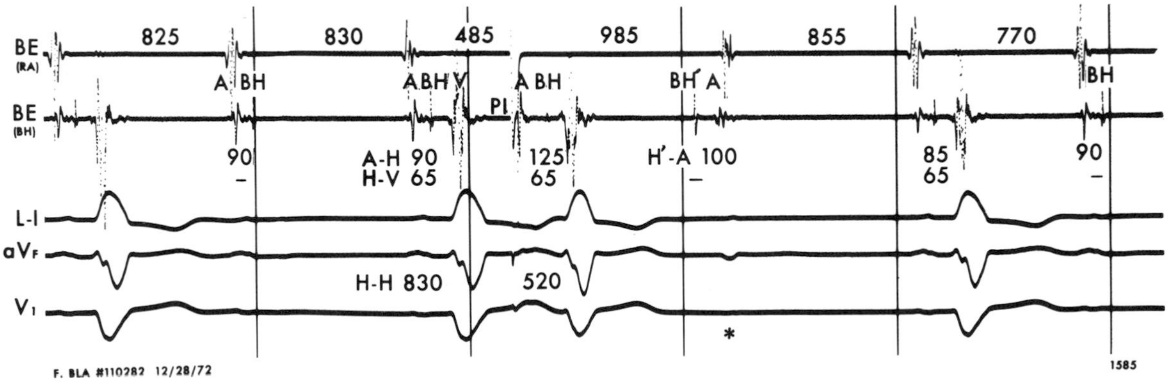

Figure 13-15. *Association of concealed His bundle extrasystoles with spontaneous second degree AV block distal to the His bundle. In additon, in the conducted beats the HV time is prolonged (65 msec). The concealed His bundle extrasystole (BN′) is blocked in antero-grade direction but results in retrograde atrial depolarization, as indicated by the inverted P wave* (asterisk) *and the sequence of atrial depolarization (fifth A wave).*

nificant AV conduction defects.[18,32] Lesions in the main His bundle proximal to its bifurcation into bundle branches do not prolong the QRS duration, and also the PR interval may not exceed 0.20 second. However, first degree AV block may be noted when marked intra-BH delays (> 40 msec) are associated with PA (45 msec) and AH (120 msec) intervals at upper limits of normal. Intra-His bundle conduction defects are frequently encountered in cases with a normal electrocardiogram and are diagnosed on the basis of (1) a wide BH deflection

(>25 msec), (2) "split" BH potentials, and (3) a prolonged HV time with a narrow QRS complex. A mild degree of intra-atrial conduction delays (PA > 45 msec) may exist despite a normal PR interval if both the AH (50 msec) and HV (35 msec) times are at lower limits of normal. Therefore, in a symptomatic patient, AV conduction defects cannot be ruled out on the basis of a normal electrocardiogram.

Therapy

Each patient should be evaluated individually, and other possible causes of syncope besides conduction abnormalities must be excluded before implantation of a permanent pacemaker. Treatment and prognosis of a patient depend on many factors, including the patient's history, symptoms, electrocardiogram, and electrophysiologic factors. The following guidelines are suggested:

1. A significantly prolonged HV time in patients with syncope and without documented AV block is an indication for pacemaker therapy, provided other possible causes for syncope have been excluded.
2. Asymptomatic patients with first degree delays in the HPS should be clinically followed at frequent intervals because of the possibility of a sudden development of type II block or CHB.
3. Irrespective of the site of block, symptomatic patients with second degree AV block are candidates for therapy. Artificial pacing is indicated in patients with HPS lesions and when drugs are ineffective in AV nodal block. Asymptomatic patients with second degree AV nodal block usually do not require therapy. However, asymptomatic patients with second degree HPS block (type I or II) should be considered for artificial pacing because these blocks are associated with sudden asystole and eventually progress to CHB.
4. Symptomatic patients with CHB, irrespective of the site of lesion, are candidates for pacemaker therapy. Asymptomatic patients with CHB localized in the AV node or in the His bundle may not require a permanent pacemaker if the subsidiary pacemaker has an adequate rate, is stable, and does not exhibit an abnormal suppression following overdrive pacing, both with and without autonomic blockade.[69] In addition, in asymptomatic patients with congenital CHB, Holter electrocardiographic recordings should be obtained in order to exclude other serious arrhythmias.[68]
5. Patients with CHB during acute myocardial infarction, irrespective of anterior or inferior wall infarction and a narrow or wide escape QRS complex, should be treated with a temporary pacemaker.[81]

Induced Atrioventricular Block

Since the first report by Gianelli and associates in 1967,[82-85] the therapeutic role of AV nodal or His bundle ablation in the management of selected patients with disabling paroxysmal supraventricular tachycardia, in whom pharmacologic agents are either ineffective or poorly tolerated, has been well established. Until recently, interruption of AV conduction necessitated surgery and thoracotomy. However, in 1981 Gonzalez and co-workers[86] reported induction of CHB by a closed chest technique that uses an electrode catheter to deliver direct current shock to ablate the His bundle. To date, this method has been applied in approximately 200 patients worldwide, each of whom received a permanent pacemaker to prevent asystole.[87-91] This technique offers a definite and significant advantage over that of thoracotomy and surgical ablation; however, it is not ideal because permanent pacemaker implantation is required and AV conduction resumes in up to 50% of patients.[89-90]

Narula has been investigating the delivery of laser energy through a catheter to interrupt or modify AV conduction in order to avoid the above-mentioned drawbacks with the direct current shock method. In 1984, we reported successful closed chest microtransection of the His bundle into proximal and distal segments ("split" His bundle potential) with laser energy delivered through a pervenous catheter (Figs. 13-16 to 13-18).[92-93]

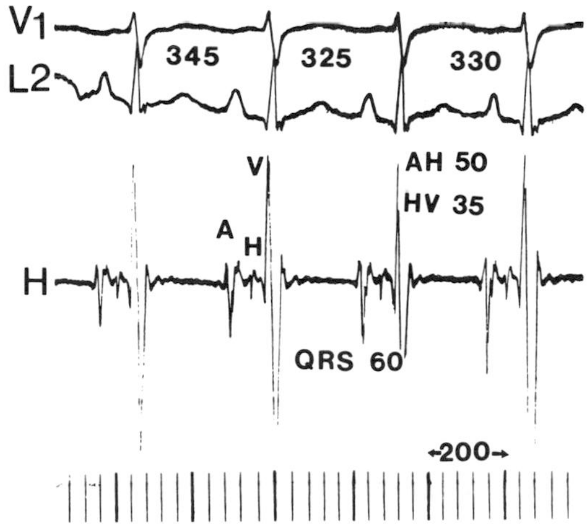

Figure 13-16. *Control His (H) bundle recordings during normal sinus rhythm. The AH and HV intervals were 50 and 35 msec, respectively. The QRS duration was 60 msec. Time lines on this and subsequent figures are 40 msec apart. (Am. J. Cardiol., 54:186–192, 1984. Reproduced with permission)*

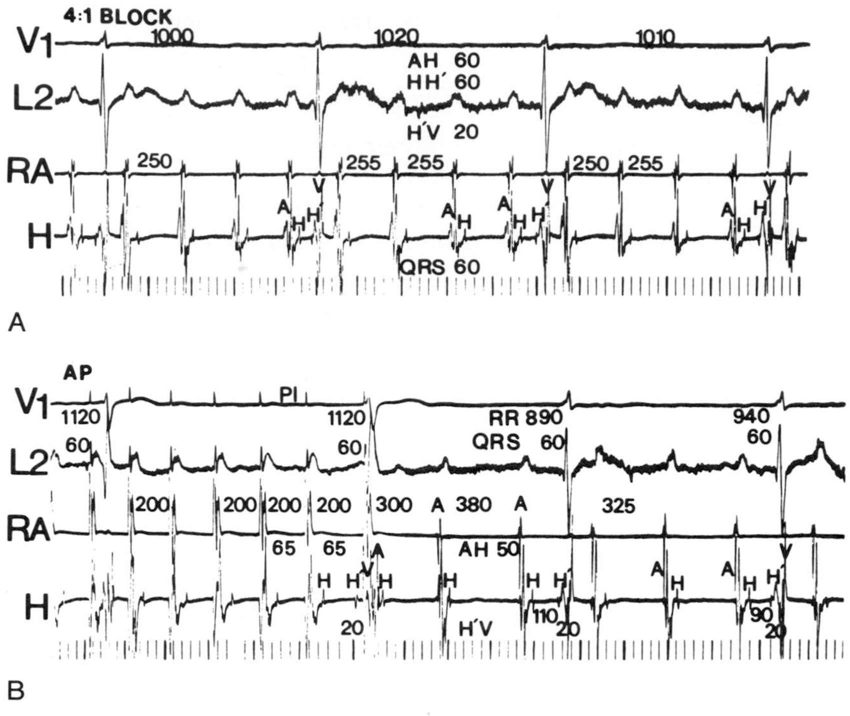

Figure 13-17. *Postlasing recordings show transient 4:1 AV conduction with an incomplete right bundle branch block in the same dog as in Figure 13-16. (A) 4:1 AV conduction with "split" His bundle potentials recorded in the conducted beats. The intra-His conduction interval (HH') is 60 msec and the H'V is 20 msec. The AH interval (60 msec) is slightly longer than in Figure 13-16 because atrial cycle length is shortened from 310 to 250 msec. Although the QRS morphology is altered, the duration is the same as that of control prelasing beats. (RA, right atrial electrogram) (B) With atrial pacing (AP) at a faster rate, the degree of AV block increased, resulting in escape of a His bundle rhythm (H'V = 20 msec) originating from the His bundle segment distal to the block. The QRS morphology in the escape His bundle beats (first two beats) is similar to that of control beats and without an incomplete right bundle branch block as seen during 3:1 and 4:1 AV conduction (last two beats). A change in atrial cycle length resulted in altered AV conduction ratios (3:1 and 4:1), RR intervals (890 to 940 msec), and the intra-His conduction time (HH' = 110 and 90 msec). Also of note is lack of fractionation of both the proximal and distal His potentials. This indicates a localized interruption of the His bundle without any injury to the adjoining His bundle fibers. (Am. J. Cardiol., 54:186–192, 1984. Reproduced with permission)*

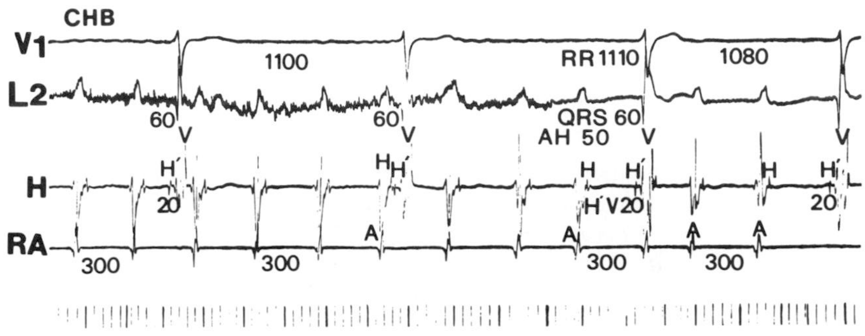

Figure 13-18. *His bundle recordings during stable complete heart block (90 minutes after lasing) in the same dog as in Figures 13-16 and 13-17 show "split" H potentials and complete AV dissociation. Each A wave is followed by an H potential, and each QRS complex is preceded by an H' potential with an H'V interval of 20 msec. The QRS complexes are similar in morphology and duration to that of control, as are the atrial cycle length and the AH interval. (Am. J. Cardiol., 54:186–192, 1984. Reproduced with permission)*

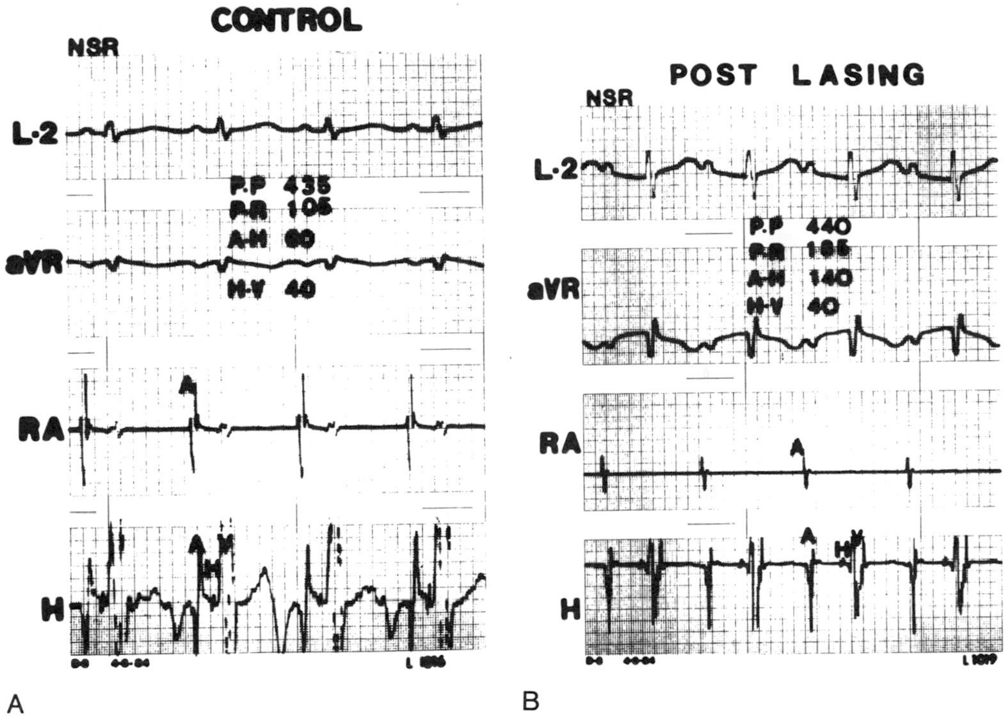

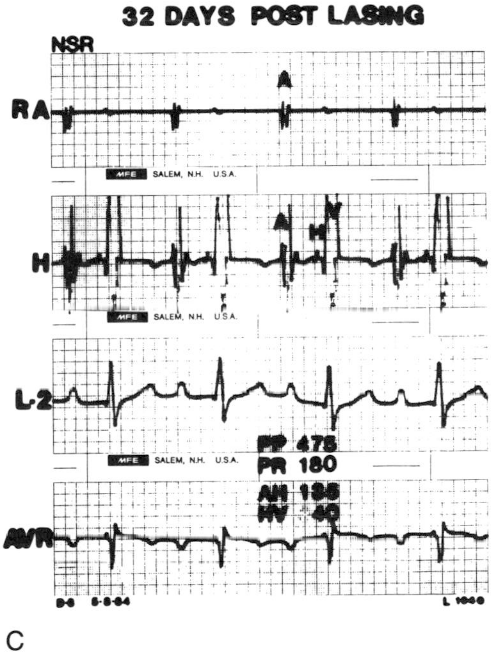

Figure 13-19. *Lasing-induced PR prolongation due to AH lengthening. These changes persisted up to 32 days. Recordings are made at 100 mm/sec speed. (A) Control His bundle (H) recordings during normal sinus rhythm. The PR and AH intervals were 105 and 60 ms, respectively. The HV time was 40 ms, and the QRS complex was narrow (60 ms). (RA, right atrial electrogram) (B) Immediate postlasing recordings show PR interval prolongation to 185 ms (versus 105 ms during control in A). This lengthening is solely contributed by AH prolongation from 60 to 140 ms. The HV time and the QRS complex remained constant. (C) Thirty days after lasing recordings show persistence of PR (180 ms) and AH (135 ms) prolongation with minimal changes (5 msec).*

These initial studies documented that laser radiation can be precisely controlled and that the degree of tissue injury can be limited to a fraction of a millimeter.[93] The latter capabilities led to our investigating the use of the laser catheter technique to alter AV nodal conduction while retaining normal sinus rhythm and 1 : 1 AV conduction.

Our experimental studies, using a pervenous laser catheter technique, have now yielded successful accomplishment of these goals of selective alteration of *AV nodal* conduction capabilities (*i.e.,* AV nodal refractioness and AV nodal conduction delays [first degree to third degree block]) in predictable and graduated steps (Figs. 13-19 to 13-22).[94] Patients with supraventricular tachyarrhythmias and rapid ventricular response may be ideally managed by induction of first or second degree AV nodal block. Clinical application of this or similar techniques holds promise and, if successful, may eliminate drug toxicity and the need for permanent pacemaker implantation.

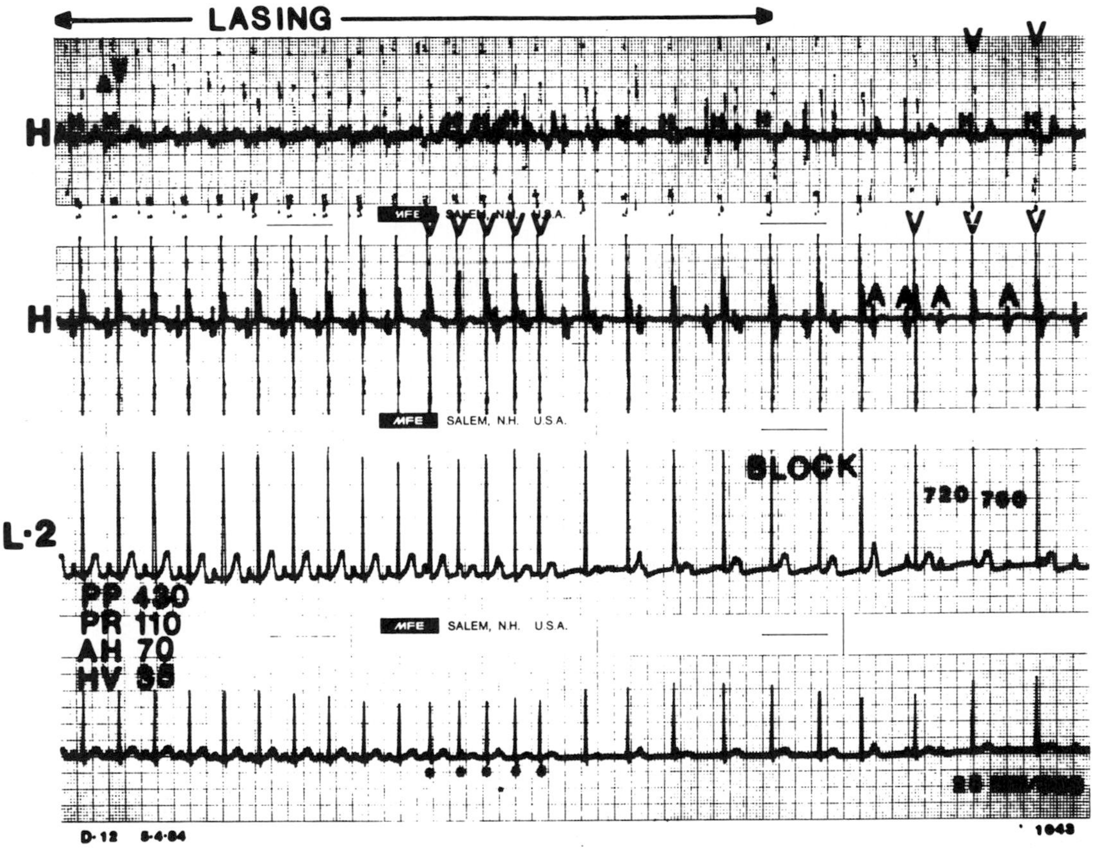

Figure 13-20. *With lasing, 1:1 AV conduction progressed through second degree block to complete heart block (last two beats) without asystole in a canine heart. The escape junctional beats are preceded by an H potential and an unchanged QRS complex.*

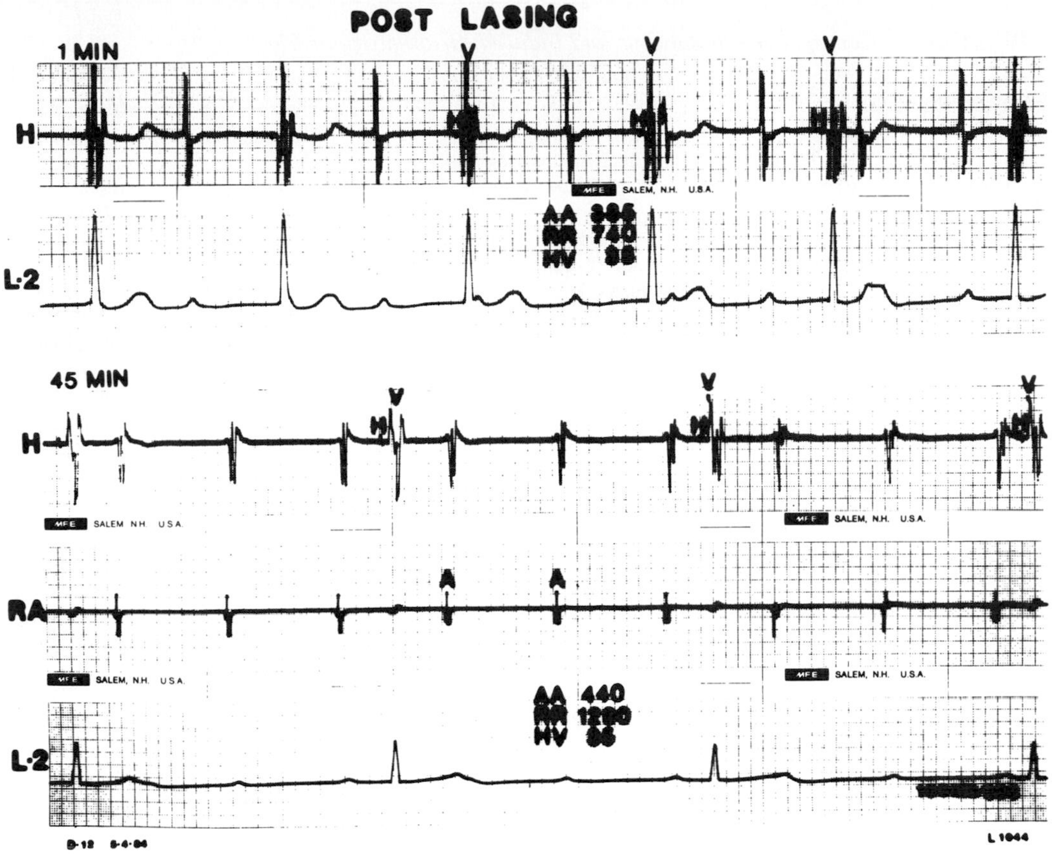

Figure 13-21. *Recordings in the same dog as in Figure 13-20 show a gradual prolongation of the cycle length of the escape junctional rhythm from 740 ms immediately after lasting* (upper panel) *to 1290 ms after 45 minutes* (bottom panel). *The QRS morphology and duration and the HV time (35 ms) remained constant and identical to normal sinus rhythm. The blocked A waves are not followed by an H potential.*

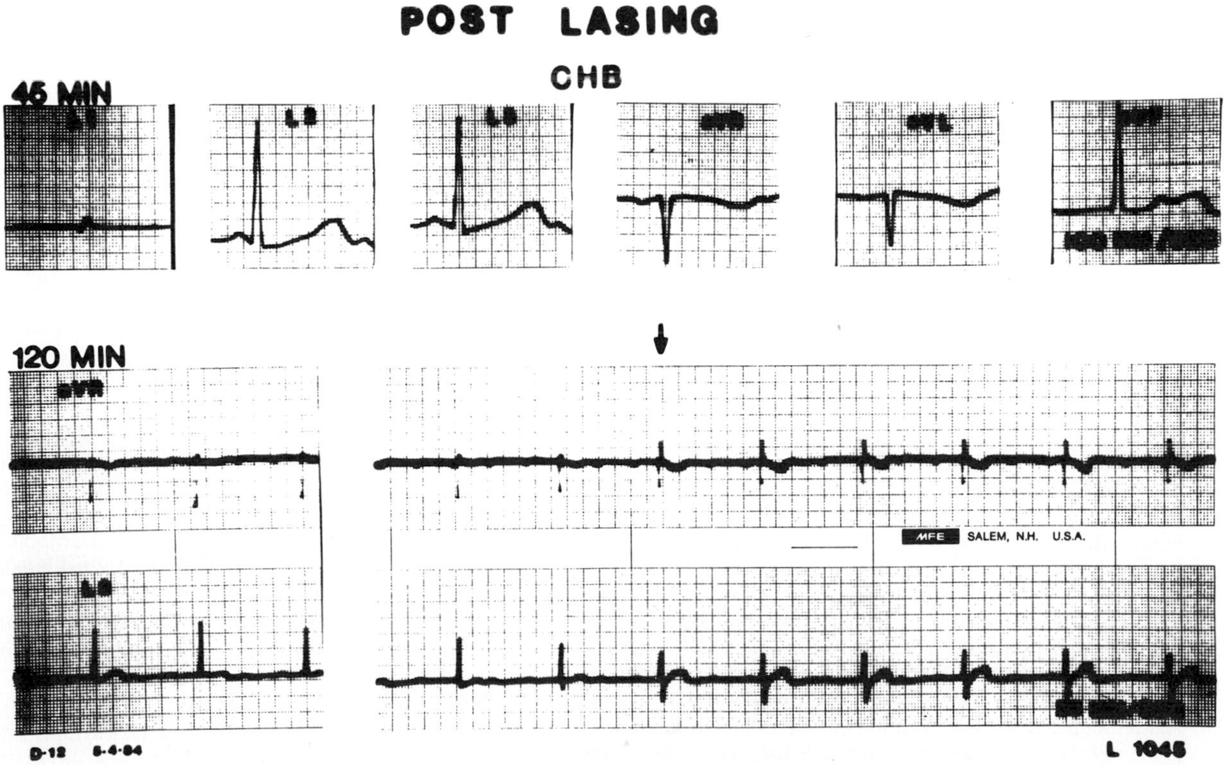

Figure 13-22. *Recordings in the same dog as in Figures 13-20 and 13-21 show a spontaneous change (2 hours after lasing) in escape rhythm from a junctional pacemaker to a distal rhythm with a wide QRS complex.*

References

1. Gaskell, W. H.: On the rhythm of the heart of the frog and the nature of the action of the vagus nerve. Philoso. Trans. R. Soc. Lond., 17:993, 1882.
2. Gaskell, W. H.: On the innervation of the heart, with special reference to the heart of the tortoise. J. Physiol. (Lond.), 4:43, 1883.
3. His, W., Jr., Die Thatigkeit des embryonalen Herzens und deren Bedeutung für die Lehre von der Herzbewegung beim Erwachsenen. Arb. Med. Klin. (Leipzig), 14, 1893.
4. Kent, A. F. S.: Researches on the structure and function of the mammalian heart. J. Physiol. (Lond.), 15:233, 1893.
5. Tawara, S.: Das Reizleitungssystem des Saugetierherzens. Jena, Fischer, 1906.
6. Aschoff, L., and Tawara, S.: Die heutige Lahre von den pathologischanatomischen Grundlagen der Herzschwache. Jena, Fisher, 1906.
7. Einthoven, W.: L'electrocardiogramme. Arch. Int. Physiol., 4:132, 1906.
8. Erlanger, J., and Blackman, J. R.: Further studies in the physiology of heart block in mammals: chronic auriculoventricular heart block in the dog. Heart, 1:177, 1909.
9. Eppinger, H., and Rotherberger, J.: Ueber die Folgen der Durchschneidung der Tawaraschen Schenkel des Reizleitungssystems. Z. Klin. Med., 70:1, 1910.
10. Mathewson, G. D.: Lesions of the branches of the auriculoventricular bundle. Heart, 4:385, 1912–1913.
11. Scherf, D., and Schookhoff, C.: Reizleitungsstorungen im Bundel: II. Mitteilung. Wien. Arch. Inn. Med., 11:425, 1926.
12. Mahaim, I.: Les Maladies Organiques du Faisceau de His-Tawara. Paris, Masson et Cie, 1931.
13. Yater, W. M., Cornell, V. H., and Clayton, T.: Auriculoventricular heart block due to bilateral bundle branch lesions. Arch. Intern. Med., 57:132, 1936.
14. Lenegre, J.: Bilateral bundle branch block. Cardiologia, 48:134, 1966.
15. Lepeschkin, E.: The electrocardiographic diagnosis of bilateral bundle branch block in relation to heart block. Prog. Cardiovasc. Dis., 6:445, 1964.
16. Narula, O. S.: His Bundle Electrocardiography and Clinical Electrophysiology. Philadelphia, F. A. Davis, 1975.
17. Narula, O. S., Cohen, L. S., Scherlag, B. J., et al.: Localization of A-V conduction defects in man by recording of the His bundle electrogram. Am. J. Cardiol., 25:228, 1970.
18. Narula, O. S.: Conduction disorders in the A-V transmission system. In Dreifus, L. S., and Likoff, W. (eds.): Cardiac Arrhythmias, 25th Hahnemann Symposium, p. 259. New York, Grune & Stratton, 1973.
19. Narula, O. S., Javier, R. P., Samet, P., and Maramba, L. C.: Significance of His and left bundle recordings from the left heart in man. Circulation, 42:385, 1970.
20. Bekheit, S., Morton, P., Murtagh, J. G., and Fletcher, E.: Comparison of sino-ventricular conduction in children and adults using bundle of His electrograms. Br. Heart J., 35:507, 1973.
21. Damato, A. N., Gallagher, J. J., Schnitzler, R. N., et al.: Use of His bundle recordings in understanding A-V conduction disturbances. Bull. N.Y. Acad. Med., 47:905, 1971.
22. Dhingra, R. C., Rosen, K. M., and Rahimtoola, S. H.: Normal conduction intervals and responses in sixty-one patients using His bundle recording and atrial pacing. Chest, 64:55, 1973.
23. Castellanos, A., Castillo, C. A., and Agha, A. S.: Contribution of His bundle recording to the understanding of clinical arrhythmias. Am. J. Cardiol., 28:499, 1971.
24. Narula, O. S.: Validation of His bundle electrograms: limitations of the catheter technique. In Narula, O. S. (ed.): His Bundle Electrocardiography, p. 65. Philadelphia, F. A. Davis, 1975.
25. Narula, O. S., and Runge, M.: A-V nodal accommodation and fatigue phenomenon in the His-Purkinje system. In Wellens, H. J. J., Lie, K. I., and Janse, M. (eds.): The Conduction System of the Heart, p. 529. Leiden, HE Stenfert Kroese, 1976.
26. Rosen, K. M.: Evaluation of cardiac conduction in the cardiac catheterization laboratory. Am. J. Cardiol., 30:701, 1972.
27. Narula, O. S., Scherlag, B. J., Samet, P., and Javier, R. P.: Atrioventricular block: localization and classification by His bundle recordings. Am. J. Med., 50:146, 1971.
28. Narula, O. S.: Atrioventricular block. In Narula, O. S. (ed.): Cardiac Arrhythmias: Electrophysiology, Diagnosis and Management. Baltimore, Williams & Wilkins, 1979.
29. Peuch, P., Grolleau, R., and Guimond, C.: Incidence of different types of A-V block and their localization by His bundle recordings. In Wellens, H. J. J., Lie, K. I., and Janse, M. (eds.): The Conduction System of the Heart, p. 467. Leiden, HE Stenfert Kroese, 1976.
30. Haft, J. I., and Levites, R.: Significance of first degree heart block (prolonged P-R interval) in bifascicular block. Am. J. Cardiol., 34:257, 1974.
31. Narula, O. S., and Samet, P.: Significance of first degree AV block. Circulation, 43:772, 1971.
32. Narula, O. S.: Current concepts of A-V block. In Narula, O. S. (ed.): His Bundle Electrocardiography and Clinical Electrophysiology, p. 139. Philadelphia, F. A. Davis, 1975.
33. Narula, O. S., Runge, M., and Samet, P.: Second degree Wenckebach type A-V block due to block within the atrium. Br. Heart J., 34:1127, 1972.
34. Leier, C. V., Meacham, J. A., and Schall, S. F.: Prolonged atrial conduction: a major predisposing factor for the development of atrial flutter. Circulation, 57:213, 1978.
35. Wenckebach, K. F.: Beitrage zur Kenntis der menschlichen Herztatigkeit. Arch. Anat. Physiol., pp. 297–354, 1906.
36. Mobitz, W.: Über die unvollstandinge Storung der Erregungsüberleitung zwischen Vorhof und Kammer des menschlichen Herzens. Z. Gesamte Exp. Med., 41:180, 1924.
37. Wenckebach, K. F., and Winterberg, H.: Die Unregelmassige Herztatigkeit. pp. 305–310. Leipzig, Wilhem Engelman, 1927.
38. Denes, P., Levy, L., Pick, A., and Rosen, K. M.: The incidence of typical and atypical A-V Wenckebach periodicity. Am. Heart J., 88:26, 1975.
39. Friedman, H. S., Gomes, J. A. C., and Haft, J. I.: An analysis of Wenckebach periodicity. J. Electrocardiol., 8:307, 1975.
40. El-Sherif, N., Aranda, J., Befler, B., and Lazzara, R.: Atypical Wenckebach periodicity simulating Mobitz II A-V block. Br. Heart J., 40:1376, 1978.
41. Halpern, M. S., Nau, G. J., Levi, R. J., et al.: Wenckebach periods of alternate beats: clinical and experimental observation. Circulation, 48:41, 1973.
42. Amat-y-Leon, F., Chuquimia, R., Wu, D., et al.: Alternating Wenckebach periodicity: A common electrophysiologic response. Am. J. Cardiol., 36:757, 1975.
43. Castellanos, A., Sung, R. J., Mallon, S. M., et al.: Effects of proximal intra-atrial Wenckebach on distal atrioventricular nodal and His-Purkinje block. With special reference to the theory of alternating Wenckebach periods. Am. Heart J., 95:228, 1978.
44. Narula, O. S., and Samet, P.: Wenckebach and Mobitz type II A-V blocks due to lesions within the His bundle and bundle branches. Circulation, 41:947, 1970.
45. Brodsky, M., Wu, D., Denes, P., et al.: Arrhythmias documented by 24 hour continuous electrocardiographic monitoring in 50 male medical students without apparent heart disease. Am. J. Cardiol., 39:390, 1977.
46. Meyles, I., Kaplinsky, E., Yahini, J., et al.: Wenckebach A-V block: a frequent feature following heavy physical training. Am. Heart J., 90:426, 1974.

47. Young, D., Eisenberg, R., Fisch, B., and Fischer, J. D.: Wenckebach AV block (Mobitz I) in children and young adults. Am. J. Cardiol., 40:393, 1977.
48. Narula, O. S.: Wenckebach type I and type II atrioventricular block (revisited). Cardiovasc. Clin., 6(3):137, 1974.
49. Langendorf, R., Cohen, H., and Gozo, E. G.: Observations on second degree atrioventricular block, including new criteria for the differential diagnosis between type I and type II block. Am. J. Cardiol., 29:111, 1972.
50. Goodfriend, M. A., and Barold, S. S.: Tachycardia dependent and bradycardia dependent Mobitz type II atrioventricular block within the bundle of His. Am. J. Cardiol., 33:908, 1974.
51. Rosen, K. M., Loeb, H. S., Gunnar, R. M., and Rahimtoola, S. H.: Mobitz type II block without bundle branch block. Circulation, 44:1111, 1971.
52. Yeh, B. K., Tao, P., and DeGuzman, N.: Mobitz type II A-V blocks as a manifestation of digitalis toxicity. J. Electrocardiol., 5:74, 1972.
53. Langendorf, R., and Pick, A.: Atrioventricular block type II (Mobitz): its nature and clinical significance. Circulation, 38:819, 1968.
54. Scherlag, B. J., El-Sherif, N., and Lazzara, R.: Experimental study of model for Mobitz type II and paroxysmal atrioventricular block. Am. J. Cardiol., 34:309, 1974.
55. Jonas, E. A., Kosowsky, B. D., and Ramaswamy, K.: Complete His-Purkinje block produced by carotid sinus massage: Report of a case. Circulation, 50:192, 1974.
56. Schuilenberg, R. M., and Durrer, D.: Problems in recognition of conduction disturbances in the His bundle. Circulation, 51:68, 1975.
57. Narula, O. S., Scherlag, B. J., Javier, R. P., et al.: Analysis of the A-V conduction defect in complete heart block utilizing His bundle electrograms. Circulation, 41:437, 1970.
58. Guimond, C., and Puech, P.: Intra-His bundle blocks (102 cases). Eur. J. Cardiol., 4:481, 1976.
59. Rosen, K. M., Dhingra, R. C., Loeb, H. S., and Rahimtoola, S. H.: Chronic heart block in adults. Arch. Intern. Med., 131:663, 1973.
60. Gupta, P. K., Lichstein, E., and Chadda, K.: Electrophysiological features of complete A-V block within the His bundle. Br. Heart J., 35:610, 1973.
61. Tricot, R., Guerot, C., Valere, P., and Coste, A.: Etude de la conduction auriculoventriculaire par enregisterment du faisceau de His dans 60 cas de block auriculoventriculaire. Arch. Mal. Coeur, 65:441, 1972.
62. Nasarallah, A. T., Gillette, P. C., and Mullins, C. E.: Congenital and surgical atrioventricular block within the His bundle. Am. J. Cardiol., 36:916, 1965.
63. Rosen, K. M., Mehta, A., Rahimtoola, S. H., and Miller, R. A.: Sites of congenital and surgical heart block as defined by His bundle electrocardiography. Circulation, 44:833, 1971.
64. Anderson, R. H., Wenick, A. C. G., Losekoot, T. G., and Becker, A. E.: Congenital complete heart block: developmental aspects. Circulation, 56:90, 1977.
65. Lev, M., Silverman, J., Fitzmaurice, F. M., et al.: Lack of connection between the atria and the more peripheral conduction system in congenital atrioventricular block. Am. J. Cardiol., 27:481, 1971.
66. Lev, M., Candros, H., and Paul, M. H.: Interruption of the atrioventricular bundle with congenital atrioventricular block. Circulation, 43:703, 1971.
67. Narula, O. S., and Samet, P.: Effect of atropine and glucagon on A-V nodal and His bundle pacemakers in man. Circulation (Suppl.), 44:II-205, 1971.
68. Levy, A. M., Camm, A. J., and Keane, J. F.: Multiple arrhythmias detected during nocturnal monitoring in patients with congenital complete heart block. Circulation, 55:247, 1977.
69. Narula, O. S., and Narula, J. T.: Junctional pacemakers in man: response to overdrive suppression with and without parasympathetic blockade. Circulation, 57:880, 1978.
70. Narula, O. S., and Samet, O.: Predilection of elderly females for intra His bundle (BH) blocks. Circulation (Suppl.), 50:III-195, 1974.
71. Pomerance, A.: Pathological and clinical study of calcification of the mitral valve ring. J. Clin. Pathol., 23:354, 1970.
72. Kelly, D. T., Brodsky, S. J., Mirowski, M., et al.: Bundle of His recordings in congenital heart block. Circulation, 45:277, 1972.
73. Rosen, K. M.: Catheter recordings of His bundle electrograms. Mod. Concepts Cardiovasc. Dis., 42:23, 1973.
74. Billette, J.: Preceding His-atrial interval as a determinant of atrioventricular nodal conduction time in the human and rabbit heart. Am. J. Cardiol., 38:889, 1976.
75. Langendorf, R., and Mehlman, J. S.: Blocked (nonconducted) A-V nodal premature systoles imitating first and second degree A-V block. Am. Heart J., 34:500, 1947.
76. Rosen, K. M., Rahimtoola, S. H., and Gunnar, R. M.: Pseudo A-V block secondary to premature non-propagated His bundle depolarizations: documentation by His bundle electrocardiography. Circulation, 42:367, 1970.
77. Grolleau, R., et al.: Les depolarizations hisiennes ectopiques non propagees. Arch. Mal. Coeur, 65:1069, 1972.
78. Fisch, C., Zipes, D. P., and McHenry, P. L.: Electrocardiographic manifestations of concealed junctional ectopic impulses. Circulation, 53:217, 1976.
79. Coumel, P., Fabiato, A., Waynberger, M., et al.: Bradycardia dependent atrioventricular block. J. Electrocardiol., 4:168, 1977.
80. Rosenbaum, M. B., Elizari, M. V., Levi, R. J., et al.: Paroxysmal atrioventricular block related to hypopolarization and spontaneous diastolic depolarization. Chest, 63:678, 1973.
81. Lie, K. I., and Durrer, D.: Conduction disturbances in acute myocardial infarction. In Narula, O. S. (ed.): Cardiac Arrhythmias: Electrophysiology, Diagnosis and Management. Baltimore, Williams & Wilkins, 1979.
82. Gianelli, S., Jr., Ayres, S. M., Gromprecht, R. F., et al.: Therapeutic surgical division of the human conduction system. J.A.M.A., 199:155–160, 1967.
83. Slama, R., Blondeau, P., Aigueperse, J., et al.: Creation chircurgicale d'un bloc auriculoventriculaire et implantation d'un stimulateur dans deux cas de troubles du rhythme irreductibles. Arch. Mal. Coeur, 60:406–422, 1967.
84. Dreifus, L. S., Nichols, H., Morse, D., et al.: Control of recurrent tachycardia of Wolff-Parkinson-White syndrome by surgical ligature of the AV bundle. Circulation, 38:1030–1036, 1968.
85. Harrison, L., Gallagher, J. J., Kasell, J., et al.: Cryosurgical ablation of the AV node–His bundle: A new method for producing AV block. Circulation, 55:463–470, 1977.
86. Gonzalez, R., Scheinman, M. M., Margaretten, W., and Rubinstein, M.: Closed-chest electrode-catheter technique for His bundle ablation in dogs. Am. J., Physiol., 241:H283–287, 1981.
87. Gonzalez, R., Scheinman, M. M., Bharati, S., and Lev, M.: Closed chest permanent atrioventricular block in dogs. Am. Heart J., 105:461–470, 1983.
88. Gallagher, J. J., Svenson, R. H., Kasell, J. H., et al.: Closed-chest ablation of the atrioventricular conduction system. N. Engl. J. Med., 306:194–200, 1982.
89. Bardy, G. H., Ideker, R. E., Kasell, J., et al.: Transvenous ablation of the atrioventricular conduction system in dogs: Electrophysiologic and histologic observations. Am. J. Cardiol., 51:1775–1782, 1983.
90. Fisher, V. J., Lee, R. J., Christianson, L. C., and Kavaler, F.: Production of chronic atrio-ventricular block in dogs without thoracotomy. J. Appl. Physiol., 21:1119–1121, 1966.
91. Scheinman, M. M., and Evans-Bell, T.: Catheter ablation of the

atrioventricular junction: A report of the percutaneous mapping and ablation registry. Circulation, 70:1024–1029, 1984.
92. Narula, O. S., Bharati, S., Chan, M. C., et al.: Laser micro transection of the His bundle: A pervenous catheter technique (abstr.). J. Am. Coll. Cardiol., 3:537, 1984.
93. Narula, O. S., Bharati, S., Chan, M. C., et al.: Micro transection of the His bundle with laser radiation via a pervenous catheter: Correlation of histological and electro-physiological data. Am. J. Cardiol., 54:186–192, 1984.
94. Narula, O. S., Boveja, B. K., Cohen, D. M., et al.: Laser catheter-induced atrioventricular nodal delays and atrioventricular block in dogs: Acute and chronic observations. J. Am. Coll. Cardiol., 5:259–267, 1985.

14

Atrioventricular Block: A Noninvasive Approach to the Problem

R. A. Massumi

This chapter does not represent a textbook treatment of atrioventricular (AV) block, nor does it contain an exhaustive review of the voluminous literature on the subject. Instead, it describes what the author considers a pragmatic noninvasive approach to the problem of localization and characterization of AV conduction disturbances. The chapter reflects the author's attempts over many years to amalgamate the anatomic characteristics of the various portions of the AV conduction pathways with their electrophysiologic and clinical peculiarities and their behavior after vagal and sympathetic influences. The remarkable contributions of noninvasive studies of vagal stimulation and inhibition and sympathetic influences to the localization of block within the AV node or the infranodal pathways will be pointed out. The views expressed are predicated on a correlation of clinical and electrophysiologic observations in over 186 patients manifesting varying grades of AV conduction disturbances and the use of vagal and sympathetic maneuvers, with subsequent documentation of the site and type of AV block by His bundle studies in over two thirds of them. Finally, emphasis is placed on the clinical analysis of the patterns and mechanisms of AV conduction disturbances, with His bundle studies introduced only for validation whenever indicated. The noninvasive approach described here has proved especially useful in the most difficult and elusive differential diagnosis between AV nodal block and main His bundle or intra-Hisian block.

Atrioventricular block consists of a slowing or complete cessation of conduction between the atria and the ventricles, reflected in the electrocardiogram by a prolonged PR interval or by failure of the P wave to be conducted to the ventricles. During atrial pacing at rates greater than 130 beats/min, an element of block is physiologic; at rates above 180 beats/min, block becomes obligatory and salutary for protection of the ventricles from unphysiologically rapid rates even though rare patients are capable of conducting 1 : 1 at rates of 200 beats/min or even higher. Conduction at such high rates may be possible in any person if sympathetic stimulation, vagal inhibition, or both are present (*e.g.,* fever, infection, blood loss, abrupt decline in cardiac output) and in the presence of the so-called accelerated AV node conduction.

The PR interval is the time required by the atrial depolarizing impulse to traverse the atrium, the AV node, the bundle of His, the intraventricular fascicles,

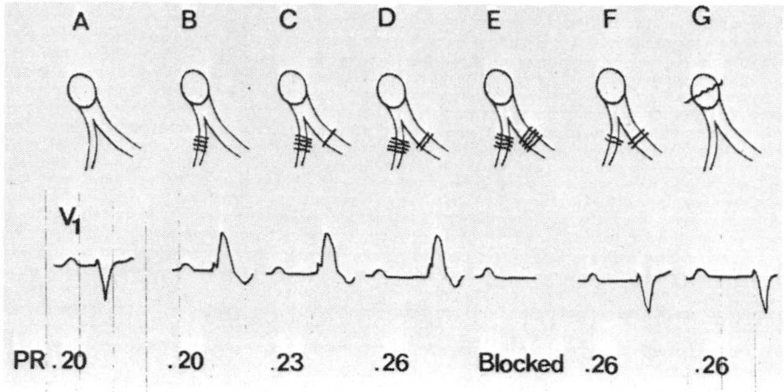

Figure 14-1. *The relationship between the pattern of conduction in the two bundle branches and the PR interval is diagramatically depicted. Drawings under the letters A to G represent the AV node and the two bundles. Lead V_1 is drawn, and the PR intervals in seconds are shown in the PR column. Horizontal lines crossing the bundle branches depict the magnitude of block under scale of 1+ to 4+. (A) No block anywhere; PR interval, 0.2 second; QRS complex, narrow. (B) Complete right bundle branch block is present. The PR interval is unchanged because conduction through the left bundle remains intact, but the QRS complex shows features of right bundle branch block. (C) Same as in B with the additional development of a mild degree of block in the left bundle, causing the PR interval to prolong. (D) Same as in C, with the only difference being a greater degree of block in the left bundle, thus making the PR interval still longer, reaching 0.26 second. Because of the greater magnitude of block in the right bundle branch than in the left bundle branch, the QRS complex retains features of right bundle branch block in B, C, and D. (E) Block in the left bundle progresses to 4+ (i.e., complete). The P wave thus cannot be conducted to the ventricles. (F) Incomplete but equal conduction delays in both bundles prolongs the PR interval to 0.26 second. However, the simultaneous depolarization of both ventricles causes the QRS complex to return to normal. (G) Incomplete block in the AV node prolongs the PR interval only, hence the similarity between F and G.*

and the Purkinje fibers and produce sufficiently large depolarization potentials within the ventricular myocardium to be recorded on the electrocardiogram. The PR interval may be significantly lengthened solely because of a conduction delay within the right atrium (*e.g.*, intra-atrial block due to extreme dilation or fibrosis). Even though the presence of intra-atrial block is usually manifested by wide and notched P waves, the surface electrocardiogram cannot differentiate delay within the right atrium and true block resulting from delay within the AV node–His-Purkinje system.

Three situations deserve special comment. The first is atrial fibrillation where the presence of AV block is suggested by a ventricular rate that is significantly slower than that expected in the presence of normal AV conduction (100 to 130 beats/min at rest, 140 beats/min or faster during physical activity, fever, or excitement). The second situation is encountered where a junctional or ventricular escape pacemaker has assumed control of the ventricles. Here, the presence of an underlying AV block is difficult or impossible to discern. This difficulty becomes compounded when 1 : 1 retrograde VA conduction is present, causing perpetual suppression of both the antegrade AV conduction and the pacemaking activity of the sinus node. Similar situations may be observed in cases of isorhythmic junctional or ventricular rhythms and during ventricular tachycardia. Since AV node function cannot be assessed during these arrhythmias, the possibility of an underlying AV block must be kept in mind before attempts are made to abolish the dominant rhythm. This is particularly true if acute myocardial infarction or digitalis intoxication is suspected. The third situation is the apparent normalization of the PR interval in cases of first degree AV block when the atrial pacemaker shifts from the sinus node to a low atrial, coronary sinus, or AV junctional focus. The apparent normalization may also occur in severe sinus bradycardia, where the AV node is afforded long intervals in which to recover normal conductivity.

Prolongation of the PR interval may have nothing to do with the AV junction and be completely accounted for by a delay in the bundle branch system. In such cases, the QRS complexes are generally wide but may be narrow if the delays within the two bundle branches become equal in length (Fig. 14-1).

Anatomic and Electrophysiologic Considerations

The site of impaired conduction may be the AV node, the main His bundle, or the intraventricular conduction system (the bundle branches or the trifascicular system). Significantly slowed conduction in the Purkinje system or the working myocardium (*e.g.*, potassium intoxication, quinidinelike drugs, severe global myocardial ischemia) may cause marked prolongation and deformity of the QRS complexes but does not cause clinical AV block except in extreme states. For the purposes of discussion, it is sufficient to view the intraventricular conduction system as a trifascicular (three-pronged) structure and not concern onself with the controversies pertaining to the middle or septal fascicle of the left bundle. The AV node is composed of conglomerates of intertwined cells, perhaps teleologically designed to impede conduction and allow for an optimal ventricular filling after atrial contraction.[1-3] The transmembrane action potentials of AV node cells are slowly inscribed, reflecting their dependency on the slow transfer of calcium ions

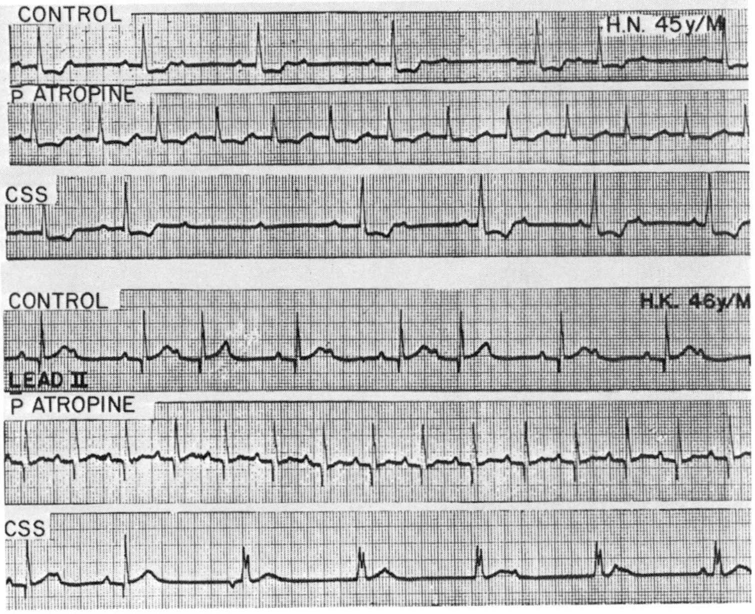

Figure 14-2. *Two cases of acute inferior wall myocardial infarction associated with incomplete block documented by His bundle electrography in the AV node. In both cases Wenckebach periods of 2:1 and 3:2 conduction ratios are present. Note that the 2:1 conduction pattern in these two cases is the shortest Wenckebach period and is really a form of Mobitz type I block. In itself, 2:1 conduction is consistent with both Mobitz type I and Mobitz type II block. However, the Mobitz type I variety is generally found in the company of 3:2 and 4:3 Wenckebach periods, whereas the Mobitz type II variety of 2:1 conduction alternates with 1:1 or 3:1 conduction. In both cases depicted in Figure 14-1, atropine reduced the magnitude of block to first degree, but carotid sinus stimulation caused complete block, thus placing block in an acetylcholine-sensitive structure, namely, the AV node. In the lower tracing, an idioventricular escape rhythm emerges when the block becomes complete. (CSS, carotid sinus stimulation)*

across the cell membrane.[4–5] Conduction within the AV node is slow and decremental, and conduction impairment becomes progressively more severe as the impulse grinds its way toward the lower pole of the node. This phenomenon results in the typical and well-known Wenckebach periodicity (Fig. 14-2). When Wenckebach periodicity occurs in the main His bundle, on the other hand, it is usually but not invariably atypical (Fig. 14-3) and probably reflects a pathologic change from sodium dependency, which is the characteristic feature of the main His bundle and the trifascicular system, to calcium dependency. These anatomic and electrophysiologic differences are further punctuated by the markedly divergent behaviors of these structures *vis-a-vis* atropine, acetylcholine, and catecholamines.[6–9] Conductivity through the AV node is exquisitely responsive to autonomic influences, accelerating with sympathetic stimulation or vagal inhibition and slowing with vagal stimulation.

The main His bundle and the bundle branch or the trifascicular conduction pathways, on the other hand, are insensitive to the direct influences of atropine, acetylcholine, and catecholamines insofar as conductivity is concerned.[6–10] Only conduction in the most proximal segment of the main His bundle adjacent to the AV node may be partially affected by autonomic influences. As a direct result of these differences, AV nodal and intra-Hisian blocks respond quite differently to vagal and other autonomic maneuvers. Thus, block of the AV node increases with carotid sinus stimulation even though the sinus rate slows concomitantly, whereas intra-Hisian block decreases or disappears with vagal stimulation (Figs. 14-4 and 14-5).[7,11] In the latter circumstance, the decrease in the number of P waves reaching the His bundle, which has not been directly influenced by vagal stimulation, enables this structure to conduct more efficiently. Physiologically, therefore, AV nodal and infranodal blocks display diametrically opposite behavior in response to physiologic body demands transmitted through the autonomic nervous system. In AV nodal block, when physiologic needs of the body demand accelerated heart rates, the sinus rate increases and the AV conduction improves. The existing Wenckebach periods and even higher grades of AV block may disappear. In intra-Hisian and trifascicular block the physiologic acceleration of the sinus rate during exertion is accompanied by an increase in the magnitude of AV block and a decrease in the effective or actual ventricular rate. This fundamental difference accounts for the markedly more benign course and the greater tolerability of the AV nodal block. The more serious symptoms and the more urgent need for pacemaker insertion in infranodal blocks in great part reflects the paradoxical response of the effective ventricular rate to body demands. Failure of the ventricular rate to increase when the body calls for faster heart rates and enhanced cardiac output not only explains the effort intolerance but also the greater frequency of ventricular irritability and fibrillation in such patients. As will be noted later in this chapter, noninvasive maneuvers have been extremely useful in differentiating AV nodal and infranodal blocks and have correctly predicted the site of block in the 14 patients with

(Text continues on p. 349.)

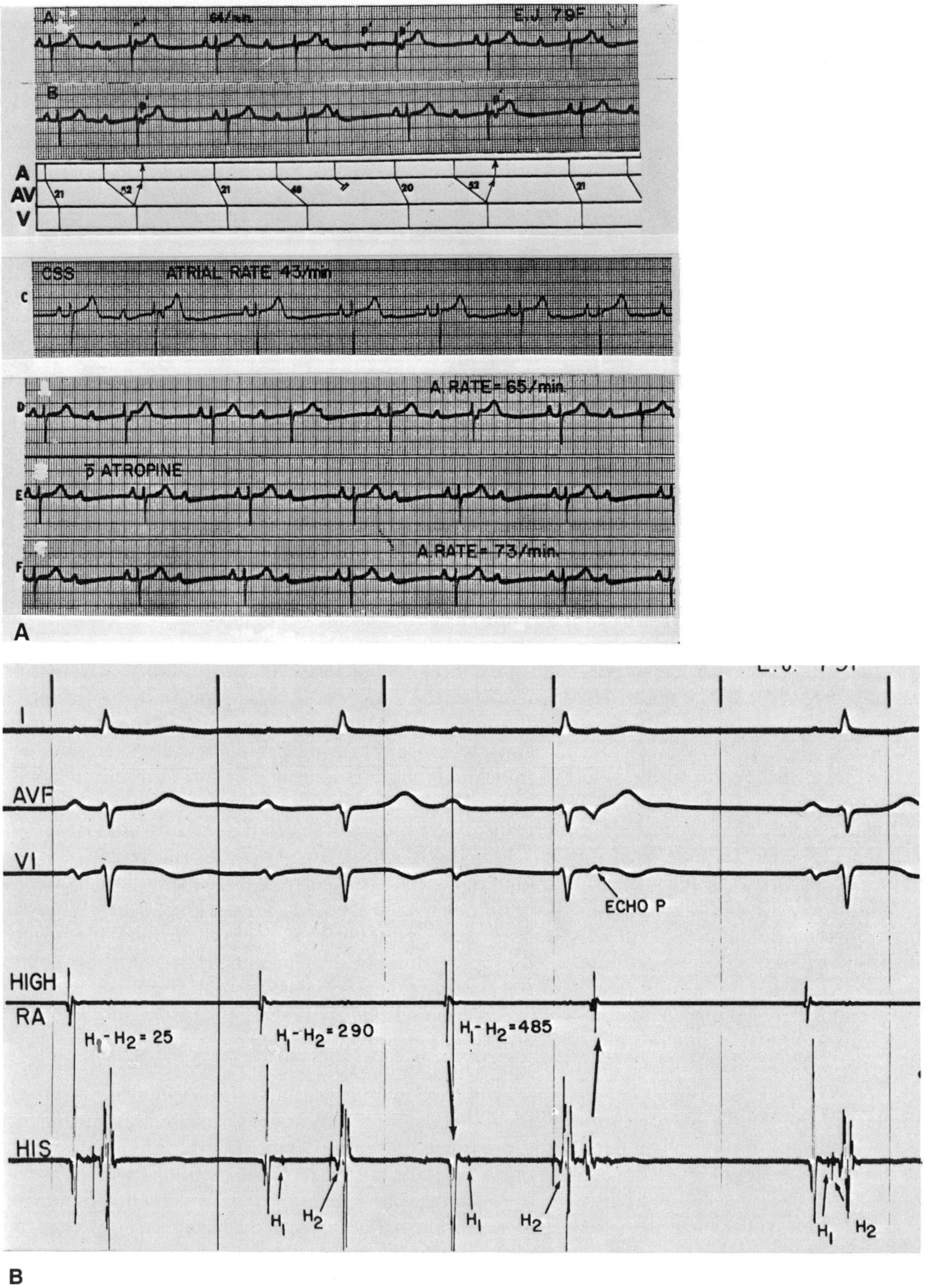

B

Figure 14-3. *(A) Rhythm strips in a woman aged 79 years with history of dizzy spells. The QRS complexes are narrow. The Wenckebach cycles begin with a PR interval of 0.2 to 0.21 second. The second P wave in the cycle is conducted with a much longer PR interval of 0.48 to 0.52 second. The increment of 0.30 second (2.5 times the first PR of the cycle) is most atypical for AV nodal–Wenckebach cycles and was considered consistent with block in the main His bundle. Slowing of the atrial rate by carotid sinus stimulation eliminated*

(Continued)

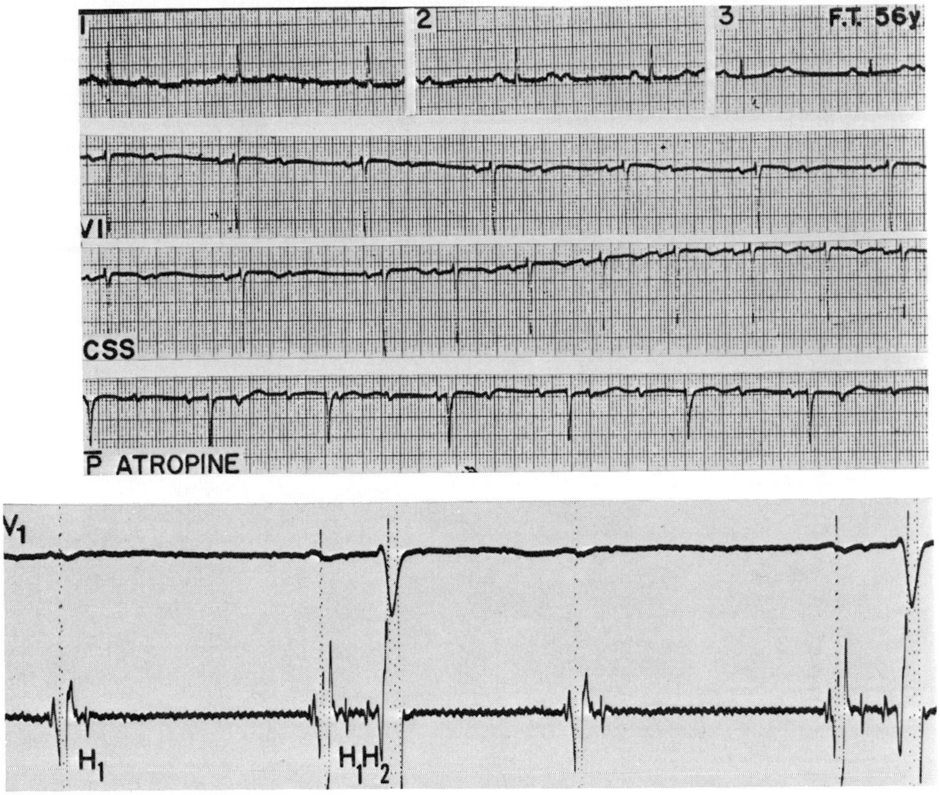

Figure 14-4. *An example of narrow QRS AV block with a fixed pattern of 2:1 AV conduction (atrial rate 92 beats/min, ventricular rate 46 beats/min) is observed in this man aged 56 years complaining of fatigue, exercise intolerance, and lightheadedness on exertion. Wenckebach periods were not found during several days of monitoring. Carotid sinus stimulation (CSS) converted the AV conduction pattern to 1:1* (third strip), *while atropine and exercise increased block to complete (*bottom strip, *atrial rate 116 beats/min, ventricular rate 48 beats/min). The ventricular rate could not keep pace with the increased sinus rate during periods of heightened physiologic demands, hence the exercise intolerance and lightheadedness. His bundle recording in the bottom panel again shows a 2:1 AV conduction pattern with two His spikes marked H_1 and H_2, with only H_1 present after the blocked P waves, thus localizing block at the level of the middle of the His bundle.*

---

block, and 1:1 AV conduction with normal PR intervals appeared. Atropine increased the magnitude of block to 2:1. Whenever the PR interval achieved a value of 0.52 second (second P wave in A and B and eighth wave in B), it was followed by a retrograde P wave. This in turn reset the sinus node, altering the basic rhythmicity. In other areas, blocked P waves were followed by retrograde (echo) P waves (sixth P wave in A). These echo P waves were in turn conducted to the ventricles and, at the same time, echoed back into the atrium. (B) His bundle recording showing split His spikes (H_1 and H_2) with the increments in H_1-H_2 intervals accounting for the entire increase in the PR intervals. After H_1-H_2 achieves a value of 485 msec, a retrograde P wave (slanted upward arrow) *ensues, indicating echo of the P wave. Note the abrupt increase of H_1-H_2 interval from 25 msec to 290 msec.*

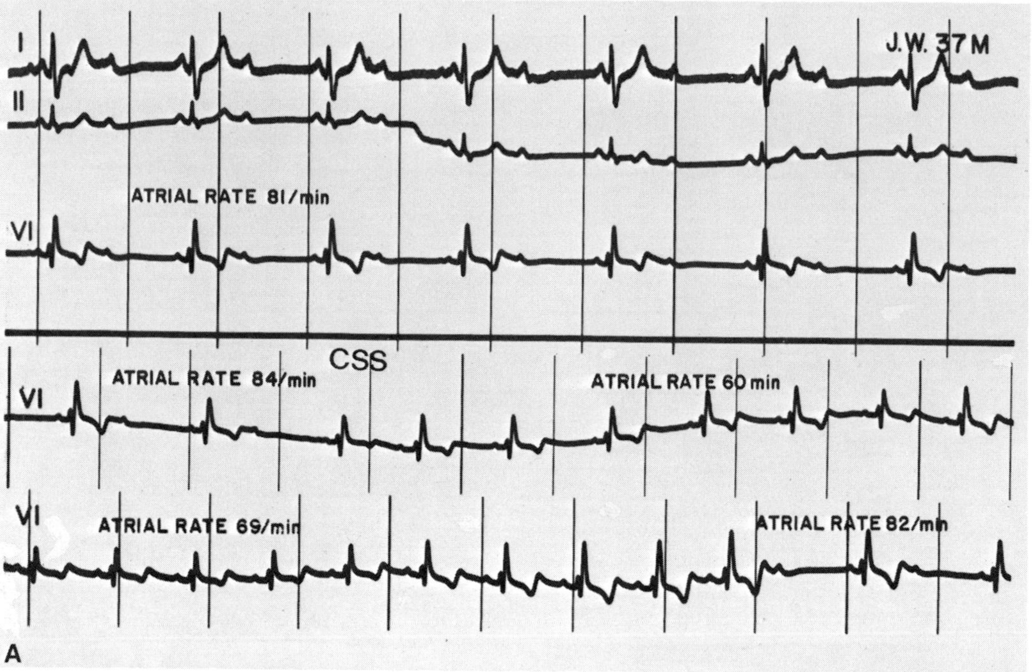

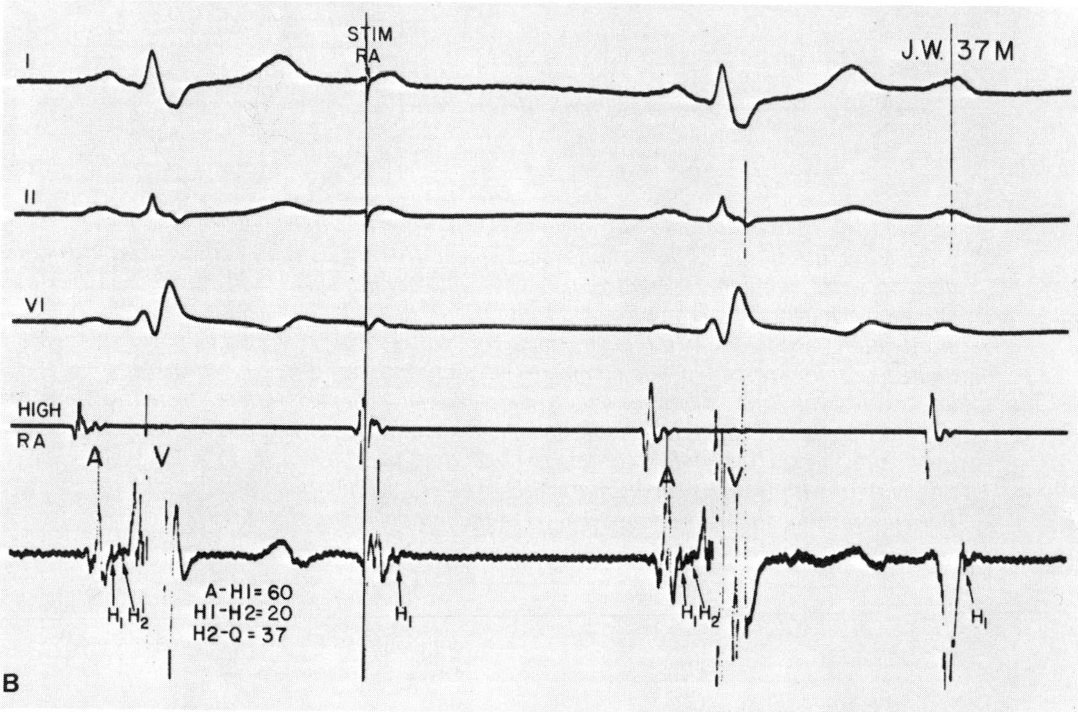

Figure 14-5. *(A) Simultaneous leads I, II, and V_1 in the top panel show a 2:1 AV conduction pattern together with right bundle branch block in which QRS duration is only 0.1 second, suggesting an incomplete variety of right bundle branch block. In the bottom panel, the two strips are continuous. The pattern of 2:1 AV conduction abruptly changes to 1:1 when the atrial rate slows from 84 beats/min to 60 beats/min following carotid sinus stimulation (CSS). As the effect of vagal stimulation wanes and the atrial rate again increases, 2:1 AV conduction suddenly returns. The change from 2:1 to 1:1 conduction pattern and again from 1:1 to 2:1 occurs abruptly, with no Wenckebach periods intervening. This behavior placed block below the AV node, either in the main His bundle or the bundle branches. However, the presence of incomplete rather than complete right bundle branch block did not favor bilateral bundle branch block and was in keeping with main His bundle block with the additional feature of incomplete right bundle branch block. (B) The first and third P waves are conducted, and the second (induced) and fourth P waves are blocked. Conducted P waves are followed by two His spikes marked H_1 and H_2, while blocked P waves are followed only by H_1, clearly placing block in the middle portion of the main His bundle.*

intra-Hisian block for whom electrophysiologic documentation was available. The same degree of specificity was observed in all cases of trifascicular block. Note, however, that in patients with sluggish or unresponsive sinus nodes, noninvasive manuevers may not be informative.

Patterns of Atrioventricular Block

Because of the distinct differences in the anatomic and electrophysiologic characteristics alluded to above, the patterns of block in the AV node differ sharply from those in the His–bundle branch system. Thus, while Mobitz type I or Wenckebach periodicity characterizes block in the AV node, impaired conduction in the main His bundle and the bundle branch (BB) system manifests itself in the form of Mobitz type II (sudden, unexpected block of a P wave) or abrupt shifts between 1:1, 2:1, 3:1, and 4:1 AV conduction ratios. These patterns are nothing more than variations of the main pattern of Mobitz type II. The diagram in Figure 14-6 illustrates the electrophysiologic phenomena underlying these various patterns of conduction and shows the differences between the gradually progressing conduction delay in Mobitz I on one hand and the abrupt appearance of block in one of the structures of His–BB system on the other. The attribute "typical" is used in relation to the Wenckebach or Mobitz I type of block when the PR intervals show the greatest increment from the first conducted P wave in the cycle to the second P wave, with the increments becoming progressively smaller (Figs. 14-6 and 14-7). This behavior gradually shortens the RR intervals before one P wave is blocked, resulting in the

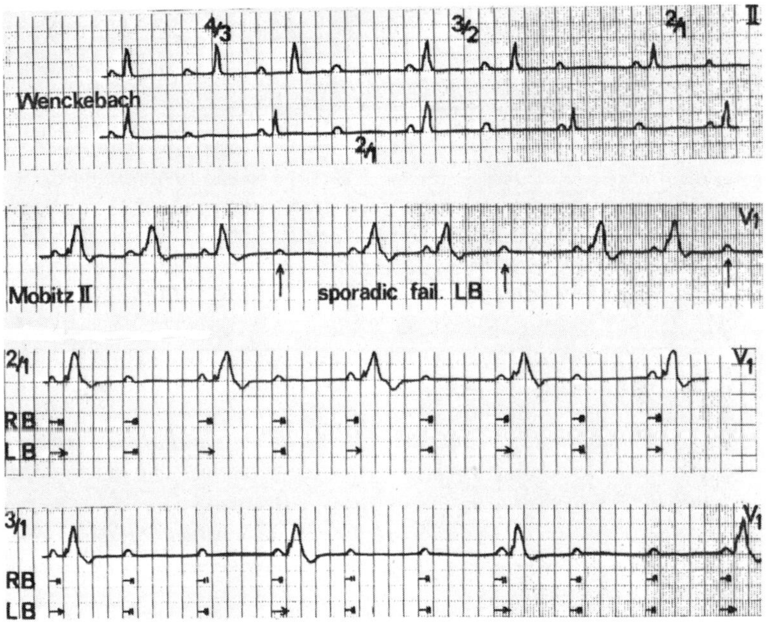

Figure 14-6. *Diagram designed to show the mechanism of typical Wenckebach cycles as they occur within the AV node* (top panel) *and Mobitz II and its variations in bilateral bundle branch block. Wenckebach cycles 4:3, 3:2, and 2:1, indicating varying and gradual grades of block in the AV node, are depicted in the top panel. The pattern of 2:1 AV conduction in this example is really a form of Wenckebach periodicity in which the increment from the first PR interval to the second goes from 0.2 second to complete failure to conduct. In the panel marked Mobitz II, PR intervals remain constant until the* fourth *and* seventh *P waves, which are inexplicably blocked. Similarly, in the panel marked 2:1, alternate P waves are conducted, while in the panel marked 3:1, two P waves are blocked and the third is conducted. The* horizontal arrows *and* double bars *indicating successful conduction and failure of conduction, respectively, depict the function of the two bundles (RB and LB). For blocked P waves, block symbols* (double bars) *are placed in both columns because both bundles fail to conduct. Conduction symbols* (arrows) *are placed in the LB column for successfully conducted P waves because these reach the ventricles through the LB. A glance at the LB columns demonstrates that the left bundle conducts 2:1 or 3:1 while the RB remains blocked throughout. The all-or-none conduction pattern of the bundles and the absence of Wenckebach cycles can be readily appreciated from the diagram.*

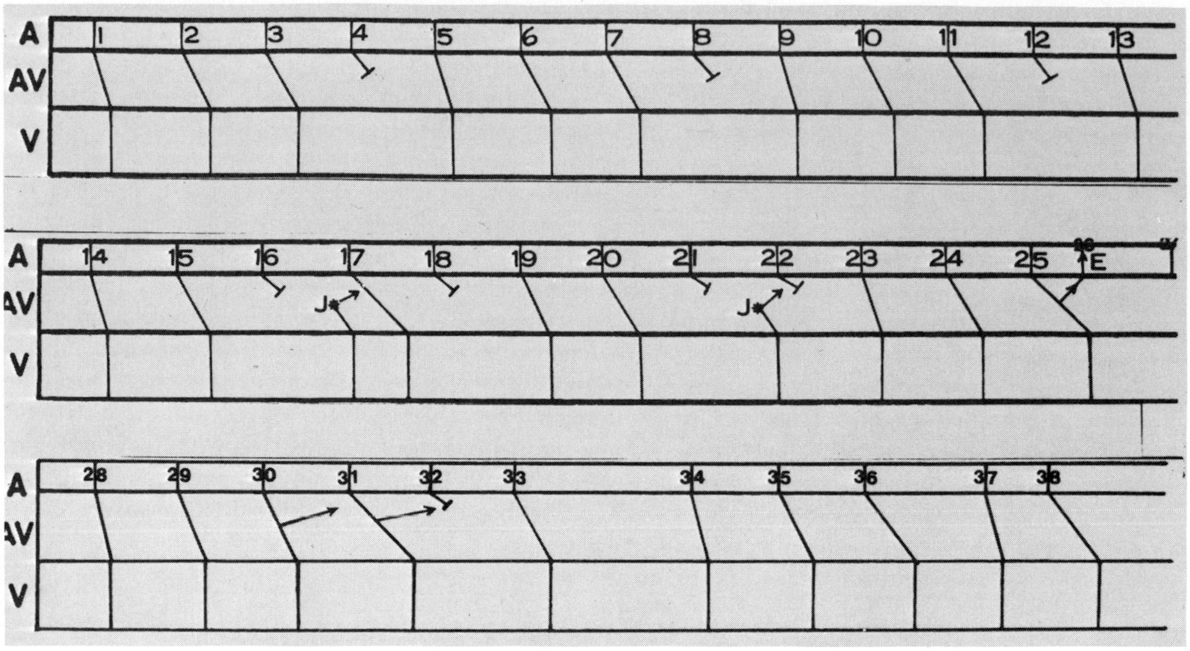

Figure 14-7. *Three ladder diagrams purporting to show a host of various and atypical features in cases of AV nodal Wenckebach. With perfectly regular sinus rhythm a typical Wenckebach of 4:3 conduction ratio is depicted* (top strip). *The PR increment is greatest from the first to the second conducted P wave (1 to 2, 5 to 6, and 9 to 10). In the middle diagram, the sinus rhythm remains perfectly regular in the Wenckebach cycles 14 to 18. The blocked P 16 is followed by a junctional escape (J) beat. The concealed conduction of this junctional discharge into the AV node causes an extraordinary prolongation of the next P 17. This in turn leads to unexpected block of the next P 18. In the Wenckebach cycle 19 to 22, a similar J beat penetrates the AV node and causes complete block of the next P 22; hence two blocked P waves occur in succession in an otherwise typical Wenckebach cycle. In the cycle 23 to 26, the markedly prolonged PR interval of P 25 occasions an echo back into the atrium, giving rise to the retrograde P 26, disturbing the normal sequence of the Wenckebach cycle and of the sinus node function. In the bottom diagram, sinus rhythm remains regular from 28 to 33. However, the markedly prolonged PR interval of P 30 occasions echo back into the AV node, further prolonging the PR interval of P 31. The echo from this long PR eventually causes complete block of P 32, after which another Wenckebach cycle begins with P 33. In the Wenckebach cycle 34 to 38, a sinus arrhythmia is present, accounting for the grossly atypical sequence of PR intervals. The PR intervals increase in the usual fashion from P 34 to P 36. The sudden prolongation of the sinus cycle 36 to 37 causes improved conduction through the AV node and return of the PR interval to a normal value. The short sinus cycle 37 to 38 again substantially prolongs the PR interval of P 38.*

pause. The first PR interval of the typical Wenckebach cycle is usually longer than 0.20 second, and the last PR interval is rarely shorter than 0.30 second. These relationships exist only when the sinus mechanism is regular. With sinus or other types of atrial arrhythmia, the PR interval is profoundly influenced by the preceding cycle length and does not follow any particular pattern (Figs. 14-7 and 14-8). Not infrequently, the beat occurring at the end of the pause is a His bundle escape beat. Penetration or concealed conduction of this beat into the AV node renders it partially or completely refractory, thus creating an incongruously long PR interval or a second blocked P wave. The return or echo P waves that may occur after very long PR intervals of the Wenckebach cycles frequently depolarize the SA node and reset it, causing a form of sinus arrhythmia interrupting the natural progression of the Wenckebach cycles (see Fig. 14-7). The QRS complexes in both the typical AV nodal Wenckebach and the atypical intra-Hisian Wenckebach are narrow. In intra-Hisian block, the disease process

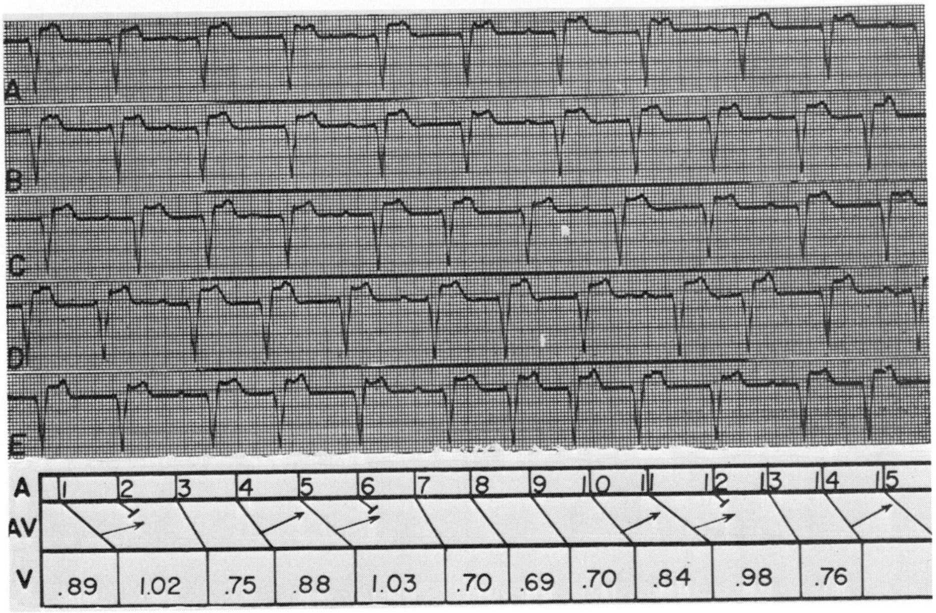

Figure 14-8. *Monitor tracings of a patient with digitalis intoxication showing a regular sinus rhythm but grossly atypical Wenckebach cycles accounted for by retrograde penetration of the AV node following the marked prolongation of the PR intervals. In E, corresponding to the ladder diagram, three blocked P waves are present, (2, 6, and 12). The next P waves, being the first in the Wenckebach cycles, are conducted with PR intervals of 0.3 second. Atypical features include (1) failure of the RR cycles to shorten progressively in the course of the Wenckebach cycles (0.7, 0.69, 0.7, 0.84 second in Wenckebach period 7 to 12), (2) the long ventricular cycles containing blocked P waves are only slightly longer than the last ventricular cycle in the course of Wenckebach cycles (1.02 versus 0.89 second; 1.03 versus 0.88 second; 0.98 versus 0.84 second), and (3) the PR interval increments become particularly striking after the first few beats of the cycle, causing the ventricular cycles to lengthen inappropriately instead of shorten.*

occasionally penetrates the origin of the right bundle branch block (RBBB) or involves those fibers in the main bundle that are destined to become the right bundle (see Fig. 14-5). Similarly, the disease process may involve the fibers of the left anterior superior fascicle. For these reasons, RBBB or left anterior superior fascicular block (LASH) may be present in the conducted beats. In our 14 cases of electrophysiologically documented main His bundle block, RBBB was present in 3 patients, and one of the three had the additional feature of LASH. As noted above, conduction in the main His bundle and the BB system is generally characterized by an all-or-none behavior. Consequently, the P waves are either conducted with a fixed PR interval or remain blocked. In contrast, in AV nodal block, conduction time varies frequently, giving rise to a host of PR intervals. The factors responsible for the constantly changing PR intervals include the autonomic influences and the intervals separating the P waves from the preceding R waves. Conduction time within the AV node is inversely related to the preceding RP interval (Fig. 14-9).

Magnitude of Atrioventricular Block

From the point of view of magnitude, block is said to be complete when evidence of conduction to the ventricles cannot be found anywhere in the tracing. Note, however, that very long rhythm strips and 24-hour ambulatory monitoring frequently reveal occasional conducted beats in patients presumed to have "complete" AV block. This situation must be differentiated from so-called supernormal conduction when a significant degree of AV block exists. In this situation, all the P waves are blocked except those occurring near the end of the T waves of the preceding ventricular complexes. This zone of enhanced conductivity corresponds to the area of negative hyperpolarization on the transmembrane action potential. All the P waves arriving in the main His bundle or the BB system at this particular time conduct successfully to the ventricles (Fig. 14-10).

In first degree AV block, PR prolongation is present but blocked P waves are not. The length of the PR inter-

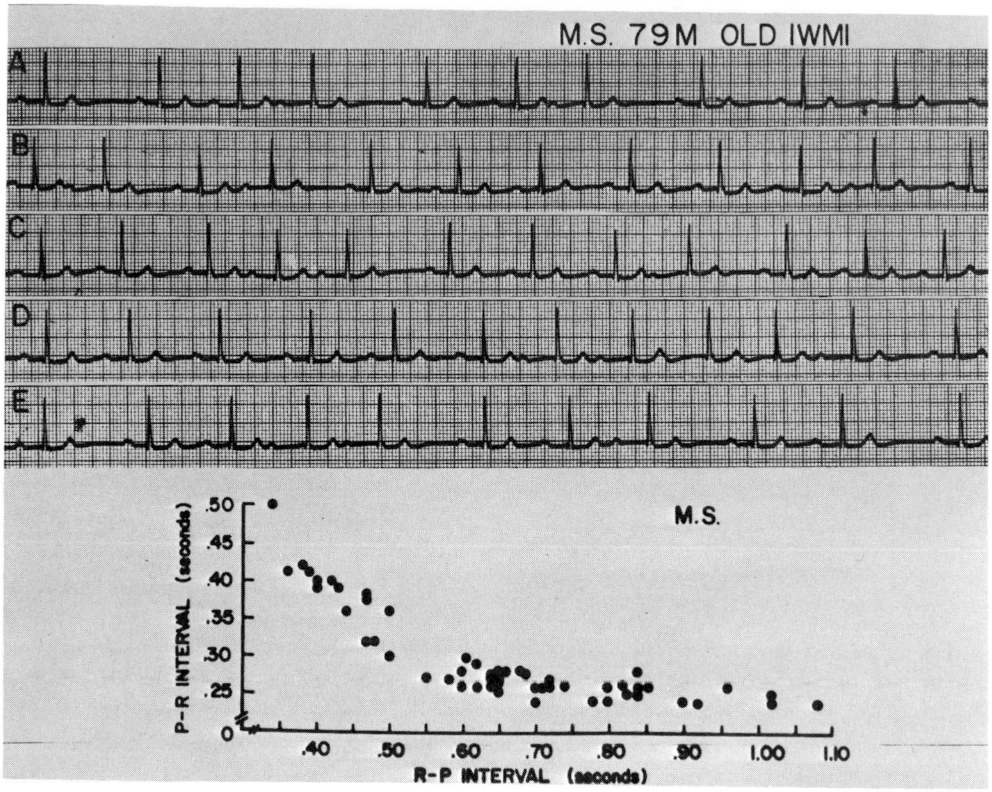

Figure 14-9. *Sequential strips of a monitor lead in a man aged 79 years with an old inferior wall myocardial infarction (IWMI) showing the remarkable dependence of the PR intervals (0.23 to 0.5 second) on the preceding RP intervals (0.35 to 1.06 second). The graph demonstrates the reverse relationship that exists between the PR intervals and the preceding RP intervals, that is, the distance separating the P wave from the preceding ventricular depolarization. Short RP intervals of less than 0.4 second are followed by very long PR intervals of 0.4 second or more because the P waves arrive within the relative refractory period of the AV node. Longer RP intervals of 0.5 to 0.7 second are associated with shorter PR intervals of 0.3 to 0.25 second. However, when RP intervals exceed 0.7 second, the AV node achieves complete recovery so that further prolongation of the RP intervals exerts no further influence on the AV node conduction. This interesting behavior of the AV node contrasts sharply with that of the His bundle and the bundle branches, which generally function in all-or-none fashion, with little dependence on the preceding RP intervals (see Fig. 14-11).*

val generally ranges between 0.2 to 0.45 second. Extremely long PR intervals of 0.6 to 0.8 second are found when the AV node is penetrated and rendered more refractory by junctional discharges or by echo P waves conducting back into the AV node (see Fig. 14-7). In incomplete or second degree AV block, successful conduction of the P waves to the ventricles is usually predictable when the AV node is the site of block, but it is sporadic and unpredictable when infranodal block is present (Fig. 14-11), except in rare cases of infranodal Wenckebach block (see Fig. 14-3). During sleep, AV nodal block tends to be more pronounced (Fig. 14-12). Infranodal blocks behave in the opposite manner.

Two phenomena peculiar to the AV node may alter the magnitude of AV conduction in an interesting and seemingly unexpected manner. One is the phenomenon of alternating Wenckebach periodicity resulting from transverse dissociation of the AV node with two different patterns of conduction in the upper and lower segments of the AV node.[12] Generally, the magnitude of block in the upper half of the AV node is greater (2:1 Wenckebach) than in the lower half (3:2 or 5:4 Wenckebach).

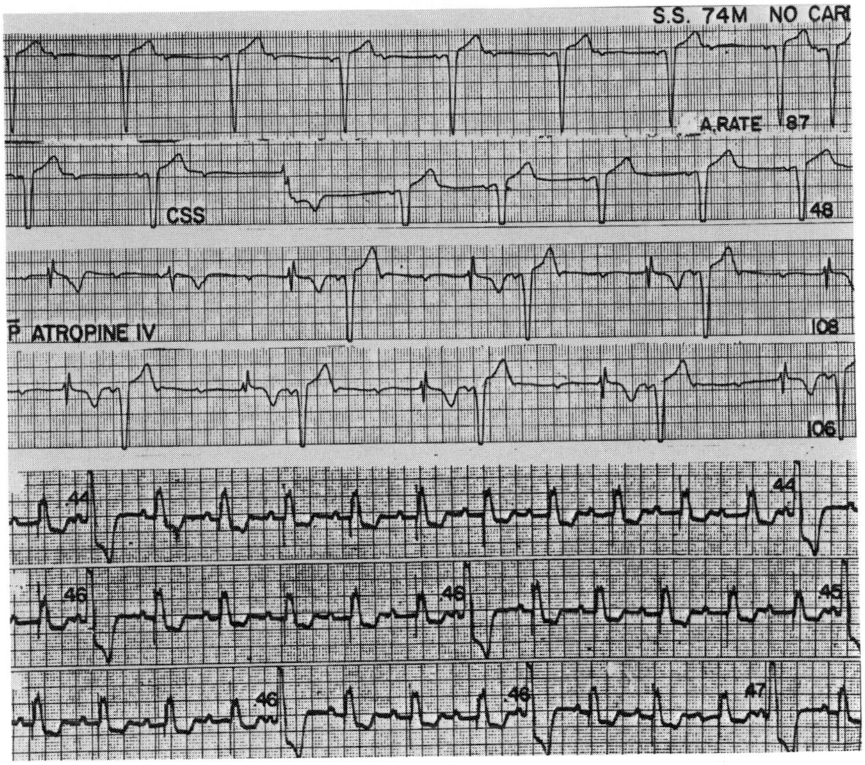

Figure 14-10. *Strips of lead V_1 in a man of 74 years with prostatic hypertrophy showing a fixed pattern of 2:1 AV conduction together with complete left bundle branch block. Vagal stimulation changes conduction abruptly from 2:1 to 1:1 as the atrial rate slows from 87 to 48 beats/min. Atropine increases block to complete for a few beats, and then an interesting pattern marked by conducted beats with a fixed PR interval of 0.16 second and the left bundle branch configuration emerges. Attention to this portion of the tracing (*third *and* fourth strips*) clearly demonstrates that conduction to the ventricles occurs when P waves appear near the end of the T waves of the preceding escape beats, with the RR intervals fixed at 0.68 second. This particular behavior strongly suggests supernormality. Following the development of complete heart block and insertion of a permanent right ventricular transvenous pacemaker, supernormal conduction of those P waves occurring shortly after the end of the T waves of the paced beats again occurs. Here, pacemaker spike-P intervals measure 0.44 second and spike-R intervals measure 0.62 to 0.65 second, closely resembling the RR intervals in the third and fourth strips. The zones of supernormal conduction are therefore almost identical before and after pacemaker insertion.*

As a result, alternate P waves are blocked in the upper region, with the lower half encountering only half of the P waves. The other phenomenon is the so-called longitudinal dissociation, or the presence of dual pathways within the AV node (Fig. 14-13).[13,14] Here, the AV node appears to contain two distinct longitudinal pathways, one possessing a long refractory period with fast conduction and the other a short refractory period with slow conduction. P waves arriving relatively early and premature atrial beats will be conducted to the ventricle through the pathway possessing shorter refractory period and longer conduction time, with long PR intervals. P waves arriving later will conduct through both pathways but will reach the ventricles earlier through the pathway with the long refractory period and fast conduction. The shift between the shorter and the longer PR intervals (0.16 to 0.22 and 0.36 to 0.45 second, respectively, in our study of 6 patients) may take place in an abrupt and unpredictable manner. However, block in one pathway and the resultant shift to the other is frequently occasioned by concealed conduction of premature atrial or ventricular beats into the first pathway (see Fig. 14-13).

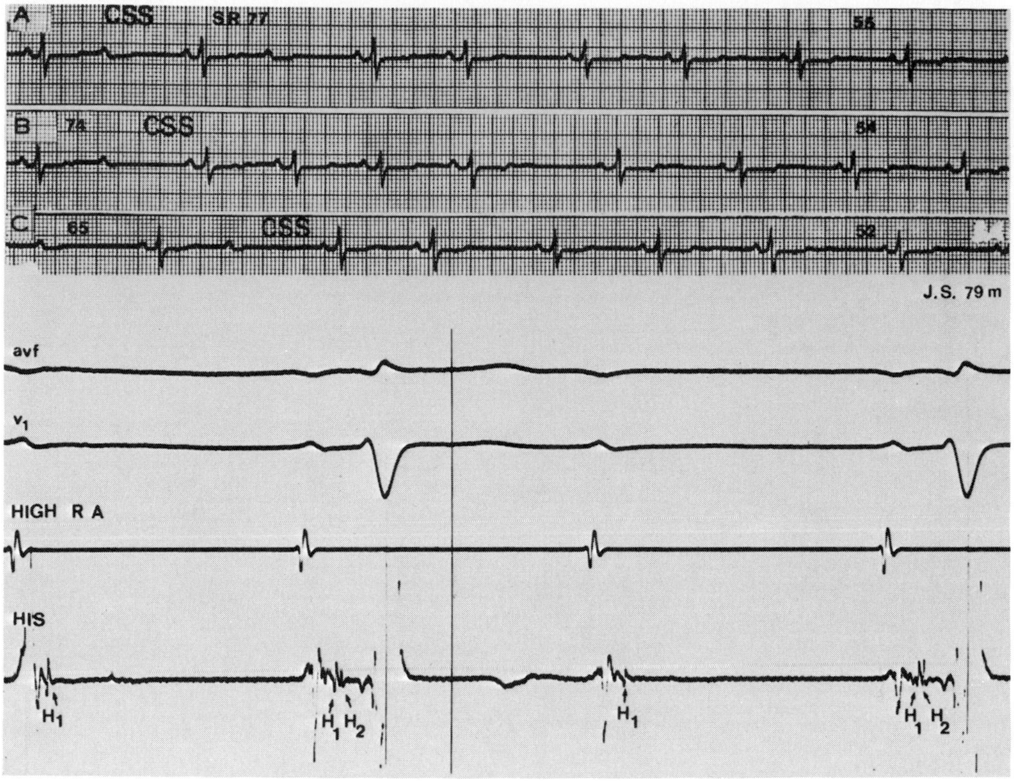

Figure 14-11. *Three rhythm strips in the top panel and His bundle recordings in bottom panel from a man of 79 years complaining of fainting and dizziness. The basic pattern of narrow QRS 2:1 AV conduction present at the beginning of strips A, B, and C, when the sinus rate is above 65 beats/min, changes abruptly to 1:1 conduction without any change in the PR intervals as the sinus rate is slowed by carotid sinus stimulation. This all-or-none behavior of AV conduction suggests an intra-Hisian block, which was subsequently documented by His bundle electrography showing split His spikes (H_1 and H_2). Only H_1 was present after blocked P waves, thus placing block in the middle of the main His bundle.*

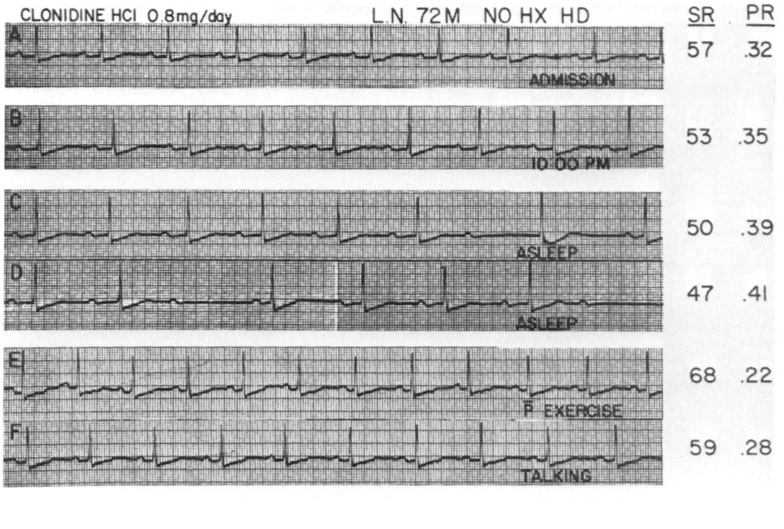

Figure 14-12. *In this hypertensive patient aged 72 receiving clonidine hydrochloride, an element of AV block marked by prolongation of the PR interval and occasional Wenckebach periods appeared (A to D). The corresponding sinus rates and PR intervals are depicted under SR and PR, respectively. The PR intervals increase and the Wenckebach periods appear as the sinus rate decreases, clearly indicating a vagal mechanism. In strips E and F the PR intervals decrease as the sinus rate accelerates with mild leg exercise in bed and talking to visitors, respectively.*

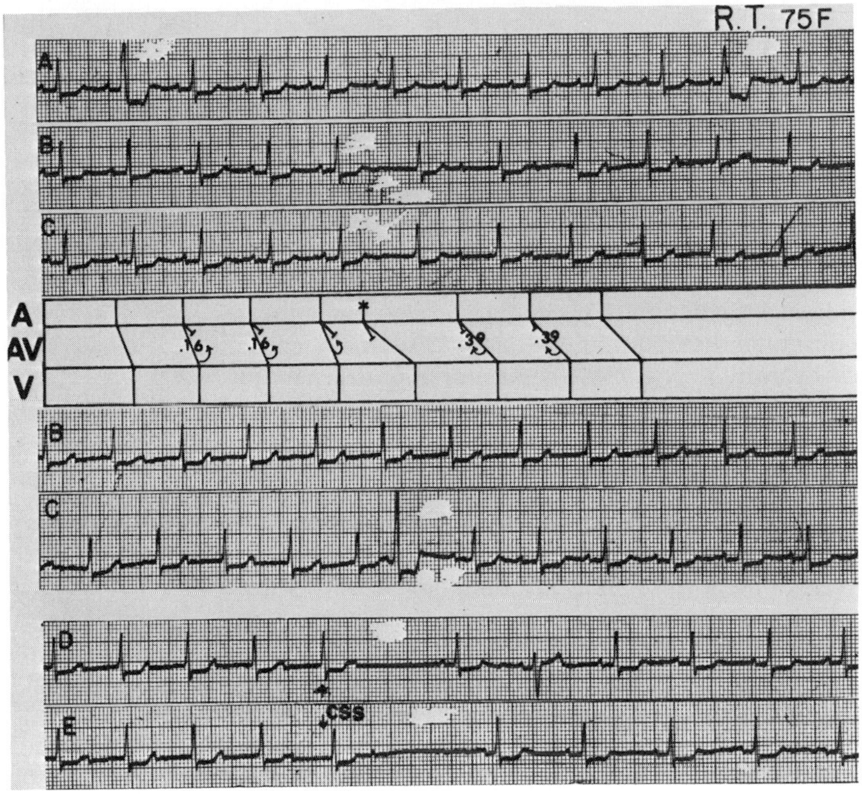

Figure 14-13. *Rhythm strips in this woman of 75 years 2 weeks after successful aortocoronary bypass surgery show two families of PR intervals of 0.16 and 0.39 second, respectively (A). In B and C, the shift from short to long PR occurs because of premature atrial depolarization* (asterisk in the ladder diagram), *the premature atrial beat, arriving early, finds the pathway with long refractory period nonconductive; it switches to the pathway with short refractory period and conducts successfully with a long PR interval. From then on, conduction proceeds down the long pathway. The persistence of conduction in only one pathway at any given time suggests retrograde concealed conduction into the nonconducting pathway every time the conducting pathway is successfully traversed. In D and E, shift from long to short PR interval is brought about by a premature ventricular beat causing retrograde concealment in the long pathway. F and G show that the slow pathway conduction in the first five beats switches to the fast pathway by vagal stimulation (CSS). At the height of vagal stimulation one P wave is completely blocked, that is, blocked in both pathways. The resultant pause enables the fast pathway to resume conduction after the pause.*

In other cases, Wenckebach type of block occurring in one pathway eventuates in block of one impulse, thus giving the other pathway the opportunity to conduct. Patients demonstrating two families of PR intervals rarely develop spontaneous AV nodal reentrant tachycardias even though the substrate for such tachycardia is always present. The most probable explanation is that both pathways are involved in antegrade conduction of the P waves, so that neither pathway is completely recovered and free for retrograde conduction and completion of the tachycardia circuit. If one of the two pathways developed antegrade unidirectional block, tachycardia circuit could be easily set up. Contrariwise, persons who are disturbed by frequent episodes of AV nodal reentrant tachycardia seldom exhibit two families of PR intervals because a unidirectional antegrade block exists in the fast pathway.

Chronology of Atrioventricular Block

In this section, the following patterns of AV block will be discussed:

1. Permanent
2. Acute or transient

3. Intermittent
4. Provoked and iatrogenic

Permanent

In permanent AV block a fixed degree of block is present in all tracings and generally reflects a fixed anatomic lesion. The site of block may be in the AV node or the main His bundle (*e.g.*, spread of calcification or fibrosis from the aortic or mitral rings, degeneration or calcification of the central fibrous body, so-called Lev's disease, congenital disruption of the main His bundle, chronic myocarditis) or in the BB system (*e.g.*, degeneration, ischemia, infiltrative processes such as amyloidosis).

Acute or Transient

Acute or transient AV block is difficult to observe unless the patient is being monitored. AV nodal block, complete or incomplete, may last but a few seconds, during which the fall in blood pressure and cardiac output activate powerful reflexes resulting in sympathetic stimulation, vagal inhibition, or both and restoration of conduction. Acute AV block occurring in the AV node is partially or completely mediated through the autonomic nervous system. The complete AV block in the first few minutes of acute inferior-posterior myocardial infarction and during the pain of Prinzmetal's angina are examples of transient AV block where the resultant bradycardia may lead to ventricular ectopy, tachycardia, and even fibrillation. Transient complete AV block occurring during contrast injection into the right coronary artery is mainly of vagal origin and can be prevented by pretreatment with atropine. Purely vagal AV block in the absence of injury to the AV node deserves special mention. The most impressive variety is that encountered in severe vasovagal reactions and during vomiting. Such blocks, occurring within the AV node, may be complete or incomplete. Also, AV block induced by carotid sinus stimulation is the prototype of vagal block, and it too may range in magnitude from first degree to complete. The so-called postural heart block occasionally observed in children is vagal and occurs usually in the supine position, disappearing with the assumption of erect posture. In certain persons with heightened vagal tone, unexplained or vasovagally mediated reflexes may lead to pronounced slowing of the sinus rate together with first and second degree AV node block. Some of these persons, especially the very old, may have been treated injudiciously with permanent pacemakers. Perhaps the most interesting variety of vagal AV block is

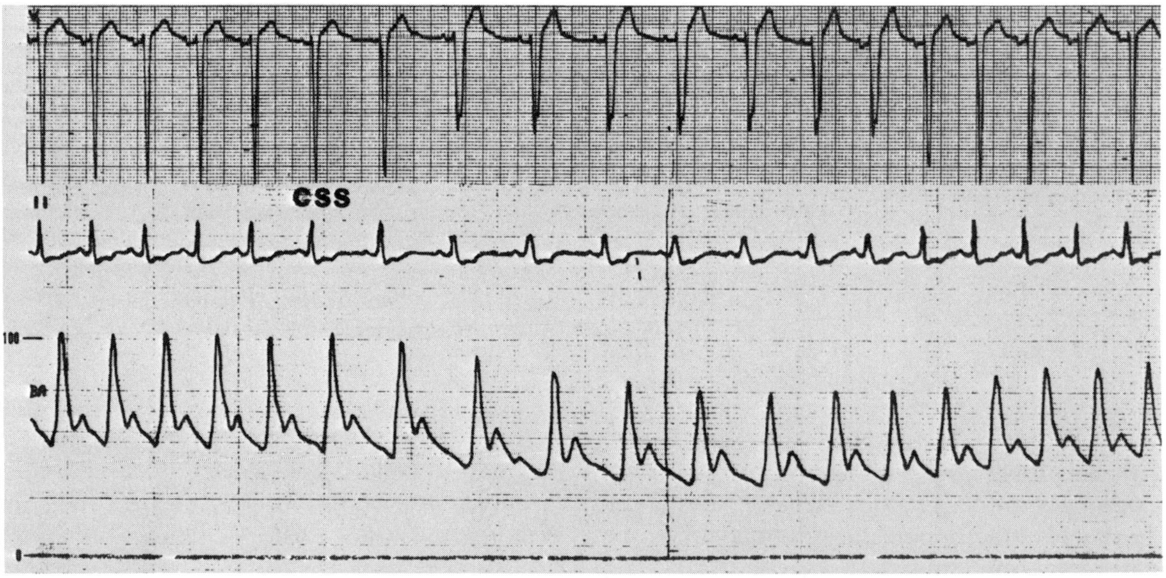

Figure 14-14. *Simultaneously recorded lead II and brachial arterial pressure* (bottom panel) *and a separate but simultaneously recorded lead V_1 in a man of 34 years with acute anterior myocardial infarction* (top panel) *are shown. Carotid sinus stimulation (CSS) is applied after the sixth beat. Slowing of the sinus rate was associated with a concurrent appearance of left bundle branch block and a significant fall in blood pressure. The fall in coronary perfusion pressure secondary to vagal stimulation was presumed the cause of failure of the left bundle branch. The slowing of the cardiac cycle and the resultant phase 4 depolarization may be incriminated. However, the slowing does not appear to be long enough (longest cycle 0.85 second) to bring about a phase 4 type of block.*

that which occurs in some patients with Cheyne-Stokes' respiration. The intense vagal stimulation present during the hyperpnea phase of Cheyne-Stokes' cycles may cause second and even third degree AV block that is reversible with atropine administration.[15]

Intermittent

Both the AV node and infranodal blocks may be intermittent. In the AV node, gradual changes in the magnitude of block are common and generally related to variations in the autonomic tone, usually with concomitant changes in the sinus rate. Here, the PR intervals remain longer than normal even when conduction is at its best (see Figs. 14-8 and 14-12). In intra-Hisian and trifascicular blocks, on the contrary, abrupt changes in the magnitude of block are the rule, and the PR intervals are frequently normal between episodes of block (see Figs. 14-3 to 14-5 and 14-11). In infranodal types of block, changes in atrial rate secondary to physiologic stimuli may bring about striking and abrupt changes in the magnitude of block and in the pattern of AV conduction (see Fig. 14-11). Similarly profound variations in the magnitude of infranodal block occur frequently in the absence of manifest stimuli. Undetectable variations in blood flow to the conduction system may be an important factor determining the pattern of conduction. Observations of the type depicted in Figure 14-14 are thought provoking in this respect. In this man of 34 years with an acute anterior wall myocardial infarction, an intermittent left bundle branch block was observed. In addition, occasional P waves unexpectedly failed to conduct to the ventricles, thus conforming to the pattern of Mobitz type II block. Also, the appearance of left bundle branch block (LBBB) corresponded with a fall in blood pressure from 110/85 to 90/70. It was reasoned that the fall in blood pressure and, consequently, in the coronary perfusion pressure was responsible for the failure of the left bundle and, at times, of both bundles. To validate this concept, blood pressure was momentarily lowered by carotid sinus stimulation. The LBBB was noted to appear with the onset of blood pressure decline and disappear with the return of blood pressure to the pre-LBBB level. The emergence and disappearance of LBBB occurred when brachial arterial pressure crossed the level of 85/60. This fundamental role of the coronary perfusion pressure in governing conduction through the bundle branches may be a more common cause of conduction disturbance in the course of acute coronary episodes than has been appreciated. Another possible manifestation of this phenomenon is the so-called postextrasystolic complete AV block. Figure 14-15 shows the emergence of complete AV block following premature atrial beats in the face of 1 : 1 AV conduction in a patient recovering from an acute inferior wall myocardial infarction complicated by RBBB. Attention to the level of brachial arterial pressure demonstrates that the arterial diastolic pressure at the time of His bundle depolarization after the first post-PAB P wave was only 58 mm Hg, presumably insufficient for normal LBB function. Although phase 4 block cannot be summarily excluded as a possibility in this and in the preceding case, the His-His intervals after the premature atrial beat were only 20 to 80 msec longer than the basal His-His intervals, probably too short to incriminate phase 4 depolarization. In Figure 14-14, LBBB disappeared several beats after the vagally induced slowing of the rate had dissipated and the heart rate had returned to the preblock level.

Provoked and Iatrogenic

First and second degree AV block have been observed in a number of patients receiving clonidine hydrocholoride for hypertension (see Fig. 14-12). We have observed cases of incomplete and even complete AV block situated at the AV node following the administration of calcium-blocking agents, particularly verapamil, in the usual doses to control the ventricular rate in atrial fibrillation. AV nodal block induced by beta-blockers is so well known that its mere mention is adequate.

The iatrogenic AV block developing in the course of right heart catheterization in patients with preexisting LBBB is well known. All patients showing LBBB in their control tracings should have a prophylactic right ventricular pacing catheter before catheterization of the right heart. A less commonly appreciated form of iatrogenic AV block is that which occurs during the 48-hour period immediately after aortocoronary bypass surgery in patients with preexisting LBBB. The 5% to 10% incidence of transient RBBB following coronary bypass surgery leads to second degree or complete AV block by adding RBBB to the already existing LBBB (Fig. 14-16).

Undoubtedly, the most interesting type of provoked AV block is that which develops as a result of the local spread of nonpropagated His bundle extrasystoles.[16] In this situation, His bundle extrasystoles fail to propagate to the ventricles but create sufficient refractoriness in the His bundle or the AV node to delay or halt conduction of the next P wave (Fig. 14-17). In our study of six patients with AV block caused by nonpropagated His bundle extrasystoles, features of His bundle parasystole were present in all. Manifest His bundle and ventricular extrasystoles also interfere with normal transit through the AV node (concealed conduction), but the reason for this kind of block is readily visible on the electrocardiogram. Atrial extrasystoles do not generally prolong or block subsequent P waves because they almost always penetrate the sinus node, reset it (noncompensatory pause), and delay the next sinus discharge, by which time the AV node has fully recovered.

(Text continues on p. 361.)

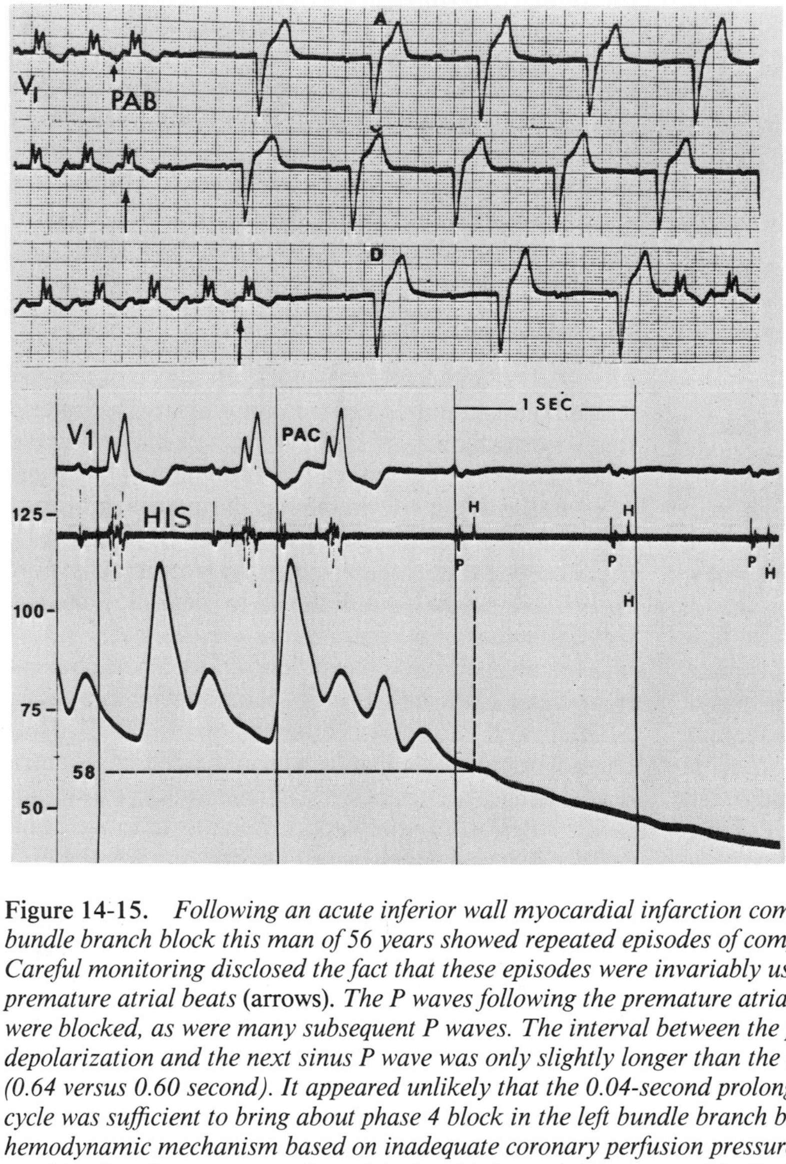

Figure 14-15. *Following an acute inferior wall myocardial infarction complicated by right bundle branch block this man of 56 years showed repeated episodes of complete AV block. Careful monitoring disclosed the fact that these episodes were invariably ushered in by premature atrial beats* (arrows). *The P waves following the premature atrial beats (PABs) were blocked, as were many subsequent P waves. The interval between the premature atrial depolarization and the next sinus P wave was only slightly longer than the basic sinus cycle (0.64 versus 0.60 second). It appeared unlikely that the 0.04-second prolongation of the cycle was sufficient to bring about phase 4 block in the left bundle branch block. The hemodynamic mechanism based on inadequate coronary perfusion pressure appeared more tenable. Simultaneous recording of the brachial arterial pressure with His bundle potentials when complete AV block emerged demonstrated first that block was infranodal (i.e., bilateral right bundle branch block) and second that the arterial pressure, which registered at 114/65 when 1:1 conduction was present, was only 80/62 with the PAB. From that level, the arterial pressure declined further and was 58 mm Hg by the time the His bundle was activated following the first post-PAB sinus P wave. It is likely that the low perfusion pressure of 58 mm Hg was not sufficient for a normal conduction through the left bundle branch block. Failure of left bundle branch conduction was thus added to that of the existing right bundle branch block and caused complete AV block. Further decline in the perfusion pressure during the long ventricular diastole accounted for block of the subsequent P waves.*

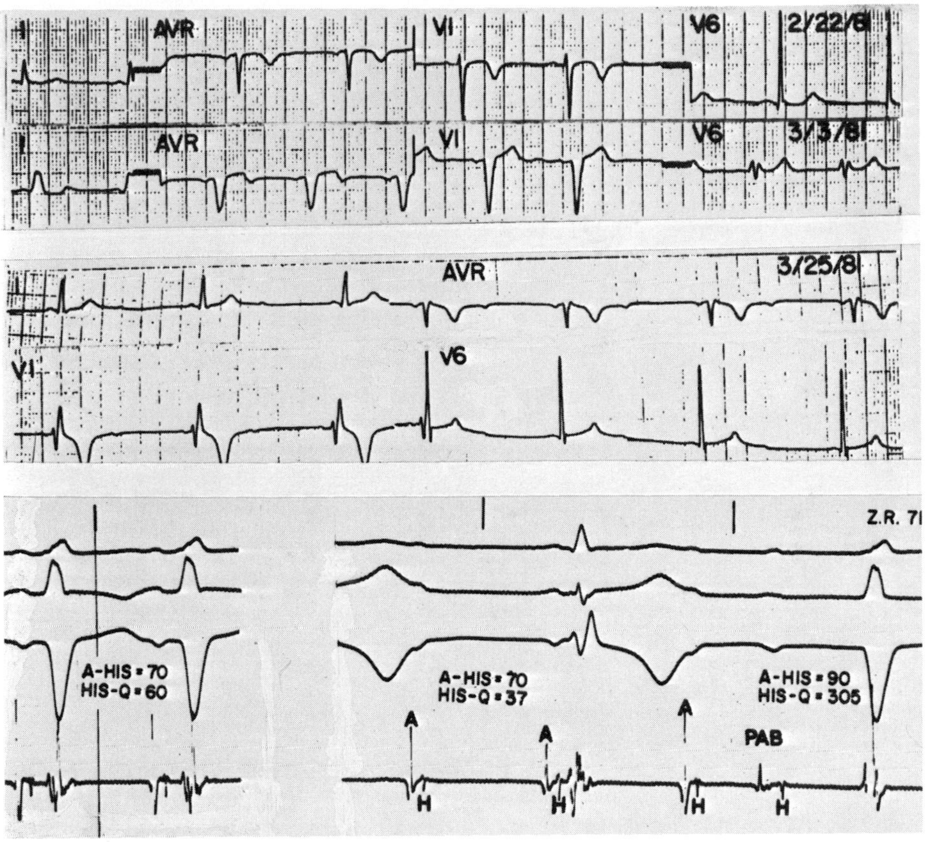

Figure 14-16. *This woman aged 71 years with coronary artery disease was admitted for aortocoronary bypass graft operation to her left anterior descending coronary artery. Preoperatively, her serial electrocardiograms showed intermittent left bundle branch block usually appearing when the sinus rate was accelerated to above 66 beats/min* (top two strips). *Postoperatively, she displayed a right bundle branch block and a 2:1 AV conduction pattern* (middle strip). *His bundle recording showed His-Q intervals of 60 msec when 1:1 conduction and left bundle branch were present. For most of the tracing, however, a 2:1 AV conduction with right bundle branch block prevailed. Block occurred below the His bundle because His spikes were present after blocked P waves. The temporary right bundle branch block that occasionally follows coronary bypass operation apparently was added to the preexisting left bundle branch block and converted 1:1 AV conduction to 2:1. The shortening of the His-Q interval in the conducted beat to 37 msec probably reflects enhanced conduction in the left bundle brought about by the slowing of the rate secondary to the 2:1 AV conduction. The premature atrial beat occurring during 2:1 AV conduction is conducted to the ventricles with a pattern of left bundle branch block. This beat is conducted through the right bundle branch but with a very long His-Q interval of 305 msec.*

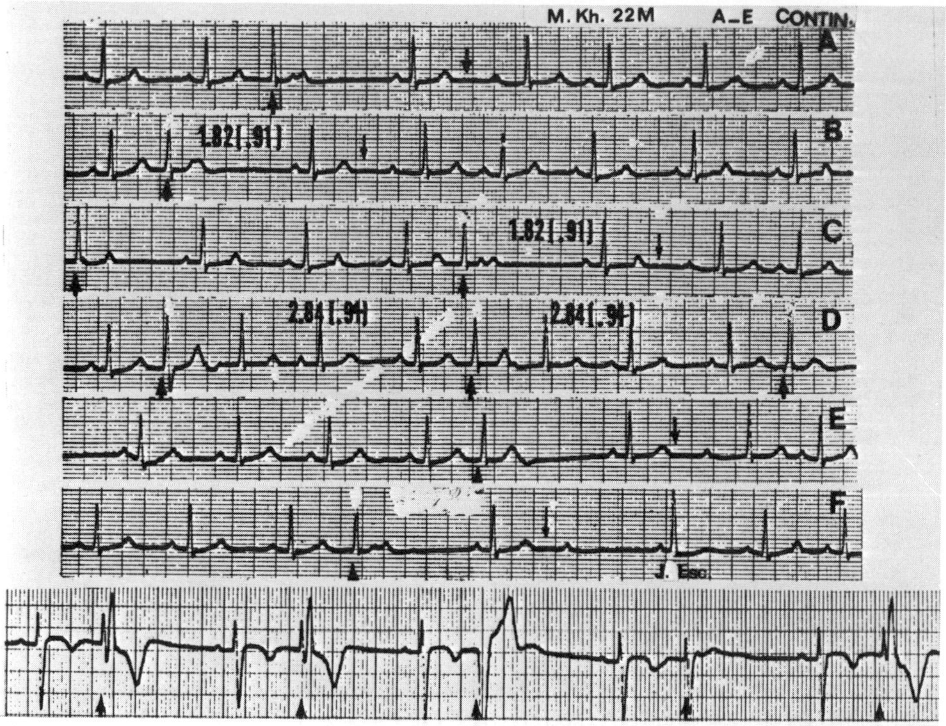
M. Kh. 22M
A_E CONTIN.
A
B
1.82(.91)
C
1.82(.91)
D
2.84(.94)
2.84(.94)
E
F
J. Esc.
A

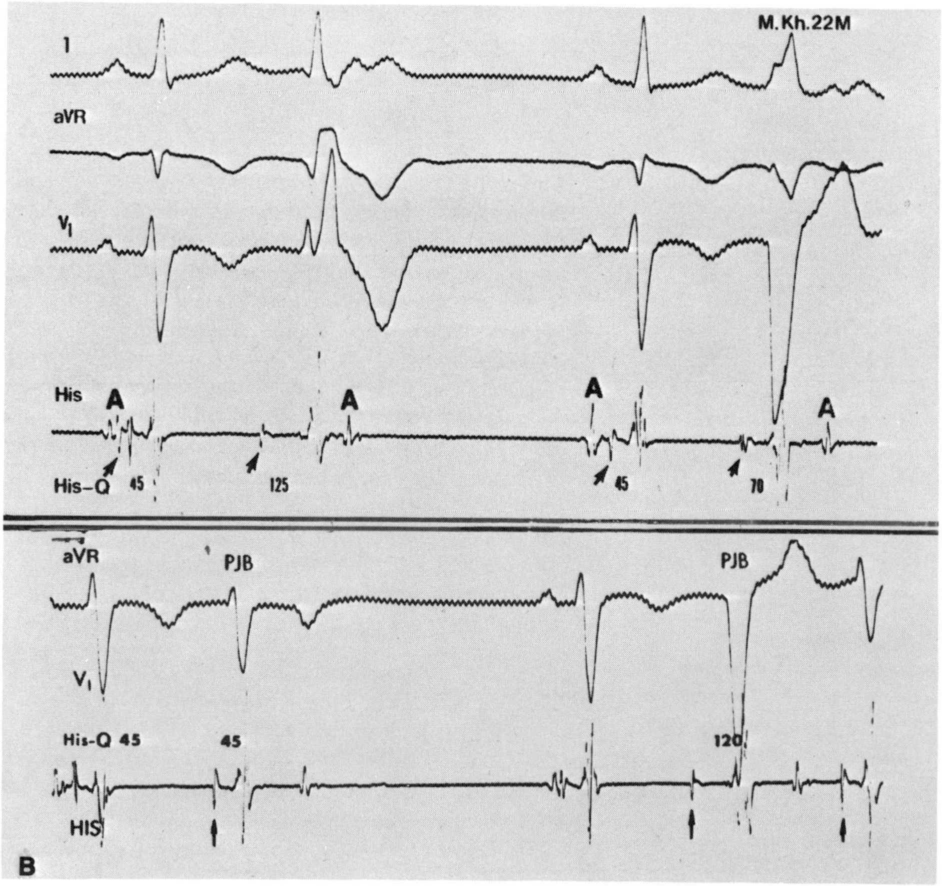
M.Kh.22M
1
aVR
V1
His
A
A
A
A
His-Q
45
125
45
70
aVR
PJB
PJB
V1
His-Q 45
45
120
HIS
B

Noninvasive Maneuvers for Determining the Site and Nature of Conduction Disturbances

The invasive electrophysiologic studies and His bundle recordings have contributed so fundamentally to understanding of intracardiac conduction as to make such studies virtually indispensable in cases of AV and IV conduction disturbances.[7] Speculation on the type and site of block without resort to His bundle electrography may thus seem an exercise in futility. However, the invasive studies of His bundle recording and atrial pacing are sometimes impractical or impossible because of medical, personal, technical, or economic reasons. First degree block situated in the AV node prolongs the A-His interval (normally 60 to 135 msec), while a completely blocked P wave is not followed by a His deflection. Noninvasive techniques can readily make the differentiation. The literature contains several reports purporting to show cases of AV nodal block that displayed a behavior characteristic of infranodal block (*i.e.*, typical Mobitz type II and sudden, unexpected shifts between 1 : 1 and 2 : 1 or complete block).[17] The AV nodal localization of block in such cases was based on the demonstration of absent His spikes after blocked P waves. However, as noted above, this finding is quite consistent with the presence of block in the upper regions of the His bundle with the electrode recording potentials from its lower regions. Occasionally repositioning the catheter will allow recording of small His potentials from the uppermost regions of the His bundle above the level of block (Fig. 14-18).[18] Blocks involving the bundle branches or the three fascicles are readily recognized through His bundle electrography because delay is between the His bundle and the ventricular myocardium, giving rise to prolonged His-Q intervals. With blocked P waves, a sharp His spike is found after the P wave. Noninvasively such cases display an increased magnitude of block when the atrial rate is accelerated and a decreased block when the atrial rate is slowed (Figs. 14-19 and 14-20).

From a clinical standpoint, the differential diagnosis between AV node and main His bundle block is of particular value and probably the most difficult. Tables 14-1 and 14-2 depict major electrophysiologic and electrocardiographic differences between the AV node and the infranodal tracts. As noted earlier, typical Wenckebach cycles are rare in the infranodal tracts. Sporadic examples of Wenckebach periodicity in one bundle branch or

(Text continues on p. 366.)

Figure 14-17. *(A) Top six strips of lead II and the bottom strip of lead V_1 were recorded from a man aged 22 years with prolapsed mitral valve. The rhythm strips showed unexplained prolongation of the PR intervals and blocked P waves scattered in an apparently sporadic fashion throughout. In addition, junctional premature beats with normal or aberrant QRS complexes were found. The P waves following the premature junctional beats were either conducted with long PR intervals or not conducted at all. Careful analysis of the relationship between the manifest junctional premature beats and the areas containing impaired AV conduction demonstrated the presence of a junctional or His bundle parasystole with a basic cycle length of 0.91 to 0.94 second corresponding to a rate of 66 beats/min. Manifest or propagated and nonpropagated junctional discharges exerted the same slowing or blocking influence on the subsequent P waves depending on their proximity. (*Upward arrows *point to junctional discharges propagated to the ventricles, resulting in manifest QRS complexes, and* downward arrows *point to the location of junctional discharges that failed to propagate to the ventricles but nevertheless exerted their influence on AV conduction by concealed conduction into the AV node). All the junctional discharges occurring within 0.48 second of the preceding QRS complexes remained nonpropagated but did penetrate the AV node and impaired conduction of the P waves. Junctional discharges appearing later than 0.48 second were successfully propagated to the ventricles, albeit with occasional aberrancy. (B) His bundle recordings in same patient as in A showing two junctional discharges (beats 2 and 4) in the top strip, one with morphologic feature of right bundle branch block and the other with left bundle branch block. No atrial depolarization can be seen preceding the His spikes* (arrows) *in these two beats, and the His-Q intervals are abnormally long, suggesting a diseased intraventricular conduction system. In the bottom strip two more junctional discharges are seen (6 and 8), one with an almost normal QRS complex and the other with left bundle branch block. The interval between these two discharges is exactly the same as between those in the top strip (His_2-His_4 and His_6-His_8 = 0.932 × 2), corresponding exactly to the shortest parasystolic interval found in A. The apparent AV block was thus entirely accounted for by nonpropagated junctional or His bundle discharges occurring in a parasystolic mode at an intrinsic rate of 66 beats/min.*

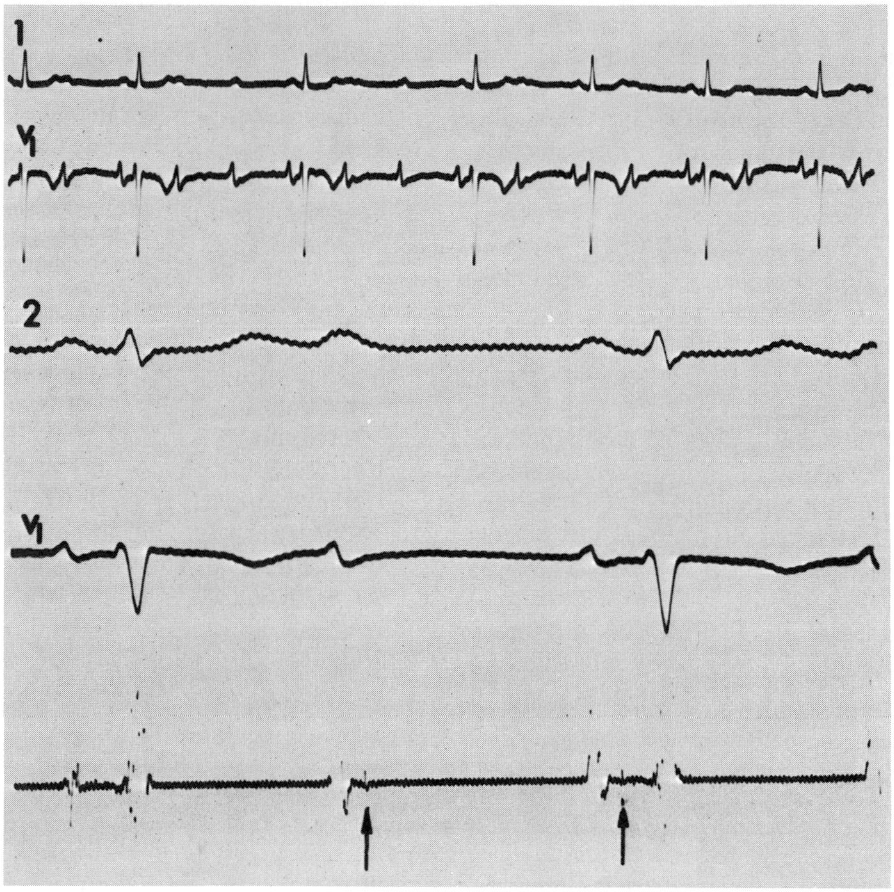

Figure 14-18. *Simultaneously recorded lead 1 and V_1* (top panel) *and His bundle recording in a woman aged 73 years with dizziness and syncopal attacks showing narrow QRS complexes with an AV conduction ratio of 2:1 or 3:1. Wenckebach periods were not observed at any time during 3 days of continuous monitoring. Notwithstanding the narrow QRS complexes, AV nodal block was excluded because of the absence of Wenckebach periods. His bundle recordings showed His spikes after blocked P waves. During the first few attempts at recording of His bundle potentials, no His spikes could be found after blocked P waves, and therefore a diagnosis of AV node block appeared inevitable. However, repeated repositioning of the catheter finally produced the tracing shown here. It was concluded that block was indeed situated in the main His bundle, involving its upper regions. The recording catheter sampling potentials from the distal His bundle could not show a His spike following blocked P waves and thus mimicked AV nodal block. Repositioning of the catheter finally allowed sampling of the uppermost regions of the His bundle proximal to the site of block.*

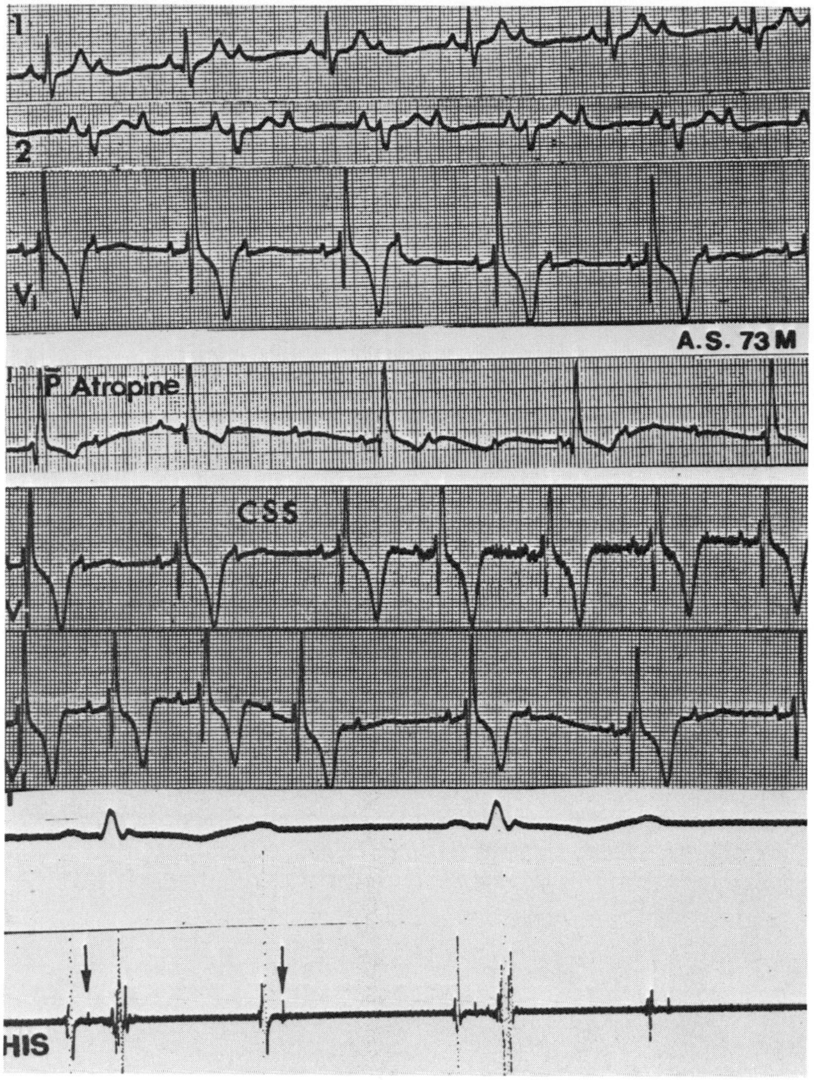

Figure 14-19. *Leads 1, II, and V_1 recorded simultaneously in this man aged 73 complaining of dizzy spells and syncope showed a fixed pattern of 2:1 AV conduction together with right bundle branch block–LAD. Atropine produced complete AV block, while vagal stimulation (CSS) normalized conduction and yielded a 1:1 AV ratio. The shifts from 2:1 to 1:1 and back were abrupt. Wenckebach cycles were never seen. The PR intervals of the conducted beats remained normal throughout, regardless of the pattern of AV conduction. His bundle recording shown in the bottom panel documents the infranodal location of the block. The pattern of conduction found in this case of trifascicular block exists uniformly in all cases of trifascicular block. The identical behavior of AV conduction in intra-Hisian, bilateral bundle branch block, and the trifascicular block is worth noting.*

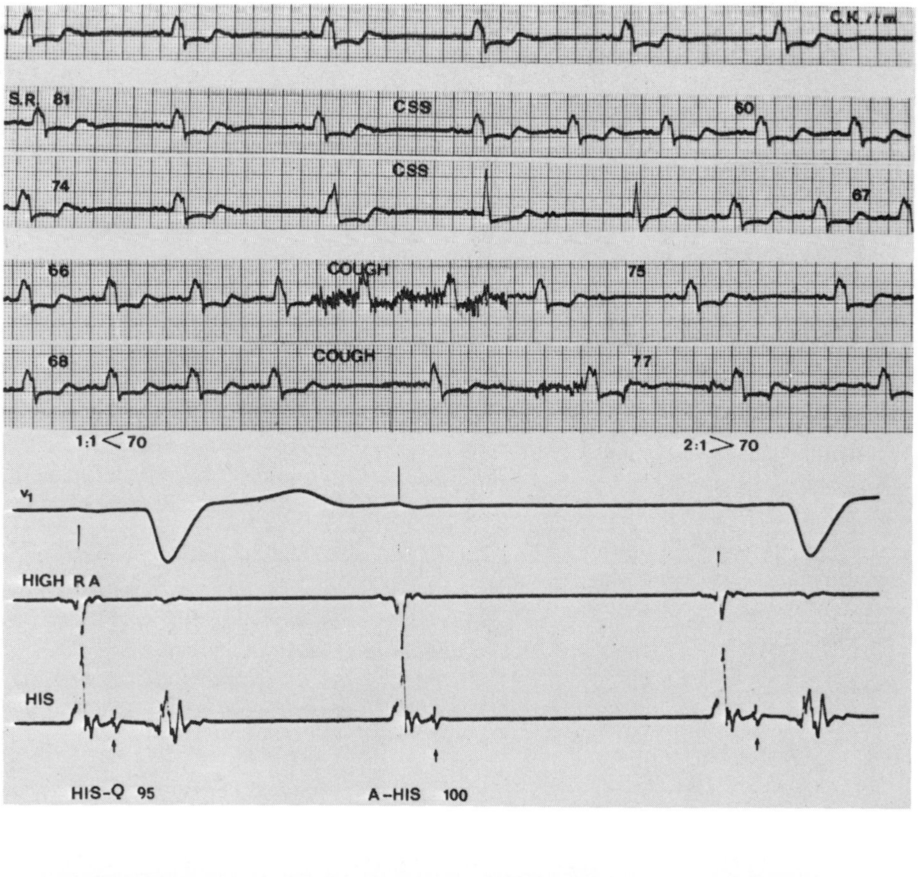

Figure 14-20. *In this example of left bundle branch block with 2:1 AV conduction, slowing of the sinus rate to below 70 beats/min abruptly established 1:1 conduction with the same PR interval present during 2:1 AV conduction. When 1:1 AV conduction prevailed, minor acceleration of the sinus rate by a few coughs changed the AV conduction ratio from 1:1 to 2:1. This behavior, typical of infranodal tracts, placed block in the bundle branches. The localization was subsequently documented by His recordings* (bottom panel).

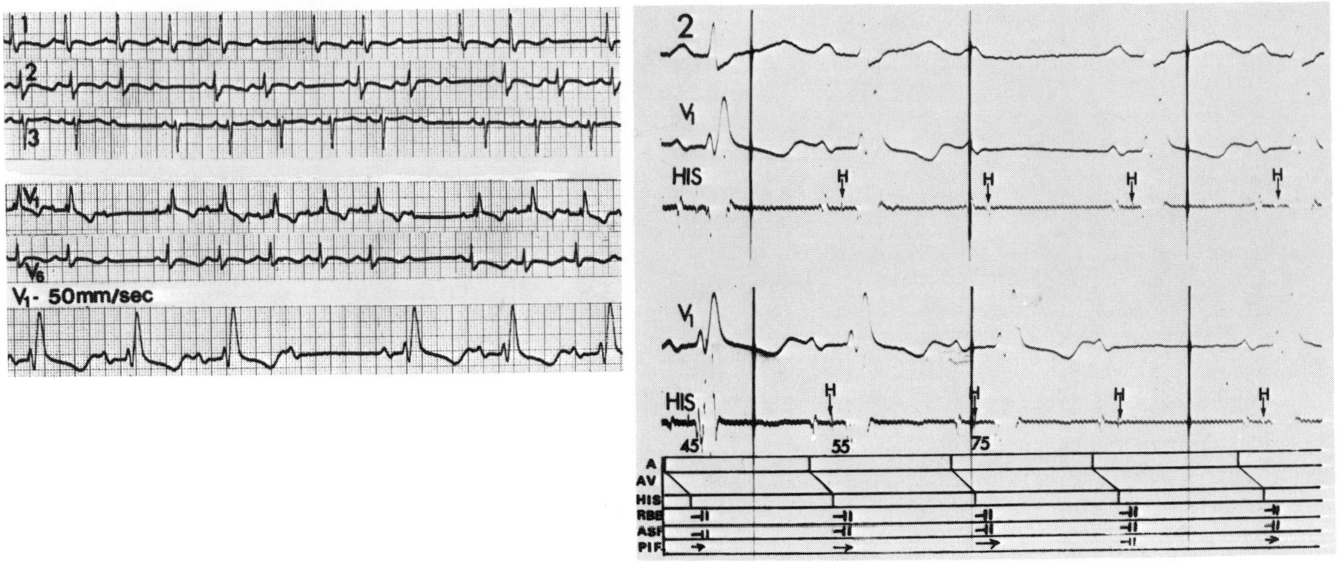

Figure 14-21. *The left panel shows 6:5 Wenckebach periods together with right bundle branch block–LAD. The Wenckebach cycle begins with a PR interval of 0.17 second and ends with a PR interval of 0.2 second, both highly atypical features for AV nodal–Wenckebach. His electrogram in the right panel demonstrates normal A-His intervals of 65 msec and His-Q intervals of 40, 45, 55, and 75 msec before the occurrence of the blocked P wave. The ladder diagram beneath the His bundle depicts the function of each fascicle and places the atypical Wenckebach in the left posterior-inferior fascicle (PIF).*

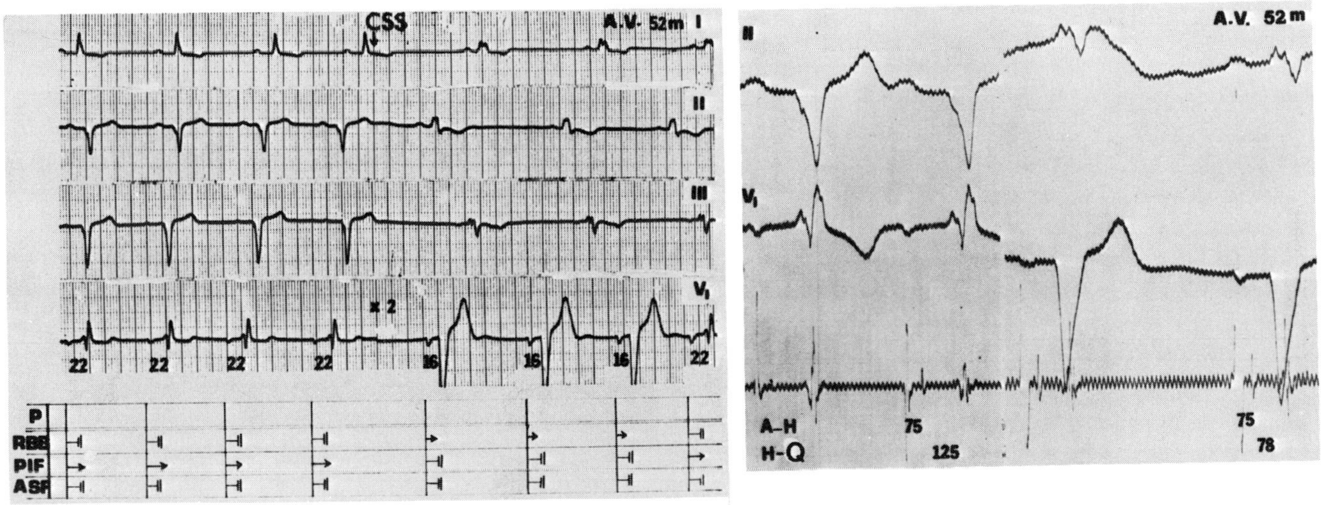

Figure 14-22. *The use of trifascicular block diagram is shown in this case of complex patterns of AV and intraventricular conduction abnormalities. This man of 58 with recent onset of angina pectoris was found to have right bundle branch (RBB) block and left axis deviation, with a normal PR interval* (left panel). *An exercise tolerance test was aborted because of the sporadic occurrence of blocked P waves. Subsequently, atropine was injected in order to reproduce events of the exercise test* (right panel). *A predominately 2:1 AV conduction with persistent RBB block, but with a normal QRS axis, was interrupted by areas of 1:1 AV conduction and changes in the QRS axis from normal to the left and then to the right. Conduction of each P wave along each of the three fascicles is depicted along horizontal lines beneath the tracing.*

In the left panel all P waves were conducted presumably through the left posterior-inferior fascicle (LPIF)—hence the arrows denoting successful conduction in the LPIF column.

(Continued)

Table 14-1. Major Anatomic and Electrophysiologic Differences Between the Atrioventricular Node and the Main His Bundle and Intraventricular Pathways

	Structure	Action Potential	Ionic Flux on Depolarization	Sensitivity of Conduction to Acetylcholine and Catecholamines	Best Role	Response to Increased Atrial Rate		Ventricular Rate When Sinus Rate Increases
						Pacing	*Autonomic or Physiologic*	
AV node	Intertwined cells	Low threshold, slow rise of phase 0	Inward calcium, slow process	++++	Slowing of AV conduction	Impaired conduction	Enhanced conduction	Increases, appropriate response
Main His bundle and IV pathways	Linearly arranged cells	High threshold, rapid rise of phase 0	Inward sodium, fast process	0	Rapid AV transmission	Impaired conduction	Impaired conduction	Decreases, inappropriate response causing symptoms and even ventricular arrhythmias

Table 14-2. Pattern of Conduction in Atrioventricular Node Versus Main His Bundle and Intraventricular Pathways

	QRS	Usual Pattern of Incomplete Block	Vagal Stimulation	Atropic and Physiologic Sympathetic Stimulation	2:1 AV Conduction Present	Circadian Variations	Phase 4 Block	Dual Pathways
AV node	Generally narrow	Typical Wenckebach	Increases block	Decreases block	Block increases to complete with vagal stimulation, disappears with atropine	Block increases during sleep	Absent	Possible
Main His bundle and IV pathways	Generally narrow, right bundle branch block or left anterior superior fascicular block in 25%	Mobitz type II, 1:1 ⇌ 2:1 ⇌ 3:1, rarely atypical Wenckebach	Decreases block	Increases block	Block decreases to 1:1 with vagal stimulation, increases to 3:1, 4:1, or complete with atropine	Block decreases during sleep	Present	None described

After atropine injection, however, RBB block persists both for conducted and for blocked P waves. Block symbols or double bars are thus placed beneath all P waves in RBB block column. Conduction through the fascicles of the left bundle, however, varies frequently. The first two conducted beats show RBB block with a normal axis, suggesting unimpeded conduction through both fascicles. Arrows indicating successful conduction are placed in the LASF and LPIF columns. The P waves between the two conducted beats fail to reach the ventricles through any of the three fascicles, hence the double bars for all the three fascicles. The fourth P wave is conducted with a pattern of RBB block and left axis deviation indicating LASF block together with RBB block. Correspondingly, double bars are placed in the appropriate columns. For the fifth P wave conduction with RBB block plus right axis deviation, block symbols are placed in the RBB and LPIF fascicle. The same process is continued throughout. Attention to each column individually shows persistent block of the right bundle, 2:1 conduction through the LASF and a pattern of 2:1, 1:1, and 3:1 conduction through the LPIF. The trifascicular nature in this pattern thus becomes obvious. Wenckebach cycles were conspicuous by their absence. Block at the AV node therefore could not be considered seriously.

one fascicle frequently exhibit atypical features (Fig. 14-21). A useful diagram for analysis of the function of each of the three fascicles is presented in Figure 14-22.

The noninvasive maneuvers have proved extremely useful in uncovering some of the most complex forms of AV block associated with changing pattern of intraventricular conduction. The most interesting contribution has been the uncovering of phase 4 block in one bundle or fascicle by vagal slowing of the rate (Fig. 14-23).

Phase 3 Versus Phase 4 Block

When a depolarizing impulse arrives early in a bundle or fascicle (*i.e.*, before complete disappearance of its refractoriness), it may be conducted slowly or be blocked completely. The term *phase 3 block* used for this phenomenon simply reflects the arrival of the impulse during phase 3 of the action potential. Impulses arriving beyond phase 3 are conducted normally. However, if the conducting structure possesses an exaggerated spontaneous phase 4 depolarizaton, usually because of disease, it cannot hold a high resting membrane potential, allowing it to drift closer and closer to the zero level, thus becoming less and less conductive. The longer the diastolic period, the greater the loss of transmembrane potential and the greater the likelihood of conduction failure. The resultant block, occurring at the end of long diastolic cycles, is commonly known as *phase 4 block.*[1] In the author's experience, phase 4 block has been a phenomenon peculiar to the intraventricular conduction system and is encountered very rarely in the AV node. Its occurrence in 13 studied cases was associated invariably with other evidence of disease in the BB–trifascicular (TF) system and has not been observed in healthy persons. For this reason, the demonstration of phase 4 depolarization in the BB-TF system may be used as strong evidence of disease in that system. The coexistence of phase 3 and phase 4 blocks in various parts of the bundle branch–trifascicular apparatus is capable of producing some of

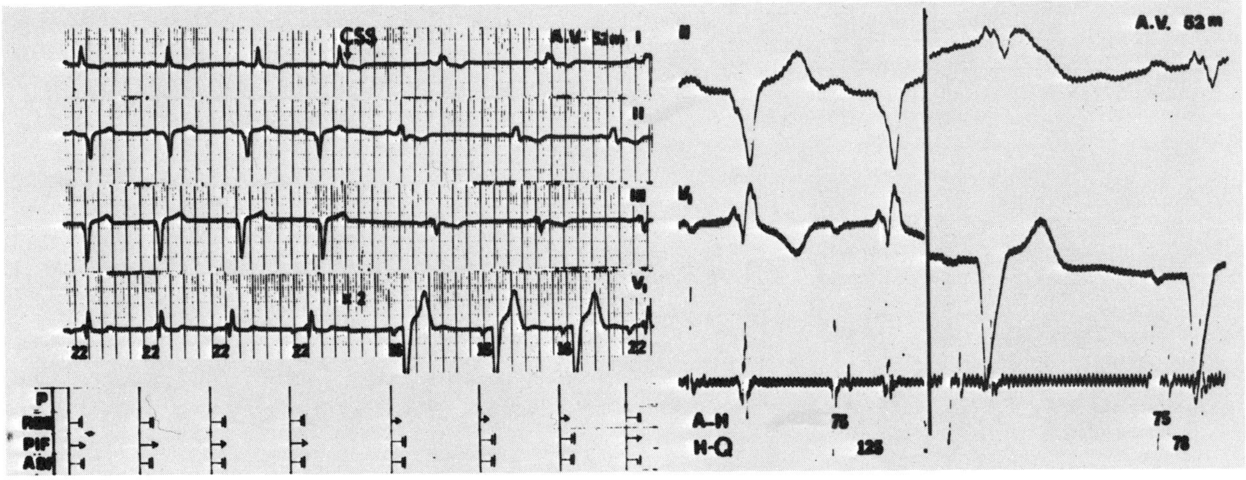

Figure 14-23. *Rhythm strips (leads I, II, III, and V_1 taken individually) and His electrogram in a man aged 52 years with documented, severe three-vessel coronary artery disease displaying shifting bundle branch block and changing QRS axis in his serial electrocardiograms. After study of many tracings right bundle branch (RBB) block–LAD together with first degree AV block were noted present at heart rates above 56 beats/min and left bundle branch (LBB)-block normal axis–normal PR intervals were present whenever heart rate was under 56 beats/min. To reproduce these rate-related phenomena, vagal stimulation (CSS) was applied in the middle of each lead reproduced in the left panel. The trifascicular block diagram pertains to lead V_1. Slowing of the rate is associated with striking changes in both the QRS morphology and the PR interval. Thus, in the basal state, with heart rate of 57 beats/min, the PR interval is 0.22 second and the QRS morphology is one of RBB block–LAD. Following vagal slowing, the rate drops below 50 beats/min. The PR interval becomes normal, and the RBB block–LAD gives its place to LBB block–normal axis. The trifascicular block diagram, showing the function of each fascicle, demonstrates a rate-related phase 3 type of block in the RBB, disappearing with vagal slowing. The LPIF develops phase 4 block after vagal slowing, while the LASF remains blocked throughout. The His electrogram in the right panel displays details of both conduction patterns. In the presence of RBB block–LAD, conduction through the LPIF is long (125 msec). Following vagal slowing, conduction proceeds solely down the RBB, with a His-Q interval of 78 msec.*

the most complex and bizarre forms of conduction disturbance (see Fig. 14-23). The possibility of phase 4 block in the postextrasystolic variety of block has already been discussed (see Figs. 14-14 and 14-15).

References

1. James, T. N., and Sherf, L.: Ultrastructure of the Human AV Node. Circulation, 37:1049–1070, 1968.
2. Watanabe, Y., and Dreifus, L. S.: Inhomogeneous conduction in the AV node. Am. Heart J., 70:505, 1965.
3. Dreifus, L., and Watanabe, Y.: Localization and significance of atrioventricular block. Am. Heart J., 82:435, 1971.
4. Cranefield, P. F.: The Conduction of the Cardiac Impulse—The Slow Response and Cardiac Arrhythmias, pp. 135–139. Mount Kisco, N.Y., Futura, 1975.
5. Zipes, D. P., Besch, H. R., Jr., and Watanabe, A. M.: Role of the slow current in cardiac electrophysiology (editorial). Circulation, 51:761–766, 1975.
6. Urthaler, F., and James, T. N.: Cholinergic and adrenergic control of the sinus node and AV junction. In Randall, W. C. (ed.): Neural Regulation of the Heart, pp. 249–288. New York, Oxford University Press, 1977.
7. Vadde, P. S., Caracta, A. R., and Damato, A. N.: Indications for HIS bundle recordings. In Augustin Castellanos, A. (ed.): Cardiac Arrhythmias—Mechanisms and Management, pp. 1–6. Philadelphia, F. A. Davis, 1980.
8. Hoffman, B. F.: Neural influences on cardiac electrical activity and rhythm. In Randall, W. C. (ed.): Neural Regulation of the Heart, pp. 291–312. New York, Oxford University Press, 1977.
9. Narula, O. S.: Electrophysiology of normal impulse propagation. In Narula, O. S. (ed.): Cardiac Arrhythmias, pp. 57–65. Baltimore, Williams & Wilkins, 1979.
10. Lister, J. W., Stein, E. M., Kosowski, B. D., et al.: Atrioventricular conduction in man. Effect of rate, exercise, isoproterenol and atropine on the PR interval. Am. J. Cardiol., 16:516–523, 1965.
11. El-Sherif, N., Scherlag, B. J., and Lazzara, R.: Conduction disorders in the canine proximal HIS-Purkinje system following acute myocardial infarction. I. The pathophysiology of intra-HIS bundle block. Circulation, 49:837–848, 1974.
12. Leon, F. A. Y., Chuquimia, R., Wu, D., et al.: Alternating Wenckebach periodicity: A common electrophysiologic response. Am. J. Cardiol., 36:757–764, 1975.
13. Moe, G. K., Mendez, C., and Han, J.: Some features of dual AV conduction system. In Dreifus, L. S., and Likoff, W., (eds.): Mechanisms and Therapy of Cardiac Arrhythmias, p. 361. New York, Grune & Stratton, 1966.
14. Pick, A., and Langendorf, R.: Interpretation of Complex Arrhythmias, pp. 222–223. Philadelphia, Lea & Febiger, 1979.
15. Massumi, R. A.: Cardiac arrhythmias associated with Cheyne-Stokes' respiratory: A note on the possible mechanisms. Dis. Chest, 54:21, 1968.
16. Rosen, K. M., Rahimtoola, S. H., and Gunnar, R. M.: Pseudo AV block secondary to premature non-propagated His bundle depolarizations. Circulation, 42:367, 1970.
17. Mangiardi, L. M., Bonamini, R., Conte, M., et al.: Bedside evaluation of atrioventricular block with narrow QRS complexes: Usefulness of carotid sinus massage and atropine administration. Am. J. Cardiol., 49:1136–1145, 1982.
18. Schilenburg, R. M., and Durrer, D.: Conduction disturbances located within the His bundle. Circulation, 45:612–628, 1972.
19. Rosenbaum, M. B., Elizari, M. V., Lazzari, J. O., et al.: Mechanisms of intermittent bundle branch block. Relationship to prolonged recovery, hypopolarization and spontaneous diastolic depolarization. Chest, 63:666–667, 1973.

15

Abberrancy: Electrophysiologic Mechanisms and Electrocardiographic Correlates

Donald H. Singer and Howard C. Cohen

The character of the QRS complex is a function of the sequence of ventricular activation, with alterations in QRS contour reflecting deviations from normal in the path of spread. This may occur in one of two general ways: (1) shift in the site of cardiac impulse formation to an ectopic focus in the ventricles or to certain types of AV nodal bypass tracts or (2) altered ventricular spread of supraventricular impulses. The latter, in turn, may result from congenital or acquired impairment of the conduction system. Alternately, it may be "functional," due to impulse conduction during periods of refractoriness.

The terms *aberrancy, aberration,* and *aberrant ventricular conduction* have, since their introduction by Sir Thomas Lewis early in this century,[1,2] come to be principally applied to functional intraventricular conduction disturbances, particularly those occurring in conjunction with changes in cycle length.[3-7] However, they apply with equal logic to the other types of intraventricular conduction disturbances. In this chapter and in Chapter 16, aberrancy will be considered within this broader context. Electrophysiologic mechanisms and clinical aspects and implications of the different types of conduction disturbances will be reviewed.

The Specialized Conducting System of the Heart

It is convenient to consider the heart as consisting of two general types of tissue (Fig. 15-1*A*): (1) ordinary atrial and ventricular myocardium that is responsible for contractile work and for inscription of the P and QRS deflections of the standard electrocardiogram and (2) a chain of "specialized" tissues[8-10] (see Chap. 2), including the SA and AV nodes and the ramifications of the His-Purkinje system.[10-13] Atrioventricular nodal bypass tracts and specialized atrial internodal tracts[9,14,15] have also been described.

The specialized tissues are responsible for normal impulse formation and for the rapid and orderly distribution of the cardiac impulse from its site of origin to the remainder of the heart. Changes in impulse formation or conduction in the specialized tissues, or both, underlie changes in heart rate in response to changing physiologic conditions as well as many dysrhythmias and conduction disturbances. The electrophysiologic characteristics of the specialized tissues are a principal determinant of

The work for this chapter was supported in part by grants-in-aid to Dr. Singer by the American Heart Association (74 1065), the Chicago Heart Association (B 74-73), the Reingold Estate, the Brinton Trust, and the Deborah M. Cooley Foundation and to Dr. Cohen by U.S.P.H.S. (HL-176648).

The authors wish to express their appreciation to Dr. John R. McCullough and Dr. James E. Rosenthal for their critical contributions and help in preparation of the manuscript; to Ms. Lillian Washington for her outstanding editorial services; to Amy Cigan, William Morrone, Vallerie Valentini, and Laura J. Moreth for their technical and artistic support; and to Ruth Singer for her patience with the whole endeavor.

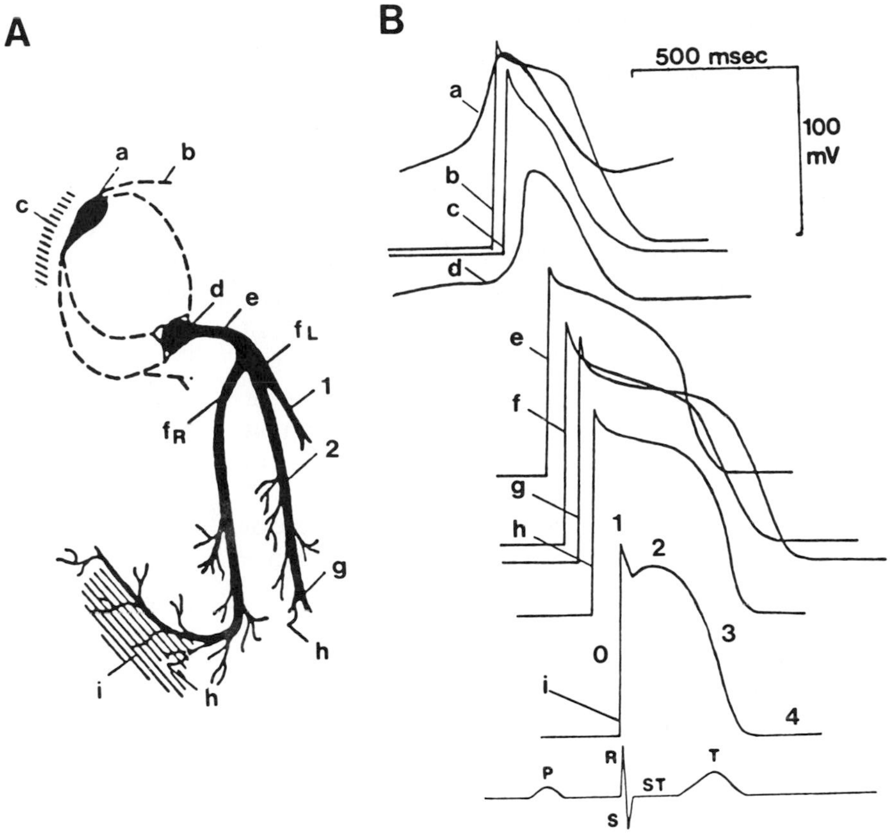

Figure 15-1. *Diagrammatic representation of the specialized cardiac conduction system (A) and transmembrane potentials from ordinary and specialized tissues of the dog heart (B) to illustrate differences in action potential characteristics at the several sites. The relationships between records indicate sequence of activation. A standard body surface electrocardiographic lead is also shown. The lower case letters a to i refer to the following: a, sinoatrial node; b, Bachmann's bundle and other specialized atrial internodal tracts (see* dashed lines *connecting sinoatrial and atrioventricular nodes); c, ordinary atrial myocardium; d, atrioventricular node; e, bundle of His; f, bundle branches;* f_R*, right bundle branch;* f_L*, left bundle branch; anterior (1) and posterior (2) divisions of the left bundle branch; g, Purkinje fiber; h, terminal Purkinje fiber at Purkinje–ventricular muscle junction; and i, ventricular muscle. The phases of ventricular muscle action potential (i) are designated by arabic numerals 0 through 4; the deflections of the surface electrocardiographic lead, by the letters P, R, S, and T. See text for discussion.*

aberrancy. Activity of the specialized tissues is not manifest on standard surface records because of their small mass relative to ordinary myocardium, a factor that has hampered electrocardiographic assessment of the underlying mechanisms.

Electrophysiologic Aspects

As noted previously, abnormalities of QRS configuration can result from a number of causes. This chapter will focus on the subgroup originally described by Sir Thomas Lewis[1,2] for which the term *aberrancy* was coined, namely, altered QRS contour of supraventricular beats occurring in conjunction with cycle length–dependent changes in conduction and refractoriness. Aberrancy represents one aspect of a larger group of cycle length–dependent conduction disturbances that includes such varied entities as *concealed conduction*,[16–18] *supernormal conduction*,[19,20] and *rate-related AV block*.[3–5] Unidirectional block and reentrant excitation[3–7] are, in a sense, also manifestations of this phenomenon.

Aberrancy will be considered in terms of cycle length

dependency of the QRS changes as proposed by Singer and Ten Eick.[21] The discussion is based on correlations between electrocardiographic material and transmembrane potential data from microelectrode studies on cardiac tissues from animals and from patients undergoing open-heart surgery.

Electrical Activity of Cardiac Cells

Understanding of the mechanisms of aberrancy depends on an understanding of the electrophysiologic basis of impulse formation and conduction in the heart and of the changes in these variables underlying development of conduction disturbances. A brief review of current concepts follows. The reader is referred to Chapter 3 as well as to numerous other textbooks of physiology[22-24] and reviews and monographs on cardiac electrophysiology[25-36] for a more comprehensive exposition.

The Normal Transmembrane Potential

Insertion of a glass microelectrode[37] into an excitable cell permits the potential difference between the cell interior and an indifferent electrode located outside the cell to be recorded. Figure 15-1*B* shows idealized transmembrane potential records from different parts of the heart, together with a simultaneously recorded surface electrocardiogram. The phases of the action potential are designated by Arabic numerals 0 to 4. During electrical diastole (phase 4), the cell interior is negative with respect to the extracellular fluid. In most normal cardiac fibers, including the ordinary atrial and ventricular myocardial cells, the potential difference during phase 4 remains constant until excitation occurs (the *"resting potential"*), normally averaging between −85 and −95 mV. On excitation, the cell undergoes rapid depolarization (phase 0) with a transient reversal of polarity, followed by a gradual repolarization process (phases 1, 2, and 3) during which membrane potential is restored to resting levels. Comparisons with the surface electrocardiogram show that phases 0 to 1 of the ventricular action potential correspond to the R and S waves and phases 2 to 3 to the ST segment and T wave, respectively (see Fig. 15-1*B*).

Transmembrane potentials recorded from ordinary and specialized fibers in different parts of the heart may differ from each other in several respects,[25] including level of diastolic potential, action potential amplitude, maximum rate of depolarization during phase 0 ($\dot{V}_{max}$), time course of repolarization, and action potential duration (see Fig. 15-1*B*). Differences in excitability, conductivity, and pacemaker capabilities also occur. Local differences in electrophysiologic properties within the His-Purkinje system[25,31-33] may be important with respect to aberrancy, as may local variability in response to various physiologic and pharmacologic factors,[25,38-47] including temperature, *p*H, rate, pCO_2, hypoxia, ischemia, inorganic cations, and a number of antiarrhythmic agents.

Membrane Mechanisms

Cardiac electrical activity originates in the movements of ions across the cell membrane.[22-36,48] Physiologic interventions and pharmacologic agents that influence impulse formation and conduction in the heart do so mainly by their ability to influence these ionic currents.[24,30,37,38-47] Figure 15-2 depicts the important ionic currents thought to underlie inscription of the action potential in Purkinje fibers. A simplified explanation for specific phenomena pertinent to considerations of aberrancy follows.

The Resting Membrane Potential. The potential difference across the cardiac cell membrane results from differences in ionic composition that exist between the cell interior and the extracellular fluid.[32,33] In the intracellular fluid, K^+ is the principal cation and phosphate and the organic acid radicals are the dominant anions. The latter are largely polyvalent ions, often associated with proteins, to which the cell membrane is impermeable. In the extracellular fluid, Na^+ and Cl^- predominate. To and fro transmembrane movements of these ions through specialized pores or channels[50] in response to changes in electrochemical gradients constitute the membrane currents[27,32-35] that underlie inscription of the action potential. The resting cell membrane is principally permeable to K^+ and relatively impermeable to the other intracellular and extracellular ions.[32] The potential difference across the resting membrane is, accordingly, largely determined by the K^+ concentration gradient.[29,31,32,48,49] Maintenance of the resting ionic and voltage differences is made possible by two factors[31,32,49]: (1) the permeability characteristics *or* conductance (g) of the membrane to these ions, which in turn reflects availability of membrane channels for use by a given ion species, and (2) the operation of various ion pumps and exchange mechanisms,[51-53] including an energy-dependent Na^+-K^+ ion exchange pump, which transports Na^+ out of and K^+ into the cell against their concentration gradients.[51,53]

The Action Potential: Depolarization. When the cell is stimulated and membrane potential lowered to a critical level, the threshold potential (*i.e.,* the potential at which a net inward current is just generated), a sequential series of changes in membrane ionic conductances and currents occurs that gives rise to inscription of the action potential[27,31,33,36] (see Fig. 15-2). In normal, well-polarized cardiac fibers, exclusive of SA and AV nodal cells,

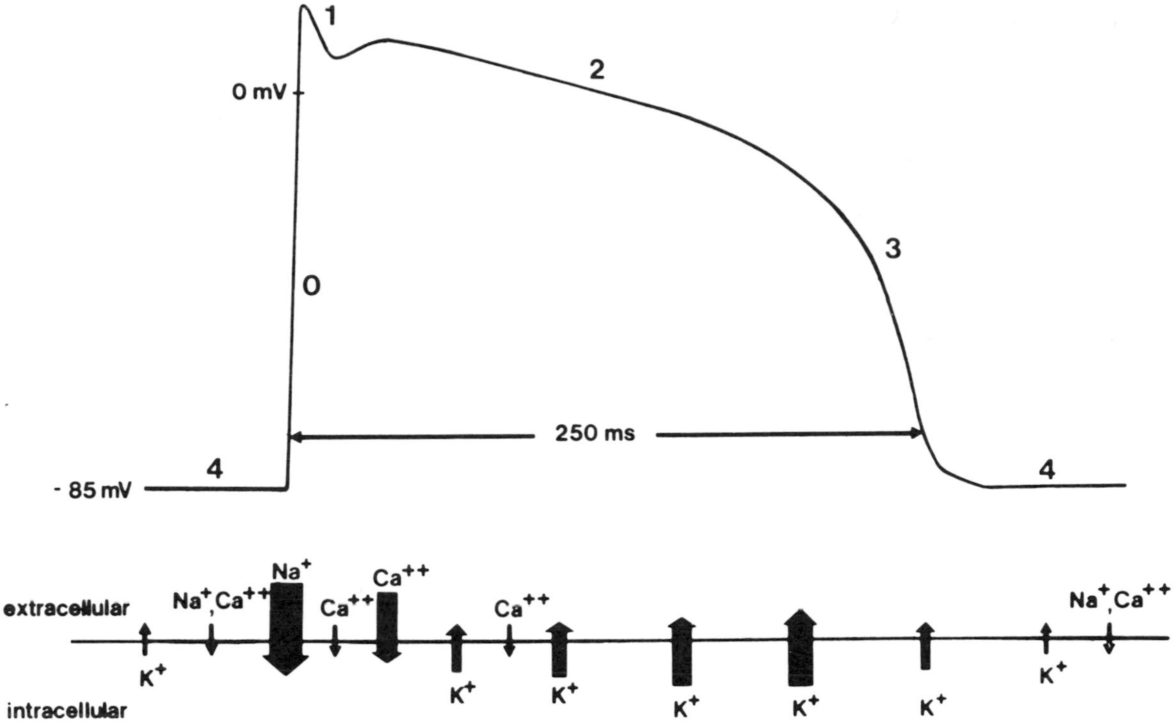

Figure 15-2. *Schematic representation of the action potential in normal ventricle depicting the direction, strength, and period of flow of the ionic currents underlying the action potential. Arrow direction and size indicate whether current is inward or outward directed and relative current strength, respectively, of the involved ion. The horizontal position of the arrow corresponds to the same moment in the time course of the action potential. See text for discussion. (After Ten Eick, R. E., Baumgarten, C. M., and Singer, D. H.: Ventricular dysrhythmia: Membrane basis of currents, channels, gates, and cables. Prog. Cardiovasc. Dis., 24:157–188, 1981)*

depolarization (phase 0) results primarily from an explosive increase in membrane conductance to Na^+ (g_{Na}) and in a rapid inward directed ionic current carried by Na^+[24,27,29,31,33,35,48] (the *fast inward Na^+ current* or *fast inward current*) in conjunction with opening of the fast Na^+ channels.

The ability of the membrane to undergo an increase in g_{Na} (*i.e.*, to open closed Na^+ channels) is related to the level of membrane potential at excitation. In general, the availability of Na^+ channels is maximal, and a maximum fast inward Na^+ current is possible, when membrane potential averages -85 to -95 mV. When membrane potential is less negative than normal, the maximum possible increase in Na^+ permeability and the magnitude of the fast Na^+ current are diminished because of decreased channel availability. If membrane potential is reduced to a low enough level, the increase in fast inward Na^+ current may be inadequate to produce a regenerative response, or even any response at all, so that the fiber becomes inexcitable.

The amplitude and maximum rate of depolarization ($\dot{V}_{max}$) during phase 0 (the upstroke) are functions of the fast inward Na^+ current. It follows that they therefore also depend on the level of membrane potential. The amplitude of well-polarized Purkinje fibers averages up to 130 mV and $\dot{V}_{max}$ is rapid, with values of 500 to 1000 V/sec being reported. Both decrease with decreases in the level of potential. Figure 15-3*A* shows the progressive decrease in amplitude and rising velocity of Purkinje fiber action potentials initiated at successively lower levels of membrane potential. The curves in Figure 15-3*B* depict the relationship between membrane potential at excitation and $\dot{V}_{max}$ of the response for two ventricular myocardial cells. This relationship, which was first defined for cardial fibers by Weidman in 1951[54] and subsequently confirmed by Hoffman and colleagues,[55] is often termed the *responsiveness relationship* and the curve termed the *responsiveness curve.*[56] Such curves are sometimes used as a rough measure of the availability of Na^+ channels.

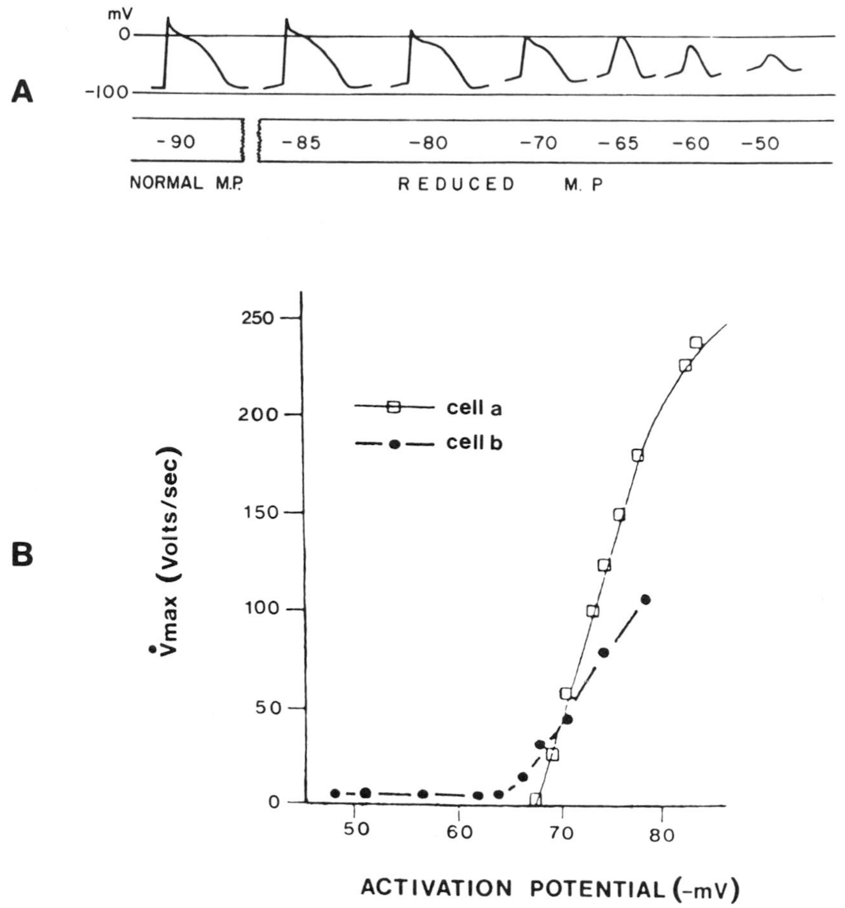

Figure 15-3. *(A) Schematic representation of the changes in the characteristics of an action potential as it propagates from a normally polarized region into one in which membrane potential (MP) is progressively reduced. The level of membrane potential, in millivolts, is indicated for selected sites along the fiber. Action potentials initiated at these sites are shown above. Note particularly the progressive diminution in amplitude and* $\dot{V}_{max}$*, which would be expected to be accompanied by progressive slowing of conduction. Also note changes in time course of repolarization and in action potential duration. (B) Curves depicting the relationship between the level of membrane potential, in millivolts, at excitation* (abscissa) *and* $\dot{V}_{max}$*, in V/sec* (ordinate), *of action potentials initiated in well-polarized cells a* ($E_m = -90$ *mV) and b* ($E_m = -79$ *mV) human ventricular muscle fibers in a specimen from a patient with coronary heart disease and ventricular aneurysm. Determinations were made on action potentials initiated at selected levels of membrane potential by stimulating the preparation at intervals during repolarization and during phase 4. Curves relating these variables are designated* responsiveness curves. *Note that the curve for cell b is shifted down and to the right in the mid-range of potential and up and to the left at the low end of the potential range. See text for discussion.*

A second inward current in heart tissue[27,29,30,33–35,57,58] is activated only at "low" levels of membrane potential, about −35 to −45 mV. This current is carried primarily by Ca^{++} ions and is of much lower density (approximately 10%) than the fast Na^+ current. The channel carrying this second current activates (turns on) and inactivates (turns off) more slowly than does the fast Na^+ channel, so that the current is slower and longer than the fast Na^+ current. Recovery from inactivation also takes longer. This current has accordingly been designated the *slow inward current.* Channels carrying the fast and slow inward currents are separable pharmacologically.[58,59] Tetrodotoxin principally blocks the fast inward Na^+ channel, whereas the slow channel is blocked by agents such as manganese (Mn^{++}), D-600, and verapamil. In normal, well-polarized cells, the slow current exerts only minimal effects on the upstroke, contributing mainly to phase 2 (the plateau) of repolarization. Depolarization of low potential nodal cells[60–64] and muscle fibers in the AV valve leaflets[66] and coronary sinus,[67] on the other hand, appears largely slow current dependent. It also becomes much more important to the depolarization of nonnodal fibers in which membrane potential is reduced.[30,33–35,66–69] This latter fact assumes particular importance in light of findings that specimens of experimentally infarcted dog heart[70–74,138,184] and human heart from patients with heart disease[21,36,76,77–90] contain large numbers of partially depolarized fibers.

The electrophysiologic properties of slow inward current-dependent fibers *(slow response fibers)* differ in a number of respects from those of fast current-dependent *(fast response)* fibers.[30,33,34,58,59] In general, *slow-response* fibers are characterized by low diastolic potential, low amplitude and slowly rising action potentials, diminished excitability, altered responsiveness, prolonged refractoriness, and slow conduction. In addition, even normally nonautomatic fibers may become capable of spontaneous impulse formation when membrane potential is reduced to levels at which the slow current becomes operative (Fig. 15-4*I*). Most of the peculiarities of SA and AV nodal activity appear explicable in terms of the behavior of the slow inward current.[25,30,61–65] This also holds for the altered electrophysiologic properties of many of the partially depolarized cells in tissues from ischemic and diseased hearts.[31,34,36,75,78,85,86,91–93]

The Action Potential: Repolarization. The increase in fast inward Na^+ current that underlies depolarization is self-limited and short (approximately a few milliseconds). Inactivation of the Na^+ channels and the consequent reduction in Na^+ current usher in repolarization, a more prolonged (up to several hundred milliseconds) and complex process involving Na^+, K^+, Ca^{++}, and Cl^- (see Fig. 15-2).[27,29,31,33,94] Specific mechanisms have not yet been completely defined. However, for repolarization to occur, a decrease in intracellular positive charge is needed. In Purkinje fibers, three clear-cut phases have been defined. The initial stage (phase 1) is rapid and results from the inactivation of the Na^+ current, an outward current carried by K^+ and, possibly, by Cl^- ions.[27,95] Following phase 1, repolarization markedly slows (the plateau, or phase 2). There is an overall reduction in membrane conductance during this phase, and the small currents that do occur more or less balance each other[27,33,94,95] (*i.e.,* the repolarizing effects of the inactivation of the Na^+ current and of activation of an outward K^+ current are counterbalanced by the depolarizing effects of the residual slow inward current). The K^+ current increases over time. This, together with the waning of the inward currents, results in an increasing net loss of positive charge, culminating in the stage of rapid repolarization (phase 3). As repolarization progresses, g_K becomes even larger, favoring additional K^+ efflux and further acceleration of repolarization. This is additionally favored by accumulation of the extruded K^+ efflux in the restricted extracellular space.[96] It has been recently suggested that electrogenic Na^+-K^+ pumping also may contribute to repolarization.[97,98] Once membrane potential is restored to about −40 to −45 mV, it falls rapidly to resting values.

Impulse Formation

Excitation and inscription of the action potential result from a flow of sufficient depolarizing current across the cell membrane to lower rapidly (*i.e.,* make less negative) the transmembrane potential to the threshold potential. The threshold potential differs for different cell types and is related to the level of maximum diastolic potential.[33,56,87,99] Excitatory (depolarizing) currents may be supplied by an external source or may arise spontaneously. Normally, they derive from local potential differences created by the propagating action potential. Certain cells, termed *automatic,* can generate such currents spontaneously and thus may undergo self-excitation and initiate impulses spontaneously (automaticity).[25]

Automaticity normally results from the cyclic occurrence of spontaneous depolarization during phase 4 in the specialized tissues of the heart[25] (see Fig. 15-1*B*). Cells with the fastest rates of spontaneous diastolic (phase 4) depolarization, normally those in the SA node, serve as the primary pacemaker; the remainder serve as latent pacemakers. Ordinarily, probably only SA nodal cells actually exhibit phase 4 depolarization (see Fig. 15-1*B*), latent ("escape") pacemakers developing the requisite changes in response to such factors as sinus slowing or AV block.

Spontaneous impulse formation can result from causes other than slow diastolic depolarization of specialized automatic cells. Since such alternate causes are not thought to develop under normal physiologic conditions, they are considered *abnormal* causes of automaticity; the resultant spontaneous activity is considered *abnormal automaticity.*[100] The term encompasses a group of diverse phenomena. Spontaneous, cyclic, pacemaker-like oscillations of the diastolic potential unrelated to a prior initiating event represent one major grouping. This type of activity is largely a phenomenon of depressed, partially depolarized fibers in which membrane potential has been reduced to levels at which the slow inward current becomes operative—hence the designation *depolarization-induced automaticity.* It appears to be evokable in most, if not all, cells, including ordinary atrial and ventricular myocardial cells, on lowering of the diastolic potential.[101–103] The phenomenon appears common in specimens of ischemic and diseased heart.[36,74,75,87,91–93] The records in Figure 15-4*I*, showing a partially depolarized, automatic, human atrial myocardial cell, are representative.

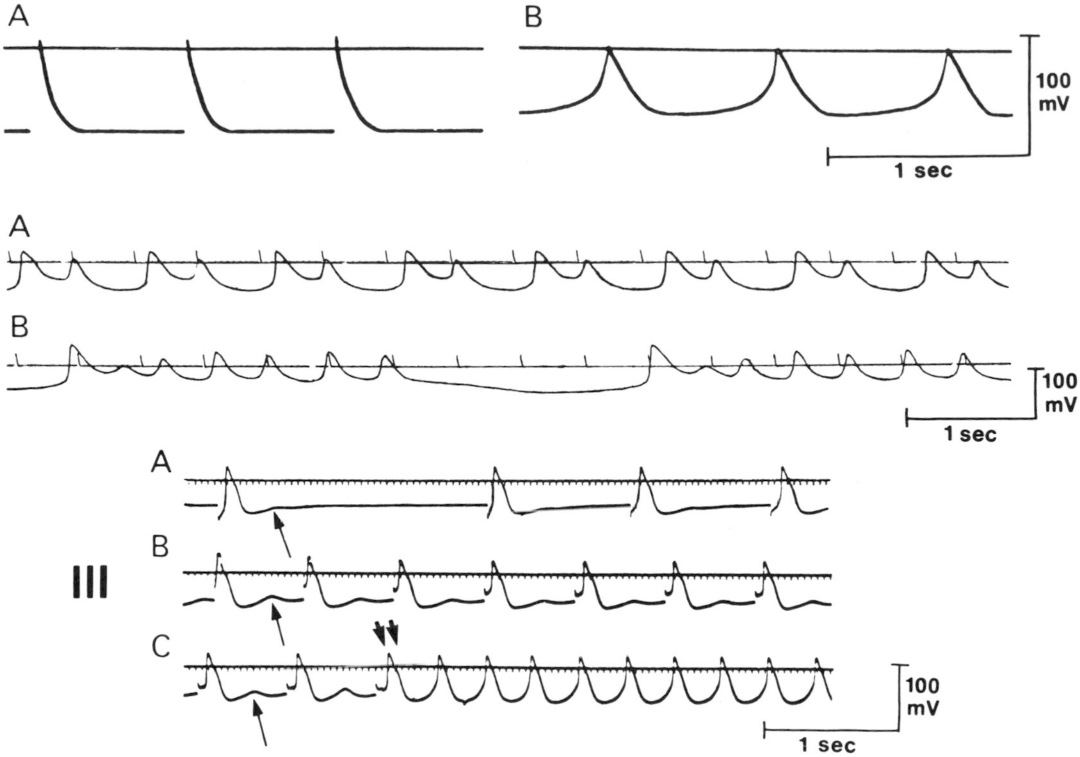

Figure 15-4. *Transmembrane potentials recorded from specimens of human atrium* (panels I and III) *and ventricle* (panel II) *to show different types of abnormal automaticity in cardiac tissues from a patient with heart disease.* (Panel I) *Transmembrane potentials from well-polarized, "fast-response" (A) and low-potential, "slow-response" (B) fibers in human right atrial appendage. Maximum diastolic potential (and amplitude) exhibited by cells A and B are −72 mV (−80 mV) and −55 mV (−55 mV), respectively. Constrast the large-amplitude, rapidly rising potentials elicited from the well-polarized fiber with the low-amplitude, slowly rising potentials from the depolarized cell. Also note that the slow response cell begins to spontaneously depolarize as soon as repolarization is complete; that is, it has become automatic (depolarization induced automaticity).* (Panel II) *Transmembrane potentials from partially depolarized, spontaneously active human papillary muscle cell from a patient with rheumatic heart disease complicated by atrial fibrillation, high-grade ventricular ectopy, and variable rate–dependent conduction disturbance. In* panel II, row A, *repolarization of each basic automatic beat is interrupted by a single early afterdepolarization type of oscillation giving rise to a bigeminal pattern. In* panel II, row B, *each basic beat is interrupted by a small oscillation followed by five larger repetitive oscillations with resultant marked prolongation of repolarization. The runs are terminated by a very low amplitude oscillation that further delays completion of repolarization of the basic beats.* (Panel III) *Induction of late afterdepolarization type of oscillations and triggered activity in an initially quiescent specimen of human atrium. The first oscillation in each panel is indicated by* (arrows). Rows A and B *as well as the initial part of* row C *show development of oscillations in conjunction with stimulation at increasing rates. Note the gradual increase in oscillation amplitude with rate increases. Eventually, oscillations reached threshold and repetitive triggered activity ensued (mid-portion,* row C*), which persisted even after discontinuation of stimulation. Although each of the examples shown occurred in partially depolarized cells, similar phenomena have been observed in well-polarized cells. See text for discussion. (After Singer, D. H., Baumgarten, C. M., and Ten Eick, R. E.: Cellular electrophysiology of ventricular and other dysrhythmias: Studies on diseased and ischemic heart. Prog. Cardiovasc. Dis., 24:97–156, 1981)*

Other types of oscillations depend on the occurrence of prior initiating action potential for their existence, that is, triggered automaticity. They may originate during or following completion of repolarization of the initiating event (see Fig. 15-4*II* and *III*). These oscillations have been accorded a number of designations, of which the most widely used is that proposed by Cranefield, who referred to them as *early* and *delayed* afterdepolarizations, respectively.[30] Early afterdepolarizations most commonly interrupt phase 2 of repolarization at plateau level potentials of −20 to −25 mV but also may occur during phase 3. They serve to prolong repolarization and refractoriness, sometimes for many seconds (see Fig. 15-4*II*). Delayed afterdepolarizations (see Fig. 15-4*III*), on the other hand, occur during phase 4 at more or less normal (−70 to −85 mV), as well as at reduced, levels of diastolic potential. Afterdepolarizations that reach threshold result in initiation of triggered rhythms (see Fig. 15-4*III*),[104] of which the best known are those due to the digitalis glycosides.

Membrane mechanisms underlying the pacemaker potential are not entirely clarified.[29,30,33] In Purkinje fibers, recent reports suggest that pacemaking activity results from activation of an inward current carried by both Na^+ and K^+.[105,106] In the SA node, there is evidence that the slow inward current also may contribute to pacemaker activity.[107–110] Ionic mechanisms underlying automatic activity in partially depolarized myocardial cells and afterdepolarization type oscillations are even less well defined.[29,30,33,34,36,102,103]

Conduction

Conduction of the cardiac impulse (action potential) is a highly complex and only imperfectly understood phenomenon. Recent monographs and reviews by Jack and co-workers,[111] Fozzard,[112] Spach and Kootsey,[113] and Cranefield[30,114] highlight the complexities. Conduction is considered to result from sequential depolarization of contiguous areas of cell membrane by local currents that arise as a result of potential differences between adjacent segments of resting (polarized) and active (depolarized) membrane and that flow from cell to cell through low resistance electrical connections. The rate at which this process proceeds (*i.e.*, conduction velocity) depends on a number of interrelated variables, including the inward current and its determinants, excitability, the passive cable properties of cardiac fibers, and fiber diameter and geometry.

The Inward Current. For normal cardiac cells outside of the SA and AV nodes, the ability of the propagating action potential to excite adjacent regions of resting membrane and therefore to conduct, as well as conduction velocity, depend on the fast inward Na^+ current and therefore on $\dot{V}_{max}$, an indirect measure of the inward current. The inward current and $\dot{V}_{max}$ are, in turn, related to membrane potential at excitation. It follows that conduction velocity also is related to the membrane potential of cells in the path of impulse spread.[54–56,112,115] Other factors being equal, the fast inward Na^+ current, $\dot{V}_{max}$, and conduction velocity are optimal in well-polarized fibers in which membrane potential is at or about −85 to −95 mV. Reduced membrane potential is associated with a decreased fast inward Na^+ current and $\dot{V}_{max}$ and with slowed conduction.[30] Conduction impairment is voltage dependent,[55,56,115] significant slowing usually first appearing at < -70 mV and failure of conduction at −50 mV or below. At such low levels of potential, the fast Na^+ current is largely inactivated and depolarization becomes increasingly slow current dependent. Figure 15-3*A* shows schematic representation of the deterioration of the action potential during propagation from a normally polarized region into one that is progressively more depolarized. Spread into the partially depolarized region is depicted as resulting in progressive reduction of amplitude and rising velocity, changes that would be expected to be associated with increasingly marked slowing of conduction.

Conduction also is influenced by the relationship between membrane potential at excitation and $\dot{V}_{max}$ of the response (responsiveness). Changes in the relationship such that the normal curve (cell *a*) depicted in Figure 15-3*B* is shifted down and to the right (cell *b* curve) depress responsiveness and slow conduction, since $\dot{V}_{max}$ of responses initiated at any given potential are decreased relative to normal. Since such a shift slows conduction at all levels of potential, it might (1) accentuate conduction disturbances resulting from reduction in membrane potential and (2) facilitate development of conduction disturbances at more normal (*i.e.*, more negative) levels of potential than usual. Changes in the responsiveness relationship such that the curve shifts up and to the left in the upper and mid-ranges of potential exert the opposite effect. Paradoxically, leftward shifts in the low range of potential (see Fig. 15-3*B*, cell *b* curve) might predispose to development of conduction disturbances, since they would facilitate generation of slowly rising, slow-conducting responses at potential levels that would otherwise be too low to support any activity at all.

Numerous cardioactive drugs, including many of the standard antiarrhythmic agents, influence conduction by affecting responsiveness.[25,30,38–44] Depressant effects of quinidine and procainamide largely reflect their actions in displacing the curve down and to the right.[116,117] Ischemia and disease also appear to affect this relationship. Studies on infarcted dog ventricle[70,71,74,75] and on diseased human heart[36,87] indicate that the curve for at least some cells appears to be shifted down and to the right in the upper and mid-regions of the voltage range up and to the left at the low end of the range (see Fig. 15-3*B*, cell *b*). The latter most probably reflects activation of the slow inward current at low potentials. Irrespective, both types of shift predispose to an increase in conduction disturbances and aberrancy.

Excitability and Conduction. Conduction also depends on membrane excitability.[118-120] The term *excitability* refers to the current required to lower membrane potential from levels extant at stimulation to the threshold potential and to initiate an action potential. It too is a complex function dependent on a number of factors, including the level of membrane potential and the threshold potential. A decrease in excitability is synonymous with an increase in current requirements for excitation and, other factors being equal, is associated with slowing of conduction. Increases in excitability have the opposite effect. Speeding of conduction in response to moderate depolarization has been explained on this basis.[118-120] Indeed, cycle length–dependent changes in excitability of depressed cells in the His-Purkinje system have been suggested as a possible cause of intermittent bundle branch block.[150] A number of physiologic and pharmacologic factors that influence conduction are thought to do so, at least in part, by affecting excitability. This appears to be true of potassium, with increases in extracellular K^+ between 2.7 to 4 mM being associated with increases in excitability and in conduction velocity. Further increases in extracellular K^+ to $>$ 7 mM depress excitability and conduction.[119] Depressive effects on conduction of lidocaine and procainamide may be related to their action in decreasing excitability.[121,122] Ischemia and disease also may depress excitability and thus influence conduction.

Cable Properties and Conduction. Cardiac fibers are considered to exhibit many of the electrical properties characteristic of a linear, coaxial cable.[23,31,111,112] Individual cells are electrically linked (coupled) by a low-resistance[123] specialization of the membrane,[124,125] the nexus or gap junction,[126] which facilitates cell-to-cell current flow and the creation of functionally long cables. The electrical properties associated with such a structure, termed *passive* or *cable* properties, include membrane resistance (the reciprocal of conduction) and capacitance *and* internal longitudinal resistance (the sum of the resistance of the cytoplasm and of the nexuses). They govern cell-to-cell current spread and are therefore also principal determinants of conduction.[23,30,36,111,112,114] Modifications of these parameters can profoundly influence conduction.[127]

Evidence suggests that drug- and disease-related changes in the cable properties may contribute to conduction disturbances in a clinical setting. Findings that toxic doses of ouabain,[128] acidosis,[129] and hypoxia and simulated ischemia,[130] all of which are associated with conduction abnormalities *in vivo,* appear to increase nexal resistance, are pertinent. Simulation studies suggest that sufficient increases in internal resistance could result in complete conduction block due to electrical uncoupling.[131] Evidence also suggests that electrical uncoupling exists in diseased human ventricular myocardium.[87] A possible role for altered cable properties in the development of slow conduction and dysrhythmia in patients with heart disease is thus suggested. The exact mechanism underlying electrical uncoupling is uncertain but appears to involve ionized Ca^{++}, as evidenced by findings that internal resistance increases when calcium is injected intracellularly.[132] A number of interventions that magnify hypoxic- ischemic-induced increases in internal resistance, including increased frequency of stimulation, also increase intracellular Ca^{++}.[133]

Conduction Disturbances in the Heart

Cardiac conduction disturbances are due to many causes. Congenital or acquired abnormalities of the specialized tissues, as well as their actual disruption due to disease, are well known.[8] In normal heart, probably the most common cause is impulse propagation in fibers in which membrane potential is low. The electrophysiologic properties of partially depolarized slow-response fibers[30,34] as well as the changes in ischemic[74,75] and diseased heart[36,87] appear pertinent with respect to the increase in aberrancy in the latter. Alterations in excitability and the cable properties of cardiac fibers due to drugs and disease[31,111,112] as well as to peculiarities of fiber geometry and temporal and spatial convergence of impulses[134,135] are also important. The discussion will focus on the membrane potential dependence of conduction disturbances.

Conduction disturbances due to low potential can occur anywhere in the heart. Numerous electrocardiographic patterns are possible, the particular pattern in a given instance reflecting the location of the depolarized fibers and the extent of membrane depolarization. If, for example, the site of involvement is the His bundle, conduction abnormalities would be manifested as AV block. If, on the other hand, the depolarized cells are located below the bifurcation, various types of intraventricular conduction defects might ensue.

The timing of the reduction in membrane potential also is critical concerning the nature of a conduction disturbance and its electrocardiographic representation.

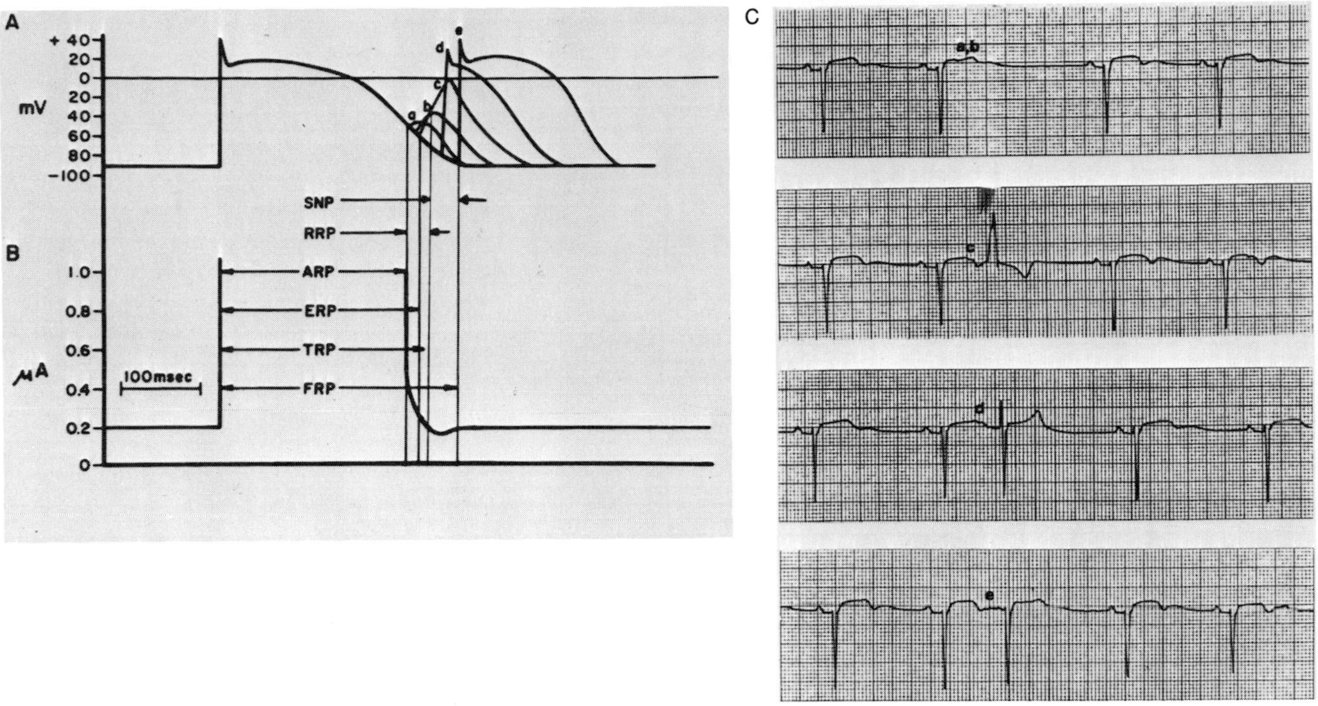

Figure 15-5. *(A) Schematic representation of a normal Purkinje fiber transmembrane action potential and of the responses elicited by premature stimulation at selected times during repolarization. The level of the threshold potential (TP) is also shown. Note that the amplitude and $\dot{V}_{max}$ of the responses are related to the level of membrane potential at stimulation. The earliest responses (a and b) arise at such low levels of membrane potential and are so small and slow rising that they cannot propagate (graded or local responses). Subsequent responses (c to e) show progressive increase in amplitude, rising velocity, and duration until completion of repolarization. The earliest propagated response (c) defines the end of the effective refractory period (ERP). The first normal response (e) defines the end of the full recovery time (FRT). Although response d arises during the end of supernormal period (SNP) of excitability, it is still smaller and rises more slowly than response e. (B) Schematic representation of the usual relationships between membrane potential and cathodal excitability. Threshold current requirements are indicated in microamperes (μA). The fiber becomes inexcitable coincident with the inscription of phase 0 of the action potential. Recovery of excitability, as indicated by changes in threshold, progresses slowly during phase 3. The diagram also illustrates the approximate duration of the absolute refractory period (ARP), effective refractory period (ERP), relative refractory period (RRP), total refractory period (TRP), full recovery time (FRT), and period of supernormal excitability (SNP). Vertical lines that connect A and B indicate the relationships between the time course of repolarization and refractoriness and excitability. Threshold potential, which becomes infinite in conjunction with rapid depolarization, is also restored to normal values during repolarization (not shown). (C) Four V_1 rhythm strips with isolated atrial premature beats initiated at different times during repolarization. The record represents an electrocardiographic "analog" of the trace in (A), atrial premature beats a, b, c, d, and e corresponding to similarly labeled responses in A. The earliest atrial premature beats (a and b) reach the AV conducting system so early during repolarization that they either do not conduct at all or else give rise to locally propagated responses that would be appreciated as a nonconducted atrial premature beat. The next two atrial premature beats (c and d) reach the conducting system somewhat later during recovery and conduct to the ventricles. However, conduction is still depressed as evidenced by the prolonged PR and altered (aberrant) QRS contour. Beat e is inscribed after completion of repolarization and conducts normally. See text for discussion.*

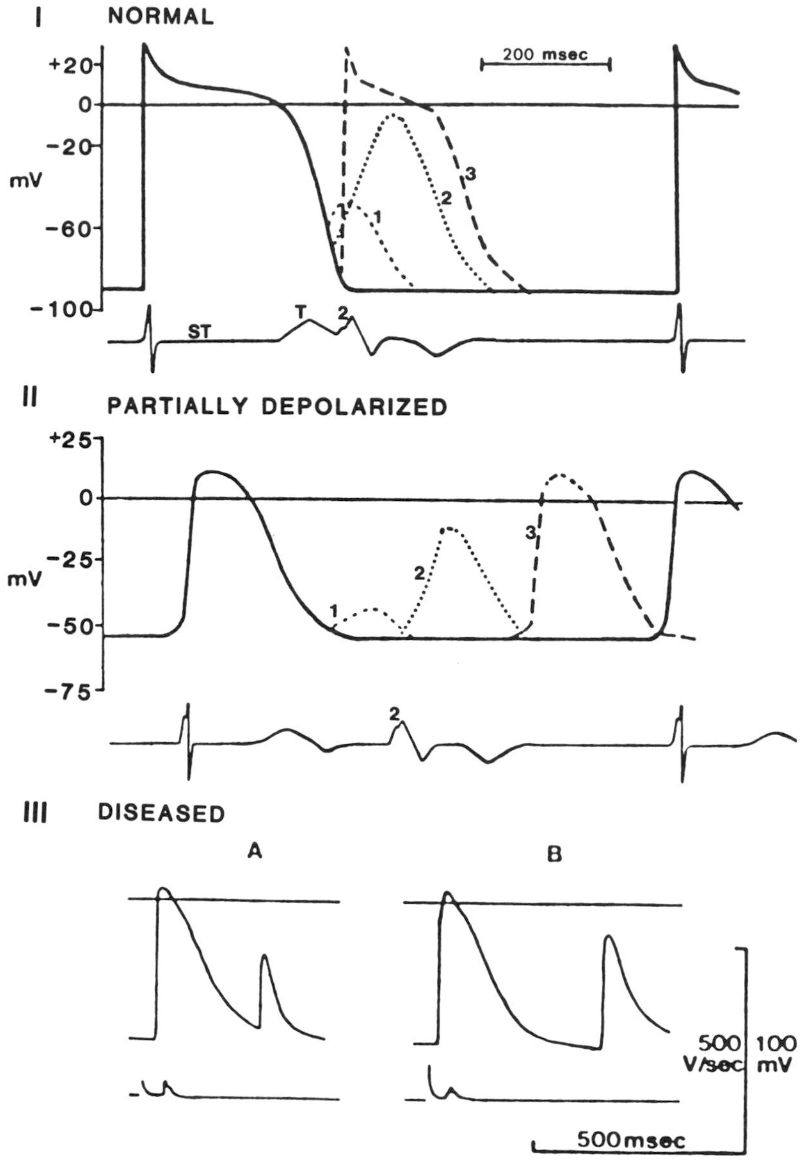

Figure 15-6. *Schematic representation of transmembrane potentials and simultaneously recorded bipolar electrograms from normal* (panel I) *and partially depolarized* (panel II) *fibers in canine right bundle branch to show time-dependent prolongation of refractoriness in the latter. Responses 1, 2, and 3 result from premature stimulation at selected times during the cycle. Response 1 is the earliest that could be elicited and defines the end of the "absolute" refractory period, 2 is the latest response to exhibit sufficient reduction in amplitude and* $\dot{V}_{max}$ *to result in an altered (aberrant) QRS contour in the electrogram, and 3 is the earliest normally configured response defining the time at which full recovery was achieved. In the normal fiber, recovery of excitability and conduction and disappearance of refractoriness virtually coincide with completion of repolarization. In the partially depolarized fiber, on the other hand, refractoriness appears to outlast repolarization, in this instance quite markedly. Time-dependent prolongation of refractoriness would increase the predisposition to aberration of even late extrasystoles.* (Panel III) *An example of postrepolarization refractoriness in a specimen of human papillary muscle obtained from a patient with chronic rheumatic heart disease complicated by congestive failure and high grade atrial and ventricular ectopy, the former with both right and left bundle branch block aberrancy. See text for discussion. (After Singer, D. H., Baumgarten, C. M., and Ten Eick, R. E.: Cellular electrophysiology of ventricular and other dysrhythmias: Studies on diseased and ischemic heart. Prog. Cardiovasc. Dis., 24:97–156, 1981)*

Two general categories can be defined. First and most common, low potential results from incomplete repolarization. Figure 15-5*A* shows a right bundle branch fiber action potential together with five premature responses initiated at different times during repolarization. The changes in action potential characteristics and conduction during repolarization, together with accompanying changes in threshold current requirements (excitability) (see Fig. 15-5*B*) and in threshold potential, comprise what is usually defined as *refractoriness.* Figure 15-5*A* shows that stimulation does not result in an active response until membrane potential has been restored to the vicinity of −50 mV. The earliest response (*a*) thus defines the end of the *absolute* refractory period and the beginning of the *relative* refractory period. The earliest responses (*a* and *b*) are, however, so small and slowly rising that they may not propagate (local or graded responses). The first propagated impulse (*c*) defines the end of the *effective* refractory period (*i.e.,* the period during which a propagated response will not occur). Amplitude $\dot{V}_{max}$, and duration of responses initiated at successively more negative levels of membrane potential increase progressively with associated improvement in conduction. An optimal response (*e*) occurs only after membrane potential is restored to −85 to −95 mV. Figure 15-5*C* shows electrocardiographic analogs.

The foregoing presumes that the recovery of excitability and conduction (*i.e.,* "functional" recovery) is strictly voltage dependent and parallels repolarization. This had been thought to be more or less true for most normal cardiac fibers except for nodal cells, in which functional recovery lags behind completion of repolarization; that is, the recovery process is time and voltage dependent.[25,30,34,61,63,64] More recent findings[136,137] indicate that this is true even for nonnodal fibers. However, the disparity is normally small, becoming appreciable only in cells with diminished levels of diastolic potential. The disparity betwen voltage and functional recovery has been termed postrepolarization refractoriness.[138]

Differences between recovery of excitability in normal and low potential fibers may be explicable in terms of differences in ionic mechanisms underlying depolarization. Depolarization of most normal fibers depends on the activitation of the fast inward Na^+ channels. Depolarization, in turn, inactivates the channels with resultant inexcitability. Removal of inactivation must occur before the channel can agan respond. By the time repolarization has progressed to about −40 to −50 mV, a sufficient number of channels have recovered to allow the cell to respond (end of the absolute refractory period). Normally, by the time the cell has repolarized to −85 to −95 mV, recovery of the fast Na^+ channels and, therefore, of excitability and conduction are virtually complete. On the other hand, as previously noted, depolarization of normally low potential fibers in the SA and AV nodes,[30,33,60–65] as well as in the AV valve leaflet and coronary sinus,[66,67] largely depend on the slow inward current. This also holds true to a variable degree for partially depolarized fibers in experimentally infarcted[30,74,75,93] and chronically diseased heart muscle.[36,78,85–87,91,92] Recovery of slow channels occurs much more slowly than does that of the fast channels, so that refractoriness may outlast completion of repolarization by up to hundreds of milliseconds. Figure 15-6*I* and *II* compares recovery in well-polarized and partially depolarized Purkinje fibers. In the well-polarized fiber, voltage and functional recovery approximate each other. In the partially depolarized fiber, on the other hand, recovery is depicted as exhibiting marked time dependency. Full functional recovery does not occur until almost mid-diastole. Under some circumstances, including exposure to certain drugs,[45,46,146–149] recovery of the fast Na^+ channels also may be slowed, so that significant postrepolarization refractoriness can occur even in well-polarized cells. Figure 15-6*III*, which shows examples of the phenomenon in a reasonably well-polarized human ventricular muscle cell, suggests that disease may exert similar effects. The changes in question would predispose to aberrant conduction of premature responses initiated during the latter stages or of repolarization as well as during diastole.

Second, membrane potential also may be reduced during electrical diastole (phase 4) due to lowering of resting potential or spontaneous diastolic depolarization of automatic cells or both. As might be predicted from the responsiveness curves in Figure 15-3*B*, reduction in diastolic potential results in changes in action potential characteristics and conduction similar to those noted during repolarization.[54,56,115] Impulse propagation in fibers with low diastolic potential could therefore be associated with slow conduction and aberrancy.

Low resting potential does not occur normally except in AV nodal cells, where it presumably contributes to slow conduction.[25,30] In contrast, low resting potential commonly occurs in experimentally infarcted hearts[74,75,93] and in diseased human heart.[76,77,87,91,92] Figure 15-7 shows examples of reduced diastolic potential and slow conduction in human ventricle. In addition, many physiologic and pharmacologic interventions to which the heart may be exposed, including stretch, ischemia, hypoxia, changes in *p*H, altered ionic milieu, and high concentrations of antiarrhythmic agents, act to lower resting potential[24,25,28–30,32,35,38–43] and cause conduction disturbances on this basis. Hyperkalemia-induced intra-atrial and intraventricular conduction disturbances represent a well-documented example.

Phase 4 depolarization of automatic cells, on the other hand, occurs even in normal heart. Automaticity of SA nodal cells is best known and may contribute to slow conduction in this tissue. Experiments on Purkinje fibers have shown that enhanced automaticity of latent pacemaker fibers can cause a broad spectrum of conduction disturbances ranging from simple slowing to complete block.[56] In addition, development of phase 4 depolarization proximal to regions of preexisting local block may further depress conduction in the latter.[150] The widespread distribution of latent pacemaker cells and the numerous environmental factors and drugs that enhance phase 4 depolarization[24,25,27–29,30,33,34,38–47] make it tempting to think that this mechanism may be a factor in human conduction disturbances. Previously alluded-to findings that ordinary myocardial cells also may become automatic (see Fig. 15-4) because of drug effects, ischemia, and disease are pertinent, since they would further predispose to conduction disturbances on this basis.

Mechanisms of Aberrancy

Aberrancy will be considered primarily in terms of impulse propagation in fibers in which membrane potential is reduced relative to normal, with the character of the disturbance being related to (1) the location of the involved cells, (2) the level of membrane potential in the path of impulse spread, and (3) the mechanism of membrane potential reduction (*i.e.*, incomplete repolarization, low resting potential, phase 4 depolarization, or combinations thereof). The effects of altered electrophysiologic properties due to disease and cardiac drugs will be considered in relation to these mechanisms.

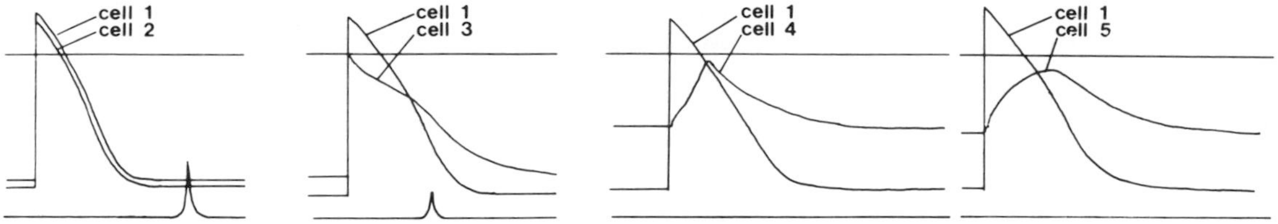

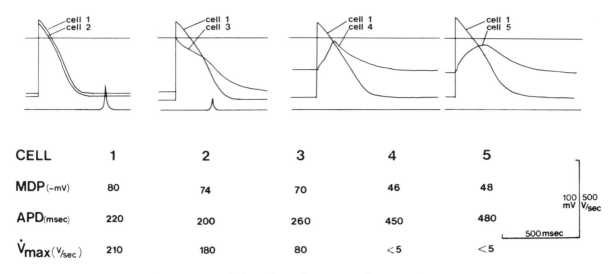

CELL	1	2	3	4	5
MDP (-mV)	80	74	70	46	48
APD (msec)	220	200	260	450	480
$\dot{V}_{max}$ (V/sec)	210	180	80	<5	<5

100 mV 500 V/sec 500 msec

Figure 15-7. *Transmembrane potentials from five cells in a papillary muscle specimen from a patient with rheumatic heart disease to show variability in diastolic potential and in action potential characteristics, together with occurrence of slow conduction and local block. Preparation was stimulated at cycle length 800 msec. Records were obtained around the margin of a small region of scar (perhaps an old microinfarct or fibrosed Aschoff body). Each panel shows simultaneous records from a well-polarized fiber (cell 1) and from one of four partially depolarized fibers (cells 2 to 5) to permit comparisons of action potential characteristics and interelectrode conduction time. $\dot{V}_{max}$ of the second cell of each pair is indicated by the differentiated spike on the bottom trace of each panel. $\dot{V}_{max}$ of cells 4 and 5 is too low to result in appreciable deflection. Values for maximum diastolic potential (MDP), action potential duration (APD) (taken as time to repolarize to −40 mV), and $\dot{V}_{max}$ of phase 0 are indicated. Note prolongation of interelectrode conduction time between cell 1 and cells 4 and 5 compared with that between cell 1 and cells 2 and 3 as evidenced by increased separation of upstrokes of responses recorded from these cells. Time and voltage calibrations are in the lower right-hand corner. See text for discussion. (After Singer, D. H., Baumgarten, C. M., and Ten Eick, R. E.: Cellular electrophysiology of ventricular and other dysrhythmias: Studies on diseased and ischemic heart. Prog. Cardiovasc. Dis., 24:97–156, 1981)*

Other possible causes of altered QRS configuration of supraventricular complexes, including impulse spread along anomalous AV communications,[3–7,139–142] disruption of the AV conducting system due to disease,[143,144] longitudinal dissociation of conduction within the AV conducting system,[151–154] asynchronous activation of the AV junction,[155] abnormalities of the "gating" mechanism of the His-Purkinje system,[156,157] impedance mismatch between fibers in different portions of the His-Purkinje system at the Purkinje–papillary muscle junction,[158] and alterations in excitability and in cable properties,[30,111–114] are outside the scope of this discussion.

Aberrancy will be classified on the basis of the cycle length dependency of the QRS changes.[21] Four major groups can be defined:

1. Short cycle aberrancy aberrancy occurring in conjunction with shortening of the cardiac cycle and increased heart rate;
2. Long cycle aberrancy aberrancy associated with prolongation of the cardiac cycle and slowed heart rate;
3. Aberrancy without significant cycle length changes
4. Mixed aberrancy

Short Cycle Aberrancy

Short cycle aberrancy, exemplified by the altered QRS contour of early supraventricular extrasystoles and of the complexes of rapid supraventricular tachyarrhythmias, is the entity for which the term was originally introduced.[1,2] Aberrancy of premature supraventricular complexes is the best known and most common form, occurring in people with clinically normal hearts as well as in those with heart disease.[3–7] The incidence of spontaneous short cycle aberrancy is not known. However, atrial pacing studies suggest that it can be induced in virtually everyone.[159–161] Aberrant complexes exhibit a right bundle branch block contour in 70% to 85% of reported clinical cases[11,162–168,179] as well as in the normal dog heart.[145,170] Left bundle branch and nonspecific intraventricular conduction defect types of aberration comprise the remainder and appear to be more common in the diseased heart, as do mixtures of the several types.

The clinical importance of short cycle aberration stems from the fact that aberrant premature supraventricular complexes, including both isolated premature complexes and bursts of tachycardia, can closely mimic isolated ventricular premature complexes and repetitive ventricular firing, including runs of ventricular tachycardia.[11,162–169,179] Aberrancy must always be considered in any differential diagnosis of wide QRS beats of undetermined type.

Figure 15-8 shows Holter monitoring records (modified V_2 surface and intra-atrial leads) obtained from a man aged 27 years with cardiomyopathy complicated by wide QRS tachycardias, which were initially suspected of being ventricular in origin in view of the left bundle branch block contour, the presence of intermediate (fusional type) complexes, and findings of clear-cut premature ventricular beats with a similar contour. The fact that the run was preceded by a supraventricular extrasystole that was normally configured despite the long preceding cycle and that the coupling interval of the latter to the preceding sinus beat differed markedly from the interval between it and the first wide QRS beat also appeared to support a possible ventricular origin for the tachycardia, as did the fact that many clear-cut supraventricular extrasystoles exhibited right bundle branch block aberrancy. Analysis of the intra-atrial lead clearly documents the supraventricular origin of the wide QRS tachycardia as well as of the aberrant beat with a right bundle branch block contour, each surface QRS complex being preceded by an atrial spike. This contrasts with the similarly configured premature ventricular beat in Fig. 15-8*II*, in which initiation of QRS precedes the atrial spike.

Numerous efforts have been made to define criteria for distinguishing between aberrant supraventricular beats from ventricular ectopic beats.[11,162–169,179] No clear-cut distinctions have as yet been found, particularly in the case of supraventricular dysrhythmias without clear-cut P waves, for example, very early atrial premature beats in which the P is superimposed on the T wave of the preceeding sinus beat, certain types of junctional rhythms, and atrial fibrillation. The latter is a particular problem. Use of esophageal or intracardiac

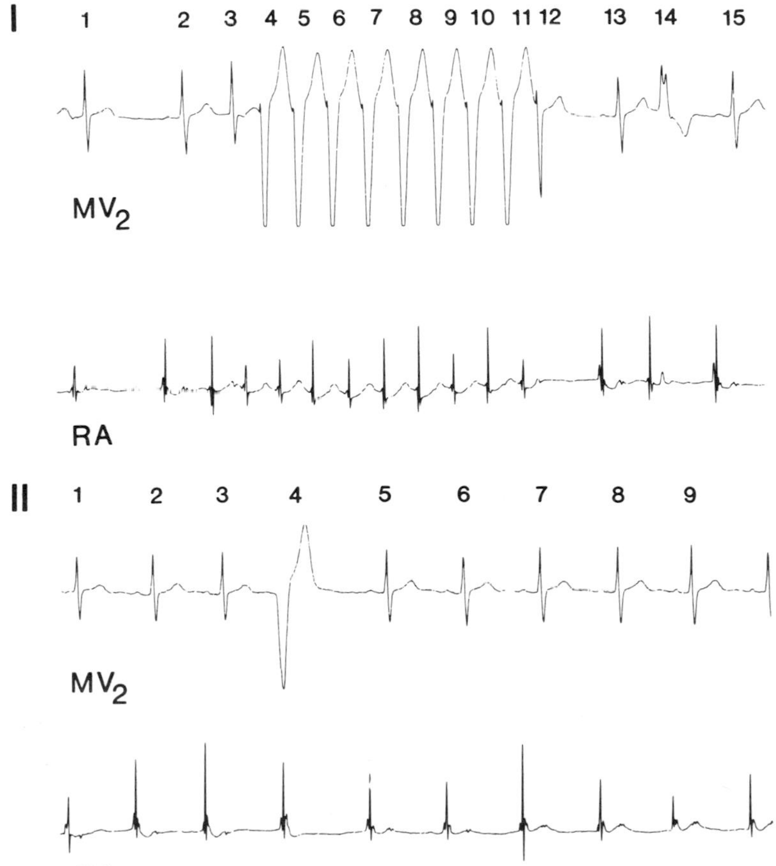

Figure 15-8. *Holter monitoring records from a man aged 27 suspected of having ventricular tachycardia in a setting of cardiomyopathy. Each panel consists of simultaneously recorded modified V_2 surface (MV_2) and intra-atrial (RA) leads.* (Panel I) *Lead MV_2 shows a nine-beat run of left bundle branch-type wide QRS tachycardia of unknown origin (beats 4 to 11) that was preceded by a normally configured supraventricular premature beat (beat 3) and terminated by an intermediate form (fusion?) beat (beat 12). Note that beat 3 did not exhibit aberrancy despite the fact that it closed a short cycle following a long cycle and that the coupling interval of the first wide QRS beat (beat 4) was shorter (0.26 second) than the interval between the last wide QRS beat and the fusional form that terminates the run (0.35 second). In addition to the beats of the tachycardia, there are also isolated premature beats exhibiting right bundle branch block (*panel I, *beat 14) and left bundle branch block (*panel II, *beat 4) configurations. The intracardiac lead shows that the wide QRS beats during the tachycardia as well as beat 14* (panel I) *were preceded by atrial deflections, thus identifying them as supraventricular with left and right bundle branch block aberration, respectively. In contrast, the onset of the QRS of left bundle branch-type beat 4* (panel II) *precedes the atrial spike, indicating a ventricular origin. See text for discussion.*

leads may be of diagnostic import in questionable cases (see Fig. 15-8).

Although some workers regard this type of aberrancy as a normal phenomenon,[174,175] others have suggested that under certain circumstances it may indicate latent conduction system disease.[11,159–161,171–173] The question is complicated by the fact that absence of clinical signs of heart disease does not necessarily preclude localized disease in a portion of the conduction system. Our own experience coincides with that of Chung,[7] namely, that occasional aberration of very early supraventricular premature complexes or of very rapid supraventricular tachycardias are physiologic. On the other hand, an unusually high incidence of aberrant beats or the occurrence of aberration at long coupling intervals, particularly of beats initiated during diastole, or at physiologic rates, are highly suggestive of underlying conduction system disease. Findings of left bundle branch block or mixed left and right bundle branch block aberrancy further increases the likelihood of underlying disease. In addition, evidence suggests an associated between short cycle aberrancy and an increased predisposition to ventricular ectopy.[176] Such an association would not be surprising from a mechanistic point of view in that impulse spread in regions of slow conduction could theoretically give rise to reentry as well as to aberrancy. High degrees of short cycle aberrancy thus might serve as a harbinger of ventricular dysrhythmia.

Electrophysiologic Mechanisms. In normal heart, short cycle aberrancy is best explained in terms of altered conduction in incompletely repolarized fibers of the His-Purkinje system, the character of the aberration being related to the location of the involved fibers and the extent to which they had repolarized by the time the impulse arrived. In general, affected fiber groups would be expected to be infra-His bundle in location, although suggestive evidence that the AV conducting system may function as a longitudinally partitioned system[151–154] could be interpreted to imply that aberrancy also may result from His bundle and possibly even AV nodal lesions.

Assume, for example, that the affected group of cells is located in the main right bundle branch. If the propagating action potential were to arrive before membrane potential were restored to about −50 mV, it might not be able to excite the cells of the right bundle branch at all, or only a local response might ensue, with resultant high-degree block in the region. The right ventricle would have to be depolarized circuitously by way of the left bundle branch, the left ventricular Purkinje system and myocardium, and, finally, the right ventricular Purkinje system and myocardium. The resultant delay in right ventricular activation would be manifest as "complete" right bundle branch block type aberrancy. If repolarization had progressed somewhat further before arrival of the impulse, conduction through the region might be slowed rather than completely blocked, and incomplete right bundle branch block aberrancy might ensue. In a similar vein, lesions in the left bundle branch system could result in left bundle branch block type conduction disturbances, and so forth. Since the rapid repolarization phase of the action potential is designated phase 3, short cycle aberrancy also has been called *phase 3 aberrancy* or *phase 3 block.*[11]

Aberrancy of Supraventricular Premature Beats

Altered QRS configuration of early supraventricular premature beats is the most common form of short cycle aberrancy. Figure 15-9 shows examples of normal and aberrantly conducted complexes in records from a woman of 43 with systemic sarcoidosis and from a man of 56 with ischemic heart disease. With one exception (see Fig. 15-9*IA*), aberrant complexes exhibit the characteristic right bundle branch block contour. Comparisons between the normally conducted and aberrant complexes demonstrate the dependence of aberration on prematurity of the complex and on the duration of the preceding cycle.[159,162–164,177,178] In general, the earlier the premature complex and the longer the preceding cycle, the more likely is aberrancy to occur and the more marked the deviation from normal. This relationship, which was described many years ago by Lewis and Master[177] and by Scherf,[178] is best exemplified by differences in QRS contour of complexes of comparable prematurity in Figure 15-9*I*. The fact that complexes *1* and *2* in Figure 15-9*IA* are aberrant whereas complex *3* exhibits a normal QRS despite its somewhat greater prematurity also is explicable in terms of differences in preceding cycle length. Beats *8* to *11* in Figure 15-9*IIC* and *D*, the most aberrant in the record, deserve comment in that at first glance they would appear to be inscribed much later than many of the nonaberrant complexes. More careful analysis shows that the complexes are, in fact, the earliest in the record but that the premature P waves are buried in the T wave of the preceding sinus complex with prolongation of PR. In a sense, PR prolongation of such early complexes may be considered aberration of AV nodal–His bundle conduction.

In Figure 15-9*I*, even the most bizarre complexes are readily identifiable as supraventricular rather than ventricular by the clear-cut preceding abnormal P waves. In Figure 15-9*II*, on the other hand, the most aberrant complexes are very difficult to distinguish from ventricular ectopic complexes, particularly during the period of bigeminy (Fig. 15-9*D*, beats *9* to *11*), the diagnosis resting on findings in the same record of other more clear-cut atrial premature complexes exhibiting intermediate degrees of aberrancy. The less than compensatory pauses

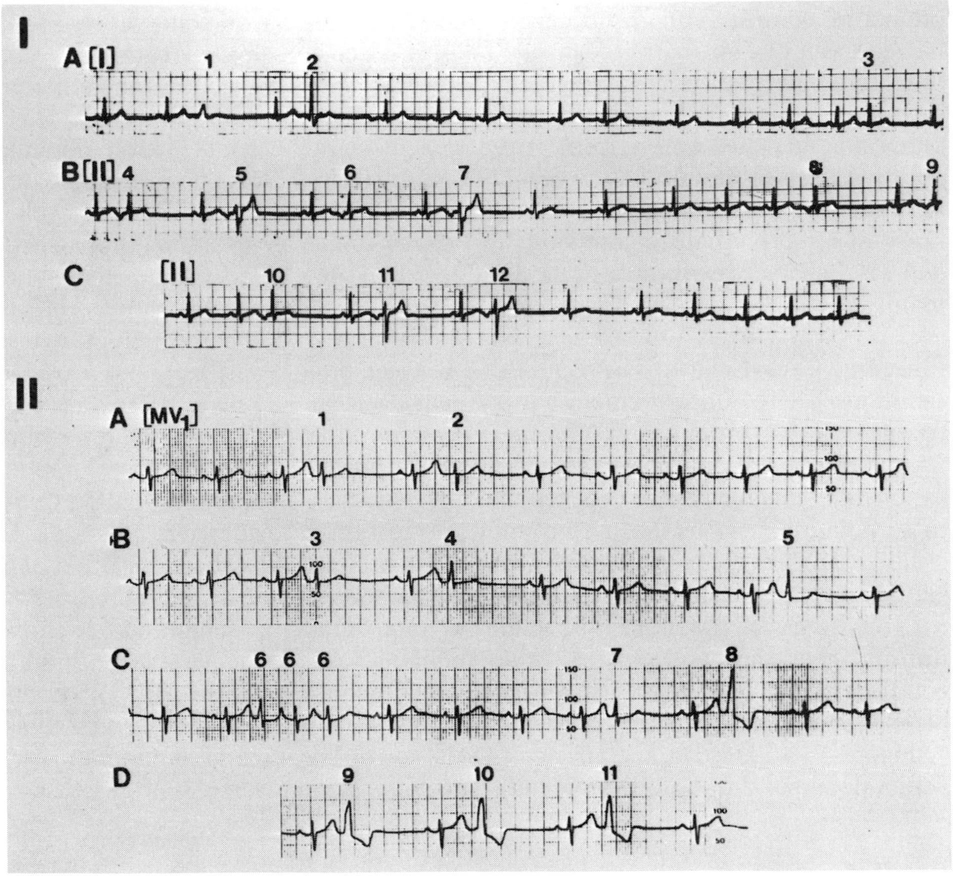

Figure 15-9. *Electrocardiographic records show varying aberrancy of atrial extrasystoles and cycle length dependence of the phenomenon.* (Panel I) *Lead I* (row A) *and lead II (*rows B *and* C*) electrocardiograms from a woman of 43 with sarcoidosis. There are 12 numbered supraventricular premature beats. Beat 1 exhibits left bundle branch block aberrancy; beats 2, 5, 7, 11, and 12, variable right bundle branch block aberrancy. The remainder of the beats are configured normally. Note the dependency of aberration on coupling interval and preceding cycle length.* (Panel II) *Modified (Holter)* V_1 *rhythm strip from a man of 54 with ischemic heart disease and high-grade atrial ectopy show the spectrum of QRS changes due to cycle length–dependent variations in short cycle aberrancy. Records contain 11 isolated atrial extrasystoles, designated by numerals 1 to 11, and a single triplet (beats 6, 6a, and 6b). Extrasystoles 2, 6a, and 6b exhibit a normal QRS contour; the remainder exhibit varying right bundle branch block aberration. In general, as was true for the records in panel I, aberration is a function of prematurity and preceding cycle length. Examination of beats 8 to 11 underscores difficulties in distinguishing between aberrant supraventricular and ventricular extrasystoles in instances in which no clear-cut ectopic P wave is discernible, due, as in this case, to superimposition on the preceding T wave or to other causes. The run of bigeminy in* row D *is particularly striking. See text for discussion.*

after the aberrant complexes also suggest a supraventricular origin.[3–7] However, this distinction is not absolute, since atrial premature complexes may give rise to fully compensatory or even longer pauses.[181–183]

Electrophysiologic Determinants

Given the relationship between membrane potential and conduction, it follows that factors that influence the level of potential encountered by the propagating premature impulse, as well as the relationship between membrane potential and $\dot{V}_{max}$, should affect the occurrence of aberrancy.

Coupling Interval. The relationship among prematurity, coupling interval, and conduction has been alluded to previously (see Fig. 15-5*A* and *C*). Other factors being equal, the earlier the complex and the shorter the coupling interval, the greater the likelihood that a given premature complex will encounter incompletely repolarized tissues in its course of spread. Thus, short coupling intervals predispose to aberrancy. However, very early premature complexes may be blocked if membrane potential has not yet repolarized to sufficiently negative levels to permit development of a regenerative response (Fig. 15-5*C*, responses *a* and *b*). Varying aberrancy of atrial premature complexes in Figures 15-5*C* and 15-7 is largely explicable in terms of degree of prematurity.

Preceding Cycle Length. The relationship between preceding cycle length and aberrancy is usually equally clear cut, at least in normal heart. With the exception of the SA and AV nodes, time course and duration of repolarization and refractoriness are a function of the frequency of stimulation.[25,145,170,184] Up to a point, decreases in cycle length shorten repolarization. Cycle length prolongation exerts the opposite effect. It follows that the longer the preceding cycle, the longer the action potential duration of the basic beat and the greater the likelihood that a complex of given prematurity will encounter incompletely repolarized fibers and conduct abnormally.

Figure 15-10*A* shows the effects of cycle length on action potential duration in a normal transitional Purkinje fiber as well as the relationships among preceding cycle length, action potential duration, and membrane potential encountered by a hypothetical complex of constant prematurity (see Fig. 15-10*B*). On the one hand, action potential duration at the longest cycle (2000 msec) is so long that the premature stimulus would occur at levels of membrane potential too low to result in a propagated response, and conduction would fail. On the other hand, action potential duration following the shortest preceding cycle (200 msec) is so short that the premature response would not be inscribed until just before or immediately following completion of repolarization and would therefore conduct normally. Action potential durations at intermediate cycles (400 msec and 630 msec) are such that the premature response would exhibit reduced amplitude and $\dot{V}_{max}$ and altered conduction. Thus, long preceding cycles predispose to aberration of premature complexes. Conversely, short preceding cycles serve to diminish aberrancy.

Figure 15-11*I* shows a transmembrane potential analog (row *A*) of the interrelationships between cycle length and QRS configuration of premature complexes (row *B*). Depressed action potential characteristics and conduction of the premature response initiated at cycle length 260 msec as compared with those at 190 msec

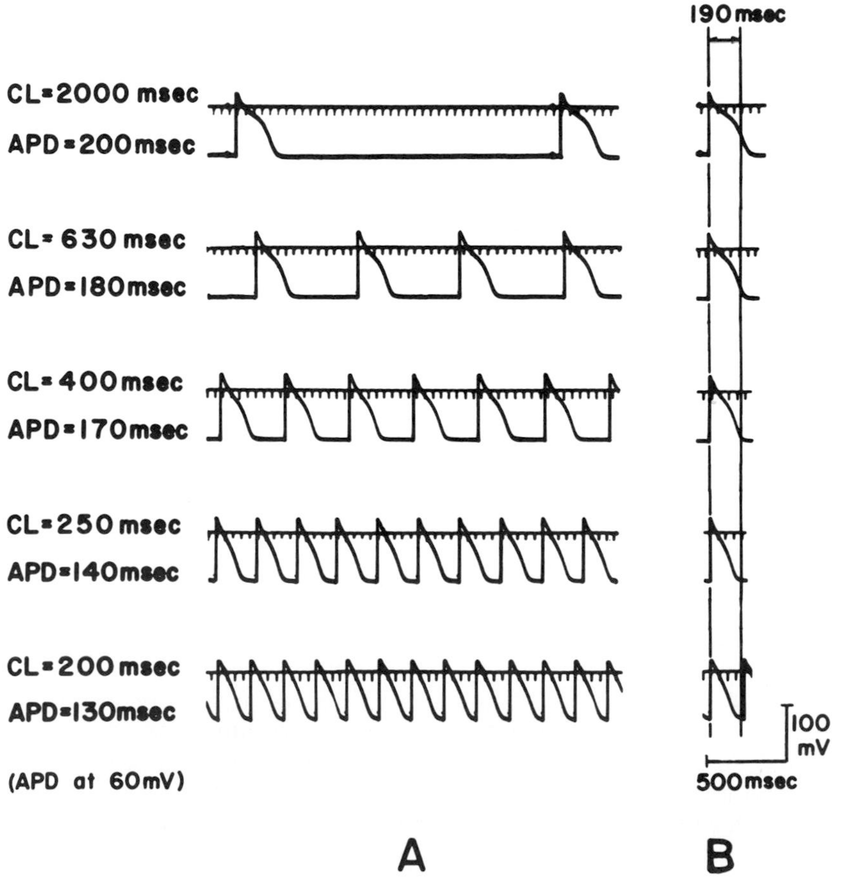

Figure 15-10. *Transmembrane potentials recorded from a normal canine Purkinje fiber show interrelationships among cycle length (CL), action potential duration (APD), and level of membrane potential encountered by a hypothetical extrasystole of constant prematurity. (A) Effects of successive abrupt rate increases frm CL 2000 to 200 msec on action potential characteristics, including APD. The CL at which the preparation was stimulated and APD, measured as the time required to repolarize to −60 mV, are indicated in milliseconds. Note progressive shortening of APD with increases in rate. (B) Normal relationships between preceding CL and membrane potential encountered by premature response. A representative action potential at each rate is shown. The upstrokes are aligned to allow better comparisons of APD. A vertical line is drawn to show level of membrane potential that would be encountered by an extrasystole having a constant coupling interval of 190 msec. Time lines are 50 msec apart. Time and voltage calibrations are in the lower right-hand corner. See text for discussion. (After Singer, D. H., and Ten Eick, R. E.: Aberrancy: Electrophysiologic aspects. Am. J. Cardiol., 28:381–401, 1971)*

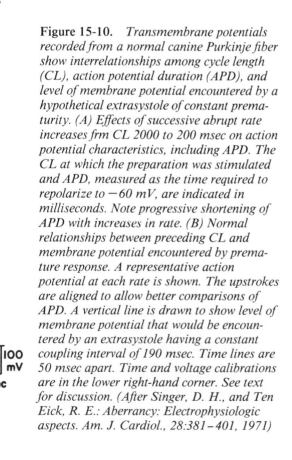

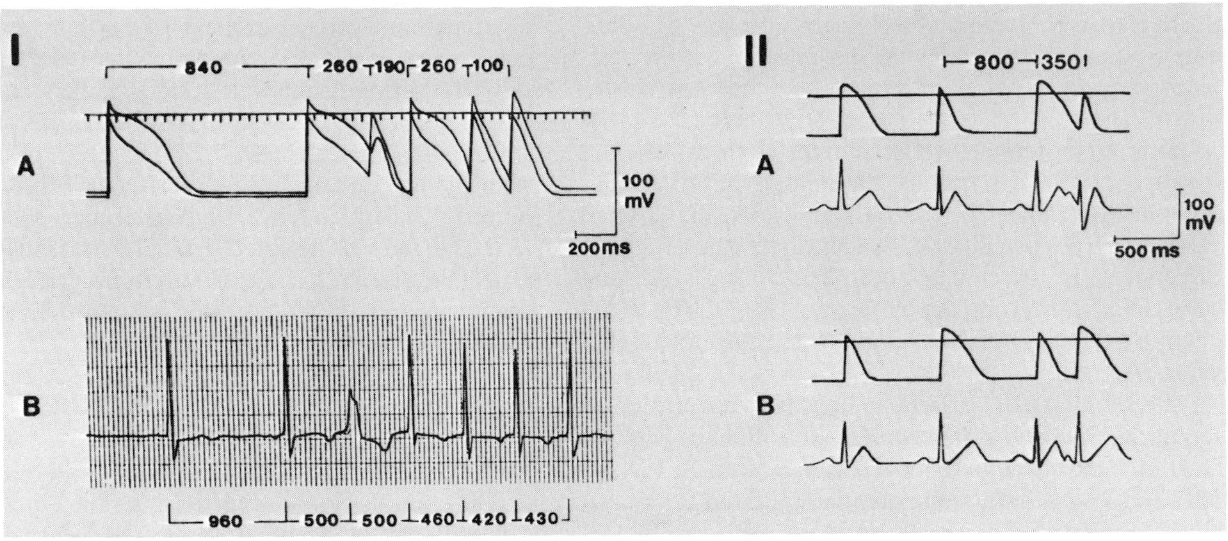

Figure 15-11. (Panel I) *Transmembrane potentials simultaneously recorded from two sites in a Purkinje fiber* (row A) *and rhythm strip from a man of 42 with high-grade atrial ectopy and short cycle right bundle branch block aberrancy* (row B) *to illustrate further the normal interrelationships among coupling interval, preceding cycle length, and conduction of premature beats. The interval between beats is indicated in milliseconds. Time and voltage calibrations for transmembrane potentials are on the lower right of each panel.* (Row A) *Effects of premature stimulation on Purkinje fiber action potential characteristics, representing a transmembrane potential analog of the cycle length-dependent changes in QRS configuration of supraventricular premature beats in* Row B. (Panel II) *Schematic surface electrocardiographic rhythm strip shows atrial extrasystoles (*rows A *and* B, *bottom trace, fourth beat) that appear to exhibit alterations in the usual relationships between QRS contour, coupling interval, and preceding cycle length. Despite identical coupling and preceding RR intervals, the extrasystole in* row A *is inscribed before completion of repolarization and is aberrant, whereas the one in* row B *occurs after repolarization is over and conducts normally. The top trace shows transmembrane potentials recorded from a specimen of diseased human papillary muscle that seek to explain the phenomenon in terms of spontaneous alteration of action potential duration of the basic beats. Associated alternation in the QT interval, if any, of the surface electrocardiogram would provide the only real clue to the nature of the electrophysiologic mechanisms in such instances. See text for discussion.*

(row *A*) are due to the longer preceding cycle, as is the more aberrant QRS contour of complexes initiated at cycle length 500 msec as compared with those initiated at cycle length 420 to 460 msec (row *B*). Figure 15-11*IA* also depicts how identically coupled premature responses may differ in amplitude, $\dot{V}_{max}$, and conduction because of differences in preceding cycle length. Compare the first and third premature responses in Figure 15-11*A*, both initiated at a coupling interval of 260 msec. Diminished amplitude and $\dot{V}_{max}$ and depressed conduction of the first response are attributable to the longer preceding cycle. Differences in QRS contour between the two complexes initiated at a coupling interval of 500 msec (row *B*) are similarly explicable. The records also show how differences in preceding cycle length can explain why even very early premature complexes sometimes conduct more normally than those with longer coupling intervals.

Exceptions to the preceding cycle length rule do, however, occur,[179,180] particularly in diseased heart and in hearts exposed to selected pharmacologic agents, including the standard antiarrhythmic agents. In part, this may reflect diminished cycle length dependence of action potential duration and of refractoriness, which has been observed *in vitro* in tissues from animal models of ischemia[74,75] and from human heart[21,87] as well as clinically.[161,180] Spontaneous variation in action potential duration at constant cycle lengths, which also has been observed in human heart muscle, represents an additional possible factor. Figure 15-11*II* shows schematic representation of two atrial premature complexes. Despite identical coupling and preceding RR intervals, the two complexes differ, the one in row *A* exhibiting an aberrant, and the one in row *B* a normal, QRS complex. Transmembrane potentials from a human ventricular muscle fiber located above each electrocardiographic sequence seek to explain the changes in terms of differences in preceding cycle length due to spontaneous alternation of action potential duration.

Membrane Potential, Action Potential Duration, and Refractoriness. Numerous physiologic interventions and pharmacologic agents to which the heart is exposed influence (*i.e.,* usually lower) diastolic potential either directly or, in the case of automatic cells, by affecting spontaneous diastolic depolarization.[25,29,30,32,33,38–47] Ischemia[74,75,93] and disease[76,87,91,92] also may lower diastolic potential.

The significance of these findings is that duration of repolarization and refractoriness are influenced by the level of membrane potential. It can be seen in Figures 15-7 and 15-14 that action potentials initiated at reduced levels of membrane potential are characterized by shortening of the early stages of repolarization (phase 2 and early phase 3). The terminal stage of phase 3, on the other hand, is relatively prolonged. This could affect conduction of premature responses in at least two ways. Shortening of phase 2 and early phase 3 might be expected to decrease the number of premature impulses that block completely. Prolongation of the terminal portion of phase 3 would increase the likelihood of any propagated premature response encountering incompletely repolarized fibers in its path of spread. Both would predispose to an overall increase in short cycle aberrancy. Prolongation of phase 3 would particularly favor development of aberrancy at longer than normal coupling intervals.

As previously noted, the level of membrane potential influences refractoriness and conduction in still other ways that might be expected to predispose to conduction disturbances and aberrancy in conjunction with premature stimulation. Development of automaticity and slow conduction in low potential cells represents one such mechanism. Prolongation of refractoriness beyond voltage recovery, and alterations in the normal cycle length dependence of action potential duration, also occur. These will be considered in relation to disease, since, except for nodal cells and possibly also cells in the AV valve leaflets and the vicinity of the coronary sinus, low diastolic potential is not seen normally.

Changes in Diseased Heart. Ischemia[30,74,75,93,187] and other experimental[186] and spontaneous[36] disease states[73–92] appear to influence profoundly the time course of repolarization and refractoriness, both directly and by reducing diastolic potential. Aside from the early stages of ischemia during which repolarization shortens, these conditions are generally associated with prolonged repolarization and refractoriness.

In part, the observed changes reflect previously alluded to findings that specimens of experimentally infarcted animal heart and spontaneously diseased human heart contain large numbers of partially depolarized cells, many of which exhibit slow response characteristics. In addition, some well-polarized fibers in such specimens appear to exhibit similar-type changes in repolarization and refractoriness.[74,83,84,87] The extent to which such changes occur in well-polarized cells is not known. However, given the vast preponderance of well-polarized cells in even diseased heart, the potential implication of the observed changes with respect to the increased frequency and altered patterns of aberration in patients with heart disease may be considerable.

Duration of Repolarization. Figure 15-7 shows records from five deep intramural cells in a papillary muscle from a patient with short cycle right bundle branch block and left bundle branch type of aberrancy in a setting of rheumatic heart disease complicated by atrial and ventricular ectopy. In contast to normal, there is considerable local variability in both diastolic potential and action potential characteristics, including, $\dot{V}_{max}$, and time course of repolarization, as well as high-grade local block. In particular, note the marked prolongation of terminal phase 3 in the partially depolarized fibers. Figure 15-14 shows similar findings. Prolongation of repolarization may be even further accentuated by early afterdepolarization type of oscillatory activity,[12–15,70–72] increases of up to many seconds having been observed.[74,83,84,87] Figure 15-4*II* shows examples in human ventricular muscle cell.

"Postrepolarization Refractoriness" and Altered Responsiveness. Partially depolarized and well-polarized fibers in infarcted dog ventricle[74,75,138,185,187] and diseased human ventricle[21,36,80,82–84,87] also may exhibit postrepolarization refractoriness and alterations in responsiveness of the type depicted by the curve for cell *b* in Figure 15-3*B*.

Figure 15-6*III* shows postrepolarization refractoriness in a slightly depolarized human ventricular muscle fiber (resting potential −70 mV). In Figure 15-6*IIIA,* note that stimulation just before the end of repolarization results in a deteriorated response even though the level of potential had been restored to nearly resting levels. In Figure 15-6*IIIB,* a second and much later response, initiated after completion of repolarization, still exhibited marked reduction in amplitude and in $\dot{V}_{max}$ at a time when full recovery should have been achieved. Similar changes in the postextrasystolic beats in Figure 15-12 are even more striking, given the long lapse (approximately 570 to 580 msec) between premature and post-extrasystolic beats. The fact that the cell in question also was only very slightly depolarized (−78 mV) shows that the phenomenon is not confined to low-potential, slow-response cells. The membrane mechanisms underlying this phenomenon are not yet defined for well-po-

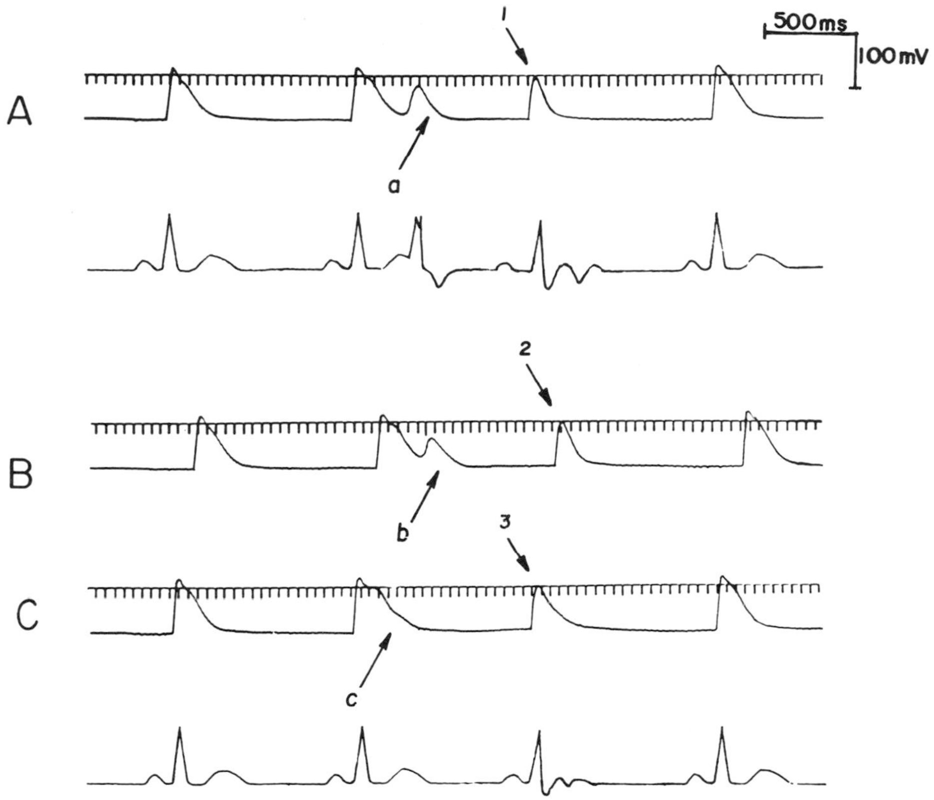

Figure 15-12. *Transmembrane potentials from human papillary muscle or transitional Purkinje fiber in specimen from patient with chronic rheumatic heart disease, together with schematic surface electrocardiogram to show how nonpropagated premature responses could result in aberration of the postectopic beat even in the absence of cycle length changes of the basic beats. The preparation was regularly stimulated at cycle length 1000 msec (60 beats/min). (*Panels A *to* C*) The basic beats were interrupted by three spontaneous early premature responses (a, b, and c). Premature response a was initiated sufficiently late to result in a propagated extrasystole, which is depicted as exhibiting typical short cycle aberrancy. Premature impulse c, on the other hand, occurred so early that only a small, nonpropagated, local (concealed) response ensued. The same was probably true of b. Note that postextrasystole beats 1, 2, and 3 exhibit marked diminution in amplitude and* $\dot{V}_{max}$ *as compared with the other basic beats, changes that could result in aberrancy. In the case of postextrasystolic beat 3, aberration would be perceived as occurring in the absence of perceptible changes in cycle length, since preceding nonpropagated local response c would not be noted electrocardiographically. Beats 1, 2, and 3 also exhibited variable alterations in time course of repolarization, which would be appreciated as postectopic T wave changes. Gross changes in amplitude and* $\dot{V}_{max}$ *did not persist beyond the first postextrasystolic beat. Changes in repolarization, on the other hand, persisted for several beats. Time marks are 50 msec apart. Time and voltage calibrations are shown on bottom right. See text for discussion. (After Singer, D. H., and Ten Eick, R. E.: Aberrancy: Electrophysiologic aspects. Am. J. Cardiol., 28:381–401, 1971)*

larized cells but may reflect, at least in part, delayed recovery of inward Na^+ channels from depolarization-induced inactivation.

The effects of the alterations in responsiveness are more complex, involving displacement of the curve down and to the right in the mid-range of potential and up and to the left at low levels of potential (see Fig. 15-3*B*). The rightward displacement results in increased generation of slowly conducting (aberrant) responses at more negative levels of potential and, therefore, later during the cycle, than normally. The leftward displacement at the low end of the range, on the other hand,

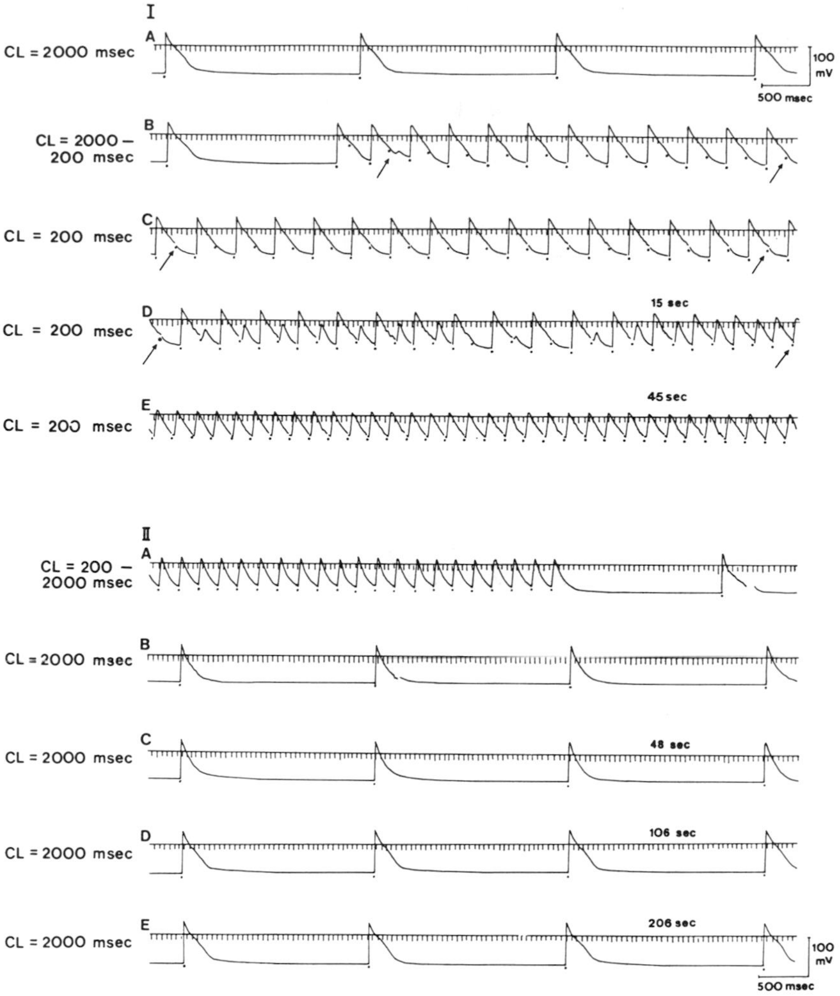

Figure 15-13. *Transmembrane potentials from well-polarized human ventricular muscle fiber in a specimen of left ventricular free wall from a patient with ventricular aneurysm to show altered cycle length (CL) dependence of action potential duration (APD) and increased time requirements to achieve new steady-state duration following rate changes.* Panel I *shows effects of an abrupt rate increase.* (Row A) *Records during stimulation at CL 2000 msec (30 beats/min). (*Rows B *to* D*): Continuous record just before and after an abrupt increase in stimulation frequency to CL 200 msec (300 beats/min). Stimulus artifacts (designated by* dots*). Initially, except for one local response (first* arrow, row B*), capture occurred with every other stimulus. Arrows at end of* row B, *the beginning and end of* row C, *and the beginning of* row D *indicate representative ineffective stimuli. Shortening of APD necessary to achieve a 1:1 response did not occur until 15 second after the rate increase (*Row D, *end). Note initial alternation of large and small responses due to differences in membrane potential at excitation. Variability persisted until APD shortened sufficiently to permit excitation of successive beats to occur at the same level of potential* (Row E). *Achieval of a new steady state required an additional 30 second for a total of 45 second (190 complexes). Also note more pronounced decrease in rising velocity of the action potential upstroke ($\dot{V}_{max}$) at CL 200 msec than in fiber from normal dog ventricle (see Fig. 15-10).* Panel II *shows effect of subsequent decrease in the frequency of stimulation back to CL 2000 msec (30 beats/min). Records in* row A *were obtained very shortly after those in* panel I, row E *and show steady-state action potentials at CL 200 msec as well as the first beat following the rate decrease. Records in* rows A *and* B *are continuous; those in* rows C *to* E *were obtained 48, 106, and 206 second, respectively, after the rate decrease. Comparisons with* panel I, row A *show that action potentials did not return to their control configuration until 206 second (103 beats) after rate decrease. Time and voltage calibrations are shown at top and bottom right. Time lines are 50 msec apart. See text for discussion.*

might increase aberration during very early recovery by facilitating generation of slowly conducting responses at potentials ordinarily too low to support any activity at all.

Altered Cycle Length Dependence of Action Potential Duration. Also pertinent are findings that the usual relationships between cycle length and action potential duration need not necessarily hold for partially depolarized or well-polarized fibers in experimentally infarcted dog ventricle[70,71,74,75] and in human heart muscle.[21,36,77,80–84,87] Some fibers may exhibit a qualitatively normal relationship, but the degree of shortening may be less than normal and may take longer to accomplish (Fig. 15-13). In other fibers, action potential duration may not change significantly with changes in cycle length, while in still others it may change contrary to normal (Fig. 15-14). Sometimes, spontaneous beat-to-beat changes in duration occur even in the absence of cycle length changes (see Fig. 15-11*II*).

Implications With Respect to Incidence and Patterns of Aberrancy of Supraventricular Extrasystoles in Diseased Heart. The foregoing changes, alone or in combination, in critical regions of the His-Purkinje system would be expected to predispose to an overall increase in aberrant conduction of premature beats, particularly those initiated during the terminal phase of repolarization and electrical diastole. They also would favor altered patterns of aberrancy. For example, to the extent that disease affects the left ventricle more than the right, the changes would favor an increase in left bundle branch block and mixed type aberrancy in diseased as compared to normal hearts. In addition, these changes might alter the usual relationships between preceding cycle length and development of aberrancy so as to make the latter much less predictable than normal and therefore more difficult to distinguish from ventricular ectopy.

The foregoing would appear to correlate well with findings in patients with organic heart disease studied by atrial pacing and His bundle recording techniques because refractory periods were found not to change, and even to increase, with increases in rate. In addition, aberrancy was largely of the left bundle branch block or mixed variety, and its development appeared unrelated to preceding cycle length.[161,179,180] Finally, insofar as disease-related changes are nonuniform,[75,80,82,87] they

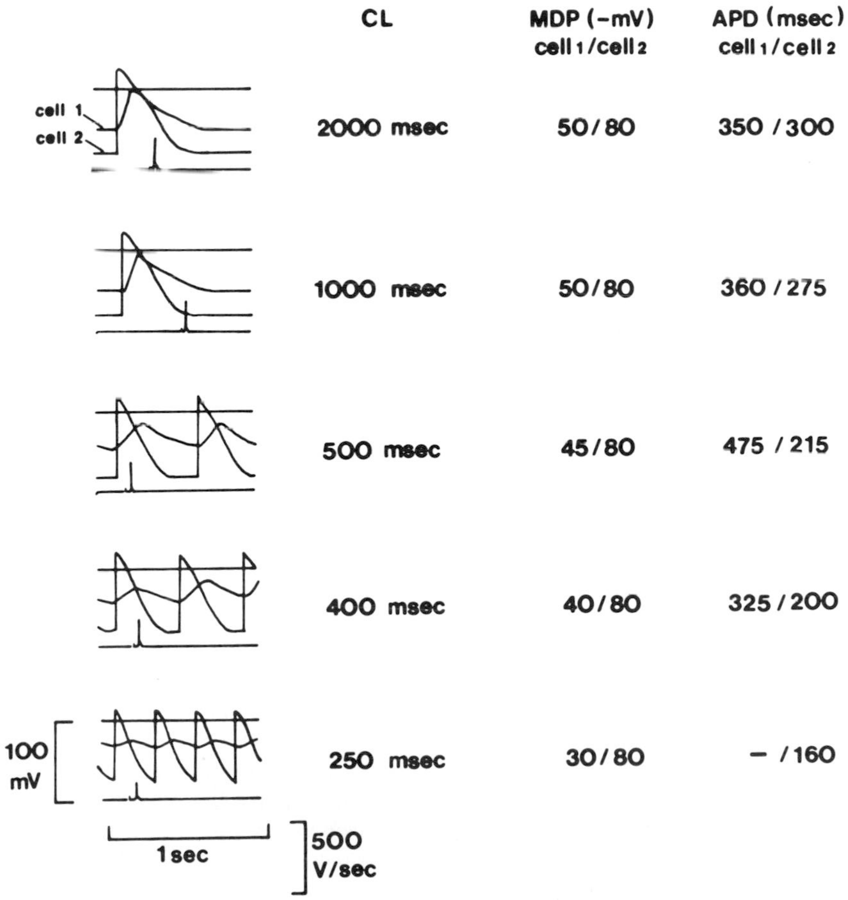

Figure 15-14. *Transmembrane potentials from well-polarized (cell 2) and partially depolarized (cell 1) fibers, in specimen of human papillary muscle from patient with severe rheumatic heart disease, to show cycle length (CL)–dependent changes in action potential characteristics, including amplitude,* $\dot{V}_{max}$, *and time course of repolarization and duration (APD). CL of stimulation, maximum diastolic potential (MDP), and APD (75% repolarization) are indicated. Amplitude of differentiated spike on bottom trace of each panel is measure of* $\dot{V}_{max}$ *of cell 2. Note that whereas APD of the well-polarized fiber decreases rapidly as rate is increased, that of the depolarized cell not only does not decrease significantly but actually increases, with the result that action potentials begin to impinge on each other at much lower rates than normally (CL = 1000 msec 60 beats/min as opposed to a CL = 250 msec [240 beats/min]). Progressive decrease in MDP and in action potential amplitude and* $\dot{V}_{max}$, *as well as progressive slowing of conduction, ensues. The fact that cell 2 is actually not entirely normal despite reasonable levels of diastolic potential is suggested by the progressive reduction in* $\dot{V}_{max}$ *with increase in rate in the absence of changes in MDP. See text for discussion.*

would increase electrical inhomogeneity and predispose to fragmentation of excitation and reentry and thus provide an additional basis for the association between aberrancy and dysrhythmia.

Characteristics of the His-Purkinje System. The electrophysiologic characteristics of the His-Purkinje system represent an additional important determinant of short cycle aberrancy. The likelihood that a supraventricular premature impulse will traverse incompletely repolarized fibers and conduct aberrantly is facilitated by the progressive increase in action potential duration between the proximal portion of the bundle of His and the peripheral Purkinje fibers (see Fig. 15-1*B*).[17,25,145,156,188] As a result, early premature impulses entering the His-Purkinje system from the AV node are likely to encounter progressively less polarized fibers during the course of distal spread, with resultant deterioration of the propagating action potential and development of conduction abnormalities. It is actually surprising that aberration does not occur more frequently than it does even in the normal heart. Presumably, many impulses that might conduct aberrantly undergo complete decrement and block as they propagate into successively less polarized regions.[17,18,145,188,189]

The predominance of right bundle branch block type aberration has been pointed out. A number of explanations have been offered.[11,170,188,190–192] Rosenbaum and co-workers[11] attributed it to the greater length of the right bundle branch. They postulated that although an early supraventricular premature complex might conduct at equal speeds in both left and right bundle branches, the greater length of the latter could result in delayed activation of the right ventricle. Peculiarities in anatomy of the right bundle branch that may render it unusually susceptible to the effects of stretch in conjunction with right ventricular dilation have also been implicated. Most investigators have, however, interpreted the findings as reflecting differences in repolarization and refractoriness between the two sides. Experimental findings have been controversial, with some workers failing to find consistent differences between the right and left sides at comparable levels.[188–191] However, the weight of recent evidence from *in vitro* studies on the dog His-Purkinje system,[156,157,192,193] as well from studies on the *in situ* dog heart,[170] and clinical electrophysiologic studies[161] indicate that the duration of repolarization and refractoriness is, in fact, somewhat longer on the right. Findings in some of the same studies[156] that action potential duration was sometimes longer on the left than on the right and that sometimes no consistent differences could be found between the two sides could explain the occasional occurrence of left bundle branch block type and mixed type aberrancy in the normal heart.

Reasons for the increase in left bundle branch block type and mixed types of aberrancy in patients with organic heart disease are, however, not yet entirely defined. One possible explanation may be found in the relatively greater involvement of the left ventricle by disease states that may lower diastolic potential and cause electrophysiologic changes that characterize depressed fibers to develop. To the extent that these processes prolong action potential duration or refractoriness of one or more portions of the left-sided conduction system beyond those on the right, they would serve to increase left bundle branch block and mixed type aberrancy.

The question of the possible site(s) at which functional conduction disturbances responsible for aberrancy occur also has been extensively studied. Theoretically, block could occur anywhere in the conducting system proximal to or at the site of maximum action potential duration in the peripheral Purkinje fibers (see Fig. 15-1*B*). Most workers have implicated the bundle branches proper and their principal proximal subdivisions.[11,17,145,170,190–195] Others, including Lewis[1,2] and, more recently, Myerburg and co-workers,[156,157] suggested that the block was peripheral. Findings that an incision into the right ventricular muscle mass can result in a right bundle branch block pattern[196] also support a peripheral site of block, since such lesions presumably damage the subendocardial Purkinje net. Still others,[160] on the basis of findings by Moore and co-workers[197] that lesions in the proximal and distal portions of the right bundle branch system give rise to complete and incomplete right bundle branch block patterns, respectively, have postulated two or more sites of block.

The concept, first proposed by Kaufman and Rothberger in 1913[151] and subsequently expanded by Scherf and James,[152] that the AV conducting system exhibits functional longitudinal dissociation, so that, for example, individual fiber bundles in the His bundle and possibly even the AV node communicate with specific portions of the right bundle branch system and others with the left bundle branch system, complicates the matter still further, since it implies that AV nodal or His bundle lesions may result in intraventricular conduction disturbances. Electrophysiologic findings suggesting the existence of dual AV nodal conduction paths in both the dog[153] and in humans[198] are pertinent, as are findings that His bundle lesions as well as electrical stimulation of the His bundle may sometimes result in electrocardiographic patterns typical of bundle branch block or fascicular block or both.[199–203] Observations in humans by Narula[154] and by El-Sherif and co-workers[204] that distal His bundle stimulation resulted in abolition of various types of preexisting intraventricular conduction defects also are supportive. Histologic studies of the His bundle[205] showing separation of the longitudinally arranged cells by poorly conducting fibrous septa with only sparse transverse connections provide a possible anatomic basis for this phenomenon. However, counterarguments based on *in vitro* electrophysiologic studies to the effect that the transverse connections, sparse though they may be, are nevertheless adequate to ensure uniform activation of the AV conducting system under normal conditions, have been presented.[200] It may be inferred from these that the occurrence of dissociation should be principally confined to instances in which the connections are damaged or destroyed by disease or environmental changes to which the diseased heart may be exposed. The preponderance of reported cases of longitudinal dissociation in patients with overt heart disease[154,200] accords with this view.

Distinctions with respect to specific sites of block and specific mechanisms of block may, however, be illusory. Considering the numerous variables that influence conduction and the extent to which they, in turn, may be affected by local environmental factors, it would not be surprising if the site, and possibly even the mechanism(s), of block varied with changing conditions.

Aberrancy of Supraventricular Tachycardias

Alterations in QRS contour during supraventricular tachyarrhythmias constitute the second major type of short cycle aberrancy. Normally, it is much less common than is aberrancy of isolated supraventricular premature beats. It also is predominantly right bundle branch block in character. Left bundle branch block, nonspecific, and multiform aberrancy, on the other hand, appear common in patients with underlying heart or conduction system disease. Aberrancy may be confined to only a few beats of a tachycardia, usually but not always the initial beats, or it may persist until the rate decreases again. Variations in the degree of aberrancy during a bout of tachycardia also occur, as do differences in the rates at which QRS changes appear and disappear.[161,179,180,207] Variable, usually minor, degrees of aberration may sometimes persist for brief periods after the rate has slowed. This, too, appears more common in patients with overt heart or conduction system disease than in those with clinically normal hearts. Aberration also occurs at lower rates and with lesser degrees of cycle length shortening in the former and may eventually appear even at normal rates and with only minimal shortening.[6,179]

Figure 15-15*A* and *B* shows examples of atrial tachycardia, at 150 to 180 beats/min, from two patients, aged 19 and 51, respectively, with a history of paroxysmal rapid heart action but without other evidence of heart disease. Despite the rapid rates, the first patient did not develop aberrancy. In the second patient, the initial six beats exhibited right bundle branch type of aberration. Subsequent beats were normally configured. Records in Figure 15-15*C* and *D* were obtained from patients with coronary artery disease and show aberrancy at successively lower rates, 90 beats/min and 60 beats/min, and with minimal cycle length shortening. In Figure 15-15*D*, aberrancy is of the left bundle branch block type. Figure 15-16 shows records from a woman aged 35 with a history of paroxysmal atrial tachyarrhythmias in a setting of rheumatic heart disease. The electrocardiograms in Figure 15-16*A* were obtained during a bout of atrial tachycardia at a rate of 140 beats/min. Despite the fact that the rate of the tachycardia was slower than those shown in Figure 15-15*A* and *B*, note that all the complexes exhibit right bundle branch block aberrancy. Restoration of sinus rhythm usually resulted in normalization of intraventricular conduction. However, sometimes minor degrees of aberration persisted for brief intervals following restoration of sinus rhythm (Fig. 15-16*B*).

The Holter monitor records in Figure 15-17, which were obtained from the same patient as those in Figure 15-8, show the wide variation in the rates at which aberrancy can occur in the same person during a 24-hour period. Aberrancy is left bundle branch block in type. Figure 15-17*A* shows an 18-beat burst of rapid (185 beats/min) paroxysmal supraventricular tachycardia (beats *3* to *18*), of which the first seven beats (beats *3* to *7*) exhibit varying left bundle branch block type of aberrancy and the last nine beats exhibit normal IV conduction even though the rate is substantially unchanged. In Figure 15-17*B*, development of aberrancy by two premature atrial beats (beats *3* and *4*) occurs at coupling intervals (0.64 to 0.68 second) equivalent to rates of 90 to 95 beats/min. In the same figure, aberration occurs at still longer intervals (0.76 to 0.80 second, rates = 75 beats/min) and in conjunction with only minimal shortening of the sinus cycle. In Figure 15-17*A* also note differences in coupling intervals at which aberrancy appears (0.44 second) and disappears (0.32 second). At other times during the same day, the patient also exhibited right bundle branch aberrancy (see Fig. 15-8).

Electrophysiologic Determinants

Aberration during supraventricular tachyarrhythmias is explicable on the same basis as for isolated premature beats, namely, conduction in incompletely repolarized fibers. The likelihood that a given rate increase will result in aberrancy as well as the magnitude and duration of the conduction disturbance depend on a number of interrelated factors, including (1) the nature of the relationship between cycle length and action potential duration and refractoriness, (2) the magnitude and abruptness of the rate change, and (3) the characteristics of the His-Purkinje system.

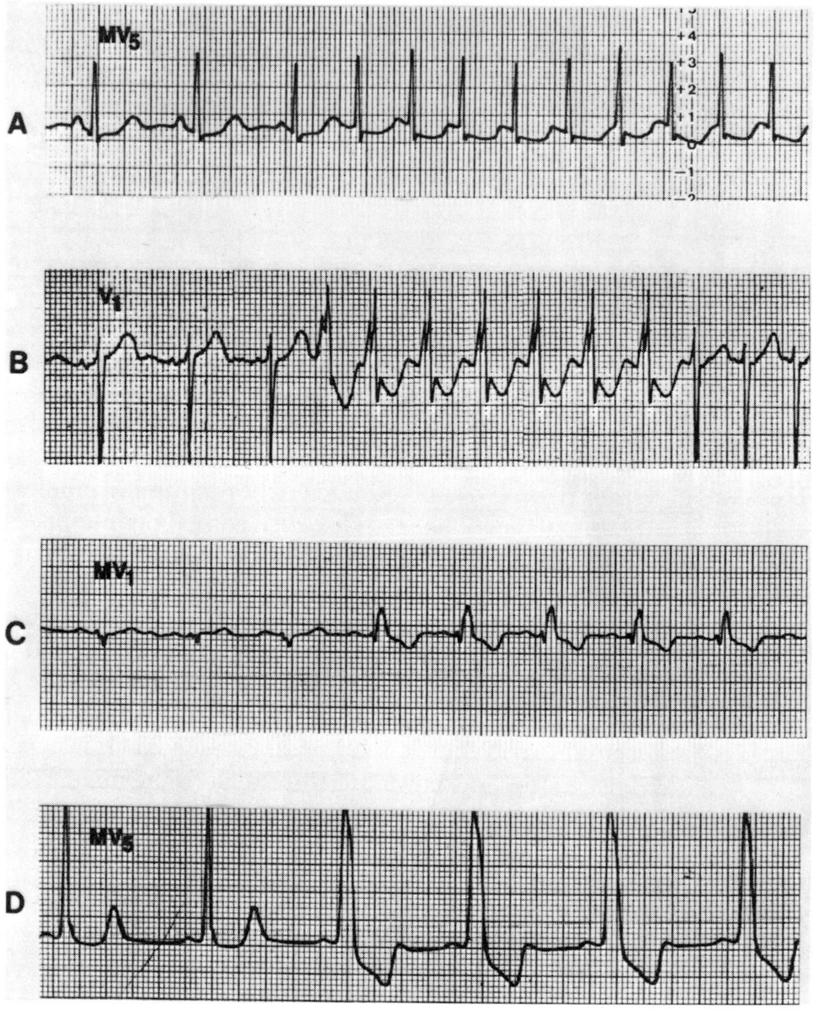

Figure 15-15. *Rhythm strips from four patients showing predisposition for aberration to occur at lower rates and with lesser degrees of cycle length shortening in patients with overt heart–conduction system disease than in those with clinically normal hearts. Eventually aberration may appear even at more or less normal rates and with minimal or imperceptible cycle length shortening. The latter is generally associated with left bundle branch block, as opposed to right bundle branch block, aberrancy. See text for discussion.*

Cycle Length Dependence of Action Potential Duration. Possible relationships between cycle length dependence of action potential duration and aberrancy of supraventricular premature complexes have been previously described. Aberration of the initial one or two beats of a supraventricular tachycardia is readily explicable on the same basis as that for premature complexes. Perpetuation of aberration for sustained periods, on the other hand, is more difficult to explain, since increases in rate are normally associated with progressive shortening of the action potential. However, the extent to which action potential duration can shorten is limited. As rate increases beyond a certain limit, shortening becomes progressively less effective in compensating for the decrease in diastole. Initiation of new action potentials before completion of the previous repolarization eventually ensues, with resultant reduction in amplitude and $\dot{V}_{max}$ and development of both intermittent and sustained conduction abnormalities, including aberrancy.

The cycle length at which action potentials begin to impinge on each other and exhibit changes associated with development of conduction disturbances varies. With the notable exceptions of SA and AV nodes,[25,30,63,64] increases to quite high rates are usually required before significant deterioration of the action potential and depression of conduction occurs normally. Figure 15-10 demonstrates the effects of step-wise rate increases on action potential duration in a normal Purkinje fiber. An increase in the frequency of stimulation from 30 to 300 beats/min was required for demonstrable diminution in action potential amplitude and rising velocity. Even at this rate the changes were still quite minimal and would not be expected to give rise to significant aberration.

The normally pronounced cycle length–dependent shortening of action potential duration makes it necessary to invoke mechanisms other than simple initiation of aberrant beats before completion of repolarization of the preceding beat in the involved region to explain perpetuation of aberrancy during supraventricular tachycardias. One view is that it reflects the effects of concealed transseptal conduction of the tachycardia

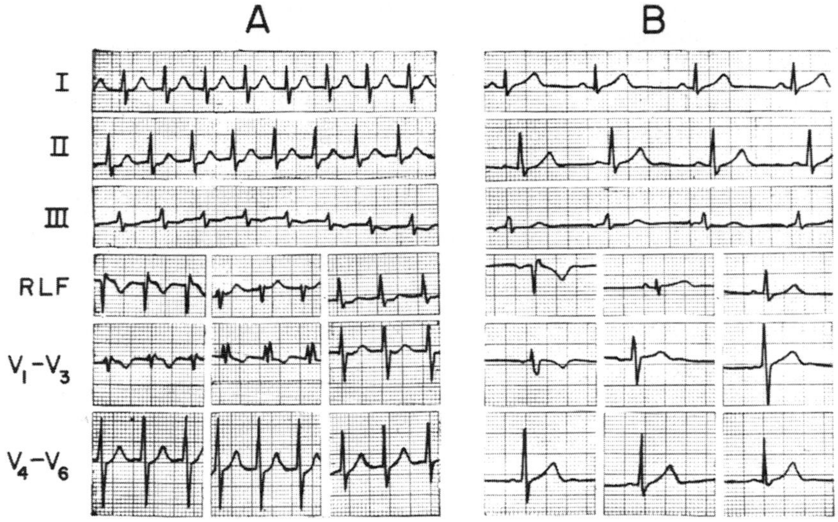

Figure 15-16. *Twelve-lead electrocardiograms from a patient aged 35 years with recurrent paroxysmal supraventricular tachycardias. (A) During tachycardia at rate of 140 beats/min. Note right bundle branch block configuration. (B) Shortly after reversion to sinus rhythm. Persistent broad S waves in limb and left chest leads represent a residual right-sided conduction delay that disappeared shortly after the record was obtained. See text for discussion.*

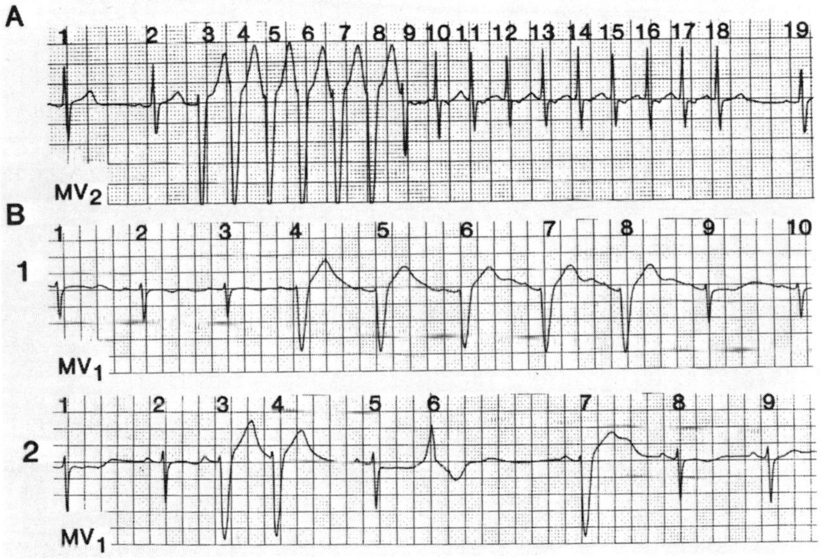

Figure 15-17. *Holter monitor records obtained to show multiple types of aberrancy during a single 24-hour monitoring period from the same patient as in Figure 15-8. (A) A 16-beat run of rapid supraventricular tachycardia (beats 3 to 18). The first seven beats exhibit varying left bundle branch block aberrancy (beats 3 to 9). The remainder are similar to the dominant beats. Note that both the coupling interval (0.52 second) and duration of the preceding cycle (0.92 second) preceding the first aberrant beat are longer than the corresponding intervals for the last aberrant beat (0.36 second and 0.34 second, respectively).* (B, row 1) *Record obtained early in the morning during a period of rest or sleep shows appearance and disappearance of left bundle branch type of aberrancy in conjunction with small cycle length changes associated with a sinus arrhythmia. Note that the interval at which aberrancy appears (0.88 second) and disappears (1 second) differ.* (B, row 2) *Records obtained 2 hours after those in* row 1 *to show examples of both short cycle left bundle branch block aberrancy of two premature atrial beats (beats 3 and 4) and long cycle left bundle branch block type aberrancy of a postectopic sinus beat (beat 7). Note that the ventricular premature beat (beat 6) exhibits a right bundle branch block contour suggestive of a left-sided origin. See text for discussion.*

impulses followed by retrograde activation of the involved bundle branch, which would maintain the latter in a refractory state.[170] Thus, repetitive right bundle branch block aberrancy would be explained in terms of concealed left-to-right transseptal conduction and retrograde activation of the right bundle branch, with the result that impulses propagating into the latter in the orthograde direction would consistently find the tissue refractory. Conversely, termination of aberrancy would be explicable in terms of block of transseptal conduction and of retrograde activation, arrival of the orthogradely conducting impulses at the bundle branch before retrograde activation, or cycle length–dependent shortening of repolarization or refractoriness. This mechanism has been implicated in a number of published cases of repetitive aberration[208–210] and documented by intracardiac electrogram[211,212] and *in vitro* microelectrode studies.[213] Irrespective, high rates are still probably required for the mechanism to operate normally.

Time to Achieve New Steady-State Action Potential Duration Following Rate Changes. Achieval of new steady-state action potential duration after abrupt rate changes is usually not immediate even in normal fibers but, rather, takes place gradually over a number of cycles.[25,214] Similar observations have been made with respect to rate-dependent changes in refractoriness in the *in situ* heart.[215] It may thus be inferred that the likelihood of premature responses being initiated before completion of repolarization of the previous beat, and therefore of aberration, is maximal immediately after the rate change and diminishes with each complex at the new rate. This explains instances in which the initial complex(es) of a tachycardia is (are) aberrant and in which aberrancy subsequently diminishes or disappears (see Fig. 15-15*B*). The number of beats needed to achieve the new steady-state action potential duration following rate increases varies, with some investigators indicating that it may normally require up to 40 to 50 beats.[214] Differences may exist with respect to the number of beats required for equilibration following increases and decreases in rate for the same fiber (see Fig. 15-13) and for the whole heart (see Fig. 15-17). However, the bulk of the change normally takes place over relatively few beats.

Changes In Diseased Heart

Findings in specimens of ischemic and diseased heart muscle suggest that the foregoing caveats need not, however, necessarily be invoked for patients with heart disease. In large measure, considerations similar to those noted in relation to aberrancy of isolated supraventricular beats apply. Two factors deserve additional comment.

Altered Cycle Length Dependence of Action Potential Duration. Findings that both partially depolarized and well-polarized fibers in such specimens may exhibit diminished action potential shortening for a given increase in rate (see Fig. 15-14) represent one such factor.[21,74,81,82,87] Other factors being equal, this would result in a greater than expected diminution in action potential amplitude and $\dot{V}_{max}$ for any given rate increase and to development of aberrancy at lower than expected rates as well as its perpetuation during bouts of tachycardia. Increased duration of repolarization (see Figs. 15-4, 15-7, and 15-14), altered responsiveness (see Fig. 15-3*B*), and time-dependent prolongation of refractoriness beyond completion of repolarization (see Fig. 15-6*III*), which also characterize fibers in diseased heart, would further accentuate this tendency. Comparisons between action potentials at comparable rates in a normal dog Purkinje fiber (see Fig. 15-10) and normal and partially depolarized fibers in diseased human ventricle (see Figs. 15-13 and 15-14) are illustrative. Note that in contrast to normal, the human ventricular muscle fibers exhibited a longer action potential duration than did the Purkinje fiber at comparable cycles. Also note that the partially depolarized fiber in Figure 15-14 exhibited much greater diminution of action potential amplitude and $\dot{V}_{max}$ in conjunction with cycle length shortening than did the well-polarized fiber in the same figure. However, the well-polarized fiber also experienced a progressive decrease in $\dot{V}_{max}$ suggestive of postrepolarization refractoriness, possibly due to delayed recovery from inactivation of the Na^+ channels or use dependent block of these channels or both.

Increased Time to Achieve Steady-State Action Potential Duration Following Rate Changes. Findings that it may take considerably longer than normal to achieve steady-state action potential after rate changes in ischemic and diseased heart muscle are the second factor.[21,36,87] Figure 15-13 shows sequential changes in action potential duration in response to an abrupt, tenfold increase (panel *I*) and decrease (panel *II*) in stimulation frequency in a well-polarized human ventricular muscle fiber from the margin of a ventricular aneurysm. Panel *I*, row *A* shows records during stimulation at cycle length 2000 msec (30 beats/min). Stimulation frequency was then increased to cycle length 200 msec (300 beats/min) (panel *I*, row *B*). An initial 2:1 response ensued. It was not until 14 seconds after the rate change that sufficient shortening of duration had occurred to permit even an abortive 1:1 response (panel *ID*). After establishment of a stable 1:1 response (panel *I*, row *E*), action potential characteristics continued to change for an additional 30 seconds before the new steady-state duration was achieved (panel *II*, row *A*). All told, equilibration required a total of 45 seconds and 190 complexes. Also note the more pronounced decrease in $\dot{V}_{max}$ at cycle length 200 msec than in a fiber from a normal dog heart (see Fig. 15-10).

Panel *II* of Figure 15-13 shows the effects of a subsequent abrupt reduction in frequency of stimulation back to 30 beats/min. The first few complexes following the rate decrease exhibited variable prolongation of action potential duration, with subsequent complexes exhibiting shortening, followed by gradual prolongation, of duration until the new steady state was reached. Equilibration time was again long, 206 seconds (103 complexes).

Implications With Respect to Incidence and Patterns of Aberrancy of Supraventricular Tachycardias in Diseased Heart. It may be inferred from the foregoing that persistent aberration during supraventricular tachycardias is unlikely to occur normally except at high rates, although not necessarily as high as those suggested by the records in Figure 15-10. Conversely, the electrophysiologic changes exhibited by fibers in ischemic and diseased heart muscle would appear to provide the necessary basis both for an overall increase in aberrancy and for its appearance at lower rates than normally. Probably, aberration of supraventricular tachycardia at physiologic rates implies that the electrophysiologic properties of the conduction system or the geometry of impulse spread, or both, have been altered by ischemia, disease, drugs, or other factors. In addition, as noted for extrasystoles, the observed changes also would favor changing patterns of aberrancy. In particular, since disease generally affects the left ventricle more than the right, the changes would favor an increase in left bundle branch block and mixed type aberrancy as compared with the right bundle branch block type ordinarily observed in normal heart. The changes also might be expected to alter the cycle length dependency of repolarization and refractoriness so as to make occurrence of aberrancy less predictable than normal and therefore more difficult to distinguish from ventricular ectopy.

Observation that achievement of a new steady-state action potential duration following abrupt rate changes may be a much more gradual process than normal in ischemic or diseased heart has other implications with respect to patterns of aberrancy. For example, local differences in equilibration time following rate decreases may help explain why aberration persists briefly after tachycardia ceases. Also, persistence of rate-related changes in action potential duration following rate slowing possibly explain posttachycardia ST-T changes. Variability in action potential duration following abrupt rate increases and before achieving the new steady state also could explain a number of other peculiarities. For example, alternation of normally configured and aberrant complexes could occur when rate changes result in an action potential alternans of the type seen in Figure 15-13*IB* and *C*. In addition, delays in achieving a 1 : 1 response in conjunction with abrupt cycle length shortening provide a possible basis for increases in the rates of initially slow supraventricular tachycardias as well as for onset of aberrancy at times other than at the beginning of a run.

Findings that the number of complexes required to reach a new steady-state action potential duration may differ following increases and decreases in rate in the same fiber (see Fig. 15-13) may underlie instances in which appearance and disappearance of short cycle type of aberrancy occur at different rates (see Fig. 15-17). Differences in preceding cycle length duration between the first aberrant (beat *3*) and nonaberrant (beat *10*) beats of a tachycardia, such as occurs in Figure 15-17*A* may also contribute. Hoffman[216] has suggested a third possible explanation on the basis of studies on impulse spread in partially depolarized regions of local block: (1) slowing of conduction in a depressed region is associated with prolonged action potential duration at its proximal margin and (2) failure of conduction, on the other hand, is associated with marked shortening of duration proximally.[134,158] Under such circumstances, abrupt rate increases would generate action potentials that are prolonged out of proportion to cycle length at the proximal margin. Rate-related block would occur at a particular cycle length. Once block develops, action potential duration shortens. On subsequent rate slowing, normal conduction will resume at shorter cycles than those at which block appeared during the prior period of acceleration. This could permit onset of aberration at lower rates than offset in conjunction with abrupt rate increases and decreases, respectively.

Abruptness of Cycle Length Change. The abruptness of a rate change also may influence aberrancy. In general, aberrancy appears more likely to occur in response to abrupt increases in rate between any two levels than if the same rate increase were made in step-wise fashion. Gradual, step-wise rate increases allow more time for shortening of action potential duration to occur and thus decrease the likelihood that the initial complexes at the new rate will be inscribed before completion of repolarization of the previous complex. This represents one possible explanation for observations that the beats of a sinus tachycardia appear less likely to become aberrant than the complexes of a paroxysmal supraventricular tachycardia at comparable rates since rate changes usually occur more gradually in the former. The phenomenon is likely to be more pronounced in normal than in diseased hearts, since changes observed in the latter, including diminished cycle length dependence of action potential duration and increased time requirements for achieval of the new steady state after rate changes, would serve to minimize differences due to abruptness of the rate change.

Electrophysiologic Characteristics of the His-Purkinje System. Certain of the conduction system characteristics that predispose to aberration of supraventricular premature complexes also favor its development during supraventricular tachycardias.

The fact that aberration of supraventricular tachycardias is not common normally is best explained in terms of the action potential shortening and concomitant reduction in the disparity of action potential duration,[157,158,170,188] both between comparable levels of the right and left ventricular components of the His-Purkinje system[157,170] and between different levels of the system,[157,158,188] that accompany cycle length shortening. In addition, Han and associates[170a] have shown that the extent of temporal dispersion of the recovery of ventricular muscle excitability is inversely related to the rate. Figure 15-11*IA* shows an example of decreased disparity in duration between action potentials simultaneously recorded from two normal Purkinje fibers on cycle length shortening.

Conversely, the increased aberration of supraventricular tachyarrhythmias in the diseased heart also could reflect diminution in the usual rate-related decreases in disparity of action potential duration in different parts of the conduction system due to such factors as (1) the decrease in cycle length dependence of action potential duration and (2) development of post-repolarization refractoriness and alterations in the responsiveness relationships of the type depicted in Figures 15-6 and 15-3*B*. The fact that the effects of ischemia and disease are not uniform tends to support this interpretation. Figure 15-14 shows increased dispersion of repolarization in a specimen of human ventricle in conjunction with cycle length shortening.

Antiarrhythmic Agents and Short Cycle Aberrancy

Many pharmacologic agents used to treat patients with heart disease,[24,25,27–29,33,38–47,117] including the standard antiarrhythmic agents and digitalis, influence time course of repolarization and refractoriness independent of any changes in diastolic potential. Procainamide and quinidine[117] are well known for their ability to slow repolarization, particularly the terminal portions of phase 3. Observations that these agents may increase aberrancy date back many years.[217] Conversely, agents such as diphenylhydantoin[218] and propranolol,[219] which shorten the time course of repolarization, may diminish aberrancy.[220]

The quinidinelike agents also influence conduction of premature complexes because they block the fast Na^+ channels.[45,46,146,221] Observations by Hoffman[118] that these agents alter the responsiveness relationship so that the curve (cell *a*) depicted in Figure 15-3*B* is shifted down and to the right in the mid- and low ranges of potential date back many years. Depressive effects on the Na^+ channel are voltage dependent, being more pronounced in low potential as compared with well-polarized cells.[46,116] These agents also appear to prolong functional recovery variably beyond completion of repolarization *(postrepolarization refractoriness),* reflecting delayed recovery from inactivation of the fast Na^+ channels.[45] Other factors being equal, these actions would be expected to increase further the likelihood that premature responses initiated during repolarization, including those initiated during late phases, and possibly even during diastole, will conduct aberrantly. The voltage dependence of the drug-induced blockade of the Na^+ channels suggests that the increase in aberrancy should be particularly prone to occur in ischemic and diseased hearts, with their large numbers of partially depolarized cells.

Insofar as supraventricular tachycardias are concerned, the aforementioned changes would be expected to predispose to an overall increase in aberrancy as well as to facilitate its development at lower than normal rates and possibly also in association with gradual, as opposed to abrupt, rate increases. Recent findings that quinidine and procainamide cause "use" (rate)-dependent block of the fast Na^+ channel[45,46,146,221] also are pertinent, since this action would serve to increase further aberration during periods of tachycardia.

Long Cycle Aberrancy

Alterations in QRS contour that appear on prolongation of the cardiac cycle and diminish or disappear on cycle length shortening represent the second major type of aberrancy. Although not as common as the short cycle variety, long cycle aberrancy is nevertheless a well-documented entity[11,151,179,222–249] that was initially described by Kaufman and Rothberger in 1913[151] and by Wilson in 1915[222] and was produced experimentally by Drury and McKenzie in 1934[244] and by Elizari and coworkers.[240] It is best exemplified by development of bundle branch block patterns on slowing of the sinus rate and by the altered QRS contour of supraventricular escapes. Although aberrant complexes may frequently exhibit a right bundle branch block contour, this does not appear to be as characteristic as with short cycle aberration.[11,179,229,232,242,243] In addition, whereas short cycle aberrancy is common in patients with both normal and impaired hearts, long cycle aberrancy appears to be more strictly confined to those with underlying conduction system pathology.[6,11,178,232,235,237,238]

The overall significance of long cycle aberrancy is in many ways similar to that described for the short cycle variety. Aberrant supraventricular complexes closing long cycles can closely mimic isolated ectopic ventricular escapes, including fusional complexes and runs of slow ventricular tachycardia. The distinction is a particular problem in records without P waves, including atrial fibrillation. Even more important, this type of aberrancy should cause the clinician to suspect intrinsic conduction system disease or functional abnormalities due to such causes as ischemia, toxic drug effects, and severe electrolyte imbalance. Suggestions that at least some types of long cycle aberrancy may be due to phase 4 depolarization of latent pacemaker cells (see below) underscore an association with increased ventricular ectopy.

Figure 15-17*B* shows a typical example of long cycle left bundle branch block type of aberrancy of a sinus beat (beat *7*) closing a 1.8-second pause following a ventricular premature beat (beat *6*). Sinus beats closing pauses <1.4 second did not exhibit the phenomenon, emphasizing long cycle dependency. Figure 15-17*A* and *B* also show examples of short cycle left bundle branch block aberration from the same patient for comparison.

The record in Figure 15-18 shows an example of long cycle right bundle branch block type aberrancy in a woman aged 78 years hospitalized for acute anteroseptal infarction. The case differs from that depicted in Figure 15-17 and is atypical in that aberration occurs with only slight prolongation in cycle length. There is prominent alternation in cycle length due to intermittent atrial bigeminy. QRS complexes closing cycles shorter than 0.76 second in duration are normal; those closing longer cycles exhibit varying degrees of right bundle branch block aberrancy. The degree of aberration is cycle length dependent; the longer the cycle, the wider the QRS complex. The phenomenon appeared on the patients' third day of hospitalization and persisted for an additional 4 days, during which time scattered early supraventricular extrasystoles exhibiting right bundle branch block type aberration also were noted. Both were superseded by fixed right bundle branch block. The latter, in turn, disappeared 3 days later, by which time all traces of long cycle aberrancy were gone. Variably coupled left bundle branch block premature ventricular beats, which had initially been present, disappeared as well.

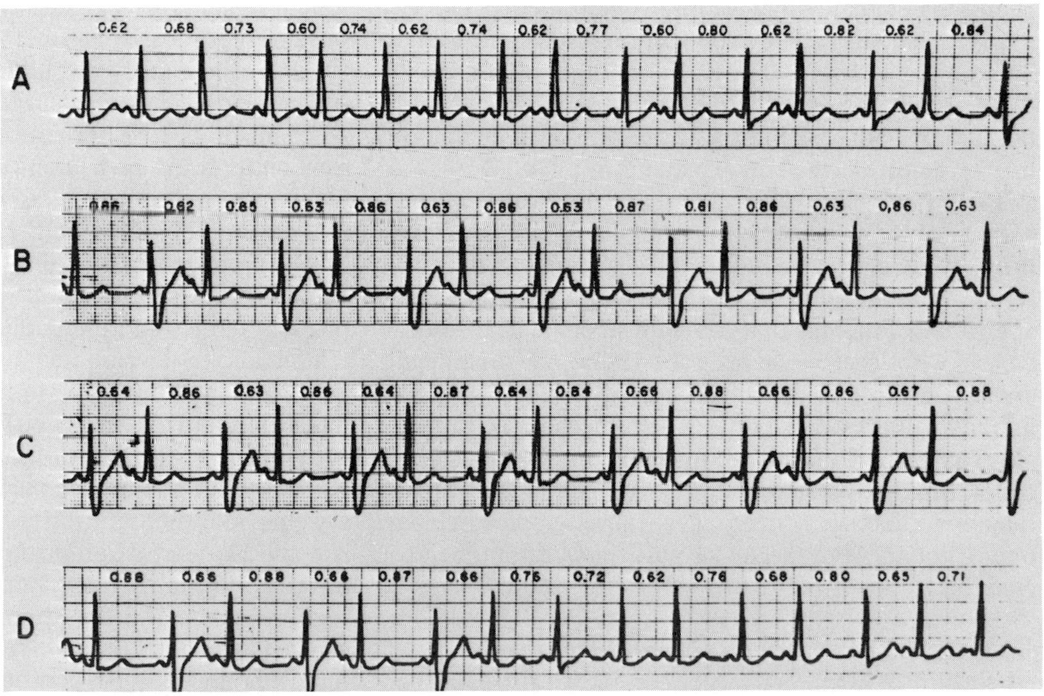

Figure 15-18. *A to D show a continuous electrocardiographic record (modified monitor lead II) obtained from a patient aged 78 years during the initial stage of acute anteroseptal myocardial infarction. QRS complexes have been retouched. RR intervals are indicated in seconds. Atrial bigeminy is present throughout most of the record. Note varying right bundle branch block aberrancy of beats closing cycles ≥0.76 second in duration, the degree of aberration generally being related to the degree of cycle length prolongation. In D, also note that of the beats closing two identical cycles of 0.76 second, one exhibits an incomplete right bundle branch block contour whereas the other is normal. See text for discussion.*

In contrast to short cycle aberrancy, the long cycle variety cannot readily be explained in terms of impulse spread in incompletely repolarized fibers, since there is more than adequate time for completion of recovery before inscription of the aberrant complex. A number of alternatives have been suggested.

"Preferential" AV Junctional Transmission of Aberrant Beats

Initial interest focused on aberration of junctional escapes. The earliest hypotheses sought to explain differences in QRS contour between normally configured sinus and aberrant junctional complexes in terms of differences in path of AV junctional spread.[151,226,233,245] Kaufman and Rothberger attributed the phenomenon to selective activation by the sinus and aberrant junctional complexes of different portions of the bundle of His,[151] a concept that implies anatomic or functional longitudinal dissociation within this structure *per se* or within the larger AV conducting system as visualized by Scherf and James.[152,245] Wellens also has invoked functional dissociation within the bundle branch system.[247] However, it is unclear why aberration due to this cause should be bradycardia dependent. In addition, to the extent that dissociation occurs at all, it would be expected to be a reasonably common phenomenon, particularly in patients with AV conduction system pathology. Since sinus bradycardia and junctional escape complexes occur frequently, it follows that long cycle aberration also should be common. Its relative rarity therefore further detracts from this explanation.

Pick[226] as well as others[230,233] have implicated spread along the paraspecific fibers of Mahaim, which run from the AV node, His bundle, and left bundle branch to septal myocardium,[140,141] as the cause of junctional aberration. Findings that Mahaim fibers appear to decrease with age[250] whereas aberration of junctional escapes is most commonly observed in older subjects detracts from this possibility, as does the lack of clear-cut electrophysiologic evidence for their functional significance. Still, the possibility that at least some instances of long cycle aberrancy may reflect impulse spread along one or the other of the AV bypass tracts cannot be excluded.

Altered Site of Origin of Aberrant Complexes

Aberration of junctional escape complexes also could be explicable in terms of an abnormal site of origin. Pick implicated the Mahaim fibers.[226] More recently, Masumi and co-workers[236] as well as Lie and co-workers[242] concluded that many such complexes were fascicular rather than junctional, originating in the anterior or posterior fascicles of the left bundle branch. Such complexes would be expected to exhibit a relatively narrow QRS with an incomplete right bundle branch block pattern, thus representing one possible cause of right bundle branch type junctional aberration. However, it would not explain left bundle branch block and nonspecific types of aberration. More important, it leaves unanswered questions concerning mechanisms of long cycle aberrancy of sinus complexes.

Vagal Mediation

Since many of the early reported cases of aberration occurred in conjunction with vagally mediated sinus slowing, the possibility that QRS prolongation resulted from direct depressive acetylcholine effects on conduction in the His-Purkinje system also was suggested.[222,223,229] Findings that acetylcholine does not depress the normal His-Purkinje system[25] and that it may actually improve conduction in depressed tissues[251] appear to obviate this explanation. In a different vein, Dressler proposed that increased vagal activity resulted in an altered QRS contour by a vagally mediated coronary vasoconstrictor reflex.[227] It would not, however, explain instances of aberration in which vagal mediation could not be invoked, for example, aberration of supraventricular complexes closing postextrasystolic pauses.

Phase 4 Depolarization

Latent Pacemaker Cells. The fact that the His-Purkinje system is composed of numerous automatic (latent pacemaker) cells capable of undergoing spontaneous diastolic depolarization suggests a fourth possible mechanism[56,238–241] for long cycle aberrancy of both slow sinus beats and junctional escapes based on the previously mentioned interrelationships between automaticity and conduction (Fig. 15-19).[56]

The cyclic lowering of diastolic potential that phase 4 depolarization entails results in a voltage- and time-dependent reduction in $\dot{V}_{max}$ and amplitude of action potentials and in development of conduction disturbances more or less comparable to those occurring in incompletely repolarized fibers (see Fig. 15-19).[56] In light of the widespread distribution of latent pacemaker cells, enhancement of phase 4 depolarization in the His-Purkinje system could theoretically result in virtually any type of AV and IV conduction disturbance, the specific nature of the abnormality being related to the location of the involved fibers and the extent of depolarization. In instances in which the involved cells are located in the bundle branches, QRS contour changes defined as aberrancy might be expected to ensue. Insofar as longitudinal dissociation of the AV conducting system occurs, it is possible that enhanced automaticity in the distal segment (NH region) of the AV node or the His bundle, which ordinarily would be expected to result in AV block, also might give rise to intraventricular conduction disturbances and aberrancy. Since aberrancy due to this cause results from lowering of membrane potential dur-

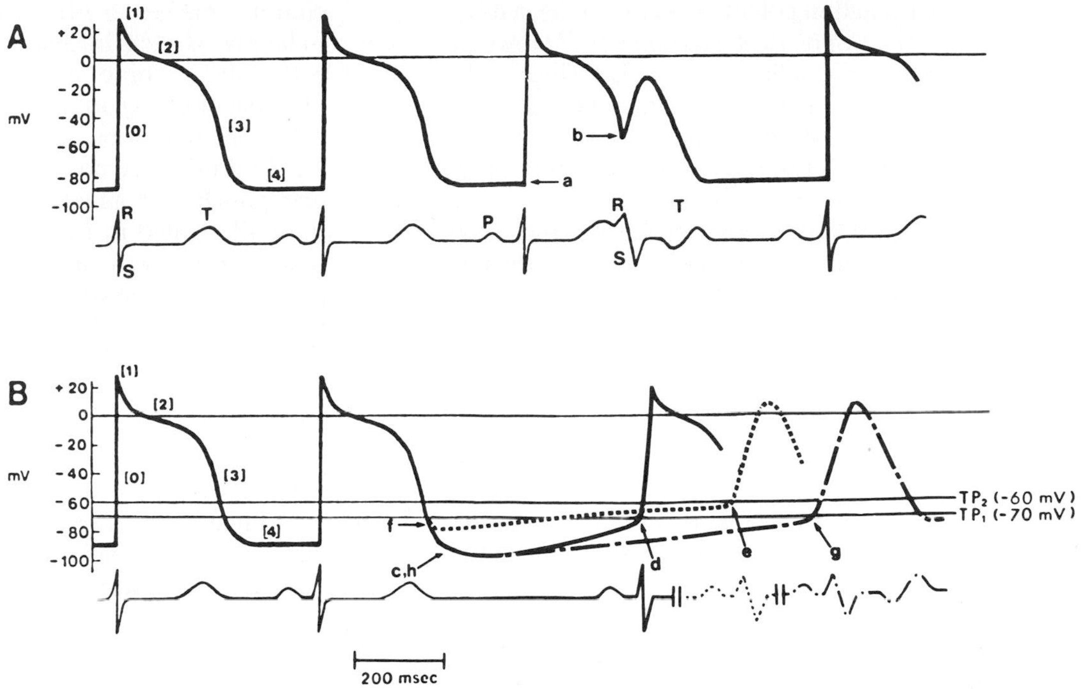

Figure 15-19. *Schematic transmembrane potentials from a latent pacemaker cell in the His-Purkinje system and simultaneous surface electrocardiogram to illustrate interrelationships between automaticity and conduction. Action potential phases are designated by arabic numerals 0 to 4; electrocardiographic deflections, by the letters P, R, S, and T. (A) During the first three beats, stimulation is sufficiently fast to suppress phase 4 depolarization, a situation analogous to that occurring during sinus rhythm. Membrane potential is normal and remains constant during diastole (phase 4). The action potentials, which are initiated at approximately −90 mV (a), also are normal, as is the electrocardiogram. Repolarization of the third beat is interrupted by a premature response initiated at approximately −60 mV (b) that exhibits marked diminution in amplitude and $\dot{V}_{max}$ and depressed conduction, as evidenced by aberrant RS contour of the electrocardiogram. (B) The initial two beats were recorded during stimulation at same rate as in A. Action potentials and electrocardiogram are normal. The third to fifth beats were evoked after development of phase 4 depolarization in response to a decrease in frequency of stimulation to a low rate. The third action potential is depicted as arising in the fiber when maximum diastolic potential (MDP, −90 mV, c) and threshold potential (approximately 70 mV, d, TP_1) are both still normal. Since the depolarization process cannot lower diastolic potential to below the threshold potential (TP), the resultant decrease in amplitude and $\dot{V}_{max}$ is not sufficient to depress conduction significantly, and the electrocardiogram remains normal. The fourth action potential depicts the effect of a shift in TP to a less negative level (TP_2). The shift allows the fourth action potential to be initiated at a much lower potential, approximately −60 mV (e), than normally. Diminution in amplitude and $\dot{V}_{max}$ and depression of conduction are correspondingly more marked. The RS complex of the electrocardiogram is aberrant. Note similarities to premature response in A, which also was initiated at approximately −60 mV. Also note that the shift in TP is associated with a decrease in MDP (f). The fifth action potential shows how responsiveness changes of the type depicted in Figure 15-3, panel B, could predispose to aberrancy due to phase 4 depolarization at more negative potentials than usual and in cells with a normal TP. Note that although this beat is initiated at approximately −70 mV (g), amplitude and $\dot{V}_{max}$ are sufficiently reduced to depress conduction and cause aberration of the RS complex. It thus resembles the fourth response, which arises at approximately −60 mV (e), more that it does the third even though the latter also is initiated at −70 mV (d). The greater than expected decrease in amplitude and $\dot{V}_{max}$ and depression of conduction for the level of potential reflect the responsiveness change. (After Singer, D. H., Lazarra, R., and Hoffman, D. S.: Interrelationships between automaticity and conduction of Purkinje fibers. Circ. Res., 21:537–558, 1967)*

ing phase 4 of the action potential, it also has been designated *phase 4 block* or *phase 4 aberrancy.*[11,238] However, this designation is not sufficiently specific, since it also applies to aberrancy due to low resting potential.

Massumi[234] has listed electrocardiographic characteristics of long cycle aberrancy. Given the nature of the proposed mechanism, it follows that progressive cycle length prolongation should be associated with increasing aberration. The records shown in Figure 15-18 are illustrative. Conversely, factors that decrease phase 4 depolarization prevent development of, and diminish or abolish preexisting, long cycle aberrancy. Shortening of the sinus cycle in conjunction with activity or by such agents as atropine *and* increasing base heart rate by pacemaker implantation in instances of bradyarrhythmia are examples, as is pharmacologic suppression of phase 4 depolarization. It further follows that interventions that manipulate sinus rate should prove useful in elucidating suspect occult cases.

In addition, patients with aberrancy due to phase 4 depolarization also might be expected to exhibit ventricular ectopic complexes originating in the region of enhanced automaticity: patients with right bundle branch block aberration should develop premature complexes exhibiting a left bundle branch block contour, and vice versa. Findings of the appropriate type of extrasystoles would support conclusions that a given case of long cycle aberration was due to enhanced automaticity. In Figures 15-17*B* and 15-18, development of left and right bundle branch block aberrancy was associated with the presence of right and left bundle branch block type ventricular ectopic beats, respectively. In addition, in Figure 15-18 both aberrancy and ventricular ectopy disappeared coincidentally.

Electrophysiologic Determinants. Aberrancy due to phase 4 depolarization would be likely to occur under circumstances that enhance automaticity of latent pacemaker cells in the His-Purkinje system, of which the two most obvious are as follows:

1. *Reduction in heart rate* due to sinus slowing or to such other causes as high-grade AV block or nonconducted atrial premature complexes. Long diastoles provide more time for phase 4 depolarization to develop, with consequent reduction in the level of diastolic membrane potential encountered by the propagating impulse (see Fig. 15-19*B*). This represents one possible explanation for aberration occurring in conjunction with decreases in heart rate to the vicinity of the intrinsic firing rate of latent AV junctional or His-Purkinje pacemakers or below (≤40 to 55 beats/min) (see Fig. 15-17*B*).
2. *Direct enhancement of latent pacemaker automaticity.* Numerous physiologic interventions, including changes in *p*H, pCO_2, and temperature, ischemia, stretch in dilated hears, alterations in extracellular ionic concentrations, and many pharmacologic agents including digitalis, act to increase the rate of phase 4 depolarization of latent His-Purkinje pacemaker cells.[25,28,38–47] It provides one possible explanation for instances such as those illustrated in Figure 15-18, in which aberrancy occurs with only modest prolongation in cycle length and at sinus rates that do not normally permit significant phase 4 depolarization of latent pacemaker cells.

It might reasonably be inferred from the widespread distribution of automatic cells and the numerous physiologic and pharmacologic factors that act to depress sinus activity or enhance latent pacemaker automaticity, or both, that this type of aberrancy is quite common. Published reports do not support this inference. This is particularly true of patients with clinically normal hearts, most reported cases occurring in a setting of organic heart disease.

Analysis of the relationships between membrane potential and conduction velocity[56,115] provides a possible explanation for this apparent paradox. As noted previously, conduction is usually well maintained and may even improve slightly until membrane potential is reduced to less than −70 mV, a finding attributed to (1) decreased current requirements for excitation (*i.e.,* increase in excitability) as membrane potential is brought closer to the threshold potential and (2) an increase in the space constant, which results from the increase in membrane resistance associated with phase 4 depolarization. Both would enhance the effectiveness of electrotonic current spread and compensate for the voltage-dependent decrease in $\dot{V}_{max}$.[56] Since the threshold potential of normal His-Purkinje fibers approximates −70 mV,[116] phase 4 depolarization cannot reduce diastolic membrane potential to less negative levels because spontaneous firing and an ectopic ventricular beat would ensue. Phase 4 depolarization is therefore unlikely to result in slow conduction and aberrancy normally (see Fig. 15-19*B*).

Phase 4 depolarization could, however, theoretically cause sufficient reduction in diastolic potential to result in significant aberration under a number of special circumstances, one of which may be operative normally. Figure 15-20 presumes that the rate of phase 4 depolarization in a latent pacemaker cell has increased to the point where its spontaneous firing rate is only fractionally lower than that of the sinus. Given a close similarity in rates, it is theoretically possible for the sinus impulse to reach the latent pacemaker cell at the time when its diastolic potential had been lowered to the vicinity of the threshold potential. Since the threshold potential is the

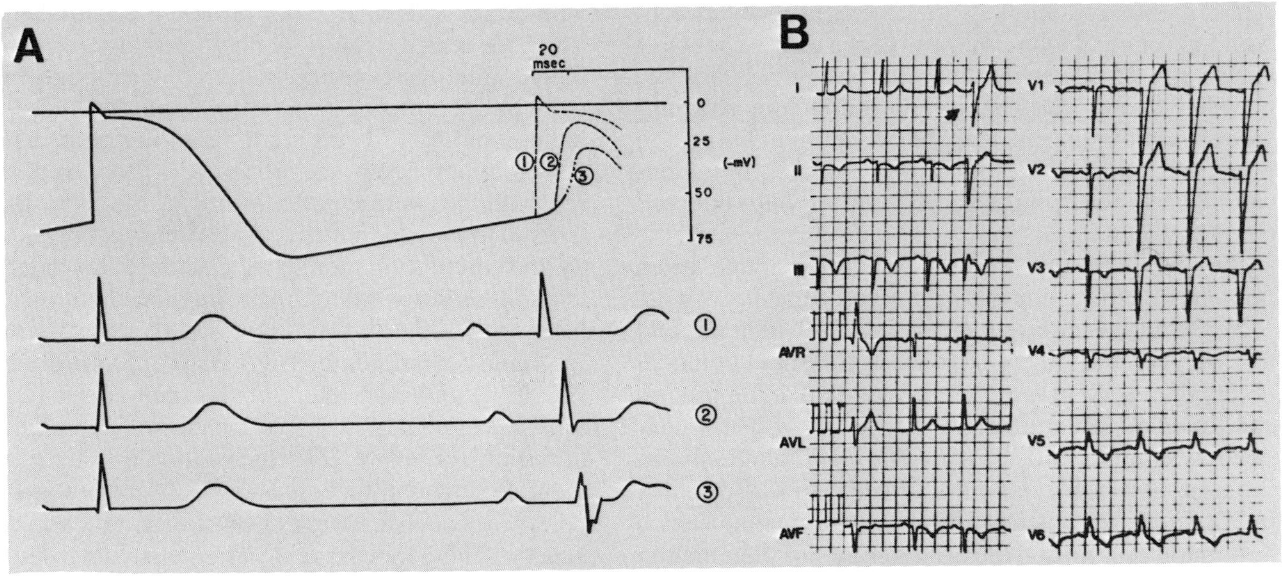

Figure 15-20. *(A) Schematic transmembrane potentials from latent pacemaker cell in the right bundle branch to show how phase 4 depolarization can result in both long cycle aberration and aberration in the absence of perceptible changes in sinus rate even in the normal heart. The rate of phase 4 depolarization in the right bundle branch cells is presumed to have increased to where it is just lower than that of the sinus. The close similarity in rates makes it possible for the propagating sinus impulse to reach the bundle branch cells at a time when diastolic potential had been lowered to the vicinity of the threshold potential. This period, the transition between phase 4 and the upstroke of the next action potential, is characterized by a rapid increase in the rate of depolarization and a large decrease in potential over a brief time (20 msec). Even slight changes in the time of arrival of the propagated impulse, due either to changes in sinus rate or in rate of diastolic depolarization of the latent pacemaker cell, would therefore be associated with marked differences in the level of potential encountered by the impulse, with resultant variability in the character and conduction of the response. Note progressive reduction in amplitude and $\dot{V}_{max}$ of the three responses (1, 2, and 3) initiated successively later during the 20-msec period, together with depressive effects on conduction (indicated by QRS changes in the electrocardiogram). Response 1 is initiated just before inscription of the threshold potential and conducts normally. Responses 2 and 3 exhibit increasing right bundle branch block aberration due to activation of the right bundle branch at successively lower potentials. The small differences in timing would not be noticeable on a standard electrocardiogram, so that variations in QRS contour would be appreciated as occurring in the absence of rate changes. This mechanism also provides a reasonable explanation for beat-to-beat changes in QRS contour of the type seen in Figure 15-18. (B) Standard 12-lead electrocardiogram from a man of 68 with coronary heart disease to show appearance and disappearance of left bundle branch block type of aberrancy in the absence of clear-cut changes in sinus rate (see leads V_1 to V_6). Findings of variably coupled, automatic-type ventricular extrasystoles exhibiting characteristics indicative of a left-sided site of origin (see beats designated by* arrow *in leads I to III) suggest that aberration may have been due to accelerated phase 4 depolarization of latent pacemakers in the left bundle branch. See text for discussion.*

transition between diastole (phase 4) and the upstroke (phase 0) of the next action potential, a rapid increase in the rate of depolarization and a large decrease in membrane potential take place over a very brief time (10 to 20 msec). Under such circumstances, even very small variations in the time of arrival of the propagated impulse, due either to changes in sinus rate or in the rate of diastolic depolarization of latent pacemaker cells, could result in marked changes in the level of membrane potential encountered by, and, therefore, in conduction of, the impulse. Accordingly, slight prolongation of the sinus cycle could result in development of considerable aberrancy. Conversely, minimal shortening might normalize conduction. In a similar vein, small changes in the rate of phase 4 depolarization of the latent pacemaker cells could affect conduction in the absence of any change in sinus rate. This mechanism would allow for virtually complex-to-complex changes in conduction and provides a possible explanation for intermittent aberration of supraventricular escapes and for differences in contour of beats occurring at closely similar escape intervals (see Fig. 15-18*D*).

Two other circumstances that might facilitate development of conduction disturbances and aberrancy deserve special mention in light of findings in ischemic and diseased heart muscle: (1) a shift in threshold potential to less than −70 mV so that the depolarization process can lower membrane potential to levels at which conduction is significantly impaired[56] and (2) alterations in the responsiveness relationship similar to that depicted in Figure 15-3*B*, which would lessen the extent to which automatic cells must depolarize before slow conduction and block ensue. In Figure 15-19*B*, for example, significant conduction disturbances might appear on depolarization to −70 rather than to −60 mV. Lesser degrees of cycle length prolongation also might suffice. It is pertinent that the experimental production of conduction disturbances due to progressive phase 4 depolarization in isolated Purkinje fibers was generally associated with changes in the voltage–time course of repolarization such that maximum diastolic potential decreased and generalized hypo-polarization ensued,[56] and by shifts in take-off potential toward zero potential.[56] Figure 15-19*B* illustrates these possibilities. Figure 15-21 *(top* and *middle panels)* seeks to explain changes in QRS configuration seen in Figure 15-18 in terms of cycle length–dependent changes in diastolic potential in latent pacemaker cells in the right bundle branch. Given the small changes in cycle length associated with the appearance and disappearance of aberrancy, the diagram presumes that phase 4 depolarization was accelerated due to ischemia and that depolarization-induced shifts in threshold potential toward zero potential or the aforementioned changes in responsiveness also have occurred. El-Sherif and co-workers,[252] on the basis of their studies of conduction disturbance in the dog His-Purkinje system following coronary ligation, further underscored the importance of these factors in the development of long cycle aberrancy. Still others have emphasized the role of cycle length–dependent changes in excitability in this regard.[150]

Oscillatory Activity. It has also been suggested that depolarization-induced and other types of oscillatory activity may give rise to conduction disturbances.[30,253] If the cyclic changes in membrane potential due to the oscillation activity are sufficiently slow to allow membrane properties to follow, they could give rise to conduction disturbances similar in type to those associated with phase 4 depolarization of latent pacemaker cells. Thus, the relatively slow oscillations associated with digitalis[253] might be expected to allow cyclic changes in $\dot{V}_{max}$ and conduction velocity during diastole. On the other hand, rapid oscillations might result in a more uniform depression of membrane properties to levels commensurate with the average potential during the oscillatory activity. This would, in turn, result in changes in excitability and conduction more typical of those associated with low resting potential than with enhanced automaticity. Findings of relatively slow oscillatory activity in many specimens of ischemic and diseased myocardium (see Fig. 15-4) and that many of the spontaneously active cells appear to exhibit changes in take-off potential[77] and in responsiveness[74,75,77,87] that would facilitate development of slow conduction underscore the potential importance of such activity as a cause of conduction disturbances. The reported association between oscillatory activity and variable local block in such specimens also is pertinent.[74,75,77,87,91–93]

Antiarrhythmic Agents and Long Cycle Aberrancy. All antiarrhythmic agents in current use act to suppress phase 4 depolarization of latent pacemaker cells and thus might be expected to influence long cycle aberrancy. However, certain caveats are in order. The actions of quinidine and procainamide are illustrative and present an interesting paradox with respect to their effects on phase 4 conduction disturbances.[40,256,257] On the one hand, therapeutic concentrations decrease or abolish automaticity of latent pacemakers. This would prevent development of, or reverse already established, aberrancy. On the other hand, the direct Na^{+} channel blocking actions of these agents[45,46,146,221] might be expected to facilitate development of or accentuate already existing aberrancy. The net effect on conduction and aberration would depend on the extent to which the beneficial effects of decreasing phase 4 depolarization would outweigh direct depressant effects. With low concentrations direct depressive effects on conduction may be so minimal that the decrease in phase 4 depolarization would result in improvement in conduction and decreased aberrancy. With high drug concentrations, on the other hand, depressive effects may prevail. In addition, with quinidine and procainamide, high drug concentrations also may lower resting potential, thus facilitating development of depolarization-induced automaticity.[40,254,255]

To the extent that the increase in phase 4 aberrancy in ischemic and diseased hearts is due to the altered electrophysiologic properties of the large numbers of partially depolarized, spontaneously active fibers contained therein, restoration of maximum diastolic potential toward more normal levels might serve to suppress automaticity and decrease aberrancy. The catechol-

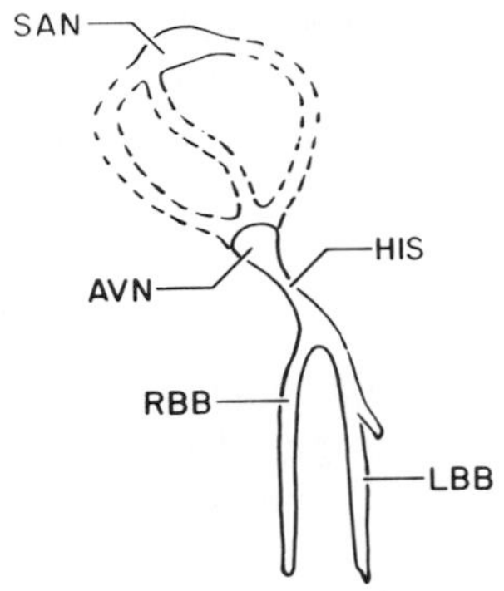

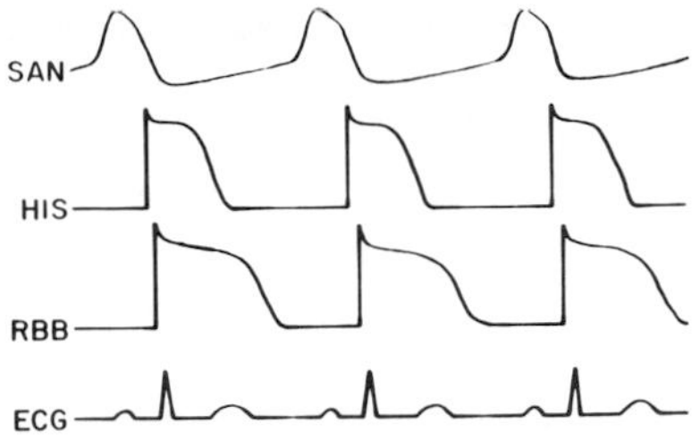

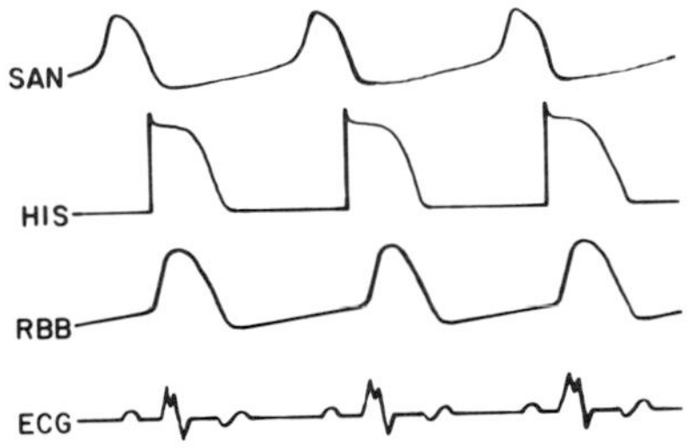

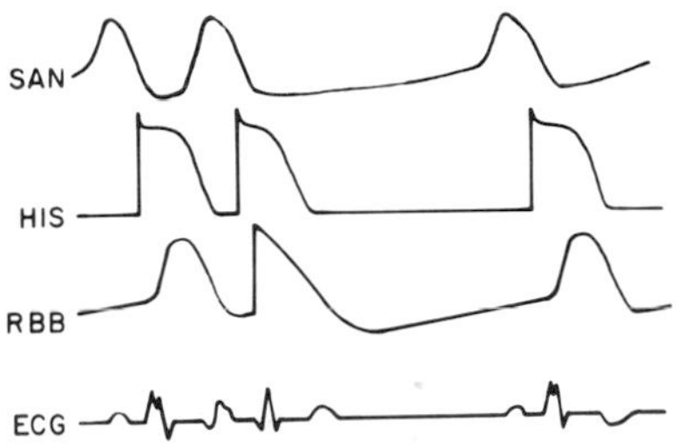

Figure 15-21. *Diagram to show an alternate mechanism whereby enhanced phase 4 depolarization of latent pacemaker cells could cause aberration in the absence of significant changes in sinus rate. A possible mechanism for "supernormal" intraventricular conduction is also shown. A simplified representation of the conduction system, similar to that in Figure 15-1A, is shown on left. Traces show transmembrane potentials from sinoatrial node* (SAN), *His bundle* (HIS), *and right bundle branch* (RBB), *together with lead II electrocardiogram. (*Top panel, *control conditions) The sinus rate is normal. Latent pacemakers in the His bundle and right bundle branch are not undergoing phase 4 depolarization. The electrocardiogram is normal.* (Middle panel) *Sinus rate is unchanged. Automaticity of latent pacemakers in right bundle branch is enhanced to where it is just less than in the sinoatrial node. Shift in threshold potential to less negative than normal levels and depressed responsiveness are assumed. As a result, amplitude and* $\dot{V}_{max}$ *of response initiated in right bundle branch cells are markedly diminished and conduction is depressed. The electrocardiogram shows right bundle branch block.* (Bottom panel) *A premature atrial extrasystole reaches the involved right bundle branch cells at the point of maximum diastolic potential. Therefore, amplitude and* $\dot{V}_{max}$ *of the premature response are greater than those of the dominant beats, with corresponding improvement of conduction in the right bundle branch relative to that of dominant beats. QRS is correspondingly less aberrant than in dominant beats (i.e., "supernormal" intraventricular conduction). See text for discussion.*

amines[56,77,254,255] act in this manner. However, they concomitantly enhance automaticity of normal latent pacemaker cells, making them less useful.

Supernormal Conduction

The concept of *supernormal intraventricular conduction* also has been invoked to explain at least some instances of long cycle aberrancy.[235,246–249] The term refers to the improvement in conduction of impulses initiated early in diastole in patients with underlying conduction disturbances.[3–5,19,20,238,241,248] A number of explanations have been offered for the phenomenon,[3–5,19,20,238,241–248] which is in a sense the reverse of aberrancy. Paradoxically, phase 4 depolarization in latent pacemaker cells in the His-Purkinje system represents one possible cause of supernormality.[56,238,241,248,258]

Since automatic cells begin to depolarize immediately on completion of repolarization, membrane potential is maximal early in the cycle and declines progressively thereafter. Action potentials initiated during the terminal phase of repolarization and immediately after its completion may therefore exhibit a greater amplitude and V_{max} and also conduct more rapidly than those initiated late in the cycle. Thus, in instances in which enhanced phase 4 depolarization causes impaired intraventricular conduction, QRS configuration of early premature beats may be more normal than those of the dominant beats. Similar-type changes in the His bundle would cause supernormal AV conduction. Figure 15-21 *(bottom panel)* depicts schematically how phase 4 depolarization could cause supernormality of IV conduction and lead to long cycle aberrancy. Notice that whereas the supernormally conducted early atrial premature complex appears normally configured, sinus complexes closing the long cycles exhibit right bundle branch block.

Aberrancy Without Significant Changes in Cycle Length

Aberrancy also may occur with only minimal or even without perceptible changes in cycle length and at normal or low heart rates. The first case was probably reported in 1913 by Sir Thomas Lewis,[259] who designated the entity *unstable* bundle branch block. *Intermittent bundle branch block, transient bundle branch block, inconstant bundle branch block, reversible bundle branch block, rate-dependent bundle branch block,* and *rate-dependent aberrancy* are other designations.[161,172,179,223,224,260–262] Although precise figures are not available, it is undoubtedly very common in diseased heart, both right and left bundle branch block type aberration having been reported.[161,172,179,180,223,224,260–263] However, in contrast to the short and long cycle varieties, left bundle branch block aberration predominates overwhelmingly. The significance of this type of aberration is substantially similar to that described for the others except that it, even more than long cycle aberrancy, indicates significant conduction system pathology and is a forerunner of fixed bundle branch block. Virtually all reported cases have occurred in patients with clinical heart disease.[161,172,179,180,223,224,260–263]

Figures 15-15*D*, 15-17*B*, 15-18*C* and *D*, 15-20*A*, and 15-22*B* show representative examples of intermittent left and right bundle branch block occurring with minimal or no change in basic cycle length and at physiologic heart rates. As noted in previous cases,[179,180] the cycle length of appearance and disappearance differed. In addition, the full-blown bundle branch block pattern usually appeared immediately, the degree of aberration varying only minimally if at all (see Figs. 15-15*D*, 15-20*A*, and 15-22*B*). In some cases, however, aberration may vary considerably. For example, of the two 0.76-second cycles in Figures 15-18*D*, one is closed by a normally configured complex and the other by a complex exhibiting a slightly delayed terminal S wave indicative of incomplete right bundle branch block. Cycle length prolongation beyond 0.76 second resulted in further increases in aberration, culminating in a complete right bundle branch block pattern (see Fig. 15-18*A* to *C*).

Electrophysiologic Determinants

Aberrancy occurring with minimal or no change in cycle length implies that the propagating impulse encounters tissues exhibiting variable refractoriness throughout much or all of the cardiac cycle. This is difficult to explain simply in terms of cycle length–dependent changes in repolarization or diastolic potential.

The physiologic and pharmacologic factors that can affect membrane potential and refractoriness independent of cycle length have been enumerated. Given the preponderant occurrence of this type of aberrancy in patients with clinical heart or conduction system disease, alterations in electrophysiologic properties associated with ischemia and disease are particularly relevant. Overall, the changes observed in ischemic and diseased cardiac tissues would predispose to increased refractoriness throughout the cardiac cycle. Findings of large pop-

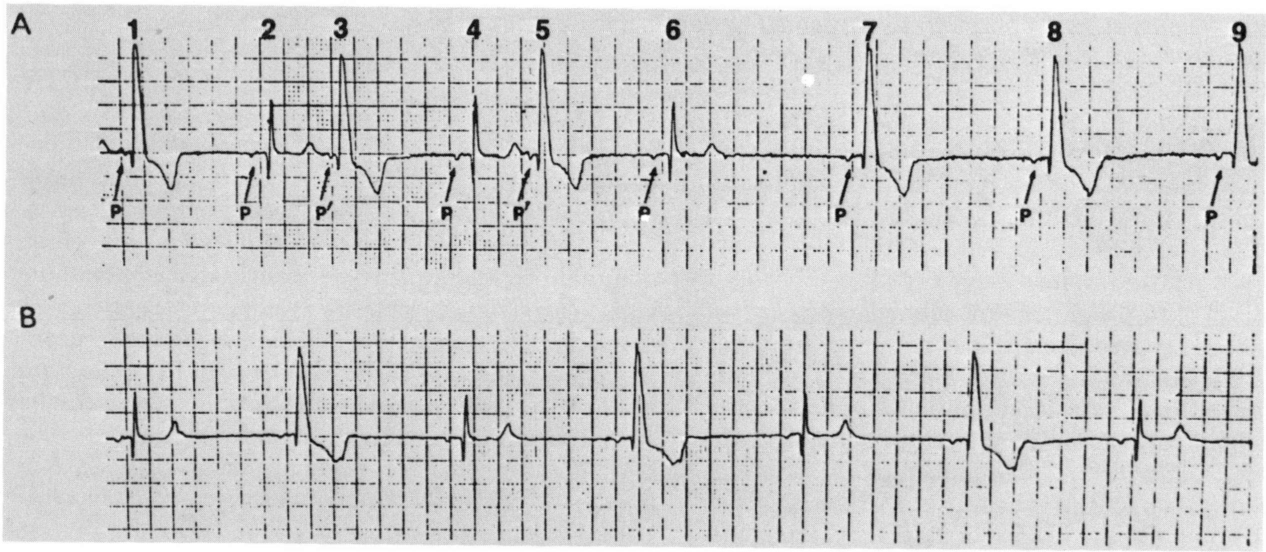

Figure 15-22. *Holter monitoring records from a patient aged 70 years with hypertensive cardiovascular disease complicated by atrial ectopy and multitype right bundle branch block aberrancy. (A) A basic sinus bradyarrhythmia and arrhythmia is interrupted by three premature atrial beats (beats 1, 3, and 5) in a bigeminal pattern. Both the beats closing the shortest cycles (beats 1, 3, and 5) and those closing the longest cycles (beats 7, 8, and 9) exhibit complete right bundle branch block. Beats closing the postectopic cycles (beats 2, 4, and 6), which are intermediate in length, exhibit incomplete right bundle branch block. (B) The sinus beats exhibit alternating incomplete and complete right bundle branch block patterns that are not clearly cycle length dependent, with differences between cycles averaging 0.04 second or less. See text for discussion.*

ulations of cells exhibiting reduced diastolic potential, enhanced automaticity, and variable prolongation of repolarization represent a case in point, since such changes facilitate traversal by the propagating impulse of regions of low potential during all phases of the cardiac cycle, irrespective of cycle length. Prolongation of refractoriness beyond completion of repolarization (see Fig. 15-6) represents an additional factor. This, together with diminished cycle length dependency of action potential duration (see Figs. 15-13 and 15-14) and an increase in the time required for establishment of new steady-state duration (see Fig. 15-13) could accentuate and prolong depressive effects on conduction and refractoriness associated with repolarization and magnify the effects of even very small rate changes. Altered responsiveness characteristics of the type depicted in Figure 15-3*B* also could be a factor in that they might predispose to development of slow conduction in conjunction with even slight lowering of membrane potential without regard to timing in the cycle.

Drug effects also are important. A number of major cardioactive drugs, including particularly high concentrations of the antiarrhythmic agents (*e.g.*, amiodarone and the quinidine-procainamide group), induce changes in action potential duration, responsiveness, conduction, and diastolic potential that predispose to aberration both during repolarization and phase 4. Waxing and waning of such changes in conjunction with varying drug concentrations could result in variations in QRS configuration independent of cycle length. These agents are principally used in patients with heart disease, underscoring their potential importance, since drug and disease-related electrophysiologic changes may act synergistically.

Figures 15-19*B*, 15-20*A*, and 15-21 show schematic diagrams of two possible mechanisms whereby phase 4 depolarization can give rise to aberration independent of cycle length. Both have been discussed in relation to long cycle aberrancy. The first involves accelerated rates of phase 4 depolarization of latent pacemaker cells in the involved tissues in combination with depressed responsiveness (see Figs. 15-19*B* and 15-21). The second presumes excitation of latent pacemaker cells at a time when they undergo large, rapid voltage changes over a brief time span (*i.e.*, in the vicinity of the threshold potential [see Fig. 15-20]) and may be operative even normally. Since these mechanisms allow conduction abnormalities to develop in the absence of significant changes in the dominant cycle, they could explain differences in QRS contour of the two complexes closing cycles of 0.76 second in Figure 15-18*D*. The fact that increases in cycle length beyond beyond 0.76 second resulted in progressively more marked aberration (see Fig. 15-18*A* to *C*) and that the patient also exhibited premature ventricular complexes with a left bundle branch block contour support contentions that differences in QRS contour between the two complexes in Figure 15-18*D* reflect changing levels of diastolic potential in the right bundle branch due to variable phase 4 depolarization. Findings that the case of intermittent left bundle branch block shown in Figure 15-19*B* was associated with premature ventricular complexes exhibiting a right bundle branch block contour suggest that it too could have been due to variable enhancement of automaticity, this time in the left bundle branch system.

The records in Figure 15-12, which were obtained from a specimen of human papillary muscle regularly stimulated at cycle length 1000 msec, show an unusual example of how altered electrophysiologic properties of diseased heart might give rise to aberration without changes in cycle length. Phase 3 of repolarization of the second beat in each of the three panels is interrupted by a spontaneously occurring premature depolarization (see Fig. 15-12, beats *a* to *c*). Premature response *a* is depicted as giving rise to an aberrantly conducted propagated response (short cycle aberrancy); *b* and *c*, on the other hand, occur at such low levels of potential that they would result in nonpropagated local responses. The postextrasystolic complexes (*1*, *2*, and *3*) also show diminished amplitude and $\dot{V}_{max}$ and might be expected to exhibit depressed conduction. If comparable changes were to occur in appropriate portions of the conducting system, aberrancy would ensue. Since premature responses *b* and *c* would not propagate to the rest of the heart and give rise to extrasystoles that would disturb the basic rhythm, alterations in QRS contour of postextrasystolic complexes *2* and *3* would be perceived as occurring in the absence of cycle length changes.

Altered QRS contour due to this cause is probably a variant of short cycle aberrancy in that the first postectopic cycle is shorter than the interval between the basic complexes because of the premature response. Although reasons for the altered characteristics of the postectopic complexes are not clear, the fact that refractoriness may considerably outlast completion of repolarization in diseased heart muscle appears to provide the best explanation in that the premature responses would serve to prolong the recovery process still further.

Mixed Type Aberrancy

The foregoing presumes that the principal types of aberrancy are explicable in terms of a unique mechanism or, at the very least, a unique primary mechanism. This generalization may hold true for most cases of short cycle aberrancy, particularly in normal heart. However, it probably does not apply to the general run of cases occurring in the absence of significant cycle length changes and to instances in which more than one type of aberration occurs in the same patient (see Figs. 15-17 and 15-22). Simultaneous operation of more than one mechanism is required.

The complex interrelationships between the several electrophysiologic variables appears to facilitate the simultaneous operation of multiple mechanisms of aberration. The interrelationships among phase 4 depolarization of automatic cells, diastolic potential, action potential duration, and conduction[56] represent a case in point. Phase 4 depolarization reduces end-diastolic potential of automatic cells with resultant decrease in amplitude and $\dot{V}_{max}$ of action potentials initiated in the involved fibers and variable depression of conduction, changes that predispose to long cycle aberrancy.[56,238–241] Since the time course of repolarization and action potential duration are also voltage dependent (see Figs. 15-3*A*, 15-7, and 15-14), it follows that reduction of diastolic potential by phase 4 depolarization may affect these variables as well (see Fig. 15-19*B*) and thus influence development of short cycle aberration. More specifically, since responses initiated in partially depolarized fibers exhibit foreshortening of the early phases and prolongation of the terminal phases of repolarization, enhanced phase 4 depolarization also might create conditions favorable to short cycle aberrancy. If phase 4 depolarization is allowed to go on unchecked and end-diastolic potential is reduced to sufficiently low levels, a change in voltage–time course of repolarization may develop such that maximum diastolic potential becomes reduced and generalized cell hypopolarization may ensue.[56] Impulses initiated in such fibers may develop slow response characteristics, with all which that entails with respect to depression of responsiveness, time-dependent prolongation of refractoriness, and diminished cycle length dependence of action potential duration. Different types of oscillatory also may develop. This combination of changes would expand the portion of the cycle during which aberration can occur. Conversely, the zone of normal conduction would increasingly be encroached on. As the zone of normal conduction is reduced, aberration becomes increasingly independent of timing in the cycle and of cycle length. Occurrence of aberrancy with only minimal or even without significant cycle length changes and, eventually, fixed bundle branch block represent the culimination of this process.

Numerous other examples can be cited of how the interrelationships between the several electrophysiologic parameters result in changes that might be expected to predispose to simultaneous operation of multiple cellular mechanisms of aberrancy. Occurrence of independent changes in two or more electrophysiologic parameters in the same or different portions of the AV conducting system, due to such causes as cardioactive drugs, ischemia and other types of disease, stretch, and so on, represent additional predisposing factors, as would changes in the cable properties of cardiac fibers. The role of the cable properties of cardiac fibers in conduction has already been mentioned. Changes in membrane resistance and capacitance and in core resistance could cause major changes in conduction velocity during all phases of the cardiac cycle. The extent to which conduction disturbances actually result from changes in the cable properties is uncertain. However, for the reasons cited previously, it is not unreasonable to suppose that changes in at least membrane and core resistance may represent significant factors underlying altered conduction due to such causes as stretch, changes in autonomic tone, altered extracellular ionic concentrations (particularly of potassium), exposure to selected cardioactive drugs, and, most important, ischemia and disease.

The concept that multiple mechanisms of aberrancy may be simultaneously operative has proved useful in explaining a number of peculiarities of conduction that are otherwise difficult to understand, including occurrence of aberration at unusual times during the cardiac cycle, aberration at normal heart rates and with minimal or no clear-cut evidence of cycle length dependency, and multiple types of (see Figs. 15-17 and 15-22) and multiform (see Figs. 15-8 and 15-9) aberrancy in a single patient. Rosenbaum and co-workers[238–240] have invoked the interrelationships between automaticity and conduction to explain cases of intermittent bundle branch block and paroxysmal AV block exhibiting both long and short cycle length dependency characteristics and transient development of fixed block. Observations by this group that many of the patients with long cycle aberrancy also exhibit the short cycle variety are readily explicable on this basis. Our own experience accords with Rosenbaum's in this regard in that we too find the combination of short and long cycle aberrancy in a single patient to be common. Records in Figures 15-17 and 15-22, which show both short and long cycle aberrancy, represent a case in point. The patient whose records are shown in Figure 15-18 represents a second case in point. She originally presented with typical long cycle, right bundle branch block type aberrancy in conjunction with acute anterior infarction and then developed short cycle right bundle branch block type aberration and finally a period of fixed right bundle branch block. Finally, it is pertinent to recall findings from *in vitro* studies showing that specimens of ischemic and diseased human cardiac tissues are characterized by a wide spectrum of electrophysiologic changes that might be expected to predispose to aberration in a number of ways since they underscore the applicability of the multiple mechanism hypothesis to considerations of clinical aberrancy.

References

1. Lewis, T.: The Mechanism and Graphic Registration of the Heart Beat, 3rd ed., p. 91. London, Shaw & Sons, 1925.
2. Lewis, T.: Observations upon disorders of the heart's action. Heart, 3:279–309, 1911.

3. Pick, A., and Langendorf, R.: Interpretation of Complex Arrhythmias. Philadelphia, Lea & Febiger, 1956.
4. Scherf, D., and Schott, A.: Extrasystoles and Allied Arrhythmias. London, William Heinemann, 1973.
5. Schamroth, L.: Disorders of Cardiac Rhythm. Oxford, Blackwell Scientific Publications, 1971.
6. Bellet, S.: Clinical Disorders of the Heart Beat, 3rd ed. Philadelphia, Lea & Febiger, 1971.
7. Chung, E. K.: Principles of Cardiac Arrhythmias. Baltimore, Williams & Wilkins, 1971.
8. Lev, M.: The conduction system. In Gould, S. F. (ed.): Pathology of the Heart and Blood Vessels, 3rd ed., pp. 180–220. Springfield, Ill., Charles C Thomas, 1968.
9. Truex, R. C.: Comparative anatomy and functional considerations of the cardiac conduction system. In Paes de Carvalho, A., De Mello, W. C., and Hoffman, B. F. (eds.): The Specialized Tissues of the Heart, pp. 22–43. Amsterdam, Elsevier, 1961.
10. Davies, M. J.: Pathology of Conducting Tissue of the Heart. New York, Appleton-Century-Crofts, 1971.
11. Rosenbaum, M. B., Elizari, M. O., and Lazzari, J. O.: The Hemiblocks. Oldsmar, Fla., Tampa Tracings, 1970.
12. Demoulin, J. C., and Kulbertus, H. E.: Left hemiblocks revisited from the histopathological viewpoint. Am. Heart J., 86:712–713, 1973.
13. Massing, G. K., and James, T. N.: Anatomical configuration of the His bundle and bundle branches in the human heart. Circulation, 53:609–621, 1976.
14. James, T. N.: The connecting pathways between the sinus node and A-V node and between the right and the left atrium in the human heart. Am. Heart J., 66:498–508, 1963.
15. Wagner, M. L., Lazzara, R., Weiss, R. M., and Hoffman, B. F.: Specialized conducting fibers in the interatrial band. Circ. Res., 18:502–518, 1966.
16. Langendorf, R.: Concealed A-V conduction: The effect of blocked impulses on the formation and conduction of subsequent impulses. Am. Heart J., 35:542–552, 1948.
17. Hoffman, B. F., Cranefield, P. F., and Stuckey, J. H.: Concealed conduction. Circ. Res., 9:194–203, 1961
18. Moe, G. K., Abildskov, J. A., and Mendez, C.: An experimental study of concealed conduction. Am. Heart J., 67:338–356, 1964.
19. Pick, A., Langendorf, R., and Katz, L.: The supernormal phase of atrioventricular conduction. I. Fundamental mechanisms. Circulation, 26:388–404, 1962.
20. Moe, G. K., Childers, R. W., and Merideth, J.: An appraisal of "supernormal" A-V conduction. Circulation, 38:5–28, 1968.
21. Singer, D. H., and Ten Eick, R. E.: Aberrancy: Electrophysiologic aspects. Am. J. Cardiol., 28:381–401, 1971.
22. Davson, H.: A Textbook of General Physiology, 4th ed., Baltimore, Williams & Wilkins, 1970.
23. Aidley, D. J.: The Physiology of Excitable Cells. Cambridge, Cambridge University Press, 1978.
24. Sperelakis, N. (ed).: Physiology and Pathophysiology of the Heart. Boston, Martinus Nijhoff, 1984.
25. Hoffman, B. F., and Cranefield, P. F.: Electrophysiology of the Heart. New York, McGraw-Hill, 1960.
26. Singer, D. H., and Ten Eick, R. E.: Electrophysiology of the heart and genesis of cardiac arrhythmias. In Conn, H. L., Jr., and Horwitz, O. (eds.): Cardiac and Vascular Diseases, vol. 1, pp. 182–213. Philadelphia, Lea & Febiger, 1971.
27. Trautwein, W.: Membrane currents in cardiac muscle fibers. Physiol. Rev., 53:793–835, 1973.
28. Weidmann, S.: Heart: Electrophysiology. Ann. Rev. Physiol., 36:155–169, 1974.
29. Noble, D.: The Initiation of the Heart Beat. Oxford, Clarendon Press, 1979.
30. Cranefield, P. F.: The Conduction of the Cardiac Impulse. The Slow Response and Cardiac Arrhythmias. Mt. Kisco, N.Y., Futura, 1975.
31. Fozzard, H. A.: Cardiac muscle: excitability and passive electrical properties. Prog. Cardiovasc. Dis., 19:343–359, 1977.
32. Sperelakis, N.: Origin of the Cardiac Resting Potential. In Berne, R. M., Sperelakis, N., and Geiger, S. R. (eds.): Handbook of Physiology, section 2. The Cardiovascular System, vol. 1, pp. 187–267. Baltimore, Williams & Wilkins, 1979.
33. Carmeliet, E., and Vereecke, J.: Electrogenesis of the action potential and automaticity. In Berne, R. M., Sperelakis, N., and Geiger, S. R. (eds.): Handbook of Physiology, section 2. The Cardiovascular System, vol. 1, pp. 269–334. Baltimore, Williams & Wilkins, 1979.
34. Zipes, D. P., Bailey, J. C., and Elharrar, V. (eds.): The Slow Inward Current and Cardiac Arrhythmias. Boston, Martinus Nijhoff, 1980.
35. Noble, D.: The surprising heart: A review of recent progress in cardiac electrophysiology. J. Physiol., 353:1–50, 1984.
36. Ten Eick, R. E., Baumgarten, C. M., and Singer, D. H.: Ventricular dysrhythmia: Membrane basis or of currents, channels, gates and cables. Prog. Cardiovasc. Dis., 24:157–188, 1981.
37. Ling, G., and Gerard, R. W.: The normal membrane potential of frog sartorius fibers. J. Cell. Comp. Physiol., 34:383–396, 1949.
38. Trautwein, W.: Generation and conduction of impulses in the heart as affected by drugs. Pharmacol. Rev., 15:277–332, 1963.
39. Singer, D. H.: Possible modes of pharmacologic regulation of disturbances of cardiac rate and rhythm. In Manning, G. W. (ed.): Electrical Activity of the Heart, pp. 163–194. Springfield, Ill., Charles C Thomas, 1968.
40. Singer, D. H., and Ten Eick, R. E.: Pharmacology of cardiac arrhythmias. Prog. Cardiovasc. Dis., 11:488–514, 1969.
41. Gettes, L. S.: The electrophysiologic effects of antiarrhythmic drugs. Am. J. Cardiol., 28:526–535, 1971.
42. Bassett, A. L., and Hoffman, B. F.: Antiarrhythmic drugs: Electrophysiological actions. Ann. Rev. Pharmacol., 11:143–170, 1971.
43. Rosen, M. R., and Hoffman, B. F.: Mechanisms of action of antiarrhythmic drugs. Circ. Res., 32:1–8, 1973.
44. Hauswirth, O., and Singh, B. N.: Ionic mechanisms in heart muscle in relation to the genesis and the pharmacologic control of cardiac arrhythmias. Pharmacol. Rev., 30:5–63, 1978.
45. Hondeghem, L. M., and Katzung, B. G.: Time- and voltage-dependent interactions of antiarrhythmic drugs with cardiac sodium channels. Biochem. Biophys. Acta, 472:373–398, 1977.
46. Carmeliet, E.: Selectivity of antiarrhythmic drugs and ionic channels: A historical overview. Ann. N. Y. Acad. Sci., 427:1–15, 1984.
47. Coraboeuf, E., Deroubaix, E., and Coulombe, A.: Acidosis-induced abnormal repolarization and repetitive activity in isolated dog Purkinje fibers. J. Physiol. (Paris), 76:97–106, 1980.
48. Hodgkin, A. L.: The ionic basis of electrical activity in nerve and muscle. Biol. Rev., 26:339–409, 1951.
49. Sperelakis, N.: Electrical properties of cells at rest and maintenance of the ion distribution. In Sperelakis, N. (ed.): Physiology and Pathophysiology of the Heart, pp. 59–82. Boston, Martinus Nijhoff, 1984.
50. Hille, B.: Ionic channels in nerve membranes. Prog. Biophys. Mol. Biol., 21:1–32, 1970.
51. Page, E., and Storm, S. R.: Cat heart muscle in vitro. VIII. Active transports of sodium in papillary muscles. J. Gen. Physiol., 48:957–972, 1965.
52. Mullins, L. J.: Ion Transport in Heart. New York, Raven Press, 1981.
53. Gadsby, D. C.: The Na/K pump of cardiac cells. Am. Rev. Biophys. Bioeng., 13:373–398, 1984.
54. Weidmann, S.: The effect of the cardiac membrane potential on

the rapid availability of the sodium carrying system. J. Physiol., 127:213–224, 1955.
55. Hoffman, B. F., Kao, C. Y., and Suckling, E. E.: Refractoriness in cardiac muscle. Am. J. Physiol., 190:473–482, 1957.
56. Singer, D. H., Lazzara, R., and Hoffman, B. F.: Interrelationships between automaticity and conduction in Purkinje fibers. Circ. Res., 21:537–558, 1967.
57. Reuter, H.: The dependence of slow inward current in Purkinje fibres on the extracellular calcium-concentration. J. Physiol., 192:479–492, 1967.
58. Reuter, H.: Properties of two inward membrane currents. Ann. Rev. Physiol., 41:413–424, 1979.
59. Kohlhardt, M., Bauer, B., Krause, H., et al.: Differentiation of the transmembrane Na and Ca channels in mammalian cardiac fibers by the use of specific inhibitors. Pfluegers Arch., 335:309–322, 1972.
60. Paes de Carvalho, A., Hoffman, B. F., and de Paula Carvalho, M.: Two components of the cardiac action potential. I. Voltage-time course and the effect of acetylcholine on atrial and nodal cells of the rabbit heart. J. Gen. Physiol., 54:607–635, 1969.
61. Wit, A. L., and Cranefield, P. F.: Effect of verapamil on the sinoatrial and atrioventricular nodes of the rabbit and the mechanism by which it arrests reentrant atrioventricular nodal tachycardia. Circ. Res., 35:413–425, 1974.
62. Zipes, D. P., and Fischer, J. C.: Effects of agents which inhibit the slow channel on sinus node automaticity and atrioventricular conduction in the dog. Circ. Res., 34:184–192, 1974.
63. Merideth, J., Mendez, C., Mueller, W. J., and Moe, G. K.: Electrical excitability of atrioventricular nodal cells. Circ. Res., 23:69–85, 1968.
64. Mendez, C., and Moe, G. K.: Atrioventricular transmission. In De Mello, W. C. (ed.): Electrical Phenomena in the Heart, pp. 263–291. New York, Academic Press, 1972.
65. Zipes, D. P., and Mendez, C.: Action of manganese ions and tetrodotoxin on atrioventricular nodal transmembrane potentials in isolated rabbit hearts. Circ. Res., 32:447–454, 1973.
66. Wit, A. L., Fenaglio, J. J. Jr., Wagner, B. M., et al.: Electrophysiologic properties of cardiac muscle in the anterior mitral valve leaflet and the adjacent atrium in the dog: Possible implications for the genesis of atrial dysrhythmias. Circ. Res., 32:731–747, 1973.
67. Wit, A. L., and Cranefield, P. F.: Triggered and automatic activity in the canine coronary sinus. Circ. Res., 41:435–445, 1977.
68. Cranefield, P. F., Wit, A. L., and Hoffman, B. F.: Conduction of the cardiac impulse. IV. Characteristics of very slow conduction. J. Gen. Physiol., 59:227–246, 1972.
69. Cranefield, P. F., Aronson, R. S., and Wit, A. L.: Effect of verapamil on the normal action potential and on a calcium dependent slow response of canine cardiac Purkinje fibers. Circ. Res., 34:204–213, 1974.
70. Solberg, L. E., Singer, D. H., and Ten Eick, R. E.: Electrophysiological study of myocardial infarction in dog (abstr.). Fed. Proc., 31:387, 1972.
71. Solberg, L., Ten Eick, R. E., and Singer, D. H.: Electrophysiological basis of arrhythmia in infarcted ventricle (abstr.). Circulation, 46(Suppl. II):116, 1972.
72. Lazzara, R., El-Sherif, N., and Scherlag, B. J.: Electrophysiological properties of canine purkinje cells in one-day old myocardial infarction. Circ. Res., 33:722–734, 1973.
73. Friedman, P. L., Stewart, J. R., Fenoglio, J. J., Jr., and Wit, A. L.: Survival of subendocardial Purkinje fibers after extensive myocardial infarction in dogs; in vitro and in vivo correlations. Circ. Res., 33:597–611, 1973.
74. Ten Eick, R. E., Singer, D. H., and Solberg, L. E.: Coronary occlusion. Effects on cellular electrical activity of the heart. Med. Clin. North Am., 60:49–67, 1976.
75. Lazzara, R., and Scherlag, R.: Cellular electrophysiology and ischemia. In Sperelakis, N. (ed.): Physiology and Pathophysiology of the Heart, pp. 443–458. Boston, Martinus Nijhoff, 1984.
76. Trautwein, W., Kassebaum, D. G., Nelson, R. M., and Hecht, H. H. Electrophysiological study of human heart muscle. Circ. Res., 10:306–312, 1962.
77. Singer, D. H., Ten Eick, R. E., and DeBoer, A. A.: Electrophysiologic correlates of human atrial tachyarrhythmias. In Dreifus, L., and Likoff, W. (eds.): Cardiac Arrhythmias, pp. 97–111. New York, Grune & Stratton, 1973.
78. Hordof, A. J., Edie, R., Malm, J. R., et al.: Electrophysiologic properties and response to pharmacologic agents of fibers from diseased human atria. Circulation, 54:774–779, 1976.
79. Ten Eick, R. E., and Singer, D. H.: Electrophysiologic properties of diseased human atrium. I. Low diastolic potential and altered cellular response to potassium. Circ. Res., 44:545–557, 1979.
80. Singer, D. H., Ten Eick, R. E., and DeBoer, A. A.: Possible electrophysiologic basis of chronic dysrhythmia. Circulation, 46(Suppl. II):90, 1972.
81. Singer, D. H., and Ten Eick, R. E.: Electrophysiologic correlates of aberrancy in diseased hearts (abstr). Am. J. Cardiol., 29:293, 1972.
82. Ten Eick, R. E., Singer, D. H., Solberg, L. E., and DeBoer, A. A.: Alterations in the electrophysiological characteristics of diseased human ventricle (abstr.). Circulation, 44(Suppl. II):9, 1972.
83. Chua, W. T., Singer, D. H., and Ten Eick, R. E.: Ventricular dysrhythmia in man: Cellular electrophysiologic aspects (abstr.). Clin. Res., 29:181, 1981.
84. Chua, W., Singer, D., Ten Eick, R., et al.: Well polarized but abnormal cells: A cause of increased heterogeneity in diseased human ventricle (abstr.). Fed. Proc., 41:1385, 1982.
85. Spear, J. F., Horowitz, L. N., Hodess, A. B., et al.: Cellular electrophysiology of human myocardial infarction. I. Abnormalities of cellular activation. Circulation, 59:247–256, 1979.
86. Talano, J. V., Singer, D. H., Ten Eick, R. E., et al.: Intractable ventricular tachyarrhythmia in post-infarction aneurysm: Clinical, electrophysiologic and electropharmacologic studies. Clin. Res., 24:242A, 1976.
87. Singer, D. H., Baumgarten, C. M., and Ten Eick, R. E.: Cellular electrophysiology of ventricular and other dysrhythmias: Studies on diseased and ischemic heart. Prog. Cardiovasc. Dis., 24:97–156, 1981.
88. Dangmann, K. H., Danilo, P., Hordof, A., et al.: Electrophysiologic characteristics of human ventricular and Purkinje fibers. Circulation, 65:362–368, 1982.
89. Gilmour, R. F., Heger, J. J., Prystowsky, E. N., and Zipes, D. P.: Cellular electrophysiologic abnormalities of diseased human ventricular myocardium. Am. J. Cardiol., 51:137–143, 1983.
90. Mary-Rabine, L., Albert, A., Pham, T. D., et al.: The relationship of human atrial cellular electrophysiology to clinical function and ultrastructure. Circ. Res., 52:188–199, 1983.
91. Spear, J. F., Horowitz, L. N., and Moore, E. N.: The slow response in human ventricle. In Zipes, D. P., Bailey, J. C., Elharrar, V. (eds.): The Slow Inward Current and Cardiac Arrhythmias, pp. 309–326. Boston, Martinus Nijhoff, 1980.
92. Rosen, M. R., and Hordof, A. J.: The slow response in human atrium. In Zipes, D. P., Bailey, J. C., and Elharrar, V. (eds.): The Slow Inward Current and Cardiac Arrhythmias, pp. 295–308. Boston, Martinus Nijhoff, 1980.
93. Lazzara, R., and Scherlag, B.: Role of the inward current in the genesis of arrhythmias in ischemic myocardium. In Zipes, D. P., Bailey, J. L., Elharrar, V. (eds.): The Slow Inward Current and Cardiac Arrhythmias, pp. 399–416. Boston, Martinus Nijhoff, 1980.
94. Noble, D., and Tsien, R. W.: The repolarization process of heart

cells. In DeMello, W. C. (ed.): Electrical Phenomena in the Heart, pp. 133–161. New York, Academic Press, 1972.
95. Kenyon, J. L., and Gibbons, W. R.: Influence of chloride potassium, and tetraethylammonium on the early outward current of sheep cardiac Purkinje fibers. J. Gen. Physiol., 73:117–138, 1979.
96. Baumgarten, C. M., and Isenberg, G.: Depletion and accumulation of potassium in the extracellular clefts of cardiac Purkinje fibers during voltage clamp hyperpolarization and depolarization. Pfluegers Arch., 368:19–31, 1977.
97. Dant, J., and Rudel, R.: The electrogenic sodium pump in guinea-pig ventricular muscle: Inhibition of pump current by cardiac glycosides. J. Physiol., 330:243–264, 1982.
98. Gadsby, D. C., and Cranfield, P. F.: Effects of electrogenic sodium extrusion on the membrane potential of cardiac Purkinje fibers. In Paes de Carvalho, A. P., Hoffman, B. F., and Lieberman, M. (eds.): Normal and Abnormal Conduction in the Heart, pp. 225–247. New York, Futura, 1982.
99. Ten Eick, R. E., and Singer, D. H.: Effect of membrane potential and potassium on threshold potential (abstr.). Fed. Proc., 28:270, 1969.
100. Hoffman, B. F., and Cranefield, P. F.: Physiologic basis of cardiac arrhythmias. Am. J. Med., 37:670–684, 1964.
101. Katzung, B. G., Hondeghem, L. M., and Grant, A. O.: Cardiac ventricular automaticity induced by current of injury. Pfluegers Arch., 360:193–197, 1975.
102. Katzung, B. G., and Morgenstern, J. A.: Effects of extracellular potassium on ventricular automaticity and evidence for a pacemaker current in mammalian ventricular myocardium. Circ. Res., 40:105–111, 1977.
103. Imanishi, S., and Surawicz, B.: Automatic activity in depolarized guinea pig ventricular myocardium. Characteristics and mechanisms. Circ. Res., 39:751–759, 1976.
104. Wit, A. L., Cranefield, P. F., and Gadsby, D. C.: Triggered activity. In Zipes, D. P., Bailey, J. C., and Elharrar, V. (eds.): The Slow Inward Current and Cardiac Arrhythmias, pp. 437–454. Boston, Martinus Nijhoff, 1980.
105. DiFrancesco, D.: A new interpretation of the pace-maker current in calf Purkinje fibres. J. Physiol., 314:359–376, 1981.
106. DiFrancesco, D.: A study of the ionic nature of the pace-maker current in calf Purkinje fibres. J. Physiol., 314:377–393, 1981.
107. Brown, H., and DiFrancesco, D.: Voltage-clamp investigations of membrane currents underlying pace-maker activity in rabbit sino-atrial node. J. Physiol., 308:331–351, 1980.
108. DiFrancesco, D., and Ojeda, C.: Properties of the current i_f in the sino-atrial node $^{i}K_2$ in Purkinje fibres. J. Physiol., 308:353–367, 1980.
109. Brown, H. F., Kimura, J., Noble, D., et al.: The ionic currents underlying pacemaker activity in rabbit sino-atrial node: Experimental results and computer simulations. Proc. R. Soc. Lond. (B) 222:329–347, 1984.
110. Irisawa, H.: General comments: Ionic currents underlying spontaneous rhythm of the cardiac primary pacemaker cells. In Bonke, F. (ed.): The Sinus Node, pp. 368–378. The Hague, Martinus Nijhoff Medical Division, 1978.
111. Jack, J. J. B., Noble, D., and Tsien, R. W.: Electric Current Flow In Excitable Cells. Oxford, Clarendon, 1975.
112. Fozzard, H. A.: Conduction of the action potential. In Berne, R. M., Sperelakis, N., and Geiger, S. R.: Handbook of Physiology, section 2, The Cardiovascular System, vol. 1, pp. 335–356. Baltimore, Williams & Wilkins, 1979.
113. Spach, M. S., and Kootsey, J. M.: The nature of electrical propagation in cardiac muscle. Am. J. Physiol., 244:H3–H22, 1983.
114. Cranefield, P. F.: Channels, cables, networks and the conduction of the cardiac impulse. Am. J. Physiol., 245:H901–910, 1983.
115. Van Dam, R. T., Moore, E. N., and Hoffman, B. F.: Initiation and conduction of impulses in partially depolarized cardiac fibers. Am. J. Physiol., 204:1133–1144, 1963.
116. Weidmann, S.: Effects of calcium ions and local anesthetics on electrical properties of Purkinje fibers. J. Physiol., 129:568–582, 1955.
117. Hoffman, B. F.: The action of quinidine and procainamide on single fibers of dog ventricle and specialized conduction systems. Ann. Acad. Bras. Cienc. 29:365–369, 1958.
118. Peon, J. Ferrier, G. R., and Moe, G. K.: The relationship of excitability to conduction velocity in canine Purkinje tissue. Circ. Res., 43:125–135, 1978.
119. Dominguez, G., and Fozzard, H. A.: Influence of extracellular K^+ concentration on cable properties and excitability of sheep cardiac Purkinje fibers. Circ. Res., 26:565–574, 1970.
120. Spear, J. F., and Moore, E. N.: Supernormal excitability and conduction in the His-Purkinje system of the dog. Circ. Res., 35:782–792, 1974.
121. Arnsdorf, M. F., and Bigger, J. T., Jr.: The effect of procainamide on components of excitability in long mammalian cardiac Purkinje fibers. Circ. Res., 38:115–122, 1976.
122. Arnsdorf, M. F., and Bigger, J. T., Jr.: The effect of lidocaine on components of excitability in long mammalian cardiac Purkinje fibers. J. Pharmacol. Exp. Ther., 195:206–215, 1975.
123. Weingart, R., Imanaga, I., and Weidmann, S.: Low resistance pathways between myocardial cells. In Fleckenstein, A., and Dhalla, N. S. (eds.): Basic Functions of Cations in Myocardial Activity, pp. 227–232. Baltimore, University Park Press, 1975.
124. McNutt, N. S., and Weinstein, R. S.: Membrane ultrastructure at mammalian intercellular junctions. Prog. Biophys. Mol. Biol., 26:45–101, 1973.
125. Sommer, J. R., and Johnson, E. A.: Ultrastructure of cardiac muscle. In Berne, R. M., Sperelakis, N., and Geiger, S. R. (eds.): Handbook of Physiology, section 2, The Cardiovascular System, pp. 113–186. Baltimore, Williams & Wilkins, 1979.
126. Dewey, M. M., and Barr, L.: Intercellular connections between smooth muscle cells: The nexus. Science, 137:670–672, 1962.
127. Clerc, L.: Directional differences of impulse spread in trabecular muscle from mammalian heart. J. Physiol., 255:335–346, 1976.
128. Weingart, R.: The actions of ouabain of intercellular coupling and conduction velocity in mammalian ventricular muscle. J. Physiol. (Lond.), 264:341–365, 1977.
129. Turin, L., and Warner, A.: Carbon dioxide reversibly abolishes ionic communications between cells of early amphibian embryo. Nature, 270:56–57, 1977.
130. Janse, M. J., VanCapelle, F. J. L., Morsink, H., et al.: Flow of "injury" current and patterns of excitation during early ventricular arrhythmias in acute regional myocardial ischemia in isolated porcine and canine hearts. Evidence for two different arrhythmogenic mechanisms. Circ. Res., 47:151–165, 1980.
131. Lieberman, M., Kootsey, J. M., Johnson, E. A., and Sawanobori, T.: Slow conduction in cardiac muscle. Biophys. J., 13:37–55, 1973.
132. DeMello, W. C.: Influence of the sodium pump on intercellular communication in heart fibres: Effect of intracellular injection of calcium and strontium on cell communication in heart. J. Physiol. (Lond.), 263:171–197, 1976.
133. Wojtczak, J.: Contractures and increase in internal longitudinal resistance of cow ventricular muscle induced by hypoxia. Circ. Res., 44:88–95, 1978.
134. Cranefield, P. F., Klein, H. O., and Hoffman, B. F.: Conduction of the cardiac impulse. I. Delay, block, and one-way block in depressed Purkinje fibers. Circ. Res., 28:199–219, 1971.
135. Cranefield, P. F., and Hoffman, B. F.: Conduction of the cardiac impulse. II. Summation and inhibition. Circ. Res., 28:220–233, 1971.
136. Gettes, L. S., and Reuter, H.: Slow recovery from inactivation of

inward currents in mammalian myocardial fibers. J. Physiol. 240:703–724, 1974.
137. Saikawa, T., and Carmeliet, E.: Slow recovery of the maximal rate of rise (V_{max}) of the action potential in sheep cardiac Purkinje fibers. Pfluegers Arch., 394(Suppl.):90–93, 1982.
138. Lazzara, R., El-Sherif, N., and Scherlag, B. J.: Ischemia of the canine His bundle. Circ. Res., 36:444–454, 1975.
139. Wood, F. C., Wolferth, C. C., and Geckeler, G. D.: Histologic demonstration of accessory muscular connections between auricle and ventricle in a case of short P-R interval and prolonged QRS complex. Am. Heart J., 25:454–462, 1943.
140. Mahaim, I.: Kent's fibers and the A-V paraspecific conduction through the upper connections of the bundle of His-Tawara. Am. Heart J., 33:651–653, 1947.
141. Lev, M., and Lerner, R.: The theory of Kent. A histologic study of the normal atrioventricular communications of the human heart. Circulation, 12:176–184, 1955.
142. James, T. N.: Morphology of the human atrioventricular node, with remarks pertinent to its electrophysiology. Am. Heart J., 62:756–771, 1961.
143. Lenegre, J.: Etiology and pathology of bilateral bundle branch block in relation to complete heart block. Prog. Cardiovasc. Dis., 6:409–444, 1964.
144. Lev, M.: The pathology of complete atrioventricular block. Prog. Cardiovasc. Dis., 6:317–326, 1964.
145. Hoffman, B. F., Moore, E. N., Stuckey, J. H., et al.: Functional properties of the atrioventricular conduction system. Circ. Res., 13:308–328, 1963.
146. Chen, C. M., Gettes, L. S., and Katzung, B. G.: Effect of lidocaine and quinidine on steady-state characteristics and recovery kinetics of $(dv/dt)_{max}$ in guinea pig ventricular myocardium. Circ. Res., 37:20–29, 1975.
147. Weld, F. M., and Bigger, J. T.: Effect of lidocaine on the early inward transient current in sheet cardiac Purkinje fibers. Circ. Res., 37:630–639, 1975.
148. Bean, B. P., Cohen, C. J., and Tsien, R. W.: Lidocaine block of cardiac sodium channels. J. Gen. Physiol., 81:613–642, 1983.
149. Hondeghem, L. M., and Katzung, B. G.: Antiarrhythmic agents: the modulated receptor mechanism of action of sodium and calcium channel-blocking drugs. Am. Rev. Pharmacol. Toxicol., 24:387–423, 1984.
150. Jalife, J., Antzelevitch, C., Lamanna, V., and Moe, G. K.: Rate-dependent changes in excitability of depressed cardiac Purkinje fibers as a mechanism of intermittent bundle branch block. Circulation, 67:912–922, 1983.
151. Kaufmann, R., and Rothberger, C. J.: Beitrage zur Entstehungsweise extrasystolischer Allorhythmien (Zweite Mitteilung). Z. Gesamte Exp. Med., 7:199–236, 1919.
152. Sherf, L., and James, T. N.: A new electrocardiographic concept: Synchronized sinoventricular conduction. Dis. Chest, 55:127–140, 1969.
153. Moe, G. K., Preston, J. B., and Burlington, H.: Physiologic evidence for a dual A-V transmission system. Circ. Res., 4:357:375, 1956.
154. Narula, O.: Longitudinal dissociation in the His bundle. Bundle branch block due to asynchronous conduction within the His bundle in man. Circulation, 56:996–1006, 1977.
155. Janse, M. J.: Influence of the direction of the atrial wave front on A-V nodal transmission in isolated hearts of rabbits. Circ. Res., 25:439–449, 1969.
156. Myerburg, R. J., Stewart, J. W., and Hoffman, B. F.: Electrophysiological properties of the canine peripheral A-V conducting system. Circ. Res., 26:361–378, 1970.
157. Myerburg, R. J., Gelband, H., and Hoffman, B. F.: Functional characteristics of the gating mechanism in the canine A-V conducting system. Circ. Res., 28:136–147, 1971.
158. Mendez, C. Mueller, W. J., Merideth, J. T., and Moe, G. K.: Interaction of transmembrane potentials in canine Purkinje fibers and at Purkinje fiber-muscle junctions. Circ. Res., 24:361–372, 1969.
159. Cohen, S. I., Lau, S. H., Haft, J. I., and Damato, A. N.: Experimental production of aberrant ventricular conduction in man. Circulation, 36:673–685, 1967.
160. Cohen, S. I., Lau, S. H., Stein, E., et al.: Variations of aberrant ventricular conduction in man: evidence of isolated and combined block within the specialized conduction system. Circulation, 38:899–916, 1968.
161. Denes, P., Wu, D., Dhingra, R. C., et al.: Electrophysiological observations in patients with rate dependent bundle branch block. Circulation, 51:244–250, 1975.
162. Ashman, R. C., and Byer, E.: Aberration in the conduction of premature ventricular impulses. J. La. State Univ. School Med., 8:62–65, 1946.
163. Gouaux, J. L., and Ashman, R.: Auricular fibrillation with aberration simulating ventricular paroxysmal tachycardia. Am. Heart J., 34:366–373, 1947.
164. Langendorf, R.: Aberrant ventricular conduction. Am. Heart J., 41:700–707, 1951.
165. Langendorf, R.: Differential diagnosis of ventricular paroxysmal tachycardia. Exp. Med. Surg. 8:228–239, 1950.
166. Sandler, I. A., and Marriott, H. J. L.: The differential morphology of anomalous ventricular complexes of RBBB type in lead V_1. Ventricular ectopy versus aberration. Circulation, 31:551–556, 1965.
167. Marriott, H. J. L., and Sandler, I. A.: Criteria, old and new, for differentiating between ectopic ventricular beats and aberrant ventricular conduction in the presence of atrial fibrillation. Prog. Cardiovasc. Dis., 9:18–28, 1966.
168. Kistin, A. D.: Problems in the differentiation of ventricular arrhythmia from supraventricular arrhythmia with abnormal QRS. Prog. Cardiovasc. Dis., 9:1–17, 1966.
169. Wellens, H. J. J., Bar, F. W. H. M., and Lie, K. I.: The valve of the electrocardiogram in the differential diagnosis of a tachycardia with a wide QRS complex. Am. J. Med., 64:27–33, 1978.
170. Moe, G. K., Mendez, C., and Han, J.: Aberrant A-V impulse propagation in the dog heart: A study of functional bundle branch block. Circ. Res., 16:261–286, 1965.
170a. Han, J., Millet, D., Chizzonotti, B., and Moe, G. K.: Temporal dispersion of recovery of excitability in atrium and ventricle as a function of heart rate. Am. Heart J., 71:481–487, 1966.
171. Carter, J. B.: The fundamentals of electrocardiographic interpretation. J.A.M.A., 99:1345–1352, 1932.
172. Shearn, M. A., and Rytand, D. A.: Intermittent bundle branch block. Observations with special reference to the critical heart rate. Arch. Intern. Med., 91:448–463, 1953.
173. Cooksey, J. D., Dunn, M., and Massie, E.,: Clinical Vectorcardiography and Electrocardiography, p. 528. Chicago, Year Book Medical Publishers, 1977.
174. Berliner, K., and Lewithin, L.: Auricular premature systole. I. Aberration of the ventricular complex in the electrocardiogram. Am. Heart J., 29:449–478, 1945.
175. White, P. D.,: Heart Disease, p. 867. New York, Macmillan, 1951.
176. Guerot, C. L., Valere, P. E., Castillo-Fenoy, A., and Tricot, R.: Tachycardie par re-entree de branche a branch. Arch. Mal. Coeur, 67:1–11, 1974.
177. Lewis, T., and Master, A. M.: Observations upon conduction in the mammalian heart: A-V conduction. Heart, 12:209–269, 1925–1926.
178. Scherf, D.: Uber intraventrikulare Storungen der Erregungsausbreitung bei den Wenckebachschen Perioden. Wein. Arch. Inn. Med., 18:403–416, 1929.
179. Fisch, C., Zipes, D. P., and McHenry, P. L.: Rate dependency aberrancy. Circulation, 48:714–724, 1973.

180. Neuss, H., Thormann, J., and Schlepper, M.: Electrophysiological findings in frequency dependent left bundle branch block. Br. Heart J., 36:888–898, 1974.
181. Klein, H., Singer, D., and Hoffman, B.: Alterations of sinus rhythm by atrial premature systoles. Circulation, 34(Suppl. III):145, 1966.
182. Klein, H. O., Singer, D. H., and Hoffman, B. F.: Effect of atrial premature systoles on sinus rhythm in the rabbit, Circ. Res., 32:480–491, 1973.
183. Bonke, F., Bouman, L., and Schopman, F.: Effects of an early atrial premature beat on activity of the sinoatrial node and atrial rhythm in the rabbit. Circ. Res., 29:704–715, 1971.
184. Moe, G. K., and Mendez, C.: Functional block in the intraventricular conduction system. Circulation, 43:949–954, 1971.
185. Downar, E., Janse, M. J., and Durrer, D.: The effect of acute coronary artery occlusion on subepicardial transmembrane potentials in the intact porcine heart. Circulation, 56:217–224, 1977.
186. Ten Eick, R. E., and Basset, A. L.: Cardiac hypertrophy and altered cellular electrical activity of the myocardium. In Sperelakis, N. (ed.): Physiology and Pathophysiology of the Heart, pp. 521–542. Boston, Martinus Nijhoff, 1984.
187. Brooks, C. McC., Gilbert, J. L., Greenspan, M. E., et al.: Excitability and electrical response of ischemic heart muscle. Am. J. Physiol., 198:1143–1147, 1960.
188. Moore, E. N., Preston, J. B., and Moe, G. K.: Durations of transmembrane action potentials and functional refractory periods of canine false tendon and ventricular myocardium: Comparisons in single fibers. Circ. Res., 17:259–273, 1965.
189. Moore, E. N.: Microelectrode studies on concealment of multiple premature atrial responses. Circ. Res., 18:660–672, 1966.
190. Elizari, M. V., Greenspan, K., and Fisch, C.: Electrophysiologic studies on intraventricular aberrant conduction. Adv. Cardiol., 14:115–124, 1975.
191. Toyami, J.: Responses of the His-Purkinje conducting system to supraventricular premature beats—in vitro and in vivo canine experiments on ventricular aberrant conduction. Jpn. Circ. J., 40:1401–1408, 1976.
192. Bailey, J. C., Lathrop, D. A., and Pippenger, D. L.: Differences between proximal left and right bundle branch block action potential durations and refractoriness in the dog heart. Circ. Res., 40:464–468, 1977.
193. Zipes, D. P., Knope, R. F., Mendez, C., and Moe, G. K.: The site of functional right bundle branch block in the intact canine heart. Adv. Cardiol., 14:105–114.
194. Damato, A. M., Lau, S. H., Berkowitz, W. D., et al.: Recording of specialized conducting fibers (A-V nodal, His bundle, and right bundle branch) in man using an electrode catheter technique. Circulation, 16:261–286, 1965.
195. Rosen, K. M., Ahahbudin, H., Rahimtoola, M. B., et al.: Bundle branch and ventricular activation in man. Circulation, 43:193–203, 1971.
196. Krongrad, E., Hefler, S. E., Bowman, F. O., Jr., et al.: Further observations on the etiology of the right bundle branch block pattern following right ventriculotomy. Circulation, 50:1105–1113, 1974.
197. Moore, E. N., Hoffman, B. F., Patterson, D. F., and Stuckey, J. H.: Electrocardiographic changes due to delayed activation of the wall of the right ventricle. Am. Heart J., 68:347–361, 1964.
198. Rosen, K. M., Mehta, M., and Miller, R. A.: Demonstration of dual atrioventricular nodal pathways in man. Am. J. Cardiol., 33:291–294, 1974.
199. Sciacca, A., and Sangiorgi, M.: Trouble de la conduction intraventriculaire droite du a la lesion du tronc common du faisceau de His. Acta Cardiol., 12:486–492, 1957.
200. Fabregas, R. A., Tse, W. W., and Han, J.: Conduction disturbances of the bundle branches produced by lesions in the nonbranching portion of the His bundle. Am. Heart J., 92:356–362, 1976.
201. El-Sherif, N., Scherlag, B. J., and Lazzara, R.: Conduction disorders in the canine proximal His-Purkinje system following acute myocardial ischemia. II. The pathology of bilateral bundle branch block. Circulation, 49:848–857, 1974.
202. Scherlag, B. J., El-Sherif, N., and Lazzara, R.: Bundle branch block due to His bundle lesions. Am. J. Cardiol., 33:169, 1974.
203. Han, J., and Fabregas, R. A.: Can His bundle lesions produce the electrocardiographic pattern of bundle branch block? J. Electrocardiol., 10:205–206, 1977.
204. El-Sherif, N., Amat-Y-Leon, F., Schonfield, C., et al.: Normalization of bundle branch block patterns by distal His bundle pacing. Clinical and experimental evidence of longitudinal dissociation in the pathologic His bundle. Circulation, 57:473–483, 1978.
205. James, T. N., and Sherf, L.: Fine structure of the His bundle. Circulation, 44:9–28, 1971.
206. Bailey, J. C., Spear, J. F., and Moore, E. N.: Functional significance of transverse conducting pathways within the canine bundle of His. Am. J. Cardiol., 34:790–795, 1979.
207. Kinoshita, S.: Variations in the critical cycle length inducing rate dependent bundle branch block. Am. Heart J., 96:54–61, 1978.
208. Wellens, H. J. J., and Durrer, D.: Supraventricular tachycardia with left aberrant conduction due to retrograde invasion into the left bundle branch. Circulation, 38:474–479, 1968.
209. Spurrell, R. A. J., Krikler, D. M., and Souton, E.: Retrograde invasion of the bundle branches producing aberration of the QRS complex during supraventricular tachycardia. Studies by programmed electrical stimulation. Circulation, 50:487–495, 1974.
210. Slama, R., Motte, A., Coumel, P. H., and Guerin, F.: Bloc de branche fonctionnel et conduction retrograde cachee sur la branche bloquee. Arch. Mal. Coeur, 63:1317–1325, 1970.
211. Cohen, S. I., Lau, S. H., Sherlag, B. J., and Damato, A. N.: Alternate patterns of premature ventricular excitation during induced atrial bigeminy. Circulation, 39:819–829, 1969.
212. Castellanos, A., Embi, A., Aranda, J., and Befeler, B.: Retrograde His bundle deflection in bundle branch re-entry. Br. Heart J., 38:301–303, 1967.
213. Bandura, J. P., and Brody, D. A.: Microelectrode study of alternating responses to repetitive premature excitation. Circ. Res., 34:406–410, 1974.
214. Carmeliet, E.: Influence du rhythme sur la duree du potentiel d'action ventriculaire cardiaque. Arch. Int. Physiol., 63:222–232, 1955.
215. Janse, M. J., van der Steen, A. B. M., van Dam, R. Th., and Durrer, D.: Refractory periods of the dog's ventricular myocardium following changes in the frequency. Circ. Res., 24:251–262, 1969.
216. Hoffman, B. F.: Electrophysiologic mechanisms for conduction abnormalities. Chest, 63:651–652, 1973.
217. Berliner, K., and Lenithin, L. P.: Auricular premature systole. I. Aberration of the ventricular complex in the electrocardiogram. Am. Heart J., 29:449–478, 1945.
218. Bigger, J. T., Bassett, A. L., and Hoffman, B. F.: Electrophysiological effects of diphenylhydantoin on canine Purkinje fibers. Circ. Res., 22:221–236, 1968.
219. Davis, L. D., and Temte, J. V.: Effects of propranolol on the transmembrane potentials of ventricular muscle and Purkinje fibers of the dog. Circ. Res., 22:661–677, 1968.
220. Bissett, J. K., De Soyza, N. D. B., Kane, J. J., and Doherty, J. E.: Effect of diphenylhydantoin on induced aberrant conduction. J. Electrocardiol., 7:65–69, 1974.
221. Johnson, E. A., and McKinnon, M. C.: The differential effect of quinidine and pyrilamine on the myocardial action potential at various rates of stimulation. J. Pharmacol. Exp. Ther., 120:460–468, 1957.
222. Wilson, F. N.: A case in which the vagus influenced the form of

the ventricular complex of the electrocardiogram. Arch. Intern. Med., 16:1008-1027, 1915.

223. Comeau, W. J., Hamilton, J. G. M., and White, P. D.: Paroxysmal bundle branch block associated with heart disease. A review and analysis of literature, with thirteen new cases and notes upon the influence of the vagus. Am. Heart J., 15:276-316, 1938.
224. Vessel, H.: Critical rates in ventricular conduction. Unstable bundle branch block. Am. J. Med. Sci., 202:198-207, 1941.
225. Hwang, W., and Langendorf, R.: Auriculoventricular nodal escape in the presence of atrial fibrillation. Circulation, 1:930-935, 1950.
226. Pick, A.: Aberrant ventricular conduction of escaped beats. Preferential and accessory pathways in the A-V junction. Circulation, 13:702-711, 1956.
227. Dressler, W.: Transient bundle branch block occurring during slowing of heart beat and following gagging. Am. Heart J., 58:760-764, 1959.
228. Goodman, R. M., and Pick, A.: An unusual type of intermittent A-V dissociation in acute rheumatic myocarditis. Am. Heart J., 61:259-263, 1961.
229. Wallace, A. G., and Lazlo, J.: Mechanisms influencing conduction in a case of intermittent bundle branch block. Am. Heart J., 61:548-555, 1961.
230. Walsh, T. J.: Ventricular aberration of A-V nodal escape beats. Comments concerning the mechanism of aberration. Am. J. Cardiol., 10:217-222, 1962.
231. Vessel, H., and Lowen, G.: Bundle branch block on cardiac slowing at a critical slow heart rate. Am. Heart J., 66:329-337, 1963.
232. Bauer, G. E., Julian, D. G., and Valentine, P. A.: Bundle branch block in acute myocardial infarction. Br. Heart J., 27:724-730, 1965.
233. Kistin, A. D.: Atrioventricular junctional premature and escape beats with altered QRS and fusion. Circulation, 34:740-751, 1966.
234. Massumi, R. A.: Bradycardia-dependent bundle-branch block. A critique and proposed criteria. Circulation, 38:1066-1073, 1968.
235. Sarachek, N. S.: Bradycardia-dependent bundle branch block. Relation to supernormal conduction and phase 4 depolarization. Am. J. Cardiol., 25:727-729, 1970.
236. Massumi, R. A., Erten, G. E., and Vera, Z.: Aberrancy of junctional escape beats. Evidence for origin in the fascicles of the left bundle branch. Am. J. Cardiol., 29:351-359, 1972.
237. Gay, R., and Brown, D. F.: Bradycardia dependent bundle branch block in acute myocardial infarction. Chest, 64:114-116, 1973.
238. Rosenbaum, M. B., Elizari, M. V., Lazzari, J. O., et al.: The mechanism of intermittent bundle branch block: relationship to prolonged recovery, hypopolarization, and spontaneous diastolic depolarization. Chest, 63:666-677, 1973.
239. Rosenbaum, M. B., Elizari, M. V., Levi, R. J., and Nau, G. J.: Paroxysmal atrioventricular block related to hypopolarization and spontaneous diastolic depolarization. Chest, 63:678-688, 1973.
240. Elizari, M. V., Nau, G. J., Levi, R. J., et al.: Experimental production of rate dependent bundle branch block in the canine heart. Circ. Res., 34:730-742, 1974.
241. Rosenbaum, M. B., Elizari, M. V., and Chiale, P.: Relationship between increased automaticity and depressed conduction in the main intraventricular conducting fascicles of the human and canine heart. Circulation, 49:818-828, 1974.
242. Lie, K. I., Wellens, H. J., Schuilenburg, R. M., and Durrer, D.: Mechanism and significance of widened QRS complexes during complete atrioventricular block in acute inferior myocardial infarction. Am. J. Cardiol., 33:833-839, 1974.
243. Cohen, H. C., D'Cruz, I., Arbel, E. R., et al.: Tachycardia and bradycardia-dependent bundle branch block alternans. Clinical observations. Circulation, 55:242-246, 1976.
244. Drury, A. M., and Mackenzie, D. W.: Aberrant ventricular beats in the dog during vagal stimulation. Q. J. Exp. Physiol., 24:237-247, 1934.
245. Sherf, L., and James, T. N.: The mechanism of aberration in late atrioventricular junctional beats. Am. J. Cardiol., 29:529-539, 1972.
246. Pick, A.: Mechanisms of cardiac arrhythmias: from hypothesis to physiologic fact. Am. Heart J., 86:249-269, 1973.
247. Wellens, H.: Unusual occurrence of nonaberrant conduction in patients with atrial fibrillation and aberrant conduction. Am. Heart J., 77:158-166, 1969.
248. Pick, A., and Fishman, A. P.: Observations in heart block. Supernormality of A-V and intraventricular conduction and ventricular parasystole under the influence of epinephrine. Acta Cardiol., 5:270-287, 1950.
249. Scherf, D., and Scharf, M. M.: Supernormal phase of intraventricular conduction. Am. Heart J., 36:621-628, 1948.
250. James T. N.: Cardiac conduction system: fetal and post natal development. Am. J. Cardiol., 25:213-226, 1970.
251. Bailey, J. C., Greenspan, K., Elizari, M. V., et al.: Effects of acetylcholine on automaticity and conduction in the proximal portion of the His-Purkinje specialized conduction system of the dog. Circ. Res., 30:210-216, 1972.
252. El-Sherif, N., Scherlag, B. J., Lazarra, R., and Samet, P.: Pathophysiology of tachycardia- and bradycardia dependent block in the canine proximal His-Purkinje system after acute myocardial ischemia. Am. J. Cardiol., 33:529-540, 1974.
253. Saunders, J. H., Ferrier, G. R., and Moe, G. K.: Conduction block associated with transient depolarizations induced by acetylstrophanthidin in isolated canine Purkinje fibers. Circ. Res., 32:610-617, 1973.
254. Hoffman, B. F., and Singer, D. H.: Appraisal of the effects of catecholamines on cardiac electrical activity. Ann. N.Y. Acad. Sci., 139:914-939, 1967.
255. Ten Eick, R. E., Singer, D. H., Parameswaran, R., and Drake, F.: Effect of catecholamines on electrical diastole in normal, acutely and chronically depolarized cardiac tissues (abstr.). Fed. Proc., 30:393, 1971.
256. Strauss, H. C., Singer, D. H., and Hoffman, B. F.: Biphasic effects of procainamide on cardiac conduction (abstr.). Bull. N.Y. Acad. Med., 43:1194, 1967.
257. Singer, D. H., Strauss, H. C., and Hoffman, B. F.: "New" mode of action of antiarrhythmic agents (abstr.). Am. J. Cardiol., 19:151-152, 1967.
258. Hoffman, B. F.: Physiology of atrioventricular transmission. Circulation, 24:506-517, 1961.
259. Lewis, T.: Certain physical signs of myocardial involvement. Br. Med. J., 1:484-489, 1913.
260. Baker, B. M., Jr.: The effect of cardiac rate and the inhalation of oxygen on transient bundle branch block. Arch. Intern. Med., 45:814-822, 1930.
261. Sandberg, A. A., Wener, J., Master, A. M., and Scherlis, L.: Intermittent and transient bundle branch block. A clinical and electrocardiographic study. Ann. Intern. Med., 35:1085-1109, 1951.
262. Bauer, G. E.: Transient bundle branch block. Circulation, 29:730-738, 1964.
263. Schuilenburg, R. M., and Durrer, D.: Rate dependency of functional block in the human His bundle and bundle branch Purkinje system. Circulation, 48:526-540, 1973.

16

Bundle Branch Block and Other Forms of Aberrant Intraventricular Conduction: Clinical Aspects

Howard C. Cohen and Donald H. Singer

The work for this chapter was supported in part by grants-in-aid to Dr. Cohen by U.S.P.H.S. (HL-176648) and by Cardiac Consultants of Chicago and to Dr. Singer by the American Heart Association (74-1065), the Chicago Heart Association (B 74-73), and the Reingold Estate.

The contour of the QRS complex reflects the directions and magnitude of the electrical potentials produced by the depolarizing cells of the ventricles. The possible number of different patterns of QRS complexes in patients is infinite, with no two patients having precisely the same 12-lead electrocardiogram. However, certain similarities allow electrocardiographic patterns of aberrant intraventricular conduction to be divided into groups according to recognizable characteristics. These groups include the bundle branch blocks (BBB), the fascicular blocks, mural blocks, the conduction defects associated with spontaneous or pacemaker-induced ectopic ventricular beats, and the several types of ventricular preexcitation.

The specialized conduction system of the heart includes the sinus node and a specialized endocardial atrial conduction system, the atrioventricular (AV) node, the His bundle (HB), which may be nonhomogeneous,[1-4] the main left bundle branch (LBB), the anterior, posterior, and possibly septal fascicles or divisions of the LBB, which may or may not be discrete,[5-7] the right bundle branch (RBB), and the Purkinje system, which spreads throughout the endocardium and is in contact with the working myocardium. The nonhomogeneity of the HB has been proved by normalization of BBB with distal HB pacing.[8]

Bundle Branch and Fascicular Block

Bundle branch block occurs in approximately 0.6% of the population and 1% to 2% of the population over 60 years of age. Organic heart disease is present in up to 80% of these patients, with coronary artery disease being present in up to 50%.[9] Conduction defects in bundle branches and fascicles diagnosed by electrocardiogram have been shown to be frequently associated with pathologic changes in the suspected locations.[10] Patients with such chronic conduction defects have a higher mortality if significant cardiac disease is present[11,12] and develop AV block and sudden death with greater frequency than patients without such defects. Mortality is also higher if premature ventricular contractions are present,[13] and the predominant cause of sudden death in these patients is ventricular arrhythmia,[14] including fibrillation.[13] The good prognosis in asymptomatic patients with BBB is due to the absence of progressive disease and perhaps in part because BBB, *per se,* at least in animals, does not decrease the fibrillation threshold.[15] In middle-aged men the 5-year mortality in those shown to have a conduction defect on a 6-hour electrocardiogram is approximately 33%.[16] Almost 33% of asymptomatic patients with intraventricular conduction defects develop clinical evidence of coronary artery disease in an average of 8 years.[17] Most patients with chronic BBB who die suddenly have coronary artery disease.[18] Patients with BBB also are more prone to hypertension, cardiomegaly and heart failure.[19] Some studies to predict prognosis, including electrode catheter recordings from the HB to diagnose the location of AV block in the presence of BBB,[20] have shown that if conduction from the HB to the ventricles (HQ interval) is markedly prolonged, the rate of progression to second degree type II AV block is high.[21] The prognosis is poor[22,23,24] in terms of progression of the conduction defect[14,25,26] and of cardiac failure[19,27] if clinically significant symptoms of cardiac disease are present when BBB is diagnosed.[28] The PR intervals may[29] or may not[22,30] be good predicters of long HQ intervals or of survival. Patients with left bundle branch block (LBBB) are more likely to have long HQ intervals than patients with right bundle branch block (RBBB),[31] at least in part because RBB conduction is normally longer than LBB conduction.[32] Although intravenous quinidine does not cause an increase in infranodal conduction time in patients with BBB,[33] intravenous procainamide[34] and disopyramide[35] have caused such increases, and drugs such as quinidine, procainamide, amiodarone,[36] ajmaline,[37] and possibly lidocaine[38] must be used with caution in these patients, especially when HQ intervals are long, to avoid producing AV block.[39] High degrees of HQ block may occur in patients with BBB and normal or almost normal HQ intervals on conducted beats.[40]

Additional studies indicate that patients with chronic BBB and prolonged conduction from the atria to the His

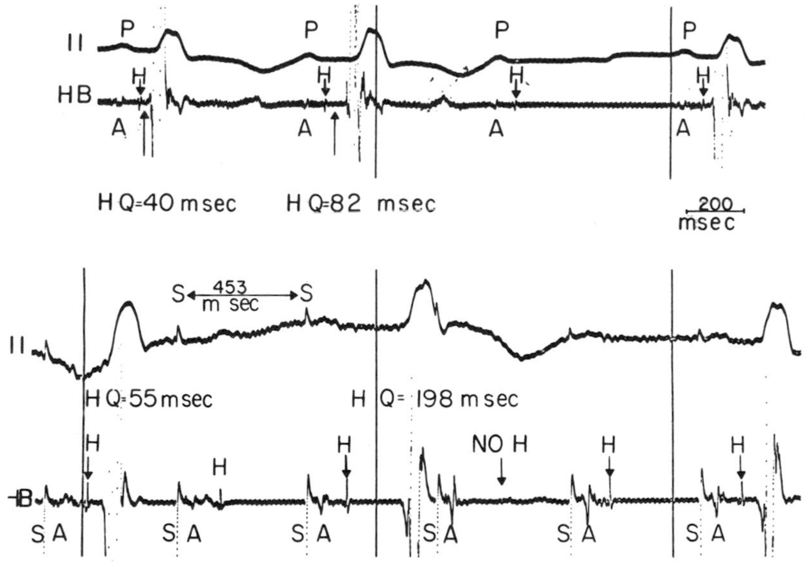

Figure 16-1. *The top panel shows lead II and a His bundle (HB) electrogram. The QRS is of left bundle branch block. The first two complexes are conducted but with a gradually prolonging His to QRS (HQ) interval going from 40 to 82 msec. The third atrial (A) wave is followed by a HB potential (H) but no QRS complex. Thus, left bundle branch block with type I second degree HQ blocks exists, possibly occurring in the right bundle branch. In the lower panel, lead II and an HB electrogram are also seen. Here, with atrial pacing (S = pacing spike) at a rate more rapid than seen in the top panel, 2:1 AV block is seen; the first complex is conducted, the second is not, and the third is conducted again. However, on the conducted beats, the HQ interval prolongs from 55 to 198 msec. The next complex that should have conducted, following the fifth pacing spike, does not reach the ventricles, although the HB potential is seen. Thus, alternate-beat type I second degree HQ block exists. Also, the fourth paced atrial beat is the only one not followed by a His potential. This beat follows the very long HQ interval (198 msec) and could be missing because there has been intra-Hisian reentry with concealed conduction moving retrogradely into the AV node, causing the subsequent atrial to His bundle (AH) block. (Abbreviations remain the same in all the figures in this chapter unless otherwise indicated.)*

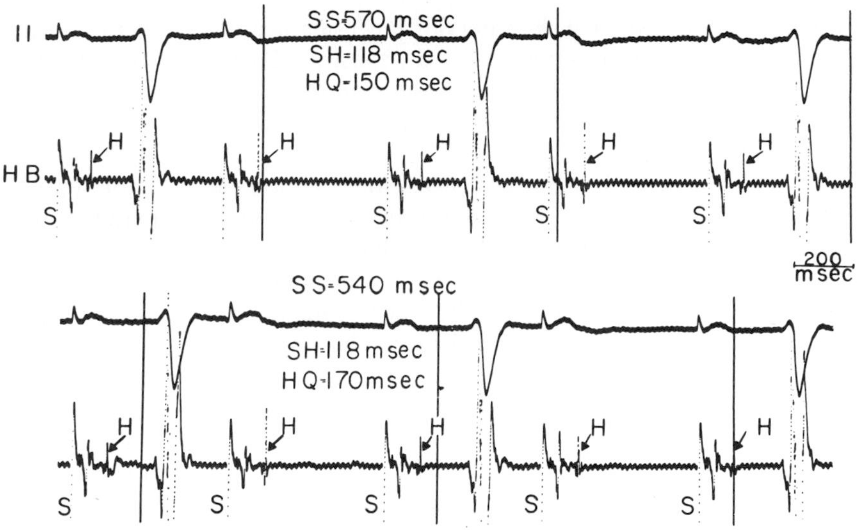

Figure 16-2. *Both the top and bottom panels show artificial pacing of the atria with 2:1 block below the His bundle. However, at the shorter pacing interval of 540 msec in the lower panel, the HQ interval has lengthened from 150 msec in the upper panel to 170 msec in the lower panel. This tendency for increasing conduction time as the rate increases is a feature of tissue capable of displaying type I second degree AV block, as shown in Figure 16-3.*

bundle (AH) interval are more likely to have significant congestive failure but have no greater mortality than patients with normal AH intervals.[41]

In the aging heart BBB appears to be a remarkably stable pattern.[42] Between 3% and 4% of patients with chronic bifascicular block develop high-degree AV block during a 5-year average follow-up study.[43] The majority of deaths are due to progression of congestive heart failure.[44]

The type and degree of AV block may indicate the most likely location of block and the general prognosis. Patients with second degree type I (Wenckebach) AV block usually have block in the AV node[45] and have a better prognosis than patients with second degree type II AV block, which is usually in the HB or the bundle branches,[46] although type I block may also occur in the HB or bundle branches[47,48] (Figs. 16-1 to 16-3). The electrocardiogram and the HB recording together give an even better indication of the location of conduction defects.[49] However, in the absence of second degree AV block, there is not yet general agreement that this information allows conclusions on the need for prophylactic artificial pacing (see above). If patients with chronic bifascicular block develop block below the HB during atrial pacing at rates of 130 beats/min or less, they are very likely to develop spontaneous AV block. The absence of such block during pacing, however, may be found in patients with long HV intervals.[50] Asymptomatic patients who have or develop BBB with no obvious heart disease are likely to have an excellent prog-

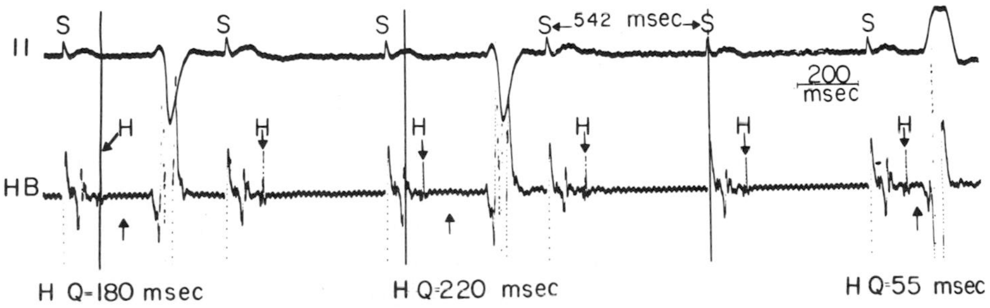

Figure 16-3. *Lead II shows left anterior fascicular block. (Lead V_1, not shown, indicated right bundle branch block simultaneously.) In the first four beats, there is a 2:1 block below the His bundle, so that the first and third H are followed by QRS complexes but the second and fourth are not. However, the HQ interval of the first conducted beat is 180 msec, and the HQ interval of the second conducted beat is 220 msec. The fifth H is not followed by the expected QRS complex, so that the pattern of alternate-beat type I second degree HQ block is seen. The sixth beat is again conducted, but now, after the long pause, the right bundle branch is recovered. Although the right bundle branch has a longer refractory period, having been blocked in previous beats, it has shorter conduction time, so that the HQ in the last beat is 55 msec and the pattern of left bundle branch block appears.*

nosis[51,52] even when HV intervals are significantly prolonged.[28] Even in patients who demonstrate RBBB and LBBB at different times, prognosis is more strongly related to associated heart disease than to the degree of AV block.[53]

Patients with BBB who have neurologic symptoms must be followed closely. However, syncope in patients with bifascicular block is usually not due to complete heart block.[19,54] AV block in these patients is likely to be associated with long HQ intervals, whereas neurologic symptoms without AV block are likely to be associated with near-normal HQ intervals.[55,56] Prophylactic permanent pacing may[56] or may not[18] protect these patients from sudden death.

Patients who have definite second degree type II AV block need permanent pacemakers.[57] The prognosis in patients with Mobitz type II AV block is probably similar to that of those with third degree AV block. In younger patients, complete heart block is frequently congenital, and although the risk of syncope is about 5% over 15 years, the risk of sudden death is probably not increased.[58] Patients with second or third degree AV block who get pacemakers are unlikely to die from pacemaker failure, but they do have an increased mortality compared with the general population, mainly because of progression of underlying heart disease.[59]

Perhaps 20% of patients admitted to a coronary care unit with definite myocardial infarction have or develop conduction defects. Of patients with definite acute myocardial infarction, complete AV block may occur in 6% of those without conduction defects, 50% of those with RBBB, 40% of those with RBBB and left anterior fascicular block (LAFB) or left posterior fascicular block (LPFB), and 20% of those with LBBB.[60] Development of LBBB, RBBB, or RBBB with fascicular block acutely at the time of a myocardial infarction indicates a poorer prognosis than the infarction without these conduction defects.[61-63] Patients with RBBB are more likely to develop cardiogenic shock, AV block, or ventricular asystole, whereas those with LBBB tend to develop ventricular arrhythmias.[64] Thirty-six percent of patients with acute myocardial infarction and BBB develop late in-hospital ventricular fibrillation.[65] Both in-hospital and out-of-hospital risk of sudden death is higher in postinfarction patients with BBB.[66,67] Ventricular tachycardia could be initiated by bundle branch reentry.[68] Even if second degree or high-degree AV block is transient, permanent pacing should be strongly considered.[19] Patients with acute conduction defects after anterior myocardial infarction have a high risk of developing complete AV block,[69-71] and a temporary artificial pacemaker should be inserted despite some evidence that such treatment may have little effect on survival.[63,72-75] Prognosis is better for patients with a normal HQ interval[76] and transient BBB.[77] The combination of BBB and congestive heart failure suggests a very poor prognosis. The prevalence of late sudden death may be high even if the BBB is transient.[19] If AV block develops and then regresses, patients are more likely to have coronary artery disease, and they have a poorer prognosis than patients with stable chronic AV block.[78] When etiologies are compared, patients with LBBB who develop AV block are likely to have coronary artery disease, whereas patients with RBB and LAFB who develop AV block are more likely to have primary conduction system disease.[79]

Bundle branch block and fascicular block may be persistent or intermittent.[53,80] These conduction defects may be tachycardia-, bradycardia-, or non-rate-dependent,[81] and they may occur on alternate beats[82] or as a BBB Wenckebach phenomenon.[83,84]

Left Bundle Branch Block

Etiology

Left bundle branch block almost always develops after birth, occasionally with no clinical evidence of heart disease,[58] and is most common in males.[85] The incidence is 1 : 100 to 1 : 10,000 in various studies.[86] Usually LBBB is associated with hypertensive heart disease,[87] coronary artery disease,[85,88] myocarditis,[89] or aortic valvular disease. Routine exercise tests may not differentiate between patients with and patients without obstructive coronary disease in the presence of LBBB,[90] but potassium and rubidium scans of the heart during exercise may show defects compatible with unsuspected old anteroseptal myocardial infarction,[91] and thallium scans may show transient ischemia, thereby delineating the possible etiology of LBBB.

Left bundle branch block is not uncommon in patients with cardiomyopathies, including the hypertrophic obstructive type.[92] Less frequently, LBBB may be associated with other cardiac or generalized conditions such as hyperkalemia,[93] rarely bacterial endocarditis,[94] or even digitalis toxicity.[95] Pathologic correlations suggest that LBBB is usually associated with fibrosis in the main LBB,[96] although electrophysiologic studies suggest that the pattern of LBBB may occur as a result of an HB lesion.[8] Left bundle branch block occurs rarely as a congenital lesion with unknown pathology.[97]

Clinical Findings

The discovery of LBBB on the electrocardiogram is usually associated with symptoms, signs, or a history compatible with clinical heart disease such as angina, old myocardial infarction, hypertension, cardiac failure, or cardiomegaly. There may be a 3-year cumulative mortality of 35% in patients with chronic LBBB.[98] On physical examination, there may be evidence of aortic valvular disease, diastolic gallops associated with heart failure, or a paradoxically split second heart sound produced by prolongation of left ventricular isometric contraction secondary to the LBBB. Also, the first heart sound may be diminished, and the preejection period may be prolonged.[99] His bundle recordings in patients with LBBB may show prolonged HQ intervals[31,100] (more commonly with hypertension than with ischemic heart disease[29] or second degree AV block (Fig. 16-4). The catheter used to record HB potentials in patients with LBBB may damage the RBB and produce complete AV block.[101,102] In general, patients with LBBB do not have as good a prognosis as patients with normal electrocardiograms because of the cardiac diseases frequently associated with this conduction abnormality. Left axis deviation may[39] or may not[30,52,103] worsen this prognosis, but additional nonspecific intraventricular conduction defects, sometimes after myocardial infarction, are independently associated with excess mortality to a significant degree.[104] Left ventricular dysfunction is more likely to be present with coronary artery disease if LBBB is present.[105] New onset LBBB in adults probably carries a poor prognosis.[58] However, the general experience is mixed. Patients with chronic LBBB and first degree AV block have a 33% yearly mortality.[15] Left bundle branch block associated with acute myocardial infarction may[106] or may not[107] affect prognosis. If new first degree AV block is associated with LBBB and acute myocardial infarction, the incidence of development of sudden AV block is higher.[108] Temporary pacemakers are usually used when new LBBB occurs with acute anteroseptal myocardial infarction, although the indication is in dispute; however, complete AV block may develop. Left bundle branch block existing before a myocardial infarction indicates an even worse prognosis, increasing the mortality to 57% acutely, compared to 29% in patients who sustain an acute myocardial infarction having had a previously normal electrocardiogram,[109] but the cause of death is usually not AV block. In the absence of associated heart disease, LBBB may be benign and without obvious hemodynamic effect,[110] even though septal motion may be abnormal on echocardiography.[111] Chronic LBBB not associated with acute myocardial infarction carries a low incidence of development of AV block and does not warrant a prophylactic permanent pacemaker.[29]

The Electrocardiogram

The electrocardiogram of LBBB (Tables 16-1 and 16-2) is generally characteristic (Fig. 16-5), with QRS complexes widening to at least 0.12 second but averaging 0.07 second greater than normal, showing slurring throughout, prolongation of the intrinsicoid deflection, and ST segment and T wave deviation away from the direction of the major QRS depolarization. QT intervals are prolonged by 0.062 second beyond normal.[112] The axis is usually normal but is sometimes leftward or even rightward, perhaps in association with LAFB or LPFB.[113] (However, the diagnosis of LAFB and LPFB is generally not used simultaneously with the diagnosis of LBBB.) There is loss of the normal Q waves in some or all of the left-sided leads (1, aV_L, V_5, and V_6) because the direction of the interventricular septal depolarization is reversed, from its normal left to right to right to left.[114] Left bundle branch block may be constant (see Fig. 16-5), intermittent (Fig. 16-6), or alternating[82] and may occur in a Wenckebach pattern.[83,84] Left bundle branch block on the electrocardiogram may in part mimic or conceal other electrocardiographic diagnoses, such as myocardial infarction.[115,116] For example, the reciprocal changes associated with the absence of Q waves in the left precordial leads are Q waves in the right precordial leads, usually in V_1 and sometimes in V_1 through V_3. Occasional cases of intermittent LBBB are associated with electrocardiograms that have QS complexes in leads V_1

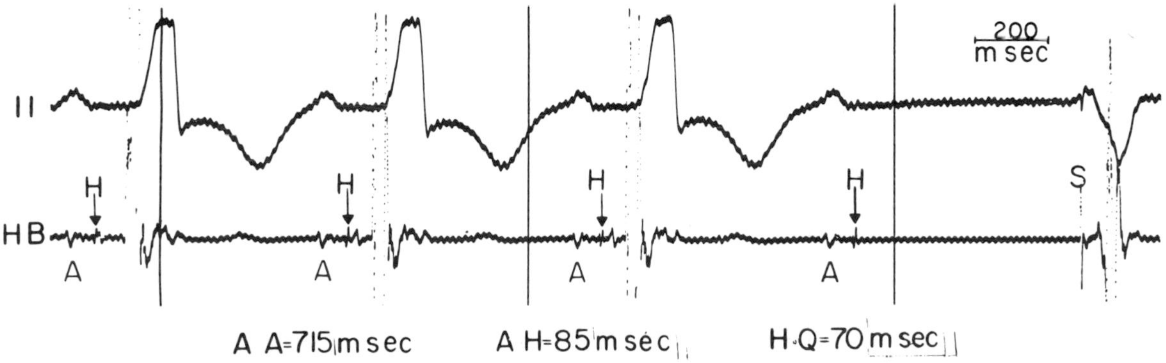

Figure 16-4. *Lead II and a His bundle recording during sinus rhythm with left bundle branch block. AH intervals are normal at 85 msec. HQ intervals are prolonged at 70 msec. Both AH and HQ intervals are fixed in the first three beats. In the fourth beat there is no QRS complex. Thus, there is second degree type II block within or below the bundle of His.*

Table 16-1. Effects of Bundle Branch and Fascicular Block on QRS Contour*

	LBBB	RBBB	IRBBB	ILBBB	LAFB	LPFB	LSFB	RBBB + LAFB	RBBB + LPFB
QRS in leads I, aV_L	Loss of Q wave	Terminal slurred S wave	Small terminal S wave	Loss of Q wave	Small Q, tall R waves	Small R, deep S waves		Small Q, tall R, terminal slurred S	Small R, deep slurred S wave
QRS in leads II, III, aV_F		Terminal slurred S or R			Small R, deep S waves	Small Q, tall R waves		Small R, deep slurred S waves	Small Q, tall R wave, slurred S wave
QRS in lead aV_R		Terminal slurred R wave	Terminal R wave		Terminal R wave	Terminal S or R wave		Terminal slurred R wave	Terminal slurred R wave
QRS in lead V_1	Mainly negative	Terminal slurred R wave	Terminal R wave	Mainly negative	May have initial Q wave		Tall R wave	Terminal slurred R wave	Terminal slurred R wave
QRS in leads V_5, V_6	Loss of Q wave	Terminal slurred S wave	Terminal S wave	Loss of Q wave	Biphasic RS wave			Biphasic R wave and slurred S	Terminal slurred S wave
May mimic RVH	No	No	No	No	No	No	No	No	Yes
May mimic LVH	Occasionally	No	No	No	Yes	No	No	Yes	No
May hide LVH	Yes	No	No	No	No	Yes	No	No	Yes
QRS duration	At least 0.12 sec or 0.07 sec greater than normal	At least 0.12 sec or 0.06 sec greater than normal	Classically 0.1–0.11 sec	0.1–0.11 sec	25 msec greater than normal (also see text)	See text		≥0.12 sec	≥0.12 sec
QRS axis	No effect	No major effect	No effect	No effect	More negative than −30°	+100° or greater	No effect	More negative than −30°	+100° or more

* RVH, right ventricular hypertrophy; LVH, left ventricular hypertrophy; LBBB, left bundle branch block, RBBB, right bundle branch block; IRBBB, incomplete right bundle branch block; ILBBB, incomplete left bundle branch block; LAFB, left anterior fascicular block; LPFB, left posterior fascicular block; LSFB, left septal fascicular block.

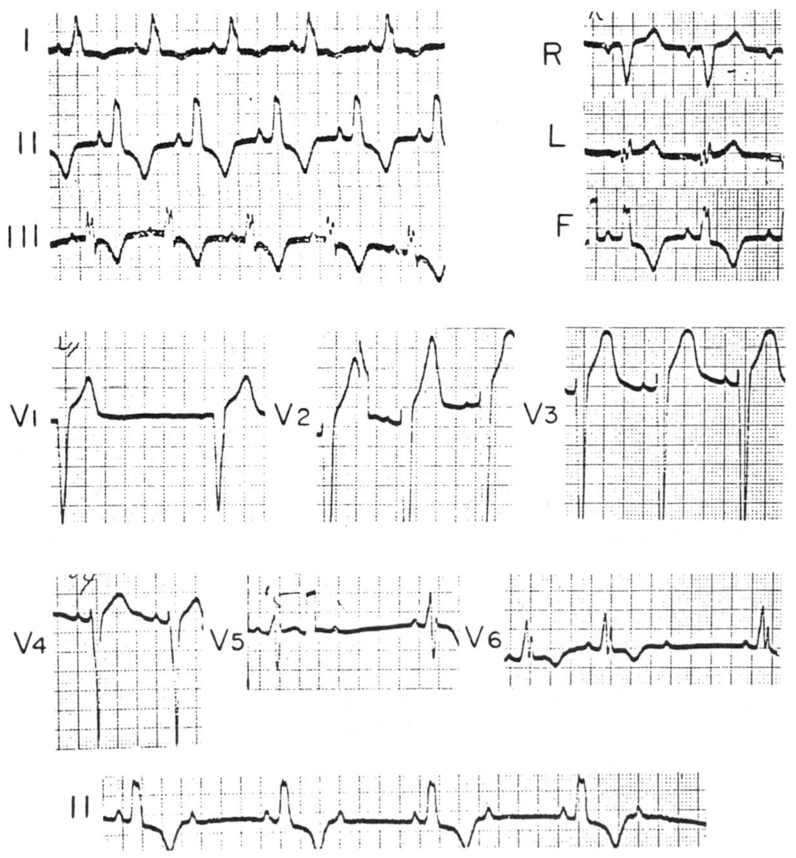

Figure 16-5. *Left bundle branch block at a sinus rate of 76 beats/min. QRS complexes are upright in lead I with no Q waves in leads I, V_5, and V_6, and they are wide and slurred throughout. Long pauses due to blocked P waves are seen in leads V_1, V_5, and V_6. PR intervals are constant in V_6. The block is second degree, type II. In the bottom strip showing lead II, 2:1 block develops at a sinus rate of 81 beats/min.*

Table 16-2. Effects of Bundle Branch and Fascicular Block on Patterns of Myocardial Ischemia

	LBBB	RBBB	ILBBB	IRBBB	LAFB	LPFB	LSFB	RBBB + LAFB	RBBB + LPFB
May mimic anteroseptal MI	Yes	No	Yes	No	Yes	No	No	Yes	No
May mimic inferior MI	Yes	No	No	No	No	Yes	No	No	Yes
May mimic lateral MI	No	No	No	No	Yes	No	No	Yes	No
May mimic true posterior MI	No	Sometimes	No	No	No	No	Yes	Sometimes	Sometimes
May hide inferior MI	Sometimes	No	Sometimes	No	Yes	No	No	Yes	No
May hide lateral MI	Yes	No	Yes	No	No	Yes	No	No	Yes
May hide true posterior MI	Yes	No	Yes	No	No	No	No	No	No
May mimic anteroseptal ischemia	No	Yes	No	Yes	No	No	Yes	Yes	Yes
May mimic inferior ischemia	Yes	No	Yes	No	No	Yes	No	No	Yes
May mimic lateral ischemia	Yes	No	Yes	No	Yes (leads I, aV_L)	No	No	No	No
May hide anteroseptal ischemia	Yes	No	Yes	No	No	No	No	No	No
May hide inferior ischemia	Sometimes	Sometimes	No	No	Yes	No	No	Yes	No
May hide lateral ischemia	No	Yes	No	Yes	Yes (leads V_5, V_6)	Yes	No	Yes (leads V_5, V_6)	Yes
May hide high lateral ischemia	No	Yes	No	Yes	No	Yes	No	Yes	Yes

LBBB, left bundle branch block; RBBB, right bundle branch block; ILBBB, incomplete left bundle branch block; IRBBB, incomplete right bundle branch block; LAFB, left anterior fascicular block; LPFB, left posterior fascicular block; LSFB, left septal fascicular block, MI, myocardial infarction.

through V_3 during LBBB but R waves in leads V_1 through V_3 during normal conduction. Thus, in the presence of LBBB, abnormal Q waves in leads V_1 through V_3 may be suggestive but not diagnostic of anteroseptal myocardial infarction. Inferior and anterolateral myocardial infarctions may be disguised by the pattern of LBBB; that is, Q or QS waves in leads II, III, and aV_F associated with inferior myocardial infarction[117] and Q waves in anterolateral precordial leads associated with anterolateral infarction may disappear with the development of LBBB. Left bundle branch block may be associated with QS complexes in leads II, III, and aV_F that truly[118] or falsely[119] suggest inferior myocardial infarction. Left bundle branch block itself produces ST segment depression and T wave inversion in leads in which QRS complexes are mainly upright and ST segment elevation in leads in which QRS complexes are mainly inverted. The superimposition of myocardial injury, ischemia, or infarction may be recognized by a changing pattern over two or several electrocardiograms and by clinical correlation[120] even in the absence of diagnostic Q waves. The changes of left ventricular hypertrophy (LVH) are also affected by the development of LBBB. Frequently a decrease in voltage occurs, causing the search for voltage criteria of LVH to be falsely negative.[121] Much less frequently voltage increases, producing false-positive criteria for LVH.[122]

Right Bundle Branch Block

Etiology

The incidence of RBBB (see Tables 16-1 and 16-2) is probably 1:4000.[58] This conduction abnormality may appear as a congenital defect unassociated with other cardiac abnormalities[123] or after surgery for pulmonary stenosis, tetralogy of Fallot, or a large ventricular septal defect (VSD).[124] Surgery for VSD in the presence of increased pulmonary vascular resistance produces less of a decrease in heart size if RBBB has developed.[125] Surgically induced RBBB may regress up to 12 years after the procedure.[126] In one study, right ventriculotomies in steps of three to seven small incisions were performed during repair of various congenital defects. Right bundle

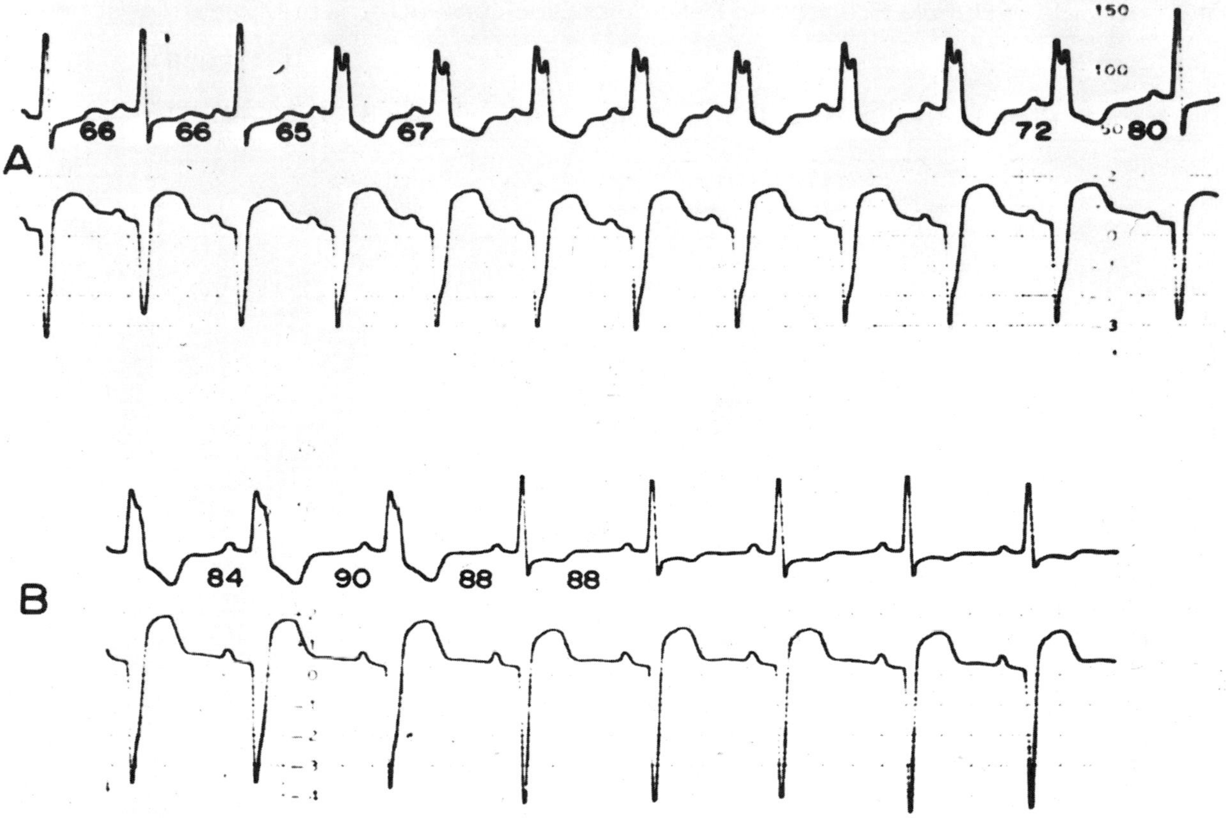

Figure 16-6. *(A) A lateral and an anterior lead during sinus arrhythmia. RP intervals are indicated in hundredths of a second. PR intervals are constant. As the RR interval decreases from 66 to 65 hundredths of a second, left bundle branch block develops and persists because of concealed transseptal retrograde conduction, even as the rate slows and RR intervals gradually change from 67 to 72 hundredths of a second. When the RR interval prolongs further, to 80 hundredths of a second, left bundle branch block disappears. (B) Left bundle branch block disappears when the RR interval goes from 90 to 88 hundredths of a second. Thus, in the upper panel, left bundle branch block is tachycardia dependent, although the rate at which it appears and the rate at which it disappears are not the same. In the lower panel the changes suggest bradycardia-dependent left bundle branch block.*

branch block developed at the time of one incision, regardless of the order of the incision, suggesting that the conduction defect was caused by disruption of a distal branch or branches of the right bundle within the right ventricle.[127] Thus, RBBB may occur with right ventricular damage. The pattern of RBBB may appear with premature supraventricular beats (Fig. 16-7), or it may be caused by hyperkalemia,[93] chest trauma,[128,129] or anteroseptal myocardial infarction. Inferior myocardial infarction may produce RBBB because a portion of the RBB is supplied by the right coronary artery.[25,60] Anteroseptal ischemia, fibrosis of the ventricular conduction system (Lenegre's disease), calcification of the root of the aorta (Lev's disease), cardiomyopathy, including the hypertrophic obstructive type,[92] and lesions within the HB may produce RBBB.[8] In patients with asymptomatic RBBB there is a 17% incidence of coronary artery disease.[58] Patients with acquired RBBB without evidence of other disease may have a benign course,[130] although the majority may have elevated left ventricular end-diastolic pressure, suggesting that they have diffuse myocardial disease.[131]

Clinical Findings

Right bundle branch block, which sometimes develops at the time of acute anteroseptal myocardial infarction or pulmonary embolus, frequently causes widely but physiologically split second heart sounds. Hemodynamic studies show right ventricular contraction to be delayed and less efficient.[132]

Right bundle branch block in children and young adults usually has no effect on prognosis when not associated with other cardiac disease, but rarely it may progress to complete AV block.[133] In older adults, RBBB

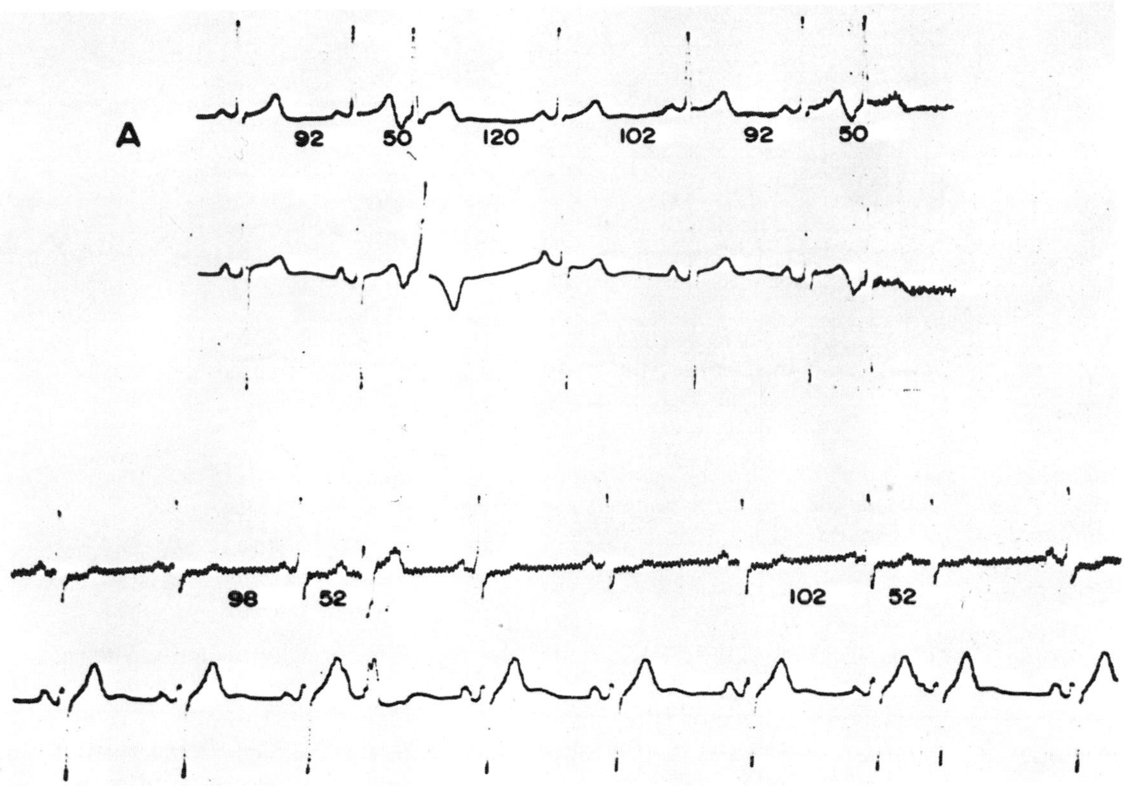

Figure 16-7. *Each panel has a lateral and an anterior lead. (A) A premature atrial beat is followed by right bundle branch block type of aberrant conduction to the ventricles. Later in A the same intervals are associated with normal conduction to the ventricles. (B) In a different patient, a premature atrial beat first does and then does not produce aberrant conduction, although the immediate cycle lengths are the same. The premature atrial beat associated with the shorter preceding cycle length of 98 hundredths of a second is the one that produces aberrant ventricular conduction. This reversal of the usual circumstances is found only in patients with significant myocardial disease.*

accompanying pulmonary disease suggests high pulmonary pressures. The vectorcardiogram may help in the presence of RBBB by demonstrating patterns either very likely or patterns unlikely to be associated with pulmonary disease or cardiac failure.[134] Right bundle branch block associated with deterioration of the specialized ventricular conduction system or with ischemic heart disease, especially at the time of acute myocardial infarction, may be the first step toward complete AV block. If RBBB is present at the time of an acute anteroseptal myocardial infarction, a temporary artificial pacemaker is indicated[135] even if the RBBB is old.[106] Patients with preexisting RBBB sustaining acute myocardial infarction are at increased risk of late sudden death.[136]

When chronic RBBB is associated with significant coronary artery disease, hypertension, or rheumatic heart disease, survival is significantly decreased.[137] Chronic RBBB found randomly is associated with a 9% progression rate to complete heart block.[138]

The Electrocardiogram

Electrocardiographic changes produced by RBBB (see Tables 16-1 and 16-2) are manifested by delayed rightward and anterior forces (Fig. 16-8), producing a slurred terminal S wave in left-sided leads (I, aV_L, V_5, and V_6). Lead V_1 shows terminal slurred R waves. The QRS duration is at least 0.12 second but averages 0.06 second longer than normal.[112] Right axis deviation in the presence of RBBB suggests right ventricular hypertrophy (RVH), associated left posterior fascicular block, loss of lateral forces secondary to myocardial infarction, or that the patient is young. Thus, ordinarily the R wave in lead I is taller than the slurred terminal S wave is deep. Occasionally, RBBB will cause the QRS to be entirely upright in lead V_1, even in the absence of RVH. The criterion, R or R′ wave in lead V_1 greater than 15 mm in the presence of RBBB, produces a high false-negative rate for RVH[139] because with RVH, RBBB decreases R wave voltage in lead V_1. On the vectorcardiogram right ventricular hy-

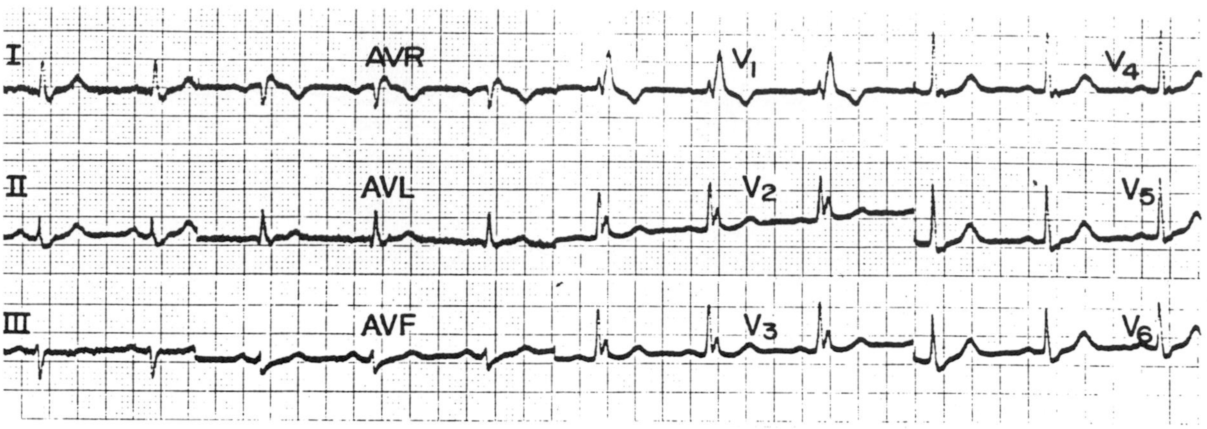

Figure 16-8. *Right bundle branch block shows terminal slurred S waves in leads I, II, aV_L, V_5, and V_6 and tall, wide, slurred R′ waves in right precordial leads V_1, V_2, and V_3. QRS duration is 0.12 second.*

pertrophy should be suspected if the 0.04 second vector and the maximum QRS vector are to the right in the horizontal plane, if the initial vector is to the left and posterior, if the maximum QRS vector in the frontal plane is greater than +110°, and if the right QRS area is greater than the left.[140] The usual criteria for LVH used in the presence of RBBB have low sensitivity. The multiple-dipole electrocardiogram may increase this sensitivity.[86]

In most cases, RBBB alone does not disturb the pattern of diagnostic Q waves due to myocardial infarction. However, cor pulmonale may be associated with RBBB and Q waves in right precordial or inferior leads that mimic myocardial infarction. With RBBB, T waves and ST segments tend to deviate in a direction opposite to that of the slurred delayed terminal forces. Thus, in leads I, aV_L, V_5, and V_6, development of RBBB may cause inverted T waves to become upright, depressed ST segments to return to baseline, and normal ST segments to become elevated. In the right precordial leads, upright T waves may become inverted, inverted T waves more inverted, elevated ST segments normal, normal ST segments depressed, and depressed ST segments more depressed. QT intervals average 0.05 second longer than normal[112] with RBBB.

Incomplete Right Bundle Branch Block

Etiology

The pattern of incomplete right bundle branch block (IRBBB) may occur as a variant of normal, especially in young adults. If the QRS complex is prolonged to 0.10 second or more, IRBBB is more likely to represent a real conduction abnormality. Such abnormalities may occur with ostium secondum type of atrial septal defects (ASD) or anomalous pulmonary venous drainage. This pattern may represent late depolarization of the crista supraventricularis in these conditions or any conditions that produce right-sided hypertension or RVH, such as pulmonary hypertension or pulmonary stenosis. When IRBBB occurs with ostium primum type of ASD, and especially with endocardial cushion defects that include VSD, there is associated LAFB.[141] Incomplete right bundle branch block may also occur as a congenital abnormality unassociated with other lesions.[142] Examination of intervals from HB potentials to right ventricular apex potentials in ASD suggests that the associated pattern of IRBBB does not represent delay in the RBBB,[143] and in animals the pattern of IRBBB may be due to variations in the thickness of the right ventricular free wall[144] or may be produced by incising the internal subdivision of the RBB (the false tendon).[145]

Clinical Findings

When IRBBB is associated with ASD, splitting of the heart sound tends to be wide and fixed. These findings may be related to the large shunt flow rather than to electrical events. The prognosis of patients with IRBBB is associated with the natural history or surgical intervention for the pathologic condition (if one exists).

The Electrocardiogram

In patients with IRBBB, there is usually a terminal S wave in some or all of the left-sided leads (leads I, aV_L, V_5, and V_6) and an R′ in right precordial leads V_1 and sometimes V_2 (see Tables 16-1 and 16-2). Right ventricular hypertrophy differs in that right axis deviation is seen, lead V_1 usually shows a QR, a QRS, or an RS, rather than an RSR′, and the QRS is narrow. QRS complex duration in patients with IRBBB is sometimes in the normal range but classically is 0.1 to 0.11 second. T waves tend to be upright and therefore opposite the abnormal S waves in the left-sided leads and are sometimes secondarily inverted and opposite the R′ waves in the right precordial leads. T wave changes on the left side tend to disguise T waves that are small or slightly inverted from other causes and, on the right side, falsely suggest an active or ischemic myocardial process.

Incomplete Left Bundle Branch Block

Etiology

Incomplete left bundle branch block (ILBBB) may represent an intermediate step along the way to "complete" LBBB and as such can be seen in the elderly without clinical evidence of other heart disease, or it may be associated with coronary artery disease, hypertensive heart disease, aortic valvular disease, or cardiomyopathy. Frequently, ILBBB is seen in association with LVH and is used by some clinicians as one electrocardiographic criterion for this diagnosis.[146]

Clinical Findings

The clinical findings and the prognosis of ILBBB are those related to the associated cardiac disease, such as hypertension with LVH.

The Electrocardiogram

QRS complexes are prolonged to 0.1 to 0.11 second, and left-sided Q waves are absent or significantly decreased in leads I, aV_L, V_5, and V_6 (Fig. 16-9; see Tables 16-1 and 16-2). The QRS complex is minimally slurred throughout. T waves become abnormally small or inverted in left-sided leads (I, aV_L, V_5, and V_6) and sometimes abnormally upright in right precordial leads. The inverted T waves in the left-sided leads may mimic the changes of anterolateral ischemia, and the changes in the right precordial leads may obliterate the electrocardiographic findings of anteroseptal ischemia.

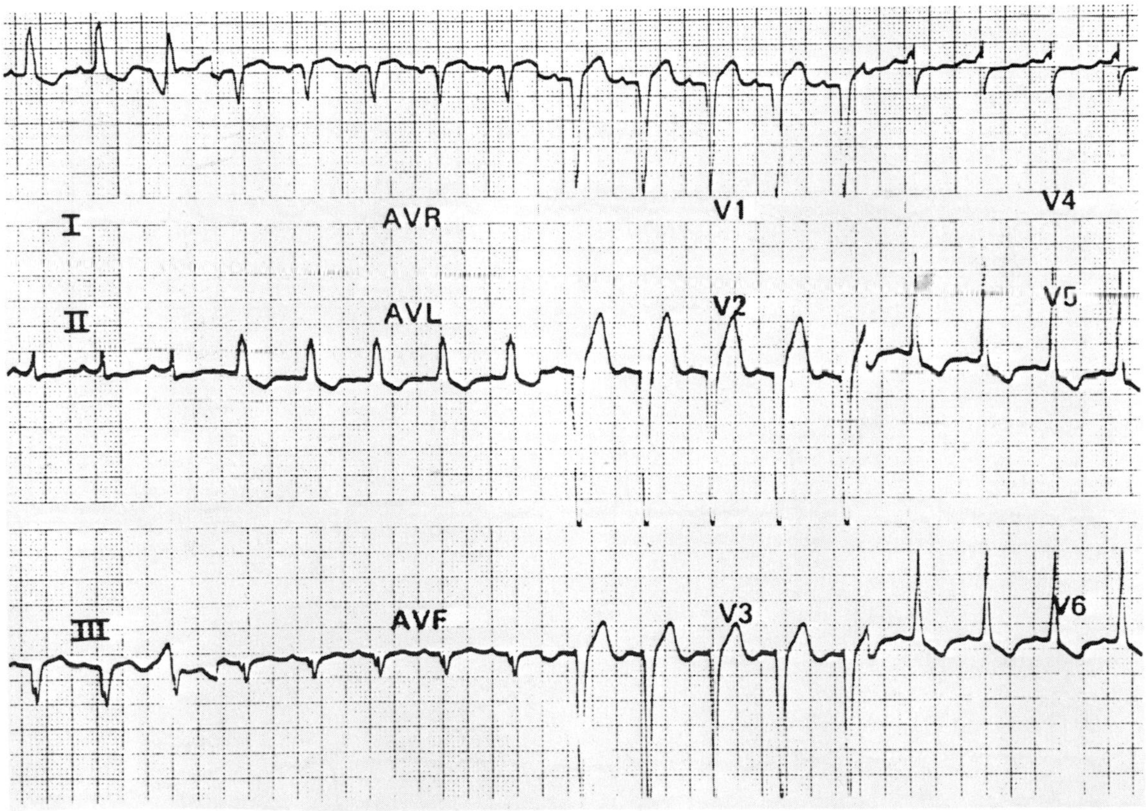

Figure 16-9. *This 12-lead electrocardiogram taken during sinus tachycardia at a rate of 114 beats/min shows incomplete left bundle branch block associated with left ventricular hypertrophy. There are no Q waves in leads I and* aV_L *or in the left precordial leads. R waves are absent or minimal in leads* V_1 *and* V_2*. QRS complexes are slurred in all leads. T waves are inverted in leads I and* aV_L *and in the left precordial leads. ST segments are depressed in the same leads and elevated in right precordial leads. QRS duration is 0.1 second.*

Left Anterior Fascicular Block

Etiology

Left anterior fascicular block (LAFB) unassociated with block in other fascicles may occur with aging without evidence of other specific cardiac disease. This conduction defect may occur secondary to a conduction defect in the HB, anterior ischemia, anterior myocardial infarction, Chagas' disease, sclerodegenerative disease, cardiomyopathy, calcific aortic valve disease,[147] hyperkalemia,[93] myocarditis, infiltrative and degenerative diseases, and trauma. The disorder is usually considered a relatively benign abnormality in adults, but one study has shown that patients with LAFB who were undergoing coronary angiography, and therefore already suspected of having coronary artery disease, had a 50% chance of having 95% or greater occlusion of the left anterior descending coronary artery.[148] Occasionally LAFB is congenital, and in an infant it often indicates either ostium primum atrial septal defect (usually with IRBB or RBBB) or tricuspid atresia.[149] However, RBBB and LAFB may be acquired conduction defects with ostium primum.[150] Left anterior fascicular block may occur in 5% of hospitalized patients. Pathologically, fibrosis has been found at autopsy in the branching portion of the LBB in patients who had LAFB. In one study fibrosis was always present in the anterior fibers but frequently was widely distributed over the anterior, mid, and posterior fibers.[151]

Clinical Findings

The physical findings associated with left anterior fascicular block are those of associated abnormalities. The prognosis of LAFB depends on the age at which it occurs and the associated cardiac diseases. There is no apparent effect on prognosis when LAFB occurs with aging, especially in the eighth decade of life, in the absence of other obvious cardiac diseases. The incidence of progression to bifascicular block is 7% and to complete AV block, 3%.[138] Also, the presence or development of LAFB does not increase mortality or complicate the course of an acute myocardial infarction.[106,152]

The Electrocardiogram

The changes of LAFB frequently find expression in most of the 12 electrocardiogram leads (Fig. 16-10; see Tables 16-1 and 16-2). In leads II, III, and aV_F, complexes tend to be rS, and in leads I and aV_L, qR.[153] These deep termi-

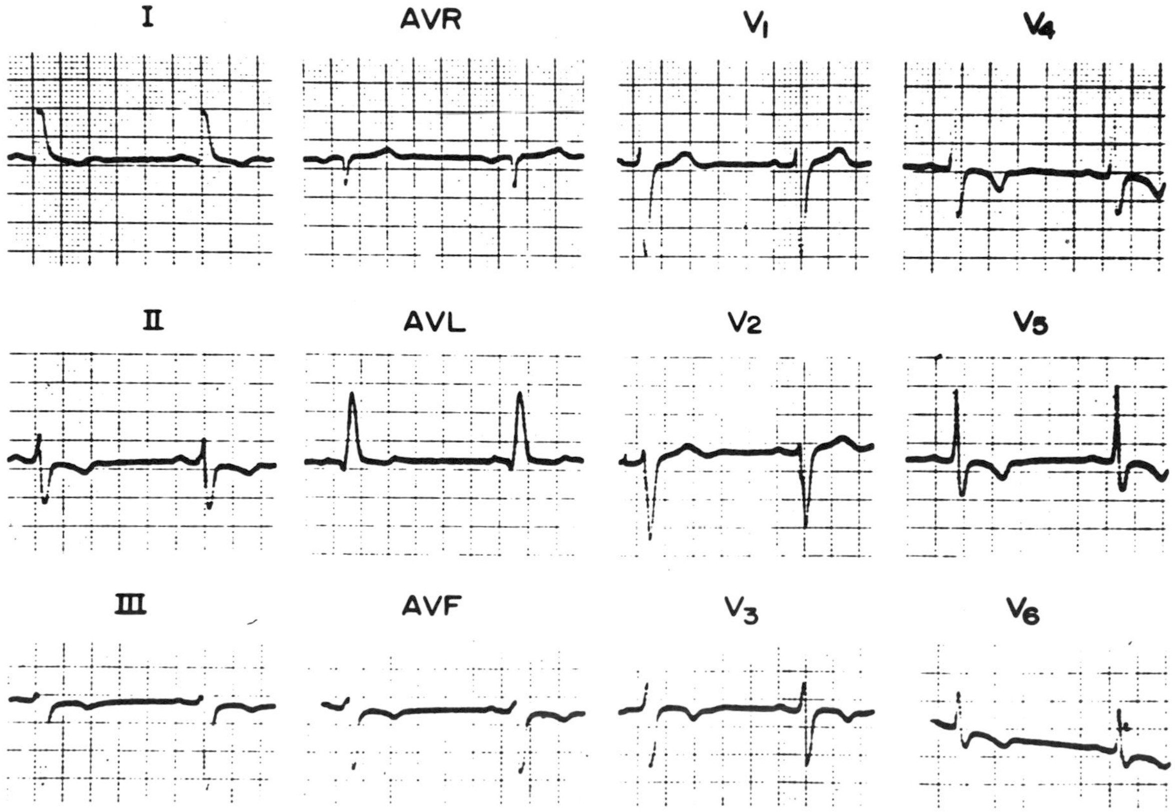

Figure 16-10. *Sinus bradycardia with left anterior fascicular block. Terminal forces are inverted in leads II, III, and aV_F, with S wave voltage greater than R wave voltage. R waves are tall in lead aV_L. There are terminal S waves in left precordial leads. QRS duration is prolonged to 0.12 second. In addition, this electrocardiogram shows inferior and anterolateral ischemia.*

nal S waves in leads II, III, and aV_F and terminal R waves in aV_R almost always mean anterior fascicular block, even in the presence of the QS complexes of inferior myocardial infarction. QRS complexes frequently become biphasic in the left precordial leads V_4 through V_6, of the RS type, and occasionally small, new Q waves may appear in the right precordial leads.[80,154] Thus, LAFB may mimic lateral myocardial or anteroseptal infarction, and new initial r waves in inferior leads may hide inferior myocardial infarction.[25] The axis is usually between $-30°$ and $-90°$ but may cross over into the right upper quadrant of the frontal plane, perhaps as far as $-110°$. R waves tend to become taller in leads I and aV_F, so that the usual criteria for left ventricular hypertrophy in these leads may not be valid in the presence of LAFB.[25] T waves may become inverted in leads I and aV_L and tend to be upright in leads II, III, and aV_L, sometimes hiding otherwise inverted T waves in the inferior leads. Likewise, T waves tend to become more upright in the left precordial leads in which the QRS complexes have become biphasic. Associated ST and T wave changes may help one differentiate between the right precordial Q waves of anteroseptal infarction and Q waves that sometimes appear in the right precordial leads secondary to LAFB. Also, the Q waves of infarction tend to be wider (≥ 0.04 second) and more slurred.

The development of LAFB is associated with slight prolongation of the QRS complex (average increase 25 msec). The more marked the left axis deviation, the greater the QRS prolongation.[155] A delay in the time of inscription of the intrinsicoid deflection in lead aV_L (greater than 50 msec) and a 10 msec longer time of inscription of the intrinsicoid deflection in lead aV_L compared to lead V_6 have also been used as criteria for LAFB,[156] as has a shift of the initial 0.02 second forces inferiorly and to the right.[157]

Left Posterior Fascicular Block

Etiology

Left posterior fascicular block (LPFB) may occur unassociated with block of other fascicles, as a result of a chronic degenerative or fibrotic process of the specialized conduction system of the ventricles, hyperkalemia, an ischemic process affecting the posterior fascicle itself or perhaps the Purkinje system or myocardium for which the posterior fascicle ordinarily serves as the specialized conduction pathway, myocarditis, infiltrative disease, Chagas' disease, and possibly acute cor pulmonale.[158]

The Electrocardiogram

Left posterior fascicular block usually produces a right axis deviation such that in lead I and usually in lead aV_L there is a small R wave and a deep S wave, while in leads II, III, and aV_F there are small Q waves and tall R waves (see Tables 16-1 and 16-2). This pattern may mimic an inferior myocardial infarction or hide a lateral myocardial infarction.[25] However, some observers suggest that right axis deviation is unusual and that the diagnosis should be made on the basis of the other described changes, including initial and terminal slurring of the QRS and delayed onset of R wave intrinsicoid deflection greater than 45 msec in lead aV_F.[159] Left precordial leads such as V_5 and V_6 sometimes display biphasic QRS complexes. The QRS complex in lead V_1 is mainly negative and thus does not suggest RVH. When LPFB is associated with a positive QRS in lead V_1 due to RBBB, RVH must be ruled out clinically. When right axis deviation is the result of the positional changes that occur with chronic pulmonary disease, R waves in leads II, III, and aV_F are not tall (as they are with LPFB), and, in general, the voltage of complexes in most of the 12 leads is decreased. In children and young adults, right axis deviation is frequently normal and differentiation between a juvenile pattern and LPFB is difficult.

T waves tend to be more upright in leads I and aV_L, and this tendency may mask pathologically small or slightly inverted T waves that would appear in these leads in the absence of the conduction defect. T waves may become inverted in leads II, III, and aV_F in patients with LPFB and may mimic an active or ischemic inferior myocardial process.

Acute cor pulmonale or anterolateral myocardial infarction may produce changes similar to those of LPFB. Thus, clinical correlation and close attention to other electrocardiographic details are necessary before LPFB can be diagnosed.

Left Septal Fascicular Block

Etiology

Left septal fascicular block (LSFB) has been anatomically demonstrated[160,161] and is most commonly found in patients with ischemic heart disease, especially when angina pectoris and papillary muscle dysfunction are present. Other etiologies include diabetes mellitus and hypertrophic cardiomyopathy. The disorder is associated with fibrosis of the septal fascicle of the LBB.[162]

Clinical Findings

Symptoms and signs in patients with LSFB are those found with the primary diseases. The cardiac findings often include a systolic murmur when papillary muscle dysfunction is associated.

The Electrocardiogram

The electrocardiogram shows prominent R waves in the right precordial leads[162] similar to those found in "true" posterior myocardial infarction or may show Q waves in these leads.[163]

Right Bundle Branch Block and Left Anterior Fascicular Block

Etiology

Among the major causes of RBBB with LAFB are sclero-degenerative disease of the specialized conduction system of the ventricles, mainly in the elderly,[147] ischemic heart disease,[164] especially myocardial infarction[165] involving the interventricular septum, hypertension,[164] and Chagas' disease (in South America). Right bundle branch block with LAFB may occur as a congenital abnormality alone[142,166] or associated with progressive ophthalmoplegia.[167] There is also a familial form associated with syncope and a high incidence of sudden death.[168-170] This conduction defect may also be associated with chest trauma,[171,172] hyperkalemia,[93] myocarditis, aortic valve disease,[147] cardiomyopathy, or granulomatous disease of the ventricles such as sarcoidosis.[173] Pathologically, many patients show fibrosis, calcification, and fatty changes in the central fibrous body, the HB, both proximal bundle branches, the intermediary portions of the RBBB, and the anterior fibers of the LBB.[3,10,22,174,175] The disorder may also occur as a result of surgical repair of tetralogy of Fallot or of VSD. Right-sided intracardiac conduction-time studies have shown that RBBB with LAFB in these circumstances indicates damage to the specialized conduction system, whereas RBBB alone indicates only a surgically induced lesion in the peripheral Purkinje system.[176] Surgically induced RBBB with LAFB may be an ominous sign requiring permanent pacing[177]; however, without evidence of fixed or transient residual trifascicular block,[178] the prognosis may be good even without pacing, at least for several years.[179] There appears to be no increase in mortality, with or without chronic coronary artery disease,[58] in the absence of fixed or transient AV block.

Clinical Findings

On physical examination, RBBB with LAFB may produce the same change in heart sounds as RBBB alone, that is, widening of the second heart sound. Phonocardiogram, carotid pulse tracings, and cardiograms show late onset and slow rise of ventricular ejection.[180] Otherwise, physical findings are related to the etiologic disease. Chronic RBBB with LAFB may carry a rate of progression to advanced AV block of 10%[181] or higher[182] in patients followed for various times and 19% in patients followed for 5 years.[58] If organic heart disease is present, the rate of progression to higher degrees of AV block ranges from 14% to 100%.[72,183,184] RBBB[185] with LAFB that develops at the time of acute anteroseptal myocardial infarction significantly changes the patient's prognosis for surviving the acute episode, especially if the HV interval on an HB recording is prolonged.[186] Complete AV block may develop, and because bifascicular block suggests that a large portion of myocardial tissue has been destroyed, the incidence of cardiogenic shock is higher than in similar patients without bifascicular block. An artificial transvenous pacemaker may not change the survival rate of patients with acute anteroseptal myocardial infarction with RBBB and LAFB. However, most cardiologists recommend insertion of a temporary ventricular pacemaker in such circumstances[187] even if RBBB was previously present.[106] If bifascicular block precedes the acute myocardial infarction, the 1-year mortality is 65%, although sudden death is unlikely.[43] If the intraventricular conduction defect persists,[187-189] and especially if transient second or third degree AV block occurs,[189,190,191] permanent pacing may prolong life.[191-193] These recommendations apply also to the development of LBBB less strongly and to the development of RBBB alone; they probably do not apply to the development of LAFB or LPFB alone at the time of myocardial infarction.

Asymptomatic ambulatory patients with chronic RBBB and LAFB have a good prognosis,[194] whereas similar hospitalized patients have a significant risk of sudden death or development of complete AV block,[195] especially if HQ intervals are markedly prolonged.[186,196] Although there is some correlation between prolonged PR intervals and long HQ intervals[197] most long HQ intervals are associated with normal PR intervals in the presence of RBBB and LAFB.[198] Patients with RBBB and LAFB who have long HQ intervals are more likely to have more severe cardiac disease with cardiomegaly and congestive heart failure as compared to patients with normal HQ intervals.[199] Pacemakers for patients with chronic RBBB and LAFB have not been shown to change statistically the risk of sudden death unless second degree AV block is present. For example, ventricular fibrillation, rather than AV block, is the cause of death in many patients who have Chagas' disease[200] with BBB. If it is not already present, second degree HQ block is not likely to occur with rapid atrial pacing[100] or during anesthesia[54,201] in patients with RBBB and LAFB without cardiac symptoms, although in one study one patient of 44 with RBBB and LAFB developed transient AV block during intubation.[202] One group has reported a 12% 3-year cardiovascular mortality in patients with bifascicular block.[98] Another showed that in patients with RBBB and LAFB and long HQ intervals, permanent pacemakers decreased the incidence of sudden death,[203] whereas the group that found a high incidence of sudden death (10% the first year, 13% the second year, and 16% the third year) in patients with chronic bifascicular block reported that monitored deaths were due to ventricular fibrillation rather than to AV block.

The Electrocardiogram

Right bundle branch block and LAFB each produce their own changes of QRS and T contour, of which some are superimposed (Fig. 16-11; see Tables 16-1 and 16-2).

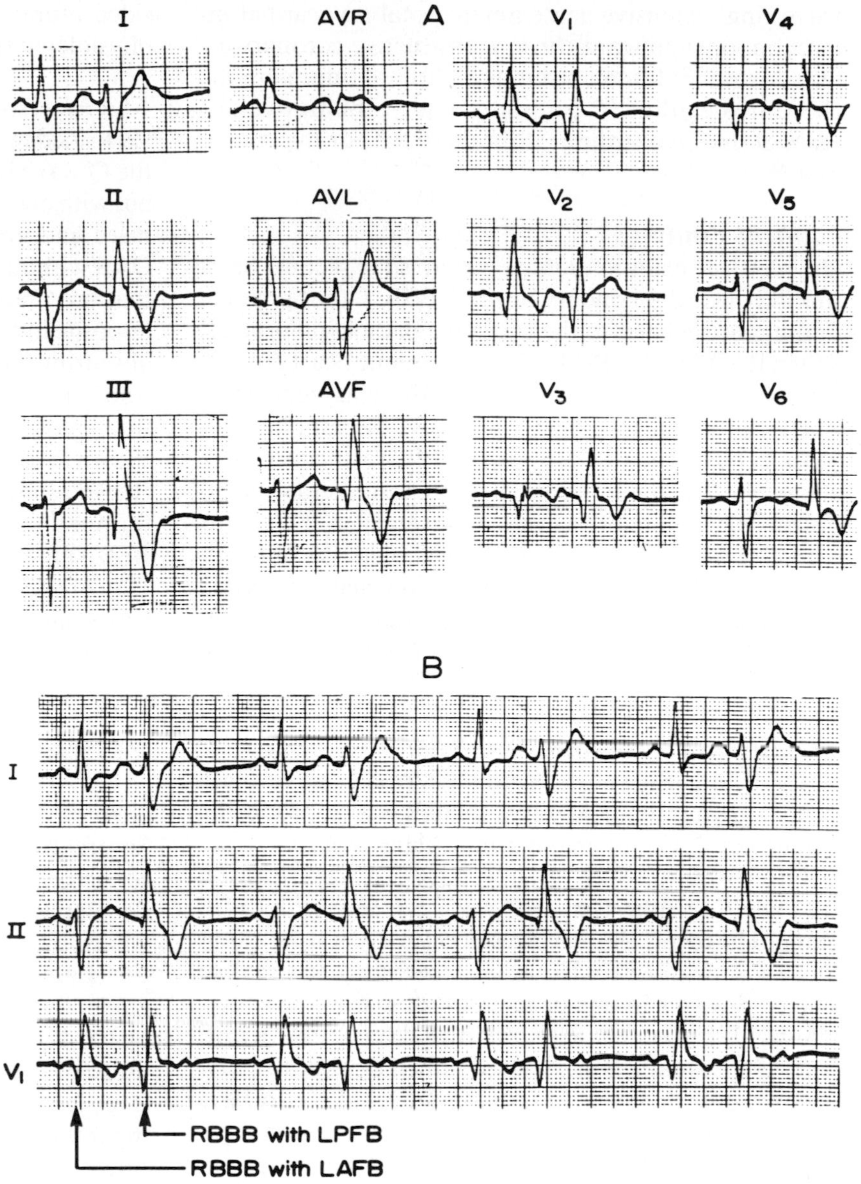

Figure 16-11. *(A) The 12-lead electrocardiogram shows two conducted P waves and one blocked P wave in each lead. (The bigeminal rhythm is best seen in the tracings in B.) In A, the first QRS complex of each pair shows right bundle branch block (RBBB) with left anterior fascicular block (LAFB). The second of each pair of QRS complexes shows RBBB with left posterior fascicular block (LPFB). The Q waves in right precordial leads in both beats indicate anteroseptal myocardial infarction. However, Q waves are present only in the second of each pair of beats in leads II, III, and aV_F, implying that LPFB may mimic inferior myocardial infarction or that LAFB may hide this abnormality. Overall, there is constant RBBB and 3:1 block in both the left anterior fascicle and the left posterior fascicle, but occurring out of phase by one beat, producing the alternate QRS pattern and the 3:2 AV block.*

Usually there is a tall R wave and a terminal slurred S wave in leads I and aV_L, and a small Q wave may be present or absent. In leads II and aV_F, small R waves and deep, widened S waves are usually seen. Lead III and sometimes leads II and aV_F shows a small R wave and either a deep, widened S wave or a deep S wave and a terminal slurred R wave. T waves tend to be more upright in leads I, aV_L, and sometimes II, III, and aV_F, sometimes obscuring small or inverted T waves that might otherwise be present. In lead V_1 and sometimes in leads V_2 and V_3 there is a terminal slurred R wave. T waves tend to be inverted, sometimes mimicking anteroseptal ischemia. Right precordial leads may also show a small Q wave and a tall, wide, slurred R or R′ wave, with an inverted T wave, and recent anteroseptal myocardial infarction must be ruled out on the basis of other clinical or electrocardiographic findings, such as the presence of only narrow Q waves or the disappearance of RBBB and LAFB simultaneously with the disappearance of anteroseptal Q waves and T wave inversions. Left precordial leads are biphasic, with terminal slurred S waves. The frontal plane axis on the basis of voltage of R and S is leftward.

Right Bundle Branch Block with Left Posterior Fascicular Block

Etiology

Right bundle branch block with LPFB may occur as a result of sclerosis of the specialized conduction system of the ventricles or, like all the other bundle branch and fascicular blocks, as a result of calcium impingement on the conduction system in the aortic valve or the mitral valve ring, extensive acute anteroseptal myocardial infarction, or significant chronic obstructive coronary artery disease.[204] It may occur as a result of trauma to the chest, myocarditis,[205] cardiomyopathy, infiltrative diseases of the myocardium, scleroderma,[206] or hyperkalemia.[93]

Clinical Findings

On physical examination, a widely split second heart sound is heard secondary to the RBBB. Other physical findings are related to the causative pathologic process. When RBBB with LPFB is due to ischemic heart disease, extensive damage to the interventricular septum is likely. The incidence of development of complete AV block is high when RBBB with LPFB is associated with acute anteroseptal myocardial infarction, a situation requiring placement of an artificial pacemaker.[207] Patients with chronic RBBB and LPFB are at high risk of developing complete AV block,[208] which is usually preceded by second degree AV block and associated with symptoms and progression of the causative pathologic process.[28]

The Electrocardiogram (See Tables 1 and 2)

Leads I and aV_L show terminal slurred S waves with voltage greater than the initial small R waves, producing a right axis deviation in the frontal plane (Fig. 16-11; see Tables 16-1 and 16-2). Usually, but not always, leads II, III, and aV_F display a small Q wave as is seen with LPFB alone. However, the R waves are usually not as tall as those seen with LPFB alone, and there may be terminal slurred S waves in one or more of these leads. The previously described changes of RBBB are present. RBBB with LPFB should be diagnosed only if right ventricular hypertrophy or lateral infarction are unlikely to have produced the right axis deviation.

Right bundle branch block with LAFB may change to RBBB with LPFB (see Fig. 16-11) suddenly[209] or gradually, the latter suggesting a Weckebach phenomenon in the left posterior fascicle.[210]

Mural Delays

Etiology

Left- and right-sided intraventricular conduction defects may occur because of damage to the muscle or the Purkinje system produced by coronary artery obstruction, cardiomyopathy,[211] infiltrative diseases such as sarcoidosis or amyloidosis, hyperkalemia, or right ventriculotomy during cardiac surgery.

Clinical Findings

Left-sided mural conduction defects may cause paradoxic splitting of the second heart sounds, and right-sided mural conduction defects may produce wide but physiologic splitting of the second heart sound.

The Electrocardiogram

Left-sided mural conduction defects may produce loss of the Q wave in leads I, aV_L, V_5, and V_6 similar to LBBB but with extreme widening of the QRS, frequently to 160 msec and greater. There may also be widening of the QRS without loss of left-sided Q waves but with forces that are mainly left and posterior. T waves tend to be opposite in direction to the main QRS forces, sometimes obscuring normal or abnormal T waves. With right-sided mural conduction defects, the electrocardiogram is frequently indistinguishable from RBBB but has been shown to differ in that QRS duration is greater than with RBBB alone.[28] Myocardial infarction may produce intramural conduction defects that are not similar to any BBB (Fig. 16-12). Intraventricular conduction defects may produce very late forces, appearing as late as the T wave and, in a reported case of right ventricular myopathy, may represent epsilon potentials.[212]

Ventricular Preexcitation

Etiology

Several bypass tracts in the human heart have been described, any one of which may cause the ventricle to be depolarized earlier than normal and all but one type of which produce a change in the QRS contour. These tracts must be operative and must demonstrate anterograde, retrograde, or bidirectional conduction to be recognized. The bundles of Kent directly connect atrial muscle to either the left posterior ventricular muscle (type A) or the right ventricular muscle (type B), producing ventricular preexcitation. It may now be more appropriate to refer to variations of accessory pathways according to location, such as left or right ventricular free wall, or to left or right septum, and even to designate high or low or anterior, posterior, or lateral ventricular wall. James' fibers connect the atrium to the HB, bypassing the AV node, allowing for short PR intervals but normal QRS complexes. However, when this type of bypass is associated with LBBB, a Kent bypass may be mistakenly suspected.[213] Mahaim fibers connect the HB to the ventricular muscle directly and, when operative, produce abnormal QRS contour without significant PR interval shortening.

Classic Wolff-Parkinson-White (WPW) syndrome is associated with an operating bundle of Kent on the right or left side that at least intermittently produces early depolarization of the ventricles associated with an initial slurred wave on the QRS (delta wave). The incidence may be 0.2%.[58] Patients with WPW syndrome have episodes of tachycardia produced either by a circus move-

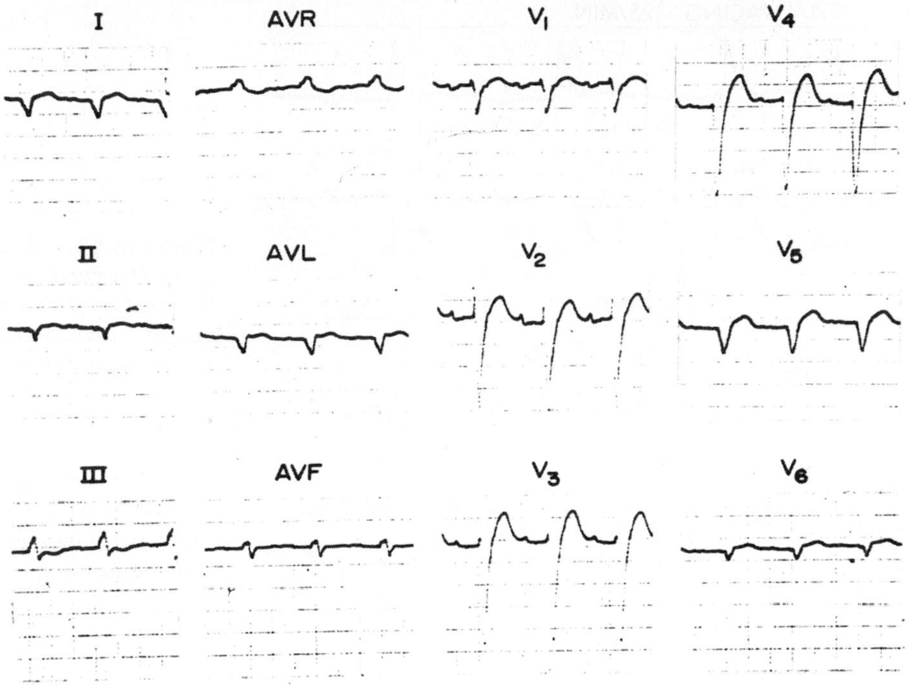

Figure 16-12. *QS complexes in leads I, II, aV_L, V_5, and V_6 are compatible with lateral myocardial infarction. QRS complexes are slightly widened and slurred, but the intraventricular conduction defect does not suggest any of the usual patterns of bundle branch block or fascicular block and is therefore a nonspecific intraventricular conduction defect secondary to the myocardial infarction.*

ment using the normal and accessory pathways or by one or several reentry beats through the accessory or the normal pathway, producing an early atrial or ventricular depolarization that provokes an atrial, reciprocating junctional, or, rarely, ventricular tachycardia.

The diagnosis of the WPW type of ventricular preexcitation may be made with greater certainty after HB recordings show short HQ intervals (Fig. 16-13) associated with delta waves, especially in patients who have demonstrated paroxysmal supraventricular tachycardias.

Clinical Findings

WPW syndrome represents the most typical set of clinical circumstances found in patients with recognized ventricular preexcitation. There is early depolarization of the ventricles through the bundle of Kent, causing a delta wave. On the physical examination, the second heart sound may be paradoxically split if the patient has ventricular preexcitation with a right-sided ventricle. The second heart sound in left-sided ventricular preexcitation is physiologically but widely split because of early depolarization of the left ventricle. Ventricular preexcitation is congenital and tends to be hereditary. One congenital lesion with a significant simultaneous occurence is Ebstein's anomaly, in which the displacement of the tricuspid valve usually causes a systolic murmur of tricuspid regurgitation and the physical findings of RVH.

Supraventricular tachycardias occur in 79% of patients with WPW syndrome, atrial fibrillation being found in 17% and atrial flutter in 40%. Long-term morbidity is slightly increased, and death may occur from rapid rates associated with paroxysmal atrial fibrillation or development of ventricular fibrillation.[58] This is more likely to occur with patients on digitalis or calcium blockers.[214] If arrhythmias are symptomatic, especially if they are life threatening and resistant to medication, surgery should be considered. Patients with ventricular rates of 200 beats/min or greater during atrial fibrillation should be considered for surgery.[215] Such high rates are more likely to be found in patients with persistent rather than intermittent preexcitation.[216] At surgery, epicardial mapping must be performed to delineate the bypass location. However, certain information should be obtained even before surgery. The 12-lead electrocardiogram may suggest the general location of the bypass tract. Ventriculoatrial conduction times may be helpful.[217] During reciprocating tachycardias using the normal conduction pathway as the anterograde tract and a free wall bypass as the retrograde tract, if BBB occurs on the side of the bypass, the ventriculoatrial interval will increase because the ventricular depolarization starts in

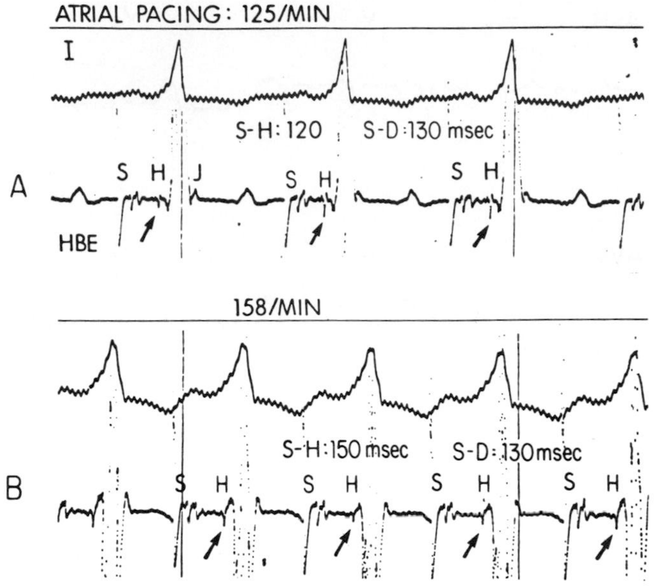

Figure 16-13. *A case of ventricular preexcitation. Lead I and a His bundle electrogram (HBE) are shown. SH intervals are 120 msec at an atrial pacing rate of 125 beats/min in A and 150 msec at a pacing rate of 158 beats/min in B. The pacing spike to the beginning of the delta wave (SD) interval remains the same at 130 msec. Thus, the conduction time through the accessory pathway remains constant at both pacing rates. However, because SH is longer at the faster pacing rate, the relationship of the H and the beginning of the delta wave changes. In A, H is almost simultaneous with the delta wave; in B, H occurs clearly after the beginning of the delta wave.*

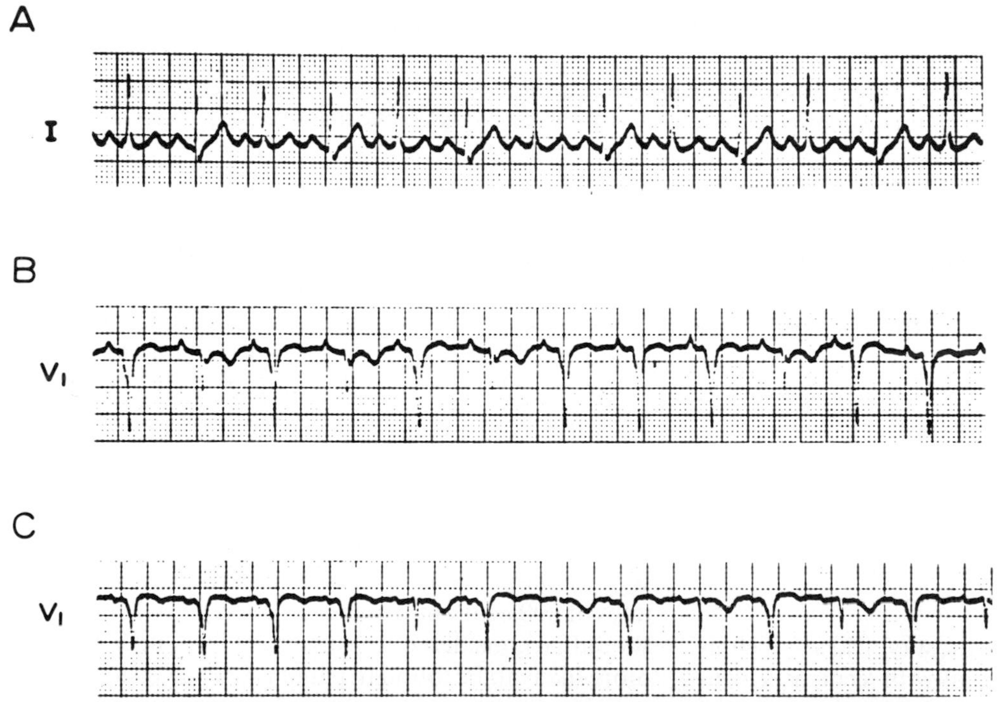

Figure 16-14. *A shows lead I during electrical alternans. Half the QRS complexes have a terminal slurred S wave and suggest incomplete right bundle branch block. Alternate complexes show disappearance of the small initial Q waves, a slightly shorter PR interval, and no terminal S wave. This occurred in a known case of ventricular preexcitation, type B. The accessory pathway goes to the right ventricle and depolarizes the area responsible for the terminal S waves in incomplete right bundle branch block. Thus, type B Wolff-Parkinson-White syndrome eliminates the findings of incomplete right bundle branch block. In B and C, lead V_1 shows clearly the shorter PR intervals associated with beats that display type B Wolff-Parkinson-White syndrome. Especially in C, the very small R′ wave suggesting incomplete right bundle branch block disappears on beats with ventricular preexcitation. The tracings in B and C are from two different patients.*

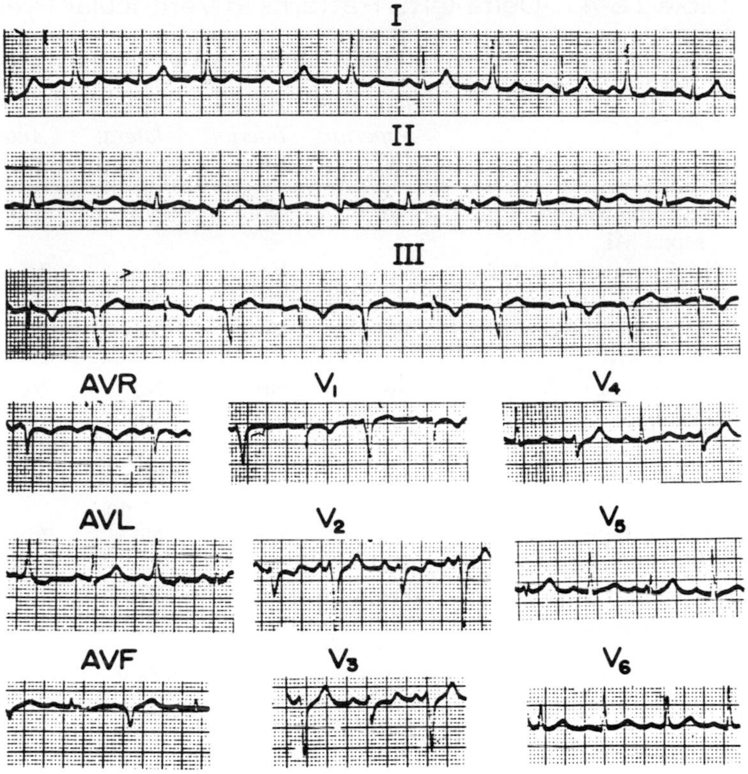

Figure 16-15. *Alternate beats are widened and slurred, especially in their initial portions, and have a short PR interval. Initial slurring is upward in leads I and aV_L and in all precordial leads, but in leads II, III, and aV_F, slurring is downward, producing wide Q waves. These features suggest ventricular preexcitation with a bypass from the atria to the left ventricle with an insertion that is to the left, posterior, and relatively inferior, so that initial forces proceed from left to right, anteriorly, and superiorly. Leads II, III, and aV_F mimic the pattern of inferior myocardial infarction.*

the ventricle opposite the bypass and must cross the septum before reaching the bypass.[218] Rarely, if the bypass cannot be selectively interrupted and arrhythmias have been unacceptably symptomatic or life threatening, complete AV block is surgically produced and a ventricular pacemaker is inserted.

The Electrocardiogram

In patients with an accessory pathway, preexcitation is sometimes intermittent, sometimes absent, sometimes constant, and sometimes found on alternate beats (Figs. 16-14 and 16-15; Tables 16-3 to 16-5).

The electrocardiogram in patients with type A (atrium to posterior left ventricular free wall bypass) WPW syndrome (Fig. 16-16) shows a slurred initial upward deflection (delta wave) in lead V_1 and usually an upright delta wave in left-sided leads such as I, aV_L, V_5, and V_6. Occasionally, the delta wave is upright in lead V_1 but inverted in leads I and aV_L (Fig. 16-17), suggesting a more superior and lateral left ventricular insertion of the

Table 16-3. Delta Waves in Ventricular Preexcitation*

	Type A: Accessory Pathway to			Type B: Accessory Pathway to
	Posterior Superior LV	*Posterior Inferior LV*	*Postero-lateral LV*	*Anterior RV*
Leads I, aV_L	Delta waves up	Delta waves up	Delta waves down	Delta Waves usually up
Leads II, III, aV_F	Delta waves up	Delta waves down	Delta waves usually up	Delta waves usually up
Lead V_1	Delta waves up	Delta waves up	Delta waves up	Delta waves down
Lead V_5, V_6	Delta waves up	Delta waves up	Delta waves down	Delta waves up

* The variation in ventricular preexcitation is greater than indicated here. These are common patterns. LV, left ventricle; RV, right ventricle.

Table 16-4. Delta-QRS Patterns in Ventricular Preexcitation*

	Type A: Accessory Pathway to			Type B: Accessory Pathway to
	Posterior Superior LV	*Posterior Inferior LV*	*Postero-lateral LV*	*Anterior RV*
May mimic antero-septal MI	No	No	No	Yes
May mimic inferior MI	No	Yes	No	No
May mimic lateral MI	No	No	Yes	No
May mimic true pos-terior MI	Yes	Yes	Yes	No
May mimic LBBB	No	No	No	Yes
May mimic RBBB	Yes	Yes	Yes	No
May hide anteroseptal MI	Yes	Yes	Yes	No
May hide inferior MI	Yes	No	Usually no	No
May hide lateral MI	Yes	Yes	No	Yes
May hide true posterior MI	No	No	No	Yes
May hide LBBB	Yes	Yes	Yes	No
May hide RBBB	No	No	No	Yes

* The variation in ventricular preexcitation is greater than indicated here. These are common patterns. LV, left ventricle; RV, right ventricle; MI, myocardial infarction; LBBB, left bundle branch block; RBBB, right bundle branch block.

accessory pathway. In type B (atrium to anterior right ventricular free wall) WPW syndrome, the delta wave is downward in lead V_1 and upward in leads I, aV_L, V_5, and V_6 (Fig. 16-18). In patients with WPW syndrome, the QRS complex usually represents a fusion beat in which a portion of the ventricle is depolarized through the accessory pathway and another portion through the normal pathway. However, if conduction through the normal pathway is prolonged or absent, the ventricle will be completely depolarized through the accessory pathway, producing complete ventricular preexcitation (Fig. 16-19*A*), either type A or type B, and complete AV block

Table 16-5. T Wave Changes in Ventricular Preexcitation*

	Type A: Accessory Pathway to			Type B: Accessory Pathway to
	Posterior Superior LV	*Posterior Inferior LV*	*Postero-lateral LV*	*Anterior RV*
May mimic anterior ischemia	Yes	Yes	Yes	No
May mimic inferior ischemia	Yes	No	Yes	Yes
May mimic lateral ischemia	Yes	Yes	No	Yes
May hide anterior ischemia	No	No	No	Yes
May hide inferior ischemia	No	Yes	No	No
May hide lateral ischemia	No	No	Yes	No

* The variation in ventricular preexcitation is greater than indicated here. These are common patterns. LV, left ventricle; RV, right ventricle.

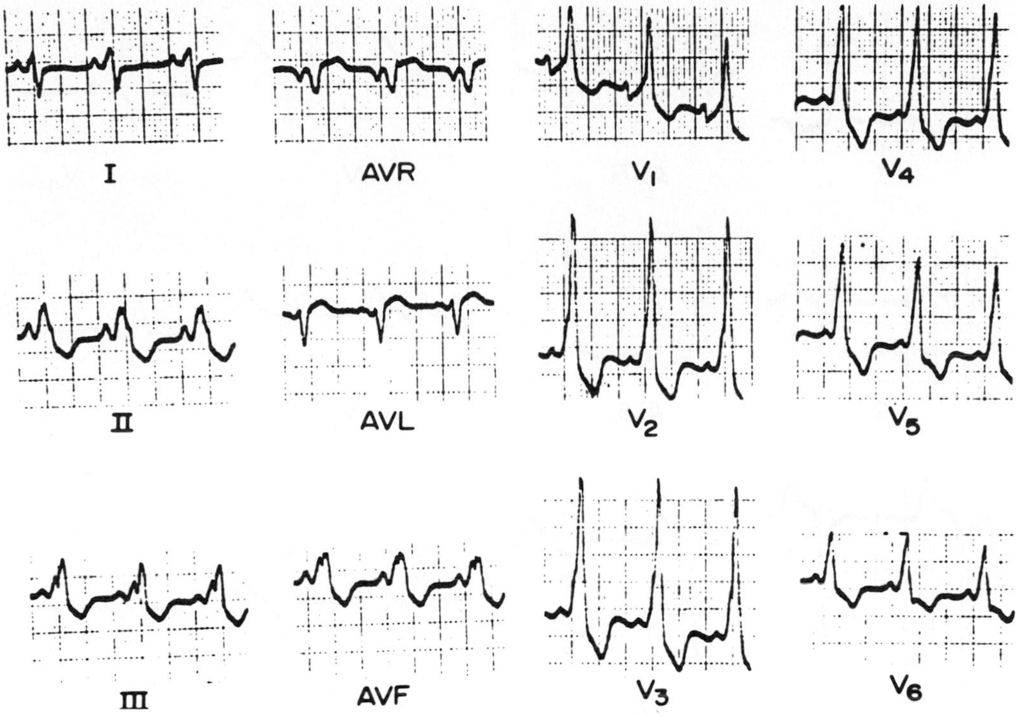

Figure 16-16. *Upright delta waves in right precordial leads. PR intervals are 0.1 second. The very wide QRS complexes, most clearly seen in leads II, III, and aV_F, the terminal S waves in lead I, and the entirely upright QRS complex in lead V_1 suggest the possibility of complete ventricular preexcitation, type A.*

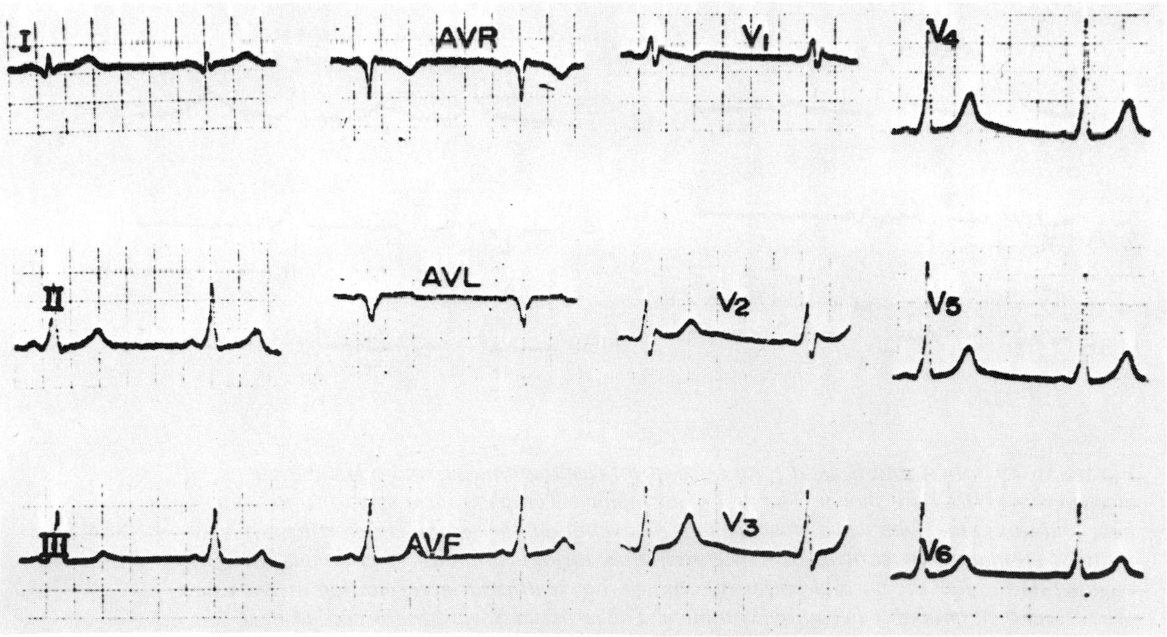

Figure 16-17. *Type A Wolff-Parkinson-White syndrome in which delta waves are upright in right precordial leads and in leads II, III, and aV_F but inverted in leads I and aV_L, mimicking high lateral myocardial infarction. There may be incomplete right bundle branch block as well.*

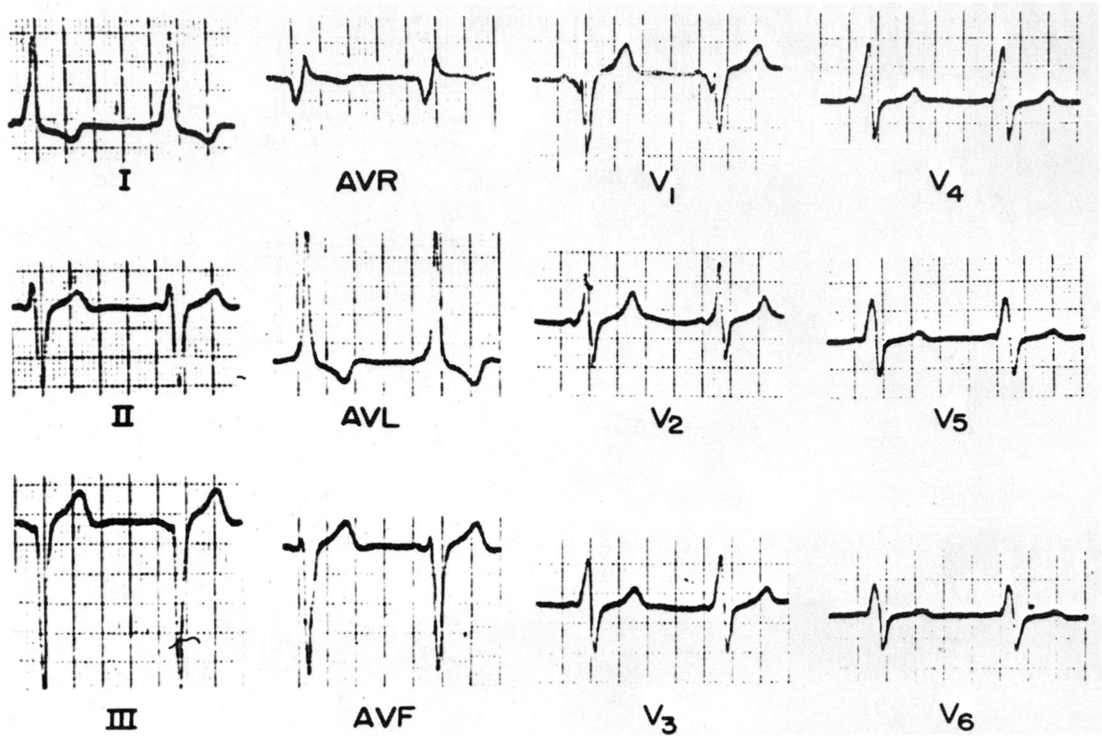

Figure 16-18. *Type B Wolff-Parkinson-White syndrome with downward-pointing delta waves in lead V_1. QRS complexes are mainly inverted in leads II, III, and aV_F, a pattern suggestive of left anterior fascicular block.*

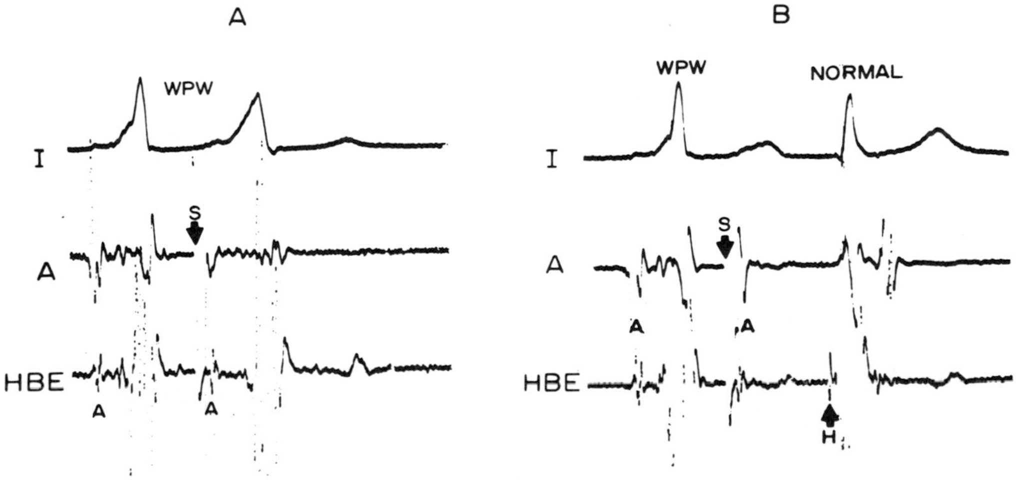

Figure 16-19. *In A and B, lead I, an intra-atrial electrogram (A), and a His bundle electrogram (HBE) are shown. The first of each pair of complexes is a spontaneous sinus beat and shows the delta wave of ventricular preexcitation; the second is an artificially induced premature atrial beat. In A, the premature atrial beat produces prolongation of conduction through the normal pathway so much that ventricular preexcitation increases on the second beat, probably becoming complete. The terminal S wave in the second beat suggests that this is type A Wolff-Parkinson-White syndrome (WPW) with a bypass to the left ventricle. In B, the atrial beat is more premature, and the wave of polarization finds the accessory pathway completely refractory, while the AV node is still relatively refractory, so that although the AH interval becomes markedly prolonged, the QRS complex is normal in contour.*

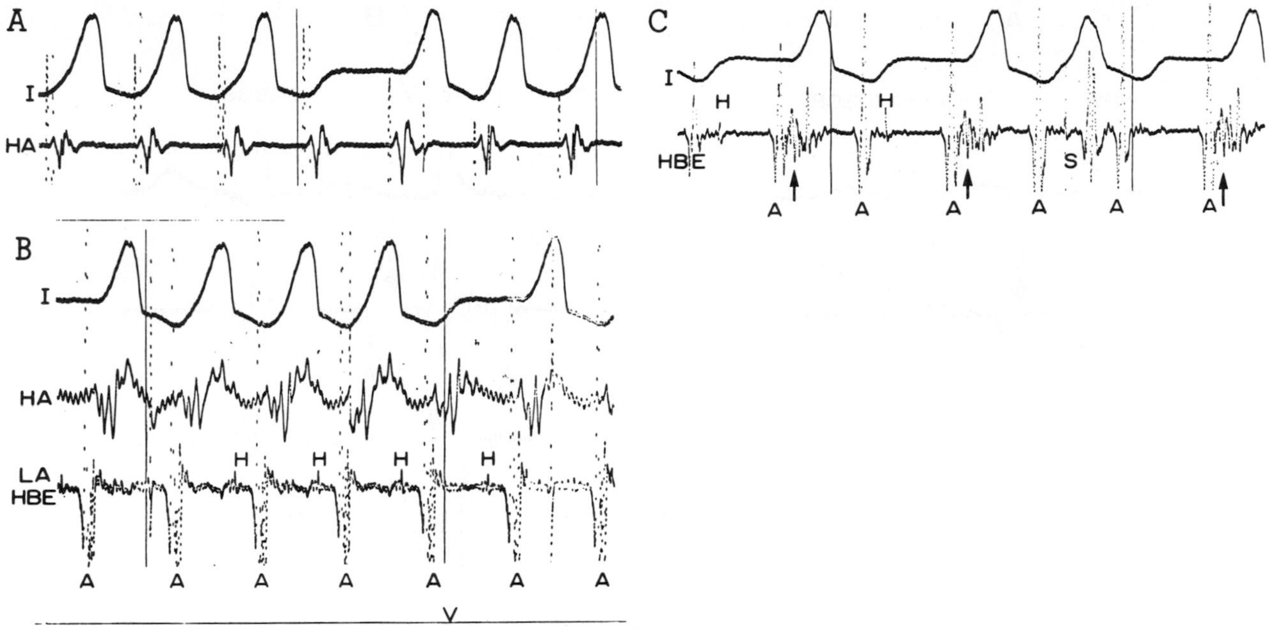

Figure 16-20. *In A, lead I and an atrial recording from the high right atrium (HA) show a regular spontaneous atrial tachycardia with slightly irregular ventricular responses, each of which shows an initial delta wave. One QRS, but no atrial complex, is missing, suggesting that although ventricular preexcitation may be present, the tachycardia is not the reciprocating type that uses the normal pathway for one leg and the accessory pathway for the other. That type of reciprocation requires involvement of the ventricles to complete the circuit, and if one ventricular beat is missing, the circuit would have been broken. B displays lead I and recordings from the HA and the low right atrium (LA) recorded at the usual location for the His bundle electrogram (HBE). Note that the His bundle appears to depolarize first, the LA second, the HA third, and the ventricles last. This would be compatible with a focal or reciprocating His bundle tachycardia using the normal AV conduction pathway retrogradely to the atria and only then using an accessory pathway anterograde to the ventricles (through James fibers). The QRS complexes in lead I all show delta waves, and the RR intervals in B progressively shorten until there is a long pause. This configuration suggests type I second degree block in the accessory pathway. Again, the pause is not associated with interruption of the atrial tachycardia. Therefore, the tachycardia cannot require the ventricle to complete the circuit. In C, lead I and an HBE are shown. An H follows each A, except the next-to-last one. Alternate A waves are followed by QRS complexes except for interruption by a premature ventricular beat (V). Additional deflections* (upward-pointing arrows) *represent depolarization of the accessory pathway in this patient with ventricular preexcitation. The atrial rhythm is not interrupted by absence of ventricular response on alternate beats or following an artificial pacemaker spike (S). In this patient, when AV conduction did not occur by the accessory pathway, it did not occur at all, suggesting complete block below the His bundle.*

in the normal pathway may be obscured.[220] If anterograde conduction in the accessory pathway fails (see Fig. 16-19*B*), and if no conduction occurs through the normal pathway, complete AV block becomes manifest (Fig. 16-20).[221]

Preexcitation may eliminate the classic features of BBB. In type B preexcitation, with a rapidly conducting bypass to the right ventricle, the portion of the heart that is last to depolarize in the presence of RBBB alone is depolarized first, so that RBBB may not be recognized.[222,223] Right bundle branch block may be diagnosed in the presence of type A WPW syndrome by showing prolongation of conduction time from the HB to the right ventricular apex[224] or by showing that the terminal portion of the QRS suggests RBBB and is the same both with and without the preexcitation (Fig. 16-21). Likewise, in type A preexcitation, with a bypass to the left side of the heart, that portion of the heart depolarized last in the presence of LBBB alone is depolarized first. Thus, type A ventricular preexcitation may obscure LBBB (Fig. 16-22).[225]

If secondary T wave changes occur with ventricular

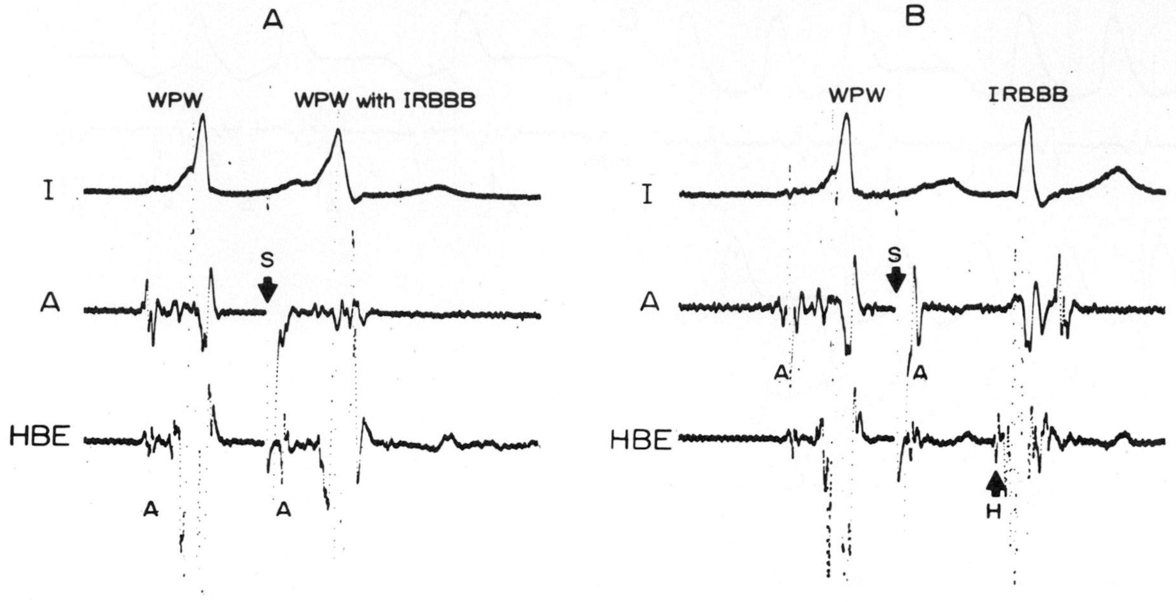

Figure 16-21. *A and B show lead I, an intra-atrial electrogram (A), and a His bundle electrogram (HBE). In A, the artificially induced premature atrial beat prolongs conduction through the normal pathway, leading to an increased degree of ventricular preexcitation. The terminal S wave is probably not related to complete ventricular preexcitation because the QRS is less wide than the one seen in Figure 16-19A (same patient). This terminal S wave is probably related to incomplete right bundle branch block (IRBBB). In B, the artifically induced atrial beat is more premature, occurring when the accessory pathway is refractory. A long AH interval is seen. However, the QRS complex shows a terminal S wave, indicating IRBBB but no ventricular preexcitation.*

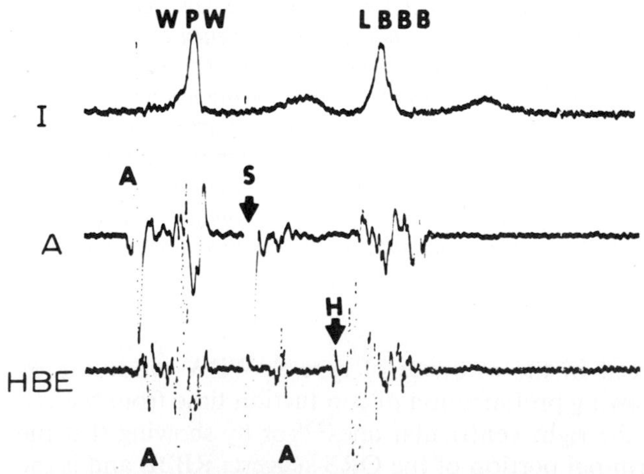

Figure 16-22. *The first complex here is a sinus beat with some degree of ventricular preexcitation, type A. The artificially induced premature atrial beat again finds the accessory pathway refractory. However, the AH interval is less long; therefore, the RR interval is shorter, and instead of incomplete right bundle branch, there is left bundle branch block (LBBB).*

preexcitation, they tend to be in the opposite direction of the delta waves. Occasionally, downward-pointing delta waves are diagnosed as myocardial infarction, for example, in atrial fibrillation where short PR intervals cannot be recognized.

Spontaneous Ectopic Ventricular Complexes

Etiology

When the spontaneous pacemaker of the ventricles lies within the Purkinje system or the ventricular muscle, or even in a bundle branch or a fascicle, depolarization of the ventricle takes place without full use of the specialized conduction system, and aberrant conduction occurs.

Ectopic ventricular complexes occur because of increased automaticity of ventricular cells, triggered responses, or because of reentry produced by microreentry or macroreentry circuits, the two legs of which must have different conduction times or different refractory periods or both and must be functionally or anatomically separate. Such circumstances may occur in patients with almost every significant cardiac disease, especially when there is marked cardiomegaly. However, ectopic ventricular beats are found on Holter monitor recordings in more than 50% of clinically normal persons, and in such a setting these beats have minimal prognostic significance. Complex ventricular ectopy with exercise in these clinically normal patients may require limitation of the highest levels of stress.[58] Excessive numbers of ectopic ventricular complexes are especially ominous in patients with ischemic heart disease, particularly following acute myocardial infarction. Ectopic ventricular complexes may be extremely difficult to control when there is marked cardiomegaly, and they are common with cardiomyopathy, with infiltrative cardiac disease such as sarcoidosis,[173] with inflammatory diseases including viral myocarditis, and with mitral valve prolapse syndrome even without cardiomegaly.

Clinical Findings

Patients with ectopic ventricular complexes frequently complain of palpitations. During auscultation of the heart or palpation of the pulse, irregularities may be recognized. Frequently, neither the patient nor the observer feels or hears the premature complexes themselves. It is the sinus beat following the pause that usually causes palpitation, a strongly felt pulse, and a loud first heart sound. During ventricular tachycardia, however, the pulse may be regular in timing. With AV dissociation, because of the changing relationship between atrial and ventricular contraction, intermittent loud first heart sounds and cannon waves in the veins of the neck may be appreciated. With slow to moderate rates of ventricular tachycardia, patients may complain of palpitations. Very rapid ventricular tachycardia may produce palpitation, dyspnea due to congestive heart failure, lightheadedness, or even syncope.

The Electrocardiogram

If the ectopic ventricular pacemaker lies in or near the posterior or anterior fascicle of the LBBB, the QRS complex will show the pattern of RBBB and LAFB or LPFB (Fig. 16-23). If the pacemaker lies in or near the main LBB, the QRS complex will demonstrate RBBB, and if the pacemaker lies in or near the RBB, the contour of the QRS complex will be that of LBBB. QRS complexes tend to be less widened if the ectopic ventricular pacemakers lie more proximal in the fascicles. Ectopic ventricular pacemakers arising in the distal Purkinje system, away from insertions of the fascicles, produce QRS complexes with contours that may not fit well into the aforementioned categories. However, pacemakers in the left ventricle produce slurred complexes with late rightward forces, whereas ectopic pacemakers arising in the right ventricle produce slurred leftward forces. Premature ventricular complexes that do not penetrate retrogradely to the atrium but that reach the AV node will cause block of the next sinus complex, such that the time between the two conducted sinus P waves that encompass the ectopic ventricular beat is equal to two sinus cycles. The pause following the ectopic ventricular beat in these circumstances is said to be *compensatory.* However, if an ectopic ventricular complex conducts back to the atrium, the SA node may be reset and no compensatory pause will occur. Thus, ectopic ventricular complexes need not

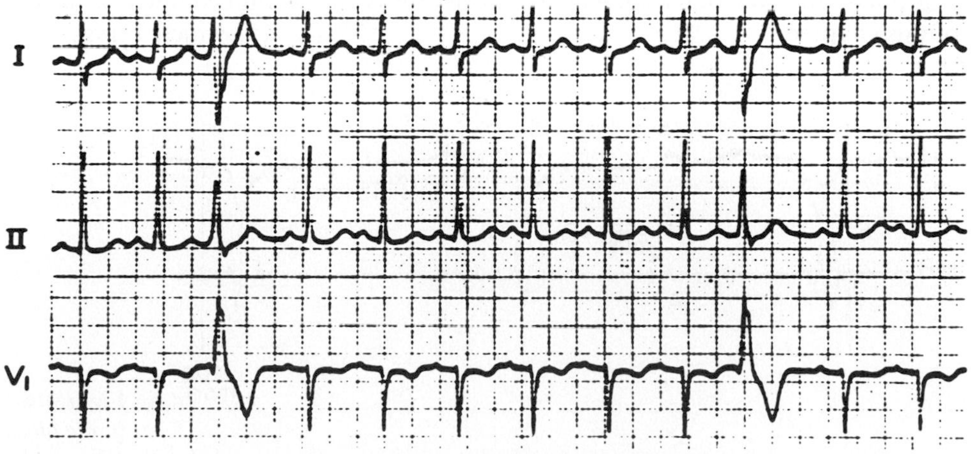

Figure 16-23. *Simultaneously recorded leads I, II, and V_1 show two premature beats. Neither is preceded by P waves, and the first has a definite compensatory pause. The pause after the second premature beat is slightly longer than compensatory. These beats are mainly inverted in lead I, upright in lead II, and upright in lead V_1, having the contour of right bundle branch block and left posterior fascicular block. If these are ventricular beats, they arise in or near the anterior fascicle of the left bundle branch.*

necessarily have compensatory pauses. Premature junctional and even atrial complexes may not reset the SA node and thus may be followed by compensatory pauses and also may be early enough to cause aberrant conduction. They may therefore appear to be ventricular because of the contour and the presence of a compensatory pause. If wide complexes do not fit the pattern of bundle branch or fascicular block, they are more likely to be ventricular. When difficulty arises in differentiating ventricular from supraventricular tachycardia with aberrant conduction, HB recordings may be necessary to differentiate one from the other.[226] At rapid rates, supraventricular tachycardia tends to be either absolutely regular or markedly irregular, whereas ventricular tachycardia, even when all complexes have the same contour, tends to be slightly irregular but usually not precisely regular or markedly irregular. Occasionally various degrees of exit block may cause ventricular tachycardia to be very irregular.

Artificially Induced Ventricular Rhythms

Etiology

Artificially induced ventricular rhythms are produced by artificial pacemakers implanted on the epicardium or into the myocardium through the epicardium or by reaching the endocardium of thc ventricles transvenously. Pacemakers are used in patients having, or having the potential for, life-threatening or symptomatic bradycardia or AV block and in patients in whom tachycardias need to be broken or suppressed. A discussion of the causes of these abnormalities and the indications for placement and type of pacemaker are beyond the scope of this chapter.

Clinical Findings

The clinical findings in patients with artificial pacemakers are the same as in patients with idoventricular rhythms at similar rates. Occasionally patients develop unacceptable palpitation when ventricular pacemakers cause AV dissociation. This problem can be solved by the use of AV sequential pacemakers.

The Electrocardiogram

Ventricular aberrancy caused by an artificial pacemaker can almost always be recognized if the artificial pacemaker spikes at the beginning of each paced QRS complex are visible (Fig. 16-24). Implanted pacemakers on the left ventricle produce complexes with RBBB similar to some of the spontaneous left ventricular pacemakers, whereas transvenous pacemakers pace the right ventricle and produce a pattern of LBBB similar to that seen with spontaneous right ventricular pacemakers (see Fig. 16-24). Usually this pattern of LBBB is associated with left axis deviation (Fig. 16-25), although a normal axis or a right axis deviation may occur. Rarely, there is alternation of the axis (Fig. 16-26), supporting the postulation that a single ectopic ventricular focus may produce QRS complexes of varying contour.

Pacemakers in the coronary sinus may pace the atria, the right ventricle, or the left ventricle[227] and thus may produce normal QRS complexes or LBBB or RBBB pattern.

Conditions Under Which Intraventricular Conduction Defects Occur

The electrophysiologic mechanisms involved in aberrant conduction have been discussed in detail in Chapter 15, which brings to date a previous review.[260] These

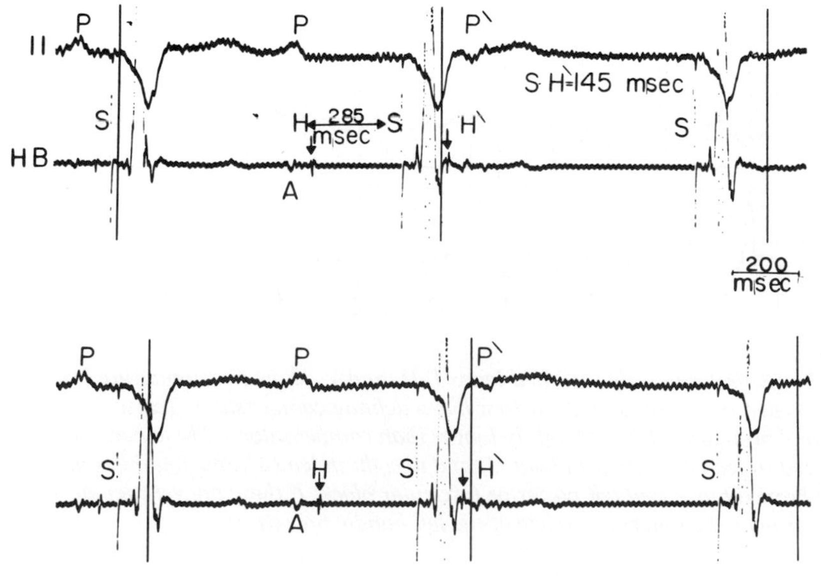

Figure 16-24. *Both panels illustrate antegrade block below the bundle of His. Each A is followed by an anterograde H but no ventricular complex. Ventricular deflections are each initiated by an artificial pacemaker spike (S), and, when the His bundle, AV node, and atria are not refractory, they are followed by a retrograde His deflection (H') and a retrograde P wave (P'). Thus, there is unidirectional block below the bundle of His.*

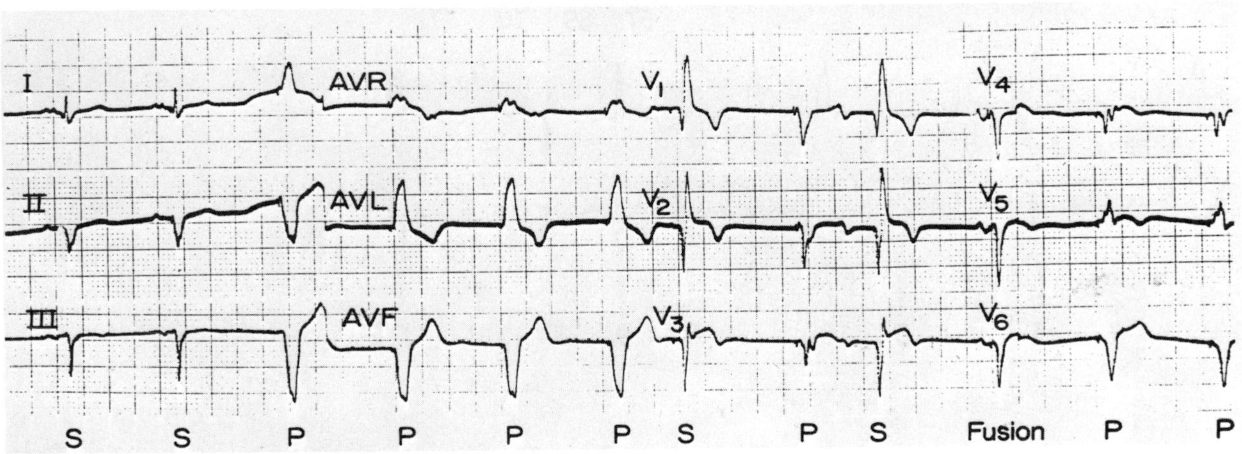

Figure 16-25. *A continuously recorded 12-lead electrocardiogram. Sinus beats are marked S and ventricular paced beats are marked P. Sinus beats show the contour of right bundle branch block, left anterior fascicular block, anteroseptal myocardial infarction, and possibly inferior infarction. Paced beats are wide, slurred, and entirely upright in leads I and aV$_L$, and therefore pacing is in the right ventricle. Paced complexes are mainly inverted in leads II, III, and aV$_F$, as is usually the case with transvenous ventricular pacing.*

mechanisms and certain additional variations are reviewed here to complete this clinical section.

Tachycardia- or Short-Cycle-Dependent Intraventricular Conduction Defects

A premature supraventricular complex may fail to depolarize a group of cells because of the refractory period produced by the preceding depolarization. When this refractory period is shortened by isoproterenol, the conduction defect may regress.[228] If such a group of cells is strategically located, for instance in the LBB, the QRS complex produced will display the features of LBBB (Fig. 16-27). In normal hearts, this is more likely to occur in the RBBB because of the longer action potential durations in the proximal RBB than the proximal LBB[229] or

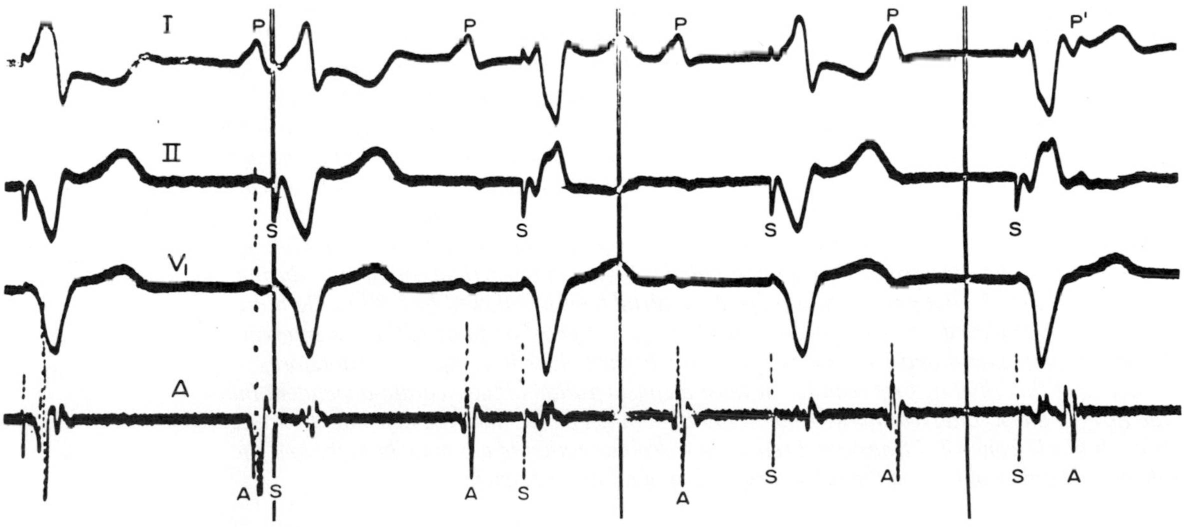

Figure 16-26. *Leads I, II, and V$_1$ and an intra-atrial electrogram (A) are recorded simultaneously. There is no antegrade conduction, all the atrial beats (P) being blocked. Retrograde conduction occurs on the last beat, with the retrograde P wave (P') seen at the end of the QRS complex. All ventricular beats begin with a pacing spike (S). QRS complexes are inverted in lead V$_1$. In leads I and II, they are alternately mainly upright and mainly inverted. Thus, artificial right ventricular pacing with a pacing catheter tip in the apex of the right ventricle produces a pattern similar to left bundle branch block, but with alternating left and right axis deviation beginning with the second QRS complex in this tracing. This suggests that a single ventricular pacemaker may produce QRS complexes of varying contours.*

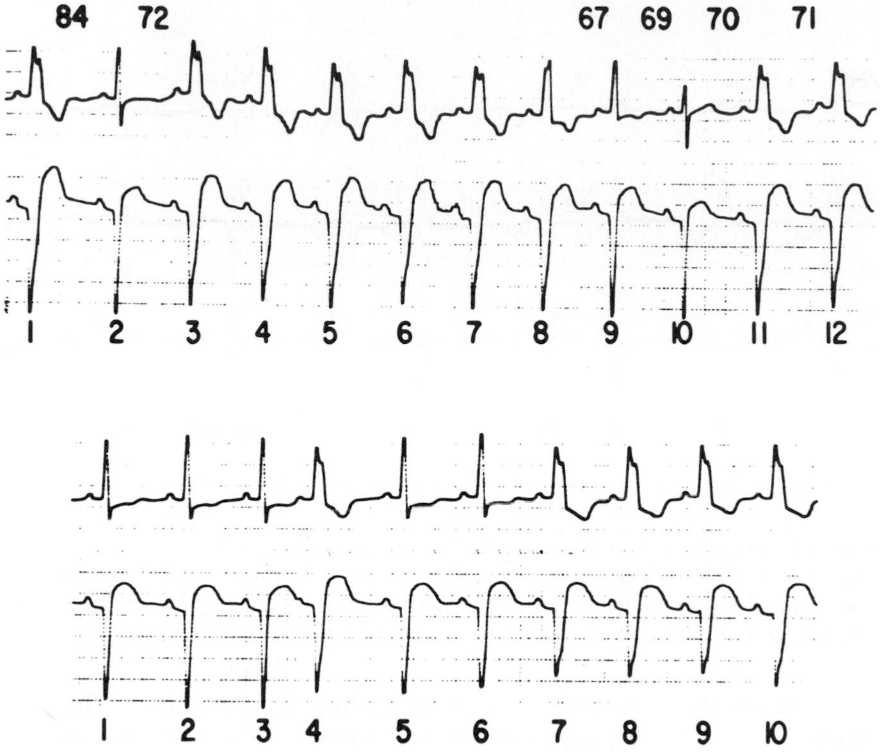

Figure 16-27. *Two panels of a consecutive electrocardiogram showing a modified lead V_5 and a modified lead V_1. The relatively long pause of 84 hundredths of a second between complexes 1 and 2 ends with a normal complex, and the next interval of 72 hundredths of a second between complexes 2 and 3 ends with tachycardia-dependent left bundle branch block. However, complex 9, ending an interval of 67 hundredths of a second, shows only incomplete left bundle branch block. The narrowing of complex 9 could be a result of the gradual shortening of the refractory period of the left bundle branch during the more rapid rhythm from complex 3 through 9, and the further decrease of left bundle branch block in complex 10 could be a result of the sudden slight sinus slowing. These findings are still compatible with tachycardia-dependent left bundle branch block. However, complex 11 follows an even longer interval of 70 hundredths of a second yet displays left bundle branch block. This could represent non-rate-dependent left bundle branch block, tachycardia-dependent left bundle branch block occurring because of a lengthened refractory period of the left bundle branch following the slight slowing seen between complexes 9 and 10, or bradycardia-dependent left bundle branch block. Complex 12, ending an interval of 71 hundredths of a second, could manifest left bundle branch block because late depolarization of the left left bundle branch has occurred following concealed transseptal retrograde conduction during complex 11. In the bottom panel, a premature atrial beat is followed by left bundle branch block that is apparently tachycardia dependent, and a slight shortening of the RR interval between complexes 6 and 7 produces left bundle branch block in complex 7. Therefore, analysis of this rhythm strip requires at least a consideration of tachycardia-dependent bundle branch block, bradycardia-dependent bundle branch block, non-rate-dependent bundle branch block, concealed transseptal retrograde depolarization of a bundle branch, and the effect of changes of rate on the refractory period of a bundle branch.*

because the RBBB is longer than the LBB. In addition, fibers more distal are more likely to be refractory because of their longer functional refractory periods.[230] The refractory period of the strategically located group of cells may be such that RBBB occurs as the rate increases, even without premature complexes, or the refractory period may be so long that abnormal conduction occurs at all rates.

The aberrancy produced by short cycle (phase III block)[231] is generally considered to partly depend on the previous cycle length, because refractory periods in the bundle branches appear to prolong at slower rates and shorten at faster rates.[25,232] However, in a group of patients with intermittent LBBB studied with pacing and HB recordings, LBB refractory periods were found not to change or to lengthen at faster pacing rates. Also, the rates at which LBBB disappeared as the atrial pacing rate slowed and the rate at which LBBB appeared as the atrial pacing frequency was increased were markedly different.[233–235]

The rate of change of pacing frequency also was a factor determining the rates at which the LBBB appeared and disappeared. Also, paradoxic improvement in conduction occurred in several instances as the rate increased, possibly related to type I, II, or III gap phenomenon.[163,236,237,238] Aberrancy sometimes does not depend on the previous cycle length.[239] Thus, tachycardia-dependent ventricular aberrancy depends on complex phenomenon (see Chap. 15).

Bradycardia- or Long-Cycle-Dependent Aberrant Ventricular Conduction

A strategically located group of cells in a ventricle may fail to conduct a wave of depolarization in a normal manner only very late after its last depolarization. Such bradycardia-dependent conduction defects occur at slow rates or after long pauses and may be associated with anterior or inferior myocardial infarction,[240,241] sclerodegenerative disease, and other diseases affecting the conduction system.[242] Bradycardia-dependent intraventricular conduction defects may be more common than tachycardia-dependent defects after acute myocardial infarction.[243] The phenomenon of bradycardia-dependent conduction defect may depend on the presence of diastolic depolarization.[244] If isoproterenol accelerates the diastolic depolarization, bradycardia-dependent BBB may appear.[228,245] Also, BBB may be present in late complexes but may disappear in very early complexes as a manifestation of supernormal conduction.[246,247] It has also been suggested that RBBB seen after long cycles may disappear after short cycles because of Wedensky facilitation.[238] Occasionally patients are reported in whom there is both tachycardia- and bradycardia-dependent BBB.[241,244–252] Bradycardia-dependent block may occur in both bundle branches simultaneously[253] and thus cause AV block. Once bradycardia-dependent AV block has occurred, it continues until the area of block is repolarized. If the AV block is unidirectional, an ectopic ventricular escape complex may fully depolarize the cells in the areas of block, allowing time to repolarize fully and once again allow anterograde conduction,[254] or the cells may depolarize to threshold potential spontaneously, fire in a concealed manner, repolarize, and conduct again.

Non-Rate- or Non-Cycle-Length-Dependent Aberrant Ventricular Conduction

If strategically located cells have been destroyed, aberrant conduction will be unrelated to rate. This may occur congenitally, because of disease or trauma, or secondary to a surgical procedure.

Aberrant ventricular conduction may also occur intermittently regardless of the direction of change in cardiac rate (see Fig. 16-7 and Chap. 15).[255]

Electrical Alternans

Tachycardia- or Short-Cycle-Length-Dependent Electrical Alternans

If an area of the ventricles has a refractory period longer than one but shorter than two cycle lengths of a given rhythm, there will be no depolarization of the cells in this area on alternate beats.[82] If this area lies in a strategic location, such as a bundle branch, alternate beats will have BBB. This BBB alternans will be tachycardia dependent because it depends on beats falling into phase III refractory period of a portion of the ventricles. The refractory period may even be longer than two cycle lengths but shorter than three, so that block will occur in two out of every three complexes (Fig. 16-28*D*). Bundle branch block alternans may occur even with irregular rhythms (Fig. 16-29).

Bradycardia-Initiated Electrical Alternans

An intraventricular conduction defect that occurs only after a long pause, possibly related to spontaneous diastolic depolarization, is bradycardia or long cycle dependent and may initiate electrical alternans, sometimes of the BBB type. Sudden bradycardia may initiate BBB alternans by prolonging the refractory period of a bundle branch.[82] The BBB that occurs is actually tachycardia dependent (see below).

Pseudo-Bradycardia-Dependent Electrical Alternans

Occasionally, electrical alternans, especially of the BBB type, changes to persistent BBB on every beat, when the rate slows (see Figs. 16-28*B* and *C*).[82] This initially suggests that the BBB is bradycardia dependent. However, with further slowing of the rate, the BBB disappears entirely (see Fig. 16-28). Under these circumstances, the electrical alternans is truly tachycardia dependent. At the faster rate, there is both anterograde and retrograde block in the abnormal bundle branch on alternate beats. At the slightly reduced rate, the "blocked" bundle branch is kept in a refractory state because of retrograde penetration on every beat. Thus, although the pattern of BBB becomes persistent, there is retrograde conduction into the abnormal bundle branch on every beat, and conduction into this bundle branch has changed from 2 : 1 to 1 : 1 (improved). With further slowing of the rate, each consecutive beat falls beyond both the anterograde and retrograde refractory periods so that all complexes are normal.

Etiology

All the diseases that produce intermittent BBB may be associated with BBB alternans. Complete anatomic in-

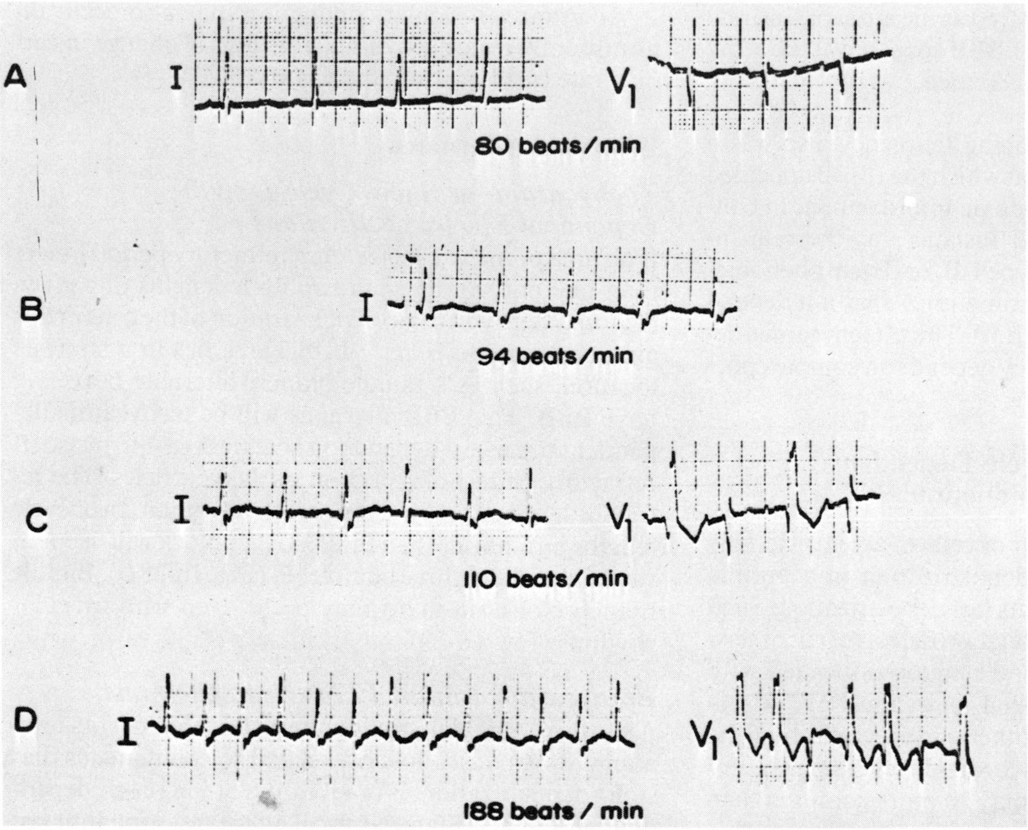

Figure 16-28. *In A, leads I and V_1 show QRS complexes of normal duration. Small terminal R waves in lead V_1 suggest the possibility of incomplete right bundle branch block. Sinus rate is 89 beats/min. In B, the sinus rate is 94 beats/min and constant right bundle branch block is seen in lead I. It must be assumed that there is transseptal retrograde conduction into the right bundle with each complex. In C, leads I and V_1 show right bundle branch block alternans. At 110 beats/min, both anterograde and retrograde refractory periods are longer than one interval but shorter than the two RR intervals, so that anterograde conduction and retrograde conduction are blocked on alternate beats. In D, leads I and V_1 show right bundle branch block in two out of every three complexes at a sinus rate of 188 beats/min. Here we assume that the right bundle branch refractory period is longer than two intervals but shorter than three. This figure shows pseudo-bradycardia-dependent bundle branch block alternans because in B there is right bundle branch block on every beat, whereas in C, at a faster rate, there is right bundle branch block on only every other beat.*

terruption of a bundle branch does not allow BBB alternans. Diseases that have been specifically associated with BBB alternans include sclerodegenerative disease of the conduction system, hypertension, ischemic heart disease, and bacterial endocarditis.[94]

Concealed Conduction Within a Portion of the Ventricles Producing Persistent or Intermittent Intraventricular Conduction

Concealed Retrograde Conduction Producing Subsequent Intraventricular Conduction Defect

The pattern of persistent BBB may occur when the apparently blocked bundle is depolarized on every complex (see Figs. 16-4 and 16-30). For instance, if an early supraventricular complex produces anterograde RBB with a QRS complex reflecting this abnormality in conduction, the refractory period of the RBBB may be over by the time there is conduction across the septum, causing retrograde conduction into the RBBB to occur. This concealed transseptal retrograde conduction causes the RBBB to remain refractory for the next regular supraventricular complex. Thus, once anterograde RBBB has occurred, retrograde conduction into that same bundle may cause the conduction defect to persist.[256,257] This phenomenon may also occur with LBBB, LAFB, LPFB, or complete ventricular preexcitation.

Concealed retrograde conduction in these circumstances may also be a step in the reentry process whereby

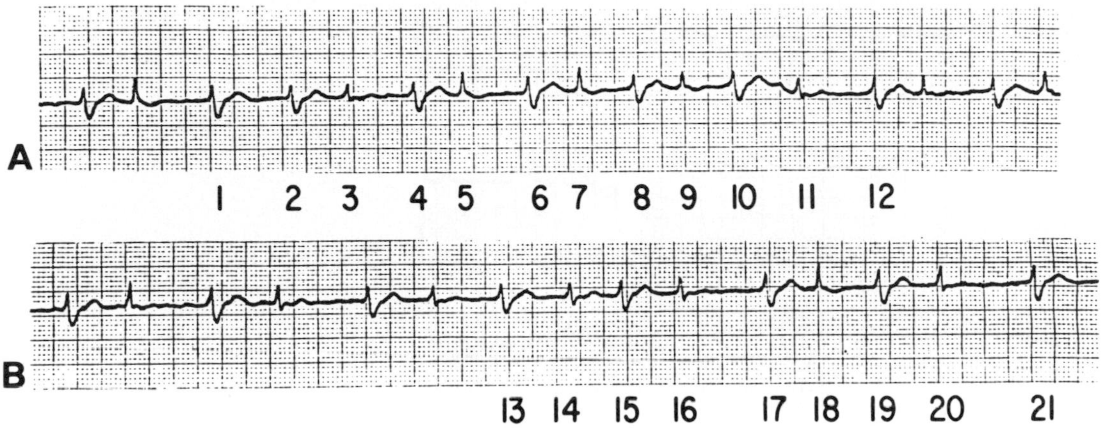

Figure 16-29. *Both A and B show lead I during atrial fibrillation. Frequent complexes show right bundle branch block producing irregular bundle branch block alternans. All longer pauses such as between complexes 1 and 2, 11 and 12, 16 and 17, and 20 and 21 show right bundle branch block, suggesting that the block is bradycardia dependent. All shorter intervals end with complexes differing from the immediately preceding complex; for example, complexes 7, 9, and 18 have no right bundle branch block, whereas complexes 8, 10, and 15 show right bundle branch block. Thus, there appears to be right bundle branch block alternans that is recognizable even though the rhythm is irregular. The alternans appears to be tachycardia dependent, whereas the right bundle branch block is bradycardia dependent. The only two consecutive long intervals end with complexes 1 and 2, both of which have right bundle branch block.*

two anatomically or functionally dissociated pathways are present, so that conduction may occur in one direction in one pathway, and, at a later time, in the opposite direction in the other pathway. Reentry may be manifest or concealed and may occur through large pathways or small ones (microreentry). Microreentry could be responsible for most coupled premature ventricular beats. Reentry has been clinically shown to occur in a ventricular fascicle (see Fig. 10-1),[47] and the conditions for reentry have been experimentally shown to be present in the RBB.[257]

Concealed Anterograde Conduction

An intraventricular conduction defect may occur not only when anterograde conduction is interrupted down a pathway into or within the ventricles, but also when there is marked delay of anterograde conduction down one of these pathways. For instance, if anterograde conduction down the RBB is very slow, both ventricles may be depolarized through LBB. This slow, delayed, anterograde conduction could also cause the RBBB to be in a refractory state for the next supraventricular complex, so that persistent intraventricular conduction defect may occur, at least for several complexes, because of concealed slow anterograde conduction. Concealed anterograde conduction discharging a bundle branch but not any other part of the ventricles may cause a subsequent conducted complex to display BBB[258] or may shorten the bundle branch cycle length and refractory period such that a subsequent short interval does not produce BBB, or it may discharge a fascicular pacemaker without reaching the rest of the ventricle.[47] Also, concealed anterograde conduction may be responsible for intermittent penetration of a proximal portion of the AV conduction system, causing curious ratios of AV conduction (Fig. 16-31).

Conclusion

In this chapter and in Chapter 15 we have examined the electrophysiologic,[259] electrocardiographic, and clinical aspects of abnormal intraventricular conduction. The cellular membrane mechanisms that mainly control single cell action potentials and impulse formation are discussed. The effects of changes at the cellular level are, in a series of steps, related to clinical examples and to implications of aberrant intraventricular conduction.

Discussion of abnormal intraventricular conduction is divided into short- and long cardiac-cycle-length-dependent and non-cycle-length-dependent aberrancy. The role of drugs as a factor in all types of aberrant conduction is included.

Finally, we have set forth a clinical compendium of the various electrocardiographic expressions of aberrant intraventricular conduction, including bundle branch

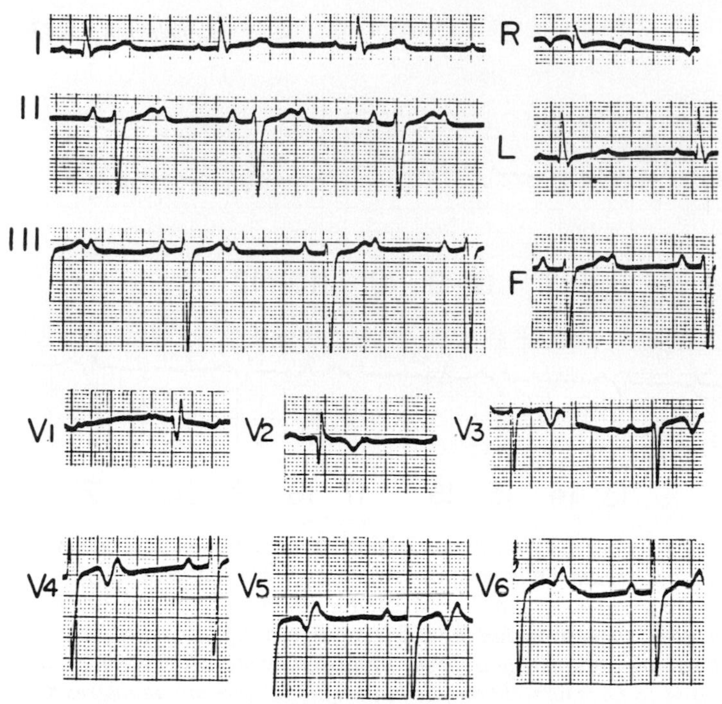

Figure 16-30. *Same patient as in Figure 16-2, at a more rapid sinus rate. In leads II, III, and aV_F, QRS complexes are mainly inverted, and there is an R′ wave in lead V_1. QRS duration is 0.12 second. These changes are compatible with right bundle branch block and left anterior fascicular block. Also, alternate beats are blocked, and PR intervals are prolonged. In the absence of digitalis, these changes suggest that the only remaining conducting fascicle (the left posterior fascicle) conducts with a prolonged interval on alternate beats and is blocked on alternate beats. Thus, conduction, although prolonged, goes through the main left bundle and the left posterior fascicle on alternate beats. Although there is the pattern of right bundle branch block, the right bundle branch must be able to conduct, as it did in the tracing in Figure 16-2 (taken several minutes earlier). Likewise, although left bundle branch block is evident in Figure 16-2, the left bundle is able to conduct, as it does in this figure. Thus, given time for recovery, either bundle can and does conduct, either in an obvious or in a concealed slow anterograde or retrograde manner. After several ventricular cycles, either bundle would have surely recovered had it not been kept refractory by concealed conduction. At this slow ventricular rate (43 beats/min), the absence of conduction down the right bundle branch with left bundle branch block pattern and a normal PR, as seen in the first portion of Figure 16-2, must be explained on the basis of a right bundle branch refractory period that has prolonged during the slow ventricular rate seen at the bottom of Figure 16-2 and in this figure.*

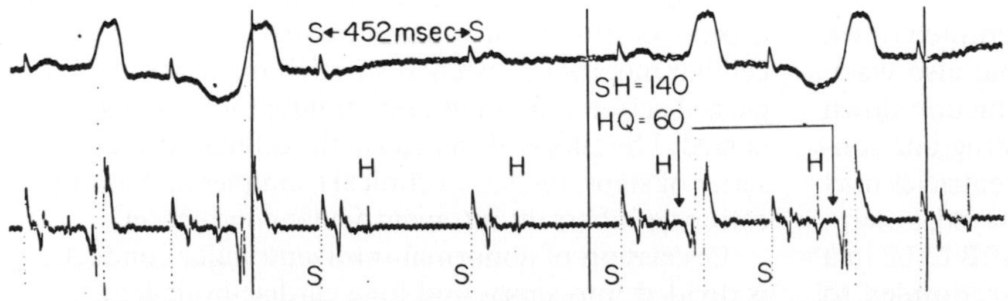

Figure 16-31. *Type II block below the bundle of His. All HQ intervals are the same in the conducted beats. Suddenly there is no conduction below the His potential following the third and fourth pacing spikes, but conduction resumes following the fifth and sixth pacing spikes with no change in HQ intervals. This 4:2 ratio can be explained by two levels of type II sub-Hisian block, the upper being 4:3 and the lower being 3:2.*

and fascicular blocks,[260] ventricular preexcitation, and spontaneous and artificial ventricular rhythms.

Descriptions and clinical implications of aberrant intraventricular conduction, such as the effect of left axis deviation on the prognosis of LBBB[261] accompany examples of the primary and secondary electrocardiographic changes.

Most of the principles included in this chapter and in Chapter 15 have been proved. Many of the explanations that accompany clinical examples of aberrant intraventricular conduction are speculative. However, the mechanistic background in these chapters and in the references should give one the tools with which to approach, and most often understand, each electrocardiogram in which intraventricular aberrancy comes into question.

References

1. Fabregas, R. A., Tse, W. W., and Han, J.: Conduction disturbances of the bundle branches produced by lesions in the nonbranching portion of His bundle. Am. Heart J., 92:356–362, 1976.
2. James, T. N., and Sherf, L.: Fine structure of the His bundle. Circulation, 44:9–28, 1971.
3. Sciacca, A., and Sangiorgi, M.: Trouble de la conduction intraventriculaire droite de la lesion du tronc commun du faisceau de His. Acta Cardiol., 12:486–492, 1957.
4. El-Sherif, N., Scherlag, B. J., and Lazzara, R.: Conduction disorders in the canine proximal His-Purkinje system following acute myocardial ischemia. II. The pathophysiology of bilateral bundle branch block. Circulation, 49:848–857, 1974.
5. Massing, G. K., and James, T. N.: Anatomical configuration of the His bundle and bundle branches in the human heart. Circulation, 53:609–621, 1976.
6. Demoulin, J. C., and Kulbertus, H. E.: Left hemiblocks revisited from the histopathological viewpoint. Am. Heart J., 86:712–713, 1973.
7. Lazzara, R., Yeh, B. K., and Samet P.: Functional transverse interconnections within the His bundle and the bundle branches. Circ. Res., 32:509, 1973.
8. El-Sherif, N., Amat-Y-Leon, F., Schonfield, C., et al.: Normalization of bundle block patterns by distal His bundle pacing. Clinical and experimental evidence of longitudinal dissociation in the pathologic His bundle. Circulation, 57:473–483, 1978.
9. McAnulty, J., and Rahimtoola, S.: Prognosis in bundle branch block. Ann. Rev. Med., 32:499–507, 1981.
10. Bharati, S., Lev, M., Dhingra, R., et al.: Pathologic correlations in three cases of bilateral bundle branch (block) disease with unusual electrophysiologic manifestations in two cases. Am. J. Cardiol., 38:508–518, 1976.
11. Singer, R. B.: Mortality in 966 life insurance applicants with bundle branch block or wide QRS. Trans. Assoc. Life Ins. Med. Dir. Am., 52:94–114, 1968.
12. Lister, J. W., Kline, R. S., and Lesser, M. E.: Chronic bilateral bundle branch block. Long-term observations in ambulatory patients. Br. Heart J., 39:203–207, 1977.
13. Denes, P., Dhingra, R. C., Wu, D., et al.: Sudden death in patients with bifascicular block. Arch. Intern Med., 137:1005, 1977.
14. Scheinman, M. M., Peters, R. W., Morady, F., et al.: Electrophysiologic studies in patients with bundle branch block. Pace, 6:1157–1165, 1983.
15. Yoon, M. S., Han, J., and Fabregas, R. A.: Effect of ventricular aberrancy on fibrillation threshold. Am. Heart J., 89:599–604, 1975.
16. Hinkle, L. E., Jr., Carver, S. T., and Stevens, M.: The frequency of asymptomatic disturbances of cardiac rhythm and conduction in middle-aged men. Am. J. Cardiol., 24:629, 1969.
17. Kannel, W. B., Kagan, A., Dawber, R. T., et al.: Epidemiology of coronary heart disease. Geriatrics, 17:675, 1962.
18. Peters, R. W., Scheinman, M. M., Modin, G. M., et al.: Prophylactic permanent pacemakers for patients with chronic bundle branch block. Am. J. Med., 66:978, 1979.
19. Fisch, G. R., Zipes, D. P., and Fisch, C.: Bundle branch block and sudden death. Prog. Cardiovasc. Dis., 23:187–224, 1980.
20. Puech, P.: Contribution of the His bundle recording to the diagnosis of bilateral bundle branch conduction defects. Adv. Cardiol., 14:178–188, 1975.
21. Aronson, A. L.: Evaluation of surface ECG findings as prodromata of type II complete heart block. Circulation, 47-48 (Suppl. IV):122, 1973.
22. Scheinman, M. M., Peters, R. W., Modin, G., et al.: Prognostic value of infranodal conduction time in patients with chronic bundle branch block. Circulation, 56:240–244, 1977.
23. Scheinman, M., and Brenman, B. A.: Clinical and anatomic implications of intraventricular conduction blocks in acute myocardial infarction. Circulation, 46:753–760, 1972.
24. Gould, L., Venkataraman, K., Mohammad, N., and Gomprecht, R. F.: Prognosis of right bundle block in acute myocardial infarction. J.A.M.A., 219:502–503, 1972.
25. Scheinman, M. M., Golschlager, N. F., and Peters, R. W.: Bundle branch block. Cardiovasc. Clin., 11:57–80, 1980.
26. Scheinman, M. M., Peters, R. W., Modin, G., et al.: Prognostic value of infranodal conduction time in patients with chronic bundle branch block. Circulation, 56:240, 1977.
27. Denes, P., Dhingra, R. C., Wu, D., et al.: HV interval in patients with bifascicular block (right bundle branch block and left anterior hemiblock). Clinical, electrocardiographic and electrophysiologic correlations. Am. J. Cardiol., 35:23–29, 1975.
28. Dhingra, R. C., Denes, P., Wu, D., et al.: Prospective observations in patients with chronic bundle branch block and marked HV prolongation. Circulation, 53:600–604, 1976.
29. Rosen, K. M., Ehsani, A., and Rahimtoola, S. H.: H-V intervals in left bundle branch block. Clinical and electrocardiographic correlations. Circulation, 46:717–723, 1972.
30. McAnulty, J. H., Kauffman, S., Murphy, E., et al.: Survival in patients with intraventricular conduction defects. Arch. Intern. Med., 128:30, 1978.
31. Berkowitz, W. D., Lau, S. H., Patton, R. D., Rosen, K. M., and Damato, A. N.: The use of His bundle recordings in the analysis of unilateral and bilateral bundle branch block. Am. Heart J., 81:340–350, 1971.
32. Castellanos, A., Jr.: HV intervals in LBBB. Circulation, 47:1133–1134, 1973.
33. Hirschfeld, D. S., Ueda, C. T., Rowland, M., et al.: Clinical and electrophysiologic effects of intravenous quinidine in man. Br. Heart J., 39:309, 1977.
34. Scheinman, M. M., Weiss, A. N., Shaftom, E., et al.: Electrophysiologic effects of procainamide in patterns with intraventricular conduction delay. Circulation, 49:522, 1974.
35. Desai, J. M., Scheinman, M. M., Peters, T. E., et al.: Electrophysiologic effects of disopyramide in patients with bundle branch block. Circulation, 59:215, 1979.
36. Santinelli, V., Chiariello, M., Ambrosio, G., et al.: Further observations on the electrophysiologic effects of oral amiodarone therapy. Chest, 82:117–120, 1982.
37. Chiale, P. A., Przybylski, J., Laino, R. A., Halpern, M. S., Nau, G. J., Sanchez, R. A., Lazzari, J. O., Elizari, M. V., and Rosen-

baum, M. B.: Usefulness of the ajmaline test in patients with latent bundle branch block. Am. J. Cardiol., 49:21–26, 1982.

38. Kunkel, F., Rowland, M., and Scheinman, M. M.: The electrophysiologic effects of lidocaine in patients with intraventricular conduction defects. Circulation, 49:894–899, 1974.
39. Gupta, P. K., Lichstein, E., and Chadda, K. D.: Lidocaine-induced heart block in patients with bundle branch block. Am. J. Cardiol., 33:487–492, 1974.
40. De Joseph, R. L., and Zipes, D. P.: Normal H-V time in a patient with right bundle branch block, left anterior hemiblock and intermittent complete distal His block. Chest, 63:564–568, 1973.
41. Dhingra, R. C., Wyndham, C., Amat-Y-Leon, F., et al.: Significance of A-H interval in patients with chronic bundle branch block. Clinical, electrophysiologic and follow-up observations. Am. J. Cardiol., 37:231–236, 1976.
42. Bhat, P. K., Watanabe, K., Rao, D. B., et al.: Conduction defects in the aging heart. J. Am. Geriatr. Soc., 22:517, 1974.
43. Wiberg, T. A., Richman, H. G., and Gobel, F. L.: The significance and prognosis of chronic bifascicular block. Chest, 71:329, 1977.
44. Graybiel, A., and Sprague, H. B.: Bundle branch block: An analysis of 395 cases. Am. J. Med. Sci., 185:395, 1933.
45. Langendorf, R., Cohen, H., and Gozo, E. G., Jr.: Observations on second degree atrioventricular block, including new criteria for the differential diagnosis between Type I and Type II block. Am. J. Cardiol., 29:111–119, 1972.
46. Dhingra, R. C., Denes, P., Wu, D., et al.: The significance of second degree atrioventricular block and bundle branch block. Observations regarding site and type of block. Circulation, 49:638–646, 1974.
47. Cohen, H. C., D'Cruz, I., and Pick, A.: Concealed intraventricular conduction in the His bundle electrogram. Circulation, 53:766–783, 1976.
48. Gray, R., Kaushik, V. S., and Mandel, W. J.: Wenckebach phenomenon occurring in the distal conducting system in a young adult. Br. Heart J., 38:204–206, 1976.
49. Akhter, M., and Damato, A. N.: Clinical uses of His bundle electrocardiography. Am. Heart J., 91:520–526, 1976.
50. Dhingra, R. C., Denes, P., Wu, D., et al.: Chronic right bundle branch block and left posterior hemiblock. Clinical, electrophysiologic and prognostic observations. Am. J. Cardiol., 36:867, 1975.
51. Smith, R. F., Jackson, D. H., Harthorne, J. W., and Sanders, C. A.: Acquired bundle branch block in a healthy population. Am. Heart J., 80:746–751, 1970.
52. Rotman, M., and Triebwasser, J. H. G.: A clinical and follow-up study of right and left bundle branch block. Circulation, 51:477, 1975.
53. Wu, D., Denes, P., Dhingra, R. C., et al.: Electrophysiological and clinical observations in patients with alternating bundle branch block. Circulation, 53:456–464, 1976.
54. Rooney, S. M., Gondiner, P. L., and Muss, E.: Relationship of right bundle branch block and marked left axis deviation in complete heart block during general anesthesia. Anesthesiology, 44:64–66, 1976.
55. Scheinman, M., Weiss, A., and Kunkel, F.: His bundle recordings in patients with bundle branch block and transient neurologic symptoms. Circulation, 48:322–330, 1973.
56. Altschuler, H., Fisher, J. D., and Furman, S.: Significance of isolated H-V interval prolongation in symptomatic patients without documented heart block. Am. Heart J., 97:19, 1979.
57. Rotman, M., Wagner, G. S., and Wallace, A. J.: Bradyarrhythmias in acute myocardial infarction. Circulation, 45:703, 1972.
58. Barrett, P. A., Peter, C. T., Swan, H. J. C., Singh, B. N., and Mandel, W. J.: The frequency and prognostic significance of electrocardiographic abnormalities in clinically normal individuals (review article). Prog. Cardiovasc. Dis., 23:299–319, 1981.
59. Simon, A. B., and Zloto, A. E.: Atrio-ventricular block. Natural history after permanent ventricular pacing. Am. J. Cardiol., 41:500–507, 1978.
60. Kones, R. J., and Phillips, J. H.: Review: Bundle branch block in acute myocardial infarction: Current concepts and indications. Acta Cardiol., 35:469–478, 1980.
61. Nimetz, A. A., Shubrooks, S. J., Hutter, A. M., and DeSanctis, R. W.: The significance of bundle branch block during acute myocardial infarction. Am. Heart J., 90:439–444, 1975.
62. Riley, C. P., Jackson, D. H., Russell, R. O., and Rackley, C. E.: Partial bilateral bundle branch block in acute myocardial infarction. Chest, 63:342–347, 1973.
63. Godman, M. J., Lassers, B. W., and Julian, D. G.: Complete bundle branch block complicating acute myocardial infarction. N. Engl. J. Med., 282:237–240, 1970.
64. Scheidt, S., and Killip, T.: Bundle-branch block complicating acute myocardial infarction. J.A.M.A., 222:919–924, 1972.
65. Lie, K. I., Liem, K. L., Schuilenburg, R. M., et al.: Early identification of patients developing late in hospital ventricular fibrillation after discharge from the coronary care unit. A 5½ year retrospective and prospective of 1897 patients. Am. J. Cardiol., 41:674–677, 1978.
66. Hindman, M. C., Wagner, G. S., JaRo, M., et al.: The clinical significance of bundle branch block complicating acute myocardial infarction. I. Clinical characteristic hospital mortality and one-year follow-up. Circulation, 58:679, 1978.
67. Hindman, M. C., Wagner, G. S., JaRo, M., et al.: The clinical significance of bundle branch block complicating acute myocardial infarction. II. Indications for temporary and permanent pacemaker insertion. Circulation, 58:690, 1978.
68. Touboul, P., Kirkorian, G., Atallah, G., and Moleur, P.: Bundle branch reentry: A possible mechanism of ventricular tachycardia. Circulation, 67:674, 1983.
69. Fenig, S., and Lichstein, E.: Incomplete bilateral bundle branch block and A-V block complicating acute anterior wall myocardial infarction. Am. Heart J., 84:38–44, 1972.
70. Rao, M. S., and Antani, J.: Prognostic profile of fascicular blocks in myocardial infarction. Jpn. Heart J., 18:406–415, 1977.
71. Nimetz, A. A., Shubrooks, S. J., Jr., Hutter, A. M., Jr., et al.: The significance of bundle branch block during acute myocardial infarction. Am. Heart J. 90:439, 1975.
72. De Pasquale, N. P., and Bruno, M. S.: Natural history of combined right bundle branch block and left anterior hemiblock (bilateral bundle branch block). Am. J. Med., 54:297–303, 1973.
73. Hunt, D., and Sloman, G.: Bundle branch block in acute myocardial infarction. Br. Med. J., 1:85–88, 1969.
74. Waters, D. D., and Mizgala, H. F.: Long-term prognosis of patients with incomplete bilateral bundle branch block complicating acute myocardial infarction. Role of cardiac pacing. Am. J. Cardiol., 34:1–6, 1974.
75. Lichstein, E., Gupta, P. K., and Chadda, K. D.: Long-term survival of patients with incomplete bundle branch block complicating acute myocardial infarction. Br. Heart J., 27:924, 1975.
76. Resnekov, L.: Pacemaking and acute myocardial infarction. Impulse, 11:1, 1978.
77. Lichstein, E., Gupta, P. K., Chadda, K. D., et al.: Findings of prognostic value in patients with incomplete bilateral bundle branch block complicating acute myocardial infarction. Am. J. Cardiol., 32:913–918, 1973.
78. Lichstein, E., Ribas-Meneclier, C., Naik, D., et al.: The natural history of trifascicular disease following permanent pacemaker implantation. Significance of continuing changes in atrioventricular conduction. Circulation, 54:780, 1978.
79. Siegman-Igra, Y., Yahini, J. H., Goldbourt, U., et al.: Intraventricular conduction disturbances. A review of prevalence, etiology, and progression for 10 years within a stable population of Israeli adult males. Am. Heart J., 96:699, 1978.

80. Rosenbaum, M. B., Elizari, M. V., Levi, R. J., et al.: Five cases of intermittent left anterior hemiblock. Am. J. Cardiol., 24:1–7, 1969.
81. Rosenbaum, M. B., Elizari, M. V., Lazzari, J. O., et al.: The mechanisms of intermittent bundle branch block. Relationship to prolonged recovery, hypopolarization and spontaneous diastolic depolarization. Chest, 63:666–677, 1973.
82. Cohen, H. C., D'Cruz, I., Arbel, E. R., et al.: Tachycardia and bradycardia-dependent bundle branch block alterans. Clinical observations. Circulation, 55:242–246, 1977.
83. Friedberg, H. D., and Schamroth, L.: The Wenckebach phenomenon in left bundle branch block. Am. J. Cardiol., 24:591–593, 1969.
84. Friedberg, H. D.: Mechanisms of the Wedensky phenomena in the left bundle branch. Am. J. Cardiol., 27:698–702, 1971.
85. Lev, M., Unger, P. N., Rosen, K. M., and Bharati, S.: The anatomic base of the electrocardiographic abnormality of left bundle branch block. Adv. Cardiol., 14:16–24, 1975.
86. Holt, J. H., Jr., Barnard, A. C. L., and Kramer, J. O., Jr.: A study of the human heart as a multiple dipole source. IV. Left ventricular hypertrophy in the presence of right bundle branch block. Circulation, 56:391–394, 1977.
87. Herbert, W. H.: Left bundle branch block and coronary artery disease. J. Electrocardiol., 8:317–324, 1975.
88. Sugiura, M., Okada, R., Ohkawa, S., and Shimada, H.: Pathohistological studies on the conduction system in 8 cases of complete left bundle branch block. Jpn. Heart J., 11:5–16, 1970.
89. Brake, C. M.: Complete left bundle branch and asymptomatic airmen. Aero. Med., 40:781–782, 1969.
90. Whinnery, J. E., Froelicher, V. F., Stewart, A. J., et al.: The electrocardiographic response to maximal treadmill exercise of asymptomatic men with left bundle branch block. Am. Heart J., 94:316–324, 1977.
91. McGowan, R. L., Welch, T. G., Zaret, B. L., et al.: Noninvasive myocardial imaging with potassium^{-43} and rubidium-81 in patients with left bundle branch block. Am. J. Cardiol., 38:422–428, 1976.
92. Chen, C. H., Sakurai, T., Fujita, M., et al.: Transient intraventricular conduction disturbances in hypertropic obstructive cardio myopathy. Am. Heart J., 101:672–674, 1981.
93. Cohen, H., Rosen, K. M., and Pick, A.: Disorders of impulse conduction and impulse formation caused by hyperkalemia in man. Am. Heart J., 89:501–509, 1975.
94. Fenichel, N. M., Jimenez, F. A., and Polachek, A. A.: 2:1 left bundle branch block in acute bacterial endocarditis with septal abscess. J. Electrocardiol., 10:287–290, 1977.
95. Singh, R. B., Agrawal, B. V., and Somani, P. N.: Left bundle branch block: A rare manifestation of digitalis intoxication. Acta Cardiol., 31:175–179, 1976.
96. Bharati, S., Lev, M., Dhingra, R. C., Chuquimia, R., Towne, W. D., and Rosen, K. M.: Electrophysiologic and pathologic correlations in two cases of chronic second degree atrioventricular block with left bundle branch block. Circulation, 52:221–229, 1975.
97. Steenkamp, W. F. J.: Familial trifascicular block. Am. Heart J., 84:758–760, 1972.
98. Dhingra, R. C., Wyndham, C., Bauernfeind, R., et al.: Significance of chronic bifascicular block without apparent organic heart disease. Circulation, 60:33, 1979.
99. D'Cunha, G. F., Friedberg, H. D., and Jaume, F.: The first heart sound in intermittent left bundle branch block. Am. J. Cardiol., 27:447–449, 1971.
100. Haft, J. I., Weinstock, M., De Guia, R., et al.: Assessment of atrioventricular conduction in left and right bundle branch block using His bundle electrogram and atrial pacing. Am. J. Cardiol., 27:474–480, 1971.
101. Jacobson, L. B., and Scheinman, M.: Catheter-induced intra-Hisian and intrafascicular block during recording of His bundle electrograms. A report of two cases. Circulation, 49:579–584, 1974.
102. Patton, R. D., Bordia, A., Ballantyne, F. et al.: Bundle-of-His recording of complete heart block during cardiac catheterization: Electrophysiologic documentation of bilateral bundle branch block. Am. Heart J., 81:108–113, 1971.
103. Haft, J. I., Herman, M. V., and Gorlin, R.: Left bundle branch block. Etiologic, hemodynamic, and ventriculographic considerations. Circulation, 43:279, 1971.
104. Coronary Drug Project Research Group: The prognostic importance of the electrocardiogram after myocardial infarction. Experience in the coronary drug project. Ann. Intern Med., 77:677, 1976.
105. Fabregas, R. A., Tse, W. W., and Han, J.: Conduction disturbances of the bundle branches produced by lesions in the nonbranching portion of the His bundle. Am. Heart J., 92:356, 1976.
106. Gann, D., Balachandran, P. K., Sherif, N. E., and Samet, P.: Prognostic significance of chronic versus acute bundle branch block in acute myocardial infarction. Chest, 67:298–303, 1975.
107. Kulbertus, H. E.: The magnitude of risk of developing complete heart block in patients with LAD-RBBB. Am. Heart J., 86:278–280, 1973.
108. Waugh, R. A., Wagner, G. S., Harvey, T. L., et al.: Immediate and remote prognostic significance of fascicular block during acute myocardial infarction. Circulation, 47:675, 1973.
109. Pell, S., and D'Alonso, C. A.: Immediate and five-year survival of employed men with a first myocardial infarction. N. Engl. J. Med., 270:915, 1964.
110. Wong, B., Rinkenberger, R., Dunn, M., and Goodyer, A.: Effect of intermittent left bundle branch block on left ventricular performance in the normal heart. Am. J. Cardiol., 39:459–463, 1977.
111. Dillon, J. C., Chang, S., and Feigenbaum, H.: Echo-cardiographic manifestations of left bundle branch block. Circulation, 49:876–880, 1974.
112. Talbot, S.: QT interval in right and left bundle branch block. Br. Heart J., 35:288–291, 1973.
113. Vera, Z., Ertem, G., and Cheng, T. O.: Left bundle branch block with intermittent right axis deviation. Evidence for left posterior hemiblock accompanying predivisional left bundle branch block. Am. J. Cardiol., 30:896–901, 1972.
114. Cannom, D. S., Wyman, M. G., and Goldreyer, B. N.: Initial ventricular activation in left-sided intraventricular conduction defects. Circulation, 62:621–631, 1980.
115. Goldman, M. J., and Pipberger, H. V.: Analysis of the orthogonal electrocardiogram and vectorcardiogram in ventricular conduction defects with and without myocardial infarction. Circulation, 39:243–250, 1969.
116. Pryor, R.: Recognition of myocardial infarction in the presence of bundle branch block. Cardiovasc. Clin., 6:255–271, 1974.
117. De Kock, J., and Schamroth, L.: Left bundle branch block associated with acute inferior wall myocardial infarction. S. Afr. Med. J., 49:397–398, 1975.
118. Horan, L. G., Flowers, N. C., Tolleson, W. J., and Thomas, J. R.: The significance of diagnostic Q waves in the presence of bundle branch block. Chest, 58:214–220, 1970.
119. Timmis, G. C., Gangadharan, V., Ramos, R. G., and Gordon, S.: Reassessment of Q waves in left bundle branch block. J. Electrocardiol., 9:109–114, 1976.
120. Chung, E. K.: Electrocardiogram of the month. Acute myocardial infarction in the presence of left bundle branch block. W. Va. Med. J., 66:20–21, 1970.
121. Petersen, G. V., and Tikoff, G.: Left bundle branch block and left ventricular hypertrophy: Electrocardiographic pathologic correlations. Chest, 59:174–177, 1971.
122. Chung, D. K., Panitch, N. M., and Chung, E. K.: A comparison

of the conventional criteria for left ventricular hypertrophy before and after the development of complete left bundle branch block. Jpn. Circ. J., 33:19–24, 1969.

123. Simonsen, E. E., and Madsen, E. G.: Four cases of right-sided bundle branch block and one case of atrioventricular block in three generations of a family. Br. Heart J., 32:501–504, 1970.
124. Gelband, H., Waldo, A. L., Kaiser, G. A., Bowman, F. O., Jr., and Hoffman, B. F.: Etiology of right bundle branch block in patients undergoing total correction of Tetralogy of Fallot. Circulation, 44:1022–1033, 1971.
125. Yasui, H., Takeda, Y., Yamauchi, S., et al.: The deleterious effects of surgically induced complete right bundle branch block on long-term follow-up results of closure of ventricular septal defect. J. Thorac. Cardiovasc. Surg., 74:210–217, 1977.
126. Mehran-Pour, M., Borkat, G., Liebman, J., and Ankeney, J.: Resolution of surgically induced right bundle branch block. Ann. Thorac. Surg., 23:139–144, 1977.
127. Krongrad, E., Hefler, S. E., Bowman, F. O., Jr., Malm, J. R., and Hoffman, B. F.: Further observations on the etiology of the right bundle branch block pattern following right ventriculotomy. Circulation, 50:1105–1113, 1974.
128. Harris, L. K.: Transient right bundle branch block following blunt chest trauma. Am. J. Cardiol., 23:884–887, 1969.
129. Kumpuris, A. G., Casale, T. B., Mokotoff, D., et al.: Right bundle branch block. J.A.M.A., 242:172–173, 1979.
130. Massing, G. K., and Lancaster, M. C.: Clinical significance of acquired complete right bundle branch block in 59 patients without overt cardiac disease. Aero. Med., 40:967–971, 1969.
131. Lancaster, M. C., Schechter, E., and Massing, G. K.: Acquired complete right bundle branch block without overt cardiac disease. Am. J. Cardiol., 30:32–36, 1972.
132. Fernandez, F., Baragan, J., Benaim, R., Seebat, L., and Lénégre, J.: Right ventricular hemodynamics in intermittent complete right bundle branch block in man. Catheterization study of one case. Acta Cardiol. (Brux.), 23:569–581, 1968.
133. Van Mieghem, W., Ector, H., Classens, J., and DeDeest, H.: Acquired complete heart block in young adults. Acta Clin. Belg., 27:506–515, 1972.
134. Fedor, J. M., Walston, A., II, Wagner, G. S., and Starr, J.: The vectorcardiogram in right bundle branch block. Correlation with cardiac failure and pulmonary disease. Circulation, 53:926–930, 1976.
135. Norris, R. M., and Croxson, M. S.: Bundle branch block in acute myocardial infarction. Am. Heart J., 79:728–733, 1970.
136. Gann, D., Balachandran, P. K., Sherif, N. E., et al.: Prognostic significance of chronic versus acute bundle branch block in acute myocardial infarction. Chest, 67:298, 1975.
137. Shreenivas, S., Messer, A. L., Johnson, R. P., et al.: Prognosis in bundle branch block. II. Factors influencing the survival period in right bundle branch block. Am. Heart J., 40:891, 1950.
138. Schneider, J. F., Thomas, H. E., Jr., Kreger, B. E., et al.: Newly acquired left bundle branch block. The Framingham study. Ann. Intern. Med., 90:303, 1979.
139. Belletti, D. A., and Gould, L.: Evaluation of the magnitude of the R′ in V1 and detecting right ventricular hypertrophy in the presence of complete right bundle branch block. Aero. Med., 40:896–897, 1969.
140. Gandhi, M. J., Rao, Y. C., and Desai, J. M.: Diagnosis of right ventricular hypertrophy in complete RBBB and electrophysiologic implications. Indian Heart J., 26:110–113, 1974.
141. MacDonald, D., Behrendt, D. M., Jochim, K. E., et al.: Electrophysiologic delineation of the intraventricular His bundle in two patients with endocardial cushion type of ventricular septal defect. Circulation, 63:225–229, 1981.
142. Husson, G. S., Blackman, M. S., Rogers, M. S., Bharati, S., and Lev, M.: Familial congenital bundle branch system disease. Am. J. Cardiol., 32:365–369, 1973.
143. Sung, R. J., Tamer, D. M., Agha, A. S., et al.: Etiology of the electrocardiographic pattern of "incomplete right bundle branch block" in atrial septal defect: An electrophysiologic study. J. Pediatr., 87:1182–1186, 1975.
144. Moore, E. N., Boineau, J. P., Patterson, D. F., et al.: Incomplete right bundle branch block. An electrocardiographic enigma and possible misnomer. Circulation, 44:678–687, 1971.
145. Hishida, H.: IRBBB pattern after incising a subdivision of the right bundle branch. Jpn. Heart J., 10:350–362, 1969.
146. Terasawa, F., Kuramochi, M., Yazaki, Y., et al.: Clinical and pathological studies on incomplete left bundle branch block in the aged. Isr. J. Med. Sci., 5:732–735, 1969.
147. Rosenbaum, M. B.: The hemiblocks: Diagnostic criteria and clinical significance. Mod. Concepts Cardiovasc. Dis., 39:141–146, 1970.
148. Kenedi, P., O'Reilly, M. V., and Goldberg, E.: Association between intraventricular conduction defects, coronary artery disease and left ventricular function. Adv. Cardiol., 16:504–506, 1976.
149. Schatz, J., Krongrad, E., and Malm, J. R.: Left anterior and left posterior hemiblock in tricuspid atresia and transposition of the great vessels. Observations and electrocardiographic nomenclature and electrophysiologic mechanisms. Circulation, 54:1010–1013, 1976.
150. Eckberg, D. L., Ross, J., Jr., and Morgan, J. R.: Acquired right bundle branch block and left anterior hemiblock in ostium primum atrial septal defect. Circulation, 45:658–662, 1972.
151. Demoulin, J. C., Simar, L. J., and Kulbertus, H. E.: Quantitative study of left bundle branch fibrosis in left anterior hemiblock: A sterologic approach. Am. J. Cardiol., 36:751–756, 1975.
152. Kincaid, D. T., and Botti, R. E.: Significance of isolated left anterior hemiblock and left axis deviation during acute myocardial infarction. Am. J. Cardiol., 30:797–800, 1972.
153. Jacobson, L. B., Lafollette, L., and Cohn, K.: An appraisal of initial QRS forces in left anterior fascicular block. Am. Heart J., 94:407, 1977.
154. McHenry, P. L., Phillips, J. F., Fisch, C., et al.: Right precordial QRS pattern due to left anterior hemiblock. Am. Heart J., 81:498, 1971.
155. Gopal, D.: Left axis deviation. A spectrum of intraventricular conduction block. Circulation, 53:917–919, 1976.
156. Horwitz, S., Lupi, E., Hayes, J., Frishman, W., Cárdenas, M., and Killip, T.: Electrocardiographic criteria for the diagnosis of left anterior fascicular block. Left axis deviation and delayed intraventricular conduction. Chest, 68:317–320, 1975.
157. Rosenbaum, M. B., Shabetai, R., Peterson, K. L., ad O'Rourke, R. A.: Nature of the conduction disturbance in selective coronary ateriography in left heart catheterization. Am. J. Cardiol., 30:334–337, 1972.
158. Scott, R. C.: The S_1Q_3 (McGinn-White) pattern in acute cor pulmonale: A form of transient left posterior hemiblock? Am. Heart J., 82:135–137, 1971.
159. Medrano, G. A., Brenes, C., Micheli, A., and Sodi-Pallares, D.: Clinical electrocardiographic and vectorcardiographic diagnosis of left posterior subdivision block, isolated or associated with RBBB. Am. Heart J. 84:727–737, 1972.
160. Demoulin, J. C., and Kulbertus, H. E.: Histopathological examination of concept of left hemiblock. Br. Heart J., 34:807, 1972.
161. Uhley, H. N.: Some controversy regarding the peripheral distribution of the conduction system. Am. J. Cardiol., 30:919, 1972.
162. Nakaya, Y., Hiasa, Y., Murayama, Y., et al.: Prominent anterior QRS force as a manifestation of left septal fascicular block. J. Electrocardiol., 11:39–46, 1978.
163. Gambetta, M., and Childers, R. A.: Rate-dependent right precordial Q waves: "Septal focal block." Am. J. Cardiol., 32:196, 1973.
164. Wei-Min, H., and Cheng-Lang, T.: Bilateral bundle branch

block. Right bundle branch block associated with left anterior fascicular block. Cardiology, 62:35–43, 1977.

165. Watt, T. B., Jr., and Pruitt, R. D.: Character, cause, and consequence of combined left axis deviation and right bundle branch block in human electrocardiograms. Am. Heart J., 77:460–465, 1969.

166. Schaal, S. F., Seidensticker, J., Goodman, R., and Wooley, C. F.: Familial right bundle branch block, left axis deviation, complete heart block, and early death. A heritable disorder or cardiac conduction. Ann. Intern. Med., 79:63–66, 1973.

167. Morriss, J. H., Eugster, G. S., Nora, J. J., and Pryor, R.: His bundle recording in progressive external opthalmoplegia. J. Pediatr., 81:1167–1170, 1972.

168. Brink, A. J., and Torrington, M.: Progressive familial heart block — two types. South Afr. Med. J., 52:6, 1977.

169. Stephen, E.: Hereditary bundle branch system defect. A new genetic entity? Am. Heart J., 97:708, 1979.

170. Evans, W.: Familial cardiomegaly. Br. Heart J., 11:68, 1949.

171. Gozo, E. G., Jr., Cohen, H. C., and Pick, A.: Traumatic bifascicular intraventricular block. Chest, 61:294–296, 1972.

172. Chuquimia, R., Ramadurai, T. S., Towne, W., and Rosen, K.: Bifascicular block due to penetrating wound of the heart: Electrophysiology studies. Chest, 66:195–197, 1974.

173. Gozo, E. G., Jr., Cosnow, I., Cohen, H. C., and Okun, L.: The heart in sarcoidosis. Chest, 60:379–388, 1971.

174. Sugiura, M., Okada, R., Hiraoka, K., and Ohkawa, S.: Histological studies on the conduction system in 14 cases of right bundle branch block associated with left axis deviation. Jpn. Heart J., 10:121–132, 1969.

175. Ohmae, M.: Correlative studies on electrocardiogram and histopathology of the conduction system. I. Right bundle branch block with left axis deviation and prolonged PR interval. Jpn. Circ., J., 41:677–686, 1977.

176. Sung, R. J., Tamer, D. M., Garcia, O. L., Castellanos, A., Myerburg, R. J., and Gelband, H.: Analysis of surgically-induced right bundle branch block pattern using intracardiac recording techniques. Circulation, 54:442–446, 1976.

177. Wolff, G. S., Rowland, T. W., and Ellison, R. C.: Surgically induced right bundle branch block with left anterior hemiblock. An ominous sign in postoperative Tetralogy of Fallot. Circulation, 46:587–594, 1972.

178. Yabek, S. M., Jarmakani, J. M., and Roberts, N.: Postoperative trifascicular block complicating Tetralogy of Fallot repair. Pediatrics, 58:236–242, 1976.

179. Cairns, J. A., Dobell, A. R. C., Gibbons, J. E., and Tessler, I.: Prognosis of right bundle branch block and left anterior hemiblock after intracardiac repair of tetrallogy of Fallot. Am. Heart J., 90:549–554, 1975.

180. Baragan, J., Fernandez, F., Coblence, B., Saad, Y., and Lénègre, J.: Left ventricular dynamics in complete right bundle branch block with left axis deviation of QRS. Circulation, 42:797–804, 1970.

181. Lasser, R. P., Haft, J. I., and Friedberg, C. K.: Relationship of right bundle branch block and marked left axis deviation (with left parietal or peri-infarction block) to complete heart block and syncope. Circulation, 37:429, 1968.

182. Ranganathan, N., Dhurandhur, R., Phillips, J. H., et al.: His bundle electrogram in bundle branch block. Circulation, 45:282, 1972.

183. Lasser, R. P., Haft, J. I., and Friedberg, C. K.: Relationship of right bundle branch block and marked left axis deviation (with left pariental or peri-infarction block) to complete left block and syncope. Circulation, 37:429, 1968.

184. Scanlon, P. J., Pryor, R., and Blount, S. G., Jr.: Right bundle branch block associated with left superior and inferior intraventricular block. Circulation, 42:1123, 1970.

185. Gould, L., Venkataraman,K., Mohammad, N., and Gomprecht, R. F.: Prognosis of right bundle branch block in acute myocardial infarction. J.A.M.A., 219:502–503, 1972.

186. Lie, K. I., Wellens, H. J., Schuilenburg, R. M., et al.: Factors influencing prognosis of bundle branch block complicating acute antero-septal infarction. Circulation, 50:935–941, 1974.

187. Aranda, J., Befeler, B., and Castellanos, A.: His bundle recordings, bundle branch block, and myocardial infarction. Ann. Intern Med., 86: 106–108, 1977.

188. Lichstein, E., Gupta, P. K., Chadda, K. D., et al.: Findings of prognostic value in patients with incomplete bilateral bundle branch block complicating acute myocardial infarction. Am. J. Cardiol., 32:913–918, 1973.

189. Atkins, J. M., Leshin, S. J., Blomqvist, G., and Mullins, C. B.: Prognosis of right bundle branch block and left anterior hemiblock: A new indication for permanent pacing (abstract). Am. J. Cardiol., 26:624, 1970.

190. Godman, M. J., Lassers, B. W., and Julian, D. G.: Complete bundle branch block complicating acute myocardial infarction. N. Engl. J. Med., 282:237–240, 1970.

191. Atkins, J. M., Leshin, S. J., Blomqvist, G., and Mullins, C. B.: Ventricular conduction blocks and sudden death in acute myocardial infarction. N. Engl. J. Med., 288:281–284, 1973.

192. Ritter, W. S., Atkins, J. M., and Blomqvist, C. G.: Permanent pacing in patients with transient trifascicular block during acute myocardial infarction: Long-term prognosis. Am. J. Cardiol., 38:205–208, 1976.

193. Resnekov, L.: Pacemaking and acute myocardial infarction. Impulse, 11 : 1, 1978.

194. Kulbertus, H. E.: Reevaluation of the prognosis of patients with LAD-RBBB. Am. Heart J., 92:665–667, 1976.

195. Watt, T. B., and Pruitt, R. D.: Character, cause and consequence of combined left axis deviation and right bundle branch block in human electrocardiograms. Am. Heart J., 77:460–465, 1969.

196. Gupta, P., Lichstein, E., and Chadda, K. D.: Followup studies in patients with right bundle branch block and left anterior hemiblock: Significance of HV interval. J. Electrocardiol., 10:221–224, 1977.

197. Levites, R., and Haft, J. I.: Significance of first degree block (prolonged P-R interval) in bifascicular block. Am. J. Cardiol., 34:259, 1974.

198. Narula, O. S., and Samet, P.: Right bundle branch block with normal, left, or right axis deviation. Am. J. Med., 51:432, 1971.

199. Denes, P., Dhingra, R. C., Wu, D., et al: H-V interval in patients with bifascicular block (right bundle branch block and left anterior hemiblock). Clinical, electrocardiographic, and electrophysiologic correlations. Am. J. Cardiol., 35:23, 1975.

200. Rosenbaum, M. B.: Chagasic myocardiopathy. Prog. Cardiovasc. Dis., 7:199, 1964.

201. Venkataraman, K., Madias, J. E., and Hood, W. B., Jr.: Indications for prophylactic preoperative insertion of pacemakers in patients with right bundle branch block and left anterior hemiblock. Chest, 68:501–506, 1975.

202. Pastore, J. O., Yurchak, P. M., Jamis, K. M., et al.: The risk of advanced heart block in surgical patients with right bundle branch block and left axis deviation. Circulation, 57:677–680, 1978.

203. Narula, O., Qazi, N., Samet, P., et al.: Ten-year prospective observations based on H-V interval in patients with right bundle branch block (RBBB) and left axis deviation (LAD). Circulation, 58 (Suppl. II):197, 1978.

204. Sugiura, M., Hiraoka, K., and Ohkawa, S.: A histological study on the conduction system in 16 cases of right bundle branch block associated with right axis deviation. Jpn. Heart J., 15:113–125, 1974.

205. Harris, R., Siew, S., and Lev, M.: Smoldering myocarditis with intermittent complete AV block and Stokes-Adams syndrome. A

histopathologic and electrocardiographic study of "trifascicular" bundle branch block. Am. J. Cardiol., 24:880–889, 1969.

206. Loperfido, F., Fiorilli, R., Santarelli, P., et al.: Severe involvement of the conduction system in a patient with sclerodermal heart disease. An electrophysiological study. Acta Cardiol., 37:31–38, 1982.
207. Varriale, P., and Kennedy, R. J.: Right bundle branch block and right axis deviation in patients with coronary artery disease. Am. Heart J., 81:291–292, 1971.
208. Castellanos, A., Jr., Maytin, O., Arcebal, A. G., et al.: Significance of complete right bundle branch block with right axis deviation in absence of right ventricular hypertrophy. Br. Heart J., 32:85, 1970.
209. Thomsen, P. E. B., Sterndorff, B., and Gøtzsche, H.: Intraventricular trifascicular block verified by His bundle electrocardiography. Am. Heart J., 92:497–500, 1976.
210. Cerquira-Gomez, M., and Teixeira, A.: Wenckebach phenomenon in the posterior division of the left branch. Am. Heart J., 82:377–381, 1971.
211. Hassan, Z. U., Mendoza, R. A., Steinke, W. E., and Propert, D. B.: Multiple conduction defects with markedly prolonged ventricular depolarization in cardiomyopathy. J. Electrocardiol., 10:275–278, 1977.
212. Angelini, P., Springer, A., Sulbaran, T., and Livesay, W. R.: Right ventricular myopathy with an unusual intraventricular conduction defect (epislon potential). Am. Heart J., 101:680–683, 1981.
213. Befeler, B., Castellanos, A., Aranda, J., et al.: Intermittent bundle branch block in patients with accessory atrio-His or atrio-AV nodal pathways. Variants of the Lown-Ganong-Levine syndrome. Br. Heart J., 38:173–179, 1976.
214. Gulamhusein, S., Ko, P., and Klein, G. J.: Ventricular fibrillation following verapamil in the Wolff-Parkinson-White syndrome. Am. Heart J., 106:145–147, 1983.
215. Morady, F., Sledge, C., Shen, E., et al.: Electrophysiologic testing in the management of patients with the Wolff-Parkinson-White syndrome and atrial fibrillation. Am. J. Cardiol., 51:1623–1628, 1983.
216. Klein, G. J., Gulamhusein, S. S.: Intermittent preexcitation in the Wolff-Parkinson-White syndrome. Am. J. Cardiol., 52:292–296, 1983.
217. Weiss, J., Brugada, P., Roy, D., et al.: Localization of the accessory pathway in the Wolf-Parkinson-White syndrome from the ventriculo-atrial conduction time of right ventricular apical extrasystoles. Pace, 6:260–267, 1983.
218. Pritchett, E. L. C., Tonkin, A. M., Dugan, F. A., et al.: Ventriculo-atrial conduction time during reciprocating tachycardia with intermittent bundle branch block in Wolff-Parkinson-White syndrome. Br. Heart J., 38:1058–1064, 1976.
219. Lichstein, E., Goyal, S., Chadda, K., and Gupta, P. K.: Alternating Wolff-Parkinson-White-(preexcitation) pattern. J. Electrocardiol., 11:81–84, 1978.
220. Seipel, L., Both, A., Breithardt, G., and Loogen, F.: His bundle recordings in a case of complete atrioventricular block combined with preexcitation syndrome. Am. Heart J., 92:623–629, 1976.
221. Massumi, R. A.: His bundle recordings in bilateral bundle branch block combined with Wolff-Parkinson-White syndrome. Antegrade type II (Mobitz) block and 1:1 retrograde conduction through the anomalous bundle. Circulation, 42:287–295, 1970.
222. Gersony, W. M., and Ekery, D. D.: Concealed right bundle branch block in the presence of type B ventricular preexcitation. Am. Heart J., 77:668–676, 1969.
223. Sobrino, J. A., Mate, I., Mũnoz, J. E., and Sobrino, N.: Disappearance of right bundle branch block with left anterior hemiblock when associated with a type B preexcitation syndrome. Am. Heart J., 87:497–500, 1974.
224. Castillo, C. A., Castellanos, A., Jr., Befeler, B., et al.: Arrival of excitation at right ventricular apical endocardium on Wolff-Parkinson-White syndrome type A, with and without right bundle branch block. Br. Heart J., 35:594–600, 1973.
225. Denes, P., Goldfinger, P., and Rosen, K. M.: Left bundle branch block and intermittent type A preexcitation. Chest, 68:356–358, 1975.
226. Brugada, P., Wylick, A. V., and Abdollah, H.: Identical QRS complexes during atrial fibrillation with aberrant conduction and ventricular tachycardia. The value of a His bundle recording. Pace, 6:1057–1061, 1983.
227. Colvard, M. C., Jr., Whalen, R. E., Johnsrude, I. and Oldham, N.: Transvenous pacing, alternate bilateral bundle branch block, and syncope. Arch. Intern. Med., 132:411–413, 1973.
228. Halpern, M., Susana, Chiale, P. A., Nau, G. J., et al.: Effects of isoproterenol on abnormal intraventricular conduction. Circulation, 62:1357–1364, 1980.
229. Bailey, J. C., Lathrop, D. A., and Pippenger, D. L.: Differences between proximal left and right bundle branch block action potential durations and refractoriness in the dog heart. Circ. Res., 40:464–468, 1977.
230. Moore, E. N., Preston, J. B., and Moe, G. K.: Durations of transmembrane action potentials and functional refractory periods of the canine false tendons and ventricular myocardium: Comparisons in single fibers. Circ. Res., 17:259, 1965.
231. Elizari, M. V., Novakosky, A., Quinteiro, R. A., et al.: The experimental evidence of phase 3 and phase 4 block in the genesis of AV conduction disturbances. In Wellens, H. J. J., Lie, K. I., and Janse, M. J. (eds.): The Conduction System of the Heart: Structure, Function and Clinical Implications, pp. 360–376. Philadelphia. Lea & Febiger, 1976.
232. Moe, G. K., Mendez, C., and Han, J.: Aberrant A-V impulse propagation in the dog heart: A study of functional bundle branch block. Circ. Res., 16:251, 1965.
233. Hoffman, B. F.: Electrophysiologic mechanisms for conduction abnormalities. Chest, 63:651–652, 1973.
234. Cranefield, P. F., Klein, H. O., and Hoffman, B. F.: Conduction of the cardiac impulse. I. Delay, block and one way block in depressed Purkinje fibers. Circ. Res., 28:199–219, 1971.
235. Mendez, C., Muller, W. J., Merideth, J., and Moe, G. K.: Interaction of transmembrane potentials in canine Purkinje fibers and at Purkinje fiber–muscle junctions. Circ. Res., 24:361–372, 1969.
236. Neuss, H., Thormann, J., and Schlepper, M.: Electrophysiological findings in frequency-dependent left bundle branch block. Br. Heart J., 36:888–898, 1974.
237. Agha, A. S., Castellanos, A., Wells, D., et al.: Type I, type II and type III gaps in the bundle branch block. Circulation, 47:325–330, 1973.
238. Gallagher, J. J., Damato, A. N., Varghese, P. J., et al.: Gap in AV conduction in man: Type I and type II. Clin. Res., 20:373, 1972.
239. Fisch, C., Zipes, D. P., and McHenry, P. L.: Rate dependent aberrancy. Circulation, 48:714–724, 1973.
240. Gay, R., and Brown, D. F.: Bradycardia-dependent bundle branch block in acute myocardial infarction. Chest, 64:114–116, 1973.
241. Rosenbaum, M. B., Elizari, M. V., Lazzari, J. O., et al.: The mechanism of intermittent bundle branch block: Relationship to prolonged recovery, hypopolarization and spontaneous diastolic depolarization. Chest, 63:666–677, 1973.
242. Massumi, R. A.: Bradycardia-dependent bundle branch block. A critique and proposed criteria. Circulation. 38:1066–1073, 1968.
243. Travazzi, L., Salerno, J. A., Chimienti, M., et al.: Tachycardia-dependent and bradycardia-dependent intraventricular conduction defects in acute myocardial infarction: Electrocardio-

graphic, electrophysiologic and clinical correlates. Am. Heart J., 102:675–685, 1981.

244. Singer, D. H., Lazzara, R., and Hoffman, B. F.: Interrelationships between automaticity and conduction in Purkinje fibers. Circ. Res., 21:537–558, 1967.
245. Suarez, L., Kreta, A., Alarez, J. A., et al.: Effects of isoproterenol on bradycardia-dependent intra-His and left bundle branch blocks. Circulation, 64:427–433, 1981.
246. Massumi, R. A., Amsterdam, E. A., and Mason, D. T.: Phenomenon of supernormality in the human heart. Circulation, 46:264–275, 1972.
247. Sarachek, N. S.: Bradycardia-dependent bundle branch block. Relation to supernormal conduction and phase 4 depolarization. Am. J. Cardiol., 25:727–729, 1970.
248. Friedberg, H. D.: Mechanism of the Wedensky phenomena in the left bundle branch. Am. J. Cardiol., 27:698–702, 1971.
249. Barold, S. S., and Schamroth, L.: Tachycardia-dependent left bundle branch block associated with bradycardia-dependent variable left bundle branch block. A case report. Circulation, 48:216–220, 1973.
250. El-Sherif, N.: Tachycardia-dependent versus bradycardia-dependent intermittent bundle branch block. Br. Heart J., 34:167–176, 1972.
251. Tanaka, H., Nuruki, K., Toyama, Y., et al.: Tachycardia- and bradycardia-dependent left bundle branch block associated with first degree AV block. A study using His bundle electrogram during carotid sinus compression. Jpn. Heart J., 17:717–726, 1976.
252. El-Sherif, N.: Tachycardia- and bradycardia-dependent bundle branch block after acute myocardial ischemia. Br. Heart J., 36:291–301, 1974.
253. Corrado, G., Levi, R. F., Nau, G. J., and Rosenbaum, M. B.: Paroxysmal atrioventricular block related to phase 4 bilateral bundle branch block. Am. J. Cardiol., 33:553–556, 1974.
254. Rosenbaum, M. B., Elizari, M. V., Chiale, P., et al.: Relationships between increased automaticity and depressed conduction in the main intraventricular conducting fascicles of the human and canine heart. Circulation, 49:818–828, 1974.
255. Patton, R. D., and Roberts, J. S.: Simultaneous intermittent right and partial left bundle branch block. Am. Heart J., 81:255–259, 1971.
256. Langendorf, R., and Pick, A.: Concealed intraventricular conduction in the human heart. Adv. Cardiol., 14:40–50, 1975.
257. Walston, A., II, Boineau, J. P., Alexander, J. A., and Sealy, W. C.: Dissociation and delayed conduction in the canine right bundle branch. Circulation, 53:605–609, 1976.
258. Mazzoleni, A., Johnson, D., Fletcher, E., and Class, R. N.: Concealed conduction in left bundle of His. Br. Heart J., 34:365–369, 1972.
259. Dhingra, R. C., Amat-Y-Leon, F., Wyndham, C., et al.: Significance of left axis deviation in patients with chronic left bundle branch block. Am. J. Cardiol., 42:551–556, 1978.
260. Singer, D. H., and Ten Eick, R. E.: Aberrancy: Electro-physiological aspects. Am. J. Cardiol., 28:381–401, 1971.
261. Fisher, M. L., Mugmon, M. A., Carliner, H. H., et al.: Left anterior fascicular block: Electrocardiographic criteria for its recognition in the presence of inferior myocardial infarction. Am. J. Cardiol., 44:645–650, 1979.

17

Electrophysiologic Mechanisms of Ischemic Ventricular Arrhythmias: Experimental-Clinical Correlation

Hrayr S. Karagueuzian and William J. Mandel

Historical Background

Sudden cardiac death due to coronary artery obstruction appears to be an ancient disease. According to von Bissing, a German Egyptologist, sudden death was depicted in pictorial scenes by an Egyptian artist on an ancient Egyptian tomb relief during the Sixth Dynasty (2625 to 2475 BC).[1] The later documentation of the presence of atherosclerotic plaques in Egyptian mummies[2] suggested to many that ischemic heart disease could, in fact, have caused sudden cardiac deaths very early in ancient civilizations.[1]

An early experimental attempt to document the relationship between interruption of blood supply to the myocardium and sudden cardiac arrest was made by Chirac in 1698 in a dog.[3] Unfortunately, however, this important pioneering experimental work did not capture the interest or the imagination of the physicians and the intelligentsia of his day. As a result, the work remained an isolated finding until some 150 years later, when interest in this field was renewed. In 1842, Dr. Marshall Hall, in his Gulstonian lecture series on "On the Mutual Relations Between Anatomy, Physiology, Pathology and Therapeutics," read at the British Association for the Advancement of Science, attributed the causes of sudden death, in many instances, to an interruption of the coronary circulation. In that same year, Ericksen[4] experimentally verified Hall's contention. He occluded coronary arteries in dogs and rabbits and reached the following conclusion:

> Any circumstance that may interfere with the passage of the blood through the coronary arteries, either directly, as in ossification of the coats of those vessels, or indirectly, by there not being sufficient blood sent out of the left ventricle, as in cases of extreme obstruction or regurgitant disease of the aortic or mitral valves, may occasion the fatal event.

In 1894, the effects of experimental coronary artery occlusion on cardiac rhythm were described in greater detail by Porter.[5] He observed irregularities of cardiac rhythm following coronary artery occlusion that commonly preceded terminal ventricular fibrillation. In 1909, Sir Thomas Lewis, in a series of elaborate experimental studies, demonstrated the relationship of paroxysmal ventricular tachycardia and coronary artery occlusion[6] (Fig. 17-1). It was of great interest to see that in 1921, Robinson and Herrman[7] extended this observa-

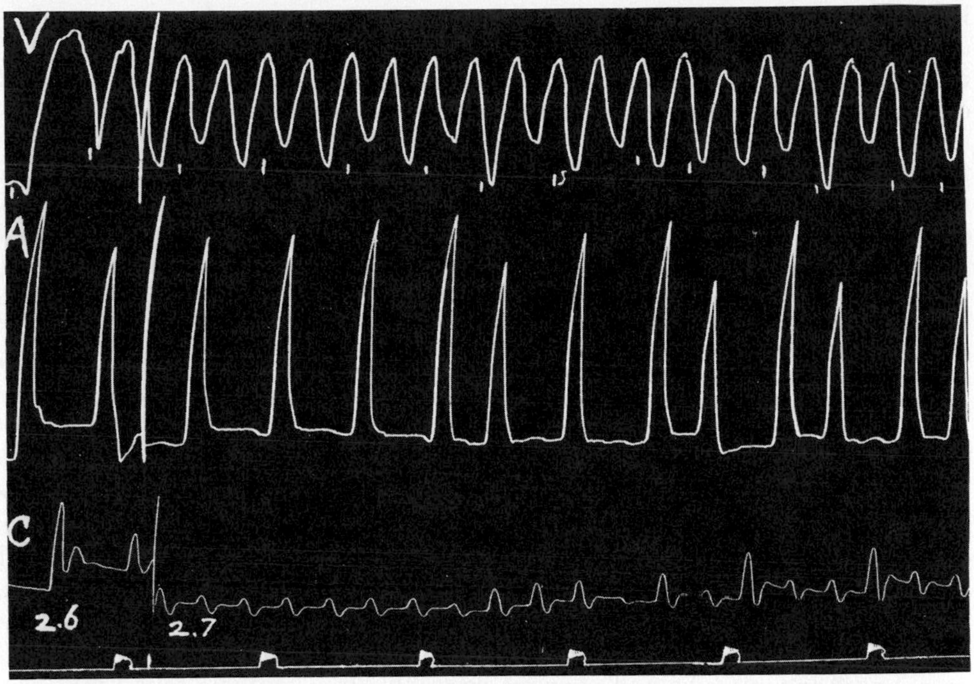

Figure 17-1. *Initiation of paroxysmal ventricular tachycardia 2 hours 6 minutes after right coronary artery occlusion in the dog. Upper recording (V) is ventricular muscle shortening; middle recording (A) is atrial muscle shortening. Both were made by special myocardiographic levers. The lower recording (C) is carotid artery pressure. The bottom tracing is time marker with 1-second intervals. The first two beats appear normal; thereafter a paroxysm of approximately 220 beats/min is initiated. Alteration is well seen in both the atrial and ventricular curves but is less marked in the carotid. At first the atrium responds to every second beat and later to two in three. With the 2:3 rhythm a periodic variation in the carotid tracing and a variation in the Vs-As intervals are seen. (Lewis, T.: The experimental production of paroxysmal tachycardia and the effects of ligation of the coronary arteries. Heart, 1:98–129, 1909)*

tion to the clinical level and established a similar relationship in humans. The increased vulnerability of the ischemic myocardium to electrical stimuli was discovered by Wiggers and associates in 1941.[8] These investigators found that ischemia caused by coronary occlusion lowered the amount of current required to induce ventricular fibrillation (reduced "fibrillation threshold") and broadened the period of the cardiac cycle during which fibrillation occurred ("vulnerable period"). Yet another novel observation of cardiac arrhythmias related to coronary occlusion was made by Harris in 1950.[9] This investigator discovered the presence of two distinct time periods (phases) after coronary occlusion in which ventricular arrhythmias were present. The first, or early, phase of arrhythmias occurred within minutes of coronary artery occlusion and often degenerated to ventricular fibrillation. The delayed, or second, phase of arrhythmias began 6 to 8 hours after occlusion and lasted for 2 to 4 days. Harris and associates[10] speculated that the electrophysiologic mechanisms of these arrhythmias operating during these two phases might differ, a speculation supported by later evidence.

The early demonstration of cardiac rhythm irregularities following experimental coronary artery occlusion and the establishment of similar relationships in humans and the demonstration of increased vulnerability of the ischemic myocardium to ventricular fibrillation during electrical stimulation of the heart laid the groundwork for the impressive and intense work during the last two decades in the area of ischemic arrhythmias.

In this chapter, we will review various electrophysiologic mechanisms of ventricular arrhythmias following experimental coronary artery occlusion and briefly evaluate the role of pharmacologic intervention designed to control these arrhythmias. Most if not all of these studies were made in dogs, and, at present, clinicians' general understanding of pathophysiologic mechanisms of ventricular arrhythmias during various phases of evolving myocardial ischemia and infarction are primarily derived from the canine model of infarction introduced by

Harris,[9] in which the left anterior descending (LAD) coronary artery is premanently occluded. Later experiments with the swine model, in which the LAD was occluded, also provided important insights. We will make every attempt, whenever evidence permits, to extrapolate experimental findings to clinical results, recognizing that experimental models may differ from clinical conditions.

Phase I or Early Ventricular Arrhythmias

Occlusion Arrhythmias

Ventricular arrhythmias that occur within minutes after complete occlusion of the LAD (the early arrhythmic phase) appear to depend primarily on the immediate effects of ischemia on working myocardial muscle cells.[11] Ventricular muscle cells depend completely on their coronary artery blood for proper supply of nutrients and oxygen; coronary occlusion therefore has a pronounced and immediate effect on the electrophysiologic, metabolic, and ultrastructural fate of the affected myocardial cells. The etiologic factors involved in alteration of the electrophysiologic properties of acutely ischemic myocardial cells include hypoxia, acidosis, elevated levels of extracellular potassium ions and intracellular calcium ions, depletion of cellular energy stores, and release of catecholamines and various mediators. The electrophysiologic consequences of the various ischemia-induced stigma on ventricular muscle cells are loss of resting membrane potential, alteration in refractoriness and excitability, and slowing of conduction with possible emergence of various mechanisms of automatic impulse initiation.

The various cellular electrophysiologic abnormalities could eventually lead to ventricular ectopic activity or ventricular tachycardia, which could degenerate into ventricular fibrillation.

Immediately after coronary occlusion, ischemia of the ventricular muscle causes the extracellular potassium ion concentration to rise.[12] Such a rise in K^+ in the extracellular space can decrease resting membrane potential, inactivating the fast inward excitatory sodium current.[13] Depending on the level of loss of resting potential, some myocardial cells will manifest depressed fast-inward currents, whereas others will only show slow-response action potentials, the results of which will be variable delay and slowing of myocardial activation in the ischemic zone. Hill and Gettes,[12] using a potassium-sensitive electrode, studied the relation between extracellular potassium rise in ischemic zones immediately after LAD occlusion in intact *in situ* porcine hearts and the pattern of myocardial activation (Fig. 17-2). These authors found that changes in myocardial activation during the early minutes of acute ischemia were quite heterogeneous and that these changes in ventricular activation paralleled quite well with the rise of extracellular K^+. A complex pattern of intramyocardial conduction slowing in an acutely ischemic segment of the canine myocardium was observed by Hamamoto and associates.[14,15] These investigators found that the acute effects of ischemia caused by coronary occlusion were highly variable and that conduction times varied depending on whether the impulse was directed toward the epicardium or the endocardium.[14] Furthermore, these

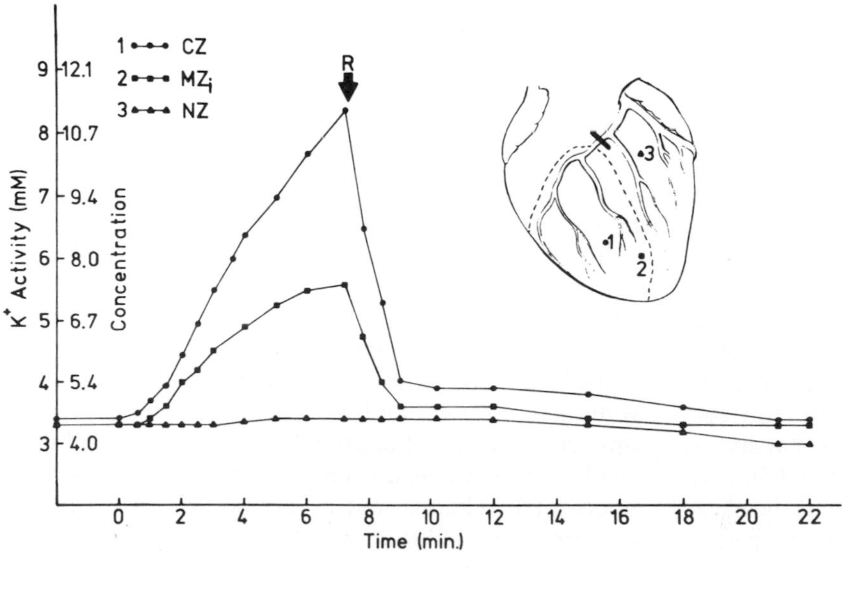

Figure 17-2. *Time course of change in midmyocardial extracellular K^+ activity (ak^+) recorded after acute occlusion of the left anterior descending (LAD) coronary artery at time zero. The diagram of the anterior surface of the heart illustrates electrode positions* (symbol *and* number), *point of LAD occlusion* (bar), *and resulting margin of cyanosis* (dashed line). *Electrode 1 was in the center of the ischemic zone (CZ), electrode 2 was within 5 mm of the inside margin of the ischemic zone (MZi), and electrode 3 was in the nonischemic zone (NZ). Release of the occlusion is indicated by the* arrow *(R). The ordinate shows both the measured ak^+ and the calculated K^+. (Hill, J. L., and Gettes, L. S.: Effect of acute coronary artery occlusion on local myocardial extracellular K^+ activity in swine. Circulation, 61:768–778, 1980. By permission of the American Heart Association, Inc.)*

authors demonstrated a disparity between antegrade and retrograde conduction times at both epicardial and endocardial ischemic sites.[15] Based on these observations, these investigators suggested that nonhomogenous abnormalities in conduction time in various regions of the ischemic myocardium can set the stage for reentrant premature excitation of the ventricles.

In an attempt to shed some light on the cellular mechanism(s) of ventricular tachyarrhythmias during the first 10 minutes after complete coronary artery occlusion, Downar and co-workers[13] recorded subepicardial transmembrane potentials from an ischemic zone after complete LAD occlusion in intact porcine hearts. During the initial 5 minutes, acute ischemia shortened action potential duration and decreased resting membrane potential, action potential amplitude, and upstroke velocity of phase zero.[13] As the duration of occlusion proceeded from 5 to 10 minutes, greater loss of resting membrane potential occurred, with long delays (100 msec) occurring between electrical stimulation and ischemic myocardial cell response (Fig. 17-3). Furthermore, before complete inexcitability of these cells was attained (10 to 12 minutes after occlusion), alternation in the amplitude of action potential progressed to 2:1 responses. These local changes in electrical response reflected the phenomenon of postrepolarization refractoriness, indicating a lengthening of effective refractory period, often greater than the basic cycle length of stimulation.[13] These local cellular electrophysiologic changes coincided with the emergence of ventricular arrhythmias. These cellular changes (conduction delays, presence of heterogenous local cellular responsiveness with variable

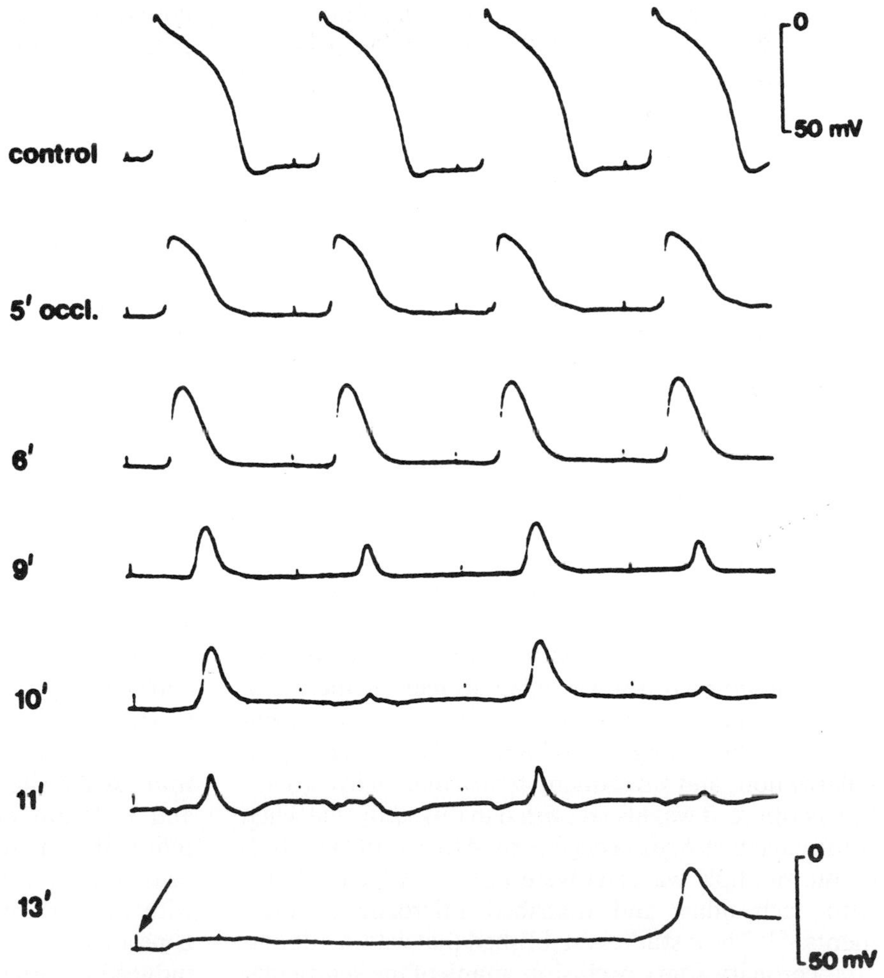

Figure 17-3. *Transmembrane action potentials recorded from the subepicardium of the left ventricle of an* in situ *pig heart before and after occlusion of the proximal left anterior descending coronary artery. (Downar, E., Janse, M. J., and Durrer, D.: The effects of acute coronary artery occlusion on subepicardial transmembrane potentials in the intact porcine heart. Circulation, 56:217–224, 1977. By permission of the American Heart Association, Inc.)*

lengthening of ischemic zone refractoriness) were taken to suggest that the early arrhythmias were caused by a reentry mechanism.[13,31]

Fujimoto and associates,[16] have suggested that the faster the rate of conduction slowing in an acutely ischemic segment of the myocardium, the higher the incidence of spontaneous initiation of ventricular fibrillation during the initial 30 minutes of complete coronary artery occlusion. These authors further suggested that conduction delay and the rate of change of conduction delay in an acutely ischemic myocardium may be used as reliable electrophysiologic markers of whether early ischemic ventricular fibrillation will develop.[16]

The relation of more complete and rapid reduction of myocardial blood flow to the incidence of ventricular fibrillation during the early postocclusion period was explored by Meesmann.[17] This investigator found that the greater the intensity of ischemia in a given region of the myocardium (*i.e.,* absence of collateral flow), the higher the incidence of ventricular fibrillation.[17] It is tempting to postulate that with more intense ischemia, electrophysiologic properties would deteriorate more rapidly, an event shown to be associated with a higher incidence of early postocclusion ventricular fibrillation.[16] In line with this suggestion are the early findings of Harris,[9] showing that gradual occlusion of the LAD (two-stage occlusion) was associated with a lesser incidence of ventricular fibrillation when compared to sudden occlusion of the same artery.

The relationship of slow conduction and unidirectional conduction block to the emergence of reentrant ventricular arrhythmias during the first few minutes after coronary artery occlusion was demonstrated by Janse and associates.[18,19] These investigators, by simultaneously recording from 60 ischemic and nonischemic sites, were able to delineate the direction and sequence of the spread of excitation during ventricular premature depolarizations. They demonstrated that the cardiac impulse was blocked when it reached the center of the ischemic zone and that two wavefronts bypassed the zone of block and invaded it retrogradely to reexcite the site of original conduction block (Fig. 17-4). This event coincided with the emergence of ventricular premature depolarizations and subsequent ventricular tachycardia.[19] Furthermore, it was also reported in this study that when ventricular tachycardia degenerated to ventricular fibrillation, multiple wavelets were present, which collided with each other and inscribed microcircus movements.[18,19] These studies established that within minutes after coronary artery occlusion, many of the ventricular tachycardias observed are caused by a macroreentrant mechanism (about 2 cm in diameter) and that ventricular fibrillation that may later develop is caused by multiple smaller or microreentrant circuits, about 0.5 cm or less in diameter.[18,19]

The possibility, however, that some sort of automatic mechanism may also cause ventricular arrhythmias during the early postocclusion period cannot be ruled out. This can be caused by the flow of an injury (depolarizing) current between ischemic and normal zones.[18] When differences in action potential duration exist in adjacent areas, current flows from the site of the longest action potential duration to that of the shorter duration. When the intensity of such a depolarizing current is large enough, it may induce threshold depolarization in adjacent cells with shorter action potential duration, causing ectopic activity.[20] The induction of pacemakerlike activity by depolarizing current pulses both in ventricular myocardial cells[20] and in Purkinje fibers[21] are well documented. Katzung[22] termed this phenomenon *depolarization-induced automaticity* (DIA) and Cranefield[21] called it *automaticity caused by early afterdepolarization* (EAD).

These descriptions simply state that if the free running course of repolarization is interrupted by an applied depolarizing current, pacemakerlike activity is induced during the entire period of applied depolarizing current. Furthermore, Katzung and colleagues[23] have shown that in *in vitro* preparations of guinea pig papillary muscle, the current that flows between cells depolarized by 145 mMK^+ and normal cells superfused with 4 mMK^+ could induce transient spontaneous activity at membrane potential levels between −70 and −50 mV in the normal cells, especially in the presence of epinephrine. The probable mechanism of the induction of pacemakerlike activity by current of injury is as follows: The membrane potentials of cells exposed to 145 mMK^+ is zero or nearly so, and the membrane potential of cells exposed to normal K^+ is approximately −80 mV. This potential gradient will set an "injury" depolarizing current to flow between the intracellular compartments of depolarized cells toward normal cells.[23] That such depolarizing current could be responsible for at least the initial beats of ventricular tachycardia and ventricular fibrillation in the intact canine and porcine hearts immediately after coronary artery occlusion was suggested by Janse and colleagues.[18] These authors estimated the intensity of the injury current and found it to be approximately 2 μA mm^3 at the site of current generation (current source) and 5 μA mm^3 at the site of current disappearance (current sink). Interestingly enough, ventricular premature beats were observed when injury currents were maximal, with the earliest activity always arising in the normal zone adjacent to an ischemic zone. Such depolarization-induced automaticity may well occur either in normal ventricular muscle fibers or in Purkinje fibers or in both as long as these fibers are adjacent to an acutely ischemic zone capable of generating enough depolarizing (injury) current to bring the potential of normal cells within the range capable of generating pacemakerlike activity.[22,25]

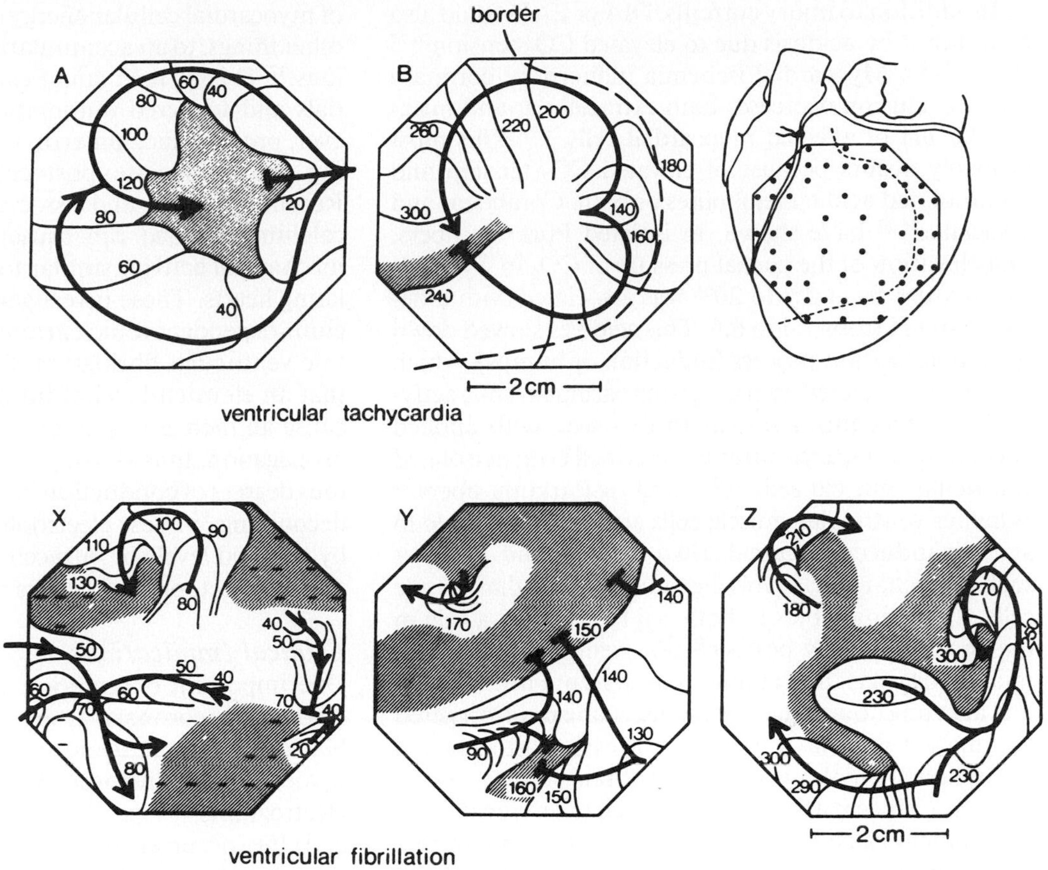

Figure 17-4. *Patterns of activation during a spontaneously occurring ventricular tachycardia that degenerated into ventricular fibrillation 4 minutes after occlusion of the left anterior descending coronary artery in an isolated pig heart. The electrode configuration is shown on the* upper right panel, *each dot indicating an electrode terminal. Direct current extracellular electrograms from these 60 terminals were recorded simultaneously. A recording period lasted for 2 seconds, during which complexes were digitalized and stored in a computer. The* dotted line *delineates the electrophysiologic border zone, that is, the zone where TQ-segment potentials of normally propagated beats became negative. In the first two ectopic beats (not shown), earliest activity was recorded in the normal myocardium close to the border. A and B (upper row) are the third and fourth ectopic beats; t = 0 was arbitrarily chosen, and isochronic lines separate areas activated within the same 20-msec interval.* Shaded areas *represent areas of conduction block.* Arrows *indicate general direction of spread of excitation; the symbol T stands for block. In A, the earliest activity is found in the normal side of the border; this wavefront is blocked in the center of the ischemic zone, but two wavefronts bypass the zone of block and invade it retrogradely to reexcite the site of origin at B after 140 msec. In B, again two semicircular wavefronts are set up, but since the 2-second recording periods ended here, it is not known how the arrhythmia continued. One second later, when the heart was fibrillating, X, Y, and Z were recorded. Multiple wavelets then were present, fusing and colliding with each other and describing microcircus movements; in the upper part of the area covered by the electrode, the reentrant wavefront describes a figure-8-shaped circus movement between 80 and 210 msec in beats X, Y, and Z. (Janse, M. J., and Kleber, A. G.: Electrophysiological changes and ventricular arrhythmias in the early phase of regional myocardial ischemia. Circ. Res., 49:1069–1081, 1981. By permission of the American Heart Association, Inc.)*

In addition to injury currents, DIA or EAD could also be induced by acidosis due to elevated CO_2 tension[26,27] (Fig. 17-5). Myocardial ischemia induced by coronary artery occlusion decreases both extracellular and intracellular *p*H of affected myocardial cells.[28,29] This most probably occurs because of elevated CO_2 tension and accumulated acidic metabolites or both. Coraboeuf and associates[26,27] have shown, in isolated Purkinje fibers, that elevation of the partial pressure of CO_2 in Tyrode's gas mixture from 3% to 20% was associated with a decrease of *p*H from 7.4 to 6.6. This acidosis slowed down the repolarization process (induction of humps), which was often associated with triggering pacemakerlike activity by a mechanism similar to that seen with applied depolarizing (injury) currents, described both in isolated ventricular muscle cells[20,22,23] and in Purkinje fibers.[21] Whether ventricular muscle cells are also susceptible to acidosis-induced pacemakerlike activity and whether such a mechanism, involving either ventricular muscle cells of Purkinje fibers or both cell types, plays a role in the genesis of early postocclusion ventricular arrhythmias in the intact heart remains to be seen. Furthermore, it is also unknown whether the mechanism of triggered automaticity[32,33] has any role in the early postocclusion ventricular arrhythmias. Such a mechanism may well be operative, since it appears to be related to an elevation of intracellular calcium ion concentration in both Purkinje fibers[34] and ventricular muscle fibers.[35,36] One of the major consequences of myocardial ischemia and hypoxia is depressed oxydative metabolism and depletion of myocardial cellular energy stores, which leads, among other things, to an accumulation of intracellular calcium ions.[37] This in turn could cause oscillatory afterpotentials and triggered automaticity to emerge.[34–36] However, proof of such an arrhythmogenic mechanism during the immediate postocclusion period is lacking. Recently, Clusin and associates[71] have suggested that calcium overload can cause fibrillatory electrical and mechanical activity similar to that recorded from fibrillating hearts. These investigators hypothesized that calcium-dependent ionic current could well mediate ischemic ventricular fibrillation. It is also important to note that an elevated level of intracellular calcium ions can cause an increase in myoplasmic resistance to impulse propagation, thus slowing conduction velocity and various degrees of conduction block due to eventual cellular decoupling.[37] These electrophysiologic changes induced by elevated levels of intracellular calcium could lead to reentrant ectopic activity, as discussed earlier.

Clinical Implications

One important observation that has resulted from occluding the coronary artery of dogs is the relationship between continuous electrical activity in the ischemic myocardium, as recorded by either bipolar extracellular electrograms[38] (Fig. 17-6) or composite electrograms,[39] and the occurrence of ventricular arrhythmias. Although it has not been possible to record this sort of electrical activity in human ventricular myocardium within the first few minutes after the onset of acute is-

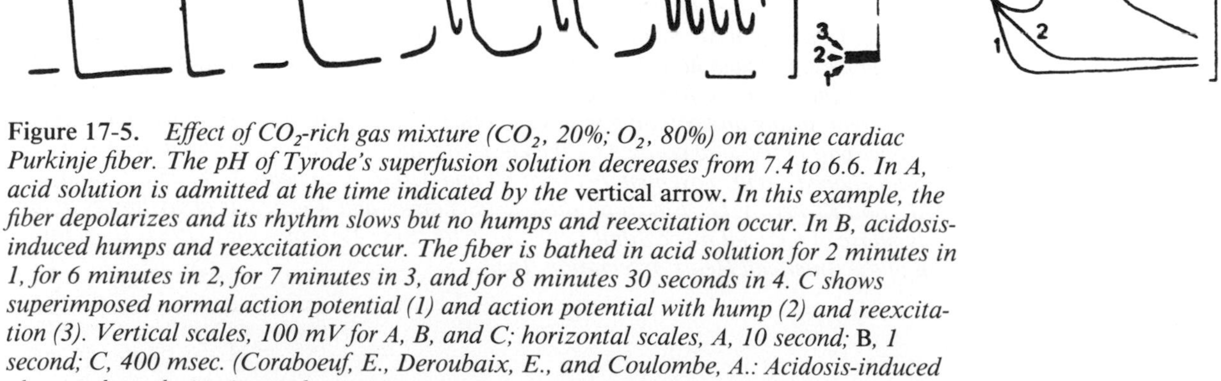

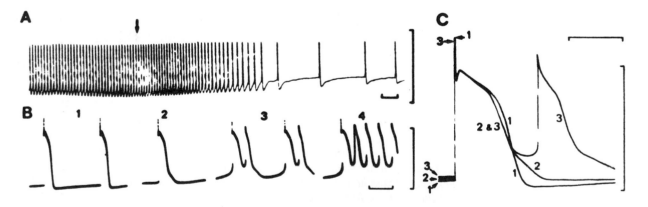

Figure 17-5. *Effect of CO_2-rich gas mixture (CO_2, 20%; O_2, 80%) on canine cardiac Purkinje fiber. The pH of Tyrode's superfusion solution decreases from 7.4 to 6.6. In A, acid solution is admitted at the time indicated by the* vertical arrow. *In this example, the fiber depolarizes and its rhythm slows but no humps and reexcitation occur. In B, acidosis-induced humps and reexcitation occur. The fiber is bathed in acid solution for 2 minutes in 1, for 6 minutes in 2, for 7 minutes in 3, and for 8 minutes 30 seconds in 4. C shows superimposed normal action potential (1) and action potential with hump (2) and reexcitation (3). Vertical scales, 100 mV for A, B, and C; horizontal scales, A, 10 second;* B, *1 second; C, 400 msec. (Coraboeuf, E., Deroubaix, E., and Coulombe, A.: Acidosis-induced abnormal repolarization and repetitive activity in isolated dog Purkinje fibers. J. Physiol. (Paris), 76:97–106, 1980)*

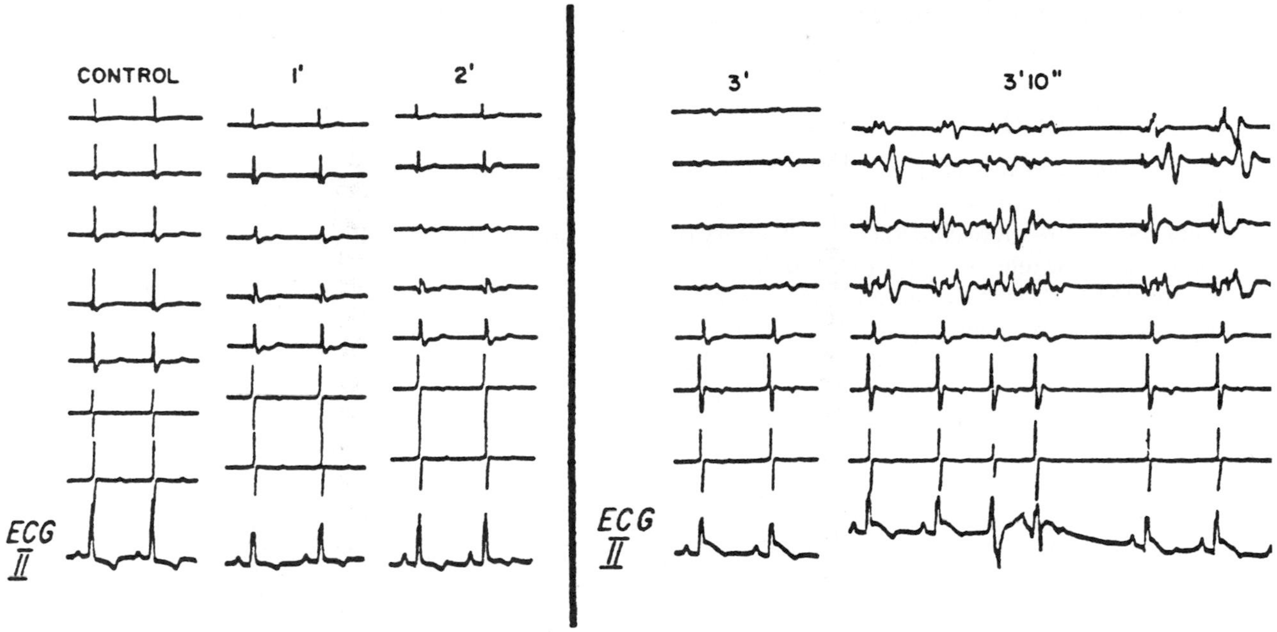

Figure 17-6. *The immediate effects of coronary artery occlusion on bipolar electrograms recorded from the epicardium of the canine heart. In each panel bipolar electrogram recordings from seven different regions are shown in the first seven traces. The* bottom trace *is a lead II electrocardiogram. The top five electrograms were recorded from the region that became ischemic after the left anterior descending (LAD) coronary artery was occluded; the sixth and seventh electrograms were recorded from nonischemic myocardium. At the left, recordings taken before coronary artery occlusion are shown (control). At all sites electrograms appear as large-amplitude spikes of short duration. To the right of the control records are records obtained 1 minute, 2 minutes, 3 minutes, and 3 minutes 10 seconds after complete occlusion of the LAD near its origin. There is a progressive decrease in amplitude and increase in duration of the electrograms recorded from the ischemic region and no change in the electrograms recorded from the nonischemic regions. ST segment changes on the electrocardiogram can be seen after 3 minutes. At 3 minutes 10 seconds the signals recorded from the ischemic region have increased amplification. Discrete spikes of electrical activity are no longer evident. In the top four traces the electrograms have become fragmented, and continuous electrical activity is evident. This is associated with the occurrence of ventricular premature depolarizations. (Waldo, A. L., and Kaiser, G. A.: A study of ventricular arrhythmias associated with acute myocardial infarction in the canine heart. Circulation, 47:1222–1228, 1973)*

chemia that causes ventricular arrhythmias, such activity has been recorded from chronic ischemic regions in aged ventricular infarcts and aneurysms (see below). This raises the possibility that such abnormal electrical activity leading to arrhythmia genesis may also occur in human ischemic ventricular myocardium immediately after the onset of an acute attack. At present, a favored hypothesis for continuous electrical activity is reentry, and this is based on the following interpretations. Continuous, low-amplitude, fragmented activity is caused by slowly conducting impulses, on one or multiple reentrant circuits in the ischemic myocardium, probably because muscle cells lose resting membrane potential and generate slowly conducting action potentials. When this occurs, continuous electrical activity, spanning the entire diastolic interval, could be recorded. The induction of this sort of continuous electrical activity is usually associated with the appearance of ventricular premature complexes and tachycardia.[38,39] However, this hypothesis, although attractive, by no means proves that reentry is occurring. Early after depolarization caused by injury currents or triggered automatic activity induced by intracellular elevation of calcium ions, the ischemic myocardium might well show a series of low-amplitude depolarizations with rapid rates of depolarizations that may show continuous electrical activity on an extracellular electrograms.[40] This might especially be the case when catecholamine levels are high, which occurs after acute coronary artery occlusion.[41] Therefore, the cellular electrophysiologic basis for cardiac electrograms showing continuous electrical activity may involve more than one mechanism.

Reperfusion Arrhythmias

Tennant and Wiggers reported in 1935[42] that ventricular fibrillation could occur when coronary blood flow was suddenly restored to an occluded coronary artery in the dog (reperfusion or release ventricular fibrillation). This early laboratory observation gained intense clinical and experimental interest when it was found that victims of sudden cardiac death (ventricular fibrillation), when resuscitated and followed carefully, did not uniformly show evidence of myocardial damage and infarction.[43] In this regard it was suggested that sudden death, in victims with no evidence of myocardial cell necrosis, was precipitated by the phenomenon of reperfusion-induced ventricular fibrillation, most likely triggered by dissolution of platelet plugs or sudden resolution of coronary artery spasm. Although the relevance of these findings to humans is uncertain, the sudden nature of reperfusion-induced ventricular fibrillation in the canine heart suggests that this model may help clinicians understand sudden cardiac death in humans. Consequently, release arrhythmias have become the subject of intense experimental studies to assess the mechanisms of reperfusion-induced ventricular fibrillation and to design effective antiarrhythmic drug regimens to prevent recurrence of sudden cardiac death. It has become clear that the duration of coronary artery occlusion before release (reperfusion) is one major factor in the induction of ventricular fibrillation. Blake and associates have studied this parameter and found that reperfusion-induced ventricular fibrillation is most likely to occur in the LAD occlusion model when the duration of occlusion is 20 to 30 minutes.[44] That the incidence of reperfusion-induced ventricular fibrillation peaks at this time may well relate to the reversibly induced ischemic myocardial damage, which is greatest at this time. Thereafter irreversible cell damage and myocardial necrosis occur.[45]

Another important parameter that influences the occurrence of ventricular fibrillation is the amount of myocardium at risk(*i.e.,* ischemic) that becomes reperfused. Austin and associates[46] described, using the logistic risk regression model, the relationship between the occurrence of ventricular fibrillation and the amount of myocardium at risk following coronary artery occlusion (Fig. 17-7). These authors found that their model could predict uniformly low and uniformly high probability of ventricular fibrillation with small and large amounts (mass) of myocardium at risk, respectively, with direct correlation for mid-range values of myocardium at risk. This study explains, to a large degree, the great variability in the incidence of reperfusion-induced ventricular fibrillation that occurs as a result of variations in the amount of myocardium at risk due to variations in the degree of collateral blood flow to the ischemic zone. In this study, however, the additional possible role of heart rate acceleration and systemic blood pressure lowering on outcome during reperfusion were not systemically evaluated. For example, increasing heart rate in dogs that sustain a smaller amount of myocardium at risk to levels comparable to dogs with large amounts of myocardium at risk could cause reperfusion-induced ventric-

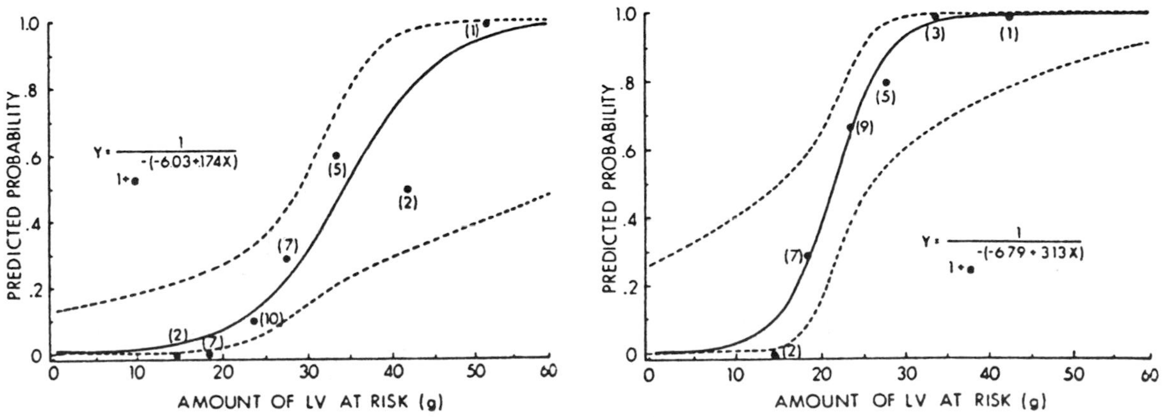

Figure 17-7. *Relationship between myocardium "at risk" and likelihood of ventricular fibrillation during occlusion* (left panel) *and after release of a 20-minute occlusion* (right panel). Solid line *is defined by equation;* hatched lines *describe 95% confidence limits. Observed incidence of ventricular fibrillation for each 5-g increment of myocardium at risk is shown with* dots. *Number of animals in each group is given in* parentheses. *(Austin, M., Wenger, T. L., Harrell, F. E., Jr., et al.: Effect of myocardium at risk on outcome after coronary artery occlusion and release. Am. J. Physiol., 243:H340–H345, 1982)*

ular fibrillation to occur more frequently. The importance of relatively faster heart rate in the genesis of ventricular arrhythmias during the initial 20 to 30 minutes of coronary artery occlusion has been stressed by Scherlag and associates.[47]

The cellular electrophysiologic mechanisms and the immediate inciting causes of reperfusion ventricular tachyarrhythmias remain questions of extreme interest and intense research. A possible explanation of reperfusion arrhythmias is that both chemical and electrical gradients caused by washout of various ions and metabolites that have accumulated in the ischemic zone may be responsible for inducing reperfusion arrhythmias. Massive washout of lactate and potassium ions were seen after reperfusion in one study.[39] The output of potassium ions into neighboring normal myocardial cells can cause partial depolarization and pacemakerlike repetitive activity of the sort described by Cranfield[21] and by Katzung and associates.[23] Such activity, if in fact present in the intact canine myocardium, can cause runs of ventricular tachycardia and ventricular fibrillation. Furthermore, the output of acidic metabolites can cause abnormal repolarization with humps during phase 3, an event described by Coraboeuf and associates[26,27] that can cause repetitive depolarizations leading to ventricular arrhythmias in the intact heart. These possibilities, however, remain just that and await experimental verification. Furthermore, potassium-induced partial depolarization of affected myocardial cells can inactivate the fast-response action potentials and leave the slow-response action potentials for impulse conduction. Such impulses conduct slowly and can lead to unidirectional conduction block. Once these events occur, reentrant premature ventricular depolarizations could emerge.[32,40] Depending on the size and the simultaneous number of wavelets that undergo reentrant premature excitation, the ventricular rhythm may manifest isolated ventricular premature complexes (single, large reentrant circuit) to ventricular fibrillation (small, multiple reentrant wavelets).[18] Therefore, as with ischemic ventricular tachyarrhythmias, both mechanisms of reentry and some sort of automatic activity may also be operative during reperfusion.[18]

Akiyama was able to record transmembrane potentials from subepicardial ventricular muscle cells in the reperfused region during reperfusion-induced ventricular fibrillation[48] (Fig. 17-8). This author found that cells in the reperfused region had depressed resting membrane potential and were sensitive to verapamil (a slow-channel blocker) but not to tetradotoxin (a fast-channel blocker). This study suggested that myocardial cells in the reperfused zone had action potentials of the slow-response type. Downar and colleagues[13] found that cells in the reperfused region had highly heterogenous transmembrane potential configurations (Fig. 17-9); some cells were inexcitable, and others were fully excitable. These properties led these authors to suggest that such heterogenous electrophysiologic substrate may well lead to reentrant type of arrhythmias. Although in these microelectrode studies automaticity was not documented,[13,48] its absence does not imply that some sort of automatic mechanism cannot be operative during the period of reperfusion ventricular arrhythmias. In fact, in a preliminary report, Ten Eick and colleagues[55] have shown that deep myocardial cells within the ischemic zone can initiate automatic impulse, suggesting that reperfused ischemic myocardial cells can generate an automatic mechanism.

Levine and associates[49] constructed strength-interval curves for both anodal and cathodal modes of stimulation within a few minutes after acute coronary artery occlusion in the dog and immediately after reperfusion during the peak incidence of ventricular arrhythmias. These authors found increased myocardial excitability that correlated well with both early occlusion and reperfusion-induced ventricular arrhythmias. Furthermore, anodal excitability correlated better with the incidence of arrhythmias than did cathodal excitability.[49] Alterations in the excitability threshold and refractoriness were also demonstrated by Elharrar and associates.[50] The prolongation of postrepolarization refractoriness (*i.e.*, inability of the cell to initiate an action potential for up to 200 msec after full repolarization) in ischemic myocardial fibers was described by Lazzara and associates,[51] as was the phenomenon of time-dependent recovery of myocardial excitability, which may have an anomalous relationship with heart rate, that is, the duration of postrepolarization refractoriness may increase as heart rate increases.[52] Such an event may well slow conduction velocity, favoring the emergence of reentrant premature excitation.

Reperfusion-induced ventricular tachyarrhythmias are complex phenomena, and multiple mechanisms may initiate and maintain reperfusion-induced arrhythmias.[53,54]

Although complex multiple mechanisms may operate during the early postocclusion and reperfusion periods, differences exist in the mechanism of ventricular arrhythmias in these two different conditions.[56,57] Coker and Parratt[67] have found that intracoronary administration of prostacyclin markedly reduced the incidence of ventricular fibrillation induced by reperfusion after a 40-minute occlusion of the LAD in dogs. These authors suggested that the release of endogenous prostacyclin may have a protective effect during reperfusion of an ischemic myocardium but could exhibit different action during occlusion arrhythmias. More studies are needed to unravel the cellular electrophysiologic differences and the precipitating factors in the induction of these potentially lethal arrhythmias in these two different settings.

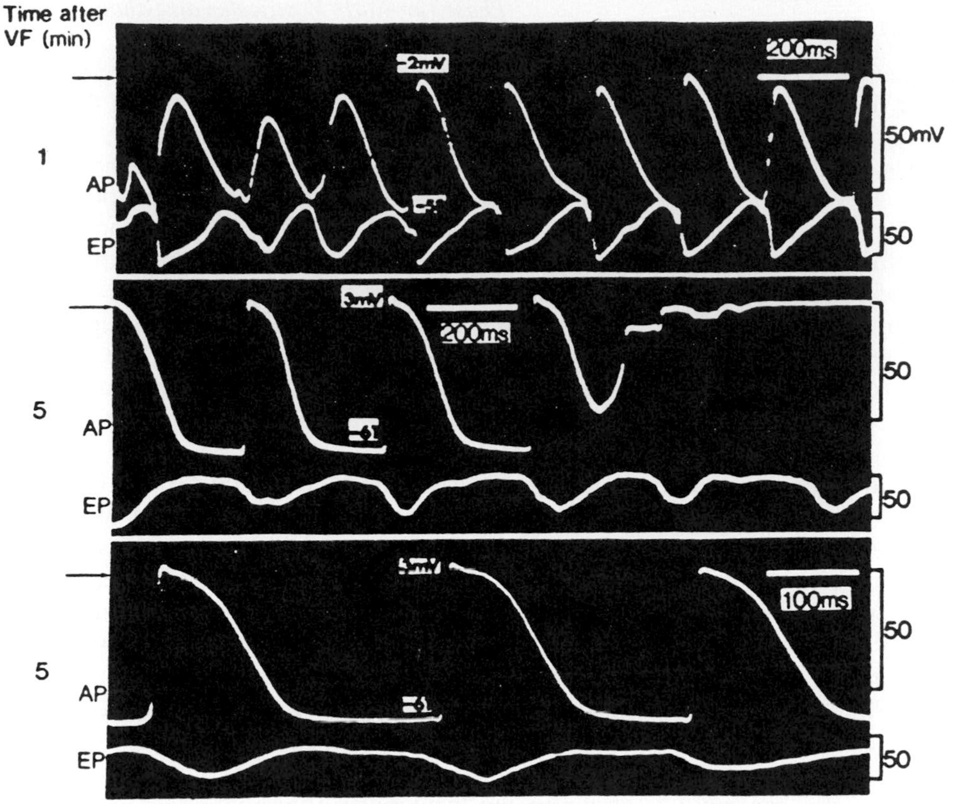

Figure 17-8. *Recording of transmembrane action potentials of subepicardial ventricular cells during ventricular fibrillation induced by reperfusion of ischemic areas. Action potentials (AP) and unipolar epicardial electrocardiograms (EP) were simultaneously recorded from reperfused areas 1 minute* (upper panel) *and 5 minutes (*middle panel *at a slower speed and* lower panel *at a faster speed) after onset of ventricular fibrillation. Zero reference level for membrane potential* (arrows, left) *is determined by withdrawing a micropipette into a thin film of Tyrode's solution covering epicardial surface inside the well* (middle panel). *At onset of ventricular fibrillation, ventricular cells discharged action potentials of various amplitudes at a fast rate of over 300 beats/min. As noted, one action potential had a maximum diastolic potential of −58 mV and overshoot potential of −2 mV* (upper panel). *Later, during ventricular fibrillation, local excitation rate slowed and remained relatively stable at about 150 beats/min, allowing membrane potential to reach a stable level during diastole. In this instance, resting potential was −61 mV and overshoot potential was 3 mV. Note increase in overshoot potential (3 mV) when local excitation rate was slower and diastolic potential before onset of upstroke reached a more negative value of −61 mV* (tracings, middle and lower panel). *(From Akiyama, T.: Inracellular recording of in situ ventricular cells during ventricular fibrillation. Am. J. Physiol., 240:H465–471, 1981)*

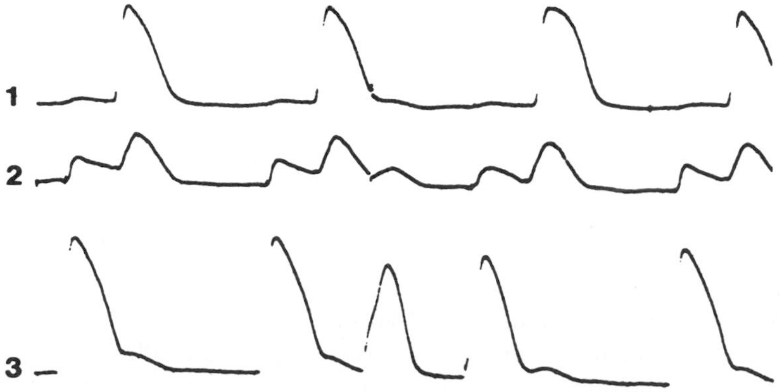

Figure 17-9. *Transmembrane action potentials recorded from the subepicardium of the left ventricle (within 1 mm of each other) of an* in situ *pig heart after left anterior descending coronary artery occlusion. Cells 1 and 2 were at the same location, but cell 1 was deeper. Action potentials from cells 3 and 1 and from cells 3 and 2 were recorded simultaneously only 1 minute apart, while stimulation pattern remained the same. Stimulating electrode was close to cell 3. All three cells were located within 1 mm of each other. Note the delay and block of the premature impulse between cells 3 and 1. (From Downar, E., Janse, M. J., and Durrer, D.: The effects of acute coronary artery occlusion on subepicardium transmembrane potentials in the intact porcine heart. Circulation, 56:217–224, 1977.)*

Pharmacologic Considerations

Pharmacologic therapy and management of early acute ischemic ventricular arrhythmias present a unique and formidable problem, since drugs have poor or no access to the site of origin of the arrhythmia. Wit and Bigger[58] suggested that if the drug can reach the site of arrhythmia origin, two mutually exclusive mechanisms must be operative for successful antiarrhythmic action. First, the drug must completely block conduction in the ischemic region; second, the drug must restore normal conduction. Furthermore, in light of newer findings, a potentially useful antiarrhythmic agent must also suppress abnormal automaticity, possibly caused by early afterdepolarizations.[23,27] Wenger and associates[59] injected procainamide intravenously in dogs, 40 minutes after complete left circumflex coronary artery occlusion, and found, depending on the severity of myocardial ischemia, progressively decreasing myocardial drug concentrations.[59] Most severely ischemic myocardial areas had the lowest myocardial drug concentration. Zito and colleagues[60] found lower myocardial lidocaine concentrations in ischemic zones in dogs given lidocaine 2 hours after LAD occlusion. Nevertheless, it appears that even such lowered levels of drug delivery to severely ischemic sites may still cause electrophysiologic effects during the early postocclusion period. The studies of Kupersmith and colleagues[61] show that lidocaine administered 2 hours after complete LAD occlusion caused a preferential increase in myocardial refractoriness in the infarcted zone, thus decreasing the disparity of refractoriness between normal and infarcted zones that was present before lidocaine administration. Furthermore, lidocaine increased the activation time in the infarcted zone but had no effect on the normal zone. In this study, however, the antiarrhythmic consequences, if any, of such local electrophysiologic effects of lidocaine on an acutely ischemic region of the myocardium were not evaluated. Moreover, the role of diminished antiarrhythmic drug delivery to an acutely ischemic zone in arrhythmia suppression is still undefined. Nattel and associates[62] have shown that introducing an antiarrhythmic agent (aprinidine) to a potentially arrhythmic region before coronary artery occlusion may lead to different regional myocardial distribution and different electrophysiologic actions and antiarrhythmic efficacy.[62] These authors, based on the frequency of arrhythmias, suggested that drug-induced further slowing in conduction in ischemic zones is likely to increase the incidence of early ventricular tachycardia and ventricular fibrillation.[62] This study demonstrated that drugs can actually exacerbate early postocclusion arrhythmias if their concentration is sufficiently raised in the ischemic zone. Further studies of this sort are needed to elaborate this important point.

As for reperfusion-induced ventricular fibrillation, most antiarrhythmic agents were found to be ineffective.[63,64] In a more recent study,[65] however, bretylium was found to reduce the incidence of reperfusion-induced ventricular fibrillation when the amount of myocardium at risk (ischemic) was taken into account during statistical computation.[65] It is refreshing to see that it is possible to introduce successfully pharmacologic agents to an acutely ischemic region of the myocardium by the coronary venous retrograde perfusion (retroperfusion) system.[68,69] Meerbaum and associates[68] lysed a thrombus in the LAD with streptokinase, administered through the great cardiac vein, which drains the perfusion bed of the LAD.[70] Whether delivery of antiarrhythmic drugs to an acutely ischemic zone by retroinfusion through cardiac veins could prevent or reduce the incidence of early arrhythmias remains to be seen. This approach, however, seems promising.[69]

Data on the mechanism(s) of early postocclusion arrhythmias in humans are difficult to study because of the extraordinary conditions under which they occur. In a preliminary report Cinca and associates[66] have compared precordial electrocardiogram recordings during the first minutes of acute myocardial infarction in humans to experimental coronary occlusion (Fig. 17-10). These authors suggested that the cellular electrophysiologic changes in humans may be similar to those in experimental animals.[66] If so, pharmacologic management of the early-phase arrhythmias will be extremely difficult. However, the possibility that similar cellular electrophysiologic abnormalities may exist in humans and in experimental ischemia emphasizes the fact that experimental studies designed to elucidate the mechanisms and pharmacologic effects of drugs might help in the management and prophylaxis of early-phase arrhythmias in humans.

Phase II Ventricular Arrhythmias

If the dog survives the early arrhythmic phase after permanent occlusion of the LAD, a relatively quiescent period ensues that may last up to 10 hours. Following this nonarrhythmic period is another prolonged interval of spontaneously occurring rapid ventricular tachycardia that may last up to 72 hours.[10,11,43,51] In the following sections, we will present experimental findings that the site(s) of origin, the cellular electrophysiologic mechanism(s), and the response of these arrhythmias to antiarrhythmic drugs differ from those arrhythmias that occur immediately after occlusion or after transient occlusion followed by reperfusion. Furthermore, we will attempt to present pertinent data showing that these arrhythmias are similar in many respects to the in-hospital phase of ventricular arrhythmias that occur in humans during the first few days after the onset of acute symptoms indicative of myocardial infarction.

The persistence of myocardial ischemia after the LAD occlusion in the dog causes myocardial cell necrosis that

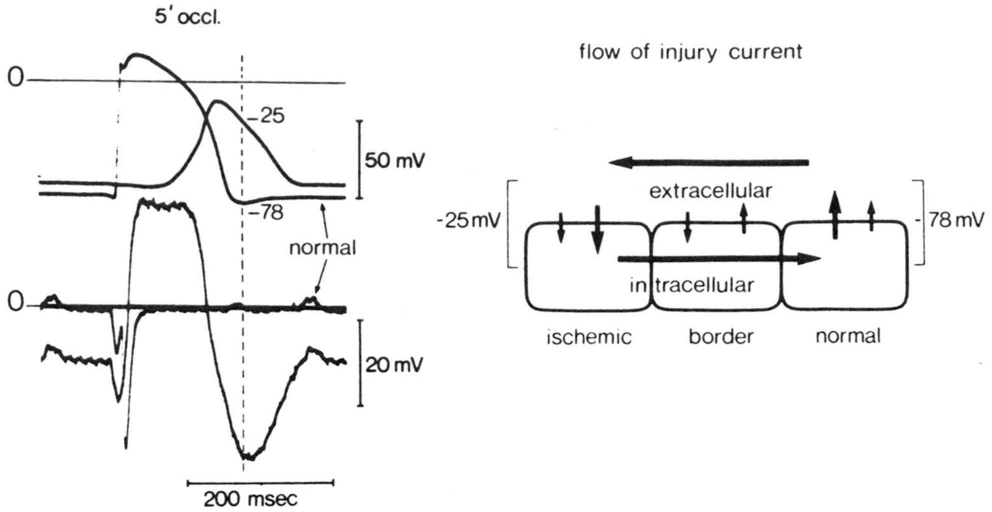

Figure 17-10. *Transmembrane and direct current extracellular potentials recorded from an* in situ *dog heart. Potentials before and 5 minutes after left anterior descending coronary artery occlusion are superimposed, using as time reference the stimulus artifact on the atrium. Note extreme delay in activation of the epicardial ischemic cell, which is depolarized when normal cells are already repolarized. The negative "T wave" in the local electrogram recorded from the ischemic zone represents the intrinsic deflection caused by the delayed activity. In the diagram, the flow of injury current at the moment indicated by the* dotted line *is schematically depicted. At the moment of the cardiac cycle, the injury current produces current sources at the nonischemic side of the border and current sinks on the ischemic side. (From Cinca, J., Janse, M. J., Morena, H., et al.: Mechanism and time course of the early electrical changes during acute coronary occlusion. An attempt to correlate the early ECG charges in man to cellular electrophysiology in pigs. Chest. 77:499-505, 1980.)*

may involve the entire left anteroseptal structures.[72,76] Usually the lateral, superior, and inferior margins of the infarct are well defined. On the epicardial surface a rim of cells, reaching in some cases one third of the left ventricular wall thickness, remain viable.[72,76] The margins at these epicardial sites are irregular and less sharply defined, and occasionally small areas of infarcted myocardium are separated from the main infarcted core by noninfarcted viable tissue.

On the endocardial surface underlying the infarcted zone, two to four layers of myocardial cells, identified as Purkinje fibers, remain viable.[74,75] The core of the infarcted myocardium (*i.e.*, within the wall of the left ventricle) manifests relatively homogeneous necrosis throughout the entire zone of infarction. In contrast, however, myocardial infarct structure produced by transient LAD occlusion followed by reperfusion differs from that produced by permanent LAD occlusion. In infarcts caused by temporary occlusions, regions of noninfarcted myocardium are found throughout the infarct. These regions of noninfarcted myocardium are either completely surrounded by infarcted myocardium or continuous with noninfarcted myocardium bordering the infarct.[76] The lateral margins of the infarct are extremely irregular, however; on both the epicardial and endocardial edges of the infarct variable layers of myocardial cells remain viable. Between 4 and 15 cell layers remain viable on the endocardial surface of the infarct, as does up to one third of the epicardium.[76] The anatomy and the pattern of myocardial cell necrosis of right ventricular infarcts caused by permanent occlusion of the right coronary artery in the dog are similar to infarcts caused by transient LAD occlusion in that necrosis is quite heterogenous, with quite irregular margins, often including viable muscle bundles within the general zone of infarction.[77] The structure of myocardial infarcts, especially infarct caused by transient LAD occlusion, demonstrates in many respects close resemblance to the structure of infarcts that occur in patients with ischemic heart disease and myocardial infarction.[78,80] The similar characteristics include (1) presence on the endocardial surface of the infarct of a zone of myocardial fibers (15 to 20 cell layers), retaining normal staining qualities and (2) normally staining bundles of myocardial cells scattered in the infarcted left ventricular wall. Such features were reported to occur in many human autopsy specimens,[78,80] more so in cases with nonocclusive coronary insufficiency involving infarction of the inner endocardial half of the wall.[81] Similarly, the structure and the pattern of myocardial cell necrosis in human right ventricular infarction[82] had many similarities to canine right ventricular infarction[77,83] in that necrosis is heterogenous and subendocardial fibers survive beneath the infarcts.

To determine the site of origins of spontaneous ventricular arrhythmias during the late phase, El-Sherif and associates[84] made multiple simultaneous bipolar recordings from the entire epicardial surface and from selected endocardial and intramural sites using a computerized multiplexing technique. These authors found that the arrhythmia had a focal origin located in the surviving subendocardial Purkinje network underlying the infarct and that frequent shift of the ectopic pacemaker occurred. Earlier studies using a limited number of biopolar recordings electrodes also indicated the subendocardial Purkinje network as a site of origin of these tachyarrhythmias.[47,74,85] Furthermore, Scherlag and coworkers[47] found that many of the ectopic beats originated from the epicardium in the infarcted zone, since electrical activity at this site preceded the Q wave of the tachycardia.[47] Both endocardial and epicardial sites of origin for late-phase spontaneous ventricular tachyarrhythmia were also suggested in the canine model by Sugi and associates[83] during myocardial infarction limited exclusively to the right ventricle. As reported by these authors, ventricular arrhythmia also occurs 24 hours after permanent right coronary artery occlusion in the dog.[83]

In addition to the spontaneous form of ventricular arrhythmia, pacing at rates above 300 beats/min could induce still another form of ventricular tachyarrhythmias in the same dogs at rates of 230 to 450 beats/min (average 345 beats/min), which is faster than spontaneous tachycardia (average 154 beats/min).[86,87] The computerized isochronal mapping studies of El-Sherif and colleagues[87] suggest that these induced rapid ventricular tachyarrhythmias arise in the surviving but apparently electrophysiologically abnormal epicardial layers of the infarcted left ventricle by a reentrant mechanism.[87] Furthermore, these induced rapid ventricular tachyarrhythmias could easily degenerate into ventricular fibrillation, especially when the rapid induced rhythm had pleomorphic ventricular rhythms and ventricular tachycardia of the torsades de pointes type.[87]

In an attempt to determine the mechanism(s) of spontaneous ventricular arrhythmias, Scherlag and associates[47] exposed ventricular "automaticity" after inducing atrial slowing by vagal stimulation. These authors found that vagal stimulation revealed a ventricular "automatic" rhythm of an average of 166 beats/min as opposed to 39 beats/min in control dogs.[47] Furthermore, such ventricular rhythm could be suppressed by rapid atrial pacing. These authors suggested the existence of an enhanced ventricular automatic mechanism as a cause for these spontaneous arrhythmias.[47] Transmembrane potential recordings from partially depolarized subendocardial Purkinje fibers isolated from the infarcted left ventricle during the late-phase arrhythmias have shown the presence of spontaneous diastolic depolarizations giving rise to automatic impulse initiation (abnormal automaticity) that could propagate and excite adjoining normal myocardial tissue[74,75,88] (Fig. 17-11). More re-

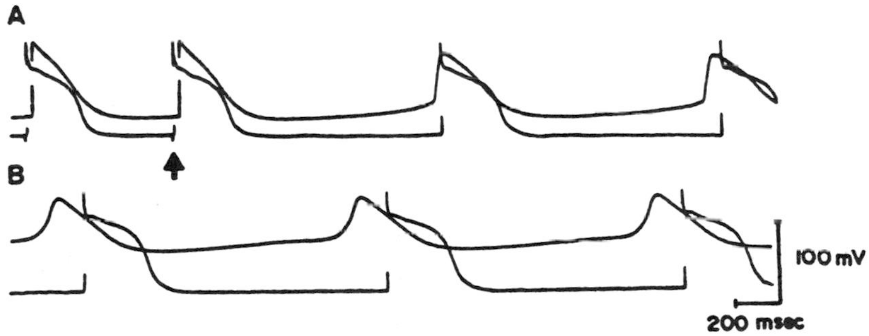

Figure 17-11. *Transmembrane potentials recorded from subendocardial Purkinje fibers in an isolated preparation of infarcted canine myocardium. The* top trace *in each panel shows action potentials recorded from a fiber on the endocardial surface of the infarct, and the* bottom trace *in each panel shows action potentials recorded from a fiber in an adjacent noninfarcted region. In A, the first two impulses are elicited by electrical stimulation of the preparation. The stimulus is turned off at the* arrow. *Spontaneous diastolic depolarization develops in the Purkinje fiber in the infarct and results in automatic firing. In B, which shows recordings from the same two cells several minutes later, impulses are arising in the automatic Purkinje fibers in the infarct* (top trace) *and conducting into the noninfarcted region. (Friedman, P. L., Stewart, J. R., Fenoglio, J. J., Jr., and Wit, A. L.: Survival of subendocardial Purkinje fibers after extensive myocardial infarction: In vitro and in vivo correlations. Circ. Res., 33:612–626, 1973)*

cently, El-Sherif and colleagues have shown that surviving subendocardial Purkinje fibers in the infarct zone, with an average resting potential of −60 mV, can develop delayed afterdepolarization and subsequent triggered automaticity by either rapid drive or by slow-background slow Purkinje fiber automaticity, which is normally present during this arrhythmic period[74,88] (Fig. 7-12).

Isolated tissue studies from dogs with isolated right ventricular infarction during the 24-hour arrhythmic period also have shown enhanced automatic activity in the surviving subendocardial Purkinje fiber network, suggesting that enhanced automaticity at this site could be responsible for the arrhythmias seen during this arrhythmic period.[83] Therefore, microelectrode studies support the idea that some sort of automatic mechanism, abnormal, triggered, or both, may be responsible for at least many of the ectopic ventricular beats that occur during the late-phase arrhythmias.

More recently Fujimoto and associates[89] have found no apparent relationship between intramyocardial conduction slowing in the ischemic zone and the emergence of late-phase ventricular arrhythmias in dogs with permanent LAD occlusion. The authors suggested abnormal automaticity as a mechanism for the late-phase ventricular arrhythmias.[89] The mechanism of induced rapid ventricular rhythm, which arises in the surviving subepicardial muscle cells, appears to be caused by a reentrant mechanism,[86,87] although the triggered automatic mechanism is possible.[84] The considerable prolongation of subendocardial Purkinje fiber action potential duration and the ability of premature stimuli to undergo conduction delay and subsequently to induce rapid nondriven

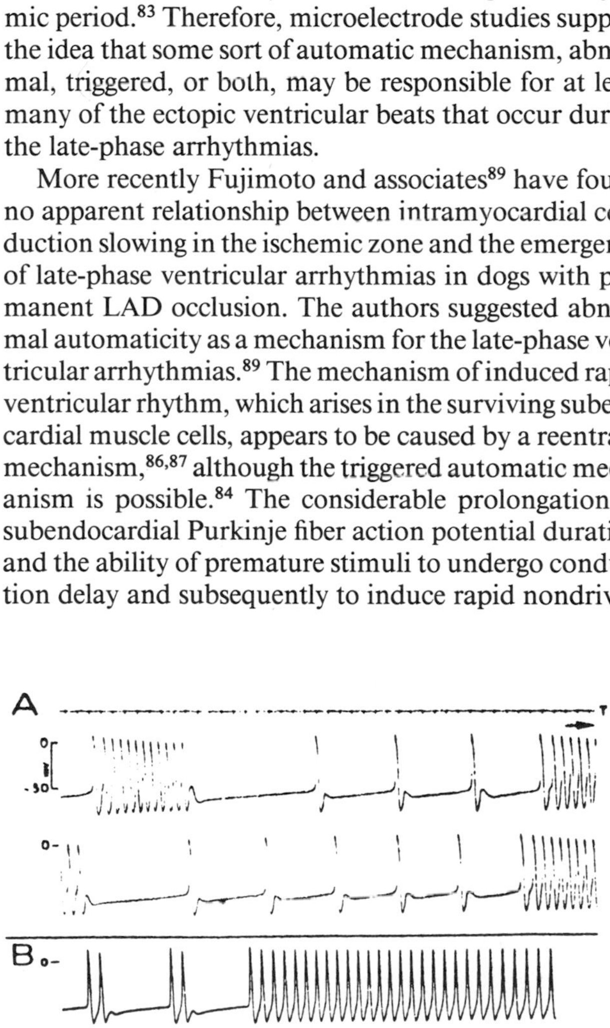

Figure 17-12. *Initiation of triggered automaticity by background slow Purkinje fiber automaticity, isolated from a canine preparation 24 hours after permanent left anterior descending coronary artery occlusion. The* upper *and* lower panels *represent transmembrane recordings from Purkinje fibers in two different infarcted endocardial preparations. The time scale (T) desigates 1-second intervals. (El-Sherif, et al.: Triggered ventricular rhythm in one day old myocardial infarction in the dog. Circ. Res., 52:566–579, 1983)*

repetitive activity in *in vitro* preparations[75,90] suggest that reentry at subendocardial sites remains a distinct potential mechanism, independent of subepicardial sites mentioned above, which could be unraveled by programmed premature stimulation during late-phase arrhythmia. Furthermore, the nature of cellular electrophysiologic properties of surviving subepicardial muscle cells and their possible role and mechanism in the induction of late-phase arrhythmias remain to be clarified.[86,87] It is therefore apparent that the mechanism(s) of the 24-hour arrhythmias are much more complex than originally thought.[9,10]

When spontaneously depolarizing Purkinje cells initiate an automatic impulse and propagate to adjacent normal ventricular muscle cells, ventricular ectopic beats and rhythms are expected to result. At times, various degrees of exit block could exist around the infarct.[90] Therefore, the rhythm that might be expected to result from at least an abnormal automatic or even a triggered mechanism could include accelerated idioventricular rhythm (AIVR), nonparoxysmal ventricular tachycardia, and noncoupled ventricular premature depolarizations. All these are common in the first few days following acute myocardial infarction in humans.[43] For instance, AIVR occurs in as many as 30% to 40% of patients with acute myocardial infarction and may very well correspond to the abnormal automaticity seen in experimental infarction.

Furthermore, histologic and ultrastructural studies have shown intact Purkinje fibers surviving on the endocardial surface of some anteroseptal human infarcts.[91] Moreover, these surviving fibers contain lipid droplets like those seen in the Purkinje fibers in canine infarcts.[72,74,75] In addition to these experimental clinical similarities, it was of great interest to see that electrophysiologic studies in the catheterization laboratory have suggested that many of the ventricular tachycardias that occur on the first day after the onset of symptoms of infarction are caused by automaticity.[92] These arrhythmias could neither be induced nor terminated by electrical stimulation of the ventricles. These findings indicate that despite the differences between experimentally and clinically occurring myocardial infarction, studies on animal models can provide meaningful information on the mechanisms of clinical arrhythmias.

Pharmacologic Considerations

Changes in myocardial site of origin and mechanisms of ventricular arrhythmias during late-phase as opposed to early-phase arrhythmia can have important pharmacologic consequences. For example, Nattel and associates[62] found that when aprinidine was administered 24 hours after LAD occlusion, it had markedly different effects on the arrhythmias than when given just after occlusion despite similar aprinidine concentrations in different myocardial zones. These authors suggested that aprinidine was more effective against the 24-hour arrhythmias than the early-phase arrhythmias because it can suppress enhanced ventricular automaticity, a mechanism responsible at least in part for late-phase arrhythmias.[62] Similarly, it was found in other studies that lidocaine and procainamide were quite effective against the 24-hour arrhythmias.[93] This was also the case with the newer investigational agents ethmozine[94] and propafenone.[95] It is worth mentioning that the response of the 24-hour experimental ventricular tachycardia to antiarrhythmic drugs is similar in many respects to the effects of drugs on humans.[43] Antiarrhythmic drugs usually control and suppress ventricular tachycardia in coronary care unit patients who have had a recent myocardial infarction.[43]

Phase III Ventricular Arrhythmias

Recurrent sustained ventricular tachycardia may occur in humans with a history of chronic ischemic heart disease and with myocardial infarcts or ventricular aneurysms.[96,97] It has been demonstrated that ventricular tachycardia similar to that occurring spontaneously can be induced in these patients by programmed electrical stimulation applied to the ventricle through an electrode catheter. Similarly, once tachycardia is initiated, it can also be terminated by electrical stimulation. It has been concluded from these clinical studies that these tachycardias that can be initiated and terminated by stimulating the ventricles are caused by reentry because it was shown in isolated preparations of cardiac tissue that reentry can be initiated and terminated in this way.[98,99] However, definite proof for such a hypothesis requires detailed mapping of the excitation pattern of the ventricles during the arrhythmia. Therefore, more detailed electrophysiologic studies on ventricular tachycardias initiated and terminated by premature depolarizations are important, since such tachycardias lead to ventricular fibrillation and sudden death and may respond to antiarrhythmic drugs differently than other types of ventricular arrhythmias. Studies designed to determine the mechanism and inciting factors of this arrhythmia can be best accomplished in animal models, since electrical recordings can be readily obtained from all regions of the ventricles and a variety of experimental interventions can be done that cannot be done in humans.[100]

The use of the experimental canine model of myocardial ischemia and infarction greatly enhanced our understanding of the pathophysiologic and pharmacologic mechanisms involved in the induction of ventricular tachyarrhythmias by the technique of programmed electrical stimulation in humans. In the following sections we will discuss some of the advances made in this field, being well aware that the present state of knowledge is by no means complete.

The importance of the structure and geometry of myocardial infarction in the induction of sustained ventricular tachycardia by a critically timed premature stimulus was stressed by Karagueuzian and associates.[76,101] These authors found that a critical mass of infarcted and ischemic myocardium, averaging 35% of the left ventricle, was needed for arrhythmia induction. Furthermore, for sustained ventricular tachycardia to occur, the structure of the infarct had to be heterogenous; that is, myocardial cell death within the zone of the infarction must not be uniform or homogenous, but numerous viable myocardial cells must be in close proximity with necrotic cells. Such structural ischemic damage conducive to arrhythmia induction could be produced by temporary coronary artery occlusion followed by reperfusion.[75,76,101] Such structural requirements for arrhythmia induction with greater ease (*i.e.*, single premature) (Fig. 17-13) and reproducibility were contrasted to myocardial infarction caused by permanent coronary artery occlusion model, in which myocardial cell death is relatively homogenous and induction of sustained ventricular tachycardia much less frequent.[76,100,101] In dogs with infarcts involving homogenous myocardial cell necrosis, only the nonsustained (less than 10 seconds duration) form of ventricular tachycardia could be induced with ease. Furthermore, since these studies were conducted in awake dogs, and each dog was studied over several consecutive days, the temporal relation between the age of the infarct and arrhythmia induction was emphasized.[76,100,101] It was found that as an infarct aged, arrhythmia could no longer be induced by premature stimuli beyond the first week of infarction, probably reflecting changing electrophysiologic properties of myocardial cells in an ischemic zone ("stabilization" of the irritable ventricle). Note however, that in studies conducted on open-chest preparations, arrhythmia induction is possible for up to 3 weeks.[102] This is probably caused by elevated circulating catecholamine levels in the open-chest model, which are known to facilitate arrhythmia induction both in experimental[94] and clinical[124] settings. It is worth mentioning that the myocardial infarction model in cats, caused by coronary artery occlusion, is associated with spontaneous ventricular arrhythmias lasting for up to 6 months after healing from acute injury.[103] Whether ventricular tachycardia could also be induced for such a long period in the feline model remains to be seen.

The importance of the size of myocardial infarction in arrhythmia induction in the coronary artery occlusion and reperfusion model was further pursued by Gang and associates.[114] These authors found in large-sized myocardial infarcts a lowered fibrillation threshold and greater ease of induction of sustained ventricular tachy-

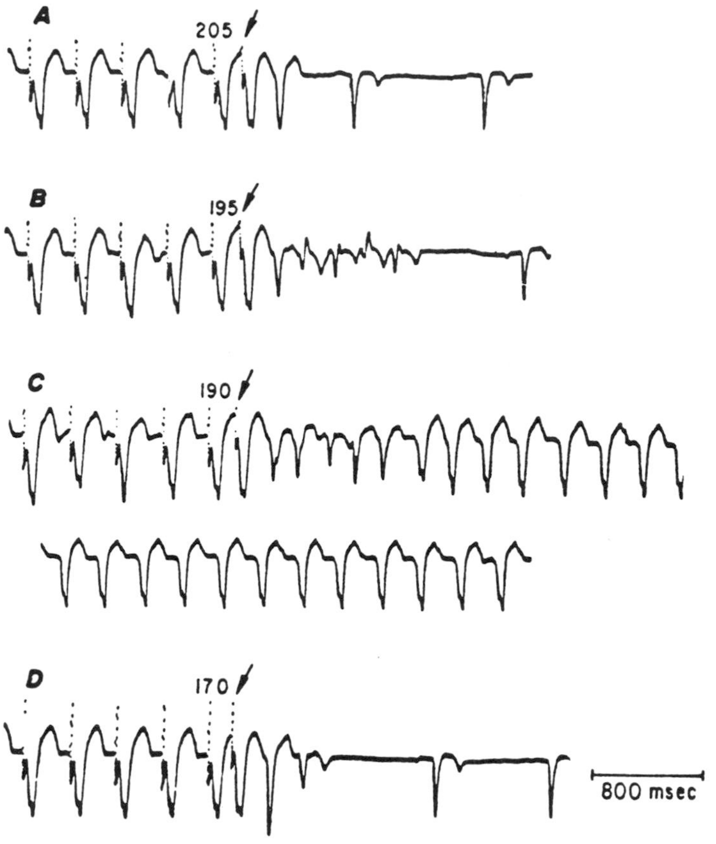

Figure 17-13. *Initiation of protracted ventricular tachycardia in a dog on the third day of reperfusion after a transient (2 hours) occlusion of the left anterior descending coronary artery. The electrocardiogram is shown in each panel. In A to D the ventricles are being driven at a cycle length of 350 msec and a single premature stimulus* (arrow) *is applied to the ventricle. In A, the coupling interval of the stimulated premature impulse is 205 msec; this is followed by a nondriven impulse. Sinus rhythm resumes after a pause of 390 msec. In B, the coupling interval of the stimulated premature impulse is 195 msec; this is followed by five nondriven impulses. The QRS morphology and the cycle length of the nondriven impulses are variable. After a pause of 720 msec, sinus rhythm reoccurs. In C, the coupling interval of the stimulated premature impulse is 190 msec; this is followed by 10 minutes of tachycardia. The lower trace in C shows the electrocardiogram 8 minutes after initiation of tachycardia. In D, a single stimulated premature impulse induced at a coupling interval of 170 msec is followed by two nondriven impulses. Sinus rhythm occurs after a pause of 760 msec. (Karagueuzian, H. S., Fenoglio, J. J., Jr., Weiss, M. B., and Wit, A. L.: Protracted ventricular tachycardia induced by premature stimulation of the canine heart after coronary artery occlusion and reperfusion. Circ. Res., 44:833–846, 1979. By permission of the American Heart Association, Inc.)*

cardia.[114] The proarrhythmic potentials of heterogenous myocardial infarcts in the canine model caused by coronary artery occlusion and reperfusion were emphasized by Michelson and colleagues.[104] These authors measured myocardial excitability and refractoriness within the heterogenous infarcted zone and found a great disparity in both excitability and refractoriness. They suggested that such disparity may well be conducive to arrhythmia induction by programmed electrical stimulation.[104] Furthermore, these authors demonstrated that the site of electrical stimulation in relation to the infarct location was important in arrhythmia induction.[105] For example, intramyocardial sites within 2 cm of the infarct had the highest success rate in arrhythmia induction with electrical stimulation.[105] Microelectrode studies were also conducted on infarcted myocardial tissues isolated from canine hearts with myocardial infarction caused by occlusion and reperfusion of the LAD. Karagueuzian and colleagues[75] studied the transmembrane potential properties of subendocardial cardiac fibers in the infarct zone. These authors found that during the period of susceptibility for tachycardia induction by electrical stimulation in the intact dog, surviving subendocardial Purkinje fibers and ventricular muscle fibers were normal or nearly so, and premature impulses did not undergo conduction delay at this site.[75] Delayed afterdepolarization and subsequent triggered automatic activity also were not seen.[75] These authors concluded that the surviving subendocardial cardiac fibers underlying the infarct could not be implicated as primary sites for arrhythmia induction.[75] Therefore other sites, namely, the intramural and subepicardial muscle cells overlying the infarct, could possibly be involved in arrhythmia genesis.[100] More recently, Spear and colleagues[106] studied the transmembrane potential properties of subepicardial muscle overlying infarcts isolated from dogs with transient coronary artery occlusion and reperfusion. These authors found that the resting potential, action potential amplitude, maximal rate of depolarization, and action potential duration at 30% repolarization were significantly reduced in the infarcted region. Furthermore, conduction velocity in the infarcted region was slowed from 0.54m/sec in normal to 0.15m/sec in the infarct zone.[106] Also, these authors found that a reduced space constant in the epicardial infarct zone was another important factor (in addition to reduced membrane responsiveness) in slowing of conduction velocity.[107] Slow conduction and depressed transmembrane potential properties of epicardial muscle cells in the infarcted zone in dogs with permanent LAD occlusion was also reported by Gessman and associates.[108]

The mechanism of induced ventricular tachycardia by electrical stimulation in the late myocardial infarction phase has been studied by several investigators.[109,110] In these studies, isochronal maps of ventricular activation were constructed during the tachycardia with bipolar electrograms recorded from multiple ventricular sites by computerized multiplexing technique. These studies attempted to identify the pattern and sequence of activation of the ventricle during the tachycardia to determine the mechanism and the site of origin of the arrhythmia. El-Sherif and colleagues[109] presented evidence that reentry occurring at the epicardial surface of the infarct was the cause of some 21% of the induced beats. Furthermore, these authors were able to present evidence for the presence of a zone of functional conduction block in the *in situ* heart, around which the activation front advanced by radial spread to cause reexcitation of the ventricle.[109] These authors also suggested that epicardial recordings were of limited value in analyzing induced ventricular beats, indicating that sites other than the epicardial infarct zone might well be involved in the process of arrhythmia induction, namely, intramural surviving muscle cells in the zone of infarction.[76,100,101] The careful studies of Wit and associates[110] using 192 simultaneous recordings from various epicardial sites also indicate that reentry is the most likely mechanism of these induced ventricular beats. As for the site of origin of these induced tachycardias, these authors suggested that the nonsustained form of the tachycardia occurred on the anterior left ventricle at the border of the infarcted region and in epicardial muscle surviving over the infarcted region, as circuitous conduction patterns in the epicardial muscle demonstrated. In contrast, however, during the sustained form of induced tachycardia, circuitous conduction pattern leading to reentry could not be seen in the surviving epicardial muscle, implying the involvement of other sites.[100,110] Recent studies by Kramer and associates[130] indicate, in fact, that intramural cells in the infarcted left ventricle may well constitute the site of origin of these reentrant ventricular tachycardias in dogs. It was of great interest to note that cooling of the reentrant circuits involved in the maintenance of induced tachycardia on the epicardial surface abruptly terminated the arrhythmia.[108,111]

It is gratifying to see that the transmembrane potential properties of surviving epicardial muscle cells, manifesting depressed action potential properties and slowed conduction velocity, can offer adequate explanation for some of the reentrant beats induced at this particular site. However, the cellular electrophysiologic basis and the precise anatomic location of induced ventricular beats not occurring at the epicardial surface remain to be determined, as in the case of induced sustained ventricular tachycardia. Earlier studies of El-Sherif and associates,[112,113] using composite electrodes to record from large areas of epicardium, interpreted the presence of continuous electrical activity bridging the entire cardiac cycle during tachycardia as evidence that reentry was occurring, even though the sequence of electrical activation of the ventricle was not determined. Wit and associates,[40,110] however, have suggested that such an electrical activity, recorded at a given site, should not be taken as evidence for reentry. These authors presented evidence from simultaneous multiple recordings and isochronal map construction that electrical activity could be recorded during the entire cardiac cycle in the absence of obvious reentry at that site.[110] Similar findings were also made by Janse and associates during the early postocclusion period.[18] Therefore, at present it seems reasonable, as suggested by Wit and associates, not to accept the occurrence of continuous electrical activity as proof of reentry, although such activity should be present in an area where reentry is occurring.[40,110]

Clinical Implications

Almost all the cellular electrophysiologic abnormalities seen in the canine model of myocardial infarction were also observed in chronic infarcted and ischemic tissues isolated from human ventricular myocardium. This indicates that the cellular electrophysiologic mechanisms of ventricular tachyarrhythmias in humans may well be analogous to canine ischemic ventricular arrhythmias.

Spear and associates[122] recorded transmembrane potentials from cardiac fibers on the endocardial surface of preparations isolated from human infarcts and aneurysms (Fig. 17-14). Although some of these potentials appear to be characteristic of Purkinje fibers, others may have been recorded from ventricular muscle cells. Some of the surviving fibers manifested phase 4 depolarization and automatic impulse initiation. These action potentials conducted slowly and were sensitive to verapamil. Furthermore, variable-amplitude action potentials ranging from normal, fast-depressed, and slow response were present in these aneurysmal tissues. These authors suggested that the heterogenous electrophysiologic profile of these surviving cells might lead to ventricular tachyarrhythmias in these patients.[122] More recently, Dangman and colleagues[123] demonstrated that human Purkinje fibers, isolated from the hearts of five patients undergoing cardiac transplantation, could manifest delayed afterdepolarization and triggered automaticity when exposed to ouabain and catecholamine, suggesting that triggered automatic mechanism can also occur in human ventricle.[116]

Pharmacologic Considerations

The response of inducible ventricular tachyarrhythmias to antiarrhythmic drugs during the chronic phase of myocardial infarction (phase III) differs from that seen during the 24-hour spontaneous ventricular arrhyth-

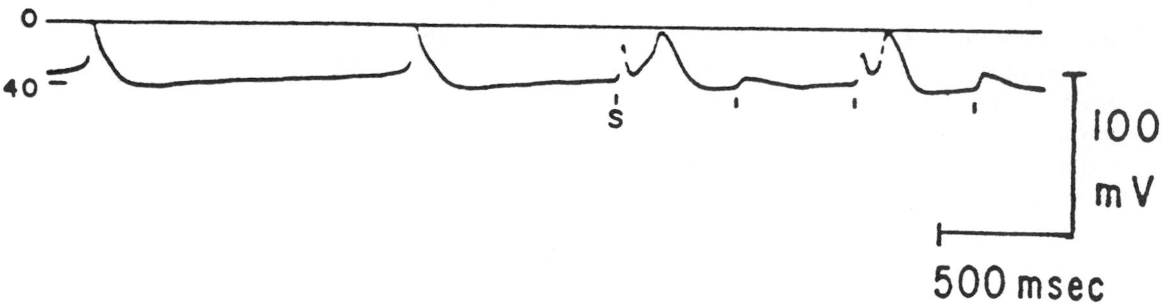

Figure 17-14. *Transmembrane potentials recorded from the endocardial surface of a human infarct. At the left, the fiber is spontaneously active and phase 4 depolarization is evident. At S, stimulation at a basic cycle length of 450 msec is begun. The first and third stimuli excite the fiber. From these records it is not possible to determine whether this is a Purkinje fiber or a ventricular muscle fiber. (Spear, J. F., Horowitz, L. N., Hodess, A. B., et al.: Cellular electrophysiology of human myocardial infarction. I. Abnormalities of cellular activation. Circulation, 59:247–256, 1979)*

mias. The chronic-phase tachyarrhythmia often manifests resistance to most pharmacologic agents.[93,104,115] This is in sharp contrast to the 24-hour arrhythmias, which could ultimately be controlled by a given antiarrhythmic agent.[93–95] The cause(s) of refractoriness to drugs remain largely undefined. In broadest terms it is not known whether the drug fails to reach the arrhythmic site and adjoining myocardial region in sufficiently high concentration (4 to 10 times that of serum levels) or whether refractoriness is a property of the site itself, relatively independent of drug concentration. The preliminary results obtained by Karagueuzian and associates[116] indicate that raising the myocardial concentration of procainamide by close coronary injection suppresses and prevents inducible ventricular tachycardia otherwise resistant to procainamide when given intravenously. In these studies, procainamide was injected through a specially designed autoinflatable balloon catheter in the great cardiac vein in dogs 3 to 8 days after permanent occlusion of the LAD.[116] Procainamide administered by the great cardiac vein (5 to 20 mg/kg) was much more effective than intravenous procainamide (35 mg/kg) in preventing and terminating inducible tachycardias. Myocardial procainamide given by the great cardiac vein had 15 to 20 times higher myocardial procainamide concentration than that obtained after intravenous injection. The need for excess levels of plasma steady-state disopyramide to terminate inducible ventricular tachyarrhythmia during the chronic phase of infarction in the canine heart was demonstrated by Patterson and associates. It was also of interest to note that bretylium was fairly effective in suppressing inducible ventricular tachycardia in the canine model,[118] an effect that may be at least partly caused by the ability of bretylium to concentrate in the myocardium and achieve myocardial levels 14 times higher than in plasma levels.[119] It is tempting to suggest that the greater efficacy of amiodarone in suppressing ventricular tachyarrhythmias (sevenfold higher in the right ventricle than in plasma) may be related to the ability of this drug to be concentrated in the myocardium.[120] However, elevation of myocardial drug concentration alone may not be sufficient to terminate the arrhythmia. It appears that a preferential increase of drug concentration at critical myocardial sites (based on the site of origin of the arrhythmia) could determine if the arrhythmia will be suppressed.[116] These considerations, however, need further clarification and experimental verification.

It is gratifying to note many similarities in the response to antiarrhythmic drugs in experimental and clinical settings. Myerburg and associates[121] have observed in patients with ischemic heart disease that higher levels of plasma procainamide concentrations were needed to control ventricular arrhythmias during the chronic phase of myocardial infarction than during the acute phase, indicating, as in canine models, a different mechanism or different site operative for arrhythmia induction during various phases of myocardial infarction.[121] Furthermore, in other studies it was found that inducible ventricular tachyarrhythmias often manifest resistance to both standard and new antiarrhythmic agents. In five reports[125–129] involving 250 patients, the majority of whom had coronary artery disease and ventricular aneurysm, refractoriness to drugs ranged from 9.5% to 47.5% (mean 26.3%). This response appears to differ from the response of ventricular tachyarrhythmias seen during the acute, in-hospital phase, where most ventricular arrhythmias can ultimately be controlled.

Conclusion

Although the experimental animal model of ischemic heart disease differs in many respects from its parallel in humans, it nevertheless has provided much important information and improved clinicians' understanding of

Table 17-1. The Nature, Time Course, Mechanism(s), Site of Origin, and Response to Drugs of Ventricular Arrhythmias After Coronary Artery Occlusion

	Phase I	Phase II	Phase III
Nature	VT/VF	VT	VT/VF
Time Course	15–30 min	6–72 hr	3–12 days
Site of Origin	Ischemic myocardial cells Purkinje fibers? Normal zone bordering the ischemic zone	Subendocardial Purkinje fibers in infarct zone Subepicardial muscle overlying the infarct	Subepicardial muscle cells overlying the infarct Surviving intramural muscle cells Purkinje fibers?
Mechanism(s)	Reentry Automaticity (early after depolarization)?	Abnormal automaticity Triggered automaticity Reentry?	Reentry Triggered automaticity?
Response to Drugs	Usually resistant	Usually suppressed	Usually resistant

VT, ventricular tachycardia; VF, ventricular fibrillation, ?, evidence uncertain. Time course refers to postocclusion period.

potentially lethal ventricular arrhythmias. Although the experimental work provided new insights into events in the clinical settings, many important questions raised in the clinical cardiac catheterization laboratory provided a stimulus for experimental work. We have outlined a few of these pathophysiologic and pharmacologic interrelationships. Surely many more important discoveries are forthcoming.

References

1. Bruetsch, W. L.: The earliest record of sudden death possibly due to atherosclerotic coronary occlusion. Circulation, 20:438–441, 1959.
2. Shattock, S. G.: A report upon the pathological condition of the aorta of King Menephtah, traditionally regarded as the pharaoh of the exodus. Proc. R. Soc. Med., 2:122, 1908–1909.
3. Chirac, P.: De motu cordis. *Adversaria Analytica,* 1698, p. 121. Cited by See, Bochefontaine, and Roussy.
4. Ericksen, J. E.: On the influence of the coronary circulation on the action of the heart. Lond. Med. Gaz., 2:561–564, 1842.
5. Porter, W. T.: On the results of ligation of the coronary arteries. J. Physiol. (Lond.), 15:121–138, 1894.
6. Lewis, T.: The experimental production of paroxysmal tachycardia and the effects of ligation of the coronary arteries. Heart, 1:98–129, 1909.
7. Robinson, G. C., and Herrman, G. R.: Paroxysmal tachycardia of ventricular origin, and its relation to coronary occlusion. Heart, 8:59–81, 1921.
8. Wiggers, C. J., Wegria, R., and Pinera, B.: The effects of myocardial ischemia on fibrillation threshold—mechanism of spontaneous ventricular fibrillation following coronary artery occlusion. Am. J. Physiol., 133:651–657, 1941.
9. Harris, A. S.: Delayed development of ventricular ectopic rhythms following experimental coronary occlusion. Circulation, 1:1318–1328, 1950.
10. Harris, A. S., Bisteni, A., Russel, R. A., et al.: Excitatory factors in ventricular tachycardia resulting from myocardial ischemia. Potassium a major excitant. Science, 119:200–203, 1954.
11. Wit, A. L., and Friedman, P. L.: The basis for ventricular arrhythmias accompanying myocardial infarction: Alterations in electrical activity of ventricular and Purkinje fibers after coronary artery occlusion. Arch. Intern. Med., 135:459–472, 1975.
12. Hill, J. L., and Gettes, L. S.: Effect of acute coronary artery occlusion on local myocardial extracellular K^+ activity in swine. Circulation, 61:768–778, 1980.
13. Downar, E., Janse, M. J., and Durrer, D.: The effects of acute coronary artery occlusion on subepicardial transmembrane potentials in the intact porcine heart. Circulation, 56:217–224, 1977.
14. Hamamoto, H., Peter, T., and Mandel, W. J.: Characteristics of conduction of premature impulses during acute myocardial ischemia and reperfusion: A comparison of epicardial and endocardial activation. Circulation, 64:190–198, 1981.
15. Hamamoto, H., Peter, T., Fujimoto, T., and Mandel, W. J.: Characteristics of conduction of premature impulses during acute myocardial ischemia and reperfusion: A comparison between antegrade and retrograde activation. Am. J. Cardiol., 49:307–316, 1982.
16. Fujimoto, T., Hamamoto, H., Peter, T., and Mandel, W. J.: Relation between conduction delay and ventricular fibrillation: Characteristics of conduction of premature impulses during acute myocardial ischemia. Am. J. Cardiol., 48:287–294, 1981.

17. Meesmann, W.: Early arrhythmias and primary ventricular fibrillation after acute myocardial ischemia in relation to pre-existing coronary collaterals. In Parratt, J. R. (ed.): Early Arrhythmias Resulting from Myocardial Ischemia, pp. 93–112. London, McMillan, 1982.
18. Janse, M. J., Van Capelle, F. J. L., Morsink, H., et al.: Flow of injury current and patterns of excitation during early ventricular arrhythmias in acute regional myocardial ischemia in isolated porcine and canine hearts. Evidence for two different arrhythmogenic mechanisms. Circ. Res., 47:151–165, 1980.
19. Janse, M. J., and Kleber, A. G.: Electrophysiological changes and ventricular arrhythmias in the early phase of regional myocardial ischemia. Circ. Res., 49:1069–1081, 1981.
20. Katzung, B.: Electrically induced automaticity in ventricular myocardium. Life Sci., 14:1133–1140, 1974.
21. Cranfield, P. E.: The Conduction of the Cardiac Impulse. Mount Kisco, N. Y., Futura, 1975.
22. Katzung, B. G.: Effects of extracellular calcium and sodium on depolarization induced automaticity in guinea pig papillary muscle. Circ. Res., 37:118–127, 1975.
23. Katzung, B. G., Hondeghem, L. M., and Grant, A. O.: Cardiac ventricular automaticity induced by current of injury. Pfluegers Arch., 360:193–197, 1975.
24. Kleber, A. G., Janse, M. J., Van Capella, F. J. L., and Durrer, D.: Mechanism and time course of S-T and T-Q segment changes during acute regional myocardial ischemia in the pig heart determined by extracellular and intracellular recordings. Circ. Res., 42:603–613, 1978.
25. Katzung, B. G., and Morgenstern, J. A.: Effects of extracellular potassium on ventricular automaticity and evidence for a pacemaker current in mammalian ventricular myocardium. Circ. Res., 40:105–111, 1977.
26. Coraboeuf, E., and Boistel, J.: L'action des taux eleves de gaz carbonique sur le tissue cardiaque, etudiee a l'aide de microelectrode intracellulaire. C. R. Soc. Biol., 147:654–658, 1953.
27. Coraboeuf, E., Deroubaix, E., and Coulombe, A.: Acidosis-induced abnormal repolarization and repetitive activity in isolated dog Purkinje fibers. J. Physiol. (Paris), 76:97–106, 1980.
28. Gerbert, A., Benzing, H., and Strohm, M.: Changes in interstitial *p*H of dog myocardium in response to local ischemia, hypoxia, hyper and hypocapnea, measured continuously by means of glass microelectrodes. Pfluegers Arch., 329:72–83, 1971.
29. Khuri, S. F., Flaherty, J. T., O'Riordan, J., et al.: Changes in intramyocardial ST segment voltage and gas tensions with regional myocardial ischemia in the dog. Circ. Res., 37:455–463, 1975.
30. Han, J.: Ventricular ectopic activity in myocardial infarction. In Springfield, H. J. (ed.): Cardiac Arrhythmias: A Symposium, p. 171. Springfield, Ill., Charles C Thomas, 1972.
31. Han, J., Goel, B. G., and Hanson, C. S.: Re-entrant beats induced in the ventricle during coronary occlusion. Am. Heart J., 80:778–784, 1970.
32. Hoffman, B. F., and Rosen, M. R.: Cellular mechanisms for cardiac arrhythmias. Circ. Res., 49:1–15, 1981.
33. Wit, A. L., and Cranfield, P. L.: Triggered activity in cardiac muscle fibers of the simian mitral valve. Circ. Res., 38:85–98, 1976.
34. Tsien, R. W., Kass, R. S., and Weingart, R.: Cellular and subcellular mechanisms of cardiac pacemaker oscillation. J. Exp. Biol., 81:205–215, 1979.
35. Karagueuzian, H. S., and Katzung, B. A.: Voltage-clamp studies of transient inward current and mechanical oscillations induced by ouabain in ferret papillary muscle. J. Physiol. (Lond.), 327:255–271, 1982.
36. Matsuda, H., Noma, A., Kurachi, Y., and Irisawa, H.: Transient depolarization and spontaneous voltage fluctuations in isolated single cells from guinea pig ventricles. Calcium-mediated membrane potential fluctuations. Circ. Res., 51:142–151, 1982.
37. De Mello, W. C.: Intercellular communication in cardiac muscle. Circ. Res., 51:1–9, 1982.
38. Waldo, A. L., and Kaiser, G. A.: A study of ventricular arrhythmias associated with acute myocardial infarction in the canine heart. Circulation, 47:1222–1228, 1973.
39. Williams, D. O., Scherlag, B. J., Hope, R. R., et al.: The pathophysiology of malignant ventricular arrhythmias during acute myocardial ischemia. Circulation, 50:1163–1172, 1974.
40. Wit, A. L., and Cranfield, P. L.: Reentrant excitation as a cause of cardiac arrhythmias. Am. J. Physiol., 235:H1–H17, 1978.
41. Ceremuzynaki, L., Staszewska-Barczak, J., and Herbaezynska-Cedro, K.: Cardiac rhythm disturbances and the release of catecholamines after acute coronary occlusion in dogs. Cardiovasc. Res., 3:190–197, 1969.
42. Tennant, R., and Wiggers, C. J.: The effect of coronary occlusion on myocardial contraction. Am. J. Physiol., 112:351–361, 1935.
43. Bigger, J. T., Jr., Dresdale, R. J., Heissenbuttel, R. H., et al.: Ventricular arrhythmias in ischemic heart disease: Mechanism, prevalence, significance, and management. Cardiovasc. Dis., 19:255–300, 1977.
44. Balke, C. W., Kaplinsky, E., Michelson, E. L., et al.: Reperfusion ventricular tachyarrhythmias: Correlation with antecedent coronary artery occlusion tachyarrhythmias and duration of myocardial ischemia. Am. Heart J., 101:449–456, 1981.
45. Jennings, R. B., Sommers, H. M., Smyth, G. A., et al.: Myocardial necrosis induced by temporary occlusion of a coronary artery in the dog. Arch. Pathol., 70:68–78, 1960.
46. Austin, M., Wenger, T. L., Harrell, F. E., Jr., et al.: Effect of myocardium at risk on outcome after coronary artery occlusion and release. Am. J. Physiol., 243:H340–H345, 1982.
47. Scherlag, B. J., El-Sherif, N., Hope, R., and Lazzara, R.: Characterization and localization of ventricular arrhythmias resulting from myocardial ischemia and infarction. Circ. Res., 35:372–383, 1974.
48. Akiyama, T.: Intracellular recording of in situ ventricular cells during ventricular fibrillation. Am. J. Physiol., 240:H465–H471, 1981.
49. Levine, H. J., Avitall, B., Pauker, S. G., and Naimi, S.: Sequential unipolar strength-interval curves and conduction times during myocardial ischemia and reperfusion in the dog. Circ. Res., 43:63–72, 1978.
50. Elharrar, V., Foster, P. R., Tirak, T. L., et al.: Alterations in canine myocardial excitability during ischemia. Circ. Res., 40:98–105, 1977.
51. Lazzara, R., El-Sherif, N., Hope, R. R., and Scherlag, B. J.: Ventricular arrhythmias and electrophysiological consequences of myocardial ischemia and infarction. Circ. Res., 42:740–749, 1978.
52. Lazzara, R., El-Sherif, N., and Schlerlag, B. J.: Disorders of cellular electrophysiology produced by ischemia of the canine His bundle. Circ. Res., 36:444–453, 1975.
53. Fujimoto, T., Peter, T., Hamamoto, H., and Mandel, W. J.: Electrophysiologic observations during the spontaneous initiation of ischemia induced ventricular fibrillation. Am. Heart J., 105:189–200, 1983.
54. Fujimoto, T., Peter, T., Hamamoto, H., and Mandel, W. J.: Electrophysiologic observations on ventricular tachyarrhythmias following reperfusion. Am. Heart J., 105:201–209, 1983.
55. Ten Eick, R., Singer, D. H., and Solberg, L. E.: Coronary occlusion. Effect on cellular electrical activity of the heart. Med. Clin. North Am., 60:49–67, 1976.
56. Corbalan, R., Verrier, R. L., and Lown, B.: Differing mechanisms for ventricular vulnerability during coronary artery occlusion and release. Am. Heart J., 92:223–230, 1976.
57. Penkoske, P. A., Sobel, B. E., and Corr, P. B.: Disparate electro-

physiological alterations accompanying dysrhythmia due to coronary occlusion and reperfusion in the cat. Circulation, 58:1023–1035, 1978.
58. Wit, A. L., and Bigger, J. T., Jr.: Electrophysiology of ventricular arrhythmias accompanying myocardial ischemia and infarction. Postgrad. Med. J., 53(Suppl. I):98–112, 1977.
59. Wenger, T. L., Browning, D. J., Masterton, C. E., et al.: Procainamide delivery to ischemic canine myocardium following rapid intravenous administration. Circ. Res., 46:789–795, 1980.
60. Zito, R. A., Caride, V. J., Holford, T., et al.: Regional myocardial lidocaine concentration following continuous intravenous infusion early and late after myocardial infarction. Am. J. Cardiol., 50:497–502, 1982.
61. Kupersmith, J., Antman, E. M., and Hoffman, B. F.: In vivo electrophysiological effects of lidocaine in canine acute myocardial infarction. Cir. Res., 36:84–91, 1975.
62. Nattel, S., Pederson, D. H., and Zipes, D. P.: Alterations in regional myocardial distribution and arrhythmogenic effects of aprinidine produced by coronary artery occlusion in the dog. Cardiovasc. Res., 15:80–85, 1981.
63. Naito, M., Michelson, E. L., Kmetzo, J. J., et al.: Failure of antiarrhythmic drugs to prevent experimental reperfusion ventricular fibrillation. Circulation, 63:70–79, 1981.
64. Rosenfeld, J., Rosen, M. R., and Hoffman, B. F.: Pharmacologic and behavioral effects on arrhythmias that immediately follow abrupt coronary occlusion: A canine model of sudden coronary death. Am. J. Cardiol., 41:1075–1082, 1978.
65. Wenger, T. L., Lederman, S., Starmer, F. C., et al.: A method for quantitating anti-fibrillatory effects of drugs after coronary reperfusion in dogs: improved outcome with bretylium. Circulation, 69:142–148, 1984.
66. Cinca, J., Janse, M. J., Morena, H., et al.: Mechanism and time course of the early electrical changes during acute coronary occlusion. An attempt to correlate the early ECG changes in man to cellular electrophysiology in the pig. Chest., 77:499–505, 1980.
67. Coker, S. J., and Parratt, J. R.: Prostacyclin—antiarrhythmic or arrhythmogenic? Comparison of the effects of intravenous and intracoronary prostacyclin and ZK36374 during coronary artery occlusion and reperfusion in anesthetized greyhounds. J. Cardiovasc. Pharmacol., 5:557–567, 1983.
68. Meerbaum, S., Lang, T. W., Povzhitkov, M., et al.: Retrograde lysis of coronary artery thrombus by coronary venous streptokinase administration. J. Am. Coll. Cardiol., 1:1262–1267, 1983.
69. Corday, E., and Meerbaum, S.: Introduction: Symposium on the present status of reperfusion of the acutely ischemic myocardium. I. J. Am. Coll. Cardiol., 1:1031–1036, 1983.
70. Friesinger, G. C., Schaefer, J., Gaestner, R. A., and Ross, R. S.: Coronary sinus drainage and measurement of left coronary artery flow in the dog. Am. J. Physiol., 206:57–62, 1964.
71. Clusin, W. T., Bristow, M. R., Karagueuzian, H. S., et al.: Do calcium-dependent ionic currents mediate ischemic ventricular fibrillation. Am. J. Cardiol. 49:606–612, 1982.
72. Fenoglio, J. J., Jr., Karagueuzian, H. S., Friedman, P. L., et al.: Time course of infarct growth toward the endocardium after coronary occlusion. Am. J. Physiol., 236:H356–H370, 1979.
73. Reimer, K. A., Louie, J. E., Rasmussen, M. M., and Jennings, R. B.: The wave-front phenomenon in ischemic cell death. I. Myocardial infarct size vs. duration of coronary occlusion in dogs. Circulation, 56:786–794, 1977.
74. Friedman, P. L., Stewart, J. R., Fenoglio, J. J., Jr., and Wit, A. L.: Survival of subendocardial Purkinje fibers after extensive myocardial infarction: In vitro and in vivo correlations. Circ. Res., 33:612–626, 1973.
75. Karagueuzian, H. S., Fenoglio, J. J., Jr., Weiss, M. B., and Wit, A. L.: Coronary occlusion and reperfusion: Effects on subendocardial fibers. Am. J. Physiol., 238:H581–H593, 1980.
76. Karagueuzian, H. S., Fenoglio, J. J., Jr., Weiss, M. B., and Wit, A. L.: Protracted ventricular tachycardia induced by premature stimulation of the canine heart after coronary artery occlusion and reperfusion. Circ. Res., 44:833–846, 1979.
77. Karagueuzian, H. S., Sugi, K., Onta, M., et al.: Inducible sustained ventricular tachycardia and ventricular fibrillation in conscious dogs with isolated right ventricular infarction: relation to infarct structure. J. Am. Coll. Cardiol., vol. 7, 1986.
78. Braunwald, E., Moroko, P. R., and Libby, P.: Reduction of infarct size following coronary occlusion. Circ. Res., 34–35(Suppl. III):192–201, 1974.
79. Edwards, J. E.: What is myocardial infarction? Circulation, 39–40(Suppl. IV):5–11, 1969.
80. Mallory, G. K., White, P. D., and Salcedo-Salazar, J.: The speed of healing of myocardial infarction. A study of the pathologic anatomy in seventy-two cases. Am. Heart J., 18:647–671, 1939.
81. Miller, R. D., Burchell, H. B., and Edwards, J. E.: Myocardial infarction with and without coronary occlusion. Arch. Intern. Med., 88:597–604, 1951.
82. Wade, W. G.: The pathogenesis of infarction of the right ventricle. Br. Heart J., 21:545–554, 1959.
83. Sugi, K., Karagueuzian, H. S., Fishbein M. C., et al.: Spontaneous ventricular tachycardia associated with isolated right ventricular infarction, one day after right coronary artery occlusion in the dog: studies on the site of origin and mechanism. Am. Heart J., 109:232–244, 1985.
84. El-Sherif, N., Gough, W. B., Zeiler, R. H., et al.: Triggered ventricular rhythms in one day old myocardial infarction in the dog. Circ. Res., 52:566–579, 1983.
85. Horowitz, L. N., Spear, J. F., and Moore, E. N.: Subendocardial origin of ventricular arrhythmias in 24-hour old experimental myocardial infarction. Circulation, 53:56–63, 1976.
86. Scherlag, B. J., Kabell, G., Brachmann, J., et al.: Mechanisms of spontaneous and induced ventricular arrhythmias in the 24-hour infarcted heart. Am. J. Cardiol., 51:207–213, 1983.
87. El-Sherif, N., Mehra, R., Gough, W. B., et al.: Ventricular activation patterns of spontaneous and induced ventricular rhythms in canine one-day old myocardial infarction. Evidence for focal and reentrant mechanisms. Circ. Res., 51:152–166, 1982.
88. Lazzara, R., El Sherif, N., and Scherlag, B. J.: Electrophysiological properties of canine Purkinje cells in one-day old myocardial infarction. Circ. Res., 33:722–734, 1973.
89. Fujimoto, T., Peter, T., Katoh, T., et al.: The relationship between ventricular arrhythmias and ischemia induced conduction delay in closed-chest animals within 24 hours of myocardial infarction. Am. Heart J., 107:201–209, 1984.
90. Friedman, P. L., Stewart, J. R., and Wit, A. L.: Spontaneous and induced cardiac arrhythmias in subendocardial Purkinje fibers surviving extensive myocardial infarction in dogs. Circ. Res., 33:612–626, 1973.
91. Fenoglio, J. J., Jr. Albala, A., Silva, F. G., et al.: Structural basis of ventricular arrhythmias in human myocardial infarction: A hypothesis. Hum. Pathol., 7:547–563, 1976.
92. Wellens, H. J. J., Lie, K. I., and Durrer, D.: Further observations on ventricular tachycardia as studied by electrical stimulation of the heart. Chronic recurrent ventricular tachycardia and ventricular tachycardia during acute myocardial infarction. Circulation, 49:647–653, 1974.
93. Davis, J., Glassman, R., and Wit, A. L.: Method for evaluating the effects of antiarrhythmic drugs on ventricular tachycardia with different electrophysiological characteristics and different mechanisms in the infarcted canine heart. Am. J. Cardiol., 49:1176–1184, 1982.
94. Danilo, P., Jr., Langan, W. B., Rosen, M. R., and Hoffman, B. F.: Effects of phenothiazine analog, EN-313, on ventricular arrhythmias in the dog. Eur. J. Pharmacol., 45:127–139, 1977.
95. Karagueuzian, H. S., Fujimoto, T., Katoh, T., et al.: Suppression of ventricular arrhythmias by propafenore, a new antiarrhythmic

agent, during acute myocardial infarction in the conscious dog. A comparative study with lidocaine. Circulation, 66:1190–1198, 1982.

96. Wellens, H. J. J., Durrer, D. R., and Lie, K. I.: Observations on mechanisms of ventricular tachycardia in man. Circulation, 54:237–244, 1976.
97. Josephson, M. E., Horowitz, L. N., Farshidi, A., and Kastor, J. A.: Recurrent sustained ventricular tachycardia in man. Circulation, 57:431–439, 1978.
98. Wit, A. L., Cranfield, P. F., and Hoffman, B. F.: Slow conduction and reentry in the ventricular conducing system. I. Return extrasystole in canine Purkinje fibers. Circ. Res., 30:1–10, 1972.
99. Sasyniuk, B. I., and Mendez, C.: A mechanism for reentry in canine ventricular tissue. Circ. Res., 28:3–15, 1971.
100. Karagueuzian, H. S., and Wit, A. L.: Studies on ventricular arrhythmias in animal models of ischemic heart disease. What can we learn? In Kulbertus, H. E., and Wellens, H. J. J. (eds.): Sudden Death, pp. 69–88. The Hague, Martinus Nijhoff, 1980.
101. Karagueuzian, H. S., Fenoglio, J. J., Jr., Hoffman, B. F., and Wit, A. L.: Sustained ventricular tachycardia induced by electrical stimulation after myocardial infarction, relation to infarct structure (abstr.). Circulation, 55–56:111–170, 1977.
102. Garan, H., Fallon, J. T., and Ruskin, J. N.: Sustained ventricular tachycardia in recent canine myocardial infarction. Circulation, 62:980–987, 1980.
103. Myerburg, R. J., Gelband, H., Nilsson, K., et al.: Long-term electrophysiological abnormalities resulting from experimental myocardial infarction in cats. Circ. Res., 41:73–84, 1977.
104. Michelson, E. L., Spear, J. F., and Moore, E. N.: Strength-interval relations in a chronic canine model of myocardial infarction. Implications for the interpretation of electrophysiologic studies. Circulation, 63:1158–1165, 1981.
105. Michelson, E. L., Spear, J. F., and Moore, E. N.: Initiation of sustained ventricular tachyarrhythmias in canine model of chronic myocardial infarction. Importance of the site of stimulation. Circulation, 63:776–784, 1981.
106. Spear, J. F., Michelson, E. L., and Moore, E. N.: Cellular electrophysiological characteristics of chronically infarcted myocardium in dogs susceptible to sustained ventricular tachyarrhythmias. J. Am. Coll. Cardiol., 1:1099–1110, 1983.
107. Spear, J. F., Michelson, E. L., and Moore, E. N.: Reduced space constant in slowly conducting regions of chronically infarcted canine myocardium. Circ. Res., 53:176–185, 1983.
108. Gessman, L. J., Agarwal, J. B., Endo, T., and Heffant, R. M.: Localization and mechanism of ventricular tachycardia by ice mapping one-week after the onset of myocardial infarction in dogs. Circulation, 68:657–666, 1983.
109. El-Sherif, N., Smith, R. A., and Evans, K.: Canine ventricular arrhythmias in the late myocardial infarction period. VIII. Epicardial mapping of reentrant circuits. Circ. Res., 49:255–265, 1981.
110. Wit, A. L., Allessie, M. A., Bonke, F. I. M., et al.: Electrophysiologic mapping to determine the mechanism of experimental ventricular tachycardia initiated by premature impulses. Experimental approach and initial results demonstrating reentrant excitation. Am. J. Cardiol., 49:166–185, 1982.
111. El-Sherif, N., Mehra, R., Gough, W. B., and Zeiler, R. H.: Reentrant ventricular arrhythmias in the late myocardial infarction period. Interruption of reentrant circuits by cryothermal techniques. Circulation, 644–656, 1983.
112. El-Sherif, N., Hope, R. R., Scherlag, B. J., and Lazzara, R.: Reentrant ventricular arrhythmias in the late myocardial infarction period. I. Conduction characteristics in the infarction zone. Circulation, 55:686–702, 1977.
113. El-Sherif, N., Hope, R. R., Scherlag, B. J., and Lazzara, R.: Reentrant arrhythmias in the late myocardial infarction period. II. Patterns of initiation and termination. Circulation, 55:702–719, 1977.
114. Gang, E. S., Bigger, J. T., Jr., and Livelli, E. D., Jr.: A model of chronic ischemic arrhythmias: The relation between electrically inducible tachycardia, ventricular fibrillation threshold and myocardial infarct size. Am. J. Cardiol., 50:469–476, 1982.
115. Glassman, R. D., Davis, J. C., and Wit, A. L.: Effects of antiarrhythmic drugs on sustained ventricular tachycardia induced by premature stimulus in dogs after coronary artery occlusion and reperfusion (Abstr.). Fed. Proc., 37:730, 1978.
116. Karagueuzian, H. S., Ohta, M., Drury, K. J., et al.: Coronary venous retroinfusion of procainamide: a new approach for the management of spontaneous and inducible sustained ventricular tachycardia during myocardial infarction, J. Am. Coll. Cardial., vol. 7, 1986.
117. Paterson, E., Gibson, J. K., and Lucchesi, B. R.: Electrophysiologic effects of disopyramide phosphate on reentrant ventricular arrhythmia in conscious dogs after myocardial infarction. Am. J. Cardiol. 46:792–799, 1980.
118. Patterson, E., Gibson, J. K., and Lucchesi, B. R.: Prevention of chronic canine ventricular tachyarrhythmias with bretylium tosylate. Circulation, 64:1045–1050, 1981.
119. Anderson, J. L., Patterson, E., Conlon, M., et al.: Kinetics of antifibrillatory effects of bretylium: Correlation with myocardial drug concentrations. Am. J. Cardiol., 46:583–592, 1980.
120. Patterson, E., Ella, B. T., Abrams, G. D., et al.: Ventricular fibrillation in a conscious canine preparation of sudden coronary death—prevention by short and long-term amiodarone administration. Circulation, 68:857–864, 1983.
121. Myerburg, R. J., Kesseler, K. M., Kiem, I., et al.: Relationship between plasma levels of procainamide, suppression of premature ventricular complexes and prevention of recurrent ventricular tachycardia. Circulation, 64:280–296, 1981.
122. Spear, J. F., Horowitz, L. N., Hodess, A. B., et al.: Cellular electrophysiology of human myocardial infarction. 1. Abnormalities of cellular activation. Circulation, 59:247–256, 1979.
123. Dangman, K. H., Danilo, P., Jr., Hordoff, A. J., et al.: Electrophysiologic characteristics of human ventricular and Purkinje fibers. Circulation, 65:362–368, 1982.
124. Reddy, C. R., and Gettes, L. S.: Use of isoproteronol as an aid to electric induction of chronic recurrent ventricular tachycardia. Am. J. Cardiol., 44:705–713, 1979.
125. Winkle, R. A., Alderman, E. L., Fitzgerald, J. W., and Harrison, D. C.: Treatment of symptomatic ventricular tachycardia. Ann. Intern. Med., 85:1–7, 1976.
126. Denes, P., Wu, D., Wyndham, C., et al.: Chronic long-term electrophysiologic study of paroxysmal ventricular tachycardia. Chest, 77:478–487, 1980.
127. Rinkenberger, R. L., Prystowsky, E. N., Jackman, W. M., et al.: Drug conversion of non-sustained ventricular tachycardia to sustained ventricular tachycardia during serial electrophysiologic studies: Identification of drugs that exacerbate tachycardia and potential mechanisms. Am. Heart J., 103:177–184, 1982.
128. Mason, J. W., and Winkle, R. A.: Electrode-catheter arrhythmia induction in the selection and assessment of antiarrhythmic drug therapy for recurrent ventricular tachycardia. Circulation, 58:971–985, 1978.
129. Waxman, H. L., Buxton, A. E., Sadowski, I. M., and Josephson, M. E.: The response to procainamide during electrophysiologic study for sustained ventricular tachyarrhythmias predicts the response to other medications. Circulation, 67:30–37, 1983.
130. Kramer, J. B., Saffitz, J. E., Witkowski, F. X., et al.: Intramural reentry as a mechanism of ventricular tachycardia during evolving canine myocardial infarction. Circ. Res., 56:736–754, 1985.

18

The Ventricular Premature Complex: Mechanisms and Significance— An Update

Nabil El-Sherif

The ubiquitous ventricular premature complex (VPC) represents one aspect of disorders of the cardiac rhythm that captures the interest of clinicians and cardiac electrophysiologists alike.

VPCs are not uncommon in an ostensibly normal population,[1,2] and their incidence tends to increase with age, paralleling the increased incidence of coronary artery disease.[1,3–8] In the absence of cardiovascular abnormalities and stigmata of coronary artery disease, VPCs may be largely innocuous.[1,4–8] Even paroxysms of ventricular tachycardia in ambulatory healthy subjects seem to have little prognostic significance.[1] The same is true for the not uncommon exercise-induced VPCs in apparently normal groups.[9–12] However, in the presence of major risk factors or evidence of coronary artery disease, frequent VPCs may be associated with an increased risk of sudden death.[1,3,4,7,13,14]

In this chapter, the electrophysiologic mechanisms, electrocardiographic patterns, and clinical significance of VPCs will be discussed with an attempt to correlate basic and clinical observations.

Electrophysiologic Mechanisms

VPCs can be caused either by pacemaker activity or by reentrant excitation. Each of these two main mechanisms has subclasses (Table 18-1). Pacemaker activity occurs when a cell or a group of closely knit cells begins to generate impulses. The mechanism can be *normal automatic activity, abnormal automatic activity, or triggered activity.*[15] Abnormal automaticity differs from normal automaticity in that it occurs at a level of transmembrane potential considerably less negative than the normal maximum diastolic potential or normal resting potential of the fibers involved. Triggered activity differs from both normal and abnormal automaticity in that it requires a prior impulse for initiation. Triggered activity is further subdivided into activity arising from early or delayed afterdepolarizations.[16] A fourth, less well-understood, subclass of pacemaker activity is *oscillatory depolarizations of membrane potential.* On the other hand, reentrant excitation occurs when the propagating impulse does not die out after complete activation of the heart, as is normally the case, but persists to reexcite the atria or ventricles after the end of the refractory period.[17] Reentrant excitation can be subdivided into *circus movement excitation* and *reflection.* In circus movement

Supported in part by the Veterans Administration Medical Research Funds and NIH grant #R01 HL 31341

Table 18-1. The Ventricular Premature Complex: Electrophysiologic Mechanisms

Pacemaker Activity
Normal automatic activity
Abnormal automatic activity
Triggered activity
Early afterdepolarizations
Delayed afterdepolarizations
Oscillatory depolarizations of membrane potential
Reentrant Excitation
Circus movement reentry
Ring model
Figure eight model
Leading circle model
Reflection

reentry, the activation wavefront encounters a site of unidirectional conduction block and propagates in a circuitous pathway before reexciting the tissue proximal to the site of block after the refractory period has ended. By contrast, in the reflection model of reentrant excitation, impulses in both directions are transmitted over the same pathway.[18]

Pacemaker Activity

Normal Automatic Activity

Automatic activity is caused by a gradual fall in membrane potential during diastole until membrane potential reaches threshold and generates an action potential. The diastolic depolarization is believed to result from an outward pacemaker current carried by K^+ that gradually declines, thereby allowing the background inward Na^+ current to depolarize the cell membrane.[19,20] A recently proposed alternative mechanism suggests that an inward Na^+ pacemaker current (I_f) increases with time, while the outward K^+ current remains constant.[21,22] Automaticity is a normal property of the sinus node, some atrial fibers, the AV junction, and the His-Purkinje system. The rate of His-Purkinje automaticity is rather slow (Fig. 18-1*A*) and characteristically decreases in a hierarchical fashion from the proximal His-Purkinje system to the distal Purkinje network. Normal His-Purkinje automaticity can account for some slow ventricular escape rhythms. However, it is difficult to envision that normal His-Purkinje automatic activity results in ventricular premature complexes. This is especially so if one remembers that normal His-Purkinje automatic activity is constantly being overdrive suppressed by the much faster supraventricular automatic activity.[23] It is possible, however, that local release of norepinephrine from sympathetic nerves en-

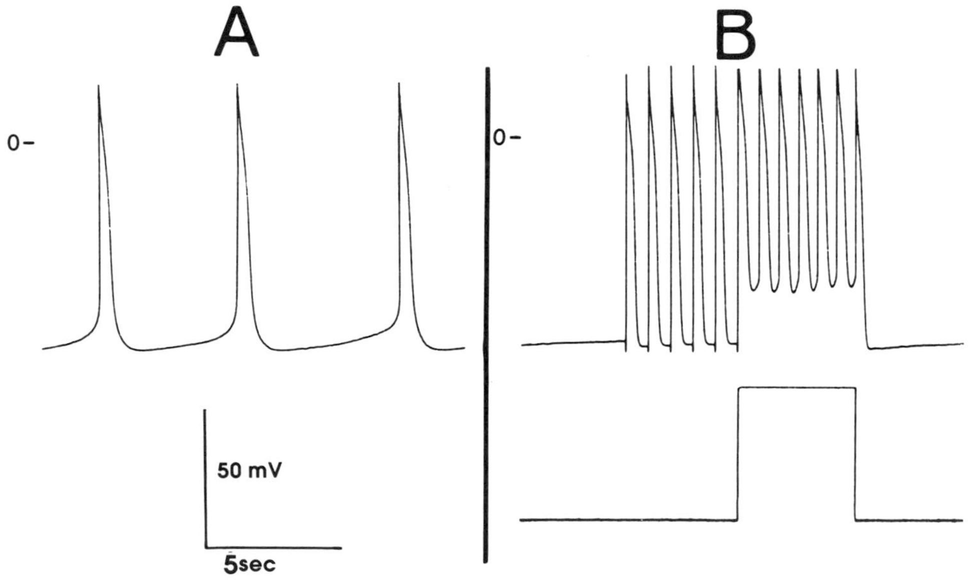

Figure 18-1. *(A) Normal automaticity in a canine Purkinje fiber with a maximum diastolic potential of −85 mV. Note the slow diastolic depolarization and the slow rate of automatic firing (9 to 12 beats/min) (B) Abnormal automaticity induced in a canine Purkinje fiber when the resting potential was reduced from −78 to −56 mV by a long-lasting current pulse injected through a suction electrode. The first six action potentials were stimulated. When the fiber was depolarized, six nonstimulated action potentials occurred. When the membrane potential was brought back to the more negative level, abnormal automatic activity terminated.*

hances the rate of normal His-Purkinje automatic activity,[24] allowing an ectopic pacemaker to reach threshold before being activated by the supraventricular impulse. It is also possible that entrance block can protect a slow normal His-Purkinje automatic focus from premature discharge by the supraventricular pacemaker, thus creating a parasystolic rhythm.[25] In this case, the ectopic discharge will capture the ventricles if it falls outside the effective refractory period.

Abnormal Automatic Activity

Impulses may be generated spontaneously by fibers in which the maximum diastolic potential has been reduced by a variety of interventions. This abnormal automaticity at a low level of diastolic potential has been demonstrated in both Purkinje and myocardial fibers.[26-28] The example studied most frequently is provided by Purkinje fibers in which the maximum diastolic potential has been decreased by experimental intervention to −50 to −60 mV rather than to −90 to −95 mV (see Fig. 18-1*B*). A likely cause of automaticity at membrane potentials of around −50 mV is deactivation of a K^+ current, called ix_i.[29] Because of the low level of membrane potential, action potential upstrokes of abnormal automaticity depend on slow inward current.[16] The reduced diastolic potential at which abnormal automaticity occurs may cause entrance block into the focus, thus creating a parasystolic rhythm.[30] Unlike normal automaticity, abnormal automaticity may not be overdrive suppressed.[31] It is therefore easier for an abnormal automatic rhythm to capture the ventricle following a brief transient slowing of the supraventricular rhythm.

Abnormal automaticity may be difficult to discern from triggered activity initiated by early afterdepolarizations as well as from triggered activity arising from delayed afterdepolarizations in partially depolarized fibers. In early studies of 1-day-old ischemic endocardial preparations, rhythmic activity at reduced levels of diastolic potential was considered the result of abnormal automaticity.[15,32,33] However, when the initiation and termination of these rhythms were carefully analyzed, the majority were found to be due to triggered activity arising from delayed afterdepolarizations in partially depolarized ischemic Purkinje fibers.[34]

Triggered Activity

Triggered activity is pacemaker activity caused by afterdepolarizations. An afterdepolarization is a second subthreshold depolarization that occurs either during repolarization (early afterdepolarization) or after repolarization is complete (delayed afterdepolarization).[35]

Early Afterdepolarization. Early afterdepolarization occurs when the fiber fails to repolarize completely after

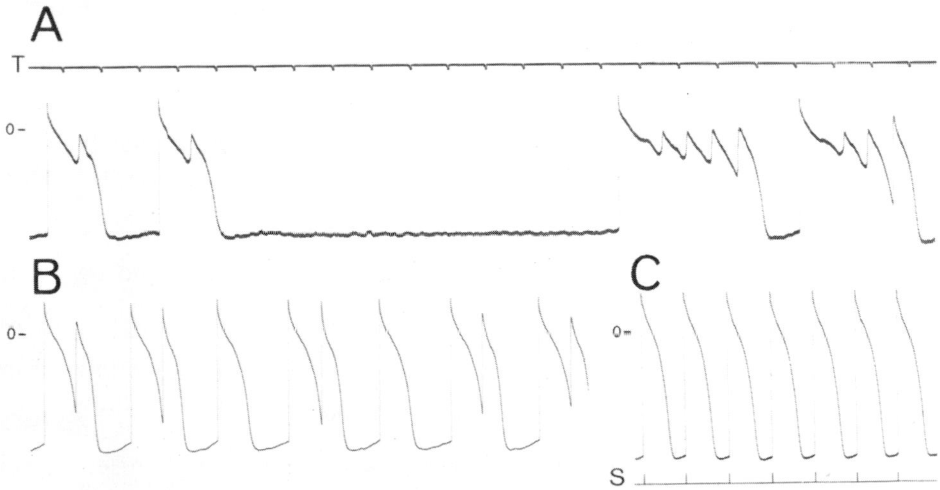

Figure 18-2. *Triggered activity due to early afterdepolarizations in canine Purkinje fibers exposed to anthopleurin-A in a concentration of 100 µg/liter. The drug prolonged the action potential duration and caused upstrokes arising from early afterdepolarizations to appear. Following a long diastolic interval in A, the action potential duration became markedly prolonged and a burst of rhythmic activity arising from a low level of membrane potential occurred. Action potentials arising from early afterdepolarizations resulted in bigeminal and trigeminal rhythms in B. In C, the preparation was paced at short cycle lengths, resulting in a shortened action potential duration and disappearance of early afterdepolarizations. This illustrates the bradycardia-dependent nature of the early afterdepolarizations. S denotes the timing of stimulation. The time scale (T) represents 1-second intervals.*

generating an action potential upstroke. As the membrane potential lingers at intermediate values, oscillatory depolarizations can occur (Fig. 18-2). Once early afterdepolarizations occur, they can attain threshold and initiate another response. Sometimes the response is followed by complete repolarization, and sometimes the first abnormal response is followed by repetitive depolarizations at a reduced level of membrane potential. Early afterdepolarizations can occur if K^+ conductance is decreased relative to the inward current conductance.[15] Many types of experimental interventions have been shown to cause early afterdepolarizations,[16] including marked and abrupt reduction of $[K^+]_o$,[36] high concentration of catecholamines,[37] and a number of drugs. Experimental drugs such as aconitine[38,39] and veratridine[40] cause early afterdepolarizations, probably by increasing steady-state Na^+ conductance during the plateau phase of the action potential. Figure 18-2 shows that another experimental drug, anthopleurin-A (AP-A), a polypeptide extracted from a sea anemone, can also prolong action potential duration and induce early afterdepolarizations. AP-A possesses several unique properties as a cardiotonic agent and causes a selective positive inotropic effect on the heart *in vivo* that is several times more powerful than digitalis.[41,42] Voltage-clamp experiments suggest that AP-A causes delayed inactivation of the fast Na^+ current.[43] Cesium is another experimental drug that prolongs action potential duration and causes early afterdepolarizations.[44] Cesium has not been shown to enhance inward current, but it is possible that the normal noninactivated Na^+ current is sufficient to cause afterdepolarizations if repolarization is sufficiently delayed and outward currents are blocked.[44]

Other clinically used drugs that markedly prolong the time course for repolarization, such as the beta-receptor blocking drug sotalol,[45] and antiarrhythmic drugs *N*-acetyl procainamide[46] and quinidine,[47] also cause early afterdepolarizations and triggered activity. As shown in Figure 18-2, both prolonged action potential duration and the early afterdepolarizations caused by AP-A are characteristically bradycardia dependent; that is, they are more pronounced at long cycle lengths (see Fig. 18-2*A*) and are markedly attenuated or abolished at short cycle lengths (see Fig. 18-2*C*). The same phenomenon has been shown with both cesium[44] and quinidine[47] and may provide a mechanism for bradycardia-dependent arrhythmias.[44,48–50]

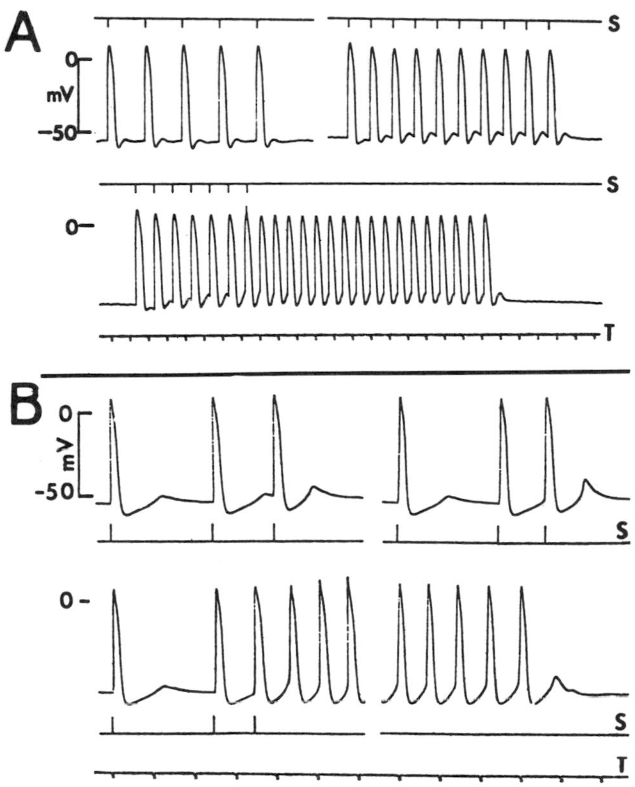

Figure 18-3. *Triggered activity arising from delayed afterdepolarizations in endocardial preparations obtained from 1-day-old canine infarction. A and B illustrate transmembrane recordings from Purkinje cells in the ischemic zone from two different preparations. In A, the preparation was stimulated at cycle lengths of 2000, 1200, and 1000 msec, respectively. Reducing the cycle length of stimulation increased the amplitude of the afterdepolarization that reached threshold and initiated triggered activity in the lower recording. The triggered rhythm terminated following a subthreshold delayed afterdepolarization. In B, the effect of premature stimulation on the amplitude of the delayed afterdepolarization is demonstrated. The preparation was paced at a basic cycle length of 2500 msec. The coupling interval of the premature stimulus was shortened from 1500 to 1200 to 1000 msec, respectively. This increased the amplitude of the afterdepolarization that reached threshold after the short coupling interval and initiated a triggered rhythm. The rhythm terminated after a subthreshold afterdepolarization. S denotes the timing of stimulation. The time scale (T) represents 1-second intervals. (After El-Sherif, N., Gough, W. B., Zeiler, R. H., and Mehra, R.: Triggered ventricular rhythm in 1-day-old myocardial infarction in the dog. Circ. Res., 52:566, 1983. By permission of the American Heart Association, Inc.)*

Delayed Afterdepolarizations. Delayed afterdepolarizations occur after phase 3 repolarization has restored maximum diastolic potential to a value somewhat less than normal. Triggered activity occurs when a delayed afterdepolarization attains threshold potential and terminates following a subthreshold afterdepolarization (Fig. 18-3). The amplitude and rate of rise of the delayed afterdepolarization are usually functions of the cycle length and number of preceding action potentials[34,51–56] (see Fig. 18-3*A*). Premature stimulation could also enhance the amplitude of delayed afterdepolarization.[34,55] A critically timed premature impulse can be followed by a delayed afterdepolarization that reaches threshold and initiates triggered activity (see Fig. 18-3*B*). The oscillatory current responsible for delayed afterdepolarizations may be normally present in Purkinje cells and can be enhanced by interventions that increase $[Ca^{2+}]_i$.[57] A model that has emerged describing the ionic mechanism responsible for delayed afterdepolarizations suggests one phenomenon common to all preparations exhibiting delayed afterdepolarizations: an increase in $[Ca^{2+}]_i$. This could be accomplished directly by increasing $[Ca^{2+}]_o$ and thereby increasing the driving force for calcium or by increasing calcium influx by increasing calcium conductance with catecholamine.[59] Indirect increases of $[Ca^{2+}]_i$ occur when Na-K ATPase is inhibited with digitalis,[60] with K-free solutions,[61] and with Na-free solutions.[62,63] When $[Ca^{2+}]_i$ is sufficiently large, subsequent action potentials initiate oscillatory calcium movements intracellularly, which in turn cause an oscillatory change in membrane conductance that permits a transient inward current.[64–66]

Delayed afterdepolarizations and triggered activity have also been shown to occur in ischemic subendocardial Purkinje fibers surviving 1-day-old canine infarct.[34] The hypoxia accompanying coronary artery occlusion inhibits the Na-K ATPase and leads to reduced pump activity and, consequently, decreased $[K^+]_i$ and increased $[Na^+]_i$.[67,68] The increase in $[Na^+]_i$ reduces the Na gradient and causes a secondary decrease in calcium extrusion by the Na-Ca exchange[62] and may promote calcium release from mitochondria,[69] eventually resulting in an increase in $[Ca^{2+}]_i$. Calcium blocking agents can inhibit triggered activity either by directly suppressing delayed afterdepolarizations or by inducing exit block around sites of triggered activity.[34]

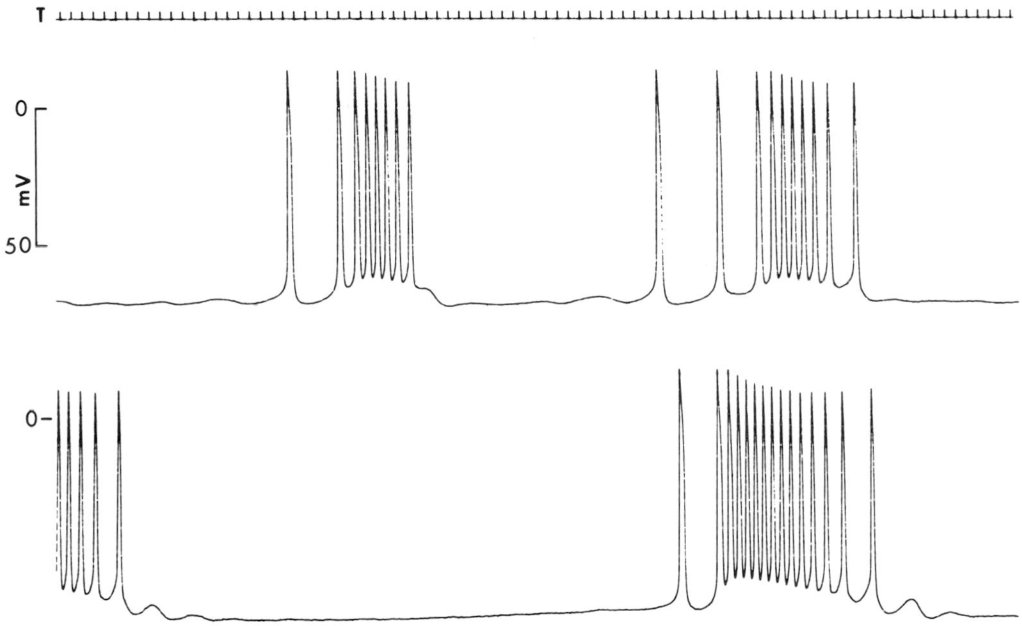

Figure 18-4. *Oscillatory depolarizations of membrane potential. Transmembrane recording from a Purkinje cell in the ischemic zone of an endocardial preparation from a 1-day-old canine infarction. These endocardial preparations commonly show triggered activity arising from delayed afterdepolarizations. The recording was obtained after the preparation was exposed to the calcium-blocking drug verapamil to suppress triggered activity and then to increased extracellular calcium (8.1 mM) to reverse the effects of verapamil. Note the presence of two types of oscillatory depolarizations of the membrane potential; those that follow the last action potential in a series of group beating progressively become smaller, like a damped oscillation, while those that precede the first action potential progressively become larger and seem to reach threshold and initiate the action potential. The second action potential in each series of group beating may be generated by a delayed afterdepolarization. However, the action potentials that follow arise before complete repolarization of the preceding action potential and may represent triggered activity from early afterdepolarizations. This activity gradually slows before termination associated with gradual increase of the maximum diastolic potential. More than one mechanism for impulse generation may contribute to the arrhythmias that follow myocardial ischemia and infarction. The time scale (T) represents 1-second intervals.*

No clinical cardiac arrhythmia has definitely been ascribed to delayed afterdepolarizations; however, some accelerated AV junctional and idioventricular rhythms as well as some of the atrial and ventricular arrhythmias caused by digitalis toxicity may be explained by delayed afterdepolarizations.[70] The spontaneous ventricular rhythms in 1-day-old canine infarct may be due to delayed afterdepolarizations and triggered activity.[71] These rhythms could be suppressed *in vivo* by verapamil following beta-adrenergic blockade resulting in cardiac quiescence. Following quiescence, the ventricular rhythms could be reinitiated (*i.e.,* triggered) only by one or more automatic or stimulated ventricular beats. Similar to the *in vitro* rhythms, the *in vivo* triggered rhythms have a focal origin from Purkinje fibers surviving the infarct.[71]

Oscillatory Depolarizations of Membrane Potential

Spontaneous impulses may arise from oscillatory changes in transmembrane potential that appear to differ from normal phase 4 depolarization (Fig. 18-4). This mechanism may not be different from delayed afterdepolarizations.[15] However, in contrast to a series of delayed afterdepolarizations that decrease progressively like a damped oscillation, oscillatory depolarizations may progressively increase, reach threshold, and initiate an action potential. Figure 18-4 illustrates both types of oscillatory potentials as well as action potentials probably generated by carly afterdepolarizations recorded from the same endocardial preparation obtained from 1-day-old canine infarction. The figure emphasizes the possibility that more than one mechanism for impulse generation may contribute to the arrhythmias that follow myocardial ischemia and infarction.

Reentrant Excitation

Circus Movement Reentry

The Ring Model of Reentry. Early experimental observations of Mayer,[72] Garrey,[73] and Mines[74,75] have shown the existence of an entrapped circuit wave (circus contractions or movement) in rings of living cardiac and other tissue cut from a variety of animals, including mammals (Fig. 18-5*A*). The presence of a fixed anatomic obstacle was considered an important requirement for circus movement to occur. Whether these experiments are related to human cardiac arrhythmias is the hypothesis first proposed by Mines. Guided by Mines' observations in rings of muscle, Thomas Lewis[76,77] tried to prove that the atrial flutter wave circulated around a natural opening in the muscles of the auricle (the vena cavae). Schmitt and Erlanger[78] suggested that a loop composed of a branching peripheral Purkinje fiber bundle and ventricular muscle might sustain a circus movement similar to rings of muscle (see Fig. 18-5*B*).

Central to the initiation of a circus movement in a ring model is the concept of unidirectional block (see Fig. 18-5*C*). Here, a stimulus will block in one direction, presumably because of nonhomogeneous refractoriness, but will continue to conduct in the other direction. A circus movement will be established if the returning wavefront finds that the site of unidirectional block has recovered excitability, thus permitting conduction to proceed uninterrupted. Although a circus movement in a Purkinje muscle loop is possible, it is difficult to demonstrate in the *in situ* heart. The only two proven examples of a ring model reentry in the intact mammalian heart are (1) the preexcitation syndrome that was suggested by Mines[75] shortly after Kent demonstrated the multiple muscular connections between auricles and ventricles in human hearts[79] and (2) circus movement involving both bundle branches (bundle branch reentry)[80] that was first suggested by the experimental observations of Moe and colleagues[81] (Fig. 18-6). What is common to the preexcitation syndrome and bundle branch reentry is that the anatomic substrate is made in large part of pathways of excitable bundles that are not connected to adjacent atrial and ventricular myocardium. A single simple circulatory wave could thus be established. The circuit could be interrupted with ease by cutting at any point along the insulated excitable bundles but most probably not at the less well-defined atrial or ventricular connections of these pathways.

The Figure Eight Model of Reentry. A fixed anatomic obstacle is not required for development of a circus movement reentry in the atria or ventricles. This was first illustrated by Allessie and colleagues, who showed that a properly timed premature stimulus can initiate a circus movement tachycardia in small pieces of atrial rabbit myocardium.[82–84] The initiation of reentry is made possible by the different refractory periods of atrial fibers in close proximity. The premature impulse that initiates reentry blocks in fibers with long refractory periods and conducts in fibers with shorter refractory periods eventually returns to the initial point of block after excitability recovers there. El-Sherif and colleagues have demonstrated circus movement reentry in the surviving electrophysiologically abnormal ischemic epicardial layer overlying canine infarction.[85–87] Ischemia was found to lengthen refractoriness with nonhomogeneous distribution, usually in the form of concentric isochrones of refractoriness, with graded increase in refractoriness going from the border zone toward the center of the ischemic zone.[88] A critically timed premature beat that succeeds in inducing reentry results in an arc of unidirectional conduction block around which the reentrant wavefront circulates. The arc of conduction block occurs between adjacent sites of short and long refractoriness, with the sites of longer refractoriness distal to the arc of block (Fig. 18-7).

A premature beat that successfully initiates reentry

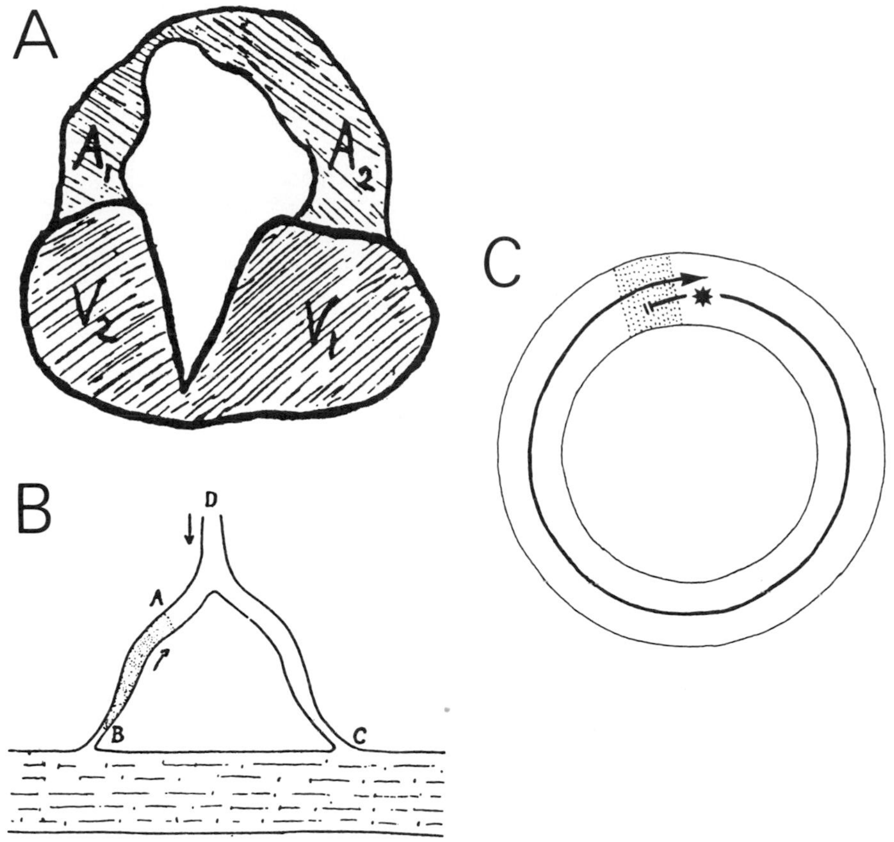

Figure 18-5. *Ring models of reentry. (A) Mines's diagram of a ring preparation composed of the auricle and ventricle of the tortoise, in which he observed reciprocating rhythm. Both connections between auricle and ventricle could transmit an excitation wave. During reciprocating rhythm, the four portions of the preparation marked V_1, V_2, A_1, and A_2, contracted in that order (from Mines, G. R.: On dynamic equilibrium in the heart. J. Physiol., 46:350–383, 1913) (B) A proposed mechanism for reentry in a Purkinje-muscle loop from the study of Schmitt and Erlanger. The diagram shows a Purkinje fiber* (bundle D) *that divides into two branches, both connected distally by ventricular muscle. Circus movement will develop if the stippled segment (A to B) is an area of unidirectional conduction. An impulse advancing from D would be blocked at A but would reach and stimulate the ventricular muscle at C through the other terminal branch. The excitation from the ventricular fiber would then reenter the Purkinje system at B and traverse the depressed region slowly so that by the time it arrived at A this site would have recovered refractoriness and would again be excited (Schmitt, F. O., and Erlanger, J.: Directional differences in the conduction of the impulse through heart muscle and their possible relation to extrasystolic and fibrillary contractions. Am. J. Physiol., 87:326–347, 1928–1929) (C) Diagrammatic illustration of the initiation of circus movement in a ring model, emphasizing the importance of unidirectional block. A properly timed stimulus* (asterisk) *will block in one direction because of nonhomogeneous refractoriness* (stippled zone) *but will continue to conduct in the ring in the other direction. A circus movement will be established if the returning wavefront finds that the site of unidirectional block has recovered excitability, thus permitting conduction to proceed uninterrupted.*

results in a longer arc of conduction block and slower conduction compared to one that fails to induce reentry. When a single premature stimulation (S_2) fails to initiate reentry, a second premature stimulation (S_3) may be necessary. S_3 usually results in a longer arc of conduction block or slower conduction around the arc. The slower activation travels around a longer, more circuitous route, thus providing time for refractoriness along the proximal side of unidirectional block to expire at one site. Reexcitation of this site will initiate reentry. The beat that initiates the first reentrant cycle, whether it is an S_2 or an S_3, results in a continuous arc of conduction block. The activation front circulates around both ends of the arc of block and rejoins on the distal side of the arc

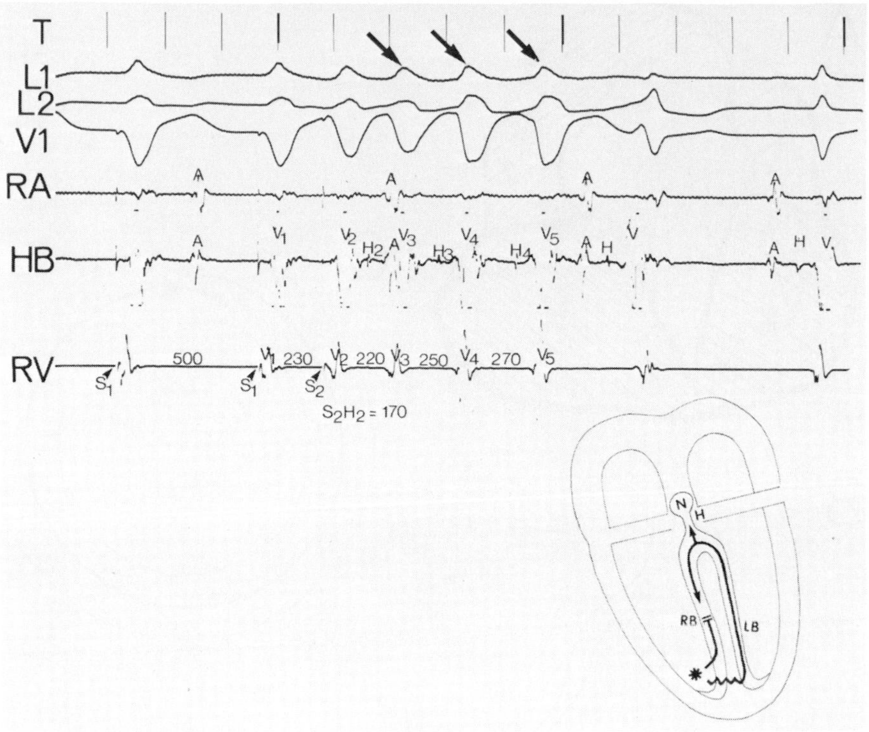

Figure 18-6. *Bundle branch reentry in the human heart. The figure was obtained from a patient aged 55 years and shows the initiation of bundle branch reentry by programmed premature stimulation. Tracings from top to bottom are surface electrocardiogram leads I, II, and V_1, high right atrial (RA) electrogram, His bundle (HB) electrogram, and right ventricular (RV) electrogram. The ventricle was paced from the right ventricular apex at a basic cycle length (S_1–S_1) of 500 msec. A single premature impulse (S_2) introduced at a coupling interval of 320 msec resulted in three nonstimulated beats* (arrows). *The QRS configuration of the induced rhythm is similar to that of the paced beats and reflects a left bundle branch block morphology. The induced rhythm was terminated by a captured sinus beat. The diagram at the bottom of the recording illustrates that the mechanism of the induced rhythm is bundle branch reentry. The premature stimulated beat, S_2, blocked retrogradely in the right bundle branch (RB)* (double bars) *but conducted slowly in the ventricular septum and engaged the left bundle branch (LB). The impulse conducted retrogradely in the LB, activated the His bundle (H), and returned back to activate the RB in an antegrade direction, thus completing the first circus movement. Activation reached the site of functional conduction block in the RB after it had recovered refractoriness and continued the circus movement reentry. The HB electrogram shows that the interval between the QRS complexes of the premature beat and the first two reentrant beats and the retrograde His deflection gradually increased, reflecting progressively greater conduction delay in the retrograde limb of the reentrant circuit. On the other hand, the interval between the retrograde His and the QRS complexes of the three reentrant beats remained constant and was equal to the HV interval of conducted sinus beats. (N, AV node)*

of block before breaking through the arc to reactivate an area proximal to the block. This splits the initial single arc of block into two separate arcs. Reentrant activation continues as a figure eight activation pattern, whereby two circulating wavefronts advance clockwise and counterclockwise, respectively, around two zones (arcs) of conduction block. During a monomorphic reentrant tachycardia, the two arcs of block and the two circulating wavefronts remain fairly stable (Fig. 18-8). On the other hand, during a pleomorphic reentrant rhythm, both arcs of block and the circulating wavefronts can change their geometric configurations while maintaining their synchrony.

The Leading Circle Model of Reentry. In the circus movement tachycardia induced by Allessie and col-

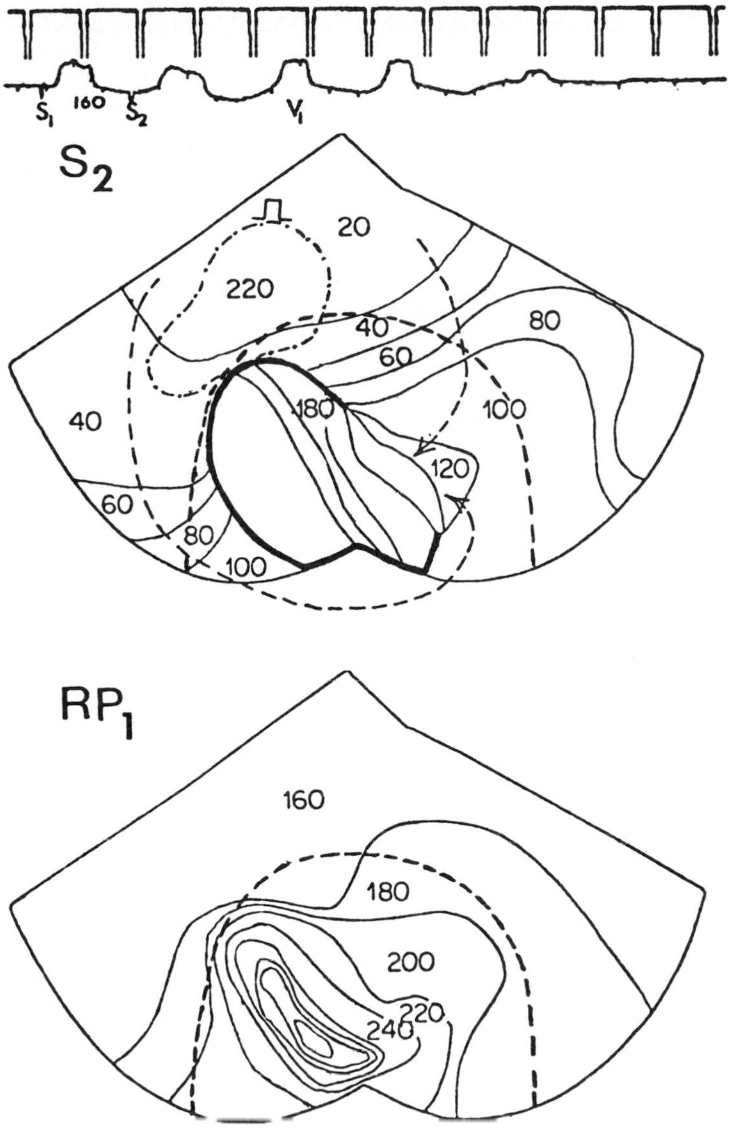

Figure 18-7. *Correlation of isochronal activation and refractory maps of circus movement reentry in the canine postinfarction heart. Recordings were obtained from a dog 4 days after ligation of the left anterior descending artery. The electrocardiogram on top shows that a single premature stimulus, S_2, at a coupling interval of 160 msec initiated a short reentrant rhythm. The epicardial activation map of S_2 is shown on the top, while the refractory map of S_1 as encountered by S_2 is shown on the bottom and labeled RP_1. Both maps were drawn at 20-msec isochrones. The border of the ischemic zone is outlined on both maps. The epicardial surface is depicted as if the ventricles were folded out after a cut was made from the crux to the apex. The top left and right borders represent the right and left AV junctions. The two curvilinear surfaces on the right and left are contiguous and extend from the posterior base to the apex of the heart. The ventricles were stimulated from the right ventricular outflow tract. The activation map shows that S_2 resulted in a long arc of functional conduction block within the epicardial border of the ischemic zone* (heavy solid line). *Epicardial activation circulated around both ends of the arc of block, coalescing into a common reentrant wavefront that conducted slowly from lateral to septal border of the ischemic zone before reactivating myocardial zones on the proximal side of the arc of block to initiate the first reentrant beat. The refractory map shows that ischemia resulted in a nonuniform refractory distribution with effective refractory periods (ERPs) of 160 and 170 msec located in the normal right and left ventricular epicardium, while the longest ERP of 320 msec was located in the center of the ischemic region. The dispersion of refractoriness was 160 msec with concentric isochrones of refractoriness producing a graded increase in ERP going from the border zone toward the center of the ischemic zone. The arc of functional conduction block encountered by S_2 developed between adjacent sites of short and long refractoriness, with the sites of longer refractoriness being distal to the arc of block.*

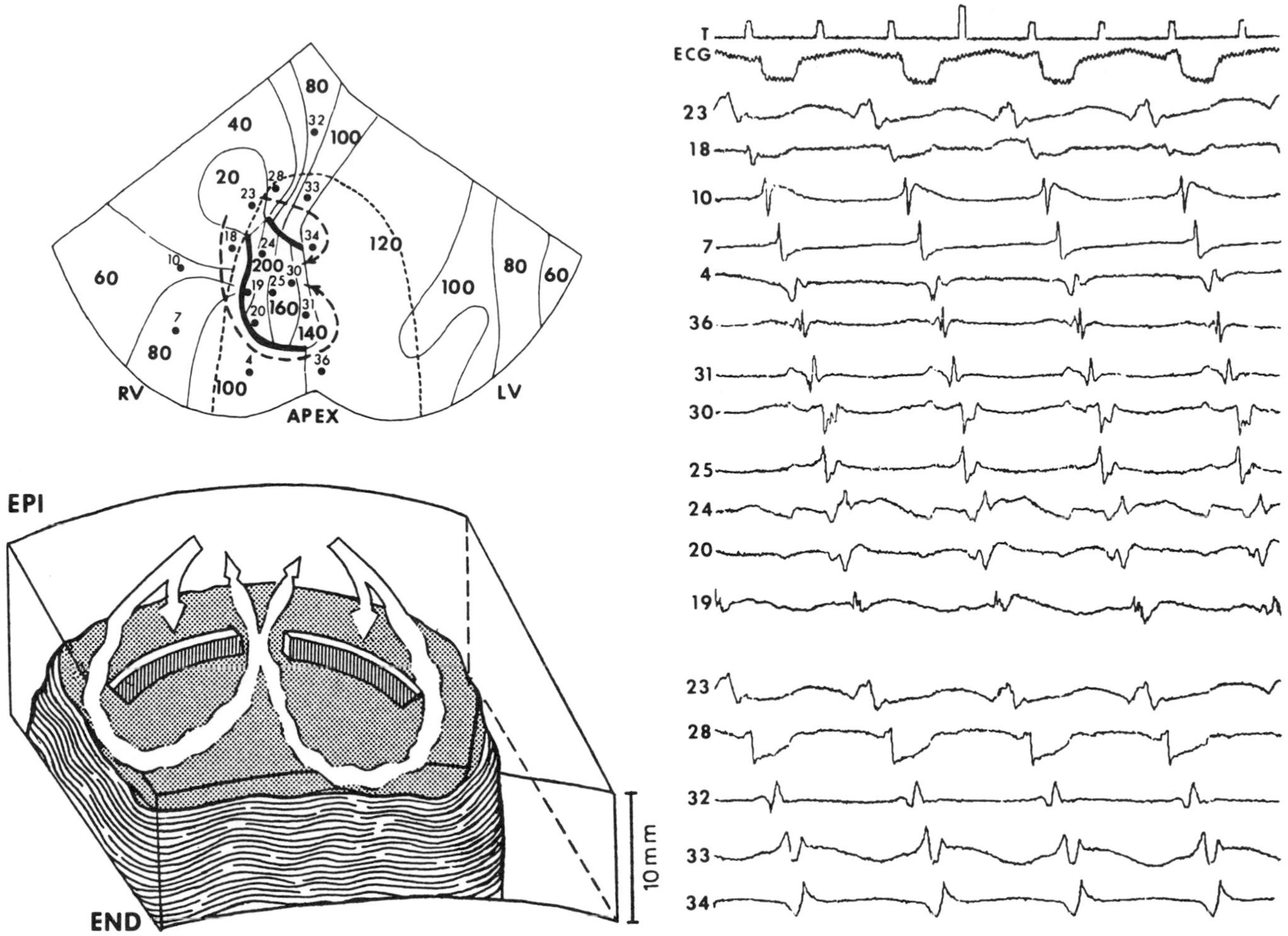

Figure 18-8. *Isochronal activation map during a monomorphic reentrant ventricular tachycardia. Recordings were obtained from a dog 4 days after ligation of the left anterior descending artery. Activation isochrones are drawn at 20-msec intervals. The reentrant circuit has a characteristic figure 8 activation pattern, whereby two circulating wavefronts advance in clockwise and counterclockwise directions, respectively, around two zones (arcs) of conduction block* (heavy solid lines). *The* right panel *shows selected simultaneous electrograms recorded along the two arcs of functional conduction block and the common reentrant wavefront and depicts the presence of diastolic bridging between reentrant beats. A tridimensional diagramatic illustration of the ventricular activation pattern during the reentrant tachycardia is shown at the* lower left corner *of the figure. In this experimental model, reentrant activation occurs in the surviving thin epicardial layer overlying the infarction. (RV, right ventricle; LV, left ventricle; EPI, epicardium; END, endocardium)*

leagues in small pieces of atrial rabbit myocardium, the center of the circuit, or the vortex, is made of excitable tissue.[82–84] However, the tissue is rendered functionally inexcitable because the center is invaded by multiple centripetal wavelets from the leading circuit outside the vortex (Fig. 18-9*C*).

A critical analysis of the leading circle model of Allessie and co-workers shows that it is indeed a special modification of the figure eight model of reentry that probably can exist only in an isolated preparation, not in the intact heart.[82–84] Figure 18-9 shows a slightly modified version of the isochronal maps of the premature beat that initiated circus movement reentry (*A*) and the first reentrant beat (*B*) in atrial muscle preparation of the rabbit.[83] (The arcs of functional block are represented by heavy solid lines instead of the double bars of the original drawing.) The S_2 map shows that a properly timed premature stimulus resulted in a continuous arc of functional conduction block. The activation wavefront circulated around both ends of the arc, coalesced, and then broke through the arc to reexcite myocardial zones on the proximal side of the arc. This split the original single arc into two separate arcs. Figure 18-9*B* shows that a circulating wavefront continued around one of the two arcs. However, the second arc of block shifted its site significantly and developed in an area that showed crowded isochrones in the S_2 map. More significantly, this arc joined the edge of the preparation, aborting a second circulating wavefront around the arc. If the preparation shown in Figure 18-9*B* was inserted in the *in situ* heart, the second aborted circulating wavefront would be activated, resulting in a figure eight activation pattern. The only situation in the *in situ* heart that would simulate the *in vitro* activation map shown in Figure 18-9*B* would be one of the two arcs of block joining the AV junction. Such an example can indeed be found in some *in vivo* maps of atrial flutter in the canine heart shown by Boineau and colleagues[89] (see Fig. 18-9*D*). In this example, a single clockwise circulating wave is seen around a zone (arc) of functional conduction block. The second potential circulating wavefront in a figure eight reentry model was prevented when the second arc of block connected to the AV junction. Thus, a figure eight pattern seems central to the occurrence of "repetitive" reentrant excitation (short of fibrillation) in the interconnected syncytial structure of the atria and ventricles. The dimension of the reentrant circuit in the ventricle could be as small as 10 mm, and, depending on the distribution of the pathologic features of the myocardium, these circuits can be located in the epicardial, intramural, or subendocardial regions.[90] The long arcs of functional conduction block that sustain large reentrant circuits in the canine postinfarction ventricle and the small vortices of functional block described by Allessie and colleagues[82–84] that sustain small reentrant circuits in rabbit atrial myocardium thus may represent two ends of a spectrum of the same electrophysiologic phenomenon.

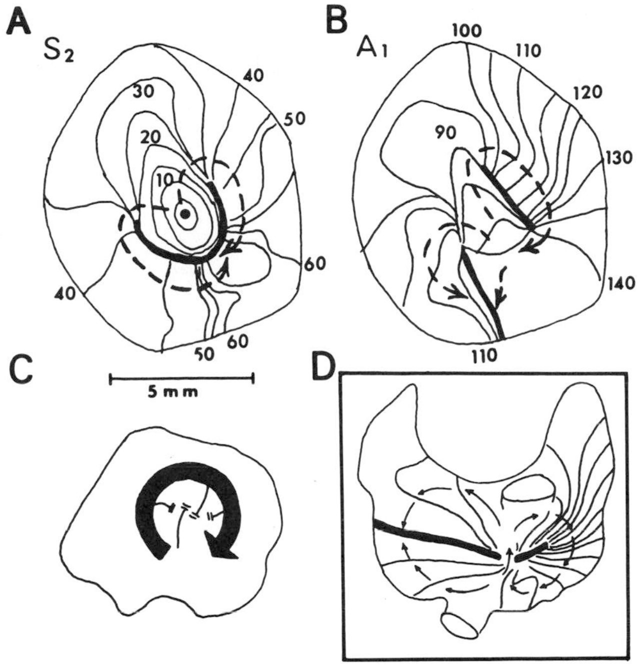

Figure 18-9. *The leading circle model of reentry. A and B are isochronal maps of activation of a premature beat (S_2) and the first reentrant beat (A_1) from an* in vitro *preparation of atrial myocardium of the rabbit. (After Allessie, M. A., Bonke, F. I. M., and Schopman, F. J. G.: Circus movement in rabbit atrial muscle as a mechanism of tachycardia. II. The role of nonuniform recovery of excitability in the occurrence of unidirectional blocks, as studied with multiple microelectrodes. Circ. Res., 39:168, 1976. With permission of the American Heart Association, Inc.) (C) Diagrammatic illustration of the leading circle model. (Allessie, M. A., Bonke, F. I. M., and Schopman, F. J. G.: Circus movement in rabbit atrial muscle as a mechanism of tachycardia. III. The "leading circle" concept: A new model of circus movement in cardiac tissue without the involvement of an anatomical obstacle. Circ. Res., 41:9, 1977. By permission of the American Heart Association, Inc.) (D)* In vivo *isochronal map of atrial activation during atrial flutter in the canine heart showing an activation pattern similar to that in B. See text for details. (After Boineau, J. B., Schussler, R. R., Mooney, C. R., et al.: Natural and evoked atrial flutter due to circus movement in dogs. Role of abnormal atrial pathways, slow conduction, nonuniform refractory period distribution, and premature beats. Am. J. Cardiol., 45:1167, 1980)*

Reflection

The term *reflection* was originally used to describe reentry in a linear bundle of conducting tissue. Longitudinal dissociation of conduction in the bundle resulting in a microreentrant circuit was thought to be the mechanism.[91] Later, Antzelevitch and colleagues described another mechanism that may cause reflection.[18,92–94] If a segment of a bundle of Purkinje fibers is inexcitable, impulses conducting along the bundle will block at this segment (Fig. 18-10*B*). However, the blocked action potential can generate axial current flow through the inexcitable segment of the bundle, which acts as a passive cable. If the inexcitable segment is sufficiently short relative to the length constant, the current flow across the gap can depolarize the excitable fibers distal to the inexcitable region and can excite an action potential (see Fig. 18-10*C*). This action potential, if sufficiently delayed, can itself cause retrograde axial current flow across the inexcitable gap. If the total time for to and fro transmission across the inexcitable gap exceeds the refractory period of the tissue proximal to the site of block, a "reflected" action potential will be generated (see Fig. 18-10*A*). Reflected reentry could perhaps occur in the damaged heart. However, it would be limited to areas where the damage to myocardial fibers was focal, since if the damage were too extensive, electrotonic transmission across the inexcitable area would fail.[95]

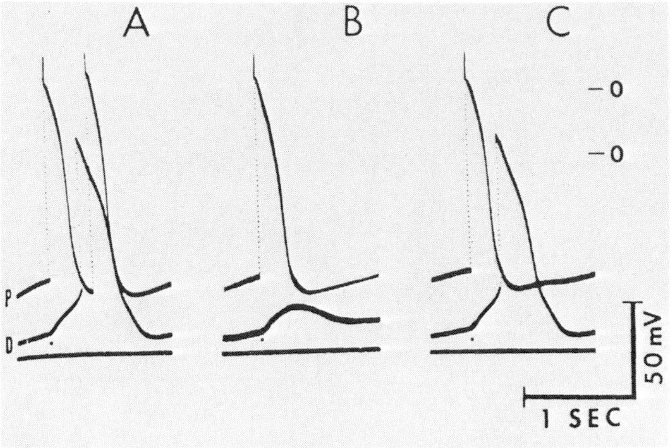

Figure 18-10. *Reflected reentry caused by electrotonic transmission across an excitable gap. Transmembrane potentials recorded from a bundle of Purkinje fibers. The* top *and* middle traces *are recordings from proximal (P) and distal (D) segments separated by an inexcitable region.* Bottom trace *is stimulus marker. In A, the first action potential in the P trace was stimulated and propagated up to the inexcitable region. Excitation occurred distal to the inexcitable region (D) because of electrotonic current flow. The delay before the distal segment was excited was long enough to allow the proximal segment to recover excitability and permitted a reflected action potential. In B, the electrotonic current flow was not sufficient to excite the fiber distal to the excitable region. In C, the distal segment was activated too quickly and reflection did not occur because the proximal segment had not yet recovered excitability. (Antzelevitch, C., Jalife, J., and Moe, G. K.: Characteristics of reflection as a mechanism of reentrant arrhythmias and its relationship to parasystole. Circulation, 61:182, 1980. By permission of the American Heart Association, Inc.)*

Electrocardiographic Patterns

According to the relationship between the VPC and the dominant cardiac rhythm, the ectopic rhythm can be classified as *extrasystolic* or *parasystolic*. In extrasystolic rhythm the VPC in some way depends on or is linked to the dominant cardiac rhythm and generally exhibits a fixed coupling interval to the dominant impulse. The parasystolic rhythm is commonly independent of the dominant cardiac rhythm, and the parasystolic VPC shows varying coupling intervals to the dominant impulse. The classification suggests that extrasystolic and parasystolic rhythms have different electrophysiologic mechanisms. As will be evident from the following discussion, this is probably an oversimplification caused primarily by the difficulty in discerning the electrophysiologic mechanisms of VPCs in clinical records.

Parasystolic Rhythm

The diagnostic criteria[96] for a parasystolic rhythm are (1) marked variation of coupling of ectopic beats during a relatively stable dominant rhythm, (2) interectopic intervals that can be reduced to a least common divisor, and (3) presence of fusion complexes. However, the last criterion is not considered necessary for diagnosis in every case. Parasystole with simple interference is diagnosed when all calculated ectopic impulses that appear at the end of the cardiac refractory period become manifest. Usually the rate of a parasystolic focus with simple interference is lower than that of the dominant rhythm (Fig. 18-11). Parasystole with exit block is suspected when the expected ectopic discharge fails to appear even though it falls outside the cardiac refractory period. Frequently, the rate of parasystolic focus with exit block is faster than that of the dominant cardiac rhythm (Fig. 18-12).

An automatic pacemaker requires entrance block to cause a parasystolic rhythm. Over the years, several mechanisms have been advanced to explain protection of an automatic parasystolic focus. Kaufmann and Rothberger assumed the presence of a zone of protective block surrounding the center in all directions.[97] Vedoya postulated two spherical zones of block surrounding the center, each one with a different refractory period.[98] Scherf argued that protection may result from excitability of the automatic center relative to the strength of the sinus impulse.[99] He also suggested that if the automatic focus has a high inherent frequency of discharge, the mere rapidity of the center will keep it refractory to the invading activation front and precludes its discharge by

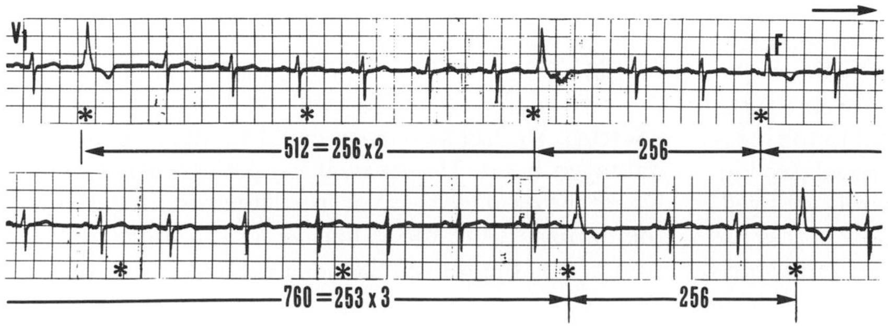

Figure 18-11. *A continuous rhythm strip showing a slow ventricular parasystolic rhythm (rate 23 beats/min) with simple interference with the dominant sinus rhythm. The* asterisks *represent the expected parasystolic discharge. Only those ectopic impulses that fall beyond the cardiac refractory period become manifest. (F, fusion beat)*

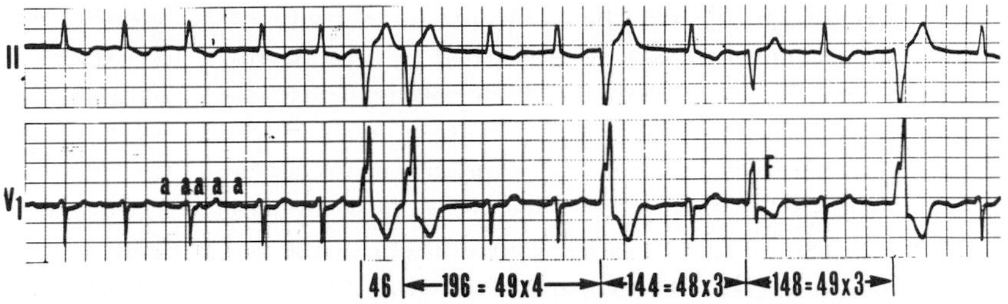

Figure 18-12. *Rapid ventricular parasystolic rhythm (rate 125 beats/min) showing exit block. Note that some expected ectopic discharges fail to appear, although they fall outside the cardiac refractory period. If the last three parasystolic beats were the only ones available for analysis, the parasystolic rate would have been misinterpreted as one third of the actual rate. On the other hand, perpetuation of consecutive ectopic discharge, as seen in the first half of the record, would have resulted in a parasystolic tachycardia. The dominant cardiac rhythm is an atrial tachyarrhythmia with varying AV block. (a, atrial deflections; F, fusion beat)*

the dominant pacemaker.[100,101] The slow diastolic depolarization of pacemaker cells was also suggested as a more plausible explanation of both entrance and exit blocks in the parasystolic focus.[102]

The original assumption of Kaufmann and Rothberger that a parasystolic pacemaker is completely independent and undisturbed by the dominant cardiac rhythm is no longer tenable. Any pacemaker connected to the surrounding tissue by a conducting pathway (entrance block, but exit conduction) is subject to some degree of modulation by the electrotonic effects of activity in that surrounding tissue.[103] The effects of electro-

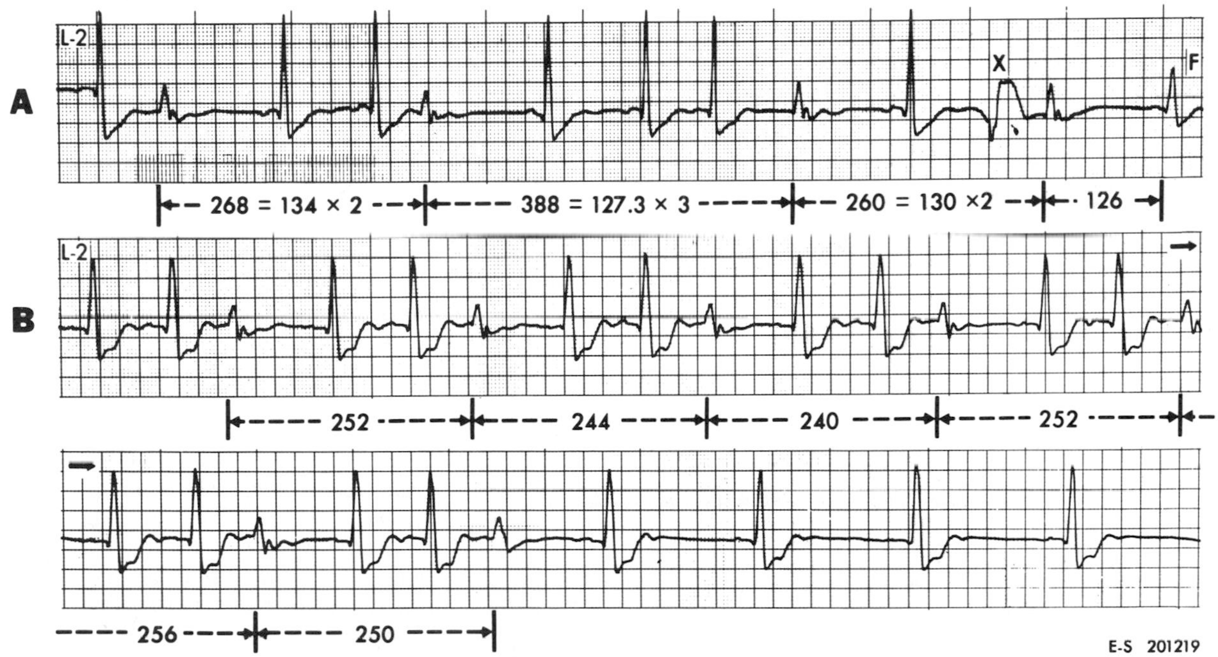

Figure 18-13. *An ectopic focus showing a parasystolic rhythm at one time and an extrasystolic rhythm at other times. The tracings in A and B were obtained from the same patient at two different times. The tracings in A show a ventricular parasystolic rhythm with a calculated rate of discharge of 46 beats/min. Tracings in B illustrate the same ectopic focus now showing a trigeminal extrasystolic rhythm with fixed coupling. Note that the coupling is constant despite slight variation of the sinus rate. In the* bottom rhythm strip, *a 2:1 AV block developed, resulting in slowing of the heart rate and immediate disappearance of the ectopic beats. This also favors an extrasystolic rhythm dependent on a critical rate of the dominant rhythm. The arrhythmia could be explained by electrotonic modulation of an automatic pacemaker.*[94]

tonic depolarizations on the spontaneous activity of automatic pacemakers can be described by a phase-response curve.[25,104] Subthreshold depolarizations induced early in a pacemaker cycle cause a delay in the next spontaneous discharge. Late depolarizations accelerate or capture the pacemaker. One of the consequences of this biphasic influence is the entrainment of the ectopic pacemaker. Because of entrainment, the automatic pacemaker discharge may exhibit fixed coupling to the dominant pacemaker impulses over a wide range of frequency.[103,105] Several clinical cases have been described where the same ectopic focus exhibited a parasystolic rhythm at one time and an extrasystolic rhythm at other times[106,107] (Fig. 18-13). Electrotonic modulation of an automatic pacemaker provides a possible explanation for these cases.[105] This mechanism can result in a continuous spectrum that can manifest as an extrasystolic rhythm, modulated (nonclassic) parasystole, or classic parasystole[103,105] (Fig. 18-14).

Electrotonic modulation of an automatic pacemaker may also explain some cases of intermittent parasystole. The arrhythmia should be suspected when a long interectopic interval is not a multiple of the calculated parasystolic cycle length, provided that an irregular or Wenckebach-type exit block from the parasystolic focus is excluded.[96,108–111] Almost all cases of intermittent parasystole have fixed coupling of the first beat of an intermittent series. This has been attributed to temporary loss of protection of the parasystolic focus, resulting in discharge and resetting of the parasystolic rhythm by beats of the dominant rhythm.[108,110] In these cases, the distance between the first parasystolic beat in a series and a preceding, presumably interrupting, beat of the dominant rhythm will be approximately equal to or a multiple of the parasystolic cycle length (Fig. 18-15). Some instances in which the fixedly coupled extrasystolic beat occurred earlier than the expected parasystolic impulse were explained by suggesting that the preceding sinus impulse "forced" premature discharge of the parasystolic focus.[108] The enhancing effect of the sinus beat on the parasystolic pacemaker was ascribed to the phenomenon of Wedensky facilitation.[112] However, Jalife and colleagues presented evidence that many published examples of intermittent parasystole may have been the result of electrotonic modulation of an ectopic pacemaker across an area of depressed excitability,[105] in line with their originally published mathematical model.[113]

The underlying electrophysiologic mechanisms for

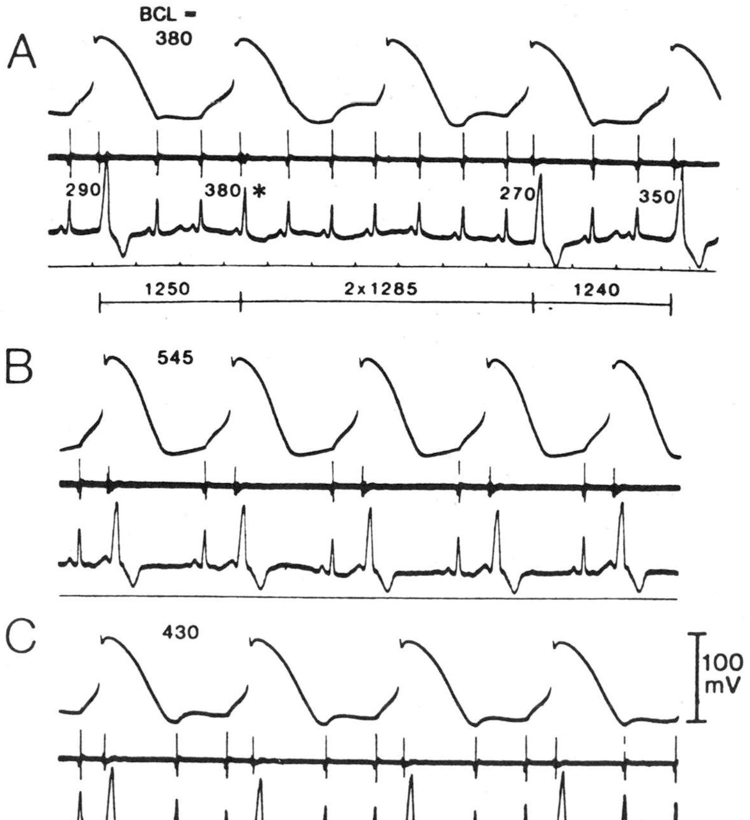

Figure 18-14. *Pacemaker modulation. The recordings were obtained from an experimental model in which a protected ectopic focus was created in tissue excised from a canine heart and was allowed to interact with the activity of the intact heart of another dog. The protected focus consisted of a Purkinje fiber in which a narrow central zone was rendered inexcitable.* Traces *from top to bottom are transmembrane potentials from the protected focus and right ventricular electrogram and lead II electrocardiogram from the* in vivo *preparation. The protected focus exhibited pacemaker activity with an intrinsic cycle length of 1530 msec. In A, atrial pacing was applied at a cycle length of 380 msec. The automatic pacemaker exhibited a parasystolic arrangement. The numbers above the electrocardiogram tracing represent the coupling intervals of the ectopic responses to the preceding normal beats in milliseconds. Note varying coupling intervals, an interectopic interval that can be reduced to a least common divisor, and a fusion beat* (asterisk), *all characteristics of a parasystolic rhythm. In B and C, atrial pacing at cycle lengths of 545 and 430 msec, respectively, resulted in typical extrasystolic rhythm with fixed coupling in a bigeminal arrangement in B and a trigeminal arrangement in C. (From Antzelevitch, C., Bernstein, M. J., Feldman, H. N., and Moe, G. K.: Parasystole, reentry and tachycardia: A canine preparation of cardiac arrhythmias, occurring across inexcitable segments of tissue. Circulation, 68:1101, 1983. With permission of the American Heart Association.)*

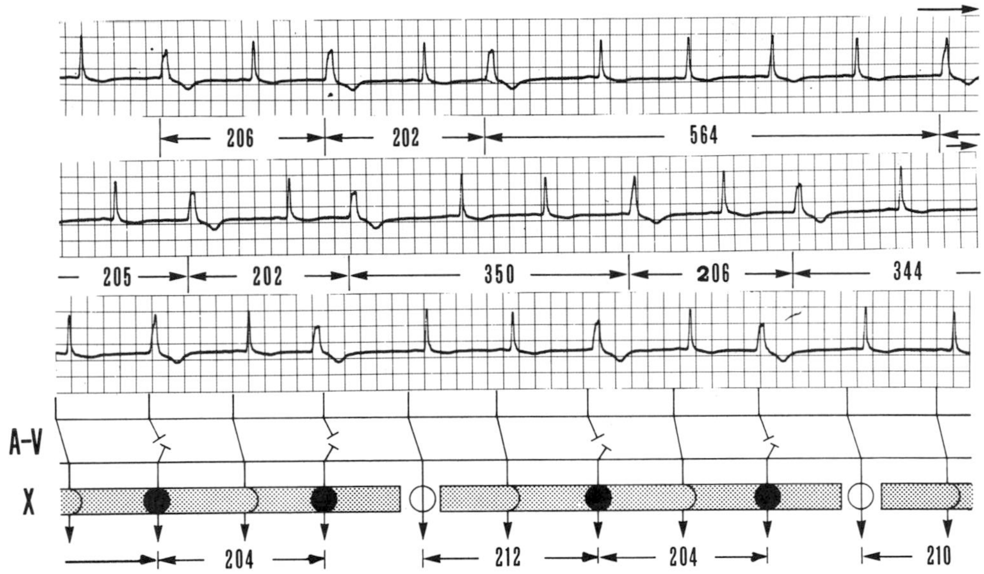

Figure 18-15. *Intermittent ventricular parasystole. This figure shows periodic bigeminal rhythm with gradual shortening of the coupling interval of consecutive ectopic beats but constant interectopic intervals establishing the parasystolic nature of the ectopic discharge. The coupling interval of the first parasystolic beat in each series is fixed at 1.04 to 1.08 second. However, interectopic intervals are not multiples of the shorter ones and have no simple common denominator. These are the characteristics of an intermittent parasystolic rhythm. The* ladder diagram *at the bottom of the figure explains the mechanism of intermittent parasystole on the basis of temporary loss of entrance block as well as the mechanism of fixed coupling of the first beat in a parasystolic series. AV indicates the atrioventricular junction. The* horizontal stippled bars *represent protection at the level of the parasystolic focus within the ventricles, and the* blank spaces *in between indicate temporary loss of the protective entrance block.* Solid circles *represent spontaneous firing of the parasystolic focus (X).* Vertical arrows *that circumvent the area of the parasystolic focus indicate sinus beats that do not interrupt the parasystolic rhythm.* Vertical arrows *transecting the blank spaces and the open circles represent sinus beats that enter, depolarize, and reset the parasystolic center. The numbers below the stippled bars indicate intervals between successive parasystolic beats or between interrupting sinus beats and the next manifest parasystolic discharge. Note that the interval between an interrupting sinus beat and the next manifest parasystolic discharge is approximately equal to the manifest parasystolic cycle length.*

the genesis of the parasystolic automatic pacemaker are difficult to discern in clinical records. It is, however, possible for normal automaticity, abnormal automaticity, and triggered activity to cause a parasystolic rhythm if the focus is protected by entrance block. Figure 18-16 illustrates a triggered rhythm arising from delayed afterdepolarizations in an ischemic endocardial preparation from 1-day-old canine infarction showing entrance block characteristic of a parasystolic rhythm. The ectopic focus also shows (1) intermittent triggered activity, (2) gradual slowing of the frequency of discharge, and (3) varying degrees of exit block including 2 : 1 block and Wenckebach conduction. The figure clearly illustrates the potential difficulties in diagnosing parasystolic rhythms in clinical records based on mathematical manipulation of interectopic intervals of manifest ectopic discharge. In addition to intermittent parasystolic pacemaker discharge, it is possible that the inherent rate of the pacemaker and the degree of exit block can vary concomitantly in response to cardiotropic drugs, electrolyte abnormalities, or autonomic impulses. This change could be responsible for the failure to unravel the exact nature of the ectopic rhythm.

Extrasystolic Rhythm

Extrasystolic VPCs exhibit fixed coupling to the dominant cardiac rhythm, which suggests that the ectopic impulse in some way depends on or is linked to the dominant rhythm. Extrasystoles may occur in repetitive patterns. One (or more) extrasystoles may follow every sinus beat (bigeminy), every other sinus beat (trigeminy), every third sinus beat (quadrigeminy), and so on. Although, by definition, extrasystoles show relatively fixed

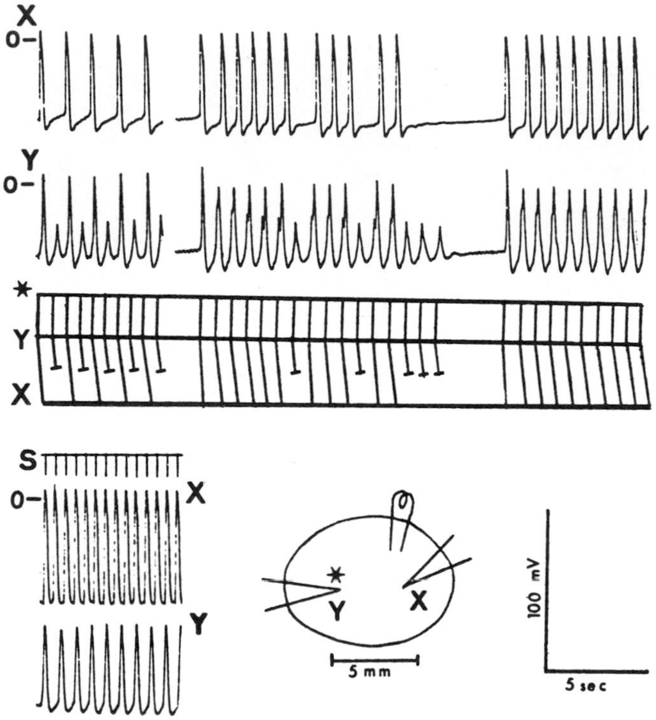

Figure 18-16. *Intermittent parasystolic rhythm due to a triggered automatic pacemaker showing both entrance and exit block. Transmembrane recordings from two Purkinje fibers (X and Y) in the ischemic zone of an endocardial preparation from a 1-day-old canine infarction (see schematic drawing). The recordings show intermittent triggered activity arising from delayed afterdepolarizations. The focus of triggered activity was probably located close to the Y recording* (asterisk), *and a varying degree of conduction delay or block or both occurred between the two sites. The Y recording showed electrotonic depolarizations that corresponded to the rhythmic discharge of the ectopic focus. Conduction delays between the two sites resulted in an electrotonic depolarization followed by a second larger upstroke in the Y recording. When conduction block occurred, the Y recording revealed only an electrotonic depolarization. In contrast to the Y recording, which could reveal the rhythmic activity of the ectopic focus, the X recording that was a few millimeters distant from the ectopic focus only showed delayed conducted action potentials. Each series of triggered activity was initiated by an action potential that was probably generated by background slow Purkinje automaticity arising from a different site in the preparation.*[34] *The exit block between the focus of triggered activity and the rest of the preparation varied from 2:1 block* (top left tracing) *to Wenckebach periodicity* (top middle tracing) *to first degree block* (top right tracing). *There was also a period of repetitive conduction block at the end of the middle series of triggered activity. Diagrammatic illustration of the conduction pattern from the ectopic focus is shown at the* bottom *of the* upper tracings. *The tracing at the* lower left corner *shows that when the preparation was stimulated (S) at a rate faster than the ectopic focus, entrance block was present. Besides the intermittence of the triggered activity and the varying degree of exit block, the tracings also show that frequency of discharge between each new series of triggered activity gradually slowed. All these factors combined can make it very difficult to diagnose parasystolic rhythms in clinical records based on mathematical manipulation of interectopic intervals of manifest ectopic discharge.*

coupling, variable coupling as well as other characteristic variations in coupling (*e.g.*, gradual lengthening of coupling of successive beats) may also be seen.[114] Several possible electrophysiologic mechanisms can account for extrasystolic VPCs, although it is difficult in clinical records to decide which mechanism is involved.

Reflected Reentry

Electrotonic depolarizations across a localized region of inexcitability, as shown in Figures 18-10 and 18-14, can give rise to extrasystolic VPCs.[18,92–94,103] The area distal to the inexcitable region may have intrinsic pacemaker characteristics. The incidence and patterns of manifest ectopic activity based on reflected reentry depend greatly on heart rate. A direct relationship between ectopic incidence and heart rate exists when conduction across the depressed zone ranges between 1 : 1 and 2 : 1 (*e.g.*, 5 : 4, 4 : 3, 3 : 2), but an inverse relationship occurs at higher level of conduction impairment (*e.g.*, 2 : 1 to 5 : 1).

Circus Movement Reentry

Extrasystolic VPCs due to circus movement reentry were directly demonstrated in the postinfarction canine heart by isochronal mapping of ventricular activation.[90] Reentrant beats with regular extrasystolic grouping are caused by characteristic tachycardia-dependent conduction disorders in a potential reentrant pathway. A bigeminal rhythm results from a 2 : 1 conduction pattern in a reentrant pathway.[114] On the other hand, a trigeminal rhythm is attributed to a 3 : 2 Wenckebach conduction sequence in the reentrant pathway (Figs. 18-17 and 18-18). A quadrigeminal rhythm could represent either a 4 : 3 Wenckebach conduction cycle or an underlying bigeminal rhythm with concealment of alternate reentrant beats, that is, concealed bigeminy (Fig. 18-19*A*). Although longer Wenckebach cycles can occasionally be seen (see Fig. 18-18), a regular pentageminy or hexageminy is rarely due to successive 5 : 4 or 6 : 5 conduction ratios, respectively. However, pentageminy is easily explained by the not uncommon regular alternation of 2 : 1 and 3 : 2 conduction cycles (see Fig. 18-19*A*). Hexageminy can be a manifestation of concealed trigeminy.[114]

Triggered Activity Due to Early Afterdepolarizations

Figure 18-2 shows that triggered action potentials arising from early afterdepolarizations can cause extrasystolic grouping (bigeminy, trigeminy) with fixed coupling to the preceding impulse. Extrasystolic beats based on early afterdepolarizations should be more pronounced at long cycle lengths and could be markedly attenuated or abolished at short cycle lengths (see Fig. 18-2). This mechanism may explain bradycardia-dependent ventricular arrhythmias seen in the setting of acute myocardial infarction[115] and in patients with high-grade AV block.[48,149] The multiform ventricular tachyarrhythmia commonly called *torsades de pointes* is also seen in patients with drug-induced prolongation of the QT (or QU) interval.[50] Figure 18-20 illustrates one example of bradycardia-dependent multiform ventricular rhythm (torsades de pointes) in a patient with quinindine toxicity that markedly prolonged the QT interval. The arrhythmia characteristically followed long cardiac cycles associated with bizarre configuration of the ST-T segment and further prolongation of the QT interval. Every episode of ventricular tachyarrhythmia was ushered in by an extrasystolic beat with fixed coupling to the preceding supraventricular beat. The extrasystolic beat seemed to arise from the terminal part of the T wave. Extrasystolic beats arising from early afterdepolarizations should characteristically exhibit a close coupling to the preceding supraventricular rhythm and represent one possible mechanism for VPCs showing the R-on-T phenomenon.

Triggered Activity Due to Delayed Afterdepolarizations

Figure 18-21*A* illustrates that triggered action potentials arising from delayed afterdepolarizations can give rise to extrasystolic grouping. In contrast to extrasystoles based on early afterdepolarizations, those resulting from delayed afterdepolarizations should characteristically occur after the end of the T wave, resulting in late coupled VPCs[70] (see Fig. 18-21*B*). Both extrasystolic beats with late coupling and accelerated ventricular rhythms that occur in the first few days following myocardial infarction may be caused by triggered activity arising from delayed afterdepolarizations in ischemic Purkinje fibers[71] (see Fig. 18-21*B*). Like other mechanisms that can cause an extrasystolic rhythm, ectopic rhythm due to delayed afterdepolarizations also depends on the cycle length of the dominant rhythm (see Fig. 18-3). Figure 18-22 illustrates a clinical record of an extrasystolic rhythm dependent on critical shortening of the sinus cycle length (*i.e.*, tachycardia dependent). The arrhythmia is an example of "extrasystolie ventriculaire ā paroxysmes tachycardiques prolongées," first described by Gallavardin.[116] The arrhythmia is intermediate between isolated VPCs and sustained ventricular tachycardia and extends from a single couplet to a nonsustained ventricular tachycardia. Several recent observations suggest that the initial extrasystole does not follow the same rules as the repetitive activity, thus favoring two different electrophysiologic mechanisms probably occurring in the same myocardial area.[117] The initial extrasystole may be due to reflected reentry or a modulated parasystolic focus, while the repetitive rhythm may result from triggered activity.

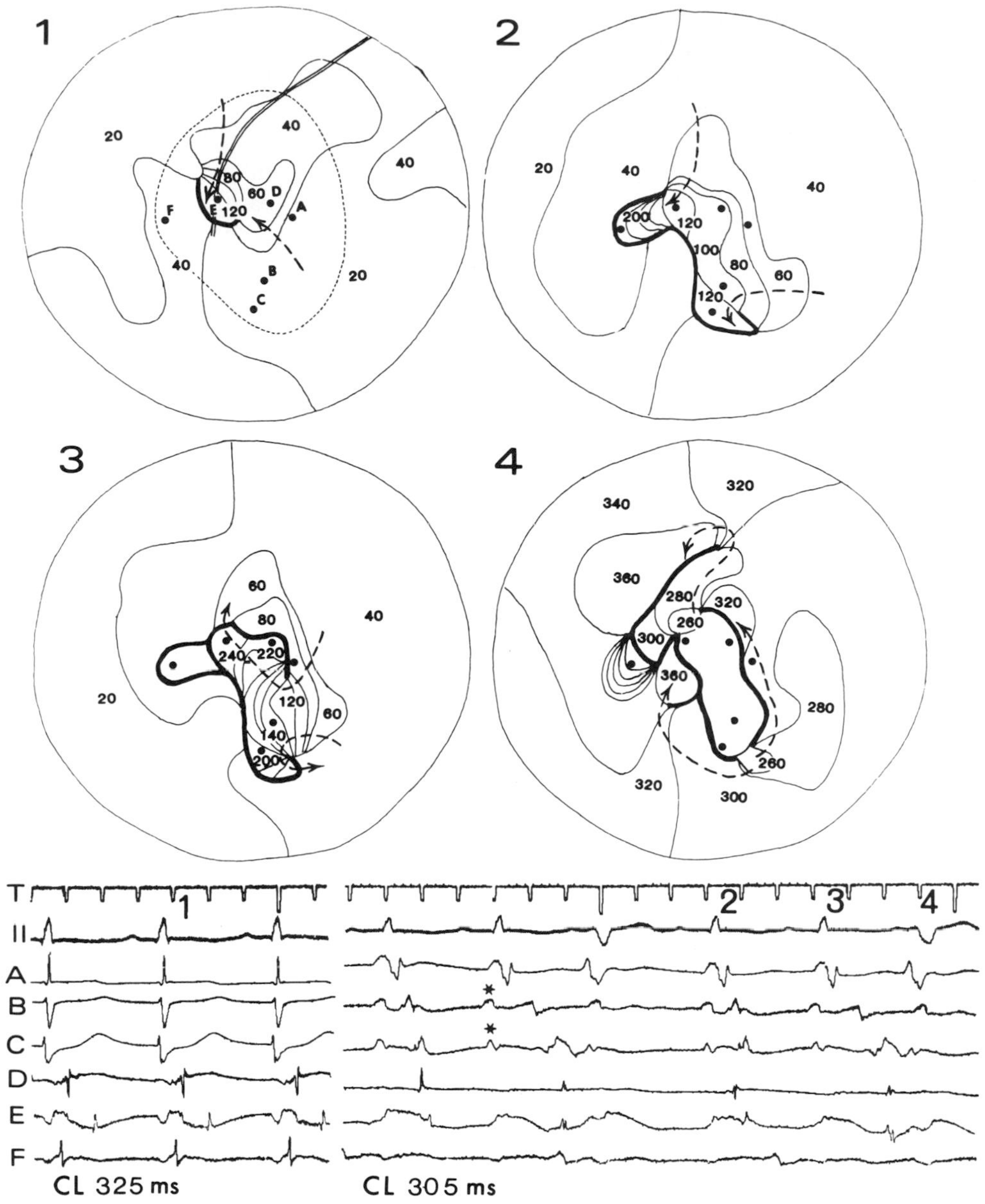

Concealed Extrasystoles

Attention was focused on the phenomenon of concealed extrasystoles when Schamroth and Marriott coined the term *concealed bigeminy.*[109] These authors noted that in electrocardiographic records containing apparently haphazard distribution of extrasystoles, the interectopic intervals always consisted of an odd number of sinus beats, that is, 3, 5, 7, and so on (2 or its multiples +1). This suggested that the bigeminal rhythm probably persisted in a concealed form. These authors later described records of concealed trigeminy, with the intervening number of sinus beats being 3 or its multiples plus 2 (*e.g.,* 5, 8, 11).[118] Other recordings that did not conform to these calculations were ascribed to fluctuation between concealed bigeminy and trigeminy. As discussed in the preceding section, the mechanisms of reflected reentry, circus movement reentry, and triggered activity can all cause concealed extrasystoles (see Fig. 18-19). Schamroth and Marriott alluded to the practical importance of the recognition of concealed extrasystoles in a clinical record, since these imply a state of greater ectopic irritability than is apparent.[118] Concealed extrasystoles, as originally described and diagnosed using rigid mathematical formulas,[109,118] are uncommon. With the recent understanding of conduction patterns across the inexcitable gap in reflected reentry as well as the conduction patterns during circus movement reentry, specifically the common alternation of 2:1 and 3:2 conduction sequences,[144] concealed extrasystoles may be a common occurrence. The prognostic significance of concealed

Figure 18-17. *Isochronal maps of a trigeminal rhythm due to circus movement reentry. The figure illustrates epicardial activation maps as well as selected electrographic recordings from a dog 4 days after infarction in which a reentrant trigeminal rhythm developed during sinus tachycardia. Epicardial activation is displayed as if the heart is viewed from the cardiac apex located at the center of the circular map. The perimeter of the circle represents the AV junction. This display is helpful in illustrating reentrant circuits located around the cardiac apex. The epicardial map of a sinus beat at a cycle length of 325 msec is labeled 1. Spontaneous shortening of the sinus cycle length to 305 msec resulted in the development of a single reentrant beat following every second sinus beat. The maps labeled 2, 3, and 4 represent the first and second sinus beats and the reentrant beat, respectively. The* dotted line *in map 1 represents the epicardial outline of the ischemic zone. The left anterior descending (LAD) artery is represented by a* double line. *During sinus rhythm at a cycle length of 325 msec there was a consistent small arc of functional conduction block near the apical region of the infarct* (heavy solid line) *and relatively slow activation of nearby myocardial zones. The activation pattern, however, was constant in successive beats, reflecting a 1:1 conduction pattern. During the reentrant trigeminal rhythm, the epicardial activation map of the first sinus beat showed the development of a longer arc of functional conduction block compared to the one during sinus rhythm at a cycle length of 325 msec. The activation front circulated around both ends of the arc of block but was not sufficiently delayed on the distal side of the arc of block. On the other hand, the activation map of the second sinus beat showed some lengthening of the arc of block at one end but, more characteristically, a much slower conduction of the two activation fronts circulating around both ends of the arc of block. The degree of conduction delay was sufficient for refractoriness to expire at two separate sites on the proximal side of the arc, resulting in two simultaneous breakthroughs close to the ends of the arc, thus initiating reentrant excitation. The leading edge of the two reentrant wavefronts coalesced but failed to conduct to the central part of the epicardial surface of the infarct (i.e., to areas showing slow conduction during the preceding cycle). This limited the reentrant process to a single cycle. It also resulted in recovery of those myocardial zones in the central part of the infarct, allowing the next sinus beat to conduct with a lesser degree of conduction delay, thus perpetuating the reentrant trigeminal rhythm. Analysis of the two electrograms recorded from each of the two reentrant pathways (B and C, and D and E, respectively) show a characteristic 3:2 Wenckebach-like conduction pattern. The* asterisks *refer to electrotonic deflections. The figure also illustrates the complexity of the conduction pattern in ischemic myocardium and the presence of a zone of dissociated conduction. This is represented by site F, which showed a 2:1 conduction pattern during the 3:2 Wenckebach cycle and reentrant trigeminal rhythm described previously. (El-Sherif, N., Gough, W. B., Zeiler, R. H., and Hariman, R.: Reentrant ventricular arrhythmias in the late myocardial infarction period. 12. Spontaneous versus induced reentry and intramural versus epicardial circuits. J. Am. Coll. Cardiol., 6:124, 1985. With permission of the American College of Cardiology)*

versus manifest extrasystoles has not been fully elucidated. However, since they may be more common than originally thought, the established practice of using the frequency of manifest VPCs in clinical records as a prognostic marker and as a guide to the efficacy of antiarrhythmic therapy may not be as useful as once believed.

Multiform VPCs

Multiform VPCs are often associated with organic heart disease, and patients with them are usually considered at high risk (see Fig. 18-13). Several early workers stressed a high incidence of sudden death in this group of patients due, presumably, to ventricular fibrillation.[99,119–121] However, in those reports, neither the electrophysiologic mechanism for the genesis of multiform ventricular ectopic rhythm nor the casual relationship of the arrhythmia to sudden death was clearly established. In a study of patients with multiform VPCs, the concurrent discharge of multiple parasystolic rhythms was found to contribute, in part, to the multiform activity.[122] Although all patients had advanced organic heart disease, and 80% of them died within 2 to 16 months, there was no sudden cardiac death and the arrhythmia did not seem directly related to mortality in any patient. Multiform ventricular rhythms are commonly seen in the first few days following myocardial infarction in both human and dogs. *In vitro* studies of endocardial preparations from 1-day-old canine infarction have shown that both entrance and exit block commonly occur around sites of triggered activity[34] (see Fig. 18-16). It is possible that

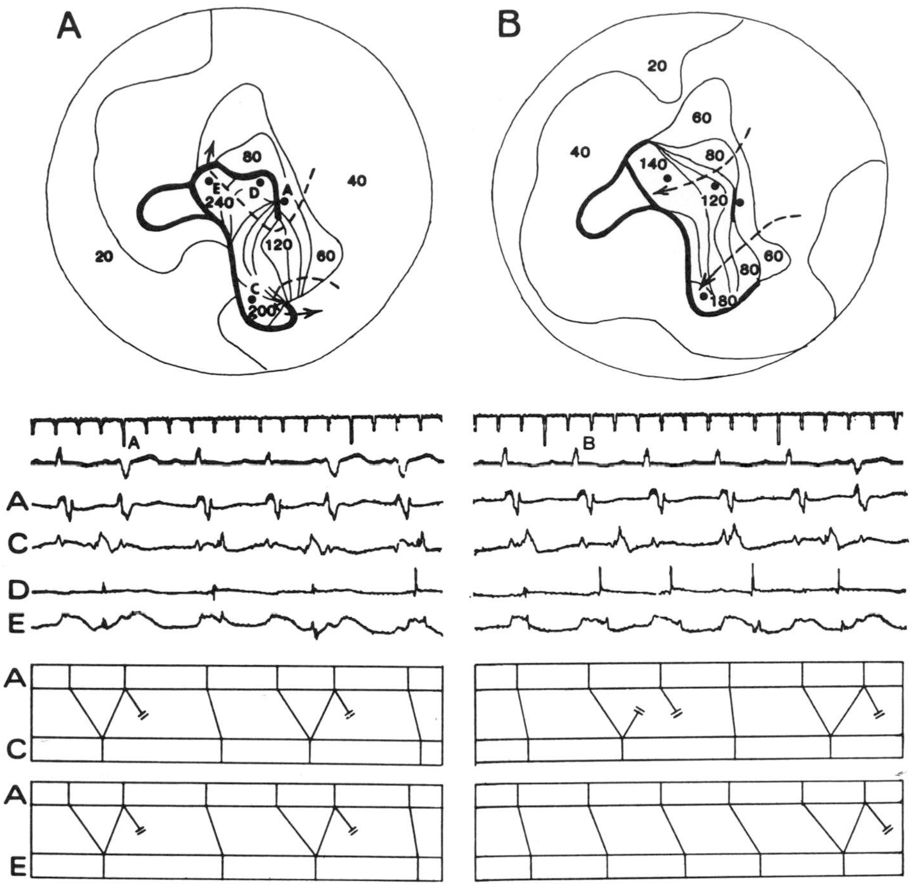

Figure 18-18. *Concealed extrasystolic rhythm due to circus movement reentry. The figure was obtained from the same experiment shown in Figure 18-17. The left side of the figure (A) shows a manifest trigeminal rhythm at a cycle length of 305 msec. Repetitive reentrant excitation is seen at the end of the recording. The epicardial activation map of the sinus beat that initiated reentry (labeled A) is shown on the top, while selected electrograms are shown on the bottom. The* ladder diagram *illustrates the conduction pattern between site A located outside the arc of functional conduction block and sites C and E within the slow conduction zone. As shown in Figure 18-17, electrograms C, D, and E illustrate a 3:2 Wenckebach conduction sequence. The right side of the figure (B) illustrates a concealed trigeminal rhythm at the same sinus cycle length during manifest reentry. The activation map of the second sinus beat that was supposed to initiate reentry (labeled B) is shown on the top. Compared to the map in* A, *the arc of functional conduction block is shorter. More important, the circulating wavefronts around the two ends of the arc show less conduction delay. The* ladder diagram *shows that a 3:2 Wenckebach conduction pattern continued during the concealed trigeminal sequence in one of the two reentrant pathways represented by electrogram C. However, the circulating wavefront arrived to site C 20 msec earlier during concealed trigeminy compared to manifest reentry. On the other hand, there was a concomitant 6:5 Wenckebach conduction sequence in the other reentrant pathway, represented by electrograms D and E. This, in addition to other sites that were, at the same time, showing a 2:1 conduction pattern (see site F in Fig. 18-17), illustrates a high degree of dissociated conduction in the ischemic zone even though the surface electrocardiogram may show a rather regular extrasystolic pattern. (El-Sherif, N., Gough, W. B., Zeiler, R. H., and Hariman, R.: Reentrant ventricular arrhythmias in the late myocardial infarction period. 12. Spontaneous versus induced reentry and intramural versus epicardial circuits. J. Am. Coll. Cardiol., 6:124, 1985. By permission of the American College of Cardiology)*

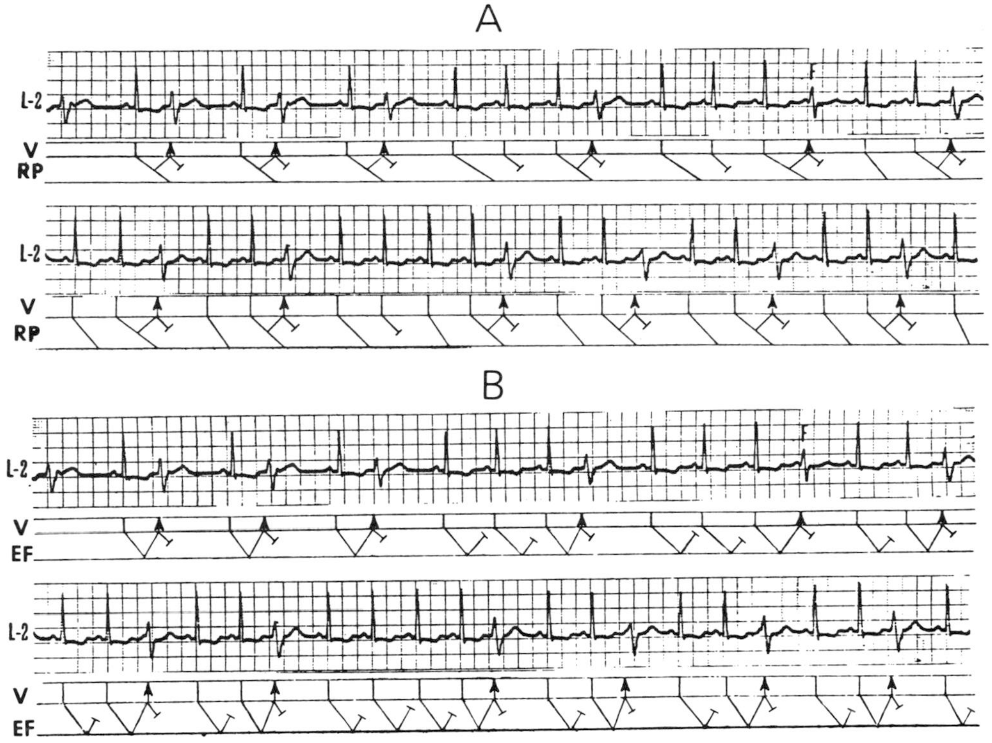

Figure 18-19. *Electrocardiographic tracings from a patient 5 days after an acute myocardial infarction showing an extrasystolic rhythm with periods of manifest bigeminy and trigeminy. The arrhythmia could be explained either by circus movement reentry (*ladder diagram *under A) or by reflected reentry or triggered activity (*ladder diagram *under B). In A, the bigeminal rhythm is explained by a 2:1 conduction pattern in the reentrant pathway (RP), while the trigeminal rhythm is due to a 3:2 Wenckebach sequence. Quadrigeminy and pentageminy could be explained, respectively, by concealed bigeminy and successive 2:1 and 3:2 Wenckebach cycles. Experimental evidence for extrasystolic rhythms based on reflected reentry and on triggered activity are shown in Figures 18-14 and 18-21, respectively. (V, ventricle; EF, ectopic focus)*

multiform ventricular rhythms in postinfarction patients are caused by triggered activity arising from multiple foci of ischemic Purkinje fibers.[71]

Clinical Significance

The three current approaches for evaluating ventricular electrical instability are discussed below.

1. *The categorization and stratification of spontaneous ventricular arrhythmias from standard surface electrocardiographic recordings including long-term ambulatory electrocardiographic monitoring.* A grading system for VPCs was first suggested by Lown.[123] Originally intended to classify VPCs in the setting of acute myocardial infarction, the grading system was soon used to classify VPCs in patients with chronic ischemic and other organic heart diseases. Although multivariate statistical techniques have suggested that frequent and complex ventricular arrhythmias may independently identify patients at high risk of sudden electrical cardiac death,[124–126] other studies have cast doubt on their usefulness.[127] A major criticism of the grading system is the apparent arbitrary assignment of high grades to certain VPC characteristics, for instance, the R-on-T phenomenon, without solid experimental or clinical evidence that these higher grades carry higher risk.[128,129] An obvious weakness of the concept of prognostic categorization of VPCs from standard electrocardiographic recordings is that it does not consider one crucial characteristic, namely, the underlying electrophysiologic mechanism.[129] Ventricular premature contractions secondary to reflected reentry, circus movement reentry, or triggered activity may not have the same prognostic significance. One more problem with the long-term ambulatory electrocardiographic recording is the great variability of spontaneous ventricular arrhythmias.[130–132]

2. *Programmed electrical stimulation.* Programmed electrical stimulation has been used in the diagnosis and

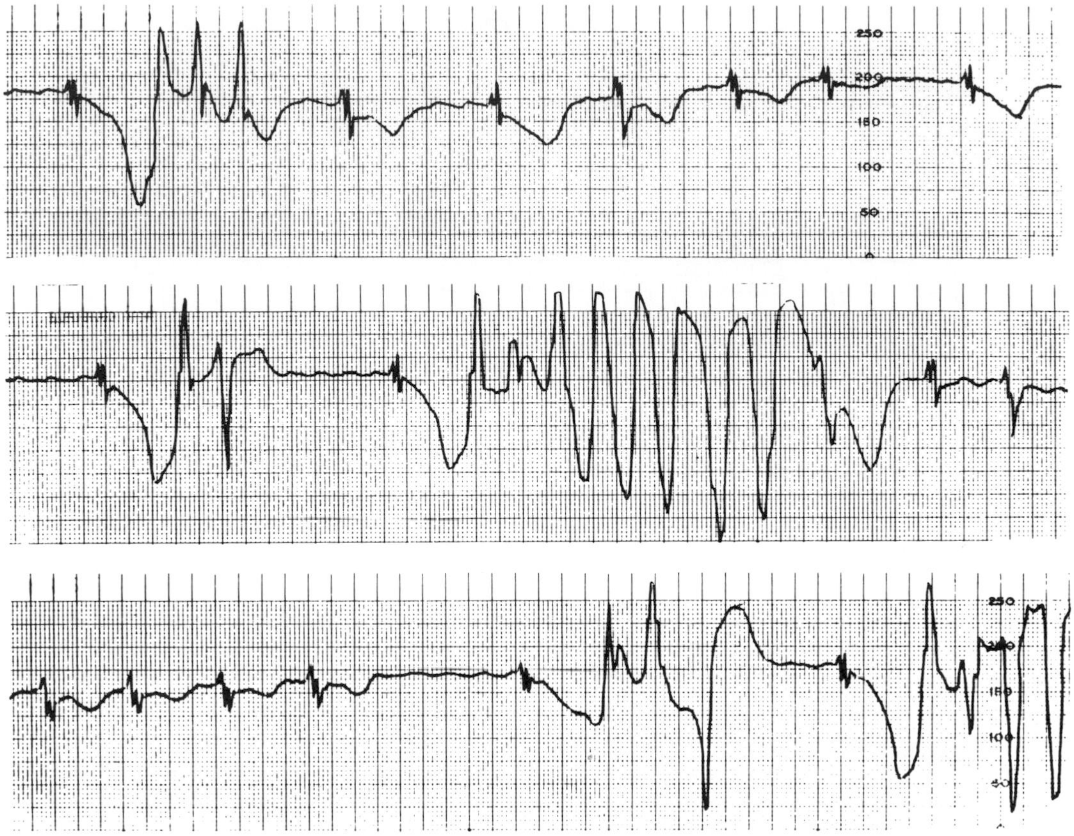

Figure 18-20. *Electrocardiographic tracings showing bradycardia-dependent multiform ventricular rhythm (torsades de pointes) in a patient aged 55 years with quinidine toxicity. The patient was receiving digoxin and quinidine sulfate to control atrial fibrillation with rapid ventricular response and ventricular ectopic beats. Note marked prolongation of the QT interval. The arrhythmia characteristically followed long cardiac cycles that resulted in further prolongation of the QT interval associated with bizarre configuration of the ST-T complex. Each episode of ventricular tachyarrhythmia was initiated by an extrasystolic beat with fixed coupling to the preceding supraventricular beat. The extrasystolic beat seemed to arise from the terminal part of the T wave (R-on-T phenomenon). The arrhythmia may be explained by triggered activity arising from early afterdepolarizations, as shown in Figure 18-2.*

management of patients with recurrent sustained ventricular tachycardia and in survivors of out-of-hospital cardiac arrest.[133–138] Ventricular tachyarrhythmias induced by programmed electrical stimulation are probably based on circus movement reentry,[138] although triggered activity arising from delayed afterdepolarizations cannot be definitely excluded.[34] Programmed cardiac stimulation can induce clinical ventricular tachyarrhythmia in approximately 75% to 90% of patients.[133,135–138] Further, antiarrhythmic agents that prevent the induction of ventricular tachyarrhythmias in the electrophysiology laboratory abolish or decrease the frequency of spontaneous tachyarrhythmias and reduce mortality in patients with out-of-hospital ventricular fibrillation. However, the clinical significance of induced nonsustained ventricular tachycardia is not clear. Both sustained and nonsustained tachycardias have been induced in patients with no documented spontaneous tachyarrhythmias.[140,141] The prognostic significance of such a finding is, again, not well established.

Ventricular premature contractions form the bulk of ventricular arrhythmias are seen in clinical practice. The significance and treatment of VPCs in patients without spontaneous ventricular tachyarrhythmia, those who suffered an out-of-hospital cardiac arrest, and those with a history of syncope remain speculative at best. A recent study suggests that programmed electrical stimulation and ventricular ejection fraction can define high- and low-risk subsets for sudden death among patients with high-grade VPCs. Patients in whom ventricular tachyarrhythmias are not inducible and those with ejection fraction of greater than 40% had a low incidence of sudden

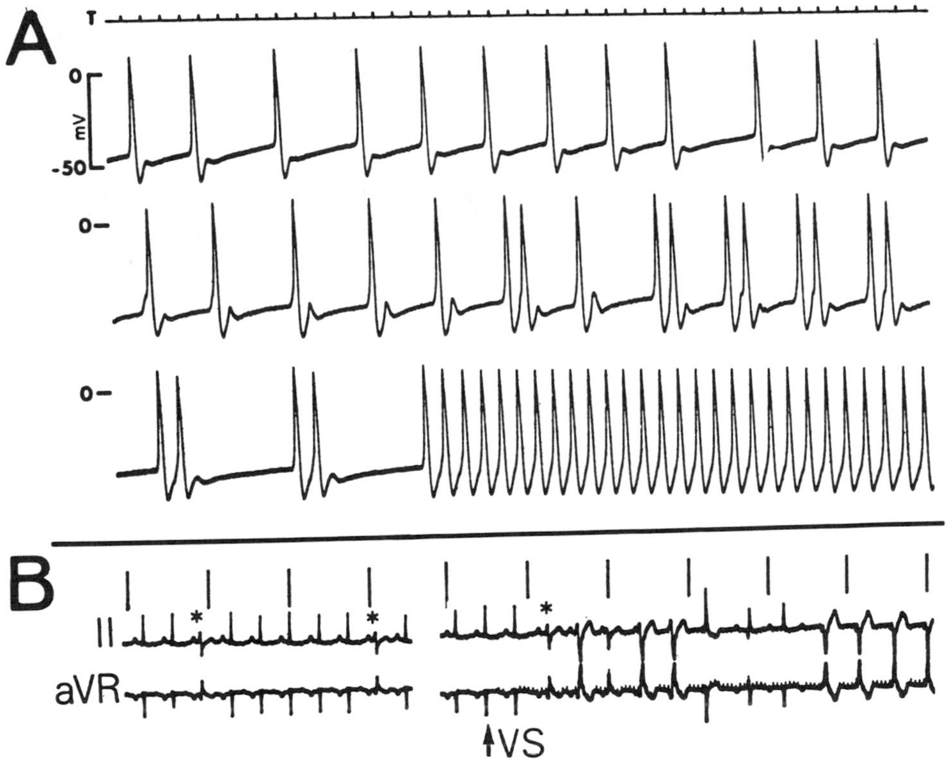

Figure 18-21. *Extrasystolic rhythm due to triggered activity arising from delayed afterdepolarizations. (A) Transmembrane recording from a Purkinje fiber in the ischemic zone of an endocardial preparation from 1-day-old canine infarction. The* upper tracing *shows a background slow automatic rhythm. Each automatic action potential is followed by a low-amplitude delayed afterdepolarization. In the* middle tracing, *the amplitude of the delayed afterdepolarization gradually increased, reached threshold, and triggered a single action potential resulting in a trigeminal rhythm followed by a bigeminal rhythm. In the* lower tracing, *a sustained triggered activity occurred when the subthreshold afterdepolarization that followed the single triggered action potential reached threshold potential. (El-Sherif, N., Gough, W. B., Zeiler, R. H., and Mehra, R.: Triggered ventricular rhythms in 1-day-old myocardial infarction in the dog. Circ. Res., 52:566, 1983. By permission of the American Heart Association, Inc.) (B) Electrocardiographic tracing obtained from a dog 1 day after ligation of the left anterior descending artery. The tracing shows sinus tachycardia and extrasystolic premature ventricular contractions with late fixed coupling* (asterisks). *Slight slowing of the sinus rhythm by vagal stimulation (VS) revealed the presence of a multiform ventricular rhythm. The extrasystolic beats and the multiform ventricular rhythm may be the result of triggered activity arising from delayed afterdepolarizations in ischemic Purkinje fibers surviving the infarct.*[71]

death and an excellent 1- to 2-year survival rate.[141] These patients may not need prophylactic antiarrhythmic therapy.

At least two major limitations of programmed electrical stimulation exist at present. First, no unanimity exists on the most sensitive and specific techniques for programmed stimulation; second, the technique is invasive and therefore less suitable for repeated follow-up evaluations.

3. *Direct recording of delayed depolarization potentials (late potentials).* Delayed activation potentials were initially described from the ischemic regions of the canine heart.[114,142–146] The relation between delayed ventricular activation in ischemic myocardial zones and ventricular arrhythmias based on circus movement of excitation in the postinfarction canine heart has been extensively investigated.[85–87,147,148] In recent years, attempts have been made to measure late potentials noninvasively in patients. The problem in identifying late potentials on the body surface is that the signal is smaller than the electrical noise produced by various sources. Two different techniques have been used to improve the

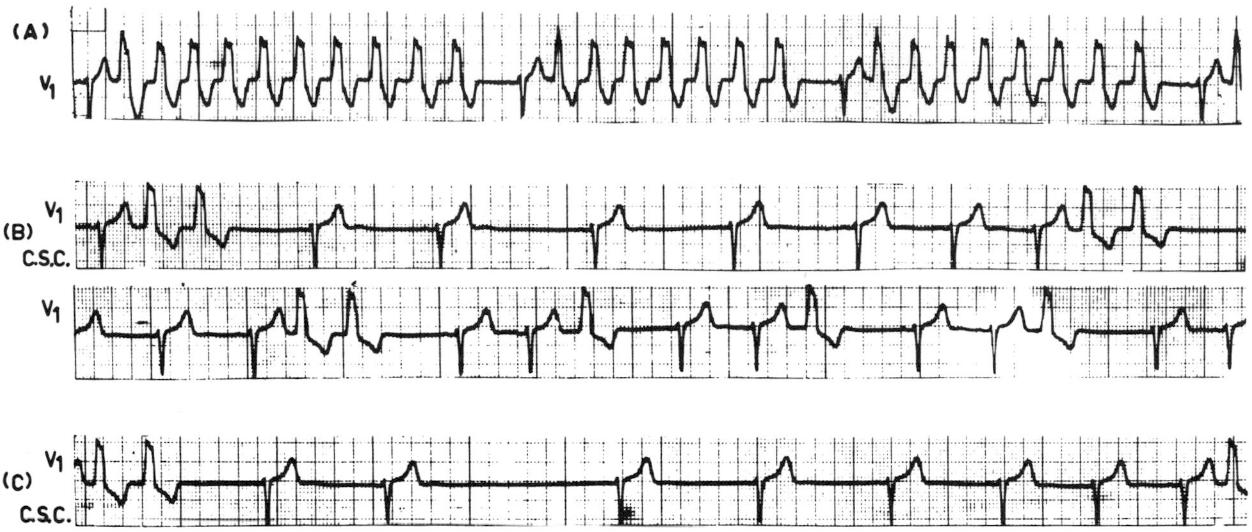

Figure 18-22. *Electrocardiographic tracings obtained from a man aged 56 years with ischemic heart disease. The tracing in A shows repetitive short runs of a monomorphic ventricular tachycardia. The initiating beats are slightly different morphologically from the beats during the tachycardia. The tracings in B and C show extrasystolic beats and couplets with the same morphologic configuration as the beats during the tachycardia. Sinus slowing by carotid sinus compression (CSC) consistently caused the extrasystolic rhythm to disappear. Following CSC, the rhythm always reappeared on gradual shortening of the sinus cycle length to a critical value of 880 to 960 msec, thus illustrating the rate dependence of the extrasystolic rhythm.*

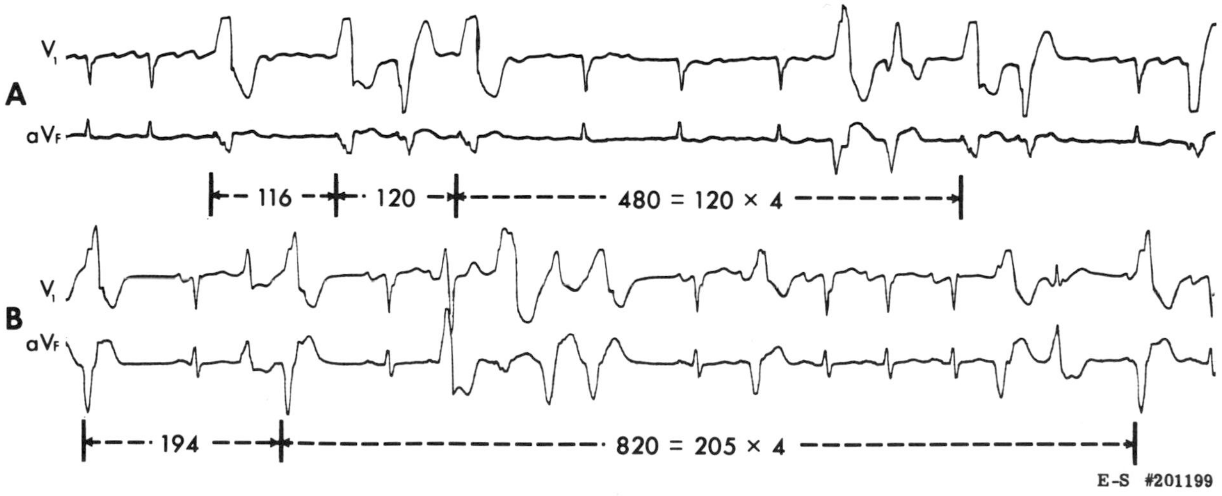

Figure 18-23. *Multiple parasystolic activity during a multiform ventricular rhythm. The electrocardiographic tracings were obtained from a man aged 65 years with ischemic cardiomyopathy and advanced congestive heart failure and reveal a complex multiform ventricular ectopic rhythm. The basic cardiac rhythm alternates between sinus rhythm and atrial fibrillation. At least three different parasystolic foci that contributed to the multiform ectopic activity are evident, two of which are shown in A and B.*

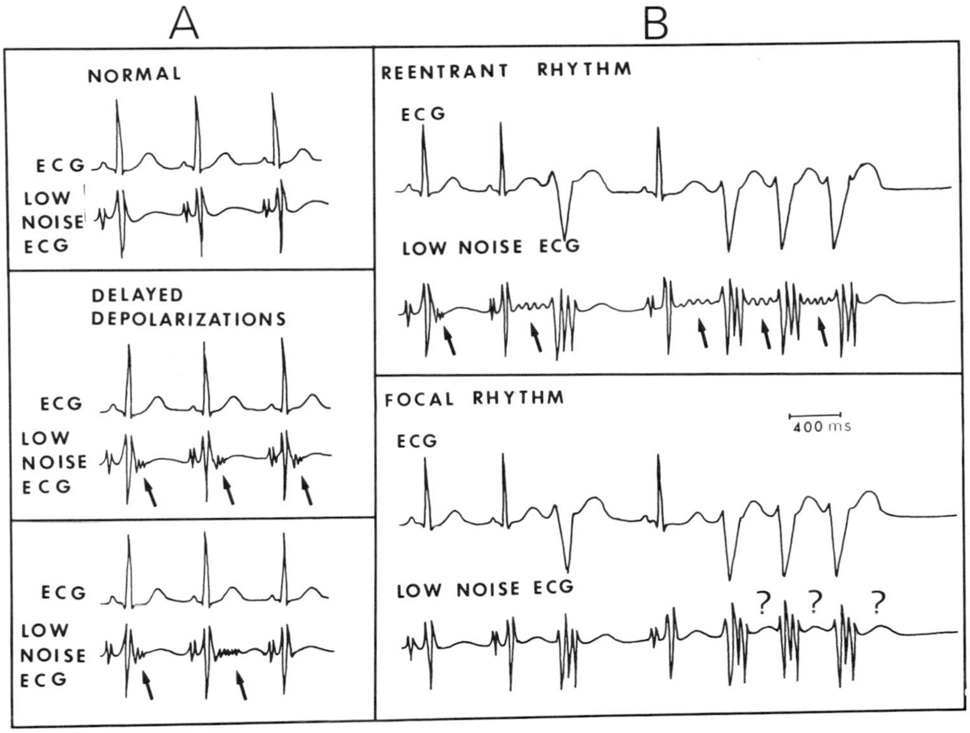

Figure 18-24. *Diagrammatic illustration of late potentials* (arrows) *during sinus rhythm (*middle *and* lower panels *in A) and preceding reentrant beats (*upper panel *in B). See text for details. (?, possible late potentials during a fast ectopic rhythm)*

signal : noise ratio: (1) ensemble averaging (routinely called signal averaging), which is applicable only to regular repetitive electrocardiographic signals and cannot detect moment-to-moment dynamic changes in the signal,[149,150] and (2) low-noise or high-resolution electrocardiography, which uses spatial averaging techniques as well as other noise-reducing measures to record the late potentials on the body surface on a beat-to-beat basis.[151–153]

Electrophysiologic Basis of Late Potentials

Figure 18-24 diagrams the electrophysiologic significance of diastolic potentials recorded on the body surface, based on data obtained from composite electrode recordings from the infarction and border zones in dogs in the late myocardial infarction period[114,145,146] as well as on more recent data on isochronal mapping of focal and reentrant ventricular arrhythmias in these dogs.[85–87,147,148] These studies show that during a regular, relatively slow rhythm (*e.g.,* the sinus rhythm), activation of some areas of the infarction zone may be delayed. If conduction maintains a regular 1 : 1 pattern, the composite electrode recording from the infarction zone will show one or more potentials in the early part of the ST-T segment that are usually continuous with the major QRS (see Fig. 18-24*A*). In some dogs, however, a more dynamic Wenckebach-like conduction pattern may develop in one or more areas of the infarction zone during a regular cardiac rhythm. This may take the form of a beat-to-beat increased delay of the late potentials followed by failure of inscription of one or more of the potentials (see Fig. 18-24*A*). On the other hand, reentrant ventricular rhythms could be induced in the postinfarction dog either by critical shortening of the cycle length of a regular rhythm or by programmed premature stimulation. In both instances, diastolic depolarizations that reflect the activation wavefronts of reentrant circuits consistently bridge the diastolic interval preceding the first reentrant beat as well as during successive reentrant beats (see Fig. 18-24*B*). In contrast, diastolic intervals that precede ventricular rhythms of focal origin usually will not show late potentials. However, a tachycardia-dependent conduction delay in ischemic myocardial zones may cause diastolic potentials to be recorded during a fast ectopic rhythm (see Fig. 18-24*B*).

The asynchronous multiphasic late potentials recorded by the composite electrode from the epicardial surface of canine infarctions closely resemble the late potentials recorded on the body surface by high-gain amplification and signal-averaging techniques in humans. Figure 18-25 illustrates that the late potentials reflect delayed activation of diseased (ischemic) myocar-

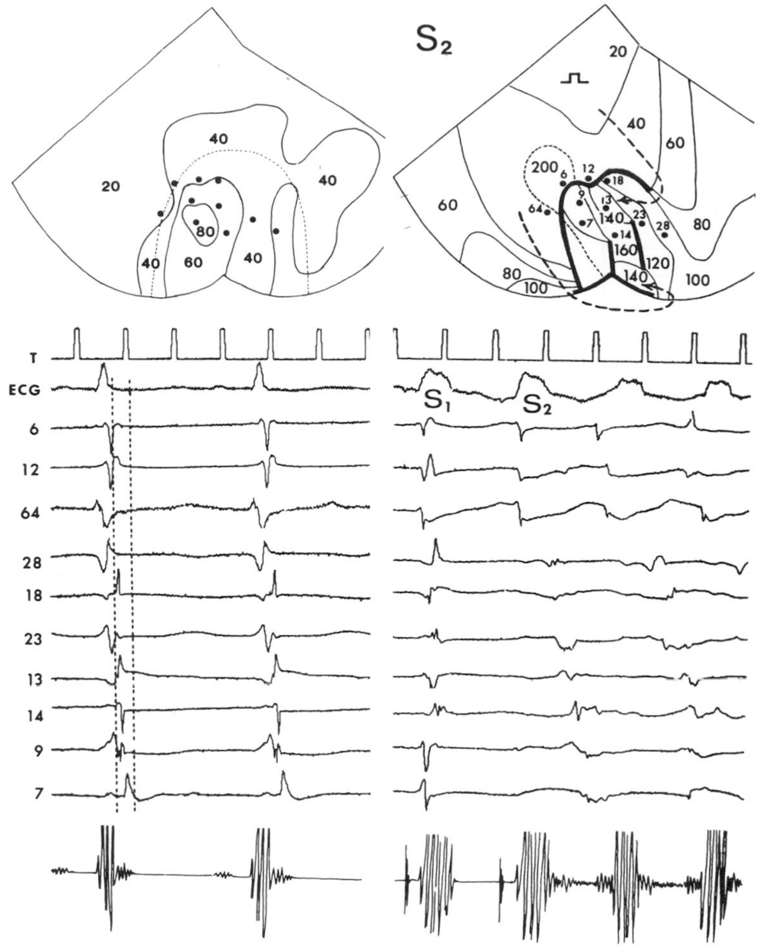

Figure 18-25. *Electrophysiologic substrate of late potentials. Isochronal maps of epicardial activation from a dog with 4-day-old infarction. The map on the* left *represents epicardial activation of a sinus beat, and the one on the* right *the S_2 beat that initiated a reentrant ventricular tachycardia. Epicardial activation is depicted as described in Figure 18-7. Selected epicardial electrograms as well as a simulated high-resolution body surface electrocardiographic recording are shown on the* bottom. *The epicardial electrograms enclosed between two* dotted lines *represent delayed activation of ischemic epicardial zones and are recorded during the early portion of the ST segment of the body surface electrocardiogram. These contribute to the late potentials in the high-resolution body surface electrocardiogram on the* bottom. *The epicardial outline of the ischemic zone is represented by the* dotted line. *See text for details.*

dial zones. The figure also illustrates the relationship of late potentials recorded during sinus rhythm and reentrant ventricular tachycardia. Recent studies have shown that after left anterior descending artery ligation in the dog, conduction delays and reentrant excitation usually occur in the surviving, although electrophysiologically abnormal, thin epicardial layer overlying the infarction.[85–87] The epicardial isochronal activation map during sinus rhythm in a dog 4 days after infarction is shown on the top left of Figure 18-25. A reentrant ventricular tachycardia can be induced by a single premature stimulation (S_2) during regular ventricular pacing (S_1). The activation map of the S_2 beat is shown on the top right of the figure. Selected epicardial electrograms as well as a simulated high-resolution body surface electrocardiographic recording are shown on the bottom. During sinus rhythm, the entire epicardial surface was activated within 80 ms, with delayed activation occurring in the central part of the epicardial ischemic zone. The QRS duration of the body surface electrocardiogram was 40 ms (the normal QRS duration in dogs is shorter than that in humans). Electrograms representing the 40 to 80 ms isochrones of delayed epicardial activation were recorded during the ST segment of the surface electrocardiogram. These represent the bioelectrical potentials generated by a relatively small mass of ischemic myocardial tissue. On the body surface, these electrocardiographic potentials are too small to be detected by routine measuring techniques. However, these signals could be detected on the body surface using high-gain amplification and appropriate noise-reduction measures. Signal averaging is one technique for improving the signal : noise ratio, but it requires that the signal of interest be repeated regularly so that multiple samples can be obtained to form an averaged signal.[149,150] The epicardial activation pattern of the premature beat (S_2) that initiated the first reentrant cycle differed markedly from that during sinus rhythm. The premature beat resulted in a long arc of functional conduction block within the epicardial border of the ischemic zone (heavy solid line). The activation wavefront circulated around both ends of the arc of block, coalesced, and advanced slowly from the lateral to septal borders of the ischemic zone. The slow common reentrant wavefront then reexcited normal myocardial zones on the septal side of the arc of block to initiate the first reentrant beat. Electrograms recorded from the reentrant pathway bridged the diastolic interval between the premature beat, S_2, and the first reentrant beat as well as between successive reentrant beats. This is clearly illustrated in the simulated highly amplified body surface electrocardiographic recording on the bottom of the figure.

Activation of the ischemic zone during sinus rhythm in Figure 18-25 followed a regular 1 : 1 pattern. This is not the case, however, in all postinfarction canine hearts. A Wenckebach conduction pattern in the ischemic myocardium may not be uncommon. Recent studies have shown that a Wenckebach conduction sequence is the initiating mechanism for "spontaneous" reentrant rhythms, that is, reentrant rhythms that occur during a regular cardiac rhythm (*i.e.*, the sinus rhythm), as contrasted with reentrant rhythms induced by one or more premature beats that interrupt an otherwise regular cardiac rhythm[88,90,114,146] (see Figs. 18-17 and 18-18). A dynamic (Wenckebach) activation pattern is not amenable to signal-averaging techniques but theoretically can be represented on the body surface in a beat-to-beat fashion using a high-resolution electrocardiographic recording.[152]

Clinical Significance of Late Potentials

In recent years, several groups of investigators have recorded low-amplitude, high-frequency signals in the terminal portion of the QRS or in the early ST segment of the signal-averaged electrocardiogram in patients with ventricular tachycardia and especially in those with ischemic heart disease.[154–161] Late potentials are rarely detected in healthy persons or in patients without complex ventricular ectopy.[154,156] The late potentials appear to correspond to delayed and fragmented ventricular activation, which has been observed in epicardial and endocardial electrograms recorded in patients and animals with ventricular tachycardia.[162,163] The loss of the ability to initiate ventricular tachycardia after successful antiarrhythmic surgery corresponded to the abolition or decrease in the duration of late potentials after surgery.[157] Although an early study suggested that late potentials are related to the presence of a ventricular aneurysm and not to the propensity to develop ventricular tachycardia,[155] this view has not been upheld in subsequent studies.

In a study by Breithardt and colleagues, late potentials were a frequent finding in patients with angiographically documented cardiac regional contraction abnormalities, both in patients with and without documented ventricular tachycardia.[156] Thus areas of ischemic diseased myocardium were considered the anatomic substrate of late potentials. Although the study suggested that the presence of late potentials was neither highly sensitive nor specific for patients with clinically evident ventricular tachyarrhythmias, it also showed the greater prevalence and longer duration of late potentials in patients with ventricular tachycardia or fibrillation.

In another study,[159] the presence of late potentials was correlated with the results of programmed ventricular stimulation in a group of patients in whom ventricular tachycardia had not been previously documented. The study showed a significant correlation between left ventricular function and the presence and duration of late potentials and between left ventricular function and the results of programmed stimulation. In contrast, late potentials and the occurrence of repetitive ventricular response or ventricular tachycardia on programmed stimulation were less closely associated. In a more recent study,[161] the overall predictive accuracy of late potentials in identifying patients with ventricular tachycardia after myocardial infarction appeared higher than the findings of long-term electrocardiographic monitoring or cardiac catheterization. This may suggest that late potentials do not simply reflect abnormalities that can be detected by other means but represent an independent characteristic of patients with postinfarction ventricular tachycardia. In a prospective multicenter study, the presence of late potentials was helpful in identifying patients prone to ventricular tachycardia or sudden death after recent acute myocardial infarction.[158] The incidence of ventricular tachycardia or sudden death was significantly less in patients without late potentials or with late potentials of less than a 20-msec duration (3.6%) compared to those with late potentials greater or equal to 20 msec (14.6%; $P < 0.01$). A recent prospective study of late potentials in the acute phase of myocardial infarction has shown that the duration of low-amplitude signals and the signal-averaged QRS vector complex was significantly longer, whereas the root mean square voltage of the terminal 40 msec of the QRS complex was significantly lower in patients with an acute infarction and ventricular tachyarrhythmias in contrast to those without tachyarrhythmias (Fig. 18-26).[164]

Electrophysiologic Limitations of the Signal-Averaged Electrocardiogram

Most technical limitations of signal averaging, such as the degree of jitter and filter ringing, can be improved by appropriate measures.[150] However, it is important to understand the following major electrophysiologic limitations of the signal-averaged electrocardiogram:

1. Since signal averaging can be applied only to regular repetitive signals, it is customarily applied to the QRS and ST-T segment of consecutive sinus beats. The recording can average delayed activation signals that occur in a regular 1 : 1 or 2 : 1 pattern but not those with a dynamic Wenckebach sequence. Thus, the prognostic significance of the "duration" of late potentials should not be overstated, since the recording may not faithfully reflect areas with marked but periodic conduction delays.

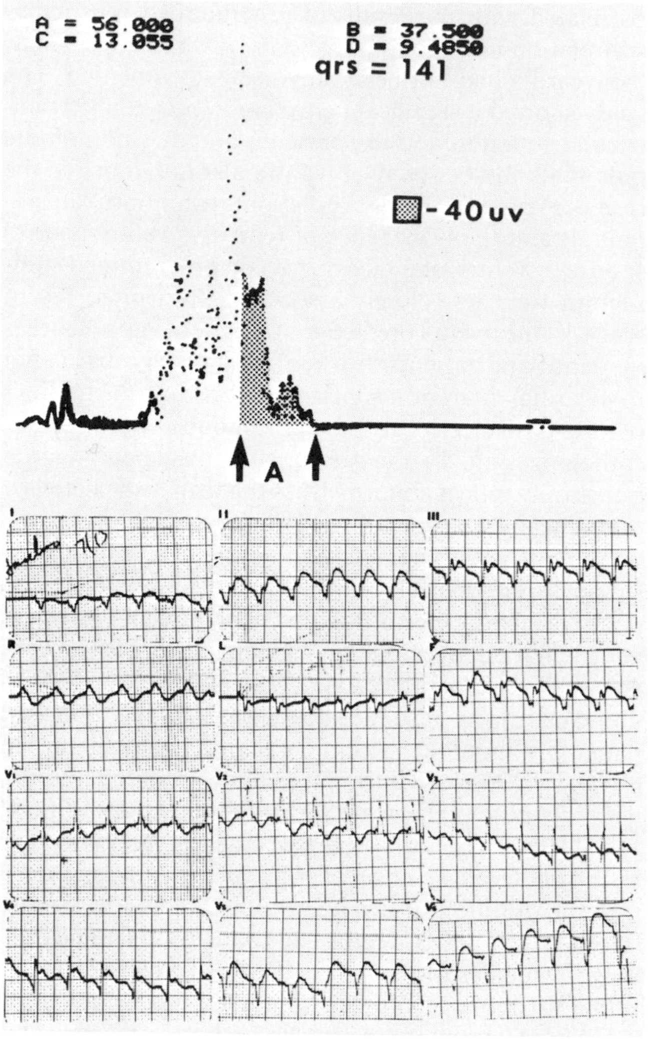

Figure 18-26. (Top tracing) *A signal-averaged QRS vector complex from a patient 4 days following acute myocardial infarction showing abnormal low-amplitude and high-frequency signals at the end of the QRS. The duration of the low amplitude signal less than 40 μV* (between the two arrows) *was 50 msec, the root mean square-voltage for the terminal 40 msec was 13 μV, and the duration of the signal-averaged QRS vector complex was 141 msec. The signal-averaged QRS vector complex is calculated from the* X, Y, and Z *electrograms as* $V = \sqrt{X^2 + Y^2 + Z^2}$ (Bottom tracing) *A 12-lead electrocardiogram from the same patient obtained 2 days later showing sustained ventricular tachycardia. (El-Sherif, N., Gomes, J. A. C., Restivo, M., and Mehra, R.: Late potentials and arrhythmogenesis. Pace, 8:440, 1985; with permission.)*

2. The relationship between myocardial zones showing conduction delay during sinus rhythm on the one hand and spontaneous or induced reentrant rhythms on the other hand is complex. Reentry requires a critical balance between the length of the zone of unidirectional block and the degree of conduction delay of the circulating wavefront. The zones of unidirectional block are not represented in the signal-averaged electrocardiogram, and the degree of conduction delay necessary for reentry may bear little relationship to the degree of conduction delay during sinus rhythm. Indeed, there may be a significant difference between reentrant rhythms that occur spontaneously and those induced by premature stimulation in the same postinfarction heart.[90] Thus, late potentials in a signal-averaged electrocardiogram during sinus rhythm at best reflect myocardial zones with conduction delays and, as such, are only indirect markers for the propensity to develop reentrant tachyarrhythmias either spontaneously or following one or more premature stimulations.
3. Although reentry commonly occurs in the postinfarction heart and most probably is the underlying electrophysiologic mechanism for ventricular fibrillation and sudden cardiac electrical death, some postinfarction ectopic rhythms may be caused by focal discharge of Purkinje fibers. A ventricular tachycardia of focal origin may occur in hearts showing late potentials during sinus rhythm and bears no relationship to these potentials.

Limitations of Prognostic Indicators of Ventricular Vulnerability

There is a significant theoretical limitation to all three currently used prognostic indicators of ventricular vulnerability (*i.e.*, spontaneous ventricular rhythms detected with long-term ambulatory electrocardiographic recording, ventricular rhythms induced by programmed electrical stimulation, and late potentials in the signal-averaged electrocardiogram during sinus rhythm). It is possible that all three indicators reflect only a fixed stable substrate of electrophysiologic abnormality. On the other hand, the eventual episode of ventricular fibrillation and sudden cardiac death may result from a *de novo* electrophysiologic perturbation totally unrelated, or only partially related, to the already present electrophysiologic abnormality. In this regard it is appropriate to question the notion that preexisting manifest VPCs in a given person can trigger a final episode of ventricular fibrillation under the proper circumstances, which can conceivably be a fresh acute ischemic episode. The crucial questions are whether an electrophysiologic derangement that culminates in ventricular fibrillation does require preexisting VPCs and what these VPCs represent in terms of deranged electrophysiology to trigger the fatal arrhythmia. In other words, is the first VPC in a bout of ventricular fibrillation part and parcel of a *de novo* electrophysiologic derangement (instability) or a preexisting culprit that takes advantage of a favorable situation, such as an acute heightening of ventricular vulnerability, to help to instigate the terminal arrhythmia? This view of the relationship between preexisting manifest VPCs and a terminal episode of ventricular fibrillation can possibly change the perspectives, goals, and expectations of antiarrhythmic therapy. In this case, the major goal of antiarrhythmic therapy will be to bolster ventricular resistance to a potential ventricular fibrillation situation. It becomes less crucial for antiarrhythmic therapy to abolish existing VPCs partially or totally unless it is proved that abolishment correlates significantly with decreased ventricular vulnerability to fibrillation. Further, the indication for antiarrhythmic therapy in given patients may not have to depend solely on the frequency and characteristics of manifest VPCs.

References

1. Hinkle, L. E., Carver, S. T., and Stevens, M.: The frequency of asymptomatic disturbances of cardiac rhythm and conduction in middle-aged men. Am. J. Cardiol., 24:629, 1969.
2. Clarke, J. M., Hamer, J., Shelton, J. R., et al.: The rhythm of the normal human heart. Lancet, 2:507, 1976.
3. Chiang, B. N., Perlman, L. V., Ostrander, L. D., Jr., and Epstein, F. H.: Relationship of premature systoles to coronary heart disease and sudden death in the Techumseh epidemiology study. Ann. Intern. Med., 70:1159, 1969.
4. Chiang, B. N., Perlman, L. V., Fulton, M., et al.: Predisposing factors in sudden cardiac death in Techumseh, Michigan: a prospective study. Circulation, 41:31, 1970.
5. Rodstein, M., Wolloch, L., and Gubner, R. S.: Mortality study of the significance of extrasystoles in an insured population. Circulation, 44:617, 1971.
6. Fisher, F. D., and Troyler, H. A.: Relationship between premature contractions in routine electrocardiography and subsequent death from coronary heart disease. Circulation, 47:712, 1973.
7. Hinkle, L. E., Carver, S. T., and Argyros, D. C.: The prognostic significance of ventricular premature contractions in healthy people with coronary heart disease. Acta Cardiol. (Suppl.), 43:5, 1974.
8. Crow, R. S., Prineas, R. J., Dias, V., et al.: Ventricular premature beats in a population sample. Frequency and association with coronary risk characteristics. Circulation (Suppl.), 51:111, 1975.
9. Blackburn, H., Taylor, H. L., and Keys, A.: The electrocardiogram in prediction of five-year coronary heart disease incidence among men aged forty through fifty-nine. Circulation (Suppl.), 41:1, 1970.
10. McHenry, P. L., Fish, C., Jordan, J. W., and Corya, B. R.: Cardiac arrhythmias observed during maximal treadmill exercise testing in clinically normal man. Am. J. Cardiol., 29:331, 1972.
11. Blackburn, H., Taylor, H. L., Hamrell, B. H., et al.: Premature ventricular complexes induced by stress testing. Their frequency and response to physical conditioning. Am. J. Cardiol., 31:441, 1973.
12. McHenry, I. L., Morris, S. N., Kavealier, M., and Jordan, J. W.: Comparative study of exercise-induced ventricular arrhythmias in normal subjects and patients with documented coronary artery disease. Am. J. Cardiol. 37:609, 1976.
13. Kotler, M. N., Tabatznik, B., Mower, M. M., and Tominaga, S.: Prognostic significance of ventricular ectopic beats with respect to sudden death in the late post-infarction period. Circulation, 47:959, 1973.
14. The Coronary Drug Project Research Group: Prognostic importance of premature beats following myocardial infarction. Experience in the coronary drug project. J.A.M.A., 223:1116, 1973.
15. Hoffman, B. F., and Rosen, M. R.: Cellular mechanisms of cardiac arrhythmias. Circ. Res., 49:1, 1981.
16. Cranefield, P. F.: The Slow Response and Cardiac Arrhythmias. Mt. Kisco, N.Y., Futura, 1975.
17. Wit, A. L., and Cranefield, P. F.: Reentrant excitation as a cause of cardiac arrhythmias. Am. J. Physiol., 235:H1, 1978.
18. Antzelevitch, C., Jalife, J., and Moe, G. K.: Characteristics of reflection as a mechanism of reentrant arrhythmias and its relationship to parasystole. Circulation, 61:182, 1980.
19. Vassalle, M.: Analysis of cardiac pacemaker potential using a "voltage clamp" technique. Am. J. Physiol., 208:770, 1965.
20. Trautwein, W.: Membrane currents in cardiac muscle fibers. Physiol. Rev., 53:793, 1973.
21. Di Francisco, D.: A new interpretation of the pacemaking current in calf Purkinje fibers. J. Physiol., 314:359, 1981.
22. Di Francisco, D: A study of the ionic nature of the pacemaker current in calf Purkinje fibers. J. Physiol., 314:377, 1981.
23. Vassalle, M.: The relationship among cardiac pacemakers: Overdrive suppression. Circ. Res., 41:269, 1977.
24. Tsien, R. W.: Effect of epinephrine on the pacemaker potassium current of cardiac Purkinje fibers. J. Gen. Physiol., 64:293, 1974.
25. Jalife, J., and Moe, G. K.: Effects of electrotonic potentials on pacemaker activity of canine Purkinje fibers in relation to parasystole. Circ. Res., 39:801, 1976.
26. Hauswirth, O., Noble, P., and Tsien, R. W.: The mechanism of oscillatory activity at low membrane potentials in cardiac Purkinje fibers. J. Physiol. (Lond.), 200:255, 1969.
27. Katzung, B. O., and Morgenstern, J. A.: Effects of extracellular potassium on ventricular automaticity and evidence for a pacemaker current in mammalian ventricular myocardium. Circ. Res., 40:105, 1977.
28. Imanishi, S., and Surawicz, B.: Automatic activity in depolarized guinea pig ventricular myocardium: Characteristics and mechanisms. Circ. Res., 39:751, 1976.
29. Noble, D., and Tsien, R. W.: The kinetics and rectifier properties of the slow potassium current in cardiac Purkinje fibers. J. Physiol. (Lond.), 195:185, 1968.
30. Ferrier, G. R., and Rosenthal, J. E.: Automaticity and entrance block induced by focal depolarization of mammalian ventricular tissues. Circ. Res., 47:238, 1980.
31. Hoffman, B. F., and Dangman, K. H.: Are arrhythmias caused by automatic impulse generation? In Normal and Abnormal Conduction in the Heart. Paes de Carvalho, A., Hoffman, B. F., and Lieberman, M. (eds.): Mt. Kisco, N.Y., Futura, pp. 152–163, 1982.
32. Friedman, P. L., Stewart, J. R., and Wit, A. L.: Spontaneous and induced cardiac arrhythmias in subendocardial Purkinje fibers surviving extensive myocardial infarction in dogs. Circ. Res., 33:612, 1973.
33. Lazzara, R., El-Sherif, N., Scherlag, B. J.: Electrophysiological properties of canine Purkinje cells in one-day-old myocardial infarction. Circ. Res., 33:722, 1973.
34. El-Sherif, N., Gough, W. B., Zeiler, R. H., and Mehra, R.: Triggered ventricular rhythms in 1-day-old myocardial infarction in the dog. Circ. Res., 52:566, 1983.
35. Cranefield, P. F.: Action potentials, afterpotentials and arrhythmias. Circ. Res., 41:415, 1977.
36. Gadsby, D., and Cranefield, P. F.: Two levels of resting potentials in cardiac Purkinje fibers. J. Gen. Physiol., 70:725, 1977.
37. Brooks, C. McC., Hoffman, B. F., Suckling, E. E., and Orias, O.: Excitability of the Heart. New York, Grune & Stratton, 1955.
38. Schmidt, R. F.: Versuche mit aconitin zum Problem der spontanen Erregungsbildung im Herzen. Pfluegers Arch., 271:526, 1950.

39. Matsuda, K., Hoshi, T., and Nameyamo, S.: Effects of aconitine on the cardiac membrane potential of the dog. Jpn. J. Physiol., 9:419, 1981.
40. Matsuda, K., Toyama, J., Hoshi, T., et al.: Veratrine induced prolongation of repolarization in the mammalian heart. Presented at the 19th International Physiology Congress (abstr.), p. 596, 1953.
41. Shibata, S., Izumi, T., Serigunchi, D. G., and Norton, T. R.: Further studies on the positive inotropic effect of the polypeptide anthopleurin-A from sea anemone. J. Pharmacol. Exp. Ther., 205:683, 1978.
42. Kodama, I., Shibata, S., Toyama, J., and Yamada, K.: Electromechanical effects of anthopleurin-A (AP-A) on rabbit ventricular muscle: Influence of driving frequency, calcium antagonists, tetrodotoxin, lidocaine and ryanodine. Br. J. Pharmacol., 74:29, 1981.
43. Low, P. A., Wu, C. H., and Narahashi, T.: The effect of anthopleurin-A on crayfish giant axon. J. Pharmacol. Exp. Ther., 210:417, 1979.
44. Brachmann, J., Scherlag, B. J., Rosenshtraukh, L. V., and Lazzara, K.: Bradycardia-dependent triggered activity: Relevance to drug-induced multiform ventricular tachycardia. Circulation, 68:846, 1983.
45. Strauss, H. C., Bigger, J. T., Jr., and Hoffman, B. F.: Electrophysiological and beta-receptor blocking effects of MJ 1999 on dog and rabbit cardiac tissues. Circ. Res., 26:661, 1970.
46. Dangman, K. H., and Hoffman, B. F.: In vivo and in vitro antiarrhythmic and arrhythmogenic effects of N-acetyl procainamide. J. Pharmacol. Exp. Ther., 217:851, 1981.
47. Roden, D. M., Arthur, M., and Woosley, R. L.: Bradycardia-dependent triggered arrhythmias in the intact heart (abstr.). J. Am. Coll. Cardiol. 5:390, 1985.
48. Schwartz, S. P.: Studies on transient ventricular fibrillation. III. The prefibrillatory mechanisms established during auriculoventricular dissociation. Am. J. Med. Sci., 192:153, 1936.
49. Langendorf, R., and Pick, A.: Causes and mechanisms of ventricular asystole in advanced A-V block. In Surawicz, B., and Pellegrino, E. E. (eds.): Sudden Cardiac Death, pp. 97–107. New York, Grune and Stratton, 1964.
50. Krikler, D. M., and Curry, P. V. L.: Torsades de pointes, an atypical ventricular tachycardia. Br. Heart J., 38:117, 1976.
51. Rosen, M. R., Gelband, H., and Hoffman, B. F.: Correlation between effects of ouabain in the canine electrocardiogram and transmembrane potentials of Purkinje fibers. Circulation 47:65, 1973.
52. Ferrier, G. R., Saunders, J. H., and Mendez, C.: A cellular mechanism for the generation of ventricular arrhythmias by acetylstrophanthidin. Circ. Res., 32:600, 1976.
53. Ferrier, G. R.: The effects of tension on acetylstrophanthidin-induced transient depolarizations and after contractions in canine myocardial and Purkinje tissues. Circ. Res., 38:156, 1976.
54. Wit, A. L., and Cranefield, P. F.: Triggered activity, in cardiac muscle fibers of the simian mitral valve. Circ. Res., 38:85, 1976.
55. Wit, A. L., and Cranefield, P. F.: Triggered and automatic activity in the canine coronary sinus. Circ. Res., 41:435, 1977.
56. Aronson, R. S.: Afterpotentials and triggered activity in hypertrophied myocardium from rats with renal hypertension. Circ. Res., 48:720, 1981.
57. Vassalle, M., and Mugelli, A.: An oscillatory current in sheep cardiac Purkinje fibers. Circ. Res., 48:618, 1981.
58. Grossman, A., and Furchgott, R. F.: The effects of various drugs on calcium exchange in the isolated guinea-pig left auricle. J. Pharmacol. Exp. Ther. 145:162, 1964.
59. Reuter, H., and Scholz, H.: The regulation of the calcium conductance of cardiac muscle by adrenaline. J. Physiol. (Lond.), 264:49, 1977.
60. Lee, K. S., and Klaus, W.: The subcellular basis for the mechanism of inotropic action of cardiac glycosides. Pharmacol. Rev., 23:193, 1971.
61. Goto, M., Yatani, A., and Tsuda, Y.: Membrane calcium current in cardiac excitation: Effects of ATP and related substances on sodium pump in bullfrog atrium. In Kobayashi, T., Sano, T., and Dhella, N. S. (eds.): Recent Advances in Studies on Cardiac Structure and Metabolism, vol. II, Heart Function and Metabolism, pp. 37–44. Baltimore, University Park Press, 1978.
62. Reuter, H., and Seitz, N.: Dependence of calcium efflux from cardiac muscle on temperature and external ion composition. J. Physiol. (Lond.), 195:451, 1968.
63. Cranefield, P. F., and Aronson, R. S.: Initiation of sustained rhythmic activity by single propagated action potentials in canine cardiac Purkinje fibers exposed to sodium-free solution or to ouabain. Circ. Res., 34:477, 1974.
64. Tsien, R. W., and Carpenter, D. O.: Ionic mechanisms of pacemaker activity in cardiac Purkinje fibers. Fed. Proc., 37:2127, 1978.
65. Kass, R. S., Lederer, W. J., Tsien, R. W., and Weingart, R.: Role of calcium ions in transient inward currents and aftercontractions induced by strophanthidin in cardiac Purkinje fibers. J. Physiol. (Lond.), 281:187, 1978.
66. Kass, R. S., Tsien, R. W., and Weingart, R.: Ionic basis of transient inward current induced by strophanthidin in cardiac Purkinje fibers. J. Physiol. (Lond.), 281:209, 1978.
67. Schwartz, A., Wood, J. M., Allen, J. C., et al.: Biochemical morphologic correlates of cardiac ischemia. I. Membrane systems. Am. J. Cardiol. 32:46, 1973.
68. Sobel, B. E.: Salient biochemical features in ischemic myocardium. Circ. Res., 35 (Suppl. III):173, 1974.
69. Carafoli, E., Tiozzo, R, Lugli, G., et al.: The release of calcium from heart mitochondria by sodium. J. Mol. Cell. Cardiol., 6:361, 1974.
70. Rosen, M. R., and Reder, R. F.: Does triggered activity have a role in the genesis of cardiac arrhythmias? Ann. Intern. Med., 94:794, 1981.
71. El-Sherif, N., Gough, W. B., Zeiler, R. H., and Mehra, R.: Ventricular rhythms in one-day-old canine infarction are due to triggered activity (abstr.). Circulation, 66 (Suppl. II):357, 1982.
72. Mayer, A. G.: Rhythmical pulsation in Scyphomedusae. II. Carnegie Institute. Papers. Washington Tortugas Lab 1:113–131, Carnegie Institute Publication No. 102, part VII, 1908.
73. Garrey, W. E.: The nature of fibrillary contraction of the heart. Its relation to tissue mass and form. Am. J. Physiol., 33:397, 1914.
74. Mines, G. R.: On dynamic equilibrium in the heart. J. Physiol.,46:350, 1913.
75. Mines, G. R.: On circulating excitations in heart muscles and their possible relation to tachycardia and fibrillation. Trans. R. Soc. Can. (series 3, section IV) 8:43, 1914.
76. Lewis, T.: The Mechanisms and Graphic Registration of the Heart Beat. London, Shaw, 1925.
77. Lewis, T., Feil, H. S., and Stroud, W. D.: Observations upon flutter and fibrillation. II. The nature of auricular flutter. Heart, 7:191, 1920.
78. Schmitt, F. O., and Erlanger, J.: Directional differences in the conduction of the impulse through heart muscle and their possible relation to extrasystolic and fibrillary contractions. Am. J. Physiol., 87:326, 1928–1929.
79. Kent, A. F. S. A.: Conducting path between the right auricle and the external wall of the right ventricle in the heart of the mammal. J. Physiol. (Lond.), 48:22, 1914.
80. Akhtar, M., Gilbert, C., Wolf, F. G., and Schmidt, D. M.: Reentry within the His-Purkinje system. Elucidation of reentrant circuit using right bundle branch and His bundle recordings. Circulation, 58:295, 1978.
81. Moe, G. K., Mendez, C., and Han, J.: Aberrant AV impulse

propagation in the dog heart: A study of functional bundle branch block. Circ. Res., 16:261, 1965.

82. Allessie, M. A., Bonke, F. I. M., and Schopman, F. J. G.: Circus movement in rabbit atrial muscle as a mechanism of tachycardia. Circ. Res., 33:54, 1973.
83. Allessie, M. A., Bonke, F. I. M., and Schopman, F. J. G.: Circus movement in rabbit atrial muscle as a mechanism of tachycardia. II. The role of nonuniform recovery of excitability in the occurrence of unidirectional blocks, as studied with multiple microelectrodes. Circ. Res., 39:168, 1976.
84. Allessie, M. A., Bonke, F. I. M., and Schopman, F. J. G.: Circus movement in rabbit atrial muscle as a mechanism of tachycardia. III. The "leading circle" concept: A new model of circus movement in cardiac tissue without the involvement of an anatomical obstacle. Circ. Res., 41:9, 1977.
85. El-Sherif, N., Mehra, R., Gough, W. B., et al.: Ventricular activation pattern of spontaneous and induced ventricular rhythms in canine one-day-old myocardial infarction. Evidence for focal and reentrant mechanisms. Circ. Res., 51:152, 1982.
86. Mehra, R., Zeiler, R. H., Gough, W. B., et al.: Reentrant ventricular arrhythmias in the late myocardial infarction period. 9. Electrophysiologic-anatomic correlation of reentrant circuits. Circulation, 67:11, 1983.
87. El-Sherif, N., Mehra, R., Gough, W. B., et al.: Reentrant ventricular arrhythmias in the late myocardial infarction period. Interruption of reentrant circuits by cryothermal techniques. Circulation, 68:644, 1983.
88. El-Sherif, N.: The figure 8 model of reentrant excitation in the canine post-infarction heart. In Zipes, D., and Jalife, J. (eds.): Cardiac Electrophysiology and Arrhythmias, pp. 363–378. New York, Grune & Stratton, 1985.
89. Boineau, J. P., Schussler, R. B., Mooney, C. R., et al.: Natural and evoked atrial flutter due to circus movement in dogs. Role of abnormal atrial pathways, slow conduction, nonuniform refractory period distribution, and premature beats. Am. J. Cardiol., 45:1167, 1980.
90. El-Sherif, N., Gough, W. B., Zeiler, R. H., et al.: Reentrant-ventricular arrhythmias in the late myocardial infarction period. 12. Spontaneous versus induced reentry and intramural versus epicardial circuits. J. Am. Coll. Cardiol., 6:124, 1985.
91. Wit, A. L., Hoffman, B. F., and Cranefield, P. F.: Slow conduction and reentry in the ventricular conducting system: I. Return extrasystole in canine Purkinje fibers. Circ. Res., 30:1, 1972.
92. Jalife, J., and Moe, G. K.: Excitation, conduction and reflection of impulses in isolated bovine and canine cardiac Purkinje fibers. Circ. Res., 49:233, 1981.
93. Antzelevitch, C., and Moe, G. K.: Electronically mediated delayed conduction and reentry in relation to "slow responses" in mammalian ventricular conducting tissue. Circ. Res., 49:1129, 1981.
94. Antzelevitch, C., Bernstein, M. J., Feldman, H. N., and Moe, G. K.: Parasystole, reentry and tachycardia: a canine preparation of cardiac arrhythmias occurring across inexcitable segments of tissue. Circulation, 68:1101, 1983.
95. Wit, A. L., and Rosen, M. R.: Cellular electrophysiology of cardiac arrhythmias. In Josephson, M. E., and Wellens, H. J. J. (eds.): Tachycardias: Mechanisms, Diagnosis and Treatment, pp. 1–27. Philadelphia, Lea & Febiger, 1984.
96. Scherf, D., Choi, K. Y., Bahadori, A., and Orphanos R. P.: Parasystole. Am. J. Cardiol. 12:527, 1963.
97. Kaufmann, R., and Rothberger, C. J.: Beitrag zur Kenntnis der Entstelungsweise estrasystolischer Allorhythmien. Z. Ges. Exp. Med., 5:349, 1917; 7:199, 1919; 9:103, 1919; 11:40, 1920; 13:1, 1922.
98. Vedoya, R.: Parasistolia. Buenos Aires, A Lopez, 1944.
99. Scherf, D., and Schott, A.: Extrasystoles and Allied Arrhythmias. London, William Heinemann, 1953.
100. Scherf, D., and Chick, F. B.: Experimental parasystole. Am. Heart J., 42:212, 1951.
101. Scherf, D., Blumenfeld, S., and Yildiz, M.: Extrasystoles and parasystole. Am. Heart J., 64:357, 1962.
102. Hoffman, B. F.: The electrophysiology of the heart muscle and the genesis of arrhythmias. In Dreifus, L. A., and Likoff, W. (eds.): Mechanism and Therapy of Cardiac Arrhythmias, p. 17. New York, Grune & Stratton, 1966.
103. Moe, G. K., Antzelevitch, C., and Jalife, J.: Premature contractions: Reentrant or parasystolic? In Harrison, D. C. (ed.): Cardiac Arrhythmias, pp. 419–427. Boston, G. K. Hall, 1981.
104. Weidmann, S.: Effect of current flow on the membrane potential of cardiac muscle. J. Physiol. 115:227, 1951.
105. Jalife, J., Antzelevitch, C., and Moe, G. K.: The case for modulated parasystole. Pace, 5:911, 1982.
106. Scherf, D., Schott, A., Reid, E. C., and Chasmai, D. G.: Intermittent parasystole. Cardiologia, 30:217, 1957.
107. Kuo, C. S., and Surawicz, B.: Coexistence of ventricular parasystole and ventricular couplets: Mechanism and clinical significance. Am. J. Cardiol., 44:435, 1979.
108. Schamroth, L., and Marriott, H. J. L.: Intermittent ventricular parasystole with observation on its relationship to extrasystolic bigeminy. Am. J. Cardiol., 7:799, 1961.
109. Steffens, T. G.: Intermittent ventricular parasystole due to entrance block failure. Circulation, 44:442, 1971.
110. Cohen, H., Langendorf, R., and Pick, A.: Intermittent parasystole. Mechanism of protection. Circulation, 48:761, 1973.
111. Kinoshita, S.: Mechanisms of ventricular parasystole. Circulation, 58:715, 1978.
112. Wedensky, N. E.: Die Erregung, Hummung und Narkose. Pfluegers Arch., 100:1, 1903.
113. Moe, G. K., Jalife, J., Mueller, M. J., et al.: A mathematical model of parasystole and its application to clinical arrhythmias. Circulation, 56:968, 1977.
114. El-Sherif, N., Lazzara, R., Hope, R. R., and Scherlag, B. J.: Reentrant ventricular arrhythmias in the late myocardial infarction period. 3. Manifest and concealed extrasystolic grouping. Circulation, 56:225, 1977.
115. Hans, J., DeTraglia, S., Millet, D., and Moe, G. K.: Incidence of ectopic beats as a function of basic rate in the ventricle. Am. Heart J., 72:632, 1966.
116. Gallavardin, L.: Extrasystolie ventriculaire à paroxysmes tachycardiques prolonges. Arch. Mal. Coeur, 15:298, 1922.
117. Coumel, P., Leclercq, J. F., and Slama, R.: Repetitive monomorphic idiopathic ventricular tachycardia. In Zipes, D. P., Jalife, J. (ed.): Electrophysiology and Arrhythmias, pp. 457–568. New York, Grune & Stratton, 1985.
118. Schamroth, L., and Marriott, H. J. L.: Concealed ventricular extrasystoles. Circulation, 27:1043, 1963.
119. Dieuaide, R. F., and Davidson, E. C.: Terminal cardiac arrhythmias. Arch. Intern. Med., 28:663, 1921.
120. Gallavardin, L.: Tachycardie ventriculaire terminale. Arch. Mal. Coeur, 19:153, 1926.
121. D'Irsay, S.: On the meaning of extrasystoles. Am. J. Med. Sci., 174:96, 1927.
122. El-Sherif, N., and Samet, P.: Multiform ventricular ectopic rhythm. Evidence for multiple parasystolic activity. Circulation, 51:492, 1975.
123. Lown, B., and Wolf, M.: Approaches to sudden death from coronary heart disease. Circulation, 44:130, 1971.
124. Geltman, E. M., Ehsani, A. A., Campbell, M. K., et al.: The influence of location and extent of myocardial infarction on long-term ventricular dysrhythmia and mortality. Circulation, 60:805, 1979.
125. Ruberman, W., Weinblatt, E., Goldberg, J. D., et al.: Ventricular premature complexes in prognosis of angina. Circulation, 61:1172, 1980.

126. Moss, A. J.: Clinical significance of ventricular arrhythmias in patients with and without coronary artery disease. Progr. Cardiovasc. Dis., 23:33, 1980.
127. Cats, V. M., Lie, K. I., vanCapele, F. J. L., et al.: Limitations of 24-hour ambulatory electrocardiographic recording in predicting coronary events after acute myocardial infarction. Am. J. Cardiol., 44:1257, 1979.
128. Bigger, J. T., Wenger, T. L., and Heissenbuttel, R. H.: Limitations of the Lown grading system for the study of human ventricular arrhythmias. Am. Heart J., 93:727, 1977.
129. El-Sherif, N.: The ventricular premature complex. Mechanisms and significance. In Mandel, W. J. (ed.): Cardiac Arrhythmias, pp. 288–320. Philadelphia, J. B. Lippincott, 1980.
130. Morganroth, J., Michelson, E. L., Horowitz, L. N., et al.: Limitations of routine long-term ambulatory electrocardiographic monitoring to assess ventricular ectopic frequency. Circulation, 58:408, 1978.
131. Winkle, R. A.: Antiarrhythmic drug effect mimicked by spontaneous variability of ventricular ectopy. Circulation, 57:1116, 1978.
132. Michelson, E. L., and Morganroth, J.: Spontaneous variability of complex ventricular arrhythmias detected by long-term electrocardiographic recording. Circulation, 61:690, 1980.
133. Fisher, J. D., Cohen, L. L., Mehra, R., et al.: Cardiac pacing and pacemakers. II. Serial electrophysiologic pharmacologic testing for control of recurrent tachyarrhythmias. Am. Heart J., 93:658, 1977.
134. Josephson, M. E., Horowitz, L. N., Farshidi, A., and Kastor, J. A.: Recurrent sustained ventricular tachycardia. I. Mechanisms. Circulation, 57:431, 1978.
135. Mason, J. W., and Winkle, R. A.: Electrode catheter arrhythmia induction in the selection and assessment of antiarrhythmic drug therapy for recurrent ventricular tachycardia. Circulation, 58:971, 1978.
136. Horowitz, L. N., Josephson, M. E., Farshidi, A., et al.: Recurrent sustained ventricular tachycardia. 3. Role of the electrophysiologic study in the selection of antiarrhythmic regimens. Circulation, 58:986, 1978.
137. Ruskin, J. N., DiMarco, J. P., and Garan, A.: Out of hospital cardiac arrest: electrophysiologic observations and selection of long term antiarrhythmic therapy. N. Engl. J. Med., 303:607, 1980.
138. Josephson, M. E., Horowitz, L., Spielman, S. R., and Greenspan, A. M.: Electrophysiologic and hemodynamic studies in patients resuscitated from cardiac arrest. Am. J. Cardiol., 46:948, 1980.
139. Wellens, H. J. J.: Value and limitations of programmed electrical stimulation of the heart in the study and treatment of tachycardias. Circulation, 57:845, 1978.
140. Gomes, J. A. C., Kang, P. S., Kahn, R., et al.: Repetitive ventricular response. Its incidence, inducibility, reproducibility, mechanism and significance. Br. Heart J., 46:152, 1981.
141. Gomes, J. A. C., Hariman, R. I., Kang, P. S., et al.: Programmed electrical stimulation in patients with high-grade ventricular ectopy: Electrophysiologic findings and prognosis for survival. Circulation, 70:43, 1984.
142. Waldo, A. L., and Kaiser, G. A.: A study of ventricular arrhythmias associated with myocardial infarction in the canine heart. Circulation 47:1222, 1973.
143. Boineau, J. P., and Cox J. L.: Slow ventricular activation in acute myocardial infarction. A source of reentrant premature ventricular contractions. Circulation, 48:702, 1973.
144. El-Sherif, N., Scherlag, B. J., and Lazzara, R.: Electrode catheter recordings during malignant ventricular arrhythmias following experimental acute myocardial ischemia. Circulation, 51:1003, 1975.
145. El-Sherif, N., Scherlag, B. J., Lazzara, R., et al.: Reentrant ventricular arrhythmias in the late myocardial infarction period. 1. Conduction characteristics in the infarction zone. Circulation, 55:686, 1977.
146. El-Sherif, N., Hope, R. R., Scherlag, B. J., et al.: Reentrant ventricular arrhythmias in the late myocardial infarction period. 2. Patterns of initiation and termination of reentry. Circulation, 55:702, 1977.
147. Janse, M. J., vanCapelle, F. J. L., Morsink, M., et al.: Flow of 'injury' current and patterns of excitation during early ventricular arrhythmias in acute regional myocardial ischemia in isolated porcine and canine hearts. Circ. Res., 47:151, 1980.
148. El-Sherif, N., Smith, R. A., and Evans, K.: Ventricular arrhythmias in the late myocardial infarction period in dog. 8. Epicardial mapping of reentrant circuits. Circ. Res., 49:255, 1981.
149. Mehra, R., and El-Sherif, N.: Signal averaging of electrocardiographic potentials: A review. Acupuncture and electrotherapeutics. Res. Int. J., 7:133, 1982.
150. Simson, M. B., Kanovsky, M., Falcone, R. A., et al.: Non-invasive methods of predicting patients at risk for malignant ventricular arrhythmias. In Josephson, M. E., Hein, J. J., and Wellen, S. (eds.): Tachycardias: Mechanisms, Diagnosis, Treatment, pp. 507–518. Philadelphia, Lea & Febiger, 1984.
151. Flowers, N. C., Shvartsman, V., Kennelly, B. M., et al.: Surface recordings of His-Purkinje activity on an every beat basis without digital averaging. Circulation, 63:948, 1981.
152. El-Sherif, N., Mehra, R., Gomes, J. A. C., et al.: Appraisal of a low noise electrocardiogram. J. Am. Coll. Cardiol., 1:456, 1983.
153. Hombach, V., Kebbel, U., Hopp, H. W., et al.: Noninvasive beat-by-beat registration of ventricular late potentials using high resolution electrocardiography. Int. J. Cardiol., 6:716, 1984.
154. Simson, M. B.: Use of signals in the terminal QRS complex to identify patients with ventricular tachycardia after myocardial infarction. Circulation 64:235, 1981.
155. Rozanski, J. J., Mortara, D., Myerburg, R. J., et al.: Body surface detection of delayed depolarizations in patients with recurrent ventricular tachycardia and left ventricular aneurysm. Circulation, 63:1172, 1981.
156. Breithardt, G., et al.: Prevalence of late potentials in patients with and without ventricular tachycardia: Correlation with angiographic findings. Am. J. Cardiol., 49:1932, 1982.
157. Breithardt, G., Seipel, L., Ostermeyer, J., et al.: Effect of surgery on late ventricular potentials recorded by precordial signal averaging in patients with ventricular tachycardia. Am. Heart J., 104:996, 1982.
158. Breithardt, G., Schwarzmaier, J., Borggrefe, M., et al.: Prognostic significance of late ventricular potentials after acute myocardial infarction. Eur. Heart J., 4:487, 1983.
159. Breithardt, G., Borggrefe, M., Quantins, B., et al.: Ventricular vulnerability assessed by programmed ventricular stimulation in patients with and without late potentials. Circulation, 68:275, 1983.
160. Denes, P., Santarelli, P., Hauser, R. G., et al.: Quantitative analysis of the high frequency components of the terminal portion of the body surface QRS in normal subjects and in patients with ventricular tachycardia. Circulation, 67:1129, 1983.
161. Kanovsky, M. S., Falcone, R., Dresden, C. A., et al.: Identification of patients with ventricular tachycardia after myocardial infarction: Signal-averaged electrocardiogram, Holter monitoring, and cardiac catheterization. Circulation, 70:264, 1984.
162. Berbari, E. J., Scherlag, B. J., Hope, R. R., et al.: Recording from the body surface of arrhythmogenic ventricular activity during the S-T segment. Am. J. Cardiol., 41:697, 1978.
163. Simson, M. B., Untereker, W. J., Spielman, S. R., et al.: The relationship between late potentials on the body surface and directly recorded fragmented electrograms in patients with ventricular tachycardia. Am. J. Cardiol., 51:105, 1983.
164. El-Sherif, N., Gomes, J. A. C., Restivo, M., and Mehra, R.: Late potentials and arrhythmogenesis. Pace, 8:440, 1985.

19

Exercise-Induced Ventricular Arrhythmias

Mary L. Dohrmann, Nora Goldschlager, and Keith Cohn

The appearance of ventricular extrasystoles following acute myocardial infarction is considered an important prognostic indicator of mortality. The Coronary Drug Project Research Group noted a twofold increase in mortality in a 3-year follow-up study of patients with ventricular extrasystoles who survived 3 months after myocardial infarction.[1] Frequent ventricular ectopy, such as pairs or runs of extrasystoles, quadruples the expected mortality in the first 3 years after infarction.[1] A similar relationship of ventricular extrasystoles to risk of sudden death and the development of symptomatic coronary disease is also suggested by the Tecumseh epidemiologic study.[2] These observations have led to the question of whether ventricular arrhythmias induced by exercise also have diagnostic or prognostic importance.

General Considerations

Prevalence

The reported prevalence of exercise-induced ventricular arrhythmias varies from 19% to 60%.[3–5] Exercise-related ventricular arrhythmias increase in frequency with subject age, and their prevalence approaches 50% in subjects over 50 years of age.[6] Prevalence of exercise-induced ventricular arrhythmias is also increased in patients with symptomatic coronary disease (Table 19-1); 19% to 38% of healthy subjects develop ventricular arrhythmias during exercise, compared to 36% to 50% of patients with coronary disease.[3,5] Exercise-induced ventricular arrhythmias in patients with coronary artery disease are commonly associated with ischemic ST segment shifts during exercise[4] and with the extent and severity of disease documented angiographically.[7] High grades of ventricular ectopy, in particular multiform extrasystoles and ventricular tachycardia, are uncommon in healthy persons undergoing exercise testing (see Table 19-1),[3–5] although they occasionally occur (Fig. 19-1). Ventricular tachycardia occurring during exercise is much more frequent in patients with known coronary artery disease, the reported prevalence generally being around 6%.[5]

Reproducibility

The occurrence of ventricular arrhythmias during serial stress tests varies.[8,9] Only in patients with known or suspected cardiovascular disease is reproducibility of arrhythmias consistent enough to be considered more than random.[6,8] In consecutively performed exercise stress tests, high grades of ventricular ectopy, in particular ven-

Table 19-1. Exercise-Induced Ventricular Ectopic Activity

	Any VEA (%)	Frequent VEA (%)	Serious VEA (Pairs, Trios, VT, VF) (%)
Normal subjects	19–38	3–11	2–6
Patients with coronary artery disease	38–50	23–37	6–15

VEA, ventricular ectopic activity; VT, ventricular tachycardia; VF, ventricular fibrillation.

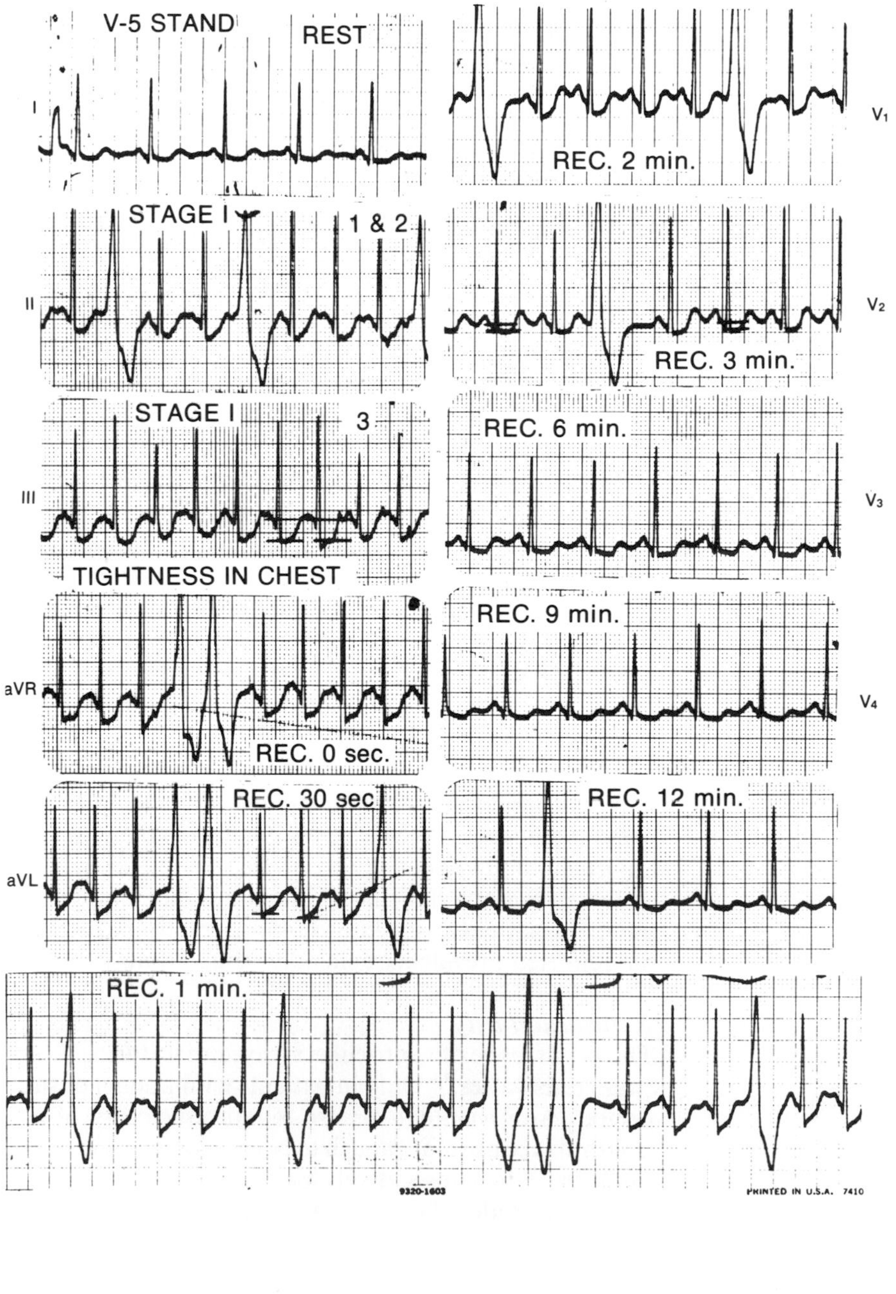

Figure 19-1. *Stress test obtained in a woman of 61 years complaining of palpitations with pairs and trios of premature ventricular beats. Selective coronary arteriography and left ventriculography were entirely normal, and there was no clinical or echographic evidence of prolapsing mitral valve.*

tricular tachycardia, appear to be more reproducible than lower grades, having a reported reproducibility of 50% to 79%.[5,10] In patients with frequent ventricular extrasystoles only, reproducibility is reported to be only 30%.[5] This inherent variation in the occurrence of exercise-induced ventricular arrhythmias in a given person makes interpretation of efficacy of antiarrhythmic therapy difficult.

Comparison of Exercise Stress Testing and Ambulatory Electrocardiographic Monitoring for Detection of Ventricular Arrhythmias

Ventricular tachycardia and other forms of high-grade ventricular ectopy are more frequently documented by ambulatory electrocardiographic monitoring than by exercise stress testing.[11] Patients with prior myocardial infarction are more likely to have ventricular ectopy noted on both exercise stress testing and ambulatory electrocardiographic monitoring, whereas patients with angina pectoris but no past infarction often demonstrate ventricular ectopy only with the latter technique.[11] The issue remains controversial, however, with some studies showing more equivalence between the two techniques.[12] Ventricular tachycardia can occasionally be induced by stress testing when it has not been documented by ambulatory electrocardiographic monitoring.[11,12] Ventricular arrhythmias noted by ambulatory electrocardiographic monitoring as well as those occurring during exercise stress testing appear to be independently predictive of the occurrence of sudden death in patients with ischemic heart disease[13]; however, the ST segment response during exercise is probably of greater value in predicting overall mortality.[14,15]

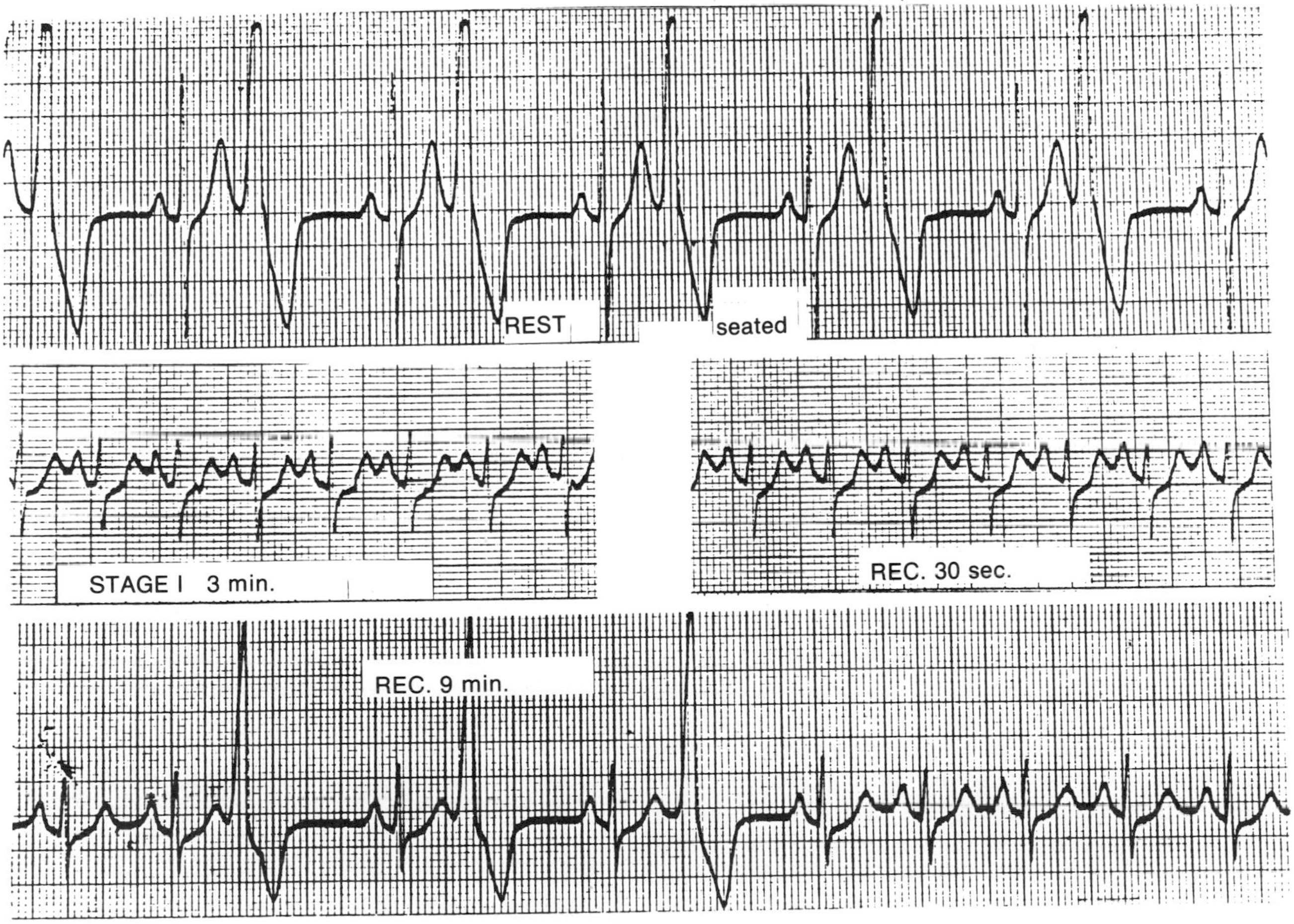

Figure 19-2. *Portions of a treadmill test performed on a man aged 57 years in whom premature ventricular complexes, occurring in a bigeminal fashion at rest, are completely suppressed during the sinus tachycardia induced by exercise and recur well into the recovery period after deceleration of sinus rate has been achieved. The patient, despite borderline ST segment alterations during exercise at a submaximal attained heart rate, had 75% stenoses in all three coronary arteries. Many patients who have ischemic cardiac pain and in whom ventricular extrasystoles are suppressed by exercise have severe coronary disease.*

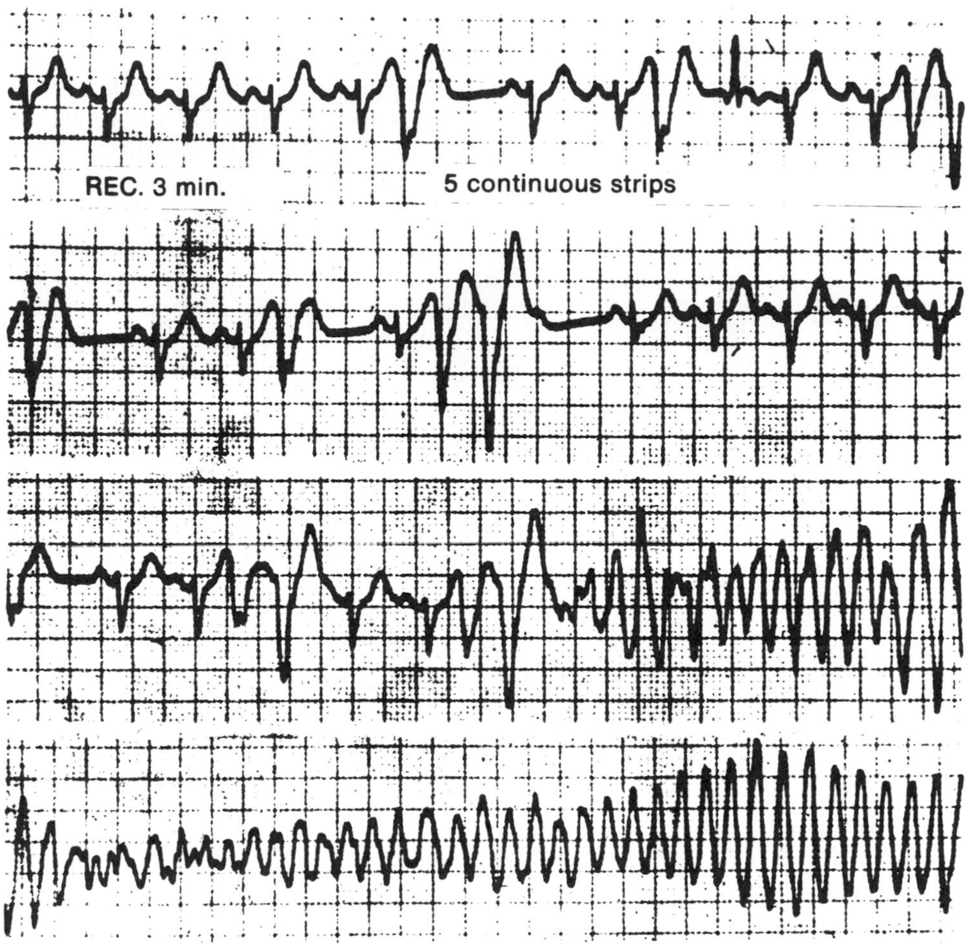

Figure 19-3. *Onset of ventricular fibrillation 3 minutes into the postexercise recovery period in a man of 55 years with exertional hypotension 1 month after he suffered an acute inferior wall myocardial infarction. After successful defibrillation, selective coronary and left ventricular angiography were performed, revealing severe triple-vessel coronary disease. Aortocoronary bypass graft surgery was accomplished, following which ventricular arrhythmias did not occur on repeat treadmill exercise testing.*

Characteristics

Ventricular arrhythmias induced by exercise frequently occur only during the postexercise recovery period, usually within the first 3 minutes.[5,7,16] It has been suggested that ventricular ectopy occurring in the recovery phase after exercise is more often observed in patients with coronary disease, whereas healthy persons are more likely to have ectopy during exercise.[5] The disappearance of resting ventricular premature beats during exercise (Fig. 19-2) does not imply that they are innocuous; in one report,[7] eight of ten such patients had triple vessel coronary artery disease. Exertional hypotension can precede exercise-induced ventricular tachycardia and fibrillation (Fig. 19-3) and was observed to occur in almost half of the 34 patients in one study.[17] Ventricular tachycardia tends to occur at heart rates of less than 150 beats/min in patients with coronary disease. Among patients with known coronary artery disease, exercise-induced ventricular arrhythmias, in particular ventricular tachycardia, tend to be associated with more severe degrees of coronary artery stenosis, double and triple vessel disease, significant left ventricular dysfunction, and ischemic ST segment depression.[7,18–20]

Exercise-Induced Ventricular Tachycardia

Ventricular tachycardia developing during exercise (Fig. 19-4) occurs much less frequently than lower grades of ventricular ectopy. In one large series of 5730 consecutive patients undergoing treadmill testing, 47 patients (0.8%) developed episodes of ventricular tachycardia.[17] In another series of 713 consecutive patients undergoing exercise testing, 12 (1.7%) developed ventricular tachycardia[16]; one fourth of these were felt to have no evidence of underlying heart disease.

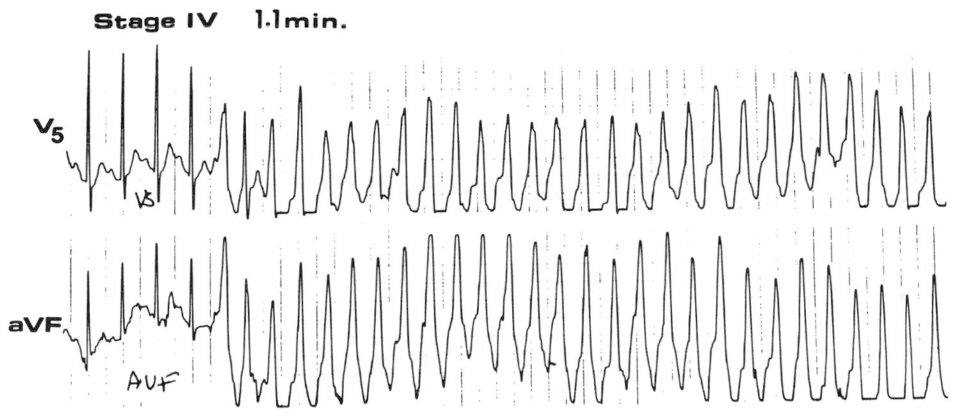

Figure 19-4. *Simultaneously recorded leads V_5 and a V_F showing the onset of ventricular tachycardia during stage IV (Bruce protocol) in a healthy man of 18 years. The tachycardia rate is 190 beats/min, and the sinus rate at its onset is 150 beats/min. The patient was treated with low doses of nadolol, which prevented the exercise-induced ventricular tachycardia.*

Mechanisms

Three mechanisms are generally accepted as underlying most cardiac arrhythmias: reentry, abnormal automaticity, and triggered activity.[21-25] These same mechanisms are thought to explain the occurrence of exercise-induced ventricular tachycardia as well.[26,27]

The requirements for *reentry* are unidirectional block and delay in impulse conduction. Regional myocardial ischemia provoked by exercise could slow conduction through the ischemic region; in this connection, variation in refractory periods of isolated Purkinje fibers has been shown to occur after experimental coronary artery occlusion.[28]

Enhanced automaticity may develop during exercise for several reasons. Experimentally induced myocardial ischemia may reduce maximum diastolic potential to between −60 and −50 mV in both Purkinje fibers and myocardium, thereby enhancing phase 4 depolarization in these tissues.[21] The high circulating catecholamine levels occurring during exercise, as well as the increased sympathetic tone, can cause myocardial ischemia through increases in heart rate and blood pressure. In addition, sympathetic stimulation can itself be arrhythmogenic, by enhancing phase 4 depolarization as well as possibly by provoking delayed afterdepolarizations.[24]

Triggered activity refers to arrhythmias that arise from oscillations in membrane potential (delayed afterdepolarizations) during phase 4 of the action potential. These membrane oscillations have two special properties: (1) they do not occur spontaneously but depend on the occurrence of previous depolarizations and (2) they are rate dependent, usually developing within a critical range of cycle lengths.[22] The amplitude of afterdepolarizations increases in the presence of catecholamines.[21] In addition, afterdepolarizations are calcium dependent, and their appearance *in vitro* can be prevented by calcium channel blocking agents such as verapamil. Afterdepolarizations and triggered activity may be provoked during exercise as a result of heightened catecholamine state as well as increased heart rate.

Electrophysiologic Studies

Electrophysiologic studies performed in patients with exercise-induced ventricular tachycardia have yielded provocative, if indefinite, information. During electrophysiologic testing, a reentry mechanism as the basis for tachycardia is suggested by initiation or termination of ventricular tachycardia with extra stimulus techniques. Catecholamine-sensitive automaticity is suggested by the ability to provoke ventricular tachycardia during or after isoproterenol infusion; abnormal automaticity is unaffected by ventricular extra stimuli. Triggered activity usually occurs only in a critical range of heart rates, and the rate of the ventricular tachycardia tends to increase as the underlying heart rate increases. Catecholamines may also play a role in triggered rhythms both by increasing heart rate and by causing afterdepolarizations. Triggered activity is assumed to be operative if verapamil can prevent the initiation of ventricular tachycardia.

Sung and associates[26] performed electrophysiologic studies in 12 patients with exercise-induced sustained ventricular tachycardia, provoking morphologically similar ventricular tachycardia in ten. Seven of the ten had findings consistent with a reentry mechanism, and three had tachycardia inducible only with isoproterenol infusion. In another study of three patients,[27] the ventricular tachycardia that could be induced with isoproterenol infusion was prevented by propranolol administration and could be terminated with verapamil.

Associated Conditions

The most common cause of exercise-related ventricular tachycardia is coronary artery disease. Disease processes other than coronary artery disease that may be associated with an increased occurrence of exercise-related ventricular arrhythmias include mitral valve prolapse, cardiomyopathy (obstructive and congestive), valvular aortic stenosis, presence of digitalis or hypokalemia, syndromes associated with prolonged QT interval (Fig. 19-5), other congenital cardiac abnormalities, and pulmonary disease (Table 19-2).[18,26,29-33]

The fairly common syndrome of mid-systolic click–late-systolic murmur, due to myxomatous degeneration of mitral valve leaflet tissue leading to prolapse of one or both leaflets, is frequently associated with ventricular ectopic activity at rest or after exercise or both. The prevalence of exercise-related ventricular arrhythmias ranges from 11% to 75%,[29-32, 34] with advanced forms of ventricular irritability often present.[32] Ventricular tachycardia has been noted to occur in 6.3% of patients with mitral valve prolapse.[29] Ventricular extrasystoles present at rest may disappear, persist, or worsen during exercise, and ventricular arrhythmias may develop *de novo* during exercise. Sudden death in patients having this syndrome, fortunately occurring only rarely, is presumably due to ventricular fibrillation. In one report, sudden death occurred without prior evidence of either rest- or effort-related ventricular arrhythmias.[34] A pro-

Table 19-2. Conditions Associated With Exercise-Induced Arrhythmias

Normal cardiovascular status
Coronary artery disease
Mitral valve prolapse
Digitalis administration
Hypokalemia
Cardiomyopathy
Left ventricular outflow obstruction
Aortic valvular stenosis
Hypertrophic subaortic stenosis
Prolonged QT interval syndromes
Idiopathic
Quinidine administration
Phenothiazine administration
Pulmonary disease

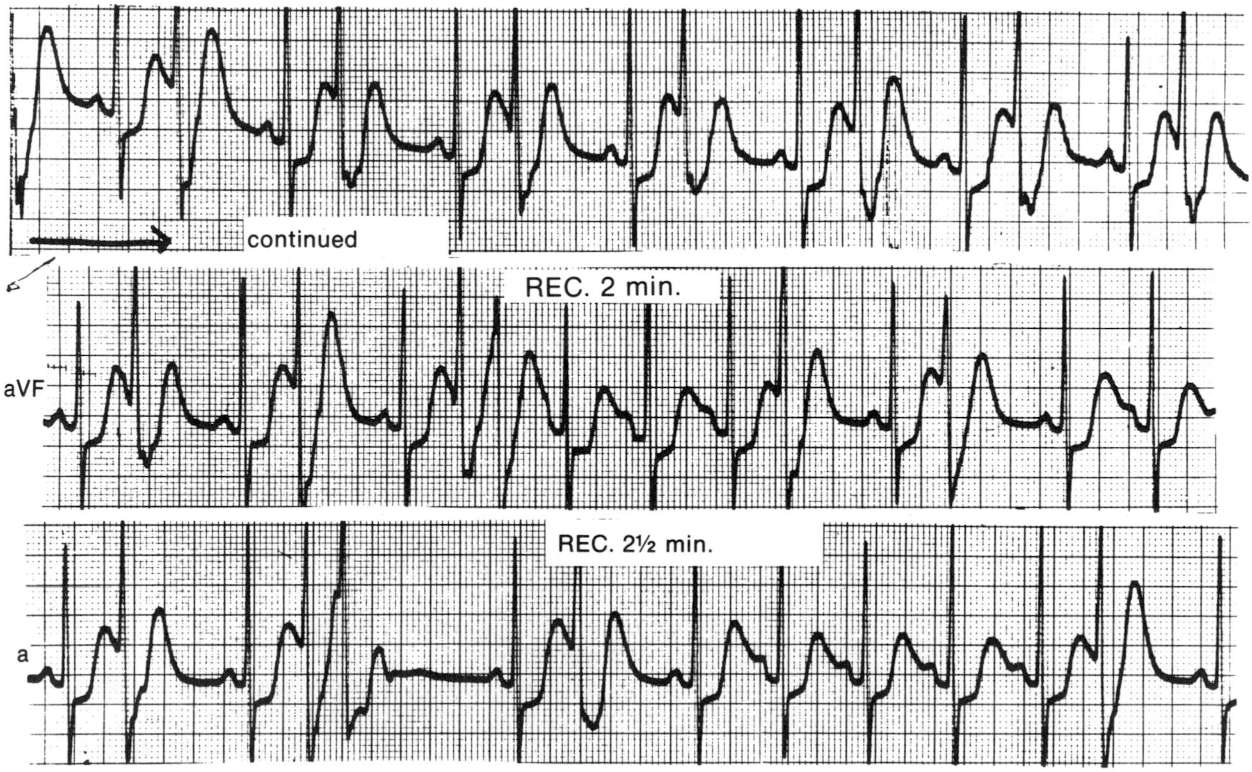

Figure 19-5. *Woman patient with QT interval prolongation, especially marked during and immediately after exercise. The QT interval measures 0.4 second with a sinus rate of 100 beats/min. J point depression, 2 mm, with slowly upsloping ST segments, is present, failing to meet criteria for a positive stress test. Ventricular ectopic activity occurs frequently, and there are occasional pairs with a short coupling interval. Exercise-induced ventricular arrhythmias in patients with long QT intervals not due to quinidine or to hypokalemia may respond favorably to propranolol.*

longed QT interval may be present in 47% of patients,[29] potentially contributing to arrhythmogenesis.

Digitalis preparations may contribute both to the uncovering of latent arrhythmias and to *de novo* arrhythmogenesis. The signs and symptoms of digitalis toxicity may not be apparent, and the ventricular arrhythmias occurring during and after exercise may be the only clue to digitalis toxicity.[33]

Prognosis

The prognosis of patients with ventricular arrhythmias occurring during exercise relates to their underlying disease and to use of specific treatment aimed at preventing the dysrhythmia. The presence of coronary artery disease and, in particular, evidence of myocardial ischemia on exercise stress testing, as well as the presence of left ventricular dysfunction, appear to be the most important prognostic indicators for risk of sudden death.[13,14] In survivors of cardiac arrest who undergo subsequent exercise stress testing, failure of the blood pressure to rise and development of angina appear to have a stronger relationship to subsequent risk of recurrent cardiac arrest than does the appearance of ventricular arrhythmias *per se.*[35] In patients who undergo coronary artery bypass surgery, the incidence of exercise-induced ventricular arrhythmias has been reported to be unchanged at 1 and 5 years following surgery.[36] However, the appearance for the first time of exercise-induced ventricular tachycardia in surgically treated patients might be predictive of recurrent sudden death.[36]

The prognosis of apparently healthy persons who experience ventricular tachycardia during exercise is much better than that of patients with symptomatic coronary artery disease. In one recent study,[37] of 11 asymptomatic persons who had exercise-related ventricular tachycardia, none had perfusion defects on thallium scintigraphy, and no heart disease, syncope, or sudden death occurred during an average 1.7-year follow-up period. It appears, therefore, that prognosis of patients with exercise-induced ventricular tachycardia may relate in part to the development of exercise-induced ischemia.

The prognosis for patients with effort-related ventricular tachycardia in conditions other than coronary disease remains virtually unknown but may depend on clinicians' ability to provide definitive antiarrhythmic therapy.

Therapy

When exercise-induced ventricular tachycardia is specifically related to myocardial ischemia, the primary treatment should be directed toward preventing the ischemia. Medical therapy with long-acting nitrates or beta- or calcium channel blocking agents or surgical therapy can be offered.

Although coronary artery bypass grafting does not appear to decrease the overall frequency of exercise-induced ventricular arrhythmias,[36] there have been reports of successful arrhythmia management by this means,[38,39] with no recurrence of arrhythmias for up to 2 years postoperatively.[39]

When exercise-induced ventricular tachycardia cannot be specifically related to myocardial ischemia, treatment should be directed at the mechanism underlying the arrhythmia, if this can be documented. Electrophysiologic testing is of specific value in this regard, since there are problems with reproducibility using serial stress testing to guide efficacy of antiarrhythmic therapy. In the series of Sung and colleagues,[26] in which electrophysiologic testing was used to guide therapy, all patients with catecholamine-sensitive automaticity responded to propranolol administered intravenously and subsequently administered orally.* Patients with reentry are usually treated successfully with procainamide or amiodarone.[26] Failure to abolish exercise-induced ventricular arrhythmias in patients without cardiac disease is not infrequent and often frustrating (Fig. 19-6).

Propranolol is of specific benefit in patients who demonstrate a relationship between the onset of exercise-induced ventricular tachycardia and a critical sinus rate. In one study,[10] of 11 patients with reproducible exercise-induced ventricular tachycardia, eight had a consistent sinus rate at the onset of ventricular tachycardia, and in all eight ventricular tachycardia was prevented by administration of acute and chronic beta-blockade medications. Propranolol is also efficacious in patients with exercise-induced ventricular tachycardia occurring in the long QT interval syndrome, although its efficacy appears to be unrelated to measured QT interval.[40] Propranolol has also been successfully used in patients with mitral valve prolapse and exercise-induced ventricular tachycardia.[30]

Intravenous verapamil appears to be highly effective in treatment of patients with exercise-induced ventricular tachycardia because it both terminates and prevents the arrhythmia.[27,41] Continued oral therapy with verapamil, however, appears to be only moderately effective in preventing exercise-induced ventricular tachycardia when compared to beta-blockade.[41] The effect of verapamil in patients with ventricular tachycardia associated with mitral valve prolapse has not been investigated, although, since afterdepolarizations have been noted in fibers from isolated simian mitral valves,[24] this would be of interest.

* Sung, R.: Personal communication.

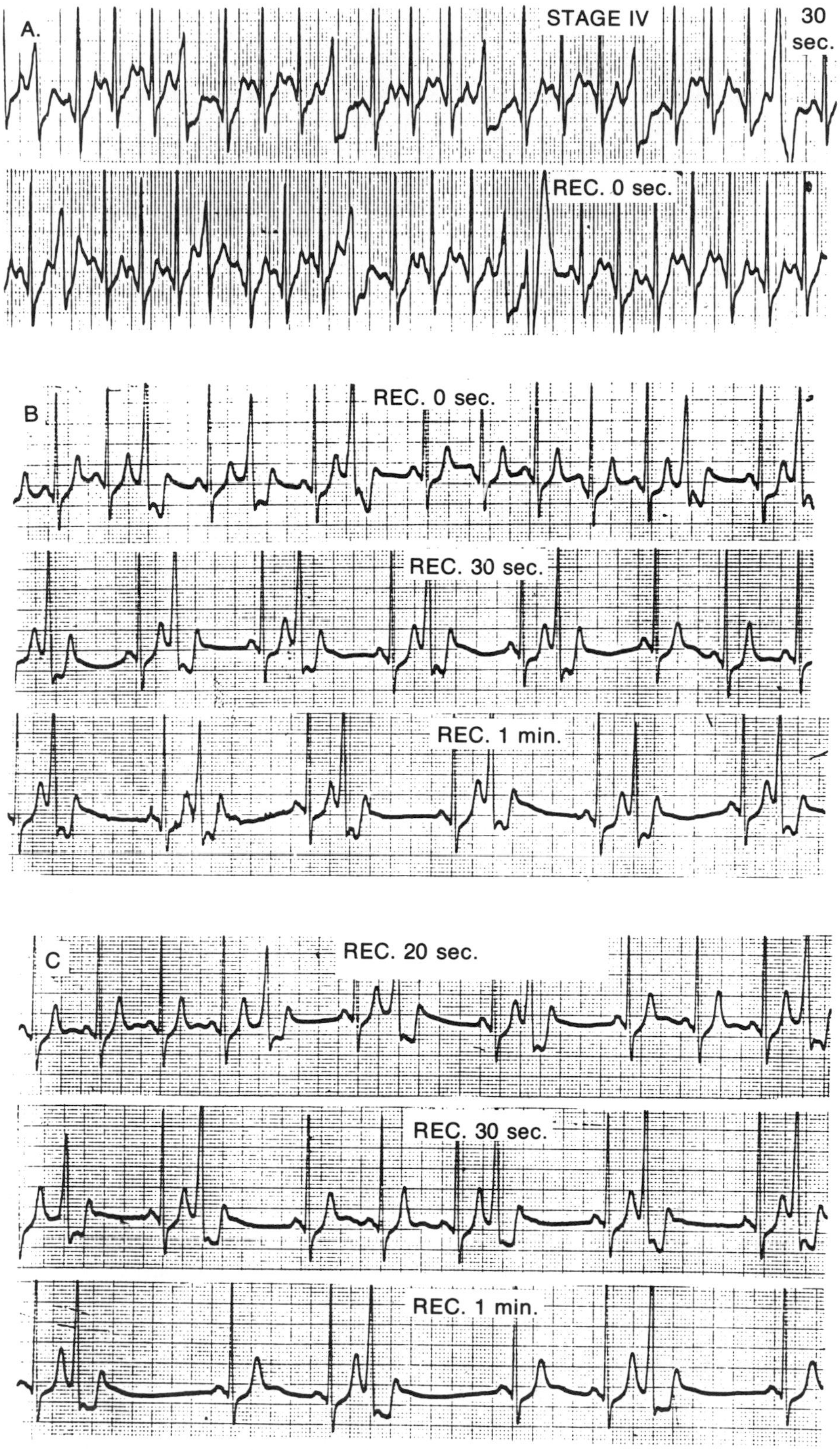

Figure 19-6. *Exercise-induced ventricular premature beats in an asymptomatic man aged 55 years whose effort tolerance was excellent. (A) Baseline treadmill stress test, illustrating closely coupled ventricular extrasystoles appearing at the height of exercise and persisting into the early recovery period, where a single pair of ventricular beats is recorded. The treadmill test is negative for myocardial ischemic changes. Although the patient had no*

(continued)

Implications for Exercise Rehabilitation Programs

The popularity of cardiac rehabilitation programs has led to two questions about patients with exercise-induced ventricular arrhythmias: what is the risk of exercise conditioning in these patients, and what is the response of the arrhythmia to physical reconditioning?

Fortunately, the risk of cardiac arrest is quite low in physician-directed cardiac rehabilitation programs.[42] However, since the risk of sudden death in patients with cardiac disease relates primarily to severity of coronary artery disease and degree of underlying left ventricular dysfunction, patients with poor left ventricular function or ongoing angina who have documented exercise-induced ventricular tachycardia should not undertake a vigorous exercise program.[43]

Physical conditioning does appear, according to one report,[44] to diminish the frequency of exercise-induced ventricular ectopy in an asymptomatic population. Nonetheless, there have been reports of sudden death in apparently healthy persons who were jogging.[45] Screening the asymptomatic person who undertakes sporadic vigorous exercise for ventricular arrhythmias is, however, probably of little overall benefit.

References

1. Coronary Drug Project Research Group: Prognostic importance of premature beats following myocardial infarction. J.A.M.A., 223:1116–1124, 1973.
2. Chiang, B. N., Perlman, L. V., Ostrander, L. D. Jr., and Epstein, F. H.. Relationship of premature systoles to coronary heart disease and sudden death in the Tecumseh epidemiologic study. Ann. Intern. Med., 70:1159–1166, 1969.
3. McHenry, P. L., Fisch, C., Jordan, J. W., and Corya, B. R.: Cardiac arrhythmias observed during maximal treadmill exercise testing in clinically normal men. Am. J. Cardiol., 29:331–336, 1972.
4. Anderson, M. T., Lee, G. B., Campion, B. C., et al.: Cardiac dysrhythmias associated with exercise testing. Am. J. Cardiol., 30:763–767, 1972.
5. Jelinek, M. V., and Lown, B.: Exercise stress testing for exposure of cardiac arrhythmia. Prog. Cardiovasc. Dis., 16:497–522, 1974.
6. Ekblom, B., Hartley, L. H., and Day, W. C.: Occurrence and reproducibility of exercise-induced ventricular ectopy in normal subjects. Am. J. Cardiol., 43:35–40, 1979.
7. Goldschlager, N., Cake, D., and Cohn, K.: Exercise-induced ventricular arrhythmias in patients with coronary artery disease. Am. J. Cardiol., 31:434–440, 1973.
8. Faris, J. V., McHenry, P. L., Jordan, J. W., and Morris, S. N.: Prevalence and reproducibility of exercise-induced ventricular arrhythmias during maximal exercise testing in normal men. Am. J. Cardiol., 37:617–622, 1976.
9. Sheps, D. S., Ernst, J. C., Briese, F. R., et al.: Decreased frequency of exercise-induced ventricular ectopic activity in the second of two consecutive treadmill tests. Circulation, 55:892–895, 1977.
10. Woelfel, A., Foster, J. R., Simpson, R. J., Jr., and Gettes, L. S.: Reproducibility and treatment of exercise-induced ventricular tachycardia. Am. J. Cardiol., 53:751–756, 1984.
11. Ryan, M., Lown, B., and Horn, H.: Comparison of ventricular ectopic activity during 24-hour monitoring and exercise testing in patients with coronary heart disease. N. Engl. J. Med., 292:224–229, 1975.
12. Kosowsky, B. D., Lown, B., Whiting, R., and Guiney, T.: Occurrence of ventricular arrhythmias with exercise as compared to monitoring. Circulation, 44:826–832, 1971.
13. Ivanova, L. A., Mazur, N. A., Smirnova, T. M., et al.: Electrocardiographic exercise testing and ambulatory monitoring to identify patients with ischemic heart disease at high risk of sudden death. Am. J. Cardiol., 45:1132–1138, 1980.
14. Kennedy, H. L.: Comparison of ambulatory electrocardiography and exercise testing. Am. J. Cardiol., 47:1359–1365, 1981.
15. Froelicher, V. E., Jr., Thomas, M. M., Pillow, C., and Lancaster, M. C.: Epidemiologic study of asymptomatic men screened by maximal treadmill testing for latent coronary artery disease. Am. J. Cardiol., 34:770–776, 1974.
16. Gooch, A. S., and McConnell, D.: Analysis of transient arrhythmias and conduction disturbances occurring during submaximal treadmill exercise testing. Prog. Cardiovasc. Dis., 13:293–307, 1970.
17. Codini, M. A., Sommerfeldt, L., Eybel, C. E., and Messer, J. V.: Clinical significance and characteristics of exercise-induced ventricular tachycardia. Cath. Cardiovasc. Diag., 7:227–234, 1981.
18. Helfant, R. H., Pine, R., Kabde, V., and Banka, V. S.: Exercise-related ventricular premature complexes in coronary heart disease. Ann. Intern. Med., 80:589–592, 1974.
19. McHenry, P. L., Morris, S. N., Kavalier, M., and Jordan, J. W.: Comparative study of exercise-induced ventricular arrhythmias in normal subjects and patients with documented coronary artery disease. Am. J. Cardiol., 37:609–616, 1976.
20. Levine, S. R., Weiner, D. A., Klein, M. D., and Ryan, T. J.: Significance of ventricular arrhythmias during exercise testing. Circulation, 68:III–76, 1983.
21. Hoffman, B. F., and Rosen, M. R.: Cellular mechanisms for cardiac arrhythmias. Cir. Res., 49:1–15, 1981.
22. Rosen, M. R., and Reder, R. F.: Does triggered activity have a role in the genesis of cardiac arrhythmias. Ann. Intern. Med., 94:794–801, 1981.
23. Spear, J. F., and Moore, E. N.: Mechanisms of cardiac arrhythmias. Ann. Rev. Physiol., 44:485–497, 1982.
24. Cranefield, P. F., and Wit, A. L.: Cardiac arrhythmias. Ann. Rev. Physiol., 41:459–472, 1979.
25. Josephson, M. E., Horowitz, L. N., Farshidi, A., and Kastor, J. A.:

symptoms, this rhythm disturbance was thought to merit suppressive treatment. (B) Repeat treadmill test performed 2 weeks later, with the patient having received propranolol, 20 mg 4 times daily. Maximum heart rate achieved is now only about 110 beats/min. Ventricular premature beats are still present and, in fact, occur more frequently. (C) A third treadmill test performed 2 weeks after that shown in B, with the patient now receiving procainamide, 375 mg every 8 hours, in addition to propranolol, 40 mg 4 times daily. Maximum attained heart rate at this time is only about 95 beats/min. This combination of antiarrhythmic medications failed to suppress the patient's ventricular ectopy.

Recurrent sustained ventricular tachycardia. Circulation, 57:431–440, 1978.
26. Sung, R. J., Shen, E. N., Morady, F., et al.: Electrophysiologic mechanism of exercise-induced sustained ventricular tachycardia. Am. J. Cardiol., 51:525–530, 1983.
27. Wu, D., Kou, H., and Hung, J.: Exercise-triggered paroxysmal ventricular tachycardia. Ann. Intern. Med., 95:410–414, 1981.
28. Sasyniuk, B. I., and Mendez, C.: A mechanism for reentry in canine ventricular tissue. Circ. Res., 28:3–15, 1971.
29. Swartz, M. H., Teichholz, L. E., and Donoso, E.: Mitral valve prolapse. Am. J. Cardiol., 62:377–389, 1977.
30. Pocock, W. A., and Barlow, J. B.: Postexercise arrhythmias in the billowing posterior mitral leaflet syndrome. Am. Heart J., 80:740–745, 1970.
31. Sloman, G., Wong, M., and Walker, J.: Arrhythmias on exercise in patients with abnormalities of the posterior leaflet of the mitral valve. Am. Heart J., 83:312–317, 1972.
32. Gooch, A. S., Vicencio, F., Maranhao, V., and Goldberg, H.: Arrhythmias and left ventricular asynergy in the prolapsing mitral leaflet syndrome. Am. J. Cardiol., 29:611–620, 1972.
33. Gooch, A. S., Natarajan, G., and Goldberg, H.: Influence of exercise on arrhythmias induced by digitalis-diuretic therapy in patients with atrial fibrillation. Am. J. Cardiol., 33:230–237, 1974.
34. Shappell, S. D., Marshall, C. E., Brown, R. E., and Bruce, T. A.: Sudden death and the familial occurrence of mid-systolic click, late systolic murmur syndrome. Circulation, 48:1128–1134, 1973.
35. Weaver, W. D., Cobb, L. A., and Hallstrom, A. P.: Characteristics of survivors of exertion- and nonexertion-related cardiac arrest: Value of subsequent exercise testing. Am. J. Cardiol. 50:671–676, 1982.
36. Lehrman, K. L., Tilkian, A. G., Hultgren, H. N., and Fowles, R. E.: Effect of coronary arterial bypass surgery on exercise-induced ventricular arrhythmias. Am. J. Cardiol., 44:1056–1061, 1979.
37. Fleg, J. L., and Lakatta, E. G.: Prevalence and prognosis of ventricular tachycardia during treadmill exercise in apparently healthy volunteers. Circulation, 68:III–75, 1983.
38. Bryson, A. L., Parisi, A. F., Schechter, E., and Wolfson, S.: Life threatening ventricular arrhythmias induced by exercise. Am. J. Cardiol., 32:995–999, 1973.
39. Codini, M. A., Sommerfeldt, L., Eybel, C. E., et al.: Efficacy of coronary bypass grafting in exercise-induced ventricular tachycardia. J. Thorac. Cardiovasc. Surg., 81:502–506, 1981.
40. Alpert, B. S., Boineau, J., and Strong, W. B.: Exercise-induced ventricular tachycardia. Ped. Cardiol., 2:51–55, 1982.
41. Woelfel, A. K., Foster, J. R., McAllister, R. G., and Gettes, L. S.: Use of verapamil in exercise-induced ventricular tachycardia. Circulation, 68:III–76, 1983.
42. Rothfield, D., Werres, R., Rommer, T. C., and Pongpoonsuksri, V.: Cardiac arrest in a physician-directed cardiac rehabilitation program. Angiology, 31:576–580, 1980.
43. Jelinek, V. M.: Exercise-induced arrhythmias: Their implications for cardiac rehabilitation programs. Med. Sci. Sports Exer., 12:223–230, 1980.
44. Blackburn, H., Taylor, H. L., Hamrell, B., et al.: Premature ventricular complexes induced by stress testing. Am. J. Cardiol., 31:441–449, 1973.
45. Kannel, W. B.: Exercise and sudden death. J.A.M.A., 248:3143–3144, 1982.

20

Ventricular Tachycardia and Ventricular Fibrillation

Dennis M. Krikler, Michael Perelman, and Edward Rowland

It clearly was very difficult for our predecessors to distinguish one arrhythmia from another until graphic methods were introduced, and even then, a century or so ago, sphygmography was insufficiently precise to allow differentiation of various tachycardias.[1] Undoubtedly Brunton[2] recognized, albeit without defining the cause, that under chloroform anesthesia some patients developed a rapid heart rate with shock and died. This observation was particularly important in light of the subsequent demonstration by Levy and Lewis[3] that ventricular tachycardia and fibrillation could be induced by chloroform. The term *paroxysmal tachycardia* can be found in a monograph by Hoffmann,[4] and, in his first book, Wenckebach[5] refers to the disorder in general, only distinguishing ventricular tachycardia from the atrial and junctional forms a decade later.[6] Although Mackenzie[7] used the term *paroxysmal tachycardia* and described cases, it is impossible to identify any of these cases as being due to paroxysmal ventricular tachycardia, and Mackenzie himself did not attempt to distinguish the site of impulse formation. In the meantime, Lewis[8] provided the essential background information to permit recognition of ventricular tachycardia, which he induced in dogs by coronary artery ligation. In his experiments, such aspects as atrioventricular dissociation, the presence or absence of ventriculoatrial conduction, lack of response to vagal maneuvers, and the development of ventricular fibrillation were carefully discussed and illustrated with electrocardiographic tracings.

Ventricular fibrillation and ventricular tachycardia are presumably the same arrhythmia as the "tremulous motion" and "tumultuous" action of the heart described under these circumstances by Erichsen.[9] Allessie[10] admirably recounts the experimental production and recordings of ventricular fibrillation by Hoffa and Ludwig, using electric currents, and also the more definitive description of ventricular fibrillation by McWilliam.[11] A clinical example by Lewis in 1911 showed atrioventricular dissociation,[12] and thereafter numerous clinical and electrocardiographic reports appeared. Better understanding of the mechanisms and causes of ventricular tachycardia and fibrillation has come in fits and starts as the importance of ischemic heart disease has become appreciated both in general and in relation to ventricular arrhythmias and as electrophysiologic techniques applied to animal preparations and those used in patients have enhanced clinicians' understanding of the mechanisms of these arrhythmias.

Definitions

Although paroxysmal ventricular tachycardia and ventricular fibrillation refer to disorders of rhythm affecting, and located in, the ventricles, a more specific definition is required. Arrhythmias associated with disturbances in the bundle of His proximal to its bifurcation are conventionally classed as supraventricular, even though this is anatomically imprecise. This is not just because they usually have narrow QRS complexes, for some focal arrhythmias arising in the bundle of His may do so eccentrically or may be conducted less well into one bundle branch than into the other, producing the appearances of aberration (Fig. 20-1). The same consideration applies, at least at present, to those few cases of tachycardia in which reciprocation occurs between an infranodal accessory pathway, a so-called Mahaim tract, and one or the other of the bundle branches.[13] The term *ventricular tachycardia* is generally meant to indicate an arrhythmia that arises within the ventricles distal to the subdivision of the bundle of His, involving either rapid discharge from an ectopic focus or reentry at a Purkinje-myocardial junction or between bundle branches or fascicles or solely within the myocardium.

Accelerated idioventricular rhythm describes the development of an independent ventricular rhythm more rapid than sinus that becomes manifest only intermittently. Semantically the arrhythmia in Figure 20-1 could be placed in this category, but a better example is seen in Figure 20-2, in which the rate is only marginally faster than sinus. Schamroth suggests a rate range of 55 to 108 beats/min.[14] Such arrhythmias often occur during acute myocardial infarction but are probably benign. It is closely linked with the lower rate limit, defined by Scherf and Schott[15] as 160/min, but even they accept that it may be as low as 110.

Electrophysiology

Arrhythmias may arise by any of a number of mechanisms: enhanced automaticity at a focal ectopic site, reentry, or triggered activity (see Chap. 3). Most early electrocardiographers believed that paroxysmal ventricular tachycardia was usually due to enhanced automaticity,[14] but more recently the evidence suggests reentry as the major cause. Intraventricular reentry is well established in animal models,[16,17] and modern electrophysiological

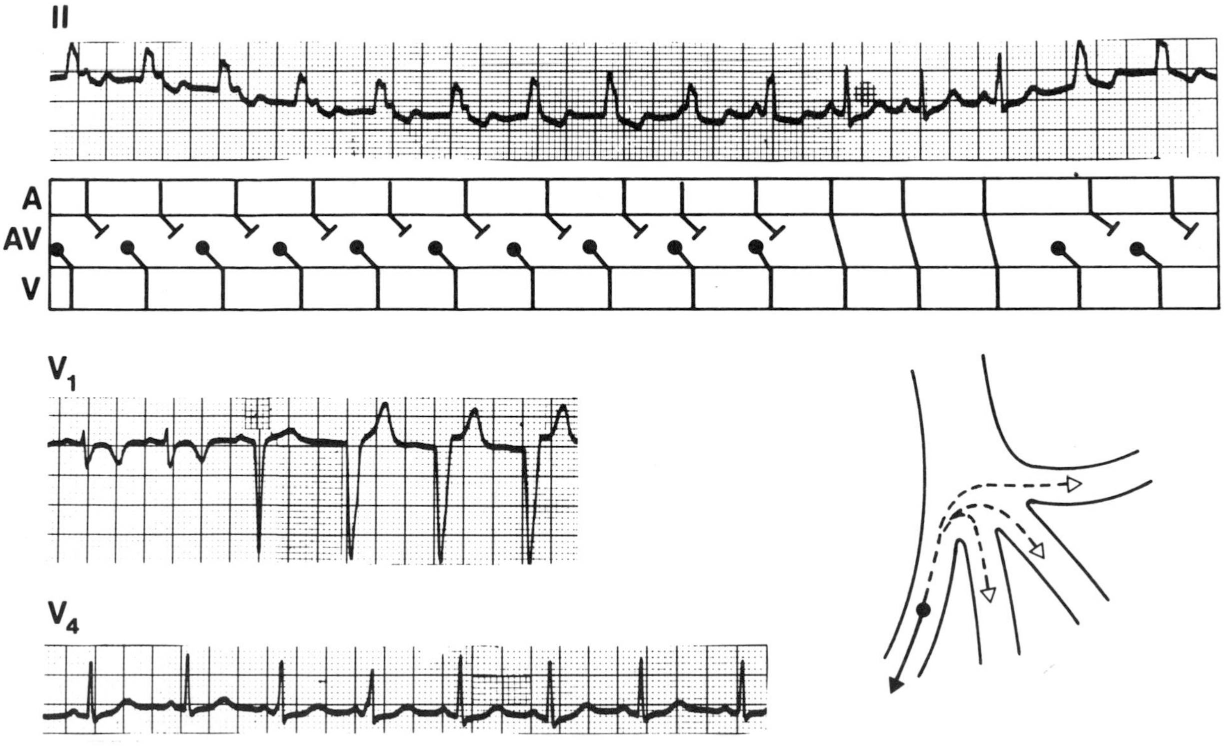

Figure 20-1. *Electrocardiograms from a woman aged 24 years with AV dissociation showing intermittent rapid discharge from an area apparently located within the proximal right bundle branch, producing, in those complexes, appearances consistent with incomplete left bundle branch block. The arrhythmia is terminated when the sinus rate increases and captures the ventricles and manifests itself as the sinus rate slows.*

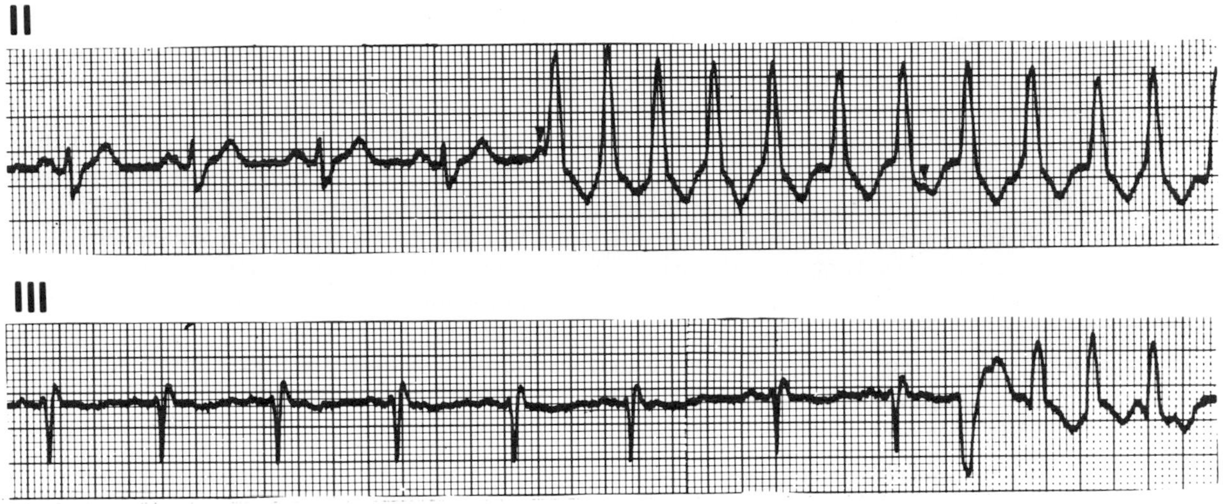

Figure 20-2. *Leads II and III electrocardiographic tracings from a patient with diffuse chronic ischemic fibrosis of the left ventricle following repeated myocardial infarcts. Uniform wide QRS complexes represent ventricular tachycardia. The arrhythmia is slightly irregular, and, in lead III, initial vectors of the QRS complex in tachycardia and sinus rhythm point in opposite directions. Selected P waves* (arrows) *help reveal the AV dissociation. In lead III, the tachycardia appears to be initiated by a QRS complex quite opposite in direction to its successors; its causative role is uncertain.*

techniques have suggested that even in humans reentry is the commonest mechanism.[18] Under appropriate circumstances one can initiate and terminate a tachycardia by suitably timed electrical impulses, suggesting a reentry loop, but current techniques may not be able to differentiate between a focal origin and reentry. The former may be due to a localized microreentry circuit occurring within an area of 30 sq mm, if studies on isolated atria can be extrapolated to the ventricles,[19] and the role of triggered activity adds a further element that is not yet well defined clinically.[20]

Propagated action potentials from myocardial cells can be induced by changes in electrolyte and acid-base balance, especially a decrease in potassium concentration, or in extracellular and intracellular *p*H, and the preliminary studies of Bouvrain and Coraboeuf may well have therapeutic implications in cardiac infarction.[21] Furthermore, the development of a stable animal model permits mapping of reentrant ventricular arrhythmias.[22] Such studies have been carried out on dogs 3 to 7 days after ligation of the anterior descending coronary artery. A specially designed composite electrode permits reentrant impulses to be mapped during their course through the infarction zone. This model has been utilized to study the patterns of initiation and termination of reentry ventricular arrhythmias and to show that ventricular fibrillation may be related to a marked delay in the reentrant pathway conduction of the beat before that apparently coupled to the premature beat (see Chap. 14).[23] Using intracellular and extracellular recordings in the dog heart *in situ,* Russell and colleagues have been able to show the development of conditions that can give rise to arrhythmias, notably slow conduction.[24] When this is accompanied by alternans of the action potential, affecting amplitude, duration, and morphology, ventricular fibrillation could be produced by occlusion of the left anterior descending coronary artery. Very similar results were reported with observations on subepicardial membrane potentials recorded from intact pig hearts by Downar and associates.[25] Both groups noted that varying degrees of localized conduction blocks (*e.g.,* 2:1 responses), as well as alternation, were important precursors of fibrillation; highly relevant to this is the way in which reentrant extrasystoles can be noted in the model by El-Sherif and co-workers.[26]

The precise importance of focal tachycardia, as opposed to macroreentry, requires reevaluation not only in persons with acute myocardial infarction but also in persons in whom other causes exist. Intracardiac studies by Brechenmacher and colleagues[27] revealed that even though surface electrocardiograms failed to disclose any evidence of reentry during sinus rhythm, a late potential could be identified with endocavitary recordings, which activated the bundle of His retrogradely and the right bundle branch anterogradely; from this localized area, obvious macroreentry developed, with typical reciprocating ventricular tachycardia. Operative endocardial and epicardial recordings have shown both continuous activity[28] and late potentials[29] in patients with ventricular tachycardia. This may also have applications to ventricular fibrillation, although focal automaticity may play a role, and indeed different electrophysiologic mechanisms may exist. Recognition of the importance of reentry in this field is growing.[30] Our own studies have shown that in those patients with underlying disorders of repolarization, electrical stimulation may lead to the form of reentry ventricular tachycardia called *torsade de pointes* (see below),[31] itself a potential forerunner of ventricular fibrillation. This indeed appears to have been the mechanism for sudden death noted during ambulatory monitoring.[32]

It is not yet appropriate in the clinical context to do more than allude to the possible role of triggered activity, a mechanism of arrhythmia well demonstrated *in vitro.*[33] Such behavior, in which a focus becomes rhythmically active only if driven at a given rate or by a critically timed premature stimulus, is thus distinguished from spontaneous automaticity; its occurrence following phase 4 depolarization due to an afterpotential is different from what is seen in the usual models for reentry. Although triggered automaticity may be responsible for experimental canine atrial arrhythmias,[34] it has yet to be linked with clinical ventricular arrhythmias, although this is an attractive explanation.[20] Indeed, Moe has shown *in vitro* that delayed reflection (type 2) can result in an extrasystole at the point of origin without the presence of pacemaker elements.[35] This work may provide an explanation for microreentry in ischemic myocardium.

It remains to be seen whether triggered automaticity is responsible for initiating one particular variety of ventricular tachycardia that can be terminated by verapamil.[36] Further support comes from Coumel, who has examined the effect of calcium channel blockers, such as verapamil, on ventricular extrasystoles.[37] Finally, the role of the autonomic nervous system in relation to the induction and termination of ventricular tachycardia and fibrillation needs reappraisal. Apparently benign chronic recurrent ventricular tachycardia can be terminated by phenylephrine,[38,39] and vagal stimulation may prevent ventricular arrhythmias, particularly in situations with high sympathetic tone,[40] such as after acute anterior myocardial infarction. That endogenous catecholamines may also be important, perhaps in increasing transmembrane calcium influx, may likewise be relevant to the initiation of ventricular arrhythmias.[39]

Electrocardiographic Features

Descriptions of the characteristics of ventricular tachycardia are, strange to say, given differently by various authorities. These should clearly be based on the existence of a rapid arrhythmia arising or existing within the ventricles distal to the bifurcation of the bundle of His,

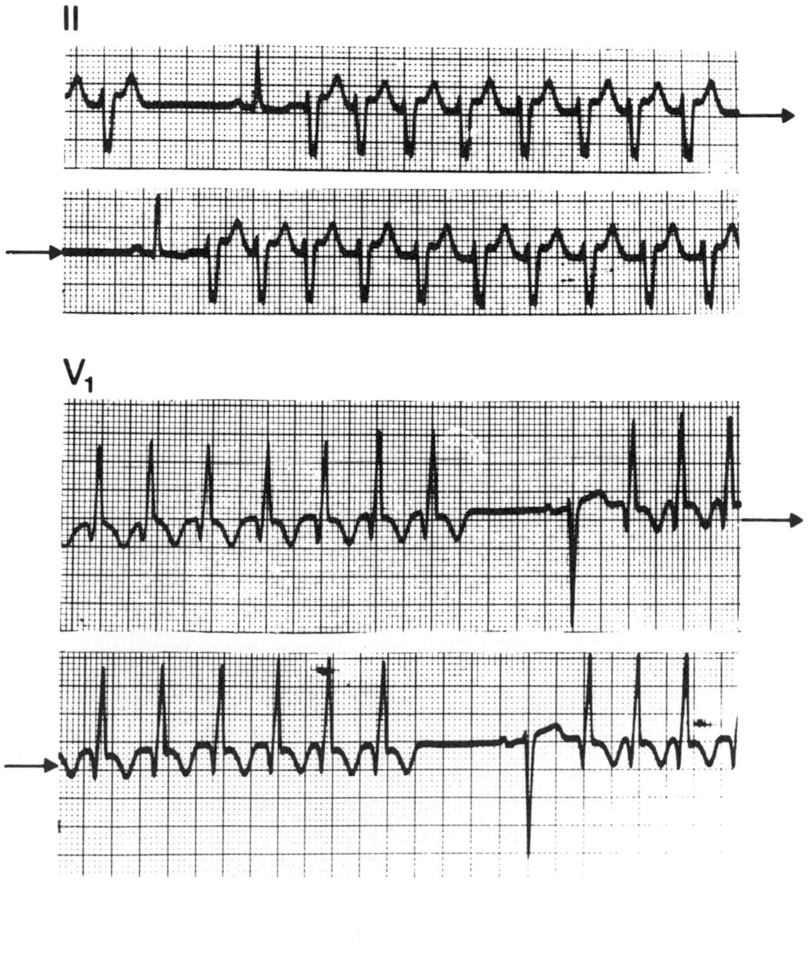

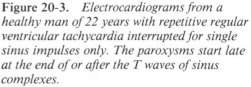

Figure 20-3. *Electrocardiograms from a healthy man of 22 years with repetitive regular ventricular tachycardia interrupted for single sinus impulses only. The paroxysms start late at the end of or after the T waves of sinus complexes.*

whether on the basis of enhanced automaticity or microscopic or macroscopic reentry. Ventricular activity is independent of that of the atria in that the atria may continue to respond to the influence of the sinus node, or they may respond to retrograde stimulation from the ventricles or be the seat of a supraventricular arrhythmia (*e.g.*, atrial fibrillation). In general terms, the QRS complex is both wider than normal and altered in appearance, the more so if the mechanism of the arrhythmia is seated further away from the bundle of His. Precisely what constitutes tachycardia in terms of number of successive complexes (Bellet[42] requires four to six, Schamroth[14] and Anderson and co-workers[43] are satisfied with three) is less important than identification of the site of the sustained rhythm disturbance; the relevance of nonsustained tachycardia must always be assessed.

Although some ventricular tachycardias do have features that may enable them to be recognized as benign, ventricular fibrillation, on the other hand, can never be pronounced as benign. Ventricular fibrillation is a disorder that leads to death unless the arrhythmia is arrested by external means, and its presence implies disease even though the precise nature may not be defined. As will be indicated below, so-called self-limited attacks of "ventricular fibrillation" usually represent torsade de pointes. In the course of the subsequent discussion, under etiologic factors, both ventricular tachycardia and fibrillation will be considered as appropriate.

Characteristically, ventricular tachycardia has a uniform aspect consisting of a series of widened QRS complexes, usually regular (Fig. 20-3) but sometimes moderately irregular (see Fig. 20-2), with appearances different from those of the basic sinus rhythm. As can be seen in Figures 20-2 and 20-3, the initial vector of the QRS complex is usually quite different from those in sinus impulses. The QRS vector may (as with total anomalous conduction in patients with the Wolff-Parkinson-White syndrome[42]) indicate that part of the ventricle first depolarized, by the forces that appear to emanate from it. Thus, in Figure 20-4, one may infer, from the marked superior axis deviation, in the frontal plane and the positive R in lead V_1, a posteroseptal origin for the ventricular tachycardia, compatible with the clinical diagnosis of mitral valve prolapse that was confirmed at operation and epicardial mapping.[45] Even though basically uniform, the QRS complexes do show some variability in morphology.

Where evident, the hallmark of ventricular tachycardia is atrioventricular dissociation. Atrial activity cannot be discerned during tachycardia in Figure 20-3, but is easier to identify in lead III in Figure 20-4 as sharper peaking of alternate T waves, possibly representing 2:1 ventriculoatrial conduction. Discrete sinus P waves, unrelated to ventricular activation, more clearly indicate atrioventricular dissociation in Figures 20-2 and 20-5, but it is sometimes necessary to record a simultaneous right atrial electrogram in order to display this phenomenon (Fig. 20-6*B*). When the P wave falls in the appropriate part of the cycle, capture as well as fusion complexes may be seen (see Fig. 20-5).

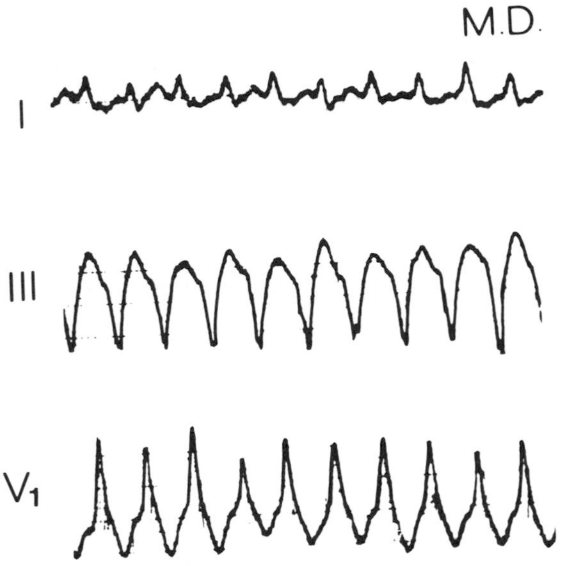

Figure 20-4. *Electrocardiograms from a patient with a floppy mitral valve, showing ventricular tachycardia with marked left axis deviation, tall R waves in lead V_1, and probable intermittent 2:1 ventriculoatrial conduction (best seen in lead III).*

In the absence of sinus rhythm (*e.g.*, when atrial fibrillation is the basic rhythm), atrioventricular dissociation can naturally not be defined in this way.

A subgroup within uniform ventricular tachycardia, in which the QRS complexes and T waves become fused in a regular and more rapid oscillation, is sometimes called *ventricular flutter*[15] and is exemplified in Figure 20-7. This type of ventricular tachycardia is generally held to indicate a poor prognosis, although in the patient shown in Figure 20-7, resuscitation and subsequent oral drug prophylaxis were successful, albeit only in the short term.

In the electrocardiogram, a frequent diagnostic difficulty is the distinction between supraventricular arrhythmias complicated by intraventricular aberration on the one hand and ventricular tachycardia on the other. The criteria of Sandler and Marriott[46] and of Wellens[47] are usually helpful; for example, characteristic right bundle branch block appearance (rSR′ in lead V_1) favors the former and a broad complex (> 140 ms) favors the latter. Figure 20-6*A* shows atrial fibrillation with a run of conducted QRS complexes showing right bundle branch block; identical changes were seen in lead V_1 in this patient when left ventricular reciprocating tachycar-

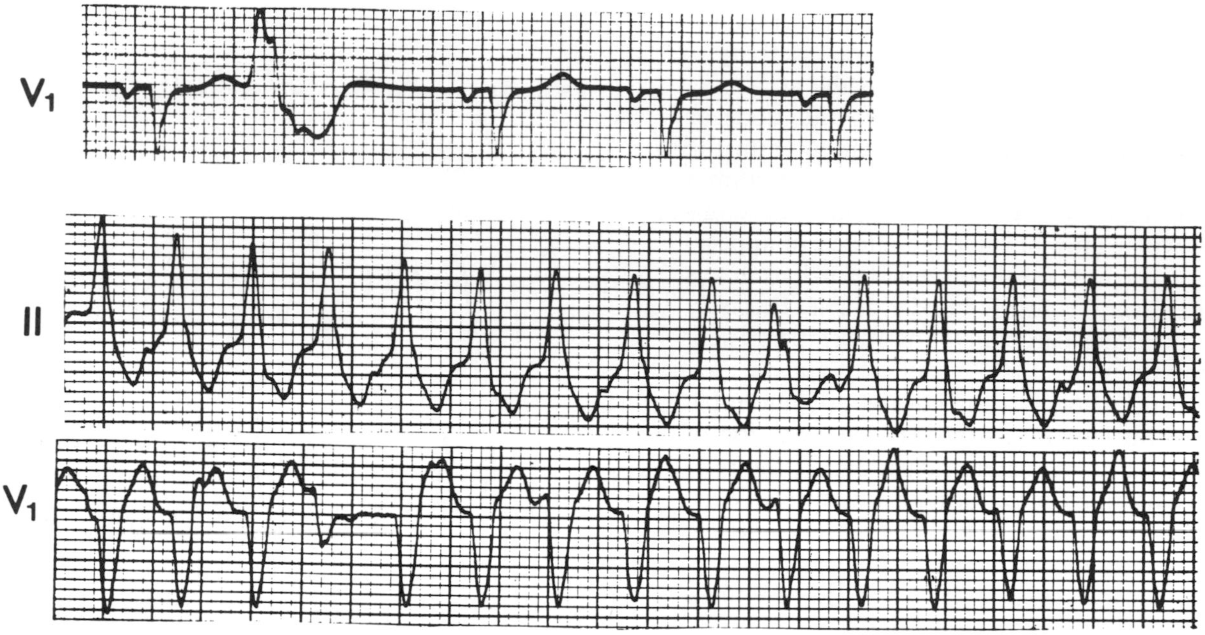

Figure 20-5. *Electrocardiograms showing (in* upper panel, *lead V_1) sinus rhythm with ventricular extrasystole that does not disturb it (normal P wave in its T).* Lower panels *(leads II and V_1) show tachycardia with broad QRS complexes; independent P waves can be discerned in some areas. The tenth QRS in lead II appears to reflect fusion; the fourth in lead V_1, capture (note similarity of latter to QRS complexes of sinus origin in* upper panel *of lead V_1).*

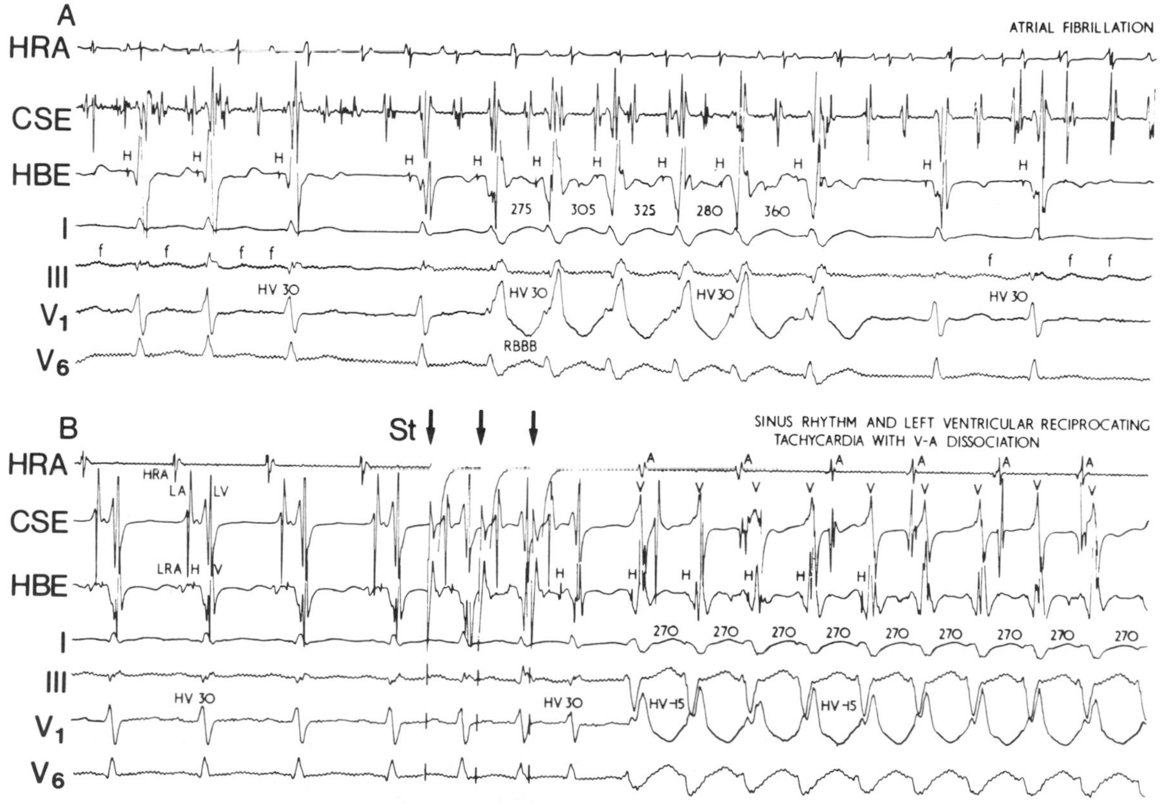

Figure 20-6. *Simultaneous intracardiac and surface electrograms from a patient with idiopathic congestive cardiomyopathy, recorded at a paper speed of 25 mm/sec. (A) During spontaneous atrial fibrillation, the HV time is normal (30 msec) whether intraventricular*

(continued)

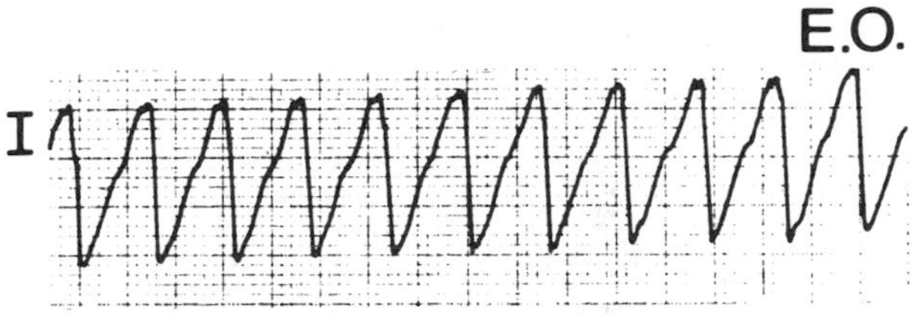

Figure 20-7. *Electrocardiogram (lead I) showing sawtooth QRS complexes merging with T waves, reflecting ventricular flutter.*

dia was induced by electrical stimulation during sinus rhythm, the diagnosis being confirmed by the presence of atrioventricular dissociation (see Fig. 20-6*B*). Where other criteria prove inadequate, intracardiac electrography (as in Fig. 20-6*B*) may be essential to establish the diagnosis of ventricular tachycardia by showing absence of activation of the ventricles from the atria.

As with ventricular extrasystoles, in uniform tachycardias the QRS configuration may suggest a right or left ventricular origin, inferred when there is a pattern suggestive of contralateral bundle branch block[48] (see Fig. 20-6), although this is by no means specific.[28] Epicardial mapping confirms this in some cases,[49,50] but right ventricular tachycardia diagnosed by these criteria may be associated with a left ventricle aneurysm,[48] raising the possibility that the reentry circuit actually arose in the diseased left ventricle and initially depolarized the healthy right ventricle. In the experience of Pietras and co-workers,[48] and from their review of the literature, left ventricular tachycardia is more consistently associated with serious organic heart disease than is right ventricular tachycardia. Our own observations, however, are mixed. More of our patients with apparently benign ventricular tachycardia have the characteristics of a right ventricular arrhythmia (Fig. 20-8), but this is by no means invariable (see Fig. 20-3). Ventricular tachycardia arising in the right ventricular outflow tract (Fig. 20-9*B*) is often benign, but ventricular tachycardia associated with a dilated right ventricular usually has malignant features. T wave inversion in the right precordial leads (see Fig. 20-9*A*) tends to indicate the presence of underlying structural right ventricle disease.[51]

In another subgroup of uniform ventricular tachycardia the QRS complex, during tachycardia, shows right bundle branch block pattern and left axis deviation.[36]

Classic ventricular tachycardia, which would be defined as above, often starts in response to a ventricular extrasystole falling during repolarization of the preceding impulse (whether of sinus or other origin), the so-called R-on-T phenomenon.[52] When this occurs, the

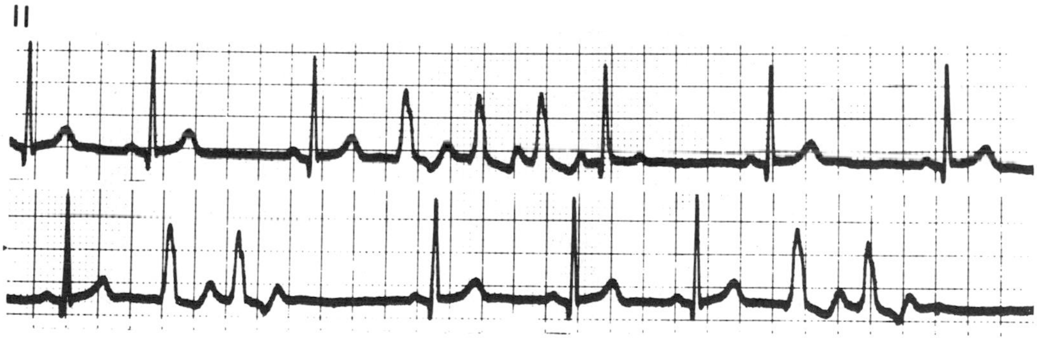

Figure 20-8. *Continuous electrocardiographic tracings (lead II) showing sinus rhythm interrupted by ventricular couplets* (lower panel) *and a three-complex episode of ventricular tachycardia* (upper panel). *The QRS complexes of the tachycardia show features consistent with what would be seen in left bundle branch block with normal conduction. There is second degree retrograde ventriculoatrial block, type I, during tachycardia, with sinus capture terminating the episode in the* upper panel.

---

conduction shows a normal pattern or right bundle branch block. (B) Sinus rhythm, with normal sequence of atrial activation in a craniocaudal, right-to-left direction, and normal HV interval. Reciprocating ventricular tachycardia at a cycle length of 270 msec was established after three successive right atrial stimuli. In tachycardia, the bundle of His was activated after the ventricle (HV is −15 msec), and AV dissociation was evident. (HRA, high right atrial electrogram; CSE, coronary sinus (left atrial) electrogram; HBE, His bundle electrogram; A, atrial activation; LA, left atrial activation; LRA, low right atrial activation; H, His bundle activation; V, ventricular action; LV, left ventricular activation; HV, intraventricular conduction time; ST and arrows, *high right atrial stimuli)*

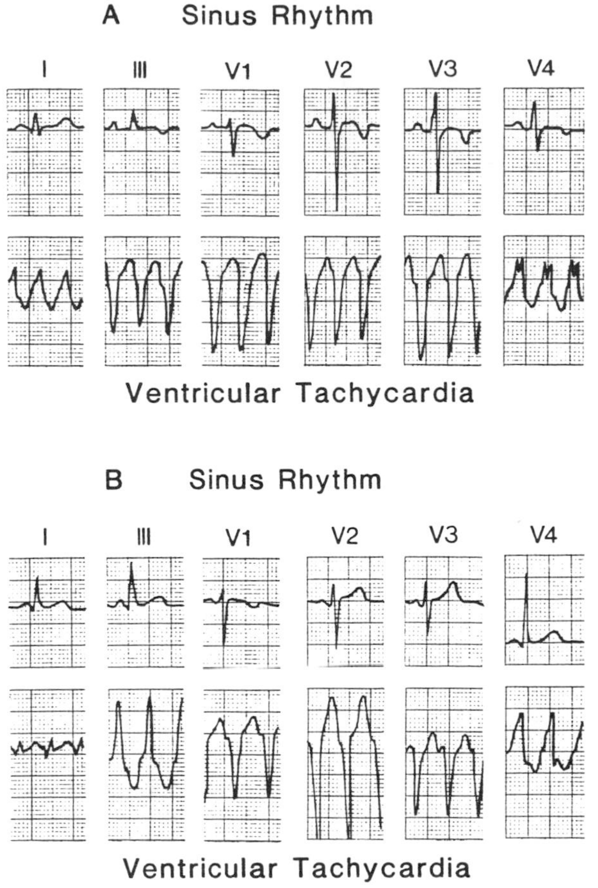

Figure 20-9. *Selected leads taken from the 12-lead electrocardiograms recorded during sinus rhythm and ventricular tachycardia in two patients who show a left bundle branch block configuration during ventricular tachycardia, suggesting a right ventricular origin. A is taken from a patient with a dilated right ventricle. During sinus rhythm there is T wave inversion in V_1 to V_4. The rate of ventricular tachycardia is 250 beats/min, and the QRS complex shows left axis deviation. B is taken from a patient with a normal right ventricle. The electrocardiogram in sinus rhythm is normal, and during ventricular tachycardia there is right axis deviation, suggesting that the tachycardia originates in the outflow tract of the right ventricle (see text).*

ventricular extrasystole usually interrupts the apex of that T wave, and a uniform tachycardia ensues in which the QRS morphology is maintained. However, the extrasystole or first complex of the tachycardia may be quite late (see Fig. 20-2) or have its effect at varying times of repolarization, but it may also not depend on this effect at all, especially in repetitive tachycardias (see Fig. 20-3). Clinically, the precise initiation sometimes cannot be defined or may vary from time to time (see Fig. 20-3), or it may have no relation whatsoever to a preceding T wave (Fig. 20-10). Initiation (and termination) by spontaneous ventricular extrasystoles favors a reentry mechanism, especially if the QRS complexes in tachycardia are of a somewhat different morphology from the extrasystoles (Fig. 20-11).[53]

Not only may spontaneous ventricular extrasystoles, early or late, initiate ventricular tachycardias (reproducible in electrophysiologic studies[31,54]), but, albeit much more rarely, suitably timed atrial extrasystoles can also be transmitted through the AV node with critical relationships and reach the ventricles when these are vulnerable and able to respond by reentry.[55] Although this is uncommon, we have observed it and have also noted its special importance in the presence of accessory atrioventricular tracts.[45] Here, of course, its significance has been seen in the induction of ventricular fibrillation by conducted impulses from the fibrillating atria in patients with the Wolff-Parkinson-White syndrome.[56] Indeed, in keeping with what we had seen when rapid atrial stimulation induced ventricular tachycardia,[45] the short RR intervals in atrial fibrillation complicating this disorder may reflect branch to branch reentry, the very initiation of ventricular arrhythmia.

Not all ventricular tachycardias are uniform, and there has been much confusion regarding the significance and terminology of such disorders. The definition of torsade de pointes has clarified much of this area[57–60] and has enabled clinicians to recognize what has previously been called by a variety of names: *transient ventricular fibrillation,*[61] *paroxysmal ventricular fibrillation,*[62] *transient recurrent ventricular fibrillation,*[63] and *cardiac ballet.*[64]

Torsade de pointes has important morphologic and etiologic facets that we have reviewed.[59,60] On the electrocardiogram one sees short runs of tachycardia in which the form and axis of the QRS complex undulate in a sinusoidal fashion around the isoelectric line (often best displayed on simultaneous tracings of several leads). Characteristically the initiating extrasystole occurs late, at the end of a prolonged QT interval (Fig. 20-12). Important etiologic factors include high degree-AV block, sinoatrial depression, electrolyte deficits, congenital QT prolongation syndromes, drugs, and extreme dietary restriction. The association with a prolonged QT interval is an important diagnostic pointer; if the QT interval is normal, then the episode, although multiform, should be

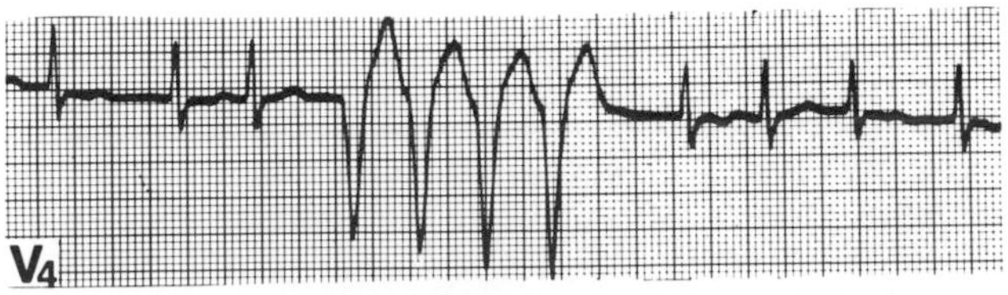

Figure 20-10. *Electrocardiogram showing atrial fibrillation as the basic rhythm. This was interrupted by four consecutive broad QRS complexes, constituting ventricular tachycardia. The patient had digitalis intoxication.*

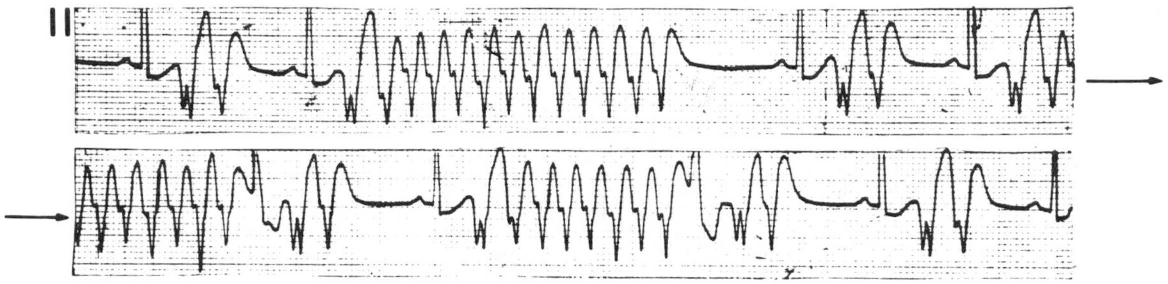

Figure 20-11. *Continuous electrocardiographic tracings from a patient during the second week after myocardial infarction. Ventricular extrasystoles interrupt T waves of sinus beats and either occur in pairs or result in runs of ventricular tachycardia with relatively narrow QRS complexes. These stopped spontaneously or were interrupted by fusion beats followed by two further extrasystoles. The appearances suggest intraventricular reentry.*

considered in the same category as the more usual uniform variety of ventricular tachycardia.[58] One cannot always assign cases into one group or the other,[58] desirable though this may be because of the different treatment that may be required.[59,60]

Torsade de pointes can easily be misdiagnosed if only a single lead is recorded, when the arrhythmia is multifocal ventricular tachycardia (Fig. 20-13), which is sometimes seen in patients with hypersensitivity to catecholamines.[65]

As already discussed in the terms of the rate definition of ventricular tachycardia, *accelerated idioventricular rhythm,* also known as *idioventricular tachycardia* and, less correctly, as slow ventricular tachycardia (a somewhat contradictory statement), can be defined as the occurrence of an independent ventricular rhythm more rapid than the sinus rate and able to manifest itself as the dominant cardiac rhythm for varying lengths of time. Semantically, it might well be justified to describe the distal junctional (right bundle branch tachycardia illustrated in Fig. 20-1) in this way; a more definite example is illustrated in Fig. 20-14, with a rate a little greater than that in sinus rhythm. It may be sustained for long periods or, as in Figures 20-1 and 20-14, may be intermittent. Often seen during acute myocardial infarction, at which time it is of uncertain significance (*i.e.,* by no means

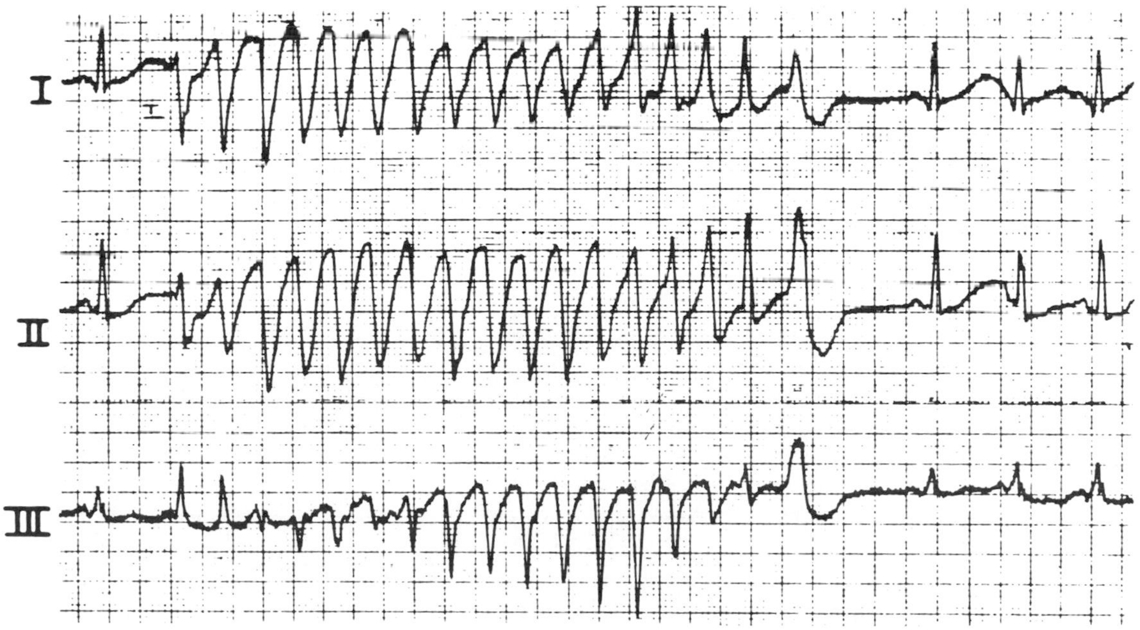

Figure 20-12. *Simultaneous recordings of leads I, II, and III from a patient with chronic hypokalemia. Sinus complexes show marked QT prolongation; note the onset of the arrhythmia toward the end of the first T waves and the alterations in the QRS axes during tachycardia.*

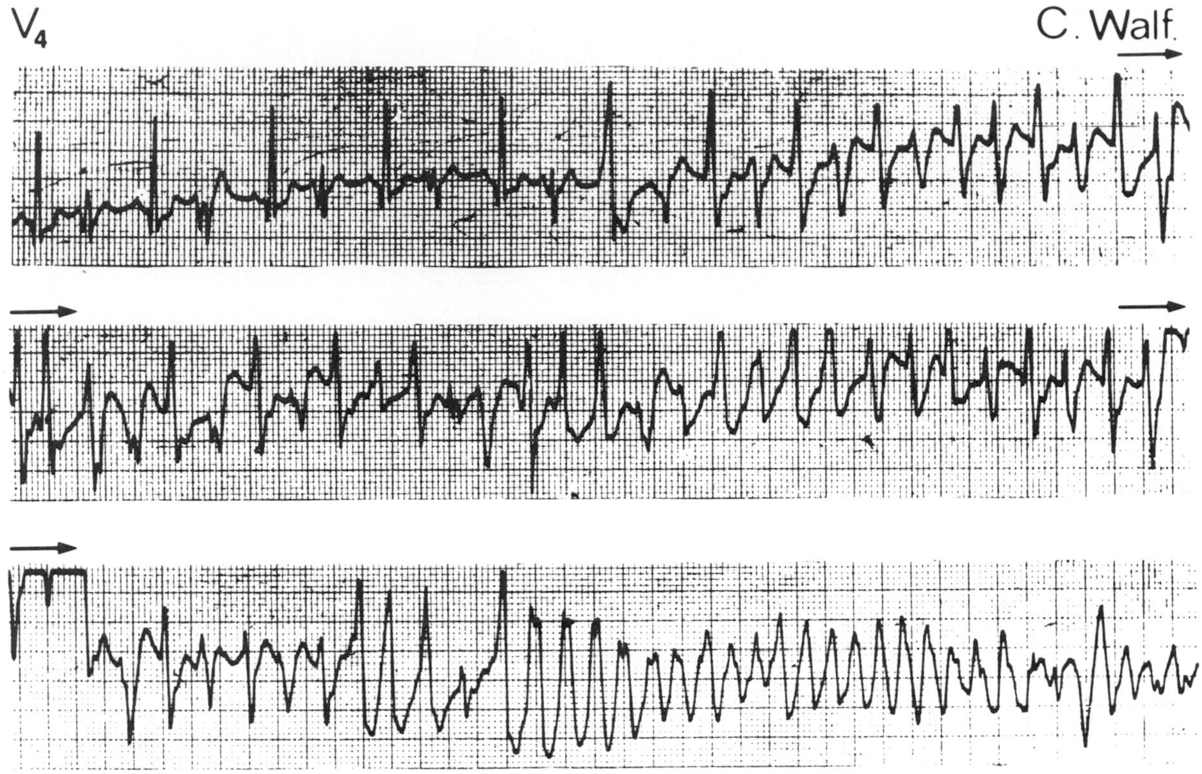

Figure 20-13. *Continuous electrocardiographic recordings (V_4) showing, at first, sinus rhythm with bigeminy due to ventricular extrasystoles. During the second part of the* upper panel, *ventricular tachycardia develops with variability in the QRS complexes that becomes grossly evident in the* second panel. *In the middle of the* third panel, *this multiform tachycardia degenerates into ventricular fibrillation for which direct current electrical defibrillation was required.*

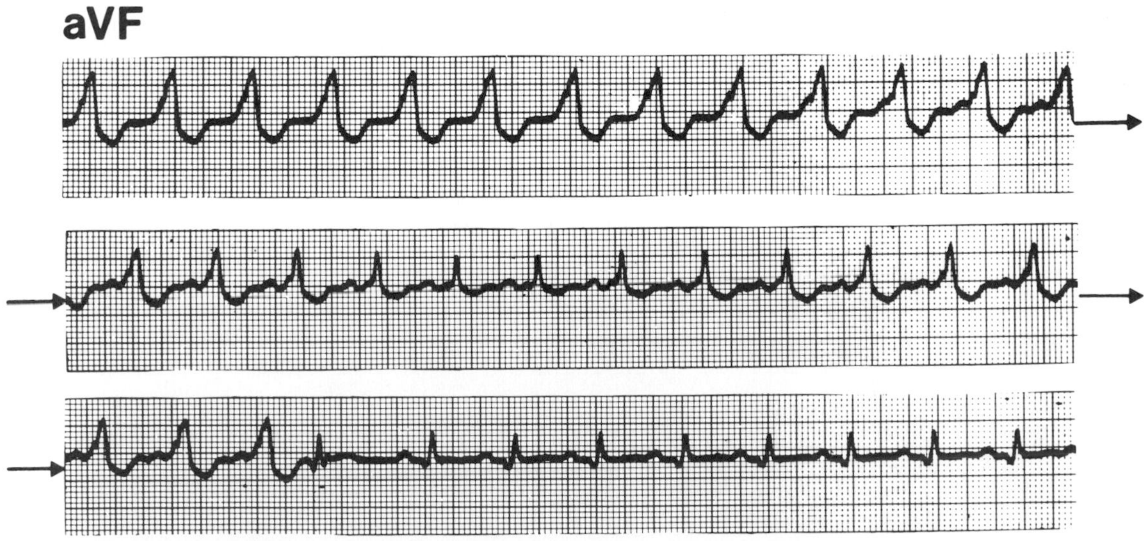

Figure 20-14. *Continuous electrocardiogram (lead a V_F) showing accelerated idioventricular rhythm only slightly faster than the inherent sinus rate, in the* upper panel, *first and last thirds of the* middle panel, *and first third of the* lower panel. *In the* second panel, *transition between "idioventricular tachycardia" and sinus rhythm shows fusion, but in the* third panel *the tachycardia appears to be terminated by a narrow extrasystole.*

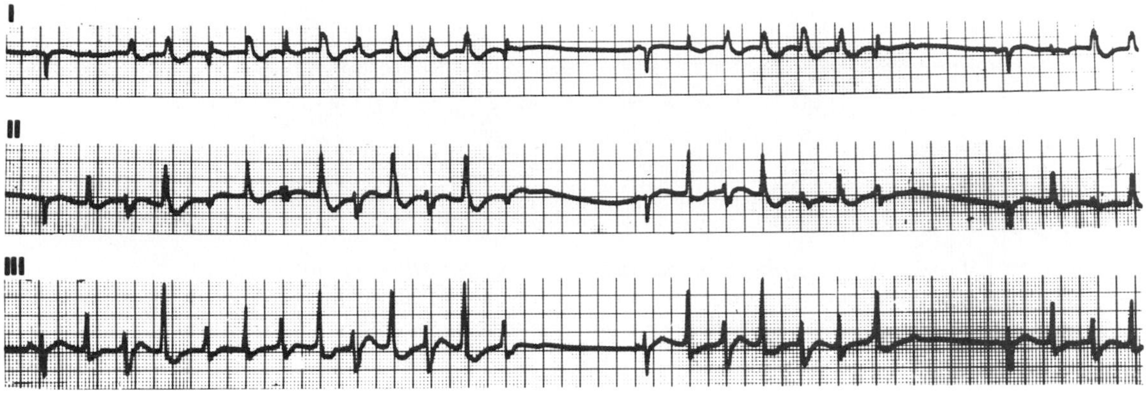

Figure 20-15. *Simultaneous electrocardiograms (leads I, II, and III) from a patient with hypokalemia due to familial periodic paralysis, showing runs of bidirectional ventricular tachycardia (most obvious in lead II).*

indicative of progression to more sinister arrhythmias), it may also, as in the patients whose electrocardiograms are shown in Figures 20-1 and 20-14, occur for no good reason, in which case it falls into the category of idiopathic repetitive ventricular tachycardias, discussed toward the end of this chapter. This particular arrhythmia is difficult to classify and, in any context, appears to have a benign prognosis. Its existence is closely linked with the lower limit of the rate defined as ventricular tachycardia of the more usual variety.

Morphologically intermediate between these uniform and the "nonuniform" arrhythmias is bidirectional ventricular tachycardia. Earlier, doubt had been cast on the existence of this entity,[14] and it was said to be a concept of historical significance only. Its reality can be confirmed not only by deductive analysis of surface electrocardiographic tracings (Fig. 20-15) but also with intracardiac recordings (Fig. 20-16). When this pattern is seen, hypokalemia—perhaps with digitalis intoxication—should be suspected. Bidirectional ventricular tachy-

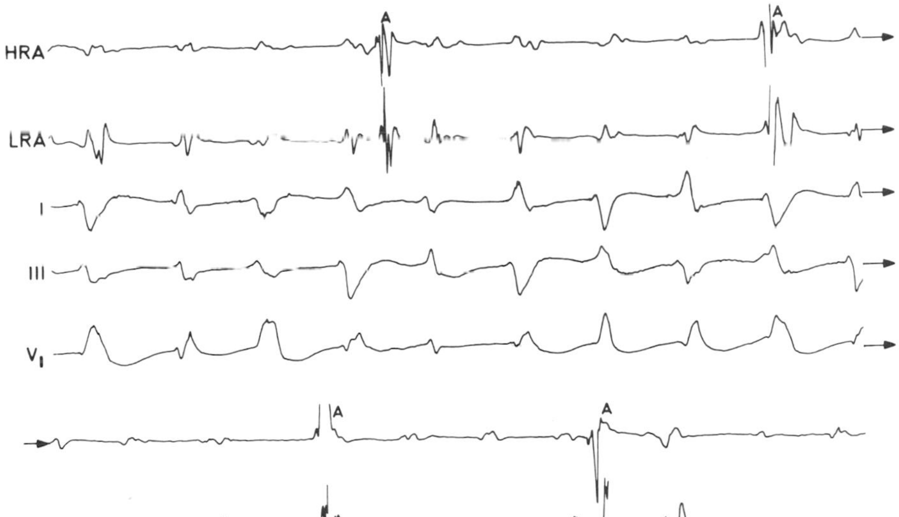

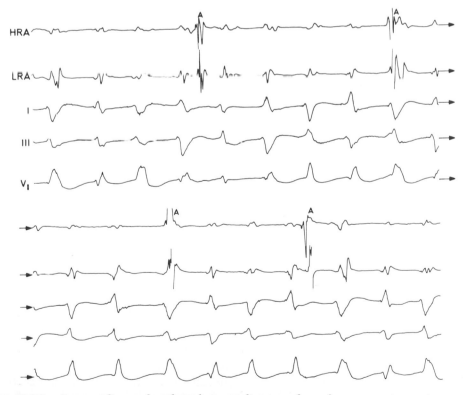

Figure 20-16. *Intracardiac and surface electrocardiograms from the same patient as in Figure 20-15. The paper speed is 100 mm/sec. Independent atrial activity (A) can be seen in the atrial electrograms. Abbreviations are the same as in Figure 20-6.*

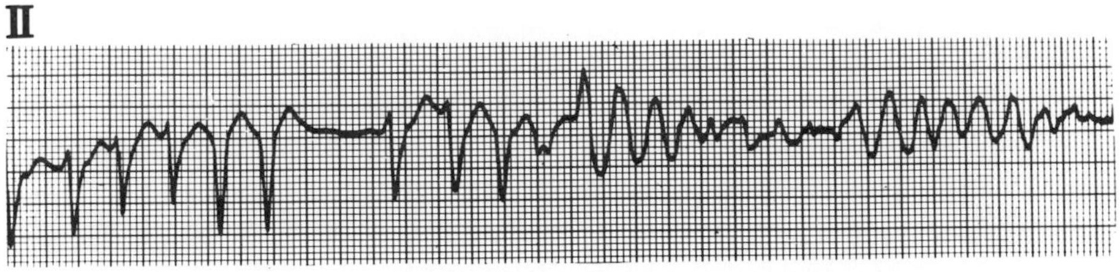

Figure 20-17. *Lead II electrocardiogram recorded from a patient with acute myocardial infarction soon after admission to the coronary care unit. Two ventricular extrasystoles, a single sinus beat, and two further ventricular extrasystoles culminate in ventricular fibrillation.*

cardia may be the forerunner of other forms of ventricular tachycardia (*e.g.*, torsade de pointes).[66]

In ventricular fibrillation, the disorganized morphologic appearances on the electrocardiogram probably reflect incoordinate localized reentry processes rather than diffuse ectopic hyperactivity and may follow from sustained ventricular tachycardia of the uniform variety, occur with the R-on-T phenomenon in previous sinus rhythm, or develop after a few beats of tachycardia (Fig. 20-17). Untreated torsade de pointes and multifocal ventricular tachycardia (see Fig. 20-13) may degenerate into ventricular fibrillation, with which they tend to be confused.

Etiologic Factors

For convenience, ventricular tachycardia (uniform or variable) and fibrillation will be considered as a single entity for the purpose of classifying underlying disease processes that may cause either or both. Only the main categories will be discussed, and it is not proposed to provide an exhaustive list of isolated causes but rather to discuss mechanisms that are of fundamental importance or to pinpoint areas where new knowledge is being acquired.

Ischemic Heart Disease

Acute Myocardial Infarction

The importance of ventricular fibrillation as a cause of sudden death or death within the first few hours after the onset of pain is well recognized and constitutes a major therapeutic challenge that still awaits resolution. From animal studies, it is possible to assess the time course of changes in ventricular fibrillation threshold and to observe its abrupt reduction immediately after acute coronary occlusion, with a return to previous levels 30 minutes later.[67] Extrapolation to the clinical situation appears reasonable, but variations among patients in a disease process preclude more categorical statements.

In this context, ventricular tachycardia in humans during the first 24 hours after myocardial infarction has been judged, by electrophysiologic techniques, to be compatible with enhanced automaticity by Wellens and Lic,[54] but these authors emphasize the relatively crude nature of such studies as can be carried out in humans and by no means exclude local reentry phenomena.[68] The clinical demonstration by Wellens and Lie[54] of reentry ventricular tachycardia late after myocardial infarction is entirely in keeping with the elegant animal mode in which this has been shown by El-Sherif and colleagues.[23] Other supporting evidence has been cited earlier in this chapter when electrophysiologic mechanisms were discussed in general. Whether triggered activity plays a role is not yet established.

Variant Angina

It is now increasingly recognized that variant angina can produce ventricular tachycardia, sometimes associated with paroxysmal AV block,[69] although this is by no means the major factor. It may be related to coronary spasm[70,71] and have appearances suggestive of torsade de pointes, although some investigators believe that such resemblance may not be of pathogenetic significance but rather reflects multifocal (multiform) tachycardia, perhaps similar to idiopathic catecholamine-induced arrhythmias,[65] discussed below.

Chronic Ischemic Heart Disease

Cardiac aneurysm forms a well-recognized anatomic basis for the occurrence of reentry ventricular tachycardia (Figs. 20-18 and 20-19), and, in sinus rhythm, the characteristic signs (usually but not always present and by no means pathognomonic of aneurysm when evident) are deep QS complexes with persistent ST segment elevation or T wave inversion after recovery from the acute infarct. The mechanism of the arrhythmia is reentry with slowed conduction across the interface between healthy and scarred myocardium. During intracardiac studies, induced extrasystoles can activate the latent circuit.[72]

Exactly similar arrhythmias may be seen with localized dyskinesia short of aneurysm formation or indeed

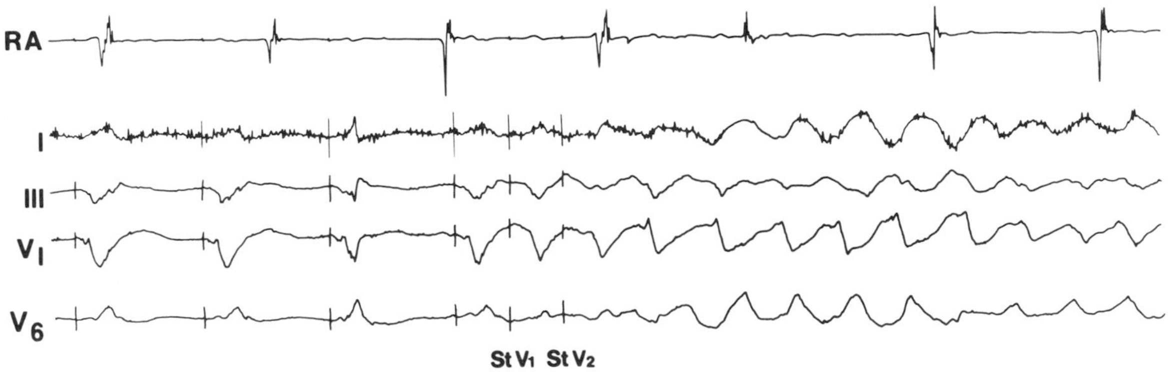

Figure 20-18. *Simultaneous right atrial (RA) electrogram and surface electrocardiographic leads from a patient with left ventricular aneurysm following myocardial infarction. Basic right ventricular pacing is being carried out* (unlabeled spikes). *The introduction of two ventricular extra stimuli (StV_1, StV_2) leads to ventricular tachycardia, but the atrial activation (RA lead) remains undisturbed (i.e., ventricular tachycardia has been induced with AV dissociation).*

without any clinically manifest scarring.[54] Strong evidence in favor of reentry has been adduced by Josephson and co-workers[28] in three cases of recurrent ventricular tachycardia after infarction; one of the patients had an aneurysm, and the other two suffered from diffuse hypokinesia. Local electrical activity was recorded from the affected area, and when it became continuous, tachycardia developed, the termination of which necessitated suppression of this activity. These findings are in keeping with the phenomenon noted experimentally by Durrer many years ago.[73] Other workers have found discrete late potentials with surface electrocardiographic signal-averaging techniques[74] and during operative endocardial mapping[29] in patients with ventricular tachycardia. Residual fibrosis after myocardial infarction may be an important factor in the occurrence of subsequent ventricular arrhythmias[75]; it is clearly essential that anatomic factors be included in any assessment of the significance of apparent "warning arrhythmias" thought possibly to signify an increased risk of sudden death, perhaps because of ventricular fibrillation.[76] This does not in any way contradict the observations of Wellens and Lie,[54] because the areas of fibrosis in their patients may have been insufficiently extensive to have been clinically detectable. In this context, observations of repolarization abnormalities in those who have survived ventricular fibrillation appear to provide further means of seeking out those at risk of recurrence.[77] The question of ventricular extrasystoles and their importance, discussed in Chapter 8, is not further dealt with here in relation to tachycardias and fibrillation.

Nonischemic Anatomic Lesions

Although posttraumatic cardiac infarction is rare, we have seen several examples of ventricular asynergy resulting from this and one patient with a discrete aneurysm. This last patient was a fit young man aged 18 who presented with ventricular tachycardia experienced while playing sports. His resting electrocardiogram showed appearances quite typical for cardiac aneurysm, and, retrospectively, a history was obtained of an extremely severe closed-chest injury 15 years previously. During one episode of palpitation, an electrocardiogram

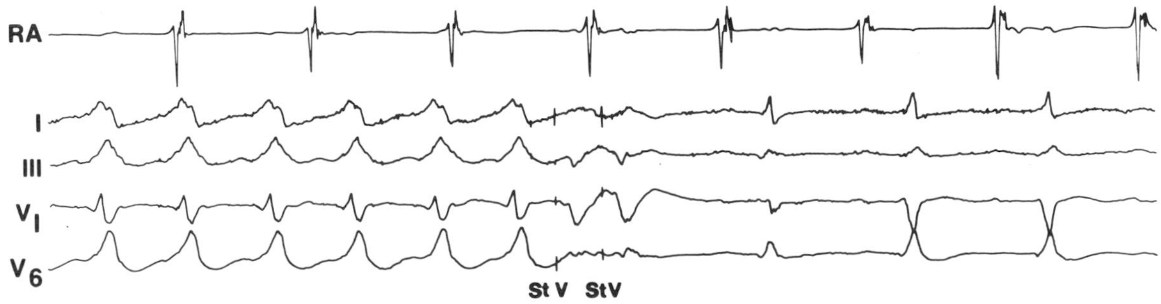

Figure 20-19. *Same patient as illustrated in Figure 20-18. At the commencement of the tracing, the patient is in ventricular tachycardia with AV dissociation. Two ventricular extra stimuli (StV) terminate the tachycardia, and the ventricles now respond to the sinus rhythm.*

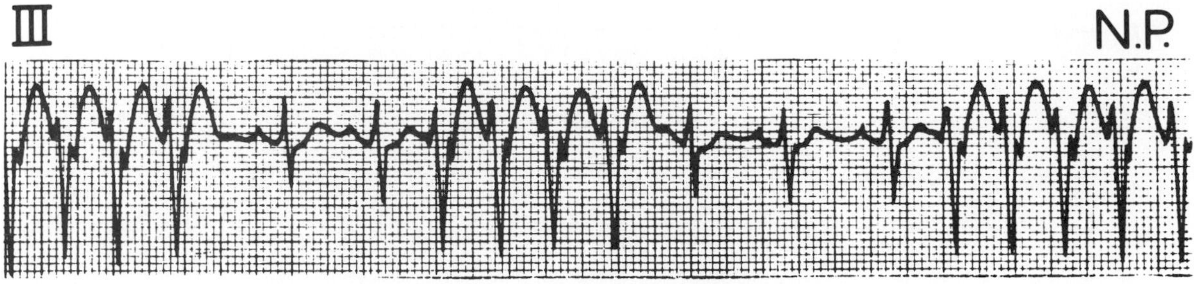

Figure 20-20. *Electrocardiogram (lead III) from a patient aged 18 years with a posttraumatic left ventricular aneurysm. Runs of ventricular tachycardia are seen at the commencement, in the middle, and at the end of the strip. There are two intervening sinus complexes between the first two episodes and three between the second.*

confirmed the presence of ventricular tachycardia (Fig. 20-20), and the aneurysm was confirmed angiographically. This study also revealed the coronary arteries to be normal. At the operation, at which the aneurysm was successfully resected, epicardial mapping during tachycardia confirmed the presence of a reentry mechanism. Similar tachycardias have also been seen in patients with a history of chest trauma but without definable cardiac aneurysm. In addition, dyskinetic areas or aneurysms may develop because of inflammatory disease, or no underlying cause may be found by full investigation of rare patients who present with ventricular tachycardia (Figs. 20-21 and 20-22).

Mitral Valve Prolapse

Although ventricular extrasystoles, as well as other arrhythmias, are common in mitral valve prolapse, they are usually benign.[78] We are aware of several cases of

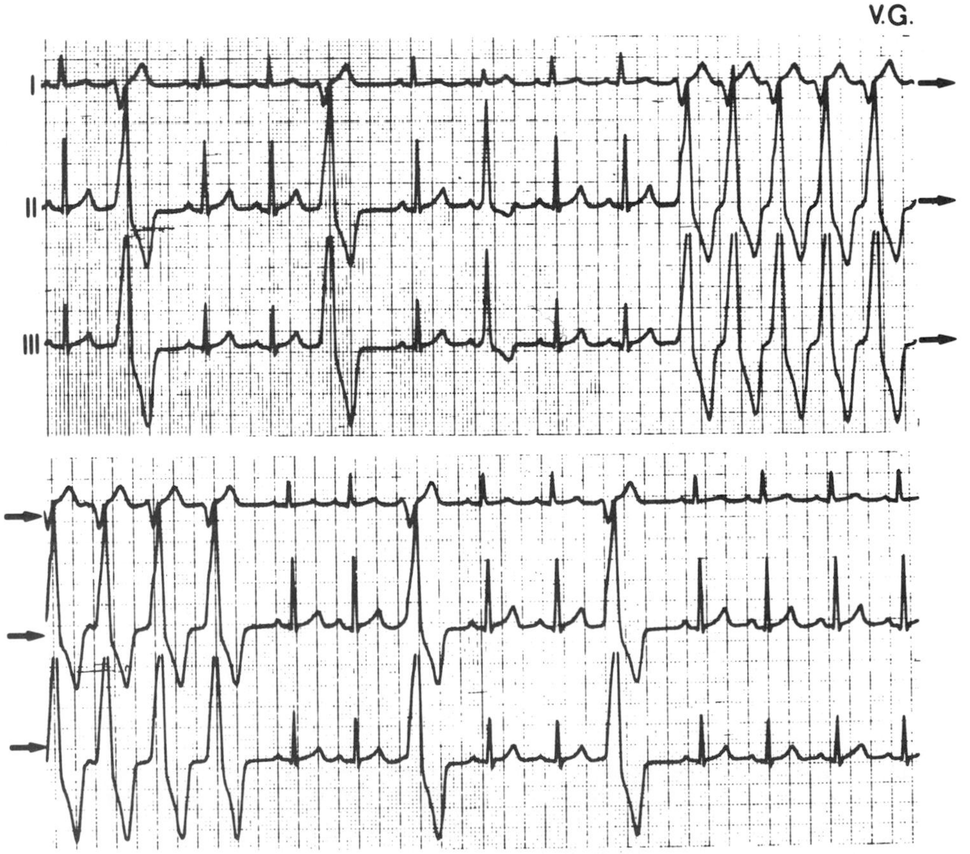

Figure 20-21. *Continuous electrocardiographic (leads I, II, and III) showing sinus rhythm with late ventricular ectopic complexes, probably parasystolic, the third of which shows fusion with the sinus activation. The fourth ectopic complex is the first of nine consecutive impulses, constituting ventricular tachycardia.*

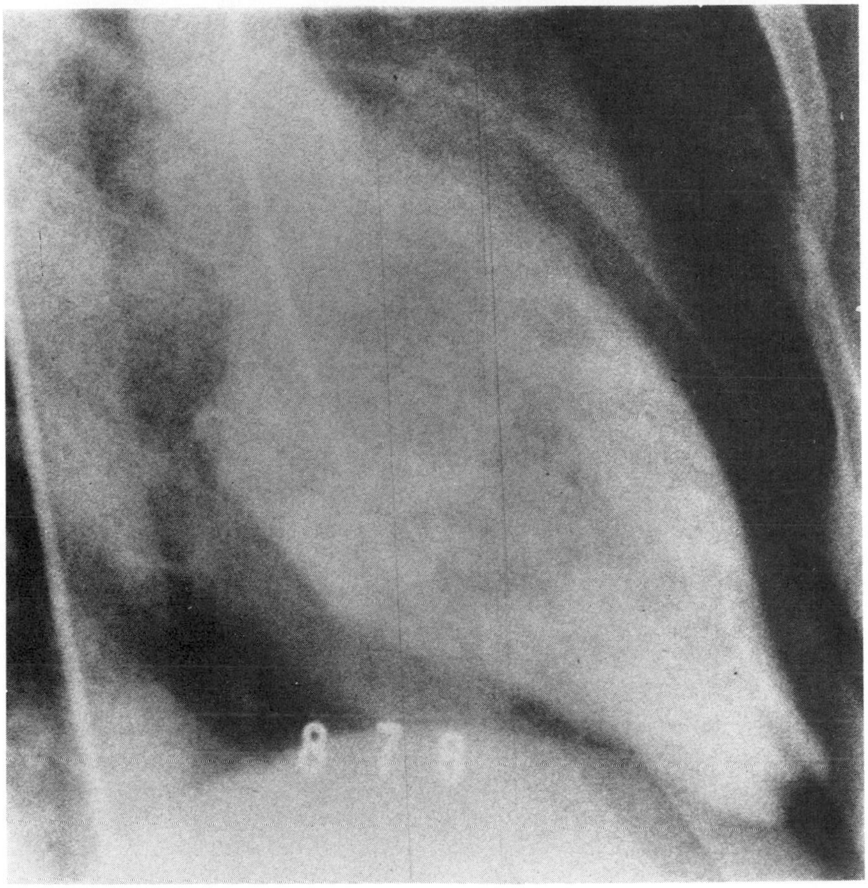

Figure 20-22. *Left ventricular angiogram (recorded in systole) from the same patient whose electrocardiogram was shown in Figure 20-21. Note dyskinetic area at the apex.*

catastrophic ventricular arrhythmias not controlled by available antiarrhythmic agents but that have been controlled by mitral valve replacement.[79,*] Indeed, we have such a patient ourselves, whose tachycardia has previously been illustrated (see Fig. 20-4). Although this patient tolerated his mild mitral incompetence well during sinus rhythm, he developed syncope during his attacks of ventricular tachycardia, undoubtedly due to the fact that under these circumstances the mitral incompetence was grossly exaggerated and transaortic blood flow minimal. At operation, reentry ventricular tachycardia identical to that seen clinically could be elicited from the posterior papillary muscle. Eight years after mitral valve replacement the patient has remained symptom free, although subsequently he required a pacemaker.

Cardiomyopathy and Myocarditis

Cardiomyopathy and myocarditis are relatively uncommon causes of ventricular tachycardia. While the inflammatory disorder is active, arrhythmias may occur.

Hypertrophic Cardiomyopathy

Ventricular tachycardia is a strong positive marker for sudden death in adults with hypertrophic cardiomyopathy.[80] Typically such episodes are slow (mean rate 142 /min) and nonsustained (mean duration eight beats) and tend to occur at night.[81] Sudden death has been attributed to the occurrence of a sustained ventricular arrhythmia, but we have full documentation of an episode of "sudden death" and successful resuscitation in one patient who remained in sinus rhythm throughout.[82] Children with hypertrophic cardiomyopathy who die suddenly have particularly marked fiber disarray,[83] a likely milieu for arrhythmias.

We have also seen one patient with hypertrophic cardiomyopathy who also had a concealed accessory pathway linking the right atrium and ventricle. This patient died as a result of ventricular tachycardia initiated by atrial stimuli during a diagnostic electrophysiologic study.[45] Although this experience has led us to avoid electrophysiologic studies in patients with hypertrophic cardiomyopathy, we would consider such studies if therapeutic value could be demonstrated; so far, this has not been the case, and ambulatory monitoring provides the only satisfactory guide in identifying those at risk.[81]

Dilated Cardiomyopathy

Ventricular arrhythmias are common in patients with dilated cardiomyopathy, but their prognostic significance is uncertain, since in many cases death is not sudden but is a gradual decline related to cardiac pump

*Yu, P. N.: Personal communication.

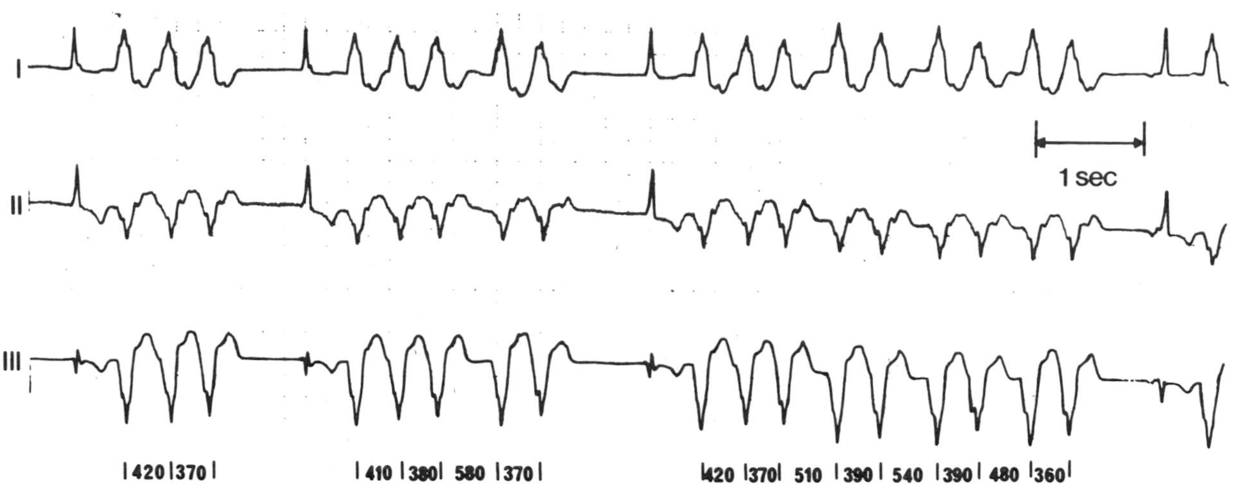

Figure 20-23. *Electrocardiogram (simultaneous recordings of leads I, II, and III) showing repetitive ventricular tachycardia interrupted by a single junctional and one atrial impulse. The numbers at the bottom indicate the RR intervals in milliseconds. These tracings were recorded from a patient with congestive cardiomyopathy.*

performance.[84] After the first year from diagnosis, sudden death becomes more common and may be arrhythmogenic, but whether drug treatment to suppress ventricular arrhythmias improves prognosis remains undetermined. In isolated cases we have seen severe ventricular arrhythmias not controlled by conventional medication (Fig. 20-23) respond to amiodarone with concomitant improvement in cardiac performance and decrease in heart size. Right ventricular dysplasia may represent one part of the spectrum of dilated cardiomyopathy in which the right ventricle bears the brunt of the disease.

QT Prolongation Syndrome

Hereditary Syndromes

There are two important and usually distinct syndromes in which a prolonged QT interval is associated with a tendency to ventricular arrhythmias. In the syndrome described first by Jervell and Lange-Nielsen,[85] there is associated deafness and the inheritance is recessive, whereas in the other form, the so-called Romano-Ward syndrome first described by Romano and co-workers,[86] there is no associated loss of hearing and the syndrome has a dominant pattern of inheritance. Patients with either variety may show uniform ventricular tachycardia (Fig. 20-24) or torsade de pointes (Fig. 20-25). Physiologically, the QT interval usually shortens with exercise; a third subset has been described in which this fails to occur and, indeed, in which the QT lengthens with exercise.[87] Unless this possibility is considered in otherwise inexplicable cases of ventricular tachycardia, the mechanism may not be appreciated. Figure 20-26 shows electrocardiograms recorded from a man aged 40 years in whom attacks of ventricular tachycardia were usually noted on exercise. As can be seen in the upper panel in this figure, the QT was slightly prolonged at rest but much more obviously so during exercise (when it should have decreased), and this was accompanied by the development of ventricular tachycardia (see Fig. 20-26*B*).

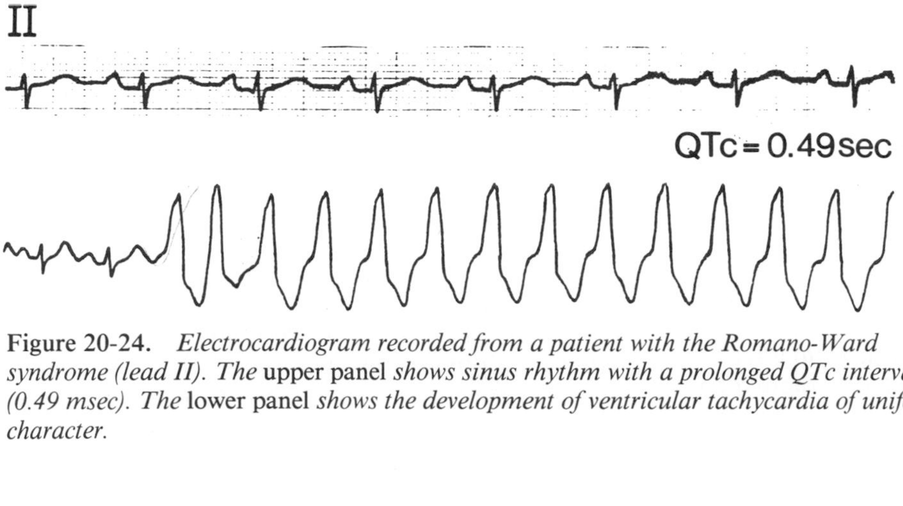

Figure 20-24. *Electrocardiogram recorded from a patient with the Romano-Ward syndrome (lead II). The* upper panel *shows sinus rhythm with a prolonged QTc interval (0.49 msec). The* lower panel *shows the development of ventricular tachycardia of uniform character.*

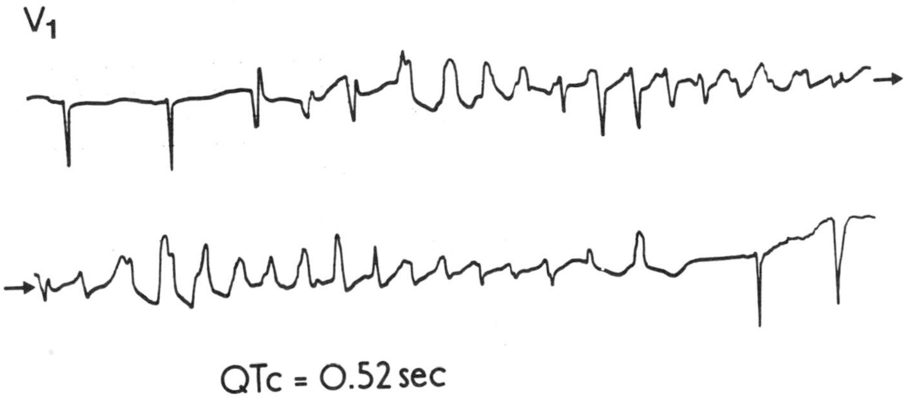

Figure 20-25. *Continuous electrocardiogram (lead V_1) from another patient with the Romano-Ward syndrome showing QTc prolongation and the development of a short run of tachycardia in which the axes of the QRS complexes appeared to rotate in keeping with* torsade de pointes.

The prognosis for patients with these syndromes is unpredictable at best, and sudden death is a recognized risk. There is only a single report of a clear-cut extrinsic autonomic defect in one member of such an affected family, with undue QT lengthening in response to small doses of isoproterenol.[88] Schwartz,[89] however, has documented through a register of persons with the long QT syndrome that prognosis is improved dramatically by left stellate sympathectomy, while beta-blockade also offers some benefit.

Acquired Syndromes

As with the congenital forms of QT prolongation, the acquired QT prolongation syndromes are associated with ventricular arrhythmias and torsade de pointes.[58] Acquired QT prolongation occurs with electrolyte disturbances (hypokalemia and apparently also hypomagnesemia and hypocalcemia), liquid protein diets, and most commonly with drugs—particularly class I antiarrhythmic agents, phenothiazines, and tricyclic antidepressants.

Catecholamine-Induced Ventricular Tachycardias

The hypothesis that ventricular arrhythmias could be induced by sensitization to epinephrine by chloroform was the subject of much work culminating in the confirmation published by Levy and Lewis,[3] and numerous instances of the direct effect of catecholamines in producing ventricular arrhythmias have subsequently ap-

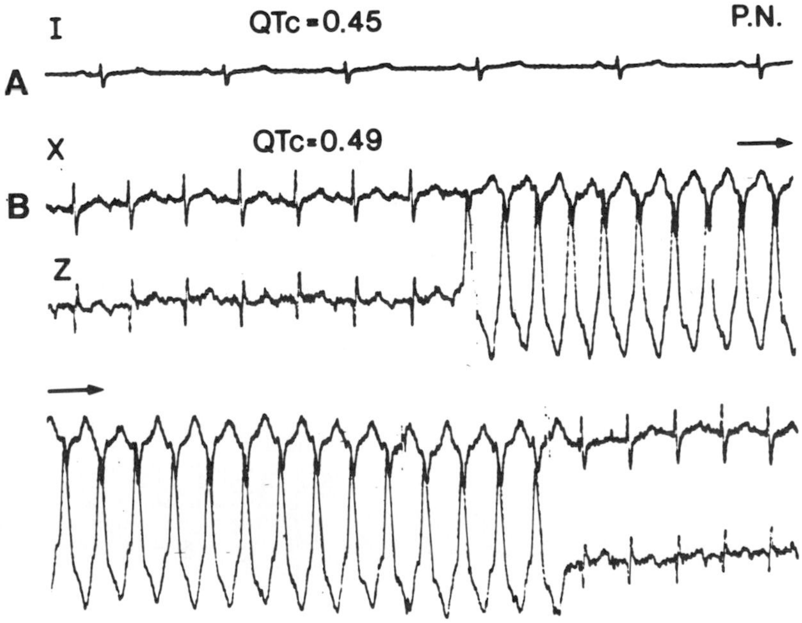

Figure 20-26. *Electrocardiograms recorded from a patient with a history of palpitations. (A) Upper panel (lead I) shows sinus rhythm with modest QTc prolongation. (B) Lower panels are continuous recordings of orthogonal X and Z leads, showing lengthening of the QT interval during exercise with the development of a self-limited episode of ventricular tachycardia.*

peared. Several years ago we studied a family* as well as sporadic cases where sensitivity to endogenous catecholamines appears to be the mechanism for ventricular arrhythmias, in some instances fatal (see Fig. 20-13); their arrhythmias can be reproduced by the infusion of small amounts of isoproterenol.[65] Therapeutic assessment is facilitated by noting the response to prophylactic beta-blockers, the dose being increased until measured exercise no longer reinduces the arrhythmia; Coumel and colleagues believe that nadolol in particular has definite benefits in this group of patients.[90]

Drug-Induced Tachycardias

Digitalis is the agent characteristically likely to produce ventricular arrhythmias because it is administered so frequently. These tachycardias are often heralded by systemic symptoms of toxicity, but the cardiac effects may come first. Sometimes bigeminy due to regular ventricular extrasystoles may be the first indication, but bidirectional tachycardia may be another warning sign. On the other hand, ventricular tachycardia may be seen without any other clinical indication of intoxication, and it may be sustained (Fig. 20-27) rather than episodic (see Fig. 20-10). A whole host of other agents may, however, be responsible, including those prone to cause torsade de pointes.[59,60] In some cases the effect is indirect, as with diuretics that produce hypokalemia, and in other cases the effect is direct, as with cardioactive agents and major tranquilizers that prolong repolarization. In our experience, the most likely offenders are quinidine, procainamide, disopyramide, phenothiazines, and tricyclic antidepressants, and whenever torsade de pointes is seen, careful inquiry should be made about the possible consumption of such medications. The calcium antagonist bepridil may cause this, especially when given to elderly, hypokalemic women[91] or if the recommended dose is exceeded.* A host of other agents have been implicated as possibly causing ventricular tachycardia,[15] but in many cases reported in the literature only single instances have been cited, and the direct relevance in each case is not always clear.

* Krikler, D., Perelman, M., and Rowland, E.: Unpublished data.

Disturbances of Impulse Formation in Conduction

The most important ventricular arrhythmia associated with either sinoatrial disease or atrioventricular block is torsade de pointes. This appears to occur in relation to the consequent disturbance of repolarization[59] and may be one of the mechanisms whereby Adams-Stokes attacks occur in either form of heart block.

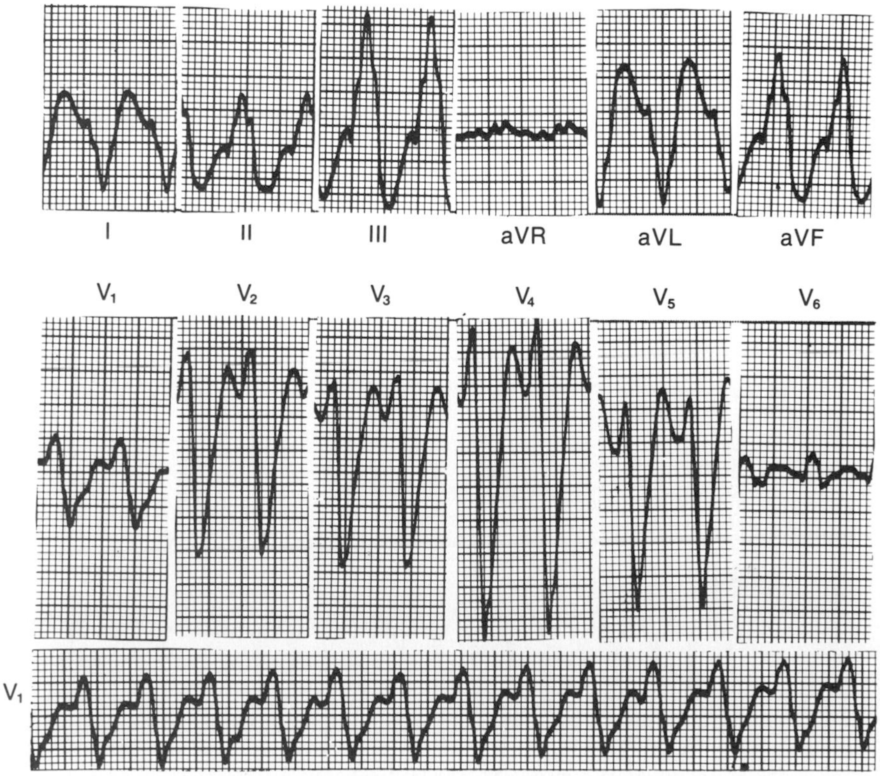

Figure 20-27. *Electrocardiogram showing ventricular tachycardia in a patient suffering from digitalis intoxication.*

Miscellaneous Causes

A whole host of disorders may be listed under miscellaneous, including collagen diseases, sarcoidosis, electrolyte disturbances, and carbon monoxide poisoning, which we have not investigated personally. The ventricular arrhythmias that occur have no specific features, and the subjects have been well reviewed elsewhere.[15] Cardiac tumors are rare but potentially treatable causes.[92]

Idiopathic Causes

A small but important group of cases can be classified as idiopathic. However, short of careful pathologic examination of the heart, it may not be possible to uphold such a diagnosis except in the short term. On the other hand, pathologic examination may be quite unhelpful, because it usually is seen in patients with, for example, QT prolongation syndromes,* although Rossi and Matturri[93] have noted nonspecific abnormalities of the conduction system in patients with this disorder.

Both Gallavardin[94] and Parkinson and Papp[95] have described patients with repetitive ventricular tachycardias in whom the prognosis has been benign in the long term. One such case is illustrated in Figure 20-8, showing electrocardiograms from a woman aged 38 years in whom the arrhythmia was noted at birth. She has been totally unaware of palpitation and leads a normal life. Electrophysiologic study and hemodynamic cardiac catheterization were normal in her case, as they usually are in others investigated in this way. Figure 20-3 shows a more impressive tachycardia in which the episodes of ventricular arrhythmia were interrupted only by single

* Davies, M. J.: Personal communication.

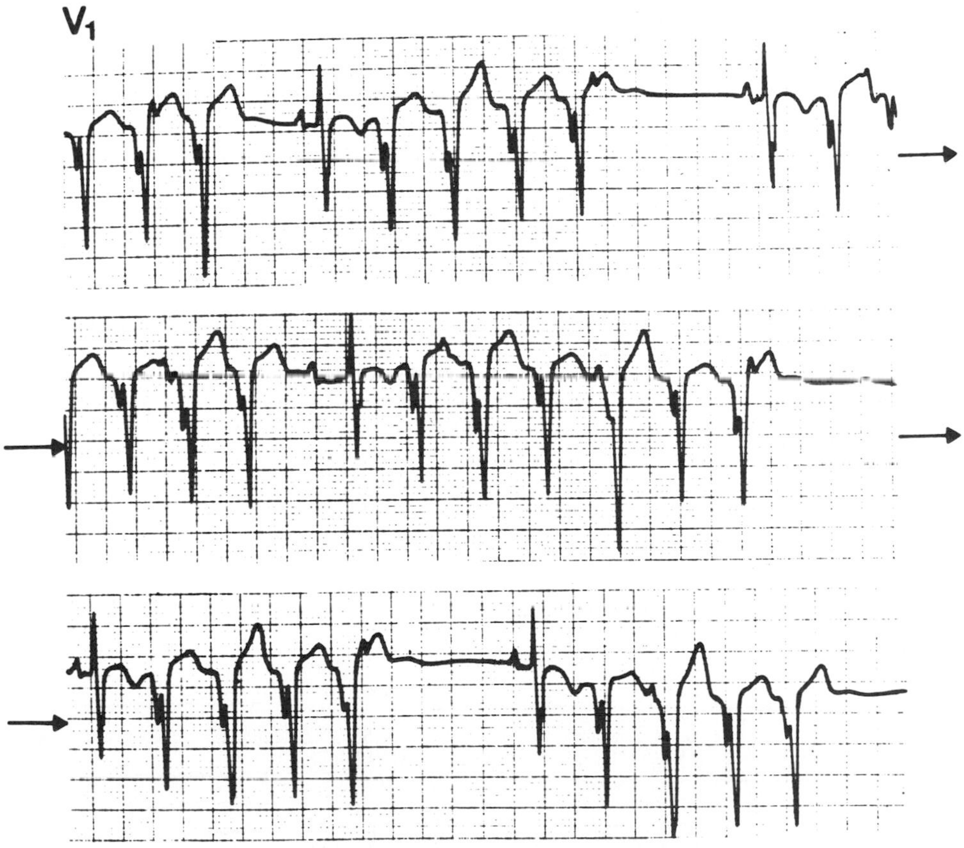

Figure 20-28. *Electrocardiogram recorded from a young man with apparently benign ventricular tachycardia (lead V_1). In tachycardia, the QRS complexes have appearances consistent with what would be seen in sinus rhythm complicated by left bundle branch block, suggesting a right ventricular origin for the tachycardia. The episodes of tachycardia are interrupted by no more than one or two sinus complexes; if two, the first one shows AV block due to concealed conduction into the AV node, which is also seen in the sinus complex interrupting the tachycardia shown in the* second panel *(PR prolongation). Atrioventricular dissociation is evident from the independent P waves.*

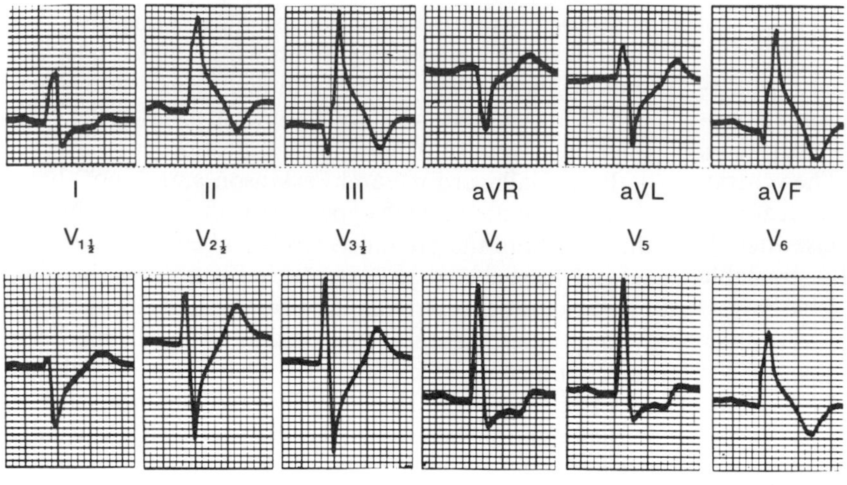

Figure 20-29. *Electrocardiogram recorded from an otherwise healthy young man suffering from ventricular tachycardia with episodes of syncope. He was not taking any medications. His electrocardiogram showed PR prolongation and broad bizarre QRS complexes with gross disturbance of the ST segment and T waves. Leads V_1, V_2, and V_3 were recorded at half voltage.*

sinus complexes; the patient was quite asymptomatic, and the arrhythmia was discovered when he was 23 years old and examined for life-insurance purposes. As is so often the case with those affected by this disorder, the arrhythmia was not suppressed by medications, and in this patient also, electrophysiologic studies showed no underlying abnormality. On the other hand, the patient aged 19 years whose electrocardiogram is depicted in Figure 20-28 and who was otherwise indistinguishable from the two previous cases, died in his sleep; electrophysiologic studies had revealed no abnormality either, and pathologic investigation was entirely negative.

A more serious view was taken in the case of the man aged 18 years whose electrocardiogram is shown in Figure 20-29. The patient had a negative family history and presented with recurrent ventricular tachycardia. He was taking no medication, and no clinical evidence of cardiac disorder was apparent. At electrophysiologic study (Fig. 20-30), the sole abnormal feature was the finding of prolonged intraventricular conduction. He was untreated and suddenly died a year later. Again, necropsy revealed no cardiac abnormalities. In both this patient and the patient discussed in Figure 20-28, the cardiac conduction system was carefully examined, but because both patients died out of hospital, autopsy was not carried out sufficiently soon after death to permit useful electron microscopic or other detailed investigations to be performed.

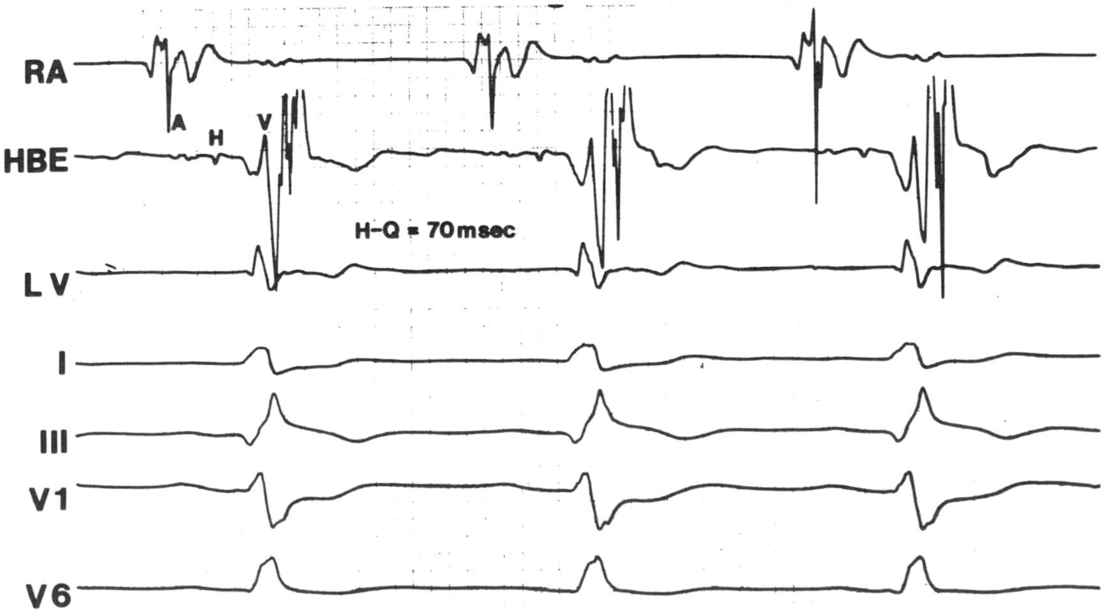

Figure 20-30. *Intracardiac and surface electrocardiograms, including left ventricular electrogram (LV) recorded at a paper speed of 100 mm/sec, from the same patient as in Figure 20-29. The sole abnormality noted on the intracardiac leads was HQ (HV) prolongation (70 msec; upper limit of normal, 55).*

Conclusion

Many reviews of ventricular tachycardia have appeared since the disorder was identified, and two aspects need consideration in determining what points arising from the large amount of data offer scope for the future. At the clinical level, the greatest difficulty in patients with chronic recurrent ventricular tachycardia is the significance and reliability of reinitiation during electrophysiologic studies.[96–98] This contentious point is dealt with in further detail elsewhere in this volume. This probably reflects the crude nature of current tools when taken in conjunction with the need to focus on what may be a very restricted area of potential reentry. The other aspect is the question of triggered activity and whether this may have implications regarding the genesis of arrhythmias.[17] One can only speculate that triggered activity might be important in some focal tachycardias, perhaps associated with the effects of catecholamines and drugs such as digoxin. However, we do not yet have the evidence that would enable us to correlate the interesting experimental electrophysiologic findings with ventricular arrhythmias that are at present little or not understood.

References

1. Lorain, T.: Etude de Médecine Clinique Faites avec l'Aide de la Methode Graphique et des Appareils Enregistreurs. Le Pouls, ses Variations et ses Formes Diverses dan les Maladies. Paris, J. B. Baillière, 1870.
2. Brunton, L.: One of the causes of death during the extraction of teeth under chloroform. Br. Med. J., 2:695, 1875.
3. Levy, A. G., and Lewis, T.: Heart irregularities, resulting from the inhalation of low percentages of chloroform vapour, and their relationship to ventricular fibrillation. Heart, 3:99, 1911–1912.
4. Hoffmann, A.: Die paroxysmale Tachycardie. Anfälle von Herzjagen. Wiesbaden, Bergmann, 1900.
5. Wenckebach, K. F.: Die Arrhythmie als Ausdruck bestimmter Funktionsstorungen des Herzens. Eine physiologisch-klinische Studie. Leipzig, Wilhelm Engelmann, 1903.
6. Wenckebach, K. F.: Die unreglmassige Herztätigkeit und ihre klinische Bedeutung. Leipzig, Wilhelm Engelmann, 1914.
7. Mackenzie, J.: Diseases of the Heart. London, Henry Frowde and Hodder & Stoughton, 1908.
8. Lewis, T.: The experimental production of paroxysmal tachycardia and the effects of ligation of the coronary arteries. Heart, 1:98, 1909–1910.
9. Erichsen, J. E.: On the influence of the coronary circulation on the action of the heart. Lond. Med. Gaz., 2:561, 1842.
10. Allessie, M. A.: Circulating Excitation in the Heart, p. 21. Maastricht, The Netherlands, Drukkerij R. U. Limburg, 1977.
11. McWilliam, J. A.: Cardiac failure and sudden death. Br. Med. J., 1:6, 1889.
12. Lewis, T.: The Mechanism of the Heart Beat. London, Shaw & Sons, 1911.
13. Coumel, P., Attuel, P., and Flammang, D.: The role of the conduction system in supraventricular tachycardias. In Wellens, H. J. J., Lie, K. I., and Janse, M. J. (eds.): Structure, Function and Clinical Implications, p. 424. Leiden, H. E. Stenfert Kroese, 1976.
14. Schamroth, L.: The Disorders of Cardiac Rhythm, pp. 13–150. London, Blackwell Scientific Publications, 1971.
15. Scherf, D., and Schott, A.: Extrasystoles and Allied Arrhythmias, 2d ed. London, William Heinemann, 1973.
16. Schmitt, F. A., and Erlanger, J.: Directional differences in the conduction of the impulse through heart muscle and their possible relation to extrasystolic and fibrillatory contractions. Am. J. Physiol., 65:125, 1928–1929.
17. Wit, A. L., Hoffman, B. F., and Cranefield, P. F.: Slow conduction and reentry in the ventricular conducting system. I. Return extrasystole in canine Purkinje fibers. Circ. Res., 30:1, 1972.
18. Wellens, H. J. J.: Value and limitations of programmed electrical stimulation of the heart in the study and treatment of tachycardia. Circulation, 57:845, 1978.
19. Allessie, M. A., Bonke, F. I. M., and Schopman, F. J. G.: Circus movement in rabbit atrial muscle as a mechanism of tachycardia. III. The "leading circle" concept: A new model of circus movement in cardiac tissue without the involvement of an anatomical obstacle. Circ. Res., 41:9, 1977.
20. Brugada, P., and Wellens, H. J. J.: The role of triggered activity in clinical ventricular arrhythmias. Pace, 7:260–271, 1984.
21. Bouvrain, Y., and Coraboeuf, E.: Pathogénie des troubles du rythme de l'infarctus aigu due myocarde. Arch. Mal. Coeur, 69:873, 1976.
22. El-Sherif, N., Scherlag, B. J., Lazzara, R., and Hope, R. R.: Reentrant ventricular arrhythmias in the late myocardial infarction period. I. Conduction characteristics in the infarction zone. Circulation, 55:686, 1977.
23. El-Sherif, N., Hope, R. R., Scherlag, B. J., and Lazzara, R.: Reentrant ventricular arrhythmias in the late myocardial infarction period. II. Patterns of initiation and termination of re-entry. Circulation, 55:702, 1977.
24. Russell, D. C., Oliver, M. F., and Wojtczak, J.: Combined electrophysiological technique for assessment of the cellular basis of early ventricular arrhythmias. Experiments in dogs. Lancet 2:686, 1977.
25. Downar, E., Janse, M. J., and Durrer, D.: The effect of acute coronary occlusion on subepicardial transmembrane potentials in the intact porcine heart. Circulation, 56:217, 1977.
26. El-Sherif, N., Lazzara, R., Hope, R. R., and Scherlag, B. J.: Re-entrant ventricular arrhythmias in the late myocardial infarction period. III. Manifest and concealed extrasystolic grouping. Circulation, 56:225, 1977.
27. Brechenmacher, C., Moussard, J. M., and Voegtlin, R.: Réentree ventriculaire permanente cachée et tachycardie ventriculaire paroxystique par mouvement circulaire. Arch. Mal. Coeur, 70:61, 1977.
28. Josephson, M. E., Horowitz, L. N., and Farshidi, A.: Continuous local electrical activity. A mechanism of recurrent ventricular tachycardia. Circulation, 57:659, 1978.
29. Klein, H., Karp, R. B., Kouchoukos, N. T., et al.: Intraoperative electrophysiologic mapping of the ventricles during sinus rhythm in patients with a previous myocardial infarction. Identification of the electrophysiologic substrate of ventricular arrhythmias. Circulation, 66:847–853, 1982
30. Antoni, H.: Electrophysiological mechanisms underlying pharmacological models of cardiac fibrillation. Arch. Pharmacol., 269:177, 1971.
31. Evans, T. R., Curry, P. V. L., Fitchett, D. H., and Krikler, D. M.: "Torsade de pointes" initiated by electrical ventricular stimulation. J. Electrocardiol., 9:255, 1976.
32. Gradman, A. H., Bell, P. A., and DeBusk, R. F.: Sudden death during ambulatory monitoring. Clinical and electrocardiographic correlations. Report of a case. Circulation, 55:210, 1977.
33. Cranefield, P. F.: Action potentials, afterpotentials and arrhythmias. Circ. Res., 41:415, 1977.

34. Wit, A. L., and Cranefield, P. F.: Triggered and automatic activity in the canine coronary sinus. Circ. Res., 41:435, 1977.
35. Rozanski, G. J., Jalife, J., and Moe, G. K.: Reflected reentry in non homogeneous ventricular muscle as a mechanism of cardiac arrhythmias. Circulation, 69:163–173, 1984.
36. Lin, F. C., Finley, C. D., Rahimtoola, S. H., and Wu, D.: Idiopathic paroxysmal ventricular tachycardia with a QRS pattern of right bundle branch block and left axis deviation: A unique clinical entity with specific properties. Am. J. Cardiol., 52:95–100, 1983
37. Coumel, Ph., Leclercq, J. F., Attuel, P., et al.: Tachycardies ventriculaires en salves. Etude electro-physiologique et theraputique. Arch. Mal. Coeur, 73:153–164, 1980.
38. Waxman, M. B., and Wald, W. R.: Termination of ventricular tachycardia by an increase in cardiac vagal drive. Circulation, 56:385, 1977.
39. Rosen, M. R., and Hoffman, B. F.: The vagus and ventricles. Circ. Res., 42:1, 1978.
40. Rardon, D. P., and Bailey, J. C.: Parasympathetic effects on electrophysiologic properties of cardiac ventricular tissue. J. Am. Coll. Cardiol., 6:1200–1209, 1983.
41. Pollack, G. H.: Cardic pacemaking: An obligatory role of catecholamines? Science, 196:731, 1977.
42. Bellet, S.: Clinical Disorders of the Heart Beat, 3rd ed., p. 532. Philadelphia, Lea & Febiger, 1971.
43. Anderson, K. P., DeCamilla, J., and Moss, A. J.: Clinical significance of ventricular tachycardia (3 beats or longer) detected during ambulatory monitoring after myocardial infarction. Circulation, 57:890, 1978.
44. Frank, R., Fontaine, G., Guiraudon, G., et al.: Corrélation entre l'orientation de l'onde delta et la topographie de la pré-excitation dans le syndrome de Wolff-Parkinson-White. Arch. Mal. Coeur, 70:441, 1977.
45. Krikler, D., Davies, M. J., Goodwin, J. F., et al.: Sudden death in hypertrophic cardiomyopathy: Associated accessory pathways. Br. Heart J., 43:245–251, 1980.
46. Sandler, I. A., and Marriott, H. J. L.: The differential morphology of anomalous ventricular complexes of right bundle branch block type in lead VI. Ventricular ectopy versus aberration. Circulation, 31:551, 1965.
47. Wellens, H. J. J., Bär, F. W. H. M., and Lie, K. I.: The value of the electrocardiogram in the differential diagnosis of a tachycardia with a widened QRS complex. Am. J. Med., 64:27–33, 1978.
48. Pietras, R. J., Mautner, R., Denes, P., et al.: Chronic recurrent right and left ventricular tachycardia: Comparison of clinical, hemodynamic and angiographic findings. Am. J. Cardiol., 40:32, 1977.
49. Gallagher, J. J., Oldham, H. N., Wallace, A. G., et al.: Ventricular aneurysm with ventricular tachycardia. Report of a case with epicardial mapping and successful resection. Am. J. Cardiol., 35:696, 1975.
50. Fontaine, G., Guiraudon, G., Frank, R., et al.: Stimulation studies and epicardial mapping in ventricular tachycardia. Study of mechanisms and selections for surgery. In Kulbertus, H. E. (ed.): Reentrant Arrhythmias, p. 334. Lancaster, MTP Press, 1976.
51. Rowland, E., McKenna, W. J., Sugrue, D., et al.: Ventricular tachycardia of left bundle branch block configuration in patients with isolated right ventricular dilatation. Br. Heart J., 51:15–24, 1984
52. Smirk, F. H.: R waves interrupting T waves. Br. Heart J., 11:23, 1949.
53. Krikler, D. M., and Curry, P. V. L.: The paroxysmal supraventricular arrhythmias. In Yu, P. N., and Goodwin, J. F. (eds): Progress in Cardiology 5, p. 291. Philadelphia, Lea & Febiger, 1976.
54. Wellens, H. J. J., and Lie, K. I.: Ventricular tachycardia: The value of programmed electrical stimulation. In Krikler, D. M., and Goodwin, J. F. (eds.): Cardiac Arrhythmias, the Modern Electrophysiological Approach, p. 182. Philadelphia, W. B. Saunders, 1975.
55. Wellens, H. J. J., Schuilenburg, R. M., and Durrer, D.: Electrical stimulation of the heart in patients with ventricular tachycardia. Circulation,46:216, 1972.
56. Dreifus, L. S., Haiat, R., Watanabe, Y., et al.: Ventricular fibrillation, a possible mechanism of sudden death in patients with the Wolff-Parkinson-White syndrome. Circulation, 43:250, 1971.
57. Dessertenne, F.: La tachycardie ventriculaire à deux foyers opposes variables. Arch. Mal. Coeur, 59:263, 1966.
58. Slama, R., Coumel, Ph., Motté, G., et al.: Tachycardies ventriculaires et torsades de pointes: Frontières morphologiques entre les dysrhythmies ventriculaires. Arch. Mal. Coeur, 66:1401, 1973.
59. Krikler, D. M., and Curry, P. V. L.: *Torsade de pointes,* an atypical ventricular tachycardia. Br. Heart J., 38:117, 1976.
60. Perelman, M., Rowland, E., and Krikler, D. M.: Torsade de pointes: A review. Int. Med., 11:126–131, 1983.
61. Schwartz, S. P., Orloff, J., and Fox, C.: Transient ventricular fibrillation. I. The prefibrillary period during established auriculoventricular dissociation with a note on the phonocardiograms obtained at such times. Am. Heart J., 37:21, 1949.
62. Loeb, H. S., Pietras, R. J., Gunnar, R. M., and Tobin, J. R., Jr.: Paroxysmal ventricular fibrillation in two patients with hypomagnesemia. Treatment by transvenous pacing. Circulation, 37:210, 1968.
63. Tamura, K., Tamura, T., Yoshida, S., et al.: Transient recurrent ventricular fibrillation due to hypopotassemia with special note on the U wave. Jpn. Heart J., 8:652, 1967.
64. Smirk, F. H., and Ng, J.: Cardiac ballet: Repetitions of complex electrocardiographic patterns. Br. Heart J., 31:426, 1969.
65. Coumel, P., Fidelle, J., Lucet, V., et al.: Catecholamine-induced severe ventricular arrhythmias with Adams-Stokes syndrome in children. Report of four cases. Br. Heart J. 40 (Suppl.):28, 1978.
66. Curry, P., Fitchett, D., Stubbs, W., and Krikler, D.: Ventricular arrhythmias and hypokalaemia. Lancet, 1:231, 1976.
67. Meesmann, W., Gülker, H., Krämer, B., and Stephan, K.: Time course of changes in ventricular fibrillation threshold in myocardial infarction: Characteristics of acute and slow occlusion with respect to the collateral vessels of the heart. Cardiovasc. Res. 10:446, 1976.
68. Scherlag, B. J., Helfant, R. H., Haft, J. I., and Damato, A. N.: Electrophysiology underlying ventricular arrhythmias due to coronary ligation. Am. J. Physiol., 219:1665, 1970.
69. Chiche, P., Haiat, R., and Steff, P.: Angina pectoris with syncope due to paroxysmal atrioventricular block: Role of ischaemia. Report of two cases. Br. Heart J., 36:577, 1974.
70. Benaim, R., Calvo, J., Seban, C., et al.: Les aspects anatomiques de l'Angine de Prinzmétal.: À propos d'une observation anatomoclinique. Arch. Mal. Coeur, 68:189, 1975.
71. Maseri, A., Mimmo, R., Chierchia, S., et al.: Coronary artery spasm as a cause of acute myocardial ischaemia in man. Chest, 68:625, 1975.
72. Hartzler, G. O., and Maloney, J. D.: Programmed ventricular stimulation in management of recurrent ventricular tachycardia. Mayo Clin. Proc., 52:731, 1977.
73. Durrer, D., et al.: Human cardiac electrophysiology. In Dickinson, C. J., and Marks, J. (eds.): Developments in Cardiovascular Medicine, pp. 53–75. Lancaster, MTP Publishers, 1978.
74. Breithardt, G., Borggrefe, M., Quantus, B. et al.: Ventricular vulnerability assessed by programmed ventricular stimulation in patients with and without late potentials. Circulation, 68:275–281, 1983
75. Califf, R. M., Burkes, J. M., Behar, V. S., et al.: Relationships among ventricular arrhythmias, coronary artery disease, and an-

giographic and electrocardiographic indicators of myocardial fibrosis. Circulation, 57:725, 1978.
76. Vismara, L. A., Amsterdam, E. A., and Mason, D. T.: Relation of ventricular arrhythmias in the late hospital phase of acute myocardial infarction to sudden death after hospital discharge. Am. J. Med., 59:6, 1975.
77. Haynes, R. E., Hallstrom, A. P., and Cobb, L. A.: Repolarisation abnormalities in survivors of out-of-hospital ventricular fibrillation. Circulation, 57:654, 1978.
78. Winkle, R. A., Lopes, M. G., Fitzgerald, J. W., et al.: Arrhythmias in patients with mitral valve prolapse. Circulation, 52:73, 1975.
79. Cobbs, B. W., Jr., and King, S. B.: Ventricular buckling: A factor in the abnormal ventriculogram and peculiar hemodynamics associated with mitral valve prolapse. Am. Heart J., 93:741, 1977.
80. McKenna, W. J., England, D., Doi, Y., et al.: Arrhythmia in hypertrophic cardiomyopathy. I. Influence on prognosis. Br. Heart J. 46:168-172, 1981.
81. McKenna, W. J.: Arrhythmia and prognosis in hypertrophic cardiomyopathy. Eur. Heart J., 4 (Suppl. F):225-234, 1983.
82. McKenna, W. J., Harris, L., and Deanfield, J.: Syncope in hypertrophic cardiomyopathy. Br. Heart J., 47:177-179, 1982.
83. Maron, B. J., and Roberts, W. C.: Quantitative analysis of cardiac muscle cell disorganisation in the ventricular septum of patients with hypertrophic cardiomyopathy. Circulation, 59:689-706, 1979.
84. Oakley, C. M.: Prognosis in dilated cardiomyopathy related to left ventricular function, conduction defects and arrhythmia. In Goodwin, J. F., Hjalmarson, A., and Olsen, E. G. J. (eds.): Congestive Cardiomyopathy, pp. 249-255. Kiruna, AB Hassle, 1980.
85. Jervell, A., and Lange-Nielson, F.: Congenital deaf-mutism, functional heart disease with prolongation of the QT interval and sudden death. Am. Heart J., 54:59, 1957.
86. Romano, C., Gemme, G., and Pongiglione, R.: Aritmie cardiocha rare dell' eta' pediatrica. Clin. Pediat. (Bologna), 45:656, 1963.
87. Von Bernuth, G., Belz, G. G., Evertz, W., and Stauch, M.: QTU-abnormalities, sinus bradycardia and Adams-Stokes attacks due to ventricular tachyarrhythmia. Acta Paed. Scand. 62:675, 1973.
88. Curtiss, E. I., Heibel, R. H., and Shaver, J. A.: Autonomic maneuvers in hereditary QT interval prolongation (Romano-Ward) syndrome. Am. Heart J., 95:420, 1978.
89. Schwartz, P. J.: The idiopathic long QT syndrome: The need for a prospective registry. Eur. Heart J., 4:529-531, 1983.
90. Coumel, Ph., Rosengarten, M. D., Leclercq, J. F., and Attuel, P.: Role of sympathetic nervous system in non-ischaemic ventricular arrhythmias. Br. Heart J. 47:137-147, 1982.
91. Leclercq, J. F., Kural, S., and Valere, P. E.: Bepridil et torsades de pointes. Arch. Mal. Coeur, 76:341-348, 1983.
92. Simcha, A., Wells, B. G., Tynan, M. J., and Waterston, D. J.: Primary cardiac tumours in childhood. Arch. Dis. Child, 46:508, 1971.
93. Rossi, L., and Matturri, L.: Histopathological findings in two cases of *torsade de pointes* with conduction disturbances. Br. Heart J., 38:1312, 1976.
94. Gallavardin, L.: Extrasystolic ventriculaire a paroxysmes tachycardiques prolonges. Arch. Mal. Coeur, 15:298, 1922.
95. Parkinson, J., and Papp, C.: Repetitive paroxysmal tachycardia. Br. Heart J., 9:241, 1947.
96. Brugada, P., Green, M., Abdullah, H., and Wellens, H. J. J.: Significance of ventricular arrhythmias initiated by programmed ventricular stimulation: The importance of the type of ventricular arrhythmia induced and the number of premature stimuli required. Circulation, 69:87-92, 1984.
97. Naccarelli, G. V., Prytowsky, E. N., Jackman, W. M., et al.: Repetitive ventricular response. Prevalence and prognostic significance. Br. Heart J., 46:152-158, 1981.
98. Gomes, J. A. C., Kang, P. S., Khan, R., et al.: Repetitive ventricular response. Its incidence, inducibility, reproducibility, mechanism, and significance. Br. Heart J., 46:159-167, 1981.

21

Electrophysiologic Studies in Patients with Ventricular Tachyarrhythmias

Daniel S. Oseran, C. Thomas Peter, and William J. Mandel

Patients with recurrent life-threatening ventricular arrhythmias have been the focus of significant clinical investigation during recent years. Intracardiac electrophysiologic studies, with programmed electrical stimulation of the heart, originally employed in patients with supraventricular tachycardia, have contributed to clinicians' understanding and treatment of patients with ventricular tachyarrhythmias. Wellens and co-workers first described, in 1972, the induction of ventricular tachycardia with programmed electrical stimulation in patients.[1] Since that time, electrophysiologic studies have assumed an increasing role in the management of patients with documented or suspected ventricular arrhythmias. These studies have been used to confirm the diagnosis of ventricular tachycardia in selected patients with wide complex tachycardias, to guide pharmacologic therapy in patients with recurrent ventricular arrhythmias, and to evaluate patients for other therapeutic modalities, such as endocardial resection or implantation of antitachycardia devices. Initially, studies were performed in patients with recurrent sustained ventricular tachycardia,[2–5] but have more recently included survivors of sudden cardiac death,[6–10] patients with nonsustained ventricular tachycardia,[11–14] patients with syncope of unknown etiology,[15–17] and survivors of myocardial infarction as means of determining prognosis.[18–21]

The relative merit of invasive electrophysiologic testing in managing patients with recurrent ventricular arrhythmias, versus other noninvasive means, is unanswered. Graboys and co-workers have reported impressive results with respect to outcome in managing patients with ventricular tachyarrhythmia using ambulatory and exercise electrocardiography to assess drug efficacy.[22] Issues of cost and patient safety and comfort, as well as therapeutic efficacy, are all factors in determining the optimal investigative approach. Undoubtedly, in some patients one approach will be a clear favorite. In this chapter we will discuss an approach to patients with ventricular arrhythmias that employs electrophysiologic techniques. We will attempt to delineate those areas where this methodology can aid in the diagnosis and management of patients with life-threatening ventricular arrhythmias.

Technical Considerations

Laboratory procedures and techniques for performing electrophysiologic studies are extensively reviewed elsewhere in this text (see Chap. 5) and will only be briefly reviewed here. Studies are performed in a cardiac catheterization laboratory or procedure room equipped with a fluoroscopic unit. The room should have an emergency cart and a defibrillator. Studies are performed with the patient in the postabsorptive state with all antiarrhythmics discontinued for at least five half-lives. Multiplepole electrode catheters are inserted percutaneously into the femoral veins and advanced to the high right atrium, right ventricular apex, and His bundle position. Catheters are occasionally positioned in other right ventricular sites, the coronary sinus, or the left ventricle for stimulation and recording (see discussion of stimulation protocols below). Quadripolar catheters are used so that two electrodes may be used for stimulation and two electrodes for recording an intracardiac electrogram. The intracardiac electrograms are filtered between 30 and 500 Hz and displayed simultaneously with at least three surface electrocardiographic levels on a multichannel oscilloscope. Recordings can be printed on hard copy or stored on FM magnetic tape for later retrieval and analysis. Stimulation is performed with one of several available devices, which should be able to deliver at least three extra stimuli.

Stimulation Protocol

The ventricular stimulation protocols used by clinical electrophysiology laboratories vary greatly. Protocols differ in the intensity, as well as the defined endpoint, of stimulation. Meaningful comparisons between the results of studies from different institutions have been hampered by the lack of a uniform stimulation protocol. Table 21-1 lists some of the variables involved in a ventricular stimulation protocol. Despite this diversity of protocols, some general comments regarding the effect of each of these variables can be made.

The endpoint sought during a ventricular stimulation protocol must be defined for the initial study and for follow-up drug studies. Three different endpoints have been used in electrophysiologic studies of patients with ventricular arrhythmias: the repetitive ventricular response, nonsustained ventricular tachycardia, and sustained ventricular tachycardia. The *repetitive ventricular response* has been defined as two or more premature ventricular depolarizations in response to a single premature ventricular stimulus delivered during sinus rhythm, atrial pacing, or ventricular pacing. It has not proved a reliable endpoint either in assessing arrhythmia risk or in evaluating drug efficacy in patients with known arrhythmias. The sensitivity of the repetitive ventricular response in patients with documented ventricular tachycardia has ranged from 15% to 92%.[18,23–26] The specificity of this endpoint has been reported to range from 57% to 90%. Some of this variability may be due to differences in techniques for eliciting the repetitive ventricular response.

Most clinical electrophysiology laboratories use *sustained ventricular tachycardia* as an endpoint in patients being evaluated for documented or suspected sustained ventricular arrhythmias. Note, however, that definitions of nonsustained and sustained ventricular tachycardia vary somewhat among centers. Definitions of sustained ventricular tachycardia vary from a tachycardia greater than 15 seconds[3] to one greater than 1 minute.[27] These differences should be kept in mind when evaluating the results of a particular laboratory. In general, most laboratories define a sustained ventricular tachycardia as one that lasts at least 30 seconds or produces loss of consciousness. In patients with previously documented sustained ventricular tachycardia, using the patient's clinical arrhythmia as the endpoint has proved both highly sensitive and specific. Similarly, in patients with suspected but not documented sustained ventricular tachycardia, the induction of sustained monomorphic ventricular tachycardia can be used as the endpoint of stimulation. There are centers, however, that use nonsustained ventricular tachycardia as the endpoint of stimulation during both initial and follow-up drug studies. There has never been a rigorous comparison of these two endpoints.

Table 21-1. Variables in a Ventricular Stimulation Protocol

Endpoints of stimulation
Repetitive ventricular response
Sustained ventricular tachycardia
Nonsustained ventricular tachycardia
Definitions of sustained and nonsustained ventricular tachycardia
Basic drive rhythm and rate (*i.e.*, sinus, atrial or ventricular paced)
Number of extra stimuli
Site of stimulation
Duration of paced pulses
Stimulus strength

Modes of Stimulation

Initiation of ventricular tachycardia with programmed ventricular stimulation depends on several variables, including the number of extra stimuli and the strength and site of stimulation. In an effort to increase the yield of inducible arrhythmias in susceptible persons and to avoid the need for left ventricular stimulation, more aggressive stimulation protocols have been developed. These protocols include the use of multiple right ventricular sites, three and four ventricular extra stimuli, and higher stimulating current. Concern exists that such aggressive protocols may produce a high incidence of nonclinical or artifactual arrhythmias. In an effort to address

Table 21-2. Stimulation Protocol Used in 91 Consecutive Patients With Documented Ventricular Arrhythmias

1. Incremental atrial pacing up to 2 : 1 AV block.
2. Single APBs during sinus rhythm and atrial pacing at 110 beats/min.
3. Incremental ventricular pacing up to 250 beats/min.
4. 1, 2, and 3 VPBs during ventricular pacing at 110 beats/min and 150 beats/min from RV apex at twice diastolic threshold.
5. 1, 2, and 3 VPBs during ventricular pacing at 150 beats/min from RV apex at five times diastolic threshold.
6. 1, 2, and 3 VPBs during ventricular pacing at 150 beats/min from RV outflow tract at five times diastolic threshold.

APB, atrial premature beat; RV, right ventricle; VPB, ventricular premature beat.

some of these issues, we evaluated a ventricular stimulation protocol that included stimulation from two right ventricular sites, with up to three extra stimuli at two and five times diastolic threshold.

Ninety-one consecutive patients referred for evaluation of ventricular arrhythmias were included in this study. Fifty-two patients were studied following one or more episodes of sustained ventricular tachycardia, and 39 patients were studied following an episode of sudden cardiac death. The majority of patients (78%) had underlying coronary artery disease. All 91 patients underwent the identical ventricular stimulation protocol (Table 21-2). Stimulation was performed in a step-wise manner and continued until sustained ventricular tachycardia was induced (longer than 30 seconds).

The results of programmed stimulation in the two patient groups are summarized in Table 21-3. In patients referred with a history of sustained ventricular tachycardia, programmed stimulation induced sustained ventricular tachycardia in 41 of 52 patients (79%) and nonsustained ventricular tachycardia in seven patients (13%). In patients with a history of sudden cardiac death, programmed stimulation induced sustained ventricular tachycardia in 21 of 39 patients (54%) and nonsustained ventricular tachycardia in seven patients (17%). One patient in each group had ventricular fibrillation induced at electrophysiologic study. There were three patients (6%) in the sustained ventricular tachycardia group who had no inducible ventricular tachyarrhythmias, as compared to ten patients (26%) in the sudden cardiac death group without inducible ventricular arrhythmias ($P < 0.02$). Overall, ventricular tachycardia was induced in 48 of 52 patients (92%) referred with a history of sustained ventricular tachycardia versus 28 of 39 patients (72%) with a history of sudden cardiac death ($P < 0.02$).

The mode of ventricular tachycardia induction is summarized in Table 21-4. In patients with a history of sustained ventricular tachycardia, atrial pacing induced ventricular tachycardia in two patients and burst ventricular pacing induced ventricular tachycardia in five patients. Single ventricular extra stimuli induced ventricular tachycardia in three patients, while double extra stimuli were required in 11 patients and triple extra stimuli were required in 19 patients. Seven patients required triple extra stimuli at five times diastolic threshold for ventricular tachycardia induction. One patient was only inducible with stimulation from the right ventricular outflow tract with triple extra stimuli at five times diastolic threshold. Ventricular fibrillation was induced in one patient by triple ventricular extra stimuli at twice diastolic threshold from the right ventricular apex.

In the sudden cardiac death group, no patients were inducible with atrial pacing. Four patients had inducible ventricular tachycardia with burst ventricular pacing. No patients had inducible ventricular tachycardia with single extra stimuli, while double extra stimuli induced ventricular tachycardia in four patients and triple extra stimuli induced ventricular tachycardia in ten patients. Six patients were inducible with triple extra stimuli at five times diastolic threshold, and four patients were inducible only from the right ventricular outflow tract with triple extra stimuli at five times diastolic threshold. Ventricular fibrillation was induced in one patient with triple extra stimuli at twice diastolic threshold from the right ventricular apex.

The cumulative yield of inducible ventricular tachycardia as a function of the mode of stimulation is shown in Figures 21-1 and 21-2. Using this step-wise protocol, 40% of patients with sustained ventricular tachycardia were inducible with a maximum of two ventricular extra stimuli. Adding a third extra stimulus increased the yield of ventricular tachycardia to 77%. The last two steps of the protocol (*i.e.*, five times diastolic threshold and stim-

Table 21-3. Results of Programmed Stimulation

	Sustained VT	Nonsustained VT	VF	None Inducible
Sustained VT (N = 52)	41(79%)	7(13%)	1(2%)	3(6%)
Sudden Cardiac Death (N = 39)	21(54%)	7(17%)	1(3%)	10(26%)

Table 21-4. Mode of Ventricular Tachycardia Induction

Group	AP	V Burst	S_1S_2	$S_1S_2S_3$	$S_1S_2S_3S_4$	5XDT	RVOT
Sustained VT (N = 48)	2	5	3	11	19	7	1
Sudden Cardiac Death (N = 28)	0	4	0	4	10	6	4

ulation of the right ventricular outflow tract) added a 15% increment in the overall yield. In patients with sudden cardiac death, adding a third extra stimulus increased the yield of inducible ventricular tachycardia from 21% to 46%. Stimulating at five times diastolic threshold and stimulating from the outflow tract increased the yield an additional 26%.

The characteristics of the induced tachycardias in the two groups of patients are shown in Table 21-5. Forty-eight patients in the sustained ventricular tachycardia group had inducible ventricular tachycardia. The mean cycle length of the tachycardias was 311 ± 59 msec. This was significantly longer than the cycle length of the tachycardias in the 28 patients in the sudden cardiac death group, who had inducible ventricular tachycardia (267 ± 56 msec, $P < 0.02$). Forty-four of the 48 inducible patients in the sustained ventricular tachycardia group had inducible monomorphic ventricular tachycardia, as compared to 19 of 28 patients in the sudden cardiac death group ($P < 0.02$). The remaining four patients in the sustained ventricular tachycardia group had inducible polymorphic ventricular tachycardia. In three of these four, conversion to a monomorphic ventricular tachycardia was obtained after a type I antiarrhythmic drug was administered. Rapid polymorphic ventricular tachycardia was induced in nine patients in the sudden

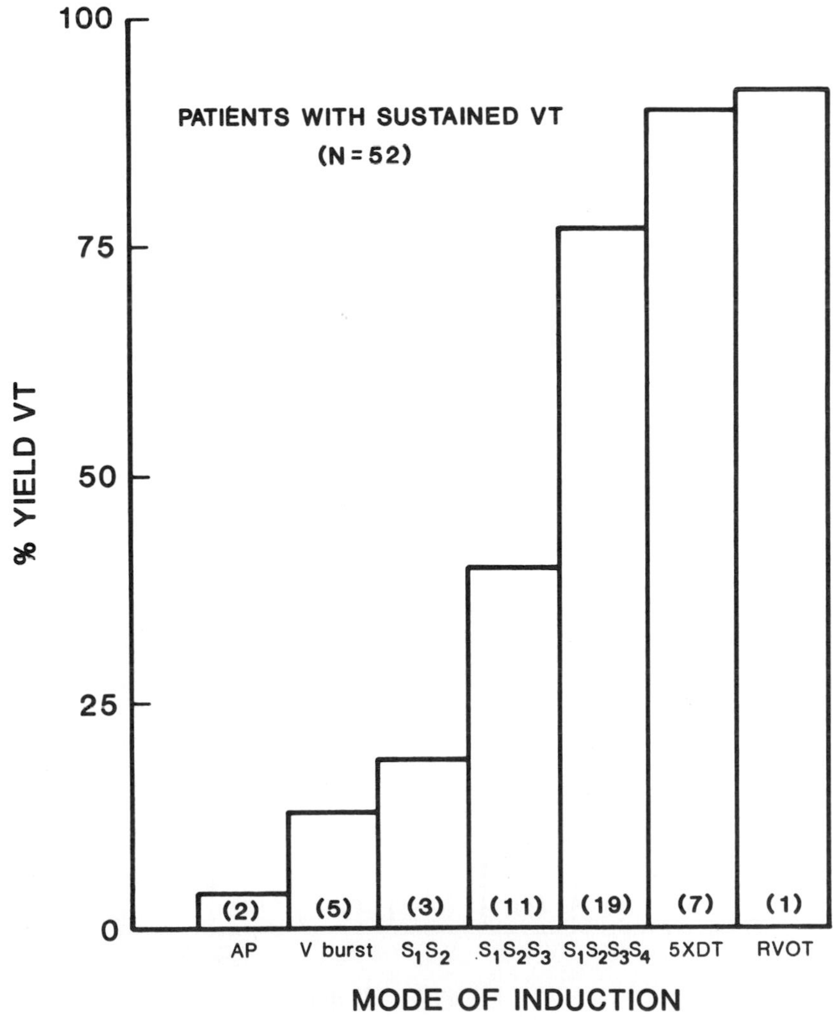

Figure 21-1. *Relation between mode of stimulation and cumulative yield of inducible ventricular tachycardia in patients with a history of sustained ventricular tachycardia. The numbers in parentheses refer to the total number of patients inducible with each mode of stimulation. (AP, atrial pacing; 5XDT, five times diastolic threshold; RVOT, right ventricular outflow tract;* S_1S_2*, single ventricular extra stimuli;* $S_1S_2S_3$*, double ventricular extra stimuli;* $S_1S_2S_3S_4$*, triple ventricular extra stimuli; V burst, ventricular burst pacing; VT, ventricular tachycardia)*

Table 21-5. Characteristics of Induced Ventricular Tachycardia

Group	Cycle Length of VT	No. of Patients	
		Monomorphic VT	*Polymorphic VT*
Sustained VT (N = 48)	311 + 59	44	4
Sudden Cardiac Death (N = 28)	267 + 56	19	9

cardiac death group. In the sustained ventricular tachycardia group, 38 patients had 12-lead electrocardiograms obtained during their spontaneous arrhythmia that were available for review. In 35 of these 38 patients, programmed stimulation induced the clinical ventricular tachycardia.

The yields for ventricular tachycardia induction in this study are comparable to those reported by other authors.[27-30] Vandepol and colleagues induced ventricular tachycardia in 91% of patients studied with a history of sustained ventricular tachycardia using a protocol that included left ventricular stimulation.[27] Using a similar protocol to the one described here, Morady and colleagues induced clinical ventricular tachycardia in 76% of patients with documented monomorphic ventricular tachycardia.[28] We found a somewhat lower rate of inducible ventricular tachycardia in the sudden cardiac death group. This finding is in agreement with other published reports of electrophysiologic studies in sudden death survivors.

This stimulation protocol allows only the cumulative yield of ventricular tachycardia induction to be deter-

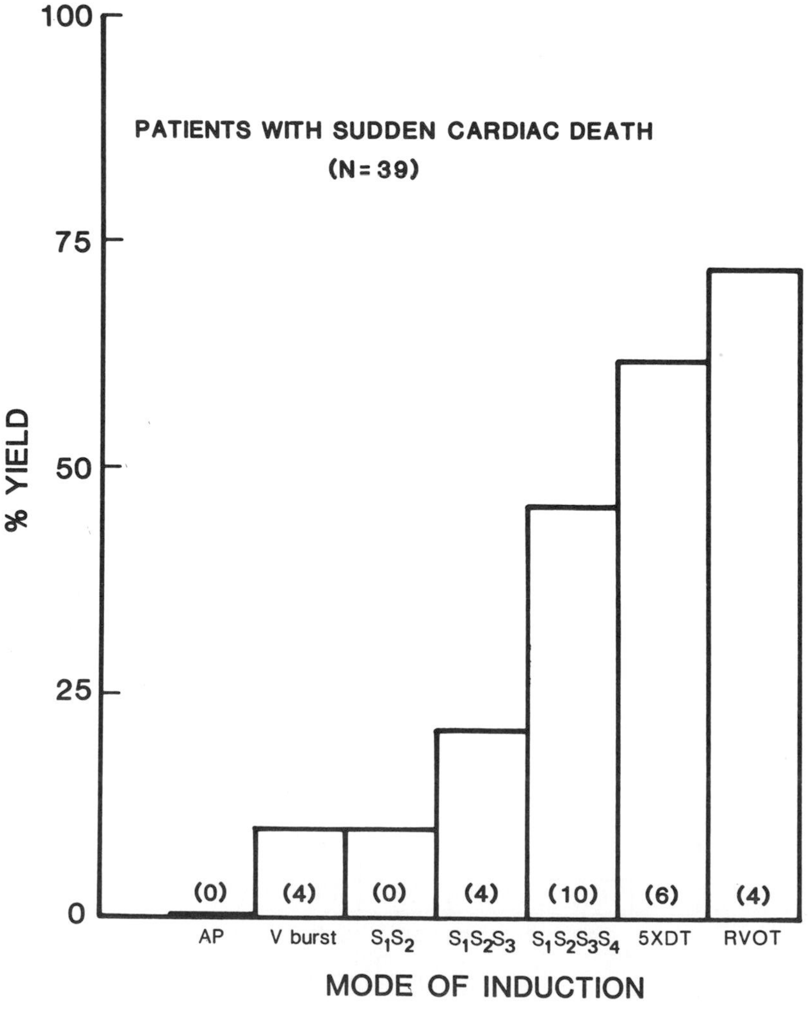

Figure 21-2. *Relation between mode of stimulation and cumulative yield of inducible ventricular tachycardia in patients with a history of sudden cardiac death. The numbers in parentheses refer to the total number of patients inducible with each mode of stimulation. (AP, atrial pacing; 5XDT, five times diastolic threshold; RVOT, right ventricular outflow tract; S_1S_2, single ventricular extra stimuli; $S_1S_2S_3$, double ventricular extra stimuli; $S_1S_2S_3S_4$, triple ventricular extra stimuli; V burst, ventricular burst pacing; VT, ventricular tachycardia)*

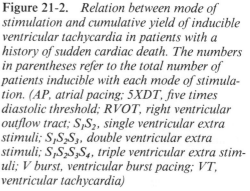

mined, rather than the absolute yield at each step in the protocol. Nonetheless, the results suggest several trends. The largest increase in yield in both groups was observed when a third extra stimulus was added, increasing the yield by 37% in patients with a history of sustained ventricular tachycardia and 25% in patients with a history of sudden cardiac death. Morady and colleagues found that a third extra stimulus was needed in 24% of patients with monomorphic ventricular tachycardia.[28] Buxton and colleagues found triple right ventricular extra stimuli induced tachycardia in 22% of patients with sustained ventricular tachycardia and in 46% of patients with sudden cardiac death.[29]

The other steps in this protocol that were evaluated were stimulation at five times threshold and stimulation from the right ventricular outflow tract. Most reported studies have used protocols in which stimulation was performed at twice diastolic threshold. In this protocol, stimulating at five times threshold increased the yield of inducible ventricular tachycardia by 13% in the sustained ventricular tachycardia group and by 15% in the sudden death group. Studies by Hamer and colleagues on normal canine myocardium showed that stimulation at five times threshold was unlikely to produce spurious ventricular fibrillation, whereas stimulation at higher levels of current produced a significantly greater incidence of ventricular fibrillation.[31] The data suggest that stimulation at five times threshold increases the yield of inducible arrhythmias without producing ventricular fibrillation.

The stimulating catheter was positioned in the right ventricular outflow tract only after stimulation had been performed at five times threshold from the right ventricular apex. Using this step-wise approach, stimulation from the right ventricular outflow tract induced ventricular tachycardia in one additional patient in the sustained ventricular tachycardia group and in four patients in the sudden death group. Thus the vast majority of inducible ventricular tachycardia in both groups was produced by stimulation from the right ventricular apex. A somewhat greater increment in yield with stimulation from the outflow tract has been reported by Doherty and co-workers.[32,33] In our protocol the use of triple extra stimuli and higher current at the right ventricular apex substantially reduced the need for stimulation from the outflow tract.

Since this stimulation protocol was not applied to a group of patients *without* a history of ventricular arrhythmias, definitive statements about specificity cannot be made. However, several observations are suggested by the data. As demonstrated by Brugada and others, the induction of non-sustained polymorphous ventricular tachycardia or ventricular fibrillation by aggressive stimulation is a nonspecific response.[34,35] Conversely, the induction of sustained monomorphic ventricular tachycardia is highly specific. We agree with these authors, and others, and suggest that the results of any individual ventricular stimulation study must be interpreted weighing not only the mode of initiation but the induced arrhythmia and patient's previous clinical history as well. For example, the initiation of non-sustained polymorphous ventricular tachycardia with triple extra stimuli in a patient without previous documentation of this arrhythmia likely represents a nonclinical arrhythmia and should not be treated. The initiation of monomorphic ventricular tachycardia in a patient with documented or suspected arrhythmias should always be considered significant, while the initiation of sustained polymorphous ventricular tachycardia or ventricular flutter in a patient with documented recurrent monomorphic ventricular tachycardia should probably be considered nonclinical. Some areas of interpretation remain unclear. For example, the significance of sustained polymorphous ventricular tachycardia in sudden death survivors is uncertain. However, it is only when these three factors are considered, namely, mode of initiation, nature of the induced arrhythymia, and the patient's clinical history, that a high degree of specificity can be obtained.

Electrophysiologic Studies as a Guide to Drug Therapy

Electrophysiologic testing has been proposed as a way to select effective antiarrhythmic drug therapy in patients with ventricular tachycardia.[2–5,36–38] This approach is based on the premise that the patient's acute or subacute response to antiarrhythmic agents as assessed by programmed ventricular stimulation predicts his or her clinical response to continued therapy. Many investigators have demonstrated that in patients with recurrent sustained ventricular tachycardia or in survivors of sudden cardiac death, the inducibility or noninducibility of ventricular tachyarrhythmias after pharmacologic interventions predicts the long-term clinical response. This approach of using inducibility of ventricular tachycardia as the endpoint in designing antiarrhythmic therapy has gained wide acceptance in clinical practice. It is important to recognize, however, that this approach depends on the definition of drug efficacy as well as the methodology of drug testing. In addition, the results of programmed stimulation may simply not predict clinical efficacy when certain antiarrhythmic agents are used.

Methodology of Serial-Day Drug Studies

Typically, a control study is performed once all antiarrhythmics have not been administered for at least five half-lives. A control study is needed because evaluation of the efficacy of subsequent interventions can best be assessed by comparison to this initial study. Further, antiarrhythmic agents can exert a proarrhythmic effect or promote inducibility in a given patient.[36,39,40] During this initial study the reproducibility of induction of ventricular tachycardia must be documented. The rate and morphology of all induced tachycardias should be noted and compared to the patient's clinical arrhythmia when possible. The level of stimulation and pacing site required to induce the tachycardia should be documented.

Following the control study, antiarrhythmic agents are tested in a serial fashion. The manner in which this is done varies among clinical electrophysiology laboratories. A drug, typically procainamide, may be infused intravenously, with repeat programmed stimulation after a therapeutic serum level is achieved. Alternatively, a drug may be administered orally for 48 to 72 hours, until steady-state concentrations are achieved, with repeat stimulation at that time. Serum drug levels are drawn during or following stimulation to document a therapeutic level, thereby ensuring that an individual drug is given a "fair chance." In this way serial agents, or combination of agents, are tested to identify an antiarrhythmic regimen that will prevent the induction of ventricular tachycardia.

As suggested earlier, the definition of drug efficacy or a positive drug response is not uniform among laboratories. In studies of patients with ventricular arrhythmias, where electropharmacologic guided therapy has been used, the criteria for drug success are often not explicitly stated. In an effort to address this issue, Swerdlow and co-workers analyzed data from 255 long-term drug trials in patients with inducible sustained ventricular tachycardia or ventricular fibrillation.[41] Arrhythmia recurrence rates on drug therapy were analyzed as a function of the number of induced ventricular complexes during initial drug testing. They found that a cut-off point between 11 and 20 beats best predicted clinical efficacy with respect to arrhythmia recurrence. At our institution, we use a cut-off point of 10 complexes as a criterion for drug efficacy in serial drug studies in patients with inducible sustained ventricular tachycardia during the control study. In patients with only nonsustained ventricular tachycardia induced during the control study, the criteria for drug efficacy are less clear.

When the effects of antiarrhythmics are tested, stimulation is performed from the same pacing site that produced that tachycardia during the control study. Some authors have suggested that an increase in the intensity of stimulation required to induce tachycardia during drug therapy indicates drug efficacy.[42,43] At our institution a drug must be effective at all levels of stimulation employed in our protocol to call a drug trial successful.

The process of serial-day drug testing can be expensive and timeconsuming. Some authors have suggested that the response to intravenous procainamide at the time of the initial electrophysiologic study predicts the response to other serial drug testing with conventional agents.[44,45] In a retrospective study of this issue, Waxman and co-workers concluded that if intravenous procainamide is ineffective in preventing the induction of ventricular tachycardia, then further testing of other antiarrhythmics is unnecessary and surgery or experimental agents such as amiodarone should be considered. To evaluate the usefulness of the response to intravenous procainamide as a "screening test," we prospectively performed drug studies on 23 patients with inducible sustained ventricular tachycardia. All patients had reproducibly inducible sustained ventricular tachycardia in a control study using the protocol described earlier in this chapter. Following the control study, patients received intravenous procainamide, 10 to 15 mg/kg over 30 minutes, with repeat stimulation. Patients were then randomly assigned to receive oral procainamide or oral quinidine with repeat stimulation after therapeutic serum levels were reached. All patients received both oral drugs in a sequential manner with programmed stimulation performed to assess drug efficacy. A positive drug response was defined as the inability to induce more than ten beats of ventricular tachycardia.

The results of programmed stimulation and the serum drug levels obtained are outlined in Table 21-6. Seven of 23 patients (30%) had a positive drug response to intravenous procainamide. Twelve of 23 patients (52%) responded to oral quinidine, and 7 of 23 patients (30%) responded to oral procainamide. There were no significant differences in serum drug concentrations between patients with positive and negative drugs response. The rates of drug efficacy, or positive drug response for intravenous and oral procainamide, are

Table 21-6. Procainamide and Quinidine Serum Levels (μg/ml)

	Positive Response	(N)	Negative Response	(N)	P
IV procainamide	10.1 + 2.2	7	11.7 + 2.1	16	NS
Oral procainamide	12.4 + 3.4	7	11.8 + 3.8	16	NS
Oral quinidine	5.4 + 0.6	12	5.4 + 1.0	11	NS

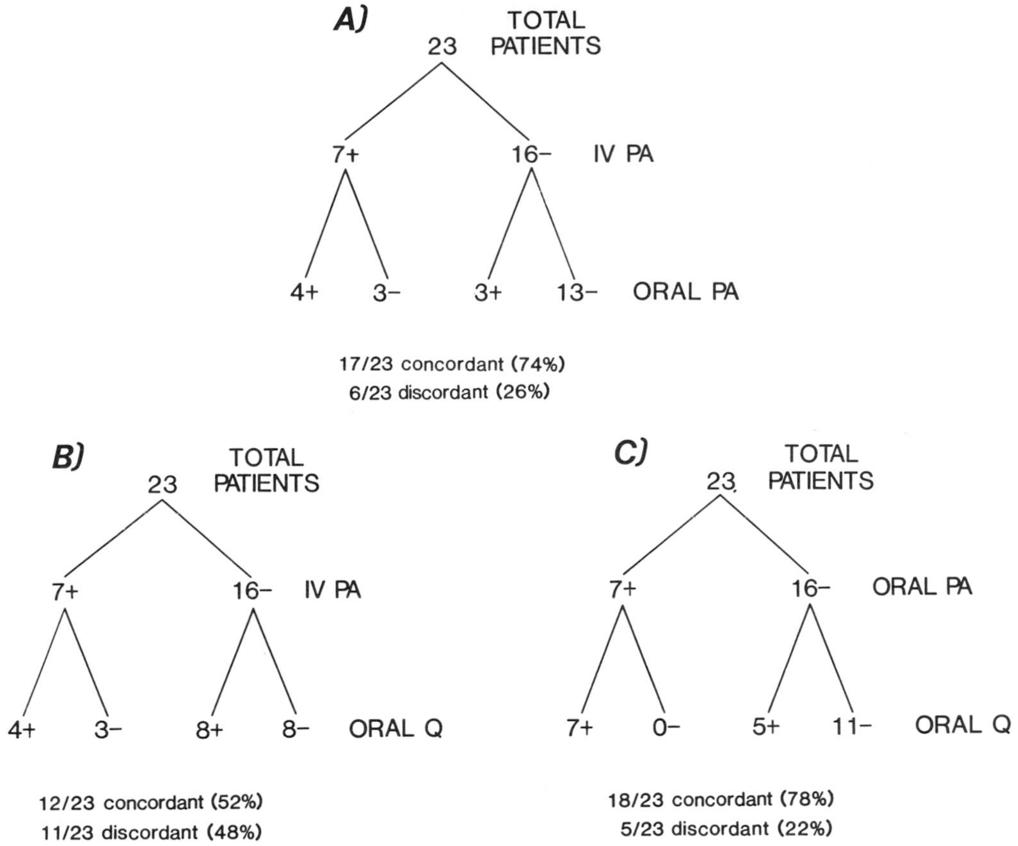

Figure 21-3. *Flowcharts illustrating the effects of intravenous procainamide (PA), oral PA, and oral quinidine (Q) on inducible ventricular tachycardia (VT) in 23 patients. (A) Intravenous PA compared with oral PA. (B) Intravenous PA compared with oral Q. (C) Oral PA compared with oral Q. (+, positive drug response defined as fewer than 10 beats of induced VT; −, negative drug response defined as greater than ten beats of induced VT)*

comparable to those reported by other authors[46–49]; however, the rate of drug efficacy for oral quinidine is higher than that reported in other studies.[50–52] We suspect that this is in part due to the substantially higher serum drug levels that were achieved in this study. This may be analogous to the efficacy of using high-dose procainamide to prevent induction of ventricular tachycardia as compared to more conventional doses.[49]

The concordance of drug response is illustrated in Figure 21-3. Seven of the 23 patients (26%) had a discordant drug response for intravenous and oral procainamide. Eleven of 23 patients (48%) had a discordant drug response for intravenous procainamide and oral quinidine. Finally, five of 23 patients (22%) had a discordant drug response for oral quinidine and oral procainamide. These data suggest that acute drug testing with intravenous antiarrhythmics in patients with ventricular tachycardia may give misleading results about the efficacy of oral agents. The presence of active metabolites, which accumulate during oral therapy, as well as myocardial concentration of drug during long-term oral therapy, may contribute to differences in drug effects between intravenous and oral therapy.[53–55] Given these moderate to high rates of drug discordance, as well as the associated toxicities of experimental agents such as amiodarone, we continue to perform serial drug testing with conventional antiarrhythmics regardless of the patient's response to intravenous procainamide.

Caveats and Considerations

As mentioned earlier, some antiarrhythmics may not be useful in studies attempting to predict long-term clinical efficacy. Initial reports of programmed ventricular stimulation in patients receiving amiodarone indicated that continued inducibility during therapy did not predict subsequent recurrent clinical arrhythmias.[56–58] Recently, other studies have demonstrated that the patient's response to programmed stimulation can predict his or her long-term clinical response to amiodarone.[59–60] Again, differences in stimulation protocols and definitions of inducibility and drug success may contribute to these disparate findings. Moreover, the complicated pharmacokinetics of amiodarone are such that the optimum time in which to evaluate drug response is still unresolved. Like others, we are uncertain of the value of electrophysiologic studies in guiding therapy in patients receiving amiodarone. The value of electrophysiologic testing for assessing drug efficacy of other investigational agents must be established on a drug by drug basis.

One final caveat with respect to electropharmacologic testing should be mentioned. It may well be that identifying an effective drug with electrophysiologic testing simply identifies patients with a better prognosis as compared to patients in whom an effective drug cannot be identified. Although some data suggest that the response to therapy during electrophysiologic study is an independent predictor of survival,[61] a prospective evaluation of this issue has not yet been published. Specifically, an antiarrhythmic that fails to prevent inducibility is rarely continued to evaluate spontaneous recurrences of tachycardia. Wellens and co-workers are apparently engaged in a protocol in which serial drug studies are performed; however, patients continue to receive antiarrhythmics irrespective of the results of programmed stimulation. Although no long-term follow-up data are available as yet, this study will help to evaluate directly the predictive value of electropharmacologic therapy in patients with recurrent ventricular tachyarrhythmias.

Electrophysiologic Studies as a Guide to Surgical and Pacing Therapy for Ventricular Arrhythmias

Surgical intervention for arrhythmia control has become an accepted mode of therapy in many centers in treating patients with ventricular tachyarrhythmias. Newer surgical techniques derived from insights gained from mapping studies have contributed to improved surgical control of arrhythmias. The majority of patients operated on for ventricular tachycardia have underlying coronary artery disease with previous infarction leading to extensive scarring and aneurysm formation. Aneurysmectomy with or without revascularization has not proved effective in controlling arrhythmias in these patients. The success rate for these procedures has been reported to be 40% to 60%.[62–66] This disappointing rate of success stems from the failure of such procedures to remove or interrupt reliably the reentrant circuit that gives rise to the tachycardia. The results of intraoperative epicardial and endocardial mapping studies suggest that the reentrant circuit is located near the ventricular endocardium at the border of the aneurysm and normal tissue.[67–69] Recent surgical techniques have been aimed at removing or interrupting this reentrant circuit.

The preoperative evaluation of these patients should include an electrophysiologic study with catheter mapping in the electrophysiologic laboratory.[70] Reference catheters are placed in the right ventricular apex, the His bundle, and, often, the coronary sinus. A mapping catheter is positioned in multiple right and left ventricular sites during sustained ventricular tachycardia. By recording electrograms from these different sites, the earliest site of electrical activation can be identified. This "earliest site" is presumed to be part of the reentrant circuit. This technique requires that the patient have a hemodynamically stable tachycardia. Antiarrhythmic drugs can be administered to slow the rate of the tachycardia so that mapping can be performed. Attempts should be made to induce and map all morphologically distinct tachycardias.

At surgery, both epicardial and endocardial mapping can be performed with a hand-held probe. Again, this mapping is typically done to locate the earliest site of electrical activity, the assumption being that this represents part of the reentrant circuit. Other techniques that have been proposed to locate the site of origin of the tachycardia include pace mapping[71,72] and endocardial mapping during sinus rhythm.[73,74]

There are several surgical approaches to removal or interruption of the reentrant circuit. Harken and Josephson have advocated a limited subendocardial resection guided by mapping in treating patients with recurrent ventricular tachycardia.[66,75–77] Other investigators have suggested more extensive endocardial resections, in which all visible endocardial scar is removed.[78] Guiraudon and co-workers introduced the encircling endocardial ventriculotomy as a technique of interrupting or isolating the reentrant circuit.[79] Finally, cryosurgery has been used alone or in conjunction with other procedures to control recurrent ventricular tachycardia.[80] In general, these procedures should be reserved for patients with drug-refractory malignant ventricular arrhythmias (See Chap. 35).

As discussed earlier in this chapter, pacing techniques can initiate ventricular tachycardia in the majority of patients who have had this arrhythmia spontaneously. A further observation drawn from the electrophysiology laboratory is that pacing techniques can terminate the induced tachycardia in the majority of instances, presumably by penetrating the reentrant circuit. This can be accomplished by a variety of pacing modalities, including underdrive, overdrive, or burst pacing, multiple extra stimuli, or a combination of these techniques.[81,82] Programmed stimulation or pacing to terminate ventricular tachycardia, however, could accelerate the rate of the tachycardia or precipitate ventricular fibrillation,[83–85] factors that have severely limited the use of pacing techniques for the long-term control or therapy of ventricular tachycardia. Antitachycardia pacemakers are either patient activated or automatic, in which case they sense the tachycardia and terminate the arrhythmia by a variety of programmable pacing settings. Before such devices are implanted, detailed electrophysiologic studies must be performed, documenting the reproducible termination of the tachycardia by the proposed pacing algorithm without acceleration of the arrhythmia. Until such pacemakers have back-up defibrillation capability, their applicability to patients with ventricular tachyarrhythmias will be limited (See Chap. 25).

Two other devices to control recurrent ventricular tachycardia or ventricular fibrillation have been proposed. Mirowski and co-workers have developed an automatic implantable defibrillator/cardioverter that can sense ventricular fibrillation or ventricular tachycardia (rates >150 beats/min) and deliver a synchronized shock of 25 to 35 J.[86] Implantation of this device requires the surgical placement of electrode patches on the left ventricle. Electrophysiologic testing must be performed when such devices are implanted to ensure appropriate sensing and defibrillation/cardioversion. A second available implantable device is a transvenous catheter system capable of cardioverting ventricular tachycardia by delivering low-energy shocks. Clinical trials with both devices are underway. Ultimately, the ideal implantable antitachycardia device for patients with recurrent drug refractory ventricular tachycardia will have the ability for cardioversion, defibrillation, and back-up pacing. Unfortunately, such a device is not currently available (See Chap. 36).

Electrophysiologic Studies in Specific Patient Subsets

As mentioned at the beginning of this chapter, electrophysiologic studies with programmed ventricular stimulation have been proposed as useful in a variety of clinical settings. As with any new technique, controversy exists regarding the sensitivity, specificity, and predictive value of such testing. One area where these studies are clearly useful is in the patient with a wide complex tachycardia of uncertain origin. Despite clues from the surface 12-lead electrocardiogram,[88] differentiation between a supraventricular rhythm with aberrant conduction and a ventricular rhythm can often be difficult. In these instances, initiating the tachycardia at the electrophysiologic study will distinguish between these two possibilities. Findings that differentiate a supraventricular tachycardia with aberrancy from ventricular tachycardia include the temporal relationship between the atrial, His, and ventricular electrograms as well as the response to atrial and ventricular stimuli during the tachycardia.

Electrophysiologic studies with programmed ventricular stimulation were first performed in patients with recurrent sustained ventricular tachycardia. As discussed, these studies can be useful in directing both pharmacologic and surgical therapy. The majority of these patients (80% to 90%) will have inducible ventricular tachycardia, usually of similar morphology to the spontaneous tachycardia. Many investigators have reported the high positive and negative predictive value of drug testing with programmed ventricular stimulation for the long-term prevention of spontaneous ventricular tachycardia.[2–5,36,37] The value of this approach in patients with nonsustained ventricular tachycardia appears to be somewhat less. Nonsustained ventricular tachycardia is often a nonspecific response to an aggressive pacing protocol, and therefore electropharmacologic testing may be much less helpful. Moreover, since the overall prognosis for this group appears to be much better than in patients with sustained ventricular tachycardia, drug testing may well have a more limited value in these patients. The use of these studies in patients with recurrent syncope is discussed in Chapter 24. It appears that in some patients with organic heart disease, electrophysiologic studies can help identify a cause of syncope, and treatment based on these findings can be implemented.[15–17]

Patients who have been resuscitated from an episode of out-of-hospital cardiac arrest have a poor prognosis, with reported mortalities of 20% to 30% at 1 year and 30% to 40% at 2 years.[89] Programmed ventricular stimulation can induce ventricular tachycardia in 30% to 75% of these patients.[6–10] Drug therapy based on the results of such testing may be an effective means of preventing recurrent ventricular arrhythmias. Moreover, the identification of patients without inducible arrhythmias may help to categorize survivors of sudden death with respect to prognosis, since data suggest that these patients have a much better prognosis than patients with inducible ventricular tachycardia.[90]

Conclusion

Electrophysiologic studies with programmed ventricular stimulation, originally employed to study the mechanisms of ventricular tachycardia, are now a firm part of the clinical tools used to diagnose and treat patients with ventricular tachyarrhythmias. Much has been learned about the sensitivity and specificity of the various pacing techniques used in these studies. The prudent application of these techniques in selected patient groups can help guide drug, surgical, and pacemaker therapy. The ability with these techniques to identify patients at high risk for sudden death following myocardial infarction is a continuing area of investigation and may add to the clinical applicability of electrophysiologic testing.

References

1. Wellens, H. J. J., Schuilenberg, R. M., and Durrer, D.: Electrical stimulation of the heart in patients with ventricular tachycardia. Circulation, 46:216, 1972.

2. Horowitz, L. N., Josephson, M. E., Farshidi, A., et al.: Recurrent sustained ventricular tachycardia. III. Role of the electrophysiological study in the selection of antiarrhythmic regimens. Circulation, 58:986, 1978.
3. Mason, J. W., and Winkle, R. A.: Electrode catheter arrhythmia induction in the selection and assessment of antiarrhythmic drug therapy for recurrent ventricular tachycardia. Circulation, 58:971, 1978.
4. Fisher, J. D., Cohen, H. L., Mehra, R., et al.: Cardiac pacing and pacemakers. II. Serial electrophysiologic-pharmacologic testing for control of recurrent tachyarrhythmias. Am. Heart J., 93:658, 1977.
5. Hartzler, G. O., and Maloney, J. D.: Programmed ventricular stimulation in management of recurrent ventricular tachycardia. Mayo Clin. Proc. 52:731, 1977.
6. Ruskin, J. N., DiMarco, J. P., and Garan, H.: Out of hospital cardiac arrest: Electrophysiologic observations in selection of long-term antiarrhythmic therapy. N. Engl. J. Med., 303:607, 1980.
7. Morady, F., Sheinman, M. M., Hess, D. S., et al.: Electrophysiologic testing in the management of survivors of out-of-hospital cardiac arrest. Am. J. Cardiol., 51:85, 1983.
8. Roy, D., Waxman, H. L., Kienzle, M. G., et al.: Clinical characteristics and long-term follow-up in 119 survivors of cardiac arrest: Relation to inducibility of electrophysiologic testing. Am. J. Cardiol., 52:969, 1983.
9. Josephson, M. E., Horowitz, I. N., Spielman, S. R., and Greenspan, A. M.: Electrophysiologic and hemodynamic studies in patients resuscitated from cardiac arrest. Am. J. Cardiol., 46:947, 1980.
10. Benditt, D. G., Benson, P. W., Klein, G. J., et al.: Prevention of recurrent sudden cardiac arrest: Role of provocative electropharmacological testing. J. Am. Coll. Cardiol., 2:418, 1983.
11. Buxton, A. E., Waxman, H. L., Marchlinski, F. E., and Josephson, M. E.: Electrophysiologic studies in non-sustained ventricular tachycardia. Relation to underlying heart disease. Am. J. Cardiol., 52:985, 1983.
12. Buxton, A. E., Waxman, H. L., Marchlinski, F. E., and Josephson, M. E.: Electropharmacology of nonsustained ventricular tachycardia: Effects of class I antiarrhythmic agents, verapamil and propranolol. Am. J. Cardiol., 53:738, 1984.
13. Swerdlow, C. D., Echt, D. S., Soderholm-Difatle, V., et al.: Limited value of programmed stimulation in patients with unsustained VT. Circulation, 66:11–145, 1982.
14. Schoenfeld, M. H., McGovern, B., Garan, H., et al.: The role of programmed stimulation in patients with nonsustained ventricular tachycardia. J. Am. Coll. Cardiol., 1:607, 1983.
15. DiMarco, J. P., Garan, H., Harthorne, J. W., and Ruskin, J. N.: Intracardiac electrophysiologic techniques in recurrent syncope of unknown cause. Ann. Intern. Med., 95:542, 1981.
16. Brandenberg, R. O., Holmes, D. R., and Hartzler, G. O.: The electrophysiologic assessment of patients with syncope. Am. J. Cardiol., 47:433, 1981.
17. Hess, D. S., Morday, F., and Scheinman, M. M.: Electrophysiologic testing in the evaluation of patients with syncope of undetermined origin. Am. J. Cardiol., 50:1309, 1982.
18. Greene, H. L., Reid, P. R., and Schaeffer, A. H.: The repetitive ventricular response in man—a predictor of sudden death. N. Engl. J. Med., 299:729, 1978.
19. Hamer, A., Vohra, J., Hunt, O., and Sloman, G.: Prediction of sudden death by electrophysiologic studies in high risk patients surviving acute myocardial infarction. Am. J. Cardiol., 50:223, 1982.
20. Richards, D. A., Cody, D. V., Deniss, A. R., et al.: Ventricular electrical instability: A predictor of death after myocardial infarction. Am. J. Cardiol., 51:75, 1983.
21. Marchlinski, F. E., Buxton, A. E., Waxman, H. L., and Josephson, M. E.: Identifying patients at risk of sudden death after myocardial infarction: Value of the response to programmed stimulation, degree of ventricular ectopic activity and severity of left ventricular dysfunction. Am. J. Cardiol., 52:1190, 1983.
22. Graboys, T. B., Lown, B., Podrid, P. J., and DeSilva, R.: Long-term survival of patients with malignant ventricular arrhythmias treated with antiarrhythmic drugs. Am. J. Cardiol., 50:437, 1982.
23. Mason, J. W.: Repetitive beating after single ventricular extrastimuli: Incidence and prognostic significance in patients with recurrent ventricular tachycardia. Am. J. Cardiol., 45:1126, 1980.
24. Ruskin, J. N., DiMarco, J. P., and Garan, H.: Repetitive responses to single ventricular extrastimuli in patients with serious ventricular arrhythmia: Incidence and clinical significance. Circulation, 63:767, 1981.
25. Farshidi, A., Michelson, E. L., Greenspan, A. M., et al.: Repetitive responses to ventricular extrastimuli: Incidence, mechanism, and significance. Am. Heart J., 100:59, 1980.
26. Livelli, F. D., Bigger, J. T., Reiffel, J. A., et al.: Response to programmed ventricular stimulation: Sensitivity, specificity and relation to heart disease. Am. J. Cardiol., 50:452, 1982.
27. Vandepol, C. J., Farshidi, A., Spielman, S. R., et al.: Incidence and clinical significance of induced ventricular tachycardia. Am. J. Cardiol., 45:725, 1980.
28. Morady, F., DiCarlo, L., Winston, S., et al.: A prospective comparison of triple extrastimuli and left ventricular stimulation in studies of ventricular tachycardia induction. Circulation, 70:52, 1984.
29. Buxton, A. E., Waxman, H. L., Marchlinski, F. E., et al.: Role of triple extrastimuli during electrophysiologic study of patients with documented sustained ventricular tachyarrhythmias. Circulation, 69:532, 1984.
30. Mann, D. E., Luck, J. C., Griffin, J. C., et al.: Induction of clinical ventricular tachycardia using programmed stimulation: Value of third and fourth extrastimuli. Am. J. Cardiol. 52:501, 1983.
31. Hamer, A. W., Karagueuzian, H. S., Sugi, K., et al.: Factors related to the induction of ventricular fibrillation in the normal canine heart by programmed electrical stimulation. J. Am. Coll. Cardiol., 3:751, 1984.
32. Doherty, J. U., Kienzle, M. G., Buxton, A. E., et al.: Discordant results of programmed ventricular stimulation at different right ventricular sites in patients with and without spontaneous sustained ventricular tachycardia: A prospective study of 56 patients. Am. J. Cardiol., 54:336, 1984.
33. Doherty, J. U., Kienzle, M. G., Waxman, H. L., et al.: Programmed ventricular stimulation at a second right ventricular site: An analysis of 100 patients, with special reference to sensitivity, specificity, and characteristics of patients with induced ventricular tachycardia. Am. J. Cardiol., 52:1184, 1983.
34. Brugada, P., Green, M., Abdollah, H., and Wellens, H. J. J.: Significance of ventricular arrhythmias initiated by programmed ventricular stimulation: The importance of the type of ventricular arrhythmia induced and the number of premature stimuli required. Circulation, 69:87, 1984.
35. Untereker, W. J., Waxman, H. L., Waspe, L. E., et al.: Programmed electrical stimulation in patients without clinical ventricular arrhythmias. Circulation, 66:II–147, 1982.
36. Horowitz, L. N., Josephson, M. E., and Kastor, J. A.: Intracardiac electrophysiologic studies as a method for the optimization of drug therapy in chronic ventricular arrhythmias. Prog. Cardiovasc. Dis., 23:81, 1980.
37. Josephson, M. E., and Horowitz, L. N.: Electrophysiologic approach to therapy of recurrent sustained ventricular tachycardia. Am. J. Cardiol., 43:631, 1979.
38. Scheinman, M. M., and Morady, F.: Invasive cardiac electrophysiologic testing: The current state of the art. Circulation, 67:1169, 1983.

39. Kang, P. S., Gomes, J. C., and El-Sherif, N.: Procainamide in the induction and perpetuation of ventricular tachycardia in man. Pace, 5:11, 1982.
40. Velebit, V., Podrid, P., Lown, B., et al.: Aggravation and provocation of ventricular arrhythmias by antiarrhythmic drugs. Circulation, 65:886, 1982.
41. Swerdlow, C. D., Winkle, R. A., and Mason, J. W.: Prognostic significance of the number of induced ventricular complexes during assessment of therapy for ventricular tachyarrhythmias. Circulation, 68:400, 1983.
42. DiMarco, J., Garan, H., and Ruskin, J.: Partial suppression of induced arrhythmias during serial electrophysiologic testing. Circulation, 62:III–261, 1980.
43. Swerdlow, C. D., Winkle, R. A., Griffin, J. C., et al.: Decreased incidence of antiarrhythmic drug efficacy at electrophysiologic study associated with the use of a third extrastimulus. Am. Heart J., 104:1004, 1982.
44. Waxman, H. L., Buxton, A. E., Sadowski, I. M., and Josephson, M. E.: Response to procainamide during electrophysiologic study for sustained ventricular tachyarrhythmias predicts response to other medications. Circulation, 67:30, 1982.
45. Ferrick, K. J., Bigger, J. T., Reiffel, J. A., et al.: Congruence in efficacy of procainamide and quinidine for induced ventricular tachycardia. Circulation, 62:II–142, 1982.
46. Marchlinski, F. E., Buxton, A. E., Vassallo, J. A. et al.: Comparative electrophysiologic effects of intravenous and oral procainamide in patients with sustained ventricular arrhythmias. J. Am. Coll. Cardiol., 4:1247, 1984.
47. Engel, T. R., Gonzalez, C., Meister, S. G., and Frankel, W. S.: Effect of procainamide on induced ventricular tachycardia. Clin. Pharmacol. Ther., 24:274, 1982.
48. Wellens, H. J. J., Bar, F. W., Lie K. I., et al.: Effect of procainamide, propranolol, and verapamil on mechanism of tachycardia in patients with chronic recurrent ventricular tachycardia. Am. J. Cardiol., 40:479, 1977.
49. Greenspan, A. M., Horowitz, I. N., Spielman, S. R., and Josephson, M. E.: Large dose procainamide therapy for ventricular tachyarrhythmia. Am. J. Cardiol., 46:453, 1980.
50. DiMarco, J. P., Garan, H., and Ruskin, I. N.: Quinidine for ventricular arrhythmias: value of electrophysiologic testing. Am. J. Cardiol., 51:90, 1983.
51. Swerdlow, C. D., Echt, D. S., Winkle, R. A., et al.: Incidence of acute antiarrhythmic drug efficacy at electrophysiologic study. Circulation, 64:IV–137, 1981.
52. Waxman, H. L., Buxton, A. E., Marchlinski, F. E., and Josephson, M. E.: Pharmacological therapy of sustained ventricular tachyarrhythmias. In Josephson, M. E., and Wellens, H. J. J. (eds.): Tachycardias: Mechanisms, Diagnosis, Treatment. Philadelphia, Lea & Febiger, 1984.
53. Engel, T. R.: The electropharmacology of acute drug testing using pacemakers. Pace, 5:577, 1982.
54. Zipes, D., Prystowsky, E. N., and Heger, J. J.: Electrophysiologic testing of antiarrhythmic agents. Am. Heart J., 103:610, 1982.
55. Woosley, R. L., and Roden, D. M.: Importance of metabolites in antiarrhthymic therapy. Am. J. Cardiol. 52:3C, 1983.
56. Hamer, A. W., Finerman, W. B, Peter, T., and Mandel, W. J.: Disparity between the clinical and electrophysiologic effects of amiodarone in the treatment of recurrent ventricular tachyarrhythmias. Am. Heart J., 102:992, 1981.
57. Heger, J. J., Prystowsky, E. N., Jackman, W. M., et al.: Amiodarone. Clinical efficacy and electrophysiology during long-term therapy for recurrent ventricular tachyarrhythmias. N. Engl. J. Med., 305:539, 1981.
58. Waxman, H. L., Groh, W. C., Marchlinski, F. E., et al.: Amiodarone for control of sustained ventricular tachyarrhythmias. Clinical and electrophysiologic effects in 51 patients. Am. J. Cardiol., 50:1066, 1982.
59. McGovern, B., Garan, H., Malacoff, R. F., et al.: Long-term outcome of ventricular tachycardia of fibrillation treated with amiodarone. Am. J. Cardiol., 53:1558, 1984.
60. Horowitz, L. N., Greenspan, A. M., Spielman, S. R., et al.: Usefulness of electrophysiologic testing in evaluation of amiodarone therapy for sustained ventricular tachyarrhythmias associated with coronary heart disease. Am. J. Cardiol., 55:367, 1985.
61. Swerdlow, C. E., Winkle, R. A., and Mason, J. W.: Determinants of survival in patients with ventricular tachyarrhythmias. N. Engl. J. Med., 308:1436, 1983.
62. Buda, A. J., Stinson, E. B., and Harrison, D. C.: Surgery for life-threatening ventricular tachyarrhythmias. Am. J. Cardiol., 44:1171, 1979.
63. Mason, J. W., Stinson, E. B., Winkle, R. A., et al.: Relative efficacy of blind left ventricular aneurysm resection for the treatment of recurrent ventricular tachycardia. Am. J. Cardiol., 49:241, 1982.
64. Sami, M., Chiltman, B. R., Bourassa, M. G., et al.: Long-term followup of aneurysmectomy for recurrent ventricular tachycardia. Am. Heart J., 96:303, 1978.
65. Mason, J. W., Stinson, E. B., and Winkle, R. A.: Surgery for ventricular tachycardia: Efficacy of left ventricular aneurysm resection compared with operation guided by electrical activation mapping. Circulation, 65:1149, 1982.
66. Harken, A. H., Horowitz, L. N., and Josephson, M. E.: Comparison of standard aneurysmectomy and aneurysmectomy with directed endocardial resection for the treatment of recurrent sustained ventricular tachycardia. J. Thorac. Cardiovasc. Surg., 80:527, 1980.
67. Josephson, M. E., Horowitz, I. N., Farshidi, A., et al.: Recurrent sustained ventricular tachycardia. II. Endocardial mapping. Circulation, 57:440, 1978.
68. Josephson, M. E., Horowitz, L. N., Spielman, S. R., et al.: Comparison of endocardial catheter mapping with intraoperative mapping of ventricular tachycardia. Circulation, 61:395, 1980.
69. Spielman, S. R., Michelson, E. L., Horowitz, L. N., et al.: The limitations of epicardial mapping as a guide to the surgical therapy for ventricular tachycardia. Circulation, 57:166, 1978.
70. Josephson, M. E., Horowitz, I. N., Spielman, S. R., et al.: Role of catheter mapping in the preoperative evaluation of ventricular tachycardia. Am. J. Cardiol., 49:207, 1982.
71. Waxman, H. L., and Josephson, M. E.: Ventricular activation during ventricular endocardial pacing. I. Electrocardiographic patterns related to the site of pacing. Am. J. Cardiol. 50:1, 1982.
72. Josephson, M. E., Waxman, H. L., Cain, M. E., et al.: Ventricular activation during ventricular endocardial pacing. II. Role of pace-mapping to localize the origin of ventricular tachycardia. Am. J. Cardiol., 50:11, 1982.
73. Klein, H., Karp, R. B., Kouchoukos, N. T., et al.: Intraoperative electrophysiologic mapping of the ventricles: During sinus rhythm in patients with a previous myocardial infarction. Circulation, 66:847, 1982.
74. Cassidy, D. M., Vassallo, J. A., Buxton, A. E., et al.: The value of catheter mapping during sinus rhythm to localize site of origin of ventricular tachycardia. Circulation, 69:1103, 1984.
75. Harken, A. H., Josephson, M. E., and Horowitz, L. N.: Surgical endocardial resection for the treatment of malignant ventricular tachycardia. Ann. Surg., 190:456, 1979.
76. Josephson, M. E., and Horowitz, L. N.: Endocardial excision: A new surgical technique for the treatment of recurrent ventricular tachycardia. Circulation, 60:1430, 1979.
77. Josephson, M. E., Harken, A. H., and Horowitz, I. N.: Long-term results of endocardial resection for sustained ventricular tachycardia in coronary disease patients. Am. Heart J., 104:51, 1982.
78. Moran, J. M., Kehoe, R. F., Loeb, J. M., et al.: Extended endocar-

dial resection for the treatment of ventricular tachycardia and ventricular fibrillation. Ann. Thorac. Surg., 34:538, 1982.

79. Guiraudon, G., Fontaine, G., Frank, R., et al.: Encircling endocardial ventriculotomy: A new surgical treatment for life-threatening ventricular tachycardias resistant to medical treatment following myocardial infarction. Ann. Thorac. Surg., 26:438, 1978.
80. Camm, H., Ward, D. E., Spurrell, R. A. J., et al.: Cryothermal mapping and cryoablation in the treatment of refractory cardiac arrhythmias. Circulation, 62:67, 1980.
81. Fisher, J. D., Kim, S. G., Furman, S., et al.: Role of implantable pacemakers in control of recurrent ventricular tachycardia. Am. J. Cardiol., 49:194, 1982.
82. Fisher, J. D., Kim, S. G., Matos, J. A., and Ostrow, E.: Comparative effectiveness of pacing techniques for termination of well-tolerated sustained ventricular tachycardia. Pace, 6:915, 1983.
83. Ruskin, J. N., Garan, H., Poulin, F., et al.: Permanent radiofrequency ventricular pacing for management of drug-resistant ventricular tachycardia. Am. J. Cardiol., 46:317, 1980.
84. Naccarelli, G. V., Zipes, D. P., Rahilly, G. T., et al.: Influence of tachycardia cycle length and antiarrhythmic drugs on pacing termination and acceleration of ventricular tachycardia. Am. Heart J., 105:1, 1982.
85. Roy, D., Waxman, H., Buxton, A. E., et al.: Termination of ventricular tachycardia: Role of tachycardia cycle length. Am. J. Cardiol., 50:1346, 1982.
86. Mirowski, M., Reid, P. R., Mower, M. M., et al.: Termination of malignant ventricular arrhythmias with an implanted automatic defibrillator in human beings. N. Engl. J. Med., 303:322, 1980.
87. Zipes, D. P., Jackman, W. M., Heger, J. J., et al.: Clinical transvenous cardioversion of recurrent life-threatening ventricular tachyarrhythmias: Low energy synchronized cardioversion of ventricular tachycardia and termination of ventricular fibrillation in patients using a catheter electrode. Am. Heart J., 103:789, 1982.
88. Wellens, H. J. J., Bär, F. W., and Lie, K. I.: The value of the electrocardiogram in the differential diagnosis of a tachycardia with a widened QRS complex. Am. J. Med., 64:27, 1978.
89. Schaffer, W. A., and Cobb, L. A.: Recurrent ventricular fibrillation and modes of death in survivors of out-of-hospital ventricular fibrillation. N. Engl. J. Med., 293:259, 1975.
90. Schoenfeld, M. H., McGovern, B., Garan, H., et al.: Long-term follow-up of patients with ventricular tachycardia or fibrillation with no inducible arrhythmia during programmed cardiac stimulation. J. Am. Coll. Cardiol., 1:606, 1983.

22

Ventricular Late Potentials: Mechanisms, Methodology, Prevalence and Potential Clinical Significance

Günter Breithardt and Martin Borggrefe

During recent years, experimental and clinical studies have provided convincing evidence that reentry plays a major role in the genesis of malignant ventricular arrhythmias.[1-5] The prerequisites for reentry are unidirectional block, slow conduction, and recovery of the tissue ahead of the wavefront of excitation.[5] In this context, one of the most compelling findings attributed to slow conduction was the detection of delayed fractionated electrical activity during diastole in regions of experimental infarctions.[1-3] Since these potentials most frequently occur in the ST segment, they have been called *late potentials.*[7] They are characterized by multiple low-amplitude spikes, sometimes separated by isoelectric intervals. The presence of such electrograms during sinus rhythm may indicate sites for potential reentrant circuits. Delayed and fractionated potentials have been observed during intraoperative epicardial and endocardial mapping (Fig. 22-1)[6-9] and endocardial catheter mapping in patients with ventricular tachycardia.[10,11]

Recently, ventricular late potentials have been recorded noninvasively using appropriate recording and filtering techniques.[7,12-19] In this chapter, the recording technologies and the presently available clinical results in patients with documented ventricular tachycardia as well as the potential role of late potentials in identifying patients at risk of ventricular tachyarrhythmias after myocardial infarction will be presented.

Electrophysiologic and Anatomic Basis of Ventricular Late Potentials

In experimental myocardial infarction, continuous electrical activity that regularly and predictably bridged the entire diastolic interval between the initiating beat and the reentrant beats, as well as between consecutive reentrant beats, was shown by El-Sherif and colleagues[1] using a specially designed composite electrode (Fig. 22-2). These findings are corroborated by the known anatomic characteristics of myocardial infarction that may show islands of relatively viable muscle alternating with areas of necrosis. Similar continuous electrical activity had previously been recorded by Waldo and Kaiser[20] during experimental myocardial infarction using bipolar electrodes. This continuous activity preceded the onset of ventricular arrhythmias.

Supported by a grant from the Sonderforschungsbereich 242 of the Deutsche Forschungsgemeinschaft, Bonn/Germany F. R., and the Ernst und Berta Grimmke-Stiftung, Düsseldorf/Germany F. R. With technical assistance from Petra Helmig (MTA) and medical candidate Sven Kielgas.

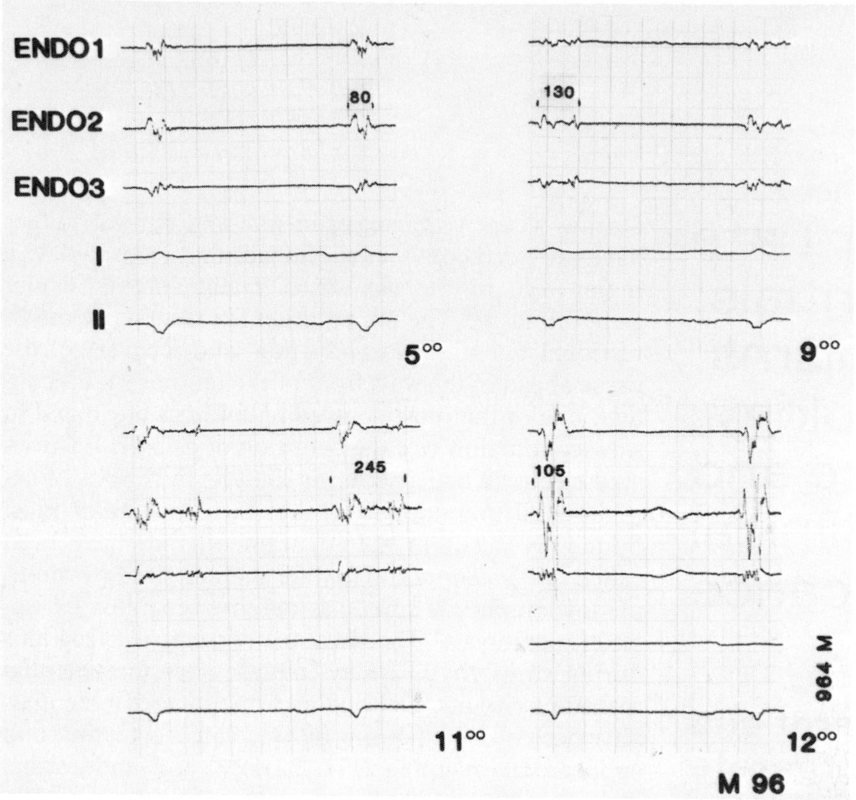

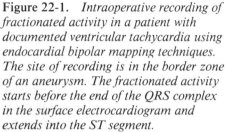

Figure 22-1. *Intraoperative recording of fractionated activity in a patient with documented ventricular tachycardia using endocardial bipolar mapping techniques. The site of recording is in the border zone of an aneurysm. The fractionated activity starts before the end of the QRS complex in the surface electrocardiogram and extends into the ST segment.*

The electrophysiologic and anatomic basis of ventricular late potentials has recently been studied in more detail. Gardner and associates[21] were able to show that slow conduction caused by depressed resting potential and action potential upstroke velocity with elevated potassium concentration in the superfusion solution were associated with a reduced electrogram amplitude and increased duration but did not cause fragmented activity. Therefore, slow conduction alone did not cause fragmented activity. Highly fractionated electrograms only occurred in preparations from chronic infarcts in which interstitial fibrosis formed insulating boundaries between muscle bundles. The individual components of fragmented electrograms therefore most likely represent asynchronous electrical activity in each of the separate bundles of surviving muscle under the electrode. The intrinsic asymmetry of cardiac activation due to fiber orientation is accentuated by infarction and may predispose to reentry.[21,22] The transmembrane potentials of muscle fibers in areas of fractionated activity in the epicardial border zone of healed canine infarcts were not depressed.[21] Instead, the slow conduction in these areas was attributed to diminished intercellular connections between muscle fibers. The low amplitude of the electrograms probably results from the paucity of surviving muscle fibers under the electrode because of the large amounts of connective tissue and not because action potentials are depressed. Therefore, the anatomic substrate for reentry seems to be present in regions where fragmented electrograms can be recorded, indicating slow, inhomogenous conduction. However, fragmented electrograms are probably found wherever myocardial fibers are separated by connective tissue, even if reentry does not occur in the region. Richards and colleagues[22] were able to show that sustained reentry may occur in areas of the epicardium showing fractionated electrograms that were as small as 5 cc.

A close correlation between the presence of continuous fractionated electrical activity and perpetuation of ventricular tachycardia was demonstrated by Garan and colleagues.[23] In these studies, ventricular pacing that captured the ventricles without affecting continuous electrical activity never terminated the tachycardia. However, transformation of continuous electrical activity into abbreviated, discrete electrograms by rapid pacing terminated ventricular tachycardia. Interruption of continuous electrical activity by a single ventricular stimulus without capture of the ventricles during ventricular tachycardia also terminated ventricular tachycardia. Surgical ablation of the site of continuous electrical activity abolished inducible ventricular tachycardia. This has also been reported in patients with previous ventricular tachycardia in whom the propensity to this arrhythmia had been successfully abolished by surgical

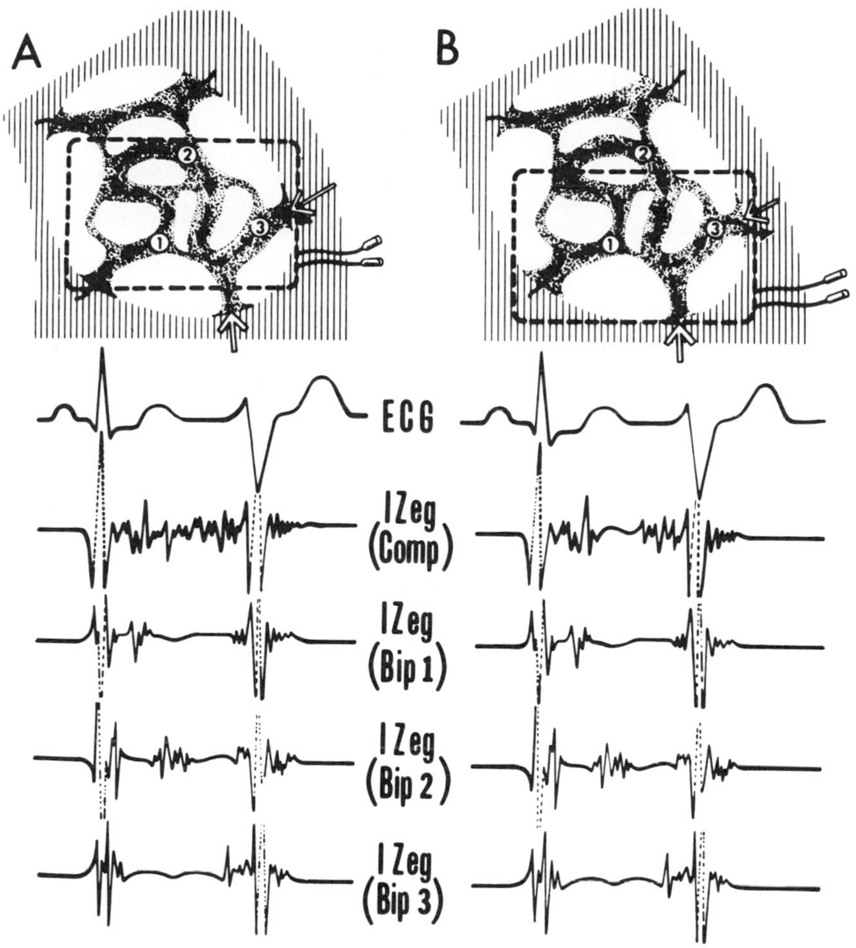

Figure 22-2. *Schematic representation of the conduction disorder in the zone of experimental infarction leading to reentry. Tracings from top to bottom represent a standard electrocardiographic lead, a composite electrode recording (Comp) with an electrogram from the ischaemic zone (IZeg), and three close bipolar recordings (IZeg [Bip], 1 to 3). The diagram in B shows that the composite electrode* (dotted line) *does not cover the entire reentrant pathway, which explains failure of the IZeg (Comp) to depict a continuous series of multiple asynchronous spikes. (El-Sherif, N., Scherlag, B. J., Lazzara, R., and Hope, R. R. Reentrant ventricular arrhythmias in the late myocardial infarction period. I. Conduction characteristics in the infarction zone. Circulation, 55:686–702, 1977)*

interventions.[24,25] These studies elegantly show the pathogenetic significance of these areas for the perpetuation of ventricular tachycardia.

It has been suggested that fractionated activity recorded in clinical studies using endocavitary electrode catheter recordings[10,11,26] might be artifacts of recording techniques caused by movement between the catheter electrodes and the tissue or distortions of the electrograms by the filtering characteristics of the amplifiers.[27] However, these fractionated electrograms can also be recorded with unipolar or bipolar electrodes from isolated superfused preparations in which mechanical movement is negligible. Since these electrodes make continuous and excellent contact with the tissue, it is obvious that these kinds of electrograms are not artifacts.

Methodological Aspects of Noninvasive Recording of Ventricular Late Potentials

The amplitude of ventricular late potentials is in the low millivolt range even if direct bipolar recordings are used. With conventional methods of electrocardiogram recording, these signals can rarely be recovered from the body surface.[28] However, these signals can be recorded from the body surface with high-gain amplification and computer-averaging techniques, as has been shown for the first time by Berbari and associates[12] in the experimental animal and by Fontaine and colleagues[7] in patients with idiopathic ventricular tachycardia. This has been confirmed by a growing number of recent reports.[13–19,29,30]

A major problem with high-gain amplification is the increasing level of noise that is generated from several sources (Table 22-1) and that makes some method of noise reduction necessary. The amplitude of these signals mostly is smaller than the electrical noise produced by the various sources. Besides careful shielding of all

Table 22-1. Causes of Noise During High-Gain Recordings of the Electrocardiogram

Environmental noise
Noise generated from the skin-electrode interface
Myotonic noise
Amplifier noise

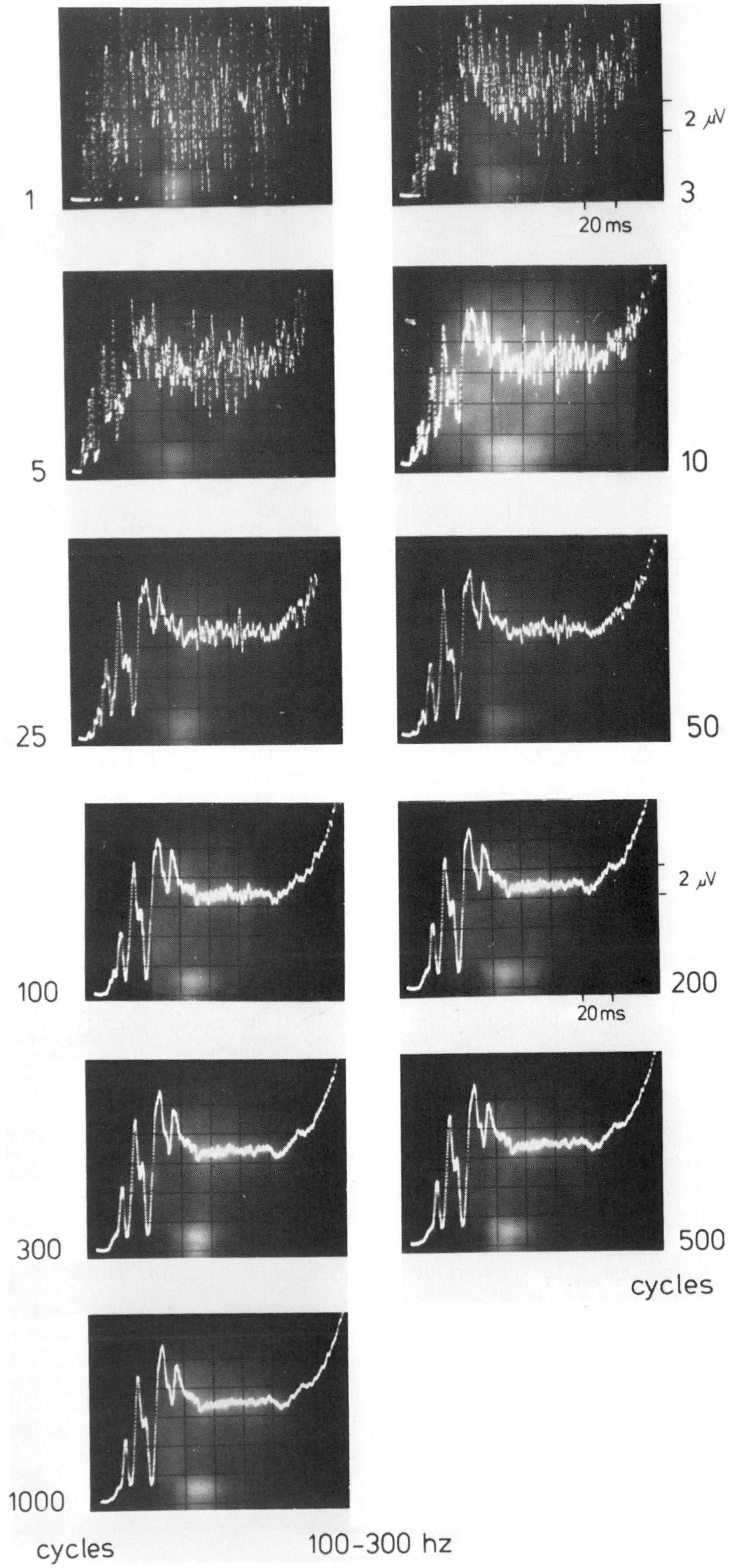

Figure 22-3. *Progress of the averaging process with evolution of the final signal depending on the number of cycles, which ranged from 1 to 1000 in a patient with left ventricular aneurysm. A circumscribed high-frequency activity represents a late potential shortly after the QRS complex in this patient with ventricular tachycardia.*

cables and the use of preamplifiers with a very high signal : noise ratio, signal averaging is used to eliminate the remaining random noise. With increasing repetition of the averaging process, randomly occurring noise is cancelled while the amplitude of the repetitively occurring "true" signal stabilizes, thus increasing the signal : noise ratio (Fig. 22-3). In our own system, 100 to 200 repetitions are sufficient to obtain a stable signal. This technique is applicable *only* to repetitive electrocardiographic signals and cannot detect moment-to-moment dynamic changes in the signal.

The sampling rate of the averaging system is determined by the frequency content of the signal. To recover a signal with good fidelity, the frequency response of the instrumentation must be commensurate with the frequency components of the signal. Ideally, there should be no frequency components of the input signal, including noise, that are higher in frequency than the sampling frequency. Input frequency components higher than half the sampling frequency cause alias frequencies that appear the same number of hertz below half the sampling frequency as the input component is above it. In our own system, alias frequencies were no problem, since the signals were filtered with a low-pass cut-off of 300 Hz and the sampling frequency was 10 kHz.[14]

One problem with high-gain amplification of biologic signals is filter ringing especially if sharp high-pass filters are used.[31] This may occur at a point of rapid transition of a higher-amplitude signal to baseline. Conventional filtering of the highly amplified QRS complex distorts the end of the signal. The degree of filter ringing increases with elevation of the high-pass cut-off. However, elimination of low-frequency components of the signal is mandatory to prevent the ST segment saturating at the extremely high amplifications used to detect late potentials and to exclude respiratory movements. Thus, in any study the characteristics of the filters used should be stated. Multiple ringing lasting for a significant time after the end of the QRS complex has been shown to occur with some filters.[18] In our own system, using single-pole filters (6 db/octave), short ringing lasting for a few milliseconds after the rapid downstroke of a rectangular signal could be demonstrated (Fig. 22-4). This, of course, might obviate short, low-amplitude signals immediately at the end of the QRS. However, it should not have a significant influence on signals appearing more than 20 ms after the rapid downstroke. A solution proposed by Simson and colleagues[18] is to use bidirectional filters that proceed backward, thus assessing the QRS complex retrogradely. This way, the low-voltage signals in the terminal QRS complex can be detected without being obscured by ringing of the filter from large-amplitude signals earlier in the QRS complex.

One of the requirements of the signal-averaging tech-

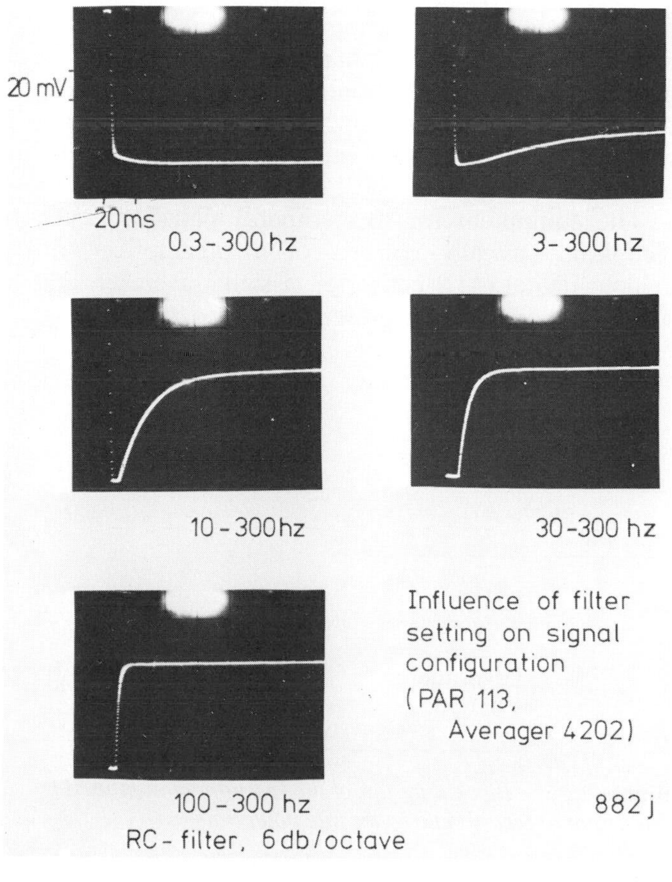

Figure 22-4. *Influence of filter setting (single-pole RC filters, 6 db/octave) on signal configuration. A rectangular signal, of which only the terminal portion is shown, was applied to the preamplifier and the averaging system using high-pass cutoffs of 0.3 to 100 Hz. The low-pass cutoff was 300 Hz. Increasing the level of high-pass cutoff leads to a pronounced depression of the horizontal portion of the signal immediately after its downstroke, making it impossible to identify signals during this short period (approximately 10 ms).*

nique is that only identical beats be averaged. Therefore, premature ventricular beats should be excluded. This can either be done simply by rejecting all beats of a given prematurity[14] or, more specifically, by passing all electrocardiographic signals through a template recognition program to reject ectopic beats and grossly noisy signals.[18] In the latter approach, an initial eight-beat template is accepted if the mean standard deviation of the signals is less than 20 μV. All subsequent beats are tested against this template and accepted if the deviation from the template is less than twice the template standard deviation. The template is updated every fourth beat.

Another prerequisite for applying the signal-averaging process is stable triggering of the signal. In case of significant jitter of the triggering point, major parts of a high-frequency signal might be cancelled, thus acting as a low-pass filter.

Equipment for Noninvasive Recording of Late Potentials

Two basic techniques are presently available for noninvasive recording of ventricular late potentials. First is the temporal signal-averaging technique, which averages a great number of identical cardiac cycles from one bipolar electrode over time.[12–19] Second is the spatial-averaging technique, which attempts to reduce the amount of noise of single beats by simultaneously recording from a great number of closely adjacent electrodes, assuming that they all depict almost identical QRS activity, whereas noise from each input is randomly distributed.[32,33]

The equipment for the temporal signal-averaging technique basically consists of a preamplifier, an analog–digital (AD) converter, a signal averager, and some method for data presentation and storage (Fig. 22-5). In addition, a trigger signal must be derived either from the same electrocardiogram source or from another lead. This trigger signal is used to initiate the averaging process at a given point within each QRS complex. To be able to record portions of the signal before the trigger point, some transient recording device may be interposed. Abnormal QRS complexes should be excluded from the averaging process as described above.

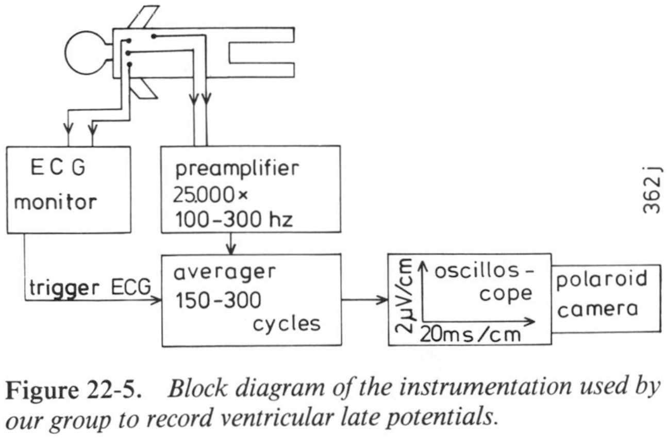

Figure 22-5. *Block diagram of the instrumentation used by our group to record ventricular late potentials.*

Some major technical differences between the various systems presently in use in several laboratories are due to lead positioning for recording, filter characteristics, and type of data presentation, storage, and evaluation. A short description of some techniques follows.

In our own recording and signal averaging system,[14] four bipolar electrodes are connected to a high-gain, low-noise, battery-powered preamplifier (Princeton Applied Research, model 113) using shielded leads. Bandpass filter settings (single-pole analog filters, 6 db/octave) are from 100 to 300 Hz. The high-pass cut-off of 100 Hz is necessary to eliminate respiratory baseline drifts and to flatten the ST segment, which otherwise would have a steep upstroke at the gain used. The low-pass cut-off of 300 Hz was chosen to eliminate any noise originating from muscular activity. The preamplified signal is connected to a dual-channel signal averager (Princeton Applied Research, Signal Averager model 4202). Both channels are combined to a single 2048 word memory. The averager is externally triggered from the QRS complex of two additional bipolar leads that are selected to yield a high-amplitude monophasic QRS signal. The threshold is adjusted for consistent triggering at the time of averaging. The jitter for triggering is ± 1.5 ms. The trigger signal initiates a sweep that, at the selected positions, lasts 204.8 ms (consisting of 2048 consecutive dwell time intervals each lasting 100 μs). In this mode of operation, the signal is digitized at a sampling rate of 10 kHz. The signal averager allows continuous monitoring of the progress of the averaging process on a storage oscilloscope. In most cases, the number of cardiac cycles averaged varies between 150 to 200. Care is taken not to include premature ventricular beats. For this purpose, a special circuit is included that automatically measures the RR intervals on a beat-to-beat basis. Premature complexes are thus eliminated from being triggered. The averaged signals are photographed with a Polaroid camera.

The system developed by Simson[18] uses the three-bipolar orthogonal leads X, Y, and Z. The high-resolution electrocardiogram is amplified 1000- to 5000-fold and prefiltered at a band width of 0.05 to 300 Hz. The signal from each lead is then passed through four-pole, 250-Hz, low-pass filters, and then AD converted to 12-bit accuracy at 1000 samples/sec. The digital information is stored on floppy disks by a Hewlett-Packard 9826 desktop computer. Each lead is sequentially recorded for 133 seconds. Only those complexes identified as normal by a template recognition program are averaged for each lead separately. To reject the low frequencies in the electrocardiogram, a bidirectional digital filter of 25 Hz (four-pole, high-pass Butterworth design) is used. The filter processes forward until 40 ms into the QRS complex. The filter is then reset and processes the signal backward up to the same position in the QRS complex. With this approach, filter ringing after the QRS complex is avoided.[18] The filtered signals for the three leads are then combined into a vector magnitude ($\sqrt{(x^2+y^2+z^2)}$) referred to as "filtered" QRS complex. The onset and the end of the total signal are automatically defined at the points where the mean amplitude of a 5-ms sample exceeds 3.5 times the voltage of the random noise. The onset and end of the total filtered QRS complex and the mean voltage of the total signal are calculated. Furthermore, the mean voltage of the last 40 and the last 50 ms of the signal are measured.[18]

Uther and co-workers[19] have used vectorcardiographic surface recordings to detect fractionated low-amplitude activity. Others[15,16] have been using a commercially available electrocardiographic recorder with the additional capabilities of signal averaging (Marquette MAC signal averager).

Since the temporal signal-averaging technique can only detect repetitive electrocardiographic signals, dynamic changes that occur on a beat-to-beat basis cannot be detected. For the latter condition, El-Sherif and associates[33] designed the technique of spatial averaging. In this technique, electronic summation of potentials recorded from multiple pairs of electrodes is performed using a specially designed volume conductor electrode. It is assumed that the electrocardiographic signal between any pair of electrodes is almost identical, whereas the noise from electromyographic sources, electrode-tissue interface, and amplifier are not completely correlated. With spatial averaging, one expects to reinforce the identical signal and to reduce the noise. Although the electrode-tissue interface and amplifier noise can be considered as completely random, electromyographic potentials are not completely incoherent.[34] The greater the distance between the electrodes, the smaller the coherence function of the electromyographic signal. However, this also reduces the coherence function of the electrocardiographic signal.

The volume conductor electrode[33] improves the ratio of electrocardiographic to electromyographic signal because the bioelectric source of the electromyographic potentials is immediately underneath the skin and the cardiac source is more distant. Both the electromyographic and electrocardiographic potentials undergo an approximate inverse square attenuation. However, because the electromyographic source is closer, it undergoes greater attenuation.

Examples of Late Potentials as Recorded with Various Techniques

The progression of the averaging process with improvement in signal quality using our approach[14] is shown in Fig. 22-3. A typical averaged recording in a normal subject exhibiting the terminal portion of the QRS complex and a part of the ST segment immediately following the QRS complex is shown in Fig. 22-6. Two repeated averaging processes were assembled on the same picture by dual exposure to demonstrate the reproducibility. There was a "smooth" transition from the high-gain QRS complex to the ST segment, which does not show any low-amplitude high-frequency signal. The small fluctuations of the baseline are due to remaining noise, the level of which is less than 1 μV. There was no filter ringing.

A typical late potential in a patient after myocardial infarction is demonstrated in Figure 22-7.

The results of signal processing using the system described by Simson[18] in a normal subject are presented in Figure 22-8. The QRS duration (DUR) is normal (86 ms); there is no low-amplitude tail at the end of the high-gain filtered QRS complex (high-pass cut-off 25 Hz); the voltage in the terminal 40 ms of the QRS complex is high (V[40] = 128.52 μV), indicating the absence of low-amplitude activity. The end of the high-amplitude, filtered QRS complex in the top tracing corresponds to the end in the standard surface leads X, Y, Z (bottom). In contrast, a low-amplitude tail appears at the end of the high-voltage part of the QRS complex in a

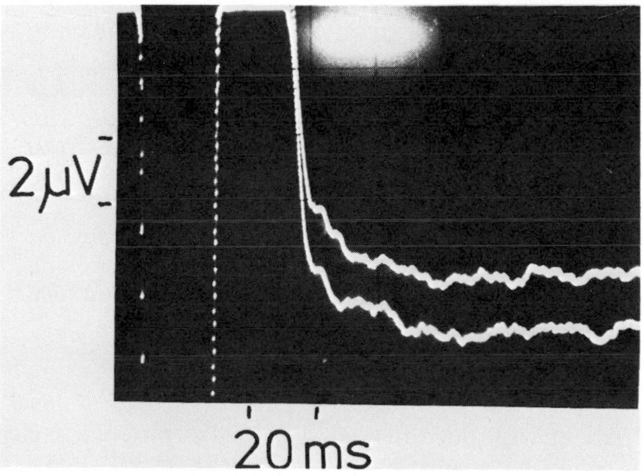

Figure 22-6. *Averaged recording of 200 cardiac cycles showing the terminal portion of the QRS complex and a part of the ST segment in a normal subject. There were no late potentials during the terminal portion of the QRS complex and ST segment. The rapid downstroke of the QRS complex showed a smooth transition to the ST segment. In order to demonstrate reproducibility, the signal was recorded twice.*

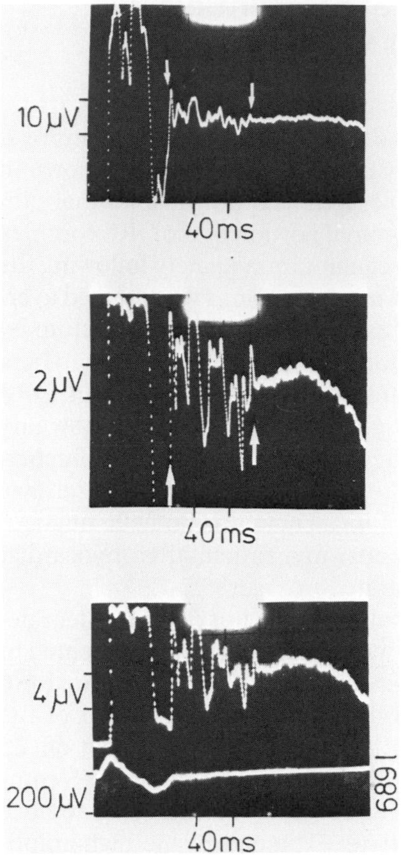

Figure 22-7. *Visual identification of a late potential at different degrees of amplification in a patient after myocardial infarction.* (Upper panel) *At low amplification (10 μV/division), a low-amplitude signal* (between arrows) *is apparent after the steep downstroke of the high-amplitude part of the QRS complex.* (Middle panel) *After rough visual identification of a late potential, a higher magnification is used (2 μV/division) to define more carefully the onset and end of the late potential. The median amplitude of the late potential is estimated from that part of the signal that has been identified at lower amplification* (upper panel). *Onset and end of the late potential are marked by* arrows. (Lower panel) *Dual-channel recording from the same patient showing the late potential* (upper tracing) *at 4 μV/division and the unfiltered terminal part of the surface electrocardiogram to demonstrate that the late potential appears within the ST segment.*

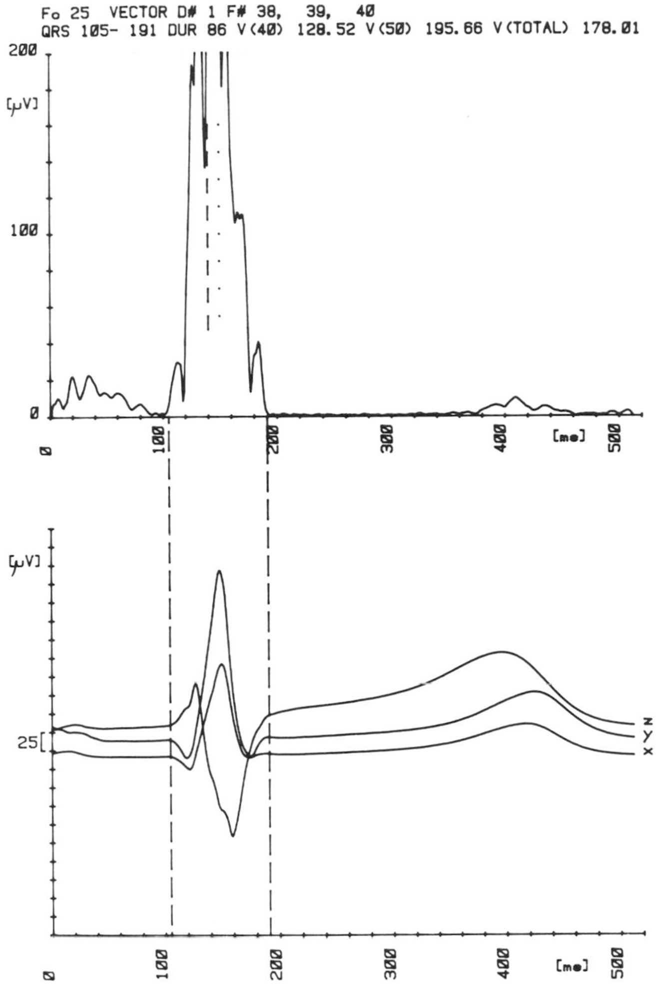

Figure 22-8. *Original recording using the system developed by M. Simson[18] in a patient with normal left ventricular function and no history of ventricular tachycardia.* (Top) *Signal-averaged and filtered beats (high-pass cutoff 25 Hz) from the body surface (lead X, Y, Z) showing the vector magnitude. There is no low-amplitude signal at the end of the filtered QRS complex.* (Bottom) *Signal-averaged leads from the body surface at lower magnification. See text for further details.*

patient with documented sustained ventricular tachycardia after myocardial infarction (Fig. 22-9). The DUR of the total filtered QRS complex was 134 ms; the voltage in the terminal 40 ms of the filtered QRS complex was low (V[40] = 3.57 μV). In Figure 22-10, the low-amplitude signal extends far into the ST segment. Using automated signal analysis, the program recently designed[40] (Fig. 22-11) identified a signal of 55 ms duration in Figure 22-9 and of 138 ms in Figure 22-10.

Definition of Ventricular Late Potentials in Surface Electrocardiogram Averaged Recordings

A schematic representation of the various approaches is presented in Figure 22-11.

In general, ventricular late potentials may be defined as low-amplitude fractionated activity appearing at the

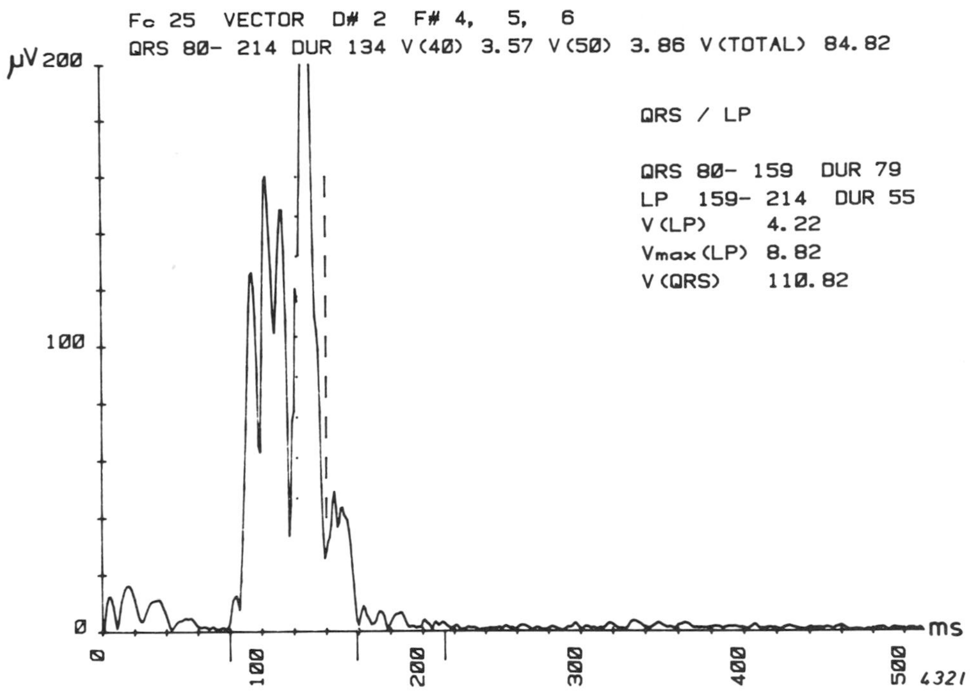

Figure 22-9. *Signal-averaged and filtered recording of leads X, Y, Z (vector magnitude) in a patient with ventricular tachycardia. QRS duration was 134 ms. The program automatically identified the end of the total QRS complex at 214 ms on the horizontal axis. The amplitude in the terminal 40 ms was low ($V[40] = 3.57\ \mu V$), which was automatically measured by the program described in the text.[18] Additionally, the onset of low-amplitude activity was automatically identified at 159 ms on the horizontal axis by the automated recognition program.[40] The latter program additionally measured the mean voltage of the late potential (V LP), the maximal voltage of the late potential (V_{max}), and the mean voltage of the true QRS complex (V QRS).*

end of the QRS complex and extending into the ST segment. At present, no universally accepted criteria for delineation of late potentials exist. One of the major issues is whether only those potentials appearing after the end of the QRS complex should be considered as such or whether any low-amplitude activity, even when appearing before the end of the surface electrocardiogram, should be termed *ventricular late potential.* We[14,35] and others[18] do not take the end of the QRS complex in the surface electrocardiogram into account (see Fig. 22-11), whereas others consider low-amplitude activity to represent a late potential only if it extends for a certain period beyond the end of the QRS complex (see Fig. 22-11). The former approach is based on findings during intraoperative endocardial mapping that demonstrate that fractionated low-amplitude activity, mostly in the border zone of an aneurysm, starts within the QRS complex. This has recently been confirmed by Simson and co-workers.[36] Therefore, in some cases the terminal part of the QRS complex in the standard surface electrocardiogram is constituted by low-amplitude activity. That is why after successful exclusion of an arrhythmogenic area after intraoperative mapping and application of semicircular subendocardial ventriculotomy[24,37,38] or subendocardial resection,[25] these potentials can no longer be recorded at the end of the QRS complex, which, at the same time, becomes shorter.[25]

Our approach includes visual identification of late potentials in the high-gain averaged recordings (see Figs. 22-7 and 22-11). No attempt is made to time the given late potential relative to the QRS complex in the standard surface electrocardiogram. If a low-amplitude signal is identified visually at the end of the high-gain QRS complex, the first step in measurement of the duration of the late potential is to define its end. The level of baseline noise (late in the ST segment) is used as a reference signal. The transition between a late potential and the level of baseline noise is at the point where the low-amplitude signal exceeds about three times the level of baseline noise. Then the onset of the late potential is identified visually by recognizing an isoelectric section between the QRS complex and the late potential. In the more frequent situations where the late potential continuously merges with the QRS signal, the onset of the late potential is visually defined as the point at which the signal amplitude markedly exceeds the mid- and termi-

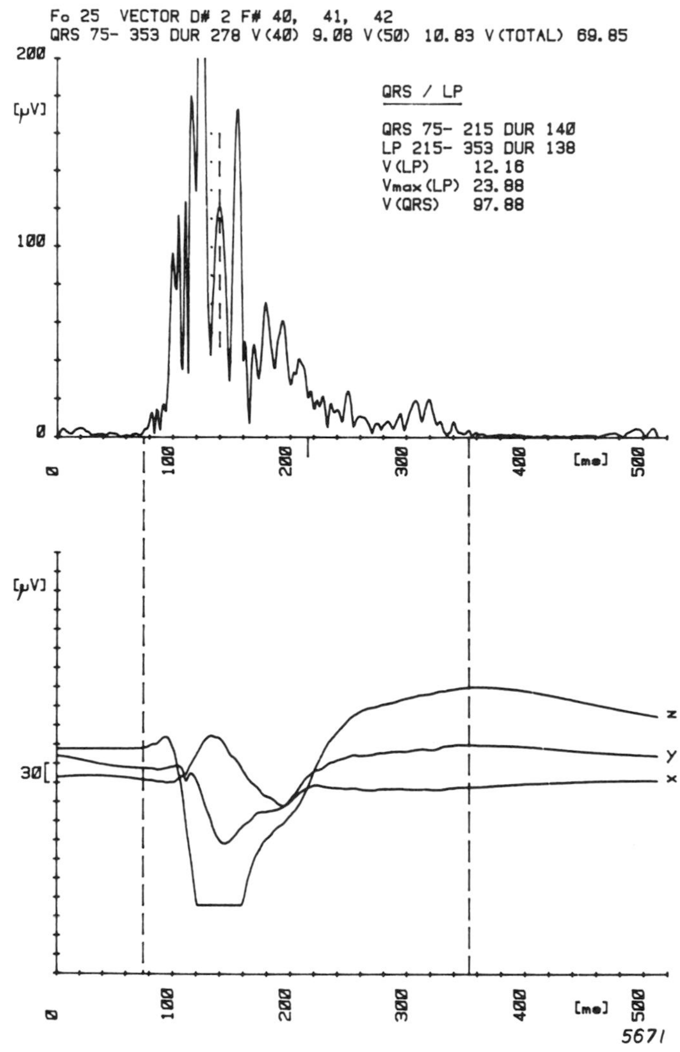

Figure 22-10. *An example that, like Figure 22-9, shows the filtered-surface electrocardiogram. In this patient, who also has sustained ventricular tachycardia and left ventricular aneurysm, a very large low-amplitude tail was identified extending into the ST segment. Some fluctuation was also seen in the surface electrocardiogram recordings.*

nal portion of the late potential. The duration of a given late potential is measured between the onset and the end of the signal as defined in this way. The minimum duration of a late potential required is 10 ms.

In contrast, Oeff and colleagues,[39] who basically use the same hardware system,[14] determine the maximum QRS width from six low-resolution reference leads (Fig. 22-12). Fragmented electrical activity that exceeds the maximum QRS duration by at least 10 ms is defined as a delayed depolarization.

Simson[18] considers delayed depolarization (late potential) to be present when the vector magnitude during the last 40 ms of the filtered and averaged QRS complex is less than 25 μV (see Figs. 22-9 and 22-10). This obviously is a more objective approach, since the measurement of amplitude in the terminal portion of the high-gain QRS complex is done by computer software.

Recently, Denes and colleagues[40] suggested identifying the point where the downstroke of the QRS complex falls short of 40 μV (see Fig. 22-11). The distance between this point and the end of the high-gain filtered and averaged QRS complex as estimated by the software developed by Simson[18] is considered to represent the late potential.

In addition to the original computer program designed by Simson,[18] we recently developed an algorithm for automated recognition of the late potential[41] (see Fig. 22-11). Since the onset and the end of the total filtered QRS complex are automatically defined by the original program, the new algorithm aims to recognize the transition point between the "true" QRS complex and the following late potential, if it exists. The terms *total* QRS, *true* QRS, and *late potential* are defined in Figure 22-13. The new program retrogradely invades the "total" QRS complex and measures the timing and the voltage of each deflection (maximum and minimum) of the signal. Specific conditions that were developed in a trial-and-

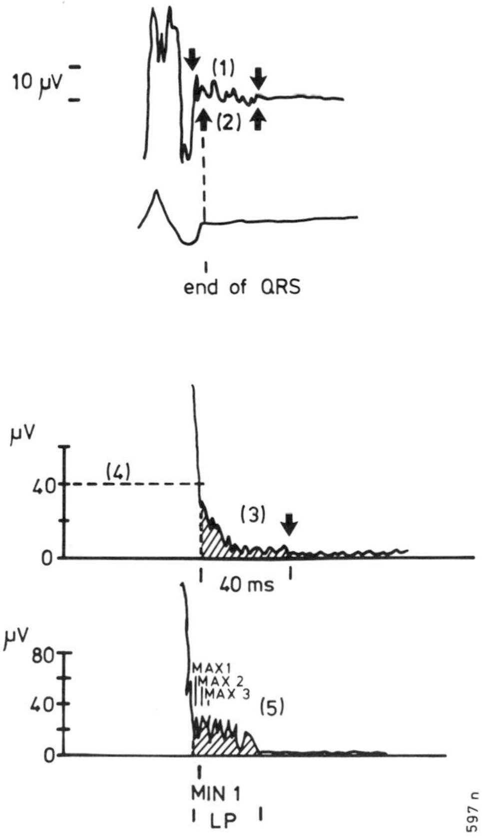

Figure 22-11. *Schematic diagram showing the various definitions of late potentials (see text).*

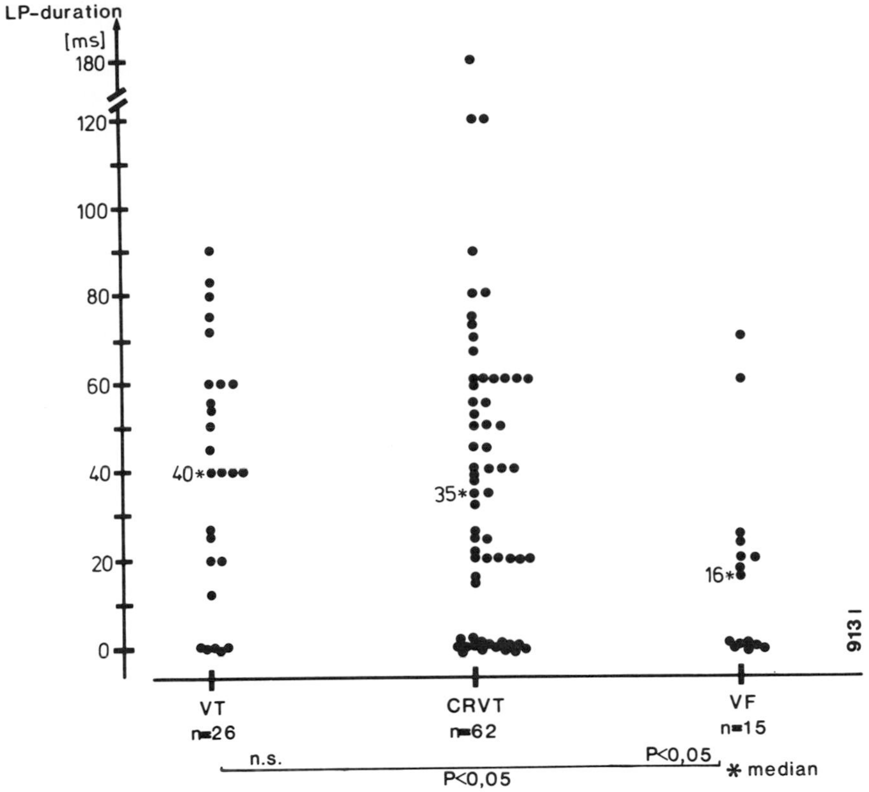

Figure 22-12. *Duration of late potentials in 26 patients with one episode of ventricular tachycardia (VT), in 62 patients with chronic recurrent ventricular tachycardia (CRVT), and in 15 patients with ventricular fibrillation outside acute myocardial infarction (VF). See text for further details.*

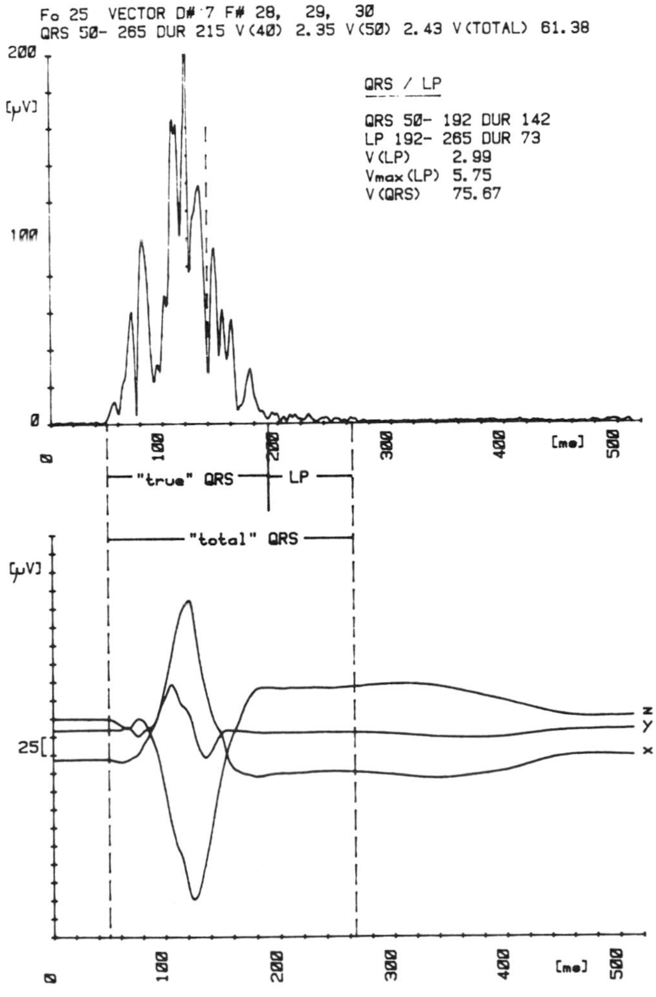

Figure 22-13. *Definition of "true" QRS, "total" QRS, and "late potential" as used for automated identification of late potentials with the software program designed by Karbenn and colleagues.[41]*

error phase must be met to consider a maximum as part of a low-amplitude, fractionated signal. These definitions that were derived during an algorithm definition phase proved reliable, objective, and well reproducible during a subsequent trial phase in a second cohort of 50 patients. As far as the presence or absence of late potentials was concerned, there was complete agreement between the results of visual analysis by three independent observers and the new computer program in 40 of 50 patients (80%), whereas there was incomplete agreement in another six patients (total 92%). In 26 of 50 patients (52%), the onset of a given late potential was indicated within ± 2 msec by both the observers and the computer program.

In comparison to visual analysis, the automated evaluation of the high-amplitude signal averaged recordings has some advantages: it is independent of the bias of observers, does not depend on personal experience, and is well reproducible. Nevertheless, the results of automated analysis should not be accepted blindly and some visual "control" may still be necessary.

Comparison of Various Methods

To evaluate the methodologic problems of noninvasive registration of ventricular late potentials, a comparative multicenter study was performed.[42] Two recording systems based on a Princeton 4202 signal averager (methods A and B), [14,39] the Marquette MAC I signal averager (method C),[15,16] and the software averaging system developed by Simson[18] (method D) were compared in the same group of 109 patients (80 with coronary artery disease, 29 with dilative cardiomyopathy). In each patient, all registrations were done within 2 hours. The main difference between methods A and B is that in method A the end of the QRS complex in the standard surface leads was taken into account.

Ventricular late potentials were recorded in 12% of patients with method A, in 21% with B, in 14% with C, and in 20% with D. Corresponding positive results were obtained in 6% and corresponding negative results in 69%. Differences in comparison with the other three methods were seen 12 times for method D, five times for method B, and two times for method A. In 10% of the patients, two methods showed the same results. Despite these differences between the various methods, detailed analysis of the tracings of patients with controversial results revealed that the differences, mainly with methods A, B, and C, were due to differences in visual interpretation. Methods that did not take into account the QRS width (methods B and D) showed a greater number of positive results than methods that did not (methods A and C). Further prospective studies must show whether delayed depolarizations occurring in the terminal portion of the QRS complex or only those that occur after the end of the QRS complex are of prognostic significance.

Incidence of Late Potentials in Patients With and Without Documented Ventricular Tachycardia

In subjects without clinically identifiable heart disease and in patients in whom coronary angiography revealed normal coronary arteries and normal left ventricular function, no late potentials were detected (Table 22-2).[35] Similarly, in patients without documented ventricular tachycardia and without a history of complex ventricular arrhythmias, no low-amplitude signal in the last 40 ms of the filtered QRS complex was seen.[18] Thus, electrical activity suggestive of slow ventricular activation cannot be or is only very rarely detected in subjects with normal left ventricular function.[15,16,39,43,44]

In contrast, patients with previously documented ventricular tachycardia or fibrillation show a high incidence of ventricular late potentials.[14,16,18,35] Of 63 patients with documented ventricular tachycardia/fibrillation, 45 (71%) had ventricular late potentials of any duration. The proportion of patients with late potentials increased to 37 of 47 patients (79%) if only patients with coronary artery disease were considered (see Table 22-2).[35] Patients with ventricular tachycardia had a low-amplitude signal in the last 40 ms of the filtered QRS complex that was not seen in the filter output from patients without ventricular tachycardia.[18] The voltage in the last 40 ms of the filtered QRS complex was found to

Table 22-2. Correlation Between Detection of Late Potentials and Angiographic Findings

	Patients Without VT/VF	Patients With VT/VF
Normal subjects	0/12	
Normal coronary arteries, normal LV	0/15	1/3
CAD, normal LV	3/17	
COCM	3/9	4/7
Diffuse hypokinesia, CAD	3/15	5/8
Regional hypokinesia, CAD	8/36	3/3
Akinesia, CAD	14/26	4/6
Aneurysm, CAD	18/43	25/30
Various findings		3/6
Mean potential duration (ms)	31 ± 15.3	51 ± 31.5

VT, ventricular tachycardia; VF, ventricular fibrillation; LV, left ventricle, CAD, coronary artery disease; COCM, congestive cardiomyopathy discriminate well between patients with and without ventricular tachycardia. Patients with ventricular tachycardia had 15 ± 14.4 μV of high-frequency signal in this segment; in contrast, patients without ventricular tachycardia had 74 ± 77.7 μV ($P < 0.0001$). The threshold used to discriminate patients with and without ventricular tachycardia in their history was 25 μV.[18] Only three of 39 patients with ventricular tachycardia (8%) exceeded 25 μV. Also, the filtered QRS voltage tended to be lower in patients with ventricular tachycardia than in those without (103 ± 30 versus 127 ± 43 μV; not significant). The QRS duration was longer in patients with ventricular tachycardia (139 ± 26 versus 95 ± 10 ms; $P < 0.0001$). Recently, Fourier analysis has shown that patients with ventricular tachycardia have a higher frequency content in their terminal QRS complex as compared to healthy subjects.[45]

There were slight differences in the incidence of late potentials in patients with documented ventricular tachyarrhythmias depending on the type of arrhythmia. In patients with chronic recurrent ventricular tachycardia, 46 of 62 patients (74%) had late potentials, a figure almost similar to patients with only one documented episode of ventricular tachycardia (21 of 26 patients; 80%). In contrast, only eight of 15 patients (53%) with a history of ventricular fibrillation without acute myocardial infarction and no previous documentation of sustained ventricular tachycardia had late potentials.[46]

The duration of late potentials may vary between 15 and 180 ms.[14,35,46] The median duration of late potentials in those patients with one (40 ms) or more (35 ms) episodes of ventricular tachycardia was longer than in those with previous ventricular fibrillation (16 ms; see Fig. 22-12). There was an inverse relation between the duration of late potentials and the rate of sustained ventricular tachycardia that, however, was not significant because of a large scatter of data. The mechanisms responsible for these findings have not yet been established. A short duration of a late potential may be due to a small area with slow fractionated conduction or to more rapid conduction in a larger area. However, because the wavefront of excitation probably travels along multiple pathways and into various directions, conduction velocity or wavelength cannot be calculated. In a recent experimental study, similar findings were reported.[22] In dogs studied 8 to 22 days after experimental anterior myocardial infarction, the duration of epicardial electrograms over the zone of infarction was significantly longer and the amplitude was significantly lower compared to control dogs during *in vivo* and *in vitro* measurements. In addition, the amplitude and duration of electrograms in dogs with inducible ventricular fibrillation were more normal than those recorded in animals with inducible ventricular tachycardia.[22]

Considering the short duration of late potentials in those patients with previous ventricular fibrillation compared to those with a history of sustained ventricular tachycardia (see Fig. 22-12), late potentials may be less suitable to identify patients at risk of sudden cardiac death than of sustained ventricular tachycardia. That this may indeed be true has been shown by our recent observations (see below on prognostic significance of late potentials).

There was no significant correlation between the induction mode of the ventricular tachyarrhythmia and the duration of late potentials, but at least some trend was apparent. The median value for the duration of late potentials in patients in whom ventricular tachycardia could be induced by single or double premature stimuli during sinus rhythm was slightly longer (60 ms) than in patients in whom it could only be induced by single or double premature stimuli at basic driven rates of 120 or more (45 and 40 ms, respectively).[46]

Ventricular late potentials cannot only be detected in patients with previously documented ventricular tachycardia but can also be detected in asymptomatic patients. This was shown in a group of 146 patients who were prospectively studied and had been referred for coronary arteriography to establish or exclude the diagnosis of coronary artery disease.[35] No patient had a history of ventricular tachycardia or fibrillation outside the acute phase of myocardial infarction. Forty-nine of these 146 patients (33.6%) had late potentials (see Table 22-2). The mean duration of late potentials was 31 ± 15.3 ms, which was significantly different ($P < 0.001$) from the mean duration of late potentials in patients with documented ventricular tachycardia or fibrillation (51 ± 31.5 ms). The mean amplitude of late potentials in these asymptomatic patients was 9 ± 10.8 μV, which did not differ from patients with documented ventricular tachycardia or fibrillation (17 ± 22.4 μV).

These data have now been extended to a total of 665 patients, also including a great number of patients after recent myocardial infarction (Table 22-3).* Of the total group of 665 patients, 405 patients (60.9%) had no late potentials in the high-gain signal-averaged recordings. In contrast, 260 patients (39.1%) had late potentials of varying duration. The mean duration of late potentials in those patients in whom they were present was 29.7 ± 12.8 ms. The prevalence of late potentials was slightly higher in patients studied within 6 months after myocardial infarction (46%) compared to those who were studied after 6 months (36%) or those without a history of myocardial infarction (25%).

In a subgroup of patients with recent myocardial infarction,[47] the prevalence of late potentials was much greater in patients with inferior wall infarction (63%) than in patients with anterior wall infarction (34%). One

* Breithardt, G., and Borggrefe, M.: Unpublished data.

Table 22-3. Prevalence of Late Potentials in 655 Patients Studied Prospectively

Absent	405		(60.9%)	
Present	260		(39.1%)	
10–19 ms		58		(8.7%)
20–39 ms		138		(20.8%)
≥40 ms		64		(9.6%)
Mean duration 29.7 ± 12.8 ms				

possible explanation for this difference might be that various left ventricular sites are activated at different times. Since the inferoposterobasal areas of the left ventricles are activated late, a late potential of a given duration from this site may clearly extend beyond the QRS complex. However, an electrogram of long duration that may even be longer than one from the inferior wall may not extend beyond the QRS and may still be hidden within it if it originates from the anterior wall and thus begins early in the QRS complex (Fig. 22-14). This explanation has been supported by data presented by Simson and colleagues.[48]

Late potentials were longer in patients with ventricular tachycardia than in those without.[35] These results are in agreement with invasive studies by Klein and colleagues[8] and by Spielman and coauthors,[10] who studied patients during open-heart surgery by epicardial and endocardial mapping or during endocardial catheter mapping. These groups found a greater incidence and extent of delayed and fragmented ventricular activity in patients with documented ventricular tachyarrhythmias compared to those without. Similar data were recently reported by Wiener and colleagues.[49] Fragmented electrograms were recorded from 33% to 58.3% of the border zone of aneurysms in patients with ventricular tachyarrhythmias but only from 0% to 16.7% of the border zone in patients without. Endocardial activity in the border zone that extended beyond the QRS complex was noted in 5 of 6 patients with ventricular tachycardia and in 1 of 5 patients without. This suggests that a critically prolonged conduction delay may favor the occurrence of reentry. Accordingly, with programmed ventricular stimulation, the incidence of inducible ventricular arrhythmias increased with increasing duration of late potentials.[50] Nevertheless, conduction delay in the present study or the previous one[35] was not long enough in any patient to reach beyond ventricular refractoriness, which would make reexcitation of normal tissue possible. Thus, it must be assumed that some "stress" is necessary to prolong regional conduction delay to a critical value.

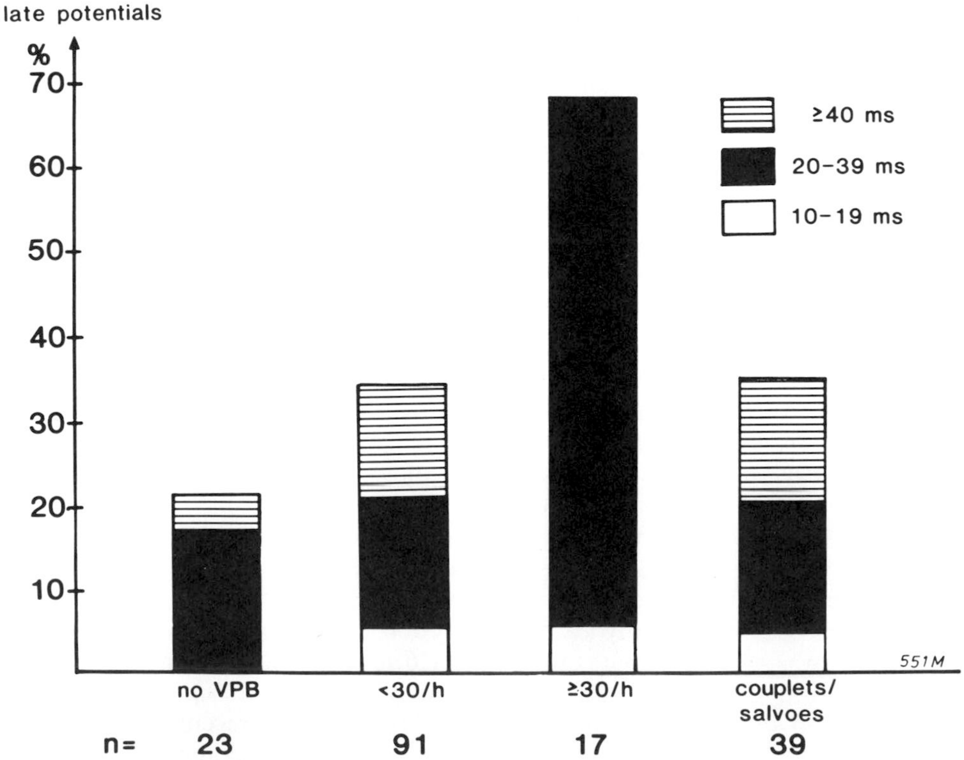

Figure 22-14. *Twenty-hour long-term electrocardiographic findings correlated to the results of signal averaging in 170 patients without documented ventricular tachycardia or fibrillation who were studied prospectively. The prevalence of late potentials and their duration are shown.*

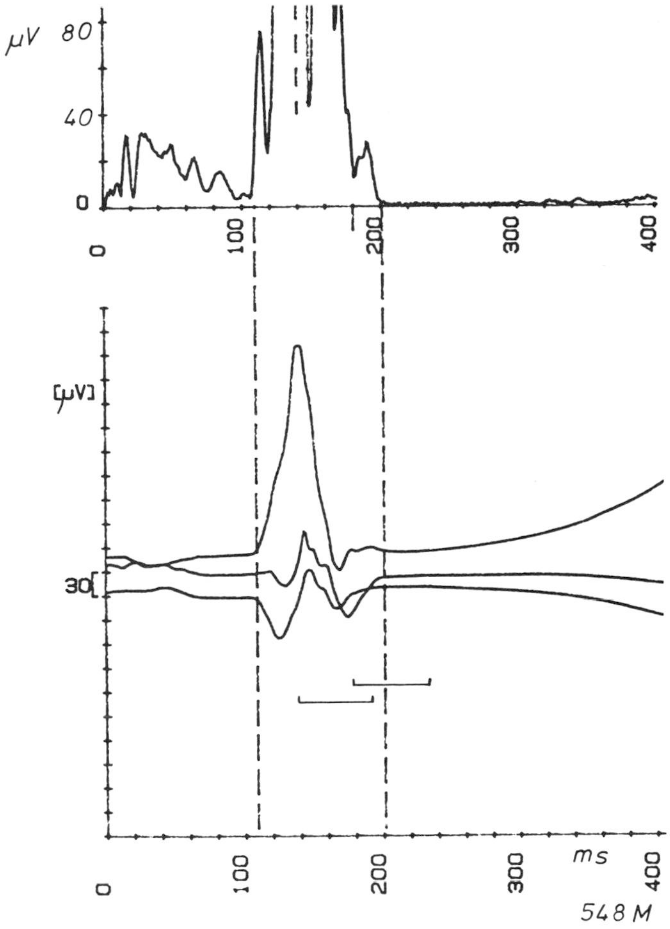

Figure 22-15. *Signal-averaged recording with schematic representation of fragmented, low-amplitude activity* (horizontal bars) *that starts at different times during ventricular excitation. A signal from an area that is activated early may be hidden within the QRS complex.*

This type of response to premature beats of regional fragmented activity has been observed in experimental myocardial infarction.[3]

Thus, the presence of late potentials proved neither highly sensitive nor specific for patients with clinically evident ventricular tachyarrhythmias. In addition, there was a large overlap in the duration of late potentials among patients with ventricular tachycardia or fibrillation and patients without a history of these arrhythmias. The longer duration of late potentials in patients with ventricular tachycardia may indicate that in these patients, regional activation is more fragmented and possibly slower than in those without previously documented ventricular tachycardia. The question arises why late potentials cannot be detected in all patients with documented ventricular tachycardia or fibrillation. Several reasons exist. First, unstable triggering may prevent the recording of late potentials, which are cancelled by the always changing timing. This seems to be of minor importance, since the jitter for triggering was relatively small in our system. Second, these signals may have amplitudes too low to be differentiated from noise. Third, fragmented activation of a certain area of the myocardium may occur so early that it is still covered within the QRS complex[35] (see Fig. 22-15). Therefore, it need not always outlast normal ventricular activation. Fourth, the signals may be too small and may occur immediately at the end of QRS, when filter ringing occurs. Last, in some patients with inducible ventricular tachycardia, the functional category for tachycardia may not be reentry but triggered automaticity.[51,52] This, however, remains speculative, since triggered automaticity as a mechanism for ventricular tachycardia has not yet been proved in humans.

Correlation Between the Presence of Late Potentials and Left Ventricular Function

In patients with documented ventricular tachycardia, the highest incidence of late potentials has been found in those with left ventricular aneurysms due to coronary artery disease. Similarly, there was a close correlation between the detection of late potentials and left ventricular function in patients without previously documented ventricular tachycardia or fibrillation (see Table 22-2).[35] On the other hand, the degree and extent of coronary artery involvement did not influence the prevalence of late potentials in patients with ventricular tachycardia or fibrillation, unless indirectly by causing left ventricular contraction abnormalities.

These correlations between presence of late potentials and left ventricular function could recently be confirmed in a larger group of 404 prospectively studied patients without documented complex ventricular arrhythmias (see Fig. 22-16).* In this group, late potentials of long duration (≥ 40 ms) were almost exclusively found in patients with hypokinesia, akinesia, or aneurysms. Moreover, about 20% of late potentials appeared in patients with left ventricles that seemed angiographically "normal" (Fig. 22-17). However, despite normal findings during left ventricular angiography, many of these patients could not be considered to have true normal left ventricular function. Most of them complained of at least atypical angina pectoris, and a great variety of abnormal findings existed, such as ST segment depression during exercise despite normal coronary arteries, an abnormal increase in pulmonary artery pressure during exercise, and perfusion defects during thallium scintigraphy.

* Breithardt, G., and Borggrefe, M.: Unpublished data.

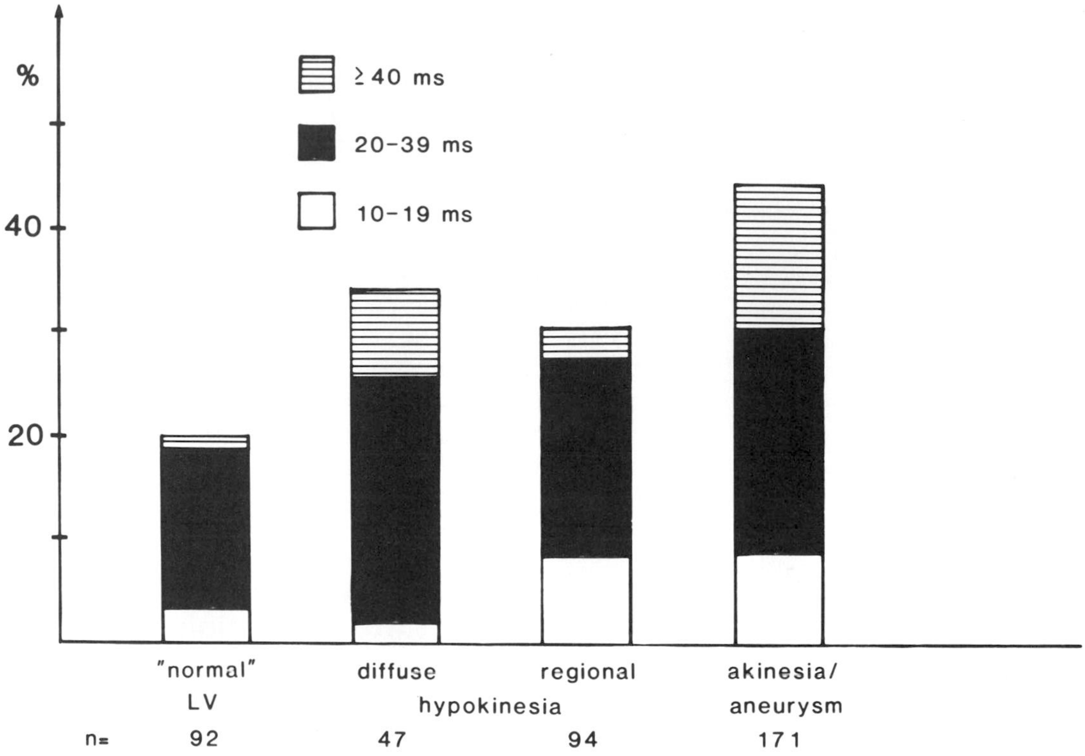

Figure 22-16. *Correlation between the presence and duration of late potentials and various types of left ventricular contraction abnormalities as estimated by left ventricular angiography.*

The fact that late potentials are found more frequently in patients with regional or diffuse ventricular contraction abnormalities (see Table 22-1 and Fig. 22-17) suggests that the anatomic substrate for late potentials is diseased tissue. Obviously, a transmural infarction may show no abnormal activation pattern because such tissue is "electrically" silent. On the other hand, tissue immediately adjacent to the infarction contains viable myocardium interspersed with fibrotic tissue.[53] Such tissue may result in fragmentation of the propagating electromotive surface with the consequent development of high-frequency components.[53–55] The border zone of old myocardial infarcts could be identified as the site of origin for delayed ventricular potentials by comparing precordial recordings using the averaging technique and intraoperative mapping techniques.[36,*] Since late potentials are abolished by subendocardial partial or complete encircling ventriculotomy[24,37,38,57] in

* Breithardt, G., and Borggrefe, M.: Unpublished data.

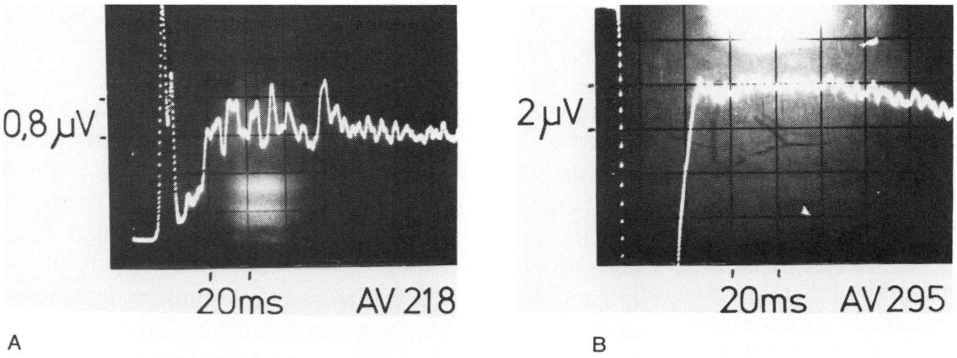

Figure 22-17. *Preoperative (A) and postoperative (B) recordings using signal averaging in a patient with sustained ventricular tachycardia whose propensity to ventricular tachycardia was successfully abolished by map-guided antitachycardiac surgery. After surgery (B), low-amplitude activity can no longer be detected.*

patients with documented ventricular tachycardia, it is very probable that they are related to the propensity to ventricular tachycardia and that they probably originate in the border zone between myocardial scars and normal myocardium.

Correlation Between Spontaneous Ventricular Arrhythmias and Late Potentials

In 170 patients, the results of 24-hour long-term electrocardiogram recordings and of signal averaging were compared (see Fig. 22-14). Although there was a significant increase in the prevalence of late potentials with increasing numbers of ventricular extrasystoles, it was also apparent that late potentials of long duration (≥ 40 ms) were not significantly correlated to spontaneous arrhythmias. They occurred in patients with either no extrasystoles or with < 30 per hour as well as in those with couplets or salvos. Thus, spontaneous ventricular extrasystolels were independent of the presence or absence of fractionated activity.

Correlation Between Late Potentials and Ventricular Vulnerability

To get more insight into the mechanisms and potential prognostic value of late potentials, 110 male patients without previously documented ventricular tachycardia or fibrillation and without a history of resuscitation or syncope were studied.[50] In addition to recording late potentials, an electrophysiologic study was performed. Programmed right ventricular stimulation included the introduction of single and double ventricular extra stimuli during sinus rhythm and paced ventricular rhythms at rates of 120, 140, 160, and 180 beats/min. A repetitive ventricular response was considered to be present if one or more nonstimulated premature depolarizations occurred after single or double premature stimulation. Since the patients studied did not have documented ventricular tachycardia, programmed ventricular stimulation was stopped as soon as four or more consecutive ventricular echo beats were induced. On the basis of the results of a previous study,[58] this response was considered abnormal. Ventricular tachycardia was defined as ten or more consecutive echo beats.

There was a significant correlation between the absence or presence of ventricular late potentials and programmed ventricular stimulation. In 70 patients in whom no late potentials could be detected from the body surface, four or more ventricular echo beats were induced less frequently than in those patients with late potentials. The incidence of abnormal responses increased in relation to the duration of late potentials ($\chi^2 = 20.97$; $P < 0.01$). Of note, 11 of 12 patients (92%) with late potentials ≥ 40 ms had four or more consecutive ventricular echo beats. Late potentials were closely associated to left ventricular function ($\chi^2 = 12.96$; $P < 0.0115$). In contrast, the association between late potentials and the results of programmed ventricular stimulation was less apparent (see Table 22-3; $\chi^2 = 5.49$; $P < 0.0643$), whereas inducible ventricular responses were significantly associated with left ventricular function ($\chi^2 = 16.24$; $P < 0.0003$).

These data show that late potentials can be considered an indicator of increased ventricular vulnerability. Patients with late potentials had more vulnerable myocardium than those without late potentials. Statistical analyses revealed left ventricular function as the predominant factor, with late potentials and repetitive ventricular responses being highly significantly correlated with it.[50] Late potentials and repetitive ventricular responses were less closely associated. However, late potentials of 40 ms duration or more predicted the inducibility of four or more consecutive ventricular echo beats with high sensitivity. Nevertheless, even in the absence of late potentials, ventricular tachycardia could be induced in 9% of patients.[50] This seeming discrepancy may be explained in different ways. First, induced ventricular tachycardia may not be related to regional slow conduction but to some other mechanism, such as triggered automaticity.[51,52] Although this cannot be excluded, another explanation seems more likely. Depending on the arrival of excitation, a given area of slow conduction may still be activated so early that it is completely hidden within the QRS complex[36] (see Fig. 22-15). Slow conduction may only extend far enough into diastole if some stress, such as premature stimulation, is exerted. In other patients, abnormal ventricular responses were not inducible despite the presence of late potentials. This may be due to the fact that only one site of stimulation was used. Using more than one site or more than two premature stimuli might have increased the number of abnormal findings. However, an extensive stimulation protocol had been applied.

Effects of Antiarrhythmic Surgery on Late Potentials

Although previous data have suggested a causal relationship between late potentials and the propensity to ventricular tachycardia, this might be coincidental. Some recent observations in patients with documented ventricular tachycardia, in whom antitachycardic surgery using a map-guided approach was successful, provide

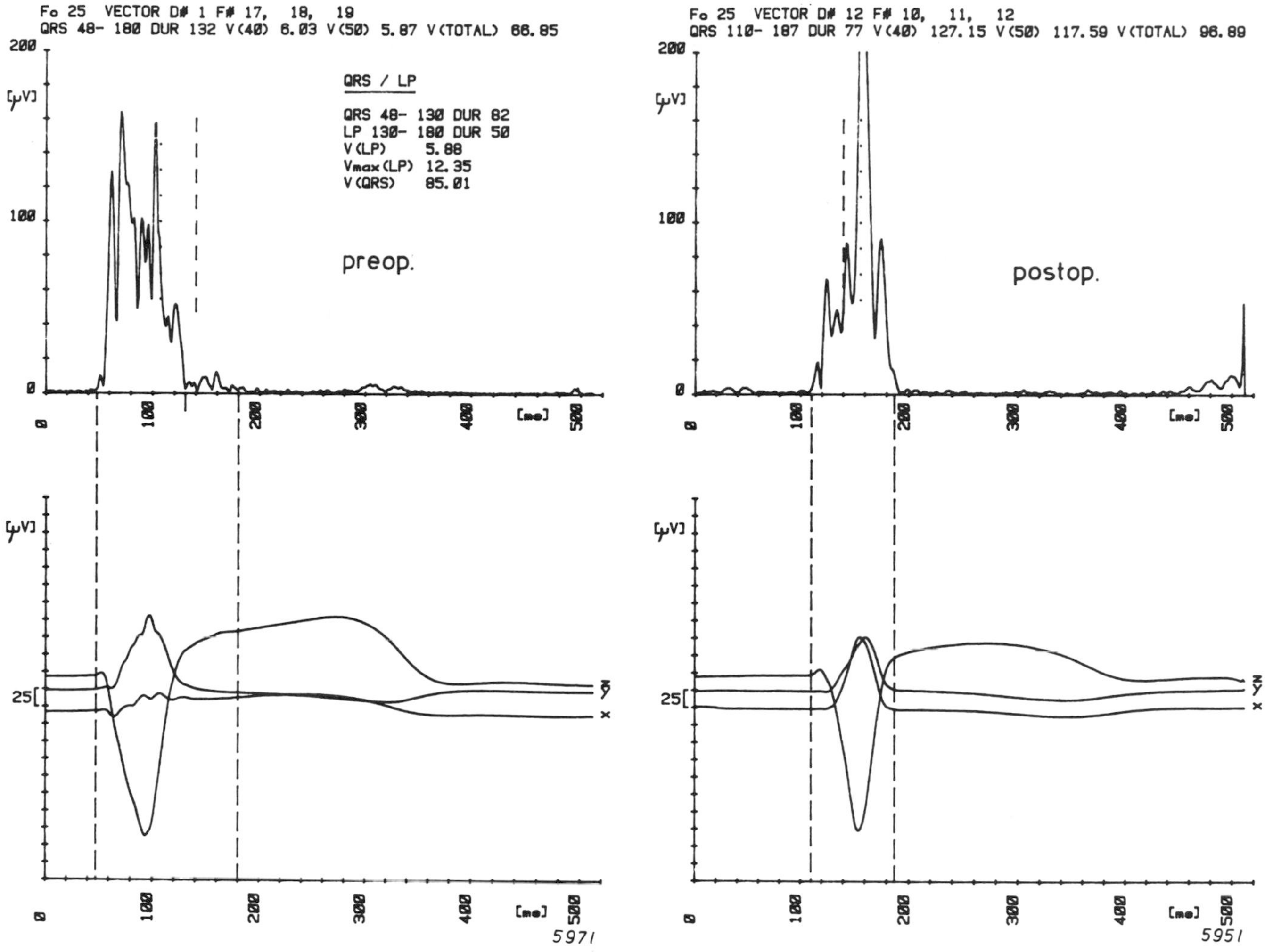

A B

Figure 22-18. *Preoperative (A) and postoperative (B) signal-averaged recording in a patient with recurrent sustained ventricular tachycardia. Before surgery (A), the amplitude in the terminal 40 ms of the filtered (total) QRS complex was low ($V\,40 = 6.03\ \mu V$); a late potential of 50 ms duration was automatically identified. After map-guided surgery (B), the amplitude in the terminal 40 ms of the QRS complex was normal ($V\,40 = 127.15\ \mu V$); there was no longer any low-amplitude tail at the end of QRS. Postoperatively, the patient was free of inducible and spontaneous ventricular tachycardia.*

new arguments in favor of the pathogenic significance of late potentials.

In almost all patients in whom late potentials were abolished or markedly reduced in duration by map-guided antitachycardic surgery, ventricular tachycardia could no longer be induced after the surgical procedure[24,25,37,38] (see Figs. 22-17 and 22-18). In contrast, if late potentials could still be detected postoperatively, ventricular tachycardia could frequently be reinduced. In contrast, long-term electrocardiographic recording did not provide clinically useful information before or after surgery.

The question arises how late potentials are abolished by surgical procedures. In the encircling endocardial ventriculotomy approach, the reentrant circuit is theoretically isolated from the pumping ventricular chamber. Thus, the reentrant arrhythmia may well persist postoperatively; however, it is prevented from engaging the normal portion of the ventricle and thus prevents hemodynamic compromise. According to this concept, one might therefore expect the late potentials in these patients to persist postoperatively. However, this was not the case in the majority of patients. One explanation might be that because of the combined surgical procedure (subendocardial encircling ventriculotomy and aneurysmectomy) used in our study, the arrhythmogenic zone is not only isolated but also devitalized.[59,60] Another explanation might be that in this zone, electrical activity still persists but is no longer synchronized to the normal heartbeat by entrance (and exit) block and thus will go undetected during averaging. Conversely, the endocardial excision approach of controlling ventricular tachyarrhythmias theoretically either damages or completely excises the reentrant circuit, and thus in patients successfully treated, late potentials should not exist postoperatively.[25]

To evaluate the success of antitachycardic surgery in patients with documented ventricular tachycardia and previous myocardial infarction, signal averaging may represent a new noninvasive approach. The method is applicable only in those patients in whom late potentials could be recorded preoperatively. Thus, the averaging technique may serve as an adjunct or even a substitute for programmed ventricular stimulation to control antitachycardic surgery. Surgical abolition of late potentials suggests that the procedure has been successful in removing abnormal tissue. However, despite persistence of late potentials, surgery might still be clinically successful by changing the milieu for initiation or perpetuation of tachycardias or by reducing at least the amount of tissue available for reentrant excitation.

Effects of Antiarrhythmic Drugs on Late Potentials

A typical action of class I antiarrhythmic drugs (quinidine-like drugs) is to slow conduction in normal and abnormal tissues. Therefore, one might expect that this group of antiarrhythmic drugs also exerts some effect on the duration of ventricular late potentials. This would provide a means for controlling antiarrhythmic effects noninvasively in patients with documented ventricular tachycardia and detectable late potentials on the body surface.

Surprisingly, no overall effects could be demonstrated with some typical representatives of class I antiarrythmic drugs. There was no significant change in the duration of late potentials before and during antiarrhythmic drug therapy, and there was no correlation between changes in inducibility of ventricular tachycardia by programmed ventricular stimulation and the response of ventricular late potentials (Table 22-4). Only in a few patients were marked changes after administration of class I antiarrhythmic drugs observed (Fig. 22-19).

Table 22-4. Response of Ventricular Late Potentials During Antiarrhythmic Therapy and Correlation to Changes in Inducibility Using Programmed Ventricular Stimulation

Change in Inducibility	Duration of Late Potentials (ms) Control	Duration of Late Potentials (ms) *During Therapy*
No Change	34 ± 30	34 ± 27
More Difficult	37 ± 55	35 ± 43
Suppressed	46 ± 50	40 ± 40

Similarly, Simson and colleagues[61] reported that ventricular tachycardia could be controlled without a change in the configuration and duration of low-amplitude activity at the end of the filtered QRS complex. Similar data have been reported by Rozanski and colleagues.[16] Also, Jauernig and associates[62] did not observe any consistent effect of antiarrhythmic drugs on late potentials during sinus rhythm. However, when changes of sinus rate induced by antiarrhythmic drugs were eliminated and heart rate was kept constant by atrial pacing at 100 or 120 beats/min, antiarrhythmic drugs consistently produced a small but significant prolongation of late potential duration. These effects were, however, unsuitable to allow an assessment of antiarrhythmic drug efficacy in preventing ventricular tachyarrhythmias.[62]

Presently, no apparent and convincing explanation exists for this lack of effect of antiarrhythmic drugs. However, with regard to the very recent data by Gardner and colleagues,[21] antiarrhythmic drugs might not affect that type of slow propagation that is produced by diminished intercellular connections, at least not at the rates studied. It might well be that by induction of early premature stimuli, more significant changes become apparent.

Prognostic Significance of Late Potentials

Although there is no doubt of the close association between ventricular late potentials and a history of sustained ventricular tachycardia, the prospective significance of the detection of late potentials in a patient who has been asymptomatic up to that time is of greater clinical significance.

Thus, a prospective study of 160 patients after recent acute myocardial infarction was initiated. Long-term follow-up study (mean ± S.D.; 7.5 ± 3.2 months) showed that the recording of late ventricular potentials from the body surface was able to predict the subsequent occurrence of symptomatic sustained ventricular tachycardia after discharge from the hospital.[47] Late potentials were a frequent finding; half the patients exhibited late potentials of varying duration at the end of or after the QRS complex. All four patients who later developed sustained ventricular tachycardia, three of whom had to be resuscitated, exhibited late potentials during their

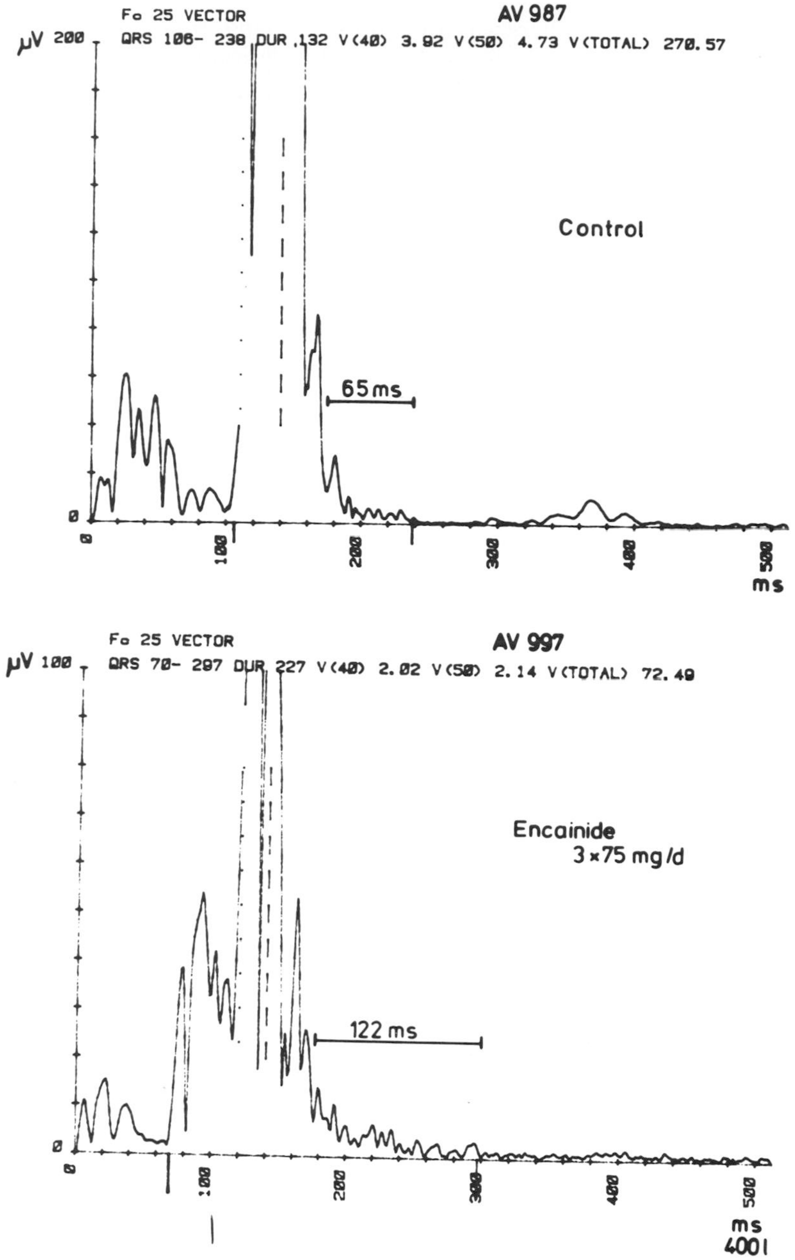

Figure 22-19. *Signal-averaged and filtered recordings of leads X, Y, Z (vector magnitude) using the recording system of M. Simson[18] in a patient with documented ventricular tachycardia. During control recording, there was low-amplitude activity of 65 ms duration, which, after long-term medication with encainide (75 mg 3 times a day) prolonged to 122 ms.*

predischarge study. Moreover, no patient without late potentials had an episode of documented symptomatic ventricular tachycardia. On the other hand, patients dying suddenly did not have a markedly greater prevalence of late potentials compared to those with an uneventful course.

These data have now been extended to a total of 511 patients in whom follow-up study (mean 18 ± 12.9 months) was greater than 6 months.* Both patients after recent acute myocardial infarction and those referred for coronary arteriography were included in this prospective study. After discharge from the hospital, 14 patients developed sustained symptomatic ventricular tachycardia. Sixteen patients died suddenly within 1 hour, and another three patients died within 24 hours. There were another 20 cardiac deaths (heart failure or reinfarction), two nonlethal reinfarctions, four noncardiac deaths, and 106 patients who were operated on, receiving coronary bypass grafts or undergoing aneurysmectomy or both.

Total mortality was low in patients without late potentials (7.2%) or with late potentials $<$ 40 ms in duration (10 to 19 ms duration 6.5%; 20 to 39 ms duration 8.4%); but in patients with late potentials $\geq$40 ms duration, total mortality was about two to three times greater (17.3%) ($\chi^2 = 5.9$; $P < 0.02$).

In patients with late potentials, the prevalence of sud-

* Breithardt, G., and Borggrefe, M.: Unpublished data.

den death (<1 hour) was about twofold higher than in those without late potentials (Fig. 22-20). Taking into account also patients dying within 24 hours, the percentage of patients dying suddenly was more than four times greater in those with late potentials ≥40 ms in duration compared to those without late potentials. The rate of sudden death (<24 hours) after 1 year was 0.95% in patients without and 3.1% in patients with late potentials. Using actuarial analysis, the differences in the rates of sudden death (<24 hours) after 1 year reached significance ($P < 0.01$, Breslow; $P < 0.02$, Mantel-Cox). However, if only patients dying within 1 hour were considered, these differences were no longer significant.

Eleven of 14 patients who later developed sustained symptomatic ventricular tachycardia had late potentials (sensitivity 78.6%). In contrast, 315 of 497 patients without ventricular tachycardia during follow-up study had no late potentials (specificity 63.3%). Of 193 patients with late potentials, 182 did not develop sustained symptomatic ventricular tachycardia (false-positive results 94.3%) during the short-term follow-up study. In eleven of 14 (78.6%) symptomatic sustained ventricular tachycardias occurred in patients who entered the study within the first 6 weeks after acute myocardial infarction. In the overall group, the predictive value of late potentials was 5.7%. It was markedly lower (2.1%) in those patients who were studied more than 6 weeks after myocardial infarction or who did not have a history of previous myocardial infarction; in contrast, the predictive value of a positive test was significantly greater (9.2%) in those who were studied within the first 6 weeks after their qualifying myocardial infarction. Furthermore, the chance of developing symptomatic sustained ventricular tachycardia depended on the duration of late potentials. It was markedly greater in those patients with late potentials ≥40 ms in duration (predictive value 15.4%) compared to those without late potentials or late potentials <40 ms in duration (see Fig. 22-20).

In a subgroup of patients with either isolated anterior or inferior wall infarction (as determined by ventricular angiography), the subsequent occurrence of sustained ventricular tachycardia depended on the site of infarction. Seven of 81 patients (8.6%) with anterior wall infarction, but only one of 52 patients (1.9%) with inferior wall infarction, developed sustained symptomatic ventricular tachycardia (Table 22-5). The prevalence of subsequent symptomatic sustained ventricular tachycardia was highest in patients included within the first 6 weeks after anterior myocardial infarction (60%; see Table 22-5).

The results of presently available prospectively designed studies on the significance of late potentials are presented in Table 22-6. A total of 1139 patients have been studied by three groups.[47,63,64] Of these patients, 332 were included within the first 6 weeks after their qualifying myocardial infarction; 518 patients entered

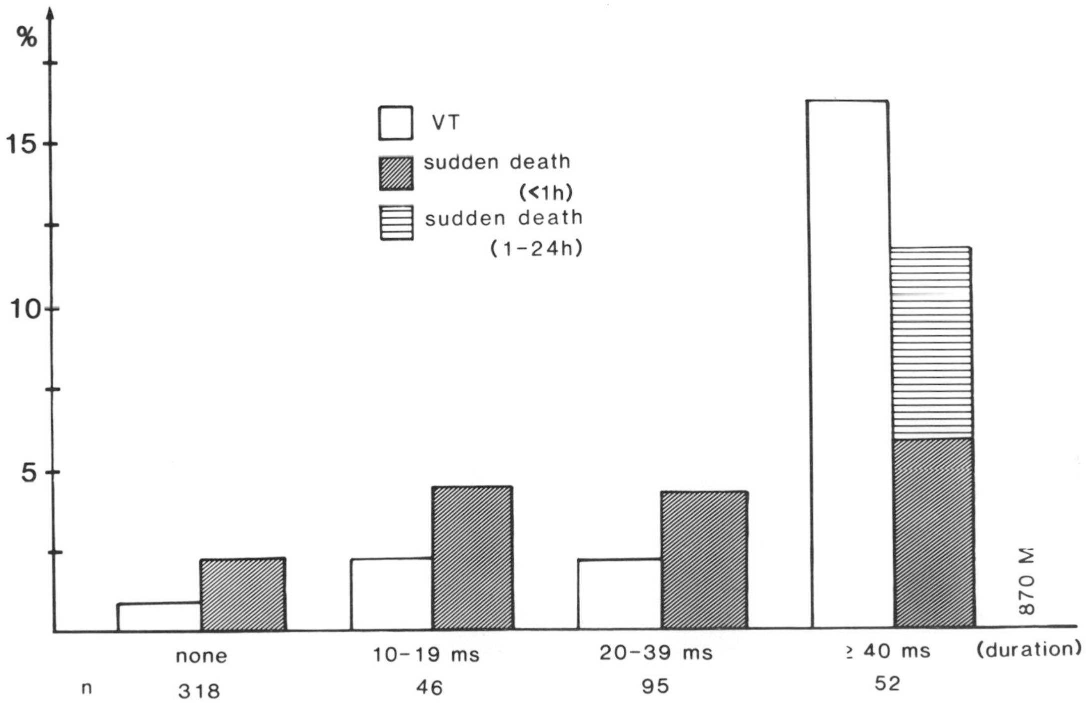

Figure 22-20. *Prognostic significance of late potentials in 511 patients studied prospectively. See text for further details.*

Table 22-5. Occurrence of Sustained Ventricular Tachycardia in Relation to Site of and Interval After Infarction

Interval After Myocardial Infarction (mo)	Site of Akinesia or Dyskinesia: *Anterior Wall* n	LP ⊕	VT	*Inferior Wall* n	LP ⊕	VT
≤1.5	31	10(32.3%)	6(60%)	21	10(47.6%)	0
>1.5	50	21(42%)	1(4.8%)	31	18(58.1%)	1(5.6%)

LP, late potentials; VT, ventricular tachycardia.

the study between 6 to 8 weeks as participants in a rehabilitation program; in 289 patients, myocardial infarction antedated the study by morc than 6 weeks or a history of myocardial infarction did not exist. The results of follow-up study were not unequivocal, since the reported endpoints for study were different (see Table 22-6). The data of Denniss and colleagues[63] as well as our data showed a significant increase in the prevalence of sustained ventricular tachycardia in patients with late potentials. With regard to total or cardiac mortality and sudden death, von Leitner and colleagues[64] and we reported an increase in mortality as a function of the presence (and duration) of late potentials. Thus, these presently available data suggest a potential role of late potentials for predicting prognosis in postmyocardial infarction patients.

One of the reasons for the different results of various studies may be that the endpoints for follow-up study were defined differently. In the present study, sudden cardiac death mostly occurring within seconds or minutes or during sleep was separated from symptomatic sustained ventricular tachycardia. However, about two thirds of those patients who were classified as having had sustained symptomatic ventricular tachycardia were in hemodynamic collapse requiring immediate intervention. Thus, it cannot be excluded that without appropriate medical or electrical therapy, these patients would have died. It may be due to this classification of deaths that there was a high prevalence of sustained symptomatic tachycardia but a relatively low incidence of sudden cardiac death.

Clinical Approach to the Evaluation of Postmyocardial Infarction Patients

From the clinical point of view, noninvasive procedures are obviously desirable for screening purposes, whereas it would be acceptable to use more aggressive, invasive techniques in certain subsets of patients. A step-wise approach using noninvasive recording of late ventricular

Table 22-6. Available Prospective Studies on the Significance of Late Potentials

Authors	No.	Interval After MI	Follow-up Duration	Prognostic Value of Late Potentials			
Present report and Breithardt *et al.*[47]	511	≤6 weeks n = 222 >6 weeks or no MI n = 289	18 ± 12.9 mo (mean ± SD)		*Total Mortality (%)*	*Sudden Death (%)*	*Sustained VT (%)*
				no LP	7.2%	2.5%	0.9%
				10–19 ms	6.5%	4.3%	2.2%
				20–39 ms	8.4%	3.2%	2.1%
				≥40 ms	17.3%	5.8%	15.4%
Von Leitner *et al.*[64]	518	6–8 weeks (rehabilitation group)	10 mo (mean)	*LP*	*Cardiac Mortality (%)*	*Sudden Death (%)*	*Sustained (%)*
				Absent	1.5	0.9	No event
				Present	7.3	3.6	
Denniss *et al.*[63]	110	7–28 days (mean 11)	2–12 mo (mean 5)	*LP*			
				Absent	No information		1.1
				Present			17.4
Total	1139						

LP, late potentials; VT, ventricular tachycardia.

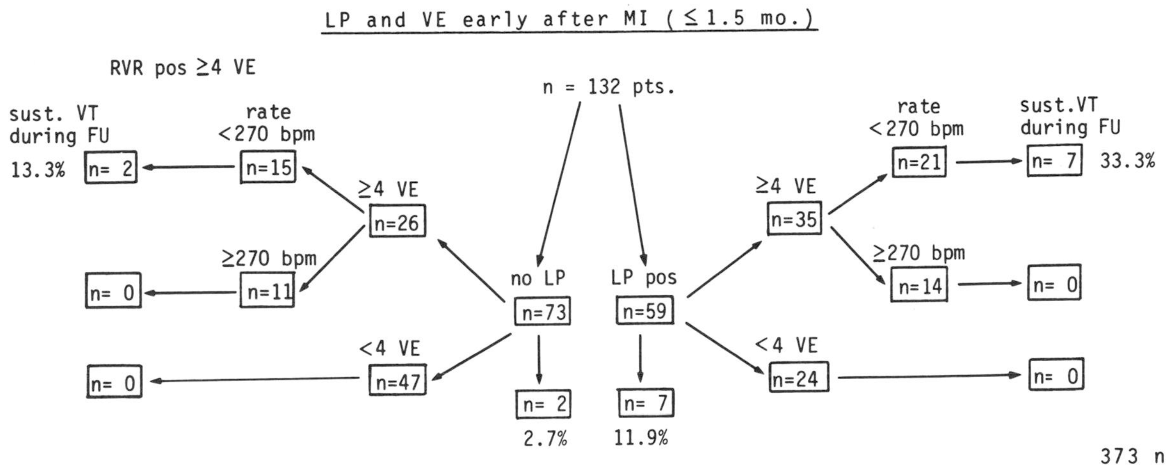

Figure 22-21. *Value of late potentials and programmed ventricular stimulation in 132 patients after recent myocardial infarction for prediction of spontaneous occurrence of sustained ventricular tachycardia. (VE, ventricular echo beat; LP, late potential; sust. VT during FU, sustained ventricular tachycardia during follow-up study)*

potentials as the initial step would allow preselection of patients for further evaluation by invasive electrophysiologic techniques. Whether this approach might be feasible was tested in 132 postmyocardial infarction patients studied prospectively.[65]

It could be demonstrated that the combined use of signal averaging and programmed ventricular stimulation helped to identify subgroups of patients at markedly different risk of developing spontaneous symptomatic sustained ventricular tachycardia (Fig. 22-21). Patients with late potentials irrespective of duration had a 4.4 times greater risk of developing symptomatic sustained ventricular tachycardia (7 of 59 patients; 11.9%) than those without (two of 73 patients; 2.7%). A further increase in the risk of ventricular tachycardia was observed in those patients with late potentials in whom an abnormal response to ventricular stimulation was observed. Ventricular tachycardia supervened in seven of 35 patients (20%) with an abnormal response to ventricular stimulation, compared to none of 24 patients with a normal response. A further important criterion was the rate of the induced ventricular arrhythmia. Only if the rate was less than 270 beats/min were there any spontaneous episodes of ventricular tachycardia. Thus, the induction of ventricular flutter or fibrillation (rate ≥270 beats/min) was of no clinical significance compared to the induction of a monomorphic and relatively slow tachyarrhythmia.

Thus, patients at highest risk of developing symptomatic sustained ventricular tachycardia after myocardial infarction were characterized by (1) the presence of late ventricular potentials, (2) an abnormal result of programmed ventricular stimulation, and (3) a rate of the induced ventricular arrhythmia less than 270 beats/min (see Fig. 22-21). With regard to establishing antiarrhythmic therapy, this might be a subgroup of postmyocardial infarction patients that would benefit most.

Provided these data are confirmed by future studies, what type of antiarrhythmic therapy to be initiated and how its effect should be controlled must be settled. Previous experience in patients with documented sustained ventricular tachycardia suggests that serial electrophysiologic testing might be an appropriate approach.[66–68] This is especially the case if patients present with a low level and grade of spontaneous ventricular ectopy in between the attacks. In those with frequent and complex ventricular ectopy, preliminary data suggest that use of antiarrhythmic drugs to suppress these spontaneous arrhythmias improves the prognoses.[69,70]

Conclusion

With respect to presently available information, signal averaging for the detection of late ventricular potentials seems to be a promising new technique for the identification of patients at risk of ventricular tachyarrhythmias. However, the relative value of this technique for the prediction of ventricular tachycardias in comparison to sudden cardiac death demands future studies. Which of the various characteristics of low-amplitude fractionated activity (duration, voltage, frequency content) is the most appropriate to predict prognosis in patients after myocardial infarction needs further evaluation. With regard to the significant number of false-positive results, which is not only the case with signal averaging but also with, for instance, long-term electrocardiographic recording, it seems unjustified to expect any one method to be able to identify a given patient at risk of sustained ventricular tachycardia or sudden death. In this context, long-term electocardiographic recording and signal averaging might prove useful as screening methods, whereas programmed ventricular stimulation might serve for further categorization by risk.

References

1. El-Sherif, N., Scherlag, B. J., Lazzara, R., and Hope, R. R.: Reentrant ventricular arrhythmias in the late myocardial infarction period. I. Conduction characteristics in the infarction zone. Circulation, 55:686–702, 1977.
2. El-Sherif, N., Scherlag, B. J., Lazzara, R., and Hope, R. R.: Reentrant ventricular arrhythmias in the late myocardial infarction period. II. Patterns of initiation and termination of reentry. Circulation, 55:702–719, 1977.
3. El-Shcrif, N., Lazzara, R., Hopc, R. R., and Scherlag, B. J.: Reentrant arrhythmias in the late myocardial infarction period. III. Manifest and concealed extra-systolic grouping. Circulation, 56:225–234, 1977.
4. Williams, D. O., Scherlag, B. J., Hope, R. R. et al.: The pathophysiology of malignant ventricular arrhythmias during acute myocardial ischemia. Circulation, 50:1163–1172, 1974.
5. Zipes, D. P.: Electrophysiological mechanisms involved in ventricular fibrillation. Circulation, 52(Suppl. III):120–130, 1975.
6. Fontaine, G., Guiraudon, G., and Frank, R.: Intramyocardial conduction defects in patients prone to ventricular tachycardia. III. The post-excitation syndrome in ventricular tachycardia. In Sandoe, E., Julian, D. G., and Bell, J. W. (eds.): Management of Ventricular Tachycardia—Role of Mexiletine, pp. 67–69. Amsterdam, Excerpta Medica, 1978.
7. Fontaine, G., Frank, R., GallaisHamonno, F., et al.: Electrocardiographie des potentiels tardifs du syndrome de post-excitation. Arch. Mal. Coeur, 71:854–864, 1978.
8. Klein, H., Karp, R. B., Kouchoukos, N. T., et al.: Intraoperative electrophysiologic mapping of the ventricles during sinus rhythm in patients with a previous myocardial infarction. Identification of the electrophysiologic substrate of ventricular arrhythmias. Circulation, 66:847, 1982.
9. Ostermeyer, J., Breithardt, G., Kolvenbach, R., et al.: Intraoperative electrophysiologic mapping during cardiac surgery. Thor. Cardiovasc. Surg., 27:260–270, 1979.
10. Spielman, S. R., Untereker, W. J., Horowitz, L. N., et al.: Fragmented electrical activity—relationship to ventricular tachycardia (abstr.). Am. J. Cardiol. 47:448, 1981.
11. Josephson, M. E., Horowitz, L. N., Farshidi, A., et al.: Sustained ventricular tachycardia:Evidence for protected localized re-entry. Am. J. Cardiol., 42:416, 1978.
12. Berbari, E. J., Scherlag, B. J., Hope, R. R., and Lazzara, R.: Recording from the body surface of arrhythmogenic ventricular activity during the ST segment. Am. J. Cardiol., 41:697–702, 1978.
13. Breithardt, G., Becker, R., and Seipel, L.: Non-invasive recording of late ventricular activation in man. Circulation, 62(suppl.):III–320, 1980.
14. Breithardt, G., Becker, R., Seipel, L., et al.: Non-invasive detection of late potentials in man—a new marker for ventricular tachycardia. Eur. Heart J., 2:1–11, 1981.
15. Hombach, V., Höpp, H.-W., Braun, V., et al.: Die Bedeutung von Nachpotentialen innerhalb des ST-Segments im Oberflächen-EKG bei Patienten mit koronarer Herzkrankheit. Dtsch. Med. Wochenschr., 105:1457–1462, 1980.
16. Rozanski, J. J., Mortara, D., Myerburg, R. J., and Castellanos, A.: Body surface detection of delayed depolarizations in patients with recurrent ventricular tachycardia and left ventricular aneurysm. Circulation, 63:1172–1178, 1981.
17. Simson, M., Horowitz, L., Josephson, M., et al.: A marker for ventricular tachycardia after myocardial infarction. Circulation, 62(Suppl.)III–262, 1980.
18. Simson, M. B.: Identification of patients with ventricular tachycardia after myocardial infarction from signals in the terminal QRS complex. Circulation, 64:235–242, 1981.
19. Uther, J. B., Dennett, C. J., and Tan, A.: The detection of delayed activation signals of low amplitude in the vectorcardiogram of patients with recurrent ventricular tachycardia by signal averaging. In Sandoe, E., Julian, D. G., and Bell, J. W. (eds.): Management of Ventricular Tachycardia—Role of Mexiletine, pp. 80–82. Amsterdam, Excerpta Medica, 1978.
20. Waldo, A. L., and Kaiser, S. G. A.: A study of ventricular arrhythmias associated with acute myocardial infarction in the canine heart. Circulation, 47:1222–1228, 1973.
21. Gardner, P. I., Ursell, P. C., Fenoglio, J. J., Jr., and Wit, A. L.: Anatomical and electrophysiological basis for electrograms showing fractionated activity. Circulation, 66(Suppl. II):78, 1982.
22. Richards, D. A., Blake, G. J., Spear, J. F., and Moore, E. N.: Electrophysiologic substrate for ventricular tachycardia: correlation of properties in vivo and in vitro. Circulation, 69:369–381, 1984.
23. Garan, H., and Ruskin, J. N.: Association of continuous electrical activity and localized reentry: Proposed criteria for causal relationship. Circulation, 66(Suppl. II):79, 1982.
24. Breithardt, G., Seipel, L., Ostermeyer, J., et al.: Effects of antiarrhythmic surgery on late ventricular potentials recorded by precordial signal averaging in patients with ventricular tachycardia. Am. Heart J., 104:996–1003, 1982.
25. Simson, M. B., Spielman, S. R., Horowitz, L. N., et al.: Effects of surgery for control of ventricular tachycardia on late potentials. Circulation, 64(Suppl.):IV–88, 1981.
26. Josephson, M. E., Horowitz, L. N., and Farshidi, A.: Continuous local electrical activity: A mechanism of recurrent ventricular tachycardia. Circulation, 57:659–665, 1978.
27. Waxman, H. L., and Sung, R. J.: Role of ventricular fragmentation in defining the mechanism of ventricular tachycardia in man. Am. J. Cardiol., 45:406, 1980.
28. Fontaine, G., Guiraudon, G., Frank, R., et al.: Stimulation studies and epicardial mapping in ventricular tachycardia: Study of mechanisms and selection for surgery. In Kulbertus, H. E. (ed).: Re-entrant Arrhythmias, Mechanisms and Treatment, pp. 333–350. Lancaster, MTP Press, 1977.
29. Höpp, H.-W., Hombach, V., Braun, V., et al.: Kammerarrhythmien und ventrikuläre Spätdepolarisationen bei akutem Myokardinfarkt (abstr.) Z. Kardiol. 70:319, 1981.
30. Simson, M., Spielman, S., Horowitz, L., et al.: Slow ventricular activation detected on the body surface in patients with ventricular tachycardia after myocardial infarction (abstr.) Am. J. Cardiol., 47:498, 1981.
31. Graene, J. G., Tobey, G. E., and Huelsman, L. P.: Operational amplifiers, p. 191. New York, McGraw-Hill, 1971.
32. Mehra, R., Restivo, M., and El-Sherif, N.: Electromyographic noise reduction for high resolution electrocardiography. In Frontiers of Engineering and Computing in Health Care—1983. Proceedings, Fifth Annual Conference, I.E.E.E. Engineering in Medicine and Biology Society, pp. 248–253.
33. El-Sherif, N., Mehra, R., Gomes, J. A. C., Kelen, G.: Appraisal of a low noise electrocardiogram. J. Am. Coll. Cardiol., 1:456–467, 1983.
34. Santipetro, R. F.: The origin and characterisation of the primary signal, noise and interface sources in the high frequency electrocardiogram. I.E.E.E. Trans. Biomed. Eng., 65:707–713, 1977.
35. Breithardt, G., Borggrefe, M., Kabenn, U., et al.: Prevalence of late

potentials in patients with and without ventricular tachycardia: Correlation with angiographic findings. Am. J. Cardiol., 49:1932–1937, 1982.

36. Simson, M. B., Untereker, W. J., Spielman, S. R., et al.: Relation between late potentials on the body surface and directly recorded fragmented electrocardiograms in patients with ventricular tachycardia. Am. J. Cardiol., 51:105, 1983.
37. Borggrefe, M., Breithardt, G., Ostermeyer, J., and Bircks, W.: Long-term efficacy of endocardial encircling ventriculotomy for ventricular tachycardia: Complete vs partial incision. Circulation, 68(suppl.):III–176, 1983.
38. Breithardt, G., Borggrefe, M., Karbenn, U., et al.: Verhalten ventrikulärer Spätpotentiale nach operativer Therapie ventrikulärer Tachykardien. Z. Kardiol., 71:381–386, 1982.
39. Oeff, M., von Leitner, E.-R., Brüggemann, T., et al.: Methodische Probleme bei der Registrierung ventrikulärer Spätpotentiale (abstr.) Z. Kardiol., 71:204, 1982.
40. Denes, P., Santarelli, P., Hauser, R. G., and Uretz, E. F.: Quantitative analysis of the high frequency components of the terminal portion of the body surface QRS in normal subjects and in patients with ventricular tachycardia. Circulation, 67:1129–1138, 1983.
41. Karbenn, U., Breithardt, G., Borggrefe, M., and Simson, M. B.: Automatic identification of late potentials. J. Electrocardiology, 18:123–134, 1985.
42. Oeff, M., von Leitner, E. R., Sthapit, R., et al.: Methods for non-invasive detection of ventricular late potentials—a comparative multicenter study. Eur. Heart J., 7:25–33, 1986.
43. Flowers, N. C., Shvartsman, V., Horan, L. G., et al.: Analysis of PR subintervals in normal subjects and early studies in patients with abnormalities of the conduction system using surface His bundle recordings. J. Am. Coll. Cardiol., 2:939, 1983.
44. Klempt, H. W., and Wulschner, W.: Die Analyse des QRS-Komplexes sowie des ST-Abschnittes mit der Signalmittelungstechnik bei Herzgesunden. Z. Kardiol., 72:369, 1983.
45. Cain, M. E., Ambos, H. D., Witowski, F. X., and Sobel, B. E.: Fast-Fourier transform analysis of signal-averaged electrocardiograms for identification of patients prone to sustained ventricular tachycardia. Circulation, 69:711–720, 1984.
46. Borggrefe, M., and Karbenn, U., Breithardt, G.: Spätpotentiale und elektrophysiologische Befunde bei ventrikulären Tachykardien. Z. Kardiol., 71:627, 1982.
47. Breithardt, G., Schwarzmaier, J., Borggrefe, M., et. al.: Prognostic significance of ventricular late potentials after acute myocardial infarction. Eur. Heart J., 4:487–495, 1983.
48. Simson, M. B., Euler, D. E., Michelson, E. L., et al.: Confirmation of a new technique for detecting slow ventricular activation on the body surface (abstr.). Am. J. Cardiol., 47:488, 1981.
49. Wiener, I., Mindich, B., Pitchon, R., et al.: Epicardial activation in patients with coronary artery disease: Effects of regional contraction abnormalities. Circulation, 65:154–160, 1982.
50. Breithardt, G., Borggrefe, M., Quantius, B., et al.: Ventricular Vulnerability assessed by programmed ventricular stimulation in patients with and without late potentials. Circulation, 68:275–281, 1983.
51. Rosen, M., Fisch, C., Hoffman, B., Knoebel, S.: Delayed afterdepolarisations as a mechanism for accelerated junctional escape rhythm. Circulation, 60(suppl.):II–253, 1979.
52. Moak, J. P., and Rosen, M. R.: Induction and termination of triggered activity by pacing in isolated canine Purkinje fibers. Circulation, 69:149–162, 1984.
53. Daniel, T., Boineau, J., and Sabiston, D.: Comparison of human ventricular activation with canine model in chronic myocardial infarction. Circulation, 44:74–89, 1971.
54. Langner, P. H., Jr., Greselowitz, D. B., and Briller, S. A.: Wide band recording of the electrocardiogram and coronary heart disease. Am. Heart J., 86:308–317, 1973.
55. Flowers, N. C., Horan, L. G., Thomas, J. R., and Tolleson, W. J.: The anatomic basis for high frequency components in the electrocardiogram. Circulation, 39:531–539, 1969.
56. Reynolds, E. W., Muller, B. F., Anderson, G. J., and Muller, B. T.: High frequency components in the electrocardiogram. A comparative study of normals and patients with myocardial disease. Circulation, 35:195–206, 1967.
57. Guiraudon, G., Fontaine, G., Frank, R., et al.: Encircling endocardial ventriculotomy. A new surgical treatment for life-threatening ventricular tachycardias resistant to medical treatment following myocardial infarction. Ann. Thorac. Surg., 26:438–444, 1978.
58. Breithardt, G., Seipel, L., Meyer, T., and Abendroth, R.-R.: Prognostic significance of repetitive ventricular response during programmed ventricular stimulation. Am. J. Cardiol., 49:693–698, 1982.
59. Ungerleider, R. M., Holman, W. L., Stanley, T. E., et al.: Encircling endocardial ventriculotomy for refractory ischemic ventricular tachycardia. II. Effects on regional myocardial blood flow. J. Thorac. Cardiovasc. Surg., 83:850–856, 1982.
60. Ungerleider, R. M., Holman, W. L., Stanley, T. E., III, et al.: Encircling endocardial ventriculotomy for refractory ischemic ventricular tachycardia. III. Effects on regional left ventricular function. J. Thorac. Cardiovasc. Surg., 83:857–864, 1982.
61. Simson, M. B., Spielman, S. R., Horowitz, L. N., et al.: Effects of antiarrhythmic drugs on body surface late potentials in patients with ventricular tachycardia (abstr.). Am. J. Cardiol., 49:1030, 1982.
62. Jauernig, R. A., Senges, J., Langfelder, W., et al.: Effect of antiarrhythmic drugs on ventricular late potentials at sinus rhythm and at constant heart rate. In Steinbach, K., Glogar, D., Laszkovics, A., et al. (eds.): Cardiac Pacing, pp. 767–772. Steinkopff Verlag Darmstadt, 1983.
63. Denniss, A. R., Cody, D. V., Fenton, S. M., et al.: Significance of delayed activation potentials in survivors of myocardial infarction (abstr.). J. Am. Coll. Cardiol., 1:582, 1983.
64. von Leitner, E. R., Oeff, M., Loock, D., et al.: Value of non-invasively detected delayed ventricular depolarizations to predict prognosis in post myocardial infarction patients. Circulation, 68(suppl.):III–83, 1983.
65. Breithardt, G., Borggrefe, M., Haerten, K., and Trampisch, H. J.: Prognostische Bedeutung der Program-mierten Ventrikelstimulation und der nichtinvasioen Registierung ventrikulärer Spätspotentiale in der Postinfarkt periode. Z. Kardiol., 74:389–396, 1985.
66. Breithardt, G., Seipel, L., Abendroth, R. R., and Loogen, F.: Serial electrophysiological testing of antiarrhythmic drug efficacy in patients with recurrent ventricular tachycardia. Eur. Heart J., 1:11–24, 1980.
67. Breithardt, G., Borggrefe, M., and Seipel, L.: Present status of serial electrophysiologic testing for predicting antiarrhythmic drug-efficacy in patients with ventricular tachycardia. In Breithardt, G., and Loogen, F., (eds.): New Aspects in the Medical Treatment of Tachyarrhythmias. Role of Amiodarone, pp. 112–126. Baltimore, Urban and Schwarzenberg, 1983.
68. Horowitz, L. N., Josephson, M. E., and Kastor, J. A.: Intracardiac electrophysiologic studies as a method for the optimization of drug therapy in chronic ventricular arrhythmia. Prog. Cardiovasc. Dis., 23:81–98, 1980.
69. Graboys, T. B., Lown, B., Podrid, P. J., and de Silva, R.: Long-term survival of patients with malignant ventricular arrhythmia treated with antiarrhythmic drugs. Am. J. Cardiol., 50:437–443, 1982.
70. Burckhardt, D., Hoffmann, A., and Follath, F.: Suppression of complex ventricular ectopic activity (VEA) and survival in chronic CAD. Eur. Heart J., E4(suppl.):244, 1983.

23

Holter Monitor Recording

William J. Mandel, C. Thomas Peter, and Selvyn B. Bleifer

Holter monitor recording means the recording on magnetic tape of all cardiac cycles for periods up to or over 24 hours. The fundamental concept of this method of electrocardiographic monitoring differs from other methods of intermittent surveillance of the electrocardiogram in which only a segment of cardiac electrical activity is recorded, and therefore these other methods cannot be considered true Holter recordings.

The ability to transmit the electrocardiogram by means of radio frequencies was first demonstrated by Holter as early as 1949 (Fig. 23-1).[1] Further development by Holter and colleagues led to the introduction of the first magnetic tape recording unit.[2-4] Subsequently, over the next two decades, a large body of investigators demonstrated the usefulness of this technique.[5-30]

The initial electronic design characteristics of the Holter monitor allowed for small recorder size and the ability to obtain electrocardiographic data over 8 hours using a rechargeable direct current power source. Subsequently, because of significant advances in electronic component design, the quality and fidelity of recordings have been improved and the size and weight of the recorders have been scaled downward. In addition, multichannel devices have become available, enabling the simultaneous recording of two or more leads with the added possibility of an additional channel for timing calibration.

Most contemporary Holter monitor systems do not absolutely meet the current standards of the American Heart Association for electrocardiography frequency response (*i.e.,* 0.05 to 100 Hz).[31] Assuming proper hookup techniques, the recordings appear to reproduce accurate rate and ST segment abnormalities. However, the entire system must be evaluated, including both the recorder and the playback system.

Holter Monitor Equipment

The Holter recorders are small and battery-operated (using either disposable or rechargeable batteries) and use standard-size cassettes or reel-to-reel tape. Recorder size varies, with small models measuring approximately 3½ by 5 by 1½ inches and several models being just slightly larger; the weight varies, with most models weighing just over one pound (Fig. 23-2*A* and *B*). This small size and weight enable the patient to carry the recorder comfortably as a harness or purse over the

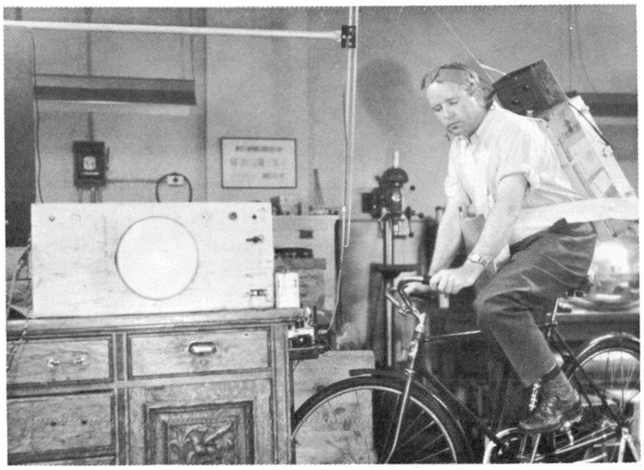

Figure 23-1. *Photograph from Dr. Holter's laboratory, showing the original electrocardiographic telemetry unit described in reference 1. (Courtesy Hoechst Pharmaceuticals, Inc.)*

shoulder or attached to a belt. Most recorders have both an event marker that the patient can activate in case of symptoms and a continuous digital time display that allows the patient to record, in a diary, the exact time of any symptom. Furthermore, time-marking channels are available in some units, enabling very accurate time definition.

Alternative Devices

A number of small ambulatory devices have been developed and marketed that record or transmit the electrocardiogram. These ambulatory devices may be grouped into (1) automatic, (2) patient-activated, and (3) telephone transmitters.

The cardiac event recorder has been available for a number of years. It contains a preprocessor that initiates the electrocardiographic recording when certain predetermined characteristics, based on rate, QRS change, or arrhythmia as defined by the program, occur. In addition to the automatic recording, the patient may initiate a recording sequence if symptoms occur. Furthermore, the instrument is programmed to automatically obtain brief recordings at regular intervals. This format includes the following limitations: (1) the recording cassette is small, and the tape may be completed before more important asymptomatic or symptomatic events occur, and (2) the reliability of the preprocessor in detecting the enormous spectrum of electrocardiographic changes remains uncertain. Difficulties encountered with computer analysis of arrhythmias in conventional electrocardiography as well as in Holter electrocardiography have shown this to be a far more difficult task than was originally anticipated.

Another alternative approach uses patient-activated or symptom-activated recording. The patient is monitored by an ambulatory tape recorder in which each recording sequence is triggered by the patient in response to symptoms or to specific instructions. However, there are several limitations to this approach; for instance, the patient may be unable, due to syncope, or incapable, due to altered mental state, to initiate the recording, or the patient's response time may be slow, and therefore the diagnostic changes may be missed, particularly the rhythm present just before symptoms appear.

Both the automatic and symptom-activated recorders fail to provide an essential characteristic of Holter recording, namely, the recording of every cardiac cycle. It is well documented that informative or diagnostic changes commonly occur without symptoms, and at present, these changes are best detected by continuous recordings. Additionally, access to quantitative data, particularly about ventricular premature complexes, requires that all such complexes be recorded. Other quantitative data such as trend records and ST segment shifts also require uninterrupted recording.

A third type of ambulatory device employs telephone transmission of the electrocardiographic signal. This device differs from Holter electrocardiography and from the two other types of devices described above because an ambulatory tape recording of the electrocardiogram is not made. Rather, an electrocardiographic signal is transmitted by telephone and reproduced directly through a strip chart recorder, with or without tape recording at the receiving end. The patient will generally transmit his electrocardiogram because of symptoms or because a signal from the device tells him that a change has occurred. This approach has not found wide acceptance because of the following logistic difficulties: (1) there must be immediate access to a telephone for the system to operate, (2) the receiving station should provide 24-hour availability to both receive the signal and provide instructions to the patient, and (3) the patient may become anxious if he is not near a telephone or if his transmission cannot be received in a clinically effective fashion. (The method is in contrast to the scheduled telephone transmission of pacemaker signals, which gained wide acceptance and provides reassurance to the patient with a pacemaker.)

Newer devices allow the patient to record the index event with the unit and then use telephone transmission at his leisure (Fig. 23-2).

Technical Aspects

Essential to the recording technique is an adequate hook-up of the recorder by the technician. Skin preparation, satisfactory electrodes (preferably silver/silver chlo-

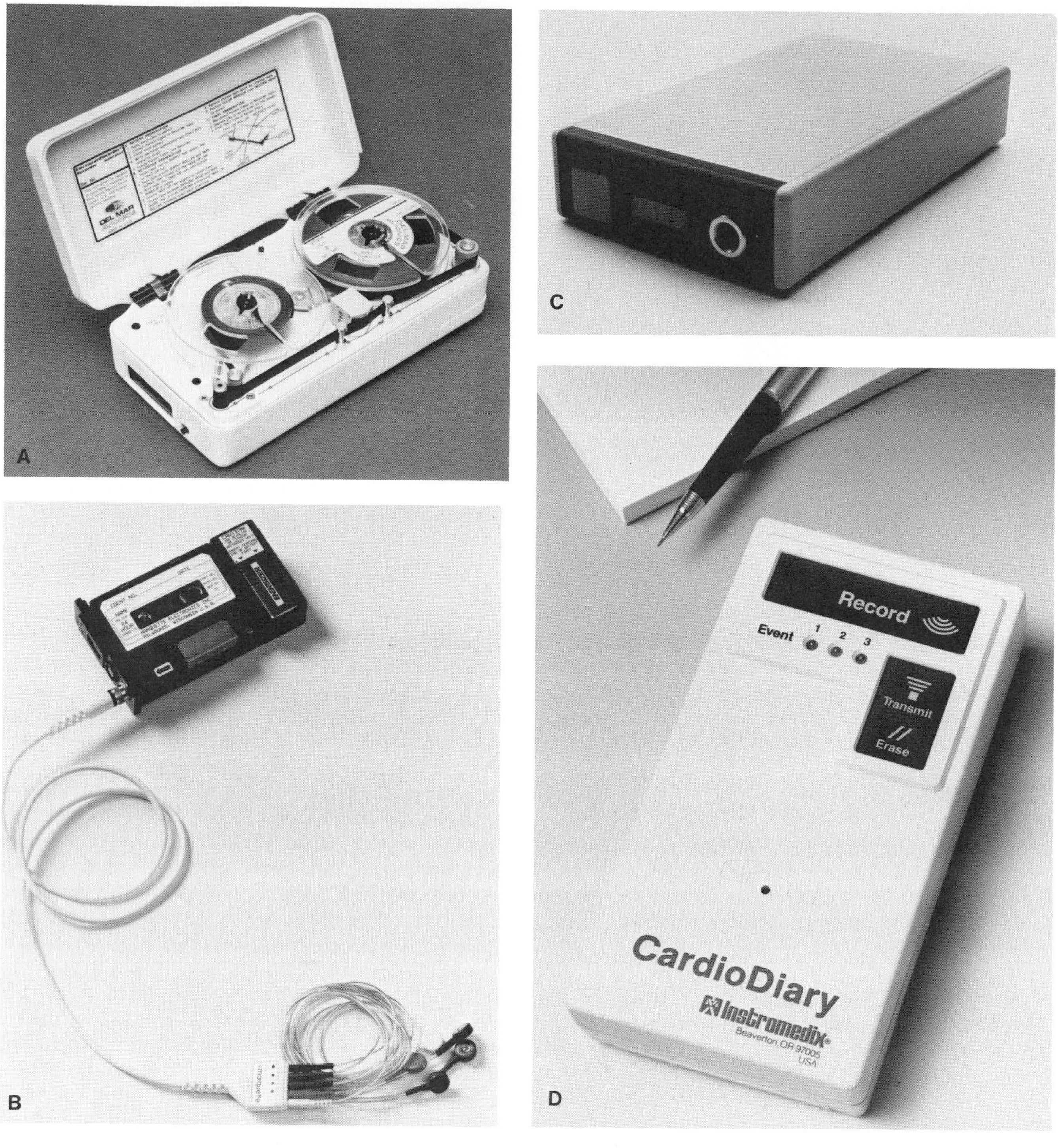

Figure 23-2. *(A and B) Contemporary Holter monitor recorder. A is a two-channel reel-to-reel tape recorder with a digital timing tract. B is a cassette recorder with three channels of electrocardiographic data plus a time channel. In C is a unit that allows for real-time preprocessing of electrocardiographic data. This unit is used with the analysis system shown in Figure 23-4C. (D) A pocket recorder capable of recording three separate 30-second events initiated at the patient's command. The data can later be played back by transtelephonic transmission.*

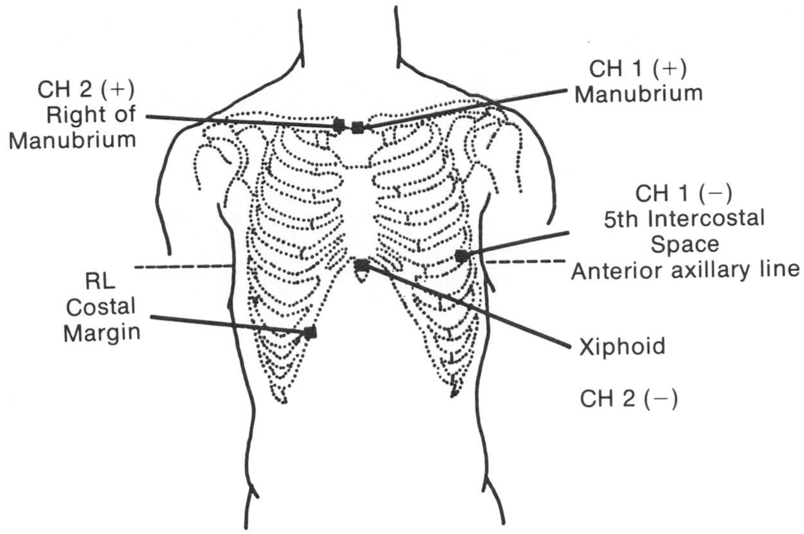

Figure 23-3. *Diagram of the typical hook-up used for standard Holter monitor recording with a five-electrode combination. Two bipolar electrode pairs are used as well as a ground electrode seen at the right lower (RL) costal margin. (CH, channel)*

ride), and secure taping of the electrodes to the chest will ensure technically adequate 24-hour recordings (Fig. 23-3).

The tape scanners or analyzers vary considerably in concept and function (Fig. 23-4*A* to *C*). The fundamental principle of tape review and documentation is the ability to perform high-speed analysis and yet detect every abnormality. The typical 24-hour recording contains over 100,000 cardiac cycles. Primary interest is directed to those episodes in the recording that contain abnormalities such as premature complexes, atrioventricular block, and paroxysmal tachycardia. Originally, visual scanning was accomplished by superimposing each P-QRS-T complex, so that a uniform, stationary image results if identical complexes are present (*i.e.*, sinus rhythm). If a complex differs from the preceding one (*i.e.*, a ventricular premature complex), the mismatched complex can readily be detected by visual inspection. The speed of playback is variable but is usually 60 to 120 times the real time of the recording. The trained observer is able to detect electrocardiographic changes that can then be documented by recording them at real time.

In some analyzer systems, an audio signal was provided in addition to the video display (*i.e.*, a constant hum), the tone of which depends on the heart rate. The faster the heart rate, the higher the pitch. A sudden tachycardia is signaled by a dramatic change in pitch, and even a single ectopic beat interrupts the constant hum. Therefore, any change in heart rate or in the morphology of the electrocardiographic complex can be detected.

"Full disclosure" systems have been introduced to allow for more rapid scanning even by technicians of limited experience. This technique permits playback of all taped data at 120 times the recorded speed and produces a report with time coordinates (Fig. 23-5). This report will allow for review of all data, albeit compressed, with ability to (1) review the quality of the recording, (2) check on technician accuracy, and (3) physically count all premature complexes. This technique can also allow for expansion of the compressed data to permit a real-time report of selected data. The visual scanning system has been updated by the addition of microprocessors that can create templates of QRS waveforms, allowing the operator to select, with greater accuracy, normal, artifact, and abnormal QRS waveforms.

These systems have been further improved with semi-automated modes of data processing. Some of these systems have central 16-byte microcomputers with hard disk. These systems filter the original electrocardiogram to eliminate voltage or frequency artifacts. Analog to digital conversion is then performed with storage on hard disk. Sophisticated algorithms are used to analyze the digitalized QRS data in a second pass through core memory.

Real-time analyzers have been developed that are digitally based and microprocessor driven. These units automatically detect arrhythmias while the patient wears them. They do not, however, analyze the P wave and may have some difficulty with ST segment analysis. These units have potential disadvantages, including reduced frequency response, higher unit cost, and inability to validate data. However, processing is much simpler and very rapid.

Sampling recorders are available in which electrocardiographic data are obtained on a prescheduled time

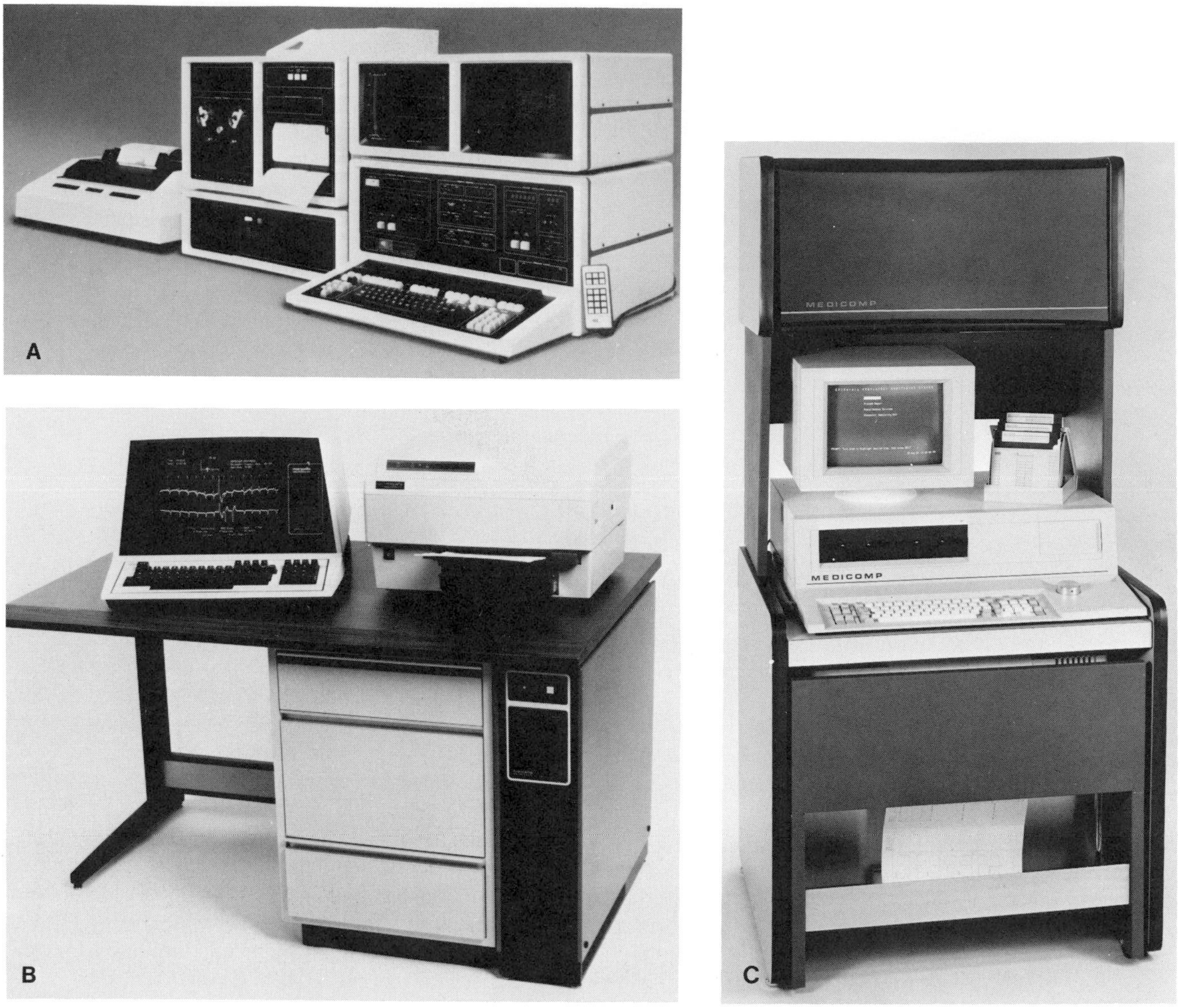

Figure 23-4. *Three contemporary analysis systems. A shows a reel-to-reel analysis system with computer-assisted hardware. B shows a cassette analysis system with a central computer with hard disk drive that allows for semiautomated analysis. C shows a central processing unit for a system using a preprocessing device, as shown in Figure 23-2C.*

format as well as when activated by the patient. The data is then replayed in real time on hard copy for analysis. This offers some advantages in patients with infrequent events who may also have silent episodes.

Indications

The clinical indications for Holter monitoring are numerous. However, in the context of this text Holter recordings are useful for documenting the presence of arrhythmias and evaluating their frequency, identifying the type of arrhythmia(s), relating pharmacologic therapy to effectiveness, identifying the possible mechanism of arrhythmias, identifying the arrhythmic etiology of clinical symptoms, and evaluating pacemaker function (Table 23-1).

Evaluation of Atrial Arrhythmias

Holter monitoring offers significant advantages in evaluating patients with suspected or documented episodes of atrial arrhythmias. The patient who presents with a history of recurrent palpitations and a normal resting electrocardiogram may require investigation by Holter monitoring; the presence of atrial premature complexes,

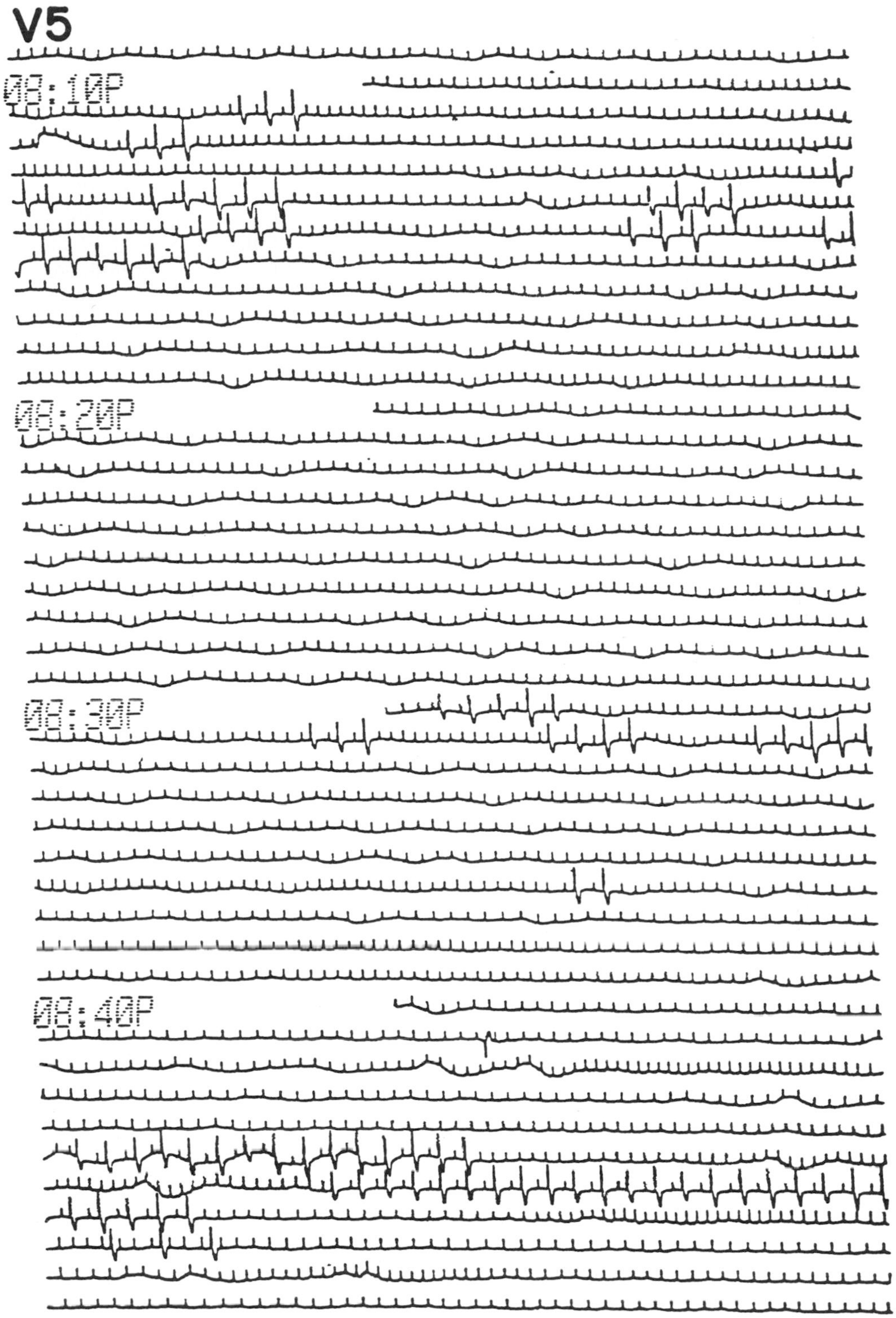

Figure 23-5. *A print-out of 40 minutes of a typical patient record, using a compressed-data system. This system allows for recording at very slow paper speed so that the entire 24-hour record can be printed out in 12 minutes at 120 times real time and compressed as shown here. Time marks are available for continuous analysis of data from a time-point reference system. Even though the data is highly compressed, it is easy to identify and count the ventricular premature complex activity. In addition, rate can be assessed by using an overlay to give accurate rate changes.*

Table 23-1. Indications for Holter Monitoring

Possible Cardiac Symptoms

Palpitations
Syncope
Chest pain
Transient central nervous system events

High Risk Patients

Conduction system disease
Sick sinus syndrome
Prolonged QT syndromes
Wolff-Parkinson-White syndrome
Ischemic heart disease
  Post myocardial infarction
Cardiomyopathy
Mitral valve prolapse
Sudden death survivors
Possible pacemaker malfunction

Antiarrhythmic Drug Evaluation

although usually considered innocuous, may indeed identify the source of the patient's clinical symptomatology. The documentation by Holter monitoring of infrequent atrial premature complexes can be reassuring. However, if frequent atrial premature complexes are noted or if unusual characteristics of the atrial premature complexes are identified, more detailed investigation may be indicated (*i.e.*, studies of thyroid function or echocardiographic evaluation). Furthermore, atrial premature complexes may be a precursor of more sustained atrial arrhythmias or perhaps may identify the earliest features of sinus node dysfunction. Of additional importance is the fact that clinical symptomatology associated with atrial premature complexes may actually not be due to the irregularity of the rhythm but to episodic, pronounced slowing of the heart rate because of nonconducted atrial premature complexes. Moreover, the documentation of atrial premature complexes allows a clearer understanding of various features of atrial electrophysiology as well as an understanding of the AV conduction characteristics in a particular patient. That a single Holter monitor recording can identify the many facets described above is clearly shown in Figure 23-6.

More sustained atrial arrhythmias cannot clearly be distinguished from frequent atrial premature complexes by a detailed history. That the Holter monitor may be critical in documenting recurrent sustained atrial arrhythmias is exemplified in Figure 23-7. Although controversy exists on the relationship between atrial premature complexes, their coupling interval, and the onset of atrial fibrillation, innumerable tracings are available from all large Holter centers demonstrating the relationship between atrial premature complexes and the initiation of atrial fibrillation. Nevertheless, these tracings do not identify the etiology, which must be more clearly evaluated by the physician (*i.e.*, catecholamine excess,

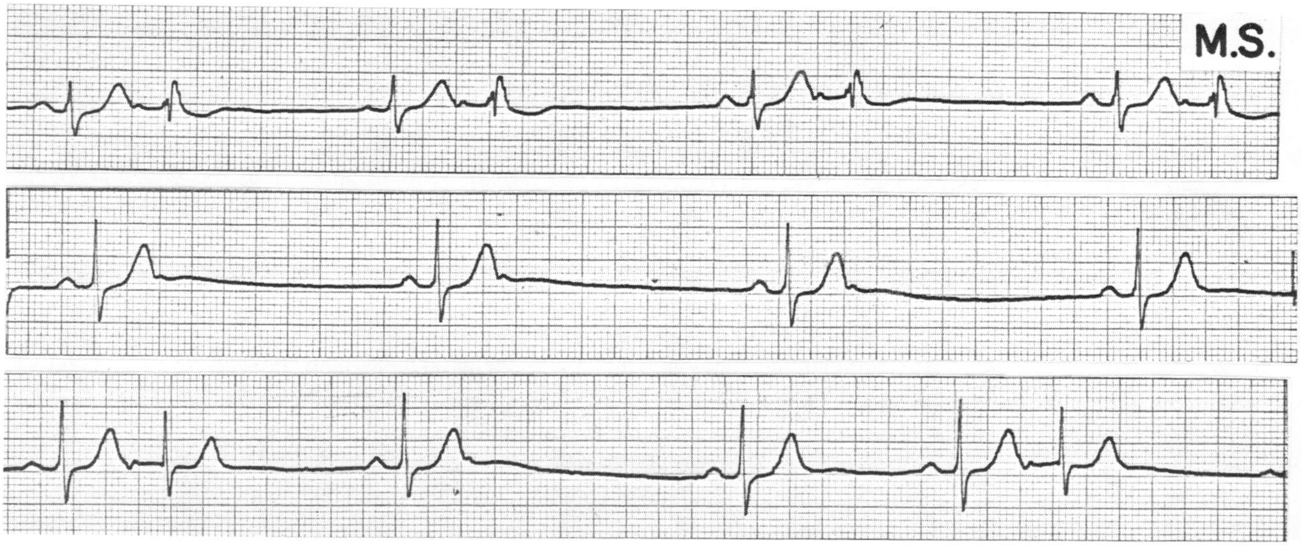

Figure 23-6. *Three Holter monitor strips obtained from a patient complaining of palpitations. The* top recording *reveals atrial premature complexes that occur in a bigeminal fashion and conduct with aberration (i.e., long–short cycle lengths) consistent with phase 3 aberration or the Ashman phenomena. In the* middle strip, *similar atrial premature complexes are noted to occur; however, they are nonconducted and lead to a dramatic slowing of the heart rate. In the* bottom strip, *atrial premature complexes occur with even later coupling intervals on occasion, which allow for conduction with normal QRS configuration. Blocked atrial premature complexes are also noted.*

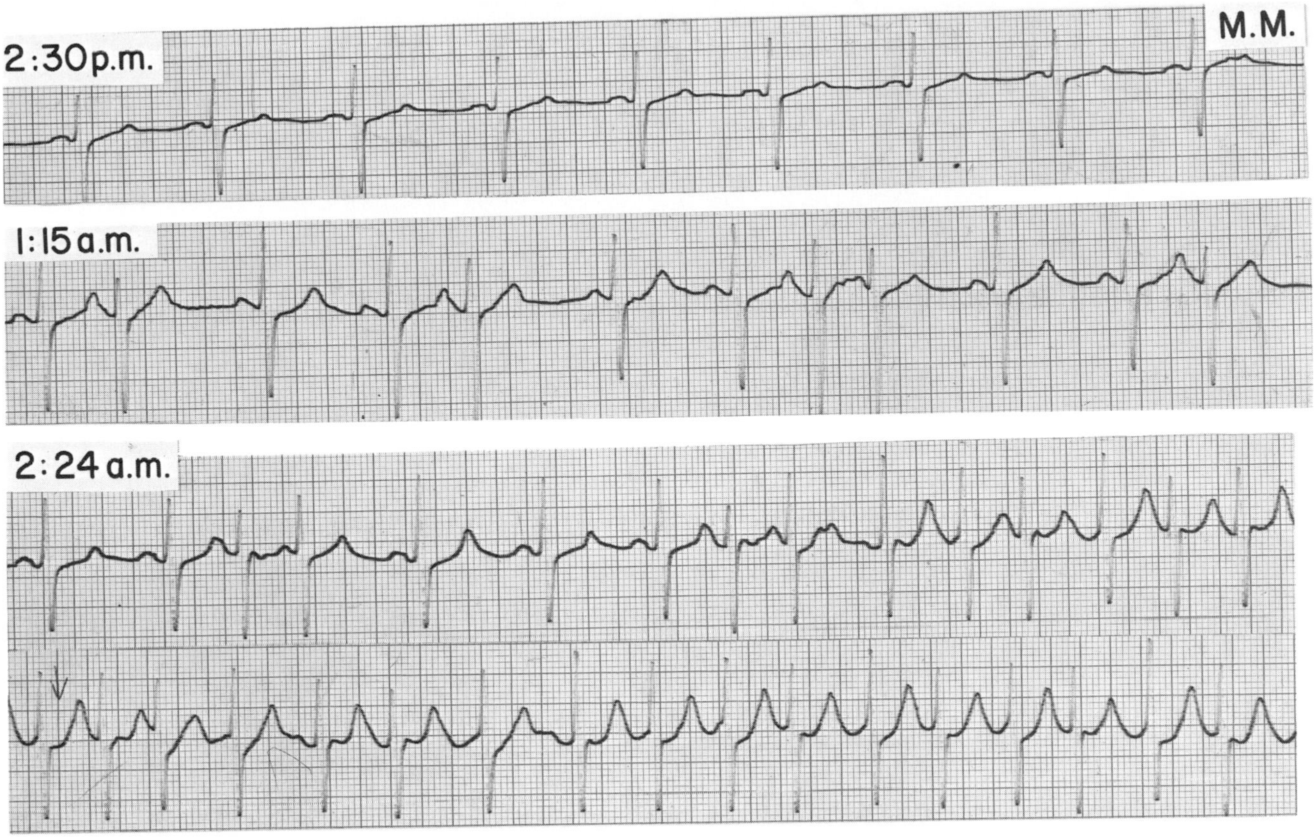

Figure 23-7. *Three representative periods during a Holter monitor recording from a patient complaining of recurrent palpitations. In the* top panel, *sinus rhythm is seen. In the* middle panel, *atrial premature complexes occur singly and in couplets. In the* bottom panel, *atrial premature complexes occur in couplets. In the later part of the* bottom strip, *three atrial premature complexes occur in a row. The last complex occurs quite early and initiates an episode of atrial fibrillation with a moderately rapid ventricular response.*

hyperthyroidism, drug-related arrhythmias, valvular dysfunction).

The onset of atrial fibrillation is usually related to atrial premature complexes in the majority of instances in which the onset of atrial fibrillation is observed on a Holter monitor recording (Figs. 23-7 and 23-8). Atrial premature complexes are frequently noted to have very short coupling intervals and may relate to initiation of atrial fibrillation by impinging upon the atrial "vulnerable period." Additional information other than the mode of onset may be obtained from such records obtained from patients who have had repeated bouts of atrial fibrillation during the course of monitoring. Dramatic alterations in rate, rhythm, and QRS morphology during such monitor recordings may frequently be observed (see Fig. 23-8). It is clear from such records and associated clinical histories that patients are occasionally unaware of dramatic changes in rhythm disturbance and may report that they have sustained palpitations throughout the day with no clear-cut relationship to rate or shift in rhythm. These phenomena may be precursors of a variant of sinus node dysfunction (*i.e.*, bradycardia-tachycardia syndrome, see below).

In some patients, regulation of the ventricular rate in atrial fibrillation may be a significant clinical problem. However, during Holter recordings, many patients with sustained atrial fibrillation may have marked variations in the ventricular response to atrial fibrillation related to changes in activity or time of day. This can result in significant difficulties with regard to developing an appropriate maintenance dose of digitalis or the use of associated AV-conduction-blocking agents such as beta-blockers. A typical example of such a patient is illustrated in Figure 23-9.

Atrial flutter on a sustained basis is a less common atrial arrhythmia. Nevertheless, its behavior mimics, to some degree, the phenomena described above in patients who have paroxysmal or sustained atrial fibrillation. Dramatic swings in the ventricular rate with atrial flutter appear to be less common than those seen with atrial

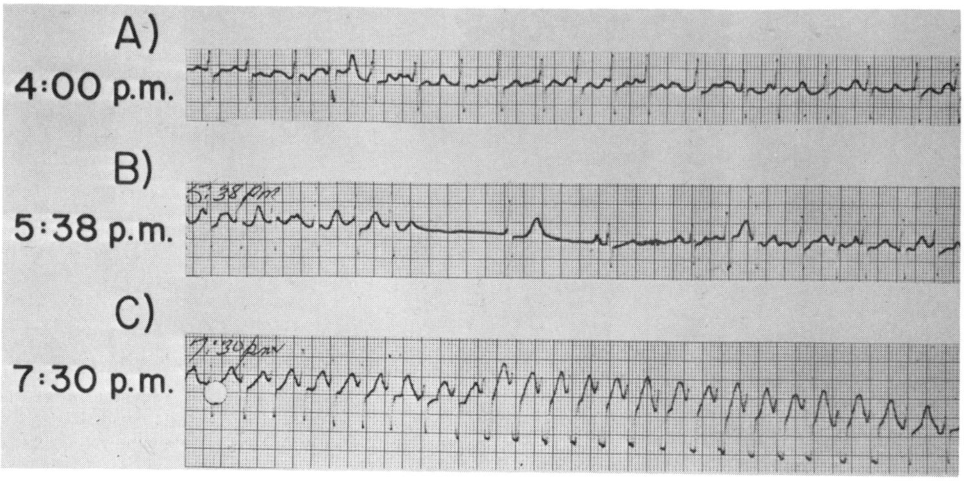

Figure 23-8. *Three representative strips from a patient with recurrent palpitations. In A, atrial fibrillation with a moderately rapid ventricular rate is noted. In B, atrial fibrillation terminates spontaneously with a junctional escape complex followed by sinus rhythm. Following the second sinus complex, an atrial premature complex initiates another episode of atrial fibrillation. In C, atrial fibrillation with a much more rapid ventricular response is noted and intermittent ventricular aberration is seen.*

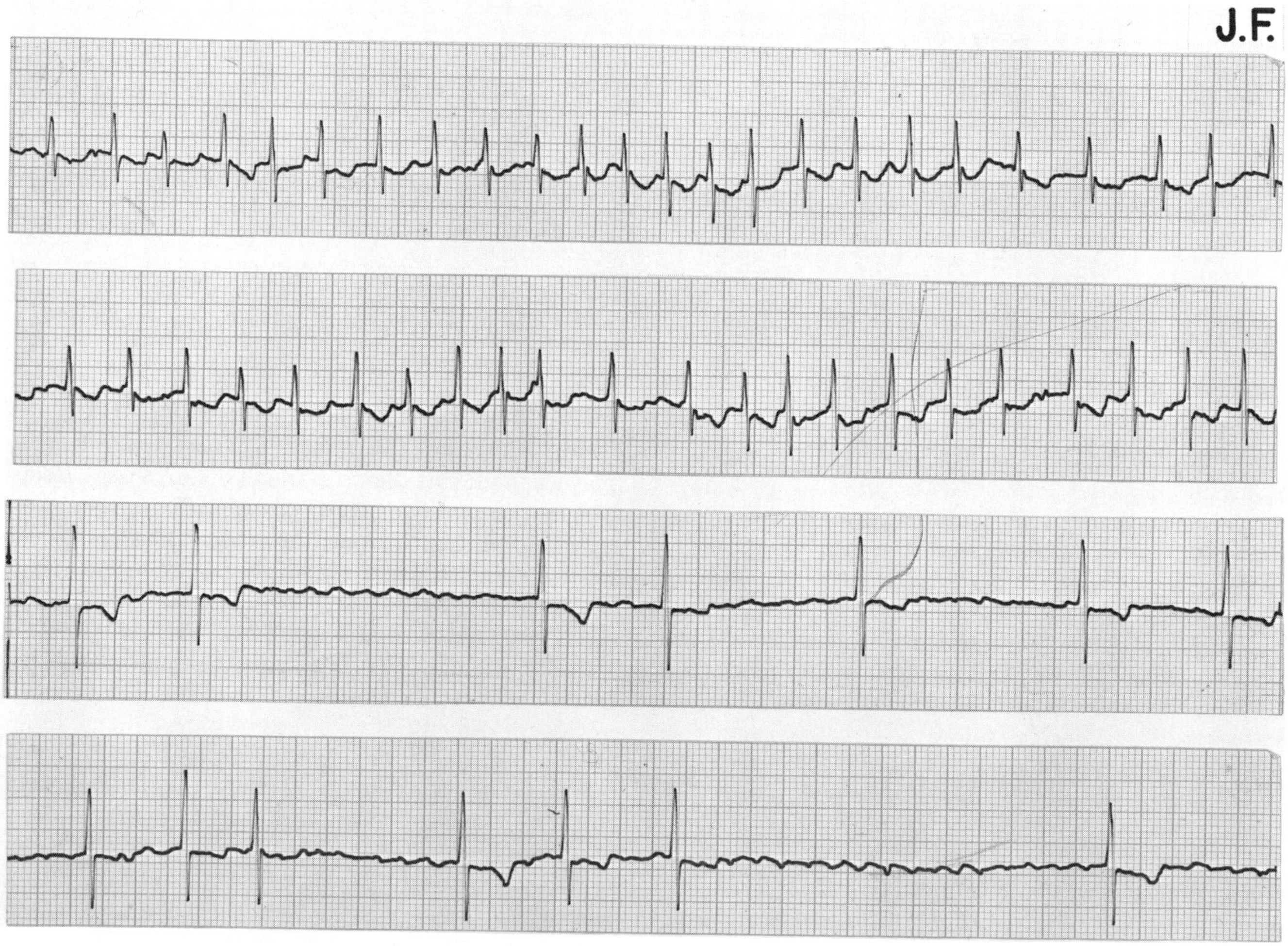

Figure 23-9. *Representative recordings taken from a patient with sustained long-standing atrial fibrillation. In the* top two panels, *atrial fibrillation is seen with ventricular rates generally in excess of 150 beats/min. The* bottom two panels, *from the same patient at a different time, show atrial fibrillation with pronounced slowing of the ventricular rate, with pauses exceeding 2 seconds seen on two occasions.*

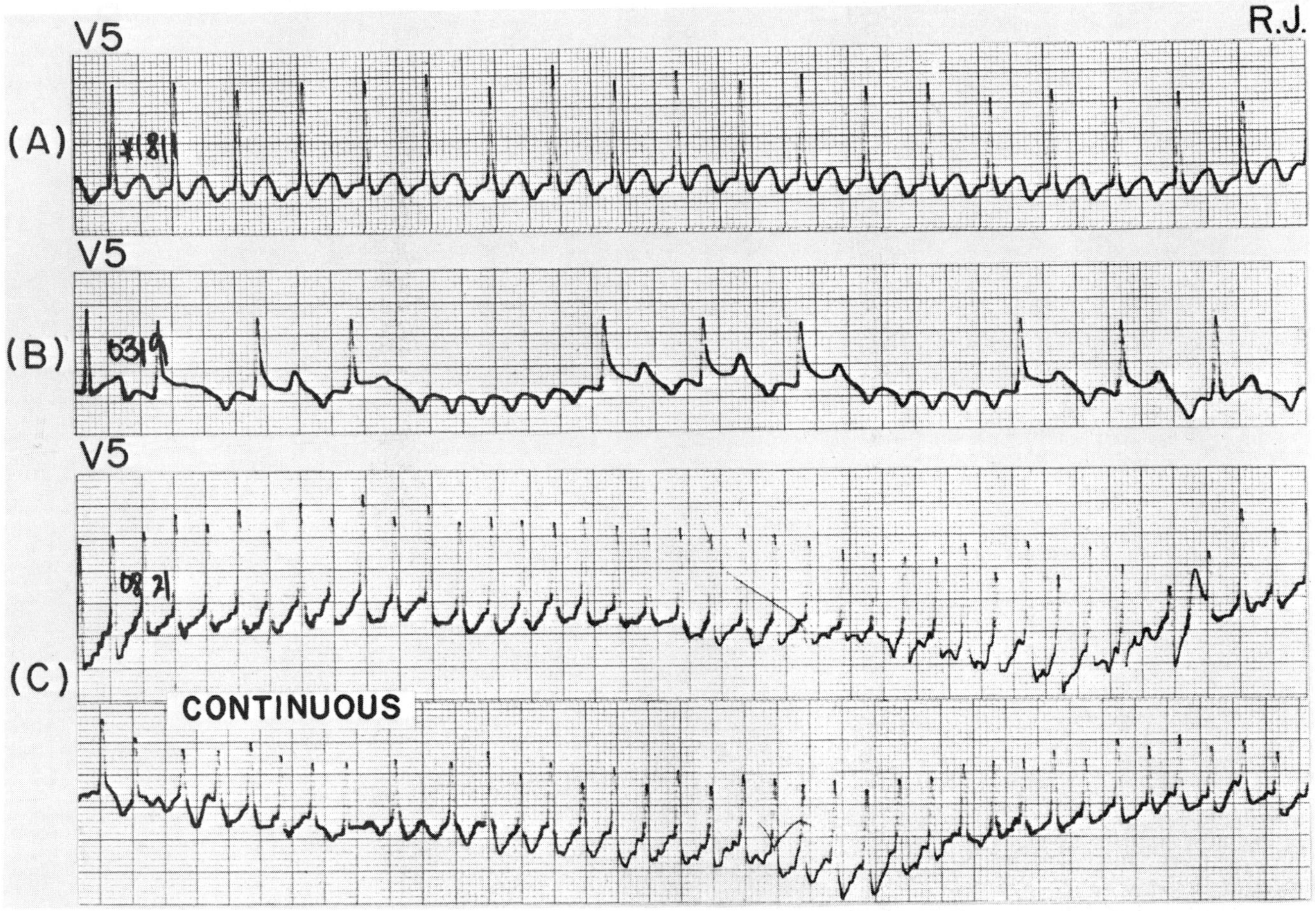

Figure 23-10. *Three representative periods obtained from a Holter recording from a patient with atrial flutter. In A, atrial flutter is seen with a 2:1 ventricular response. Later, in B, the patient is in atrial flutter with a controlled ventricular rate in which long pauses are seen. In C, during an episode of sustained dizziness, the patient is in atrial flutter but with 1:1 conduction, with a ventricular response of approximately 300 beats/min.*

fibrillation. Nevertheless, such events occur and may produce dramatic clinical symptomatology. This is clearly illustrated in Figure 23-10.

In many instances, the onset of atrial flutter, like the onset of atrial fibrillation, appears to be related to the presence (and prematurity) of atrial premature complexes. In patients with recurrent palpitations, intermittent atrial flutter should be considered among the differential diagnoses. The presence of palpitations associated with dizziness suggests that the ventricular rate may in fact be rapid. On rare occasions, very rapid ventricular rates are indeed noted with the onset of atrial flutter (Fig. 23-11).

Atrial flutter may be a sustained arrhythmia and, in

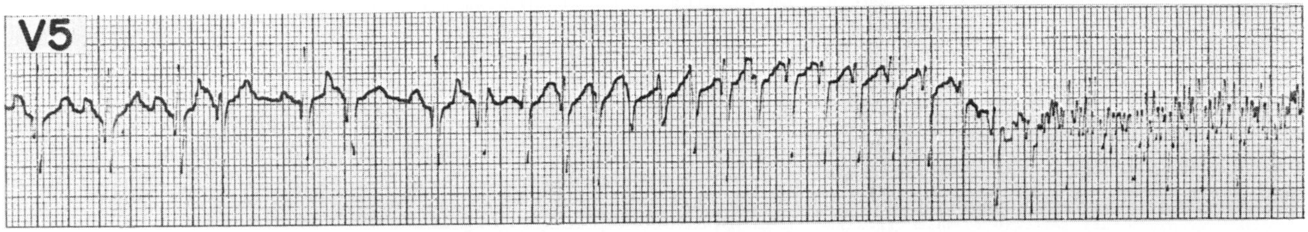

Figure 23-11. *Onset of atrial flutter in a patient with a history of recurrent palpitations. The beginning of the strip shows premature complexes as isolated events. The third atrial premature complex initiates a sustained episode of atrial flutter with a 1:1 ventricular response and with a ventricular rate of approximately 300 beats/min.*

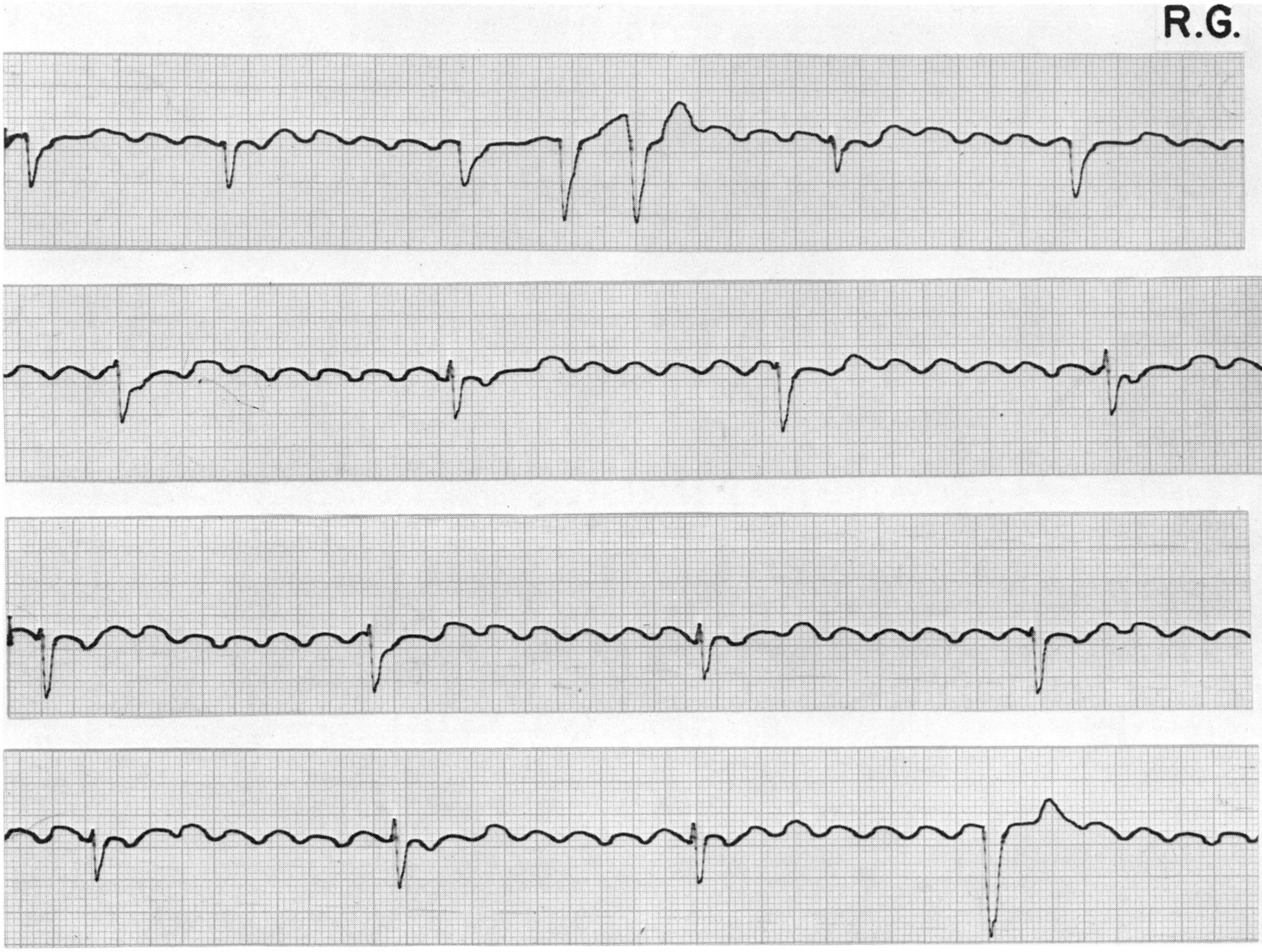

Figure 23-12. *Strips obtained from a Holter recording in a patient with sustained atrial flutter. Throughout the recording, the patient demonstrates atrial flutter with a profound degree of AV conduction disturbance. Ventricular premature complexes are seen, and a possible ventricular escape complex is also noted in the last strip.*

general, requires larger maintenance doses of digitalis than does atrial fibrillation, sometimes with the additional use of ancillary agents to depress AV conduction. The use of higher doses of digitalis with or without adjuvant agents may depress AV conduction more than necessary for clinical effectiveness. This phenomenon is exemplified in Figure 23-12.

Episodic tachyarrhythmias or palpitations or both may be documented by a Holter monitor recording and yet may not fit into the classic categories of atrial arrhythmias (Fig. 23-13). Once these unusual atrial arrhythmias (*e.g.,* paroxysmal atrial tachycardia with block, multifocal atrial tachycardia, ectopic atrial tachycardia) are documented, they may explain the difficulty in managing such patients with routine therapeutic agents.

Recurrent supraventricular tachycardias such as described above may on occasion be associated with alternating periods of bradyarrhythmias. If ventricular rates are not dramatically different from those observed during sinus rhythm, limited (if any) symptomatology may be recounted by the patient. Nevertheless, these arrhythmias may be dramatic and may be precursors of more pronounced degrees of supraventricular arrhythmias. Exaggerated versions of the above alternation of tachycardia and bradycardia may be associated with clinical symptomatology of cerebral hypoperfusion. Figures 23-14 and 23-15 offer dramatic examples of such instances.

Palpitations may be reported as clinical symptoms of minor magnitude or of major clinical significance. Holter recordings can identify clinically insignificant episodes or episodes associated with major clinical problems. Furthermore, these recordings can offer some significant insight into the mechanism of the tachyarrhythmias as well as insight into the function of the sinus and

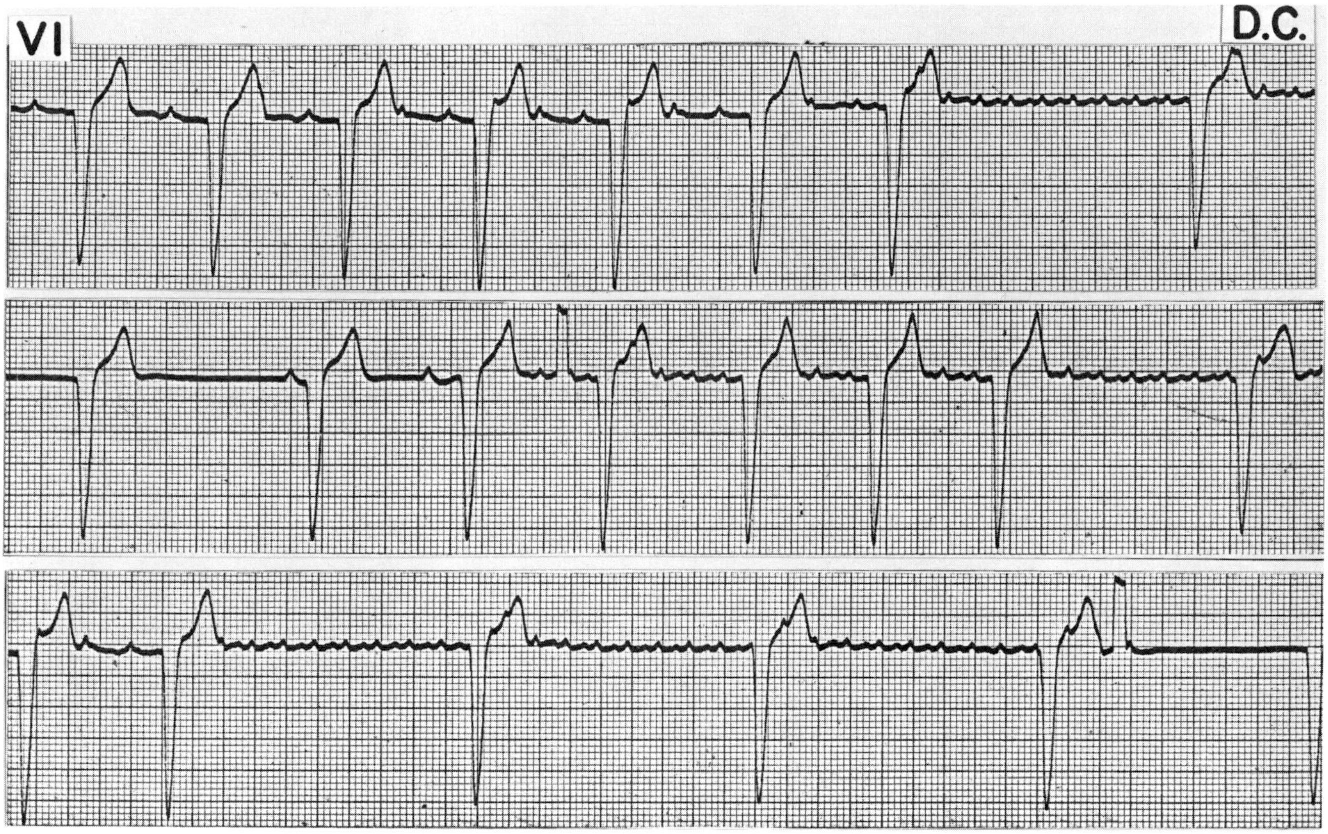

Figure 23-13. *An unusual recording obtained from a patient complaining of recurrent palpitations. In these representative Holter strips, several unusual arrhythmias are noted. In the* top strip, *atrial tachycardia with variable conduction delay is initiated by an atrial premature complex. The atrial tachycardia suddenly converts into an episode of apparent atrial flutter with peculiar flutter waves and with an atrial flutter rate of approximately 300 beats/min. The flutter terminates spontaneously, with resultant junctional escape complex and then restoration of sinus rhythm. In the* middle strip, *following restoration of sinus rhythm, the atypical atrial flutter is initiated again and ultimately results in termination and restoration of junctional escape rhythm in the last complex of the* bottom strip.

AV nodes. These features are illustrated in Figures 23-16 and 23-17.

Detection and Quantitation of Ventricular Arrhythmias

Holter monitoring has been a mainstay in the detection and quantitation of ventricular arrhythmias, especially ventricular premature complexes. Extensive recent studies have emphasized very clearly that spontaneously occurring fluctuations in the ventricular premature complex frequency are such that brief periods of recording may give an extremely erroneous impression of the frequency of arrhythmias as well as the success or failure of antiarrhythmic drug therapy. Studies by Morganroth and co-workers and Winkle and co-workers have adequately emphasized the importance of longer-duration recordings.[32,33] Spontaneous variability is such that in the findings of both of these groups, variability in the ventricular premature complex frequency is so great as to mimic the effects of antiarrhythmic drug therapy (Fig. 23-18). Furthermore, these studies have emphasized (Fig. 23-19) that the spontaneous incidence of ventricular arrhythmias may in large part depend on daytime or nighttime recordings, such that during sleep the ventricular arrhythmias may be nearly abolished. Finally, the spontaneous day-to-day variability is such (Fig. 23-20) that on three different days the number of ventricular premature complexes may vary from as few as 70 to as many as 700 per hour. This variability may greatly inhibit accurate evaluation of antiarrhythmic drug therapy and may be a critical point with regard to the long-term management of patients with ventricular arrhythmias. These authors have emphasized clearly that statistically significant reductions in ventricular premature complex activity cannot be observed at the 5% confidence limit

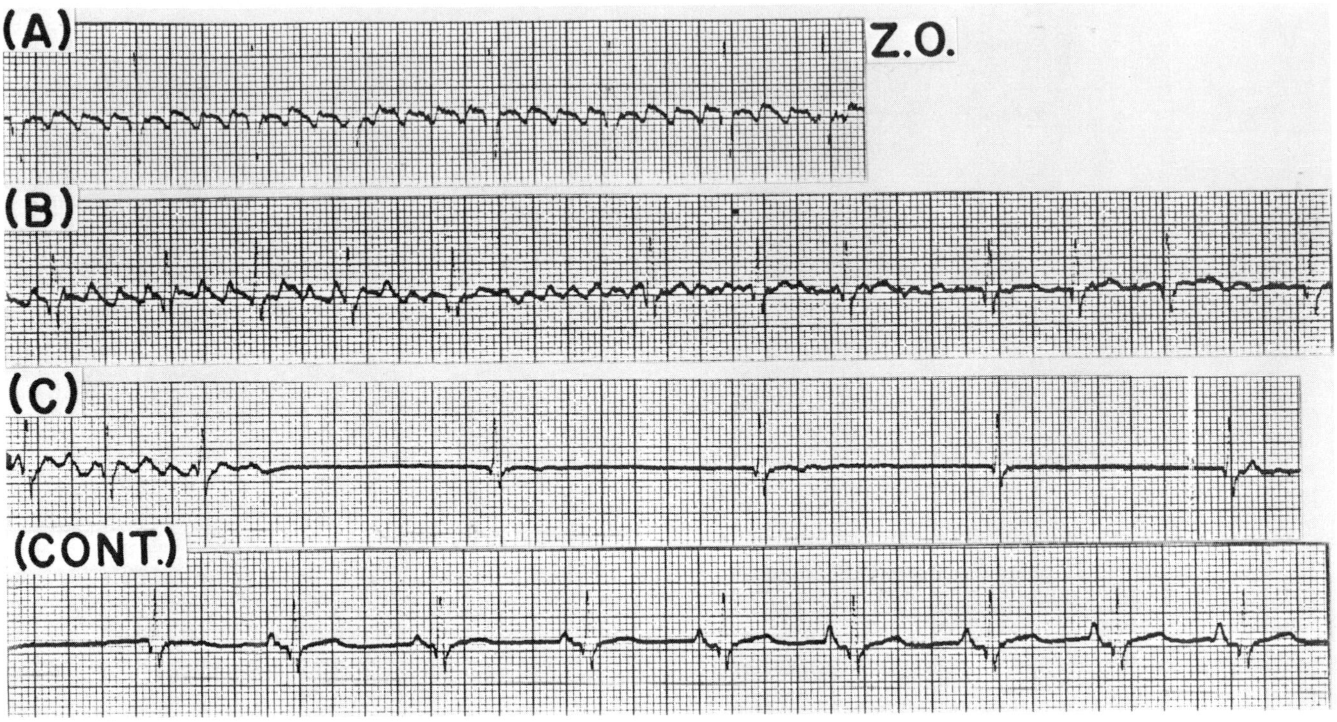

Figure 23-14. *Representative Holter strips from a recording in a patient with recurrent tachycardia alternating with bradycardia. In A, atrial flutter is seen with typical flutter waves both in rate and in configuration. The ventricular response is controlled. In B, the flutter waves change in configuration in the early portion of the record and then convert into atrial fibrillation with a controlled ventricular response. In C (continuous strip), atrial fibrillation terminates and is followed by junctional bradycardia. Subsequently, sinus rhythm is restored, with normal heart rate and normal AV conduction seen in the later portion of C.*

unless there is a 90% reduction in ventricular premature complex activity over 24 hours. Longer periods will allow for statistical comparison with less of a reduction in ventricular premature complex activity.[32,33] The random electrocardiogram may identify the presence of ventricular premature complexes and may clarify the mechanism of patient-related symptomatology (*i.e.,* the sensation of palpitation). Albeit controversial, the use of grading systems for evaluation of the nature of ventricular arrhythmias nevertheless suggests that a more detailed evaluation of the frequency and nature of the ventricular premature complex activity be obtained. This necessitates, as described above, the need for more protracted periods of electrocardiographic observation. During such observation, it would not be uncommon to determine episodic complex ventricular arrhythmia activity without sustained ventricular tachycardia, as exemplified in Figure 23-21. (In this regard, it is necessary to point out the importance of two-channel recordings. The very nature of the premature complex may not be obvious without two separate electrocardiogram channels; see Fig. 23-22.)

Recent studies by Pratt and co-workers[34] have identified that the variability of complex ventricular arrhythmias is significantly higher in patients with (rather than without) coronary artery disease. This is especially true in patients with runs of ventricular tachycardia. The importance of variability has been further emphasized by recent studies by Kennedy and colleagues[35] in asymptomatic healthy subjects with frequent and complex ectopy. This study identified that the long-term prognosis in this group is similar to that in a cohort of healthy patients and that no increased incidence of death should be anticipated.

Age may appear to predispose to cardiac arrhythmias. Fleg and Kennedy[36] have studied an elderly (60 to 85 years) population without clinical cardiac disease. These patients demonstrated a significant prevalence of supraventricular and ventricular premature complexes, isolated and complex. However, marked bradycardia, sinus arrest, or high degrees of AV block were not noted.

More sustained episodes of ventricular arrhythmias may occur and yet may be unrelated to clinical symptomatology. Accelerated idioventricular rhythm (AIVR)

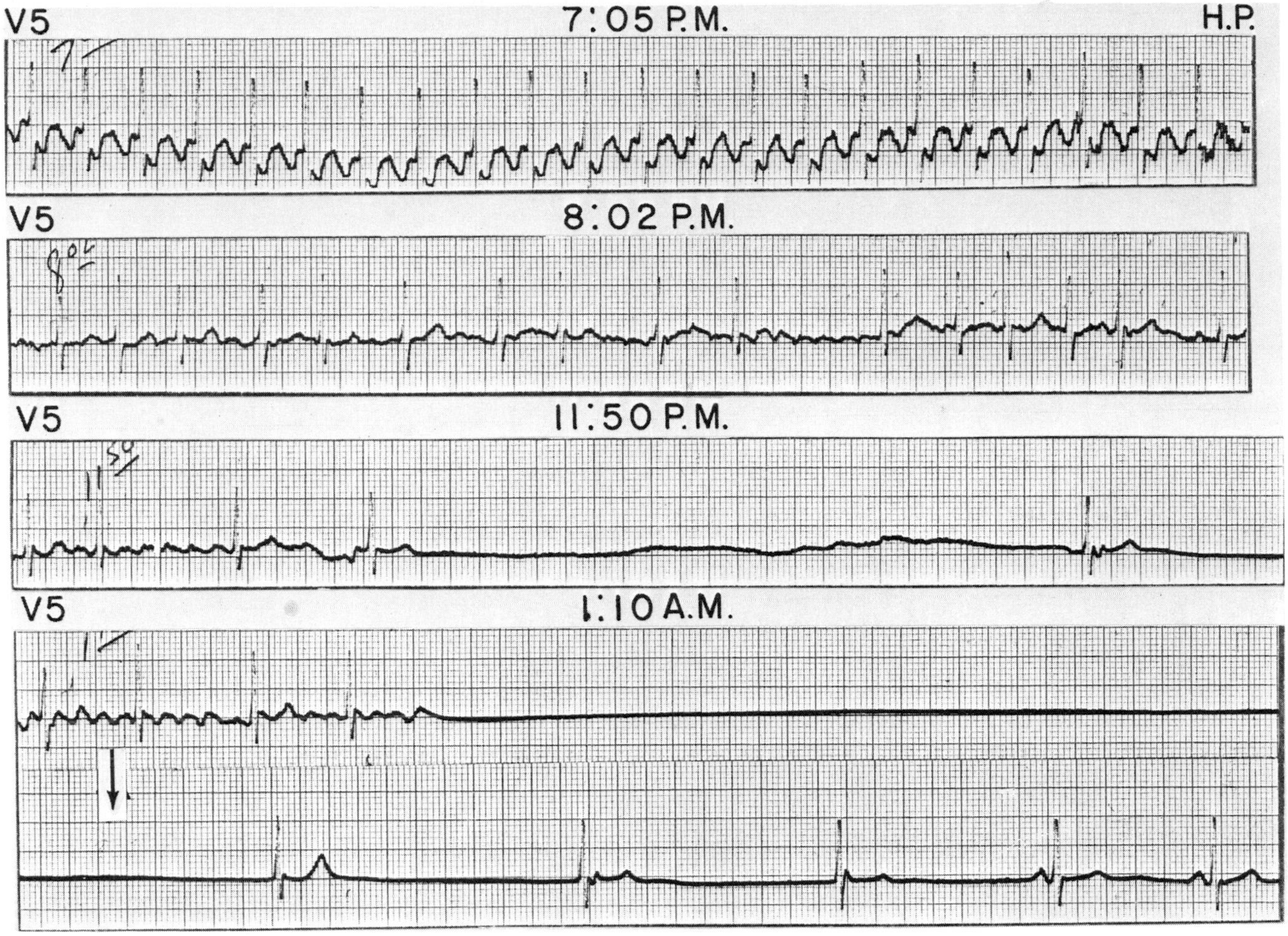

Figure 23-15. *Representative Holter strips from a patient with recurrent tachycardia and bradycardia. In the first strip (at 7:05 PM), atrial flutter with 2:1 ventricular response is noted. Approximately 1 hour later (the second strip, at 8:02 PM), atrial fluter has converted to atrial fibrillation with a moderately rapid ventricular response. In the third strip (at 11:50 PM), atrial fibrillation terminates spontaneously with a profound sinus arrest terminated by a junctional escape complex. In the final strips (at 1:10 AM), atrial flutter/fibrillation terminates spontaneously with a dramatic sinus arrest terminated by three junctional escape complexes followed by restoration of sinus rhythm.*

may occur in patients without obvious clinical evidence of heart disease; AIVR may be of brief duration associated with sinus arrhythmia (Fig. 23-23), or it may occur on a more sustained basis, usually in patients with significant organic heart disease (Fig. 23-24). The ventricular rate seen during AIVR is, by definition, less than 100 beats/min. This, in large part, explains the general lack of symptomatology associated with the presence of intermittent short-lived or even sustained episodes of AIVR.

Symptomatic ventricular arrhythmias can occur in patients without overt cardiovascular disease, but, in the vast majority of instances, organic cardiovascular disease is present. In clinical practice, the most common background for the development of ventricular arrhythmias is ischemic heart disease. The presence of intermittent ischemia may play a substantive role in the development of short or more sustained episodes of ventricular tachycardia. This is exemplified by the findings in Figure 23-25, which identify that the development of ST segment depression associated with clinically important ischemia was associated with the development of ventricular tachycardia.

Sustained episodes of ventricular tachycardia generally are associated with clinical symptomatology such as palpitations, lightheadedness, dizziness, or frank syncope. However, the development of sustained ventricular tachycardia may occur at rates below 150 beats/min and may be associated only with the sensation of mild palpitations (Fig. 23-26). That ventricular tachycardia

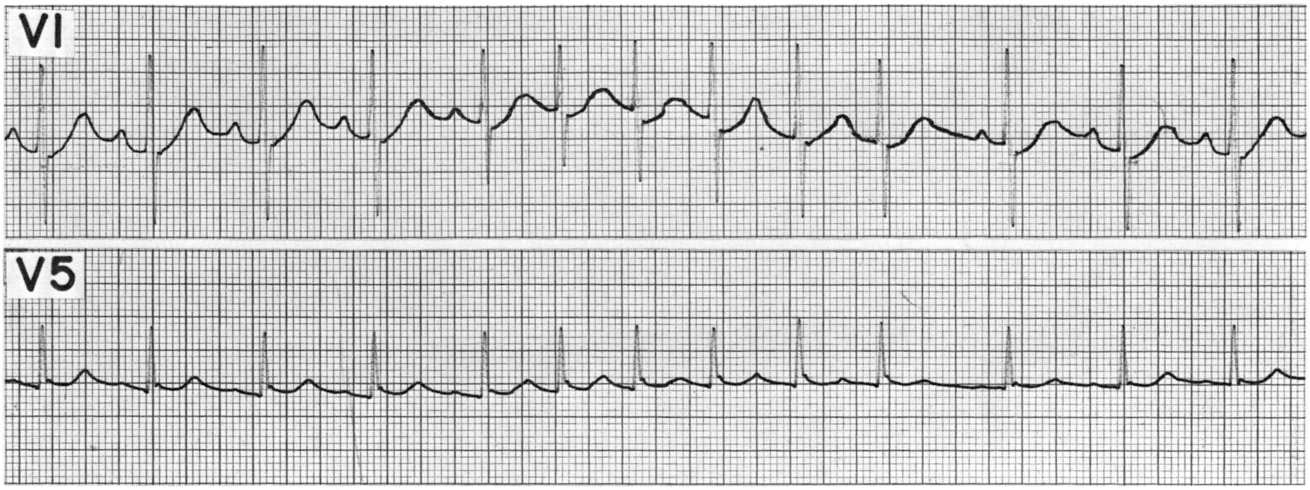

Figure 23-16. *Representative two-channel Holter monitor strips from a patient with a recurrent history of palpitations. In the middle portion of this recording, a short burst of supraventricular tachycardia lasting for five complexes is seen with a ventricular rate of approximately 130 beats/min. Following the burst of tachycardia, sinus rhythm is restored with a normal sinus node recovery time. Throughout the 24-hour period of this recording, the patient had repeated short bursts of supraventricular tachycardia. Documentation by electrocardiography had never been made in previous examinations.*

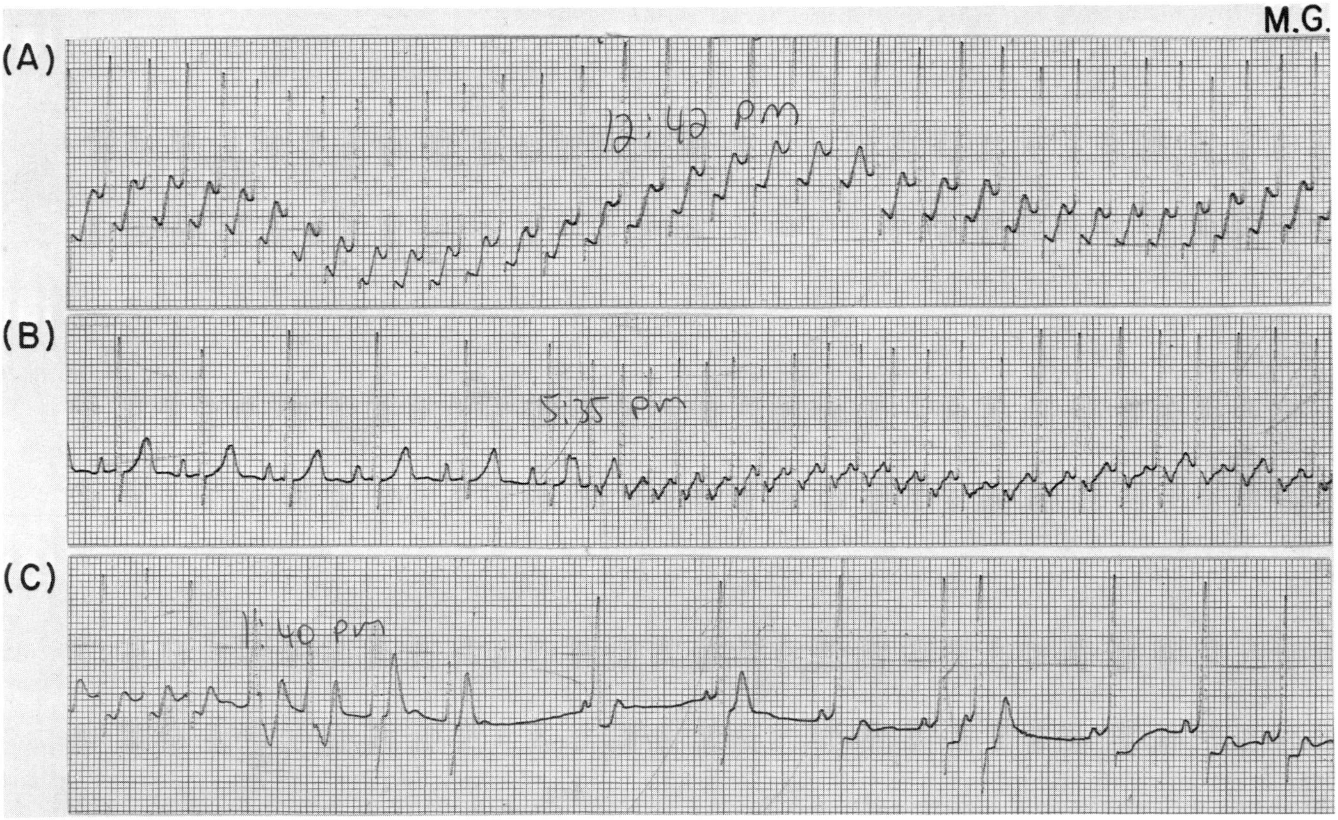

Figure 23-17. *Representative Holter strips from a patient with recurrent paroxysmal supraventricular tachycardia. In A (at 12:42* AM*), the patient had a sustained episode of supraventricular tachycardia with a ventricular rate in excess of 220 beats/min. Atrial activity following the QRS appears to be present. In B (at 5:35* PM*), the onset of supraventricular tachycardia is observed in the same patient. The tachycardia is initiated by an atrial premature complex with modest prolongation of the PR interval followed by atrial activation after the QRS complex. In C (at 1:40* PM*), an episode of supraventricular tachycardia terminates, with bizarre complex activity, possibly ventricular in origin, seen just before termination.*

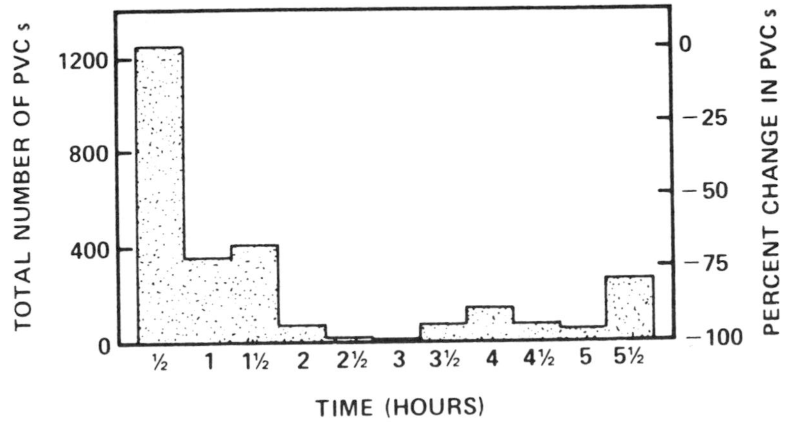

Figure 23-18. *Graph demonstrating the highly variable nature of ventricular premature complex activity seen in one patient's Holter recording over a 5½-hour time span. The patient was not receiving antiarrhythmic drugs at the time of the Holter recording. (Winkle, R. A.: Antiarrhythmic drug effect mimicked by spontaneous variability of ventricular ectopy. Circulation, 57:1116, 1978. By permission of the American Heart Association, Inc.)*

can occur at slow rates even in the presence of organic heart disease is clinically evident. In the setting of relatively normal ventricular function, the presence of ventricular tachycardia at rates below 150 beats/min should not lead to significant hemodynamic compromise and, therefore, may not be clinically evident by review of the patient's history. In contrast to the findings listed above, more rapid ventricular rates in patients with impaired hemodynamic function invariably lead to significant hemodynamic compromise (Fig. 23-27).

Therapy with antiarrhythmic agents is used in many instances in patients with significant ventricular arrhythmias. Unfortunately, the initiation of therapy with antiarrhythmic agents may precipitate rather than prevent ventricular arrhythmias. This is particularly true with quinidine. During the early stages of therapy with quinidine, QT prolongation may occur without suppression of ventricular arrhythmias and may lead to enhanced vulnerability and to the development of sustained ventricular arrhythmias (*i.e.*, quinidine syncope). An example is demonstrated in Figure 23-28.

Other conditions also predispose to the development of sustained ventricular arrhythmias. If these conditions are not readily recognized, historical features of syncope may be associated with Holter-documented severe ventricular arrhythmias. This has been most clearly demonstrated in the situation of hereditary QT prolongation syndromes in which syncope and near syncope are asso-

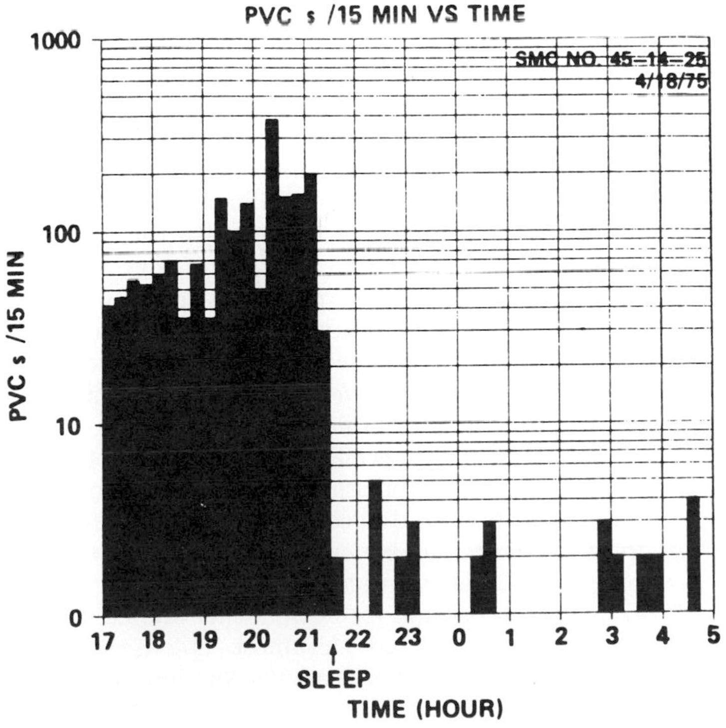

Figure 23-19. *The horizontal axis shows the time during a 24-hour span, and the vertical axis shows the number of premature ventricular contractions (PVCs) per 15 minutes. Note the dramatic reduction in PVC frequency when the patient falls asleep. (Winkle, R. A.: Antiarrhythmic drug effect mimicked by spontaneous variability of ventricular ectopy. Circulation, 57:1116, 1978. By permission of the American Heart Association, Inc.)*

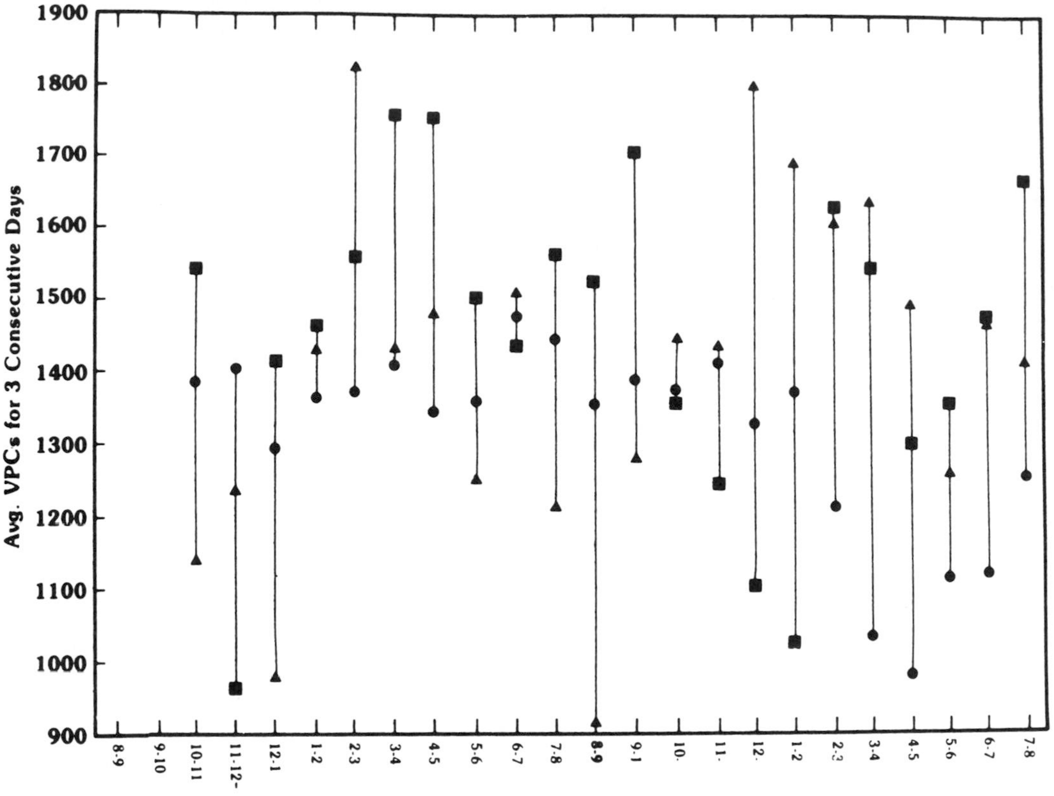

Figure 23-20. *One-hour time periods are plotted on the horizontal axis, and the average numbers of premature ventricular contractions (PVCs) seen on 3 consecutive days are shown on the vertical axis. Note the dramatic swings in PVC frequency relative to the days the Holter recording was taken. (Morganroth, J., Michelson, E. L., Horowitz, L. N., et al.: Limitations of routine long-term electrocardiographic monitoring to assess ventricular ectopic frequency. Circulation, 58:408, 1978. By permission of the American Heart Association, Inc.)*

ciated with the presence of sustained ventricular arrhythmias and even episodic ventricular fibrillation. A typical example is shown in Figure 23-29.

Most recently, another iatrogenic cause of sustained ventricular arrhythimas has been noted in patients who have developed a QT prolongation associated with dietary therapy using liquid-protein supplementation. Serious and even life-threatening arrhythmias, associated with a significant QT prolongation, have been documented to occur in such patients. These patients frequently demonstrated *torsade de pointes* and even episodes of ventricular flutter/fibrillation (Fig. 23-30).

An additional area of application for Holter monitoring is related to prophylactic aspects of ventricular arrhythmias. Over the past decade, attempts have been made to categorize certain patients as high risk for the development of serious ventricular arrhythmias. Such high-risk population groups include patients who have had myocardial infarction, especially those patients with bundle branch block and those patients who have had open-heart surgery. It has been suggested that Holter recordings should be obtained in all such patients before discharge and then serially for at least 6 months. In this way, ventricular arrhythmias can be identified, circumventing episodes of sudden cardiac death.

Diagnosis of Atrioventricular Block

In clinical practice, the electrocardiographic diagnosis of AV block seldom requires the additional use of Holter monitor recording. Moreover, Holter recordings generally play only a limited role in the clinical management of asymptomatic patients with first degree AV block. In general, second degree AV block of the type II (Mobitz) variety also should be managed with permanent pacing without the need for Holter recordings. However, in the setting of second degree AV block of the type I (Wenckebach) variety, Holter recordings may give the clinician much needed data. This is especially the case in asymptomatic patients without evidence of acute or chronic cardiac disease who are not receiving cardioactive drugs. Recently,[37] data have accumulated that have identified a

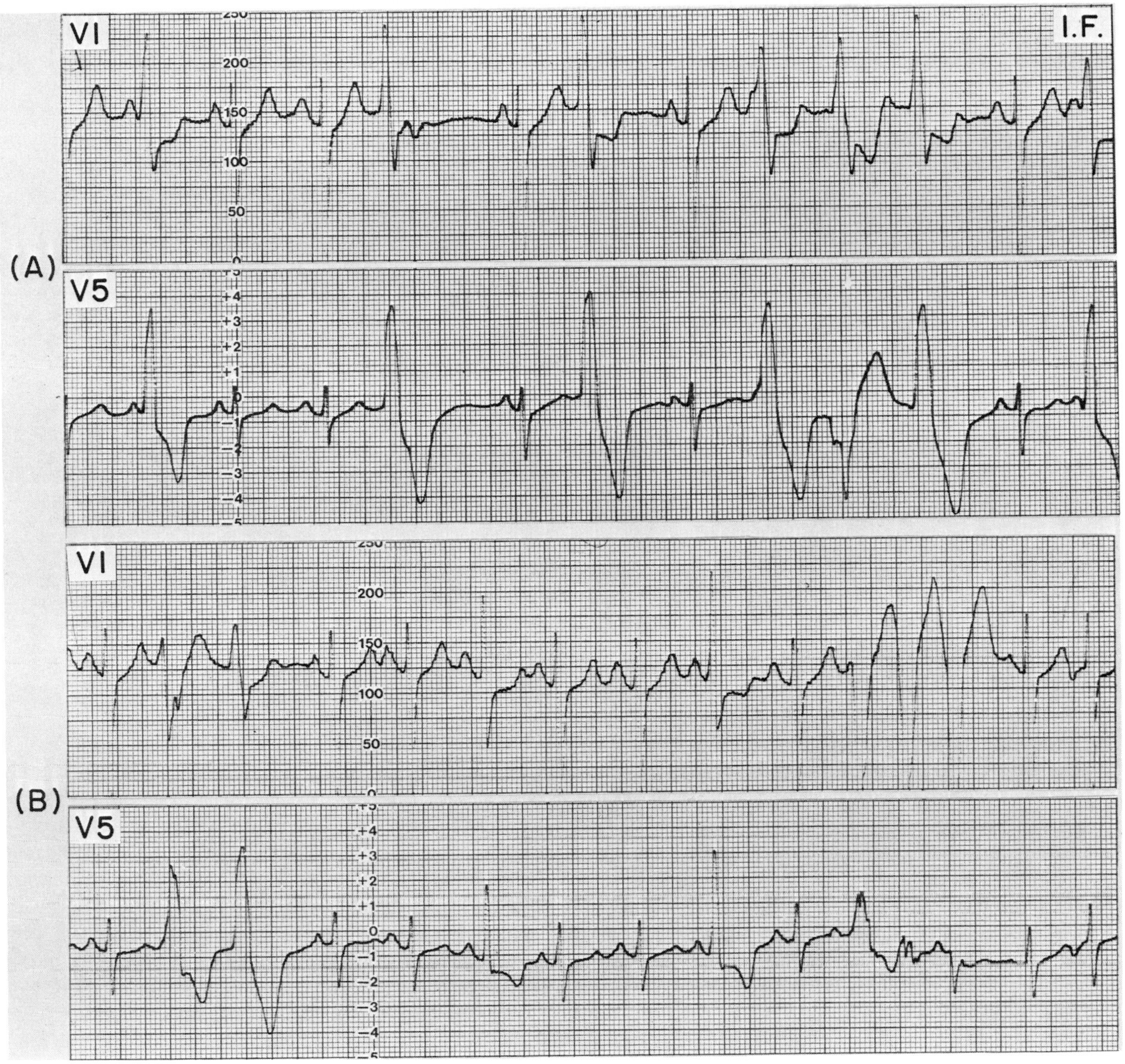

Figure 23-21. *Representative two-channel Holter monitor recordings from a patient with a cardiomyopathy and a history of palpitations. Multiform frequent ventricular premature complexes are noted occurring as isolated events and in groups of up to three premature ventricular contractions in a row.*

category of younger patients (under 40 years of age) with second degree AV block with no evidence of underlying heart disease or central nervous system symptoms. Conduction studies in these patients have identified that AV nodal "dysfunction" secondary to altered response to parasympathetic tone appears to be the pathophysiologic basis. In these patients, exercise and atropine reduce or eliminate second and first degree AV block. Figure 23-31*A* shows an episode of second degree AV block of the Wenckebach type that is followed, in Figure 23-31*B*, by sinus tachycardia with a normal PR interval. This recording was obtained from a man aged 30 years without symptoms who, at rest, had persistent second degree AV block (type I). Conduction studies identified the site of block at the AV nodal level. Atropine administration as well as exercise abolished the block. Although the long-term prognosis of these patients is uncertain, repeated Holter recordings appear necessary to follow their clinical status.

In patients with a history of features of intermittent

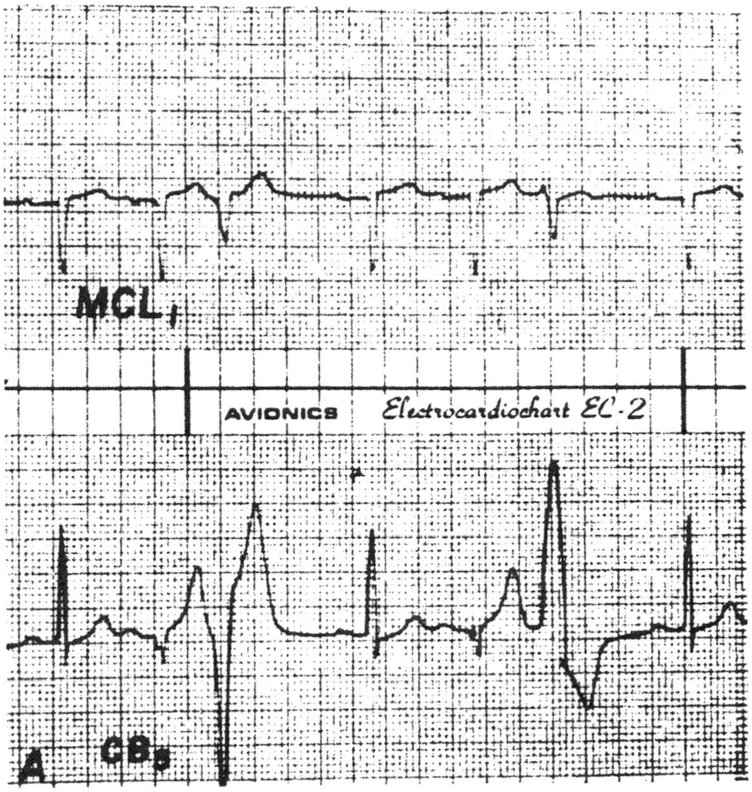

Figure 23-22. *Two-channel Holter monitor recording demonstrating the importance of a two-channel recording system to define the nature of premature complexes. In the* top strip, *using only the upper channel, premature complexes are noted, but the exact nature is uncertain. In the* bottom strip, *a simultaneous record demonstrates multiform configurations of the premature ventricular complexes.*

syncope or near syncope, Holter recordings can be invaluable. The documentation of paroxysmal advanced AV block in patients with intermittent central nervous system symptoms may prove lifesaving. Nevertheless, persistence on the part of the clinician may be of paramount importance, especially in the patient with infrequent symptoms. An example of this clinical problem is shown in Figure 23-32. The record in this figure was obtained from a woman aged 50 years with a 5-year history of seizures of the grand mal type. The patient had previously been investigated by three neurologists who had been unsuccessful in eliminating her "seizures" despite extensive neurologic evaluation and pharmacologic therapy. The patient was hospitalized by her physician for further studies, during which time she was noted to have an electrocardiogram with right bundle branch

(Text continues on p. 600.)

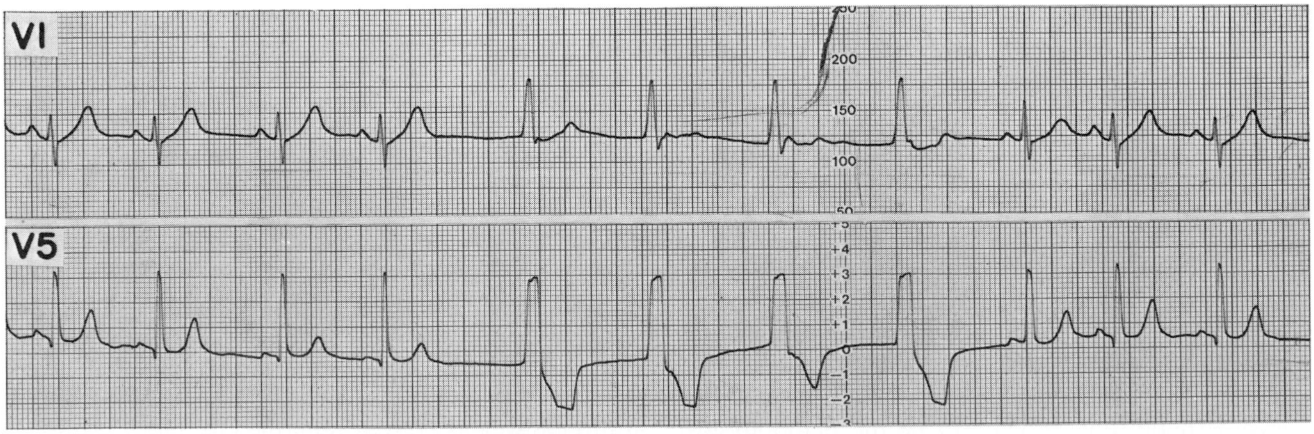

Figure 23-23. *Two-channel Holter monitor recordings obtained from a patient without clinical symptoms. In the middle of the recordings, note that the significant sinus arrhythmia was terminated by the appearance of accelerated idioventricular rhythm lasting four complexes. Subsequently, sinus rhythm is restored.*

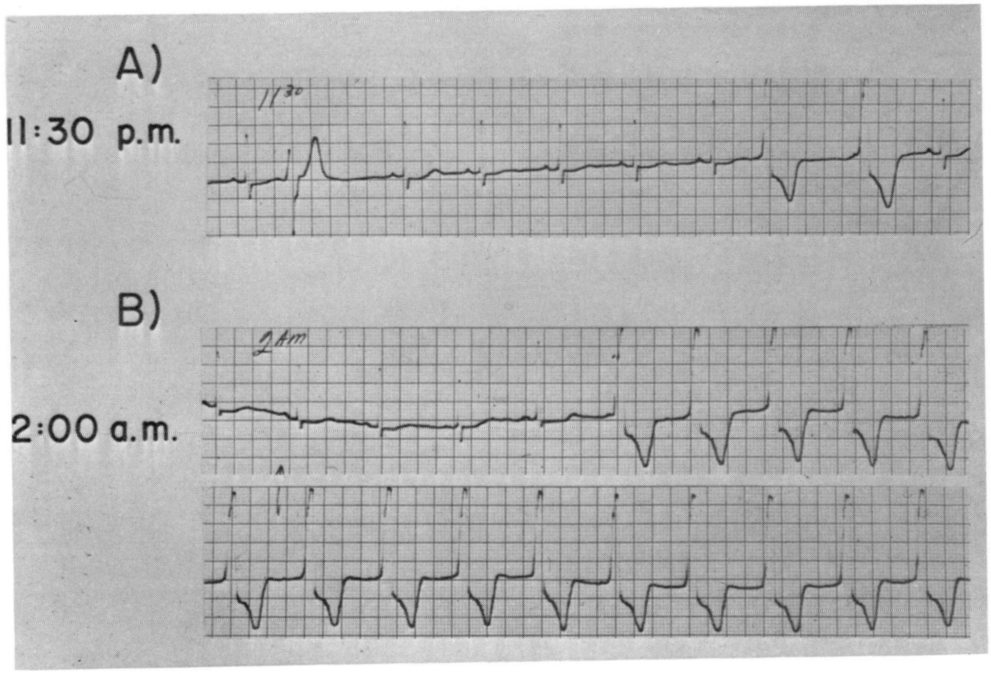

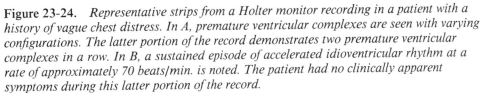

Figure 23-24. *Representative strips from a Holter monitor recording in a patient with a history of vague chest distress. In A, premature ventricular complexes are seen with varying configurations. The latter portion of the record demonstrates two premature ventricular complexes in a row. In B, a sustained episode of accelerated idioventricular rhythm at a rate of approximately 70 beats/min. is noted. The patient had no clinically apparent symptoms during this latter portion of the record.*

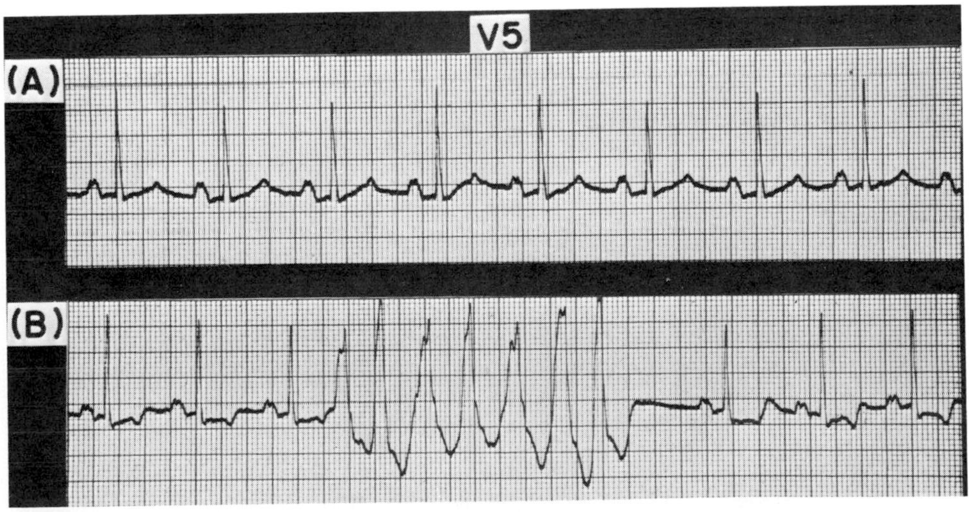

Figure 23-25. *Representative single-channel Holter monitor recordings from a patient with ischemic heart disease and a history of palpitations. In A, during a time when the patient was free from pain, normal ST segments are noted and the patient has no ventricular arrhythmias. In B, during an episode of significant angina, the patient complained of palpitations. ST segment depression of significant degree is noted associated with a short run of ventricular tachycardia, lasting seven complexes.*

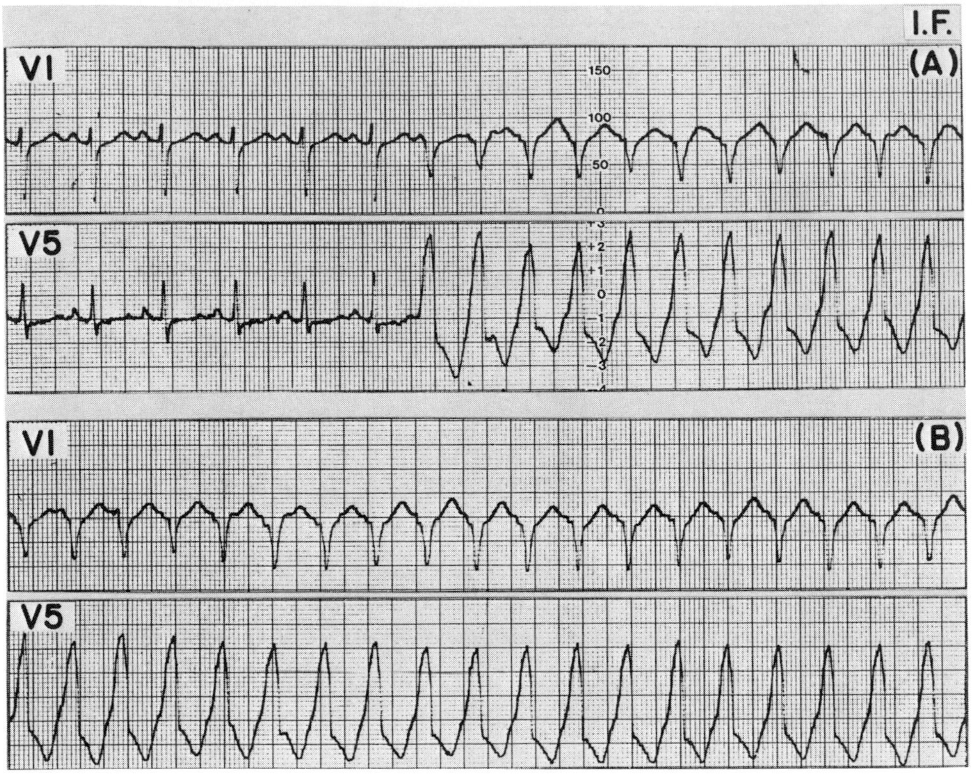

Figure 23-26. *Paroxysms of ventricular tachycardia are not always recognized by the patient even though the ventricular rates during such tachycardia episodes are over 100 beats/min. This is illustrated by the recordings shown in this figure. In A, the onset of ventricular tachycardia at a rate of approximately 140 beats/min. is noted. A sustained episode of the ventricular tachycardia is observed in B. The patient had a history of palpitations but was unaware of this episode despite the relatively rapid rate.*

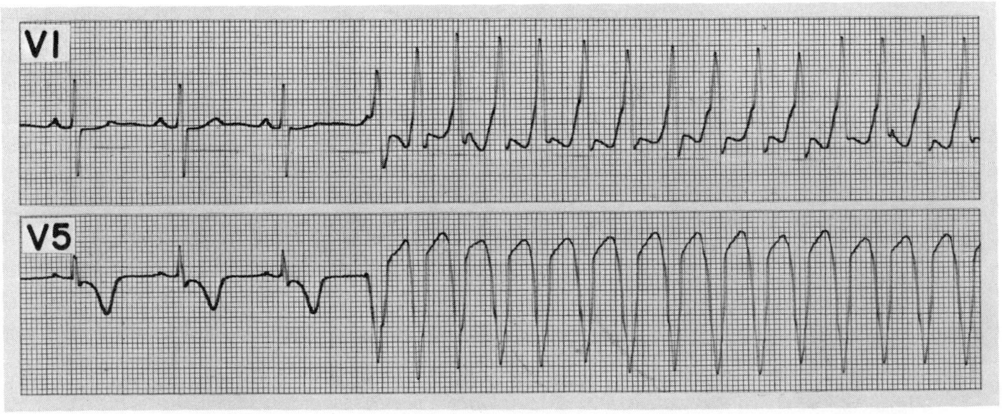

Figure 23-27. *Two-channel Holter monitor recordings obtained from a patient with recurrent palpitations and near-syncopal episodes. The onset of ventricular tachycardia is clearly observed. The ventricular tachycardia rate is approximately 170 beats/min. After the tachycardia began, the patient was clinically symptomatic and had a near-syncopal episode.*

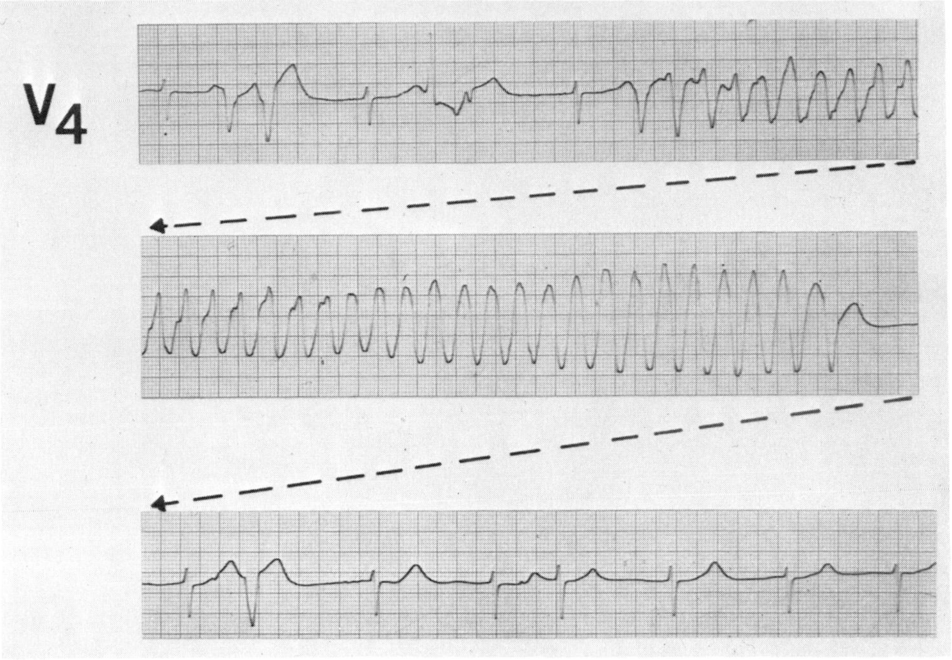

Figure 23-28. *Recordings obtained from a patient with recurrent near-syncopal episodes following institution of quinidine therapy. Note that multiform premature ventricular complexes are present at the beginning of the* top strip. *A sustained burst of ventricular tachycardia is observed initiated by a ventricular premature complex that interrupts the T wave in a complex with a markedly prolonged QT interval. The ventricular tachycardia/ flutter terminates spontaneously with restoration of sinus rhythm.*

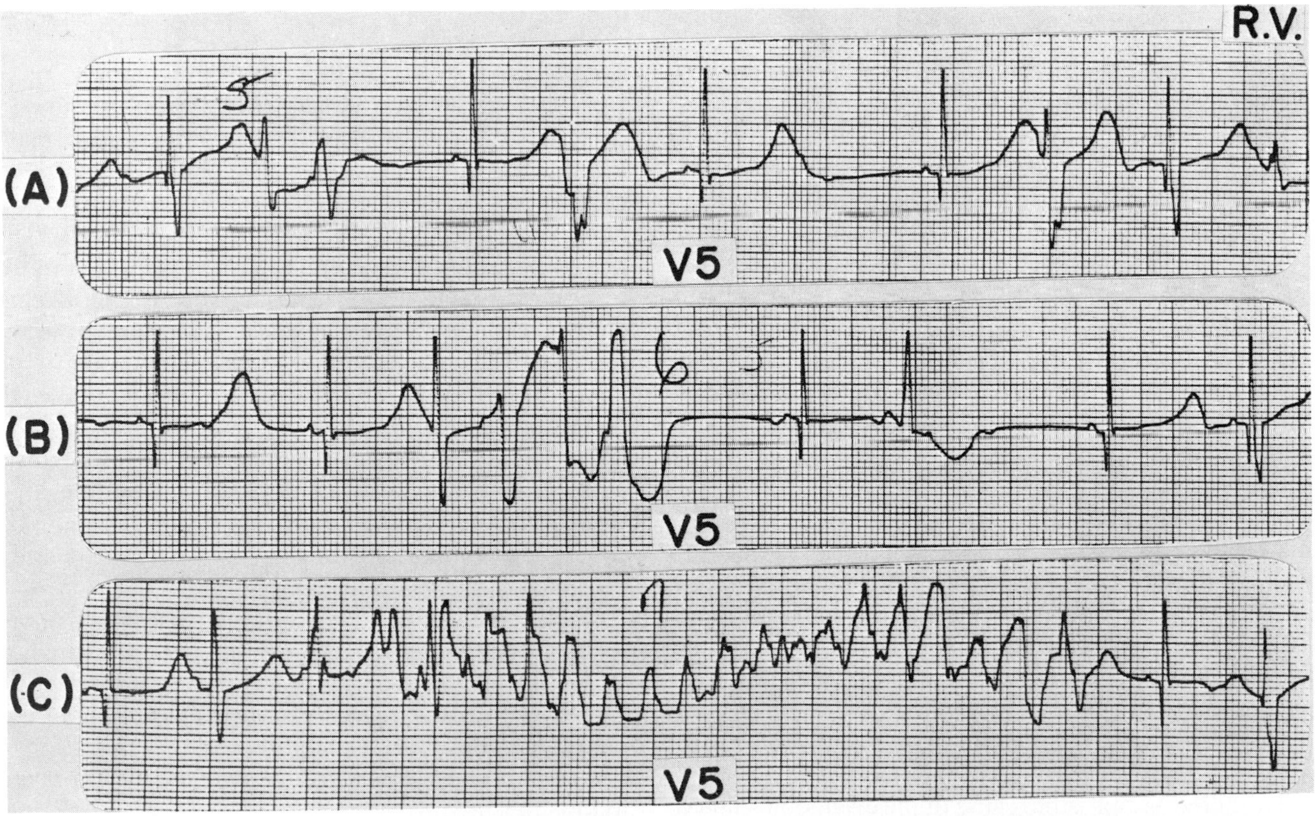

Figure 23-29. *Holter monitor strips obtained from a girl aged 7 years with recurrent syncopal episodes. In A and B, the patient demonstrates multiform premature ventricular complexes, sometimes occurring in short bursts. In C, a ventricular premature complex initiates a burst of ventricular tachycardia with features suggestive of* torsade de pointes. *This patient had a hereditary QT prolongation syndrome.*

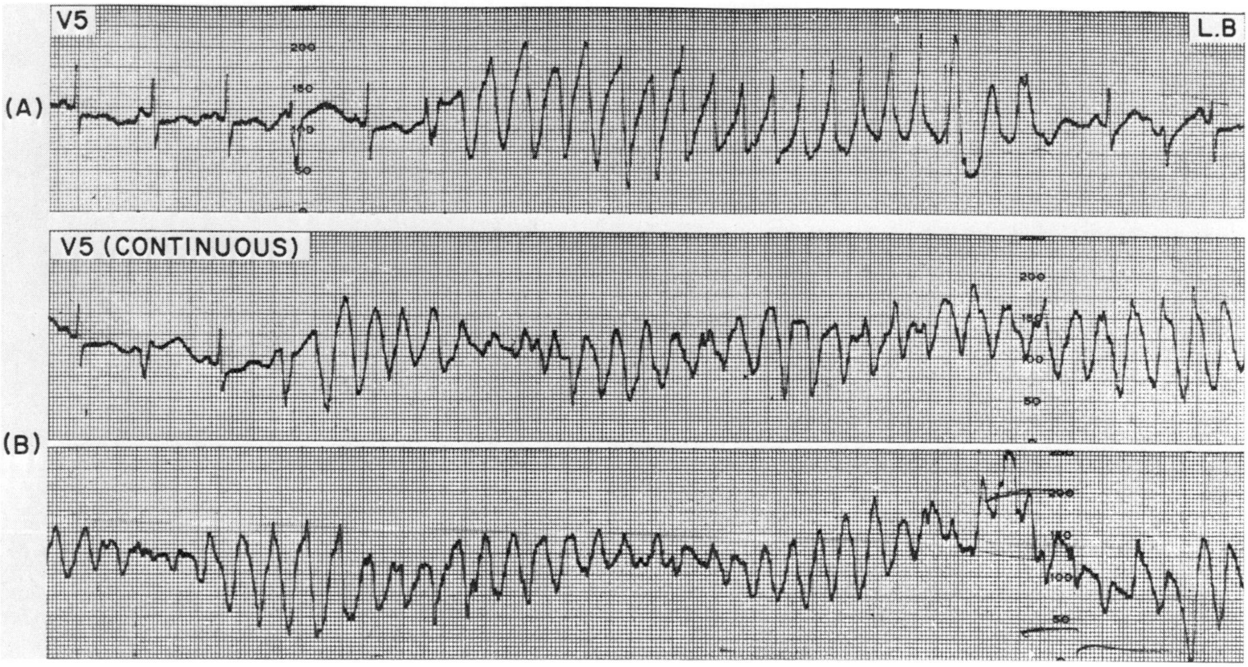

Figure 23-30. *Two representative strips from a patient who had been taking a liquid protein mixture without medical supervision to lose weight. In A, a burst of ventricular tachycardia is noted with characteristic features of* torsade de pointes. *In B, a continuous episode of ventricular tachycardia/flutter/fibrillation is observed.*

block, left anterior superior fascicular block, and first degree AV block. The patient was to undergo conduction studies but had a Holter recording before the catheterization. The Holter recording shown in Figure 23-32 was obtained during this study and shows an episode of paroxysmal AV block during a "seizure" episode. The patient subsequently had a permanent pacemaker implanted, with complete cure of her "seizure" disorder.

These examples, albeit unusual, point out the benefits of Holter recording in patients with onset of suspected paroxysmal AV block. Pacemaker therapy may be justifiably withheld or urgently implemented based on the results of such studies.

Sudden Cardiac Death

Holter monitoring has been very useful in identifying the arrhythmic mechanism(s) of sudden cardiac death. The original documentation of sudden death during Holter monitoring by Bleifer and colleages[14] has been followed by observation from multiple centers.[38–43]

Denes and associates, in their observations on five patients, identified increase in the QT_c possibly related to quinidine as a possible cause of the events.[44] Detailed analysis of premonitory data in other reports has further aided in clinicians' understanding the premorbid charges in ventricular arrhythmias that may herald sudden death. Nikolic and co-workers[45] identified in six patients complex ventricular arrhythmias, variations of cycle length, and the R-on-T phenomenon as major events. Lewis and co-workers,[46] in 12 patients, further confirmed (1) an increase in premature complexes or complexity preceding the terminal event, (2) R-on-T phenomenon, and (3) repolarization abnormality for several hours before the termination event. They did not confirm changes in cycle length as an important factor. Finally, Pratt and co-workers,[47] in their study of 15 patients, confirmed (1) an increase in ventricular arrhythmia (number and complexity) and (2) ventricular fibrillation preceded by ventricular tachycardia in all patients. R-on-T phenomenon and QT prolongation were not significant factors. In contrast, Roelandt and colleagues[48] found that no specific arrhythmic pattern predicted sudden cardiac death

Vlay and colleagues[49] have found that Holter monitoring 1 month following the index event in patients who survive sudden cardiac death has important prognostic value. If ventricular tachycardia (asymptomatic) persisted (≥3 beats, ≥120 beats/min) at that time, 42% of the patients had syncope or sudden death by 700 days of follow-up study.

Patients who have sustained an acute myocardial infarction are a much larger group who may be at risk for sudden cardiac death. Prior studies have sought to iden-

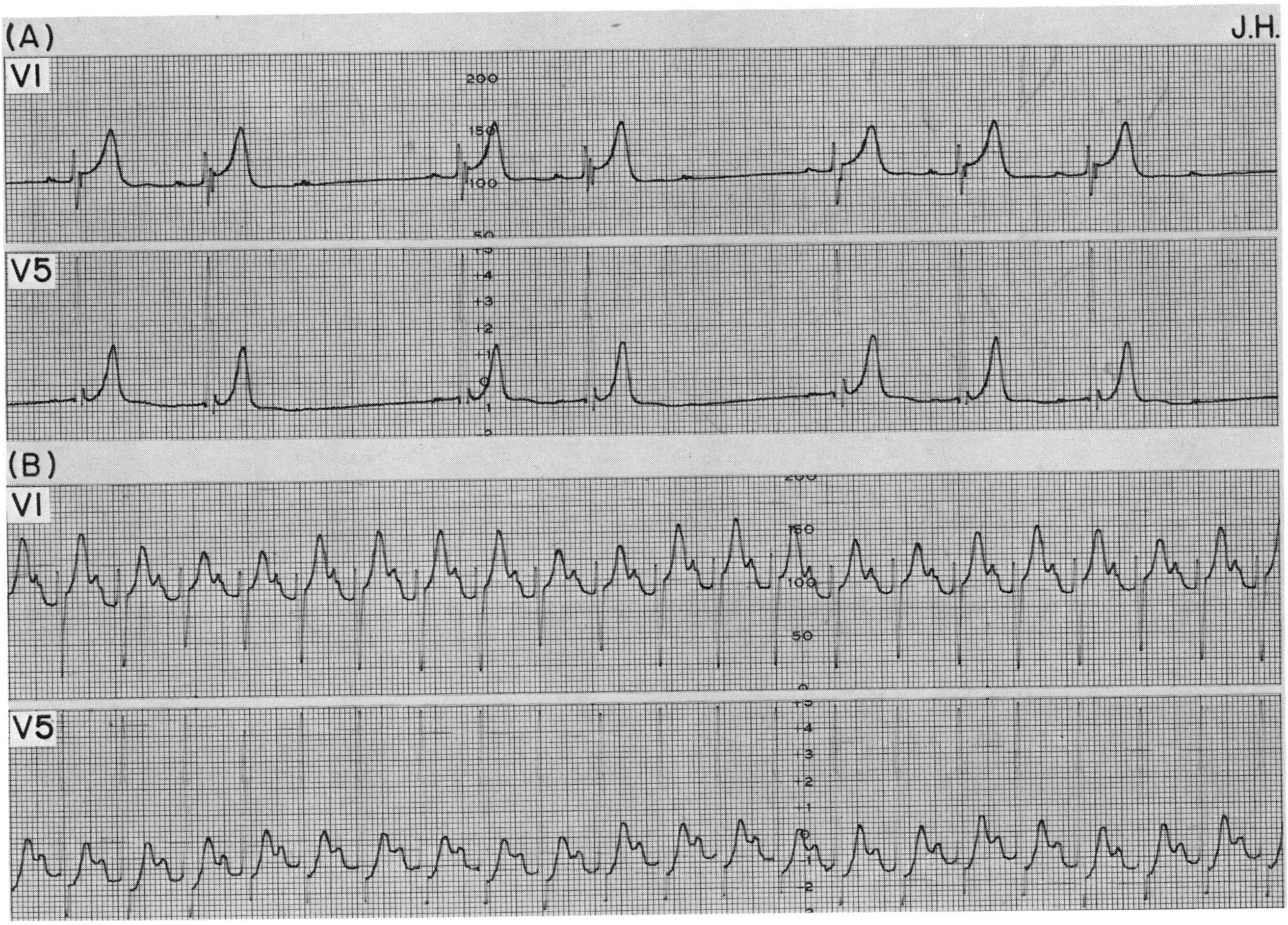

Figure 23-31. *Representative Holter monitor two-channel recordings from a patient with episodic second degree AV block. In A, typical group-beating episodes are seen with characteristic features suggestive of AV nodal Wenckebach phenomenon. In B, during an episode of vigorous activity, 1:1 AV conduction is noted with a PR interval that is within the normal range.*

tify whether ventricular arrhythmias alone or by special category are of value for predicting which patients will have sudden death. These studies have been criticized for a variety of flaws in design. Recently, in a carefully designed prospective cooperative study on 766 patients evaluated using multivariate analysis, Bigger and coworkers identified that ventricular arrhythmias *are* an independent risk related to mortality.[50]

Electrophysiologic studies have been considered the hallmark for evaluation of the treatment for patients who have had recurrent ventricular tachycardia or ventricular fibrillation. Many centers have now undertaken prospective studies attempting to evaluate the comparative worth of noninvasive Holter monitoring versus invasive evaluation by electrophysiologic testing. Recent studies by Platia and Reed[51] identified that the electrophysiologic studies had a better long-term predictive accuracy than Holter monitoring.

Hypertrophic Cardiomyopathy

Patients with hypertrophic cardiomyopathy are noted to have a significant incidence of syncope and sudden death. Holter monitoring has been used as a tool to assess the incidence and complexity of ventricular arrhythmias in this patient population. Maron and colleagues[52] have determined that 66% of a cohort of 99 patients had "high-grade" ventricular arrhythmias, including 19% with asymptomatic ventricular tachycardia. This latter group appears to identify a subset of patients who are at high risk for sudden death.

Digitalis-Induced Arrhythmias

The relationship between digitalis administration, serum digoxin levels, and the incidence of arrhythmias considered to represent digitalis intoxication was studied

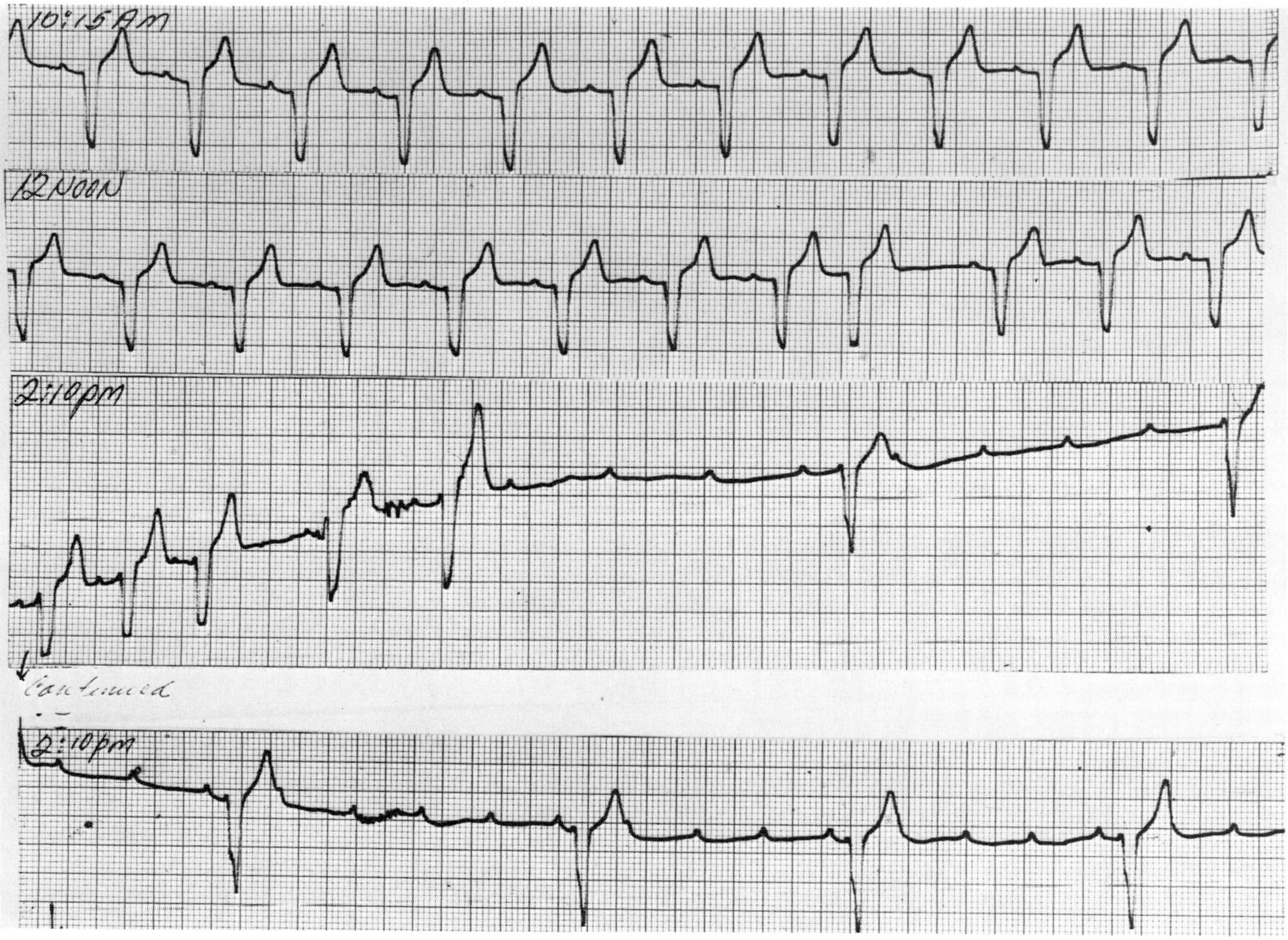

Figure 23-32. *Holter monitor strips obtained from a patient with recurrent epileptic "seizures" who had, on a standard electrocardiogram, right bundle branch block with anterior superior fascicular block and first degree AV block. The* two lower strips *demonstrate the features seen during a typical "seizure" in which paroxysmal AV block occurred.*

in a prospective manner by Goren and Denes.[53] These authors noted that digitalis-provoked arrhythmias were demonstrated in 10 of 69 patients undergoing Holter monitoring. There was *no* relationship between these arrhythmias and the digoxin level. It was concluded that rhythm disorders considered typical for digitalis intoxication do not always reflect clinically evident toxicity.

Cardiac Surgery

Patients subjected to cardiac surgery are frequency noted to have atrial and ventricular arrhythmias in the perioperative period. Dewar and associates[54] have reported on a detailed preoperative, intraoperative, and postoperative Holter monitoring study in 52 adult patients undergoing cardiac surgery. Their investigations identified (1) a high incidence of arrhythmias associated with anesthesia induction and thoracotomy, (2) a lack of correlation between peak creatinine kinase (MB) and arrhythmias, and (3) a higher incidence of arrhythmias in valve replacements.

In children undergoing cardiac surgery, arrhythmias have been well documented, especially in patients who have undergone repair of an atrial septal defect or a Mustard procedure. Potentially more important is the group that includes patients having repair for tetralogy of Fallot in whom ventricular arrhythmias and sudden death have been documented. In a prospective study, Ringel and colleagues[55] evaluated 65 patients with Holter recordings preoperatively as well as early (1 to 10 days) and late (3 to 12 months) postoperatively. The preoperative data indicated a 25% incidence of supraventricular and a 39% incidence of ventricular arrhythmias. These percentages were increased dramatically in the early postoperative state and were still above preoperative values in the later postoperative period.

Pacemaker Evaluation

Implantations of permanent pacemakers have increased at a dramatic rate since their introduction into the armamentarium of the cardiologist. Over the past two decades, electronic circuitry and design have improved at a spectacular rate, allowing pacemaker manufacturers to develop smaller and much more reliable units. These developments have been paralleled by the development of new power sources that have increased the longevity of the devices severalfold. Moreover, new units have been developed that allow for the addition of new pacemaker functions, making the implanted unit an even more highly specialized electronic instrument. External programmability of multiple parameters, sensing and pacing of multiple chambers, multiple pacing modes for the same unit, and especially the DDD pacemaker have introduced a complexity into the evaluation of unit function that requires specialized knowledge. The use of pacemakers has necessitated that a sophisticated system of follow-up study of the functional integrity of the entire system (generator, power source, electrodes) be made available. The development in many cardiologic centers of pacemaker evaluation units designed solely to analyze pacemaker function has proved invaluable in the long-term follow-up study of pacemaker patients. Critical rate analysis, rhythm strip interpretation, waveform analysis, and so on have been inherent in the evaluation of these patients. Nevertheless, some patients have intermittent pacemaker malfunction that escapes detection even with the sophisticated analysis outlined above. The electrocardiographic surveillance used in most pacemaker clinics requires the recording of a short (30-second to 2-minute) rhythm strip directly or transtelephonically. This limited database may fail to reveal any significant intermittent malfunctions, which may also not be detected by rate or waveform analysis. The use of Holter monitor recordings has been invaluable in evaluating intermittent pacemaker malfunction in symptomatic patients. In addition, Holter monitor recordings may prove to be invaluable in the detection of pacemaker malfunction that has not, as yet, been significant enough to be associated with clinical complaints.

It is not suggested that Holter monitoring replace the present mode of pacemaker evaluation but rather that it be used as an important ancillary tool to evaluate pacemaker patients. In this regard, this chapter demonstrates the usefulness of Holter monitor recording by illustrating a variety of examples of intermittent pacemaker failure. In Figure 23-33, a 24-hour Holter record was recorded in a patient with a permanent ventricular demand (VVI) pacemaker who complained of the recent onset of palpitations. Rhythm strip analysis at the time of follow-up study had revealed rare premature ventricular complexes that were appropriately sensed and suppressed by the pacemaker unit. However, during the course of the 24-hour recording, numerous examples of both failure to pace and failure to sense were recorded, which resulted in the replacement of the unit. The observations in such patients have led Kelen and colleagues to develop a Holter scanning system that will enable the technician to evaluate even rare episodes of failure to sense or capture.[56] Their circuitry allows for isolation of pacemaker artifact from the QRS, with quantification of both waveforms, analog display, and statistical presentation. This system will much more clearly enable the Holter monitor to serve as a tool in evaluating potential pacemaker malfunction.

The pacemaker patient with recurrent dizzy episodes postimplantation may be a frustrating clinical problem. Noncardiac causes must be evaluated in detail, but pacemaker malfunction must also be considered. Detailed pacemaker function analysis may, as described above, fail to identify any significant abnormality. Figure 23-34 was recorded from a patient with recent onset of recurrent near-syncopal episodes. The 24-hour Holter recording did not demonstrate any prolonged pauses but did show occasional isolated premature ventricular complexes (see Fig. 23-34*A*) that were sensed appropriately. However, occasional irregular firing was noted (see Fig. 23-34*B*). The initial impression was that "concealed" premature ventricular complexes were being sensed, resulting in recycling of the pacemaker, but antiarrhythmic therapy failed to suppress these pauses. In this patient with a unipolar unit, significant pectoralis muscle exercise produced total suppression of the device and thereby duplicated the patient's symptoms. In retrospect, the artifact seen in Figure 23-34*B* indicated minor muscle artifact that was sensed by the unit, resulting in partial suppression. The unipolar device was converted to a bipolar unit, with total elimination of the patient's symptoms.

A somewhat similar clinical situation is illustrated in Figure 23-35, which shows the Holter monitor recordings from a patient with the sick sinus syndrome and a permanent atrial pacemaker (AOO). This patient also complained of recurrent dizzy episodes postimplantation; however, pacemaker clinic evaluation was normal. A 24-hour Holter recording was done, which showed, during the dizzy spells, multiple episodes of pacemaker failure. In retrospect, the patient revealed that she only had symptoms while in certain positions. Subsequent evaluation revealed a partial lead fracture in this patient. Implantation of a new lead restored normal pacemaker function.

Holter monitor recording is not only useful for evaluation of pacemaker malfunction but can also identify unusual causes of pacemaker-associated problems.

A 24-hour Holter recording was obtained in a patient with a newly implanted ventricular demand (VVI) unit

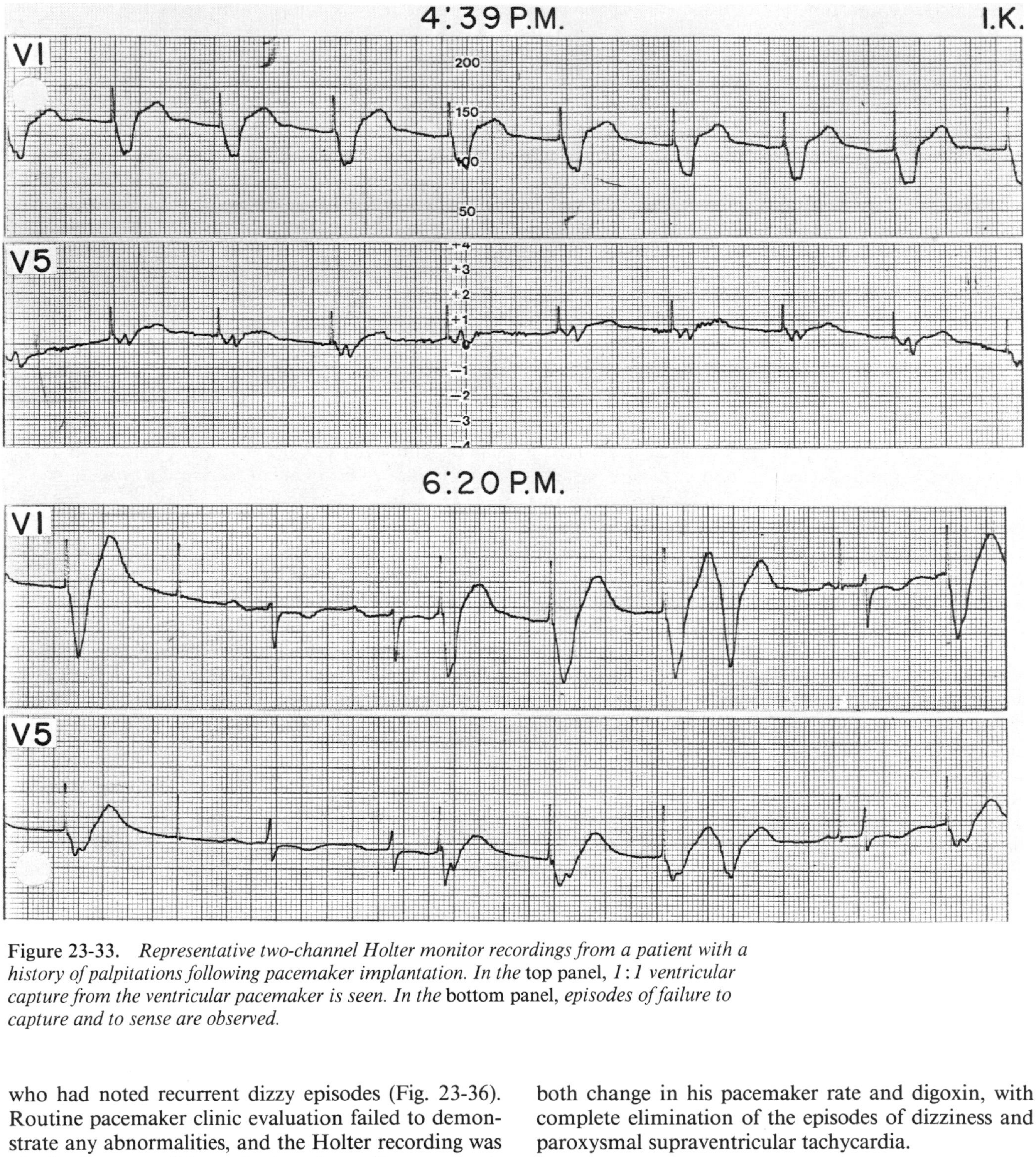

Figure 23-33. *Representative two-channel Holter monitor recordings from a patient with a history of palpitations following pacemaker implantation. In the* top panel, *1:1 ventricular capture from the ventricular pacemaker is seen. In the* bottom panel, *episodes of failure to capture and to sense are observed.*

who had noted recurrent dizzy episodes (Fig. 23-36). Routine pacemaker clinic evaluation failed to demonstrate any abnormalities, and the Holter recording was obtained as part of the patient work-up. Recurrent episodes of paroxysmal supraventricular tachycardia were demonstrated during this 24-hour recording. AV dissociation was present, and with an appropriately timed P wave, sinus capture occurred. However, if the P waves were appropriately positioned, significant anterograde delay occurred, allowing sustained AV nodal reciprocating tachycardia to develop. This patient was treated with both change in his pacemaker rate and digoxin, with complete elimination of the episodes of dizziness and paroxysmal supraventricular tachycardia.

Artifacts in Holter Monitoring

The previous sections have discussed the use of Holter recordings in the evaluation and management of cardiovascular patients. However, it is essential that both the technician and the physician be aware of the many pit-

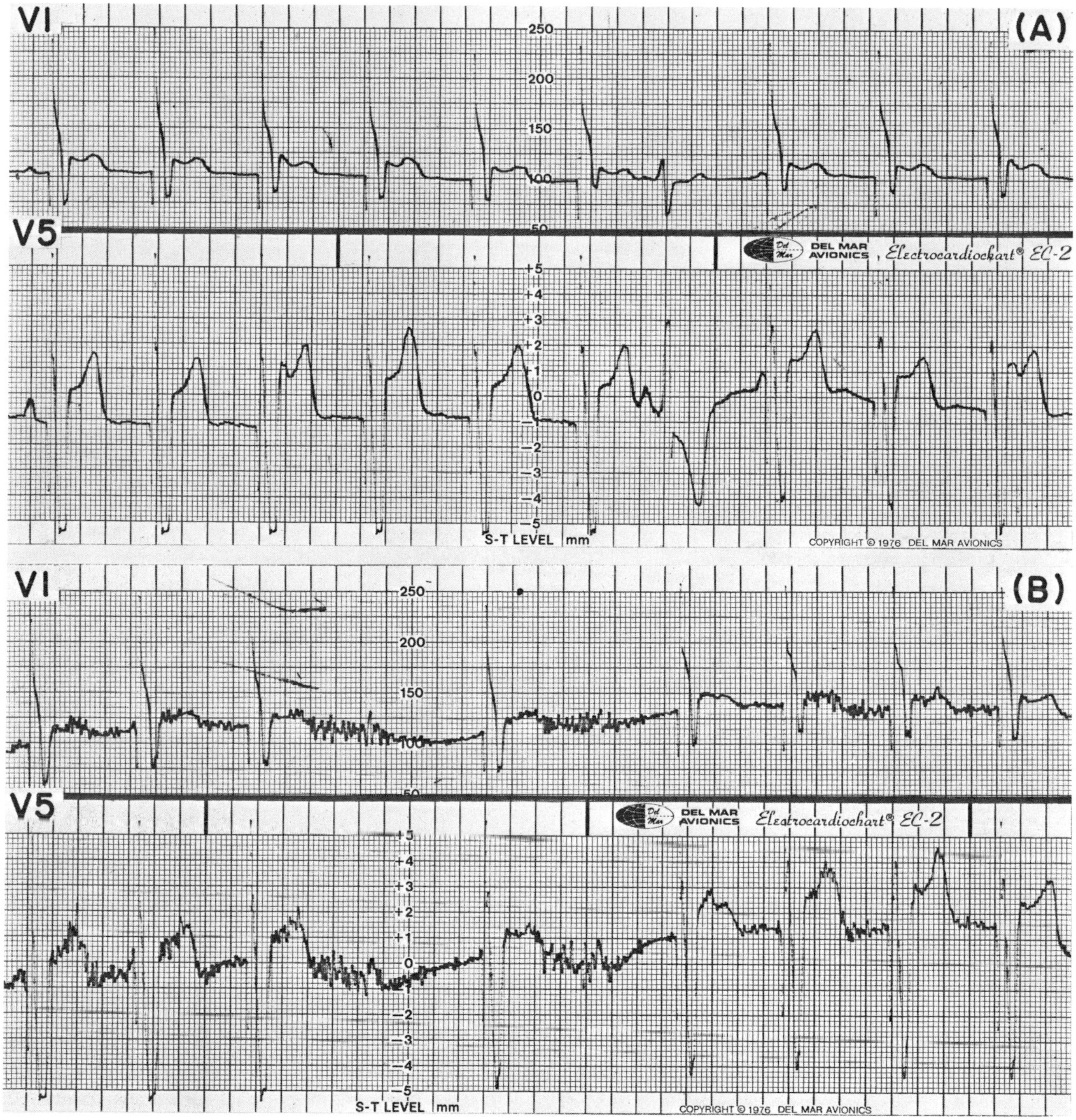

Figure 23-34. *Two representative Holter recordings from a patient who had an aortic valve replacement and an implanted permanent ventricular demand pacemaker. The patient complained of a recent onset of near-syncopal episodes. In A, a premature complex is sensed by the pacemaker. In B, irregular firing of the ventricular pacemaker is noted without premature complexes being observed. The artifacts seen on the electrocardiogram represent somatic muscle noise. The original interpretation of this tracing was that concealed ventricular premature complexes were producing recycling of the pacemaker. On further examination, when the patient voluntarily produced pectoralis muscle activity, the pacemaker was suppressed, indicating myopotential sensing by the unipolar pacemaker. The pacemaker was converted to a bipolar mode, and no more syncopal or near-syncopal episodes occurred.*

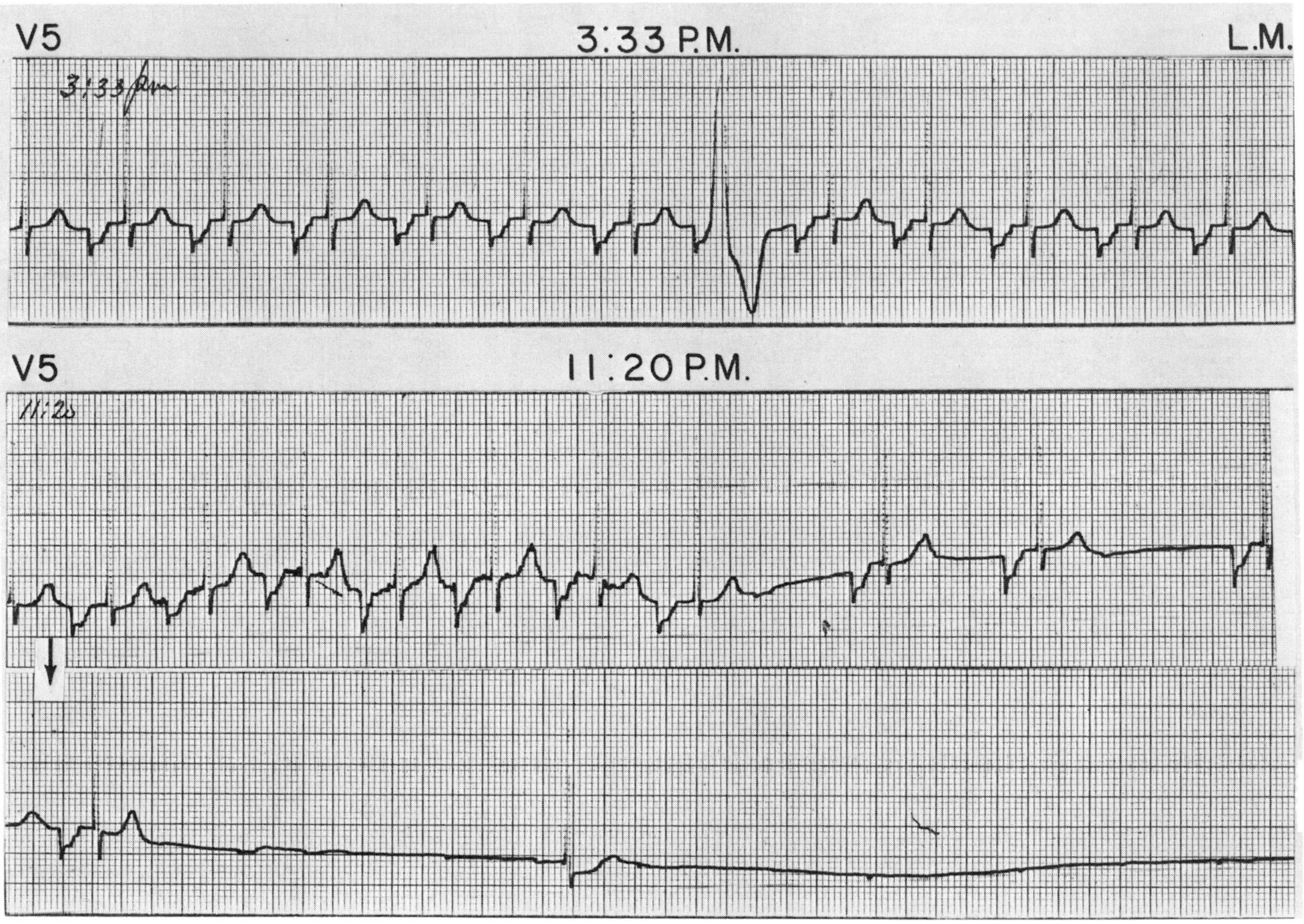

Figure 23-35. *Two representative strips obtained from a Holter monitor recording in a patient with an atrial pacemaker who complained about recurrent syncopal episodes. In the* upper panel, *atrial pacing was noted with one ventricular premature complex seen. In the* lower strip, *when the patient turned abruptly onto her left side, the atrial pacemaker became irregular and finally ceased to fire. Further detailed evaluation revealed that the patient had a fractured lead wire. The pacemaker functioned appropriately once the lead was replaced.*

falls that may occur with the use of 24-hour recorders and playback units.[57,58] It is critical to the patient's well-being that inappropriate interpretation of inaccurate data be prevented from influencing the patient's medical management. Although the Holter recording may be invaluable in the clinical care of many patients, errors in evaluation may be equally costly. This section will identify many of the technical problems that, when recognized, will clarify the appropriate clinical decision-making process.

Technical problems with the recorders, playback amplifier(s), or stylus may be manifest in a variety of ways that may result in inability to evaluate the electrocardiographic events. Excessive damping, inappropriate calibration, saturation of the amplifier, and poorly adjusted stylus are just several of many potential examples that may render the final report worthless for interpretation (Figs. 23-37 and 23-38).

Vacillation in QRS or T wave morphology may frequently be noted related to change in respiration or body position. Recognition of these frequently observed variations is essential for proper interpretation of Holter recordings, especially in patients with suspected ischemic heart disease (Fig. 23-39).

Inappropriate display or inappropriate mounting of the tape during playback, if not recognized, will lead to misdiagnosis, with significant associated clinical implications. In Figure 23-40, the electrocardiographic signal has been displayed in an inverted fashion, which results in an electrocardiographic record with an inverted P wave, a prominent Q wave, and an inverted T wave. Because of this inversion, the inappropriate diagnosis of ectopic atrial or junctional rhythm and repolarization abnormalities could clearly have been made.

In Figure 23-41, the initial impression of this record might be of first degree AV block with short QT interval

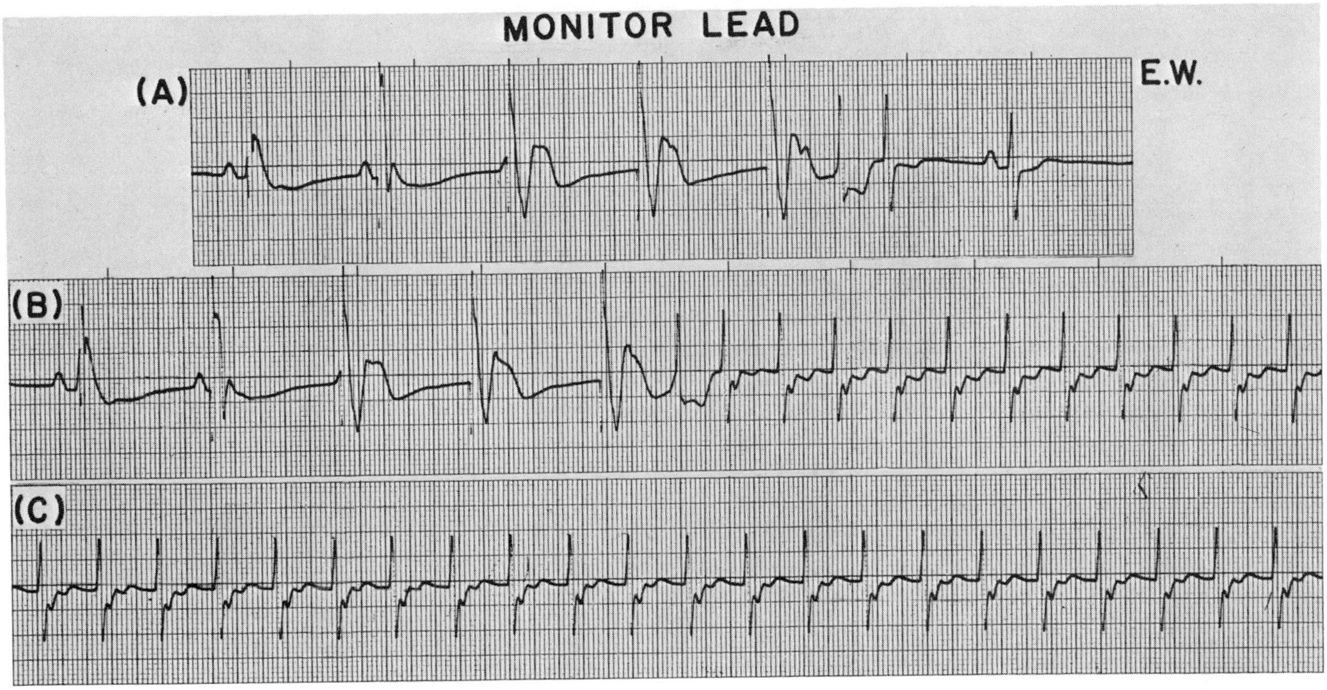

Figure 23-36. *Representative records from a Holter monitor recording in an elderly patient who had a permanent ventricular demand pacemaker implanted because of bradycardia associated with near syncope. Following the implantation of the pacemaker, the patient continued to have syncopal episodes. In A, the Holter monitor record demonstrates the presence of AV dissociation and supraventricular captures. In B, AV dissociation is again noted, with a sinus complex occurring at a time that allows for capture of the ventricle but with an extremely long PR interval. Supraventricular tachycardia is then initiated, resulting in sustained reentrant tachycardia associated with severe central nervous system symptomatology in this elderly patient with diminished cardiovascular reserve.*

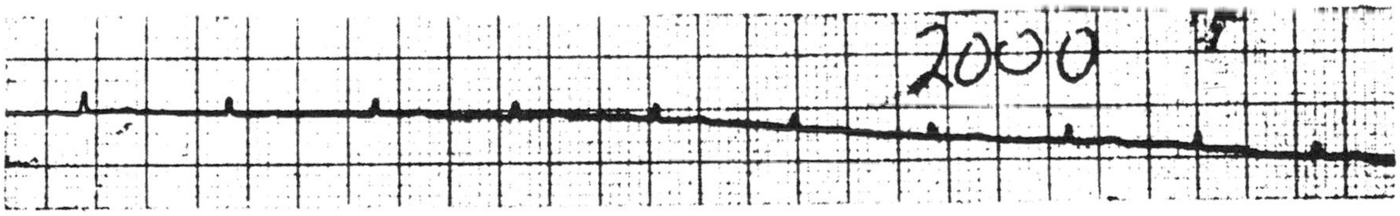

Figure 23-37. *This record demonstrates the influence of partial battery failure on Holter monitor recordings. Note the predominant voltage reduction. (Krasnow, A. Z., and Bloomfield, D. K.: Artifacts in portable electrocardiographic monitoring. Am. Heart J., 91:349, 1976)*

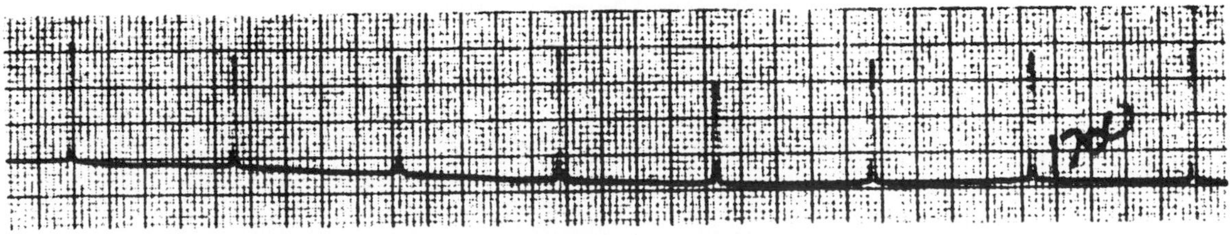

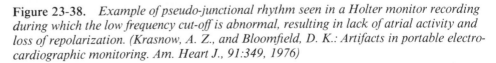

Figure 23-38. *Example of pseudo-junctional rhythm seen in a Holter monitor recording during which the low frequency cut-off is abnormal, resulting in lack of atrial activity and loss of repolarization. (Krasnow, A. Z., and Bloomfield, D. K.: Artifacts in portable electrocardiographic monitoring. Am. Heart J., 91:349, 1976)*

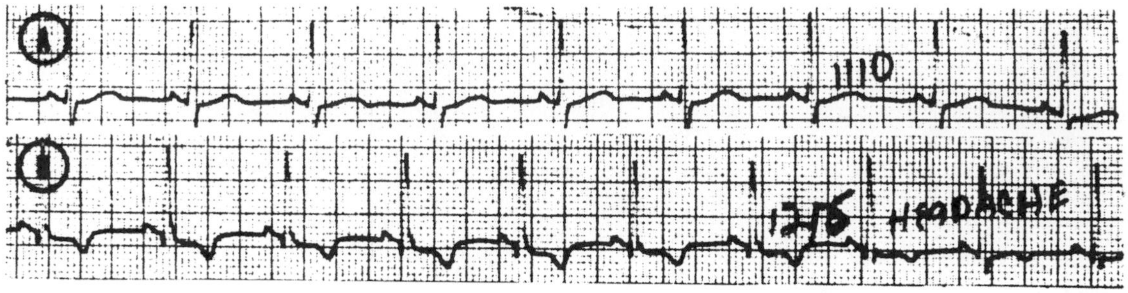

Figure 23-39. *Positional changes in the ST-T wave and the QRS seen in this tracing are commonly noted in Holter monitor recordings in patients without significant cardiac disease. (Krasnow, A. Z., and Bloomfield, D. K.: Artifacts in portable electrocardiographic monitoring. Am. Heart J., 91:349, 1976)*

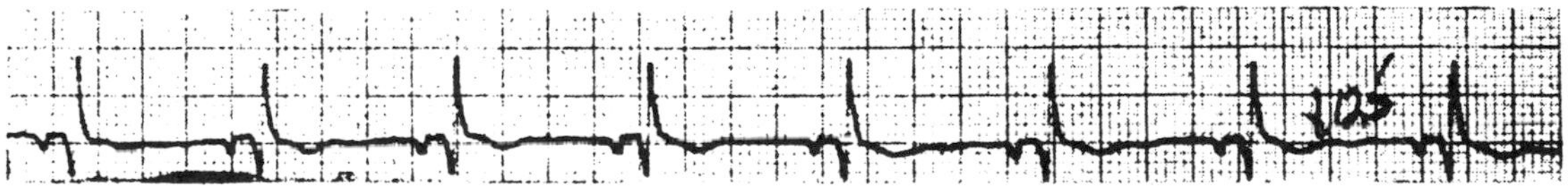

Figure 23-40. *Recording in which reversed polarity is obtained, with inversion of the P, QRS, and T because of improper lead placement. (Krasnow, A. Z., and Bloomfield, D. K.: Artifacts in portable electrocardiographic monitoring. Am. Heart J., 91:349, 1976)*

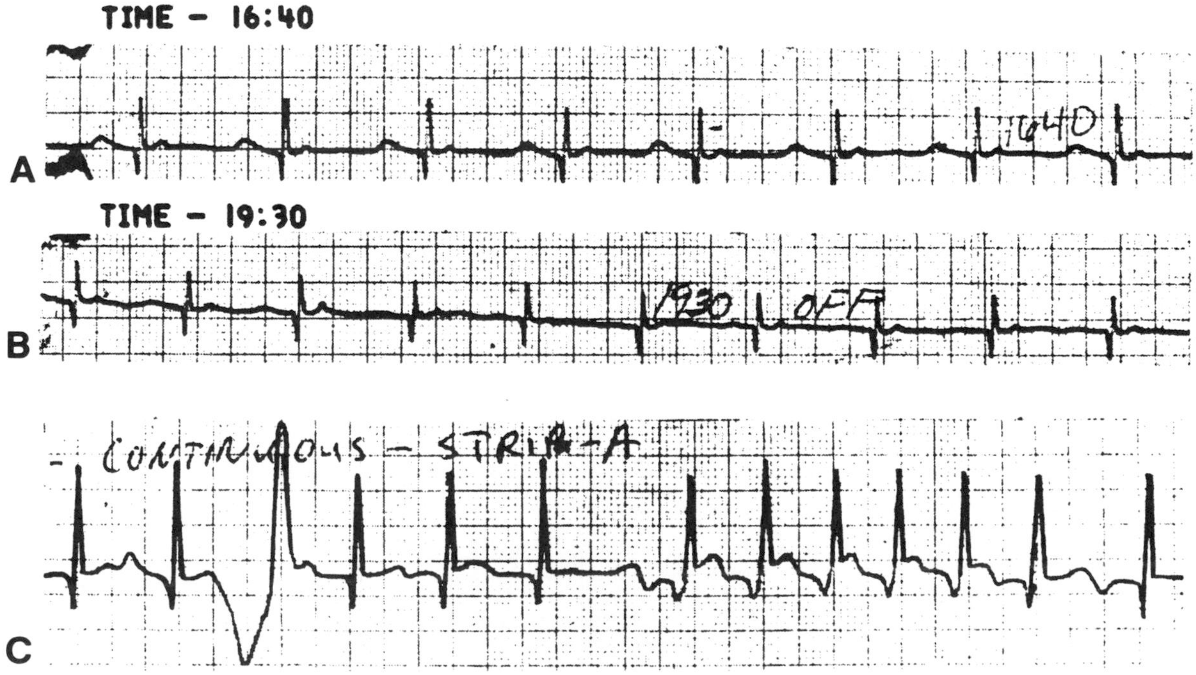

Figure 23-41. *Strips in this recording demonstrate prolonged PR interval, short QT interval, and ST segment elevation. In reality, these strips represent a mirror image sequence in which the tape has been run in a reversed fashion. (Krasnow, A. Z., and Bloomfield, D. K.: Artifacts in portable electrocardiographic monitoring. Am. Heart J., 91:349, 1976)*

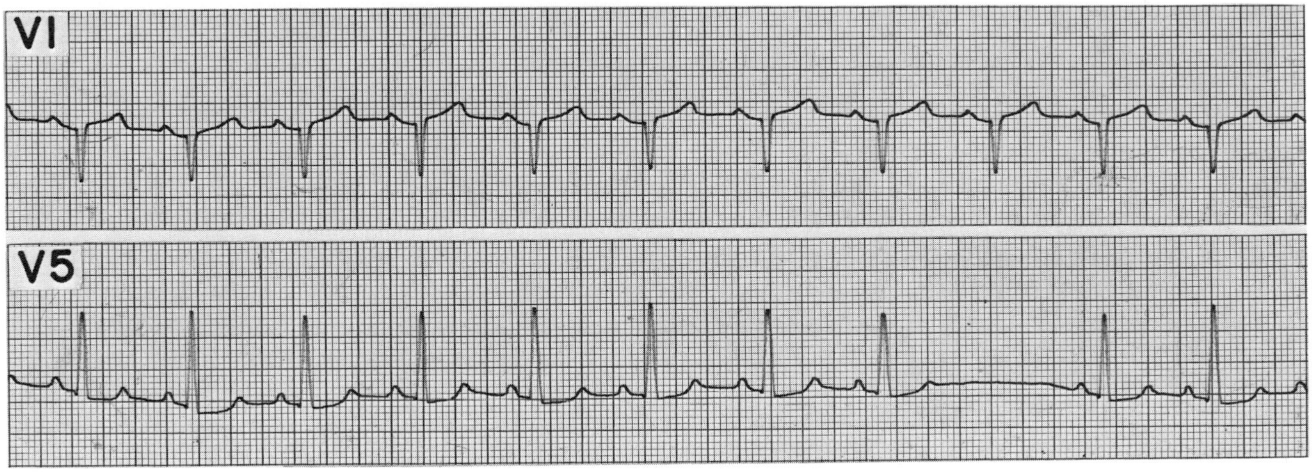

Figure 23-42. *The advantages of a two-channel system are clearly demonstrated by looking at the simultaneously obtained lead V_1 and lead V_5 recordings. In lead V_5, an episode of what appears to be 2:1 sinoatrial block is, in reality, loss of signal on the V_5 electrode during a time at which the patient was clearly in sinus rhythm.*

(see Fig. 23-41*A* and *B*) and ST segment elevations with a premature ventricular complex during tachycardia of possible supraventricular origin. More careful analysis of the tracing reveals that the tape has been analyzed in a reverse fashion, with the resultant electrocardiogram showing T, QRS, and P; the ST segment "elevation" is, in fact, ST depression.

The use of two-channel recorders has previously been emphasized (see Fig. 23-22) with regard to documenting the potential origin of premature complexes. Of equal importance is the significance of two-channel recordings in evaluating artifacts, which, if only single-channel data were available, might lead to erroneous clinical decisions. In Figure 23-42, lead V_5 identifies a sudden pause that is a multiple of the sinus rate, suggesting 2:1 sinoatrial block. However, in lead V_1, the "absent" sinus complex was clearly recorded, thereby identifying that the sinoatrial block was, in fact, a lead artifact.

More protracted technical artifacts can lead to the clinical decision for urgent permanent pacing even if the patient remains asymptomatic. In Figure 23-43, such an example is seen in which, despite the use of a two-channel Holter monitor, transient recording failure has produced a short pause (MV_1) followed by a long pause. The clue to the artifactual nature of this record is the absence of the pause in the first portion of the record (MV_5) and the irregular nature of the second and longer pause in the MV_1 and the MV_5.

In Figures 23-42 and 23-43, sudden pauses were apparent that were multiples of the basic sinus cycle length. These technical artifacts were due to lead electrode artifacts or electronic artifacts. However, another form of

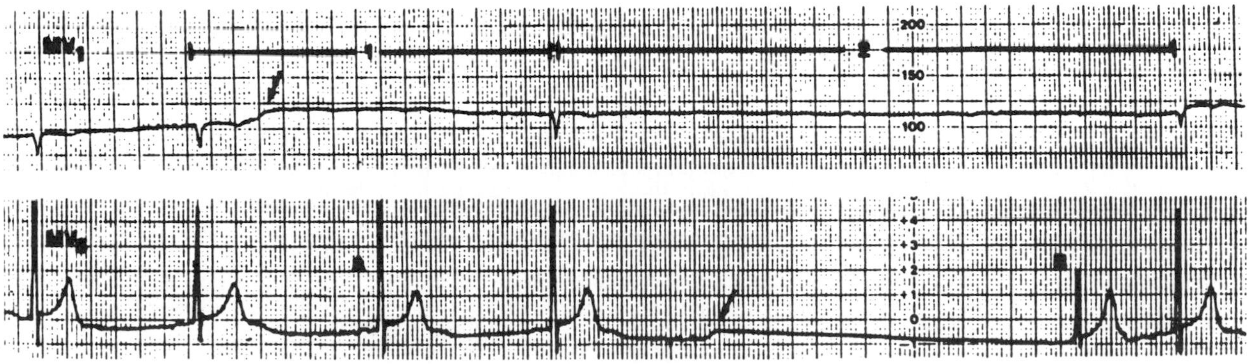

Figure 23-43. *A more dramatic example of the events illustrated in Figure 23-42. This two-channel recording identifies repeated loss of signal in the* upper strip *and intermittent loss of signal in the* lower strip. *The above data suggest marked sinus node dysfunction but in reality are artifactual secondary to signal loss. (Gardin, J. M., Belic, N., and Singer, D. H.: Pseudoarrhythmias in ambulatory ECG monitoring. Arch. Intern. Med., 139:809, 1979)*

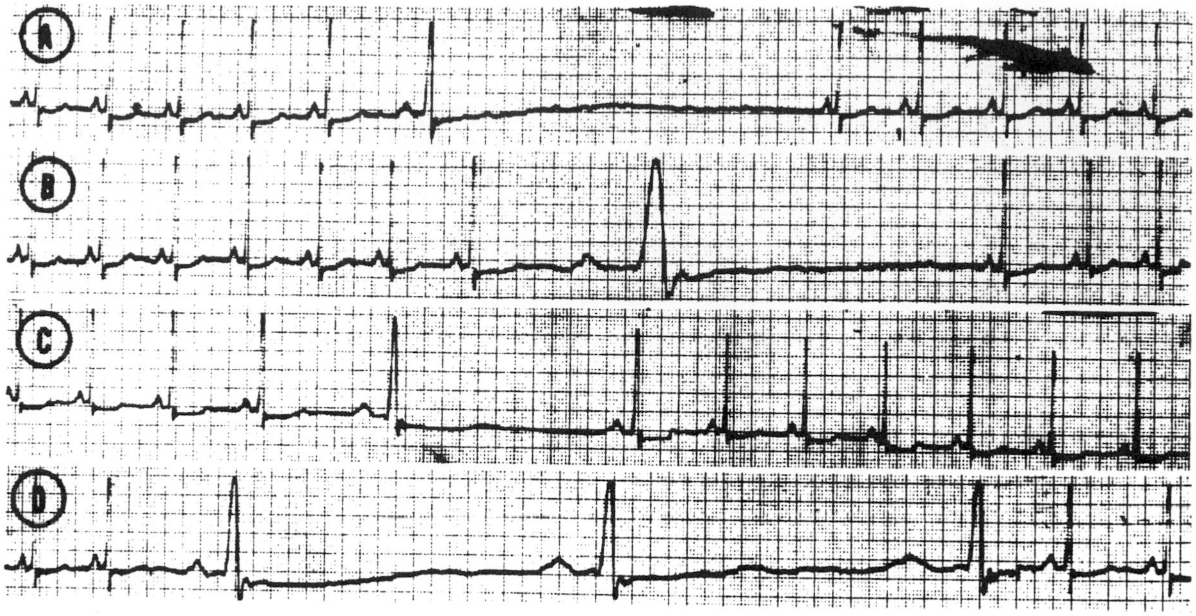

Figure 23-44. *Episodes suggestive of pseudo-sinus arrest that are, in reality, due to marked alterations in tape speed or tape stretching or both. The patient had no demonstrable abnormalities of sinus function. Note the marked prolongation of the PR interval and QRS interval, especially well seen in B and D. (Krasnow, A. Z., and Bloomfield, D., K.: Artifacts in portable electrocardiographic monitoring. Am. Heart J., 91:349, 1976)*

artifacts may result in dramatic rate changes that can be misinterpreted as sinus arrest, with a resultant clinical decision for urgent pacemaker therapy. This artifact is dramatically illustrated in Figure 23-44. In this recording, marked sinus arrest and sinus slowing are noted. Closer inspection of the record reveals that PR, QRS, and QT prolongation of varying degrees can be identified before, during, and following the pauses. This record should be properly identified as artifact secondary to stretching of the tape and subsequent distortion of the analogue waveforms and associated PP intervals.

Pseudoarrhythmias may also occur secondary to technical artifact. In a very minor fashion, their misinterpretation may not lead to clinical changes, but recurrent "arrhythmias" may result in serious errors in clinical management. In Figure 23-45*A*, an example of pseudoatrial premature complexes is seen. These premature complexes occur because of sudden, momentary

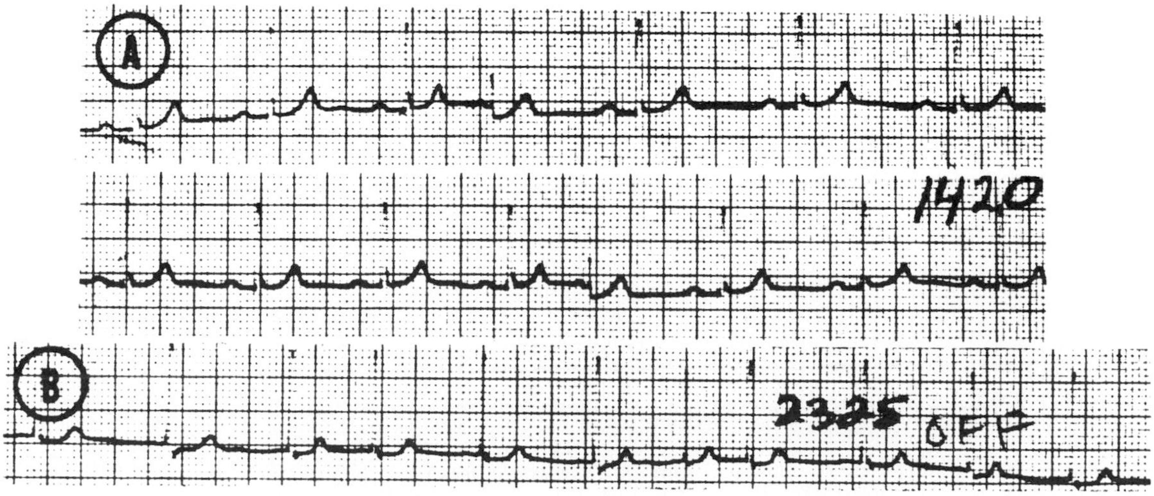

Figure 23-45. *Pseudoextrasystoles due to tape sticking are demonstrated. This tape sticking results in "premature complexes" with extremely short PR and QRS duration. (Krasnow, A. Z., and Bloomfield, D. K.: Artifacts in portable electrocardiographic monitoring. Am. Heart J., 91:349, 1976)*

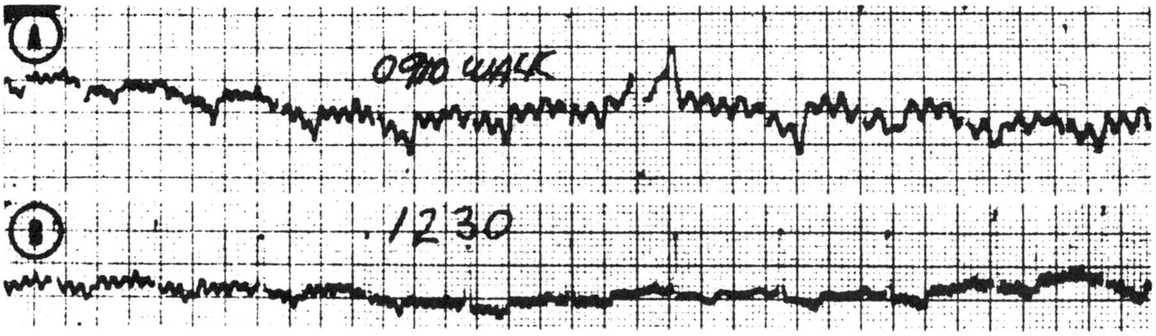

Figure 23-46. *(A) Pseudo-atrial fibrillation/flutter. B demonstrates clear-cut sinus rhythm which, in retrospect, is the circumstance seen in A. This patient's records showing pseudo-atrial fibrillation/flutter are due to electrode noise and are not associated with patient tremor or atrial flutter. (Krasnow, A. Z., and Bloomfield, D. K.: Artifacts in portable electrocardiographic monitoring. Am. Heart J., 91:349, 1976)*

changes in tape transport speed. In Figure 23-45*B*, an example of a "junctional" rhythm with supraventricular premature complexes is seen. This also is artifact and results from a combination of amplifier artifact (see Fig. 23-38) and tape transport distortion.

Artifact outside of the recorder-playback system may also result in an inappropriate rhythm diagnosis. Figure 23-46*A* shows an apparent episode of atrial flutter with a controlled ventricular rate. On closer inspection, in Figure 23-46*B*, the initial portion of the record shows "atrial flutter" that disappears as the baseline changes. This is an example of sinus rhythm with extraneous surface electrode noise mimicking a paroxysmal episode of atrial flutter.

Episodes of paroxysmal tachycardia also can be a manifestation of technical artifact. Variations in the degree of artifact can produce subtle or overt manifestations of this event. Figure 23-47*A* shows sinus rhythm with narrow PR, QRS, and QT intervals. In Figure 23-47*B*, at a time when the battery was near depletion, there is an apparent sinus tachycardia. Closer inspection reveals that there is not only an increase in heart rate but also a decrease in the PR, QRS, and QT intervals, indicating a significant change in tape transport speed. A more dramatic example of this phenomenon is illustrated in Figure 23-48. In the upper panel, intermittent decrease in battery output results in sudden "acceleration" of heart rate; this phenomenon is both more sustained and increased in rate in the lower panel. The heart rate of approximately 300 beats/min in the lower panel mimics atrial flutter with 1 : 1 conduction but is clearly artifact for the reasons outlined above.

Artifacts can also mimic ventricular arrhythmias; this has important clinical implications if they are misinterpreted by the reviewing physician. This is dramatically illustrated by the Holter monitor strips shown in Figure 23-49. In Figure 23-49*A*, sinus rhythm is seen with normal PR, QRS, and QT intervals. Moments later, as de-

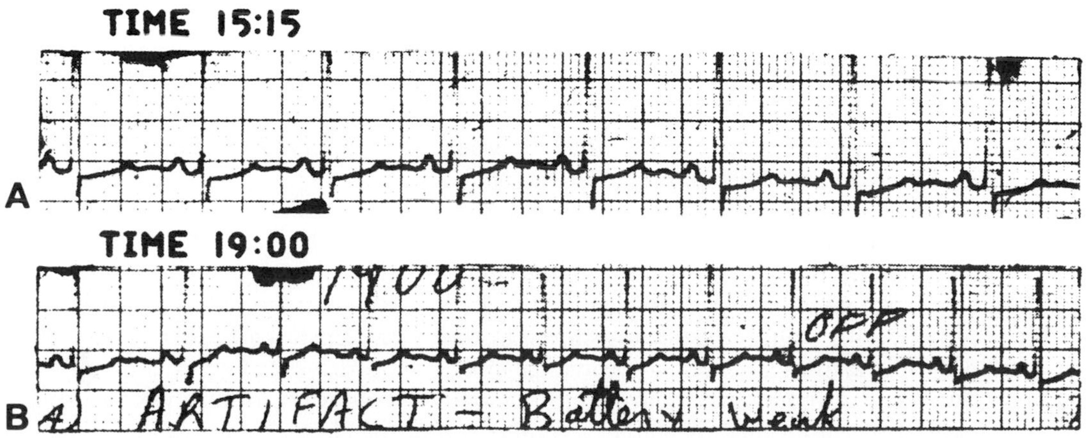

Figure 23-47. *Paroxysmal pseudo-sinus tachycardia. B demonstrates increase in the heart rate, suggestive of sinus tachycardia. Note the shortening of the PR, QRS, and QT intervals, consistent with early battery failure. (Krasnow, A. Z., and Bloomfield, D. K.: Artifacts in portable electrocardiographic monitoring. Am. Heart J., 91:349, 1976)*

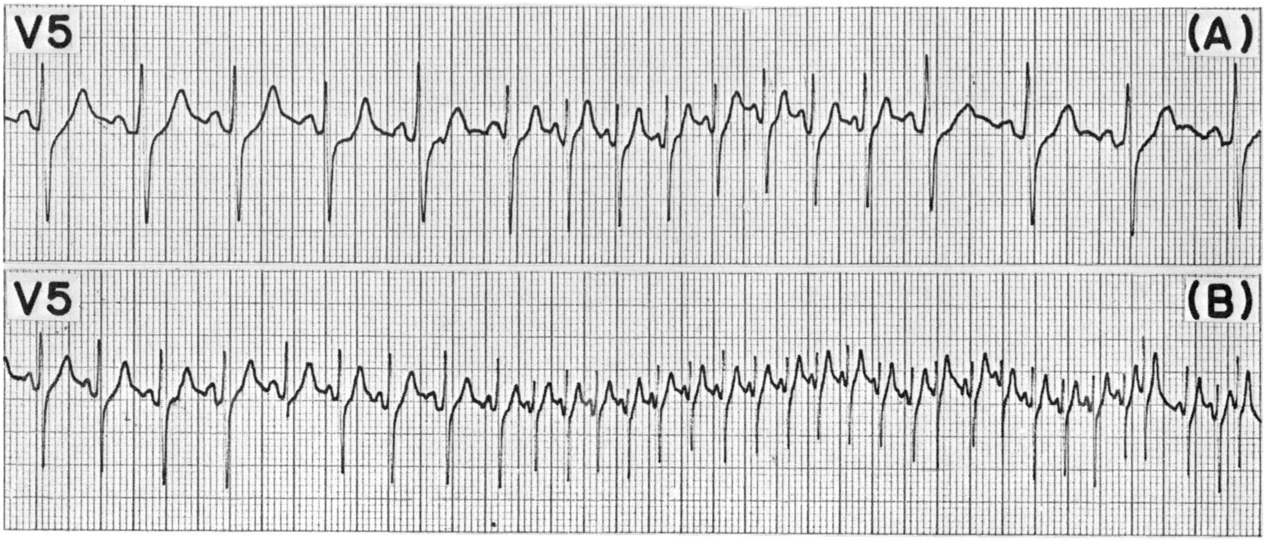

Figure 23-48. *Two representative strips from a patient's Holter monitor recording during which time battery failure occurred. In A, a short period of diminished battery output apparently accelerates the heart rate. In B, more prominent battery failure results in apparent supraventricular "tachycardia" at rates of nearly 300 beats/min.*

picted in Figure 23-49*B,* the recording shows a marked increase in heart rate associated with a wide "QRS" complex. On close inspection, a regular QRS can be discerned among the bizarre "QRS" complexes at a rate of approximately 120 beats/min. This recording represents electrode artifact during exercise in a patient with sinus tachycardia.

Conduction defects can also be simulated by artifacts. These "defects" in conduction may have minor clinical implications, or they may result in significant but inappropriate clinical decisions with regard to permanent pacing. A dramatic example with substantial clinical implications is evident in the tracings shown in Figure 23-50. Episodic second degree AV block (Mobitz II) appears to be present in *A,* which progresses to a more advanced degree of AV block in *B.* More careful inspection of the records reveals that, in fact, the "nonconducted P waves" represent distorted QRS complexes secondary to amplifier artifact.

Decisions to implant permanent pacemakers based on inadequate data or misinterpretation must be avoided. However, on occasion, the Holter monitor recording may demonstrate evidence of normal "pacemaker function" in the absence of any pacemaker, temporary or permanent. This is graphically illustrated In Figure 23-51. This continuous record shows, in the lower strip, a rapid artifact similar to a pacemaker spike. In fact, however, this represents electrode motion artifact in a patient in whom there is neither a temporary nor a permanent pacemaker.

The ultimate artifactual arrhythmia is illustrated in Figure 23-52. In this case, two distinct QRS types suggest two independent supraventricular sites of origin (*e.g.,* sinus and "junctional" parasystole). The true explanation of this most unusual rhythm is, in fact, readily apparent when one discovers that this tracing was obtained from a tape that had previously been used for another Holter recording. This resulted in the recording of the present patient's electrocardiogram (small QRS) superimposed upon the previous patient's electrocardiogram (large QRS). This has been described as the "siamese-twin" effect.

Miscellaneous

There is a variety of uncategorized areas in which Holter monitoring can be invaluable in the evaluation and management of cardiac patients. This section will illustrate some aspects of a potpourri of clinical situations in which long-term electrocardiographic monitoring may be of clinical usefulness.

In Figure 23-53, a record obtained from a patient with a history of recurrent tachycardias is shown. The upper panel shows sinus rhythm with first degree AV block, yet in the lower panel, with a decrease in the sinus rate, the PR shortens and QRS complexes with initial slurring of the upstroke appear. These latter complexes only appeared at slow sinus rates with a fixed PR associated with a uniform, bizarre QRS during such times. Therefore, the Holter recording identified that this patient had ventricular preexcitation with a long bypass refractory period. His tachyarrhythmias could thus be explained, and a more critical formulation of antiarrhythmic therapy

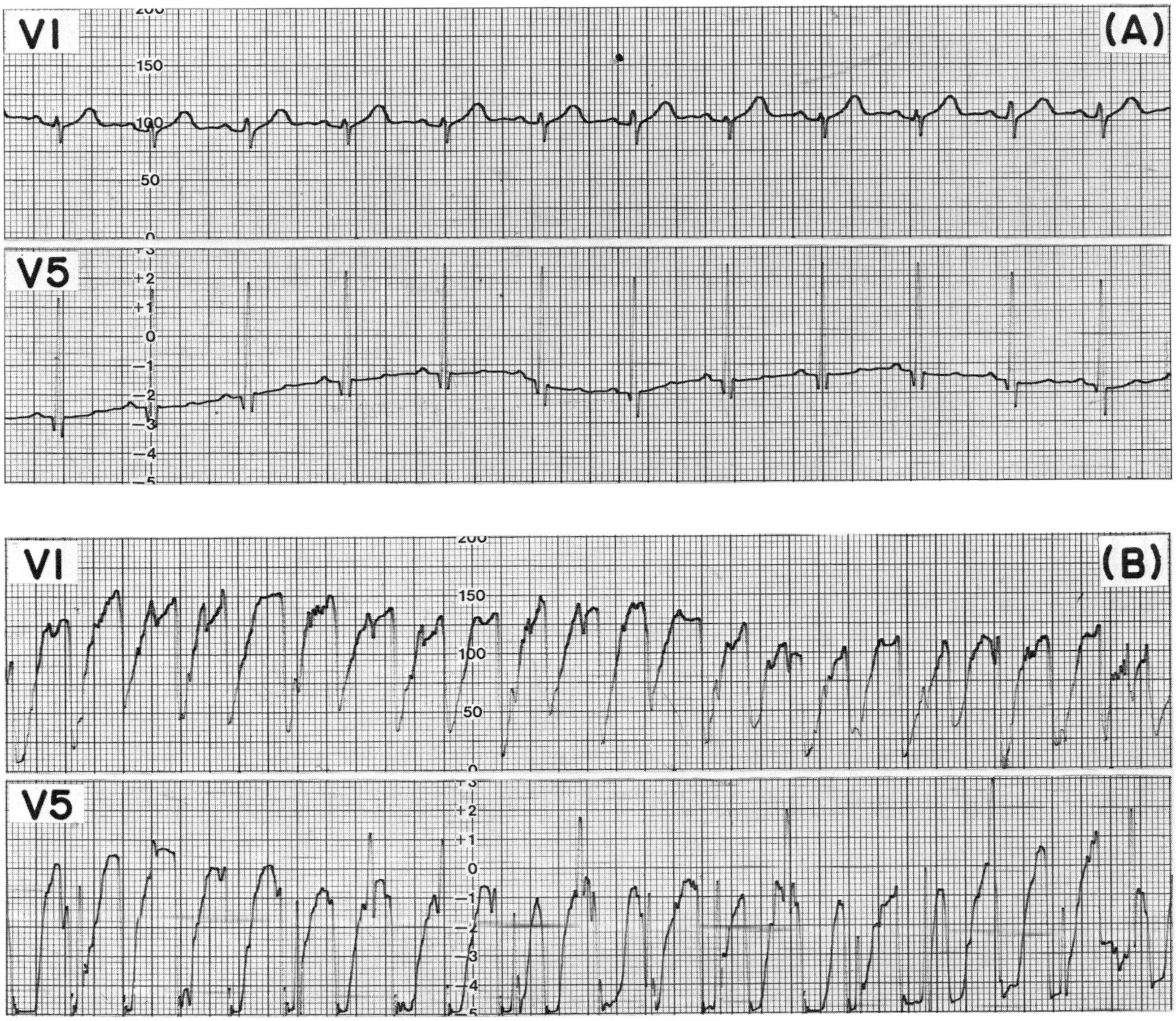

Figure 23-49. *Pseudo-ventricular tachycardia is illustrated in this record obtained from a patient without significant palpitations. In A, sinus rhythm is demonstrated. In B, bizarre regular activity is noted in both V_1 and V_5 electrode leads. More careful inspection of the record demonstrates sinus tachycardia with narrow QRS complexes seen interspersed between the bizarre waveforms. Marked electrode artifact is demonstrated.*

could be designed. (Prior studies in patients with Wolff-Parkinson-White syndrome have documented tachyarrhythmias without symptoms and symptoms without tachyarrhythmias.[59,60])

Patients with ischemic heart disease have, on many occasions, a prominent variability in clinical symptomatology. Nevertheless, there are times when patients may not manifest clinical complaints and yet have electrocardiographic evidence of "ischemia" with a potential for significant ventricular arrhythmias. This vacillation in the electrocardiographic manifestations of ischemia (*i.e.,* ST segment depression) is clearly illustrated by the records (Fig. 23-54) obtained over a 24-hour period in a patient with intermittent angina. That ST segment depression can occur during sleep, unassociated with clinical symptoms, is clearly illustrated (see also Fig. 23-25).

An equally important use of Holter monitoring may be in the patients with clinically atypical but angina-like chest pain. These patients may represent variant angina, and electrocardiographic recordings during episodes of chest pain may be crucial to their diagnosis and management. The patients may present not only with histories of chest distress but also with a history of palpitations. The Holter recordings will allow for clear documenta-

(Text continues on p. 617.)

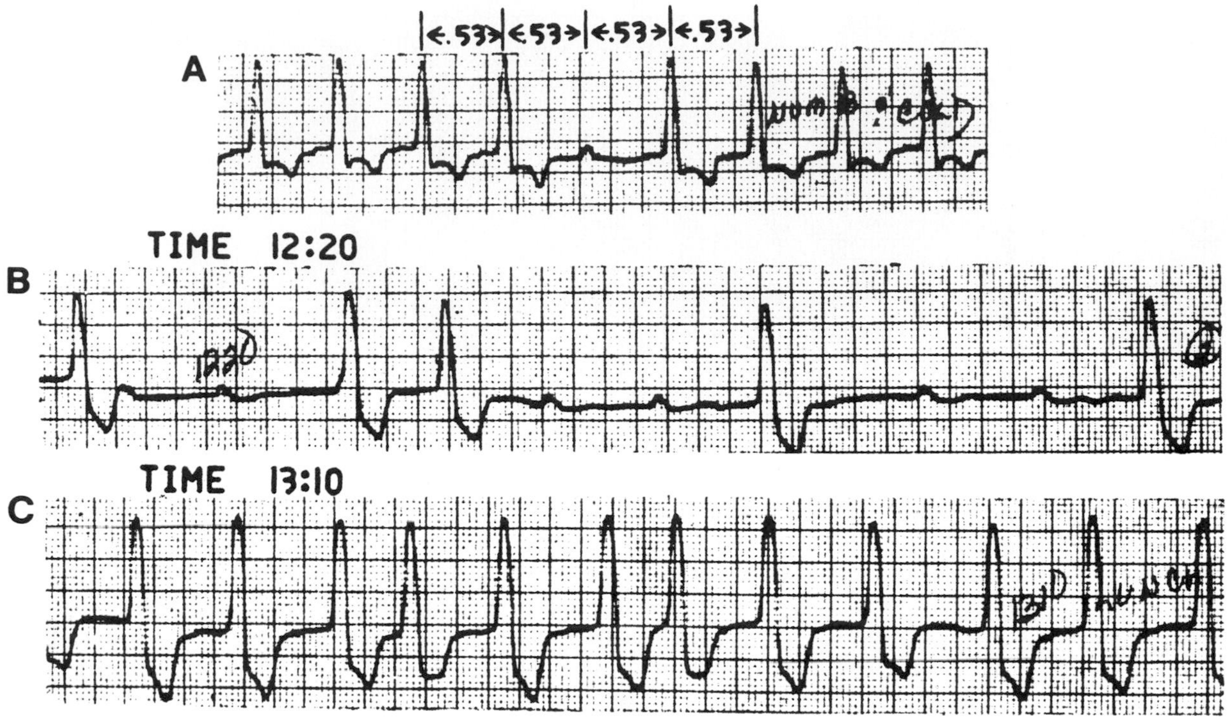

Figure 23-50. *Pseudo-AV block is illustrated in this record obtained from a patient without a history of syncope but with an intraventricular conduction defect of the left bundle branch block type. Episodes of apparent second degree AV block with nonconducted sinus complexes are seen in A and B. The small complexes initially interpreted as atrial activity are, in fact, normal QRS complexes that are damped by amplifier artifact. (Krasnow, A. Z., and Bloomfield, D. K.: Artifacts in portable electrocardiographic monitoring. Am. Heart J., 91:349, 1976)*

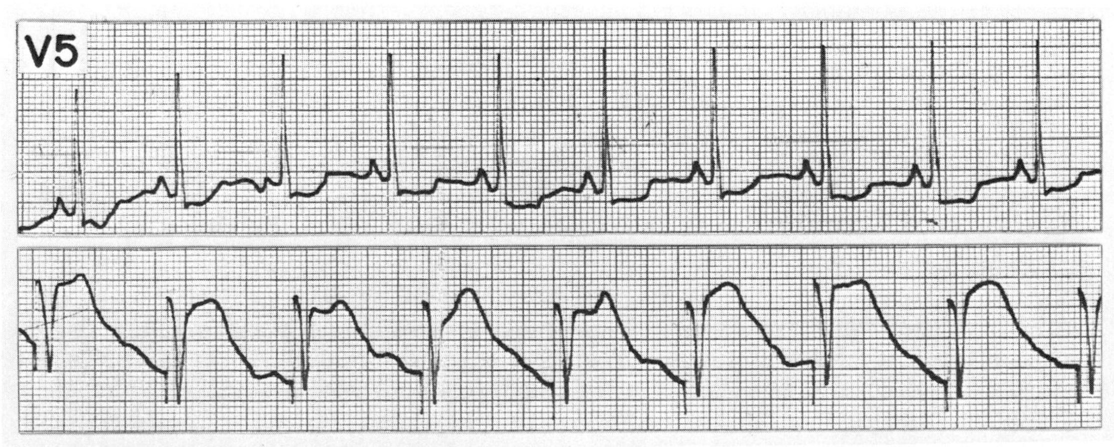

Figure 23-51. *Pseudo-pacemaker activity in a continuous record from a single-channel recording. Marked amplifier and electrode artifact mimics the presence of a demand pacemaker.*

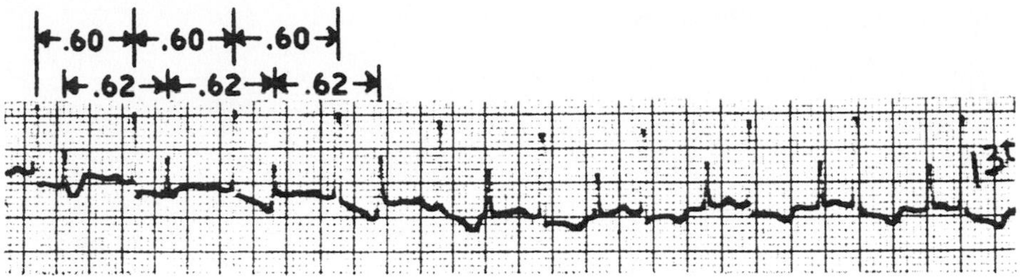

Figure 23-52. *Pseudo-electrical alternans due to the presence of a "siamese-twin" effect. This record illustrates the ultimate complex arrhythmia in Holter recording. The electrocardiograms of two patients have been recorded on the same tape, accounting for the bizarre arrhythmia seen in this tracing. (Krasnow, A. Z., and Bloomfield, D. K.: Artifacts in portable electrocardiographic monitoring. Am. Heart J., 91:349, 1976)*

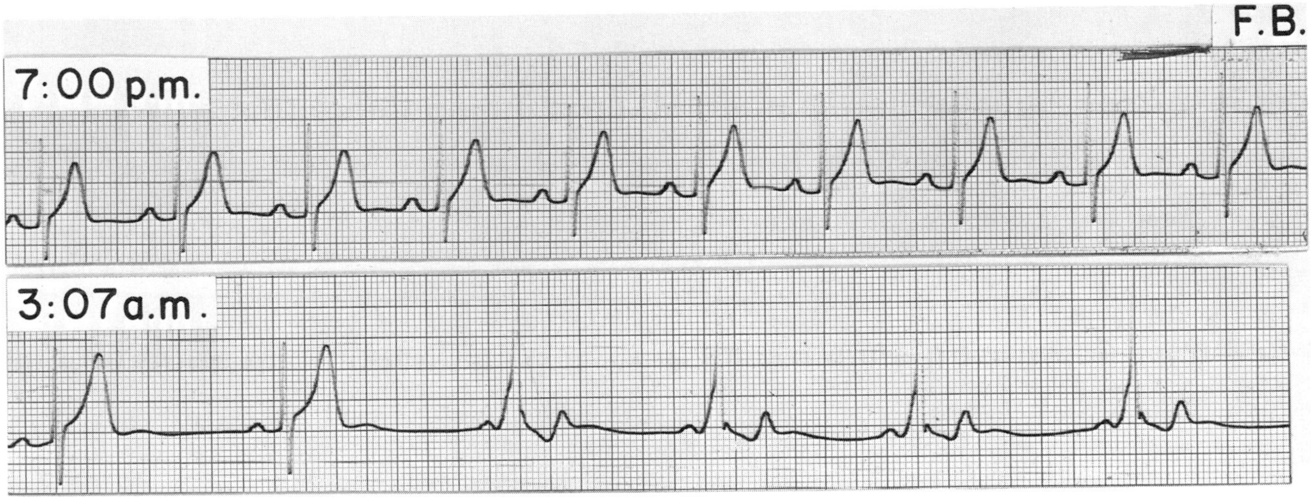

Figure 23-53. *Two representative strips from a patient with a history of tachycardia. In the* top strip, *sinus rhythm with normal AV conduction is noted. In the* bottom strip, *during the sinus bradycardia, ventricular preexcitation is now noted.*

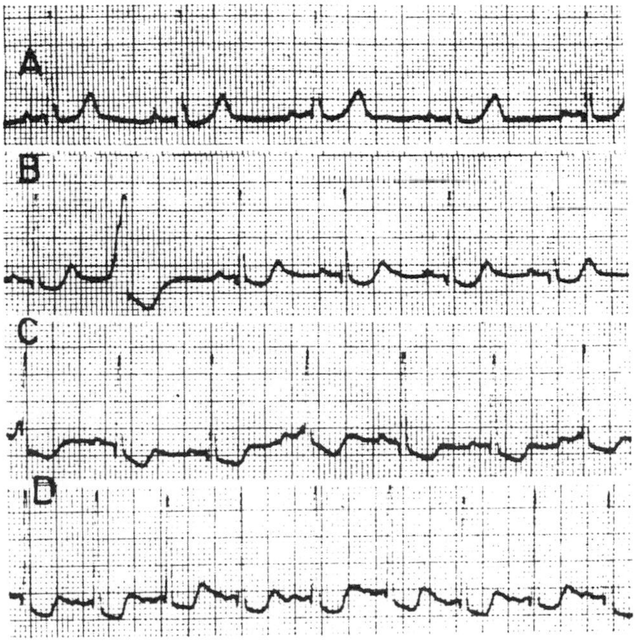

Figure 23-54. *Marked variation in ST segment displacement seen at various times of the day but unassociated with significant clinical symptomatology in a patient with coronary artery disease. (Stern, S., and Tzivoni, D.: The dynamic nature of ST-T segment in ischemic heart disease. Am. Heart J., 91:820, 1976)*

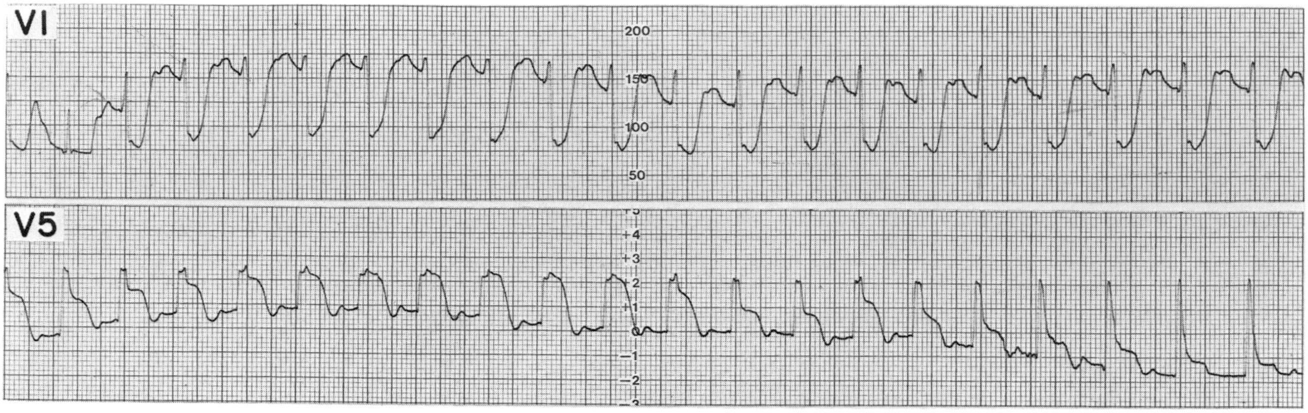

Figure 23-55. *Recording obtained from a patient with recurrent episodes of chest pain of an atypical variety but suggestive of reflux esophagitis. During an episode of chest pain, marked ST segment elevation is seen in lead V_5, consistent with Prinzmetal's variant angina.*

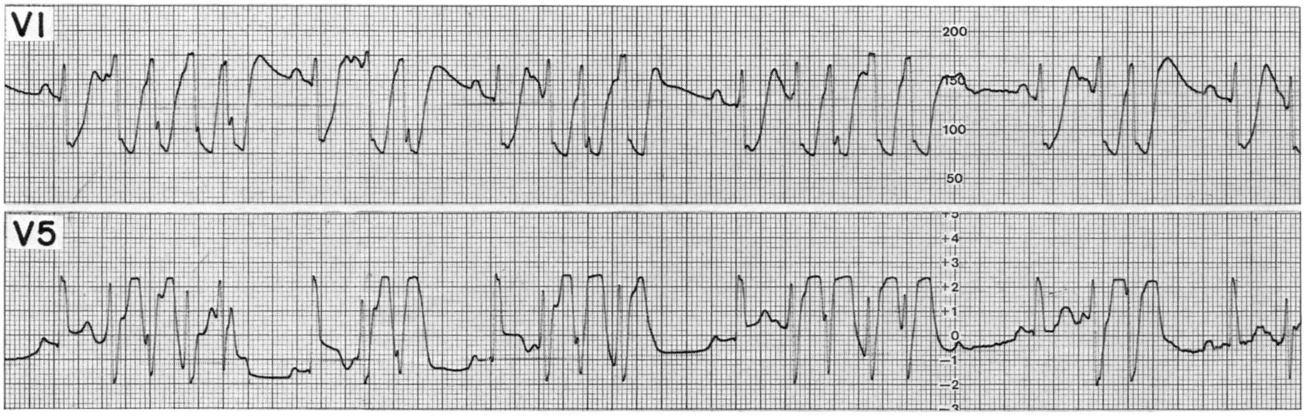

Figure 23-56. *Another portion of the recording from the same patient as in Figure 23-55. This portion of the recording was obtained during a period when the patient had both palpitations and chest pain. Noe the prominent ST segment elevation and the burst of ventricular premature complexes.*

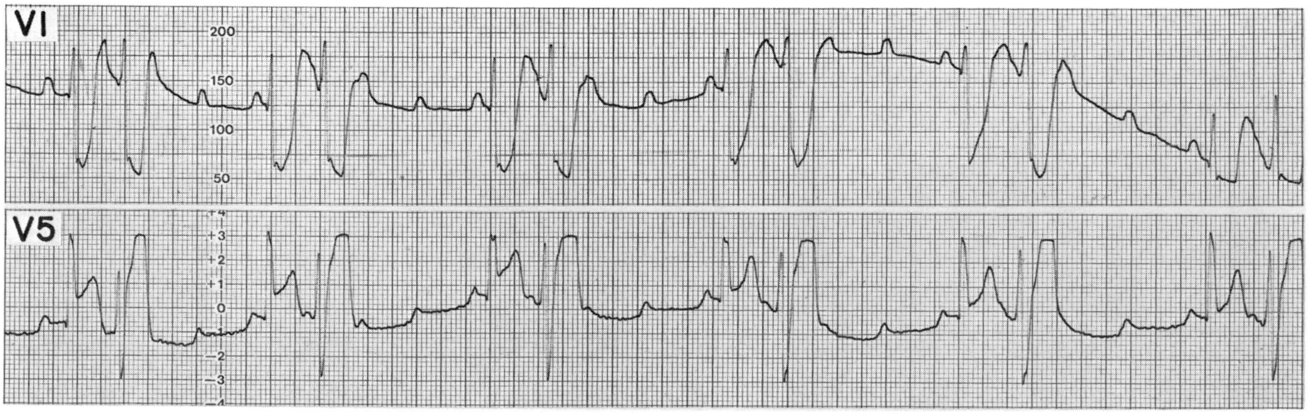

Figure 23-57. *Another portion of the Holter recording obtained from the same patient as in Figures 23-55 and 23-56, illustrating another period during which the patient complained of palpitations and chest pain. Note the presence of marked ST segment elevation, AV block, and ventricular premature complexes.*

tion of the basis for these symptoms. The spectrum of such a clinical situation is illustrated in Figures 23-55 to 23-57 obtained from a woman aged 48 years with burning epigastric pain of recent onset occurring at rest and unrelated to food intake. Her internist could not control the episodes of pain (more than 15 per day) with routine antacid therapy. A gallbladder series was negative, and an upper gastrointestinal series demonstrated a small hiatus hernia. The patient was referred to a gastroenterologist for further work-up. His evaluation was inconclusive, but he felt the pain was not gastrointestinal in origin. A Holter monitor was ordered because the patient also admitted that she experienced palpitations during some of those episodes of pain. In Figure 23-55, obtained during an episode of pain, dramatic ST segment elevation is seen in lead V_5. These electrocardiographic events were repeatedly documented during all episodes of pain that the patient experienced during the 24-hour recording. On several occasions, the patient had complained of palpitations, and in Figure 23-56, a recording shows repetitive short bursts of probable ventricular tachycardia that were documented on multiple oc-

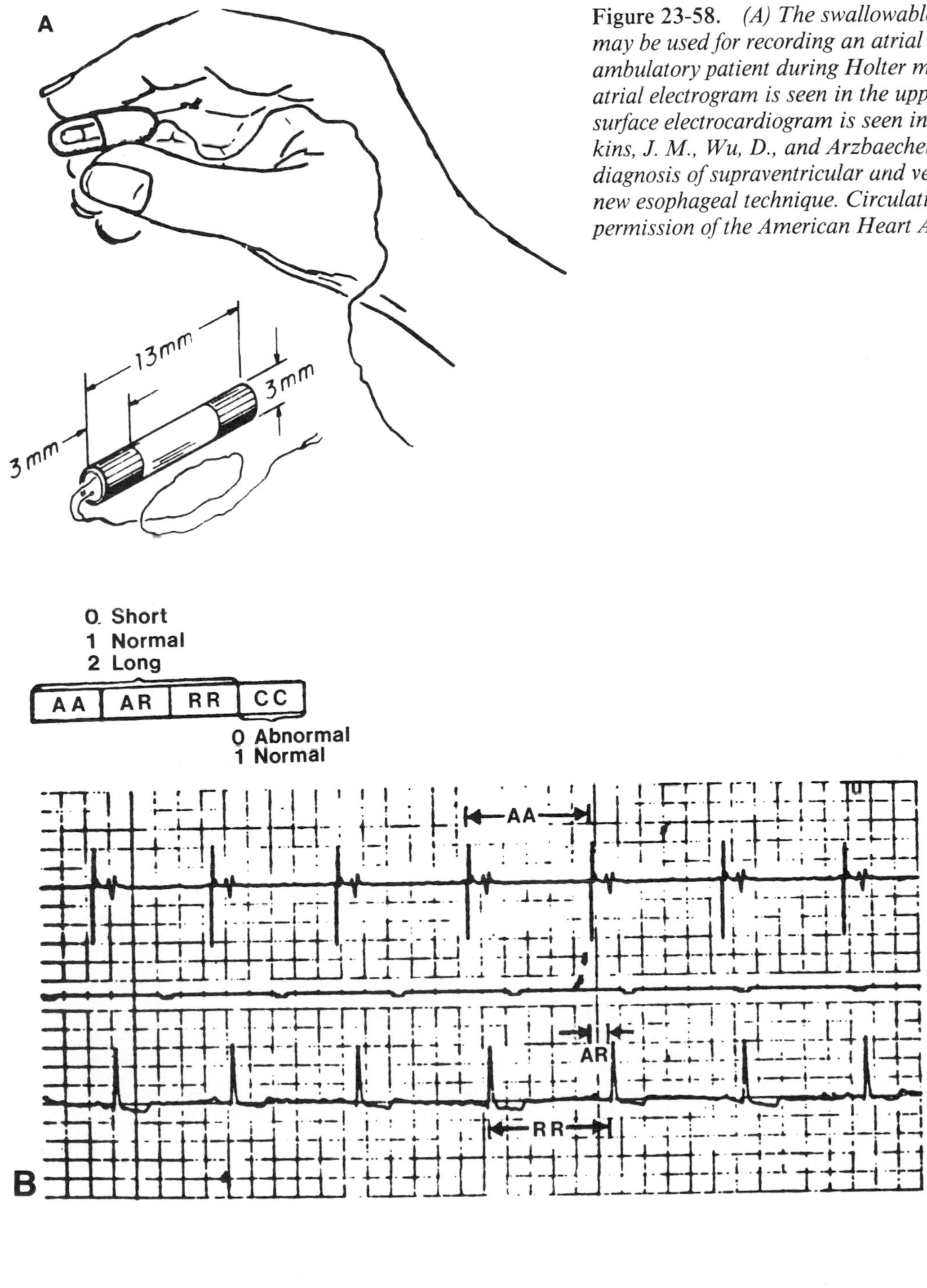

Figure 23-58. *(A) The swallowable bipolar electrode that may be used for recording an atrial electrogram in an ambulatory patient during Holter monitor recording. (B) The atrial electrogram is seen in the upper channel, and the surface electrocardiogram is seen in the lower channel. (Jenkins, J. M., Wu, D., and Arzbaecher, R. L.: Computer diagnosis of supraventricular and ventricular arrhythmias. A new esophageal technique. Circulation, 60:977, 1979. By permission of the American Heart Association, Inc.)*

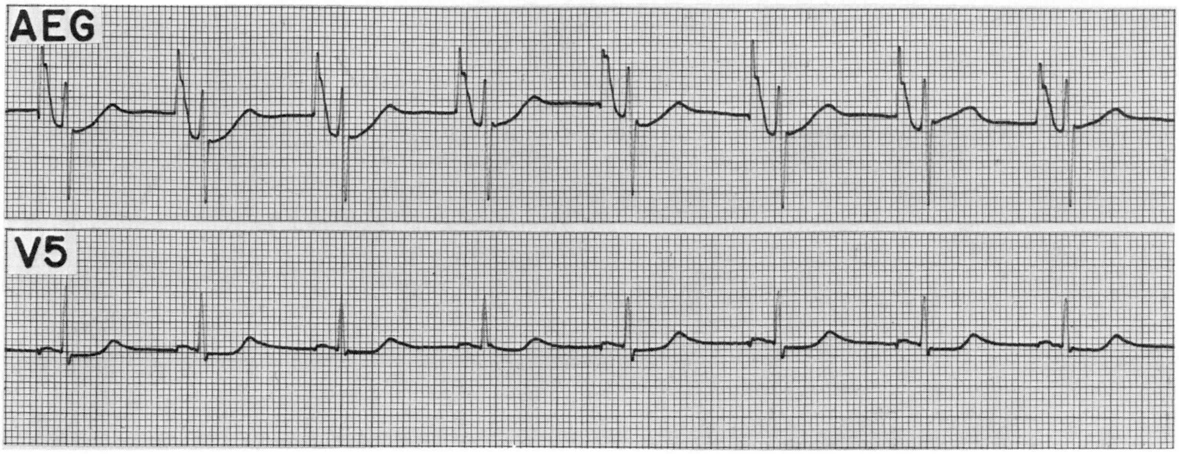

Figure 23-59. *Atrial electrodes implanted at cardiac surgery were used to obtain an atrial electrogram during recording with the two-channel Holter monitor. In the* top strip, *the atrial electrogram was recorded with a prominent atrial spike as well as a QRS spike. The surface electrocardiogram in the* bottom strip *was obtained during sinus rhythm.*

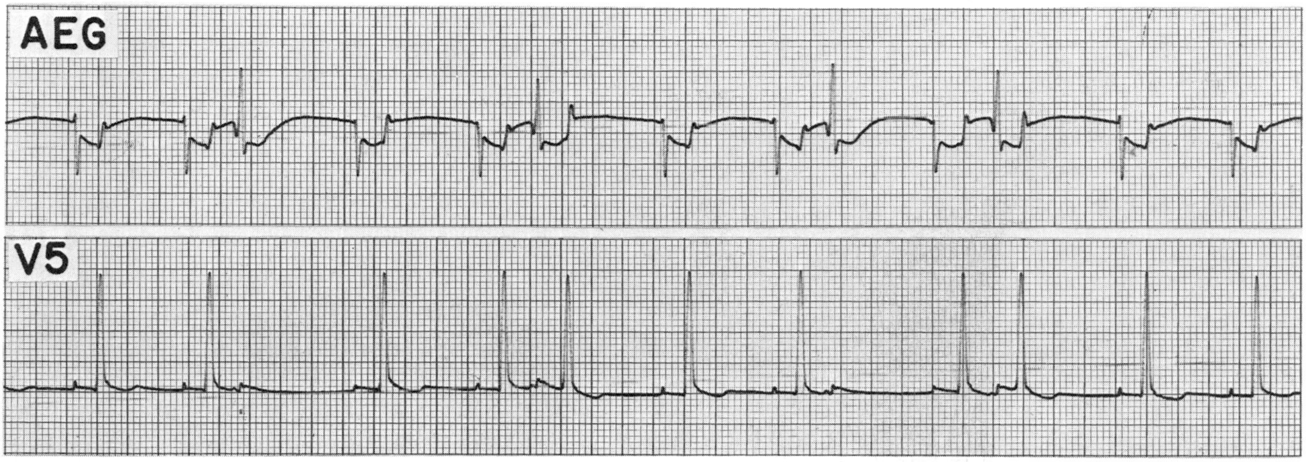

Figure 23-60. *Using the technique discussed in Figure 23-59, a record is obtained during standard Holter monitor recording in a postoperative cardiac surgical patient. The* top strip *demonstrates the atrial electrogram, and the* bottom strip *demonstrates a surface electrocardiogram. Note the presence of premature complexes that are clearly atrial in origin as demonstrated by the prominent P waves seen both during the nonconducted complexes as well as during the conducted complexes.*

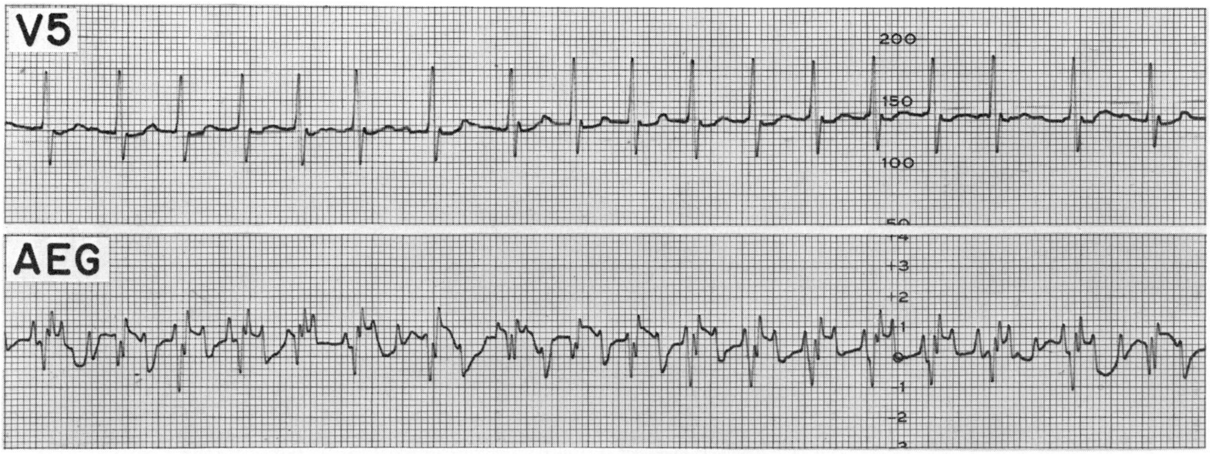

Figure 23-61. *A representative recording from a patient following cardiac surgery, during which time recurrent supraventricular tachycardia was noted on Holter monitoring. The* bottom strip *shows the atrial electrogram, which clearly identifies the presence of two atrial complexes for each QRS complex (i.e., atrial flutter with 2:1 ventricular response).*

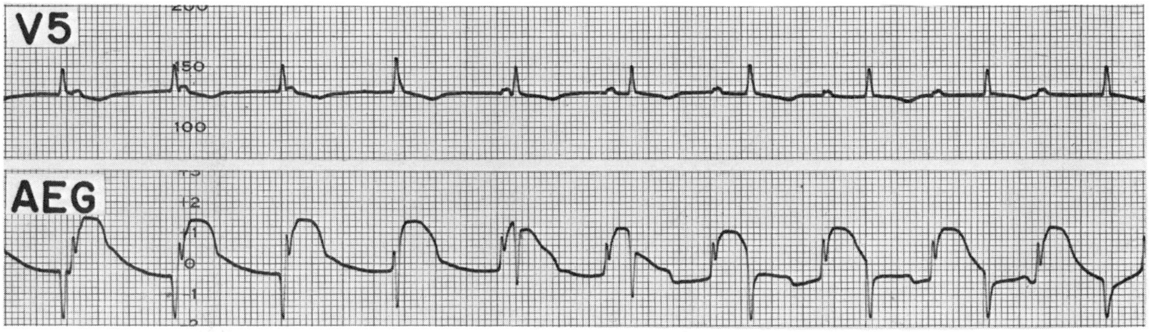

Figure 23-62. *A two-lead Holter monitor recording from a patient following cardiac surgery; during the recording, the lower channel was used to record the atrial electrogram. Note the presence of AV dissociation, clearly seen in the atrial electrogram, with varying QRS and P wave rates.*

casions associated with clinical complaints of chest pain and palpitations. However, these were not the only events documented during such periods of chest pain and palpitations. On several other occasions, the patient had recordings obtained during which paroxysmal AV block occurred during complaints of chest pain and palpitations (see Fig. 23-57). Therefore, in this patient, the gamut of phasic ST segment elevation, ventricular arrhythmias, and AV block were all recorded during episodes of chest pain. The diagnosis of variant angina was established, and appropriate medical therapy was initiated. Therefore, Holter recordings such as those shown in these figures may be an invaluable tool in evaluating patients with suspected or documented ischemic heart disease.

Ideally, in many patients with cardiac arrhythmias, magnification of atrial activity would offer significant diagnostic (and potentially therapeutic) advantages. The use of various lead placement changes can, on occasion, enhance atrial activity on the surface electrocardiogram (*i.e.,* Lewis lead). Nevertheless, even with the use of dual-channel systems and novel lead placements, Holter recordings may not always allow for accurate rhythm interpretation.

Jenkins and co-workers have demonstrated that a bipolar electrode can be introduced per os for continuous recording of an atrial electrogram on one channel of a dual-channel recorder (Fig. 23-58*A*).[61] This swallowable bipolar esophageal electrode has been shown by Jenkins and colleagues to give adequate atrial recording satisfactory for the use of computerized techniques for arrhythmia analysis (Fig. 23-58*B*).

In studies from our institution, we have identified that a similar-quality atrial recording can be obtained over 24-hour periods with the use of atrial wires implanted at cardiac surgery (Fig. 23-59). Adequate atrial signals can

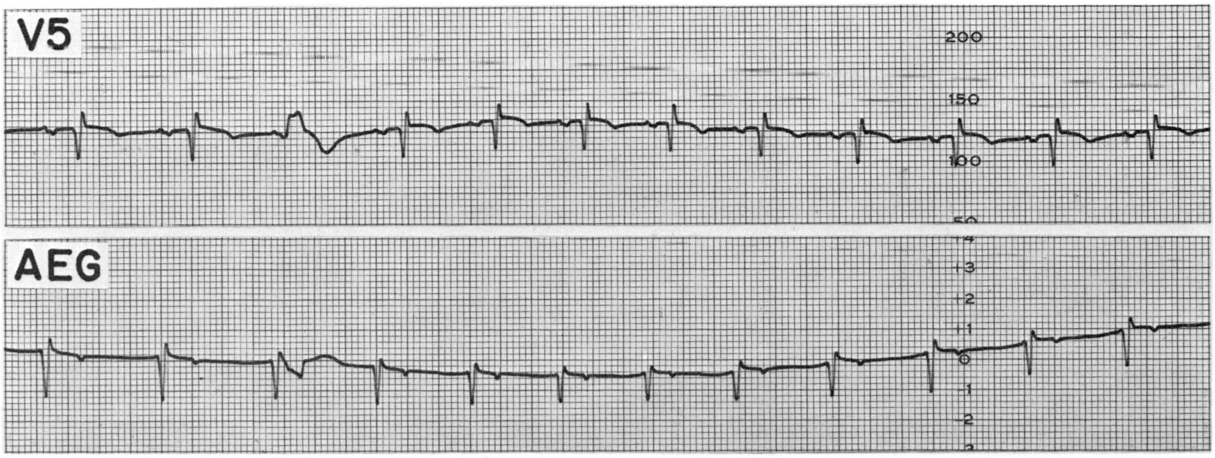

Figure 23-63. *A two-lead Holter monitor recording during which one channel was used to record an atrial electrogram in a patient following cardiac surgery. Note the presence of the premature complex unassociated with a change in sinus rate (i.e., suggesting ventricular origin).*

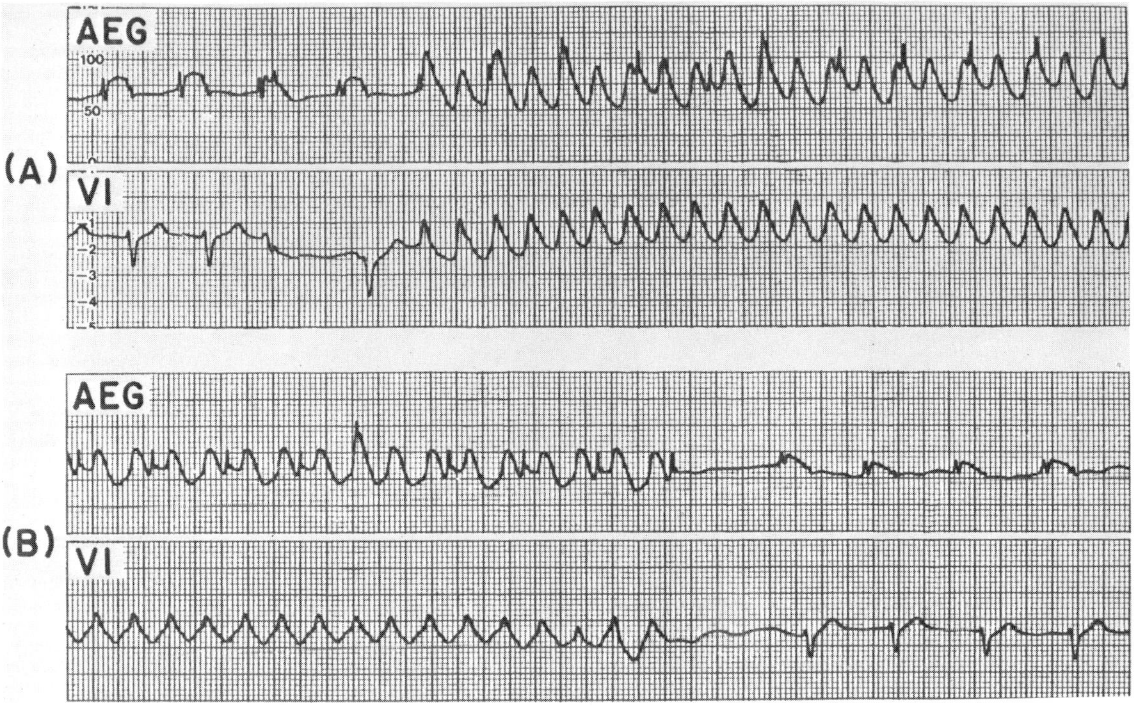

Figure 23-64. *A two-channel Holter monitor recording obtained from a postoperative cardiac surgical patient during an episode of tachycardia. The upper tracing in both A and B is an atrial electrogram. The lower tracings are lead V_1 surface electrocardiograms. In A, the onset of a wide QRS rapid tachycardia is noted. Inspection of the atrial electrogram recordings clearly demonstrates AV dissociation, indicating a very high likelihood of ventricular origin of the tachycardia.*

be continuously recorded on one of the two channels of the Holter recorder to allow for accurate evaluation of many transient or more persistent arrhythmias. Atrial arrhythmias such as isolated atrial premature complexes or atrial flutter can be clearly documented (Figs. 23-60 and 23-61). AV dissociation, premature ventricular complexes, and ventricular tachycardia also can readily be diagnosed (Figs. 23-62 to 23-64). The techniques described above can be anticipated to extend significantly the usefulness of Holter recording devices.

References

1. Holter, N. J., and Gengerelli, J. A.: Remote recording of physiologic data by radio. Rocky Mt. Med. J., 46:79, 1949.
2. Holter, N. J.: Radioelectrocardiography: new technique for cardiovascular studies. Ann. N.Y. Acad. Sci., 65:913, 1957.
3. Holter, N. J.: New method for heart studies. Science, 134:1214, 1961.
4. Gilson, J. S., Holter, N. J., and Glascock, W. R.: Continuous ambulant electrocardiograms and their analysis—clinical observations using the electrocardiocorder and AVsep analyzer. Circulation, 24:940, 1961.
5. Gilson, J. S., Holter, N. J., and Glascock, W. R.: Clinical observations using electrocardiocorder and AVsep continuous electrocardiographic system. Am. J. Cardiol., 14:204, 1964.
6. Sanders, J. S., and Martt, J. M.: Dynamic electrocardiography at high altitude. Am. J. Cardiol., 14:287, 1964.
7. Corday, E., Bazika, V., Lang, T-W., et al.: Detection of phantom arrhythmias and evanescent electrocardiographic abnormalities. J.A.M.A., 193:417, 1965.
8. Hinkle, L. E., Meyer, J., Stevens, M., et al.: Tape recording of the ECG of active men: limitations and advantages of the Holter-Avionics instruments. Circulation, 36:752, 1967.
9. Walter, P. F., Reid, S. J., Jr., and Wenger, N. K.: Transient cerebral ischemia due to arrhythmias. Ann. Intern. Med., 72:471, 1970.
10. Karpman, H. L., Bleifer, S. B., and Bleifer, D. F.: Clinical applications of dynamic electrocardiography. Chest, 58:283, 1970.
11. Crook,B. R. M.,Cashman, P. M. M., Stott, F. D., et al.: Tape monitoring of the electrocardiogram in ambulant patients with sinoatrial disease. Br. Heart J., 35:1009, 1973.
12. Crawford, M., O'Rourke, R., Ramakrishna, N., et al.: Comparative effectiveness of exercise testing and continuous monitoring for detecting arrhythmias in patients with previous myocardial infarction. Circulation, 50:301, 1974.
13. Kleiger, R. E., and Senior, R. M.: Long-term electrocardiographic monitoring of ambulatory patients with chronic airway obstruction. Chest, 65:483, 1974.
14. Bleifer, S. B., Bleifer, D. J., Hausmann, D. R., et al.: Diagnosis of occult arrhythmias by Holter electrocardiography. Prog. Cardiovasc. Dis., 16:569, 1974.
15. Stein, I. M.: Ambulatory long-term electrocardiography—the "LCG." Am. Heart J., 88:37, 1974.
16. Ryan, M., Lown, B., and Horn, H.: Comparison of ventricular ectopic activity during 24-hour monitoring and exercise testing in

patients with coronary heart disease. N. Engl. J. Med., 292:224, 1974.
17. Winkle, R. A., Lopes, M. G., Fitzgerald, J. W., et al.: Arrhythmias in patients with mitral valve prolapse. Circulation, 52:73, 1975.
18. Coumel, P.: Continuous electrocardiographic recording. Clinical, diagnostic and therapeutic value. Arch. Mal. Coeur, 68:941, 1975.
19. Harrison, D. C., Fitzgerald, J. W., and Winkle, R. A.: Ambulatory electrocardiography for diagnosis and treatment of cardiac arrhythmias. N. Engl. J. Med., 294:373, 1976.
20. Vismara, L. A., Pratt, C., Miller, R. R., et al.: Correlation of standard electrocardiogram and continuous ambulatory monitoring in detection of ventricular arrhythmias in coronary patients. Circulation, 53:27, 1976.
21. Stern, S., and Tzivoni, D.: The dynamic nature of the ST-T segment in ischemic heart disease. Am. Heart J., 91:820, 1976.
22. Schroeder, J. S.: Ambulatory electrocardiographic monitoring—technique and clinical indications. J.A.M.A., 236:494, 1976.
23. Romero, C. A.: Holter monitoring in diagnosis and management of cardiac rhythm disturbances. Med. Clin. North Am., 60:299, 1976.
24. Johansson, B. W.: Long term ECG in ambulatory clinical practice. Analysis and two year follow-up of 100 patients studied with a portable ECG tape recorder. Eur. J. Cardiol., 5:39, 1977.
25. Brodsky, M., Wu, D., Denes, P., et al.: Arrhythmias documented by 24 hour continuous electrocardiograph monitoring in 50 male medical students without apparent heart disease. Am. J. Cardiol., 39:390, 1977.
26. Kennedy, H. L.: Ambulatory electrocardiography. Ann. Intern. Med., 87:729, 1977.
27. Fletcher, G. F., and Cantwell, J. D.: Continuous ambulatory electrocardiographic monitoring. Use in cardiac exercise programs. Chest, 71:27, 1977.
28. McLeod, A. A., and Jewitt, D. E.: Role of 24 hour ambulatory electrocardiographic monitoring in a general hospital. Br. Med. J., 1:1197, 1978.
29. Michelson, E. L., Morganroth, J., and MacVaugh, H., III: Postoperative arrhythmias after coronary artery and cardiac valvular surgery detected by long-term electrocardiographic monitoring. Am. Heart J., 97:442, 1979.
30. Gradman, A. H., Bell, P. A., and DeBusk, R. F.: Sudden death during ambulatory monitoring. Circulation, 55:210, 1977.
31. Winkle, R. A., Rodriguez, I., and Bragg-Remschel, D. A.: Technological status and problems of ambulatory electrocardiographic monitoring. Ann. N.Y. Acad. Sci., 432:108–116, 1984.
32. Morganroth, J., Michelson, E. L., Horowitz, L. N., et al.: Limitations of routine long-term electrocardiographic monitoring to assess ventricular ectopic frequency. Circulation, 58:408, 1978.
33. Winkle, R. A.: Antiarrhythmic drug effect mimicked by spontaneous variability of ventricular ectopy. Circulation, 57:1116, 1978.
34. Pratt, C. M., Slymen, D. J., Wierman, A. M., et al.: Analysis of the spontaneous variability of ventricular arrhythmias: Consecutive ambulatory electrocardiographic recordings of ventricular tachycardia. Am. J. Cardiol., 56:67–72, 1985.
35. Kennedy, H. L., Whitlock, J. A., Sprague, M. K., et al.: Long-term follow-up of asymptomatic healthy subjects with frequent and complex ventricular ectopy. N. Engl. J. Med., 312:193–197, 1985.
36. Fleg, J. L., and Kennedy, H. L.: Cardiac arrhythmias in a healthy elderly population. Chest, 81:3,302–307, 1982.
37. Lightfoot,P. R., Sasse, L., Mandel, W. J., et al.: His bundle electrograms in healthy adolescents with persistent second degree AV block. Chest, 63:358–362, 1973.
38. Hinkle, L. E., Argyros, D. C., Hayes, J. C., et al.: Pathogenesis of an unexpected sudden death: role of early cycle ventricular premature contractions. Am. J. Cardiol., 39:873, 1977.
39. Gradman, A. H., Bell, P. A., and DeBusk, R. F.: Sudden death during ambulatory monitoring. Circulation, 55:210, 1977.
40. Pool, I., Kunst, K., and Van Wermeskerken, J.: Two monitored cases of sudden death outside hospital. Br. Heart J., 40:627, 1978.
41. Lahiri, A., Balasubramanian, V., and Raferty, E. B.: Sudden death during ambulatory monitoring. Br. Med. J. 1:1676, 1979.
42. Bissett, J. K., Watson, J. W., Scovil, J. A., et al.: Sudden death in cardiomyopathy: Role of bradycardia-dependent repolarization changes. Am. Heart J., 99:625, 1980.
43. Salerno, D., Hodges, M., Graham, E., et al.: Fatal cardiac arrest during continuous ambulatory monitoring. N. Engl. J. Med., 305:700, 1981.
44. Denes, P., Gabster, A., and Huang, S. K.: Clinical, electrocardiographic and follow-up observations in patients having ventricular fibrillation during Holter monitoring: Role of quinidine therapy. J. Am. Coll. Cardiol., 48:9–16, 1981.
45. Nikolic, G., Bishop, R. L., and Singh, J. B.: Sudden death recorded during Holter monitoring. Circulation, 66:218–225, 1982.
46. Lewis, B. H., Antman, E. M., and Graboys, T. B.: Detailed analysis of 24 hour ambulatory electrocardiographic recordings during ventricular fibrillation or Torsade de Pointes. J. Am. Coll. Cardiol., 2:426–436, 1983.
47. Pratt, C. M., Francis, M. J., Luck, J. C., et al.: Analysis of ambulatory electrocardiograms in 15 patients during spontaneous ventricular fibrillation with special reference to preceding arrhythmic events. J. Am. Coll. Cardiol., 2:789–797, 1983.
48. Roelandt, J., Klootwijk, P., Lubsen, J., and Jansen, M. J.: Sudden death during longterm ambulatory monitoring. Eur. Heart J., 5:7–20, 1984.
49. Vlay, S. C., Kallman, C. H., and Reid, P. R.: Prognostic assessment of survivors of ventricular tachycardia and ventricular fibrillation with ambulatory monitoring. Am. J. Cardiol., 54:87–90, 1984.
50. Bigger, T. J., Jr., Fleiss, J. L., Kleiger, R., et al.: The relationships among ventricular arrhythmias, left ventricular dysfunction, and mortality in the 2 years after myocardial infarction. Circulation, 69:250–258, 1984.
51. Platia, E. V., and Reid, P. R.: Comparison of programmed electrical stimulation and ambulatory electrocardiographic (Holter) monitoring in the management of ventricular tachycardia and ventricular fibrillation. J. Am. Coll. Cardiol., 4:493–500, 1984.
52. Maron, B. J., Savage, D. D., Wolfson, J. K., and Epstein, S. E.: Prognostic significance of 24 hour ambulatory electrocardiographic monitoring in patients with hypertrophic cardiomyopathy: A prospective study. J. Am. Coll. Cardiol., 48:252–257, 1981.
53. Goren, C., and Denes, P.: The role of Holter monitoring in detecting digitalis-provoked arrhythmias. Chest, 79:555–558, 1981.
54. Dewar, M. L., Rosengarten, M. D., Bundell, P. E., and Chiu, R. C. J.: Perioperative Holter monitoring and computer analysis of dysrhythmias in cardiac surgery. Chest, 87:593–598, 1985.
55. Ringel, R. E., Kennedy, H. L., Brenner, J. I., et al.: Detection of cardiac dysrhythmias by continuous electrocardiographic recording in children undergoing cardiac surgery. J. Electrocardiol. 17:1–6, 1984.
56. Kelen, G., Bloomfield, D., and Hardage, M.: Holter monitoring the patient with an artificial pacemaker—a new approach. Amb. Electrocardiol. 1:1, 1978.
57. Krasnow, A. Z., and Bloomfield, D. K.: Artifacts in portable electrocardiographic monitoring. Am. Heart J., 91:349, 1976.
58. Gardin, J. M., Belic, N., and Singer, D. H.: Pseudoarrhythmias in ambulatory ECG monitoring. Arch. Intern. Med., 139:809, 1979.
59. Isaeff, D. M., and Harrison, D. C.: Tachyarrhythmias in patients with Wolff-Parkinson-White syndrome in long-term Holter monitoring. Chest, 58:282, 1970.
60. Hindman, M. C., Last, J. H., and Rosen, K. M.: Wolff-Parkinson-White syndrome observed by portable monitoring. Ann. Intern. Med., 79:654, 1973.
61. Jenkins, J. M., Wu, D., and Arzbaecher, R. L.: Computer diagnosis of supraventricular and ventricular arrhythmias. A new esophogeal technique. Circulation, 60:977, 1979.

24

Electrophysiologic Testing in the Management of Patients with Unexplained Syncope

Fred Morady

Syncope, defined as transient loss of consciousness with spontaneous recovery, can be caused by a variety of metabolic, neurologic, and cardiac causes. In some patients, for example the patient who has a "fainting spell" during phlebotomy, syncope is a benign condition of little or no prognostic significance. On the other hand, if syncope is due to ventricular tachycardia, it may be a harbinger of sudden death. It is therefore always important to establish the cause of syncope.

The most common causes of syncope are listed in Table 24-1. The patient who experiences syncope should be evaluated initially with a thorough history, physical examination, and electrocardiogram. Several potential causes of syncope can be diagnosed on the basis of this initial evaluation, for example, classic vasodepressor syncope, orthostatic hypotension, carotid sinus hypersensitivity, obstructive cardiac lesions, and high-degree atrioventricular (AV) block. Depending on clues obtained from the history, physical examination, and electrocardiogram, it may be appropriate for the patient to have a thorough neurologic evaluation, echocardiogram, exercise treadmill test, or cardiac catheterization. Unless the cause of syncope is apparent, the evaluation should always include electrocardiographic monitoring, preferably on a prolonged, continuous, ambulatory basis, to look for potential arrhythmic causes of syncope.

It has been reported that the cause of syncope can be determined by history, physical examination, or noninvasive evaluation in 52% to 87% of unselected patients who are hospitalized with syncope.[1,2] However, in a significant proportion of patients, the cause of syncope remains unclear despite a thorough metabolic, neurologic, and noninvasive cardiac evaluation. In these patients, the sporadic and infrequent nature of the syncopal episodes may make it difficult to establish whether an arrhythmia is the cause of syncope. Although ambulatory electrocardiographic monitoring offers the potential for demonstrating an arrhythmic etiology of syncope, experience indicates that it is uncommon for syncope to occur while the patient is undergoing ambulatory monitoring. Gibson and Heitzman found that among 1512 patients who underwent ambulatory electrocardiographic monitoring because of syncope, only 15 patients (1%) had syncope during the monitoring period.[3] It is more often the case that ambulatory monitoring demonstrates arrhythmias, such as short episodes of nonsustained ventricular tachycardia or a sinus pause, that are not associated with cerebral symptoms. In these patients,

Table 24-1. The Most Common Causes of Syncope

I. Metabolic
  A. Hypoxema
  B. Hypoglycemia
  C. Hypocapnia, alkalosis
II. Neuropsychiatric
  A. Syncopal migraine
  B. Akinetic temporal lobe seizure
  C. Partial complex seizure
  D. Posterior circulation transient ischemic attack
III. Cardiovascular
  A. Vagally-mediated (cardioinhibitory or vasodepressor)
    1. Common faint
    2. Carotid sinus hypersensitivity
    3. Postmicturition syncope
    4. Swallow syncope
    5. Cough syncope
  B. Orthostatic hypotension
    1. Drug induced
    2. Hypovolemia
    3. Idiopathic
  C. Obstructive lesions
    1. Aortic stenosis
    2. Hypertrophic obstructive cardiomyopathy
    3. Atrial myxoma
    4. Pulmonary vascular disease
  D. Arrhythmias
    1. Sick sinus syndrome
    2. Atrioventricular block
    3. Supraventricular tachycardia
    4. Ventricular tachycardia

it cannot be assumed that the observed asymptomatic arrhythmia is the cause of syncope.

This chapter shall review the usefulness of electrophysiologic testing in establishing the cause of syncope in patients with unexplained syncope. Electrophysiologic testing may be helpful in uncovering the following potential arrhythmic causes of syncope: sinus node dysfunction, supraventricular tachycardia, AV block, and ventricular tachycardia.

Indications for Electrophysiologic Study

Syncope does not recur in a significant proportion of patients who experience an episode of it.[4,5] Electrophysiologic testing should therefore generally be considered only for patients in whom syncope has been demonstrated to be a recurrent, unexplained problem. However, in some patients it may be appropriate to perform electrophysiologic testing after only one episode of unexplained syncope. For example, if a patient suffers a severe injury as a result of a syncopal episode, a thorough evaluation including electrophysiologic testing may be indicated in order to minimize the possibility of additional injury. An electrophysiologic study should be considered in patients with one episode of unexplained syncope who are at risk of sudden death, for instance, patients with a cardiomyopathy or coronary artery disease and a history of myocardial infarction who have asymptomatic complex ventricular ectopic activity[6-8]; in these patients, one must consider the possibility that the syncope was caused by ventricular tachycardia and that the next episode might be fatal.

Evaluation of Sinus Node Function

Sinus node function is evaluated during electrophysiologic testing by determining the sinus node recovery time,[9,10] sinoatrial conduction time, [11,12] and sinus node refractory period.[13] Sinus node recovery time (SNRT) is determined by pacing the right atrium at various cycle lengths (*e.g.*, 600 to 300 msec in 50-msec decrements) for 30 to 60 seconds. The SNRT is defined as the interval between the last paced atrial depolarization and the first spontaneous atrial depolarization resulting from sinus node discharge. The SNRT is corrected for the patient's spontaneous cycle length simply by subtracting the spontaneous cycle length from the SNRT. The upper limits of normal of the corrected SNRT is approximately 550 msec. The normal response after the first sinus recovery beat is a gradual return to the baseline spontaneous cycle length after three to four beats. A secondary pause has been defined as an inappropriately long cycle length among the nine beats following the first sinus recovery beat following atrial overdrive pacing.[14] Evaluation of secondary pauses increases the sensitivity of the SNRT in the detection of sinus node dysfunction.[15]

The sinoatrial conduction time can be measured indirectly by the extrastimulus[11] or the overdrive[12] technique. Recently, Reiffel and colleagues described a catheter technique for recording the sinus node electrogram in humans, allowing direct measurements of the sinoatrial conduction time.[16]

Sinus node refractoriness can be determined in humans with an extrastimulus technique and has been reported to more clearly differentiate patients with and without sinus node dysfunction than does the SNRT or sinoatrial conduction time.[13]

Most patients with the sick sinus syndrome will demonstrate evidence of sinus node dysfunction during prolonged, continuous, ambulatory electrocardiographic recordings.[17,18] In published reports on the results of electrophysiologic testing in patients with unexplained syncope, patients have been screened for evidence of sinus node dysfunction during ambulatory electrocardiographic monitoring. It is therefore not surprising that sinus node dysfunction has been an infrequent finding among patients with unexplained syncope who underwent electrophysiologic testing. DiMarco and colleagues found a prolonged SNRT in only one of 25 patients with recurrent, unexplained syncope who underwent electrophysiologic testing.[19] Akhtar and associates found that four of 30 patients with recurrent unexplained syncope had a corrected SNRT greater than 800 msec.[20] Morady and co-workers reported that only two of 53 patients with recurrent, unexplained syncope had evidence of sinus node dysfunction—a prolonged SNRT in one patient and an abnormal sinoatrial conduction time in another.[21] Therefore, among a total of 108 patients with recurrent, unexplained syncope who did not have evidence of sinus node dysfunction during ambulatory monitoring and who underwent complete electrophysiologic testing, only seven patients (6%) were found to have sinus node dysfunction as the potential cause of syncope.

Because the presence of sinus node dysfunction may in some patients be an incidental finding unrelated to syncope, demonstration of an abnormal SNRT or sinoatrial conduction time during electrophysiologic testing does not guarantee that syncope will resolve after a permanent pacemaker is implanted. For example, Akhtar and colleagues reported that syncope recurred in 2 of 4 patients with unexplained syncope who were found to have a prolonged SNRT.[20] The clinical significance of a prolonged SNRT appears to be at least in part related to the degree of prolongation. Symptoms are most likely to resolve with pacemaker implantation when the SNRT is greater than 2 seconds (Figure 24-1).[22] If the patient's symptoms are reproduced during a postpacing pause, this may indicate that the cause of the patient's symptoms has been identified. On the other hand, the significance of a mildly prolonged SNRT in a patient with unexplained syncope and no evidence of sinus node dysfunction during ambulatory electrocardiographic monitoring is unclear. The decision to implant a permanent pacemaker in such patients remains a matter of clinical judgement.

In elderly patients with cerebral symptoms, ambulatory electrocardiographic recordings will not infrequently demonstrate asymptomatic sinus bradycardia. In these patients, symptoms cannot be assumed to be related to the sick sinus syndrome unless there is documentation that the symptoms are related to the bradyarrhythmia. Electrophysiologic testing may be helpful in evaluating these patients. Gann and colleagues reported that an abnormal SNRT was useful in selecting patients with chronic sinus bradycardia and dizziness or syncope for pacemaker therapy.[23] Among a group of 36 patients with a history of syncope and sinus bradycardia, 16 of 18 patients who had an abnormal SNRT had a permanent pacemaker implanted, and all subsequently remained asymptomatic; the two patients with an abnormal SNRT who refused pacemaker implantation remained symptomatic. Among the remaining 18 patients who had a normal SNRT, nine of ten patients without pacemakers became asymptomatic, while two of eight patients who underwent pacemaker implantation continued to have syncope. Therefore, a prolonged SNRT appeared to predict a response to pacemaker implantation. However, Gann, and colleagues did not take into account the degree of prolongation of the SNRT. The

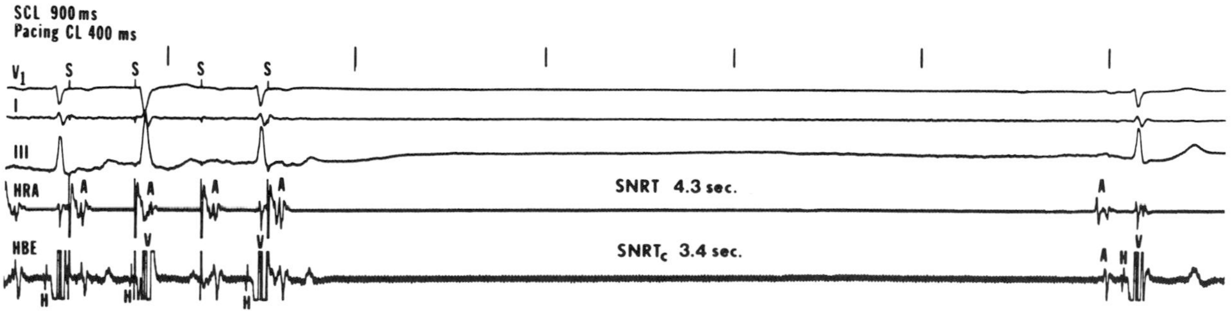

Figure 24-1. *A markedly prolonged sinus node recovery time (SNRT) in a patient with recurrent, unexplained syncope. From top to bottom are electrocardiographic leads V_1, I, and III, a high right atrial (HRA) electrogram, and the His bundle electrogram (HBE). Upon cessation of atrial pacing at a cycle length (CL) of 400 msec, there is a 4.3-second pause between the last paced atrial depolarization and the first spontaneous atrial depolarization resulting from sinus node discharge. Subtracting the spontaneous cycle length (SCL) of 900 msec yields a corrected sinus node recovery time ($SNRT_c$) of 3.4 seconds. Syncope did not recur after a permanent pacemaker was implanted. Time lines in this and subsequent figures represent 1-second intervals. (A, atrial depolarization; H, His bundle depolarization; S, pacing stimulus; V, ventricular depolarization)*

same considerations regarding the clinical significance of a prolonged SNRT apply in patients with syncope and chronic sinus bradycardia as apply in patients with syncope and no evidence of sinus node dysfunction during ambulatory monitoring. The clinical significance of a mildly prolonged SNRT should be interpreted with great caution.

Although the sinoatrial conduction time is a sensitive indicator of sinus node disease, it lacks a high degree of specificity and has been of limited value in evaluating the need for a permanent pacemaker.[24] For example, Morady and colleagues reported that a patient with recurrent unexplained syncope who had an abnormal sinoatrial conduction time and no other abnormalities during electrophysiologic testing had recurrent syncope despite implantation of a permanent pacemaker.[21]

Measurement of sinus node refractoriness using an extrastimulus technique has been found to increase the sensitivity of diagnosis of patients with sinus node dysfunction when compared to the SNRT and sinoatrial conduction time.[13] However, the usefulness of this measure of sinus node function in selecting patients with unexplained syncope who will benefit from pacemaker implantation has not been assessed.

Supraventricular Tachycardia

Although supraventricular tachycardia may cause syncope, this is uncommon unless the patient has underlying heart disease or the rate of the tachycardia is extremely rapid. In many patients, syncope or near-syncope may occur at the onset of an episode of supraventricular tachycardia because of an initial drop in blood pressure, especially if the patient is standing; compensatory mechanisms, that is, peripheral vasoconstriction, and assumption of a supine position then result in an increase in blood pressure and cerebral perfusion and the patient often regains consciousness although the tachycardia persists. Many patients with syncope due to supraventricular tachycardia do not experience syncope with every episode of tachycardia. For these reasons, patients who have syncope due to supraventricular tachycardia often do not present a diagnostic problem. However, an occasional patient with supraventricular tachycardia may have sporadic episodes of syncope as the only manifestation of the tachycardia. Repeated ambulatory electrocardiographic recordings may be unrevealing except in the unlikely event that the patient has an episode of syncope during the monitoring period. Electrophysiologic testing may be helpful in demonstrating the cause of syncope in these patients.

Electrophysiologic testing in patients with unexplained syncope should include incremental atrial and ventricular pacing and programmed atrial and ventricular stimulation with one extrastimulus to uncover the presence of an accessory pathway,[25,26] dual AV nodal pathways,[27,28] and enhanced AV nodal conduction.[29,30] Attempts should be made to induce AV nodal reentrant tachycardia, AV reciprocating tachycardia using an overt or concealed accessory pathway,[31] atrial tachycardia, and atrial fibrillation/flutter. The aggressiveness of the stimulation protocol used to induce these tachycardias should be guided by the clinical picture. In patients with recurrent, unexplained syncope who have repeated ambulatory electrocardiographic recordings that do not reveal symptomatic or asymptomatic supraventricular tachycardia, it is unlikely that electrophysiologic testing will demonstrate supraventricular tachycardia as the potential cause of syncope. Accordingly, among 108 patients with recurrent, unexplained syncope and negative ambulatory electrocardiographic recordings who underwent electrophysiologic testing, only one patient was found to have a supraventricular tachycardia felt to be the cause of syncope (atrial flutter with a ventricular rate of 205 beats/min).[19–21] However, if the patient is an otherwise healthy person who describes a prodome of rapid palpitations in association with syncope or if ambulatory electrocardiographic recordings demonstrate short runs of supraventricular tachycardia, then supraventricular tachycardia is more likely to be the cause of syncope and the electrophysiologic study should include vigorous attempts to induce the tachycardias described above (Fig. 24-2). If supraventricular tachycardia cannot be induced in the baseline state, atrial and ventricular stimulation repeated during an infusion of isoproterenol may be helpful in inducing a symptomatic supraventricular tachycardia (Fig. 24-3).[32,33]

In patients with the Wolff-Parkinson-White syndrome, the arrhythmias most likely to cause syncope are atrial fibrillation or flutter with a rapid ventricular response or AV reciprocating tachycardia. However, if these arrhythmias are not inducible during electrophysiologic testing, or if they are not rapid and associated with hypotension, a complete evaluation should be performed to look for other causes of syncope. Lloyd and colleagues reported on five patients with ventricular preexcitation and syncope who, based on the results of electrophysiologic testing, were found to have ventricular tachycardia rather than supraventricular tachycardia as the cause of syncope.[34]

Supraventricular tachycardia may at times be inducible during electrophysiologic testing in patients who have never had spontaneous episodes of supraventricular tachycardia. An induced tachycardia is unlikely to be the cause of syncope unless it is rapid and associated with a significant fall in blood pressure. In patients who have had syncope in association with supraventricular tachycardia, syncope usually does not occur when the supraventricular tachycardia is induced during electrophysio-

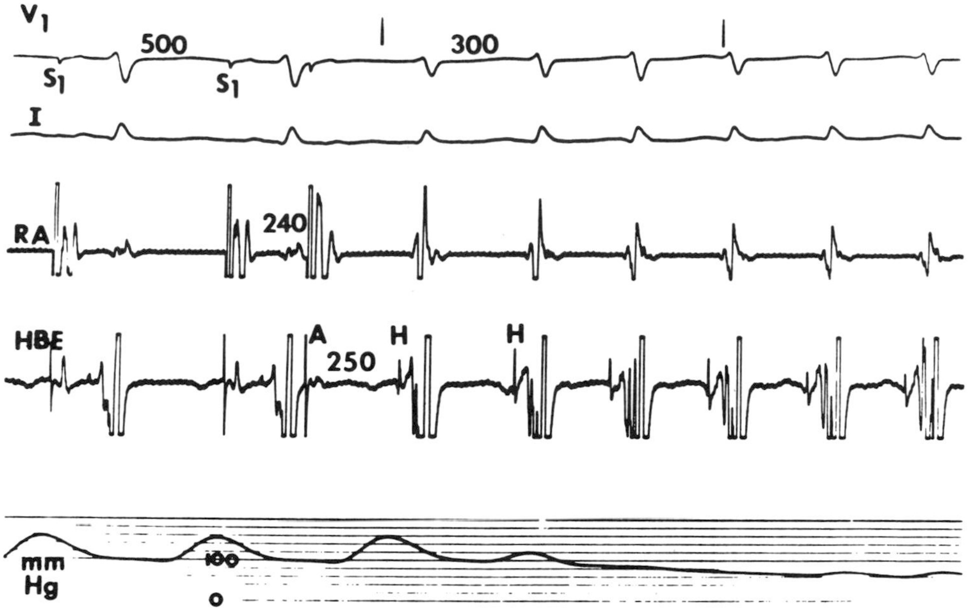

Figure 24-2. *Supraventricular tachycardia induced during electrophysiologic testing in a woman aged 36 years with a several-year history of paroxysmal palpitations, on one occasion associated with syncope. From top to bottom are electrocardiographic leads V_1 and I, a right atrial (RA) electrogram, the His bundle electrogram (HBE), and a recording of arterial blood pressure on a scale of 200 mm Hg. Right atrial programmed stimulation at a drive cycle length (S_1–S_1) of 500 msec with a single atrial extrastimulus (coupling interval 240 msec) induced AV nodal reentrant tachycardia, cycle length 300 msec. The systolic blood pressure fell rapidly from 160 to 70 mm Hg, and the patient experienced rapid palpitations and lightheadedness, similar to the symptoms she experienced before her episode of syncope. Propranolol was effective in suppressing the induction of this tachycardia, and no further episodes of palpitations or syncope occurred while the drug was given.*

logic testing in the supine position; however, the patient will often experience dizziness or near-syncope. Supraventricular tachycardia is probably not the cause of syncope if it is not associated with a fall in blood pressure or cerebral symptoms when induced in the electrophysiology laboratory. For example, Akhtar and associates found that AV nodal reentrant tachycardia could be initiated in three of 30 patients with recurrent, unexplained syncope who underwent electrophysiologic testing.[20] The rate of the tachycardia was 146 to 158 beats/min, and in none of the patients was the tachycardia associated with a significant fall in blood pressure or symptoms of dizziness. Despite treatment aimed at preventing the supraventricular tachycardia, these three patients continued to have syncope during the follow-up period, indicating that the supraventricular tachycardia was most likely an incidental finding.

Atrioventricular Block

Some patients with syncope caused by intermittent high-degree AV block may have normal AV conduction between episodes of AV block. Because syncope may be quite infrequent and unpredictable in these patients, it may not be possible to demonstrate the intermittent high-degree AV block despite repeated ambulatory electrocardiographic recordings. Electrophysiologic testing may be helpful in evaluating these patients.

Evaluation of AV conduction during electrophysiologic testing includes determining the baseline AV nodal to His bundle conduction time (AH interval) and the His bundle to ventricular conduction time (HV interval). Atrioventricular conduction is assessed by incremental atrial pacing, and AV nodal and His-Purkinje refractory periods are determined by the extrastimulus technique.[35]

Because it is uncommon for AV nodal block to be associated with severe bradycardia or syncope, the finding of a prolonged AV nodal refractory period may not necessarily be clinically significant. A complete evaluation for other potential causes of syncope should be performed before attributing the patient's syncope to intermittent second or third degree AV nodal block. If the only abnormality found during electrophysiologic testing in a patient with unexplained syncope is prolongation of AV nodal refractoriness, implantation of a permanent pacemaker is usually not indicated unless a

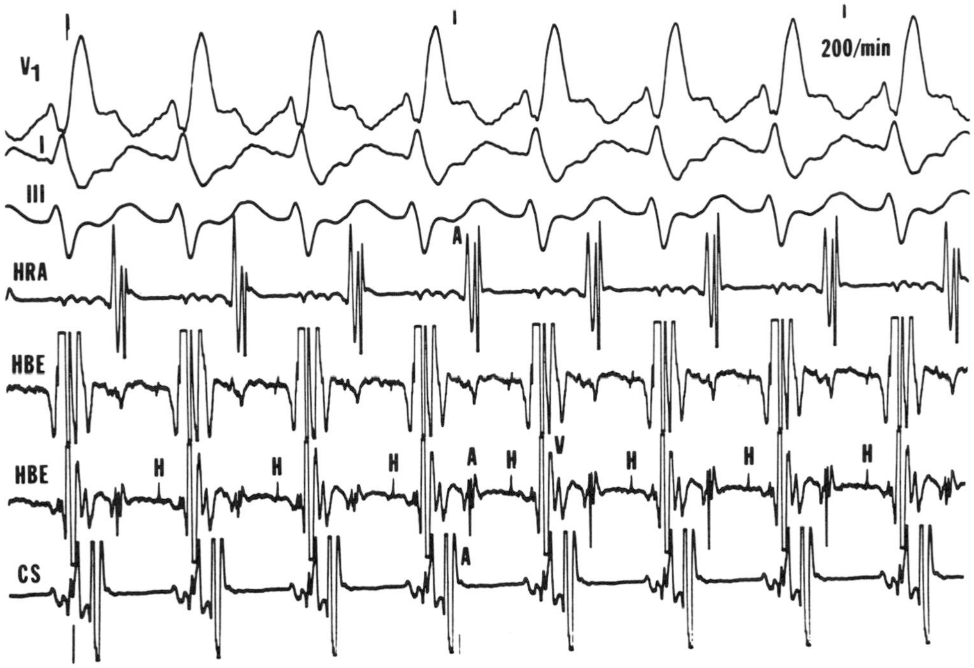

Figure 24-3. *Orthodromic reciprocating tachycardia induced during an infusion of isoproterenol. From top to bottom are leads V_1, I, and III, high right atrial (HRA) electrogram, two His bundle electrograms (HBE), and a distal coronary sinus (CS) electrogram. The patient had a concealed left-sided accessory pathway. Before the infusion of isoproterenol, only single echo beats were induced by atrial programmed stimulation. During infusion of isoproterenol, 2 μg/min, sustained orthodromic reciprocating tachycardia (rate 200 beats/min) was induced. Note the eccentric pattern of atrial activation, with earliest activation recorded in the distal coronary sinus, consistent with retrograde conduction over a left-sided accessory pathway. Abbreviations as in Figure 24-1.*

symptomatic bradyarrhythmia is documented during repeated ambulatory electrocardiographic recordings.

The clinical usefulness of the HV interval in patients with unexplained syncope has been controversial. Because patients with bundle branch block are much more likely to have a prolonged HV interval than are patients without bundle branch block, most published studies on the clinical significance of a prolonged HV interval have been conducted with patients with bundle branch block.

Dhingra and co-workers evaluated the clinical significance of the HV interval in a prospective study of 517 patients with bundle branch block, the majority of whom did not have syncope.[36] The HV interval was normal in 319 patients and prolonged (> 55 msec) in 198 patients. The cumulative 7-year incidence of high-degree AV block was 3% in the patients with a normal HV interval and 12% in the patients with a prolonged HV interval. These authors concluded that the HV interval is useful for evaluating patients with bundle branch block and that a prolonged HV interval in patients with bundle branch block and syncope implicates intermittent high-degree AV block as the cause of symptoms.

McAnulty and colleagues also conducted a prospective study of patients with bundle branch block, most of whom did not have syncope.[37] The HV interval was normal in 161 patients and prolonged in 190 patients. The mean followup period was 42 ± 8 months (±SD). In contrast to the findings of Dhingra and colleagues,[36] these authors found that patients with a prolonged HV interval did not have a statistically increased risk of high-degree AV block as compared to patients with a normal HV interval (4.9% versus 1.9%, $P > 0.05$). McAnulty and colleagues therefore concluded that the HV interval cannot be used to determine which patients with bundle branch block are at increased risk of developing AV block.

In the studies of Dhingra and colleagues[36] and McAnulty and associates,[37] patients with a prolonged HV interval were not categorized according to the degree of HV prolongation. Scheinman and co-workers performed a prospective study of 313 patients with bundle branch block (60% of whom did not have syncope) in which patients with a prolonged HV interval were categorized according to the degree of HV interval prolongation: normal in 97 patients, 55 to 69 msec in 99 patients, and ≥70 msec in 117 patients.[38] The mean follow-up period was approximately 3 years. The progression to high-degree AV block was greater in the group with an

HV interval ≥70 msec (12%) than in the other groups (2% to 4%). Of note is that high-degree AV block occurred in 4 of 17 patients (24%) with an HV interval ≥100 msec. Scheinman and associates concluded that an HV interval ≥70 msec is an independent risk factor for progression to high-degree AV block and that an HV interval ≥100 msec identifies a subgroup at particularly high risk.[38] These authors recommended pacemaker implantation in patients with bundle branch block and unexplained transient neurologic symptoms who have an HV interval ≥70 msec, particularly if the HV interval is ≥100 msec.

In applying the results of the above large-scale studies to the management of patients who undergo electrophysiologic testing because of unexplained syncope, one is faced with a significant limitation: both symptomatic and asymptomatic patients with bundle branch block were included in these studies, and the majority of patients did not have a history of syncope. In the studies summarized above, the prognostic significance of HV interval prolongation was not analyzed in the subgroup of patients who had syncope. It cannot be assumed that the results obtained by analyzing all patients with bundle branch block can be applied to patients with bundle branch block who have had syncope.

Of interest is a study by Altschuler and colleagues in which the significance of HV interval prolongation was assessed in a group of patients who all had either dizziness or syncope.[39] Eighteen patients who had a normal HV interval (<55 msec) did not undergo pacemaker implantation. Among 35 patients with HV interval prolongation (≥60 msec), 18 underwent pacemaker implantation and 17 did not. The decision to implant a pacemaker was left to the referring physician. Over a mean follow-up period of 22 ± 17 months, none of the patients with a normal HV interval died or developed AV block. Among the 17 patients with prolonged HV interval who did not receive a pacemaker, after a mean follow-up period of 6 ± 5 months, three patients had died suddenly, three had progressed to high-degree AV block requiring a pacemaker, and nine remained symptomatic. In contrast, among the 18 patients who received a pacemaker, after a mean follow-up period of 23 ± 13 months, none of the patients had died suddenly and only two remained symptomatic with syncope or dizziness. These results suggested that symptomatic patients with a prolonged HV interval were at increased risk of dying suddenly and that the incidence of both sudden death and symptoms could be diminished by pacemaker implantation. Altschuler and co-workers therefore concluded that patients with unexplained transient neurologic symptoms whose HV interval is ≥60 msec should receive a permanent pacemaker.[39]

The principal limitations of this study are the relatively small number of patients in the various subgroups and the nonrandom fashion in which pacemakers were implanted in the patients with a prolonged HV interval. Although the study of Altschuler and associates[39] does not provide definitive proof that patients with HV interval prolongation and syncope have an improved outcome with pacing, their results do suggest that pacemaker implantation should be considered for patients with recurrent, unexplained syncope whose only abnormality during electrophysiologic testing is a prolonged HV interval. In light of the findings of Scheinman and colleagues,[38] a permanent pacemaker would appear to be particularly appropriate in patients with unexplained syncope who have a markedly prolonged HV interval (≥100 msec) (Fig. 24-4). However, although there is a correlation between the degree of HV interval prolongation and the risk of high-degree AV block, a normal or mildly prolonged HV interval does not exclude the possibility of intermittent high-degree AV block in a patient with unexplained syncope (Fig. 24-5).

An uncommon finding in patients with bundle branch block, but one that is helpful when found, is infranodal block during atrial pacing. However, "pathologic" infranodal block must be distinguished from "functional" infranodal block.[40] Pathologic infranodal block during atrial pacing occurs when AV nodal conduction is intact (Fig. 24-6). Functional infranodal block during atrial pacing occurs when there is AV nodal Wenckebach; failure of impulse propagation in the AV node results in a pause that lengthens refractoriness in the His-Purkinje system such that the second beat in the next Wenckebach cycle blocks in or distal to the His bundle ("long-short" phenomenon, Fig. 24-7). Dhingra and colleagues reported that patients with functional infranodal block had a benign prognosis when left untreated, whereas among 15 patients with pacing-induced infranodal AV block during intact AV nodal conduction, eight patients developed AV block over a mean follow-up period of 3.4 years.[40] The electrophysiologic evaluation of patients with unexplained syncope should therefore include an assessment of the response to atrial pacing. Because of the high risk of AV block in patients with pathologic infranodal block induced by atrial pacing, pacemaker implantation is indicated in patients in whom no other apparent cause of syncope is found.

In patients who develop AV nodal Wenckebach block during atrial pacing at a long cycle length (≥450 msec), it may not be possible to assess conduction adequately within the His-Purkinje system. In these patients, it may be helpful to perform incremental atrial pacing after the administration of atropine (0.5 to 1 mg intravenously). A shortening of the cycle length at which AV nodal Wenckebach periodicity occurs allows one to subject the His-Purkinje system to greater stress and may uncover infranodal block. However, if infranodal block occurs only at a very short atrial pacing cycle length (<300

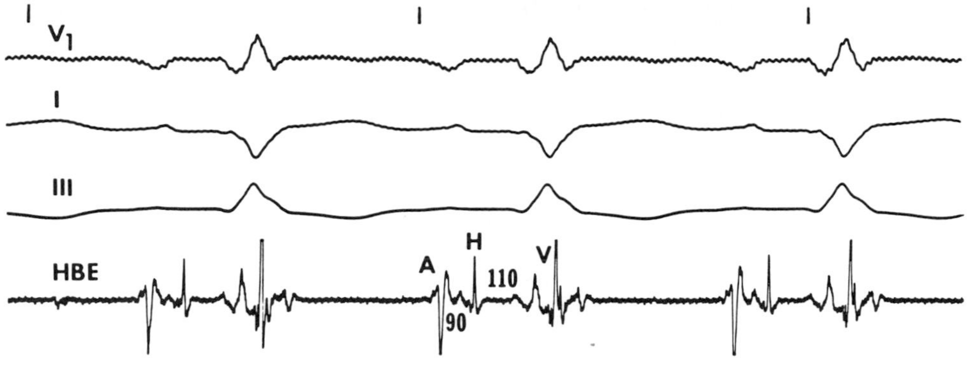

Figure 24-4. *A markedly prolonged HV interval. From top to bottom are electrocardiographic leads V_1, I, and III and a His bundle electrogram (HBE). This patient with recurrent, unexplained syncope had a right bundle branch block, a normal AH interval of 90 msec, and a markedly prolonged HV interval of 110 msec (upper limits of normal = 55 msec). Ventricular tachycardia was not inducible. The patient had no further syncope after a permanent pacemaker was implanted. Abbreviations as in Figure 24-1.*

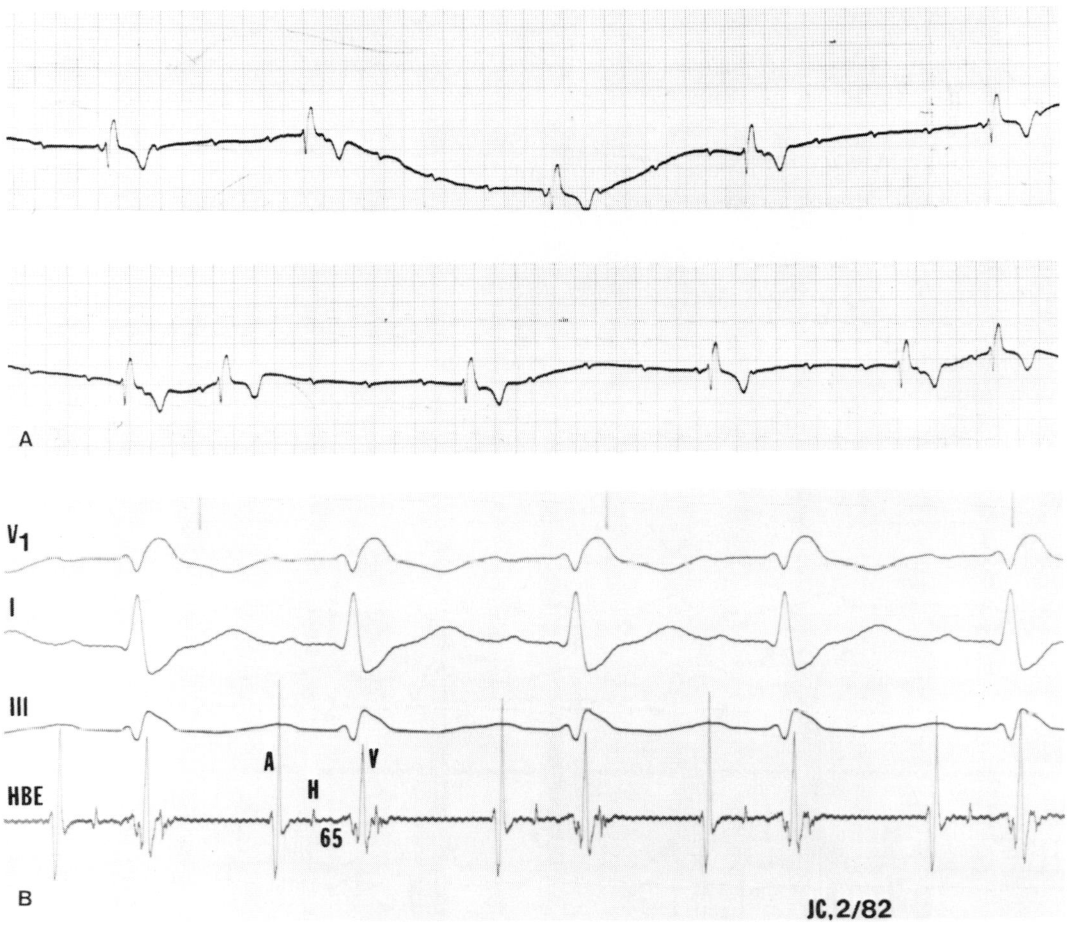

Figure 24-5. *An example of high-degree AV block in a patient with an HV interval that was only mildly prolonged. (A) The patient had a history of recurrent syncope. During a syncopal episode that occurred during hospitalization, an electrocardiogram demonstrated high-degree AV block with an average ventricular rate of 30 beats/min. Shown is a continuous recording of lead V_1. (B) A His bundle electrogram (HBE) recorded at permanent pacemaker implantation, when there was 1 : 1 AV conduction, demonstrated an HV interval of 65 msec. This example shows that a mildly prolonged HV interval does not rule out the possibility that syncope is due to intermittent high-degree AV block.*

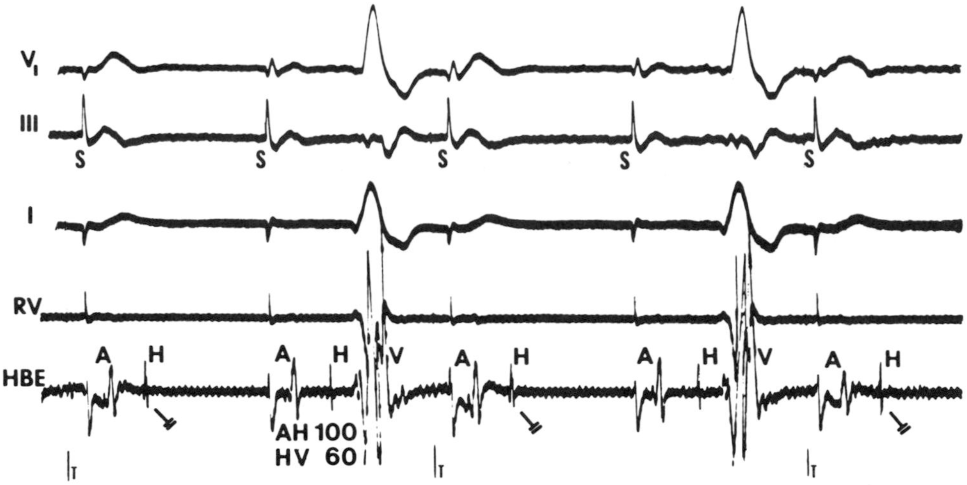

Figure 24-6. *Pathologic infranodal AV block during atrial pacing. From top to bottom are leads V_1, III, and I, a right ventricular (RV) electrogram, and a His bundle electrogram (HBE). The atrial pacing cycle length is 500 msec. There is intact AV nodal conduction, with an AH interval of 100 msec. Two-to-one infra-Hisian block is seen. This abnormality is associated with a high risk of high-degree AV block. Abbreviations as in Figure 24-1.*

msec), this may not be an abnormal response and is not necessarily an indication for pacemaker implantation in the patient with unexplained syncope.

Ventricular Tachycardia

Several studies have demonstrated that thc most common abnormality in patients with recurrent, unexplained syncope who undergo electrophysiologic testing is ventricular tachycardia.[19–21] The prevalence of inducible ventricular tachycardia in patients with recurrent, unexplained syncope has ranged from 36% to 53%.[19–21] However, it cannot be assumed that ventricular tachycardia is always the cause of syncope in these patients. Programmed ventricular stimulation is helpful in evaluating patients with unexplained syncope only to the extent that it results in the induction of clinical forms of ventricular tachycardia, that is, ventricular tachycardia that a patient has had spontaneously. Because pro-

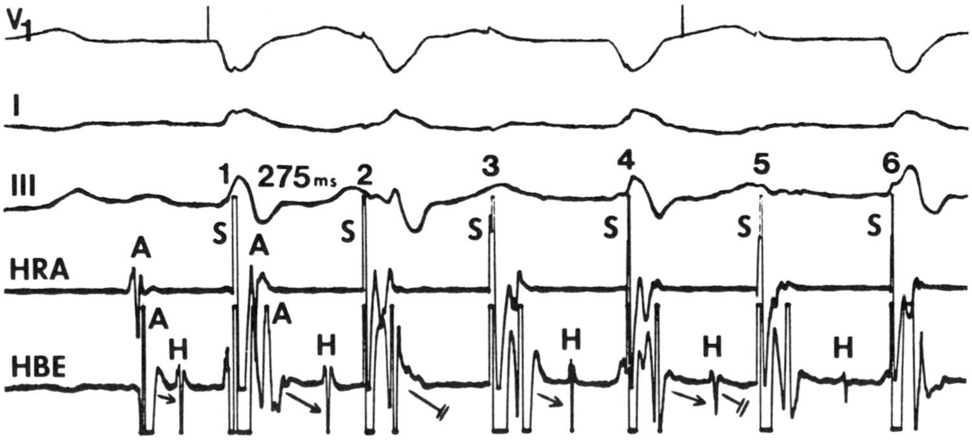

Figure 24-7. *Functional infranodal AV block during atrial pacing. From top to bottom are leads V_1, I, and III, a high right atrial (HRA) electrogram, and a His bundle electrogram (HBE). The atrial pacing cycle length is 275 msec. There is AV nodal Wenckebach block, with AV nodal block following stimulus number 2. The HH interval preceding stimulus number 4 is therefore lengthened, prolonging refractoriness in the His-Purkinje system. This accounts for the infra-Hisian block following stimulus number 4. This type of functional infranodal block is not associated with an increased risk of high-degree AV block. Abbreviations as in Figure 24-1.*

grammed ventricular stimulation may result in the induction of nonclinical forms of ventricular tachycardia, and because the "clinical" ventricular tachycardia (if there is one) in a patient with unexplained syncope has not been documented, it may be unclear whether an induced episode of ventricular tachycardia is clinically significant. A judgement on the clinical significance of induced ventricular tachycardia in a patient with unexplained syncope must be based on knowledge of the sensitivity and specificity of the particular stimulation protocol being used, the type of ventricular tachycardia induced, and the results of therapy reported in published studies.

Nonclinical forms of ventricular tachycardia are induced infrequently when the stimulation protocol includes only single and double extrastimuli.[41,42] However, recent studies have demonstrated that triple extra stimuli are often required to induce the clinical form of ventricular tachycardia in patients with documented ventricular tachycardia.[43,44] Unfortunately, although the sensitivity of programmed ventricular stimulation increases when triple extrastimuli are used, the specificity falls. When the ventricular stimulation protocol includes triple extrastimuli, ventricular tachycardia can be induced in 37% to 45% of patients who have no documented or suspected history of ventricular tachycardia.[44–47] The nonclinical episodes of ventricular tachycardia induced in these patients are usually polymorphic, rapid (cycle length <230 msec), and unsustained[44–47] and are more commonly induced in patients who have structural heart disease than in those who do not.[47] In contrast, sustained, unimorphic ventricular tachycardia is rarely inducible in patients who have not had spontaneous ventricular tachycardia.[44–47]

Based on the results of studies that have assessed the specificity of ventricular stimulation protocols, it can be predicted that in patients with unexplained syncope, sustained unimorphic ventricular tachycardia induced during electrophysiologic testing is more likely to be clinically significant than is polymorphic, nonsustained ventricular tachycardia. This is borne out by the results of a study by Morady and colleagues in which 53 patients with unexplained, recurrent syncope underwent electrophysiologic testing, including ventricular stimulation with up to triple extrastimuli.[21] Nonsustained ventricular tachycardia (usually polymorphic) was induced in 15 patients (28%), sustained ventricular tachycardia (usually unimorphic) was induced in nine (17%), and ventricular fibrillation was induced in four (8%). In the majority of patients, sustained ventricular tachycardia, nonsustained ventricular tachycardia, and ventricular fibrillation were induced by triple extrastimuli. These patients were treated with antiarrhythmic drugs selected on the basis of the results of electropharmacologic testing. The recurrence rate of syncope was 40% over 22 ± 6 months of follow-up study in patients with inducible nonsustained ventricular tachycardia, 0% over 30 ± 12 months of follow-up study in patients with inducible sustained ventricular tachycardia, and 25% over 21 ± 10 months of follow-up study in patients with inducible ventricular fibrillation. The excellent response rate in patients treated for sustained ventricular tachycardia implies that the cause of syncope was correctly identified and treated (Fig. 24-8). However, the 25% to 40% recurrence rate in the patients with induced polymorphic unsustained ventricular tachycardia or ventricular fibrillation suggests that at least in some patients, the induced arrhythmia may have been a nonspecific response to an aggressive stimulation protocol, unrelated to syncope (Fig. 24-9).

Because of the uncertainty that may arise regarding the clinical significance of ventricular tachycardia induced during electrophysiologic testing in patients with unexplained syncope, it is important to use a stimulation protocol that is sensitive in detecting ventricular tachycardia but that has maximum specificity. Multiple variables exist in a stimulation protocol (*e.g.*, stimulus strength, number of extrastimuli, number of basic drive rates, number of right ventricular stimulation sites, and the use of left ventricular stimulation). The ideal stimulation protocol, taking into account all these variables, has yet to be determined. However, based on available data, it seems prudent to use a relatively low current strength (between twice diastolic threshold and 5 mA), at least two right ventricular stimulation sites, at least two basic drive rates, and left ventricular stimulation only if ventricular tachycardia is not induced by right ventricular stimulation and if the patient has structural heart disease. The latter recommendation is based on the observation that the yield of inducible ventricular tachycardia in patients with unexplained syncope who do not have structural heart disease is exceedingly small[19–21]; the additional time and potential morbidity involved in performing left ventricular stimulation does not seem warranted in these patients.

Ventricular stimulation during an isoproterenol infusion increases the sensitivity of electrophysiologic testing,[48] but its effect on specificity has not been determined. Isoproterenol should be used as an additional provocative maneuver particularly in patients in whom syncope occurred in the setting of elevated catecholamine levels (*e.g.*, during or immediately after exercise).

As to the number of extrastimuli to use, because single and double extrastimuli induce nonclinical forms of ventricular tachycardia less often than do triple extrastimuli, it seems prudent to perform ventricular stimulation at two or more sites with single and double extrastimuli, reserving the use of triple extrastimuli for patients who do not have inducible ventricular tachycardia with fewer extrastimuli. This type of stimulation

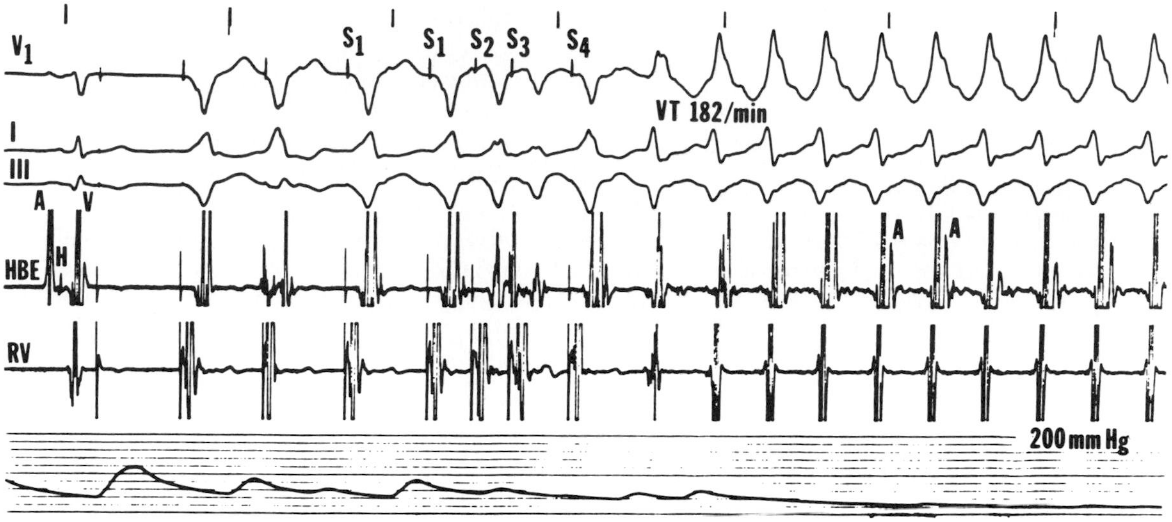

Figure 24-8. *Sustained unimorphic ventricular tachycardia (VT) induced in a patient with recurrent, unexplained syncope who had coronary artery disease, a history of myocardial infarction, and occasional ventricular premature depolarizations during prolonged ambulatory electrocardiographic monitoring. From top to bottom are leads V_1, I, and III, a His bundle electrogram (HBE), a right ventricular (RV) electrogram, and a recording of arterial blood pressure on a scale of 200 mm Hg. Triple extrastimuli (S_2, S_3, S_4) introduced during ventricular drive (S_1–S_1) induced VT, rate 182 beats/min. Systolic blood pressure fell rapidly from 120 to 0 mm Hg. The patient lost consciousness, and the VT was terminated by direct current countershock. Based on the results of electropharmacologic testing, the patient was treated with procainamide and has no further episodes of syncope. Sustained unimorphic VT has high diagnostic value when induced in a patient with unexplained syncope. Abbreviations as in Figure 24-1.*

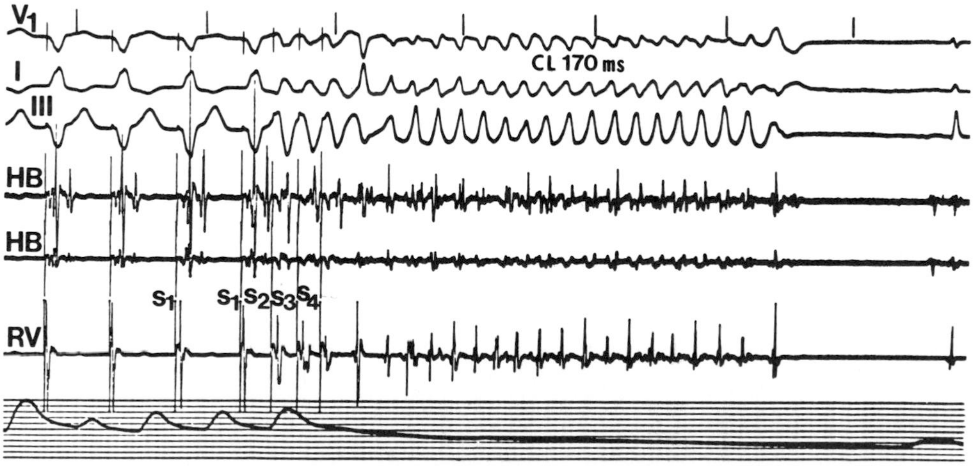

Figure 24-9. *Polymorphic, unsustained ventricular tachycardia, cycle length 170 msec, induced by triple extrastimuli (S_2, S_3, S_4) in a patient who had mitral valve prolapse and recurrent, unexplained syncope. From top to bottom are leads V_1, I, and III, two His bundle electrograms (HBE), a right ventricular (RV) electrogram, and an arterial blood pressure recording on a scale of 200 mm Hg. The patient was monitored and was documented to be in sinus rhythm during a typical episode of syncope that occurred after the electrophysiologic study. The VT induced in this patient was therefore most likely a laboratory artifact unrelated to syncope. This type of polymorphic, unsustained VT is often a nonspecific response to programmed stimulation with triple extrastimuli.*

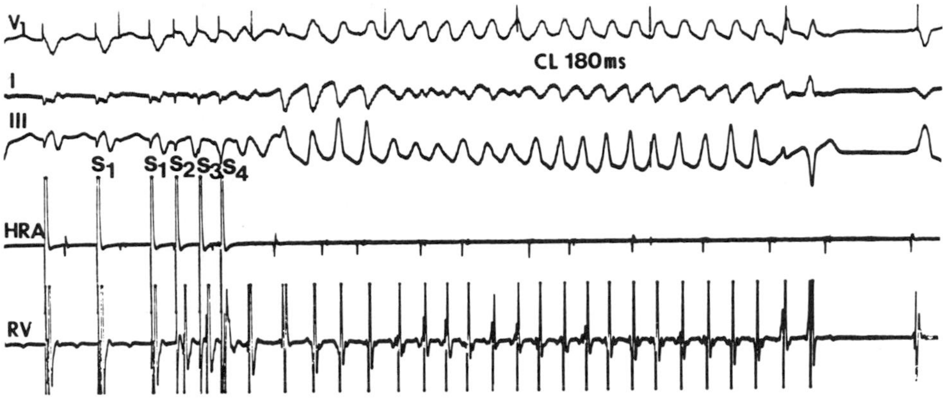

Figure 24-10. *Polymorphic, unsustained ventricular tachycardia, cycle length (CL) 180 msec, induced by triple extrastimuli (S_2, S_3, S_4) in a patient with a congestive cardiomyopathy and recurrent syncope and presyncope. Ambulatory electrocardiographic recordings demonstrated bursts of rapid, polymorphic ventricular tachycardia, CL 200 msec, associated with presyncope. From top to bottom are leads V_1, I, and III, a high right atrial (HRA) electrogram, and a right ventricular (RV) electrogram. In this patient, polymorphic, unsustained ventricular tachycardia induced by triple extrastimuli appeared to be a clinically significant arrhythmia. However, if the patient had not been found to have similar episodes of ventricular tachycardia during ambulatory monitoring, the polymorphic, unsustained tachycardia might have mistakenly been thought to be a nonspecific response to an aggressive stimulation protocol, as was the case in the example presented in Figure 24-9.*

protocol has been demonstrated to minimize the yield of nonclinical forms of ventricular tachycardia and to maximize the yield of clinical forms of ventricular tachycardia.[49]

Although unimorphic ventricular tachycardia is more likely than is polymorphic ventricular tachycardia to be a clinically significant arrhythmia when induced in a patient with unexplained syncope, the clinical significance of polymorphic ventricular tachycardia in a given patient may be difficult to assess. In some patients, polymorphic ventricular tachycardia is a laboratory artifact, while in others it is the cause of syncope; the dilemma is how to distinguish the two (Fig. 24-10). Based on available data regarding the specificity of ventricular tachycardia induction protocols, the probability that polymorphic ventricular tachycardia is the cause of syncope appears to be inversely related to the number of extrastimuli needed to induce the ventricular tachycardia; that is, the greater the number of extrastimuli needed to induce the polymorphic ventricular tachycardia, the less likely it is to be the cause of syncope. If no other potential cause for syncope is found, a clinical trial of antiarrhythmic drug therapy aimed at suppressing polymorphic ventricular tachycardia may be indicated. If syncope recurs despite antiarrhythmic drug therapy predicted to be efficacious on the basis of electropharmacologic testing, polymorphic ventricular tachycardia may not be the cause of syncope.

Particular mention should be made of patients with bundle branch block who have unexplained syncope. Ezri and colleagues found that ventricular tachycardia was inducible in four of 13 patients with bundle branch block and unexplained syncope.[50] In a group of 32 patients with bundle branch block and unexplained syncope, Morady and associates reported that unimorphic ventricular tachycardia was inducible in nine (28%); one of these patients (who was noncompliant) died suddenly, while the other eight patients, who were treated with antiarrhythmic drugs directed at suppressing ventricular tachycardia, did not have recurrent syncope.[51] Of note is that four of the nine patients had an HV interval ≥70 msec, indicating a second potential cause of syncope, namely, intermittent AV block. These results demonstrate that patients with bundle branch block and unexplained syncope should undergo programmed ventricular stimulation even when a prolonged HV interval indicates that AV block may be a cause of syncope. Some patients with bundle branch block may be found to have two potential causes of syncope and may require more than one form of therapy (*i.e.*, a pacemaker plus antiarrhythmic drugs).

Patients Most Likely to Have a Positive Electrophysiologic Study

The diagnostic yield of electrophysiologic testing has been found to be higher in patients with unexplained syncope who have structural heart disease than in those who do not. Akhtar and co-workers reported that an inducible arrhythmia that could have accounted for syncope was found in 16 of 18 patients who had structural heart disease, compared to only one of 12 patients who did not have structural heart disease.[20] Gulamhusein and colleagues performed electrophysiologic testing in 34 patients who had unexplained syncope or presyncope and no clinical evidence of organic heart disease.[52] A diagnostic abnormality was found in only four patients (12%).

Morady and colleagues analyzed the correlation between several clinical variables and the finding of inducible ventricular tachycardia in patients with unexplained syncope.[21] The absence of structural heart disease was independently associated with the lack of inducible ventricular tachycardia. The following variables had no independent effect on the outcome of electrophysiologic testing: age, frequency of ventricular premature depolarizations during ambulatory electrocardiographic monitoring, previous myocardial infarction, congestive heart failure, and an abnormal electrocardiogram.

These findings suggest that, as expected, patients without structural heart disease are less likely to have a serious arrhythmia as the cause of syncope than are patients who have structural heart disease. However, among patients who have structural heart disease, it cannot be predicted on the basis of simple clinical variables which patients will have a positive or negative electrophysiologic study.

Implications of a Negative Electrophysiologic Study

In a group of 34 patients without organic heart disease who had unexplained syncope or presyncope, Gulamhusein and associates reported that 15 of 28 patients (44%) who had a normal electrophysiologic study had no recurrence of syncope over a mean of 15 months of follow-up study (range 2 to 44 months).[52] Morady and colleagues also found a high spontaneous remission rate in patients with a normal electrophysiologic study; 7 of 10 patients (70%) who received no therapy had no recurrence of syncope over 31 ± 10 months of follow-up study.[21] In a group of 32 patients with bundle branch block and unexplained syncope, no diagnostic abnormalities were found during electrophysiologic testing in eight patients; only one of these eight patients had a recurrence of syncope over a mean of 18 months follow-up study (range 6 to 41 months).[51] Therefore, it appears that patients with unexplained syncope who have a negative electrophysiologic study may have a low incidence of recurrent syncope.

The explanation for the high spontaneous remission rate among patients who have a negative electrophysiologic study is unclear. The apparent remission may be due to spontaneous fluctuations in frequency; syncope may eventually recur with longer follow-up study. Some of these patients may have a psychiatric or hysterical basis for syncope and benefit from a placebo effect associated with undergoing an electrophysiologic study.

A normal electrophysiologic study does not rule out the possibility of an arrhythmic etiology for a patient's syncope. Patients with bundle branch block and intermittent high-degree infranodal AV block may at times have a normal HV interval between episodes of AV block.[53,54] If syncope is caused by ventricular tachycardia that is due to abnormal automaticity rather than reentry, the ventricular tachycardia will usually not be inducible by programmed ventricular stimulation and may not be provoked by isoproterenol either. In some patients with coronary artery disease, syncope due to ventricular tachycardia may occur only in the setting of myocardial ischemia; these patients may not have inducible ventricular tachycardia if ischemia is not present during electrophysiologic testing. Therefore, although a normal electrophysiologic study decreases the likelihood that syncope is caused by an arrhythmia, it does not rule out the possibility.

Also, a benign prognosis is not guaranteed by an electrophysiologic study that does not demonstrate any diagnostic abnormalities. Among 12 patients with unexplained syncope and a negative electrophysiologic study who were treated empirically with an antiarrhythmic drug because of ventricular premature depolarizations, two patients (both of whom had coronary artery disease) died suddenly.[21] Unfortunately, the mechanism of sudden death and whether antiarrhythmic drug therapy contributed to it is unclear.

What is the most appropriate management of the patient with unexplained syncope who has frequent ventricular premature depolarizations or nonsustained ventricular tachycardia without associated symptoms during ambulatory electrocardiographic monitoring *and* a normal electrophysiologic study? The asymptomatic ventricular ectopy may be an incidental finding, or the ventricular ectopy may be a clue that the patient's syncope is caused by ventricular tachycardia that is not inducible by programmed stimulation. Although no definitive recommendations can be made, it seems reasonable to attempt to suppress the ectopy with antiarrhythmic drugs in patients who, irrespective of their syncope, may be at increased risk of sudden death, for example, patients with coronary artery disease or dilated cardiomyopathy who have complex forms of ventricular ectopy.[6–8] In patients with unexplained syncope, complex but asymptomatic ventricular arrhythmias, and a normal electrophysiologic study who do not fall into a "high-risk" subgroup, for example, patients without identifiable structural heart disease, an empiric trial of antiarrhythmic drug therapy becomes a matter of clinical judgement. The potential toxicity and expense of chronic antiarrhythmic drug treatment must be weighed against the risk of symptomatic ventricular tachycardia or sudden death; the latter risk appears to be small in patients without identifiable heart disease.[55]

Is there a role for empiric pacemaker implantation in the patient with recurrent, unexplained syncope who has a normal electrophysiologic study? Gulamhusein and colleagues reported that there was no recurrence of syncope in seven patients with syncope or presyncope who had a normal electrophysiologic study and underwent pacemaker implantation.[52] However, these authors also found a high remission rate in patients with a normal electrophysiologic study who received no therapy. Morady and colleagues found that syncope recurred in two of three patients with recurrent syncope and a normal electrophysiologic study who received a permanent pacemaker.[21] It seems that there is little or no role for pacemaker implantation in patients with unexplained syncope who have no abnormalities demonstrated by electrocardiographic monitoring or electrophysiologic testing. However, it may be appropriate to institute an empiric trial of permanent pacing in the patient who has recurrent, unexplained syncope that causes injury and who is found to have a borderline abnormal but asymptomatic bradyarrhythmia during electrocardiographic monitoring (*e.g.*, a 1.7-second sinus pause).

Conclusions

Electrophysiologic testing in the evaluation of patients with unexplained syncope is associated with several important limitations. Diagnosis of the cause of syncope based on the results of electrophysiologic testing is inferential. Electrophysiologic testing may demonstrate abnormalities that are not related to the patient's syncope. A normal electrophysiologic study does not rule out an arrhythmic cause of syncope. These limitations must be kept in mind when selecting patients to undergo electrophysiologic testing and when interpreting the results.

Among patients with unexplained syncope who do not have organic heart disease, an arrhythmic cause of syncope is unlikely, and therefore the diagnostic yield of electrophysiologic testing is very low. Unless there is a specific reason to suspect an arrhythmic cause of syncope (*e.g.*, abrupt onset of rapid palpitations before syncope), electrophysiologic testing is unlikely to be of value in these patients.

On the other hand, electrophysiologic testing can uncover an abnormality that is likely to be the cause of syncope in a significant percentage of patients with organic heart disease. Probably the most significant contribution of electrophysiologic testing in the evaluation of patients with organic heart disease who have unexplained syncope is to demonstrate whether ventricular tachycardia may be the cause of syncope. Electrophysiologic testing is therefore particularly appropriate in patients who belong to subgroups demonstrated to be at increased risk of sudden death.

The following abnormalities have the highest diagnostic value: inducible unimorphic ventricular tachycardia, a markedly prolonged SNRT (>3 seconds), inducible supraventricular tachycardia that is rapid and causes hypotension, a markedly prolonged HV interval (≥ 100 msec), and pacing-induced infranodal AV block during intact AV nodal conduction. The diagnostic value of these abnormalities is enhanced if the induced arrhythmia reproduces the patient's symptoms.

A mildly prolonged SNRT, an abnormal sinoatrial conduction time, a moderately prolonged HV interval (70 to 100 msec), and inducible polymorphic ventricular tachycardia or ventricular fibrillation may be related to the cause of syncope in some patients; however, in many patients these may be incidental findings or laboratory artifacts unrelated to syncope.

Despite its limitations, electrophysiologic testing can make an important contribution to the diagnosis and treatment of selected patients with unexplained syncope.

References

1. Day, S. C., Cook, E. F., Funkenstein, H., Goldman, L.: Evaluation and outcome of emergency room patients with transient loss of consciousness. Am. J. Med., 73:15–23, 1982.
2. Kapoor, W. N., Karpf, M., Wieand, S., et al.: A prospective evaluation and follow up of patients with syncope. N. Engl. J. Med., 309:197–204, 1983.
3. Gibson, T. C., and Heitzman, M. R.: Diagnostic efficacy of 24-hour electrocardiographic monitoring for syncope. Am. J. Cardiol., 53:1013–1017, 1984.
4. Dhingra, R. C., Denes, P., Wu, D., et al.: Syncope in patients with chronic bifascicular block. Significance, causative mechanisms, and clinical implications. Ann. Intern. Med., 81:302–306, 1974.
5. Peters, R. W., Scheinman, M. M., Modin, G., et al.: Prophylactic permanent pacemakers for patients with chronic bundle branch block. Am. J. Med., 66:978–985, 1979.
6. Meinertz, T., Hofmann, T., Wolfgang, K., et al.: Significance of ventricular arrhythmias in idiopathic dilated cardiomyopathy. Am. J. Cardiol., 53:902–907, 1984.
7. Ruberman, W., Weinblatt, E., Goldberg, J. D., et al.: Ventricular premature complexes and sudden death after myocardial infarction. Circulation, 64:297–305, 1981.
8. Bigger, J. T., Jr., Fleiss, J. L., Kleiger, R., et al.: The relationships among ventricular arrhythmias, left ventricular dysfunction, and mortality in the 2 years after myocardial infarction. Circulation, 69:250–258, 1984.
9. Mandel, W. J., Hayakawa, H., Danzig, R., and Marcus, H. S.: Evaluation of sinoatrial node function in man by overdrive suppression. Circulation, 44:59–66, 1971.
10. Narula, O. S., Samet, P., and Javier, R. P.: Significance of the sinus node recovery time. Circulation, 45:140–158, 1972.
11. Strauss, H. C., Saroff, A. L.,. Bigger, J. T., and Giardina, E. G. V.:

Premature atrial stimulation as a key to the understanding of sinoatrial conduction in man. Presentation of data and critical review of the literature. Circulation, 47:86–93, 1973.
12. Narula, O. S., Shantha, N., Vasquez, M., et al.: A new method for measurement of sinoatrial conduction time. Circulation, 58:706–714, 1978.
13. Kerr, C. R., and Strauss, H. C.: The measurement of sinus node refractoriness in man. Circulation, 68:1231–1237, 1983.
14. Benditt, D. G., Strauss, H. C., Scheinman, M., et al.: Analysis of secondary pauses following termination of rapid atrial pacing in man. Circulation, 54:436–441, 1976.
15. Scheinman, M. M., Strauss, H. C., Abbott, J. A., et al.: Electrophysiologic testing in patients with sinus pauses and/or sinoatrial exit block. Eur. J. Cardiol., 8:51–60, 1978
16. Reiffel, J. A., Gang, E., Gliklich, J., et al.: The human sinus node electrogram: a transvenous catheter technique and a comparison of directly measured and indirectly estimated sinoatrial conduction time in adults. Circulation, 62:1324–1334, 1980.
17. Moss, A. J., and Davis, R. J.: Brady-tachy syndrome. Prog. Cardiovasc. Dis., 16:439–454, 1974.
18. Scheinman, M. M., Peters, R., Hirschfeld, D. S. et al.: The sick sinus ailing atrium. West. J. Med., 121:473–481, 1974.
19. DiMarco, J. P., Garan, H., Harthorne, J. W., and Ruskin, J. N.: Intracardiac electrophysiologic techniques in recurrent syncope of unknown cause. Ann. Intern. Med., 95:542–548, 1981.
20. Akhtar, M., Shenasa, M., Denker, S., et al.: Role of cardiac electrophysiologic studies in patients with unexplained recurrent syncope. Pace, 6:192–201, 1983.
21. Morady, F., Shen, E., Schwartz, A., et al.: Long-term follow-up of patients with recurrent unexplained syncope evaluated by electrophysiologic testing. J. Am. Coll. Cardiol., 2:1053–1059, 1983.
22. Scheinman, M. M., Strauss, H. C., and Abbott, J. A.: Electrophysiologic testing for patients with sinus node dysfunction. J Electrocardiol., 12:211–216, 1979.
23. Gann, D., Tolentino, A., and Samet, P.: Electrophysiologic evaluation of elderly patients with sinus bradycardia. A long-term follow-up study. Ann. Intern. Med., 90:24–29, 1979.
24. Dhingra, R. C., Amat-Y-Leon, F., Wyndham, C., et al.: Clinical significance of prolonged sinoatrial conduction time. Circulation, 55:8–15, 1977.
25. Durrer, D., Schoo, L., Schuilenburg, R. M., and Wellens, H. J. J.: The role of premature beats in the initiation and the termination of supraventricular tachycardia in the Wolff-Parkinson-White syndrome. Circulation, 36:644–662, 1967.
26. Sung, R. J., Castellanos, A., Mallon, S. M., et al.: Mode of initiation of reciprocating tachycardia during programmed ventricular stimulation in the Wolff-Parkinson-White syndrome: With reference to various patterns of ventriculoatrial conduction. Am. J. Cardiol., 40:24–31, 1977.
27. Denes, P., Wu, D., Dhingra, R. C., et al.: Demonstration of dual A-V nodal pathways in patients with paroxysmal supraventricular tachycardia. Circulation, 48:549–555, 1973.
28. Rosen, K. M., Mehta, A., and Miller, R. A.: Demonstration of dual atrioventricular nodal pathways in man. Am. J. Cardiol. 33:291–294, 1974.
29. Benditt, D. G., Pritchett, E. L., Smith, W. M., et al.: Characteristics of atrioventricular conduction and the spectrum of arrhythmias in Lown-Ganong-Levine syndrome. Circulation, 57:454–465, 1978.
30. Moleiro, F., Mendoza, I. J., Medina-Ravell, V., et al.: One to one atrioventricular conduction during atrial pacing at rates of 300/minute in absence of Wolff-Parkinson-White syndrome. Am. J. Cardiol., 48:789–796, 1981.
31. Farshidi, A., Josephson, M. E., and Horowitz, L. N.: Electrophysiologic characteristics of concealed bypass tracts: Clinical and electrocardiographic correlates. Am. J. Cardiol., 41:1052–1060, 1978.
32. Przybylski, J., Chiale, P. A., Halpern, M. S., et al.: Unmasking of ventricular preexcitation by vagal stimulation or isoproterenol administration. Circulation, 61:1030–1036, 1980.
33. Hariman, R. J., Gomes, J. A. C., and El-Sherif, N.: Catecholamine-dependent atrioventricular nodal reentrant tachycardia. Circulation, 67:681–682, 1983.
34. Lloyd, E. A., Hauer, R. N., Zipes, D. P., et al.: Syncope and ventricular tachycardia in patients with ventricular preexcitation. Am. J. Cardiol., 52:79–82, 1983.
35. Josephson, M. E., and Seides, S. F.: Clinical Cardiac Electrophysiology: Techniques and Interpretations, pp. 23–59. Philadelphia, Lea & Febiger, 1979.
36. Dhingra, R. C., Palileo, E., Strasberg, B., et al.: Significance of the HV interval in 517 patients with chronic bifascicular block. Circulation, 64:1265–1271, 1981.
37. McAnulty, J. H., Rahimtoola, S. H., Murphy, E., et al.: Natural history of "high-risk" bundle-branch block. Final report of a prospective study. N. Engl. J. Med. 307:137–143, 1982.
38. Scheinman, M. M., Peters, R. W., Sauve, M. J., et al.: Value of the H-Q interval in patients with bundle branch block and the role of prophylactic permanent pacing. Am. J. Cardiol., 50:1316–1322, 1982.
39. Altschuler, H., Fisher, J. D., and Furman, S.,: Significance of isolated H-V interval prolongation in symptomatic patients without documented heart block. Am. Heart J., 97:19–26, 1979.
40. Dhingra, R. C., Wyndham, C., Bauernfeind, R., et al.: Significance of block distal to the His bundle induced by atrial pacing in patients with chronic bifascicular block. Circulation, 60:1455–1465, 1979.
41. Vandepol, C. J., Farshidi, A., Spielman, S. R., et al.: Incidence and clinical significance of induced ventricular tachycardia. Am. J. Cardiol., 45:725–731, 1980.
42. Livelli, F. D., Jr., Bigger, J. T., Jr., Reiffel, J. A., et al.: Response to programmed ventricular stimulation: sensitivity, specificity and relation to heart disease. Am. J. Cardiol., 50:452–458, 1982.
43. Mann, D. E., Luck, J. C., Griffin, J. C., et al.: Induction of clinical ventricular tachycardia using programmed stimulation: Value of third and fourth extrastimuli. Am. J. Cardiol., 52:501–506, 1983.
44. Buxton, A. E., Waxman, H. L., Marchlinski, F. E., et al.: Role of triple extrastimuli during electrophysiologic study of patients with documented sustained ventricular tachyarrhythmias. Circulation, 69:532–540, 1984.
45. Brugada, P., Abdollah, H., Heddle, B., and Wellens, H. J. J.: Results of a ventricular stimulation protocol using a maximum of 4 premature stimuli in patients without documented or suspected ventricular arrhythmias. Am. J. Cardiol., 52:1214–1218, 1983.
46. Brugada, P., Green, M., Abdollah, H., and Wellens, H. J. J.: Significance of ventricular arrhythmias initiated by programmed ventricular stimulation: the importance of the type of ventricular arrhythmia induced and the number of premature stimuli required. Circulation, 69:87–92, 1984.
47. Morady, F., Shapiro, W., Shen, E., et al.: Programmed ventricular stimulation in patients without spontaneous ventricular tachycardia. Am. Heart J., 107:875–882, 1984.
48. Reddy, C. P., and Gettes, L. S.: Use of isoproterenol as an aid to electric induction of chronic recurrent ventricular tachycardia. Am. J. Cardiol., 44:705–713, 1979.
49. Morady, F., DiCarlo, L., Winston, S., et al.: A prospective comparison of triple extrastimuli and left ventricular stimulation in ventricular tachycardia induction studies. Circulation, 70:52–57, 1984.
50. Ezri, M., Lerman, B. B., Marchlinski, F. E., et al.: Electrophysio-

logic evaluation of syncope in patients with bifascicular block. Am. Heart J. 106:693–697, 1983.

51. Morady, F., Higgins, J., Peters, R. W., et al.: Results of electrophysiologic testing in patients with bundle branch block and unexplained syncope. Am. J. Cardiol., 54:587–591, 1984.
52. Gulamhusein, S., Naccarelli, G. V., Ko, P. T., et al.: Value and limitations of clinical electrophysiologic study in assessment of patients with unexplained syncope. Am. J. Med., 73:700–705, 1982.
53. DeJoseph, R. L., and Zipes, D. P.: Normal HV time in a patient with right bundle branch block, left anterior hemiblock and intermittent complete distal His block. Chest, 63:564–568, 1973.
54. McKenna, W. J., Rowland, E., Davies, J., and Krikler, D. M.: Failure to predict development of atrioventricular block with electrophysiological testing supplemented by ajmaline. Pace, 3:666–669, 1980.
55. Montague, T. J., McPherson, D. D., MacKenzie, B. R., et al.: Frequent ventricular ectopic activity without underlying cardiac disease: analysis of 45 subjects. Am. J. Cardiol., 52:980–984, 1983.

25

Pacemaker-Induced Arrhythmias

Agustin Castellanos, Richard M. Luceri, Victor A. Medina-Ravell, and Robert J. Myerburg

In the years since the first edition of this book was published, so many medical, technologic, and geopolitical changes have occurred that a drastic revision of this chapter appeared mandatory. In 1980 the pulse generator used most often was the VVI pacemaker.[1] DVI pacemakers then became popular. Lately, there has been a dramatic increase in the use of DDD pacemakers. Although we think that DDD pacemakers should be the pacemaker of choice (except when specific contraindications exist), DVI pacing will also be described, since DDD pacemakers sometimes still must be programmed in this mode. Moreover, various reasons (*e.g.,* cost, availability) will probably make it necessary for clinicians to use VVI pacemakers in certain instances. Therefore, this chapter discusses the arrhythmias produced by all three types of pacemakers. The term *arrhythmia* refers to any rhythm produced (initiated and sustained) by the pacemakers when they are functioning as programmed.

To understand fully normal and abnormal modes of pacemaker operation, one must be familiar with the five-position identification code introduced by the Pacemaker Study Group of the Inter-Society Commission for Heart Disease Resources (ICHD) in 1983 (Table 25-1)[1] The reader is encouraged to study this code carefully. Henceforth, the various pacemakers will be referred to in this "language" rather than in the now obsolete nomenclature based on older usage or generic descriptions.[1] The ICHD has made it clear that the electrocardiographer should be provided with adequate information, including pacemaker model number, programmed mode, and *latest* programmed settings. Because nearly all pacemakers are programmable, it is important to recognize that the rates, output parameters, refractory periods, and mode may differ not only in devices from various manufacturers but in pacemakers made by the same manufacturer. This, and rapid advances in the pacemaker field, make it essential for the interpreter to check the brochure supplied by the manufacturer when attempting to interpret the electrocardiographic manifestations of pacemaker arrhythmias.

This chapter should be viewed as having a didactic orientation. The pacemaker parameters given are supplied as examples, since some or all of the prototype descriptions that follow may not apply by the time this book is published.

Table 25-1. Inter-Society Commission for Heart Disease Five-Position Pacemaker Code

Position	I	II	III	IV	V
Category	Chamber(s) paced	Chambers(s) sensed	Modes of response(s)	Programmable functions	Special antitachyarrhythmia functions
Letters used	Ventricle (V)	Ventricle (V)	Triggered (T)	Programmable (rate or output) (P)	Bursts (B)
	Atrium (A)	Atrium (A)	Inhibited (I)	Multiprogrammable (M)	Normal rate competition (N)
	Double (D)	Double (D)	Double (D)*	Communicating (C)	Scanning (S)
			None (0)		
		None (0)	Reverse (R)	None (0)	External (E)
Manufacturer's designation only	Single chamber(s)	Single chamber(s)		↓ , Comma optional here	

(Parsonnet, V., Furman, S., Smyth, N. P. D., and Belitch, M.: Optimal resources for implantable cardiac pacemakers. Circulation, 68:227, 1983)
* Triggered and inhibited response.

VVI Pacemakers

Pacemaker Intervals

The *automatic interval* is the interval between two consecutive spikes while the pacemaker is functioning in its VVI mode.[2] The *escape interval* is the interval between a natural beat and the subsequent spike.[2] Escape intervals are measured from the beginning of a sensed ventricular complex (or other electrical signal) to the subsequent spike.[3] Theoretically, the escape interval should equal the automatic interval.[2,3] This can be determined when ectopic right ventricular beats arise very close to the sensing electrodes (Fig. 25-1).

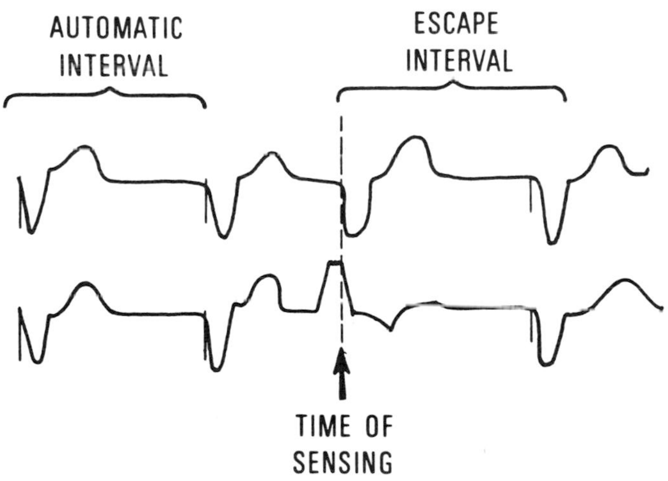

Figure 25-1. *Diagrammatic representation of the duration of escape intervals in a patient with an implanted VVI pacemaker whose leads were properly positioned in the right ventricular apex. Escape intervals following right and left ventricular extrasystoles are shown in the* top *and* bottom diagrams, *respectively. The escape intervals measured from surface lead V_1 are similar* (top) *and longer* (bottom) *than the automatic interval. Nevertheless, the actual time of sensing* (arrow pointing to vertical broken line) *was the same within the pulse generator.*

In practice, most escape intervals are *longer* than the automatic intervals, because sensing does not occur at the very onset of the QRS complex recorded at the body surface but depends on the various factors influencing the signals perceived by the sensing electrodes. The moment of arrival of excitation at the sensing electrodes (in relation to the onset of the QRS complex) also plays a role.[2–7] This is well illustrated in patients with sinus rhythm and complete right bundle branch block, or with left ventricular ectopic beats, when arrival of excitation at the right ventricular apical sensing electrodes occurs at least 50 msec after the onset of ventricular depolarization (see Fig. 25-1). This interval, which represents the minimal left septal to right ventricular apex conduction time, can even be longer (up to 120 msec) when ectopic beats originate in the posterosuperior wall of the left ventricle. In addition, escape intervals may be (by design) *significantly longer* than automatic intervals. This feature, called *rate hysteresis,* is shown in Figure 25-2.[8]

Escape intervals can also be shorter than the automatic intervals. According to Barold and Keller, the term *partial sensing* implies that electrical signals appearing at any moment of the cycle produce escape in-

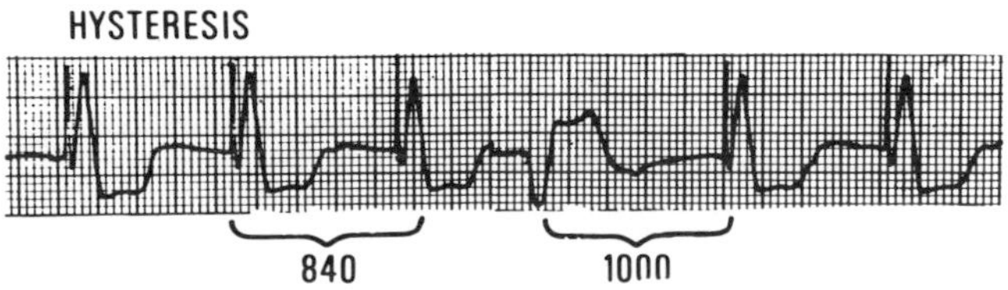

Figure 25-2. *Rate hysteresis. Note that the escape interval was significantly longer than the automatic interval.*

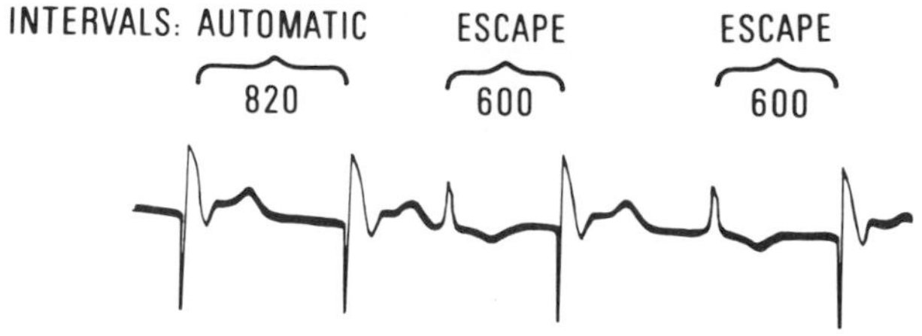

Figure 25-3. *Partial sensing (shorter-than-normal escape intervals occurring after natural ventricular beats falling in* different *moments of the cycle) in a patient with a VVI pacemaker.*

tervals shorter than automatic intervals (Fig. 25-3).[9] This phenomenon has been attributed to signals of borderline amplitude or poor slew rate. On the other hand, the term *partial recycling* is used when the shorter escape intervals are related to the timing of the electrical signals. Partial recycling is usually produced by spikes falling during the relative refractory period of the pacemaker, which occurs at the end of the absolute refractory period (Fig. 25-4).

Partial sensing of implanted pacemakers is, in our experience, almost invariably due to malfunction of the pacing system (generally electrode displacement). Partial recycling, however, is a normal electronic feature of some VVI pacemakers.[9]

Pacemaker Refractory Periods

The *delivery refractory period* follows the emission of a spike, and the *sensing refractory period* follows the sensing of a spontaneous beat or a signal generated by external chest wall stimulation.[9] The duration of the sensing and delivery refractory periods can differ in some pulse generators.[9]

Most pacemakers have an *absolute* as well as a *relative* refractory period. During the absolute refractory period, electric signals occurring early in the cycle (following either a paced or a sensed beat) will not be sensed (see Fig. 25-4). This does *not* imply pacemaker system malfunction. Thus, the clinician must know the duration of the refractory period of each pulse generator to differentiate between non-sensing due to normal pacemaker refractoriness and non-sensing related to malfunction. The relative refractory period, occurring after the absolute refractory period, has two electrocardiographic expressions. First, in some units, early sensing requires a much larger signal than later sensing. If signals of normal or slightly greater than normal amplitude are not sensed because of pacemaker relative refractoriness, the pacemaker absolute refractory period appears to be abnormally prolonged, falsely suggesting pacing system malfunction. Second, in other units, signals that with the same amplitude result in full (normal) recycling later in the cycle will produce partial recycling (escape intervals

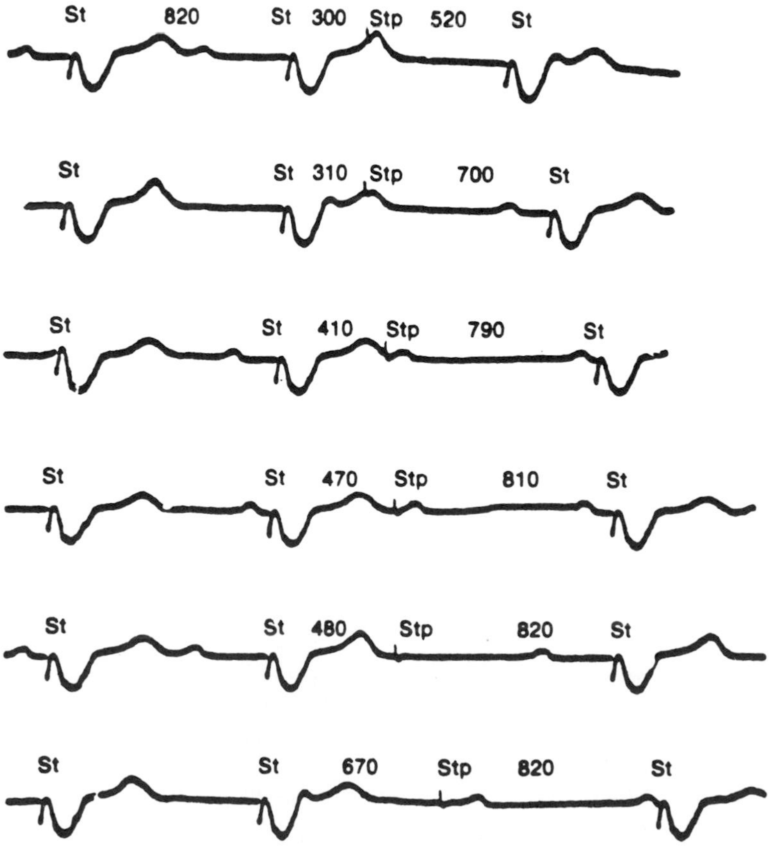

Figure 25-4. *Partial recycling of VVI pacemaker exposed by premature external chest wall stimuli (Stp). The automatic interval measured 820 msec. In the* second, third, *and* fourth strips *premature chest wall stimuli with coupling intervals of 310, 410, and 470 msec, respectively, caused partial pacemaker recycling in which the escape intervals (Stp-St) (700, 790, and 810 msec, respectively) were shorter than the automatic interval (820 msec).*

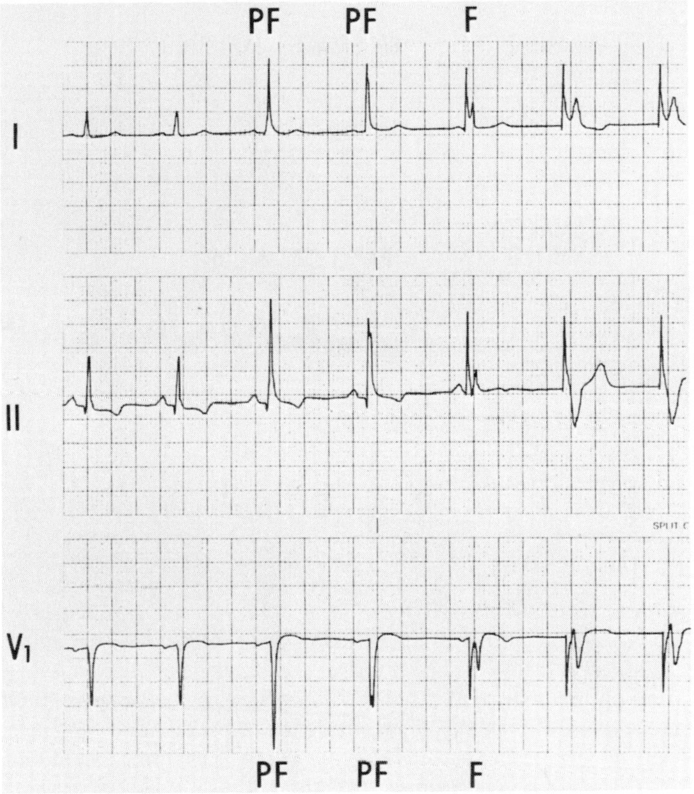

Figure 25-5. *Fusion (F) and pseudofusion (PF) beats produced by normally functioning VVI pacemaker. The three leads were recorded simultaneously.*

of shorter than normal duration) during the pacemaker relative refractory period.[9,10]

Ventricular Fusion and Pseudofusion Beats

True *fusion beats* occur when the ventricles are activated, in part by the natural complex and in part by the pacemaker-initiated ventricular depolarization (Fig. 25-5). *Pseudofusion beats* result from the superimposition (on the surface electrocardiogram) of an ineffective ventricular spike on a QRS complex (Fig. 25-5).[7] They occur because, as previously stated, the initial part of the QRS complex (recorded at the body surface) may be inscribed before the moment of sensing.

VOO Pacing

Few pacemakers are implanted to provide VOO pacing. In practice, this mode of stimulation is most frequently produced when the physician, usually attempting to evaluate pacemaker function, applies an external magnet over the pulse generator. Spontaneous VOO stimulation is seen in the presence of electromagnetic interference (see below) because the pacemaker reverts to its noise rate or interference mode. The latter does not imply pacing system malfunction. However, spontaneous VOO stimulation may also occur when pacing system malfunction characterized by failure to sense occurs.

Electromagnetic Interference

Electromagnetic interference arose when sensing circuits, required to avoid the competition that occurred with VOO pacemakers, were developed. However, VVI pacemakers can be inhibited not only by natural electrical activity but also by electromagnetic influences from other sources, either extrinsic (environmental) or intrinsic (skeletal muscle potentials). Because of this potential hazard, manufacturers introduced various remedial changes including shielding, filtration of extraneous signals, and incorporation of a noise rate or interference mode during which the pacemaker reverted to a continuous asynchronous mode (Fig. 25-6).[11-20] Despite these changes, absolute protection may not be possible, specifically in a highly industrialized environment where technologic advances are rapid (Fig. 25-7). In a previous study[21] dealing with the way in which VVI pacemakers responded to simulated electromagnetic interference, we observed reversion to continuous VOO pacing (see Fig. 25-6) and to an irregular and erratic ventricular stimulation mode (Fig. 25-8). Although electromagnetic interference will be discussed below, suffice it to say here that myopotential inhibition is the major source of electromagnetic interference affecting VVI pacemakers. This problem has been encountered with *unipolar* VVI pacemakers. A unipolar pacemaker is subjected to myopotential inhibition because of the difference in voltage

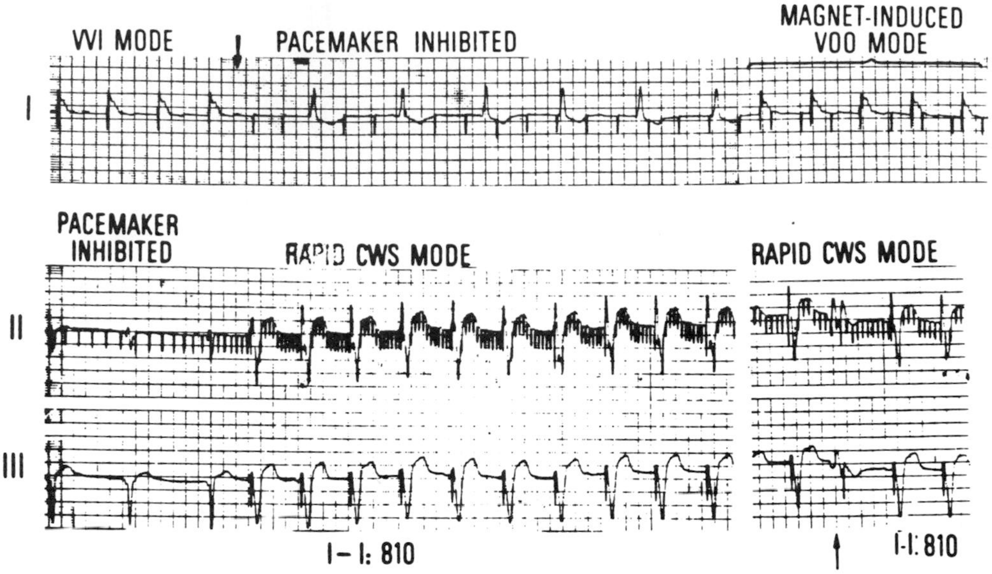

Figure 25-6. *Normally functioning VVI pacemaker. Control VVI (QRS-inhibited) mode of operation* (beginning of upper strip), *temporary inhibition by slow external chest wall stimulation* (arrow in upper strip), *and magnet-induced VOO (fixed-rate) mode of operation* (end of upper strip). *Note that the duration of the (automatic) interstimulus intervals (I-I) of the implanted pacemaker was designed to be the same (810 ms) during both VVI and magnet-induced VOO modes of operation. The* lower two *(simultaneously recorded)* strips *show reversion to electromagnetic interference, in this case rapid external chest wall stimulation (CWS) mode. That this mode was VOO could be corroborated by noting that a premature QRS complex* (arrow) *did not recycle the pacemaker. Note that external stimuli did not distort QRS complexes in lead III. This shows why electromagnetic interference is best seen when simultaneous leads are recorded.*

between indifferent electrode (plate of the pulse generator) and the intracardiac electrodes, which are located on opposite sites of contracting muscle.[19] Also, myopotentials undergo low-pass filtering in the body, making the pacemaker more prone to be affected by them. Furthermore, amplitude and frequency analysis of skeletal muscle potentials from the pectoral muscles have large enough amplitudes (and maximal derivatives) to inhibit pacemaker function.[19] However, although their amplitude usually does not exceed 4 mV, that of the natural intraventricular electrogram is generally around 10 mV. Hence, several authors have stated that using 4 mV as the lowest sensitivity should reduce the incidence of myopotential inhibition without creating a significant risk of undersensing of the natural intraventricular electrograms.[19]

Finally, myopotential inhibition has been shown to occur with bipolar electrical systems.[14,19,22–25] In many cases, this may have been due to defective insulation of the catheter electrodes or to penetration (or perforation), which in turn could have allowed myopotentials from the diaphragm to be picked up by the sensing electrodes. The latter implies pacing system malfunction.

Changes in the Electrical Axis of the Pacemaker Spike

Although a change in amplitude and polarity of a pacemaker spike can be seen normally in one single lead when the spike is perpendicular to the lead, a change in more than one lead is usually considered a sign of pacing system malfunction (*e.g.,* partial electrode fracture, defective electrode insulation or short-circuiting of bipolar electrodes). However, a spatial (three-lead) change, resulting in variations in the electrical axis (in standard leads), amplitude, and polarity (in all leads) of the spike may be produced factitiously by a digital electrocardio-

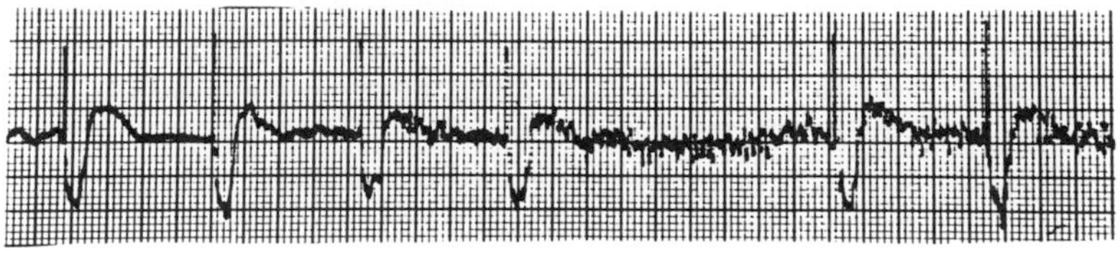

Figure 25-7. *Myopotential inhibition of normally functioning VVI pacemaker.*

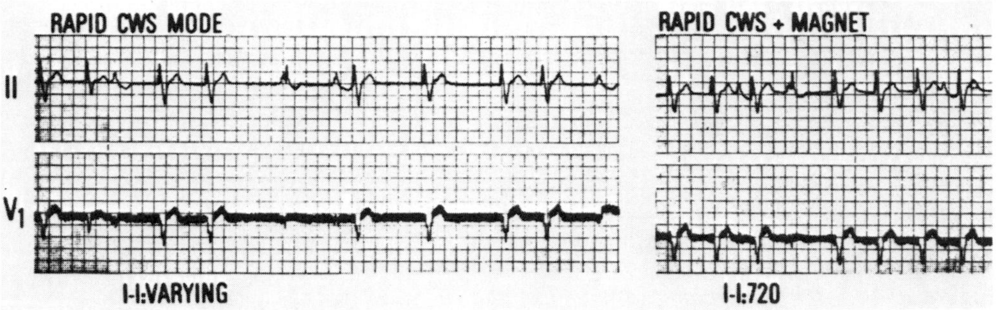

Figure 25-8. *Irregular interstimulus intervals occurring after 1 minute of simulated electromagnetic interference (A) and magnet-induced VOO mode of operation during simulated electromagnetic interference (B).*

graphic machine.[26] The phenomenon illustrated in Figure 25-9 is an electrocardiographic artifact due to the digital "roll-over" effect. In digital numeric systems, the largest possible positive number and largest negative number are adjacent. Hence, if the amplitude of the input signal exceeds the maximum positive value, a negative number may be recorded. Conversely, if the input is greater than the negative value, a positive number may be recorded. In Figure 25-9 the amplitude of the pacemaker spike (large when measured by oscilloscope) caused intermittent digital roll-over that produced variations in spike polarity. Furthermore, beat-to-beat differences in the point from which the spike was sampled resulted in marked variability in pulse amplitude. Recording the same signal, not only with an oscilloscope but with a conventional (analog) electrocardiographic machine, confirmed the artifactual nature of the varying spatial orientation of the ventricular spike.[26]

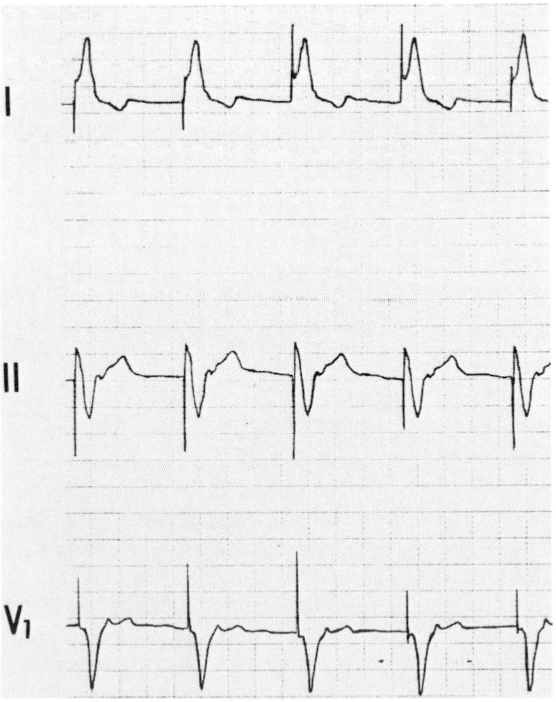

Figure 25-9. *Spatial (three-lead) artifactual alternation of electrical axis, amplitude, and polarity of the pacemaker spikes.*

DVI Pacemakers

Without "Committed" Ventricular Stimulation

Pacemaker Intervals

In DVI pacemakers without committed stimulation, the *atrial escape interval*[27–38] is the time elapsing between a ventricular spike, or sensed ventricular beat, and subsequent atrial spike (Fig. 25-10). The *ventricular escape interval*[37] is the time elapsing between a ventricular spike, or sensed ventricular beat, and subsequent ventricular spike (see Fig. 25-10). The artificial AV sequential interval is the difference between atrial, and ventricular, escape intervals (see Fig. 25-10). The natural AV interval is the time elapsing between an atrial spike and a ventricular beat sensed before the ventricular spike is expected to occur. Artificial and natural AV intervals coexist when the ventricular spike is emitted after the onset of a ventricular beat but before sensing occurs within the QRS complexes recorded at the body surface. In these cases the interval between atrial and ventricular spikes equals the artificial AV interval. In pacemakers with so-called semicommitted ventricular stimulation, a ventricular beat sensed between 12 and 110 msec after an atrial spike will cause a ventricular spike to be emitted at an artificial AV interval of 110 msec. Magnet application also shortens the artificial AV interval in some pacemaker models.

Pacemaker Refractory Periods

The *atrial refractory period* is very short because DVI models do not sense the atria. After an atrial spike the

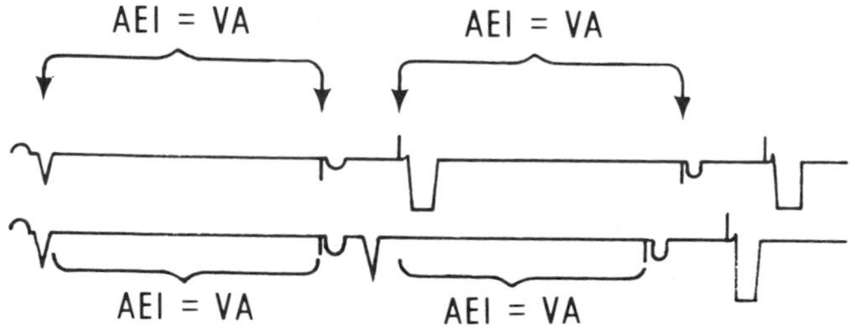

Figure 25-10. *DVI pacemaker without "committed" ventricular stimulation. Diagrammatic representation of atrial escape intervals (AEI). Following a sensed ventricular beat the AEI equals the ventriculoauricular (VA) interval given by the time elapsing between the moment of sensing and the subsequent atrial spike* (upper *and* lower left). *After a paced ventricular beat, the VA interval is given by the time elapsing between the ventricular spike and the atrial spike immediately following* (upper right).

ventricular amplifier is disabled for a short time (around 12 msec) to prevent an atrial spike being sensed as a ventricular event. The interval after a paced or sensed ventricular event, of which 60% is another ventricular blanking period and 40% is a noise-sampling period, is a *ventricular refractory period.* An event sensed during a noise-sampling period initiates a new ventricular refractory period without resetting the basic rate time.

With "Committed" Ventricular Stimulation

Pacemaker Intervals

DVI pacemakers with committed ventricular stimulations initiate an atrial escape interval after an atrial spike (not after a ventricular spike, as do DVI pacemakers without committed ventricular stimulation) and following a sensed ventricular beat.[38] Thus, in Figure 25-11 the first atrial escape interval is given by the interval between the first and second atrial spikes (not the VA interval), whereas the escape interval following the sixth, sensed, QRS complex is given by the interval between this ventricular beat and the atrial spike (VA interval) immediately following.

The pacemaker is obliged to deliver a ventricular spike after having emitted an atrial spike. In other words, in contrast to DVI pacemakers without committed stimulation, either both spikes are seen or no spike is seen (see Fig. 25-11).

Pacemaker Refractory Periods

The pacemaker refractory period starts when an atrial spike is delivered and lasts roughly 330 msec (longer than the artificial AV interval); it explains why the pacemaker is "committed" to emit a ventricular spike.

As previously stated, in patients with right bundle branch block or left ventricular extrasystoles, sensing may occur late in the QRS complex recorded at the body surface. This atrial spike appearing within the terminal parts of such (wide) ventricular complexes can be followed by a ventricular spike falling on the ascending part of the T wave (see Fig. 25-11).

Fusion, Pseudofusion, and Pseudofusion Beats

Fusion and *pseudofusion* beats are seen in patients not only with VVI but also with DVI pacemakers.[37,38] In addition, in patients with DVI pacemakers, pseudopseudofusion beats can occur when an ineffective atrial spike (see Fig. 25-11) falls on a QRS complex.

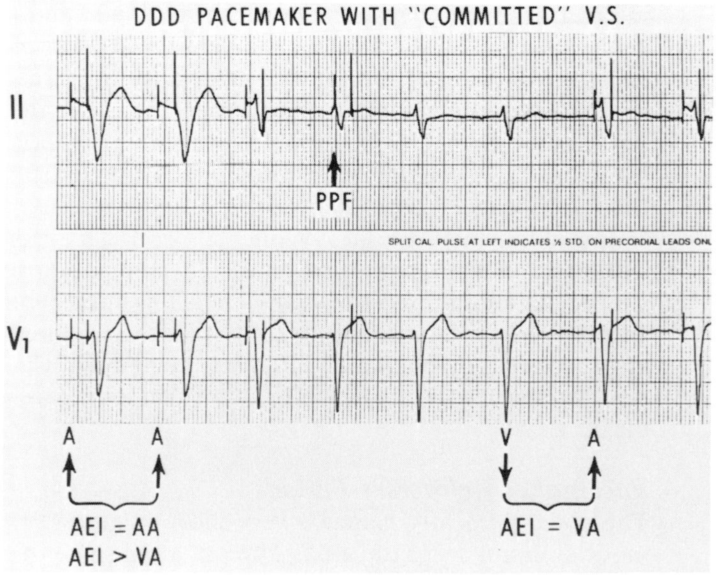

Figure 25-11. *DVI pacemaker with "committed" ventricular stimulation in a patient with transient atrial fibrillation. When two paced beats occurred in succession* (left), *the atrial escape interval (AEI) equaled the (AA) interval between two consecutive atrial spikes. On the other hand, after a sensed ventricular beat, the atrial escape interval was given by the time elapsing between the moment of sensing and the subsequent atrial spike (VA interval). Because of the committed ventricular stimulation, some of the ventricular spikes occurred after the end of the QRS complexes. (PPF, pseudopseudofusion beat)*

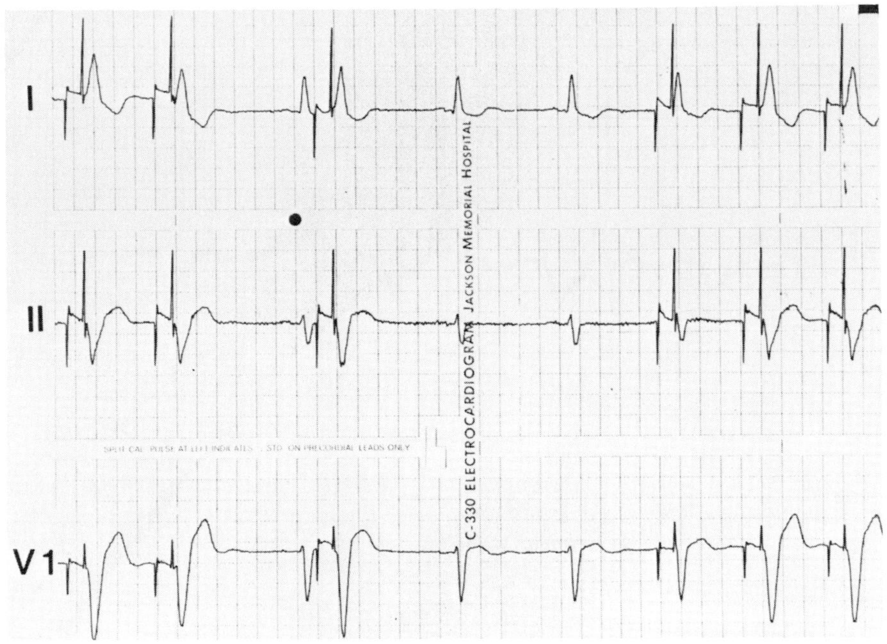

Figure 25-12. *Myopotential inhibition of DVI pacemaker with "committed" ventricular stimulation.*

DOO Pacing

DOO pacing usually occurs when the physician applies an external magnet over the pulse generator.

The Letter D in Position 1 of the ICHD Five-Position Pacemaker Code

The letter D means that both chambers can be paced. From the orthodox point of view it does not necessarily mean that the chambers *must* be paced "sequentially." That is, the D would apply if both chambers were to be paced simultaneously. In practice, however, all pacemakers capable of stimulating the atria as well as the ventricles do so sequentially, although the AV intervals may vary significantly.

Myopotential Inhibition

Myopotential inhibition is more frequent with unipolar systems, and most cases of it have been reported in patients with DVI pacemakers with committed ventricular stimulation (Fig. 25-12).[39]

DDD Pacemakers

Although DDD pacemakers, whether unipolar or bipolar, may be programmed to VVI and DVI modes, the following discussion applies to the DDD mode, which is the most versatile.[40–49] DDD pacemakers from different manufacturers do not operate in exactly the same way; moreover, even pacemakers from the same manufacturer may change as needs dictate. Further modifications will no doubt have occurred between the writing and the publication of this edition. To reiterate, physicians and paramedical personnel should *routinely* consult the brochures supplied by the manufacturers to determine such modifications.

Pacing Rates and Intervals

In the absence of spontaneous atrial activity for the preselected time, DDD pacemakers provide AV sequential pacing (Fig. 25-13). When the natural atrial rates range between the programmed lower rate and the programmed upper rate, the pacemaker provides P wave–triggered pacing (see Fig. 25-13). Theoretically, the interval between atrial and ventricular spikes should be the same as the P-to-spike interval. The latter, however, may seem longer than the artificial AV interval when measured from the beginning of the P wave, because sensing does occur at the onset of the atrial depolarization as recorded by the surface electrocardiogram.

The AV sequential pacing seen in patients with most DDD pacemakers has been referred to as *semicommitted.* This means that a ventricular beat, or artifact interpreted as such, sensed between 12 and 110 msec after an atrial spike, will cause a ventricular spike to be emitted at the end of an (artificial) AV interval of 110 msec (Fig. 25-14).[47–50] Since most programmed artificial AV intervals exceed this value, it is not infrequent to see, in the same rhythm strip, artificial AV interval with two different values (see Fig. 25-14). Moreover, in some models, magnet application results in DOO pacing with artificial

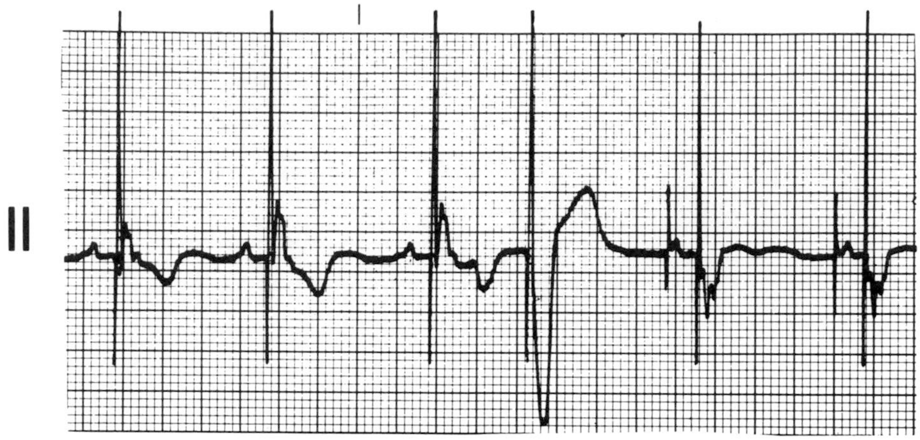

Figure 25-13. *Normally functioning DDD pacemaker providing (when the sinus rate was fast enough, and after a premature atrial beat) P wave–triggered pacing* (left), *and (when the sinus rate slowed) AV sequential pacing* (last two beats).

AV intervals that can also be shorter than the programmed artificial AV intervals (Fig. 25-15).

The function of this pacemaker when the atrial rate is faster than the programmed upper rate is described below.

Atrial Refractory Periods

The *atrial refractory period* starts with a ventricular event (postventricular refractory atrial refractory period). However, the total atrial refractory period is usually composed of the sum of two parts: the AV interval and the postventricular atrial refractory period. As discussed below, in some models, after a ventricular extrasystole, the postventricular atrial refractory period is automatically extended for variable periods, regardless of the programmed setting.[50–51]

Ventricular Blanking Period Following an Atrial Impulse

After an atrial impulse, the ventricular sensing amplifier is turned off for approximately 12 msec to prevent the atrial impulse from inhibiting the ventricular output.

Ventricular Refractory Period

Following a ventricular spike or a sensed ventricular beat, the *ventricular refractory period* lasts for around 225 msec. This period is composed of an initial 125-msec ventricular blanking period followed by a terminal 100-msec noise-sampling period. When a ventricular ectopic beat appears so that two ventricular events occur without any sensed atrial activity, the noise-sampling period is lengthened to 220 msec. Consequently, the refractory period increases to 345 msec in some models and can be extended further in other models.

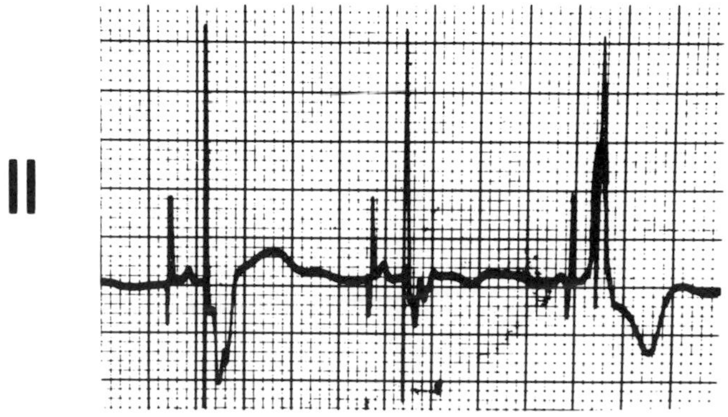

Figure 25-14. *DDD pacemaker providing AV sequential pacing with the programmed AV intervals of 150 msec* (left) *and with the shorter artificial AV interval (100 msec) resulting from the so-called semicommitted stimulation* (right).

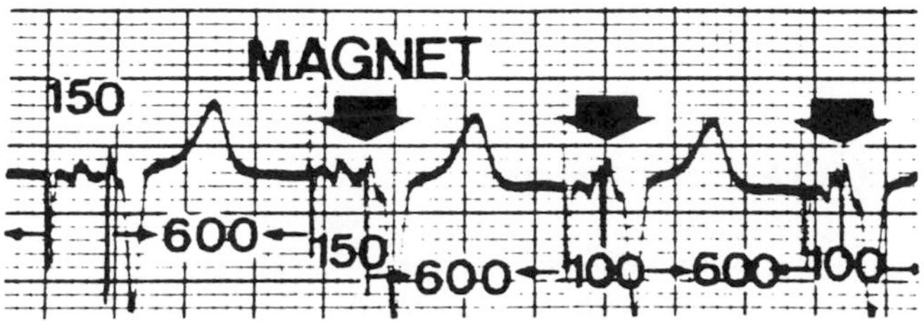

Figure 25-15. *DDD pacemaker providing AV sequential pacing with the programmed AV interval of 150 msec and with the shorter (100 msec) AV intervals resulting from the DOO mode induced by magnet application.*

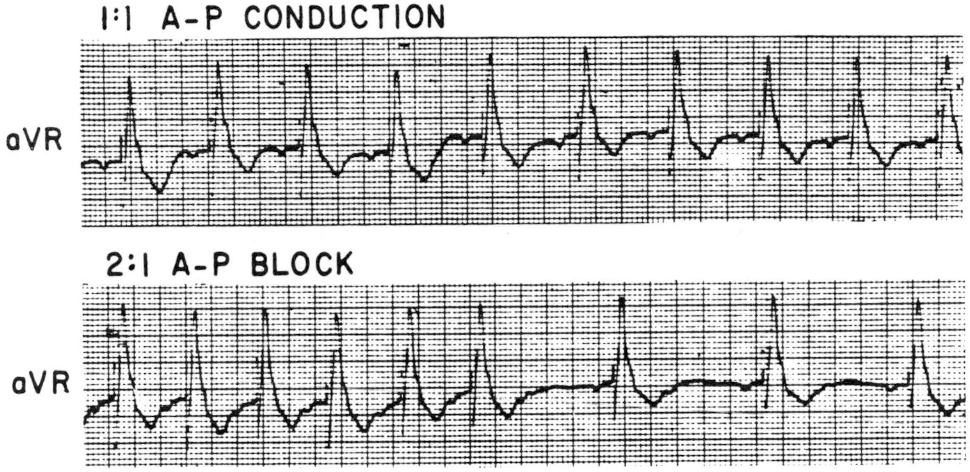

Figure 25-16. *One-to-one P wave–triggered pacing* (top strip *and* first part of the bottom strip) *with sudden onset of 2:1 block* (end of bottom strip).

Modes of Operation When Spontaneous Atrial Rates are Faster than Programmed Upper (Ventricular) Rates

If the atrial rate increases so much that the AA intervals are shorter than the atrial refractory period, only every other P wave will be sensed during an abrupt halving of the ventricular rate. This will cause sudden 2:1 block, as shown in Figure 25-16.[52]

The fastest ventricular rate possible is determined by the programmed upper rate.[52] Regardless of how early a P wave is sensed (and regardless of the AV interval), the ventricular spike will not be emitted until after the end of the programmed upper cycle length. For example, in Figure 25-17 the atrial rate was slightly faster (130 beats/min, cycle length 460 msec) than the programmed upper rate (125 beats/min, cycle length 480 msec). Under these circumstances, the atrial refractory period, although always ending 155 msec after a ventricular spike, was gradually extended (because of the progressive increase in AV intervals). Note that, because of the previously mentioned difference in atrial and ventricular rates, P waves 2 to 8 yielded progressively longer AV intervals but coexisted with constant VV intervals. Finally, P wave 8 occurred close to the ventricular spike, thus falling within the atrial refractory period. It thus did not trigger a ventricular spike, and the Wenckebach-like period ended. Thereafter, the pacemaker synchronized its output to the next, sensed, P wave (9) at the programmed AV interval.

The differences between the natural AV nodal Wenckebach and the artificial Wenckebach-like periods are as follows[53]: (1) the VV intervals are not constant, tending (in general) to decrease as the cycles progress, and (2) the nonconducted P wave is blocked because of the refractory period of the AV node, not of the atrium.

Interestingly, historical developments in the pacemaker field show that when generations with programmable atrial refractory periods capable of being increased for variable intervals after a sensed ventricular event were introduced, an unexpected event occurred, namely, Wenckebach-like periods became less frequent. This happened because the relationship between the duration of the total atrial refractory period and the programmed upper cycle length determined whether the upper rate response would be 2:1 or Wenckebach-like AV block. Simply stated, if (1) the total atrial refractory period (AV

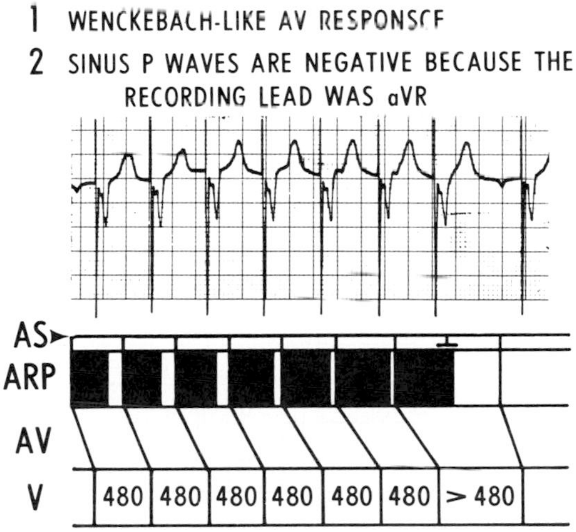

Figure 25-17. *8:7 Wenckebach-like period occurring during the normal function of a DDD pacemaker. AS indicated the moment where atrial sensing occurred. Black squares at the atrial refractory period (ARP) level represented pacemaker* total *ARP.* Oblique lines *at the AV level show an association between a P wave and a ventricular spike. Numbers (480 msec) between vertical lines at the V level correspond to the programmed upper cycle length.*

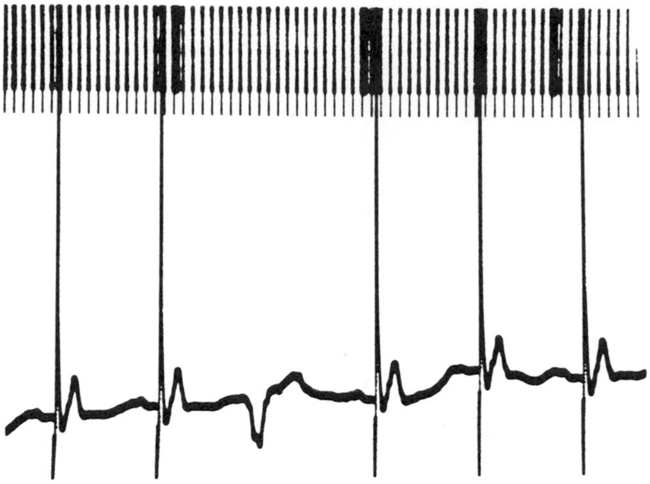

Figure 25-18. *DDD pacemaker with P wave–triggered pacing, both before and after a ventricular extrasystole with retrograde conduction to the atria.*

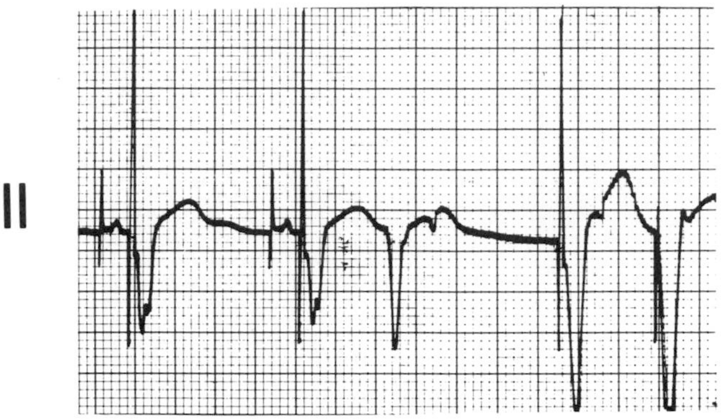

Figure 25-20. *Early generation of DDD pacemaker in which a ventricular (pacemaker) escape occurred after a ventricular extrasystole with retrograde conduction to the atria. The retrograde conduction of the paced ventricular beat initiated an "endless loop" tachycardia.*

interval plus postventricular atrial refractory period) is greater than the programmed upper rate, the response will be AV block, and if (2) the total atrial refractory period is less than the programmed upper cycle length, some degree of Wenckebach will result, with the maximal prolongation of the AV interval (over control values) being the difference between the total atrial refractory period and the programmed upper cycle length.

Modes of Operation Following a Ventricular Premature Beat

Knowing what the pacemaker does after a ventricular premature beat is important because the way it operates after a ventricular extrasystole may lead to arrhythmias sustained by the pacemaker itself (Figs. 25-18 to 25-20). During pacemaker development over the years the following modifications have been made: no change in the atrial refractory period, the delivery of a ventricular spike at a given interval after the ventricular extrasystole, automatic extension of the atrial refractory period, the delivery of an obligatory AV paced beat (DDX mode),[50] and automatic extension of both atrial and ventricular refractory periods.

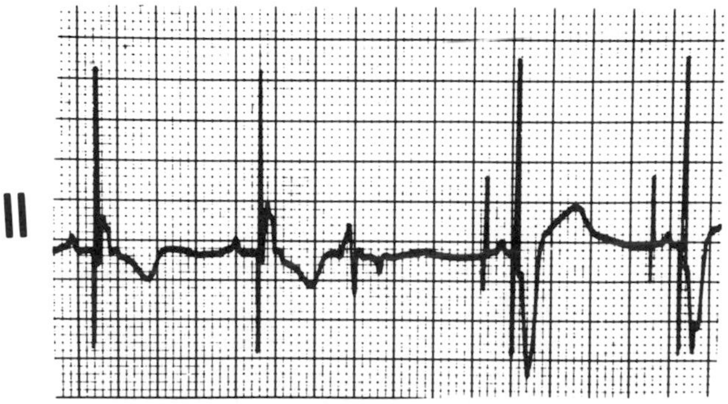

Figure 25-19. *DDD pacemaker providing AV sequential pacing after a ventricular extrasystole with retrograde conduction to the atria.*

Endless Loop Tachycardia

The duration of the atrial refractory period of DDD pacemakers varies depending on the manufacturer and on the programmed interval after sensed (sinus or ectopic) ventricular beats. If a retrograde P wave from an ectopic ventricular beat is sensed by the atrial amplifier, it initiates an AV delay.[54] Consequently, a ventricular spike is emitted at an interval that cannot exceed the programmed upper cycle length. If the paced ventricular beat also has retrograde conduction and the corresponding P wave is sensed, the process repeats itself. This arrhythmia was called *endless loop tachycardia* by Furman and Fisher, in an analogy to a computer program that repeats itself *ad infinitum.*[45] Although it can be initiated by a spontaneous or paced impulse, it is always sustained by pacemaker participation (Figs. 25-21 to 25-23). Once started, the pacemaker limits the maximum rate but not its duration.[45–49,55–57] Termination requires external intervention or spontaneous variability of natural conduction; therefore, efforts have been made to prevent its induction. This arrhythmia, whose occurrence was predicted in 1969,[54] can also be seen in patients with implanted VDD (atrial triggered–ventricular inhibited) pacemakers.[58–60]

Endless loop tachycardia requires not only retrograde conduction through a natural AV pathway but also a VA conduction time greater than the postventricular atrial refractory period. Thus, programming of the latter has decreased the frequency of this arrhythmia. In different

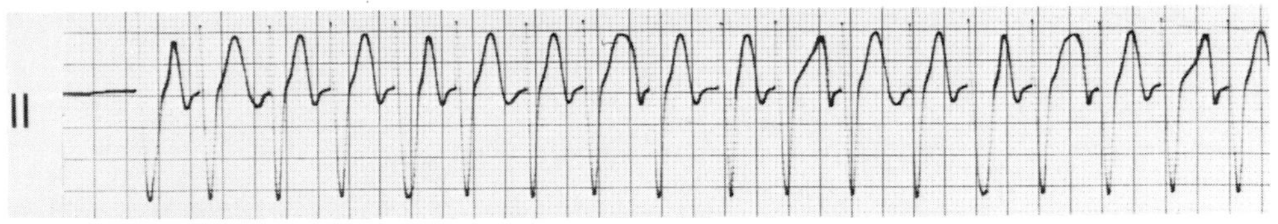

Figure 25-21. *"Endless loop" tachycardia initiated by the retrograde conduction to the atria of a paced ventricular beat without any antecedent P wave.*

generations of DDD pacemakers, endless loop tachycardia has been variously initiated by (1) premature ventricular contractions with VA conduction, (2) ventricular escape beats with VA conduction, (3) premature atrial contractions triggering a ventricular spike after a long delay with the corresponding paced ventricular beat having retrograde atrial conduction, and (4) magnet-induced DOO pacing with the first atrial spike falling in the atrial refractory period so that the first ventricular spike can produce a QRS complex with retrograde conduction. Abolishment of endless loop tachycardia requires spontaneous occurrence of VA block or external intervention such as carotid sinus massage. Magnet application by producing DOO pacing abruptly inhibits atrial sensing and interrupts the arrhythmia. Prevention is the best approach for the problems created by the occurrence of endless loop tachycardia. Extension of the atrial refractory period (in beats other than extrasystolic) limits the programmed upper rate. If the latter is too low, for example 100 per min, it may not be ideal for a younger patient, who may need faster atrial rates with 1 : 1 AV conduction. One possible solution would be one in which the pacemaker itself could discriminate between sinus and retrograde P waves. Because a perfect solution does not yet exist, the following approaches have been tried:

1. The tachycardia termination algorithm.[61] This approach detects continued pacing at the ventricular tracking rate, allows it to proceed for 15 consecutive paced events, and inhibits the 16th ventricular output pulse, thus breaking the reentry loop.[61]
2. The "fall-back" response. In this approach, as the atrial rate exceeds the programmed upper rate, up to four P wave–triggered pacing pulses are allowed. After a pause, there is a shift to VVI pacing for 36 seconds or so until the programmed "fall-back" rate is achieved. If an atrial rate below the programmed upper rate is apparent, this modality of response is discontinued so that P wave triggered–pacing can be resumed.[62]
3. Atrial stimulation synchronous with a premature ventricular beat.[62,63]

It seems that prophylaxis lies in the ability to extend the postventricular atrial refractory period (through programming) beyond the VA conduction time. The previously mentioned automatic extension of the postventricular atrial refractory period after a ventricular extrasystole has been most helpful in this respect. Conceptual extension to infinity may be associated with the obligatory delivery of an AV sequentially paced beat.

Pseudo Endless Loop Tachycardia

Pseudo endless loop tachycardia was first used by Amikam and colleagues to refer to electrocardiographic findings that at first glance appeared to have resulted from endless loop tachycardia but in further evaluations were seen to have mimicked the latter.[64] This arrhythmia resembled endless loop tachycardia because it appeared after a premature ventricular contraction, its rate approached the upper rate limit, and the P wave was difficult to discern. A careful analysis revealed that the mechanism of this arrhythmia was different than that of endless loop tachycardia, since regular sinus P waves continued at their own rate. There was a combination of

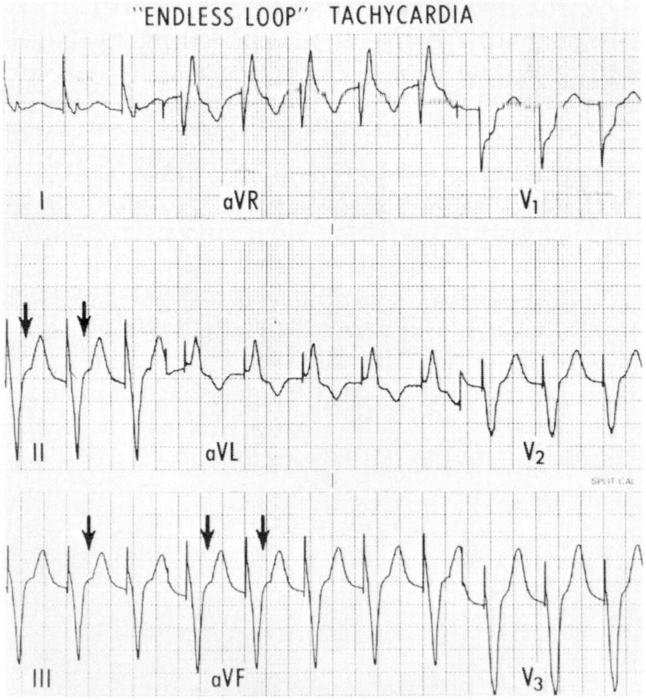

Figure 25-22. *Twelve-lead electrocardiogram in a patient with an "endless loop" tachycardia.* Arrows *indicate retrograde P waves.*

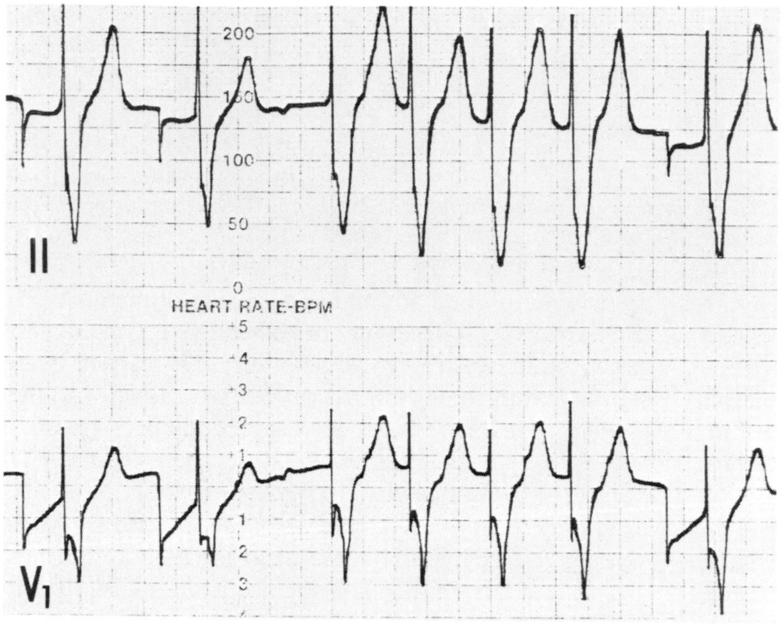

Figure 25-23. *A premature atrial beat triggered a ventricular spike after a long artificial AV delay. The resulting paced ventricular beat had retrograde conduction to the atria and initiated an "endless loop" tachycardia.*

interference by a ventricular extrasystole of the regular sequence of normally conducted ventricular complexes and the pacemaker commitment to maintain an upper rate limit by prolonging the artificial AV interval. In summary, because retrograde (VA) conduction from the extrasystole did not exist, "true" endless loop tachycardia did not occur (Fig. 25-24).

Electromagnetic Interference

The presence of two sensing (atrial and ventricular) circuits in the unipolar DDD pacemakers enhances the possibility of interference between myopotentials and pacemaker. Whenever sensing of myopotential by the atrial channel is interpreted as intrinsic atrial activity, the ventricular rate increases to the programmed upper rate (see Fig. 25-22). The resulting atrial arrhythmia can also be considered as pseudo endless loop tachycardia. Although one such episode may be interpreted as such, careful analysis will reveal the absence of retrograde P waves, without which endless loop tachycardia cannot be present (see Fig. 25-24).[64,65] Interestingly, Smyth and colleagues reported rapid firing of an atrial synchronous ventricular pacemaker induced by the electromagnetic field generated by a weapons detector.[66] On the other hand, when myopotentials are interpreted by the ventricular channel as ventricular signals, ventricular input is inhibited, so that atrial spikes are not followed by ventricular spikes. Reversion to continuous asynchronous mode (DOO or VOO) may also occur.

As with VVI and DVI pacemakers, the problems created by myopotentials in particular, and by external magnetic fields in general, will probably decrease with the use of bipolar leads; however, as previously stated, they will not be eliminated in the near future. Technologic advances in medicine must be counteracted by advances in pacemaker technology. Since the former cannot be foreseen, the latter must evolve as medical technology is applied. For example, magnetic fields produced by nuclear magnetic resonance may adversely affect pacemakers.[50] The same is true of cobalt machines and linear accelerators used for cancer treatment and therapeutic diathermy.[50] However, there is no evidence that routine *diagnostic* x-ray procedures can damage a pulse generator. Furthermore, physicians should be aware that electrosurgical cautery in the vicinity of the leads may result in ventricular fibrillation and iatrogenic

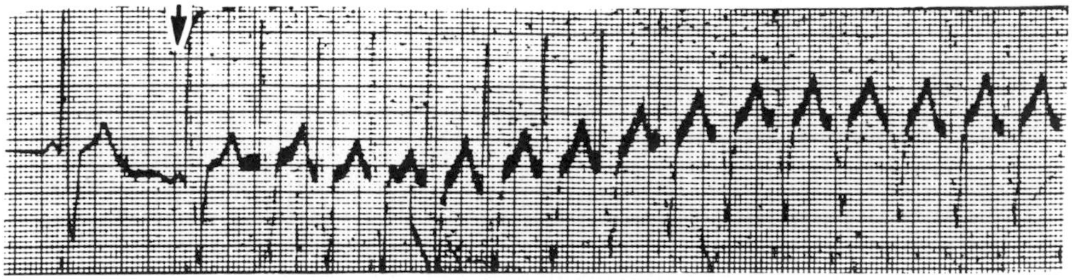

Figure 25-24. *"Pseudoendless loop" tachycardia triggered by myopotential interference.*

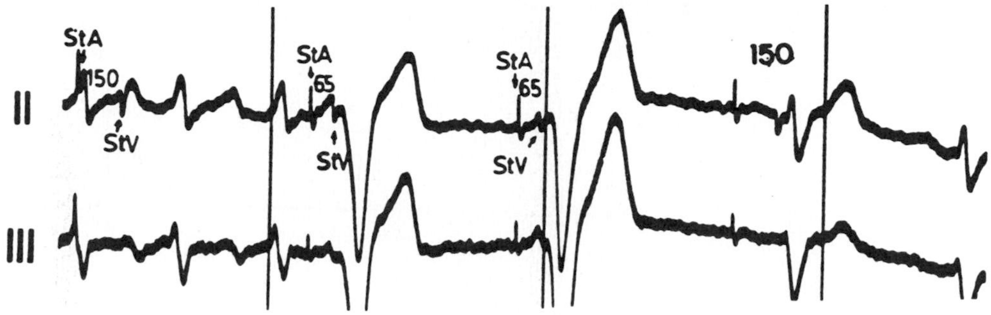

Figure 25-25. *"Eccentricity"[43] of DVI,MN pacemaker. In this patient with an AV reciprocating tachycardia, the first (spontaneous) artificial AV interval, delivered during tachycardia, measured 150 msec. The second (which stopped the arrhythmia) and third AV intervals measured 65 msec. Finally, the last artificial AV interval, delivered after the tachycardia was abolished again, was 150 msec.*

reprogramming.[50] Finally, high-energy countershock may damage the pacemaker or cause spontaneous reprogramming. At present, internal shocks, delivered for internal cardioversion catheter ablation of specific anatomic structures, and internal defibrillation have as-yet-undetermined effects on pacemaker function.

DDD Pacemakers With Antitachycardia Function

Since DDD pacemakers with antitachycardia function are discussed elsewhere in this book, our comments will deal only with certain modes of operation used to treat patients with drug-resistant AV reciprocating tachycardia. There is no doubt that in regarding the antitachycardia function of dual chamber pacemakers, incorporation of this feature into DDD pacemakers profited from the experience obtained with the use of pulse generators capable of providing burst stimulation and underdrive AV sequential pacing.[67–71] Some authors implanted DVI,MN pacemakers that automatically detected the tachycardia and thereafter provided underdrive AV stimulation (with short AV intervals) only until the arrhythmia was terminated (Fig. 25-25).[71] Some of the DDD pacemakers can do this when programmed to the DDD,MN mode (Fig. 25-26). They are also capable of providing atrial burst pacing (Fig. 25-27). Antitachycar-

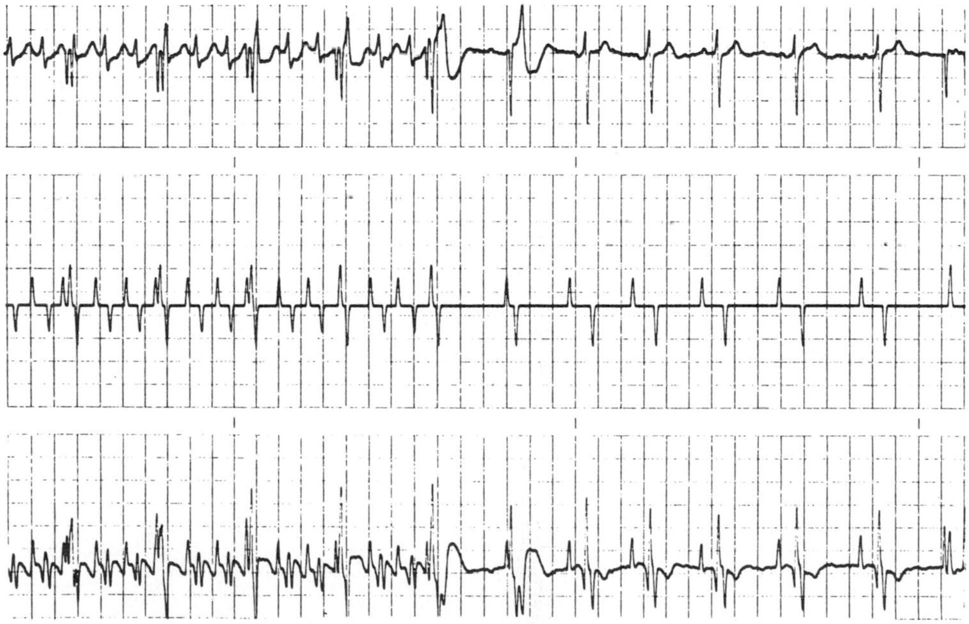

Figure 25-26. *Recordings obtained during termination of AV tachycardia in a patient with a DDD,MN pacemaker. From top to bottom are surface lead II, "marker" channel, and intracardiac electrocardiogram from atrial lead.*

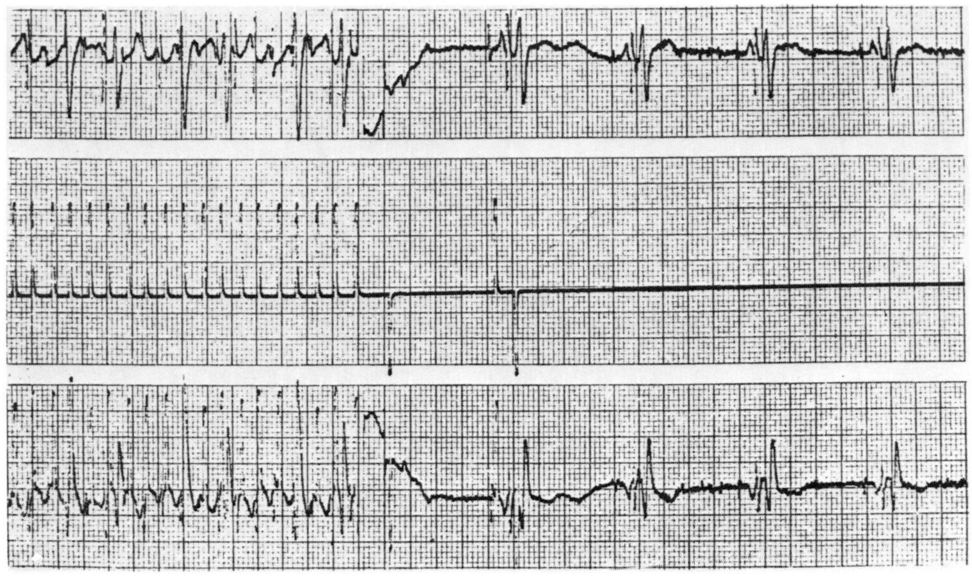

Figure 25-27. *Termination of AV reciprocating tachycardia by burst atrial pacing in a patient with an antitachycardia DDD pacemaker. Surface leads* (top *and* bottom) *and marker channel* (middle) *were recorded simultaneously.*

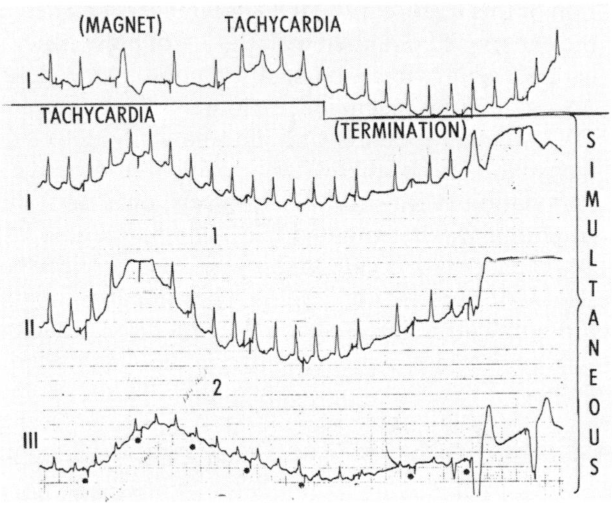

Figure 25-28. *Records obtained from a patient with drug-resistant recurrent sustained AV reciprocating tachycardia in whom a DVI,MN pacemaker was implanted. The* top panel *(long strip of lead I) shows the induction of the arrhythmia by DOO stimulation (with short AV intervals) induced by magnet application. This occurred when an atrial spike paced the atria (and was conducted to the ventricles with a long AV conduction time to initiate the tachycardia) while the ventricular spike fell during the ventricular effective refractory period. The arrhythmia was terminated by automatically induced AV pacing toward the right of the* bottom panel *(simultaneously recorded leads I, II, and III).*

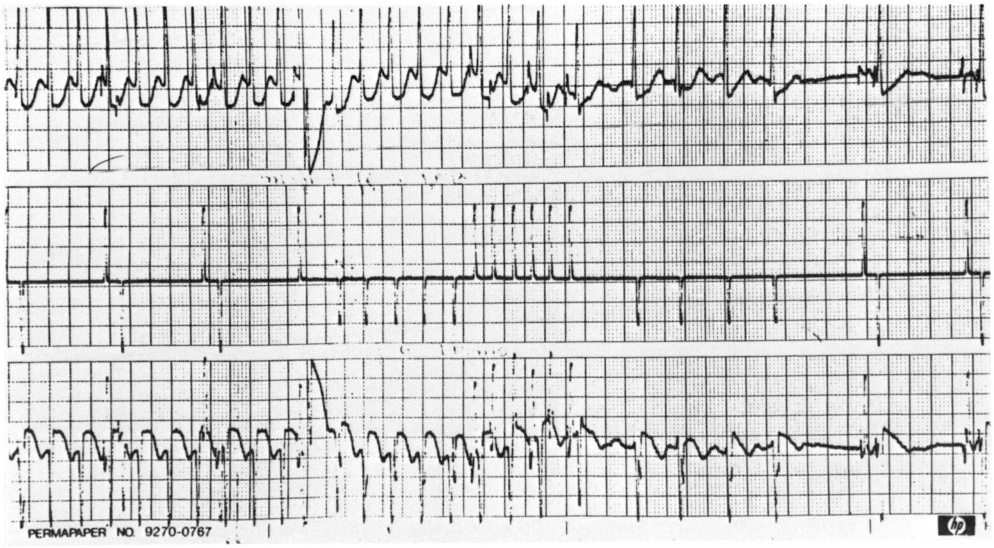

Figure 25-29. *Induction of short run of atrial fibrillation by burst of atrial stimuli (delivered during AV reciprocating tachycardia) in a patient with a DDD,MB pacemaker.*

dia pacemakers can also produce arrhythmias.[71] This is not an undesirable feature, since it has been used to test the antitachycardia function of the pacemaker. Induction of an AV reciprocating tachycardia (by the DOO pacing produced by magnet application) in a patient with a DVI,MN pacemaker is shown in Figure 25-28. A short burst of atrial fibrillation during DDD,MB pacing is shown in Figure 25-29. Finally, electromagnetic interference on these pacemakers may activate the programmed antitachycardia mode (either burst atrial pacing or underdrive AV sequential stimulation).

References

1. Parsonnet, V., Furman, S., Smyth, N. P. D., and Bilitch, M.: Optimal resources for implantable cardiac pacemakers. Circulation, 68:227, 1983.
2. Barold, S. S., and Gaidula, J. J.: Evaluation of normal and abnormal sensing function of demand pacemakers. Am. J. Cardiol., 28:201, 1971.
3. Lemberg, L., Castellanos, A., and Berkovits, B.: Pacing on demand in A-V block. J.A.M.A., 191:12, 1965.
4. Kastor, J. A., Berkovits, B. V., and DeSanctis, R.: Variations in discharge rate of demand pacemaker not due to malfunction. Am. J. Cardiol., 25:344, 1970.
5. Vera, Z., Mason, D., Awan, N. A., et al.: Lack of sensing by demand pacemakers due to intraventricular conduction defects. Circulation, 51:815, 1975.
6. Furman, S., Hurzeler, D., and DeCaprio, V.: Cardiac pacing and pacemakers. III. Sensing the cardiac electrogram. Am. Heart J., 93:794, 1977.
7. Barold, S. S.: Fusion, Pseudo Fusion and Confusion Beats, pp. 1–6. St. Paul, Minn., Impulse, Cardiac Pacemaker, Inc., 1972.
8. Castellanos, A., Jr., and Lemberg, L.: Pacemaker arrhythmias and electrocardiographic recognition of pacemakers. Circulation, 47:1382, 1973.
9. Barold, S. S., and Keller, J. W.: Sensing problems with demand pacemakers. In Samet, P. (ed.): Cardiac Pacing. New York, Grune & Stratton, 1973.
10. Sung, R. J., Castellanos, A., Thurer, R. J., and Myerburg, R. J.: Partial pacemaker recycling of implanted QRS-inhibited pulse generators. Pace, 1:189, 1978.
11. Parker, B., Furman, S., and Escher, D. J. W.: Input signals to pacemakers in a hospital environment. Ann. N. Y. Acad. Sci., 167:823, 1969.
12. Chatterjee, K., Harris, A., and Leatham, A.: The risk of pacing after infarction, and current recommendations. Lancet, 2:1061, 1969.
13. Wirtzfeld, A., Lampadius, M., and Ruprecht, E. O.: Unterdrückung von Demand-Schrittmachern durch Muskelpotensiale. Stsch. Med. Wochenschr., 97:61, 1972.
14. Mymin, D., Cuddy, T. W., Sinha, S. N., et al.: Inhibition of demand pacemakers by skeletal muscle potentials. J.A.M.A., 223:527, 1973.
15. Piller, L. W., and Kennelly, B. M.: Myopotential inhibition of demand pacemakers. Chest, 66:418, 1974.
16. Ohm, O.-J., Brulnov, D. H., Pedersin, O. M., et al.: Interference effect of myopotentials on function of unipolar demand pacemakers. Br. Heart J., 36:77, 1974.
17. Anderson, S. T., Pitt, A., Whitford, J. A., et al.: Interference with function of unipolar pacemaker due to muscle potentials. J. Thorac. Cardiovasc. Surg., 71:698, 1976.
18. Ohm, O.-J., Hammer, E., and Mörkrid, L.: Biological signals and their characteristics as a cause of pacemaker malfunction. In Watanabe, Y. (ed.): Cardiac Pacing, p. 401. Amsterdam, Excerpta Medica, 1976.
19. Breivik, K., and Ohm, O.-J.: Myopotential inhibited (VVI) pacemakers assessed by ambulatory Holter monitoring of the electrocardiogram. Pace, 3:470, 1980.
20. Berger, R., and Jacobs, W.: Myopotential inhibition of demand pacemakers: Etiologic, diagnostic and therapeutic conclusions. Pace, 2:596, 1979.
21. Castellanos, A., Bloom, M. G., Sung, R. J., et al.: Modes of operations induced by rapid external chest wall stimulation in patients with normally functioning QRS inhibited (VVI) pacemakers. Pace, 2:2, 1979.
22. Widlandsky, S., and Zipes, D. P.: Suppression of a ventricular inhibited bipolar pacemaker by skeletal muscle activity. J. Electrocardiol., 7:371, 1974.
23. Barold, S. S., Ong, L. S., Falkoff, M. D., et al.: Inhibition of bipolar demand pacemaker by diaphragmatic myopotentials. Circulation, 56:679, 1977.
24. Amikam, S., Peleg, H., Lemer, J., et al.: Myopotential inhibition of a bipolar pacemaker caused by electrode insulation defect. Br. Heart J., 39:1279, 1977.
25. El Gamal, M., and Van Gelder, B.: Suppression of an external demand pacemaker by diaphragmatic myopotentials: A sign of electrode perforation? Pace, 2:191, 1979.
26. Engler, R. L., Goldberger, A. L., Bhargava, V., and Kapelusznik, D.: Pacemaker spike alternans: An artifact of digital signal processing. Pace 5:748, 1982.
27. Berkovits, B. V., Castellanos, A., Jr., and Lemberg, L.: Bifocal demand pacemaker. Circulation, 39 and 40 (Suppl. III):40, 1969.
28. Castillo, C. A., Berkovits, B. V., Castellanos, A., Jr., et al.: Bifocal demand pacing. Chest, 59:360, 1971.
29. Fields, J., Berkovits, B. V., and Matloff, J. M.: Surgical experience with temporary and permanent AV sequential demand pacing. J. Thorac. Cardiovasc. Surg., 66:865, 1973.
30. Furman, S., Reicher-Reiss, H., and Escher, D. J. W.: Atrioventricular sequential pacing and pacemakers. Chest, 63:783, 1973.
31. Zucker, R. I., Parsonnet, V., and Gilbert, L.: A method of permanent implantation of an atrial electrode. Am. Heart J., 85:195, 1973.
32. Dreifus, L. S., Berkovits, B. V., Kimbiris, D., et al.: Use of atrial and bifocal cardiac pacemakers for treating resistant dysrhythmias. Eur. J. Cardiol., 3:257, 1975.
33. Levy, S., Jausseran, J. M., Boyer, C., et al.: La stimulation séquentielle auriculoventriculaire par stimulateur bifocal implantable. Arch. Mal. Coeur, 69:1285, 1976.
34. Salvador-Mazenq, M., Graulle, A., Laborde, G., et al.: Résultats à court terme de la stimulation bifocal. Stimucoeur, 21:67, 1978.
35. Bognolo, D. A., Vijayanagar, R. R., and Eckstein, P. E.: Atrial and atrioventricular sequential pacing. Rationale and clinical experience. J. Florida Med. Assoc., 66:1028, 1979.
36. Sutton, R., and Citron, P.: Electrophysiological and hemodynamic basis for application of new pacemaker technology in sick sinus syndrome and atrioventricular block. Br. Heart J., 41:600, 1979.
37. Barold, S. S., Falkoff, M. D., Ong, L. S., et al.: Characterization of pacemaker arrhythmias due to normally functioning AV demand (DVI) pulse generators. Pace, 3:712, 1980.
38. Barold, S. S., Falkoff, M. D., Ong, L. S., and Heinle, R. A.: Interpretation of electrocardiograms produced by a new unipolar multiprogrammable "committed" A-V sequential demand (DVI) pulse generator. Pace, 4:692, 1981.
39. Echeverria, H. J., Luceri, R. M., Thurer, R. J., and Castellanos, A.: Myopotential inhibition of unipolar AV sequential (DVI) pacemaker. Pace, 5:20, 1982.

40. Funke, H. D.: Une experience clinique de frois annés avec la stimulation sequentielle optimisée du coeur. Stimucoeur, 9:26, 1981.
41. Redd, R., Messenger, J., and Castellanet, M.: Early experience with DDD pacing (Medtronic SP 0060). Clin. Res., 30:18A, 1982.
42. Versatrav II Model 7000A Universal AV pacemaker: Minneapolis, Medtronic, 1981.
43. Furman, S.: Pacemaker eccentricity. Pace, 4:261, 1981.
44. Furman, S.: Arrhythmias of dual chamber pacemakers. Pace, 5:469, 1982.
45. Furman, S., and Fisher, J. D.: Endless loop tachycardia in an A-V universal (DDD) pacemaker. Pace, 5:486, 1982.
46. Dendulk, K., Lindemans, F. W., Bar, F. W., and Wellens, H. J. J.: Pacemaker related tachycardia. Pace 5:476, 1982.
47. Hauser, R. G.: The electrocardiography of A-V universal DDD pacemakers. Pace 6:399, 1983.
48. Luceri, R. M., Castellanos, A., Zaman, L., and Myerburg, R. J.: The arrhythmias of dual-chamber cardiac pacemakers and their management. Ann. Intern. Med., 99:354, 1983.
49. Funke, H. D.: Cardiac pacing with the universal DDD pulse generator. Technological and electrophysiological considerations. In Barold, S. S. (ed.): The Third Decade of Cardiac Pacing, pp.191–223. Mount Kisco, N. Y., Futura, 1982.
50. Technical Manual 7007/7008 Universal A-V Telemetric Pacemaker with Tachyarrhythmia Control: Minneapolis, Medtronic, 1982.
51. Levine, P.: Postventricular atrial refractory periods and pacemaker mediated tachycardias. Clin. Prog. Pacing Electrophys., 1:394, 1983.
52. Furman, S.: Retreat from Wenckebach. Pace, 7:1, 1984.
53. Castellanos, A., Medina-Ravell, V., Berkovits, B. V., et al.: Atrial demand and AV sequential pacemakers. In Dreifus, L. S., (ed.): Pacemaker Therapy, pp. 149–164. Cardiovascular Clinics, Philadelphia, F. A. Davis, 1983.
54. Castellanos, A., and Lemberg, L.: Electrophysiology of Pacing and Cardioversion, p. 76. New York, Appleton-Century Crofts, 1969.
55. Furman, S.: Arrhythmias of dual chamber pacemakers. Pace, 5:469, 1982.
56. Duek, K. D., Lindemans, F. W., Bar, F. W., and Wellens, H. J. J.: Pacemaker related tachycardias. Pace, 5:476, 1982.
57. Johnson, C. D.: AV Universal (DDD) pacemaker-mediated reentrant endless loop tachycardia initiated by a reciprocal beat of atrial origin. Pace, 7:29,1984.
58. Tolentino, A. O., Javier, R. P., Byrd, C., and Samet, D.: Pacemaker induced tachycardia associated with an atrial synchronous ventricular inhibited (ASVIP) pulse generator. Pace, 5:251, 1982.
59. Freedman, R. A., Rothman, M. T., and Mason, J. W.: Recurrent ventricular tachycardia induced by an atrial synchronous ventricular-inhibited pacemaker. Pace, 5:490, 1982.
60. Bathen, J., Gundersen, T., and Forfang, K.: Tachycardias related to atrial synchronous ventricular pacing. Pace 5:471, 1982.
61. Gelder, L. M., El-Gamal, M. I. H., Baker, R., and Sanders, R. S.: Tachycardia-termination algorithm: a valuable feature for interruption of pacemaker mediated tachycardia. Pace, 7:283, 1984.
62. Van Mechelen, R., Hagemeijrer, F., De Jong, J., and De Boer, H.: Responses of an AV Universal (DDD) pulse generator (Cordis 233D) to programmed single ventricular extrastimuli. Pace, 7:215, 1984.
63. Elmgvist, H.: Letters to the editor (reply). Pace, 7:304, 1984.
64. Amikam, S., Andrews, C., and Furman, S.: "Pseudo-endless loop" tachycardia in an AV Universal (DDD) pacemaker. Pace, 7:129, 1984.
65. Quintal, R., Dhurandhar, R. W., and Jain, R. K.: Myopotential interference with a DDD pacemaker—report of a case. Pace, 7:37, 1984.
66. Smyth, N. P. P., et al.: Effect of an active magnetometer on permanently implanted pacemakers. J.A.M.A., 221:162, 1972.
67. Lister, J. W., Cohen, L. S., Bernstein, W. H., and Samet, P.: Treatment of supraventricular tachycardias by rapid atrial stimulation. Circulation, 38:144, 1968.
68. Fischer, J. D., Cohen, H. L., Mehra, R., et al.: Cardiac pacing and pacemakers. II. Several electrophysiologic-pharmacologic testing for recurrent tachyarrhythmias. Am. Heart J., 93:658, 1977.
69. Hartzler, G. O., Holmes, D. R., and Osborn, M. T.: Patient-activated transvenous cardiac stimulation for the treatment of supraventricular tachycardia. Am. J. Cardiol., 47:903, 1981.
70. Castellanos, A., Waxman, H. L., Moleiro, F., et al.: Preliminary studies with an implantable multimodal A-V pacemaker for reciprocating atrioventricular tachycardias. Pace, 3:257, 1980.
71. Portillo, B., Medina-Ravell, V., Portillo-Leon, N., et al.: Treatment of drug resistant AV reciproeating tachycardias with multiprogrammable dual demand AV sequential (DVI,MN) pacemakers. Pace, 5:814, 1982.

26

The Use of Electrophysiologic Testing in Pediatric Patients

Paul C. Gillette, Bertrand Ross, Derek A. Fyfe, Ashby B. Taylor, Alexander J. Zinner, and Vicki L. Zeigler

Cardiac dysrhythmias, which used to be considered rare in children, are now recognized quite frequently, probably because of three factors: (1) increased awareness, (2) improved detection techniques, and (3) a true increase in incidence secondary to successful cardiac surgical procedures.

The tools with which clinicians may detect and treat these dysrhythmias have improved manyfold. Noninvasive techniques such as ambulatory, transtelephonic, and exercise electrocardiography and inpatient telemetric monitoring have been very useful.[1] Invasive electrophysiologic testing, however, has been the most important both in improving clinicians' understanding of mechanisms of dysrhythmias and in their day-to-day management.[2] The techniques of electrophysiology testing are very similar in children and adults, but equipment, techniques, and indications do differ.

In this chapter, we will attempt to highlight these differences while giving an overall picture of pediatric electrophysiologic studies (EPS).

Techniques

Electrophysiologic studies are carried out by the percutaneous sheath technique.[3] Most catheters are introduced into the femoral veins. The same percutaneous sheath technique is used to introduce a catheter into the coronary sinus by way of the brachial or cephalic vein[4] (Fig. 26-1). Subclavian, internal jugular, and axillary venipuncture have also been used but may carry a greater risk and are usually reserved for patients in whom the more distal veins are not usable. Anticoagulation is used only in patients with right to left shunts or when catheters are positioned in the left atrium or ventricle. Antibiotic prophylaxis is not used.

Sedation is necessary for pediatric EPS. Each sedative has an effect on the patient's electrophysiology.[5] We have usually used meperidine and promethazine for premedication and ketamine for additional sedation. Ketamine is advantageous because it is short acting and does not depress respiration. Standard recording equipment, freeze oscilloscope tape recorders, and stimulators can be used (Fig. 26-2).

Catheters

The catheters used for pediatric EPS differ in French size and electrode spacing. We use Nos. 4, 5, and 6 French

We would like to thank Mrs. Donna Nash for her excellent secretarial assistance.

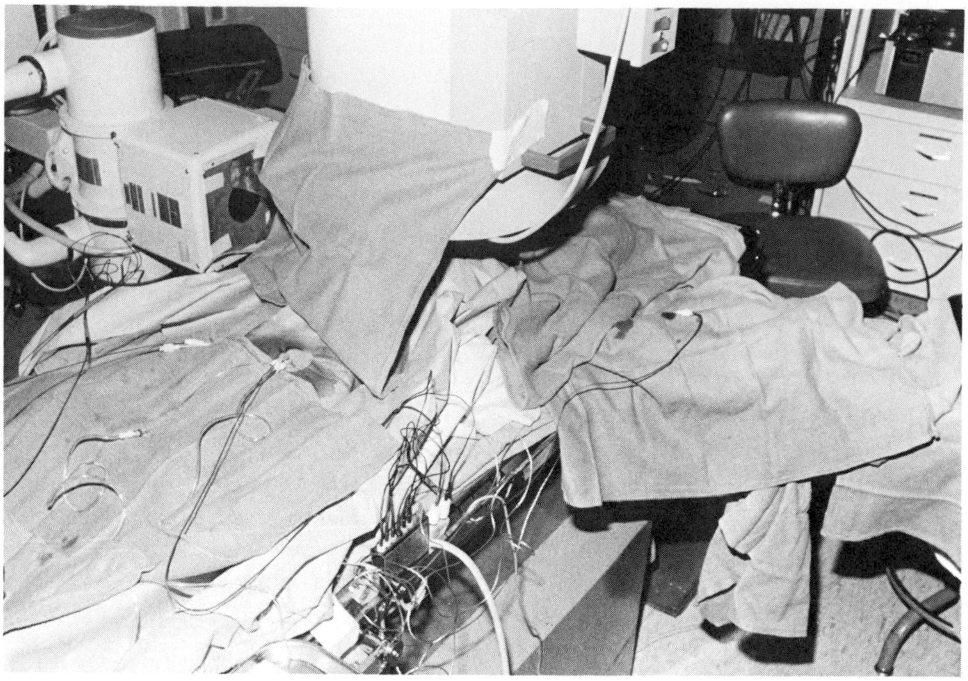

Figure 26-1. *Photograph of a pediatric patient undergoing an electrophysiologic study. The photograph is taken from the patient's left foot. Two electrode catheters have been introduced from the right femoral vein, one from the left femoral vein and one from the left brachial vein. A plastic cannula is in the left femoral artery. Posteroanterior and lateral x-ray equipment is shown.*

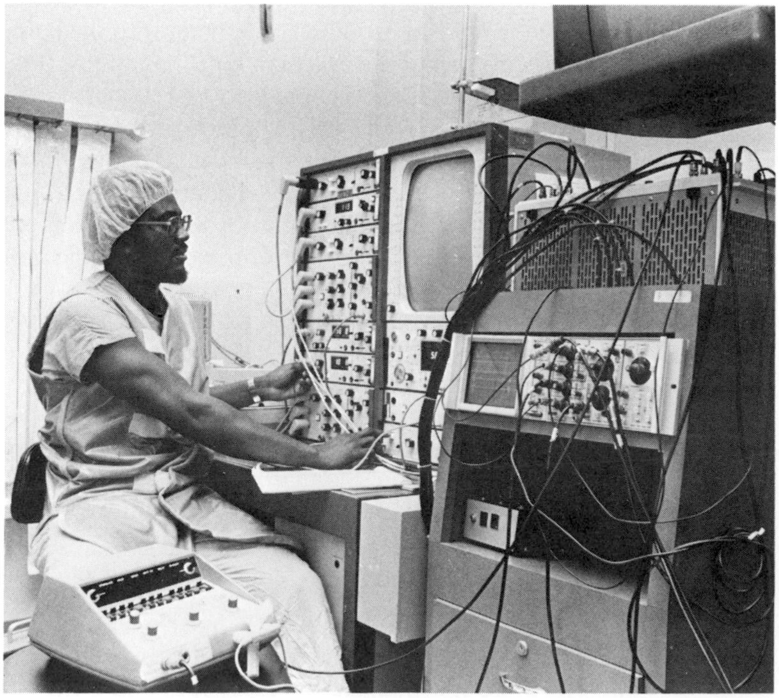

Figure 26-2. *Recording equipment used in pediatric electrophysiologic studies. A multichannel oscilloscopic recorder is used together with a six-channel storage oscilloscope and an eight-channel tape recorder. A programmable stimulator is in the foreground.*

catheters with 2- to 5-mm electrode spacing. For mapping we prefer six French catheters with up to 14 electrodes spaced 2, 5, 2, 5, and 2, 5 mm. We record between the 2-mm spacing in a bipolar fashion. Since the catheters do not have lumens, we use one side-arm sheath one French size greater than its catheter. A small plastic arterial cannula is used in each patient for blood pressure monitoring and arterial blood sampling.

Standard commercially available junction boxes are used to connect the patient to a standard 16-channel oscilloscopic recorder. A paper recording is made of each maneuver, and an FM tape recorder is used to catch any transient events. Biplane fluoroscopy is used to position the catheters, and biplane cinefluoroscopy is used to document catheter positions for later comparisons to EPS recordings.

Full resuscitation equipment is present and is tested frequently. R-2 pads are applied to patients considered at high risk for ventricular tachycardia or fibrillation, making rapid cardioversion possible.

Electrophysiologic studies are frequently carried out concomitant with hemodynamic catheterization and angiography. Pressures and oxygen saturation are frequently performed before EPS but angiography is always deferred because of its possible effect on the patient's physiology.

Automation

Each of our stimulation and measurement protocols is now carried out by an automated system that we have designed (Medtronic Dysrhythmia Research Instrument and Digital Equipment Corporation, DEC 11–23).[6–8] Patient information is typed in, and the initial protocol is selected (*e.g.*, sinus node recovery time). The initial stimulation cycle length and decrement cycle length are selected, and the protocol automaticity is carried out and measured. The recorder and a storage oscilloscope are automatically controlled. The results are presented in tabular and graphic form immediately. Tachycardia or bradycardia is automatically detected, and treatment options are presented to the operator.

Each new protocol is begun by the operator. The measured points on electrograms that were selected by the system are shown to the operator for confirmation (Fig. 26-3). Measurements are made of the same points that were hand measured (Fig. 26-4). At the end of the procedure a report is prepared and put on the patient's chart.

This system has greatly shortened the time required for our studies and has improved their reproducibility.

Indications

An EPS should be performed when any information that is clinically needed cannot be obtained by noninvasive means. Patients with recurrent supraventricular tachycardia are the most frequently studied in our laboratory.[9] The mechanisms of supraventricular tachycardia are more varied in pediatric patients. Wolff-Parkinson-White syndrome makes up 44% of all cases; atrial automatic focus, 10%; and junctional automatic focus, 4%.[10] Atrioventricular nodal reentry makes up only 30% of our supraventricular tachycardia cases. Determination of the mechanism not only directs our drug therapy but often clarifies the choice of pacemaker, surgical, or catheter ablative procedures.

Ventricular tachycardia makes up only 20% of pediatric tachycardias seen in the electrophysiology laboratory.[11] Three situations account for most cases: (1) in-

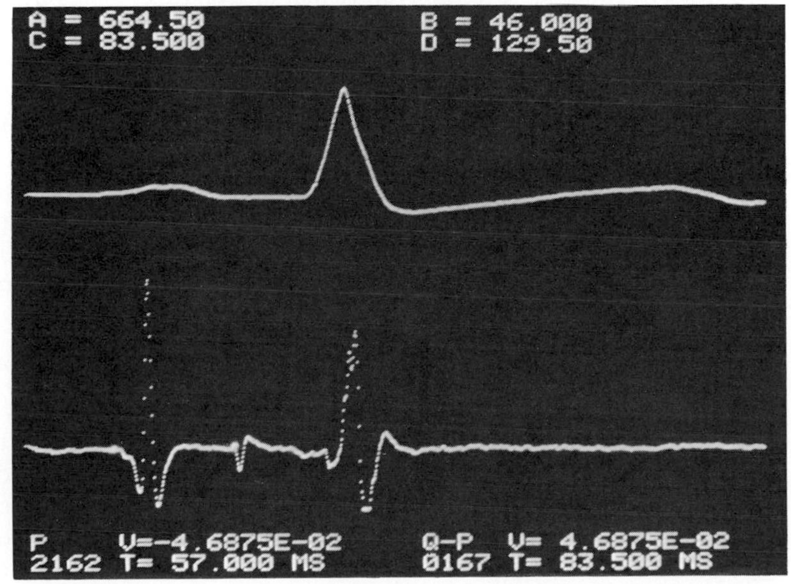

Figure 26-3. *Oscilloscope screen from an automated measuring device. A lead II surface electrocardiogram and a His bundle recording are displayed. The device has automatically selected the beginning of the low septal right atrium and His bundle* (bright spots).

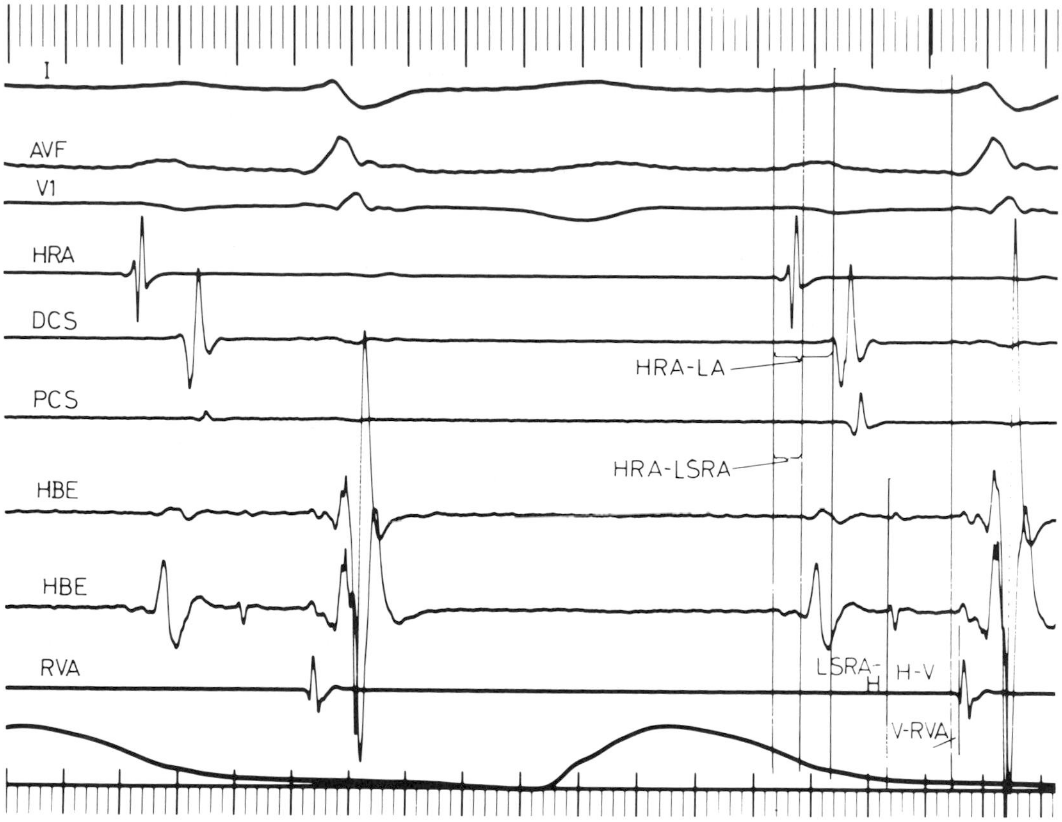

Figure 26-4. *Three surface electrocardiographic leads recorded simultaneously with intracardiac electrograms showing points of measurement of high right atrium (HRA) and left atrium (LA) from the coronary sinus, low septal right atrium (LSRA), His bundle (H), ventricle, and right ventricular apex (RVA).*

fants with tumors, (2) adolescents who have undergone surgery for congenital heart disease, and (3) patients with arrhythmogenic right ventricular dysplasia.[12–14] Angiography is a part of almost all these studies but often is not performed in patients with supraventricular tachycardia if two-dimensional and Doppler echocardiograms are normal.

In each tachycardia study, a thorough evaluation of sinus node, atrial, AV nodal, and His-Purkinje function is performed first. Tachycardia induction protocols are very similar to those in adults. We induce only two premature ventricular contractions (PVCs) in patients who have never had documented ventricular tachycardia. In those with previously documented tachycardia, we use up to three PVCs and carefully compare induced ventricular tachycardia to clinical ventricular tachycardia.

Drugs such as atropine and isoproterenol may be necessary to induce tachycardia. Other drugs, such as digoxin and propranolol, may be given in an attempt to predict clinical efficacy.[15] Repeat drug studies are done by reinducing catheters on another day rather than by leaving them in.

Mapping is done with up to 15 channels using closely spaced bipolar and sometimes unipolar electrograms displayed on the storage oscilloscope and paper recorder (Fig. 26-5). The catheter positions are recorded by biplane cinefluoroscopy.

Functional and anatomic properties of the arrhythmogenic focus or reentrant circuit are considered together with the patient's previous clinical course and any other heart disease.[16–18] During the procedure the best treatment, be it medication, pacing, catheter ablation, or surgery, is tentatively identified. If pacing or ablation is chosen and parental permission has been obtained, treatment may be done at that time. If pharmacologic therapy is chosen, a drug may be given intravenously and arrhythmia induction again attempted.

Syncope

Patients with syncope require a complete evaluation including testing of their sinus nodes and conduction systems and inducibility of supraventricular or ventricular tachydysrhythmias. Even if one possible cause for syncope is found, evaluation should be completed. Once the study is completed, the treatment of choice can be identified.

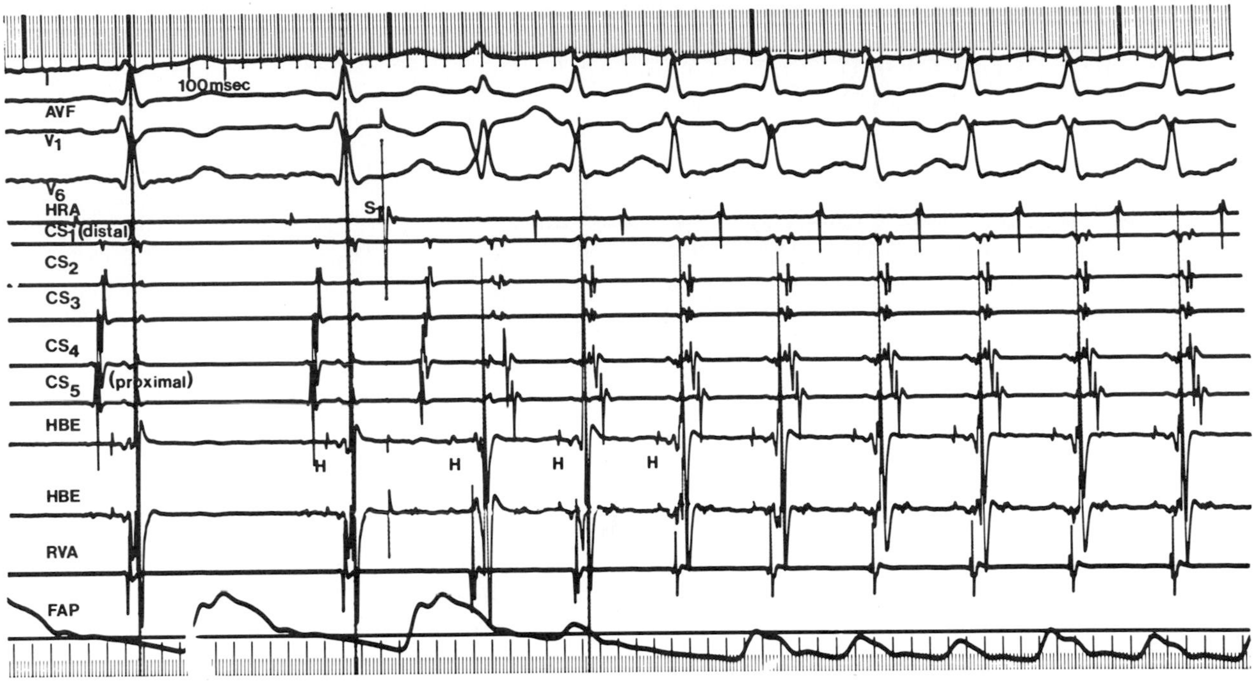

Figure 26-5. *Recordings from a tachycardia mapping study showing early activation of the coronary sinus (CS).*

Postoperative Management

Patients who have had certain major open-heart repairs of congenital cardiac defects should undergo postoperative EPS.[19–21] These include tetralogy of Fallot, truncus arteriosus, endocardial cushion defect, ventricular septal defect with pulmonary hypertension, and Mustard, Senning, and Fontan repairs. Each of these defects carries the significant possibility of sudden death within 5 years postoperatively.

These deaths are felt to be due to abnormalities of impulse initiation or conduction or tachydysrhythmias. It is likely that more than one factor plays a role in a single patient. For example, sinus bradycardia coupled with prolonged intra-atrial conduction may predispose patients who have undergone atrial repairs to atrial flutter or fibrillation.

Since the exact mode of death in these patients is speculative, a complete evaluation should be performed in each. Data are presently available to suggest what constitutes a normal versus an abnormal response in the postoperative situation (Fig. 26-6). Although most patients who require treatment are symptomatic, some asymptomatic patients probably should be treated. The induction of a sustained monomorphic ventricular tachycardia by two or fewer PVCs in a patient after repair of tetralogy of Fallot is such a situation. The induction of sustained atrial flutter in a patient who has undergone a Mustard procedure is another. A mildly prolonged HV interval ($\leq$90 msc) has been a benign finding in our almost 10 years of follow-up study. Sinus node recovery time 50% greater than normal is frequently found and does not seem to be of adverse prognostic significance. Splitting of the His bundle potential, block below the His bundle, and single ventricular reentrant beats using the conduction system likewise seem to be benign findings.

Wolff-Parkinson-White Syndrome

Patients with the Wolff-Parkinson-White syndrome, even those without tachycardia, should be considered for study. In some patients, the first symptom is sudden death. Patients who are resuscitated from sudden death and who are found to have the Wolff-Parkinson-White syndrome almost always have short antegrade refractory periods of their accessory connections. Since accessory pathways with the shortest refractory periods are the least sensitive to medication, and since patient compliance is known to be poor, we recommend surgical division of these pathways.

Conclusion

Electrophysiologic testing is now an internal part of the practice of pediatric cardiology, as it is within adult cardiology. It has allowed clinicians to care for the increasing number of patients with dysrhythmias. Together with noninvasive testing, it has allowed clinicians to treat those patients who require treatment and withhold treatment from those who do not. Surgical and catheter

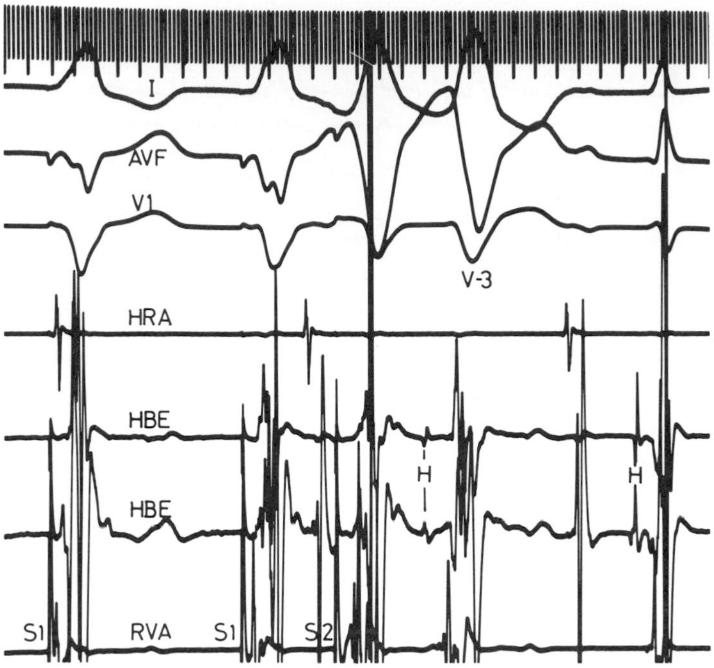

Figure 26-6. *Recording shows macroreentry within the His-Purkinje system. After the premature ventricular beat, the His bundle (H) is reactivated and reexcites the ventricles (V_3).*

treatment allows physicians to "cure" some patients without the need for lifelong treatment. The use of pacemakers, including antitachycardia pacemakers, may be lifesaving for some patients and may simplify treatment for others.

References

1. Hesslein, P. S.: Noninvasive diagnosis of dysrhythmias. In Gillette, P. C., and Garson, A., Jr. (eds.): Pediatric Cardiac Dysrhythmias. New York, Grune & Stratton, 1981.
2. Gillette, P. C., and Garson, A., Jr.: Intracardiac electrophysiologic studies: Use in determining the site and mechanism of dysrhythmias. In Gillette, P. C., and Garson, A., Jr. (eds.): Pediatric Cardiac Dysrhythmias. New York, Grune & Stratton, 1981.
3. Gillette, P. C., Reitman, M. J., Gutgesell, H. P., et al.: Intracardiac electrography in children and young adults. Am. Heart J., 89:36–44, 1975.
4. Gillette, P. C., and Garson, A., Jr.: Pediatric Cardiac Dysrhythmias, pp. 77–404. New York, Grune & Stratton, 1981.
5. Clapp, S. K., Driscoll, D. J., Mitrani, I., et al.: The comparative effects of age and sedation on sinus node automatically and atrioventricular conduction. Dev. Pharmacol. Ther., 2:180–187, 1981.
6. Zinner, A., Gillette, P. C., and Combs, W.: Totally automated electrophysiologic testing of sinus node function. Am Heart J., 108:1024–1028, 1984.
7. Gillette, P. C., Garson, A., Zinner, A., and Kugler, J. D.: Continuous computer automated measurement of electrophysiologic data during cardiac catheterization. Comput. Cardiol., 1981.
8. Gillette, P. C., Garson, A., Jr., Zinner, A., et al.: Automated online measurement of electrophysiologic intervals during cardiac catheterization. Pace, 3:456–460, 1980.
9. Garson, A., Jr.: Supraventricular tachycardia. In Gillette, P. C., and Garson, A., Jr. (eds.): Pediatric Cardiac Dysrhythmias. New York, Grune & Stratton, 1981.
10. Gillette, P. C.: The preexcitation syndromes. In Gillette, P. C., and Garson, A., Jr. (eds.): Pediatric Cardiac Dysrhythmias. New York, Grune & Stratton, 1981.
11. Garson, A., Jr.: Ventricular Dysrhythmias. In Gillette, P. C., and Garson, A., Jr. (eds.): Pediatric Cardiac Dysrhythmias. New York, Grune & Stratton, 1981.
12. Garson, A., Jr., Gillette, P. C., Titus, J. L., et al.: Surgical treatment of ventricular tachycardia in infants: Infant ventricular tachycardia surgery. N. Engl. J. Med. 310:1443–1445, 1984.
13. Garson, A., Jr., Kugler, J. D., Gillette, P. C., et al.: Control of last postoperative ventricular arrhythmias with phenytoin in young patients. Am. J. Cardiol., 46:290–294, 1980.
14. Dungan, W. T., Garson, A., Jr., and Gillette, P. C.: Arrythmogenic right ventricular dysplasia: A cause of ventricular tachycardia in children with apparently normal hearts. Am. Heart J., 102:745–750, 1981.
15. Jedeikin, R., Gillette, P. C., Garson, A., Jr., et al.: Effect of ouabain on the antegrade effective refractory period of accessory atrioventricular connection in children. J. Am. Coll. Cardiol., 1:869–872, 1983.
16. Gillette, P. C., Garson, A., Jr., Porter, C. J., et al.: Junctional automatic ectopic tachycardia: New proposed treatment by transcatheter His bundle ablation. Am. Heart J., 106:619–623, 1983.
17. Silka, M. J., Gillette, P. C., Garson, A., Jr., and Zinner, A.: Transvenous catheter ablation of a right atrial automatic ectopic tachycardia. Am. Coll. Cardiol., 5:999–1001, 1985.
18. Gillette, P. C., Wampler, D. G., Garson, A., Jr., et al.: Treatment of atrial automatic tachycardia by ablation procedures. J. Am. Coll. Cardiol., 6:405–409, 1985.
19. Garson, A., Jr., Porter, C. J., Gillette, P. C., and McNamara, D. G.: Induction of ventricular tachycardia during electrophysiology study after repair of tetralogy of Fallot. J. Am. Coll. Cardiol., 1:1493–1502, 1983.
20. Gillette, P. C., El-Said, G. M., Sivarajan, N., et al.: Electrophysiologic abnormalities after Mustard's operation for transposition of the great arteries. Br. Heart J., 36:186–191, 1974.
21. El-Said, G. M., Gillette, P. C., Cooley, D. A., et al.: Protection of the sinus node in Mustard's operation. Circulation, 53:788–791, 1976.

27

Diagnosis and Treatment of Arrhythmias Following Open-Heart Surgery

Albert L. Waldo

This work was supported in part by U.S. Public Health Service NHLBI Program Project Grant HL11,310 and SCOR on Ischemic Heart Disease Grant 1P17HL17667 and by a grant-in-aid from the American Heart Association.

Abnormalities of cardiac rhythm and conduction are remarkably common following open-heart surgery. Fortunately, in most instances, these arrhythmias are transient and amenable to standard modes of therapy discussed elsewhere in this book. What is unique about the postoperative open-heart surgical patient is that, at operation, temporary wire electrodes can be placed on the epicardium of both the atria and the ventricles. These wire electrodes can then be brought out through the anterior chest wall for diagnostic and therapeutic use in the postoperative period.[1-21] At the University of Alabama in Birmingham, a pair of atrial stainless steel wire electrodes and at least one and often two ventricular stainless steel wire electrodes are routinely placed in all open-heart surgical patients at operation. The use of these electrodes in the management of patients with arrhythmias following open-heart surgery has proved invaluable. Not only can they be used with great effectiveness both diagnostically and therapeutically, but the techniques for their use are safe, easy to implement, reliable, and rapid.[1-21]

In this chapter, the diagnostic and therapeutic use of the temporary atrial wire electrodes will be especially emphasized. These electrodes can be used diagnostically in two ways. First, they can be used to record atrial electrograms, that is, electrical activity recorded directly from the atria. The ability to record atrial electrograms provides a clear record of atrial activity and is particularly valuable in the diagnosis of arrhythmias in which the nature of atrial activation or the relationship of atrial activation to ventricular activation is unclear from the standard electrocardiogram (Fig. 27-1). Second, they can be used to pace the heart to assist in the diagnosis of an arrhythmia. For example, atrial pacing may be required to diagnose a narrow QRS complex tachycardia with a regular RR interval and a 1 : 1 AV relationship at a rate of 150 beats/min, and it may also be used to assess AV conduction. In addition, these temporary epicardial atrial electrodes can be used in the effective pacing treatment of virtually all abnormalities of rhythm and conduction with the exception of atrial fibrillation, type II atrial flutter, and ventricular fibrillation. Thus, atrial pacing may be used to suppress premature atrial or ventricular beats, terminate tachyarrhythmias, increase heart rate as treatment of bradyarrhythmias, or override or suppress undesirable rhythms with continuous rapid atrial pacing.

The great value of temporary atrial epicardial wire

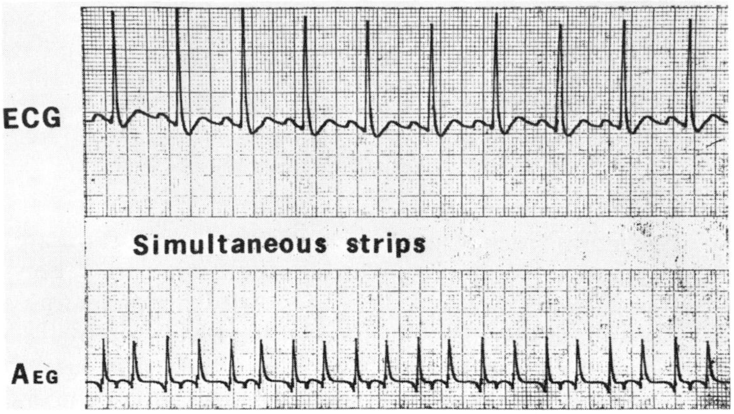

Figure 27-1. *Monitor electrocardiogram (ECG) recorded simultaneously with a bipolar electrogram (A_{EG}) demonstrating ectopic atrial tachycardia with 2:1 AV conduction. This rhythm was recorded from a patient who previously had demonstrated an ectopic atrial tachycardia with variable AV block. The rhythm then became regular at a rate of about 100 beats/min. The routine monitor ECG suggested that a sinus rhythm had developed, but the simultaneous recording of the bipolar atrial electrogram with the ECG clearly demonstrated that the ectopic atrial tachycardia was still present. Finally, note the irregularity of the beat-to-beat cycle length evident in the recorded atrial electrograms. This is a common, although not invariable, characteristic of this rhythm. See text for discussion. (Waldo, A. L., MacLean, W. A. H., Cooper, T. B., et al.: Use of temporarily placed epicardial atrial wire electrodes for the diagnosis and treatment of cardiac arrhythmias following open heart surgery. J. Thorac. Cardiovasc. Surg., 76:500–505, 1978)*

electrodes has been amply documented in various reports.[1-21] However, to assess both the incidence and risk of their use, we recently selected a 1-month period at random and analyzed the use of these electrodes during this time in 70 consecutive patients on one of the cardiovascular surgical services at the University of Alabama Medical Center.[16] As summarized in Table 27-1, atrial wire electrodes were used diagnostically or therapeutically in 57 patients a total of 139 times and were not used for any reason in only 13 patients. In none of these patients was either their use or removal associated with morbidity or mortality. Parenthetically, over the past 7½ years, we have routinely placed temporary atrial wire electrodes in over 9000 patients without experiencing any clinically significant morbidity and without any mortality.

Table 27-1. Use of Temporarily Placed Epicardial Atrial Wire Electrodes in 70 Consecutive Surgical Patients

	No. of Patients
Used in 57 patients	
Only to record an atrial electrogram	8
Only to pace the atria	23
To record an atrial electrogram and pace the atria	26
Used on two or more separate occasions	13
Not used	13

(Waldo, A. L., MacLean, W. A. H., Cooper, T. B., Kouchoukos, N. T., and Karp, R. B.: Use of temporarily placed epicardial atrial wire electrodes for the diagnosis and treatment of cardiac arrhythmias following open heart surgery. J. Thorac. Cardiovasc. Surg., 76:500–505, 1978)

Table 27-2 demonstrates the incidence and indications for use of atrial wire electrodes in the same group of patients as in Table 27-1. Atrial electrograms were recorded 63 times in 34 patients, 41 times to establish the rhythm diagnosis and 22 times to confirm the rhythm diagnosis. They were not used for diagnostic purposes in 36 patients. As shown in Table 27-3, atrial pacing was used to treat abnormalities of rhythm and conduction 75 times in 49 of the 70 patients. It is clear from assessment of this study that the frequent use of the technique not only reflects its clinical usefulness, but also its safety, reliability, speed, and accuracy.

Temporary ventricular epicardial wire electrodes are also of great value. Although they are rarely of use diagnostically, they are of great use therapeutically, particularly in the treatment of various bradyarrhythmias, especially forms of AV block, and for the treatment of serious tachyarrhythmias such as AV junctional tachycardia or recurrent ventricular tachycardia.

In sum, by having wire electrodes available in the postoperative period, arrhythmia diagnosis is greatly facilitated. Furthermore, because of the clinical advantages of cardiac pacing, it becomes the treatment of choice for many, if not most, postoperative arrhythmias.

Table 27-2. Diagnoses Obtained By Use of Atrial Wire Electrodes in 70 Consecutive Surgical Patients

	Diagnosis	
Rhythm	*Primary*	*Confirm*
Premature atrial beats	2	0
Premature ventricular beats	5	1
Atrial fibrillation	5	6
Atrial flutter	6	1
PAT, Atrial tachycardia	3	0
Aberrant AV conduction	1	0
AV junctional rhythm	5	1
Ventricular tachycardia	1	0
AV dissociation	2	2
Normal sinus rhythm	5	8
AV block*	2	0
Other†	4	3
Totals‡	41	22

PAT, paroxysmal atrial tachycardia; AV, atrioventricular.
* Atrial pacing used to assess AV conduction.
† Sinus bradycardia, atrial bigeminy, sinus tachycardia, and atrial standstill.
‡ Thirty-six patients had no indication for recording an atrial electrogram. Thirteen patients had two or more indications for recording an atrial electrogram.
(Waldo, A. L., MacLean, W. A. H., Cooper, T. B., Kouchoukos, N. T., and Karp, R. B.: Use of temporarily placed epicardial atrial wire electrodes for the diagnosis and treatment of cardiac arrhythmias following open heart surgery. J. Thorac. Cardiovasc. Surg., 76:500–505, 1978)

Table 27-3. Reasons for Pacing Treatment Using Wire Electrodes in 70 Consecutive Surgical Patients

Rhythm Disturbance	Atrial Pacing	Ventricular Pacing*
Sinus bradycardia (<80 beats/min)	24	1
Premature atrial beats	11	0
Premature ventricular beats	22	2
AV junctional rhythm	3	1
Atrial flutter†	6	0
Paroxysmal atrial tachycardia†	2	0
Atrial tachycardia†	1	0
Ventricular tachycardia	2	2
AV dissociation	2	1
Second degree AV block	2	1
Totals‡	75	8

* Demand mode ventricular pacing excluded.
† Rapid atrial pacing to interrupt arrhythmia, or continuous rapid atrial pacing to suppress recurrent arrhythmia.
‡ Twenty-one patients had no indication for cardiac pacing. Eighteen patients had two or more indications for cardiac pacing.
(Waldo, A. L., MacLean, W. A. H., Cooper, T. B., Kouchoukos, N. T., and Karp, R. B.: Use of temporarily placed epicardial atrial wire electrodes for the diagnosis and treatment of cardiac arrhythmias following open heart surgery. J. Thorac. Cardiovasc. Surg., 76:500–505, 1978)

Cardiac pacing therapy has the following clinical advantages:

1. It is immediate in onset and effect.
2. It frequently avoids the need for drugs and their attendant undesirable toxic and side-effects.
3. It frequently avoids the need for direct current cardioversion.
4. It is associated with virtually no discomfort.
5. When pacing therapy is no longer desirable, it can be terminated promptly.
6. Pacing may provide a period of effective therapy during which time antiarrhythmic drugs that may be needed to provide effective chronic suppression of arrhythmias can be administered.

Placement of Temporary Epicardial Wire Electrodes at Surgery

Atrial Wire Electrodes

I recommend placing at least one pair of atrial wire electrodes for two important reasons. First, if the wire electrodes are placed high in the right atrium, and the interelectrode distance is 0.5 to 1 cm, the bipolar atrial electrogram will primarily demonstrate only atrial activation (*i.e.*, little or virtually no ventricular complex will be present). This is particularly important in the diagnosis of various arrhythmias in which atrial activation may coincide with ventricular activation. In such a circumstance, if only one atrial wire is placed, or if the interelectrode distance is so wide that both atrial and ventricular activation are recorded, atrial activation may be masked within the ventricular complex. The second reason for placing a pair of wire electrodes is that during bipolar atrial pacing, the stimulus artifact is narrow and does not distort the electrocardiogram, whereas if only one atrial wire has been placed, the unipolar stimulus artifact usually will completely distort the atrial complex in the electrocardiogram. This distortion becomes particularly important when using rapid atrial pacing techniques to treat supraventricular tachycardias, because it precludes clear identification of atrial activation in the electrocardiogram and may prevent recognizing whether atrial capture has been obtained.

Ventricular Electrodes

We recommend the routine placement of at least one temporary epicardial ventricular electrode, and, if possible, two. Because the need to record bipolar ventricular electrograms, or in fact any ventricular electrogram, is very infrequent, and because unipolar ventricular pacing is quite easy, effective, and safe, the need to place two ventricular wire electrodes is not as clear as the need to place two atrial wire electrodes. However, the advantage of two ventricular electrodes is that during bipolar pacing, the stimulus artifact is narrow, and therefore failure to obtain ventricular capture is easily appreciated in the electrocardiogram. The latter may not be appreciated with unipolar pacing because a unipolar stimulus artifact itself may mimic a QRS complex, thereby suggesting that ventricular capture has occurred when it has not. Additionally, in unipolar ventricular pacing, the indifferent electrode may have to be a wire placed subcutaneously, with its attendant discomforts.

Technique of Placement

Following completion of cardiopulmonary bypass and before surgical closure of the chest, a pair of Teflon-coated wire electrodes are secured to the epicardium high in the free wall of the right atrium. Each wire is first bared of Teflon for approximately 0.5 to 1 cm at its tip, and this bared end is then bent in the form of a J hook.[16,17] A superficial stitch of 5-0 cardiovascular silk is then placed in the atrial epicardium to form a loop. The Teflon-free end of one wire electrode is secured to the atrial epicardium by placing it through the loop and tying the suture. A second wire electrode is placed in the same manner about 0.5 to 1 cm from the first wire electrode. Each of these wires is then brought out through the anterior chest wall, and the distal end of each wire is bared of Teflon for about 0.5 cm to permit either recording of atrial electrograms or atrial pacing.

For each patient, one or a pair of wire electrodes should be routinely placed on the free wall of the right ventricle according to the above method or alternatively by implanting the electrode(s) into the right ventricular muscle using the atraumatic round needle that is attached to most commercially available wire electrodes. After having been placed, the ventricular wire electrode(s) is brought out through the anterior chest wall and treated in the same manner described above for the atrial wire electrodes.

Finally, the placement of the wire electrodes is designed so that they may be removed easily. Therefore, a stay suture should be placed in the skin close to the site where each wire electrode exits the chest wall to anchor each one to the anterior chest wall. This helps to secure the electrodes so that during use they are not inadvertently pulled free from the heart.

Care of Epicardial Wire Electrodes

Because the epicardial wire electrodes provide a direct electrical circuit from outside the body to the heart, great care must be taken to ensure that the Teflon-free portion of the wire that is outside the chest wall is electrically isolated at all times. One way to do this is to encase the Teflon-free portion of the wire with electrically inert plastic tape when the electrode is not in use. The tape can be removed easily whenever the wire is to be used. When in use, the wire electrodes will be electrically isolated if during cardiac pacing the cardiac pacemaker is a battery-powered device and if during recording electrograms the recording device is electrically isolated.

We suggest that the wire electrodes be left in place until the night before the patient's discharge from the hospital. All wire electrodes should be easy to remove with a gentle tug after removal of the skin stay suture. Removing the wire electrodes in this fashion has been associated with no complications and only negligible discomfort. I have had only three instances in which a wire electrode could not be pulled out because it could not be pulled through the chest wall.[16,17] In each instance, removal was accomplished by simply cutting the wire at the skin where it exited the chest wall and permitting the distal end to fall back into the chest, following which there were no further complications. When removing ventricular wire electrodes that have been imbedded within the ventricular myocardium, one must be alert to the rare possibility of causing pericardial tamponade.

Recording Atrial Electrograms

It is usually preferable to record a bipolar atrial electrogram simultaneously with an electrocardiogram for purposes of arrhythmia diagnosis. This, of course, requires at least a two-channel recording machine. However, a single-channel recording machine is often adequate, because the sequential recording of an electrocardiogram and either a bipolar or unipolar atrial electrogram usually provides the needed information. To record an atrial electrogram using a single-channel electrocardiograph recorder, the right and left leg leads should be connected to the patient and the right and left arm leads should each be attached to one of the atrial wire electrodes. This can be done by using alligator clips to interface with each limb lead and each electrode (Fig. 27-2). Since lead I is a bipolar recording between the right arm and left arm leads, by moving the electrocardiogram lead selector to the lead I position, a bipolar atrial electrogram will be recorded. By moving the electrocardiogram lead selector either to the lead II or lead III position, a unipolar atrial electrogram will be recorded, because in each instance the recording will be made between an atrial wire electrode and the left leg, that is, the right arm lead attached to a wire electrode and the left leg (lead II) or the left arm lead attached to a wire electrode and the left leg (lead III).

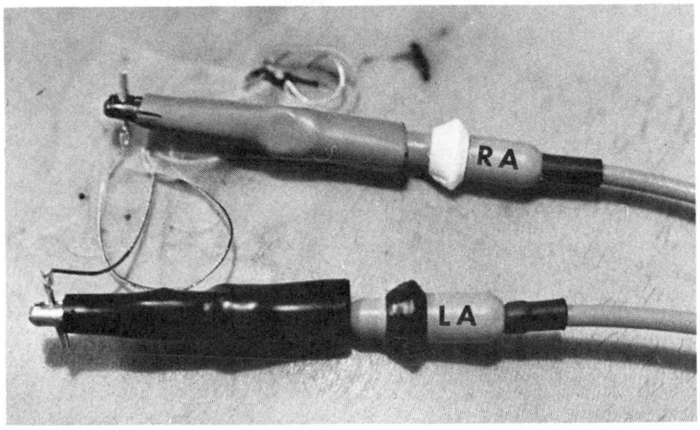

Figure 27-2. *The right (RA) and left (LA) arm leads of the patient cable from a standard electrocardiogram machine are attached with alligator clips to the exteriorized, Teflon-coated atrial wire electrodes. The Teflon-free end of each wire has been trimmed and crimped. The leg leads of the patient cable are attached to the patient in the usual manner. Now, standard lead I can be used to record a bipolar atrial electrogram, and either standard lead II or III can be used to record a unipolar atrial electrogram. (Waldo, A. L., and MacLean, W. A. H.: The Diagnosis and Treatment of Arrhythmias Following Open Heart Surgery—Emphasis on the Use of Epicardial Wire Electrodes. Mt. Kisco, N.Y., Futura, 1980)*

Pacing the Heart

A standard, demand-mode, battery-powered, external cardiac pacemaker should be available. Most standard battery-powered cardiac pacemakers can achieve rates of only 150 to 180 beats/min. Although these pacing rates are adequate for the pacing treatment of some cardiac arrhythmias, many arrhythmias require cardiac pacing at far faster rates, including some as fast as 450 beats/min.[13] Therefore, a cardiac pacemaker capable of generating rates up to 600 to 800 beats/min should be available. In addition, a pacemaker that can perform paired pacing should be available.[12,17,18] This latter technique is particularly important for some of the rare instances of tachyarrhythmias originating below the AV node and, on occasion, may even be important in treating or suppressing supraventricular arrhythmias. Also, a pacemaker capable of performing sequential or coordinated AV pacing should be available, primarily for patients who have developed heart block in association with the cardiovascular surgical repair.

Diagnosis and Treatment of Postoperative Arrhythmias

Bradycardias

Sinus bradycardias (rates less than 60 beats/min) and relative sinus bradycardias (rates between 60 and 75 or 60 and 80 beats/min) are common postoperative arrhythmias.[16] They are often associated with a low cardiac output and rate-related supraventricular and ventricular arrhythmias. Ventricular extrasystoles that would not be present at a more rapid heart rate are the most obvious examples. By pacing the atria or ventricles at a more rapid rate than the spontaneous rate, it is possible to increase the cardiac output solely by this rate augmentation and at the same time suppress the ventricular arrhythmia. If AV conduction is intact, this is best accomplished by overriding the spontaneous heart rate with atrial pacing at an appropriate rate, often as fast as 100 to 110 beats/min.

If the bradycardia is the result of second or third degree AV block, ventricular pacing at an appropriate rate, virtually always in a demand mode, is indicated. If the cardiac output during ventricular pacing in the face of second or third degree AV block is less than satisfactory, it may be desirable to initiate AV sequential pacing to include the atrial contribution to cardiac output. This is particularly important in treatment of complete heart block that results following surgical repair of congenital heart disease in infants.

Supraventricular Tachycardias

Atrial Fibrillation

Diagnosis. Atrial fibrillation is a common postoperative arrhythmia in adults, regardless of the preoperative rhythm or the nature of the cardiac surgery. For patients who had sinus rhythm preoperatively and develop atrial fibrillation postoperatively, the arrhythmia is usually transient.

Although this arrhythmia usually is easily diagnosed from an electrocardiogram, the recording of an atrial electrogram for diagnostic purposes may be quite helpful and in fact is sometimes necessary. Bipolar atrial electrograms recorded from patients with atrial fibrillation are characterized by complexes having a myriad of sizes, shapes, polarities, and amplitudes as well as a broad range of rates and beat-to-beat intervals.[15] In fact, based on recorded bipolar atrial electrograms, the hallmark of atrial fibrillation is the characteristic beat-to-beat variability of these parameters.

On the basis of the morphology of the bipolar atrial electrogram and the nature of the baseline between the atrial electrogram complexes, atrial fibrillation can be divided into four distinct types.[15] *Type I atrial fibrillation* is characterized by atrial electrograms with discrete complexes of variable morphology, polarity, amplitude, and cycle length separated by an isoelectric baseline free of perturbation (Fig. 27-3). *Type II atrial fibrillation* is characterized by discrete beat-to-beat atrial electrogram complexes of variable morphology, polarity, amplitude, and cycle length, but differs from type I atrial fibrillation in that the baseline is not isoelectric, having perturba-

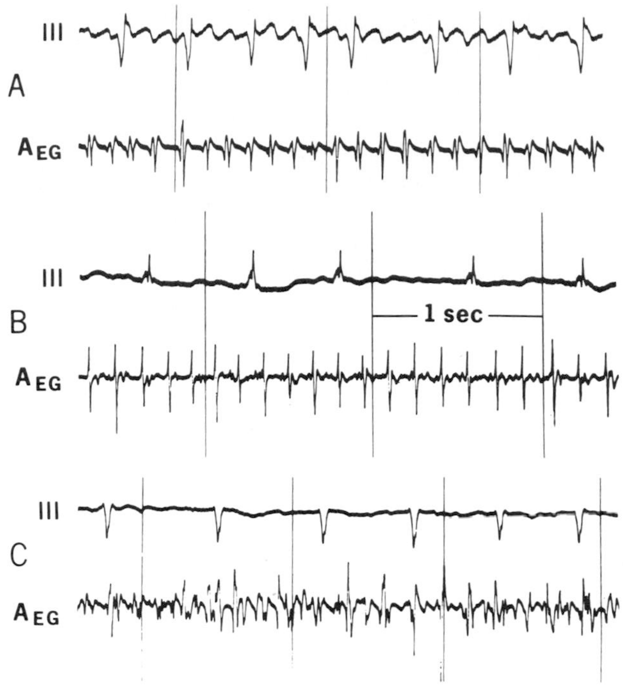

Figure 27-3. *In each of the three panels in this figure, electrocardiographic lead III has been recorded simultaneously with a bipolar atrial electrogram (A_{EG}). A demonstrates the characteristic atrial electrogram for type I atrial fibrillation, B for type II atrial fibrillation, and C for type III atrial fibrillation. Note that the electrocardiogram in A mimics atrial flutter, but careful examination of the recorded bipolar atrial electrogram clearly demonstrates that the rhythm is atrial fibrillation. Time lines are at 1-second intervals. (After Wells, J. L., Jr., Karp, R. B., Kouchoukos, N. T., et al.: Characterization of atrial fibrillation in man. Studies following open heart surgery. Pace, 3:965–980, 1978)*

tions of varying degrees (see Fig. 27-3). *Type III atrial fibrillation* is characterized by atrial electrograms that appear chaotic and that fail to demonstrate either discrete complexes or isoelectric intervals. *Type IV atrial fibrillation* is characterized by atrial electrograms consistent with type III, alternating with periods of atrial electrograms consistent with type I or II (Fig. 27-4).

It is clear from the recordings in Figures 27-3 and 27-4 that despite the fact that the atrial electrograms recorded during atrial fibrillation are characterized by variability in morphology, polarity, amplitude, and cycle length, not all atrial fibrillation is of the chaotic type manifested by type III. Some types of atrial fibrillation appear to be rather well ordered. This fact is even reflected in the electrocardiogram shown in Figure 27-3*A*, in which coarse, rather discrete atrial complexes can be seen. Furthermore, although the atrial rates as measured from atrial electrograms recorded during atrial fibrillation range widely, surprisingly low rates (in fact, as low as 263 beats/min) have been documented during atrial fibrillation.[15] Also, it is not unusual to find atrial rates associated with type I or II atrial fibrillation within the range associated with atrial flutter.[15,19] Thus, should the rate of atrial fibrillation be relatively slow and the atrial electrogram be relatively organized, atrial fibrillation may mimic atrial flutter (see Fig. 27-3). In such instances, it is important to identify the rhythms properly, because classic atrial flutter can be treated effectively with rapid atrial pacing whereas atrial fibrillation cannot be so treated.[11,13–17,19] While it remains to be seen whether the identification of four types of atrial fibrillation on the basis of the recorded bipolar atrial electrogram has any mechanistic implications, this characterization is clinically useful in distinguishing atrial fibrillation (particularly types I and II) from atrial flutter.

Treatment. The drug treatment of atrial fibrillation in the postoperative period does not differ from the standard therapy of this arrhythmia. However, there is one consideration in treatment that is somewhat different: direct current cardioversion is rarely indicated in the immediate period following development of this arrhythmia, because although it usually will be successful in converting the rhythm to sinus rhythm, the milieu that contributed to the development of the arrhythmia remains unchanged and will almost always lead to its redevelopment. However, for patients who develop atrial fibrillation postoperatively and in whom the arrhythmia does not spontaneously revert to sinus rhythm (with or without drug therapy), direct current cardioversion one or two days before hospital discharge and before removal of the temporary wire electrodes is recommended.

Atrial Flutter

Diagnosis. For rhythms with rapid ventricular rates, the differential diagnosis often includes atrial flutter. However, it may be difficult to identify the atrial flutter waves in the electrocardiograms especially if one of the flutter waves is masked within the QRS complex. In such cases, by recording a bipolar atrial electrogram, atrial activation is readily identified and the nature of the atrial rate and rhythm is usually easily established. Thus, the recording of a bipolar atrial electrogram is extremely helpful in making the diagnosis of atrial flutter, and this probably should be done even when the electrocardiogram clearly suggests this diagnosis.

Recent studies in patients following open-heart surgery have identified two types of atrial flutter, labeled type I (classic) and type II.[19] Both types of atrial flutter resemble each other in that they are rapid, regular atrial rhythms. The bipolar atrial electrogram recorded during each type of atrial flutter characteristically is of uniform morphology, polarity, and amplitude, has a remarkably regular beat-to-beat interval, and has an isoelectric inter-

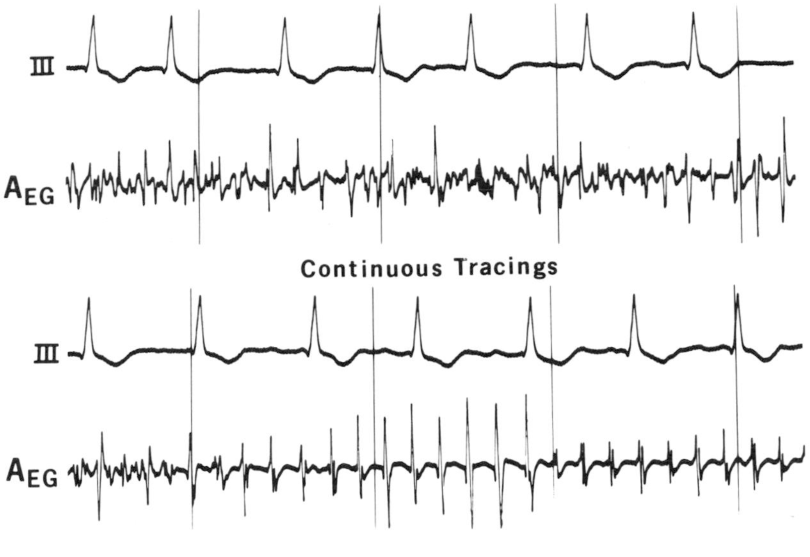

Figure 27-4. *Electrocardiographic lead III recorded simultaneously with a bipolar atrial electrogram demonstrating the atrial electrogram characteristic of type IV atrial fibrillation. Time lines are at 1-second intervals. (Wells, J. L., Jr., Karp, R. B., Kouchoukos, N. T., et al.: Characterization of atrial fibrillation in man. Studies following open heart surgery. Pace, 3:965–980, 1978)*

val between the discrete electrogram complexes (Fig. 27-5).[16,17,19] Occasionally, the recorded bipolar atrial electrogram in each type of atrial flutter demonstrates a beat-to-beat electrical alternans (Fig. 27-6), and sometimes the latter is also associated with an alternans in the beat-to-beat cycle length.

The two types of atrial flutter differ from each other in that type I atrial flutter can always be influenced by rapid atrial pacing from the high right atrium (*i.e.*, from the usual atrial location of the temporary, epicardial atrial wire electrodes), whereas type II atrial flutter cannot be so influenced.[14,19] They also differ in their range of atrial rates, the range of type I atrial flutter being about 230 to

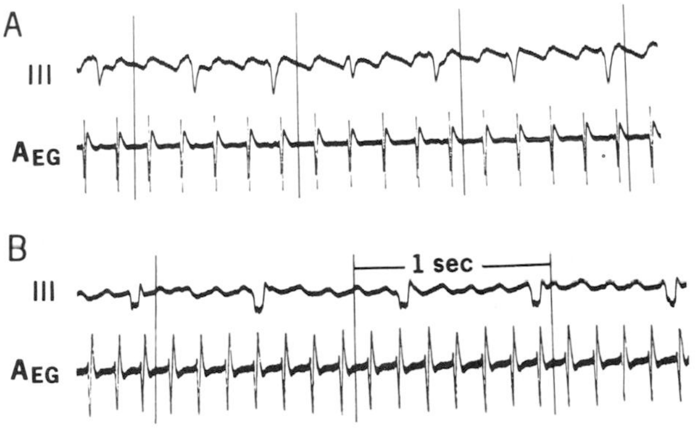

Figure 27-5. *(A) Electrocardiographic lead III recorded simultaneously with a bipolar atrial electrogram (A_{EG}) from a patient demonstrating the atrial electrogram characteristic of type I (classic) atrial flutter. (B) Electrocardiographic lead III recorded simultaneously with a bipolar atrial electrogram from another patient demonstrating the atrial electrogram characteristic of type II atrial flutter. Time lines are at 1-second intervals. (After Wells, J. L., Jr., MacLean, W. A. H., James, T. N., and Waldo, A. L.: Characterization of atrial flutter. Studies in man after open heart surgery using fixed atrial electrodes. Circulation, 60:665–673, 1979)*

340 beats/min and the range of type II atrial flutter being about 340 to 433 beats/min, the upper and lower limits for each being somewhat variable. In fact, there is almost certainly overlap of rates between the upper range of type I atrial flutter and the lower range of type II atrial flutter.

Treatment of Type I (Classic) Atrial Flutter. Rapid atrial pacing is the treatment of choice for patients who develop type I atrial flutter following open-heart surgery. We currently recommend a ramp atrial pacing technique, in which bipolar atrial pacing at a rate about 10 beats faster than the spontaneous atrial rate is begun and electrocardiogram lead II is recorded continuously. When it is demonstrated that the atrial rate has increased to the pacing rate, the atrial pacing rate is gradually increased until the atrial complexes (flutter waves) in lead II, which previously had been negative, become frankly positive. When this occurs, the atrial pacing may be abruptly terminated or the pacing rate may be quickly slowed. The latter permits control of the atrial rhythm until a desirable atrial rate, such as 100 to 110 beats/min, is achieved. A representative example is illustrated in Figures 27-7 and 27-8.

In another pacing technique, the constant-rate technique, rapid atrial pacing is initiated at a rate faster than the spontaneous rate. Pacing at this rate is continued for 30 seconds and then is either abruptly terminated or rapidly slowed to a desirable atrial rate. Because we have found that the most successful rate for interruption of type I atrial flutter is approximately 120% to 130% (range 111% to 135%) of the spontaneous atrial rate, using this second technique, one could start pacing at a rate within this range of the spontaneous atrial flutter rate (*e.g.*, 125% of the spontaneous rate) and pace either for 30 seconds or until the atrial complexes in electrocardiogram lead II change from negative to positive. If pacing at the initial rate does not interrupt atrial flutter, the

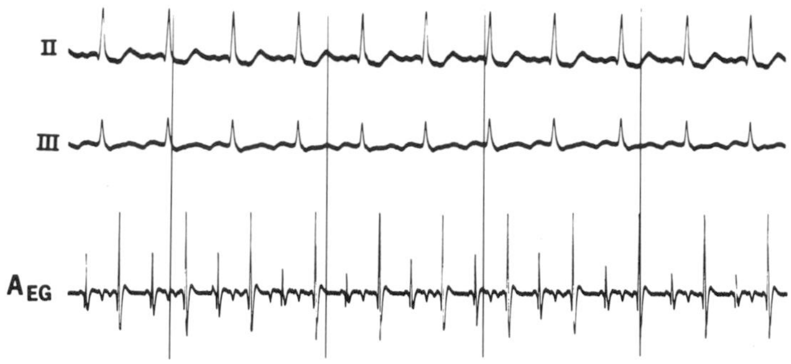

Figure 27-6. *Electrocardiographic leads II and III recorded simultaneously with a bipolar atrial electrogram (A_{EG}) from a patient demonstrating type I (classic) atrial flutter, illustrating an example of electrical alternans of the atrial electrogram. Time lines are at 1-second intervals. (Wells, J. L., Jr., MacLean, W. A. H., James T. N., and Waldo, A. L.: Characterization of atrial flutter. Studies in man after open heart surgery using fixed electrodes. Circulation, 60:665–673, 1979. By permission of the American Heart Association, Inc.)*

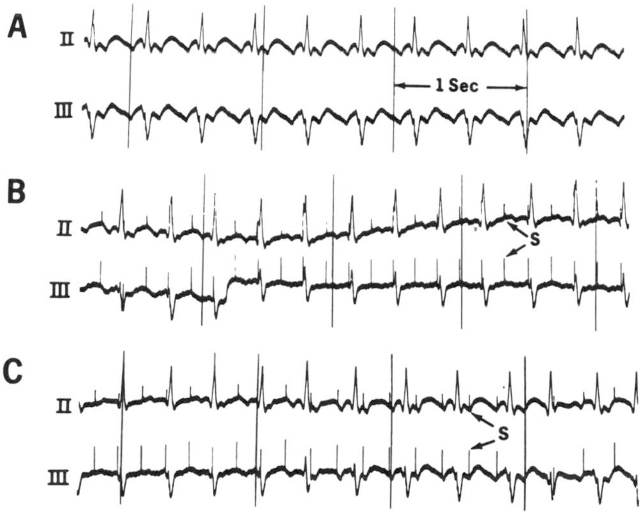

Figure 27-7. *Electrocardiographic leads II and III recorded from a patient with type I (classic) atrial flutter. A demonstrates that the atrial flutter rate is about 300 beats/min. Atrial pacing was initiated at a rate of 310 beats/min. Then, using the ramp pacing technique, the pacing rate was gradually increased. B demonstrates that as the atrial pacing rate was increased from about 342 to 350 beats/min, the morphology of the flutter waves changed in lead II from negative to biphasic and in lead III from negative to flat. The record in C is continuous with that in B and demonstrates that when the pacing rate was decreased to a rate slower than that of the spontaneous atrial flutter, the atrial flutter recurred. This is clearly evident at the end of the tracings in C, where the atrial flutter waves reappeared at a rate faster than the pacing rate. Thus, despite pacing at rates faster than the atrial flutter, the atrial flutter was not interrupted. Time lines are at 1-second intervals. (S, stimulus artifact) (After Waldo, A. L., MacLean, W. A. H., Karp, R. B., et al.: Entrainment and interruption of atrial flutter with atrial pacing. Studies in man following open heart surgery. Circulation, 56:737–745, 1977)*

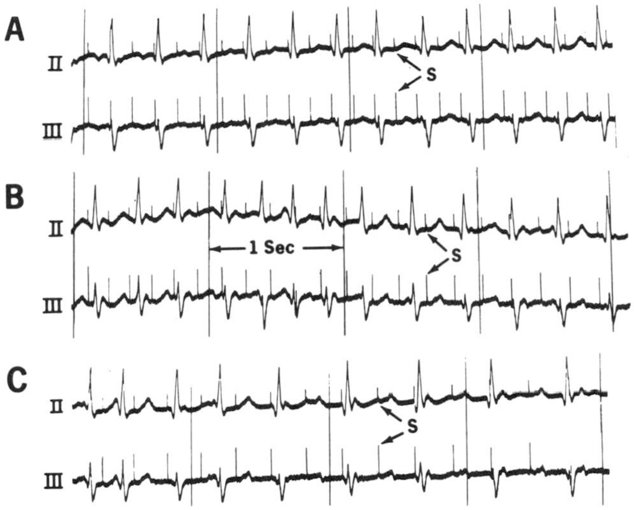

Figure 27-8. *Electrocardiographic leads II and III recorded from the same patient as in Figure 27-7. The rapid atrial pacing was repeated, but this time the atrial pacing rate was increased above that demonstrated in the previous figure. As the pacing rate was increased from 350 beats/min to a high of 382 beats/min, the atrial complexes became completely positive in leads II and III. In fact, close observation of the records in A reveals that this occurred at a pacing rate of about 370 beats/min. Now, when the pacing rate was slowed, atrial capture was maintained (B) and (C). Note at the end of B at a pacing rate of 270 beats/min (*i.e.*, a rate much slower than that of the previous spontaneous atrial flutter) the P waves remained positive, and as the pacing rate was decreased further, the atrial flutter did not recur (C). In fact, atrial capture was maintained as the pacing rate was decreased to 110 beats/min. Thus, in this patient, the atrial flutter finally was interrupted by the rapid atrial pacing when an appropriate pacing rate was achieved. The hallmark of the appropriate pacing rate was the appearance of positive atrial complexes in leads II and III. Time lines are at 1-second intervals. (S, stimulus artifact) (After Waldo, A. L., MacLean, W. A. H., Karp, et al.: Entrainment and interruption of atrial flutter with atrial pacing. Studies in man following open heart surgery. Circulation, 56:737–745, 1977)*

atrial pacing rate may be increased in increments of 5 to 10 beats/min until the atrial flutter has successfully interrupted. A representative example is illustrated in Figures 27-9 through 27-11.

With either of the above two pacing techniques, whenever the atria are paced at rates faster than the spontaneous rate, but when such pacing does not interrupt the atrial flutter despite the fact that the atrial rate increased to the pacing rate (see Figs. 27-7, 27-9, and 27-10),[14] this should not be considered evidence that rapid atrial pacing will be unsuccessful. Rather, it provides evidence that pacing at a more rapid rate is required to interrupt the atrial flutter.[14] Also, as illustrated in Figure 27-11, when using the constant-rate technique to interrupt the atrial flutter, a critical duration of pacing at the critical rate is required.[14]

Occasionally, pacing rates of over 400 beats/min may be required to interrupt type I atrial flutter when using either the ramp or constant-rate pacing technique.[14,17] In a small percentage of patients, rapid atrial pacing produces atrial fibrillation. This usually occurs when the atrial pacing rate required to interrupt the atrial flutter is greater than 135% of the spontaneous atrial flutter rate. Atrial fibrillation precipitated by rapid atrial pacing is almost always transient, lasting seconds to minutes before spontaneously converting to sinus rhythm. For those few patients in whom the atrial fibrillation persists, it is usually a more desirable rhythm than the continuation of type I atrial flutter because atrial fibrillation is almost always associated with a slower ventricular response rate than that during atrial flutter.[13,14,16,17] Also, in almost all instances the ventricular response rate to atrial fibrillation can be quite easily controlled with digitalis. For those patients in whom type I atrial flutter recurs despite its interruption by rapid atrial pacing, continuous rapid atrial pacing to precipitate and sustain atrial fibrillation may be indicated (see Pacing to Produce Desirable Supraventricular Tachyarrhythmias, below.)

Treatment of Type II Atrial Flutter. Because type II atrial flutter cannot be interrupted with rapid atrial pacing techniques, at least when pacing from high in the right atrium, this rhythm must be treated much as one would treat atrial fibrillation with a rapid ventricular

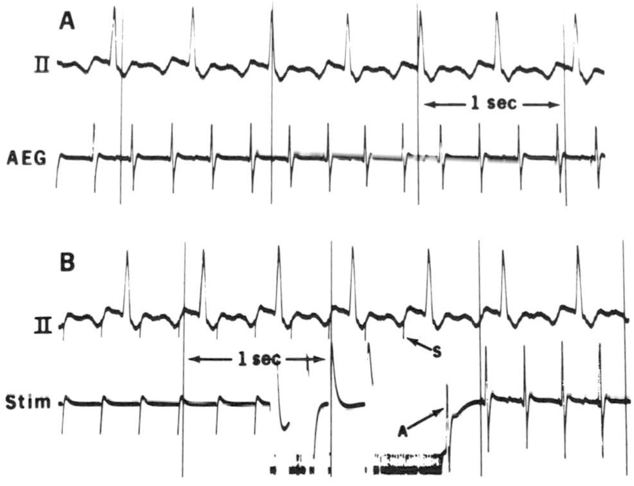

Figure 27-9. *(A) Electrocardiographic lead II recorded simultaneously with a bipolar atrial electrogram demonstrating type I (classic) atrial flutter at a cycle length of 264 msec. (B) Recordings from the same patient after 30 seconds of rapid atrial pacing at a cycle length of 254 msec. Note that despite the fact that the atrial rate increased to the pacing rate during the rapid atrial pacing, the morphology of the atrial complexes during the rapid pacing was essentially unchanged when compared to that during the spontaneous rhythm. Time lines are at 1-second intervals. (S, stimulus artifact; A, atrial electrograms) (After Waldo, A. L., MacLean, W. A. H., Karp, R. B., et al.: Entrainment and interruption of atrial flutter with atrial pacing. Studies in man following open heart surgery. Circulation, 56:737–745, 1977)*

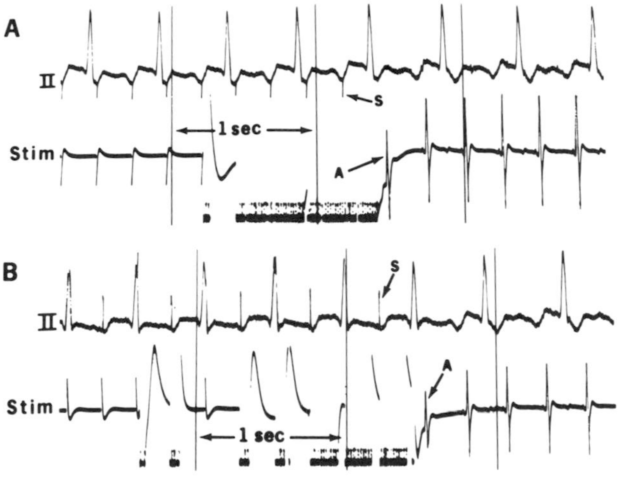

Figure 27-10. *A and B were recorded from the same patient as in Figure 27-9. A was recorded at the termination of 30 seconds of atrial pacing and at a cycle length of 242 msec; B, at the termination of 30 seconds of atrial pacing at a cycle length of 232 msec. Once again, note in each panel that the atrial rate increased to the atrial pacing rate during the rapid atrial pacing, yet following termination of the pacing the atrial flutter returned promptly. Furthermore, note that the morphology of the atrial complexes during the atrial pacing in A was virtually identical to that of the spontaneous atrial flutter, and in B it was only minimally changed from that of the spontaneous atrial flutter. Thus, during the rapid atrial pacing, the atrial rate increased to the pacing rate, but the atrial flutter was not interrupted. Time lines are at 1-second intervals. (S, stimulus artifact; A, atrial electrogram) (After Waldo, A. L., MacLean, W. A. H., Karp, R. B., et al.: Entrainment and interruption of atrial flutter with atrial pacing. Studies in man following open heart surgery. Circulation, 56:737–745, 1977)*

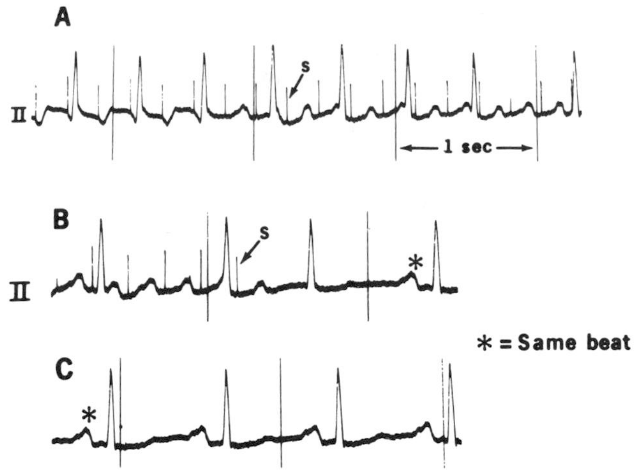

Figure 27-11. *Electrocardiographic lead II recorded from the same patient as in Figures 27-9 and 27-10 during atrial pacing at a cycle length of 224 msec. In A, note that with the seventh atrial beat, and 22 seconds after the onset of atrial pacing at this cycle length, the morphology of the atrial complexes in the electrocardiogram suddenly changed from the negative complex characteristic of the spontaneous atrial flutter to a positive complex characteristic of pacing from the high right atrium (the site that was the location of the temporarily fixed epicardial atrial wire electrodes). B was recorded several seconds after the tracing in A and demonstrates that now when atrial pacing was abruptly terminated, a spontaneous sinus rhythm developed. The first beat in C (*asterisk*) is identical to the last beat in panel B (*asterisk*). Thus, this figure illustrates both the critical pacing rate and critical duration of pacing to interrupt type I atrial flutter. Time lines are at 1-second intervals. (S, stimulus artifact) (After Waldo, A. L., MacLean, W. A. H., Karp, R. B., et al.: Entrainment and interruption of atrial flutter with atrial pacing. Studies in man following open heart surgery. Circulation, 56:737–745, 1977)*

response rate. Thus, aggressive use of digitalis to slow the ventricular rate is important. If the ventricular rate remains unacceptably rapid despite vigorous therapy with digitalis, either propranolol or verapamil therapy should be added. Rarely, direct current cardioversion will be required.

Paroxysmal Atrial Tachycardia

Diagnosis. The diagnosis of paroxysmal atrial tachycardia usually should be suspected from examination of the standard electrocardiogram particularly when a 1 : 1 AV relationship is established during a regular rhythm with a narrow QRS complex at rates between 180 to 200 beats/min. However, the range of rates of paroxysmal atrial tachycardia is quite broad (about 130 to 220 beats/min), and the differential diagnosis for regular rhythms with rates in this range includes several arrhythmias. To establish the diagnosis, the recording of a bipolar atrial electrogram is quite helpful because it clearly identifies atrial activation and its relationship to ventricular activation. For instance, during a tachycardia with a regular ventricular rate of 150 beats/min, a bipolar atrial electrogram recording demonstrating a rate of 150 beats/min would quickly eliminate atrial flutter as the underlying rhythm. However, the rhythm could still be a sinus tachycardia, an AV junctional tachycardia, paroxysmal atrial tachycardia, a sinus node reentrant tachycardia, and, in the presence of a wide QRS complex, a ventricular tachycardia. If the atrial electrogram were recorded simultaneously with or just after the QRS complex, it would make a sinus node reentrant rhythm most unlikely. The diagnosis is further assisted by the response of the arrhythmia to rapid atrial pacing. If the rhythm were successfully interrupted by rapid atrial pacing in the presence of a narrow QRS complex, the rhythm would almost certainly have to be paroxysmal atrial tachycardia. Thus, rapid atrial pacing would be both diagnostic and therapeutic, permitting the diagnosis to be established and also providing effective therapy.

Treatment. Paroxysmal atrial tachycardia probably is the simplest tachyarrhythmia to interrupt with atrial pacing, and in patients who have undergone open-heart surgery, atrial pacing is the treatment of choice. Several acceptable methods of cardiac pacing can interrupt this arrhythmia.[17,20,21] Paroxysmal atrial tachycardia can often be interrupted with an appropriately timed premature atrial beat. Therefore, one can initiate atrial pacing at a rate significantly slower than the paroxysmal tachycardia, for example, 100 beats/min, and interrupt the faster rhythm because the random occurrence of a premature atrial beat at an appropriate interval following a spontaneous atrial beat often will interrupt this reentrant rhythm. However, since paroxysmal atrial tachycardia can always be interrupted with atrial pacing at a rate faster than the spontaneous rate, this simple and more predictable method of pacing therapy is recommended. Using this latter technique, the atria are paced at a rate about 10 beats/min faster than the spontaneous rate of the tachycardia. After achieving atrial capture, atrial pacing may be abruptly terminated (Fig. 27-12), or the atrial pacing rate may be slowed rapidly to a predetermined pacing rate (*e.g.*, 100 to 110 beats/min). Occasionally, overdrive pacing to interrupt paroxysmal atrial tachycardia may require pacing at rates 20 to 50 beats/min faster than the spontaneous rate of the paroxysmal atrial tachycardia.[17] For those patients in whom paroxysmal atrial tachycardia recurs despite its successful interruption by rapid atrial pacing, continuous rapid atrial pacing techniques may be required to suppress the arrhythmia and to control ventricular rate (see Pacing to Produce Desirable Supraventricular Tachyarrhythmias, below).

Of course, standard antiarrhythmic drug therapy

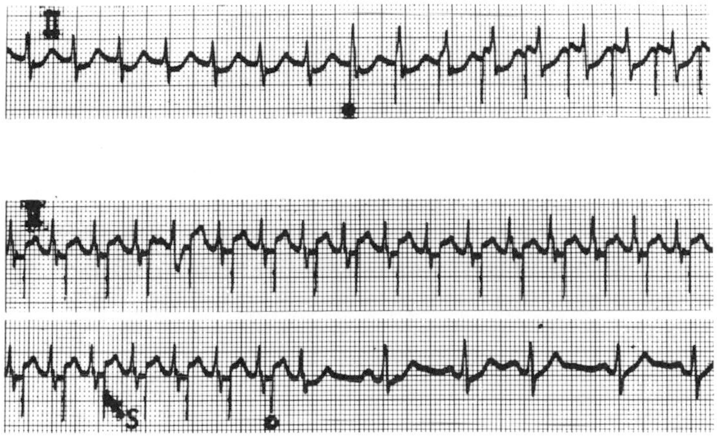

Figure 27-12. *The top tracing shows electrocardiographic lead II recorded during an episode of paroxysmal atrial tachycardia at a rate of 150 beats/min. Rapid atrial pacing at a rate of 165 beats/min was initiated at the eighth beat in this tracing (*solid circle*). In the middle tracing, which begins 12 seconds after the top tracing, atrial capture is clearly demonstrated. In the bottom tracing, which is continuous with the middle tracing, sinus rhythm appears when atrial pacing is terminated abruptly (*open circle*). (S, stimulus artifact) (Cooper, T. B., MacLean, W. A. H., and Waldo, A. L.: Overdrive pacing for supraventricular tachycardia. A review of theoretical implications and therapeutic techniques. Pace, 1:196–221, 1978)*

should be initiated to suppress recurrent paroxysmal atrial tachycardia. Effective medications include digitalis, quinidine, and procainamide. In patients whose arrhythmias are persistently resistant to effective suppression with standard drug therapy, electrophysiologic studies during cardiac catheterization should be performed, in particular to look for AV bypass pathways that only function in a retrograde direction.

Ectopic (Nonparoxysmal) Atrial Tachycardia

Diagnosis. Ectopic atrial tachycardia is a poorly understood rhythm that is generated in the atria and is characterized by an atrial rate ranging from about 130 to 240 beats/min. When the atrial rate is greater than 160 beats/min, it is usually characterized by second degree AV block (see Fig. 27-1). The latter is particularly helpful in differentiating this rhythm from paroxysmal atrial tachycardia. Another frequent, although not constant, characteristic of this rhythm that helps differentiate it from other supraventricular tachycardias with similar atrial rates is a remarkable beat-to-beat variability in atrial cycle length, easily discerned from the bipolar atrial electrogram (see Fig. 27-1). This arrhythmia occurs not uncommonly in adult patients immediately following open-heart surgery and in this circumstance is virtually never a consequence of digitalis toxicity. This latter point bears emphasis, because in other circumstances, this arrhythmia is a common manifestation of digitalis toxicity.

Treatment. When present, ectopic atrial tachycardia is commonly associated with 2 : 1 AV conduction such that, despite rapid atrial rates (*e.g.,* 200 beats/min), the ventricular rate of 100 beats/min is clinically quite acceptable. Thus, therapy to interrupt the arrhythmia may not be required. Usually, the rhythm will spontaneously revert to the preoperative rhythm (*e.g.,* sinus rhythm or atrial fibrillation) over 1 or 2 days. However, because the degree of AV conduction may be variable and therefore often rapid, atrial pacing may be used to interrupt the rhythm. The pacing technique is similar to the constant pacing rate technique described for type I atrial flutter. With the atrial wire electrodes, atrial pacing at a rate 10 beats/min faster than the intrinsic rate of the arrhythmia should be initiated. Pacing should be continued for at least 30 seconds and then should either be abruptly terminated or quickly slowed to a desirable atrial pacing rate (*e.g.,* 100 beats/min). Should the rapid atrial pacing fail to interrupt the arrhythmia, rapid atrial pacing should be reinitiated, increasing the pacing rate in five-to ten-beat increments, until the arrhythmia has been interrupted.

Overdrive rapid atrial pacing of this arrhythmia may have one of three outcomes: (1) the arrhythmia may be interrupted with return to sinus rhythm, (2) the arrhythmia may be converted to atrial fibrillation, or (3) the arrhythmia may be converted to atrial flutter, usually type I. Should the latter occur, this new rhythm should be treated as any type I atrial flutter. During rapid atrial pacing to interrupt ectopic atrial tachycardia, the arrhythmia commonly is transiently entrained to the pacing rate until a sufficiently rapid pacing rate is achieved to which the arrhythmia cannot be entrained. Therefore, failure to interrupt the arrhythmia with rapid pacing at rates faster than the pacing rate should not be interpreted as indicating that this rhythm is not interruptable by pacing.[21] Also, for some patients, continuous rapid atrial pacing to achieve and maintain 2 : 1 AV conduction may be required to control the ventricular rate (see Pacing to Produce Desirable Supraventricular Tachyarrhythmias, below).

Interruption of this arrhythmia with drug therapy usually is quite unsuccessful in the postoperative period. Rapid atrial pacing and time seem most effective. However, if the patient is receiving procainamide, it should be discontinued, because the drug seems to potentiate rather than alleviate ectopic atrial tachycardia. Of course, should digitalis toxicity be suspected, the drug should be discontinued and the diagnosis confirmed by obtaining a serum digoxin level.

Spontaneous Sinus and Atrioventricular Junctional Automatic Tachycardia

Diagnosis. Generally, sinus and AV junctional automatic tachycardias in the postoperative period are transient and benign and do not require special attention apart from seeking the etiology of the tachycardia (*e.g.,* fever, anemia, cardiac tamponade, or hypovolemia for sinus tachycardia) and initiating appropriate therapy. Sinus and AV junctional automatic tachycardias are not readily amenable to therapy with standard atrial pacing techniques. Although they can be overdriven, as soon as the external pacemaker is turned off or its rate is slowed to a rate less than that of the spontaneous rate, the spontaneous automatic tachycardia again becomes the rhythm of the heart. In fact, these latter characteristics are used to help establish the diagnosis of the tachycardia when it is uncertain. Both these rhythms demonstrate overdrive suppression during rapid pacing of the appropriate chamber (atrium for sinus tachycardia and either atrium or ventricle for AV junctional tachycardia).[22] With abrupt cessation of the overdrive pacing, both rhythms demonstrate a warm-up period.[22] When it is not clear whether a tachyarrhythmia is a sinus tachycardia with first degree AV block or an AV junctional tachycardia with 1 : 1 retrograde AV conduction, the relationship of atrial to ventricular activation following abrupt termination of pacing should differentiate between these two rhythms. The persistence of atrial activation preceding ventricular activation indicates a sinus mechanism, and the opposite indicates an AV junctional mechanism.

Treatment of Atrioventricular Junctional Tachycardia. Usually an AV junctional tachycardia occurring in the postoperative period is secondary to trauma in the AV junction associated with the surgical procedure. Thus, the arrhythmia usually will subside spontaneously over several days. It has not been established whether drug therapy speeds this process or helps in any way. However, a trial with virtually any of the standard antiarrhythmic drugs except propranolol (which may increase AV block and make atrial pacing ineffective) may be helpful because they all suppress ectopic automaticity.[12] Digitalis is probably contraindicated because it enhances automaticity of the AV junctional pacemaker.

On occasion, it may be desirable to overdrive an AV junctional tachycardia to provide an atrial contribution to cardiac output. This usually may be accomplished simply by pacing the atria at a rate just faster than the AV junctional rate (Fig. 27-13). On occasion, the enhanced AV junctional pacemaker responsible for the spontaneous tachycardia may be associated with a significant degree of anterograde AV block, such that an atrial impulse produced by pacing the atria at a rate faster than that of the AV junction will block proximal to the focus of the AV junctional pacemaker and thus will not overdrive the AV junctional rhythm. In such circumstances, it may be desirable to initiate AV sequential pacing. This is performed by pacing the atria at a rate appropriately faster than the AV junctional rate and then, utilizing the ventricular wire electrode, pacing the ventricles after an appropriate delay (*i.e.,* creating a PR interval).

Whenever an automatic AV junctional tachycardia becomes life threatening, generally because of marked hypotension and low cardiac output, ventricular paired pacing may be required and should be effective.[12,17,23–25] With this mode of therapy, the ventricles are paced rapidly but every other beat is deliberately premature. In effect, ventricular pacing with ventricular bigeminy is produced. However, each premature ventricular beat is introduced early enough so that although ventricular activation occurs, the ventricles do not eject blood because their contraction is ineffective. With this mode of therapy, although the heart rate will still be quite rapid, the effective heart rate will be halved because every other beat will be mechanically ineffective. For example, during ventricular paired pacing at a rate of 240 beats/min, while the electrical rate will be 240 beats/min the mechanical rate will be 120 beats/min, a rate that should be hemodynamically satisfactory. An example of the use of this technique is illustrated in Figure 27-14. This mode of therapy is potentially quite hazardous because, if inappropriately applied, it may not effectively halve the mechanical rate, thus resulting in a ventricular rate even faster than the spontaneous rate or in ventricular fibrillation. Also, primarily in adults, if applied for a prolonged period, it may be difficult to wean the patient from the ventricular paired pacing because cessation of the pacing may be associated with marked hypotension and impaired cardiac output.

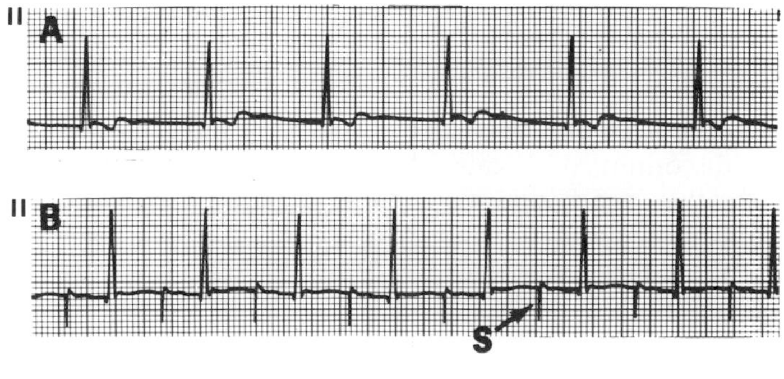

Figure 27-13. *Electrocardiographic lead II recorded from the same patient in both A and B. A demonstrates a spontaneous AV junctional rhythm with retrograde AV conduction at about 65 beats/min. B demonstrates that when atrial pacing at 90 beats/min was initiated, 1 : 1 anterograde AV conduction was obtained. (S, stimulus artifact(Waldo, A. L., and MacLean, W. A. H.: The Diagnosis and Treatment of Arrhythmias Following Open Heart Surgery—Emphasis on the Use of Epicardial Wire Electrodes. Mt. Kisco, N. Y., Futura, 1980)*

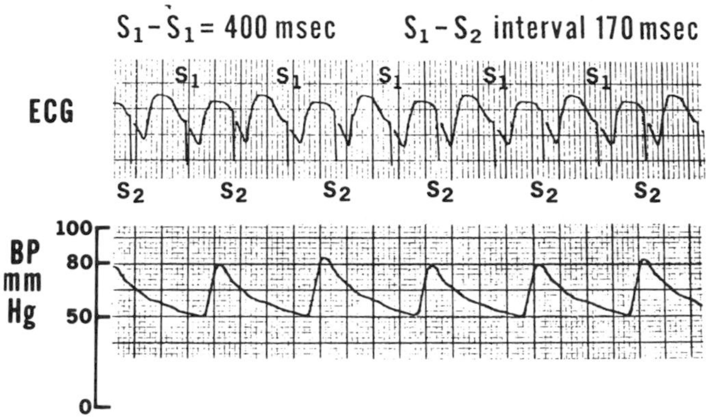

Figure 27-14. *These tracings were recorded from a patient aged 4 months in the immediate postoperative period following a Mustard procedure for the repair of transposition of the great vessels. The patient had developed a spontaneous AV junctional tachycardia at a rate of 285 beats/min with 2:1 retrograde conduction to the atria. This was associated with a mean aortic pressure of 40 mm Hg and anuria and was refractory to standard modes of therapy. Ventricular paired pacing was initiated to control the rapid ventricular heart rate in this patient. The top panel demonstrates the recorded electrocardiogram during ventricular paired pacing at an S_1-S_1 interval of 400 msec and an S_1-S_2 interval of 270 msec. The* bottom trace *records the blood pressure from a catheter in the femoral artery. These tracings were monitored simultaneously but were recorded sequentially. Note that in the* bottom tracing *there was only one pressure pulse for every two QRS complexes. Thus, despite the fact that the ventricles were being paced at a rate of 300 beats/min, the effective ventricular rate was 150 beats/min, considerably less than the spontaneous rate. With this pacing technique, the mean aortic pressure quickly rose to 60 to 65 mm Hg, and normal urine output resumed. The ventricular paired pacing provided a stable rhythm and stable hemodynamic state. Ventricular paired pacing was maintained for 14.5 hours, at which time it was stopped because the patient's spontaneous rhythm, which remained AV junctional, provided a hemodynamically stable state. The AV junctional rhythm resolved spontaneously, and the patient was discharged from the hospital with a normal sinus rhythm. (Waldo, A. L., Kron grad, E., Kupersmith, J., et al.: Ventricular paired pacing to control rapid ventricular heart rate following open heart surgery. Observations on ectopic automaticity. Report of a case in a four-month-old patient. Circulation, 53:176–181, 1976. By permission of the American Heart Association, Inc.)*

Treatment of Sinus Tachycardia. Atrial paired pacing may be used to slow the effective ventricular rate during sinus tachycardia.[21,26,27] The technique relies on block in the AV node to slow the ventricular rate. However, clinical experience with this atrial pacing technique is lacking during sinus tachycardias at rates above 130 beats/min. For instance, it is possible that at the more rapid sinus rates, the factors that have generated an increase in the sinus rate may also affect the refractory period of the AV node such that its effective refractory period will be too short to permit effective use of this technique. Therefore, this technique cannot be recommended until more data become available regarding its therapeutic efficacy.

Pacing to Produce Desirable Supraventricular Tachyarrhythmias

Continuous Rapid Atrial Pacing to Precipitate and Sustain Atrial Fibrillation. On occasion, some arrhythmias that have been successfully interrupted with rapid atrial pacing techniques may recur despite their successful interruption. In these instances, particularly when these arrhythmias are associated with rapid ventricular rates, it may be desirable to precipitate and sustain atrial fibrillation by pacing the atria continuously at 450 beats/min.[13,17] The ventricular response rate may be

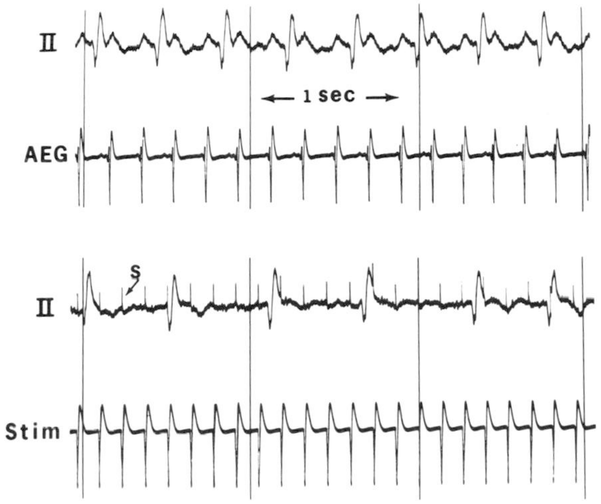

Figure 27-15. *The* top panel *shows electrocardiographic lead II recorded simultaneously with a bipolar atrial electrogram (A_{EG}) during atrial flutter at a rate of 320 beats/min with 2:1 AV conduction, producing a ventricular rate of 160 beats/min. The atrial flutter had been interrupted successfully on several occasions with rapid atrial pacing, but it recurred each time. Therefore, as shown in the* bottom panel, *continuous rapid atrial pacing at 450 beats/min was initiated. Pacing at this rate precipitated and sustained atrial fibrillation and was associated with a slowing of the ventricular response rate to about 120 beats/min. Digoxin was administered to slow the ventricular response rate further. Quinidine was also administered. Continuous rapid atrial pacing to sustain atrial fibrillation for control of the ventricular rate was required for 26 hours in this patient. Earlier termination of rapid pacing resulted in recurrence of the atrial flutter. When the rapid atrial pacing was finally terminated, atrial fibrillation was transiently present, converting spontaneously to sinus rhythm within several minutes. Time lines are at 1-second intervals. (S, stimulus artifact) (Waldo, A. L., MacLean, W. A. H., Karp, R. B., et al.: Continuous rapid atrial pacing to control recurrent or sustained supraventricular tachycardias following open heart surgery. Circulation, 54:245–250, 1976. By permission of the American Heart Association, Inc.)*

clinically acceptable without need for additional drug therapy, but if it is too rapid, it can virtually always be easily controlled with drug therapy.

One indication for the use of this technique is recurrent type I atrial flutter. If type I atrial flutter recurs twice following its successful interruption with rapid atrial pacing, and if the arrhythmia is associated with a rapid ventricular response rate, rapid atrial pacing at a rate of 450 beats/min should be initiated and maintained so that atrial fibrillation will be precipitated and sustained.[13,17] In almost all instances, this will permit effective control of the ventricular response rate (Fig. 27-15). Should additional slowing of the ventricular rate be desirable, digitalis or, in rare instances, digitalis plus propranolol should be administered. Either quinidine or procainamide usually should be administered, because they are the most effective drugs available for suppression of atrial flutter. After an appropriate period, the rapid atrial pacing should be terminated on a trial basis. If the atrial flutter recurs, continuous rapid atrial pacing should be resumed. If the atrial flutter does not recur, usually the atrial fibrillation will convert spontaneously to sinus rhythm within a short period. Occasionally, atrial fibrillation may persist in a patient, and direct current cardioversion may be required to obtain sinus rhythm. We have never had to perform continuous rapid atrial pacing to sustain atrial fibrillation for more than 72 hours, the average period of pacing being about 24 hours.

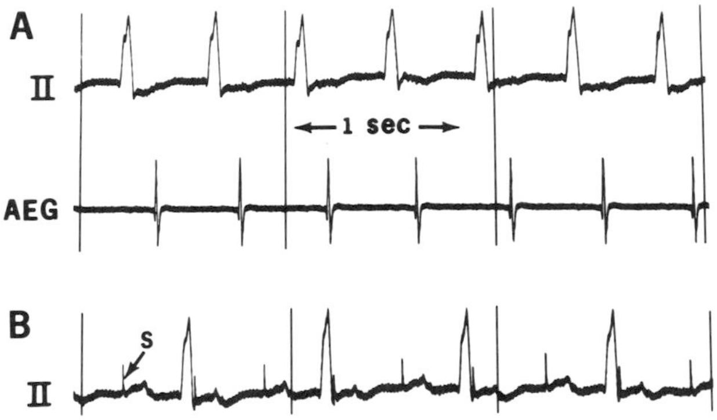

Figure 27-16. *(A) Electrocardiographic lead II recorded simultaneously with a bipolar atrial electrogram (A_{EG}) demonstrating an ectopic atrial tachycardia at a rate of 140 beats/min with 1:1 conduction. Overdrive atrial pacing suppressed the arrhythmia, but rapid atrial pacing at rates just short of precipitating atrial fibrillation failed to interrupt it. Therefore, as shown in B, continuous rapid atrial pacing at 180 beats/min was initiated. This produced 2:1 AV conduction with a clinically satisfactory rate of 90 beats/min. The arrhythmia resolved spontaneously in 24 hours. Time lines are at 1-second intervals. (S, stimulus artifact) (Cooper, T. B., MacLean, W. A. H., and Waldo, A. L.: Overdrive pacing for supraventricular tachycardia. A review of theoretical implications and therapeutic techniques. Pace, 1:196–221, 1978)*

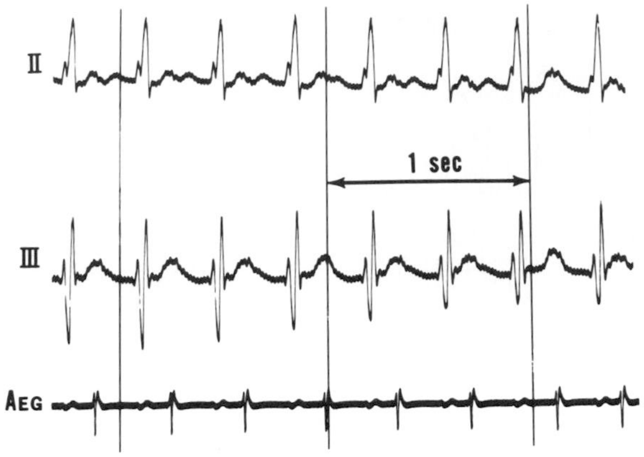

Figure 27-17. *Electrocardiographic leads II and III recorded simultaneously with a bipolar atrial electrogram (A_{EG}) during an episode of paroxysmal atrial tachycardia. The atrial and ventricular rates are 175 beats/min. Time lines are at 1-second intervals. (Waldo, A. L., MacLean, W. A. H., Karp, R. B., et al.: Continuous rapid atrial pacing to control recurrent or sustained supraventricular tachycardias following open heart surgery. Circulation, 54:245–250, 1976. By permission of the American Heart Association, Inc.)*

Rapid Atrial Pacing to Produce 2:1 Atrioventricular Conduction. In the event of recurrent paroxysmal atrial tachycardia following its interruption with rapid atrial pacing or any other technique, or in the event of ectopic (nonparoxysmal) atrial tachycardia with 1:1 AV conduction in which rapid atrial pacing short of producing atrial fibrillation has not interrupted the rhythm, rapid atrial pacing in the range of 180 to 230 beats/min can be initiated to slow the ventricular rate by producing a paced atrial tachycardia with a 2:1 AV response.[13] Thus, as illustrated in Figure 27-16, for an ectopic (nonparoxysmal) atrial tachycardia at a rate of 140 beats/min with 1:1 AV conduction, continuous rapid atrial pacing at a rate of 180 beats/min produced 2:1 AV conduction with a ventricular rate of 90 beats/min. Figures 27-17 to 27-19 illustrate a similar example for a patient with recurrent paroxysmal atrial tachycardia. In each of these examples, the ventricular rate was decreased very significantly simply by pacing the atria rapidly and taking advantage of functional AV block. We have never had to perform continuous rapid atrial pacing to sustain 2:1 AV conduction for more than 72 hours, the average period of pacing being about 21 hours.

Ventricular Tachyarrhythmias

Ventricular Tachycardias

Diagnosis. Ventricular tachycardia must always be suspected in the presence of a wide QRS complex tachycardia. The differential diagnosis, of course, includes a supraventricular tachycardia with aberrant ventricular conduction. When the diagnosis is unclear, and if the

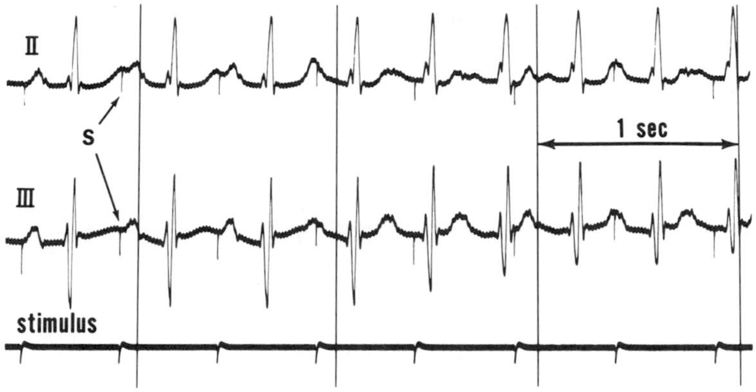

Figure 27-18. *Electrocardiographic leads II and III recorded simultaneously with the stimulus artifact during atrial pacing at a rate of 120 beats/min in the same patient as Figure 27-17. In the time interval between the records in Figures 27-17 and 27-18, atrial pacing at a rate of 180 beats/min had successfully interrupted the paroxysmal atrial tachycardia. With cessation of the rapid pacing, the rhythm returned to a sinus rhythm with frequent premature atrial beats. Atrial pacing at rates of 100, 110, and 120 beats/min failed to suppress the premature atrial beats. As illustrated in this figure, a premature atrial beat (fourth beat) precipitated another episode of paroxysmal atrial tachycardia that was not interrupted by continued atrial pacing at 120 beats/min. Time lines are at 1-second intervals. (S, stimulus artifact) (Waldo, A. L., MacLean, W. A. H., Karp, R. B., et al.: Continuous rapid atrial pacing to control recurrent or sustained supraventricular tachycardias following open heart surgery. Circulation, 54:245–250, 1976. By permission of the American Heart Association, Inc.)*

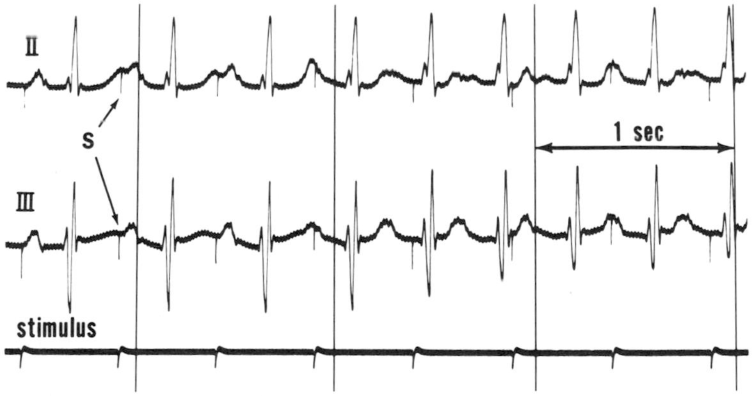

Figure 27-19. *Electrocardiographic leads II and III recorded simultaneously with the stimulus artifact from the same patient as in Figures 27-17 and 27-18 during atrial pacing at a rate of 220 beats/min. Pacing at this rate produced 2 : 1 AV conduction and a clinically acceptable ventricular rate, with complete suppression of the premature atrial beats and therefore suppression of the paroxysmal atrial tachycardia. During the rapid atrial pacing, digitalis and procainamide were administered. After about 20 hours of continuous rapid atrial pacing, cessation of the pacing resulted in sustained normal sinus rhythm. Earlier termination of the rapid atrial pacing was associated with reprecipitations of the paroxysmal atrial tachycardia. Time lines are at 1-second intervals. (S, stimulus artifact) (Waldo, A. L., MacLean, W. A. H., Karp, R. B., et al.: Continuous rapid atrial pacing to control recurrent or sustained supraventricular tachycardias following open heart surgery. Circulation, 54:245–250, 1976. By permission of the American Heart Association, Inc.)*

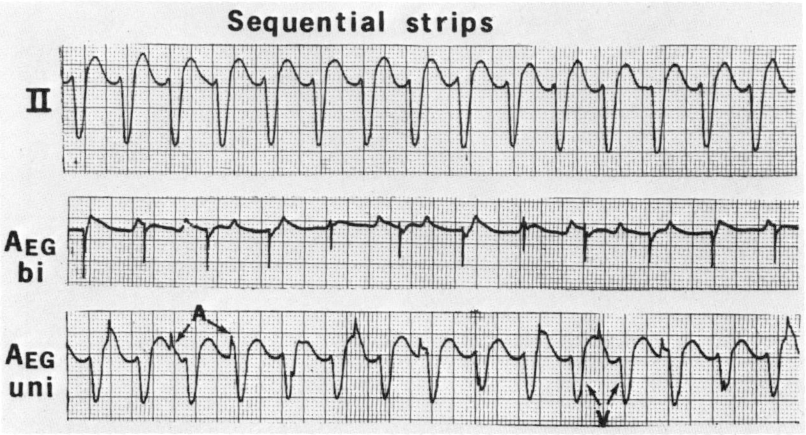

Figure 27-20. *The* top tracing *demonstrates a regular, wide QRS complex tachycardia at 130 beats/min and presents the classic problem of the differential diagnosis of such a tachycardia. A bipolar atrial electrogram (*middle tracing*) was then recorded and demonstrated a regular rate of 100 beats/min, clearly establishing the presence of AV dissociation and making the diagnosis of ventricular tachycardia virtually certain. However, the diagnosis of an AV junctional tachycardia with aberrant conduction was still possible, although unlikely. The* bottom tracing *demonstrates a unipolar atrial electrogram and is presented to illustrate that although the diagnosis of AV dissociation could be made from the unipolar atrial electrogram, the diagnosis is infinitely easier and more certain from the recording of the bipolar atrial electrogram. (A, atrial complex; V, ventricular complex) (Waldo, A. L., MacLean, W. A. H., Cooper, T. B., et al.: Use of temporarily placed epicardial atrial wire electrodes for the diagnosis and treatment of cardiac arrhythmias following open heart surgery. J. Thorac. Cardiovasc. Surg., 76:500–505, 1978)*

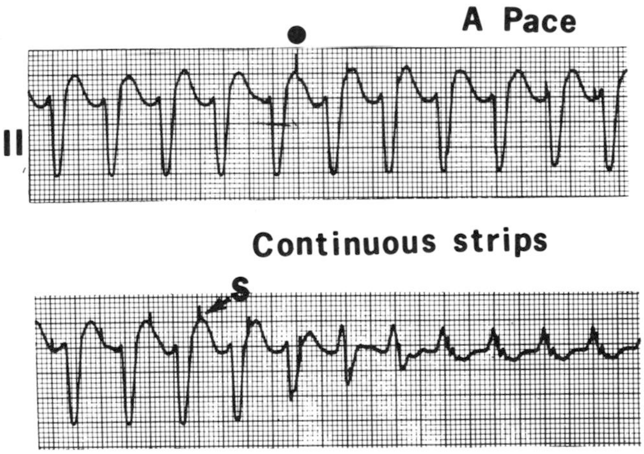

Figure 27-21. *Electrocardiographic lead II recorded from the same patient whose electrocardiographic tracings are illustrated in Figure 27-20. The* solid circle *in the* top strip *marks the onset of atrial pacing at a rate just faster than that of the spontaneous tachycardia. The* bottom strip, *which is continuous with the* top strip, *illustrates that the ventricular rate increases to the atrial pacing rate. More important, the appearance of fusion beats (fifth through seventh beats) permits the diagnosis of ventricular tachycardia to be established with certainty. (S, stimulus artifact) (Waldo, A. L., MacLean, W. A. H., Cooper, T. B., et al.: Use of temporarily placed epicardial atrial wire electrodes for the diagnosis and treatment of cardiac arrhythmias following open heart surgery. J. Thorac. Cardiovasc. Surg., 76:500–505, 1978)*

patient's clinical status permits it, either recording or pacing through the bipolar atrial wire electrodes usually will enable the diagnosis to be established. Recording of a bipolar electrogram may document AV dissociation (see Fig. 27-20). In the presence of a wide QRS complex tachycardia with a 1 : 1 AV relationship, if atrial pacing at a rate just faster than that of the tachycardia results in production of a fusion beat or a narrow QRS complex, the diagnosis is established (Figs. 27-21 and 27-22).

Treatment. Either intravenous lidocaine therapy or direct current cardioversion is generally the treatment of choice for ventricular tachycardia. However, this arrhythmia, when not induced by a spontaneous automatic pacemaker, may be effectively treated by rapid ventricular or even rapid atrial pacing.[17,18,28] Atrial pacing will only be successful if 1 : 1 AV conduction of each atrially paced beat occurs. The method of pacing is similar to the pacing technique described for type I atrial flutter. When the situation permits it, pacing at a rate at least ten beats faster than the spontaneous ventricular rate should be initiated, and after 15 to 30 seconds, pacing should be abruptly terminated. If the ventricular tachycardia has not been interrupted, the pacing should be repeated, increasing the pacing rate by increments of 5 to 10 beats/min. Generally, pacing at rates between 115% to 125% of the intrinsic rate are required to interrupt the tachycardia, although rates as high as or higher

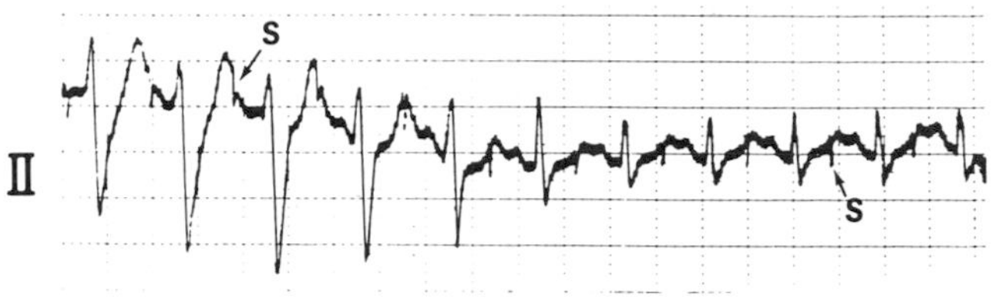

Figure 27-22. *Electrocardiographic lead II recorded from a patient who developed a wide QRS complex tachycardia at a rate of 150 beats/min with a 1:1 AV relationship. It was uncertain whether this was in a supraventricular rhythm with aberrant conduction or a ventricular tachycardia with retrograde conduction to the atria. Atrial pacing at a rate of 160 beats/min was initiated. As illustrated in this figure, the ventricular rate increased to the atrial pacing rate with the demonstration of fusion beats (third through seventh beats). The latter established the rhythm as ventricular tachycardia. (Waldo, A. L., MacLean, W. A. H., and James, T. N.: Utilization of the cardiac catheterization laboratory for the diagnosis and treatment of cardiac arrhythmias and conduction disturbances. Ala. J. Med. Sci., 11:120–128, 1974)*

than 140% of the intrinsic rate have been reported.[18,28] Rapid pacing at rates faster than the intrinsic rate of the tachycardia that fail to interrupt the tachycardia have merely transiently entrained it (Fig. 27-23).[18] Despite the fact that the ventricular rate increased to the pacing rate, this should not be considered evidence that the rapid pacing will be unsuccessful. Rather, as with rapid atrial pacing to interrupt type I atrial flutter, ventricular pacing to interrupt ventricular tachycardia must achieve a critical rate to interrupt the ventricular tachycardia that cannot be entrained (see Fig. 27-23).[17,18,28] On occasion, ventricular paired pacing may be required to interrupt or control this arrhythmia.[17,18] It must be emphasized that whenever rapid ventricular pacing techniques are being used to treat ventricular tachycardia, one must be prepared to initiate prompt direct current cardioversion should ventricular fibrillation be precipitated.

Ventricular Fibrillation

Ventricular fibrillation is incompatible with life and cannot be treated with ventricular pacing. Rapid treatment with direct current cardioversion is mandatory and should be performed as quickly as possible.

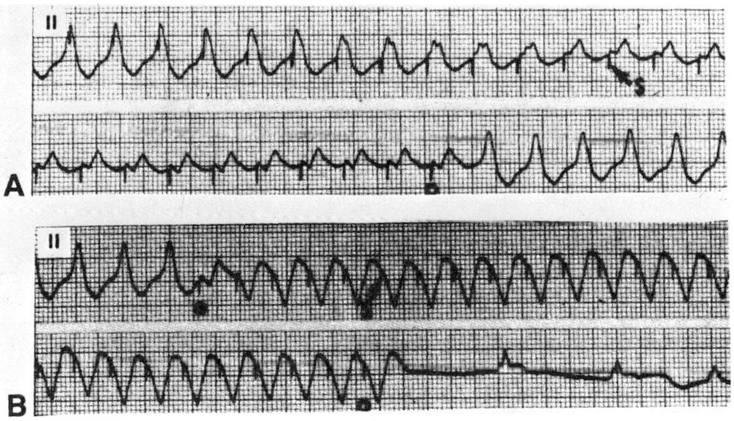

Figure 27-23. *A and B were recorded from a patient who had developed ventricular tachycardia at a rate of 150 beats/min. A demonstrates ventricular pacing at 160 beats/min. On cessation of pacing (*open circle*), the ventricular tachycardia resumed at its previous rate. Note that during the pacing, the ventricular rate was entrained to the pacing rate. Also, note the change in QRS morphology associated with entrainment. This change in morphology represents a fusion between the morphology of the QRS complex of the ventricular tachycardia and the morphology of the QRS compiex associated with ventricular pacing from that site. In B, the pacing rate has been increased to 195 beats/min. The* solid circle *marks the onset of pacing at this rate. With cessation of pacing (denoted by the* open circle*), the ventricular tachycardia has been interrupted. Note that the QRS morphology during the ventricular pacing at the rate that successfully interrupted the ventricular tachycardia differs considerably from the fusion morphology demonstrated in A during entrainment of the ventricular tachycardia with ventricular pacing at a slower rate. (S, stimulus artifact) (MacLean, W. A. H., Cooper, T. B., and Waldo, A. L.: Use of cardiac electrodes in the diagnosis and treatment of tachyarrhythmias. Cardiovasc. Med., 3:965–980, 1978)*

Extrasystoles

Diagnosis. The ability to record a bipolar atrial electrogram is especially helpful in establishing the chamber of origin of a premature beat, particularly when the premature beat is associated with a wide QRS complex and identification of atrial activation in the electrocardiogram is uncertain. Also, on occasion, it may be desirable to introduce premature atrial beats by the atrial electrodes to establish whether they are associated with aberrant ventricular conduction manifesting a QRS morphology that was previously recorded but that could not be diagnosed as ventricular or supraventricular.

Treatment. Ventricular extrasystoles are often easily suppressed simply by increasing the heart rate with atrial or ventricular pacing.[16,17] When rate augmentation alone is ineffective in suppressing the ventricular extrasystoles, the addition or substitution of either lidocaine, procainamide, quinidine, disopyramide, or diphenylhydantoin is necessary. Also, one of the latter four drugs may be required for chronic suppression of the arrhythmia.

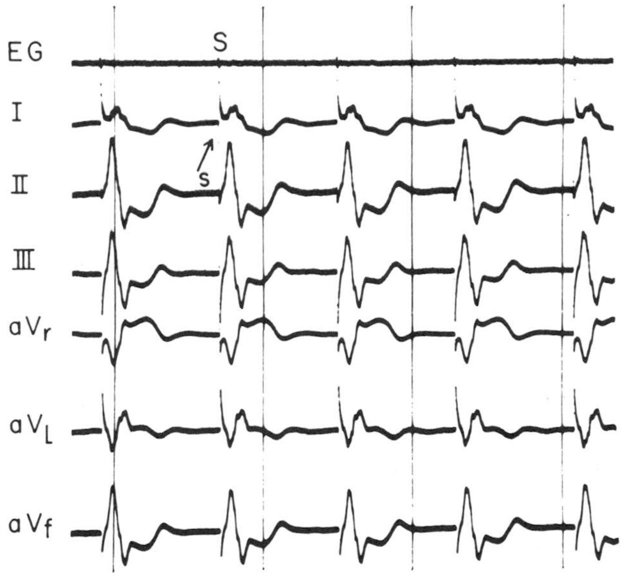

Figure 27-24. *Bipolar atrial electrogram (EG) recorded simultaneously with the standard and augmented electrocardiographic leads from a patient following open-heart surgery. The ventricles were being paced through a ventricular electrode placed during surgery because the spontaneous AV junctional rhythm was too slow. The absence of P waves in the electrocardiogram and the absence of any atrial activity in the atrial electrogram demonstrate atrial standstill and suggest atrial quiescence. The diagnosis of atrial quiescence was established when stimuli delivered through the atrial wire electrodes failed to capture the atria. Time lines are at 1-second intervals. (S, stimulus artifact) (Waldo, A. L., Vitikainen, K. J., Kaiser, G. A., et al.: Atrial standstill secondary to atrial inexcitability (atrial quiescence). Circulation, 46:690–697, 1972. By permission of the American Heart Association, Inc.)*

Atrial extrasystoles also may be suppressed simply by increasing the atrial rate with atrial pacing.[17] It is often desirable to suppress atrial extrasystoles if they are frequent, since they are the harbingers of atrial fibrillation, paroxysmal atrial tachycardia, ectopic atrial tachycardia, and atrial flutter. Usually the combination of atrial pacing and either procainamide or quinidine administration is required for satisfactory suppression of the atrial extrasystoles. For some patients in whom it is judged important to suppress the premature atrial beats, it may be necessary to pace the atria at very rapid rates. This usually requires atrial pacing at rates between 180 and 230 beats/min because these rates are most effective in suppressing the premature atrial beats and also will produce 2 : 1 AV conduction with a clinically acceptable ventricular rate.[13,16,17]

Atrial Quiescence

Diagnosis. Atrial quiescence is a form of atrial standstill in which there is no spontaneous activity and in which the atria cannot be paced (*i.e.*, the atria are inexcitable).[9] During this rhythm, the ventricles are usually depolarized from an AV junctional pacemaker. Because the ensuing ventricular rate is usually less than 60 beats/min, ventricular pacing is required. The incidence of this arrhythmia following open-heart surgery is not known, largely because it usually goes unrecognized and because it is usually transient, most often lasting not more than 24 hours. However, it is easily diagnosed when there are no P waves in the electrocardiogram, an atrial electrogram cannot be recorded, and the atria cannot be paced (Fig. 27-24).[9,17]

Treatment. Administration of intravenous isoproterenol at a rate of about 1 μg/min has been shown to restore atrial excitability with return of spontaneous atrial activity (Fig. 27-25).[9] The atria may then be paced to increase cardiac output, treat bradyarrhythmias, and suppress extrasystoles or tachyarrhythmias, thereby improving cardiac performance.

Drug Therapy for Supraventricular Tachycardias

Prophylaxis. Soon after the advent of cardiac surgery, observations from multiple centers documented a significant incidence of supraventricular arrhythmias in the early postoperative period.[29–31] Subsequent studies have identified that from 15% to 100% of patients undergoing a variety of cardiac procedures have supraventricular arrhythmias.[32–34] This variability in large part relates to the method of arrhythmia detection. In one study, with 100% of patients having supraventricular arrhythmias,

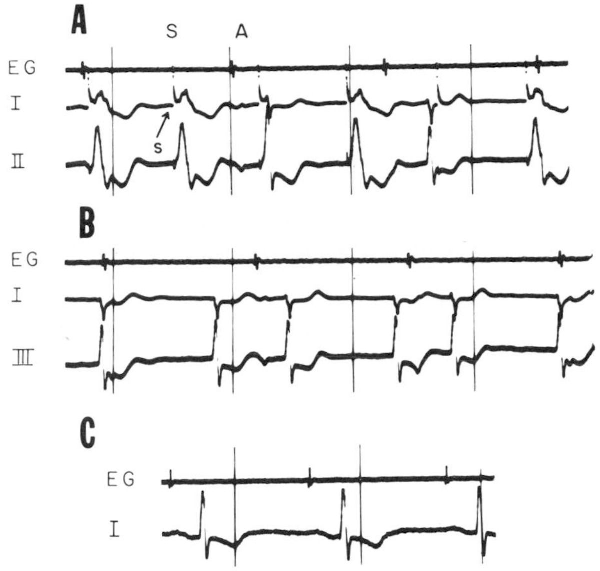

Figure 27-25. *Tracings from the same patient as in Figure 27-24. An infusion of isoproterenol, 1 μg/min, was initiated after the demonstration of atrial quiescence. In about 10 minutes, evidence of spontaneous atrial activity appeared. A shows the rhythm about 15 minutes after the initiation of isoproterenol therapy. A spontaneous atrial rate of about 30 beats/min is present, and anterograde AV conduction, as evidenced by the fusion beat (third QRS complex), has returned. The external ventricular pacemaker was then turned off, and a spontaneous AV junctional rhythm with atrial capture beats appeared (B). Atrial pacing was then initiated with successful atrial capture with 1:1 AV conduction. Atrial pacing was maintained for several hours until no longer required. C shows the patient's spontaneous rhythm several hours after the recording in B, documenting the pressence of sinus rhythm. Time lines are at 1-second intervals. (S, stimulus artifact; A, atrial electrogram) (Waldo, A. L., Vitikainen, K. J., Kaiser, G. A., et al.: Atrial standstill secondary to atrial inexcitability (atrial quiescence). Circulation, 46:690–697, 1972. By permission of the American Heart Association, Inc.)*

24-hour Holter monitoring was performed for 1 day before and for 7 days after surgery.[34]

This high incidence of symptomatic arrhythmias prompted a variety of studies designed to see if any prophylactic drug regimen could significantly reduce the incidence of these arrhythmic events. One major group of studies relates to the prophylactic effect of beta-blockade drugs. Most studies identified a significant reduction in supraventricular arrhythmias with propranolol administration,[35–37] but some centers did not observe any significant change.[38] The most comprehensive study involved protracted periods of continuous electrocardiographic monitoring with the beta-blocker timolol being given intravenously and then orally. Although only involving 41 patients, this study showed beta-blocker therapy to be of significant benefit.[34]

Another series of studies was directed toward the effect of prophylaxis achieved with digitalis therapy. Selzer and colleagues cautioned against the prophylactic use of digitalis in patients undergoing cardiac surgery.[39] However, a decade later, Johnson and co-workers found that prophylactic use of digitalis was beneficial in a group of coronary revascularization patients.[40] However, in 1977, Tyras and colleagues found that prophylactic use of digitalis did not prevent supraventricular tachycardia in such patients.[41] A more recent study by Csiscko and colleagues in 1981 evaluated 407 patients undergoing coronary revascularization.[33] These authors identified a supraventricular arrhythmic incidence of 2% in the 137 patients who received digitalis and a 15% incidence in the 270 control patients.[33] Whether digitalis is useful in the postoperative cardiac surgical patient remains unclear.

In light of the above findings, another tack was taken by Roffman and Fieldman,[42] who compared three groups of patients undergoing coronary revascularization:

1. A control group (63 patients)
2. A group given prophylactic digitalis (59 patients)
3. A group given prophylactic digitalis and propranolol (50 patients)

There was a significant difference between groups 1 and 3 but no significant difference between groups 1 and 2. Mills and co-workers, in a subsequent paper, confirmed the benefit of a combination of digitalis and a beta-blockade agent in preventing supraventricular arrhythmias in 179 patients undergoing coronary artery revascularization surgery.[43] However, neither group clarified whether digitalis alone was effective.

Treatment. Newer therapies have become available for the rapid pharmacologic treatment of supraventricular arrhythmias associated with cardiac surgery. The slow channel blocking group of drugs has gained widespread acceptance. Although this class of drugs has been widely used for urgent treatment of a variety of supraventricular arrhythmias, it was not systematically studied in the postoperative cardiac surgical patient until 1982, when Gray and colleagues reported on their experience with 22 postoperative open-heart surgical patients.[44] These authors found that intravenous verapamil rapidly and safely controlled the ventricular rate but only infrequently restored sinus rhythm. Another agent of the same class, diltiazem, has also been found effective when given intravenously.[45]

Beta-blocking agents have been demonstrated to be effective in reducing the incidence of supraventricular arrhythmias following open-heart surgery (see above). Recently an ultra-short-acting ($t\frac{1}{2} = 9$ minute) beta blocker (esmolol) has become available. This agent has been studied in the postoperative open-heart surgical patient with supraventricular arrhythmias. Esmolol proved effective for rapid rate control and caused a higher rate of conversion to sinus rhythm than that observed with verapamil.[46]

Preliminary data have been presented identifying the use of intravenous adenosine and adenosine triphosphate as agents for rapid conversion or rate control of supraventricular tachycardia.[47,48] Adenosine produced a very rapid effect (*i.e.,* less than 30 seconds). However, the systemic side-effects included sinus arrest, AV block, flushing, and malaise. Intravenous amiodarone has also proved effective in more resistant supraventricular tachycardias, especially in patients with bypass tracts.[49] It not only treats the existing arrhythmia, but acts to prevent future arrhythmias as well.

References

1. Harris, P. D., Singer, D. H., Malm, J. R., and Hoffman, B. F.: Chronically implanted cardiac electrodes for diagnostic, therapeutic, and investigational use in man. J. Thorac. Cardiovasc. Surg., 54:190–198, 1967.
2. Harris, P. D., Malm, J. R., Bowman, F. O., Jr., et al.: Epicardial pacing to control arrhythmias following cardiac surgery. Circulation, 37(Suppl. 2):178–183, 1968.
3. Litwak, R. S., Kuhn, L. A., Gadboys, H. L., et al.: Support of myocardial performance after open cardiac operations by rate augmentation. J. Thorac. Cardiovasc. Surg., 56:484–496, 1968.
4. Woodson, R. D., and Starr, A.: Atrial pacing after mitral valve surgery. Arch. Surg., 97:894–990, 1968.
5. Beller, B. M., Frater, R. W. M., and Wulfsohn, N.: Cardiac pacemaking in the management of postoperative arrhythmias. Ann. Thorac. Surg., 6:68–78, 1968.
6. Hodam, R. P., and Starr, A.: Temporary postoperative epicardial pacing electrodes. Their value and management after open heart surgery. Ann. Thorac. Surg., 8:506–510, 1969.
7. Iwa, T., Sugiki, K., Todo, K., et al.: Atrial pacemaker III. Jpn. J. Thorac. Surg., 24:796–802, 1971.
8. Waldo, A. L., Ross, S. M., and Kaiser, G. A.: The epicardial electrogram in the diagnosis of cardiac arrhythmias in the postoperative patient. Geriatrics, 26:108–112, 1971.
9. Waldo, A. L., Vitikainen, K. J., Kaiser, G. A., et al.: Atrial standstill secondary to atrial inexcitability (atrial quiescence). Circulation, 46:690–697, 1972.
10. Mills, N. L., and Ochsner, J. L.: Experience with atrial pacemaker wires implanted during cardiac operations. J. Thorac. Cardiovasc. Surg., 66:878–886, 1973.
11. Pittman, D. E., Gay, T. C., Patel, I. I., and Joyner, C. R.: Termination of atrial flutter and atrial tachycardia with rapid atrial stimulation. Angiology, 36:784–802, 1975.
12. Waldo, A. L., Krongrad, E., Kupersmith, J., et al.: Ventricular paired pacing to control rapid ventricular heart rate following open heart surgery. Observations on ectopic automaticity. Report of a case in a four-month-old patient. Circulation, 53:176–181, 1976.
13. Waldo, A. L., MacLean, W. A. H., Karp, R. B., et al.: Continuous rapid atrial pacing to control recurrent or sustained supraventricular tachycardias following open heart surgery. Circulation, 54:245–250, 1976.
14. Waldo, A. L., MacLean, W. A. H., Karp, R. B., et al.: Entrainment and interruption of atrial flutter with atrial pacing. Studies in man following open heart surgery. Circulation, 56:737–745, 1977.
15. Wells, J. L., Jr., Karp, R. B., Kouchoukos, N. T., et al.: Characterization of atrial fibrillation in man. Studies following open heart surgery. Pace, 3:965–980, 1978.
16. Waldo, A. L., MacLean, W. A. H., Cooper, T. B., et al.: Use of temporarily placed epicardial atrial wire electrodes for the diagnosis and treatment of cardiac arrhythmias following open heart surgery. J. Thorac. Surg., 76:500–505, 1978.
17. Waldo, A. L., and MacLean, W. A. H.: The Diagnosis and Treatment of Arrhythmias Following Open Heart Surgery—Emphasis on the Use of Epicardial Wire Electrodes. Mt. Kisco, N.Y., Futura, 1980.
18. MacLean, W. A. H., James, T. N., and Waldo, A. L.: Entrainment and interruption of ventricular tachycardia in man with rapid pacing. Pace, *in press.*
19. Wells, J. L., Jr., MacLean, W. A. H., James, T. N., and Waldo, A. L.: Characterization of atrial flutter. Studies in man after open heart surgery using fixed atrial electrodes. Circulation, 60:665–673, 1979.
20. MacLean, W. A. H., Cooper, T. B., and Waldo, A. L.: Use of cardiac electrodes in the diagnosis and treatment of tachyarrhythmias. Cardiovasc. Med., 3:965–980, 1978.
21. Cooper, T. B., MacLean, W. A. H., and Waldo, A. L.: Overdrive pacing for supraventricular tachycardia. A review of theoretical implications and therapeutic techniques. Pace, 1:196–221, 1978.
22. Vassalle, M.: The relationship among cardiac pacemakers. Overdrive suppression. Circ. Res., 41:269–277, 1977.
23. Cranefield, P. F.: Paired pulse stimulation and postextrasystolic potentiation of the heart. Prog. Cardiovasc. Dis., 8:446–460, 1966.
24. Cranefield, P. F., and Hoffman, B. F.: The physiologic basis and clinical implications of paired pulse stimulation of the heart. Dis. Chest, 49:561–567, 1966.
25. Resnikov, L.: Electrical slowing of the heart and postextrasystolic potentiation. Med. Clin. North Am., 54:247–259, 1970.
26. Langendorf, R., and Pick, A.: Observations on the clinical use of paired electrical stimulation of the heart. Bull. N.Y. Acad. Med., 41:535–540, 1965.
27. Lister, J. W., Damato, A. N., Kosowsky, B. D., et al.: The hemodynamic effects of slowing the heart rate by paired or coupled stimulation of the atria. Am. Heart J., 73:362–368, 1967.
28. Fisher, J. D., Mehra, R., and Furman, J.: Termination of ventricular tachycardia with bursts of rapid ventricular pacing. Am. J. Cardiol., 41:94–102, 1978.
29. MacCuish, R. K.: Cardiac arrhythmias following mitral valvulotomy. Acta Med. Scand., 160:125, 1958.
30. Sasaki, R., Theilen, E. O., January, L. E., and Ehrenhaft, J. L.: Cardiac arrhythmias associated with the repair of atrial and ventricular septal defects. Circulation, 18:909, 1958.
31. Rabbino, M. D., Dreifus, L. S., and Likoff, W.: Cardiac arrhythmias following intracardiac surgery. Am. J. Cardiol., 7:681–689, 1961.
32. Michelson, E. L., Morganroth, J., and MacVaugh, H.: Post operative arrhythmias after coronary artery and cardiac valvular surgery detected by long-term electrocardiographic monitoring. Am. Heart J. 97:442, 1979.
33. Csicsko, J. F., Schatzlein, M. H., and King, R. D.: Immediate postoperative digitalization in the prophylaxis of supraventricular arrhythmias following coronary artery bypass. J. Thorac. Cardiovasc. Surg. 81:419–422, 1981.
34. White, H. D., Antman, E. M., Gyna, M. A., et al.: Efficiency and safety of timolol for prevention of supraventricular tachyarrhythmias after coronary artery bypass surgery. Circulation, 70:479–484, 1984.
35. Stephenson, L. W., MacVaugh, H., III, Tomasello, D. N., and Josephson, M. E.: Propranolol for prevention of postoperative cardiac arrhythmias: A randomized study. Ann. Thorac. Surg., 29:113–116, 1980.

36. Mohr, R., Smolinsky, A., and Goor, D. A.: Prevention of supraventricular tachyarrhythmia with low-dose propranolol after coronary bypass. J. Thorac. Cardiovasc. Surg., 81:840–845, 1981.
37. Williams, J. B., Stephenson, L. W., Holford, F. D., et al.: Arrhythmia prophylaxis using propranolol after coronary artery surgery. Ann. Thorac. Surg., 34:435–438, 1982.
38. Ivey, M. F., Ivey, T. D., Bailey, W. W., et al.: Influence of propranolol on supraventricular tachycardia early after coronary artery revascularization. J. Thorac. Cardiovasc. Surg., 85:214–218, 1983.
39. Selzer, A., Kelly, J. J., Jr., Gerbade, F., et al.: Case against routine use of digitalis in patients undergoing cardiac surgery. J.A.M.A., 195:141, 1966.
40. Johnson, L. W., Dickstein, R. A., Fruehan, C. T., et al.: Prophylactic digitalization for coronary artery surgery. Circulation, 53:819–822, 1976.
41. Tyras, D. H., Stothert, J. C., Jr., Kaiser, G. C., et al.: Supraventricular tachyarrhythmias after myocardial revascularization: A randomized trial of prophylactic digitalization. J. Thorac. Cardiovasc. Surg., 77:310–313, 1977.
42. Roffman, J. A., and Fieldman, A.: Digoxin and propranolol in the prophylaxis of supraventricular tachydysrhythmias after coronary artery bypass surgery. Ann. Thorac. Surg., 31:496–501, 1981.
43. Mills, S. A., Poole, G. V., Jr., Breyer, R. H., et al.: Digoxin and propranolol in the prophylaxis of dysrhythmias after coronary artery bypass grafting. Circulation, 68 (Suppl II):222–225, 1983.
44. Gray, R. J., Conklin, C. M., Sethna, D. H., et al.: Role of verapamil in supraventricular tachyarrhythmias after open heart surgery. Am. Heart J. 104:799–802, 1982.
45. Betriv, A., Chaitman, B. R., Bourassa, M. G., et al.: Beneficial effect of intravenous diltiazem in the acute management of paroxysmal supraventricular tachyarrhythmias. Circulation, 67:88–94, 1983.
46. Gray, R. J., Bateman, T. M., Czer, L. S., et al.: Esmolol: A new ultra short acting beta-adrenergic blocking agent for rapid control of heart rate in postoperative supraventricular tachyarrhythmias. J. Am. Coll. Cardiol., 5:1451–1456, 1985.
47. DiMarco, J. P., Sellers, T. D., Berne, R. M., et al.: Adenosine: Electrophysiologic effects and therapeutic use for terminating supraventricular tachycardia. Circulation, 68:1254–1262, 1983.
48. Belhassen, B., and Pelleg, A.: Acute management of paroxysmal supraventricular tachycardia: Verapamil, adenosine triphosphate or adenosine? Am. J. Cardiol., 54:225–227, 1984.
49. Alboni, P., Shantha, N., Pirani, R., et al.: Effects of amiodarone on supraventricular tachycardia involving bypass tracts. Am. J. Cardiol., 53:93–98, 1984.

28

Digitalis Toxicity: An Overview

William J. Mandel, Hrayr S. Karagueuzian, and Thomas W. Smith

In 1785, William Withering first described the clinical use of digitalis.[1] Since then, extraordinary research efforts have been directed toward understanding the mechanism of action of this compound. Although it is beyond the scope of this chapter to discuss in detail the cellular mechanisms of digitalis relative to the contractile process, its action potential appears to trigger the release of calcium ions stored in the sarcoplasmic reticulum (SR) through the calcium current. The transient release of calcium into the cytoplasm permits the calcium ion to interact with troponin C, blocking the interaction of the contractile proteins, actin and myosin. Relaxation occurs when calcium dissociates from troponin and is again taken up into the SA. Force development appears to be related to (1) the magnitude of the calcium current, (2) the amount of calcium stored in and released from the SR, and (3) the sensitivity of actin and myosin to the calcium ion.[2]

Another important facet of digitalis action is the interrelationship between calcium and sodium ions and the role of intracellular sodium levels in modulating contractility through the Na-Ca exchange mechanism.[3] The primary mechanism by which the digitalis glycosides produce their cellular effects is believed to be binding to sodium-potassium (Na-K) ATPase, inhibiting the sodium pump (Fig. 28-1). Interaction of digitalis with the sodium pump is reduced in the presence of elevated extracellular potassium levels and is enhanced in the presence of lowered potassium levels. When digitalis inhibits the Na-K ATPase system the intracellular sodium level increases, leading to an increased intracellular calcium level through Na-Ca exchange, thus producing a positive inotropic effect.[4]

Cardiac Electrophysiology

Preliminary investigations of the cellular electrophysiologic manifestations of digitalis intoxication were conducted by Woodbury and colleagues in the early 1950s.[5,6] They found that exposure to digitalis first prolonged and then accelerated repolarization and decreased the amplitude of the action potential without altering the resting potential (Fig. 28-2). Over the next decade, numerous studies dealt with the effects of digitalis glycosides on the various segments of the cardiac conducting system. Decreased membrane potentials were noted in atrioventricular (AV) nodal cells, Purkinje

Dr. H. S. Karagueuzian is the recipient of Research Career Development award HL 01293-03 from the National Heart, Lung, and Blood Institute, Bethesda, MD.

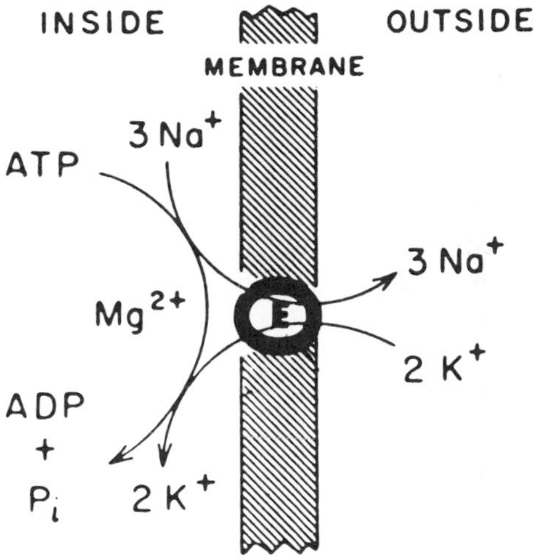

Figure 28-1. *Schematic diagram of reactions catalyzed by the sodium pump. (Horackova, M., and Vassort, G.: Sodium–calcium exchange in regulation of cardiac contractility. Evidence for an electrogenic, voltage-dependent mechanism. J. Gen. Physiol., 73:403–424, 1979.)*

fibers, and atrial and ventricular myocardial cells after exposure to toxic concentrations of digitalis glycosides. These findings were associated with decreases in action potential amplitude and upstroke velocity ($\dot{V}_{max}$), and repolarization was accelerated in all cardiac cell types studied. However, perhaps the most profound effect of toxic doses of digitalis compounds was the development or acceleration of spontaneous phase 4 depolarization (Fig. 28-3). This was readily seen in AV nodal and Purkinje fibers but not in ordinary working myocardial fibers. The latter point emphasizes that digitalis exhibits a "hierarchy" of effects, since the conducting system is more sensitive to the drug than is myocardial tissue. Finally, if exposure to toxic doses of digitalis was prolonged, electrical quiescence occurred.[7–10]

The cellular mechanism by which toxic doses of digitalis produce such effects has been felt to be related to the accumulation of extracellular potassium, with a concomitant rise in intracellular sodium ion concentration[11] due to the inhibition of Na-K ATPase (see above). Furthermore, the reduction in intracellular potassium and the increase in extracellular potassium relate directly to a loss in resting membrane potential, which is further exacerbated by loss of a part of the electrogenic Na-K pump current contribution to membrane polarization. The elevated extracellular potassium increases membrane conductance of potassium, accelerating repolarization and depressing the action potential plateau (phase 2). The depression of upstroke velocity and amplitude and the loss of resting potential can all be directly related to a slowing of or block in conduction. Digitalis, along with its ability to enhance acetylcholine release (see below), causes a more noticeable depression in conduction in tissues more sensitive to parasympathetic influence (*i.e.*, the sinoatrial (SA) and AV nodes as well as the atrium). Tachyarrhythmias due to digitalis excess may in some cases be related to an increase in the slope of phase 4 depolarization (see Fig. 28-3 and Table 28-1).[8–10] To some degree, this enhancement of phase 4 depolarization may be augmented by increased efferent sympathetic traffic to the heart due to central nervous system actions of digitalis (see below).

Over the past decade, data have accumulated suggesting that in addition to altering phase 4 depolarization, digitalis can induce oscillatory activity, that is, delayed afterdepolarizations or oscillatory afterpotentials (see Figs. 28-3 and 28-4 and Table 28-1).[10,12,13] These delayed afterdepolarizations seem to result from a sequence of events starting with inhibition of the Na-K ATPase system. The resulting increase in intracellular calcium through Na-Ca exchange appears to trigger a transient inward current carried predominantly by sodium ions through a tetrodotoxin-insensitive sodium channel (*i.e.*, a channel different from the fast sodium channel).[14] The latter current appears to be the major factor underlying

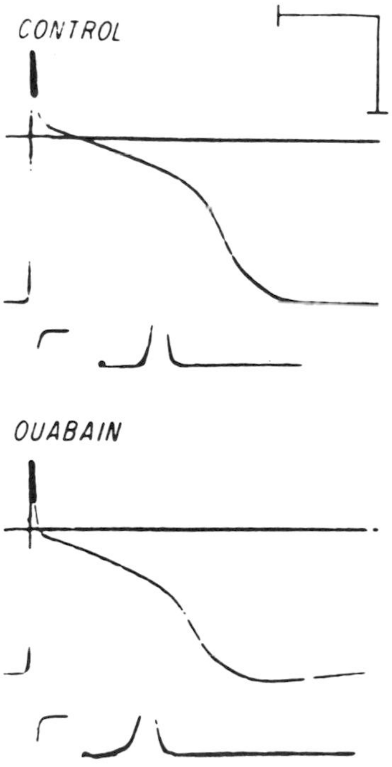

Figure 28-2. *Typical effects of exposure to toxic concentrations of digitalis on a canine Purkinje fiber action potential. Note: (1) Decrease in resting potential; (2) decrease in amplitude; (3) acceleration of voltage-time course of repolarization; (4) decrease in $\dot{V}_{max}$; and (5) increase in phase 4 slope. (Katz, A. M.: Effects of digitalis on cell biochemistry; sodium pump inhibition J.A.C.C., 5:16–21A, 1985.)*

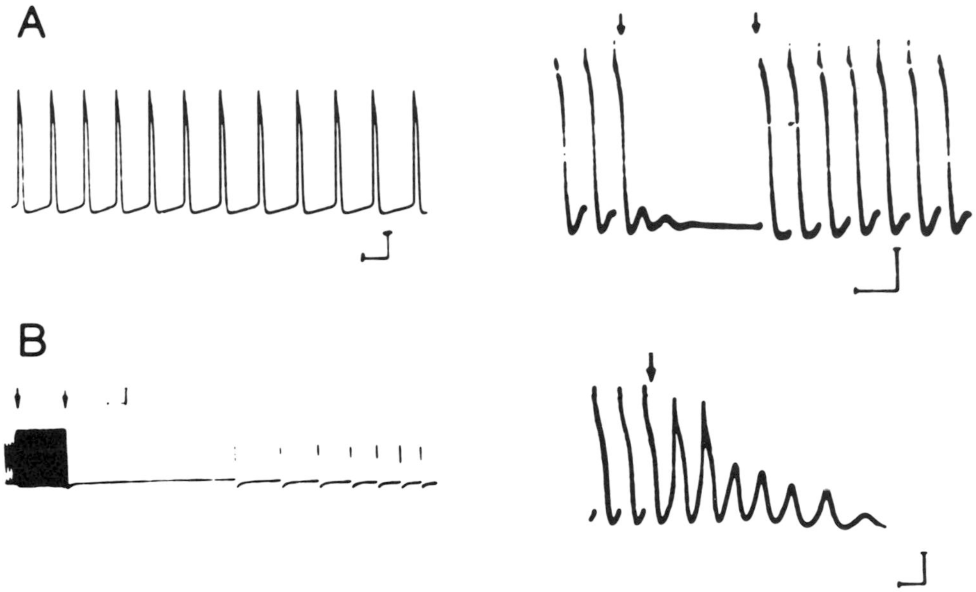

Figure 28-3. *Comparison of automatic activity to delayed afterdepolarizations in canine Purkinje fiber. In A, an automatic fiber with phase 4 depolarization (left) is compared with a fiber exposed to toxic concentrations of digitalis. After the first arrow, the drive is stopped, and a series of oscillations is seen. Drive is resumed at the second arrow, and several beats are needed before the delayed afterdepolarizations achieve full amplitude. In B, the panel to the left shows the effect of overdrive on an automatic rhythm. Rapid pacing starts at the first arrow and stops at the second arrow. Hyperpolarization occurs with overdrive. After overdrive, a long pause is observed before automatic firing resumes. At the right of B, pacing is stopped after three cycles, and two action potentials follow secondary to delayed afterdepolarizations reaching threshold. Subsequently, nonthreshold afterdepolarizations occur until they also cease. (Rosen, M. R.: Cellular electrophysiology of digitalis toxicity. J.A.C.C., 5:22–34A, 1985.)*

these afterdepolarizations. In humans, delayed afterpolarizations may play a specific role in the development of arrhythmias unrelated to digitalis intoxication. However detailed electrophysiologic studies in isolated tissues suggest that the delayed afterdepolarizations are the most likely mechanism underlying many tachyarrhythmias associated with digitalis toxicity (see Table 28-1).

Alterations in extracellular potassium clearly modify the electrophysiologic events occurring in digitalis intoxication. Low levels of extracellular potassium enhance the likelihood that digitalis will bind receptors. In addition, low extracellular potassium enhances the development of spontaneous phase 4 depolarization and automatic rhythms apart from its interaction with car-

Table 28-1. Comparison of Digitalis-Induced Repetitive Ventricular Responses in Intact Animals and Delayed Afterdepolarizations in Isolated Tissues

Repetitive Ventricular Responses	Delayed Afterdepolarizations
Initiated by premature beat during T wave (after vulnerable period) or early diastole	Initiated most readily at short drive cycle lengths or by premature depolarizations occurring at short coupling intervals
With increasing degree of digitalis toxicity, the electrical current needed to induce repetitive ventricular responses decreases	With increasing degree of digitalis toxicity, the electrical current required to bring delayed afterdepolarizations to threshold potential decreases
With increasing digitalis toxicity, there is a greater likelihood of longer trains of repetitive ventricular responses	With increasing digitalis toxicity, the trains of tachyarrhythmias induced by delayed afterdepolarizations tend to get longer

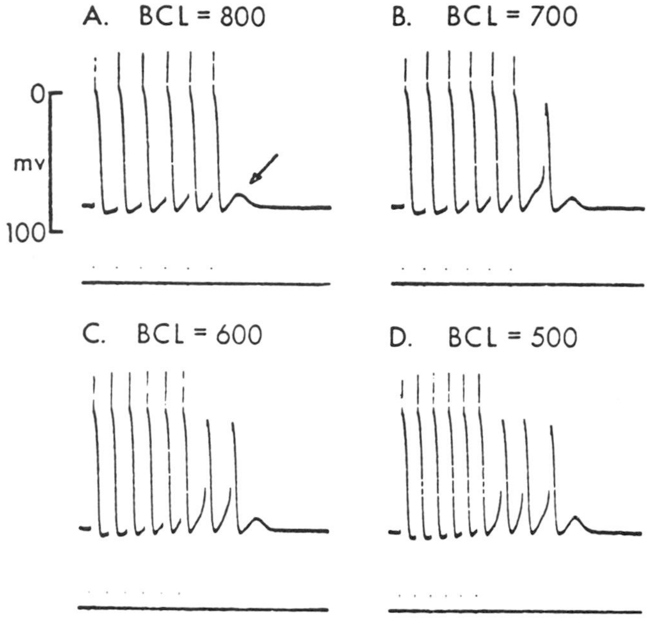

Figure 28-4. *The effect of heart rate on the magnitude of delayed afterdepolarizations and triggered automaticity in canine Purkinje fibers exposed to toxic doses of digitalis. The bottom portion of each panel shows a train of six stimuli. Note that as the cycle length (BCL) decreases, the number of suprathreshold afterdepolarizations increases, therefore increasing the number of triggered action potentials. (Smith, T. W., Antman, E. A., Friedman, P., Blatt, C. M., and Marsh, J. D.: Digitalis glycosides: mechanisms and manifestations of toxicity. Prog. Cardiovasc. Dis., 26:413–441, 26:495–523, 27:21–56, 1984.)*

diac glycosides. In contrast, as extracellular potassium increases, potassium tends to diminish cardiac glycoside binding, inhibiting the Na-K ATPase system. At levels above the upper limit of normal, however, elevated extracellular potassium accelerates repolarization and decreases the resting potential and the amplitude and upstroke velocity of the action potential. Ultimately this can reduce conduction velocity significantly.[10] Any shift from the normal range of extracellular potassium concentration, in association with digitalis excess, may precipitate or worsen conduction disturbances and hasten the emergence of ectopic activity in the atria, ventricles, or both.

Another ion altering digitalis responses is calcium. Elevations in extracellular calcium can reduce the threshold potential and, perhaps more important, augment the transient inward current associated with delayed afterdepolarizations. In contrast, a reduction in extracellular calcium tends to increase the threshold potential and thus augments excitability.[10]

Thus, above-normal extracellular concentrations of potassium and calcium ions can produce detrimental effects in the setting of digitalis intoxication, and vigorous efforts to maintain normal levels of these electrolytes, and magnesium, are indicated.

Age appears to modify the electrophysiologic effects of digitalis. Previous experimental studies have shown that in neonatal hearts, higher concentrations of digitalis were needed to produce the typical effects of digitalis excess. In contrast, in heart preparations from older animals, digitalis effects were seen more readily.[15] Finally, the diseased heart appears to be the most sensitive to digitalis glycosides, and toxicity develops more readily.[16]

Autonomic Nervous System

Note that important effects of cardiac glycosides stem from their influence on the autonomic nervous system.[17,18] Digitalis clearly enhances vagal tone and, hence, acetylcholine release. This is especially evident in the atria, where parasympathetic enervation is most prominent. Enhanced acetylcholine release hyperpolarizes atrial and SA nodal fibers, thus decreasing the slope of phase 4 and the rate of discharge of pacemaker cells.

Autonomic nervous system effects of digitalis glycosides are multifaceted. In the parasympathetic system, digitalis glycosides have both central and peripheral effects. Afferent as well as efferent activity is altered, as is primary central nervous system processing of impulses. The afferent impulses seem to be related predominantly to baroreceptors and chemoreceptors, especially in the carotid sinus and aortic arch.[17] Apparently the myocardium also appears to have receptors that mediate increases in afferent impulses in the presence of digitalis. Efferent activity is enhanced after digitalis administration, possibly as a result of enhanced ganglionic transmission. Of additional importance is the fact that digitalis potentiates cardiac vagal responses, especially in the SA and AV nodes.[19]

The influence of digitalis in the sympathetic nervous system under clinical circumstances remains to be clarified but seems evident only at higher levels.[17] First, efferent sympathetic activity is affected generally in association with clearly toxic doses of digitalis. Second, digitalis, in excess, appears to cause the release of catecholamines from sympathetic nerve terminals or to prevent catecholamine uptake. Catecholamine release may potentiate digitalis toxicity, apparently as a result of increasing automaticity of ectopic pacemakers, at least in part by increasing the magnitude of delayed afterdepolarizations.

Pharmacokinetics

Chemically, cardiac glycosides consist of a combination of an aglycone (also called a genin) with one to four sugar

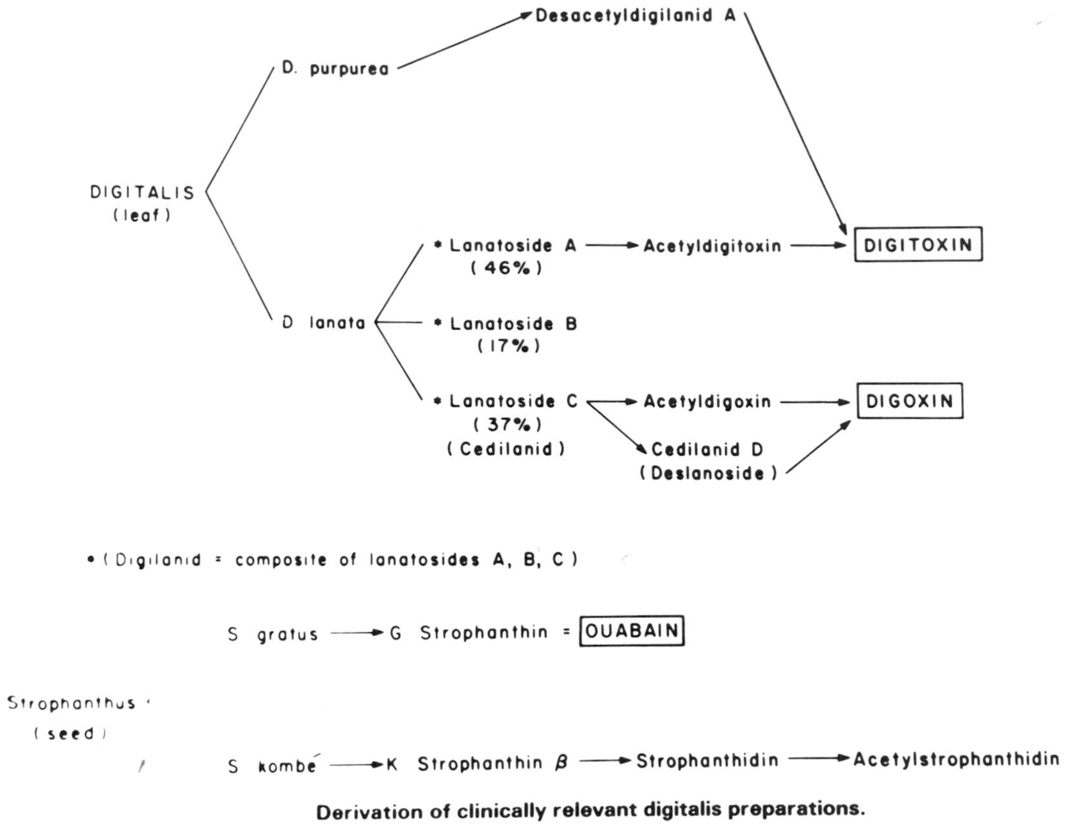

Figure 28-5. *Schematic of the derivation of digoxin, digitoxin, and ouabain.*

residues attached. Pharmacologic properties reside in the genin, while factors influencing pharmacokinetics are related to the sugar moieties (Fig. 28-5).

Pharmacokinetic studies have shown that digoxin fits well into a two-compartment model (Fig. 28-6), with the distribution (or alpha) phase having a half-time of approximately 30 minutes and the exertion (or beta) phase having an average half-time of 36 hours in healthy persons with normal renal function. Intravenous administration is the most rapid way to give loading doses; intramuscular administration is not recommended.[20] Digoxin is generally excreted in its unchanged form, but some patients (about 10%) excrete relatively large amounts of cardioinactive reduced metabolites.[21]

Digitalis preparations are passively absorbed from the gastrointestinal tract, with rate and completeness of absorption inversely related to the polarity of the compound.[22] About 85% of digoxin is absorbed when it is given as an elixir, and about 60% to 75% is absorbed when it is given in standard tablet form. About 20% binds to plasma proteins normally, and only the free portion is pharmacologically active.[23]

A steady state is achieved with digoxin only after approximately four to five excretory half-lives have been reached (*i.e.*, about 1 week in patients with normal renal function).[24] Note that in obese patients, digoxin pharmacokinetics change little with significant loss of adipose tissue; only lean body weight should be considered when one is calculating the dose.[25]

The major pool for digoxin in the body is the skeletal muscle, but concentrations per gram of tissue are considerably higher in the kidney and heart. Although renal excretion is the dominant route of elimination, in some patients digoxin is appreciably metabolized to dihydrodigoxin and dihydrodigoxigenin. The quantity of these metabolites is related both to bioavailability of the drug and bacterial flora of the gastrointestinal tract. Therefore, if antibiotic therapy that alters the gut flora is being used concurrently, the amount of "effective drug" may be increased even though there has been no change in the dose of digoxin.[26]

Since digoxin crosses the placental barrier, fetal umbilical cord levels are similar to those in maternal venous blood. In infants, the usual dose recommendations are based on calculations of milligrams per kilogram of body surface area and are generally higher than those for adults; such a schedule is usually associated with higher blood levels.[27]

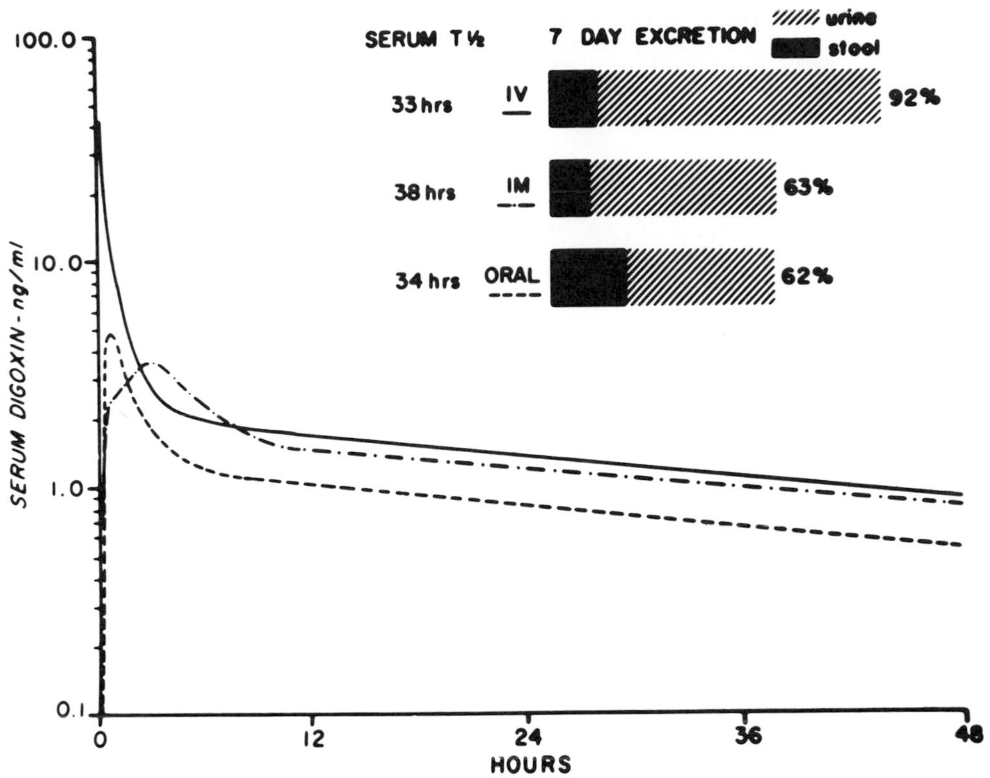

Figure 28-6. *Pharmacokinetic comparison of intravenous, intramuscular, and orally administered digoxin. (Doherty, J. E., deSoyza, N., Kane, J. J., et al.: Clinical pharmacokinetics of digitalis glycosides. Prog. Cardiovasc. Dis., 21:141–158, 1978.)*

Bioavailability

Over the past decade, studies comparing the bioavailability of digoxin tablets from a variety of manufacturers have indicated that the range of dissolution rates may be wide, which would lead to significant variability in bioavailability and hence in serum digoxin levels.[28] Malabsorption syndromes may alter bioavailability. Ingesting digoxin along with or shortly after meals also decreases its peak serum or plasma levels but has relatively little effect on the total amount of drug absorbed by the normal gastrointestinal tract. Drugs that reduce gastrointestinal tract motility may enhance drug absorption. Agents such as cholestyramine, kaolin-pectin, and nonabsorbable antacids can reduce absorption (Tables 28-2 and 28-3). Problems with bioavailability can be reduced by the use of a digoxin gel solution in capsule form (Lanoxi-Caps, a formulation that approximates the elixir in bioavailability).[29]

Serum Levels of Digitalis

Serum digitalis measurements are obtained in most institutions by radioimmunoassay.[30] The variety of technical problems this assay presents includes potential errors caused by the presence in serum or plasma of diagnostic radioisotopes for nuclear medical studies. Although there appears to be a significant and direct relationship between serum levels and the pharmacologic effects of digitalis, it may vary in patients with pulmonary or cardiac diseases or in the elderly (see below). *No specific serum level* can be used to differentiate with certainty between toxic and nontoxic concentrations of digoxin.[31]

From the hemodynamic standpoint, digoxin levels of 1 to 1.5 ng/ml appear to provide significant benefit. However, conventional "therapeutic" levels of digoxin often fail to produce optimal heart rate control during exercise in patients with atrial fibrillation. Serum digoxin levels of equal to or greater than 2.5 ng/ml were necessary to produce a controlled ventricular response in 39% of patients in the study of Goldman and colleagues.[32] Improved rate control can often be achieved by judicious coadministration of beta-blockers or verapamil.

Drug Interactions With Digitalis

In 1978, it was first reported that the administration of quinidine to digitalized patients led to an approximate doubling of the serum digoxin concentration.[33] The

Table 28-2. Pharmacokinetic Drug Interactions With Digoxin

Drug	Mechanism of Interaction: Effect on Digoxin	Mean Magnitude of Interaction (%)*	Suggested Intervention
Cholestyramine	Adsorption of digoxin	↓ 25	1. Give digoxin 8 hours before cholestyramine 2. Use solution or capsule form of digoxin
Antacids	Unclear	↓ 25	Temporal separation of time of administration
Kaolin-pectate	Adsorption of digoxin	?	1. Give digoxin 2 hours before kaolin-pectate 2. ? Use solution or capsule form of digoxin
Bran	Adsorption of Digoxin	↓ 20	Temporal separation of time of administration
Neomycin Sulfasalazine PAS	Unknown	↓ 28 ↓ 18 ↓ 22	Increase dose of digoxin
Erythromycin Tetracycline (in < 10% of subjects)	↑ Bioavailability by ↑ intestinal metabolism of digoxin by certain gut flora	↑ 43 to 116	1. Measure serum digoxin concentration 2. Decrease digoxin dose 3. Use solution or capsule form of digoxin
Quinidine	? ↓ Bioavailability ↓ volume of distribution, ↓ renal and nonrenal clearance	↑ 100	1. Decrease dose by 50% 2. Measure serum digoxin concentration
Amiodarone	↓ Renal and nonrenal clearance	↑ 70 to 100	Same as for quinidine
Verapamil	↓ Renal and nonrenal clearance	↑ 70 to 100	Same as for quinidine
Diltiazem	? ↓ Renal clearance	↑ 22	None
Nicardipine	Unknown	↑ 15	None
Tiapamil	Unknown	↑ 60	Same as for quinidine
Spironolactone	↓ Renal and nonrenal clearance	↑ 30	Measure serum digoxin concentration
Triamterene	↓ Nonrenal clearance	↑ 20	Measure serum digoxin concentration
Indomethacin (preterm infants)	? ↓ Renal clearance	↑ 50	Decrease dose by 25%

mechanism underlying this effect is multifaceted and includes (1) a decrease in the volume of distribution of digoxin, possibly reflecting displacement of digoxin binding by quinidine, and (2) a quinidine-related reduction in renal and nonrenal clearance of digoxin. This latter factor appears to be related in large part to a decrease in the tubular secretion of digoxin.[34,35] The increase in serum digoxin levels is directly but not linearly related to the dose of quinidine. It has also been observed that quinine, the dextroisomer of quinidine, increases the half-life of digoxin.

Other antiarrhythmic drugs, such as amiodarone, have been associated with a significant increase in serum digoxin levels.[36] This interaction appears to be due to decreased renal and nonrenal clearance with a consequent increase in the half-life; no change in the volume of distribution of digoxin has been documented with amiodarone. Agents including procainamide, disopyramide, mexilitine, flecainide, and ethmozine do not appear to interact with digoxin pharmacokinetically,[37] but pharmacodynamic interactions (*e.g.*, depression of conduction) must be watched for carefully.

The calcium channel blocking drug verapamil has demonstrated a dose-dependent interaction with digoxin due to decreases in both renal and extrarenal clearance; the renal factor appears to be due to inhibition of tubular secretion.[38] Other slow channel blocking agents, such as diltiazem, seem to have a less prominent (if any) effect, and nifedipine appears to have no pharmacokinetic interaction with digoxin.

Diuretics constitute another class of cardiovascular drugs that may interact with digoxin. Nevertheless, data conflict regarding digoxin levels in patients taking these agents as well as the mechanisms involved in such an

Table 28-3. Certain Factors Modifying Digitalis Tolerance

Possible Reasons for Increased Sensitivity	Possible Reasons for Increased Tolerance
Cardiac	Decreased automaticity of ectopic pacemakers
Increased automaticity of ectopic pacemakers	High potassium*
Heart disease*	Antiarrhythmic drugs†
Heart surgery*	Vagal stimulation
Low potassium*	Decreased vagal or increased sympathetic activity
Chronic lung disease (?)	Fever, infection, hypoxia, hyperkinetic states (?)
Catecholamines and sympathetic stimulation†	Hyperthyroidism*
Impaired SAN function and AV conduction	Normal infants and young children
Increased vagal activity	Decreased absorption or unusual losses
Decreased sympathetic activity	Malabsorption
Heart disease*	Dialysis (?)
Heart surgery*	Cardiac bypass (?)
Low potassium*	
High potassium	
Impaired degradation or excretion	
Hypothyroidism*	
Renal disease*	
Liver disease	
Premature infants*	
Old age (?)	
Interaction with drugs	
Extracardiac	
Allergy and hypersensitivity	
CNS disorders	
Low weight	

* Factors that appear to be of greatest practical importance. † Variable effects. (?) Inconclusive evidence. AV, atrioventricular; CNS, central nervous system; SAN, sinoatrial node.

interaction. Apart from effects on serum potassium levels, diuretics may reduce digoxin excretion by reducing glomerular filtration rate if excessive diuresis with reduced vascular volume occurs. Potassium-sparing diuretics such as spironolactone may inhibit renal tubular secretion of digoxin and therefore elevate serum digoxin levels. Triamterene reduces extrarenal but not renal clearance of digoxin, while amiloride increases renal clearance but decreases extrarenal clearance of digoxin.[37]

Several other drugs may alter digoxin pharmacokinetics, including indomethacin, which increases digoxin levels in premature infants. Rifampin significantly reduces digoxin levels in patients receiving dialysis. The explanation for this may relate to increased biotransformation or to decreased absorption or increased biliary excretion.[37]

Factors Modifying Digitalis Dosage

Renal excretion of digoxin depends greatly on the glomerular filtration rate.[31] In patients with impaired renal function, elimination of digoxin parallels creatinine clearance. The amount of digoxin removed during peritoneal dialysis is small; extracorporeal dialysis removes digoxin at a rate of only 10% of that expected when renal function is normal.[39,40]

During cardiopulmonary bypass, loss of digoxin into the pump oxygenator is small. Some evidence suggests that cardiovascular sensitivity to digoxin increases in the first 24 hours after cardiopulmonary bypass, increasing the risk of toxic rhythm disturbances.[41,42]

As noted earlier, the effect of the interaction of potassium and digitalis on AV conduction is complex. Both elevated and depressed levels of serum potassium may depress AV conduction, so that one cannot easily predict the net effects of mild to moderate hyperkalemia in patients receiving digitalis. Moderate hyperkalemia may either further depress or enhance AV conduction. Hypokalemia can also worsen AV block induced by digitalis excess; moreover, hypokalemia enhances automaticity, further augmenting ectopic automaticity enhancement by digoxin.[43]

The effect of elevated serum calcium in digitalized patients is controversial, but reports have suggested that administering calcium to these patients may precipitate life-threatening arrhythmias.[44,45]

Cardiac toxicity may also develop in digitalized pa-

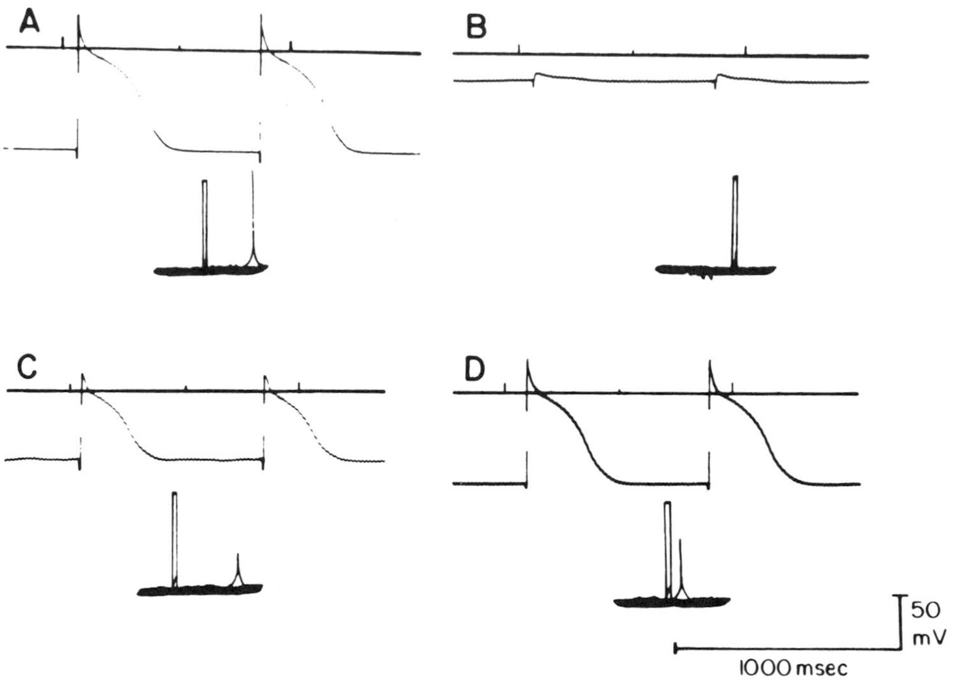

Figure 28-7. *Reversal of digoxin-induced toxicity in a canine Purkinje fiber. A shows control action potentials with dV/dT ($\dot{V}_{max}$) at the bottom. B shows near electrical quiescence after exposure to 120 min of 1×10^{-7}M digoxin. Digoxin-specific antibody (DSA) was then superfused for 15 min (C) and for 60 min (D). Nearly normal electrical characteristics resulted from DSA exposure. (Mandel, W. J., Bigger, J. T., Jr., and Butler, V. P., Jr.: The electrophysiologic effects of low and high digoxin concentrations on isolated mammalian cardiac tissue: reversal by digoxin-specific antibody. J. Clin. Invest., 51:1378–1387, 1972.)*

tients with hypomagnesemia. Patients with arrhythmias associated with digitalis intoxication have been reported to benefit from receiving magnesium sulfate.[43]

Anesthetic agents such as cyclopropane and suxamethonium may enhance automaticity; decreased tolerance to digitalis may also be seen with halothane anesthesia.[43]

Although direct current synchronized countershock has been reported to precipitate supraventricular and ventricular premature complexes and arrhythmias in the digitalized patient,[46] this finding has recently been challenged in the case of patients receiving conventional doses with no evidence of toxicity.[47]

In the setting of acute myocardial infarction it re-

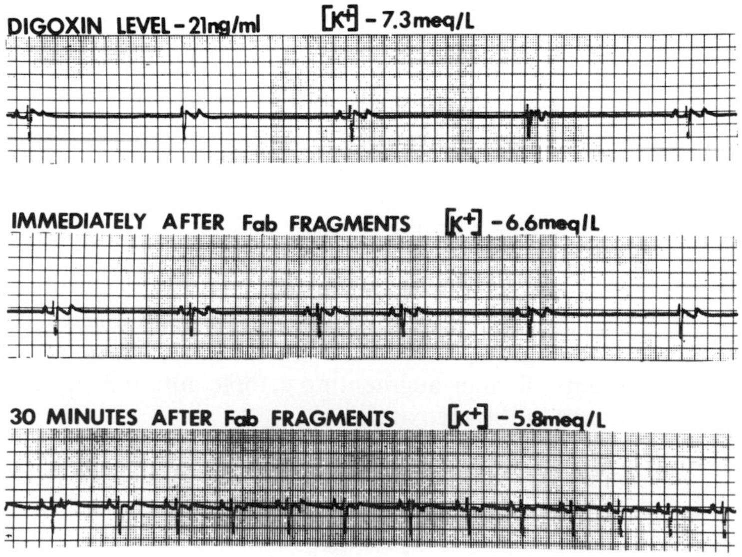

Figure 28-8. *Time course of reversal of bradycardia and hyperkalemia in a 22-year-old man who had ingested 100 tablets of 0.25-mg digoxin. (Spiegel, A., and Marchlinski, F. E.: Time course for reversal of digoxin toxicity with digoxin-specific antibody fragment. Am. Heart J., 109:1397–1399, 1985; by permission of the American Heart Association, Inc.)*

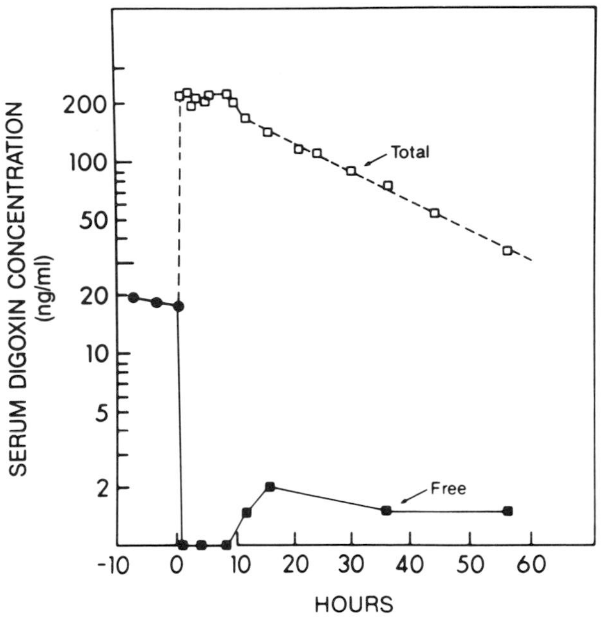

Figure 28-9. *Time course of serum digoxin concentrations before (filled circles), and total (empty squares) and free (filled squares) digoxin concentration after treatment with digoxin-specific Fab fragments begun at 0 hours. (Wenger, T. L., Butler, V. P., Jr., Haber, E., and Smith, T. W.: Treatment of 63 severely digitalis-toxic patients with digoxin-specific antibody fragments. J.A.C.C., 5:118–123A, 1985.)*

mains unclear whether therapeutic doses of digoxin enhance the incidence of ventricular arrhythmias. Patients with chronic pulmonary disease do seem to have increased propensity to develop cardiac arrhythmias, but whether digitalis toxicity is a causal factor is not entirely clear.[43]

Hypothyroid patients are usually considered to be more sensitive to digoxin, whereas hyperthyroid patients are less sensitive. Overall, such sensitivity can be attributed in part to slower renal elimination of digoxin in the hypothyroid group and faster renal elimination in the hyperthyroid group.[43] In addition, however, true changes in sensitivity to digitalis clearly occur in the presence of thyroid dysfunction.[31]

Electrocardiographic Manifestations of Digitalis Intoxication

The major manifestations of digitalis intoxication relate to depression of pacemaker function, depression of conduction, or development of ectopic rhythms.[57] Table 28-4 summarizes the major rhythm disturbances associated with digitalis excess.

Ectopic arrhythmias in the setting of digitalis excess appear to be due to enhancement of automaticity, development of reentry, or emergence to "triggered" arrhythmias associated at the cellular level with oscillatory afterpotentials (see above). Alterations in automaticity would be the more likely mechanism in the setting of nonparoxysmal junctional tachycardia (Fig. 28-10) and junctional escape rhythms as well as the rare bidirectional ventricular tachycardia (Fig. 28-11). In the clinical setting, the automatic origin of arrhythmias would be suggested by the gradual appearance and disappearance of the arrhythmia associated with fusion complexes and evidence of "protection." Arrhythmias such as atrial fibrillation, ventricular premature complexes, and ventricular flutter are less specifically indicative of digitalis toxicity and are likely to be due to reentrant mechanisms, whatever their cause. Atrial tachycardia with block (Fig. 28-12), an arrhythmia that shows a high clinical correlation with digitalis intoxication, has not been clearly defined in terms of mechanism (*i.e.*, reentry versus enhanced automaticity).

Although depression of the sinus node with marked sinus slowing, sinus arrest, or SA exit block is not an uncommon manifestation of digitalis intoxication, much more common is the development of conduction disturbances. The manifestation of conduction disturbance is usually related to AV transmission or exit block. Intraventricular conduction disturbances are rarely seen in the setting of digitalis excess. In sinus rhythm, first degree or second degree AV block (almost always of the Wenckebach type) is a frequent manifestation of digitalis intoxication. Third degree AV block is uncommon when the patient is in sinus rhythm; when the patient is in atrial fibrillation, however, advanced AV block with

Table 28-4. Major Rhythm Disturbances Associated with Digitalis Excess

1. Ectopic rhythms due to reentry or enhanced automaticity or both (atrial tachycardia with block, atrial fibrillation, atrial flutter, nonparoxysmal junctional tachycardia, reciprocation, ventricular premature complexes, ventricular tachycardia, ventricular flutter and fibrillation, "bidirectional" ventricular tachycardia, parasystolic ventricular tachycardia, ectopic rhythms from multiple sites of the specialized conducting tissue)
2. Depression of pacemakers (SA arrest)
3. Depression of conduction (SA block, AV block, exit block)

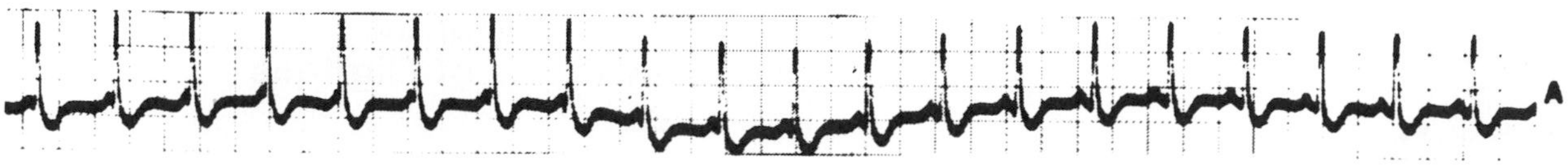

Figure 28-10. *Nonparoxysmal junctional tachycardia. AV dissociation is noted. (After Fisch, C., and Knoebel, S. B.: Digitalis cardiotoxicity. J.A.C.C., 5:91–98A, 1985.)*

junctional or another escape pacemaker phenomenon is seen much more often. High-grade AV block is quite common with massive suicidal or accidental digitalis ingestion.[51]

Various manifestations of exit block may be seen with digitalis intoxication. These can occur at the SA level or as arrhythmias involving the AV junctional and distal conducting system (Fig. 28-13). Electrophysiologically, the mechanism does not appear to be related to the intrinsic properties of the pacemaker cell(s) but rather to disturbances of conduction between pacemaker sites and surrounding tissue.

Another relatively specific form of arrhythmia seen with digitalis intoxication is the development of more than one accelerated rhythm, especially in combination with depressed conduction (*e.g.,* simultaneous junctional and ventricular rhythms or atrial tachycardia with block) (Fig. 28-14).

As previously discussed in this chapter, in the experimental electrophysiology laboratory, delayed afterdepolarizations have often been seen as manifestations of digitalis excess. Thus, "triggered automatic" arrhythmias would be expected to occur in the clinical setting as well. However, the specific diagnosis of this mechanism in patients is difficult. One clinical arrhythmia potentially related to triggered automaticity is accelerated junctional rhythm occurring after a premature complex (Fig. 28-15). Ventricular premature depolarizations or sustained ventricular tachycardia could also occur by this mechanism, but clinical proof is difficult to obtain.

Treatment of Patients With Digitalis Intoxication

In the setting of digitalis-induced ventricular tachyarrhythmias, lidocaine or diphenylhydantoin have been found to be effective. It is mandatory to measure serum potassium levels and to administer potassium to any patient who is overtly hypokalemic; potassium supplementation may also be useful in patients with low normal serum potassium levels. Other antiarrhythmic agents have been used but appear to offer less specific benefit or greater risk of depressing conduction in the setting of digitalis intoxication. In the presence of bradyarrhythmias such as SA block, sinus arrest, or significant AV block, temporary pacing is essential unless there is an excellent response to intravenous atropine. As noted above, potassium must be administered with great caution because of the risk of exacerbating conduction disturbances.

Digoxin Antibodies

Antibodies to digoxin were first produced by Butler and Chen in 1967 to facilitate the measurement of serum digoxin concentrations.[49] A few years later, Schmidt and Butler demonstrated that such antibodies could be used to reverse life-threatening arrhythmias in an animal model.[50] Not only do they appear to bind digoxin in the extracellular fluid and decrease the effective free digoxin

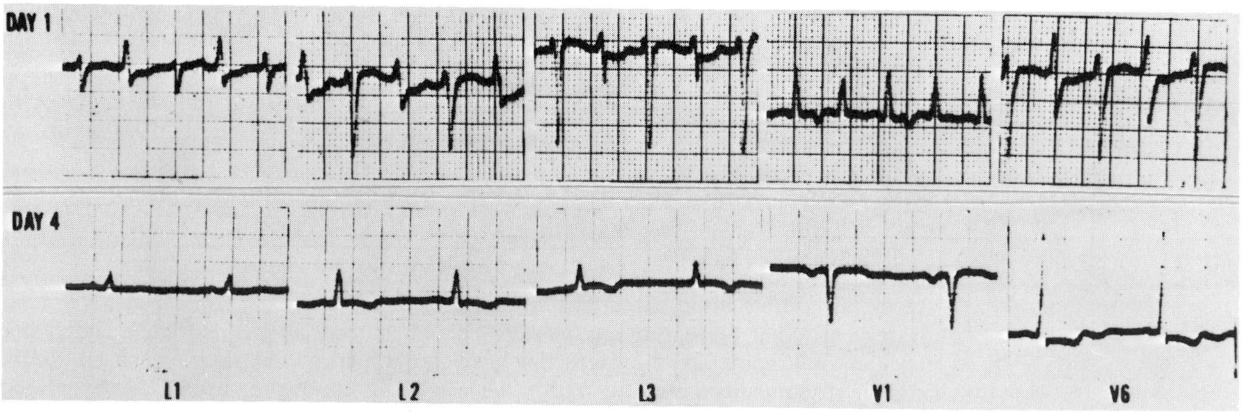

Figure 28-11. *Bidirectional ventricular tachycardia compared with sinus rhythm 4 days later. (After Fisch, C., and Knoebel, S. B.: Digitalis cardiotoxicity. J.A.C.C., 5:91–98A, 1985.)*

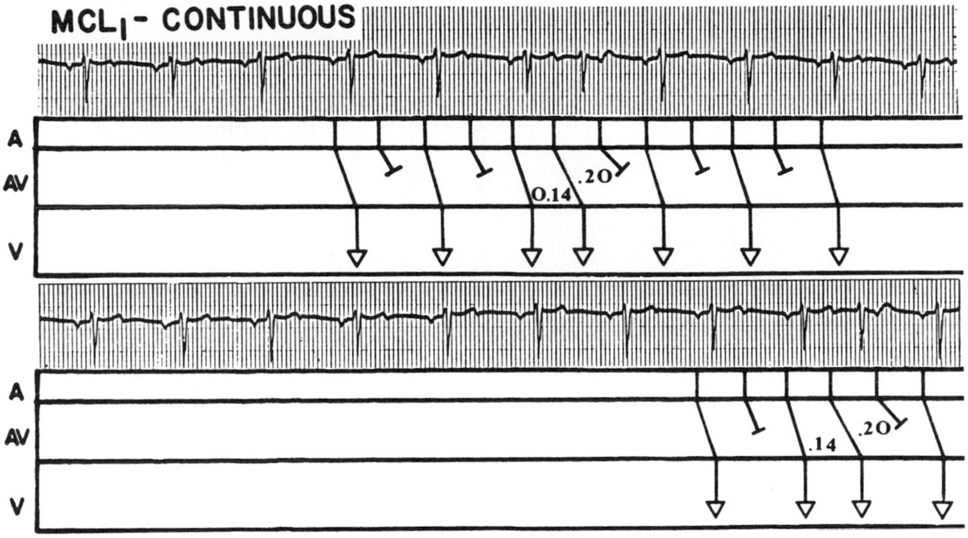

Figure 28-12. *Nonparoxysmal junctional tachycardia with exit block simulating high-degree AV block. The basic rhythm is atrial fibrillation, with the RR intervals being multiples of the basic RR cycle. (After Fisch, C., and Knoebel, S. B.: Digitalis cardiotoxicity. J.A.C.C., 5:91–98A, 1985.)*

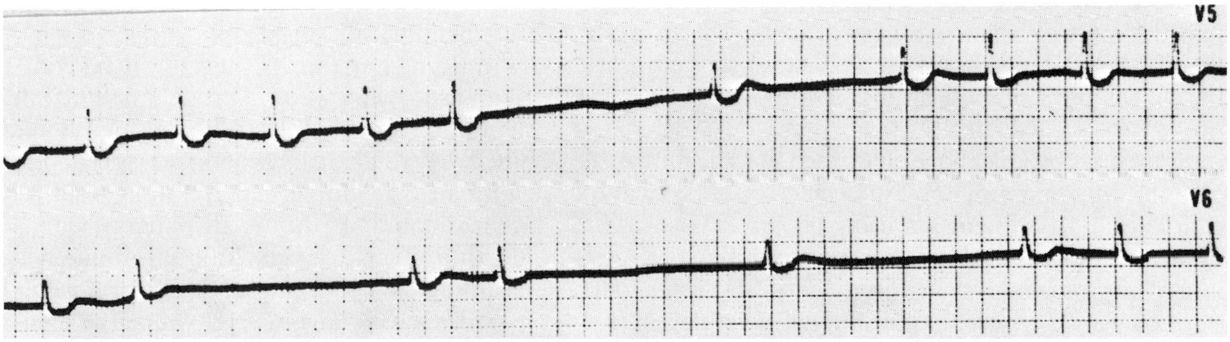

Figure 28-13. *Atrial tachycardia with block. The atrial rate is 150/min. AV Wenckebach alternates with 2:1 AV conduction.*

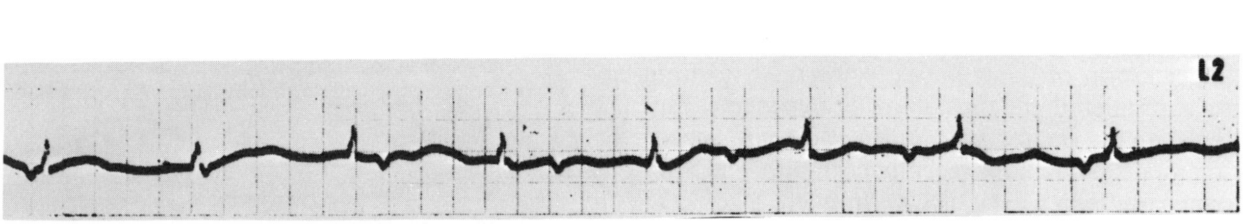

Figure 28-14. *Double junctional rhythm; RR = 0.96, PP = 1.08 sec. (After Fisch, C., and Knoebel, S. B.: Digitalis cardiotoxicity. J.A.C.C., 5:91–98A, 1985.)*

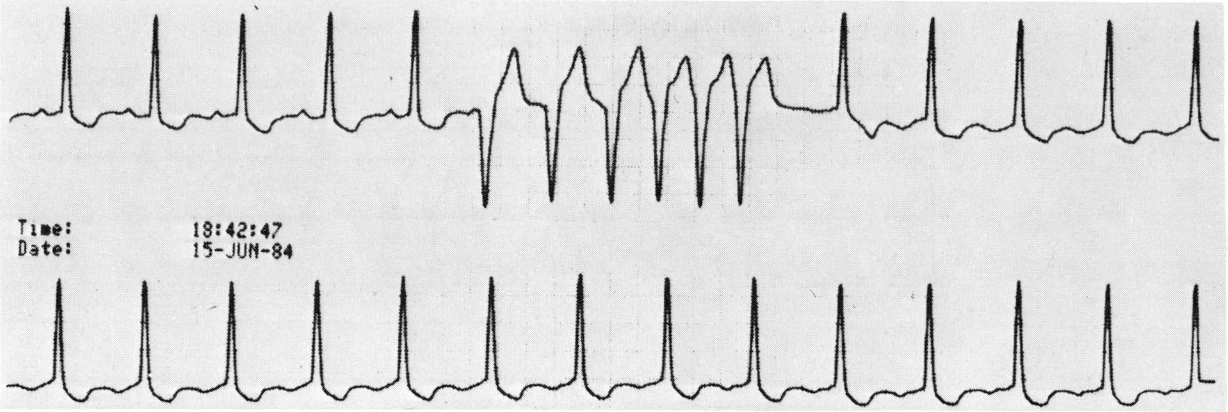

Figure 28-15. *Possible triggered automaticity. A burst of nonsustained ventricular tachycardia is followed by a junctional tachycardia. (After Fisch, C., and Knoebel, S. B.: Digitalis cardiotoxicity. J.A.C.C., 5:91–98A, 1985.)*

level, but they also produce a concentration gradient that further dissociates digoxin from receptor sites.[51] These digoxin-specific antibodies were shown able to reverse various drug effects, including ion transport in erythrocytes, positive inotropic effects in isolated muscle preparations, and digitalis-induced ventricular tachyarrhythmias.[50,52]

Electrophysiologic studies in isolated tissue from both Purkinje fibers and AV nodal tissue confirmed that digoxin-specific antibodies could promptly reverse the toxic membrane effects of excessive doses of digoxin (see Fig. 28-4).[53] These effects were very rapid, in contrast to the slower effect of these antibodies on cardiac contractility.[31]

Subsequent studies have confirmed that the immunoglobulin (digoxin antibody) molecule could be cleaved into Fab and Fc fragments using papain.[52] One of the main advantages of using Fab fragments is that this form is less immunogenic when injected intravenously.[55] The purified Fab fragment has additional advantages; it is small, which allows for more rapid distribution and distribution into a larger volume, thus facilitating rapid reversal of toxicity. In addition, the Fab fragment can be excreted relatively rapidly through glomerular filtration.[55]

Based on these studies, a clinical protocol has been designed for treating patients with severe digoxin intoxication with the Fab fragment. The first clinical report, in 1976,[56] has been followed by subsequent studies on a larger group of patients (see below). At no time have toxic or allergic manifestations been observed in any of the patients treated with purified digoxin-specific Fab fragments. Data have recently been published summarizing results in 63 patients with severe digoxin toxicity who were treated with digoxin-specific antibody fragments.[51] Digoxin levels ranged from 2.4 to over 100 ng/ml, with an average concentration of 14.1 ng/ml. The response was dramatic and rapid (*i.e.,* within about 30 minutes in most patients) (see Fig. 28-8). Free digoxin levels measured in a small number of patients were markedly reduced within 2 minutes of administration of the antibody fragments. In contrast, there was an increase in the total serum digoxin concentration to 10 to 20 times the pretreatment level. Nearly all the drug was bound to antibody fragments and thus was pharmacologically inactive (Fig. 28-9). A significant reduction in serum potassium level was also associated with this treatment, with levels dropping on average from 5.8 to 4.4 mEq/liter, within 4 hours, due to reversal of Na^+ and K^+ transport inhibition. Throughout the clinical trial, no significant or obvious adverse manifestations were noted. The digoxin-Fab complex appears to be rapidly eliminated by glomerular filtration, with a half-life of approximately 16 hours in patients with good renal function. To date, very little information is available regarding the elimination half-life of the Fab fragments in patients who have severely impaired renal function.

References

1. Withering, W.: An account of the Foxglove and some of its medical uses; with practical remarks on dropsy and other diseases. 1785.
2. Fozzard, H. A., and Sheets, M. F.: Cellular mechanism of action of cardiac glycosides. J.A.C.C., 5:10–15A, 1985.
3. Horackova, M., and Vassort, G.: Sodium–calcium exchange in regulation of cardiac contractility. Evidence for an electrogenic, voltage-dependent mechanism. J. Gen. Physiol. 73:403–424, 1979.
4. Katz, A. M. Effects of digitalis on cell biochemistry: sodium pump inhibition. J.A.C.C., 5:16–21A, 1985.
5. Woodbury, L. A., and Hecht, H. H.: Effects of cardiac glycosides upon the electrical activity of single ventricular fibers of the frog heart, and their relation to the digitalis effect on the electrocardiogram. Circulation, 6:172–182, 1952.
6. Fingl, E., Woodbury, L. A., and Hecht, H. H.: Effects of innerva-

tion and drugs upon direct membrane potentials of embryonic chick myocardium. J. Pharmacol. Exp. Ther., 104:103–114, 1951.
7. Watanabe, Y., and Dreifus, L.: Electrophysiologic effects of digitalis on A–V transmission. Am. J. Physiol., 211:1461–1466, 1966.
8. Vassalle, M., Karis, J., and Hoffman, B. F.: Toxic effects of ouabain on Purkinje fibers and ventricular muscle fibers. Am. J. Physiol., 203:433–439, 1962.
9. Hoffman, B. F., and Singer, D. H.: Effects of digitalis on electrical activity of cardiac fibers. Prog. Cardiovasc. Dis., 7:226–260, 1964.
10. Rosen, M. R.: Cellular electrophysiology of digitalis toxicity. J.A.C.C., 5:22–34A, 1985.
11. Lin, C. I., and Vassalle, M.: Role of sodium in strophanthidin toxicity of Purkinje fibers. Am. J. Physiol., 234:H477–H486, 1978.
12. Rosen, M. R., Gelband, H., Merker, C., and Hoffman, B. F.: Mechanisms of digitalis toxicity: effects of ouabain on phase 4 of canine Purkinje fiber transmembrane potentials. Circ. Res., in press.
13. Ferrier, G. R., Saunders, J. H., and Mendez, C.: Cellular mechanism for the generation of ventricular arrhythmias by acetylstrophanthidin. Circ. Res., 32:600–609, 1973.
14. Tsien, R. W., Kass, R. S., and Weingart, R.: Cellular and subcellular mechanism of cardiac pacemaker oscillations. J. Exp. Biol., 81:205–215, 1979.
15. Rosen, M. R., Hordof, A. J., Hodess, A., et al.: Ouabain induced changes in electrophysiologic properties of neonatal, young and adult canine cardiac Purkinje fibers. J. Pharmacol. Exp. Ther., 194:255–263, 1973.
16. Brennan, J. F., and Bonn, J. R.: Effects of ouabain on the electrophysiological properties of subendocardial Purkinje fibers surviving in regions of acute myocardial infarction. Am. Heart J., 100:201–212, 1980.
17. Gillis, R. A., and Quest, J. A.: The role of the nervous system in the cardiovascular effects of digitalis. Pharmacol. Rev., 31:19–97, 1980.
18. Watanabe, A. M.: Digitalis and the autonomic nervous system. J.A.C.C., 5(5):35A–42A, 1985.
19. Toda, N., and West, T. C.: The influence of ouabain on cholinergic responses in the sinoatrial node. J. Pharmacol. Exp. Ther., 153:104–113, 1966.
20. Doherty, J. E., deSoyza, N., Kane, J. J., et al.: Clinical pharmacokinetics of digitalis glycosides. Prog. Cardiovasc. Dis., 21:141–158, 1978.
21. Peters, U., Falk, L. C., and Kalman, S. M.: Digoxin metabolism in patients. Arch. Intern. Med., 138:1074–1076, 1978.
22. Haass, A., Lüllmann, H., Peters, L.: Absorption rates of some cardiac glycosides and portal blood flow. Am. J. Pharmacol., 19:366–370, 1979.
23. Storstein, L.: Studies on digitalis V. The influence of impaired renal function, hemodialysis, and drug interaction on serum protein binding of digitoxin and digoxin. Clin. Pharmacol. Ther., 20:6–13, 1976.
24. Marcus, F. L., Burkhalter, L., Cuccia, C., et al.: Administration of tritiated digoxin with and without a loading dose—a metabolic study. Circulation, 34:865–874, 1966.
25. Abernethy, D. R., Greenblatt, D. J., and Smith, L. W.: Digoxin disposition in obesity: clinical pharmacokinetic investigation. Am. Heart J., 102:740–744, 1981.
26. Lindenbaum, J., Rund, D. G., Butler, V.P., et al.: Inactivation of digoxin by the gut flora: reversal by antibiotic therapy. N. Engl. J. Med., 305:789–794, 1981.
27. Rogers, M. C., Willerson, J. T., Goldblatt, A., et al.: Serum digoxin concentrations in the human fetus, neonate and infant. N. Engl. J. Med., 287:1010–1013, 1972.
28. Greenblatt, D. J., Smith L. W., and Koch, W. J.: Bioavailability of drugs: the digoxin dilemma. Clin. Pharmacokinet., 1976.
29. Smith, T. W.: Pharmacokinetics, bioavailability and serum levels of cardiac glyosides. J.A.C.C., 5(5):43A–50A, 1985.
30. Smith, T. W., Butler, B. P., Jr., and Haber, E.: Determination of therapeutic and toxic serum digoxin concentrations by radioimmunoassay. N. Engl. J. Med., 281:1212–1216, 1969.
31. Smith, T. W., Antman, E. A., Friedman, P., Blatt, C. M., and Marsh, J. D.: Digitalis glycosides: mechanisms and manifestations of toxicity. Prog. Cardiovasc. Dis., 26:413–441, 26:495–523, 27:21–56, 1984.
32. Goldman, S., Probst, P., Selzer, A., et al.: Inefficiency of "therapeutic" serum levels of digoxin in controlling the ventricular rate in atrial fibrillation. Am. J. Cardiol., 35:651–656, 1975.
33. Ejvinsson, G.: Effect of quinidine on plasma concentrations of digoxin. Br. Med. J., 1:279–280, 1978.
34. Pedersen, K. E., Christiansen, B. D., Klitgaard, N. A., and Nielsen-Kudsk, F.: Effect of quinidine on digoxin bioavailability. Am. J. Clin. Pharmacol., 24:41–47, 1983.
35. Schenck-Gustafsson, K., and Dahlquist, R.: Pharmacokinetics of digoxin in patients subjected to the quinidine digoxin interaction. Br. J. Clin. Pharmacol., 11:181–186, 1981.
36. Moysey, J. O., Jaggarao, N. S. V., Grundy, E. N., and Chamberlain, D. A.: Amiodarone increases plasma digoxin concentrations. Br. Med. J., 282:272, 1981.
37. Marcus, F. I.: Pharmacokinetic interactions between digoxin and other drugs. J.A.C.C., 5:82–90A, 1985.
38. Pedersen, K. E., Dorph-Pedersen, A., Hvidt, S., Klitgaard, N. A., and Nielsen-Kudsk, F.: Digoxin–verapamil interaction. Clin. Pharmacol. Ther., 30:311–316, 1981.
39. Doherty, J. E., Perkins, W. H., and Wilson, M. C.: Studies with tritiated digoxin in renal failure. Am. J. Med., 37:536–544, 1964.
40. Bloom, P. M., and Nelp, W. B.: Relationship of the excretion of tritiated digoxin to renal function. Am J. Med. Sci., 251:133–144, 1966.
41. Beall, A. C., Johnson, P. C., Driscoll, T., et al.: Effect of total cardiopulmonary bypass on myocardial and blood digoxin concentration in man. Am. J. Cardiol., 11:194–200, 1963.
42. Austen, W. B., Ebert, P. A., Greenfield, L. J., and Morrow, A. G.: The effect of cardiopulmonary bypass on tissue digoxin concentrations in the dog. J. Surg. Res., 2:85–89, 1962.
43. Surawicz, B.: Factors affecting tolerance to digitalis. J.A.C.C., 5:69–81A, 1985.
44. Surawicz, B.: Use of the chelating agent, EDTA, in digitalis intoxication and cardiac arrhythmias. Prog. Cardiovasc. Dis., 2:432–443, 1960.
45. Smith, P. K., Winkler, A. W., and Hoff, H. E.: Calcium and digitalis synergism: the toxicity of calcium salts injected intravenously into digitalized animals. Arch. Intern. Med., 64:322–429, 1939.
46. Kleiger, R., and Lown, B.: Cardioversion and digitalis II. Clinical studies. Circulation, 33:878–886, 1966.
47. Ditchey, R. V., and Curtis, G. P.: Effects of apparently nontoxic doses of digoxin on ventricular ectopy after direct current electrical shocks in dogs. J. Pharmacol. Exp. Ther., 218:212–216, 1981.
48. Haber, E.: Antibodies and digitalis: the modern revolution in the use of an ancient drug. J.A.C.C., 5:111–117A, 1985.
49. Butler, V. P., Jr., and Chen. J. P.: Digoxin-specific antibodies. Proc. Natl. Acad. Sci. USA, 57:71–78, 1967.
50. Schmidt, D. H., and Butler, V. P., Jr.: Reversal of digoxin toxicity with specific antibodies. J. Clin. Invest., 50:1738–1744, 1971.
51. Wenger, T. L., Butler, V. P., Jr., Haber, E., and Smith, T. W.: Treatment of 63 severely digitalis-toxic patients with digoxin-specific antibody fragments. J.A.C.C., 5:118–123A, 1985.
52. Curd, J., Smith, T. W., Jaton, J. C., and Haber, E.: The isolation of digoxin-specific antibody and its use in reversing the effects of digoxin. Proc. Natl. Acad. Sci. USA, 68:2401–2406, 1971.

53. Mandel, W. J., Bigger, J. T., Jr., and Butler, V. P., Jr.: The electrophysiologic effects of low and high digoxin concentrations on isolated mammalian cardiac tissue: reversal by digoxin-specific antibody. J. Clin. Invest., 51:1378–1387, 1972.
54. Smith, T. W.: Discussion paper: use of antibodies in the study of the mechanism of action of digitalis. Ann. N.Y. Acad. Sci., 242:731–736, 1974.
55. Smith, T. W., Lloyd, B. L., Spicer, N., and Haber, E.: Immunogenicity and kinetics of distribution and elimination of sheep digoxin-specific IgG and Fab fragments in the rabbit and baboon. Clin. Exp. Immunol., 36:384–396, 1979.
56. Smith, T. W., Haber, E., Yeatman, L., and Butler, V. P., Jr.: Reversal of advanced digoxin intoxication with Fab fragments of digoxin-specific antibodies. N. Engl. J. Med., 294:797–800, 1976.
57. Fisch, C., and Knoebel, S. B.: Digitalis cardiotoxicity. J.A.C.C., 5:91–98A, 1985.

29

Antiarrhythmic Drugs: Mode of Action, Pharmacokinetic Properties, and Clinical Application

Hrayr S. Karagueuzian, Bramah N. Singh, and William J. Mandel

Cardiac arrhythmias are thought to be caused by abnormalities of cellular electrophysiologic properties of cardiac cells in a given region of the heart.[1,2] The rational use of antiarrhythmic drugs for the management and prevention of these arrhythmias is based on (1) knowledge of cellular electrophysiologic mechanisms leading to the genesis of arrhythmias, (2) knowledge of cellular electropharmacologic properties of antiarrhythmic drugs on cardiac cells at their presumed site of origin, and (3) appreciation of the pharmacokinetic properties of antiarrhythmic drugs. Although at present these requirements are still far from complete, the last decade or so has witnessed significant advances in clarifying arrhythmia mechanisms, electropharmacology, and drug assays in biologic samples. Appreciation of differential electropharmacologic properties of a given antiarrhythmic drug on normal versus diseased myocardium and elucidation of the profound influence exerted by extracellular ions, such as H^+ and K^+, on the action of antiarrhythmic drugs has opened new avenues for a more rational approach to arrhythmia management and prevention. The introduction in clinical cardiology of programmed electrical stimulation of the heart to induce arrhythmias to test antiarrhythmic drug efficacy has provided new insight into effective drug therapy. In this chapter the cellular electrophysiologic mechanisms of antiarrhythmic drugs are discussed in relation to the cellular mechanisms of cardiac arrhythmias. The clinical pharmacokinetic profile of various drugs and their clinical applications will be examined.

Electrophysiologic Basis For Cardiac Electrical Activity

To understand better the cellular mechanisms responsible for cardiac arrhythmias, one must understand the normal cellular mechanisms responsible for cardiac electrical activity (see Chap. 3). Much of the present information has been obtained by recording of transmembrane potential of cardiac fibers with the microelectrode technique and studying the nature and properties of transmembrane flow of ionic current using voltage-clamp studies, ion replacement, and various pharmacologic agents.

Cardiac fibers maintain a transmembrane resting potential because of the dominant permeability of the membrane to potassium ions (K). If this permeability

Dr. H. S. Karagueuzian is the recipient of Research Career Development award HL 01293-03 from the National Heart, Lung, and Blood Institute, Bethesda, MD.

were extremely high compared to the permeability of other ions, the resting membrane potential (Er) would equal the equilibrium potential for K ions (Ek), as governed by the Nernst equation. However, this does not occur because Er usually approaches but is not quite equal to EK because residual background ionic currents carried by other ions are present.[3]

Action potentials are inscribed because of sequential changes in the conductance (permeability) of transmembrane ionic currents, which allows ions to move across the membrane in a direction and at a rate determined by concentration and voltage gradients. Inward currents correspond to a net entry of positive charges, that is, of cations into the cell, and outward currents correspond to a net positive charge leaving the cell. Ionic currents responsible for generating action potentials are not the same for all cardiac fibers. Atrial, ventricular, and Purkinje fibers maintain a relatively high Er (close to Ek) and have many similarities in their processes of depolarization and repolarization. The cells of the sinoatrial node and certain parts of the AV node are special in that they maintain a much lower Er (less negative, that is, approximately −50 mV), and in that their excitatory (depolarizing) currents differ from those of atrial and ventricular fibers. These electrophysiologic differences have important pharmacologic implications, as will be discussed later in the chapter.

In the absence of excitation, atrial and ventricular fibers not engaged in pacemaker activity sustain a steady resting potential (phase 4). On excitation (depolarizing pulses), transmembrane action potential is inscribed. Rapid depolarization (phase 0) carries the membrane potential from −90 to +40 mV. Phase 0 is generated whenever resting potential is rapidly reduced to threshold potential. This occurs because threshold depolarization increases conductance of the fast sodium channel (GNa), a process referred to as *activation of the fast sodium channel.* Inward, depolarizing (excitatory) sodium current carries the membrane potential toward the sodium equilibrium potential (ENa), but before this goal is attained, GNa decreases again, a process referred to as *inactivation of the fast sodium channel.* Both activation and inactivation depend on membrane potential. Repolarization does not immediately follow depolarization, as in nerve and muscle. A plateau (phase 2) region precedes rapid repolarization (phase 3) because of two factors. Depolarization activates another depolarizing channel, called the *secondary, or slow inward, current* (Isi). This channel permits calcium and probably some sodium to enter the cell (inward current) and keep membrane potential fairly constant during phase 2 (plateau). Toward the end of phase 2, Isi decreases because of inactivation, causing a decrease in inward current. At this time another conductance (IX1) is fully activated, which permits rapid outward current carried by K^+ to repolarize the cell (phase 3) and shifts membrane potential back to the resting state. When this occurs, the depolarizing conductances, GNa and Isi, are restored and available again for reactivation (reactivation phase). In sinoatrial and AV nodal cells the fast inward current is absent because the normally present low resting potential inactivates the fast sodium channels. In these cells, the excitatory inward current depends solely on Isi.[3]

Automaticity

Most specialized cardiac cells can develop action potentials in the absence of external stimuli. This is known as *automaticity.* At the end of repolarization (phase 3), the transmembrane potential decreases slowly (spontaneous phase 4 depolarization) until threshold potential and then initiates an action potential. The pacemaker current responsible for spontaneous depolarization and automatic impulse initiation is brought about by decay of time-dependent potassium currents (that differ in various tissues) in the presence of an inward background current, carried mainly by sodium and calcium ions.[4] The conditioning role of the inward background current in spontaneous diastolic depolarization is due to the fact that in the absence of inward background current the potential would nearly equal EK, where a decrease in time-dependent potassium conductance alone would fail to depolarize the cell. In normal Purkinje fibers, the pacemaker current, also known as IK_2, is fully activated at −50 mV and deactivated at −90 mV. In the sinus node the pacemaker current also seems to arise from deactivation of a potassium current that is activated at +20 mV and deactivated at −50 mV. Pacemaker activity can also occur in myocardial fibers when long depolarizing pulses are applied, a mechanism known as *depolarization-induced automaticity* (DIA) or automaticity caused by early afterdepolarization. This form of pacemaker activity is perhaps caused by the deactivation of the IX1 current. The range of activation is −30 to +20 mV, and deactivation occurs at −90 mV. In Purkinje fibers depolarized to −60 mV or less, and manifesting pacemaker activity (abnormal automaticity), the pacemaker current also seems to be brought about by a decay of the slow outward current.[4]

Triggered Automaticity

Triggered automatic impulses, as their name indicates, are a direct result of prior electrical activity. One or multiple impulses initiate (trigger) one impulse or sustained rhythmic activity.[5,6] This occurs because after full repolarization, the triggerable fiber (*e.g.,* atrial, ventricular, mitral valve, Purkinje fiber) develops one or more small depolarizations. These postrepolarization potentials, called *transient depolarizations* (TDs) or *delayed afterdepolarizations* (DAD), are oscillatory afterpotentials (OAPs) that can reach threshold potential and initiate one or more triggered automatic impulses. The pacemaker current responsible for triggered automaticity, known as TI, is activated in the range of −20 to +40 mV and does not follow the characteristic Hodgkin-Huxley kinetics described for other ionic currents. The reversal potential of this current is −5 to −8 mV.[7,8] The TI emerges by various procedures that elevate intracellular calcium ions. The current seems to be carried by sodium and perhaps by calcium ions in both Purkinje and ventricular muscle cells.[7,8]

Cellular Mechanisms of Cardiac Arrhythmias and Effects of Antiarrhythmic Drugs

Cardiac arrhythmias result from abnormalities of impulse initiation, impulse conduction, or both.[9]

Normal Automatic Mechanism and Effects of Antiarrhythmic Drugs

Arrhythmias caused by normal automatic mechanism may arise if impulse initiation in the sinus node is too slow or too fast or if the automaticity of latent pacemakers (atrial, junctional, or ventricular) increases and is faster than the sinus rate. These abnormalities in automatic rates can lead to single, multiple, or sustained ectopic rhythms (tachycardia). Quinidine, procainamide, lidocaine, diphenylhydantoin, disopyramide, aprindine, mexiletine, tocainide, propafenone, and cibenzoline (class I) and beta-blocker (class II) antiarrhythmic agents depress spontaneous phase 4 depolarization of Purkinje fibers in a concentration-dependent manner[10,11] (Table 29-1).

Abnormal Automatic Mechanism and Effects of Antiarrhythmic Drugs

Arrhythmias resulting from abnormal (spontaneous) automaticity (*i.e.,* Er about −60 mV) are resistant to "therapeutic" concentrations of all the above-mentioned antiarrhythmic agents but are suppressed promptly by verapamil (a calcium channel blocker). Similar electropharmacologic profiles are applicable to arrhythmias caused by triggered automatic mechanism and by depolarization-induced automaticity. Verapamil, a secondary inward (slow) channel blocking agent (class IV agent), promptly suppresses both these arrhythmogenic mechanisms (see Table 29-1).

Arrhythmias Caused by Abnormal Conduction (Reentry) and Effects of Antiarrhythmic Drugs

It is now established that both unidirectional conduction block and slow conduction are required for reentrant excitation to occur. Perhaps the most definitive example is provided by the reentrant arrhythmias in the Wolff-Parkinson-White (WPW) syndrome, in which an anomalous accessory pathway exists between the atrium and the ventricle. If in such a heart there is unidirectional

Table 29-1. Comparative Mechanisms of Action of Antiarrhythmic Drugs*

Class	Agent	Depression of Phase 0 and Fast Response	Effect on Action Potential Duration	Sympatholytic Effect	Depression of the Slow Response	Extracardiac Actions
I	Quinidine	++++	Lengthen+	+(Noncompetitive antagonism)	0	Anticholinergic; peripheral vasodilation
	Procainamide	++++	Lengthen+	0	0	
	Lidocaine	++++	Shorten+	0	0	Local anesthetic
	Diphenylhydantoin	++++	Shorten+	0	0	Anticonvulsant
	Disopyramide	++++	Lengthen+	0	0	Anticholinergic
	Aprindine	++++	0	0	+	Anticonvulsant
	Mexiletine	++++	0	0	0	Anticonvulsant
	Tocainide	++++	0	0	0	Local anesthetic
II (β-adrenoceptor blocking drugs)	Propranolol	+	Shorten+	++++(Competitive inhibition)	0	Insignificant
III	Bretylium	Increases phase 4	Lengthen++++	Neuron blockade+	0	Hypotensive
	Amiodarone	Decreases phase 4 only	Lengthen++++	Noncompetitive blockade+	0	Coronary vasodilator
IV	Verapamil	Phase 4 only	Lengthen phases 1 and 2	Noncompetitive blockade+	++++	Coronary vasodilator

* Classification based on electrophysiologic actions[8,36,34]. ++++, principal electrophysiologic action; +, subsidiary effect; 0, no effect in presumed therapeutic plasma concentrations. Propafenone, mexiletine, encanide, flecainide, lorcainide, cibenzoline, ajmaline, and aprinidine are considered class I, and sotalol is considered class III.

conduction block in either the normal or the abnormal AV pathway, reentrant excitation of both the ventricles and the atria may result from continuous and circulatory propagation of the wave of excitation. For example, if anterograde conduction block exists in the abnormal pathway, the impulse propagates from atria to ventricles over the normal AV nodal route and then, if permitted by atrial refractoriness, returns from the ventricles to the atria over the abnormal pathway. It may then propagate once again to the ventricles over the normal pathway.[9] In such a setting prolongation of the refractory period of either antegrade or retrograde direction with, for example, amiodarone (*i.e.,* a class III agent) could be quite useful.

Unidirectional block and slow conduction are highly likely to occur in any part of the heart, causing atrial, junctional, or ventricular reentrant rhythms. Theoretically, all antiarrhythmic drugs at appropriate myocardial concentrations can change the refractoriness or conduction properties of affected cells, with two possible outcomes. First, the fine balance between conduction and refractoriness, necessary to perpetuate reentry, may be altered and reentrant activity promptly terminated. Second, drug-induced changes in conduction and refractoriness may facilitate reentrant excitation.[12] Examples of drug-induced aggravation of arrhythmias are ample. At present, it is impossible to predict accurately whether an antiarrhythmic drug will successfully terminate a reentrant arrhythmia because (1) the cellular electrophysiologic basis for reentry in the intact human heart or in an animal model is unknown and (2) it is not known how a given drug will interact with affected (diseased) myocardial cells engaged in the genesis of reentrant excitation. Normal and diseased cells may respond differently to a given antiarrhythmic agent. Recent intense research aimed at elucidating these electrophysiologic and electropharmacologic peculiarities is encouraging, and further studies should provide a more rational framework for successful pharmacotherapy of reentrant arrhythmias in humans.

Arrhythmias Caused by Simultaneous Abnormalities of Impulse Formation and Impulse Conduction: Effects of Antiarrhythmic Drugs

Under a number of conditions, both impulse formation and impulse conduction may be abnormal.[9,13] Since phase 4 depolarization (normal, abnormal, or oscillatory afterpotential) shifts membrane potential toward zero, there will be partial inactivation of the fast inward depolarizing channel, slowing conduction and favoring reentry. A drug able to stabilize phase 4 is likely to improve conduction velocity, a property that may terminate reentrant excitation. Other examples of coexisting abnormalities of conduction and automaticity are provided by parasystolic foci and discussed elsewhere in this volume.

Basic Pharmacokinetic Principles and Antiarrhythmic Drug Efficacy

A working knowledge of basic pharmacokinetic principles is vital for effective management and control of patients with cardiac arrhythmias. This is so because of the narrow therapeutic ratio (*i.e.,* narrow range between minimum effective and toxic plasma concentration), which requires skillful dose adjustment to prevent undesirable side-effects.[14,15] The ability of an antiarrhythmic drug to suppress reliably or at times even exaggerate an arrhythmia is usually related to drug plasma concentration, which indirectly reflects drug concentration in the vicinity of the site of action in the myocardium. (Amiodarone, however, is an exception.) Later we will discuss the time course of plasma drug concentration and show how various factors can modify blood level curves; at present, we would like to stress that a general knowledge of pharmacokinetic properties of antiarrhythmic drugs is but a guide for instituting initial therapy and that subsequent doses must be adjusted strictly in relation to the patient's clinical course.

Time Course of Plasma Drug Concentration

Rapid Intravenous Injection

When a drug is rapidly injected (bolus injection) into the plasma, it undergoes many physiologic processes (*e.g.,* metabolism, distribution, elimination), all of which reduce the plasma concentration of the drug until the plasma becomes free of the drug. Plasma decay of the drug is often found to be exponential, and experience has shown that simple mathematic transformation, that is, a plot of log plasma concentration (ln Cp) versus time, results in a straight line (monoexponential), which can be of great use to clinicians (Fig. 29-1). A monoexponential decay is expressed by the formula $Cp = Cp_o e^{-K_e t}$, or simply by

$$\ln Cp = \ln Cp_o - Ket \qquad \text{(Eq. 29-1)}$$

in which Cp is plasma drug concentration at time t, K_e is the elimination rate constant ($time^{-1}$), and Cp^o is plasma drug concentration at time zero, obtained by extrapolating the line relating ln Cp versus time to time zero. If the time course of a drug is linear (ln Cp versus time), it is said that the drug behaves according to a one-compartment model (first-order plot). Usually all antiarrhythmic drugs show a plasma decay consistent with two-compartment systems, with the initial, rapid phase of decline corresponding to the rapid distribution of the drug in the

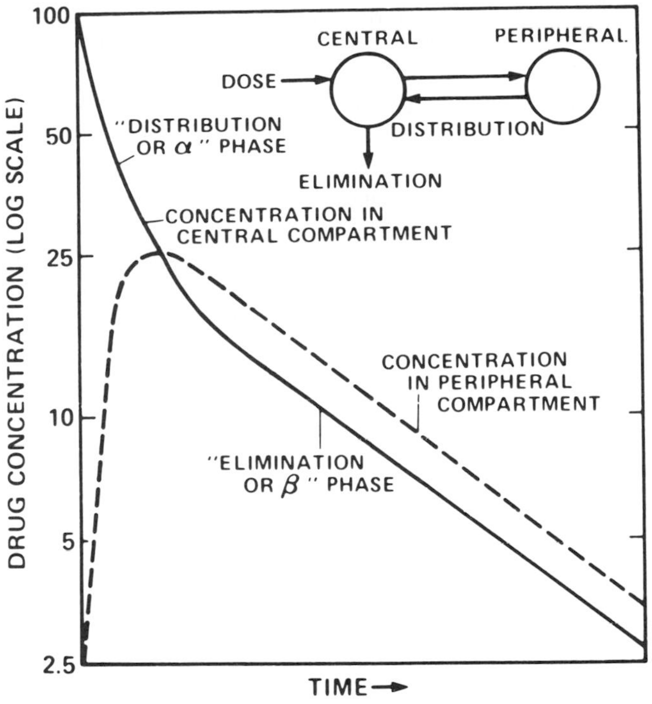

Figure 29-1. *Drug concentrations at various times following a bolus dose, when the body has the characteristics of a one-compartment model. The* inset *shows the same information with concentration plotted on a logarithmic scale. (Harrison, D. C., Meffin, P. J., and Winkle, R. A.: Clinical pharmacokinetics of antiarrhythmic drugs. Prog. Cardiovasc. Dis., 20:217–242, 1977)*

body (central compartment) and the slower compartment corresponding to drug elimination and distribution to a more slowly accessible (peripheral) compartment (Fig. 29-2). Note that most antiarrhythmic drugs are eliminated from the body by renal excretion and hepatic biotransformation, an elimination that proceeds as a first-order process.[14,15] The linear first-order plot offers many useful pharmacokinetic drug properties.

Half-Life. The half-life ($t_{1/2}$) of a drug is defined as the time required for any given plasma concentration to decrease to half, that is,

$$\ln Cp/\ln Cp_o \text{ becomes } 1/2 \text{ in Eq. 29-1}$$

$$\ln 1/2 = 0.693 = K_e t \qquad \text{(Eq. 29-2)}$$

Contrary to a first-order process, a zero-order process does not have a constant half-life. A zero-order process continues at a constant rate independent of the fraction of the process already completed. The following formula describes a zero-order process:

$$t_{1/2} = \frac{0.5 \times Cp^o}{Ko}$$

In such a case, it is inappropriate to discuss half-life for that particular drug, because, as shown in the above equation, the zero-order rate constant (Ko) in the denominator represents a constant value, so that the larger the initial concentration (Cp^o), the longer the apparent half-life will be. Therefore, drugs behaving in this man-

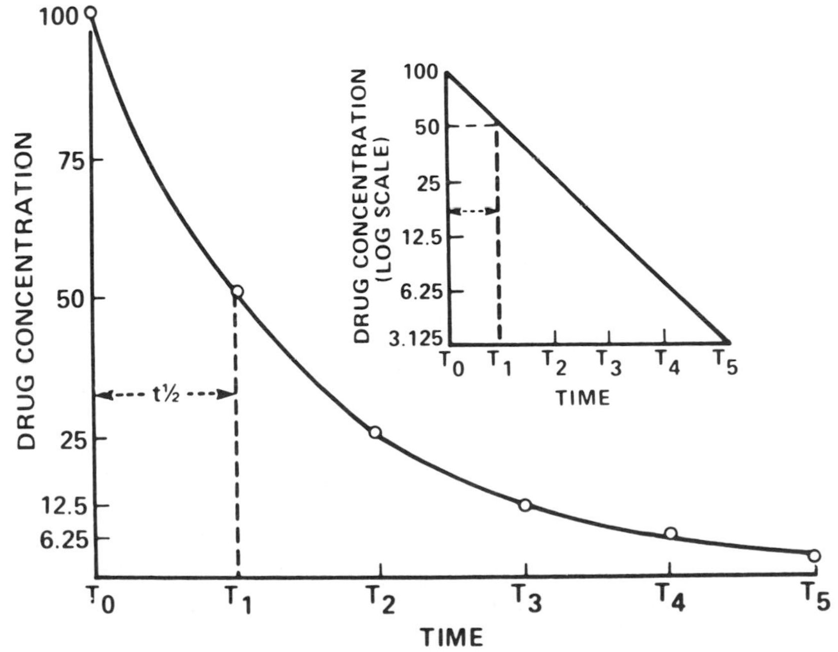

Figure 29-2. *The conceptual representation of a two-compartment model showing reversible distribution between a rapidly equilibrating peripheral compartment. Also shown are the concentrations of drug at various times, both in the central and peripheral compartments, following an intravenous bolus into the central compartment. (Harrison, D. C., Meffin, P. J., and Winkle, R. A.: Clinical pharmacokinetics of antiarrhythmic drugs. Prog. Cardiovasc. Dis., 20:217–242, 1977)*

ner appear to have half-lives that increase with increased dose. Although commonly referred to as *nonlinear kinetics,* this is a misnomer because the plot is linear on ordinary graph paper. The concept refers to *dose-dependent kinetics.* As one increases the dose of such a drug, the kinetic data may change from those of apparent first order (state of no metabolic [enzyme] saturation) to apparent zero order (state of metabolic [enzyme] saturation). Thus, plasma levels of such drugs may not be a linear function of the dose. It is for this reason that their kinetics are termed *nonlinear.* Of the conventional antiarrhythmic drugs, diphenylhydantoin is one drug that manifests this pharmacokinetic behavior.

Volume of Distribution. The volume of distribution or, more properly termed, the *apparent volume of distribution* (Vd), is determined by dividing the concentration of the drug at time zero (extrapolation, see above) to the total amount of the drug administered intravenously (M). This term, often confusing, defines the volume of blood into which the total amount of the drug must be diluted to result in a plasma concentration at time zero:

$$Vd = \frac{M}{Cp_o} \qquad \text{(Eq. 29-3)}$$

where M is the amount of drug administered (*e.g.,* $\underline{X}$ mg and Cp_o plasma drug concentration at time zero [mg/liter]). Note that Vd has the unit of volume and is best considered as a factor that will convert plasma concentration (Cp) to total amount in the body at any desired time (*i.e.,* amount in the body = Cp × Vd).

Continuous Intravenous Infusion. When a drug is continuously infused, the plasma level increases until a constant or steady-state plasma level is achieved. During the steady state (*i.e.,* the period during which the plasma level of the drug is maintained constant), the rate of drug infusion (input) is equal to the rate of elimination (output). Equation 29-4 describes this relation:

$$Ki = Cp_{ss} \times Cl \qquad \text{(Eq. 29-4)}$$

where Ki is the rate of infusion of the drug (such as milligrams per minute), and Cp_{ss}, plasma drug concentration at steady state, and Cl, total body clearance of the drug (milliliters per minute). Equation 29-4 can be rewritten using the parameter of Vd as follows:

$$Cl = K_e \times Vd \qquad \text{(Eq. 29-5)}$$

where K_e is the apparent first-order elimination rate constant ($time^{-1}$). Substituting Equation 29-5 for clearance in Equation 29-4 yields:

$$K_i = Cp_{ss} \times K_e \times Vd \qquad \text{(Eq. 29-6)}$$

Since for the one-compartment model of plasma drug decay (linear semi-logarithmic plot) Ke = $0.693/t_{1/2}$ (Eq. 29-2) Equation 29-6 becomes

$$Ki = \frac{Cp_{ss} \times 0.693 \times Vd}{t_{1/2}} \qquad \text{(Eq. 29-7)}$$

Consequently, if one knows either the clearance (Cl) or the volume of distribution (Vd) and the half-life ($t_{1/2}$) or the elimination rate constant (Ke), Equations 29-4 and 29-7 can be used to calculate the required intravenous infusion rate to achieve any desired steady-state plasma level of a drug. If one accepts 90% of the plasma steady state as a reasonable estimate of the desired therapeutic concentration, then 3.3 half-lives are required for onset of drug action. Therefore, for a drug with a half-life of 2 hours, 6.6 hours are needed to achieve 90% of the desired steady-state plasma drug concentration. It is therefore apparent that slow continuous intravenous infusion will not lead to a rapid therapeutic effect (arrhythmia suppression). This problem is often overcome by the rapid administration of a single dose (*i.e.,* a loading dose). A loading dose is a rapid intravenous injection of a calculated amount of a drug to provide a plasma steady-state amount in the body. This amount can be calculated from Equation 29-3 by substituting the desired steady-state plasma concentration (Cp_{ss}) for the value of C_p.

When steady-state plasma drug concentration is attained by multiple intermittent intravenous doses (D) of a drug, clearance (Cl) and dose (D) become the principal determinants of the average drug concentration (C_{av}), and of the area under the plasma concentration versus time curve:

$$AUC = \frac{D}{Cl} \qquad \text{(Eq. 29-8)}$$

where AUC is the area under the plasma concentration versus time curve. Furthermore, the average plasma drug concentration (C_{av}) can be equated to D and Cl:

$$C_{av} = \frac{D}{Cl \times t} \qquad \text{(Eq. 29-9)}$$

where t is the time interval between intravenous doses.

Oral Drug Administration

When a drug is administered orally or by a route requiring absorption (*e.g.,* buccal, intramuscular, subcutaneous, topical), the time course of the plasma drug concentration will initially increase (input > output), then the concentration will reach a maximum (input = output), and finally it will decay (output > input). The terminal portion of the blood level curve becomes linear (semi-logarithmic plot), and when absorption is sufficiently fast, the slope of this curve will represent the rate constant for elimination; therefore the half-life of the drug can be calculated from Equation 29-2 ($t_{1/2}$ = 0.693/Ke). However, if absorption of the drug is sufficiently slow, the terminal slope of such a plot does not represent Ke, since absorption is still occurring while part of the drug is being eliminated. Therefore, the true half-life of a given drug should be regarded as the one determined by rapid intravenous administration, showing linear kinetics. When the observed half-life of a drug after oral administration is longer than that reported by rapid intravenous administration, a slow rate of absorption is present.

Bioavailability

For complete and total absorption, drug molecules must be fully available for absorption at the absorption site. However, this is often not possible, and one should differentiate between *labeled* and *bioavailable* dose. The labeled dose, for example, the amount per tablet, is the actual chemical content of the dose form, and the bioavailable dose is the amount of the drug that actually enters the blood stream on administration. The bioavailable fraction, F, is the fraction of the labeled dose that is absorbed and enters the blood stream. For example, if 200 mg was absorbed from a tablet containing 250 mg of a given drug, the bioavailable fraction F is

$$\frac{200}{250} = 0.8$$

In intravenous dosing, F = 1 because all the drug is delivered directly to the blood stream. How can one determine the amount of drug that reaches the blood stream after oral administration? Since in Equation 29-8, D is the bioavailable dose, F × D (note F is 1 because of intravenous administration), by rearranging it one obtains

$$AUC = \frac{F \times Dose}{Cl}$$

and thus

$$F = \frac{AUC \times Cl}{Dose} \qquad \text{(Eq. 29-10)}$$

This equation states that the fraction of the drug absorbed may be calculated from a knowledge of the AUC following the oral dose, along with the clearance for that drug and the size of the dose administered. Furthermore, F can also be calculated as the fraction of a drug absorbed orally by the formula

$$F = \frac{AUC_0^{\infty}\,(oral)}{AUC_0^{\infty}\,(IV)} \times \frac{Dose\,(IV)}{Dose\,(oral)} \qquad \text{(Eq. 29-11)}$$

AUC_0^{∞} is the area under the curve from time equals zero to time equals infinity. Some of the antiarrhythmic drugs in which bioavailability problems have been of clinical significance include diphenylhydantoin, procainamide, and quinidine.

Intestinal and First-Pass Metabolism

First-pass metabolism takes its name from the fact that an absorbed drug, after oral administration, passes directly to the liver before reaching the systemic blood circulation. This can result in increased metabolism of the drug and reduced blood levels. For example, the area under the blood level–time curve for lidocaine is significantly greater when the drug is infused into a peripheral vein than when an equal amount is infused into the portal vein in the dog. Introducing the drug directly into the portal vein may be analogous to the pathway after oral administration. Thus, the area under the curve is reduced because the drug is exposed to the liver before it is sampled to determine bioavailability. Furthermore, an intravenous dose is distributed to other parts of the body simultaneously with passage of blood through the liver. Drugs initially distributed to other organs may be temporarily protected from metabolism by the liver. Other mechanisms by which drugs can be metabolized before reaching the systemic circulation may exist. Unless the actual mechanism for metabolism is clearly identified (*i.e.,* first-pass metabolism), it would be more appropriate to refer to such metabolic loss of drug as *presystemic metabolism.* The presystemic, or first-pass, elimination occurs with lidocaine and propranolol (*i.e.,* high hepatic clearance); therefore, alterations of hepatic blood flow will have a major impact on the clearances of these drugs. Because first-pass drug metabolism may be subject to saturation (zero-order), it is possible to observe a nonlinear dependency for the area under the curve (AUC) as a function of the oral dose. Since the drug-metabolizing enzyme will be saturated with increasing oral doses of the drug, more drug will enter the blood stream in intact (unmetabolized) form and thus raise the blood level abruptly (positive deviation form linearity).

Absorption and Diseased States

Physiologic and pathologic differences between persons or in a given person at different times can affect gastrointestinal absorption of drugs. In general, most antiarrhythmic drugs are well absorbed from the small intestine, and absorption from the stomach is relatively insignificant. As a result, any factors that delay the rate of gastric emptying potentially reduce the rate of absorption of orally administered drugs and prevent attainment of peak plasma concentration in the blood, resulting in failure of arrhythmia suppression. Remember that the patient's physiologic state, including level of physical activity and presence or absence of food components forming poorly absorbable complexes with antiarrhythmic drugs, can affect gastrointestinal motility and may alter the bioavailability of antiarrhythmic agents.

Antiarrhythmic Drugs

In the following sections we will discuss the mode of action, pharmacokinetic properties, and clinical use of standard and new investigational antiarrhythmic agents.

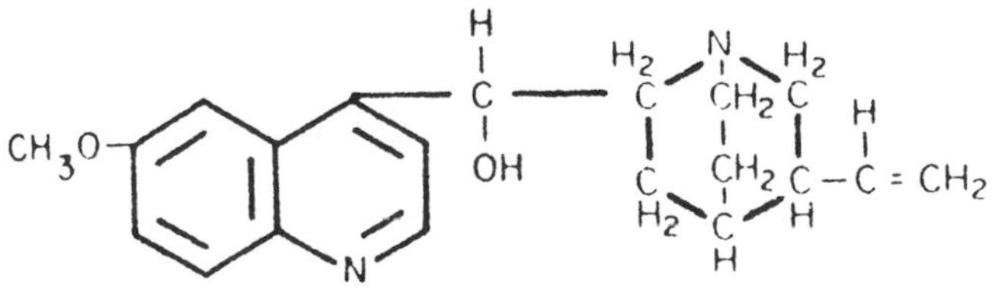

Figure 29-3. *Quinidine.*

Standard Agents

Quinidine

Mode of Action. Microelectrode studies on isolated superfused cardiac preparations have shown that quinidine (Fig. 29-3), at concentrations considered clinically effective, decreases the slope of spontaneous phase 4 depolarization in Purkinje fibers, which arise from a resting potential of −90 to −70 mV, thus decreasing the rate of automatic impulse initiation.[16] In cardiac fibers manifesting abnormal or triggered automatic mechanism, quinidine has no significant effect. The drug causes a concentration-dependent decrease in the maximum rate of depolarization ($\dot{V}_{max}$) and in the overshoot potential and markedly prolongs action potential duration and effective refractory period, with no significant change in resting membrane potential.[16-18] The increase in refractoriness caused by quinidine is greater than the increase in action potential duration (*i.e.,* ratio of ERP/APD is greater than 1), and the effect indicates delay in the reactivation kinetics of the fast sodium channel.[17] In addition, quinidine decreases excitability of atrial and ventricular fibers (*i.e.,* a higher stimulus intensity is needed to elicit an action potential).[18] These electrophysiologic effects might terminate arrhythmias caused by enhanced normal automaticity or by reentry due to changes in refractoriness and, possibly, conduction (depression of $\dot{V}_{max}$).[12,16] Moreover, the decrease in excitability resulting from a shift of threshold potential to a more positive value might significantly decrease the likelihood that a premature impulse would propagate.

More recently it has been emphasized that the degree of depression ($\dot{V}_{max}$) is increased as the rate of stimulation is increased (use-dependent block).[17,18] In addition, greater binding of quinidine to the cardiac sodium channel and thus greater depression of $\dot{V}_{max}$, occurs in partially depolarized cardiac muscle and Purkinje fibers.[17] These observations led Hondeghem and Katzung to suggest that quinidine might selectively slow conduction in partially depolarized "sick" myocardial cells engaged in a reentrant circuit, thus terminating reentrant arrhythmias.[17] Membrane-depressant effects of quinidine (decrease in $\dot{V}_{max}$) and prolongation of effective refractory period are potentiated by an elevated extracellular potassium concentration.[20] Dreifus and associates found that a return to normal values of $\dot{V}_{max}$ and action potential amplitude occurred in the presence of lowered potassium ion concentration.[20] The direct depressant effects of quinidine are masked by its indirect vagolytic and antiadrenergic effects on the heart and vasculature.[19,21] The vagolytic action of the drug may increase heart rate; its antiadrenergic property tends to reduce it. Therefore quinidine administration in unanesthetized humans causes either no change or a slight acceleration in the sinus rate.[22] In situations such as thyrotoxicosis or general anesthesia, where excessive sympathetic activity is present, quinidine almost invariably produces bradycardia.

The interaction between the direct and indirect (autonomic) effects of quinidine have great clinical significance. Josephson and associates found that quinidine prolonged His-Purkinje and intraventricular conduction time in humans.[23] In addition, the refractory periods of the atria and His-Purkinje systems were prolonged, while the effective refractory period of the AV node was consistently shortened. Furthermore, quinidine consistently slowed conduction and increased refractoriness in the accessory pathways in various preexcitation syndromes,[24] a property found quite effective in reducing the ventricular rate in patients with the WPW syndrome complicated by atrial flutter or fibrillation.[25] Heissenbuttel and Bigger[26] have attempted to correlate the electrophysiologic effects of quinidine to its plasma concentration in humans. They found increased QRS duration with increased quinidine plasma concentration ($r = .56$, $P < 0.0001$). The correlation of the QT_c interval with plasma quinidine level was, however, not as high as the QRS ($r = .28$, $p < 0.01$). More consistent prolongation of the QT_c interval was found with toxic plasma concentrations of quinidine. It has been suggested that a nonhomogenous prolongation of refractoriness by quinidine (*i.e.,* temporal dispersion of excitability) favors the development of ventricular fibrillation or atypical ventricular tachycardia known as *torsade de pointes*.[27] These arrhythmias are thought to be the basis of quinidine syncope in many patients.[28] It is worth mentioning that in some patients, torsade de pointes has been observed with quinidine plasma levels considered well below those usually considered toxic.[29,30]

Metabolism and Pharmacokinetics. Quinidine is usually administered orally, occasionally intrasmuscularly, and infrequently intravenously.[22] In humans, quinidine is metabolized (up to 85%) in the liver to two metabolites (hydroxylated compounds) with very little antiarrhythmic activity. These metabolites and the remainder (15% to 20%) of unchanged quinidine are excreted in the urine. The amount of unchanged quinidine recovered in the urine varies inversely with urine *p*H. In alkaline urine quinidine excretion is decreased. These findings are based on recent specific quinidine assay methods.[31] Plasma clearance averaged 4.7 ml/kg/min (range 1.5 to 7.1 ml/kg/min), with a half-life of 6.3 hours (range 3.6 to 8.2 hours). The low clearance of the drug in relation to liver blood flow indicates poor hepatic extraction and explains the good bioavailability of the drug (76%). The intravenous route is not recommended because of profound circulatory depression caused by a large single dose. However, very slow infusion of quinidine has been found safe in patients studied to date.[22,32]

In humans, quinidine is well absorbed orally, mainly in the small intestine. Gastric acidity does not influence quinidine bioavailability; however, gastrointestinal motility and the presence of food in the gut can influence its rate of absorption.[33] Quinidine can be detected in serum within 15 minutes of an oral dose; its onset of action begins within 30 minutes, and peak effects are attained in 1 to 3 hours. Several different oral quinidine salt preparations are prescribed. Quinidine sulfate is rapidly absorbed (peak levels at about 1 to 2 hours), with 60% to 100% of the salt being available for systemic circulation. In contrast, quinidine gluconate is more slowly absorbed, with peak blood levels attained about 4 hours after administration. This salt is less available, and absorption is more erratic (40% to 90%) than with the sulfate salt.[34] The slower absorption rate of gluconate salt allows less frequent administration of quinidine than the sulfate salt (8 to 12 hours as opposed to 4 to 6 hours). The slower absorption process, however, results in lower peak plasma levels of quinidine. The principle of prolonging absorption, with no concomitant change in elimination half-life, is used commercially to increase the duration of action of quinidine in slow-release preparations of sulfate, gluconate, and polygalacturonate. Note that these various salts of quinidine contain different amounts of quinidine base. For example, the sulfate contains 83% of the base, the gluconate 62%, and the polygalacturonate 60%.[14] About 80% of plasma quinidine is bound to albumin.

Although the bound fraction of quinidine does not diffuse out of the vascular compartment, quinidine is still extensively and rapidly distributed to various body tissues. Ueda and colleagues[31] studied the time course of quinidine plasma concentration after intravenous injection and described its disposition by a two-compartment model system. A rapid phase of distribution (*i.e.*, central compartment [alpha phase]) is followed by slower plasma decline (distribution to the peripheral compartment [beta phase]). The volume of the central compartment was 0.9 ± 0.11 liter/kg, and the steady-state volume of distribution was 3.03 ± 0.25 liter/kg. The initial rapid phase of distribution half-life ($t_{½alpha}$) was 7.2 ± 0.7 minutes, and the apparent elimination half-life ($t_{½beta}$) was $6.3 + 0.47$ hours. After an intravenous injection $t_{½beta}$ was similar to $t_{½beta}$ obtained after both oral and intramuscular injections. Concentrations of 1.5 to 6 μg/ml are generally considered therapeutic, and levels of 7 μg/ml and above are associated with an increased incidence of toxicity.

Effects of Renal, Hepatic, and Cardiac Failure on Quinidine Pharmacokinetics. Kessler and associates[35] analyzed the kinetics of quinidine in patients with renal failure by determining quinidine levels using two different assay methods. They concluded that quinidine doses should not be reduced in patients with renal failure, a recommendation consistent with the minor role played by the kidney in eliminating quinidine. No data are available on the effects of liver disease on the kinetics of quinidine. In patients with congestive heart failure,[35] however, the volume of distribution of quinidine and its absorption rate appear to be reduced, with no change in the elimination half-life. These effects should tend to increase plasma quinidine levels. The clinical significance of such an increase remains unknown in light of known large variations in quinidine plasma levels among patients.

Drug Interactions with Quinidine

Quinidine was shown to potentiate the muscle-relaxing effects of certain neuromuscular junction blocking agents[36] and of aminoglycoside antibiotics such as gentamicin, kanamicin, and streptomycin.[37] Because urine *p*H can influence quinidine elimination (in alkaline urine, excretion is decreased), coadministration of drugs that acidify (*e.g.*, acetazolamide, ascorbic acid) or alkalinize (*e.g.*, sodium bicarbonate) the urine are expected to alter the clearance of quinidine. Displacement of quinidine from protein-binding sites with drugs increases the likelihood of toxicity (cinchonism).[38] Koch-Weser[39] observed a potentiation of the anticoagulant effect of warfarin with quinidine, possibly caused by displacement of warfarin from its protein-binding sites. Finally, when quinidine is given to patients taking digoxin, the serum digoxin concentration increases.[40–42] In patients receiving constant glycoside maintenance doses, the addition of quinidine to digoxin therapy resulted in a mean 2.5-fold increase in digoxin plasma levels (from 0.98 ± 0.37 to 2.47 ± 0.7 ng/ml).[40] Although the clinical significance of an increased digoxin level is not clear, patients receiving quinidine and digoxin simultaneously should be closely monitored for a possible reduction in digoxin dose to prevent digitalis-induced toxic arrhythmias.[40] A 30% to 40% reduction of digoxin has been suggested.[40]

Therapeutic Action, Dose, and Side-Effects. Quinidine, the oldest primary antiarrhythmic drug in clinical use, was first described by Wenckebach in 1918.[19] However, as early as 1749, a French physician, Jean-Baptiste de

Senac of Paris,[43] used quinidine successfully in the management of patients with a rhythm disorder that he referred to as *rebellious palpitation* (most likely atrial fibrillation). He described the usefulness of quinidine as follows[44]:

> Of all the stomachic remedies the one whose effects have appeared to be the most constant and the most prompt in many cases is quinidine mixed with a little rhubarb. Long and rebellious palpitation have ceded to this febrifuge seconded with a light purgative.

This interesting and important observation was overlooked for more than two centuries. Even Wenckebach and Frey, who were responsible for the modern use of quinidine,[19] were unaware of de Senac's early important findings.

Quinidine is used to treat a wide variety of arrhythmias of atrial, junctional, and ventricular origin, and it is thus classified as a "broad-spectrum" antiarrhythmic drug. Used alone or in combination with beta-blockers or digoxin, it is of great value in terminating atrial flutter and fibrillation. In patients with AV nodal reentrant supraventricular tachycardia, quinidine alone may not be effective because it does not slow AV nodal conduction. However, it may be successfully used in patients with premature atrial or ventricular depolarization, which may be responsible for initiating the tachycardia. However, quinidine is frequently effective in atrial tachycardia, with or without WPW syndrome.[24,25] Before initiating quinidine therapy in patients with atrial tachycardia, either digoxin or a beta-blocker should be administered to prevent sudden acceleration of the ventricular rate. This occurs because quinidine, because of its vagolytic action, can facilitate AV transmission and can progressively slow the atrial rate of depolarization and may remove concealed AV conduction, allowing more atrial impulses to propagate successfully through the AV node, thereby increasing the ventricular rate. Although quinidine is effective in suppressing most types of ventricular arrhythmias, it is usually not effective in controlling digitalis-induced arrhythmias. In these settings lidocaine and diphenylhydantoin are quite effective. The drug has potentially proarrhythmic effects, perhaps by prolonging the QTc interval. In this context, it has been reported that quinidine can convert nonsustained to sustained ventricular tachycardia[45] and induce torsade de pointes.[30]

A number of methods have been suggested for rapidly achieving and maintaining therapeutic plasma levels of quinidine. For example, quinidine sulfate has often been given orally in 200- to 400-mg doses every 2 hours, followed by maintenance therapy of up to 2.4 g/day. The 2-hourly dose regimen is particularly useful in the chemical conversion of atrial fibrillation. An initial loading dose, which is twice the maintenance dose, has also been recommended for rapid attainment of a plateau plasma concentration, and in this way a single oral dose of 600 mg has been administered safely.[46] If rapid attainment of therapeutic plasma levels is not essential, the maintenance dose of the drug (200 to 400 mg every 6 hours) may be commenced and a steady-state plasma concentration achieved after at least five eliminating half-lives have been exceeded. Adjustment in dose should be dictated by (1) patient response, (2) serum levels, and (3) toxic manifestations. The doses of quinidine gluconate and quinidine polygalacturonate are larger than that of sulfate. A 324-mg tablet of the gluconate is equivalent to 240 mg of quinidine sulfate, and a 275-mg tablet of the polygalacturonate is equivalent to 200 mg of quinidine sulfate. Quinidine, as mentioned earlier, can be given intravenously; if so, 6 to 10 mg/kg of the gluconate should be administered slowly (*i.e.,* 30 to 50 mg/min) with careful and continuous monitoring of the patient's clinical status, blood pressure, and electrocardiogram.[47] Quinidine is potentially very toxic, and its kinetics are highly variable, making plasma level monitoring highly desirable.

Quinidine toxicity (*i.e.,* cinchonism) is characterized by various symptoms ranging from tinnitus, temporary deafness, headache, and blurred vision to diplopia, photophobia, vertigo, confusion, delirium, and, in severe cases, psychosis. Anorexia, nausea, vomiting, diarrhea, and abdominal colic occur frequently (*i.e.,* 20%) in patients taking oral quinidine. These gastrointestinal disturbances, probably due to local irritation, have been reported to be less severe when the polygalacturonate or a slow-release formulation of the sulfate was used.[48] Hypersensitivity reaction to quinidine is not common, but drug fever, urticaria, maculopapular rash, and exfoliative dermatitis have all been reported. Of the other allergic manifestations, anaphylactic reactions are rare, although a variety of hematologic effects have developed during protracted oral quinidine therapy, of which thrombocytopenia is the best known.

Electrocardiographic monitoring of patients receiving maintenance quinidine therapy can detect early signs of toxicity with characteristic widening of the QRS and the QTc intervals, the QRS widening occurring at a lower concentration.[26] In advanced toxicity, the P wave becomes widened and deformed and the sinus rate slows, eventually leading to intra-atrial conduction block and atrial arrest. Simultaneous intraventricular conduction abnormalities may cause ventricular tachycardia and fibrillation (quinidine syncope and sudden death).[28]

Procainamide

Mode of Action. The cellular electrophysiologic properties of procainamide (Fig. 29-4) in isolated cardiac preparations, in both intact animals and humans, are fairly similar to those of quinidine. Microelectrode studies

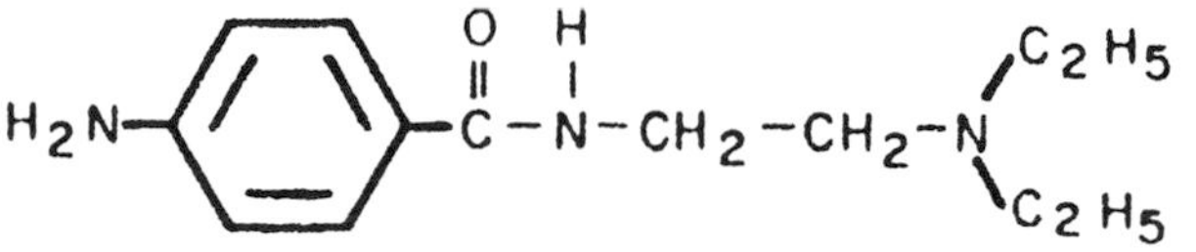

Figure 29-4. *Procainamide.*

have shown that the drug prolongs action potential and refractory period, decreases the rate of automatic impulse initiation and the rate of rise of phase zero ($\dot{V}_{max}$), and slows conduction.[19,49,50] Arnsdorf and Bigger[51] have shown, in isolated Purkinje fibers, that therapeutic concentrations of procainamide shifted threshold potential to a less negative value and shifted the nonnormalized strength duration curve upward and to the right, indicating decreased excitability and increased refractoriness. The decrease in excitability induced by procainamide was not, however, uniform; rather, it depended on the relative contribution of procainamide-induced changes in both passive and active membrane properties.[51] Furthermore, these authors suggested that these findings may explain the conflicting results of cardiac excitability both in clinical and experimental studies, an effect that may also explain the proarrhythmic potential of procainamide in some patients. Procainamide-induced slowing of conduction can further delay retrograde conduction in the depressed segment of a reentry loop, an effect that could convert unidirectional conduction block to bidirectional block. Once this occurs, a reentrant premature depolarization can be terminated. Giardina and Bigger[52] studied the effects of intravenous procainamide in patients with frequent premature ventricular depolarizations. As plasma procainamide concentration was increased (2 to 7 μg/ml), the coupling interval of the premature complexes progressively increased until the premature beat was suppressed.

In humans, procainamide produces a dose-dependent prolongation of the PR, QRS, and QT intervals. Clinical electrophysiologic studies have shown prolonged refractory periods in the atrium, ventricle, and His-Purkinje system and slowed conduction in the His-Purkinje system as indicated by a 10% to 30% prolongation of the HV interval.[53] All these effects, however, along with effects on heart rate and AV conduction, are quite variable because of the vagolytic actions of procainamide on the heart.[19] Vagal inhibition induced by procainamide offsets its direct myocardial depressant actions. Note that procainamide shifts the strength interval curve of the right ventricular endocardium in humans upward and to the right as in isolated cardiac tissue preparation.[54]

Metabolism and Pharmacokinetics. Absorption of oral procainamide is rapid and virtually complete. Koch-Weser[55] studied the gastrointestinal absorption of the hydrochloride salt of procainamide in fasting healthy subjects. After a 15- to 20-minute "lag time," first-order absorption kinetics were seen with a $t_{1/2}$ of absorption of 20 to 30 minutes. In healthy subjects peak plasma levels are reached in 1 hour. Graffner and colleagues,[56] using titrated procainamide, found that the area under the plasma concentration curve (AUC) after a single oral dose was 75% of that observed after intravenous injection of the same dose. These authors estimated that the "first-pass," or presystemic, elimination was approximately 15%. The extent of oral procainamide absorption in patients, however, is more variable. In patients with severe heart failure or myocardial infarction, intestinal absorption of procainamide is usually delayed and produces lower peak plasma levels.[57] An initial intravenous administration of procainamide in such patients was suggested as being more effective. Absorption of procainamide from sustained-release preparations is slower, which could lead to less fluctuation in plasma procainamide levels.[58] Absorption after intramuscular injection is fast and complete; peak levels are reached within 20 to 30 minutes.[59] However, intramuscular injections are painful and may raise plasma creatine phosphokinase and produce peak plasma levels fairly slowly, especially in patients with low cardiac output.

Procainamide is rapidly and extensively distributed to various body tissues. The highest concentrations occur in the liver, lungs, kidneys, and heart. The ratio of myocardial tissue to plasma procainamide concentration is about 4.[49,59,60] Fifteen percent of procainamide is bound to serum albumin. The apparent volume of distribution of procainamide in subjects with normal renal, hepatic, and cardiac function ranges between 1.7 to 2.2 liter/kg and is smaller in patients with low cardiac output (1.5 to 1.8 liter/kg). The rate of distribution of procainamide after intravenous administration is rapid (alpha phase) (average half-life about 5 minutes)[58,61–67]; it is complete within 20 minutes. After an initial rapid distribution, elimination half-life ($t_{1/2\ beta}$) of procainamide is between 2.2 and 3.7 hours in subjects with normal kidney and liver function. First-order elimination kinetics are observed over a wide range of plasma concentrations (0.5 to 26 μg/ml), indicating that the elimination of procainamide is not a saturable process in this range.

Procainamide is metabolized in the liver through the action of polymorphic enzyme *N*-acetyltransferase, with conversion of the parent product to *N*-acetylprocainamide (NAPA). Dreyfuss and colleagues[69] were the first to discover NAPA in the urine of rhesus monkeys and, later, in the pooled urine of four humans. The rate and extent of procainamide acetylation depends on the genetically determined "acetylator phenotype."[63–65, 69–71] Renal clearance is the major route of elimination of procainamide, with some 40% to 54% of the administered dose appearing in the urine. The 24-hour urinary excretion of NAPA under steady-state conditions varies between 6% and 25% of the administered dose. Between 2% and 10% of the administered dose is hydrolyzed to para-aminobenzoic acid.

The electrophysiologic and antiarrhythmic properties of NAPA are similar to those of procainamide.[49,61] When plasma monitoring of NAPA and procainamide is performed simultaneously to assess drug efficacy, NAPA, in contrast to its parent compound, is almost entirely eliminated by the kidney, with a lower clearance (180 ml/min).[62,64] The half-life of elimination of NAPA in patients with normal renal function is about twice that of procainamide (6 to 8 hours); its apparent volume of distribution is 1.38 liter/kg, and it appears to be well tolerated to levels as high as 40 μg/ml.

Renal insufficiency prolongs the plasma half-life of both procainamide and NAPA. Urinary excretion of these agents correlates very well with creatine clearance. Gibson and colleagues[64] found the half-life ($t_{½beta}$) of procainamide to increase 11.3 to 16 hours in patients with renal failure. Urinary *p*H can influence the elimination of procainamide. Renal clearance of procainamide increases with decreasing urine *p*H (aciduria) and decreases with increasing urine *p*H (alkaluria). This can be explained by the phenomenon of ion trapping. As the free base, procainamide, enters the urine from the plasma by passive diffusion, it becomes charged (protonated) in acid urine. This charged form cannot reenter the plasma (ion trapping) and is therefore eliminated in the urine.

Therapeutic Action, Dosage, and Side-Effects. Procainamide is effective in preventing and suppressing both ventricular and supraventricular arrhythmias. It is of particular value in patients with life-threatening ventricular arrhythmias who fail to respond to lidocaine.[72] Procainamide therapy is also effective in patients with the WPW syndrome[24,25,73]; however, this effect does not seem to be uniform.[72] Intravenous procainamide produces somewhat less cardiovascular depression than quinidine, although its negative inotropic effects are not negligible. Giardina and co-workers[74] found that 100 mg of the drug can be safely given intravenously every 5 minutes to a total of 1 g. However, during intravenous administration of procainamide, both blood pressure and electrocardiogram should be monitored continuously and the rate of drug administration should not exceed 50 mg/min.[55] The average patient requires 50 mg/kg/day of oral procainamide to achieve and maintain an acceptable therapeutic plasma level of 4 to 8 μg/ml.[55,58] The intramuscular route offers little advantage over the oral route in most instances. It may be necessary to adjust the dose of procainamide to take into account plasma NAPA concentrations, since this metabolite has antiarrhythmic efficacy and a longer half-life. The patient who is a fast or slow "acetylator" may be unmasked by monitoring plasma levels of both compounds.

The limitations of procainamide therapy are largely caused by potentially troublesome side-effects, which often occur after prolonged use of high doses of the drug. Toxic cardiac effects of procainamide manifested by progressive lengthening of the QTc interval and QRS duration are in general similar to those of quinidine and appear with a plasma concentration over 12 μg/ml. However, sudden death or recurrent syncope due to ventricular tachycardia or ventricular fibrillation is less common than with quinidine use. During chronic oral administration, gastrointestinal side-effects such as anorexia, nausea, vomiting, or diarrhea are common, especially with high doses. Hematologic complications such as leukopenia and agranulocytosis have been reported.[74] A syndrome resembling systemic lupus erythematosus may appear in up to 40% of patients chronically treated with procainamide.[76] The initial symptoms of this syndrome may appear as early as 2 weeks after the start of therapy up to several years later and include fever, rash, myalgia, arthralgia, arthritis, pericarditis, pleuritis, hepatosplenomegaly, and occasionally pericardial tamponade. This syndrome is associated with high antinuclear titers and is more likely to occur in patients who are slow acetylators of procainamide.[77] These drug-induced symptoms fortunately disappear when procainamide is discontinued. If they persist, corticosteroid therapy may be helpful in eliminating them.

Disopyramide

Disopyramide (Norpace) (Fig. 29-5) has been approved for general clinical use since 1977.

Mode of Action. The cellular electrophysiologic properties of disopyramide (Fig. 29-6) are fairly similar to those of quinidine and procainamide. Disopyramide, in isolated Purkinje fibers, increases action potential duration and refractory periods with a concomitant decrease in

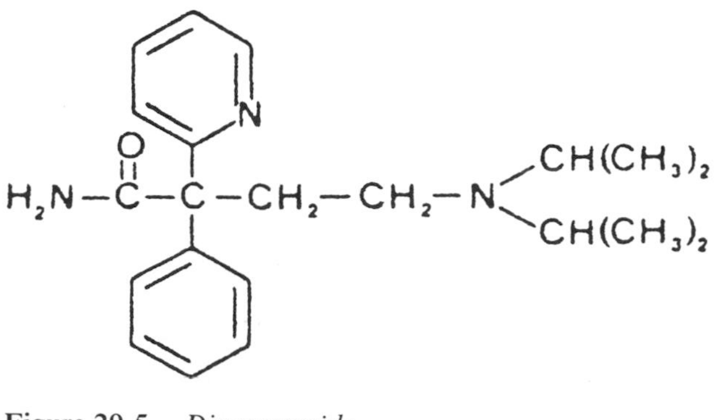

Figure 29-5. *Disopyramide.*

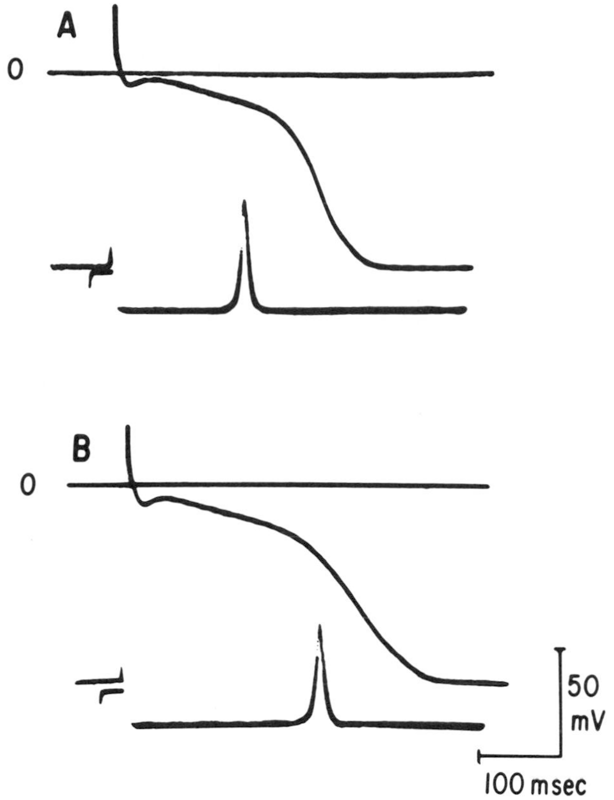

Figure 29-6. *Effect of disopyramide, 10^{-5} M, on Purkinje fiber action potential (cycle length = 500 msec; T = 37° C). In A and B, the top trace is a reference, zero potential; the middle trace is an action potential recorded using an intracellular glass microelectrode; and the bottom trace is the electronically differentiated upstroke of a sawtooth wave, with a rate of rise of 200 V/sec followed by the differentiated phase 0 upstroke of the action potential, $\dot{V}_{max}$. A is a control. B shows effects of disopyramide, 10^{-5} M. Note the decrease in action potential amplitude and $\dot{V}_{max}$ and the prolongation of the voltage-time course of repolarization. (Danilo, P., and Rosen, M. R.: Cardiac effects of disopyramide. Am. Heart J., 92:532–536, 1976)*

action potential amplitude and maximum rate of rise of phase zero and conduction velocity; it does not affect resting membrane potential[78] (see Fig. 29-6). Disopyramide has no appreciable effect on slow-response action potentials but suppresses the slope of spontaneous diastolic depolarization in Purkinje fibers with high resting membrane potentials.[79] Lowering the extracellular potassium concentration tends to reverse the membrane-depressant effects of the drug.[20] In addition, disopyramide has important anticholinergic (atropinelike) properties[21] that often offset its direct membrane-depressant effects on the myocardium. For example, its depressant effect on AV conduction is nullified or even reversed so that the PR interval may be little altered or even shortened.[80] Pretreatment with atropine (0.02 mg/kg) allows more uniform inducement of the depressant effects of disopyramide, namely, prolonged AH interval and functional refractory period of the AV node, prolonged sinus nodal recovery time, and slowed heart rate.[81] Recently, Katoh and associates[82] have shown, using the microelectrode technique on isolated rabbit sinoatrial preparations, that disopyramide depresses sinus nodal automaticity at upper therapeutic and toxic levels during cholinergic blockade; its acelearoty action on the sinus node appears at a much lower concentration and only during cholinergic stimulation. These results indicate that earlier observations of disopyramide, which reported variable effects on conduction and sinus rate, could have been due to its inhibitory effects on vagal tone. However, in high doses, direct depressant effects predominate, including widening of the QRS and QT intervals and slowing of the sinus rate.

Metabolism and Pharmacokinetics. At present, the metabolism and pharmacokinetic disposition of disopyramide have not been completely determined,[83] particularly in various disease states. Ward and Kingham[84] reported that postinfarction patients achieved about a twofold lower concentration of disopyramide after oral administration of 100 mg than did healthy subjects, who attained a peak level of about 3 μg/ml. Orally administered disopyramide phosphate is well absorbed, albeit relatively slowly, with a bioavailability of approximately 90%.[85,86] Peak serum concentrations generally occur 2 to 3 hours after administration and may be maintained for several hours, since the terminal half-life ($t_{½beta}$) of disopyramide is 5 to 6 hours in healthy persons.[84–87] Total disopyramide clearance is approximately 1.5 ml/min/kg, and its apparent volume of distribution is 0.8 liter/kg. Serum binding of disopyramide decreases with increasing serum concentration; at therapeutic concentration range (2 to 6 μg/ml) about 30% to 50% of the drug in the serum is free.[86–88] In this concentration range the free fraction varies relatively little, and no important clinical consequences related to the protein binding of disopyramide have been reported. Note that because the clearance of the drug depends on its free levels and because the level of free drug increases as the concentration of disopyramide is increased (protein unbinding), disopyramide displays nonlinear pharmacokinetics with respect to total drug concentration. For this reason, there is less than proportional increase in total drug concentration as the dose is increased. With multiple doses, however, the free concentration does not increase linearly with dose. The major metabolite of disopyramide, the N-dealkylated form, has some antiarrhythmic efficacy (about 50% of the parent drug); it is formed in the liver and excreted in the urine.

Therapeutic Action, Dose, and Side-Effects. Disopyramide is effective in suppressing premature depolarizations and tachycardias of both supraventricular and ventricular origin.[89–91] Its ability to prolong conduction time and refractory period of the accessory pathway in patients with WPW syndrome may also be quite useful in the management of arrhythmias associated with the preexcitation syndrome.[92] In patients with supraventricular arrhythmias, disopyramide has been used to prevent recurrences of atrial fibrillation after direct current conversion to sinus rhythm. Disopyramide was also found to terminate paroxysmal supraventricular tachycardia, atrial flutter, and atrial fibrillation of recent onset.[91] However, the atropinelike actions of disopyramide make the drug of limited value in the management of patients with paroxysmal atrial tachycardias resulting from AV nodal reentry. Moreover, facilitation of AV conduction in susceptible patients may actually increase the ventricular response rate in atrial flutter and fibrillation.

In a large multicenter study,[93] disopyramide was found to suppress ventricular arrhythmias effectively. Furthermore, in a double-blind comparative study with quinidine, disopyramide was found to have similar efficacy in suppressing ventricular premature depolarizations, with an overall decrease of about 88% with disopyramide and 93% with quinidine.[94] The incidence of side-effects, however, was higher with quinidine. Recent studies have also indicated that disopyramide may be of value in the prophylaxis of ventricular arrhythmias in patients with recent myocardial infarction.[95,96] Rangno and colleagues[97] showed that in postinfarction patients the drug had a somewhat reduced clearance and prolonged half-life of about 12 hours, presumably due to impaired renal function. These authors suggested that a suitable intravenous regimen would be 2 mg/kg over 15 minutes, then 2 mg/kg over the next 45 minutes, followed by a maintenance infusion of 0.4 mg/kg/hr. Such a regimen would yield a plasma level of about 4 μg/ml in patients with an average clearance level of 57 ml/min. These doses should be reduced in patients who show greater reductions in creatinine clearance.

In most patients, plasma levels of disopyramide within a 2 to 4-μg/ml range can be achieved with daily divided doses of 400 to 1200 mg. If rapid attainment of therapeutic levels is desired, a loading dose of the drug (200 to 300 mg) can be given, followed by maintenance doses every half-life (5 to 6 hours). Recently a sustained-release preparation (Norpace CR®) has become available, allowing a 12-hour dosage schedule. Intravenous disopyramide (2 mg/kg) exerts mild negative inotropic action on the heart, an effect less apparent after oral administration. Although disopyramide is well tolerated after oral administration, 10% to 40% of patients reported side-effects due to anticholinergic activity of the drug, including dry mouth, urinary hesitancy, constipation, blurred vision, and dry eyes, nose, and throat.[94] Although the drug is similar to quinidine in many respects, disopyramide-induced "syncope" (ventricular tachycardia and ventricular fibrillation) or marked QTc prolongation have not been reported with usual maintenance doses of disopyramide.

Observations in patients with recent myocardial infarction have suggested that the drug exerts more profound negative inotropic effects in this patient group.[98] The exact etiology of this effect in the setting of acute myocardial infarction is unclear.

Lidocaine

Mode of Action. Microelectrode studies on isolated cardiac tissue preparations have shown that lidocaine (Fig. 29-7) invariably shortens action potential duration and refractoriness but delays the reactivation process of excitability.[17,19,99,100] Maximum rate of rise of phase zero ($\dot{V}_{max}$) is decreased in a concentration-dependent manner with a depression of membrane responsiveness.[17] These effects are more pronounced in the presence of 4 to 5.4 mM extracellular potassium concentration and are negligible or nonexistent when extracellular potassium concentration is lowered to 2.7 mM.[100–102] These membrane-depressant effects, when present, are expected to slow conduction velocity and could thus theoretically convert areas of unidirectional conduction block into bidirectional block, thus terminating reentrant arrhythmias.[12,20] Lidocaine seems to exert a preferentially greater membrane-depressant effect on ischemic and hypoxic myocardial cells than on normal cardiac fibers.[17] Isolated tissue studies with microelectrodes have shown a greater degree of depression of $\dot{V}_{max}$ and conduction velocity as well as slower recovery from the process of inactivation with lidocaine in acidic and hypoxic media.[107,108] Lidocaine at therapeutic concentrations can abolish tetrodotoxin-sensitive depressed fast responses in depolarized tissues that still depend on the sodium channel.[104,105]

More recently, Lamenna and colleagues[106] have shown that lidocaine impairs conduction through potassium-depolarized isolated Purkinje fibers, an effect these authors suggest is caused by suppression of a background sodium current.[106] This may impart to lidocaine signifi-

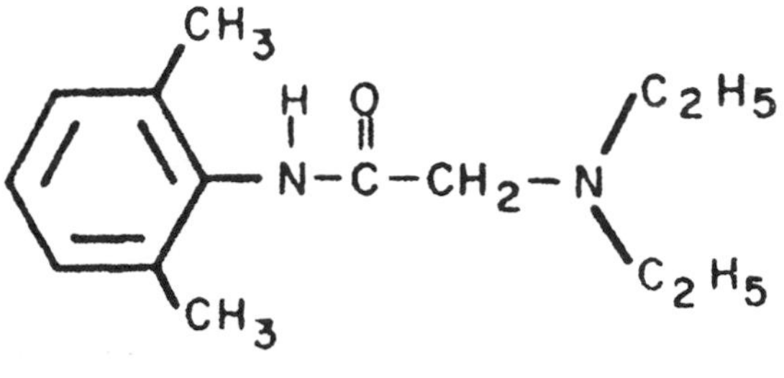

Figure 29-7. *Lidocaine.*

cant antiarrhythmic properties in a setting of ischemic arrhythmias.[12,20] The degree of shortening of action potential duration and refractoriness of Purkinje fibers by lidocaine is related to the particular location of the Purkinje fiber cell, since the most pronounced effect is seen at a site close to where the free running strands insert into the ventricular myocardium. Furthermore, lidocaine causes the greatest changes in action potential duration and refractoriness in normal Purkinje fibers, in which these parameters are very long to begin with.[100] Lidocaine suppresses spontaneous diastolic depolarization and automatic impulse initiation at membrane potentials between −90 and −70 mV. This occurs at lidocaine concentrations that do not affect sinus node automaticity.[109] Lidocaine was also found to decrease the amplitude of ouabain-induced delayed afterdepolarization in Purkinje fibers[110]; however, such an effect was not seen in ventricular fibers.[111] In long mammalian Purkinje fibers superfused with lidocaine containing 4 mM of potassium, Arnsdorf and Bigger[99,112] found that lidocaine shifted the nonnormalized strength-duration curve toward higher current levels to elicit an action potential without altering resting membrane or threshold potential. These effects differ from those of procainamide in that lidocaine does not shift membrane threshold potential to less negative values, as does procainamide; rather, it increases threshold current primarily by increasing subthreshold membrane conductance. More recently, Karagueuzian and associates[113,114] have shown that lidocaine had no effect on the strength-interval curve of the right ventricular endocardium in intact dogs.

Metabolism and Pharmacokinetics. Lidocaine is primarily eliminated by metabolism in the liver, which is extremely efficient in removing the drug from the circulation. As a result of this very high hepatic extraction, the clearance of lidocaine approaches hepatic blood flow.[14,115] Furthermore, lidocaine clearance and lidocaine plasma concentration are greatly influenced by alteration in liver blood flow.[115] A large number of metabolites of lidocaine have been identified, and two metabolites that have some pharmacologic action have undergone clinical experimental investigations, namely, the monoethylglycine xylidide metabolite (MEGX), which has some antiarrhythmic efficacy,[116] and the glycine xylidide (GX), which potentiates the convulsant action of both lidocaine and MEGX. Lidocaine is not recommended orally because of high presystemic (hepatic) elimination of some 80% of the dose.[14] When doses four to five times higher are administered in an attempt to achieve therapeutic plasma levels similar to procainamide, considerable toxic side-effects ensue. In addition, gastric irritation becomes a major clinical problem. Attempts have been made to develop congeners of lidocaine that are less efficiently extracted by the liver so that they could be orally effective. Tocainide and mexiletine seem useful in this regard (see below).

Disposition of lidocaine may be explained on the basis of the linear two-compartment model. In healthy persons the $t_{½alpha}$ of the rapid phase of distribution is about 8 minutes, and the $t_{½beta}$ of elimination from the peripheral compartment is around 100 minutes. The volume of the central compartment is approximately 0.44 liter/kg, and the volume of distribution (steady state) is 1.11 liter/kg, with a total body clearance averaging 10 ml/min/kg. Very little (> 3%) lidocaine is excreted unchanged in the urine; thus renal function impairment has no significant effect on lidocaine pharmacokinetics. However, in patients with heart failure, lidocaine clearance is reduced to about 60% because of reduced liver blood flow. Consequently, some 60% reduction in the maintenance dose of lidocaine should be contemplated in these patients to avoid toxic side-effects. Similar considerations should also apply in patients with liver disease and reduced hepatic blood flow.[14]

Therapeutic Action, Dose, and Side-Effects. Lidocaine is very effective against ventricular arrhythmias of diverse clinical etiologies (*e.g.*, surgery, ischemic heart disease, digitalis toxicity). It is considered the drug of choice for the emergency intravenous therapy of patients with ventricular arrhythmias[117] because it is relatively devoid of toxic side-effects and because antiarrhythmic plasma concentration can be rapidly achieved by intravenous titration.[14] Intravenous prophylactic lidocaine given for 48 hours after the onset of symptoms indicating acute myocardial infarction was found to be of value in preventing primary ventricular fibrillation.[118-120] In rare cases lidocaine may aggravate arrhythmias and may even be lethal.[121] These "paradoxic" effects of lidocaine require further investigation. Lidocaine is considered relatively ineffective in the management of patients with supraventricular arrhythmias.[117,122] The lesser sensitivity of atrial fibers to lidocaine was attributed by Kabela[123] to a smaller efflux of potassium ions from atrial fibers than from ventricular muscle and Purkinje fibers. However, lidocaine may be quite useful against supraventricular tachyarrhythmias in patients with WPW syndrome, in whom atrial impulses conducting antegradely over an AV bypass tract may be slowed.[124]

The therapeutic range of plasma lidocaine levels is 1.6 to 5 μg/ml.[14] As discussed earlier, the infusion rate at steady state is equal to the desired steady-state plasma concentration multiplied by the clearance. For example, if a 3 μg/ml steady-state plasma lidocaine level is desired, with a clearance of 10 ml/kg/min, the infusion rate of lidocaine should be 30 μg/kg/min. If in patients with heart failure the clearance is reduced by 50%, the infusion rate then becomes 15 μg/kg/min.

In patients with relatively normal weight and cardiac

output, a total of about 175 mg of lidocaine should be given in the first 10 to 15 minutes. This dose is given as a single intravenous injection over 5 to 10 minutes or as a series of small injections several minutes apart.[125] If arrhythmias recur during this initial phase, a small (25 to 50 mg) bolus injection should be given while a constant infusion of 2 to 4 mg/min, initiated after the loading dose, is continued. When breakthrough arrhythmias occur after steady-state conditions have been attained, a further small bolus and a temporary increase in infusion rate become necessary.

Lidocaine is considered relatively safe and free from adverse hemodynamic side-effects. The most commonly reported adverse effects are related to central nervous system toxicity, including dizziness, paresthesias, confusion, delirium, stupor, seizure, and coma. The drug normally has minimal depressant effects on the cardiac conducting system.[124] Larger doses, however, may produce heart block due to a preexisting abnormally long His-Purkinje conduction time.[126] Life-threatening increases in ventricular rates have been reported after lidocaine administration in patients with atrial tachyarrhythmia and rapid ventricular response.[121] However, clinically significant adverse hemodynamic effects rarely occur. Note that when propranolol is administered with lidocaine, clearance is decreased and plasma level of lidocaine increases because propranolol decreases hepatic blood flow.[14,127]

Diphenylhydantoin

Diphenylhydantoin (DPH), formerly known as phenytoin (Fig. 29-8), has a limited role in the management of patients with cardiac arrhythmias, since it is both devoid of potent inherent antiarrhythmic effects and associated with a wide range of toxic side-effects.

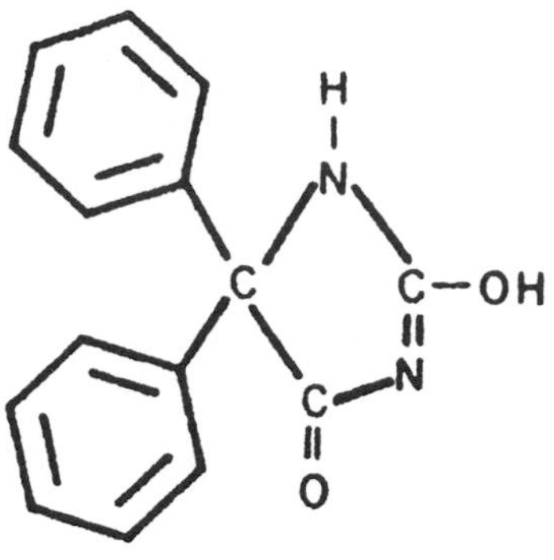

Figure 29-8. *Diphenylhydantoin.*

Mode of Action. Microelectrode studies have shown that DPH depresses the slope of both spontaneous phase 4 depolarization and the amplitude of ouabain-induced afterdepolarizations in Purkinje fibers,[128-130] slowing automatic impulse initiation and eventually suppressing ectopic automatic foci. Like lidocaine, DPH depresses the maximum rate of phase zero depolarization in a concentration-dependent manner (2 to 25 μg/ml), that is, depending on extracellular potassium concentration.[131] With a low potassium level (3 mM), the membrane-depressant effect of DPH is minimal. The drug markedly shortens action potential duration and delays reactivation kinetics of the fast sodium inward current, as do other antiarrhythmic drugs.[17,19] This effect leads to delay in excitability.

It has been suggested that some of the antiarrhythmic properties of DPH may be mediated through its central nervous system depressant actions.[11,19] Since AV nodal cells are highly innervated, DPH-induced effects on the AV transmission may be at least partly explained by the initial state of autonomic tone and the nature and extent of interaction of DPH with sympathetic or parasympathetic components of the autonomic nervous system.

Metabolism and Pharmacokinetics. Diphenylhydantoin is eliminated almost entirely by metabolism by hepatic microsomal enzyme systems, which convert DPH to 5-phenylhydantoin by parahydroxylation.[132] The elimination of DPH is an example of zero-order kinetics (nonlinear); that is, the metabolism (elimination) becomes a saturated process over the therapeutic range of plasma concentration (10 to 20 μg/ml). Once the process of elimination becomes saturated, the clearance of DPH becomes progressively reduced and its half-life prolonged as dose increases.[132-134] Most patients can metabolize at least 10 mg/kg/day[135]; however, this may change with disease states and administration of other drugs. Bishydroxycoumarin, chloramphenicol, isoniazide, chlorpromazine, prochlorperazine, chlordiazepoxide, and diazepam inhibit DPH metabolism by competing for hepatic enzymes, whereas carbamazepine and phenobarbital stimulate DPH metabolism, mostly through microsomal enzyme induction.[14] The dose at which metabolism becomes saturated varies quite widely among patients, and at best the clinician can only approximate average pharmacokinetic values. Therefore, continuous plasma monitoring of DPH levels is highly desirable. An average half-life value of 22 hours can be used as a guide.[14] Thus three to five half-lives (3 to 4 days) are required to reach a steady state.

In healthy subjects, 90% of DPH is protein bound, mostly to albumin,[136] but this can be altered by various disease states. Decreased binding was seen in patients with renal failure, hypoalbuminemia, the nephrotic syndrome, and hyperbilirubinemia as well as those receiving phenylbutazone and salicylic acid. These situations therefore tend to increase the concentration of free DPH, causing toxic side-effects. However, with the availability of greater free to bound DPH ratios, greater metabolism of DPH should be expected if microsomal enzymes are not yet saturated. The importance of those considerations is that similar total DPH plasma concentration may be associated with quite variable free, unbound plasma DPH levels. Therefore, total DPH plasma levels should not be used for accurate monitoring; free DPH levels should be considered instead. Finally, DPH metabolism can be altered significantly by a genetically determined defect in parahydroxylation.[137] Such patients can be expected to maintain higher DPH levels for a given dose, with an attendant decrease in clearance and prolonged half-life.

Therapeutic Action, Dose, and Side-Effects. The use of DPH as an antiarrhythmic agent is usually limited to the management of patients with atrial and ventricular arrhythmias caused by digitalis toxicity.[138] Ventricular arrhythmias associated with other disease processes respond much less frequently to DPH.[138–141] Some success has been noted in the management of patients with ventricular arrhythmias associated with general anesthesia, cardiac surgery, and direct current cardioversion of atrial tachyarrhythmias.[122] The drug is not considered effective in the management of atrial arrhythmias *not* caused by digitalis toxicity. It is generally given orally, 750 to 1000 mg in divided doses for loading, followed by 300 to 400 mg daily. If given intravenously, small doses (30 to 50 mg/min) are injected to avoid hypotension, until toxicity develops (nystagmus) or 1000 mg is reached.[141] For oral maintenance, appropriate allowances should be made for other drugs being given and for the state of the patient's hepatic function.

Intravenous DPH can cause severe hypotension, especially in the elderly. This effect is dose related and occurs with rapid intravenous loading. It is, however, transient, rarely lasting more than 20 minutes. The most common manifestations of DPH toxicity relate to central nervous system effects, including nystagmus, dizziness, ataxia, stupor, and coma. Adverse electrophysiologic effects are rare. Diphenylhydantoin may cause sinus node depression and bradycardia, increased ventricular response to atrial flutter or fibrillation (facilitation of AV conduction), or even AV block.[130]

A number of unusual syndromes with unknown etiology may also develop in patients receiving chronic oral DPH therapy. Salient among these is gingival hyperplasia, which may develop in up to 40% of patients. Other complications include systemic lupus erythematosus, pseudolymphoma, osteomalacia, peripheral neuropathy, megaloblastic anemia, and a variety of dermatologic disorders including pigmentation and hirsutism. The development of lymphadenopathy is often diagnostically confusing but disappears when DPH is withdrawn.

Propranolol

Mode of Action. The antiarrhythmic properties of propranolol (Fig. 29-9) are brought about by (1) beta-adrenergic receptor blocking properties, which occur at low

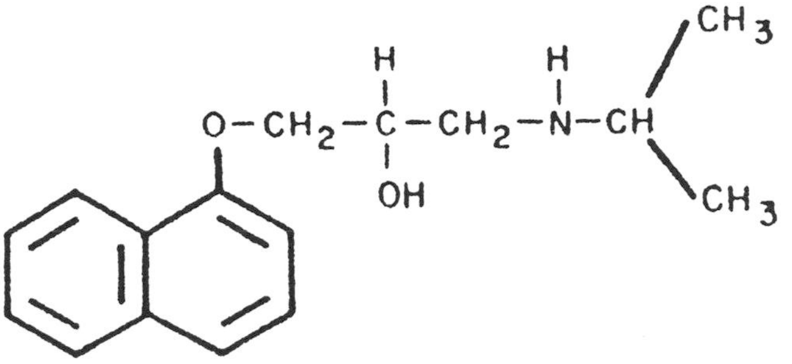

Figure 29-9. *Propranolol.*

plasma levels (25 to 500 ng/ml) and by (2) direct "membrane-depressant" actions, which occur at higher plasma levels.

On isolated cardiac tissue preparations, microelectrode studies have shown that beta-blocking concentrations of propranolol have little or no effect on transmembrane potential properties. However, such beta-blocking concentrations effectively decrease the slope of spontaneous phase 4 depolarization and the rate of automatic impulse initiation in both sinus nodal and ectopic pacemakers, especially when automaticity is promoted by catecholamines or ouabain.[142] Therefore, arrhythmias caused by enhanced automaticity with sympathetic hyperactivity are likely to respond to beta-adrenergic blockade. At higher concentrations, propranolol exerts membrane-depressant effect (like lidocaine) on Purkinje fibers (*i.e.,* decrease in membrane responsiveness). Action potential duration and refractoriness both are shortened, although the latter is not shortened as much as the former. This effect is similar to that of lidocaine[17] because propranolol delays the reactivation kinetic of the fast medium current, thereby delaying recovery of excitability.[19,141] Beta-blocking effects of propranolol can be expected to increase AV nodal refractoriness and to slow conduction velocity (removal of sympathetic facilitation effect), both of great value in suppressing supraventricular tachycardia using the AV node as a reentry pathway. This action of propranolol on the AV node can also be of value in decreasing ventricular response rate during atrial tachycardias, particularly when used in combination with digitalis.[20,122,142]

Metabolism and Pharmacokinetics. Propranolol is eliminated almost entirely by hepatic metabolism. Bioavailability of a single oral dose of propranolol is very low because of presystemic elimination caused by high hepatic extraction ratio. Large variations in peak plasma levels (up to 20-fold)[14] occur in patients given the same oral dose of propranolol. These variabilities may be at least in part related to the level of hepatic blood flow, the ability of hepatic microsomal enzyme to metabolize propranolol, and the dose. At low propranolol concentrations, virtually all the drug is removed by the liver.

The major metabolite of propranolol is 4-hydroxypropranolol. Its role in arrhythmia suppression is not defined. During chronic oral therapy, the hepatic extraction ratio of propranolol falls to almost 65% as hepatic microsomal sites become saturated. Plasma propranolol levels under these conditions become a function of the administered dose. The clearance of propranolol, like lidocaine, is limited by hepatic blood flow. Half-life of elimination is between 2 and 5 hours (3.2 hours after a single oral dose and 4.6 hours after chronic therapy). The clearance of propranolol is approximately 1 liter/min, and its apparent volume of distribution is 3 liter/kg. About 90% of the drug is bound to protein. Patient variations in plasma propranolol levels reflect variations in hepatic blood flow.[14,142,143]

Although pharmacokinetic interaction with other drugs has not been described in clinical reports, drugs that stimulate microsomal enzymes, such as phenobarbital, probably decrease the half-life of propranolol; drugs that inhibit these enzymes, such as chlorpromazine, tend to increase its half-life and plasma level, causing toxic side-effects.

Therapeutic Action, Dose, and Side-Effects. The ability of propranolol to slow conduction and increase refractoriness in the AV node has made it quite useful in the management and prevention of paroxysmal supraventricular tachycardia. When prophylaxis is considered, propranolol in combination with digitalis is particularly useful. Exercise-induced arrhythmias and those associated with pheochromocytoma, thyrotoxicosis, and anesthesia with cyclopropane or halothane, which are largely due to excess sympathetic nervous activity, can be suppressed with propranolol.[144,145] Patients with resistant arrhythmias after myocardial infarction may respond well to propranolol. Propranolol and other beta-blockers may reduce the incidence of sudden cardiac death in survivors of myocardial infarction.[146–148] Propranolol is the drug of choice in the treatment of arrhythmias associated with prolonged QT interval.[142] Similarly, propranolol is also helpful in treating patients with arrhythmias associated with mitral valve prolapse.[149,150]

Propranolol may be administered orally or intravenously. An average plasma level of 50 ng/ml can be expected when 160 mg/day of propranolol is given orally, but the scatter in the plasma levels is so large that this figure is at best an approximation.[150] Individual titration of the dosing schedule is therefore necessary. Reduction of resting heart rate to 50 to 55 beats/min after propranolol administration may reflect achievement of adequate sympathetic blockade. If arrhythmias fail to respond to propranolol, daily doses of up to 640 mg should be considered, unless side-effects limit this regimen.

When intravenous propranolol is indicated, doses of 0.1 to 0.15 mg/kg can be administered slowly at a rate not exceeding 1 mg/min. McAllister[151] proposed a single dose of 11.4 mg (2 mg/min) followed by an infusion at a rate of 0.055 mg/min. This regimen will cause a steady-state plasma propranolol level of 38 ng/ml after 30 minutes. Continuous hemodynamic and electrocardiographic monitoring during intravenous propranolol infusion is mandatory, especially in patients with cardiac decompensation.

The most common side-effects of propranolol include worsening of asthmatic attacks, congestive heart failure, and depression of sinus node function and AV nodal conduction. Among insulin-dependent diabetics, propranolol may increase the risk of hypoglycemia. Impaired sexual activity (impotence) and easy fatigability occur with chronic propranolol therapy. Symptoms probably related to sympathetic supersensitivity have been observed after abrupt withdrawal from chronic (*i.e.*, 12 weeks) propranolol therapy.[153–154] Diarrhea may also be a problem. Sympathetic supersensitivity to the chronotropic effect of isoproterenol has been demonstrated among patients with essential hypertension abruptly withdrawn from propranolol therapy. Therefore, gradual reduction of propranolol doses should be considered to avoid withdrawal symptoms, which may include unstable angina, myocardial infarction, and even sudden death. Even gradual withdrawal has at times been associated with failure.[156]

Verapamil

In 1982 verapamil (Fig. 29-10), a slow channel blocking agent, became available for clinical use in the United States, mainly for the management of patients with supraventricular tachyarrhythmias.

Mode of Action. Microelectrode studies in isolated cardiac tissue have shown that the electrophysiologic effects

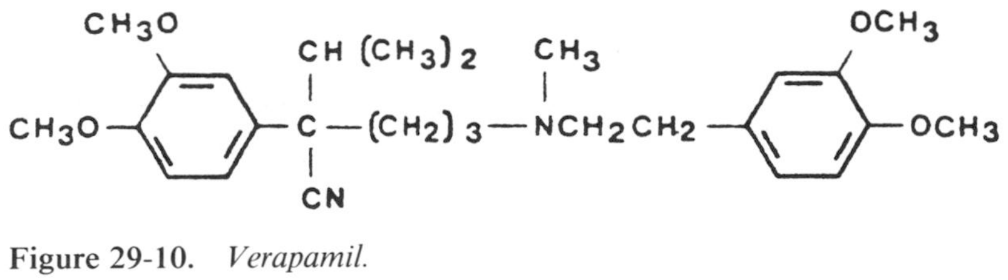

Figure 29-10. *Verapamil.*

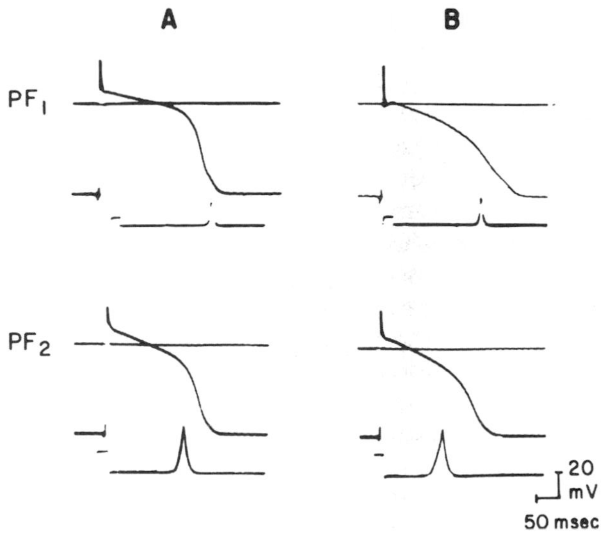

Figure 29-11. *Effects of verapamil on normal canine cardiac Purkinje fibers. The* upper tracing *is the action potential, and the* lower tracing *shows a 200-V/sec calibration followed by electronic differentiation of the maximum rate of rise of phase O ($\dot{V}_{max}$). A is a control record of two Purkinje fiber potentials: PF_1 and PF_2. B shows the same action potentials 30 minutes after onset of superfusion with verapamil, 1 mg/liter. Note that this concentration of verapamil has no effect on action potential amplitude or $\dot{V}_{max}$ or on resting membrane potential. However, the voltage at which the plateau originates is decreased and the slope of phase 2 repolarization is increased by verapamil. These changes are consistent with the block of a slow inward current such as that by calcium ion. (Rosen, M. R., Wit, A. L., and Hoffman, B. F.: Electrophysiology and pharmacology of cardiac arrhythmias. VI. Cardiac effects of verapamil. Am. Heart J., 89:665–673, 1975)*

of verapamil differ from those of other antiarrhythmic agents. At concentrations considered therapeutic, verapamil exerts little or no effect on normal Purkinje fibers except for minor acceleration of phase 2 repolarization and a slight depression of the plateau[157] (Fig. 29-11). Moreover, in depressed fibers (resting potential less negative than −60 mV) and sinus nodal fibers, verapamil suppresses the excitatory depolarizing current, which is mainly carried by calcium and sodium ions.[157–159] In depressed fibers (atrial or ventricular) manifesting spontaneous automatic activity or delayed afterdepolarization with the potential for triggered automatic activity, verapamil can terminate such ectopic automatic foci (Fig. 29-12). Therefore, it seems that verapamil could terminate reentrant arrhythmias by further reducing the slow conduction in one limb of a reentry circuit as well as arrhythmias caused by abnormal automatic mechanisms or triggered automatic activity. Because all these arrhythmic mechanisms use the secondary or slow inward current to initiate and maintain cardiac arrhythmias, verapamil, which suppresses this current, can eliminate these arrhythmic mechanisms. Although verapamil can suppress triggered automaticity in both Purkinje[110] and ventricular[111] muscle fibers, its role in the management of patients with ventricular tachycardia is still controversial.

Metabolism and Pharmacokinetics. Verapamil is eliminated largely by metabolism in the liver; only 5% is found in urine in the unchanged form. The major metabolite with pharmacologic activity has been identified as N-demethyl verapamil, or norverapamil.[160] The large hepatic capacity to metabolize verapamil is consistent with its relatively low bioavailability (35%),[160] which is largely due to presystemic (first-pass) hepatic elimination (metabolism). Therapeutically, the effective plasma

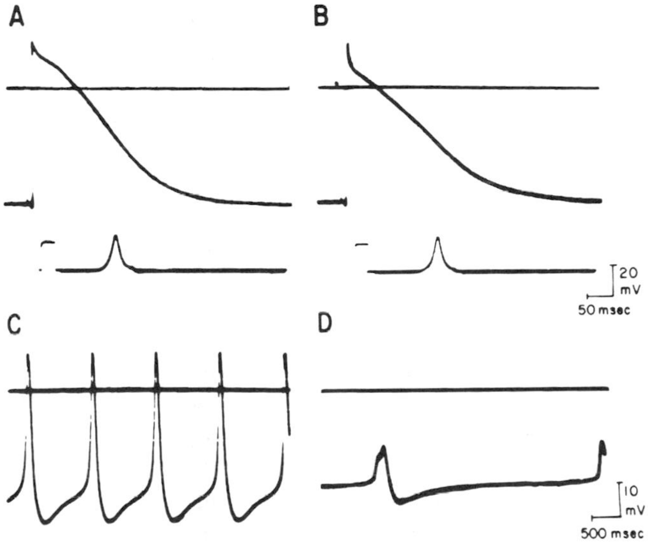

Figure 29-12. *Effects of verapamil on specialized conducting fibers from normal and diseased human atria. A and B are from a segment of normal human atrium stimulated at a cycle length of 800 msec. A is a control. In B, after 30 minutes of superfusion with verapamil, 1 mg/liter, resting membrane potential, action potential amplitude, and $\dot{V}_{max}$ are unchanged. However, the voltage at which the plateau originates is decreased and the slope of phase 2 is increased. C and D were recorded from an isolated sample of diseased human atrium. C is a control record of the spontaneous rhythm occurring in this tissue. In D, following 7 minutes of superfusion with verapamil, 1 mg/liter, the maximum diastolic potential, the slope of phase 4, and the spontaneous rate have decreased and action potential amplitude is markedly diminished. Within 1 minute the preparation became quiescent. Both samples were obtained from human right atria as part of the routine procedure for cardiac bypass. (Rosen, M. R., Wit, A. L., and Hoffman, B. F.: Electrophysiology and pharmacology of cardiac arrhythmias. VI. Cardiac effects of verapamil. Am. Heart J., 89:665–673, 1975)*

verapamil concentration is 0.1 to 0.3 μg/ml. The half-life of the drug is related to dose. After a single oral dose of verapamil, mean $t_{1/2}$ was 6 hours (range 2 to 15 hours,)[160] but this figure increased to 12 hours (range 9 to 25 hours) 10 to 12 weeks after daily oral maintenance therapy with verapamil.[161,162] Similar prolongation of $t_{1/2}$ was seen with norverapamil, when $t_{1/2}$ increased from 10 to 16 hours.[161,162] Although the mechanism of such slowing of elimination is not clear, reduced hepatic flow and subsequent reduced clearance of verapamil might be responsible. These findings are crucial for a rational and effective design of maintenance oral verapamil therapy. A reduction in the maintenance dose of verapamil or less frequent administration of the drug becomes mandatory to avoid or minimize toxic side-effects. In a recent report, oral verapamil was found ineffective in preventing spontaneously occurring paroxysmal supraventricular tachycardia in patients in whom intravenous verapamil had previously suppressed tachycardia induction by programmed electrical stimulation.[163] Such a discrepancy may occur because (1) the antiarrhythmic effects of verapamil are transient (*i.e.*, exhibit tachyphylaxis) and (2) oral verapamil is less potent (*i.e.*, requires higher plasma concentration for a given effect) than intravenous verapamil. McAllister and Kirsten[164] have shown that two to three times higher plasma verapamil concentrations were needed after oral verapamil was given to prolong the PR interval as much as an intravenous bolus injection. Similar results were also obtained by Reiter and colleagues,[165] who found that plasma verapamil concentration corresponding to a 10% prolongation of the PR interval was 36 ng/ml after intravenous bolus, 132 ng/ml after an oral dose, and 85 ng/ml after steady intravenous infusion. Maximum PR prolongation in this study, however, was comparable for the three methods of administration. Why an intravenous bolus injection of verapamil is more effective is not clear. Although an antagonistic role of norverapamil is not the reason, intravenous verapamil has similar effects on the PR interval when appreciable plasma levels of norverapamil are present.[165] The fact that oral verapamil causes appreciable slowing through the AV node implies that it should be effective, at least in patients with paroxysmal supraventricular tachycardia.[166,167] However, more work is needed to determine the mechanism of the apparent differences between oral and intravenous verapamil.

The clearance of verapamil is 13 ml/min/kg, and its steady-state volume of distribution is 4.3 liter/kg.[160] Woodcock and associates[168] have demonstrated a reduction in the elimination of single doses of verapamil in patients with liver disease or compromised left ventricular function, which could conceivably be explained by differences in hepatic flow and subsequent hepatic clearance of verapamil. About 90% of verapamil is bound to plasma protein.

Therapeutic Action, Dose, and Side-Effects. The antiarrhythmic properties of verapamil are caused mainly by its ability to suppress slow-response action potentials, which are initiated by the secondary or slow inward current and carried mainly by calcium and sodium ions. Abnormal automaticity and triggered automatic activity, mechanisms that depend on the slow inward current, are also suppressed by verapamil.

Intravenous verapamil is highly effective in treating patients with paroxysmal supraventricular tachycardias.[163] In this respect, it may well become the drug of choice in reverting acute episodes of supraventricular tachycardia to normal sinus rhythm. Furthermore, it has a very fast onset of action (usually less than a minute). Successful and prompt conversion of this arrhythmia has been reported to be 80% to 100% following intravenous administration.[169] Conversion of atrial fibrillation to normal sinus rhythm with verapamil is uncommon; however, verapamil can slow ventricular rate during atrial flutter and fibrillation by slowing conduction velocity and increasing AV nodal refractoriness. Verapamil has minimal effect on antegrade and retrograde conduction and on refractoriness in the anomalous pathway in patients with WPW syndrome. Therefore, it is unlikely to be of value in the management of this syndrome complicated by atrial flutter or fibrillation, and, in some instances, it may be associated with a paradoxic increase in the ventricular rate. Ventricular arrhythmias frequently fail to respond to verapamil,[170] but a good response to verapamil was observed in patients with ventricular arrhythmias during halothane anesthesia.[171] Overall, the role of verapamil in the management of patients with ventricular arrhythmias has not been conclusively established. For the conversion of atrial arrhythmias, the most commonly used dosage is a single bolus intravenous injection of 10 to 15 mg over a 1-minute period. If there is no response, an additional 5 to 10 mg of verapamil can be administered 20 to 40 minutes later. Although not customary, continuous intravenous infusion can also be instituted after a bolus. An infusion rate of 5 to 10 mg/hr can be used, with adjustment dependent on clinical response.

An oral regimen of verapamil is generally 80 to 120 mg every 6 to 8 hours. Rarely, higher doses are used. However, with chronic oral therapy, subsequent adjustments may be necessary because clearance of the drug decreases with time.

Verapamil is generally well tolerated. Side-effects are not common, and they are mainly limited to the cardiovascular system. Verapamil may cause mild congestive heart failure because it depresses myocardial contractility and thus should not be used in the presence of frank heart failure. Nevertheless, it may, through its peripheral vasodilation effects, increase cardiac output in some patients. Verapamil causes sinus bradycardia and depresses AV nodal conduction (*i.e.,* PR prolongation); it therefore is contraindicated in patients with the sick sinus syndrome. Intravenous verapamil has rarely been associated with severe hypotension, severe bradycardia, and, in some instances, asystole. Continuous monitoring in this setting is mandatory. Unlike beta-blockers, verapamil does not increase airway resistance and therefore can be given to patients with bronchial asthma. Constipation, headache, gastrointestinal upset, vertigo, dizziness, and nervousness are uncommon but have been reported to occur with oral verapamil.

New Agents

None of the available antiarrhythmic drugs is ideal, and a substantial number of patients do not respond to "therapeutic" doses of the antiarrhythmic agents discussed above. These considerations have led investigators to search for new agents with higher toxic to therapeutic ratios. Although no such agent is currently available, many drugs have recently been introduced to control and prevent life-threatening arrhythmias. These new agents, which admittedly are not perfect, nevertheless offer the alert clinician alternatives, which, if prescribed cautiously under strict scrutiny, can well be useful. The following sections discuss some of the newer antiarrhythmic agents being used clinically: amiodarone, mexiletine, tocainide, aprindine, sotalol, propafenone, bretylium, ethmozin, flecainide, lorcainide, encainide, ajmaline, and cibenzoline.

Amiodarone

Recently amiodarone has been approved by the FDA, and marketed under the brand name of Cordarone for the management of ventricular arrhythmias.

Mode of Action. Amiodarone (Fig. 29-13) differs in a major way from all other antiarrhythmic drugs by its very slow onset of action requiring weeks to months before full antiarrhythmic efficacy is manifest. At present no clear explanation is available for such peculiar behavior. Microelectrode studies on isolated cardiac preparations obtained from rabbits and dogs receiving daily doses of amiodarone for up to 6 weeks have shown considerable prolongation of action potential duration of atrial, ventricular muscle, and Purkinje fibers, with no significant alteration in other transmembrane potential properties.[172,173] Microelectrode studies have also shown slowed sinus nodal automaticity by depression of phase 4 depolarization and prolongation of action potential duration, actions that slow sinus rate.[174] Recently Ohta and associates[175] have shown that amiodarone reduces the amplitude of DAD and subsequent triggered automaticity in isolated rabbit ventricular myocardium. Furthermore, it was found in this study that chronic therapy

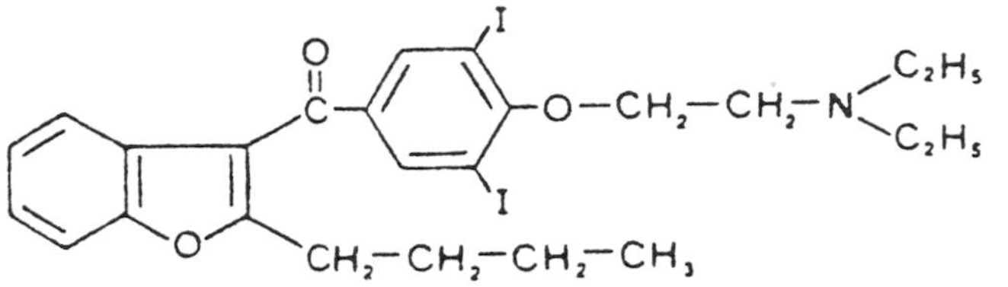

Figure 29-13. *Amiodarone.*

was more effective than acute (superfusion) therapy.[175] In intact dogs, amiodarone, 10 mg/kg administered intravenously, had maximum electrophysiologic effects between 5 and 10 minutes. The sinus rate was slowed by 36%, and atrial and ventricular monophasic action potentials and refractory periods were prolonged, as was AV node conduction time.[176]

In unanesthetized dogs with complete heart block, intravenous amiodarone had no effect on the ventricular escape rhythm.[177]

In dogs with coronary artery occlusion, Patterson and colleagues[178] have demonstrated that both short-term intravenous amiodarone and long-term (24 days) oral amiodarone significantly reduced the incidence of ventricular fibrillation. Long-term oral amiodarone, however, was more effective against ventricular fibrillation and caused greater prolongation of effective refractory period and the QT segment of the right ventricle.[178]

Metabolism and Pharmacokinetics. Amiodarone is a unique antiarrhythmic agent in both its pharmacokinetic and pharmacologic properties. Only recently have data on the pharmacokinetic and metabolic fate of amiodarone become available, with the development of new high-pressure liquid chromatographic assay techniques.[179–181] The full spectrum of the disposition kinetic of the drug remains poorly understood.

The salient pharmacologic feature of amiodarone (*i.e.,* delay in onset of antiarrhythmic action) has been attributed to slow accumulation of the drug in the myocardium and to extensive uptake by adipose tissue, causing slow attainment of steady-state plasma drug concentration with sufficient myocardial tissue amiodarone uptake.[179–181] Recent data suggest that the slow development of metabolic alterations in thyroid hormone activity may have an antiarrhythmic implication in the efficacy of long-term amiodarone therapy.[182] Long-term oral amiodarone increases plasma concentrations of reverse triiodothyronine (T_3) and thyroxine (T_4), changes that parallel the onset and magnitude of QT prolongation and suppression of ventricular premature depolarizations.[182] Finally, desmethylamiodarone, a major metabolite of amiodarone occurring with long-term amiodarone therapy, and a possible antagonism of the sympathetic nervous system by both amiodarone and its major metabolite may influence the ability of this drug to suppress arrhythmias. At present, the full pharmacologic spectrum of activity of amiodarone is unresolved.

Oral absorption of amiodarone is relatively slow, and peak serum concentration after an oral dose of 800 mg is reached after 5.2 hours, with a half-life of absorption of 1.62 hours.[179] The maximum serum concentration after a single oral dose of 800 mg is reported to be 1.7 μg/ml (range 0.6 to 3.2 μg/ml).[179] The half-life of amiodarone after a single oral dose is 4.62 hours. Oral bioavailability of amiodarone (Cordarone) is 35%.[181] Preliminary results* indicate that the half-life after a single intravenous dose (5 mg/kg) is similar to that after a single oral dose. However, with chronic oral therapy, the half-life of amiodarone is considerably prolonged, up to 30 days. The mechanism of this prolongation is unknown but could reflect amiodarone tissue distribution (slow process) and perhaps formation of metabolites that slow clearance of the parent drug.[180] No amiodarone, or its pharmacologically active metabolite desmethylamiodarone, is found in the urine for 24 hours after a single oral dose.[179-181] Animal studies have also failed to show amiodarone in feces after intravenous administration.[179] It appears that amiodarone has a strong ability to concentrate in various tissues. The preliminary studies of Haffajee and associates[179] have shown that amiodarone can concentrate to values up to 385 times that of plasma amiodarone concentration in the fatty mesenteric tissue and up to 36 times in the heart.

In the dog, mean right ventricular amiodarone concentration following long-term oral administration (28 days) was 13 μg/g, representing a sevenfold uptake; it was 54 μg/g for desmethylamiodarone, representing a 20-fold uptake.[178] How amiodarone becomes so concentrated in various tissues is unknown. One important electrophysiologic consequence of such concentrating ability in myocardial tissue is a lack of any apparent correlation between plasma amiodarone levels and antiarrhythmic efficacy. Many responders to amiodarone had plasma amiodarone levels lower than those of nonresponders.[179] This may well reflect lower myocardial uptake of amiodarone in the nonresponders, assuming that amiodarone has the necessary antiarrhythmic properties. Clearly these considerations need further research and experimental verification. Recently, Wellens and associates[183] have shown that oral amiodarone had different electrophysiologic effects than intravenous amiodarone. Whereas oral amiodarone prolonged the effective refractory period of the atrium and the ventricle and the HV interval, intravenous amiodarone had no effect on these parameters. Despite these differences in electrophysiologic responses, it was intriguing to see that intravenous amiodarone predicted outcome with oral amiodarone in preventing inducible tachycardia.[179] If similar observations are to be made on a larger patient population,[184] additional electrophysiologic mechanisms on the heart are then needed (other than the simple prolongation of refractory period) by which amiodarone suppresses tachycardia.

Therapeutic Action, Dose, and Side-Effects. The ability of amiodarone to prolong refractoriness of almost all cardiac tissues makes it quite useful in the clinical management of patients with supraventricular and ventricular arrhythmias as well as arrhythmias associated with the WPW syndrome.[179,184-190] Amiodarone is often effective in the management of these arrhythmias when conventional antiarrhythmics fail to correct the rhythm disorder. There appears to be general agreement that it requires days, and sometimes weeks, for the full antiarrhythmic efficacy of oral amiodarone to become manifest. The considerable prolongation of its half-life of elimination seems to be the result of accumulation in various body tissues. Such "body stores" may, at least in part, explain the persistence, in some cases, of its antiarrhythmic efficacy for at least 30 to 40 days after complete discontinuation. Intravenous amiodarone 5 mg/kg, may be used by administering the agent at a rate of 30 to 50 mg/min in a central line. Most commonly the drug is given orally, usually with a loading dose of 800 to 1800 mg/day during the first week, followed by daily maintenance dose of 200 to 800 mg/day. Amiodarone seems to be well tolerated by most patients; however, with its increasing use, several unwanted side-effects have been recognized.[191] Of the side-effects that complicate amiodarone therapy, pulmonary fibrosis is the most serious.[192] Unfortunately, no reliable test can predict the likelihood of this troublesome complication. The frequency (approximately 5%) can, however, be reduced by lowering the maintenance dose. A recent multicenter study has shown pulmonary toxicity to occur in up to 45% of patients over a 4-year period with a daily maintenance dose of 500 mg amiodarone.* The most consistent complication of amiodarone therapy is corneal microdeposits (lypofuscin), which appear as peculiar yellow-brown granular pigmentation in the cornea.[191] This may cause photophobia. Fortunately, these symptoms disappear within weeks or months after amiodarone is discontinued. Amiodarone may also cause thyroid dysfunction, and patients may manifest either hypothyroidism or hyperthyroidism.[191] In the long term (generally over 1 year) amiodarone therapy may occasionally cause a peculiar bluish or slate-gray discoloration of the skin, which may take several weeks or even months to disappear when the drug is stopped. This discoloration generally begins nasally and then spreads to encompass

* Kannan, R.: Personal communication.

* Mason, J.: Personal communication.

the entire face. It may not clear completely for months to years following discontinuation of the drug. Approximately 5% of patients must discontinue amiodarone because of more serious and even life-threatening side-effects. These include refractory heart failure, pulmonary fibrosis, central nervous system side-effects such as tremor, ataxia, paresthesias, headache, and nightmares, sinus arrest, aplastic anemia, and exacerbation of ventricular tachycardia. Amiodarone interacts with several drugs with important clinical implications; chief among these interactions is potentiation of the anticoagulant effect of warfarin.[193] Although increases in prothrombin time vary, the maintenance dose of warfarin should be reduced by one third to one half in patients receiving amiodarone.[193] Torsade de pointes has been observed when quinidine, propafenone, or mexiletine is given with amiodarone.[194] Adding amiodarone to maintenance digoxin therapy causes a progressive increase (up to 70%) in serum digoxin concentration, with the emergence of symptoms compatible with digoxin toxicity.[194] Finally, amiodarone may interact with beta-blockers and certain calcium channel antagonists (verapamil and diltiazem) to cause severe sinus bradycardia and even sinus arrest, especially in patients with the sick sinus syndrome.[194]

Mexiletine

Mexiletine, a structural analog of lidocaine (Fig. 29-14), shares many of its electrophysiologic effects on the transmembrane potential of cardiac fibers. Mexiletine differs from lidocaine in that it is effective orally and is not eliminated by first-pass hepatic metabolism. Recently mexiletine has been approved by the FDA, and released under the brand name of Mexitil® for the management of ventricular arrhythmias.

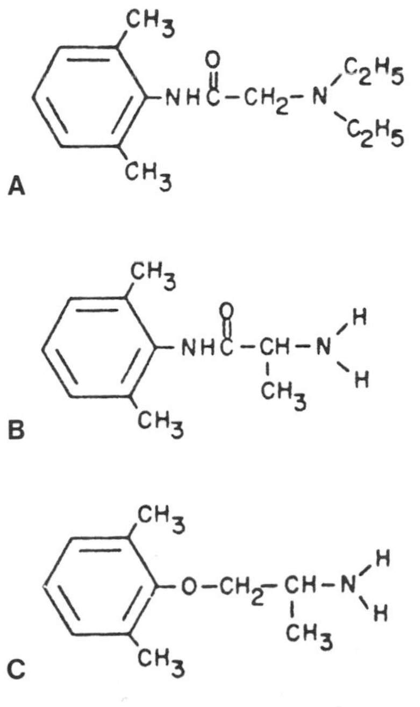

Figure 29-14. *(A) Lidocaine. (B) Tocainide. (C) Mexiletine.*

Mode of Action. Microelectrode studies on isolated Purkinje fibers have shown that mexiletine decreases the maximum rate of phase-zero depolarization and membrane responsiveness and shortens the effective refractory period more than it shortens action potential duration.[195–199] Mexiletine suppresses normal, abnormal, and triggered automatic mechanisms in Purkinje fibers at concentrations that have little or no effect on sinus nodal automaticity.[197] In isolated guinea pig hearts, mexiletine was effective against reperfusion arrhythmias after a period of ischemia and hypoxia.[198] Furthermore, in isolated Purkinje fibers, mexiletine decreased the amplitude of delayed afterdepolarizations and triggered automaticity induced by either barium or strophantidin.[197,198]

Mexiletine does not appear to have any effect on the slow response[200]; however, on partially depolarized Purkinje fibers manifesting spontaneous automatic activity (abnormal automaticity), mexiletine at concentration 0.4 to 2 μg/ml depressed phase 4 depolarization and reduced the rate of automatic impulse initiation.[197] Furthermore, when partially depolarized Purkinje fibers showing phase 4 depolarization were electrically driven, the application of mexiletine rendered the maximum diastolic potential more negative, with a concomitant decrease of pacemaker slope and an increase in the $\dot{V}_{max}$ of the phase-zero action potential.[197] In Purkinje fibers with normal resting potential, mexiletine decreases the rate of automatic impulse initiation by shifting the threshold potential to less negative values.[197]

In humans, mexiletine increases the functional refractory period of the AV node and the relative and effective refractory periods of the His-Purkinje system and prolongs the HV interval. These findings are not always uniform, however. Differences may reflect differences between patients or between therapeutic regimens. Harper and associates[201] found that mexiletine had no effect on the duration of endocardial right ventricular monophasic action potentials in humans, nor did it alter the effective refractory period of this site when the ventricles were regularly driven at cycle lengths of 500 to 600 msec. However, mexiletine did prolong the monophasic action potential duration of early premature ventricular beats.[201] These authors concluded that this property of the drug may be related to its antiarrhythmic activity. Furthermore, these authors have shown that mexiletine abolished the supernormal conduction phase, which occurs immediately after repolarization, presumably as a result of phase 4 depolarization in the cells of the specialized conducting system.[201] The antiarrhythmic significance of such an effect is still undefined.

Metabolism and Pharmacokinetics. Mexiletine is rapidly and well absorbed after oral administration in healthy volunteers.[202] However, absorption is incomplete and delayed in patients with myocardial infarction and in patients receiving narcotic analgesics that retard gastric emptying. Mexiletine is eliminated largely by liver metabolism, with only less than 10% excreted by the kidneys unchanged. Renal clearance of mexiletine decreases as urinary *p*H increases.[202] The half-life of elimination is around 12 hours, and therapeutic plasma concentrations (1 to 2 μg/ml) can be maintained with 200- to 300-mg oral doses every 6 to 8 hours. The half-life of mexiletine increases in patients treated in the coronary care unit, and careful monitoring for dose readjustment is needed. About 70% of the drug is protein bound.[202]

Therapeutic Actions, Doses, and Side-Effects. Mexiletine can be given orally, 100 to 400 mg every 6 to 8 hours. For urgent therapy, the intravenous route may be considered, with 200 to 250 mg over 5 minutes followed by an infusion of 60 to 90 mg/hr. Mexiletine is effective in suppressing ventricular arrhythmias, and its relatively long half-life is beneficial for patient compliance.[203–205] Its definite role in controlling ventricular arrhythmias remains undefined. Most side-effects are seen during the initial period of therapy and disappear during maintenance therapy; most are of central nervous system origin. They include tremor, nystagmus diplopia, dizziness, dysarthria, paresthesias, ataxia, and confusion. Gastrointestinal side-effects are common and include nausea, vomiting, and dyspepsia. Thrombocytopenia and positive antinuclear antibody occur rarely but have been reported. Side-effects are more likely to occur at mexiletine plasma concentrations over 1.5 to 2 μg/ml, which is very close to the therapeutic level. Cardiovascular effects of mexiletine are infrequent and include hypotension, bradycardia, and exacerbation of arrhythmias. The drug is generally well tolerated.

Tocainide

Tocainide, only recently released for clinical use (Tonocard®) another lidocaine analog (see Fig. 29-14), has many electrophysiologic similarities to mexiletine. It also resembles mexiletine in that it is active orally and does not undergo presystemic elimination by first-pass hepatic degradation.

Mode of Action. Microelectrode studies have shown that tocainide has similar electrophysiologic effects to those of lidocaine on resting and action potential.[206,207] Its effects on $\dot{V}_{max}$ are potassium dependent. At normal extracellular potassium concentration (3 to 5 mM), tocainide slightly reduces $\dot{V}_{max}$. However, at elevated potassium concentration, at which $\dot{V}_{max}$ is already depressed, tocainide has a much greater depressant effect.[206,207] Furthermore, microelectrode studies on isolated Purkinje fibers have demonstrated that tocainide increases, in a concentration-dependent manner, the amount of current necessary to evoke an action potential by intracellular current injection, an indication of decreased excitability.[206] Tocainide decreases the amplitude and plateau phase of the action potential in a concentration-dependent manner, thereby decreasing time to 50% repolarization.[206] However, tocainide had no effect on total duration of action potential, maximal action potential amplitude, or resting membrane potential. Although the drug had no consistent effect on the effective refractory period of Purkinje fibers, the ratio of effective refractory period to action potential duration was consistently increased in a concentration-dependent manner after tocainide superfusion.[206] Tocainide completely suppresses ventricular tachycardia induced by ouabain intoxication in dogs, with an average plasma level of 18 μg/ml. Similarly, tocainide suppresses the 24-hour ventricular arrhythmias induced by coronary artery occlusion in the dog, with an average plasma level of 42 μg/ml (range 28 to 67 μg/ml).[206] With lower plasma levels of tocainide (mean 18 μg/ml), these ischemic ventricular arrhythmias were suppressed by about 50%. Tocainide increased the ventricular fibrillation threshold, with a maximum increase of about 150% achieved with a plasma tocainide concentration of 48 μg/ml.[206]

Metabolism and Pharmacokinetics. Tocainide is rapidly and predictably well absorbed by the oral route and has a high system bioavailability.[208–209] Plasma tocainide levels are highly predictable after an oral dose. The drug undergoes hepatic degradation (40% and 60%); the remainder is eliminated by the kidney unchanged. The half-life of elimination of tocainide is 12 hours (range 10 to 17 hours), and it is 50% bound to plasma protein. Tocainide clearance is 2.2 ml/min/kg, and its steady-state volume of distribution is 1.6 liter/kg. Renal elimination of tocainide is reduced with an increase in urinary *p*H.[208,209]

Therapeutic Action, Dose, and Side-Effects. A number of clinical studies have shown that tocainide can decrease the frequency of ventricular premature depolarizations and has variable effects on ventricular tachycardias.[210–211] The precise role of tocainide, and the clinical setting in which it may eventually be used, remain undefined. It appears that tocainide exerts its antiarrhythmic efficacy at plasma concentrations above 6 μg/ml, if at all. The oral regimen for tocainide is usually 400 to 600 mg every 8 hours. Tocainide is generally well tolerated. Side-effects include central nervous system disorders such as tremor, headache, sweating, altered hearing, dizziness, nervousness, hot flashes, paresthe-

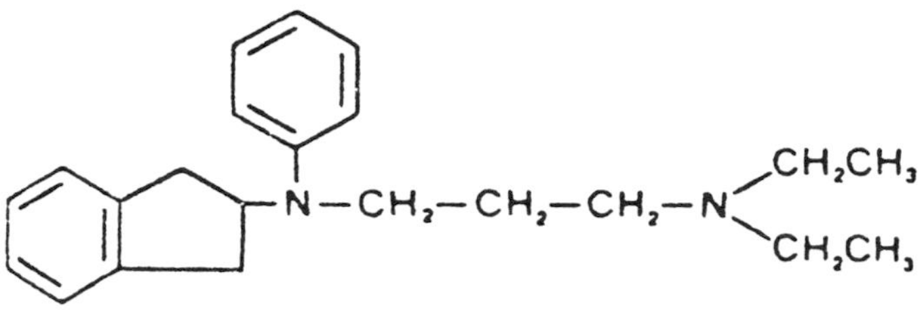

Figure 29-15. *Aprindine.*

sias, blurred vision of diplopia, anxiety, and lightheadedness. Gastrointestinal complaints are more common and include anorexia, vomiting, nausea, abdominal pain, and constipation.[211] Tocainide was recently approved by the FDA, and released in the market (Tonogard® MSD) for the management of ventricular arrhythmias.

Aprindine

Aprindine, developed in Belgium, has important local anesthetic effects. It is still an investigational agent in the United States.

Mode of Action. On isolated canine Purkinje fibers and atrial ventricular muscle fibers, aprindine (Fig. 29-15) shortens action potential duration and, to a lesser extent, effective refractory period.[212–215] Therefore, the ratio of effective refractory period shortening to action potential duration shortening is greater than 1.[212–214] The effects of the drug on Purkinje fibers occur at lower concentrations than on atrial and ventricular fibers. Aprindine depresses maximum rate of rise of phase zero of action potential in a frequency-dependent manner; greater depression occurs at faster rate of drive.[212–215] Membrane responsiveness is shifted to the right with aprindine superfusion in a concentration-dependent manner. Aprindine also decreases the slope of spontaneous phase 4 depolarization of Purkinje fibers with high resting membrane potential (normal enhanced automaticity), thereby decreasing the rate of automatic impulse initiation and eventually arresting automaticity.[212–215] In anesthetized dogs, aprindine injected into the sinus node artery slows sinus discharge rate; when injected into the AV nodal artery, it prolongs conduction time and the functional refractory period of the AV node.[216] These nodal effects are independent of indirect autonomic nervous system influences. Furthermore, aprindine prolongs both atrial and ventricular effective refractory periods.[216]

Aprindine suppresses transient depolarization and subsequent triggered automatic activity induced by ouabain in Purkinje fibers.[215] However, it does not have any effect on transmembrane potential properties of "slow-response" Purkinje fibers induced with a 22-mM potassium superfusion in the presence of isoproterenol.[215] Aprindine (2.8 mg/kg) administered intravenously completely eliminated accelerated idioventricular rhythm induced by ouabain in all 14 dogs studied, an effect not seen with other antiarrhythmic agents,[217] and significantly reduced the frequency of premature ventricular depolarization 24 hours after permanent coronary artery occlusion in dogs.[218] The precise cellular ionic mechanisms by which aprindine suppresses digitalis arrhythmias are still uncertain. The reduction in the amplitude of delayed afterdepolarizations and suppression of subsequent triggered automatic activity may well be one operative mechanism.

Metabolism and Pharmacokinetics. Aprindine is active orally and has high systemic bioavailability, with a rapid rate of oral absorption. Pharmacokinetic parameters of aprindine are still not defined. In healthy volunteers, clearance of aprindine was 2.55 ml/min/kg, and its half-life of elimination was 30 hours, with a steady-state volume of distribution of 3.6 liters/kg. Less than 1% of the dose is excreted unchanged in the urine. Therapeutic plasma levels (1 to 2 μg/ml) of aprindine overlap with toxic side-effects (*i.e.,* low toxic : therapeutic ratio), and 8% to 95% of the drug is protein bound.[219,220]

Therapeutic Action, Dose, and Side-Effects. Aprindine appears to be very effective against both supraventricular and ventricular arrhythmias of various etiologies.[219] It has been used orally in a loading dose of 200 to 300 mg followed by a daily maintenance dose of 147 mg/day. This dosage regimen achieved mean plasma aprindine levels of 1.7 μg/ml. Its slowing effect of conduction through the AV node and its ability to increase atrial refractoriness make it potentially useful in the management of patients with WPW syndrome.[219,221] Electrophysiologic studies in such patients have demonstrated that aprindine increased refractoriness of the accessory pathway in both an anterograde and retrograde direction in most of them.[219,221]

Unfortunately, the potential usefulness of aprindine is severely limited by its narrow toxic : therapeutic ratio, which is particularly evident during the initial loading period. It is advisable, when therapy permits, to initiate therapy without an initial loading dose, since this may well decrease the incidence of side-effects. The central nervous system is the major site of toxic side-effects, the most common being tremor. With high plasma levels (1.5 to 2.5 μg/ml) dizziness, intention tremor, ataxia, nervousness, hallucinations, diplopia, memory impairment, or seizures may also occur. These neurologic disorders are minimal or absent with aprindine plasma levels of less than 1 μg/ml.[219,220] Gastrointestinal side-effects, which are less common, include nausea and occasional diarrhea. Agranulocytosis has been reported to occur in 5% of patients and is manifest idiosyncratically.

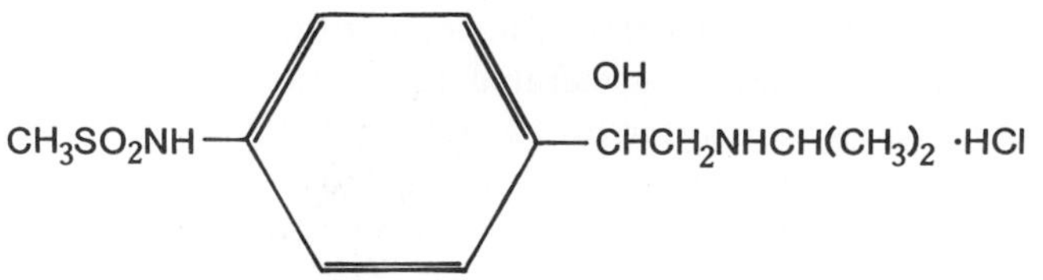

Figure 29-16. *Sotalol.*

Sotalol

Sotalol (Fig. 29-16) is a beta-adrenergic blocking agent that differs from propranolol in that it prolongs considerably both action potential duration and effective refractory period.

Mode of Action. Microelectrode studies on isolated tissue preparations have shown that sotalol considerably prolongs action potential duration and effective refractory period more so in Purkinje fibers than in ventricular muscle.[222,223] Sotalol, however, had no appreciable effect on other transmembrane potential properties, namely, resting membrane potential, action potential amplitude, and maximum rate of rise of phase zero of action potential.[222,223] Automaticity in sinus node cells and in normal Purkinje fibers is not altered, although some slowing in automaticity occurs at higher sotalol concentrations. Sotalol, however, antagonizes, in a concentration-dependent manner, isoproterenol-induced sinus acceleration. In partially depolarized Purkinje fibers, sotalol terminated abnormal automatic mechanism, suppressing spontaneous phase 4 depolarization.[222] In intact dogs with induced AV block, sotalol (2 mg/kg intravenously) slowed the rate of idioventricular rhythm and the idioventricular escape interval.[222] Recently sotalol was found to prevent or slow the rate of induced reentrant ventricular tachycardia in 11 of 19 dogs with coronary artery occlusion.[224] This effect of sotalol was found to be superior to that of metoprolol, which led Cobbe and colleagues to suggest that its greater efficacy might well be caused by its ability to prolong both action potential duration and effective refractory period.[224]

The acute electrophysiologic effects of sotalol have also been studied in humans.[225–227] These studies have shown, as predicted by animal studies, that sotalol significantly increases the refractory period of ventricular myocardium. An increase in the atrio-His conduction time, effective refractory period of the AV node, and AV nodal functional refractory period were also observed. Later studies by Nathan and colleagues[228] found that sotalol prolongs the effective refractory period of both atrial and ventricular tissue. It thus appears that sotalol prolongs refractoriness uniformly in all cardiac tissues.

Metabolism and Pharmacokinetics. Schnelle and colleagues found that after an intravenous dose of sotalol in healthy subjects, its elimination half-life was 6 to 8 hours.[229] The drug was excreted mainly by glomerular filtration, and metabolites were not found.[229]

Plasma concentration of sotalol was measured after oral administration of increasing doses to healthy subjects.[230] Plasma levels 2 hours after an oral dose of 400 and 800 mg showed a fourfold variation among subjects. This may be caused by differences in presystemic elimination (perhaps first-pass hepatic metabolism) causing variations in systemic bioavailability. Peak plasma levels of sotalol after oral administration are reached within 2 to 3 hours. Plasma time course of sotalol decays in a biexponential manner; the apparent half-life of the first phase ($t_{\frac{1}{2}alpha}$, the distribution phase) is 6.5 hours, and the slower phase ($t_{\frac{1}{2}beta}$, the elimination phase) has a half-life of approximately 13 hours. In patients with renal failure, the half-life of sotalol is considerably prolonged, since this drug appears to be eliminated mainly by glomerular filtration.[231] Tjandramaga and colleagues[231] reported a sotalol half-life of 42 hours in patients with renal failure. Considerable prolongation of half-life in anuric patients has been reported in more recent studies.[232]

Propafenone

Propafenone (Fig. 29-17), an investigational drug, has been used with a variety of success in the management of patients with supraventricular and ventricular arrhythmias and arrhythmias associated with the WPW syndrome.

Mode of Action. Microelectrode studies on isolated cardiac tissues have shown that propafenone decreases the maximum rate of depolarization of phase zero action potential without changing the resting membrane potential of atrial and ventricular muscle and Purkinje fibers.[233,234] The decrease in $\dot{V}_{max}$ that the drug induces is rate dependent (*i.e.*, $\dot{V}_{max}$ is depressed more quickly at a faster rate of stimulation).[234]

Propafenone shortens action potential duration more than it shortens the effective refractory period, making the ratio of decrease in effective refractory period to action potential shortening greater than 1.[233] Propafenone also decreases the slope of spontaneous phase 4 depolarization in Purkinje fibers with relatively high resting membrane potential (−75 mV), causing a decrease in the rate of automatic impulse initiation. The antiautomatic concentrations of propafenone on Purkinje fibers have no appreciable effect on sinus nodal automaticity.[233] Thus it appears that propafenone has no, or a mild, blocking effect on the sinus nodal pacemaker current. On ventricular and atrial tissue, propafenone prolonged action potential duration and elevated diastolic excitability threshold.[233,235] In studies involving dogs with coronary artery occlusion, propafenone suppressed

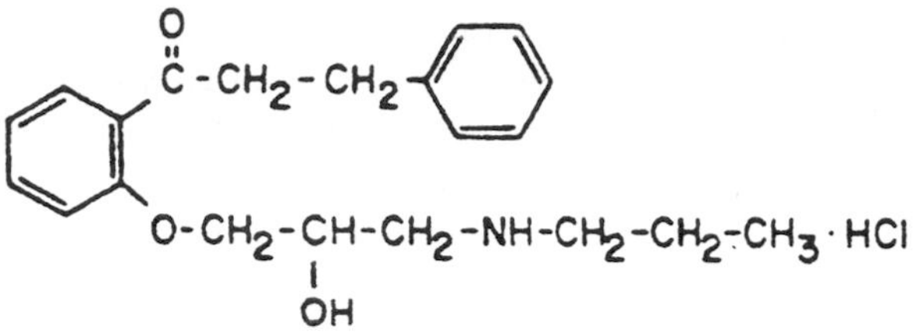

Figure 29-17. *Propafenone*

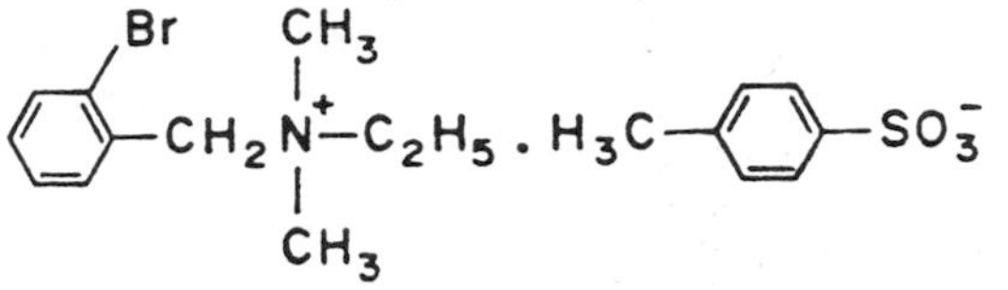

Figure 29-18. *Bretylium tosylate.*

ventricular arrhythmias promptly during the 24-hour postocclusion arrhythmic period, an effect superior to that of lidocaine.[113] Electrophysiologic studies in humans have shown that propafenone slows both AV nodal and intra-atrial conduction and prolongs QRS duration and QT interval. Both atrial and ventricular effective refractory periods were prolonged.[237]

Metabolism and Pharmacokinetics. Propafenone seems to be well absorbed orally, but considerable patient variation exists in its half-life of elimination.[237,239] Keller and associates[240] found peak plasma propafenone levels of about 2.4 μg/ml after an oral dose of 900 mg, with a mean half-life of 3.6 hours. More recent studies by Connolly and associates[239] found large patient variability in elimination half-life (range 2.4 to 11.8 hours). These authors dismissed liver disease, age, heart failure, and the presence or absence of concomitant medication as factors that could conceivably interfere with elimination of propafenone, suggesting instead that patient differences in metabolism cause the differences seen in its elimination half-life. Furthermore, in this study, great variability was found in the steady-state mean propafenone concentration in different patients receiving the same dose of propafenone. Although some of these variabilities can be explained by differences in elimination half-life, no strong correlation between half-life and steady-state concentration could be found, indicating the involvement of other factors. One such possible factor, the role of which is still ill defined, is systemic bioavailability and presystemic elimination (first-pass metabolism). A nonlinear relationship between dose and steady-state concentration was seen; that is, a large increase in plasma propafenone level followed a small increase in propafenone dose.[239] The mechanism of such plasma elevation of propafenone concentration is unknown but could conceivably be caused by saturation of the first-pass metabolic process. More work is needed to elucidate fully the pharmacokinetic behavior of propafenone.

Therapeutic Action, Dose, and Side-Effects. Propafenone has been reported to be very effective against premature ventricular depolarizations,[238] paroxysmal supraventricular tachycardia,[240] and arrhythmias associated with the WPW syndrome.[236,242] The drug is not as effective against inducible ventricular tachycardia[237,238]; in this setting it is comparable to other antiarrhythmic drugs. Thus, determination of its efficacy and role against inducible ventricular tachycardia awaits further studies involving a larger patient population with a variety of underlying heart diseases. In a recent study, propafenone was found to be fairly effective against ventricular arrhythmias judged by exercise testing, since 70% of patients responded to propafenone therapy.[235] Intravenous injections of propafenone, 1 to 2 mg/kg followed by 0.3 to 0.5 mg/min constant infusion, achieved impressive results in patients with torsade de pointes. Torsade de pointes ceased even during bolus injections.[243]

Propafenone is usually given orally, 150 mg to 300 mg every 8 hours. A therapeutic window of propafenone has not yet been established, but the drug appears to exert its antiarrhythmic efficacy in the plasma level range of 0.5 to 1.8 μg/ml.[239] Side-effects include potential block of AV transmission, requiring caution in the use of propafenone in patients with preexisting AV conduction abnormalities.[239] Propafenone may also aggravate ventricular arrhythmias.[235,238] Neurologic disorders are not uncommon and may include weakness and disorientation, dry mouth, metallic taste, and sometimes nausea, not often necessitating discontinuation of the drug.[236,237] Propafenone must be employed with caution in patients with congestive heart failure or evidence of conduction abnormalities.[235]

Bretylium

Bretylium (Fig. 29-18) has recently been approved for clinical use in the United States for the treatment of recurrent life-threatening ventricular arrhythmias, such as seen in postmyocardial infarction patients. It is marketed under the brand name of Bretylol.

Mode of Action. The antiarrhythmic mechanism(s) of action of bretylium is still not fully understood. It has been suggested that arrhythmia suppression may result from the ability of bretylium to interact with the sympathetic nervous system and from its direct effects on the transmembrane potentials of cardiac fibers or by a combination of these mechanisms. *In vitro* studies on isolated papillary muscle preparations have shown that bretylium, at clinically relevant concentrations, causes a concentration-dependent increase in the force of contraction.[244] Pretreating animals with reserpine to produce catecholamine depletion or adding propranolol to the superfusion chamber prevents this positive inotropic effect, suggesting that it is not direct but indirect, mediated through myocardial catecholamine release.[244,245] Although other studies ascribe a direct effect to increased force of contraction, there is little doubt that the primary action of bretylium on myocardial force of contraction results from release of catecholamine from adrenergic nerve endings.[245]

Microelectrode studies on isolated cardiac fibers have shown that bretylium in concentrations up to 20 μg/ml has no effect on resting membrane potential, upstroke velocity, or action potential amplitude in Purkinje and ventricular myocardial fibers.[246,247] However, the drug may transiently increase resting potential (make it more negative) and upstroke velocity, with an attendant increase in conduction velocity. These effects may be caused by release of norepinephrine from nerve endings.[245,246] At concentrations above 20 μg/ml, bretylium exerts a direct membrane-depressant effect, decreasing upstroke velocity and action potential amplitude and slowing conduction velocity.[245] Bretylium prolongs the duration of action potential and effective refractory period of both ventricular and Purkinje fibers.[245–247] The considerable prolongation of action potential duration and refractory period may be one major mechanism by which bretylium can suppress life-threatening ventricular arrhythmias during acute myocardial infarction. Furthermore, bretylium-induced prolongation of action potential duration is greater in regions of the heart where action potentials are shortest.[245–247] Cardinal and Sasyniuk have shown that bretylium prolonged action potential duration of subendocardial Purkinje fibers in the normal zone more than in ischemic Purkinje fibers in the infarcted zone, where the action potential duration was already considerably prolonged (due to ischemia) before bretylium superfusion.[248] Such a differential effect on action potential duration and, presumably, on refractoriness decreases the disparity in the repolarization process, thereby decreasing the likelihood of reentrant premature excitation.

The antiarrhythmic effects of bretylium may be delayed after parenteral administration, sometimes for more than 1 hour. Animal studies have shown that myocardial bretylium concentrations, after intravenous (6 mg/kg) injection (over 1 minute), rise slowly and reach a peak 1.5 to 6 hours after injection.[249] The ratio of myocardial to serum drug concentration reaches 7 at 12 hours after injection.[249] It is tempting to postulate that the delay required for development of full antiarrhythmic efficacy is caused by the slowly rising myocardial bretylium concentration. The antifibrillatory effect of bretylium was demonstrated by Wenger and colleagues.[250] In a canine model of ischemic ventricular fibrillation caused by transient occlusion followed by coronary artery reperfusion, bretylium decreased the incidence of ventricular fibrillation during reperfusion.[250] Bretylium is one of the few antiarrhythmic drugs that significantly reduces the incidence of ventricular fibrillation in dogs after release of an acute coronary artery occlusion. Most of the commonly used antiarrhythmic drugs, including amiodarone, are ineffective against reperfusion-induced ventricular fibrillation in the canine model.[253]

Metabolism and Pharmacokinetics. Bretylium can be administered by the oral, intramuscular, or intravenous route, although the oral route is not preferred because bretylium has a poor and erratic pattern of absorption.[220] Similar considerations apply for the intramuscular route. The pharmacokinetic desposition of bretylium is not yet fully described. The drug is mainly eliminated by the kidneys unchanged and is not metabolized significantly. Bretylium maintenance doses should be reduced in patients with renal failure.

Therapeutic Action, Dose, and Side-Effects. The major clinical use of bretylium is the emergency treatment of life-threatening drug-resistant ventricular tachycardia and ventricular fibrillation.[245,249–253] Bretylium tosylate has also been used orally in the management of patients with ventricular tachycardia, with 200 to 400 mg given every 8 hours. Although orthostatic hypotension may develop in the initial stages of oral drug administration, tolerance usually develops without loss of antiarrhythmic efficacy. Much of the reported clinical experience is, however, with parenterally administered bretylium. A suitable regimen is a loading dose of 600 to 900 mg (5 to 10 mg/kg) intramuscularly with incremental doses of 200 mg every 1 to 2 hours, until the arrhythmia is controlled or about 2 g of drug has been given. The recommended maintenance dose is 5 mg/kg every 6 to 8 hours. During intravenous infusion, bretylium should be diluted in 50 to 100 ml of 5% dextrose in water, and the loading dose (5 to 10 mg/kg) administered slowly over 15 to 30 minutes. This regimen may be followed by a constant infusion of 1 to 10 mg/min. The initial release of catecholamines induced by bretylium results in increased heart rate and blood pressure. Arrhythmias may be aggravated.

The most common adverse effect is hypotension, usually postural.[98] Nausea and vomiting have occasionally been reported. Parotid enlargement commonly develops after 2 to 4 months of oral bretylium therapy. The consequences of bretylium-induced beta-adrenergic blockade, which usually follows an initial activation, include exacerbation of AV conduction slowing, congestive heart failure, and asthmatic attacks. Caution must

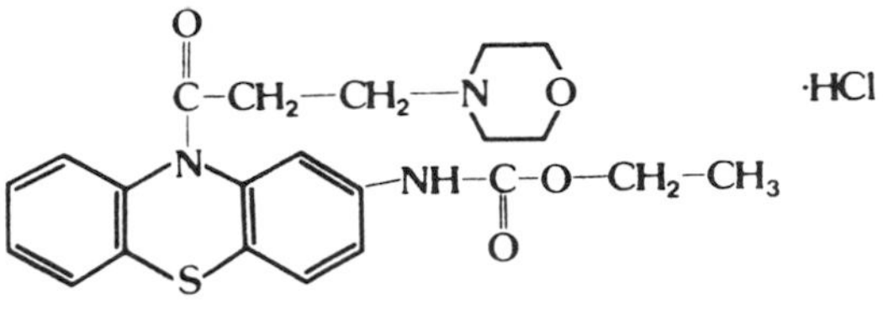

Figure 29-19. *Ethmozin.*

be exercised when catecholamine administration is sought to counteract the effects of bretylium because of supersensitivity reactions due to blockade of norepinephrine uptake by adrenergic nerve endings. It has been suggested that bretylium not be used in combination with other antiarrhythmic drugs, because complete nullification of either drug may result from combination therapy.[20]

Ethmozin

Ethmozin (Fig. 29-19), a phenothiazine derivative (10-[3-morpholinopropionyl]- phenothiazine-2-carbamic acid), has been used clinically in the Soviet Union for the management of patients with atrial and ventricular arrhythmias associated with a variety of heart diseases.[259] Its clinical use in the United States began during the late 1970s, and at present only scanty data are available on its clinical use, efficacy, and indications.[254,257,258]

Mode of Action. Microelectrode studies on isolated Purkinje fibers have shown that ethmozine decreases the $\dot{V}_{max}$ of phase zero and amplitude of the action potential, with a concomitant shortening of action potential duration.[254,255] These effects are concentration dependent. Voltage-clamp studies on isolated frog atrial muscle preparations have shown that ethmozin decreases the fast inward sodium current by decreasing the maximum conductance of sodium (GNa), without affecting the kinetics of activation, inactivation, and reactivation.[259] Such an effect, if also present in mammalian cardiac fibers, differs from that of other antiarrhythmic agents, which almost always delay the reactivation kinetic of the fast sodium inward current. Ethmozin does not seem to affect slow-response action potentials, since in the results obtained in open-chest anesthetized canine studies, ethmozin did not change spontaneous sinus node cycle length or AV conduction time when selectively injected into the sinus nodal artery and the posterior septal artery, respectively.[256] Right and left ventricular diastolic excitability threshold levels are increased following intravenous (4 mg/kg) administration. Although the drug decreases Purkinje fiber action potential duration, intact canine studies have shown that ethmozin increases both the right and left ventricular muscle cell refractory period.[256]

Further studies are needed to elucidate the mode of action of this potentially useful antiarrhythmic agent. Ethmozin appears to be effective against spontaneously occurring ventricular arrhythmias 24 hours after coronary artery occlusion in dogs as well as against ventricular arrhythmias induced by epinephrine 2 to 5 days after coronary artery occlusion.[255]

Metabolism and Pharmacokinetics. Little information has been published on the pharmacokinetics of ethmozin in humans. The drug appears to be well absorbed when given orally, and only small amounts of the agent (¼1%) appears unchanged in the urine and feces, suggesting extensive metabolism.[254,257,259] The elimination half-life of ethmozin in five healthy volunteers after an oral dose of 500 mg was 4 hours, with a range of 2.1 to 5.1 hours.[254] Plasma levels of ethmozin associated with significant antiarrhythmic effect were 244 to 1300 ng/ml. Atrial premature depolarization appeared to be suppressed with lower ethmozin plasma levels than did ventricular premature depolarization.[254,257]

Therapeutic Action, Dose, and Side-Effects. Ethmozin is very well tolerated by patients receiving up to 600 mg daily. The drug has almost no adverse effects.[254,256] A good control of premature ventricular complexes was achieved with a 600-mg, total daily oral dose of ethmozine (200 mg three times daily). In a recent preliminary report, including a double-blind, placebo-controlled, crossover study involving 27 patients, oral ethmozin (250 mg three times daily) was found to be more effective than oral disopyramide in controlling complex ventricular arrhythmias. Furthermore, ethmozin was associated with minimal side effects.[258] The almost complete absence of toxic side-effects makes ethmozin an attractive alternative antiarrhythmic agent; however, its value and effectiveness in the control of life-threatening ventricular arrhythmias remain to be seen.

Flecainide

Flecainide (Fig. 29-20) has recently been approved by the FDA and marketed (Tambocor®) for the management of life-threatening ventricular arrhythmias.[260]

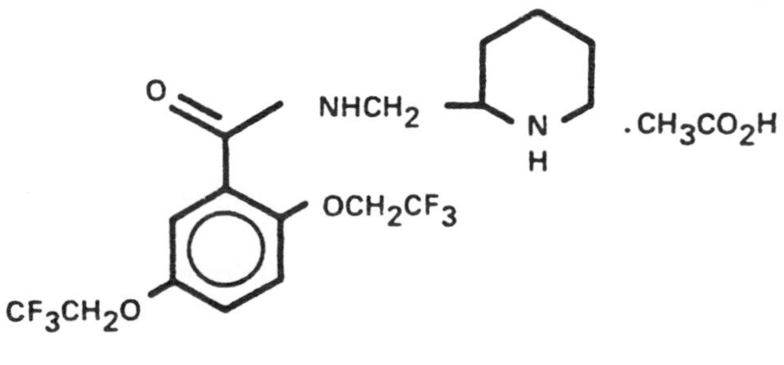

Figure 29-20. *Flecainide acetate.*

Mode of Action. Microelectrode studies on isolated tissue preparations have shown that flecainide decreases $\dot{V}_{max}$ of the upstroke of canine Purkinje and ventricular muscle cells in a concentration-dependent manner.[261] Ventricular muscle action potential duration was increased and Purkinje fiber duration decreased. Furthermore, flecainide depressed Purkinje fiber automaticity by elevating threshold potential.[262] These effects were considered relevant for the antiarrhythmic actions of the drug.

Metabolism and Pharmacokinetics. In anesthetized open-chest canine preparations, intravenous flecainide infusion, 0.1 to 0.25 mg/kg/min with plasma levels of 0.5 to 6.5 μg/ml, caused a concentration-dependent prolongation in atrial effective refractory periods and AV nodal functional and relative refractory periods.[260,262] At a lower flecainide concentration (0.7 μg/ml), the drug significantly reduced ventricular rate during atrial fibrillation and appeared to increase the ventricular fibrillation threshold.[262] Pretreatment with flecainide (2 mg/kg intravenously) appeared to reduce the incidence of ventricular fibrillation in open-chest swine preparations during the first 30 minutes of partial ischemia caused by 75% reduction in flow in the left anterior descending coronary artery.[263] However, flecainide had no effect on the incidence of ventricular fibrillation after complete occlusion of this artery.[263] Furthermore, flecainide depressed myocardial contractility (LV dP/dt max), caused hypotension, and increased QRS duration in a concentration-dependent manner.[260,263] Similar antiarrhythmic and electrophysiologic effects were also seen in humans. Prolonged PR and QT intervals and QRS widening were seen after flecainide administration.[264-267] Furthermore, flecainide appeared to be quite effective in suppressing premature ventricular complexes of various etiologies.[264-267]

Therapeutic Action, Dose, and Side-Effects. In most patients, an oral regimen of 200 mg twice daily was quite effective; a few patients required 300 mg twice daily. The half-life of flecainide is approximately 20 hours, with average effective flecainide concentrations of 650 ng/ml (range 200 to 800 ng/ml), which can be achieved with the above oral dosing schedule. In a preliminary report, intravenous flecainide (2 mg/kg over 5 minutes) was found to be effective in patients with the WPW syndrome because it increased both anterograde and retrograde effective refractory periods of the accessory pathway.[260,268] In addition, intravenous flecainide (2 mg/kg) suppressed premature ventricular complexes.[269] Flecainide seems to be well tolerated. Its side-effects include dizziness, blurred vision, headache, and nausea.[260,264-267] Some patients experience abnormal taste sensations, flushing, tinnitus, sleepiness, and paresthesias.[264]

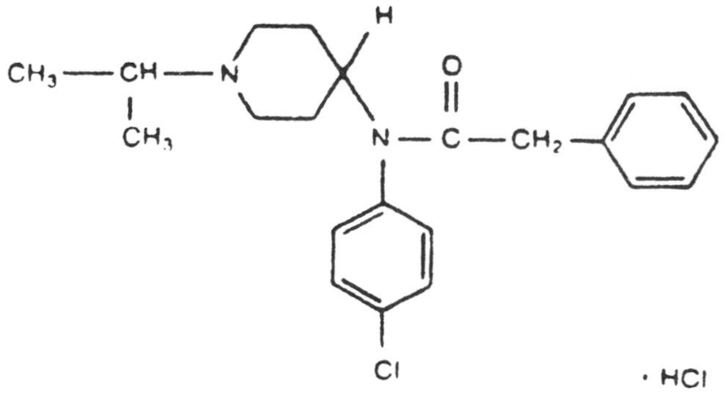

Figure 29-21. *Lorcainide.*

Lorcainide

Mode of Action. Carmeliet and Zaman[270,271] evaluated the effects of lorcainide (Fig. 29-21) on the transmembrane potential characteristics of isolated tissue preparations with microelectrodes. The drug decreased the $\dot{V}_{max}$ of the action potential of Purkinje fibers and prolonged the effective refractory periods of both Purkinje and ventricular muscle fibers. Slow-response action potentials were unaffected by lorcainide concentrations of up to 5 μg/ml.[271] Lorcainide decreases conduction velocity and automaticity in isolated normal Purkinje fibers[271] and causes a concentration-dependent slowing in the HV interval in both basic and premature impulses in the intact guinea pig hearts.[272] Experimental ventricular arrhythmias caused by left anterior descending coronary artery occlusion during the 24-hour arrhythmic phase, as well as arrhythmias caused by ouabain toxicity, respond well to lorcainide.[272]

Electrophysiologic studies in humans have shown that lorcainide consistently prolongs HV interval in a dose-dependent manner and is thus, contraindicated in patients with preexisting intraventricular conduction abnormalities.[272] Lorcainide has a variable effect on the AV nodal effective and functional refractory periods and the effective refractory period of the right ventricle. Most studies, however, found prolonged PR, QRS, and QT intervals.[272] Furthermore, lorcainide prolonged both antegrade and retrograde conduction times and effective refractory periods of the accessory pathway in patients with WPW syndrome; it therefore can be quite useful in this patient population.[273]

Metabolism and Pharmacokinetics. Lorcainide is rapidly distributed to well-perfused tissues, with very early decline in plasma lorcainide concentrations, necessitating a three-compartment model system to describe the kinetics adequately, at least in patients with ventricular arrhythmias.[274] The volume of distribution of lorcainide at steady state is 6.3 liter/kg, and its terminal half-life is 7.8 hours.[274] Clearance of lorcainide is extremely high and approximates normal blood flow.[272,274] The drug is

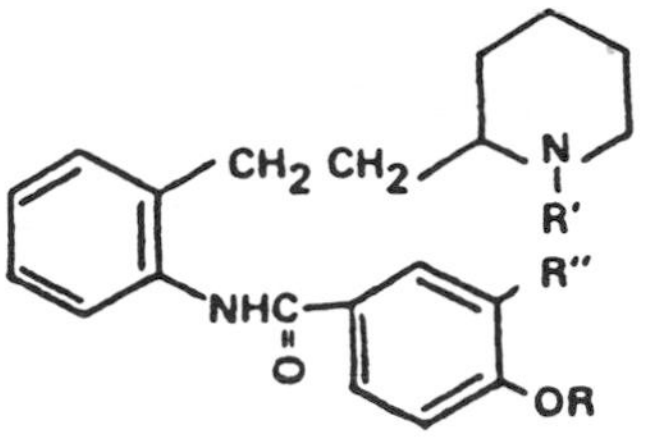

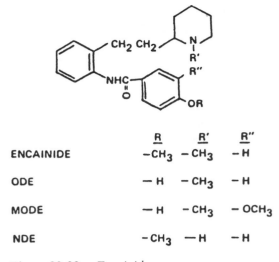

	R	R'	R''
ENCAINIDE	$-CH_3$	$-CH_3$	$-H$
ODE	$-H$	$-CH_3$	$-H$
MODE	$-H$	$-CH_3$	$-OCH_3$
NDE	$-CH_3$	$-H$	$-H$

Figure 29-22. *Encainide.*

83% bound to protein, with significantly lower binding in patients with congestive heart failure.[272] Oral bioavailability of lorcainide increases with higher and long-term oral doses and ranges from 2% to 4% after a single oral dose of 100 mg to 100% after 200 mg of long-term oral administration.[273,275] This occurs because of a saturable presystemic elimination of lorcainide, primarily caused by first-pass metabolism.[275] Only 2% of lorcainide is excreted unchanged in the urine. The major metabolite of lorcainide is norlorcainide, which has potent antiarrhythmic efficacy.[272] Its elimination half-life is 26.8 hours after 1 week of oral lorcainide administration in patients with ventricular arrhythmias.[274] Plasma concentration of lorcainide associated with effective suppression of ventricular arrhythmias seems to be variable but usually ranges between 150 and 400 ng/ml, a concentration range usually achieved with 100 mg twice or three times daily.[272,276] The complete elimination of lorcainide by hepatic metabolism indicates that hepatic function and blood flow could influence the disposition kinetics of this drug. Klots and associates[277] have shown that the half-life of lorcainide increases from 7.7 to 12.5 hours in patients with alcoholic cirrhosis. Furthermore, in patients with congestive heart failure, half-life increased from 7.7 to 15.6 hours, with a concomitant decrease in clearance from 1000 to 385 ml/min, probably caused by a decrease in hepatic blood flow.[277,278]

Therapeutic Action and Side-Effects. Lorcainide appears to suppress effectively ventricular prematures depolarizations[279] and to prevent induction of sustained ventricular tachycardia by programmed electrical stimulation in most patients.[279,280] The agent also appears to be effective in patients with the preexcitation syndrome[272,273] but relatively ineffective against atrial arrhythmias.[272] The most common side-effect, occurring at the start of therapy, is sleep disturbances,[272,279,280] characterized by frequent awakening, hot flashes, and vivid dreams. It appears, however, that patients do not complain of fatigue during the day.[279] Other side-effects include metallic taste during therapy, gastrointestinal distress, headache, nausea, and excessive perspiration.[272,279] The long-term efficacy and adverse effects of this agent remain to be seen.

Encainide

Mode of Action. Encainide (4-methoxy-2′[2-(1 methyl-2-piperidyl) ethyl] benzanilide hydrochloride) (Fig. 29-22) seems to be an effective and potent antiarrhythmic agent orally and intravenously.[281] Isolated tissue studies with microelectrodes have shown that encainide decreases the $\dot{V}_{max}$ of the action potential of Purkinje fiber in a rate-dependent manner and shortens action potential duration of Purkinje but not ventricular muscle fibers.[282,283] Encainide also suppresses normal Purkinje fiber automaticity but has no effect on abnormal automaticity initiated in partially depolarized Purkinje fibers induced by high extracellular potassium or depolarizing current injections.[282] Thus, the drug appears not to affect slow-response action potentials. Furthermore, encainide decreases excitability (increased current threshold) by shifting threshold voltage to less negative values.[284] Note that a metabolite of encainide, o-demethyl encainide, has more potent cellular electrophysiologic effects in *in vitro* studies[282] and higher antiarrhythmic activity in rat model of arrhythmias induced by aconitine[289] than the parent drugs.

Metabolism and Pharmacokinetics. In anesthetized open-chest dogs encainide prolonged the refractory period and the duration of monophasic action potential duration in both atrial and right ventricular endocardial tissues, with a more pronounced increase in the atrium.[285] Furthermore, in this study, encainide also caused an increase in the AH, HV, QRS, and QTc intervals. O-demethyl encainide abolished spontaneously occurring ventricular arrhythmias in dogs 48 hours after a 2-hour left anterior descending coronary artery occlusion followed by reperfusion.[286] However, o-demethyl encainide appears to facilitate initiation of ventricular fibrillation by brief right ventricular pacing at 200 beats/min, which could not be defibrillated in the majority of dogs studied.[286] The experimental studies of the electrophysiologic, antiarrhythmic, and proarrhythmic properties of encainide and its major metabolite, o-demethyl encainide, seem to corroborate well with the clinical findings. Encainide prolonged AH, HV, and QRS intervals in humans.[287,288] Prolongation of the QT interval, however, was noted only during long-term therapy, possibly due to accumulation of the active metabolite.[290]

Oral absorption of encainide is highly variable. Bioavailability ranges between 7.4% and 82% (mean 42%).[291] Such variability may be due to presystemic elimination.[281] The half-life after intravenous dosing was 3.3 ± 1.68 hours (range 2 to 6.9 hours), and it tended to be shorter after oral dosing, averaging 2.4 hours (range 1.5 to 3.7 hours).[291] Clearance also varied widely, ranging from 210 to 1790 ml/min (average 1157 ml/min). The time to peak plasma concentration after oral dosing was 1.5 to 3 hours (average 1.6 hours).[291] The major route of elimination of encainide is hepatic metabolism, which should be taken into account when long-term oral encainide therapy is contemplated, because the metabolites have important antiarrhythmic efficacy.[290,292,299]

Therapeutic Action, Dose, and Side-Effects. Encainide was found to be fairly effective against frequent and complex premature ventricular depolarizations[291,293] and arrhythmias associated with the WPW syndrome.[298] Encainide appears to be more effective and better tolerated than quinidine in patients with premature ventricular complexes.[295] Minimal antiarrhythmic plasma concentration after intravenous dosing is higher than after oral dosing (39 versus 14 ng/ml), suggesting the presence of an active metabolite after the latter.[291,297] Note that in a patient who did not respond to encainide, no o-demethyl encainide was found in the plasma. Subsequent studies have shown 6% to 10% of patients cannot metabolize encainide.[290] It is not clear if nonresponders lack the capacity to metabolize encainide and whether such deficiency in metabolism may cause arrhythmias in the WPW syndrome.[298] Dose schedule should carefully be reevaluated in each patient on the basis of drug ability to suppress arrhythmias or widen the QRS interval. Daily oral doses of encainide are between 75 to 300 mg, given in divided doses every 4 to 6 hours. Peak plasma level after an intravenous dose of 75 mg is 996 ng/ml; after an oral dose it is 241 ng/ml.[291]

The most troublesome side-effect of encainide therapy is aggravation of ventricular arrhythmias, including induction of ventricular fibrillation.[291,295,296] A common type of arrhythmia induced by encainide seems to be polymorphic ventricular tachycardia, resulting in cardiac arrest.[296] Such an arrhythmia aggravation appears to differ from other drug-induced arrhythmias with quinidinelike drugs in that encainide-induced rhythm disorders were not associated with marked QT prolongation and usually did not self-terminate.[296] The risk of encainide-induced ventricular tachyarrhythmias was 11% in 90 patients receiving the drug for recurrent sustained ventricular tachycardia or ventricular fibrillation and was 2.2% in 47 patients receiving the drug for chronic complex premature ventricular depolarizations.[295] Rhythm aggravation occurs 17 to 48 hours after the start of chronic oral maintenance dosing with encainide.[296] Patients with a history of recurrent sustained ventricular tachycardia and ventricular fibrillation should receive encainide therapy only in a hospital with continuous electrocardiographic monitoring and personnel skilled in cardiopulmonary resuscitation. In a more recent report, encainide was associated with the highest incidence of aggravating ventricular arrhythmias of nine different antiarrhythmic drugs.[300]

Ajmaline

Ajmaline (Fig. 29-23), a tertiary indoline alkaloid, was first isolated from the root of *Rauwolfia serpentina,* an Indian plant, by Siddiqui and Siddiqui in 1932.[301] Unlike the reserpinelike alkaloids, the ajmalinelike alkaloids isolated from the plant do not seem to affect adrenergic nerve terminals. Microelectrode studies on isolated cardiac tissues have shown that ajmaline (1 μg/ml) had no effect on resting membrane potential but decreased $\dot{V}_{max}$, action potential amplitude, and overshoot of canine atrial Purkinje and ventricular muscle fibers.[302] Furthermore, it shortened Purkinje fiber action potential but prolonged both atrial and ventricular muscle action potential duration.[302] Similar findings were observed by Dreifus and colleagues[20] on partially depolarized (resting membrane potential about −60 mV) ventricular muscle fibers when superfused with 3 μg/ml of 17-monochloroacetyl ajmaline hydrochloride. Furthermore, ajmaline decreased excitability of both canine atrial and ventricular tissues.[302] Ajmaline also decreases normal Purkinje fiber automaticity by decreasing the slope of phase 4 depolarization and slows linear conduction velocity in isolated strands of canine Purkinje fibers.[303]

Ajmaline is effective against digitalis-induced ventricular arrhythmias in dogs.[302,304] However, this drug is most effective against aconitine-induced atrial tachyarrhythmias.[302] Electrophysiologic studies in both anesthetized and conscious dogs demonstrated a significant depression of intraventricular conduction with QRS widening but without significant prolongation of the AH interval.[305] In addition, ajmaline was effective against ventricular arrhythmias that occur 24 hours after left anterior descending coronary artery occlusion in the dog.[305] Early clinical studies indicate that ajmaline can be of some value in the management of paroxysmal supraventricular tachycardia.[302,318] Bojorges and associates[302] have shown that 1 mg/kg of ajmaline given over 5 minutes suppressed these arrhythmias in 30 of 36 patients. In a more recent study,[318] intravenous administration of ajmaline (50 mg) was found to be effective in 10 patients with paroxysmal supraventricular tachycardia mediated by dual AV nodal pathways. Furthermore, ajmaline was found to be relatively ineffective against arrhythmias of ventricular origin.[302] Wellens and colleagues[306] found that ajmaline caused complete antegrade block in the accessory pathway in 32 of 59 patients

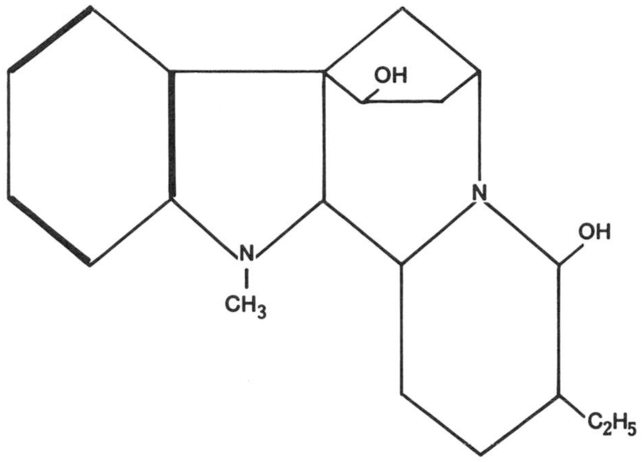

Figure 29-23. *Ajmalin.*

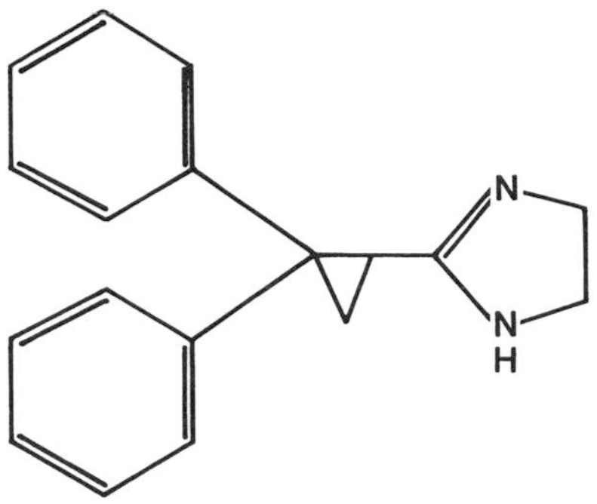

Figure 29-24. *Cibenzoline.*

with the WPW syndrome. Furthermore, failure of ajmaline to produce complete anterograde block appeared to be related to a shorter (less than 270 msec) refractory period of this pathway.

The role of ajmaline in the long-term management of arrhythmias of various etiologies, and the role, if any, of its metabolite, remain to be seen. The drug does not seem to be associated with serious side-effects.[306] Mild side-effects include flushing, nausea, and blinking of eyes. However, severe toxicity can cause worsening of congestive heart failure, shock, sinoatrial block, and even ventricular tachycardia and ventricular fibrillation.[306,318] The drug should be used with caution in patients with conduction disturbances of the AV node and the His–Purkinje system. Hypotension may develop during intravenous administration; it is therefore imperative to infuse the drug slowly, 1 mg/kg over 3 to 5 minutes.[302,306]

Cibenzoline

Mode of Action. Cibenzoline, a new antiarrhythmic drug of imidazoline derivation (2-[2,-diphenyl-cyclopropyl]) (Fig. 29-24), is not related chemically to any other known antiarrhythmic drug. The succinate salt is used. Preliminary clinical trials indicate the potential usefulness of this agent to suppress ventricular premature depolarizations[307] and arrhythmias associated with the WPW syndrome.[308]

Microelectrode studies on isolated cardiac tissue have shown that cibenzoline prolongs the action potential duration of atrial and ventricular muscle cells; no such effect or shortening of action potential duration occurs in Purkinje fibers.[309–311] Furthermore, this agent appears to prevent action potential shortening during hypoxia.[310] Cibenzoline decreases $\dot{V}_{max}$ in atrial and ventricular tissues[309–311] and slows conduction velocity in isolated ventricular preparations.[310] The drug does not interfere with sinus nodal automaticity[309] but causes a concentration-dependent prolongation of sinus node cell action potential duration, which tends to decrease the rate of sinus firing.[309,310] Cibenzoline decreased the slope of phase 4 depolarization in normal Purkinje fibers, causing a decrease in the rate of automatic impulse initiation.[309] However, such an effect was not observed in Dangman's studies,[311] but in his study, cibenzoline depressed automaticity in normal Purkinje fibers induced by isoproterenol by a mechanism independent of beta-adrenergic receptor blockade.[311] Cibenzoline was found to depress abnormal automatic mechanism (resting potential −60 to 40 mV) in Purkinje fibers induced by barium ions.[311] Note that in this study cibenzoline induced early afterdepolarizations and triggered activity in Purkinje fibers.[311] This observation may explain, at least in part, the proarrhythmic properties of this agent in certain experimental[319] and clinical settings.[312]

In clinical studies, cibenzoline increased the PR, HV, and QTC intervals, with QRS widening following oral or intravenous administration.[313,314] Cibenzoline suppressed or decreased the frequency of premature ventricular depolarizations of many etiologies.[307,312,313] In patients in whom ventricular tachycardia was induced by electrical stimulation, cibenzoline prevented tachycardia induction in 40% to 58% (total of 17 patients in two studies).[313,314] Cibenzoline appears to be ineffective in patients with sustained ventricular tachycardia or ventricular fibrillation but quite effective in patients with symptomatic premature ventricular depolarizations or nonsustained ventricular tachycardia.[316]

Cibenzoline is well absorbed after oral administration (92% bioavailability), with maximum plasma levels occurring 1 hour and 36 minutes after drug ingestion.[315] Its half-life is 4 hours in healthy persons[315] and is prolonged up to 22 hours in persons with kidney failure[312] because elimination is mainly renal. Clearance of cibenzoline correlates well with creatinine clearance, with an average rate of 495 ml/min.[315] Finally, 60% of the drug is excreted unchanged in the urine, and approximately 60% is protein bound.[316]

The average oral dose of cibenzoline is 65 mg, 4 times daily, with 1 to 2 mg/kg given intravenously. Effective plasma cibenzoline concentrations appear to be 215 to 400 ng/ml. The drug appears to be well tolerated, with side-effects including epigastric burning, blurred vision, nausea, vomiting, and potential arrhythmia aggravation.

References

1. Wit, A. L., Rosen, M. R., and Hoffman, B. F.: Electrophysiology and pharmacology of cardiac arrhythmias. II. Relationship for normal and abnormal electrical activity of cardiac fibers to the genesis of arrhythmias. B. Reentry sec. 1. Am. Heart J., 88:664–670, 1974.
2. Wit, A. L., Rosen, M. R., and Hoffman, B. F.: Electrophysiology and pharmacology of cardiac arrhythmias. II. Relationship of normal and abnormal electrical activity of cardiac fibers to the genesis of arrhythmias. B. Reentry sec. 2. Am. Heart J., 88:798–806, 1974.
3. Coraboeuf, E.: Ionic basis of electrical activity in cardiac tissues. Am. J. Physiol., 234:H101–H116, 1978.
4. Vassalle, M.: Electrogenesis of the plateau and pacemaker potential. Ann. Rev. Physiol., 41:425–440, 1977.
5. Cranefield, P. F.: Action potentials and arrhythmias. Circ. Res., 41:415–423, 1977.
6. Wit, A. L., and Cranfield, P. F.: Triggered and automatic activity in the canine coronary sinus. Circ. Res., 41:435–445, 1977.
7. Tsien, R. W., Kass, R. S., and Weingart, R.: Cellular and subcellular mechanisms of cardiac pacemaker oscillations. J. Exp. Biol. 81:205–215, 1979.
8. Karagueuzian, H. S., and Katzung, B. G.: Voltage-clamp studies of transient inward current and mechanical oscillations induced by ouabain in ferret papillary muscle. J. Physiol. (Lond.) 327:255–271, 1982.
9. Hoffman, B. F., and Rosen, M. R.: Cellular mechanisms of cardiac arrhythmias. Circ. Res. 49:1–15, 1981.
10. Vaughn Williams, E. M.: Classification of antiarrhythmic drugs. J. Pharmacol. Ther., 1:115–138, 1975.
11. Singh, B. N., and Hauswirth, O.: Comparative mechanisms of action of antiarrhythmic drugs. Am. Heart J., 87:367–382, 1974.
12. Rosen, M. R.: Effects of pharmacological agents on mechanisms responsible for re-entry. In Kulbertus H. E. (ed.): Reentrant Arrhythmias. Mechanisms and Treatment, pp. 283–294. Baltimore, University Park Press, 1976.
13. Anzelevitch, C., Bernstein, M. J., Feldman, H. N., and Moe, G. K.: Parasystole reentry and tachycardia: A canine preparation of cardiac arrhythmia occurring across inexcitable segment of tissue. Circulation, 68:1101–1115, 1983.
14. Woosley, R. L., and Shand, D. G.: Pharmacokinetics of antiarrhythmic drugs. Am. J. Cardiol., 41:986–995, 1978.
15. Harrison, D. C., Meffin, P. J., and Winkle, R. A.: Clinical pharmacokinetics of antiarrhythmic drugs. Prog. Cardiovasc. Dis., 20:217–242, 1977.
16. Hoffman, B. F., Rosen, M. R., and Wit, A. L.: Electrophysiology and pharmacology of cardiac arrhythmias. VII. Cardiac effects of quinidine and procainamide. Am. Heart J., 90:117–122, 1975.
17. Hondeghem, L. and Katzung, B. G.: Test of a model of antiarrhythmic drug action. Effects of quinidine and lidocaine on myocardial conduction. Circulation, 61:1217–1224, 1980.
18. Weld, F. M., Coromilas, J., Rottman, J. N., and Bigger, J. T., Jr.: Mechanisms of quinidine-induced depression of maximum upstroke velocity in ovine cardiac Purkinje fibers. Circ. Res., 50:369–376, 1982.
19. Hoffman, B. F., and Bigger, J. T., Jr.: Antiarrhythmic drugs. In Dipalma, J. R. (ed.): Drill's Pharmacology in Medicine, pp. 824–852. New York, McGraw-Hill, 1971.
20. Dreifus, L. S., Watanabe, Y., Dreifus, H. N., and Azevedo, I. D.: The effect of antiarrhythmic agents on impulse formation and impulse conduction. In Wellens, H. J. J., Lie, K. I., and Janse, M. J., (eds.): The Conduction System of the Heart, pp. 182–206. Philadelphia, Lea & Febiger, 1976.
21. Mirro, M. J., Manalan, A. S., Bailey, J. C., and Watanabe, A. M.: Anticholinergic effects of dysopyramide and quinidine on guinea pig myocardium. Mediation by direct muscarinic receptor blockade. Circ. Res., 47:855–865, 1980.
22. Ochs, H. R., Grube, E., Greenblatt, D. J., et al.: Intravenous quinidine: pharmacokinetic properties and effects on left ventricular performance in human. Am. Heart J., 99:468–475, 1980.
23. Josephson, M. E., Seides, S. E., Battsford, W. P., et al.: The electrophysiological effects of intramuscular quinidine on the atrioventricular conducting system in man. Am. Heart J., 87:55–64, 1974.
24. Seller, T. D., Campbell, R. W. F., Bashore, T. M., and Gallagher, J. G.: Effects of procainamide and quinidine sulphate in the Wolff-Parkinson-White syndrome. Circulation, 55:15–22, 1977.
25. Wellens, H. J., and Durrer, D.: Effect of procainamide, quinidine, and ajmaline in the Wolff-Parkinson-White syndrome. Circulation, 50:116–120, 1974.
26. Heissenbuttel, R. H., and Bigger, J. T., Jr.: The effect of oral quinidine on intraventricular conduction in man: Correlation of plasma quinidine with changes in QRS duration. Am. Heart J., 80:453–462, 1970.
27. Krikler, D. M., and Curry, P. V. L.: Torsades de pointes, an atypical ventricular tachycardia. Br. Heart J., 38:117–120, 1976.
28. Selzer, A., and Wray, H. W.: Quinidine syncope: Paroxysmal ventricular fibrillation occurring during treatment of chronic atrial fibrillation. Circulation, 30:17–26, 1964.
29. Karen, A., Tzivoni, D., Gavish, D., et al.: Etiology, warning signs and therapy of torsades de pointes. A study of 10 patients. Circulation, 64:1164–1174, 1981.
30. Jenger, H. R., and Hagemaijer, F.: Quinidine syncope: Torsades de pointes with low quinidine plasma concentrations. Eur. J. Cardiol., 4:447–453, 1976.
31. Ueda, C. T., Hirschfeld, D. S., Scheinman, M. M., et al.: Disposition kinetics of quinidine. Clin. Pharmacol. Ther., 19:30–36, 1976.
32. Hirschfeld, D. S., Veda, C. T., Rowland, M., et al.: Clinical and electrophysiological effects of intravenous quinidine in man (abstr). Circulation, 50 (Suppl. III): III–230, 1974.
33. Khorsandian, R., Chaplan, R. F., Feinberg, J. F., and Bellet, S.: Plasma quinidine content levels following single oral doses of quinidine polygalacturonate. Am. J. Med. Sci., 245:311–319, 1963.
34. Greenblatt, D. J., Pfeifer, H. J., Ochs, H. R., et al.: Pharmacokinetics or quinidine in humans after intravenous, intramuscular and oral administration. J. Pharmacol. Exp. Ther., 202:365–378, 1977.
35. Kessler, K. M., Lowenthal, D. T., Warner H., et al.: Quinidine elimination in patients with congestive heart failure or poor renal function. N. Engl. J. Med., 290:706–709, 1974.
36. Miller, R. D., Way, W. L., and Katzung, B. G.: The potentiation of neuromuscular blocking agents by quinidine. Anesthesiology, 28:1036–1041, 1972.
37. Aviado, D. M., and Salem, H.: Drug action, reaction and interaction. I. Quinidine for cardiac arrhythmia. J. Clin. Pharmacol., 15:447–483, 1975.

38. Blout, R. E.: Management of chloroquine resistant falciparum malana. Arch. Intern. Med., 119:557–561, 1967.
39. Koch-Weser, J.: Quinidine induced hypoprothrombinemia hemorrhage in patients on chronic warfarin therapy. Ann. Intern. Med., 68:511–517, 1968.
40. Doering, W.: Quinidine-digoxin interaction. Pharmacokinetics, underlying mechanism, and clinical implication. N. Engl. J. Med., 301:400–404, 1979.
41. Bigger, J. T., Jr.: The quinidine-digoxin interaction. What do we know about it? N. Engl. J. Med., 301:779–781, 1979.
42. Hirsh, P. D., Weiner, H. J., and North, R. L.: Further insights into digoxin-quinidine interaction. Lack of correlation between serum digoxin concentration and inotropic state of the heart. Am. J. Cardiol., 46:863–868, 1980.
43. de Senac, J. B.: Traite de la structure du coeur, de son action et de ses maladies. Paris J Vincent, 2:504, 1749.
44. Willius, F. A., and Keys, T. E.: A remarkably early reference to the use of cinchona in cardiac arrhythmias. Staff meetings of the Mayo Clinic, pp. 294–296, May 13, 1942.
45. Rinkenerger, R. L., Prystowsky, E. N., Jackman, W. M., et al.: Drug conversion of nonsustained ventricular tachycardia to sustained ventricular tachycardia during serial electrophysiologic studies: Identification of drugs that exacerbate tachycardia and potential mechanisms. Am. Heart J., 103:179–184, 1982.
46. Gaughan, C. E., Lown, B., Lanigan, J., et al.: Acute oral testing for determining antiarrhythmic drug efficacy. I. Quinidine. Am. J. Cardiol., 38:677–684, 1976.
47. Hirschfeld, D. S., Veda, C. T., Rowland, M., et al.: Clinical and electrophysiological effects of intravenous quinidine in man. Br. Heart J., 37:309–316, 1977.
48. Torok, E., Bajkay, G., Gulyas, A., and Maklary, E.: Comparative study of a long acting quinidine preparation and quinidine sulphate in chronic atrial fibrillation. Pharmacol. Clin., 2:90–93, 1970.
49. Bagwell, E. E., Walle, T., Drayer, D. E., et al.: Correlation of the electrophysiological and antiarrhythmic properties of the N-acetyl metabolite of procainamide with plasma and tissue drug concentrations in the dog. J. Pharmacol. Exp. Ther., 197:38–48, 1976.
50. Rosen, M. R., Gelband, H., and Hoffman, B. F.: Canine electrocardiographic and cardiac electrophysiologic changes induced by procainamide. Circulation, 46:528–536, 1972.
51. Arnsdorf, M. F., and Bigger, J. T.: The effect of procainamide on components of excitability in long mammalian cardiac Purkinje fibers. Circ. Res., 38:115–122, 1976.
52. Giardina, E. C., and Bigger, J. T.: Procaine amide against reentrant ventricular arrhythmias. Lengthening R-V intervals of coupled ventricular premature depolarization as an insight into the mechanism of action procaine amide. Circulation, 48:959–968, 1973.
53. Josephson, M. E., Caracta, A. R., Ricciutti, M. A., et al.: Electrophysiologic properties of procainamide in man. Am. J. Cardiol., 33:596–603, 1974.
54. Camardo, J. S., Greenspan, A. M., Horowitz, L. N., et al.: Strength-interval relation in the human ventricle: Effect of procainamide. Am. J. Cardiol., 45:856–860, 1980.
55. Koch-Weser, J., and Klein, S. W.: Procainamide dosage schedules, plasma concentrations and clinical effects. J.A.M.A., 215:1454–1460, 1971.
56. Graffner, C., Johnsson, G., and Sjogren, J.: Pharmacokinetics of procainamide intravenously and orally as conventional slow-release tablets. Clin. Pharmacol. Ther., 17:414–423, 1975.
57. Shaw, T. R. D., Kumana, D. R., Royds, R. D., et al.: Use of plasma level in evaluation of procainamide dosage. Br. Heart J., 36:265–269, 1974.
58. Giardina, E. G. V., Fenster, P. E., Bigger, J. T., Jr., et al.: Efficacy, plasma concentrations and adverse effects of a new sustained release procainamide preparation. Am. J. Cardiol., 46:855–862, 1980.
59. Koch-Weser, J.: Pharmacokinetics of procainamide in man. Ann. N. Y. Acad. Sci., 179:370–382, 1971.
60. Wenger, T. L., Browning, D. J., Masterton, C. E., et al.: Procainamide delivery to ischemic canine myocardium following rapid intravenous administration. Circ. Res., 46:789–795, 1980.
61. Wenger, T. L., Masterton, C. E., Abou-Donia, M. B., et al.: Relationship between regional myocardial procainamide concentration and regional myocardial blood flow during ischemia in the dog. Circ. Res., 42:846–851, 1978.
62. Elson, J., Strong, J. M., Lee, W.-K., et al.: Antiarrhythmic potency of N-acetylprocainamide. Clin. Pharmacol. Ther., 17:137–140, 1975.
63. Strong, J. M., Dutcher, J. S., Lee, W.-K., et al.: Pharmacokinetics in man of the N-acetylated metabolite of procainamide. J. Pharmacokinet. Biopharm. 3:223–235, 1975.
64. Gibson, T. P., Matusik, J., Matusik, E., et al.: Acetylation of procainamide in man and its relationship to isonicotinic acid hydrazide acetylation phenotype. Clin. Pharmacol. Ther. 17:395–399, 1975.
65. Gibson, R. P., Matuski, E. J., and Briggs, W. A.: N-acetylprocainamide levels in patients with end-stage renal failure. Clin. Pharmacol. Ther., 19:206–212, 1976.
66. Galeazzi, R. L., Sheiner, L. B., Lockwood, T., et al.: The renal elimination of procainamide. Clin. Pharmacol. Ther., 19:55–61, 1976.
67. Weily, H. S., and Genton, E.: Pharmacokinetics of procainamide. Arch. Intern. Med., 130:366–369, 1972.
68. Collste, P., and Karlsson, E.: Arrhythmias prophylaxis with procainamide plasma concentrations in relation to dose. Acta Med. Scand., 194:405–411, 1973.
69. Dreyfuss, J., Bigger, J. T., Jr., Cohen, A. I., and Schreiber, E. C.: Metabolism of procainamide in rhesus monkey and man. Clin. Pharmacol. Ther., 13:366-371, 1972.
70. Giardina, E. G. V., Dreyfuss, J., Bigger, J. T., Jr., et al.: Metabolism of procainamide in normal and cardiac subjects. Clin. Pharmacol. Ther., 17:339–351, 1976.
71. Reidenberg, M. M., Drayer, D. E., Levy, M., et al.: Polymorphic-acetylation of procainamide in man. Clin. Pharmacol. Ther., 17:722–730, 1975.
72. Bigger, J. T., Jr., and Heissenbuttel, R. H.: The use of procainamide and lidocaine in the treatment of cardiac arrhythmias. Prog. Cardiovasc. Dis., 11:515–534, 1969.
73. Mandel, W. J., Laks, M. M., Obayashi, K., et al.: The Wolff-Parkinson-White syndrome: Pharmacologic effects of procaine amide. Am. Heart J., 90:744–754, 1975.
74. Giardina, E. G. V., Heissenbuttel, R. H., and Bigger, J. T., Jr.: Intermittent intravenous procainamide to treat ventricular arrhythmias. Ann. Intern. Med., 78:183–193, 1973.
75. Inouye, M., Millar, J., and Townsend, J. H.: Agranulocytosis following maintenance dosage of pronestyl. Report of severe case with recovery. J.A.M.A., 147:652–653, 1951.
76. Blomgren, S. E., Condemi, J. J., and Vaughan, J. H.: Procainamide-induced lupus erthematosus. Clinical and laboratory observations. Am. J. Med., 52:338–348, 1972.
77. Woosley, R. L., Drayer, D. E., Reidenburg, M. M., et al.: Effect of acetylator on the rate at which procainamide induces antinuclear antibodies and the lupus syndrome. N. Engl. J. Med., 298:1157–1159, 1978.
78. Danilo, P., and Rosen, M. R.: Cardiac effects of disopyramide. Am. Heart J., 92:532–536, 1976.
79. Danilo, P., Hordof, A. J., and Rosen, M. R.: Effects of disopyramide on electrophysiologic properties of canine cardiac Purkinje fibers. J. Pharmacol. Ther., 201:701–710, 1977.
80. Josephson, M. E., Caracta, A. R., Lau, S. R., et al.: Electrophysio-

logical evaluation of disopyramide in man. Am. Heart J., 86:771–780, 1973.
81. Birkhead, J. S., and Vaughan William, E. M.: Dual effect of disopyramide on atrial and atrioventricular conduction and refractory periods. Br. Heart J., 39:657–660, 1977.
82. Katoh, T., Karagueuzian, H. S., Jordan, J., and Mandel, W. J.: The cellular electrophysiologic mechanism of the dual actions of disopyramide on rabbit sinus node function. Circulation, 66:1216–1224, 1982.
83. Hinderling, P. H., and Garrett, E. R.: Pharmacokinetics of the antiarrhythmic disopyramide in healthy humans. J. Pharmacokinet. Biopharm., 4:199–229, 1976.
84. Ward, J. W., and Kinghom, C. R.: The pharmacokinetics of disopyramide following myocardial infarction with special reference to oral and intravenous dose regimen. J. Intern. Med. Res., 4 (Suppl 1):49–53, 1976.
85. Bryson, S. M., Whiting, B., and Lawrence, J. R.: Disopyramide serum and pharmacologic effect kinetics applied to the assessment of bioavailability. Br. J. Clin. Pharmacol., 6:409–419, 1978.
86. Dubetz, D. K., Brown, N. N., Hooper, W. D., et al.: Disopyramide pharmacokinetics and bioavailability. Br. J. Clin. Pharmacol., 6:279–281, 1976.
87. Hinderling, P. H., and Garrett, E. R.: Pharmacokinetics of the antiarrhythmic disopyramide in healthy humans. J. Pharmacokinet. Biopharm., 4:199–230, 1976.
88. Cunningham, J. L., Shen, D. D., Shudo, I., et al.: The effects of urine pH and plasma protein binding on the renal clearance of disopyramide. Clin. Pharmacokinet., 2:373–383, 1977.
89. Hartel, G., Louhua, A., and Konttinen, A.: Disopyramide in the prevention of recurrence of atrial fibrillation after electroconversion. Clin. Pharmacol. Ther., 15:551–555, 1974.
90. Vismara, L. A., Vera, Z., Miller, R. R., et al.: Efficacy of disopyramide phosphate in the treatment of refractory ventricular tachycardia. Am. J. Cardiol., 39:1027–1034, 1977.
91. Koch-Weser, J.: Disopyramide. N. Engl. J. Med., 300:957–962, 1979.
92. Spurrell, R. A. J., Thorburn, C. W., Camm, J., et al.: Effects of disopyramide on electrophysiological properties of specialized conduction system in man and on accessory atrioventricular pathway in Wolff-Parkinson-White syndrome. Br. Heart J., 37:861–867, 1975.
93. Investigational brochure: Norpace (disopyramide phosphate), an antiarrhythmic drug. Searle Laboratories, May 1977.
94. Heel, R. C., Brogden, R. N., Speight, T. M., and Avery, G. S.: Disopyramide: A review of its pharmacological properties and therapeutic use in treating cardiac arrhythmias. Drugs, 15:331–368, 1978.
95. Jennings, G., Model, D. G., Jones, M. B. S., et al.: Oral disopyramide in prophylaxis of arrhythmias following myocardial infarction. Lancet, 1:51–54, 1976.
96. Zainal, N., Carmichael, D. J. S., Griffiths, J. W., et al.: Oral disopyramide for the prevention of arrhythmias in patients with acute myocardial infarction admitted to open wards. Lancet, 2:887–889, 1977.
97. Rangno, R. E., Warnica, W., Ogilvie, R. I., et al.: Correlation of disopyramide pharmacokinetics with efficacy in ventricular tachyarrhythmias. J. Intern. Med. Res., 4 (Suppl): 4:54–60, 1976.
98. Block, P. J., and Winkle, R. A.: Hemodynamic effects of antiarrhythmic drugs. Am. J. Cardiol., 52:146–236, 1983.
99. Arnsdorg, M. F., and Bigger, J. T., Jr.: The effect of lidocaine on membrane conductance in mammalian Purkinje fibers. J. Clin. Invest., 51:2252–2263, 1972.
100. Bigger, M. T., Jr., and Mandel, W. J.: Effect of lidocaine on conduction in canine Purkinje fibers and at the ventricular muscle Purkinje fiber junction. J. Pharmacol. Exp. Ther., 174:487–499, 1970.
101. Singh, B. N., and Vaughan Williams, E. M.: Effect of altering potassium concentration on the action of lidocaine and diphenylhydantoin on rabbit and ventricular muscle. Circ. Res., 29:286–297, 1971.
102. Rosen, M. R., Merker, C., and Pippenger, C. E.: The effects of lidocaine on the canine ECG and electrophysiological properties of Purkinje fibers. Am. Heart J., 91:191–202, 1976.
103. Kupersmith, J., Antman, E. M., and Hoffman, B. F.: In vivo electrophysiologic effects of lidocaine in canine acute myocardial infarction. Circ. Res., 36:84–91, 1975.
104. Brennan, F. J., Cranfield, P. F., and Wit, A. L.: Effects of lidocaine on slow response and depressed fast response action potentials of canine Purkinje fibers. J. Pharmacol. Exp. Ther., 204:312–324, 1978.
105. El-Sheriff, N., Sherlag, B. J., Lazzara, R., and Hope, R. R.: Reentrant ventricular arrhythmias in the late myocardial infarction period. Mechanism of action of lidocaine. Circulation, 56:395–402, 1977.
106. Lamanna, V., Antzelevitch, C., and Moe, G. K.: Effects of lidocaine on conduction through depolarized canine false tendons and on O model of reflected reentry. J. Pharmacol. Exp. Ther., 221:353–371, 1982.
107. Kimura, S., Nakaya, H., and Kanno, M.: Effects of verapamil and lidocaine on changes in action potential characteristics and conduction time induced by combined hypoxia, hyperkalemia and acidosis in canine ventricular myocardium. J. Cardiovasc. Pharmacol., 4:658–667, 1982.
108. Grant, A. O., Strauss, L. J., Wallace, A. G., and Strauss, H. C.: The influence of PH on the electrophysiological effects of lidocaine in guinea pig ventricular myocardium. Circ. Res., 47:542–550, 1980.
109. Mandel, W. J., and Bigger, J. T., Jr.: Electrophysiologic effects of lidocaine on isolated canine and rabbit atrial tissue. J. Pharmacol. Exp. Ther., 185:438–446, 1973.
110. Rosen, M. R., and Danilo, P., Jr.: Effects of tetrodotoxin, lidocaine, verapamil, and AHR-2666 on ouabain induced delayed after depolarizations in canine Purkinje fibers. Circ. Res., 46:117–124, 1980.
111. Karagueuzian, H. S., and Katzung, B. G.: Relative inotropic and arrhythmogenic effects of five cardiac steroids in ventricular myocardium: Oscillatory after potentials and the role of endogenous catecholamines. J. Pharmacol. Exp. Ther., 218:348–356, 1981.
112. Arnsdorf, M. F., and Bigger, J. T., Jr.: The effect of lidocaine on components of excitability in long mammalian cardiac Purkinje fibers. J. Pharmacol. Exp. Ther., 195:206–215, 1975.
113. Karagueuzian, H. S., Fujimoto, T., Katoh, T., et al.: Suppression of ventricular arrhythmias by propafenone, a new antiarrhythmic agent, during acute myocardial infarction in the conscious dog. A comparative study with lidocaine. Circulation, 66:1190–1198, 1982.
114. Karagueuzian, H. S., Katoh, T., McCullen, A., et al.: Electrophysiologic and hemodynamic effects of propafenone, a new antiarrhythmic agent, on the anesthetized, closed-chest dog: comparative study with lidocaine. Am. Heart J., 107:418–424, 1984.
115. Stenson, R. E., Constantino, R. T., and Harrison, D. C.: Interrelationships of hepatic bloodflow, cardiac output, and blood levels of lidocaine in man. Circulation, 43:205–211, 1971.
116. Blumer, J., Strong, J. M., and Atkinson, A. J.: The convulsant potency of lidocaine and its N-dealkylated metabolites. J. Pharmacol. Exp. Ther., 186:31–36, 1973.
117. Rosen, M. R., Hoffman, B. F., and Wit, A. L.: Electrophysiology and pharmacology of cardiac arrhythmias. V. Cardiac antiarrhythmic effects of lidocaine. Am. Heart J., 89:526–536, 1975.

118. Noreman, J. W., and Rogers, J. F.: Lidocaine prophylaxis in acute myocardial infarction. Medicine, 57:501, 1978.
119. Lie, K. I., Wellens, H. J., Van Capelle, F. J., et al.: Lidocaine in the prevention of primary ventricular fibrillation. N. Engl. J. Med., 291:1324–1326, 1974.
120. Harrison, D. C.: Should lidocaine be administered routinely to all patients after acute myocardial infarction. Circulation, 58:581, 1978.
121. Marriott, H. J. L., and Bieza, C. F.: Alarming ventricular acceleration after lidocaine administration. Chest, 61:682–683, 1972.
122. Nattel, S., and Zipes, D. P.: Clinical pharmacology of old and new antiarrhythmic drugs. In Castellanos, A. (ed.): Cardiac Arrhythmias, Mechanisms and Management, pp. 221–248. Philadelphia, F. A. Davis, 1980.
123. Kabela, E.: The effects of lidocaine on potassium efflux from various tissues of thc hcart. J. Pharmacol. Exp. Ther., 184:611–618, 1973.
124. Rosen, K. M., Barwolf, C., Ehsani, A., and Rahimtoola, S.: Effects of lidocaine and propranolol on the normal and abnormal pathways in patients with pre-excitation. Am. J. Cardiol., 30:801–803,1972.
125. Harrison, D. C., and Alderman, E. L.: The Pharmacology and Clinical Usc of Lidocaine as an Antiarrhythmic Drug. Modern Treatment Monograph No. 9. Hagerstown, Md., Harper & Row, 1972.
126. Gupta, P. K., Lichstein, E., and Chadda, K. D.: Lidocaine-induced heart block in patients with bundle branch block. Am. J. Cardiol., 33:487–492, 1974.
127. Fccly, J., Wade, D., McAllister, C. B., et al.: Effect of hypertension on liver blood flow and lidocaine disposition. N. Engl. J. Med., 307:866–869, 1982.
128. Strauss, H. C., Bigger, J. T., Jr., Basset, A. L., and Hoffman, B. F.: Actions of diphenylhydantoin on the electrical properties of isolated rabbit and canine atria. Circ. Res., 23:463–477, 1968.
129. Rosen, M. R., Danilo, P., Alonso, M. B., and Pippenger, C. E.: Effect of therapeutic concentrations of diphenylhydantoin on transmembrane potentials of normal and depressed Purkinje fibers. J. Pharmacol. Exp. Ther., 197:594–604, 1976.
130. Wit, A. L., Rosen, M. R., and Hoffman, B. F.: Electrophysiology and pharmacology of cardiac arrhythmias. VIII. Cardiac effects of diphenylhydantoin. Am. Heart J., 90:397–404, 1975.
131. Singh, B. N., and Vaughan Williams, E. M.: Explanation for the discrepancy in reported cardiac electrophysiological actions of diphenylhydantoin and lidocaine. Br. J. Pharmacol., 41:385–386, 1971.
132. Butler, T. C.: The metabolic conversion of 4,5-diphenylhydantoin to 5-(p-hydroxyphenyl)5 phenylhydantoin. J. Pharmacol. Exp. Thcr., 119:1–11, 1957.
133. Glazko, A. J., Chang, T., Baukema, J., et al.: Metabolic disposition of diphenylhydantoin in normal human subjects following intravenous administration. Clin. Pharmacol. Ther., 10:498–504, 1969.
134. Houghsen, G. W., and Richens, A.: Rate of elimination of tracer doses of phenytoin at different steady-state serum phenytoin concentrations in epileptic patients. Br. J. Clin. Pharmacol., 1:155–161, 1974.
135. Kutt, H.: Biochemical and genetic factors regulating dilantin metabolism in man. Ann. N.Y. Acad. Sci., 179:704–722, 1971.
136. Lunde, P. K. M., Rane, A., Yaffe, S. I., et al.: Plasma protein binding of diphenylhydantoin in man: Interaction with other drugs and the effect of temperature and plasma dilution. Clin. Pharmacol. Ther., 11:846–855, 1970.
137. Kutt, H., Wolk, M., Scherman, R., et al: Insufficient parahydroxylation as a cause of diphenylhydantoin toxicity. Neurology, 14:542–548, 1964.
138. Bigger, J. T., and Strauss, H. C.: Digitalis toxicity: Drug interactions promoting toxicity and the management of toxicity. Semin. Drug Treat., 2:147–172, 1972.
139. Mercer, E. N., and Osborne, J. A.: The current status of diphenylhydantoin in heart disease. Ann. Intern. Med., 67:1084–1107, 1967.
140. Stone, N., Klein, M. D., and Lown, B.: Diphenylhydantoin in the prevention of recurring ventricular tachycardia. Circulation, 43:420–427, 1971.
141. Bigger, J. T., Schmidt, D. H., and Kult, H.: Relationship between one plasma level of diphenylhydantoin sodium and its cardiac antiarrhythmic effects. Circulation, 38:363–374, 1968.
142. Wit, A. L., Hoffman, B. F., and Rosen, M. R.: Electrophysiology and pharmacology of cardiac arrhythmias. IX. Cardiac electrophysiologic effects of beta adrenergic receptor stimulation and blockade. Am. Heart J., 90:665–675, 1975.
143. Shand, D. G., Nuckolls, E. M., and Oates, J. A.: Plasma propranolol in adults. Clin. Pharmacol. Ther., 11:112–120, 1970.
144. Davis, L. D., Temte, J. V., and Murphy, Q. R.: Epinephrine-cyclopropane effects on Purkinje fibers. Anesthesiology, 36:369, 1969.
145. Nixon, J. V., Pennington, W., Ritter, W., et al.: Efficacy of propranolol in the control of exercise-induced or augmented ventricular ectopic activity. Circulation, 57:115–122, 1978.
146. Lemberg, L., Castellanos, A., and Arcebal, A. G.: The use of propranolol in arrhythmias complicating acute myocardial infarction. Am. Heart J., 80:479, 1970.
147. Multicentre International Study: Improvement in prognosis of myocardial infarction by long-term beta adrenoreceptor blockade using practolol. Br. Med. J., 3:735–740, 1975.
148. Singh, B. N.: B-adrenoreceptor blocking drugs and acute myocardial infarction. Drugs, 15:218–223, 1978.
149. Barlow, J. R., Bosman, C. K., Pocock, W. A., et al.: Late systolic murmurs and non-ejection ("mid-late") systolic clicks. Br. Heart J., 30:203, 1968.
150. Nies, A. S., and Shand, D. G.: Clinical pharmacology of propranolol. Circulation, 52:6–15, 1975.
151. McAllister, R. G.: Intravenous propranolol administration: A method for rapidly achieving and sustaining desired plasma levels. Clin. Pharmacol. Ther., 20:517–523, 1976.
152. Miller, R. R., Olson, H. G., Amsterdam, E. A., et al.: Propranolol-withdrawal rebound phenomenon. N. Engl. J. Med., 293:416–418, 1975.
153. Mizgala, H. F., and Counsell, J.: Acute coronary syndromes following abrupt cessation of oral propranolol therapy. Can. Med. Assoc. J., 114:1123, 1976.
154. Nattel, S., Shanks, J., and Rangno, R. E.: Propranolol withdrawal. Ann. Intern. Med., 89:288, 1978.
155. Nattel, S., Rangno, R. E., and Van Loon, G.: Mechanism of propranolol withdrawal phenomena. Circulation, 59:1158–1163, 1979.
156. Nattel, S., and Rangno, R. E.: Failure of gradual withdrawal of propranolol to prevent beta adrenergic supersensitivity. Circulation, 57, 58 (Suppl. III):103, 1978.
157. Cranefield, P. F., Aronson, R. S., and Wit, A. L.: Effect of verapamil on the normal action potential and on a calcium-dependent slow response of canine cardiac Purkinje fibers. Circ. Res., 34:204–213, 1974.
158. Wit, A. L., and Cranefield, P. F.: Effect of verapamil on the sinoatrial and atrioventricular nodes of the rabbit and the mechanism by which in arrests reentrant atrioventricular nodal tachycardia. Circ. Res., 35:413–425, 1974.
159. Zipes, D. P., and Fischer, J. C.: Effects of agents which inhibit the slow channel on sinus node automaticity and atrioventricular conduction in the dog. Circ. Res., 34:184–192, 1974.
160. Kates, R. E., Keefe, D. L. D., Sehwatz, J., et al.: Verapamil

disposition: Kinetics in chronic atrial fibrillation. J. Clin. Pharmacol. Ther., 30:44–51, 1981.

161. Schwartz, J. B., Keefe, D. L., Kirsten, E., et al.: Prolongation of verapamil elimination kinetics during chronic oral administration. Am. Heart J., 104:198–203, 1982.

162. Shand, D. G., Hammil, S. C., Aanosen, L., and Pritchett, E. L. C.: Reduced verapamil clearance during long-term oral administration. Clin. Pharmacol. Ther., 30:701–703, 1981.

163. Rikenberger, R. L., Prystowsky, E. N., Heger, J. J., et al.: Effects of intravenous and chronic oral verapamil administration in patients with supraventricular tachyarrhythmias. Circulation, 62:996–1010, 1980.

164. McAllister, R. G., and Kirsten, E. B.: The pharmacology of *verapamil IV kinetic* and dynamic effects after single intravenous and oral doses. Clin. Pharmacol. Ther., 31:418–426, 1982.

165. Reiter, M. J., Shand, D. G., and Pritchett, E. L. C.: Comparison of intravenous and oral verapamil dosing. Clin. Pharmacol. Ther., 32:711–720, 1982.

166. Klein, G. J., Gulamhusein, S., Prystowsky, E. N., et al.: Comparison of the electrophysiologic effects of intravenous and oral verapamil in patients with paroxysmal supraventricular tachycardia. Am. J. Cardiol., 49:117–124, 1982.

167. Mauriston, D. R., Winnifold, M. D., Walker, W. S., et al.: Oral verapamil for paroxysmal supraventricular tachycardia. A long-term, double-blind randomized trial. Ann. Intern. Med., 96:409–412, 1982.

168. Woodcock, B. G., Reitbrock, I., Vohringer, H. F., and Reitbrock, N.: Verapamil disposition in liver disease and intensive care patients. Kinetics, clearance and apparent blood flow relationships. Clin. Pharmacol. Ther., 29:27–32, 1981.

169. Singh, G. N., Ellrodt, G., and Peter, C. T.: Verapamil: A review of its pharmacologic properties and therapeutic use. Drugs, 15:169–197, 1978.

170. Wellens, H. J. J., Bar, F. W., Lie, K. I., et al.: Effect of procainamide, propranolol and verapamil on mechanism of tachycardia in patients with chronic recurrent ventricular tachycardia. Am. J. Cardiol., 40:579–585, 1977.

171. Brichard, G., and Zimmerman, P. E.: Verapamil in cardiac dysrhythmias during anesthesia. Br. J. Anaesthesiol., 42:1005–1011, 1970.

172. Singh, B. N., and Vaughan Williams, E. M.: The effects of amiodarone, a new antianginal drug, on cardiac muscle. Br. J. Pharmacol., 39:657, 1970.

173. Rosenbaum, M. B., Chiale, P. A., Halpern, M. S., et al.: Clinical efficacy of amiodarone as an antiarrhythmic agent. Am. J. Cardiol., 38:934–944, 1966.

174. Gooupil, N., and Lenfant, J.: The effects of amiodarone on sinus node activity of the rabbit heart. Eur. J. Pharmacol. 39:23–31, 1976.

175. Ohta, M., Karagueuzian H. S., McCullen, A., et al.: Effect of amiodarone on delayed after depolarization and triggered automaticity in isolated rabbit ventricular muscle. (Abstract) J. Am. Coll. Cardiol., 5:492, 1985.

176. Cabasson, J., Puch, P., Mellet, J. M., et al.: Analyse des effets electrophysiologigues de l'amiodarone par l'enregistrement simultane' des potentiels d'action monophasiques et da faisceau de His. Arch. Mal. Coeur, 7:691–698, 1976.

177. Boucher, M., and Duchene-Marullaz, P.: Comparative effects of amiodarone perhexilline and bepridil on the cardiac rhythms of the unanesthetized dog in the chronic heart block. Arch. Intern. Pharmacodyn. Ther., 233:65–72, 1978.

178. Patternson, E., Eller, B. T., Abrams, G. D., et al.: Ventricular fibrillation in a conscious canine preparation of sudden coronary death—prevention by short-and-long-term amiodarone administration. Circulation, 68:857–864, 1983.

179. Haffajee, C. T., Love, J. C., Canada, A. T., et al.: Clinical pharmacokinetics and efficacy of amiodarone for refractory tachyarrhythmias. Circulation, 67:1347–1355, 1983.

180. Siddoway, L. A., McAllister, C. B., Wilkinson, G. R., et al.: Amiodarone dosing: A proposal based on its pharmacokinetics. Am. Heart J., 106:951–956, 1983.

181. Zipes, D. P., Prystowsky, E. N., and Heger, J. J.: Amiodarone: Electrophysiologic actions, pharmacokinetics and clinical effects. J. Am. Coll. Cardiol., 3:1059–1071, 1984.

182. Nademanee, K., Singh, B. N., Hendrickson, J. A., et al.: Pharmacokinetics significance of serum reverse T_3 levels during amiodarone treatment: A potential method for monitoring chronic drug therapy. Circulation, 66:202–211, 1982.

183. Wellens, H. J. J., Brugada, P., Abdollah, H., and Dassen, W. R.: A comparison of the electrophysiologic effects of intravenous and oral amiodarone in the same patients. Circulation, 69:120–124, 1984.

184. Hamer, A. W., Finnerman, W. B., Peter, T., and Mandel, W. J.: Disparity between the clinical and electrophysiologic effects of amiodarone in the treatment of recurrent ventricular tachycardias. Am. Heart J., 102:992–1001, 1981.

185. Feld, G. K., Nademanee, K., Weiss, J., et al.: Electrophysiologic basis for the suppression by amiodarone of orthodromic supraventricular tachycardia complicating pre-excitation syndromes. J. Am. Coll. Cardiol., 3:1298–1307, 1984.

186. Nademanee, K., Handrickson, J., Cannom, D. S., et al.: Control of refractory life-threatening ventricular tachyarrhythmias by amiodarone. Am. Heart J., 101:759–768, 1981.

187. Heger, J. J., Prystowsky, E. N., and Zipes, D. P.: Clinical efficacy of amiodarone in the treatment of recurrent ventricular tachycardia and ventricular fibrillation. Am. Heart J., 106:887–894, 1983.

188. Graboys, T. B., Podrid, P. J., and Lown, B.: Efficacy of amiodarone for refractory supraventricular tachyarrhythmias. Am. Heart J., 106:870–876, 1983.

189. Wellens, H. J. J., Brugada, P., and Abdollah, H.: Effect of amiodarone in paroxysmal supraventricular tachycardia with and without WPW syndrome. Am. Heart J., 106:876–880, 1983.

190. Hamer, A. W. F., Mandel, W. J., Zaher, C. A., et al.: The electrophysiological basis for the use of amiodarone for treatment of cardiac arrhythmias. Pace, 6:784–794, 1983.

191. Harris, L., McKenna, W. J., Roland, E., et al.: Amiodarone: Side effects of long-term therapy. Circulation, 67:45, 1983.

192. Rakita, L., Sobol, S. M., Mostow, N., and Vrobel, T.: Amiodarone pulmonary toxicity. Am. Heart J., 106:906–916, 1983.

193. Hamer, A., Peter, T., Mandel, W. J., et al.: The potentiation of warfarin anticoagulation by amiodarone and anticoagulant treatment. Circulation, 65:1025–1029, 1982.

194. Marcus, F. I.: Drug interactions with amiodarone. Am. Heart J., 106:924–930, 1983.

195. Singh, B. N., and Vaughan Williams, E. M.: Investigations of the mode of action of a new antidysrhythmic drug (KO 1173). Br. J. Pharmacol., 44:1, 1972.

196. Yamaguchi, I., Singh, B. N., and Mandel, W. J.: Electrophysiological actions of mexiletine on isolated rabbit atrial and canine ventricular muscle and Purkinje fiber. Cardiovasc. Res., 13:288, 1979.

197. Weld, F. M., Bigger, J. T., Swister, D., et al.: Electrophysiological effects of mexiletine (KO 1173) on ovine cardiac Purkinje fibers. J. Pharmacol. Exp. Ther., 210:222–228, 1979.

198. Amerini, S., Carbonin, P., Cerbai, E., et al.: Electrophysiological mechanisms for the antiarrhythmic action of mexiletine on digitalis-, reperfusion-, and reoxy-generation–induced arrhythmias. Br. J. Pharmacol., 86:805–815, 1985.

199. Arita, M., Masayosi, G., Nagamoto, Y., and Saikawa, T.: Electrophysiological actions of mexiletine (KO 1173) on canine Pur-

kinje fibers and ventricular muscle. Br. J. Pharmacol., 67:143–152, 1979.
200. Carmeliet, E.: Mechanisms of arrhythmias and of antiarrhythmic activity with special reference to mexiletine. Acta Cardiol., 25 (Suppl.):5, 1980.
201. Harper, R. W., and Olsson, B.: Effect of mexiletine on conduction of premature ventricular beats in man: a study using monophasic action potential recordings from the right ventricle. Cardiovasc. Res., 13:311–319, 1979.
202. Prescott, L. F., Pottage, A., and Clements, J. A.: Absorption, distribution and elimination of mexiletine. Postgrad. Med. J., 53 (Suppl. I):50–55, 1977.
203. Hegger, J. J., Nattel, S., Rinkenberger, R. L., and Zipes, D. P.: Mexiletine therapy in 15 patients with drug-resistant ventricular tachycardia. Am. J. Cardiol., 45:627–632, 1980.
204. Duff, H. J., Roden, D., Prim, R. K., et al.: Mexiletine in the treatment of resistant ventricular arrhythmias: Enhancement of efficacy and reduction of dose related side effects by combination with quinidine. Circulation, 67:1124–1128, 1983.
205. Podrid, P. J., and Lown, B.: Mexiletine for ventricular arrhythmias. Am. J. Cardiol., 47:895–902, 1981.
206. Moore, E. M., Spear, J. F., Horowitz, L. N., et al.: Electrophysiologic properties of a new antiarrhythmic drug—tocainide. Am. J. Cardiol., 41:703–709, 1978.
207. Oshita, S., Sada, H., Kojima, M., and Ban, T.: Effects of tocainide and lidocaine on the transmembrane action potentials as related to external potassium and calcium concentrations in guinea pig papillary muscles. Arch. Pharmacol., 314:62–71, 1980.
208. Winkle, R. A., Meffin, P. J., Fitzgerald, J. W., et al.: Clinical efficacy and pharmacokinetics of a new orally effective antiarrhythmic—tocainide. Circulation, 54:884–889, 1976.
209. Lalka, D., Meyer, M. B., Duce, B. R., et al.: Kinetics of oral antiarrhythmic lidocaine congener—tocainide. Clin. Pharmacol. Ther., 19:767–768, 1976.
210. Lewinter, M. M., Engler, R. L., and Karliner, J. S.: Tocainide therapy of ventricular arrhythmias: Assessment with ambulatory electrocardiographic monitoring and treadmill exercise. Am. J. Cardiol., 45:1045–1052, 1980.
211. Pottage, A.: Clinical profiles of newer class I antiarrhythmic agents—tocainide, mexiletine, encainide, flecanide, and lorcainide. Am. J. Cardiol., 52:24C–31C, 1983.
212. Carmeliet, E., and Verdonck, F.: Effects of aprindine and lidocaine on transmembrane potentials and radioactive K efflux in different cardiac tissues. Acta. Cardiol. (Brux.), 18:73–81, 1974.
213. Verdonck, F., Vereecke, J., and Vleugels, A.: Electrophysiological effects of aprindine on isolated heart preparations. Eur. J. Pharmacol., 26:338–346, 1974.
214. Steinberg, M. I., and Greenspan, K.: Intracellular electrophysiological alterations in canine conducting tissue induced by aprindine and lidocaine. Cardiovasc. Res., 10:236–244, 1976.
215. Elharrar, V., Bailey, J. C., Lathrop, D. A., and Zipes, D. P.: Effects of aprindine on slow channel action potentials and transient depolarizations in canine Purkinje fibers. J. Pharmacol. Exp. Ther., 205:410–417, 1978.
216. Elharrar, V., Foster, P. R., and Zipes, D. P.: Effects of aprindine *HCL* on cardiac tissue. J. Pharmacol. Exp. Ther., 195:201–205, 1975.
217. Foster, P. R., King, R. M., Dehnicoll, A., and Zipes, D. P.: Suppression of ouabain-induced ventricular rhythms with aprindine *HCL*: A comparison with other antiarrhythmic agents. Circulation, 53:315–321, 1976.
218. Zipes, D. P., Elharrar, V., Gilmour, R. F., Jr., et al.: Studies with aprindine. Am. Heart J., 100:1055–1062, 1980.
219. Reid, P. R., Greene, H. L., and Varphese, P. J.: Suppression of refractory arrhythmias by aprindine in patients with the WPW syndrome. Br. Heart J., 39:1353–1360, 1977.
220. Ronfeld, R. A.: Comparative pharmacokinetics of new antiarrhythmic drugs. Am. Heart J., 100:978–983, 1980.
221. Zipes, D. P., Gaum, W. E., Foster, P. R., et al.: Aprindine treatment of supraventricular tachycardia, with particular application to Wolff-Parkinson-White syndrome. Am. J. Cardiol., 40:586–596, 1977.
222. Strauss, H. C., Bigger, J. T., Jr., and Hoffman, B. F.: Electrophysiological and beta-receptor blocking effects of *MJ* 1999 on dog and rabbit tissue. Circ. Res., 26:661–678, 1970.
223. Singh, B. N., and Vaughan Williams, E. M.: A third class of antiarrhythmic action. Effect on atrial and ventricular intracellular potentials, and other pharmacological actions on cardiac muscle of MJ 1999 and AH-3474. Br. J. Pharmacol., 39:675–682, 1970.
224. Cobbe, S. M., Hoffman, E., Ritzenhoff, A., et al.: Action of sotalol on potential reentrant pathways and ventricular tachyarrhythmias in conscious dogs in the late postmyocardial infarction phase. Circulation, 68:865–871, 1983.
225. Edvardson, N., Hirsch, I., Emanuelsson, H., et al.: Sotalol induced delayed ventricular repolarization in man. Eur. Heart J., 1:335–342, 1980.
226. Echt, D. S., Berte, L. E., Clusin, W. T., et al.: Prolongation of the human cardiac monophasic action potential by sotalol. Am. J. Cardiol., 50:1082–1086, 1982.
227. Bennett, D. H.: Acute prolongation of myocardial refractoriness by sotalol. Br. Heart J., 47:521–526, 1982.
228. Nathan, A. W., Hellestrand, K. I., Bexton, R. S., et al.: Electrophysiological effects of sotalol—just another beta blocker? Br. Heart J., 47:515–520, 1982.
229. Schnelle, K., Klein, G., and Schinz, A.: Studies on the pharmacokinetics and pharmacodynamics of the beta-adrenergic blocking agent sotalol in normal man. J. Clin. Pharmacol., 19 11:516–522, 1979.
230. Investigator's Brochure MJ 1999, Sotalol. Evansville, IN: Bristol-Myers Company, March 31, 1983, rev. June 24, 1983.
231. Tjandramaga Thoma, T., Verbeeck, R., Venbeselt, R., et al.: The effect of end-stage renal failure and haemodialysis on the elimination kinetics and sotalol. Br. J. Clin. Pharmacol., 3:259–265, 1976.
232. Berglund, G., Descamps, R., and Thomis, S.: Pharmacokinetics of sotalol after chronic administration to patients with renal insufficiency. Eur. J. Clin. Pharmacol., 18:321–326, 1980.
233. Karagueuzian, H. S., Katoh, T., Sugi, K., et al.: Electrophysiologic effects of propafenone, a new antiarrhythmic drug, on isolated cardiac tissue. Circulation, 66 (Suppl II): II–378, 1982.
234. Ledda, F., Mantella, L., Manzini, S., et al.: Electrophysiologic effects of propafenone in isolated cardiac preparations. J. Cardiovasc. Pharmacol., 3:1162–1173, 1981.
235. Podrid, P. J., and Lown, B.: Propafenone: a new agent for ventricular arrhythmias. J. Am. Coll. Cardiol., 4:117–125, 1984.
236. Karagueuzian, H. S., Mandel, W. J., and Peter, T.: Propafenone. In Scriabine, A. (ed.): New Drugs Annual: Cardiovascular Drugs, Vol. 3. New York: Raven Press, 1985, pp. 285–299.
237. Connolly, S. J., Katz, R. E., Lebsack, C. S., et al.: Clinical efficacy of oral propafenone for ventricular tachycardia. Am. J. Cardiol., 52:1203–1213, 1983.
238. Shen, E. N., Sung, R. J., Morady, F., et al.: Electrophysiologic and hemodynamic effects of intravenous propafenone in patients with recurrent ventricular tachycardia. J. Am. Coll. Cardiol., 3:1291–1297, 1984.
239. Connolly, S. J., Katz, R. E., Lebsack, C. S., et al.: Clinical pharmacology of propafenone. Circulation, 68:589–596, 1983.
240. Keller, K., Meyer-Estorg, G., Beck, O. A., and Hochrein, H.: Correlation between serum concentration and pharmacological effect on the atrioventricular conduction time of the antiarrhyth-

mic drug propafenone. Eur. J. Clin. Pharmacol., 13:17–20, 1978.

241. Waleffe, A., Mary-Rabine, L., DeRijbel, R., et al.: Electrophysiological effects of propafenone studied with programmed electrical stimulation of the heart in patients with recurrent supraventricular tachycardia. Eur. Heart J., 2:345–352, 1981.
242. Rudolph, W., Petri, H., Kafka, W., et al.: Effects of propafenone on the accessory pathway (AP) in patients with WPW syndrome (abstr.). Am. J. Cardiol., 43:430, 1979.
243. Zilcher, H., Glogar, D., and Kaindl, F.: Torsades de pointes: Occurrence in myocardial ischemia as a separate entity. Multiform ventricular tachycardia or not? Eur. Heart J., 1:63–69, 1980.
244. Hammermeister, K. E., Boerth, R. C., Warbasse, J. R.: The comparative inotropic effects of six clinically used antiarrhythmic agents. Am. Heart J., 84:643–652, 1972.
245. Heissenbuttel, R. H., and Bigger, J. T.: Bretylium tosylate: A newly available antiarrhythmic drug for ventricular arrhythmia. Ann. Intern. Med., 91:229–238, 1979.
246. Bigger, J. R., and Jaffe, C.: The effect of bretylium tosylate on the electrophysiological properties of ventricular muscle and Purkinje fibers. Am. J. Cardiol., 27:82–92, 1971.
247. Wit, A. L., Steiner, C., and Damato, A. N.: Electrophysiologic effects of bretylium tosylate on single fibers of the canine specialized conducting system and ventricle. J. Pharmacol. Exp. Ther., 173:344–356, 1970.
248. Cardinal, R., and Sasyniuk, B. I.: Electrophysiological effects of bretylium tosylate on subendocardial Purkinje fibers from infarcted canine hearts. J. Pharmacol. Exp. Ther., 204:159–174, 1978.
249. Anderson, J. C., Patterson, E., Conlon, M., et al.: Kinetics of antifibrillatory effects of bretylium: Correlation with myocardial drug concentration. Am. J. Cardiol., 46:583–592, 1980.
250. Wenger, T. C., Lederman, S., Starmer, F. C., et al.: A method for quantitating antifibrillatory effects of drugs after coronary reperfusion in dogs: Improved outcome with bretylium. Circulation, 69:142–148, 1984.
251. Bernstein, J. G., and Koch-Weser, J.: Effectiveness of bretylium tosylate against refractory ventricular arrhythmias. Circulation, 45:1024–1034, 1972.
252. Bacaner, M. B.: Quantitative comparison of bretylium with other antifibrillatory drugs. Am. J. Cardiol., 21:504–512, 1968.
253. Naito, M., Michelson, E. L., Kmetz, J. J., et al.: Failure of antiarrhythmic drug to prevent experimental reperfusion ventricular fibrillation. Circulation, 63:70–79, 1981.
254. Morganorth, J., Pearlman, A. S., and Dunkman, W. B.: Ethmozin: A new antiarrhythmic agent developed in the USSR. Efficacy and tolerance. Am. Heart J., 98:621–628, 1979.
255. Denilo, P. J., Lanfan, W. B., Rosen, M. R., and Hoffman, B. F.: Effects of the phenothiazine analog, EN-313, on ventricular arrhythmias in the dog. Eur. J. Pharmacol., 45:127–139, 1977.
256. Ruffy, R., Rozenshtraukh, Elharrai, V., and Zipes, D. P.: Electrophysiological effects of ethmozin on canine myocardium. Cardiovasc. Res., 13:354–363, 1979.
257. Podrid, P. J., Lyakishev, A., Lown, B., and Mazur, N.: Ethmozin: A new antiarrhythmic drug for suppressing ventricular premature complexes. Circulation, 61:450–457, 1980.
258. Pratt, C. M., English, L. J., Yepsen, S. C., et al.: Double-blind placebo control crossover trial of ethmozin and dispyramide in the suppression of complex ventricular arrhythmias (abstr.). Circulation, (Suppl III):1659, 1983.
259. Zipes, D. P., and Troup, P. J.: New antiarrhythmic agents. Amiodarone, aprinidine, disopyramide, ethmozin, mexiletine, tocainide, verapamil. Am. J. Cardiol., 41:1005–1024, 1978.
260. Holmes, B., and Heel, R. C.: Flecainide: A preliminary review of its pharmacodynamic properties and therapeutic efficacy. Drugs, 29:1–33, 1985.
261. Ikeda, N., Singh, B. N., Davis, L. D., and Hauswirth, O.: Effects of flecainide on the electrophysiological properties of isolated canine and rabbit myocardial fibers. J. Am. Coll. Cardiol., 5:303–310, 1985.
262. Hodess, A. B., Follansbee, W. P., Spear, J. F., and Moore, E. W.: Electrophysiological effects of a new antiarrhythmic agent, flecainide, on the intact canine heart. J. Cardiovasc. Pharmacol., 1:427–439, 1979.
263. Verdouw, P. D., Deckers, J. W., and Connad, G. J.: Antiarrhythmic and hemodynamic actions of flecainide acetate (R-818) in the ischemic porcine heart. J. Cardiovasc. Pharmacol., 1:473–486, 1979.
264. Anderson, J. L., Stewart, J. R., Perry, B. A., et al.: Oral flecainide acetate for the treatment of ventricular arrhythmias. N. Engl. J. Med., 305:473–477, 1981.
265. Duff, H. J., Roden, D. M., Maffucci, R. J., et al.: Suppression of resistant ventricular arrhythmias by twice daily dosing with flecainide. Am. J. Cardiol., 48:1133–1140, 1981.
266. Hodges, M., Haugland, M., and Granrud, G.: Suppression of ventricular ectopic depolarizations by flecainide acetate, a new antiarrhythmic agent. Circulation, 65:879–885, 1982.
267. The Flecainide-Quinidine Research Group: Flecainide versus quinidine for treatment of chronic ventricular arrhythmias. A multicenter clinical trial. Circulation, 67:1117–1123, 1983.
268. Hellestrand, K. J., Nathan, A. W., Bexton, R. S., and Camm, A. J.: Effect of flecainide on anomalous pathways and reentrant junctional tachycardia (abstr.). Circulation, 66 (Suppl. II):II-273, 1982.
269. Abitbol, H., Califano, J. E., and Abate, C., et al.: Use of flecainide acetate in the treatment of premature ventricular contractions. Am. Heart J., 105:227–230, 1983.
270. Carmeliet, E., Jansen, P. A. J., Marsboom, R., et al.: Antiarrhythmic electrophysiologic and hemodynamic effect of lorcainide. Arch. Intern. Pharmacodyn. Ther., 231:104–130, 1978.
271. Carmeliet, E., and Zaman, M. Y.: Comparative effects of lignocaine and lorcainide on conduction in the hangendorff-perfused guinea pig heart. Cardiovasc. Pharmacol., 13:439–440, 1979.
272. Eriksson, C. E., and Brogden, R. N.: Lorcainide, a preliminary review of its pharmacodynamic properties and therapeutic efficacy. Drugs, 27:279–300, 1984.
273. Kasper, W., Treese, N., Meinertz, T., et al.: Electrophysiologic effects of lorcainide on the accessory pathway in the Wolff-Parkinson-White syndrome. Am. J. Cardiol., 51:1618–1622, 1983.
274. Kates, R. E., Keefe, D. L., and Winkle, R. A.: Lorcainide disposition kinetics in arrhythmia patients. Clin. Pharmacol. Ther., 33:28–34, 1983.
275. Jahnchen, E., Bechtold, H., Kasper, W., et al.: Lorcainide. I. Saturable presystemic elimination. Clin. Pharmacol. Ther., 26:187–195, 1979.
276. Meinertz, T., Kasper, W., Kersting, F., et al.: Lorcainide. II. Plasma concentration-effect relationship. Clin. Pharmacol. Ther., 26:196–204, 1979.
277. Klotz, U., Fischer, C., Muller-Scydlitz, P., et al.: Alterations in the disposition of differently cleared drugs in patients with cirrhosis. Clin. Pharmacol. Ther., 26:221–227, 1979.
278. Klotz, U.: Disposition and anti-arrhythmic effects of lorcainide. Inter. J. Clin. Pharmacol. Biopharm., 17:152–158, 1979.
279. Keefe, D. L., Peters, F., and Winkle, R. A.: Randomized double-blind placebo controlled crossover trial documenting oral lorcainide efficacy in suppression of symptomatic ventricular tachyarrhythmias. Am. Heart J., 103:511–518, 1982.
280. Saksena, S., Rothbart, S. T., Capello, G., et al.: Clinical and electrophysiological effects of chronic lorcainide therapy in refractory ventricular tachycardia. J. Am. Coll. Cardiol., 2:538–544, 1983.
281. Pottage, A.: Clinical profiles of newer class 1 antiarrhythmic

agents. Tocainide, mexiletine, encainide, flecainide and lorcainide. Am. J. Cardiol., 52:24c–31c, 1983.

282. Elharrar, V., and Zipes, D. P.: Effects of encainide and metabolites (MJ 14030 and MJ 9444) on canine, cardia Purkinje and ventricular fibers. J. Pharmacol. Exp. Ther., 220:440–447, 1982.
283. Gibson, J. K., Somani, P., and Bassett, A. L.: Electrophysiologic effects of encainide (MJ 9067) on canine Purkinje fibers. Eur. J. Pharmacol., 52:161–169, 1978.
284. Schmidt, G., Sawicki, G. J., and Arnsdorf, M. F.: Effects of encainide on components of excitability in cardiac Purkinje fibers (abstr.). Circulation, 64 (Suppl. IV): 1037, 1981.
285. Samuelsson, R. G., and Harrison, D. C.: Electrophysiologic evaluation of encainide with use of monophasic action potential recording. Am. J. Cardiol., 48:871–876, 1981.
286. Dawson, A. K., Duff, H. J., and Woosley, R. L.: Paradoxical response to o-demethyl encainide in a canine infarction model (abstr.). Circulation, 64 (Suppl. IV):1039, 1981.
287. Jackman, W. M., Zipes, D. P., Naccarelli, G. V., et al.: Electrophysiology of oral encainide. Am. J. Cardiol., 49:1270–1278, 1982.
288. Sami, M., Mason, J. W., Peters, F., and Harrison, D. C.: Clinical electrophysiologic effects of encainide, a newly developed antiarrhythmic agent. Am. J. Cardiol., 44:526–532, 1979.
289. Roden, D. M., Duff, H. J., Altenberg, D., and Woosley, R. L.: Antiarrhythmic activity of the o-demethyl metabolite of encainide. J. Pharmacol. Ther., 221:552–557, 1982.
290. Woosley, R. L., and Roden, D. M.: Importance of metabolites in antiarrhythmic therapy. Am. J. Cardiol., 52:3c–7c, 1983.
291. Winkle, R. A., Peters, F., Kates, R. E., et al.: Clinical pharmacology and antiarrhythmic efficacy of encainide in patients with chronic ventricular arrhythmias. Circulation, 64:290–296, 1981.
292. Kates, R. E., Harrison, D. C., Winkle, R. A.: Metabolite cumulation during long-term oral encainide administration. Clin. Pharmacol. Ther., 31:427–432, 1982.
293. Roden, D. M., Reele, S. B., Higgins, S. B., et al.: Total suppression of ventricular arrhythmias by encainide. N. Engl. J. Med., 302:877–882, 1980.
294. Mason, J. W., and Peters, F.: Antiarrhythmic efficacy of encainide in patients with refractory recurrent ventricular tachycardia. Circulation, 63:670–675, 1981.
295. Sami, M., Harrison, D. C., Kramer, H., et al.: Antiarrhythmic efficacy of encainide and quinidine: Validation of a model for drug assessment. Am. J. Cardiol., 48:147–156, 1981.
296. Winkle, R. A., Mason, J. W., Griffin, J. C., and Ross, D.: Malignant ventricular tachyarrhythmias associated with the use of encainide. Am. Heart J., 102:857–864, 1981.
297. Duff, H. J., Dawson, A. K., and Roden, D. M.: Electrophysiologic actions of o-demethyl encainide: An active metabolite. Circulation, 68:385–391, 1983.
298. Prystowsky, E. N., Klein, G. J., Rinkenberger, R. L., et al.: Clinical efficacy and electrophysiologic effects of encainide in patients with Wolff-Parkinson-White syndrome. Circulation, 69:278–287, 1984.
299. Carey, E. L., Duff, H. J., and Roden, D. M.: Encainide and its metabolites: Comparative effects in man on ventricular arrhythmias and electrocardiography intervals. J. Clin. Invest., 73:539–547, 1984.
300. Posen, R., Lombardi, E., Podrid, P., and Lown, B.: Aggravation of induced arrhythmias with antiarrhythmic drugs during electrophysiological testing (abstr.). Am. J. Cardiol., 1:709, 1983.
301. Siddiqui, S., and Siddiqui, R. H.: The alkaloids of Rauwolfia serpentina. J. Indian Chem. Soc., 9:539–544, 1932.
302. Bojorges, R., Pastelin, G., Sanchez-Perez, S., et al.: The effects of ajmaline in experimental and clinical arrhythmias and their relation to some electrophysiological parameters of the heart. J. Exp. Pharmacol. Ther., 193:183–193, 1975.
303. Obayashi, K., and Mandel, W. J.: Electrophysiological effects of ajmaline in isolated cardiac tissue. Cardiovasc. Res., 10:20–24, 1976.
304. Bazika, V., Lang, T. W., Pappelbaum, S., and Corday, E.: Ajmaline, a Rauwolfia alkaloid for the treatment and digitalis arrhythmias. Am. J. Cardiol., 17:227–231, 1966.
305. Obayashi, K., Hagasawa, K., Mandel, W. J., et al.: Cardiovascular effects of ajmaline. Am. Heart J., 92:487–496, 1976.
306. Wellens, H. J. J., Bar, F. W., Gorgel, A. P., and Vanagt, E. J.: Use of ajmaline in patients with the Wolff-Parkinson-White syndrome to disclose short refractory period of the accessory pathway. Am. J. Cardiol., 45:130–133, 1980.
307. Herpin, D., Gaudeau, B., Amid, A., et al.: Etude de l'activite et de la tolerance d' un nouvel anti-arythmique la cibenzoline (Cipralan) administre par voie orale. Acta Cardiol., 36:131–148, 1981.
308. Thebaut, J. F., Archard, F., de Langenhagen, B.: Etude electrophysiologique chez l'homme d'un nouvel antiarythmic, la cibenzoline, dans de syndrome de Wolff-Parkinson-White. L'Inform. Cardiol., 4:393–402, 1980.
309. Ohta, M., Sugi, K., McCullen, A., et al.: Electrophysiologic effects of cibenzoline, a new antiarrhythmic drug, on isolated cardiac tissue (abstr.). Circulation, 68 (Suppl. III):III–220, 1983.
310. Millar, J. S., Vaughan William, E. M.: Effects on rabbit nodal atrial ventricular and Purkinje cell potentials of a new antiarrhythmic drug, cibenzoline, which protects against action potential shortening in hypoxia. Br. J. Pharmacol., 75:469–478, 1982.
311. Dangman, K. H.: Cardiac effects of cibenzoline. J. Cardiovasc. Pharmacol. 6:300–311, 1984.
312. Brazzell, R. K., Aogaichi, K., Meger, J. J., Jr., et al.: Cibenzoline plasma concentration and antiarrhythmic effect. Clin. Pharmacol. Ther., 35:307–316, 1984.
313. Browne, K. F., Hegger, J. J., Zipes, D. P., et al.: Clinical and electrophysiologic effects of cibenzoline in patients with ventricular arrhythmias (abstr.). J. Am. Coll. Cardiol., 1:699, 1983.
314. Miura, D. S., Karen, G., Siegel, L., et al.: Effect of cibenzoline in suppressing ventricular tachycardia induced by programmed electrical stimulation (abstr.). J. Am. Coll. Cardiol., 1:699, 1983.
315. Canal, M., Flouvat, B., Tremblay, D., and Disfour, A.: Pharmacokinetics in man of a new antiarrhythmic drug: Cibenzoline. Eur. J. Clin. Pharmacol., 24:509–515, 1983.
316. Brown, K. F., Prystowsky, E. N., Zipes, D. P., et al.: Clinical efficacy and electrophysiologic effects of cibenzoline therapy in patients with ventricular arrhythmias. J. Am. Coll. Cardiol., 3:857–864, 1984.
317. Cibenzoline (RO 22-7796) Investigational Brochure: Hoffman-LaRoche Inc., Nutly, N.J., 1982.
318. Sethi, K. K., Jaishankar, S., and Gupta, M. P.: Salutary effects of intravenous ajmaline in patients with paroxysmal supraventricular tachycardia mediated by dual atrioventricular nodal pathways: Blockade of the retrograde fast pathway. Circulation, 70:876–883, 1984.
319. Karagueuzian, H. S., Sugi, K., Ohta, M., et al.: The efficacy of cibenzoline and propafenone against inducible sustained and non-sustained ventricular tachycardia in conscious dogs with isolated chronic right ventricular infarction: A comparative study with procainamide. Am. Heart J., 1986 (In press).

30

High-Energy Electrical Current in the Management of Cardiac Dysrhythmias

Leon Resnekov

The pharmacologic management of patients with cardiac rhythm disturbances, although time honored, may have the following serious limitations when used clinically:

1. There is no standard dose for any specific drug, the amounts given usually vary among patients.
2. The margin between therapeutic and toxic dosages is often small.
3. Because it is necessary to titrate the dose given against the effects obtained, the patient must be observed closely throughout pharmacologic therapy, which may last several days.
4. Many of the drugs used have important negative inotropic effects that may further compromise disturbed heart action. In addition, important dromotropic effects may emerge.
5. The toxic effects of a drug may be more serious than the effects of the rhythm disturbance.
6. Many drugs may suppress the normal sinus mechanism and inhibit reversion to sinus rhythm.

In contrast, an electrical shock momentarily depolarizes the majority of heart fibers, terminates the ectopic rhythm, and permits the sinus node to be reestablished as the pacemaker of the heart (Fig. 30-1). Such treatment is now known to be both successful and safe, provided careful adherence to detail is maintained.

Historical Highlights

Ventricular fibrillation was described first by Hoffa and Ludwig in 1850.[1] Shortly thereafter, fatalities as a result of electrocution were reported, but the realization that an electrical shock could also terminate ventricular fibrillation came about only many years thereafter. In 1898, Prevost and Battelli[2] observed that a direct current shock across a dog's heart in ventricular fibrillation caused sinus rhythm to return. This important fact was ignored or unrecognized until the effects of electrical current on the heart were restudied by Kouwenhoven and colleagues in a series of experiments over many years[3] and by Ferris and co-workers[4] at almost the same time. Between 1927 and 1935, the following important conclusions on the effects of electricity on the heart were arrived at:

1. Current rather than voltage is the proper criterion for shock intensity.

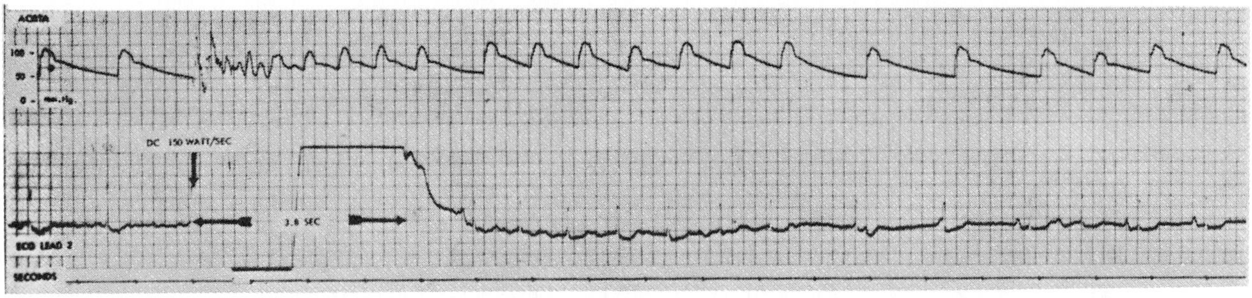

Figure 30-1. *Electroversion of atrial fibrillation. Shown are central aortic pressure (*top*) and lead II of the electrocardiogram (*bottom*). Immediately following delivery of 150 watt-sec (J), atrial fibrillation is followed by ectopic beats recorded on the aortic tracing when electrical interference causes the electrocardiographic signal to be lost for 3.8 seconds. Subsequently, sinus rhythm with a prolonged PR interval and junctional beats are recorded before sinus rhythm is established.*

2. Ventricular fibrillation may be caused by the passage of an electrical current across the heart even in the absence of recognizable myocardial damage.
3. Ventricular fibrillation will cause death within a few minutes unless it is treated successfully by a second shock of appropriate intensity.

Not all electrical shocks will produce ventricular fibrillation, and King[5] was able to show that those shocks delivered close to the apex of the T wave of the electrocardiogram were more likely to do so.

Pioneer work using direct current electrical discharge clinically was undertaken by scientists in the U.S.S.R.[6] These early attempts are regarded as an important inspiration for later investigators, including Peleška (Czechoslovakia), Tsukerman (U.S.S.R.), and Lown and coworkers (United States).[7]

Electrical Defibrillation of the Heart

A high-energy impulse of short duration is delivered between two concave paddles applied closely to the heart (internal defibrillation) or through the chest wall using two flat paddles (external defibrillation).

External defibrillation both for direct and alternating currents depends not only on the electrical current used but also on the resistance of the heart, of the bony cage, and of the skin. A current of at least 1 amp is needed to bring all heart fibers instantaneously to the same refractory point.[8] To achieve a current of 1 amp across the myocardium usually requires 100 v at a power of 100 watts. The usual duration for an *alternating current* shock for defibrillation is 200 msec; thus the energy needed for internal defibrillation is about 20 J. Because of the increased resistance, external alternating current defibrillation requires a sixfold increase in current and voltage rating, 1800 watts for 0.2 second producing 500 J. Note that the waveform for alternating current defibrillation is standard and is produced at the electrical generating station as a sinusoidal impulse with a frequency of 60 Hz.

Direct current defibrillators discharge a single or bank of capacitors that have been charged previously for 2 to 10 seconds by line current and a step-up transformer. The duration of the delivered impulse is much shorter than for alternating current defibrillators, usually being in the range of 1.5 to 4 msec. An infinite variety of waveforms is obtained following a capacitor discharge. When unmodified, a spike discharge with a very abrupt rise in voltage and current to a sharp peak, followed by an exponential decay to the baseline, is obtained. This unmodified waveform can be shaped by adding varying amounts of inductance to the circuit. Experimental evidence has shown that defibrillation is safer and more likely to succeed when an inductance-modified waveform is used.[9] Inductance reduces the rate of rise of the current and voltage waveform to round off the peak and to prolong the down slope. As more inductance is introduced into the circuit, undesirable oscillations in the tail of the waveform occur. Many commercial direct current defibrillators produce a monophasic, slightly underdamped current and voltage waveform, obtained by charging a capacitor of 16 μf to a maximum of 7000 v and discharging it across an inductance of 100 mh. The average duration of the waveform is 3.5 msec, and when maximally charged, 329 J of electrical energy is delivered. The current is about 19 amp, and the power is 133,000 watts. The waveform is shown in Figure 30-2.

Important variables relating to the safe clinical use of direct current shock are the capacitance of the conductors and the inductance of the circuit. The rise time of the waveform should not exceed 500 μsec, and absence of ringing of its tail should be ensured. Many different waveforms have been investigated, and the two that are

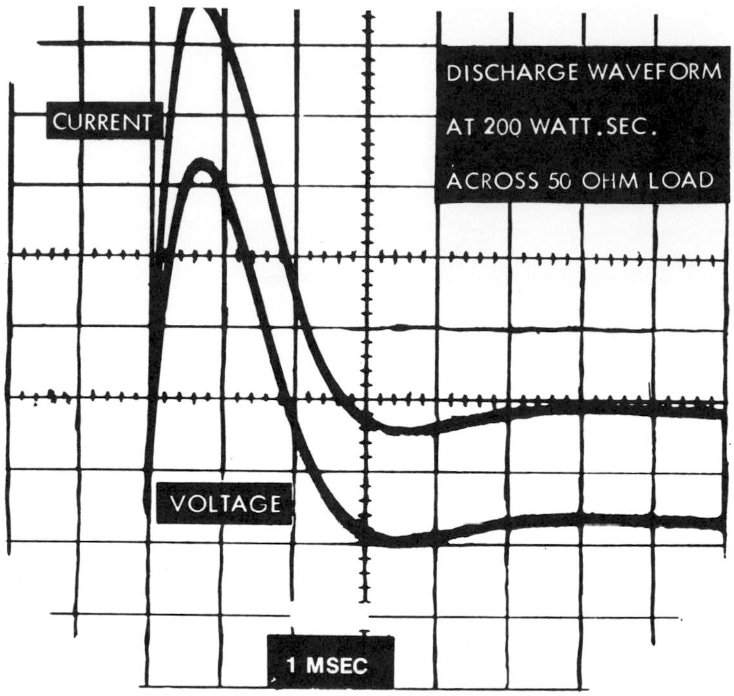

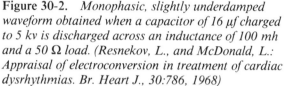

Figure 30-2. *Monophasic, slightly underdamped waveform obtained when a capacitor of 16 μf charged to 5 kv is discharged across an inductance of 100 mh and a 50 Ω load. (Resnekov, L., and McDonald, L.: Appraisal of electroconversion in treatment of cardiac dysrhythmias. Br. Heart J., 30:786, 1968)*

most used in clinical practice are the damped sinusoidal (see Fig. 30-2) and the trapezoidal.

Note that the energy setting on the moving-coil meter of the defibrillator apparatus reflects the energy delivered to the skin. The true energy delivered to the heart muscle, however, is influenced by the resistance of the skin and deeper tissues. Nevertheless, a short-duration direct current monophasic pulse allows the transmyocardial passage of 1.5 amp or more. Shaping the electrical pulse by using an inductor in series permits the electrical energy to be delivered to the heart muscle without causing undue damage.

Alternating or Direct Current

Although direct current develops many times the power of alternating current, less energy is delivered because the shock persists only for 3 to 4 msec. Alternating current shocks are more harmful to the myocardium and cause greater deterioration in ventricular function.[10]

Beck and coauthors[11] were the first to defibrillate a human heart electrically using an alternating current discharge, and for many years thereafter, alternating current defibrillation was the standard method. The waveforms of direct current discharges are so dissimilar as to make any true comparison difficult. Why then did direct current discharge become the preferred method? Two important clinical observations stimulated its use: (1) alternating current frequently failed to defibrillate the heart in the presence of acute myocardial infarction and (2) electrical conversion of rhythms other than ventricular fibrillation was needed.

A certain amount of experience had already been obtained in treating organized atrial and ventricular dysrhythmias with electrical current,[12] and although this was occasionally successful, alternating current used in this way could precipitate ventricular fibrillation and even death.[13] Nachlas and co-workers[14] were able to demonstrate that direct current was unmistakably superior even in terminating ventricular fibrillation. Therefore, it seems reasonable to conclude from the above that alternating current is feasible and successful for treating ventricular fibrillation in the clinical setting but that direct current is more effective. However, under no circumstances should alternating current be used for treating atrial rhythm disturbances or ventricular tachycardia because of the high risk of precipitating ventricular fibrillation.

Is Synchronization Needed?

Despite the use of electrical circuits that produce acceptable waveforms, a transmyocardial or transthoracic direct current shock occasionally precipitates ventricular fibrillation. For many years, a vulnerable period of ventricular excitability has been postulated in a wide variety of animals.[15] Wiggers and Wegria[16] showed this period to be 27 msec before the end of ventricular systole in the dog, and a similar period of vulnerability has also been demonstrated for the atrium.[17] The vulnerable period of the ventricle occurs just before the apex of the T wave of the electrocardiogram, at which time recovery from the refractory state is not uniform, thus allowing reentry of the depolarization wave, which favors self-sustained ac-

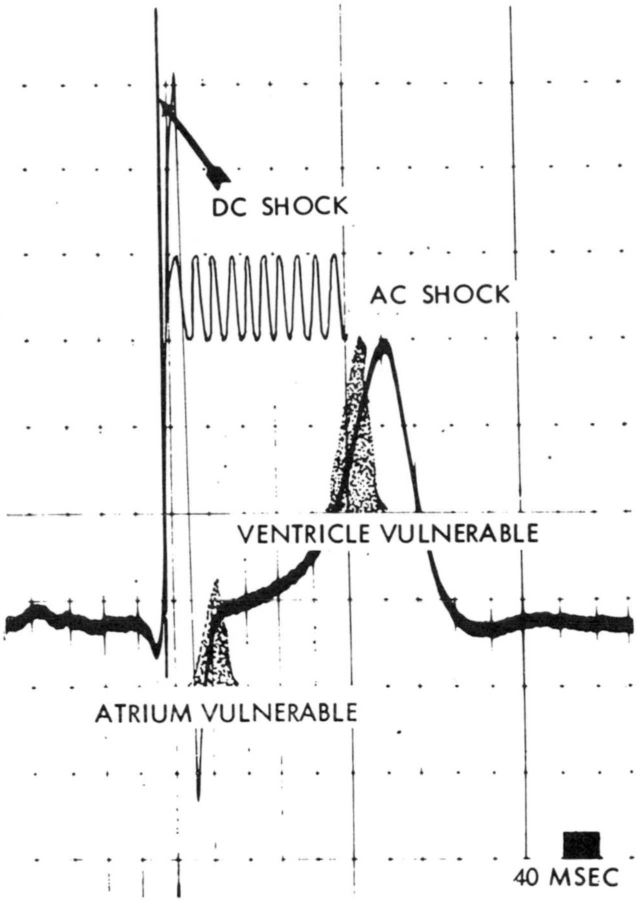

Figure 30-3. *Vulnerable phases of the cardiac cycle for fibrillation of the atrium and ventricle. R wave synchronization of a 3-msec direct current (DC) shock avoids the phases of vulnerability. Alternate current (AC) shocks, which persist for 100 to 250 msec, cannot be safely phased in this way. (Resnekov, L., and McDonald, L.: Appraisal of electroconversion in treatment of cardiac dysrhythmias. Br. Heart J., 30:786, 1968)*

tivity. That a similar phenomenon also occurs in the human heart has been demonstrated by Castellanos and colleagues.[18] The time relationship of vulnerability in the ventricle and atrium for both alternating and direct current shocks is shown in Figure 30-3.

One can conclude, therefore, that in the treatment of rhythm disturbances other than ventricular fibrillation, the risk of inducing ventricular fibrillation is lessened by timing the direct current shock to avoid the apex of the T wave. It is almost impossible to avoid the ventricular phase of vulnerability when alternating current shocks are used (see Fig. 30-3), and most direct current defibrillators incorporate a synchronizer that permits triggering of the shock by the R or S wave of the electrocardiogram. When ventricular fibrillation is treated, the synchronizer should be switched out of the circuit. The chance of ventricular fibrillation following randomized unsynchronized shocks is approximately 2%.[19] Kreus and co-workers[20] deliberately did not use a synchronizer in clinical practice, without dire consequences. When a synchronizer is not used, sufficient energy must be delivered so that a current of at least 1.5 to 2 amp flows across the heart; smaller energies may cause ventricular fibrillation and are dangerous. Therefore, when no synchronizer is used, increased levels of energy settings are mandatory.

Physiology of Electroversion

There is as yet no general agreement on the mechanism of ventricular fibrillation, and it is small wonder that the mechanism of electrical defibrillation remains in doubt. The subject has been reviewed by Antoni.[21] If a circus movement or reentry mechanism is assumed to be the cause of the fibrillation, the main effect of the direct current defibrillation pulse might be synchronous stimulation of a normally refractory myocardium. If, on the other hand, defibrillation is thought to reduce the activity of a heterotopic focus, some other mode of action must be assumed, for example, direct inhibition of the heterotopic pacemaker. Experimental findings on isolated myocardial preparations have shed some light on the problem.[22] Both the above mechanisms seem important in direct current defibrillation, but a significantly higher electrical energy is needed to cause transient inhibition of the heterotopic focus, allowing the sinus node to resume its normal role as pacemaker.

Clinical Use of Electroversion

Capacitor discharge with inductance in series was first used clinically by Lown and co-workers to treat patients with refractory ventricular tachycardia.[7] The technique has sometimes been called *countershock*[23] or *cardioversion*,[7] although some have preferred the term *electroversion*.[24] Many thousands of patients have now been treated successfully both for atrial and ventricular dysrhythmias, and the combined experience has completely justified the high initial hopes for, and confidence in, the method. The overall success rate for terminating atrial and ventricular rhythm disturbances is 90%.[25,26] It has also been shown that there is a success rate of more than 85% even when determined efforts at pharmacologic conversion of dysrhythmias have failed.[27] The correct choice of patients and meticulous attention to detail, including correction of electrolyte imbalance if present, postponing treatment in the presence of overdigitalization, proper synchronization, and the choice of antidysrhythmic agents immediately before and following treatment ensure both immediate success and the absence of a high incidence of complications.[25] The importance of meticulous attention to detail, however, cannot be overemphasized and is summarized below.

Technique

The Apparatus

Up to 7000 v may be needed to charge the capacitors to deliver 400 J. Furthermore, commercial apparatuses are either "isolated" or "nonisolated." In the former case, the output is isolated from earth (ground); with the nonisolated type, one paddle is grounded. The following monthly checks of the apparatus must be made:

1. A general examination for electrical safety .
2. The waveform produced should be inspected critically following discharge across a 50-ohm load in the laboratory.
3. The actual electrical energy of the discharge should be measured and compared with the setting on the apparatus. Most apparatuses provide a moving-coil meter that is calibrated in joules (watt-seconds), but models are still in use in which the desired energy is obtained by depressing a labeled switch, a highly undesirable feature.

During the shock, it is most important that assisting personnel do not touch the patient or the bed, because with both isolated and nonisolated circuits, a large electrical field is created that results in a shock to any person in contact. In addition, the nonisolated unit has an added risk; if the paddle on the patient's chest conducts poorly, there is an electrical pathway between the "hot" paddle and the electrocardiographic electrode at earth potential (right leg), and an electrical burn may result.

Synchronization Test

Synchronization is a safety feature that should be used routinely unless ventricular fibrillation is being treated. Defibrillators now provide visual demonstration of synchronization by a superimposed "blip" on the electrocardiographic signal being monitored on the oscilloscope. Synchronization should always be tested before administering the first shock to the patient by charging the capacitor to a low energy (5 J), attaching the electrocardiographic cables to the patient, and then discharging the capacitor, holding the two paddles in close apposition away from the patient while the connecting lead of the electrocardiogram is applied to the two cables from the paddles. In this way, a "blip" is induced on the electrocardiogram and can be easily recorded on any electrocardiogram that is being used to monitor the electroversion (Fig. 30-4).

Paddles

Paddles of adequate size should always be used, because during ventricular fibrillation the heart is subdivided into a large number of fibrillating segments. To be successful, defibrillation must simultaneously depolarize the majority of myocardial fibers. It can be shown that

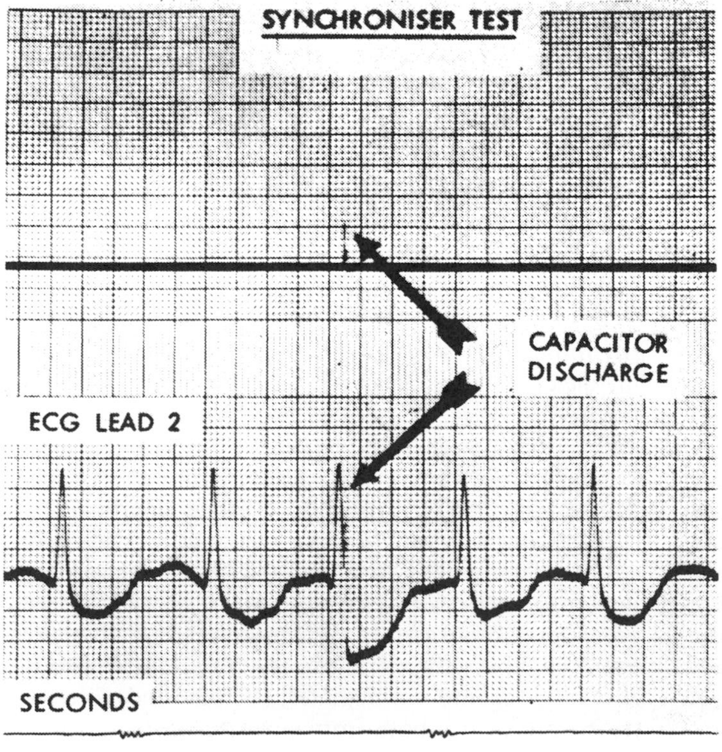

Figure 30-4. *Test of synchronization. Note the small spike (*upper tracing*) superimposed on the electrocardiographic recording of lead II (*lower tracing*). See text for details. (Resnekov, L., and McDonald, L.: Appraisal of electroconversion in treatment of cardiac dysrhythmias. Br. Heart J., 30:786, 1968)*

the current density is 20 times greater between the paddles than at the margins of the heart when small electrodes are used, and this can produce myocardial damage because of a high interelectrode current density.[29] In addition, defibrillation may well fail because of the inadequate myocardial effect at some distance from the paddles. In contrast, when large-sized paddles are used, even the cardiac margins receive up to 42% of the total current discharge, and the risk of myocardial damage is less and the chance of successful defibrillation is greater. A diameter of 9.5 cm is recommended for adults, and a diameter of 4.5 cm is recommended for children. For both adults and children, spoon-shaped paddles of appropriate size are available for internal defibrillation. When an external direct current shock is used, two anterior paddles or, alternatively, an anterior and a posterior paddle may be employed. The latter is more convenient because the patient lies on the flat posterior one, and it is only the anterior paddle that must be held by the operator (an important safety measure, especially when an apparatus in which one paddle is grounded is being used). Lown and co-workers[30] reported that using the anterior-posterior paddle position significantly lowered the energy required for electroversion, but others could not confirm this finding.[26] Indeed, experimental work[14] has shown that the anterior positioning of the paddles, as originally suggested by Kouwenhoven,[31] results in delivering 2.5 times more current to the heart. It is likely that the failure to note more striking clinical differences with variations in paddle placement results from the excess amounts of electrical energy that are consistently used to achieve electroversion. This being the case, the added safety of a flat posterior paddle, untouched by the operator and supported only by the weight of the patient, is advantageous, and the anteroposterior position is therefore recommended.

More recently, self-adhesive electropads for defibrillation have been suggested.[32] These obviate many of the disadvantages of traditional hand-held paddle-shaped electrodes applied to the skin's surface with the prior application of electrocardiographic gel or saline-soaked pads to the skin surface. If the coupling agent inadvertently spreads across the chest, less electrical energy will be delivered to the heart. In addition, hand-held electrodes are often incorrectly placed, particularly when speed is needed, as, for example, in treating ventricular fibrillation. Incorrect paddle placement was noted in 35% of patients treated for ventricular fibrillation.[33] The self-adhesive electropads could have a high electrical impedance, since no pressure is applied to them; indeed, in animal studies this was found to be the case.[34] A clinical study using the self-adhesive pads in 80 patients, however, demonstrated that the transthoracic impedance was 75 ± 21 ohms, which compared very favorably with the expected transthoracic impedance of 67 ± 36 ohms with standard hand-held electrode paddles.[35] The advantage of not having to hold the paddles during the electrical discharge of the shock is obvious, and self-adhesive electrodes can be recommended.

Drugs

If at all possible, digoxin or any other digitalis preparation should be withheld for 24 to 48 hours before treatment. When treatment cannot be postponed and must be undertaken in the presence of heavy digitalization, the initial energy setting should be markedly reduced (5 to 10 J), and an intravenous injection of 100 mg of lidocaine should precede the shock. Many physicians use quinidine or some other antidysrhythmic agent orally, intramuscularly, or even intravenously routinely before direct current shock,[36] but the efficacy of these drugs in reducing energy requirements or in helping to maintain sinus rhythm thereafter is questionable.[26] It is possible, however, that an antidysrhythmic drug such as quinidine could help in preventing premature beats immediately following direct current shock,[37] which could precipitate a return to the dysrhythmia immediately after successful electroversion (see below).

Anticoagulants

The incidence of embolism following electroversion varies from 1.4 to 2.4%, a figure quite similar to that following the quinidine conversion of cardiac dysrhythmia.[38] The need for anticoagulant protection was the subject of much debate in the absence of any well-controlled study, but such a study has now been reported,[39] and a statistically significant benefit in the group of patients who received electroversion under anticoagulant control has been shown. When there is a clear risk of embolism or thrombosis, as in patients with recent myocardial infarction, coronary heart disease, mitral valve disease, cardiomyopathy, prosthetic heart valves, or a previous history of embolism, prior anticoagulant therapy with a warfarin derivative should be given or heparin used when the need for direct current shock is urgent. Because the risk of reverting back to the rhythm disturbance is highest during the first month of treatment (see Figs. 30-9 and 30-10), anticoagulant therapy should be maintained for at least 4 weeks even after successful direct current shock, after which it may be discontinued unless the underlying heart disease requires its continuance.

Anesthesia

General anesthesia is not required,[40,41] but amnesia, which follows an intravenous injection of 5 to 10 mg of diazepam, is recommended.[42] Muscle relaxants, especially halothane, which is known to predispose to ventricular rhythm disturbances, should not be used with electroversion.[43] Although diazepam is a reasonably safe drug, it must be given cautiously to those patients with congestive cardiac failure. Because diazepam is both safe and has a rapid action, the skilled help of an anesthesiologist is not mandatory, nor is elaborate anesthetic equipment needed. The anesthesia for direct current shock has been reviewed by Gilston and coauthors.[44]

The Treatment Room

Electroversion should only be undertaken in an area fully equipped for cardiac monitoring and resuscitation, if needed, including emergency pacemaking. The heart rate should be displayed throughout on a tachometer, if available. A technically satisfactory electrocardiographic lead should be clearly visible on an oscilloscope throughout, and provision should be made for recording the electrocardiogram in several leads as needed.

Routine Preparation

The method of treatment should be carefully explained to the patient and any anxiety relieved. For subsequent comparison, a short strip of lead V_1 of the electrocardiogram should be recorded just before the shock because P waves can be difficult to detect immediately after direct current shock even when the patient is in sinus rhythm. The skin of the chest should be carefully prepared by liberally applying electrocardiogram paste, which should be rubbed in well to reduce electrical resistance and to prevent painful superficial skin burns. It is important that no conductive material be allowed to run between the two paddles because current, which takes the path of least resistance, will be diverted away from the heart, possibly resulting in failure of treatment.

Electrical Energies

Small energies should be used first, and if these are unsuccessful, repeated shocks can be given at an increased energy-level setting. For an adult, an initial setting of 25 to 50 J is satisfactory, increasing the setting in 25- to 50-J increments. If heavy digitalization is present, an initial setting of 5 to 10 J is appropriate. If extrasystoles follow the first shock, and as a routine before treating a patient known to be heavily digitalized, 100 mg of lidocaine should be given intravenously before continuing to a higher energy setting. The initial setting for a child is 5 to 10 J delivered across appropriately sized pediatric paddles and then increased in 5- to 10-J increments. There should be great reluctance to exceed an energy setting of 300 J in an adult being treated for a chronic rhythm disturbance. However, where an acute dysrhythmia causes serious hemodynamic effects, maximum energies (400 J) should be used if needed. The initial setting for ventricular fibrillation (no synchronizer in circuit) is 200 J, increasing thereafter to 300- or 400-J settings if needed. Energy settings for internal defibrillation (internal paddles) are 20 to 100 J in 20-J increments.

Immediately After the Shock

With the reinstitution of sinus rhythm, or if sinus rhythm fails to occur after optional energies have been delivered, the amnesic drug is discontinued and a 12-lead electrocardiogram recorded. The electrocardiogram should be monitored on an oscilloscope for the next 24 hours or longer if needed, records of the blood pressure should be taken every half hour until the control value before the shock is regained, and serum enzyme levels should be obtained routinely 8 hours after the shock and repeated at appropriate intervals if the initial values are raised.

Specific Rhythm Disturbances

Atrial Fibrillation

Atrial fibrillation remains the commonest organized rhythm disturbance treated by electroversion, and its cause is frequently rheumatic or coronary heart disease. Among other causes of atrial fibrillation, the lone or idiopathic variety requires special mention because the success rate of its electroversion is low, the incidence of complications is high, and the length of time during which sinus rhythm persists is disappointingly short.[45] For atrial fibrillation as a result of rheumatic heart disease, the initial success rate of treatment by electroversion is 90%, but for idiopathic atrial fibrillation it is less than 75%.[26,28]

Success of electroversion is not related to the patients' age or sex, the type of heart disease (idiopathic atrial fibrillation excepted), or even to overall body size. However, an important factor is the duration of the rhythm disturbance.[28] When atrial fibrillation has been present for 5 years or longer, the rate of success is only 50% (Fig. 30-5). The overall size of the heart and selective enlargement of the left atrium also lessen the chance of success.[28]

Every patient with chronic atrial fibrillation requires individual assessment to determine whether treatment is really worthwhile. Despite this, there is no doubt that hemodynamic benefit can be achieved by successful electroversion.[46] Certain patients can be maintained free of cardiac failure only by repeated electrical termination of atrial fibrillation because their ventricular function requires the booster action of atrial systole to achieve an optimal output.

Although it is usually easy to achieve open-chest electroversion at heart surgery, reversion to atrial fibrillation in the immediate postoperative period is almost universal. Atrial fibrillation with the ventricular rate controlled by digoxin is preferred to rapidly changing cardiac rhythms in the postoperative state, and it is therefore recommended that the electroversion of these patients be postponed until they are convalescent following open- or closed-heart valve surgery.[28,47]

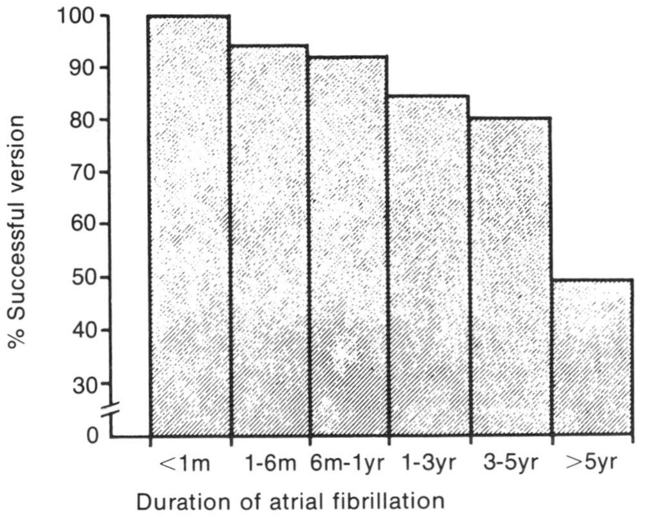

Figure 30-5. *Percentage of successful electroversion and duration of atrial fibrillation in 147 patients before treatment (idiopathic atrial fibrillation excluded). (m, month; yr, year) (Resnekov, L., and McDonald, L.: Appraisal of electroconversion in treatment of cardiac dysrhythmias. Br. Heart J., 30:786, 1968)*

The following groups of patients are, in general, unsuitable for electroversion unless special circumstances exist:

1. Patients with idiopathic or lone atrial fibrillation.
2. Patients with coronary heart disease and atrial fibrillation with a slow ventricular response even in the absence of digoxin.
3. Patients unable to maintain sinus rhythm for more than a brief period even when receiving suitable antidysrhythmic drugs.
4. Patients presenting with atrial rhythm disturbances in rapid succession.
5. Patients in the tachycardic phase of the tachycardia-bradycardia syndrome unless emergency pacemaking is at hand, because dangerous asystole may well follow a transmyocardial shock in this condition.
6. Patients with long-standing atrial fibrillation (more than 5 years) with considerable enlargement of the heart (cardiothoracic ratio of more than 50%), unless successful cardiac surgery has been performed.
7. Patients with atrial fibrillation in association with conduction disturbances.

Atrial Flutter

A 95% success rate for converting atrial flutter is common.[28] The electrical energy setting needed is much lower than for atrial fibrillation, the average being 50 J. In contrast to idiopathic atrial fibrillation, atrial flutter not associated with a detectable heart disease may still be successfully reverted by direct current shock with low-energy settings, and sinus rhythm may even be maintained for significantly long periods.[46]

Paroxysmal Atrial Tachycardia

The rate of successful electroversion of paroxysmal atrial tachycardia varies from 75% to 80% and depends on the underlying cause; even so, electrical reversion is preferable to pharmacologic therapy.[28] Direct current should not be used for digitalis-induced supraventricular or junctional tachycardia, except under the most unusual circumstances, because of the very high risk of precipitating ventricular fibrillation.[48]

Ventricular Tachycardia

The initial success rate for electroversion of ventricular tachycardia exceeds 97%, and electrical energies needed are low.[28] Direct current shock should be avoided if ventricular tachycardia is digitalis induced, except under unusual circumstances.

Ventricular Fibrillation

Experimental animal studies have shown the superiority of direct current electrical defibrillation over alternating current electrical defibrillation for the treatment of patients with ventricular fibrillation.[14] In clinical practice, successful resuscitation, as judged by the patient's leaving the hospital, can be achieved in some 60% of patients using direct current shock and well-conducted principles of resuscitation.[49] However, without meticulous attention to the latter, electrical defibrillation universally fails.

Complications of Electroversion

Complications following electroversion are not as rare as initially predicted, nor do they relate only to drugs given to maintain sinus rhythm.[50] The incidence of complications among 220 patients treated with electroversion has been reported to be 14.5%.[24] (These do not include minor complications such as superficial burns due to poor preparation of the skin or transient rhythm disturbances immediately after shock.)

Complications are related to the energy-level settings used (Fig. 30-6). When a setting of 150 J was employed, there was a 6% incidence of complications, which increased to more than 30% at 400 J.[24] It is frequently patients being treated for atrial fibrillation who require higher energy-level settings, particularly when the dysrhythmia has persisted for more than 3 years and in whom the rhythm disturbance is associated with cardiomyopathy or coronary heart disease. Similarly, patients with idiopathic atrial fibrillation require high energy-level settings.

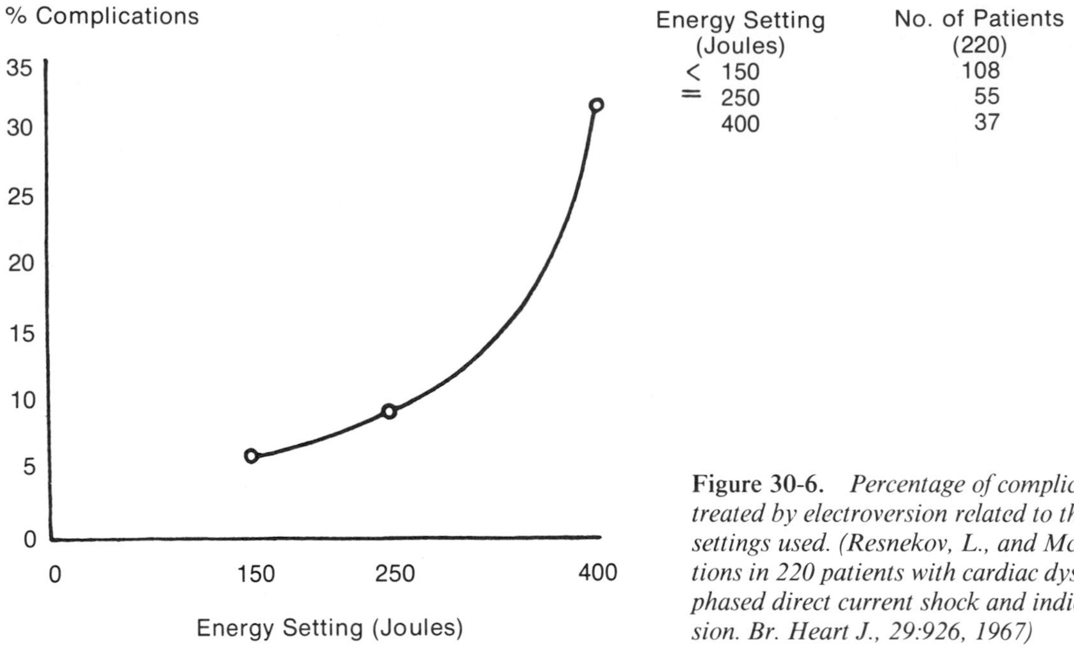

Figure 30-6. *Percentage of complications in 220 patients treated by electroversion related to the maximal energy settings used. (Resnekov, L., and McDonald, L.: Complications in 220 patients with cardiac dysrhythmias treated by phased direct current shock and indications for electroconversion. Br. Heart J., 29:926, 1967)*

From these facts, one can conclude that to prevent unnecessary complications, there rarely is an indication for exceeding settings of 300 J in patients who present with long-standing atrial fibrillation, and great caution must be advised in treating those patients who are heavily digitalized, those whose dysrhythmia is due to cardiomyopathy or coronary heart disease, and those whose atrial fibrillation is of the lone or idiopathic variety.

The origin of the raised serum enzyme levels following electroversion is still debated, and many consider damage to skeletal muscle to be the cause.[51] Other signs of myocardial damage frequently coexist,[28] suggesting that some of the elevation is due to release of enzymes from the damaged myocardium into the general circulation.[60]

The incidence of raised levels of serum enzymes is 10%.

Hypotension

Following electroversion, a fall in blood pressure not related to the anesthetic is more common when higher electrical energies are used. Hypotension may persist for several hours but usually requires no particular therapeutic intervention. Patients should, however, be carefully monitored until the control blood pressure level is regained.

The incidence of hypotension following electroversion is 3%.

Electrocardiographic Evidence of Myocardial Damage

Electrocardiographic changes following electroversion may be recorded even in the absence of any untoward symptoms (Fig. 30-7). Patterns of myocardial infarction may persist for several months and are commonest following treatment at higher energy level settings.

The incidence of electrocardiographic evidence of myocardial damage following electroversion is 3%.

Pulmonary and Systemic Emboli

Embolism following electroversion indicates the need for prior anticoagulant administration (see above). The incidence of this complication is 1.4%.

Ventricular Dysrhythmia

Following electroversion, ventricular rhythm disturbances are common at low-energy settings if the patient is digitalized and at high energies even in the absence of digoxin. Their emergence requires an intravenous antidysrhythmic drug before the energy-level setting is increased for a further shock.

Increase in Heart Size and Pulmonary Edema

Increase in heart size and pulmonary edema (Fig. 30-8), when they occur, are seen within 1 to 3 hours of electroversion, and these complications are unlike all others in that they are found only in patients successfully converted to sinus rhythm. (Their usual incidence is 3%.) Although Lown[25] considered pulmonary emboli as the cause, others believe that following electroversion, there is considerable depression of mechanical function of the heart,[52] which in the presence of any additional obstruction to flow across the mitral valve or associated left ventricular dysfunction may result in pulmonary edema. As with the other complications, the incidence of

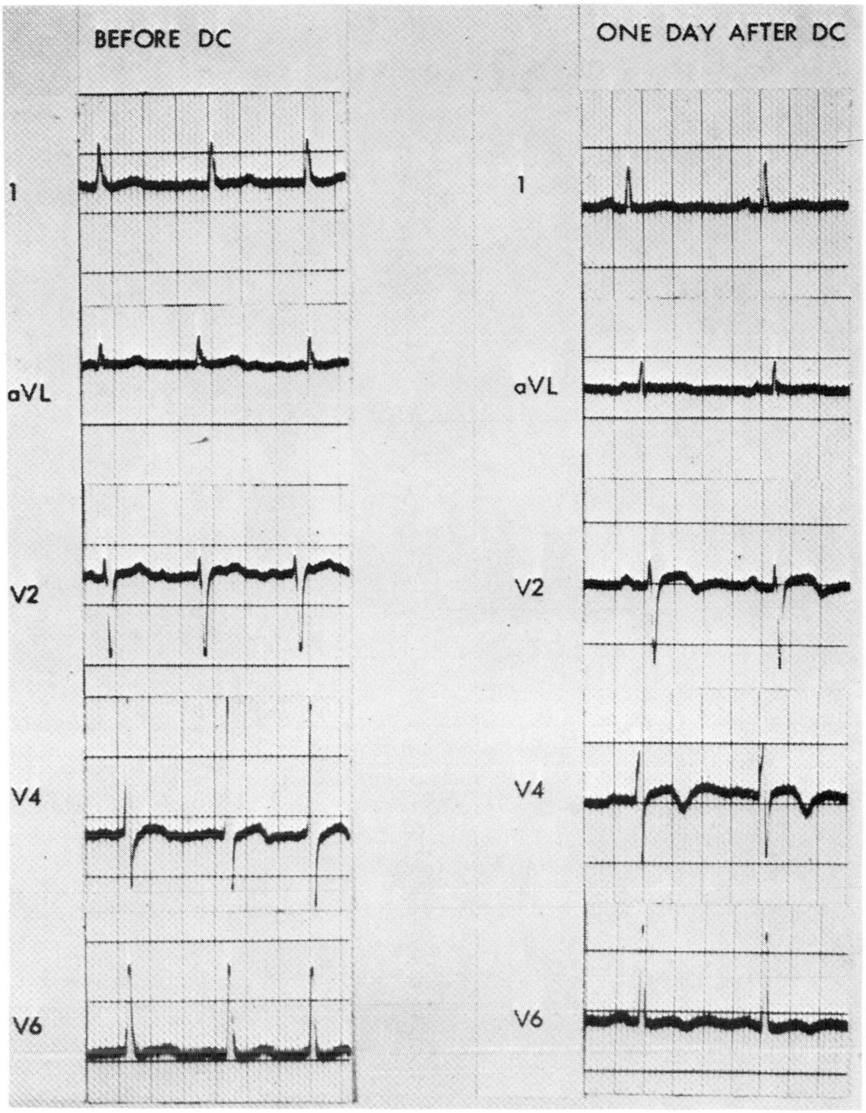

Figure 30-7. *Electrocardiogram immediately before (left) and 1 day after (right) the electroversion of idiopathic atrial fibrillation using 300 J. In sinus rhythm a pattern of nontransmural infarction is shown, which was associated with a diagnostic elevation of serum enzymes. The electrocardiographic abnormalities persisted for more than 6 months. (Resnekov, L., and McDonald, L.: Complications in 220 patients with cardiac dysrhythmias treated by phased direct current shock and indications for electroconversion. Br. Heart J., 29:926, 1967)*

these two findings is greatest following higher energy-level settings.

Follow-Up Studies

Electroversion is very successful in the treatment of rhythm disturbances, but the number of patients remaining in sinus rhythm is disappointingly small, particularly when patients with atrial fibrillation are treated.[26,28] A 36-month follow-up study involving 183 patients who were successfully brought into sinus rhythm shows that less than 30% remained in sinus rhythm.[26] The highest incidence of reverting occurs by the end of the first month of the treatment (Fig. 30-9), but the incidence is actually highest within the first 24 hours of successful electroversion (Fig. 30-10). Patients with significant underlying heart disease and radiographic evidence of cardiac enlargement are particularly prone to revert to the original rhythm disturbance,[26,28] and in any patient in whom atrial fibrillation is of long duration (3 years or longer), a 70% chance of reverting back to that rhythm can be expected (Fig. 30-11).

Pharmacologic Therapy and Electroversion

Digitalis Preparation

In the presence of heavy digitalization, Lown and coworkers[53] found that the direct current threshold for ventricular tachycardia in the dog fell by some 2000%, to 0.2 J. The importance of this observation in clinical

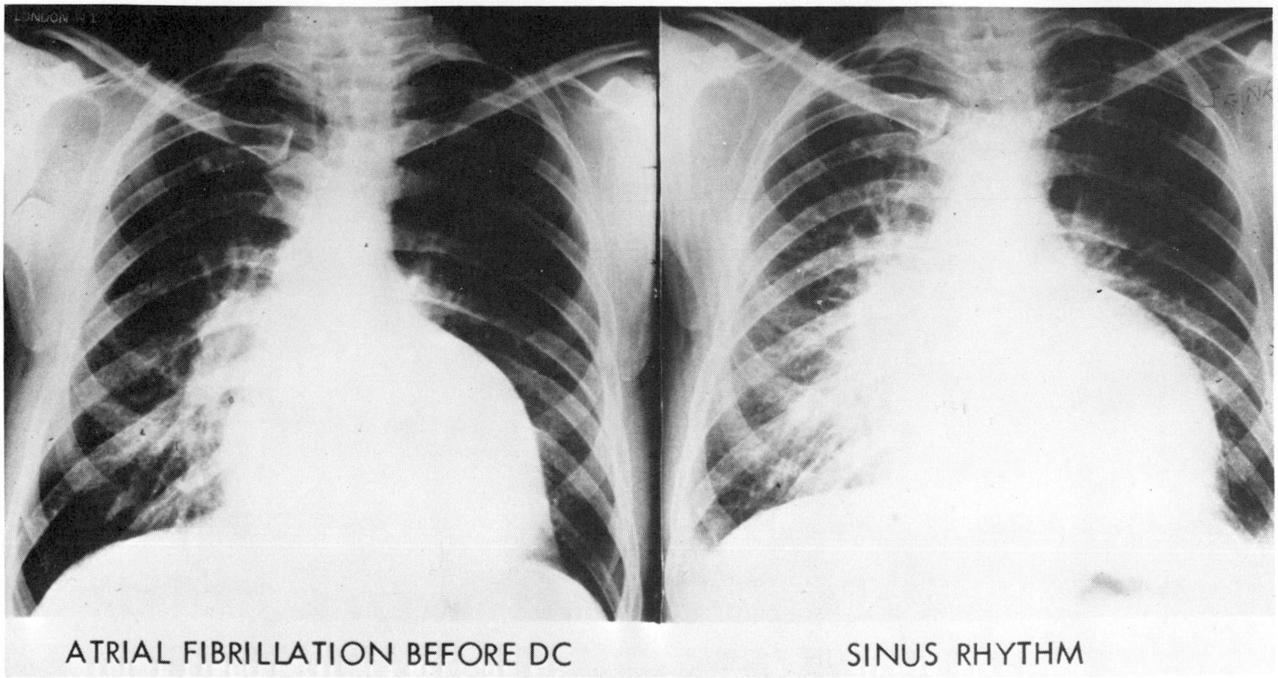

Figure 30-8. *Chest radiograph (posteroanterior) immediately before (left) and 12 hours after (right) the electroversion of atrial fibrillation (200 J) in a patient with corrected transposition of the great vessels. Note the marked increase in size of the heart and obvious pulmonary edema in sinus rhythm. (Resnekov, L., and McDonald, L.: Complications in 220 patients with cardiac dysrhythmias treated by phased direct current shock and indications for electroconversion. Br. Heart J., 29:926, 1967)*

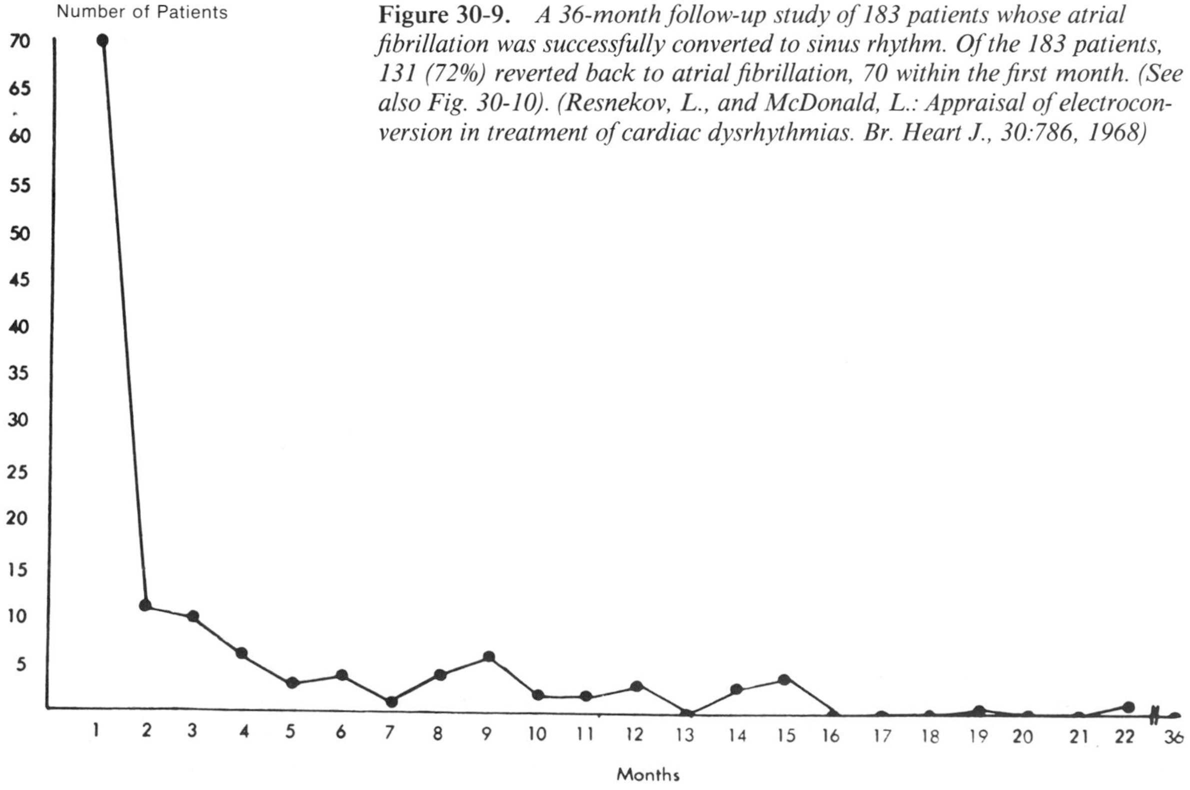

Figure 30-9. *A 36-month follow-up study of 183 patients whose atrial fibrillation was successfully converted to sinus rhythm. Of the 183 patients, 131 (72%) reverted back to atrial fibrillation, 70 within the first month. (See also Fig. 30-10). (Resnekov, L., and McDonald, L.: Appraisal of electroconversion in treatment of cardiac dysrhythmias. Br. Heart J., 30:786, 1968)*

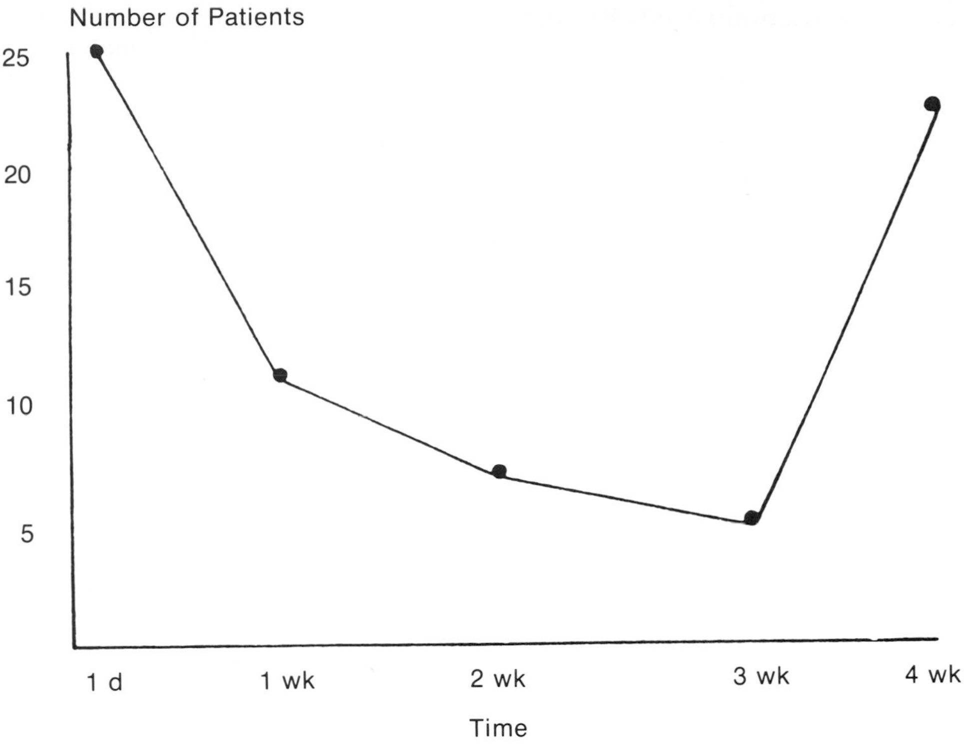

Figure 30-10. *Of the 70 patients who reverted to atrial fibrillation within the first 4 weeks (see Fig. 30-9), 25 did so within the first day of electroversion. (d, day; wk, week) (Resnekov, L., and McDonald, L.: Complications in 220 patients with cardiac dysrhythmias treated by phased direct current shock and indications for electroconversion. Br. Heart J., 29:926, 1967)*

practice is that although digitalis effects may not be clinically apparent, they can be unmasked by an electrical shock, and any associated myocardial cell potassium deficit enhances this effect. Conversely, the administration of potassium may reverse the undesirable effects. The higher the electrical energy used, the higher the risk of emergence of serious ventricular dysrhythmias, and death has been reported as a result.[54] As already indicated, electroversion should rarely be used for the management of a known digitalis-induced rhythm disturbance. Despite the occasional reported success,[55] fatal ventricular fibrillation may follow even when the shock is properly synchronized.[48] If electroversion is needed in a patient known to be heavily digitalized, an intravenous injection of an antidysrhythmic drug should always precede the shock, and the energy-level setting should be significantly reduced, as previously indicated.

Propranolol may be helpful in reducing the dangerous myocardial sensitivity to a high-energy level of electrical current. If used, however, it should be combined with intravenous atropine[56] to protect the patient against cardiac arrest, which may follow direct current shock in patients primed with propranolol.[57]

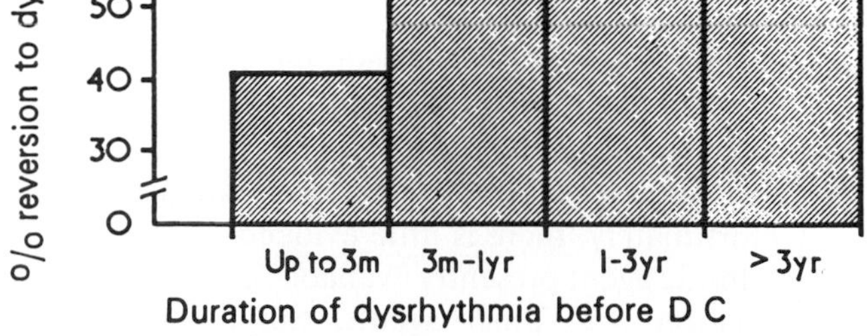

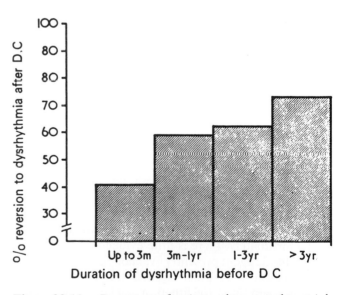

Figure 30-11. *Percentage of patients who reverted to atrial fibrillation related to the duration of the dysrhythmia before electroversion (excluding idiopathic atrial fibrillation). (m, month; yr, year; DC, direct current) (Resnekov, L., and McDonald, L.: Complications in 220 patients with cardiac dysrhythmias treated by phased direct current shock and indications for electroconversion. Br. Heart J., 29:926, 1967)*

Drugs to Maintain Sinus Rhythm

For electroversion to succeed, an energy-level setting sufficient to depolarize instantaneously the majority of heart fibers is needed. For sinus rhythm to follow, the sinoatrial node must function adequately and must not be diseased or fibrosed. Ectopic beats should be kept to a minimum immediately after a shock.[42] Excess electrical energies can be harmful, and any interruption of the rhythm disturbance by the direct current shock is good evidence that depolarization of the heart did occur and that the level of electrical energy used was adequate. Should sinus rhythm fail to emerge or be short lived despite adequate electrical energies, it is likely that either the sinus node cannot function as the pacemaker or that ectopic rhythms were precipitated by a vagal surge or by a sudden release of catecholamine following the electrical discharge.

To improve pacemaker function following direct current shock, atropine, 1 to 2 mg intravenously, should be routinely administered to patients in whom atrial fibrillation has been present for 5 years or longer, although the chance of these chronic dysrhythmic patients converting easily or maintaining sinus rhythm for any length of time thereafter is small.[26] Similarly, any bradycardia after direct current shock will enhance the likelihood of atrial ventricular premature beats.[25] Note that although they are successful in suppressing ectopic beats, antidysrhythmic drugs such as quinidine, procainamide, lidocaine, and propranolol may depress pacemaker function. Furthermore, since there is already a likelihood of intense parasympathetic stimulation immediately after direct current shock,[58] the *routine* use of these drugs is not advised because they may well precipitate dangerous asystole.

Isolated ventricular premature beats or ventricular tachycardia immediately after direct current shock frequently result from overdigitalization, from the effects on the heart of the shock itself, and from a lowered myocardial potassium content. As previously indicated, such patients should be protected by postponing treatment if possible, by ensuring an adequate serum and myocardial potassium level, and by using antidysrhythmic drugs immediately before the shock, which should be delivered at a reduced energy-level setting.

Unfortunately, there is little evidence that any antidysrhythmic agent presently available, either alone or in combination with other agents, can maintain sinus rhythm when sinoatrial function is at fault, when serious underlying myocardial or valvular heart disease is present, or when atrial fibrillation has existed for 5 years or longer. Nevertheless, sinus rhythm may be hemodynamically important in certain patients. Under these circumstances, quinidine or procainamide may be used in an attempt to maintain sinus rhythm over a prolonged period. If cardiac failure is not too severe, it may be possible to maintain sinus rhythm by a combination of quinidine and propranolol,[59] which will permit reducing the dose of quinidine and thus lessening the chance of toxicity.

General Aspects of the Use of High-Energy Electrical Current

The refinement of high-energy electrical current has been a very great advance in the management of cardiac dysrhythmias. Provided meticulous attention to detail is adhered to, the method is efficient, successful, and relatively free of complications. Nevertheless, important questions about its actual use in clinical practice remain, particularly regarding the possibility of causing myocardial damage. Closely allied is the level of energy to be used and its recommended upper limit, beyond which complication rates become forbiddingly high.

Complications following synchronized direct current shock are often multiple.[24] Changes in the levels of serum enzymes are the commonest complication reported, and Ehsani and co-workers[60] were able to show that in patients suffering acute myocardial infarction, high-energy electrical current discharge to the heart was followed by a release of creatine phosphokinase (CPK) into the peripheral blood, with a substantial rise in the MB, or cardiac fraction. In patients without acute myocardial infarction, the same energy-level setting resulted in an increase in total CPK made up almost entirely of the MM, or skeletal muscle fraction. Earlier work by Dahl and co-workers[61] had shown that myocardial damage was caused by direct current shock, particularly at high energy–level settings. Myocardial damage is related to the energy level delivered, the size of the electrodes, and the time between shocks; careful attention to all these factors should help minimize its occurrence.

In 1961, Peleška[62] showed that myocardial damage could result from capacitor discharge. The important electrical variables that relate to the safe clinical use of high-energy electrical current include the capacitance of the condensors, the value of inductance of the circuit, the resistance between the patient electrodes, and the rise time of the current waveform. If a defibrillation apparatus is considered in terms of a direct current–resistive circuit, the resistance between the inductance and the body may alter significantly because of a change in total body impedance, and this may well be responsible for changes in the discharge-current waveform flowing across the heart.

Using trapezoidal current waveforms for external ventricular defibrillation, Tacker and co-workers[63] reported that the effectiveness of treatment decreased as body weight increased. At present, there is a regrettable lack of certainty regarding the optimal characteristics for duration, peak current, and other parameters needed for effective and safe defibrillation. Nevertheless, high-output defibrillators have already been designed and are being recommended.[64] Much of the present argument regarding the need for higher-energy defibrillators in clinical use relates particularly to animal studies,[65] backed by as yet inadequate clinical investigations.[66]

In an attempt to resolve this question, Pantridge and associates undertook a prospective study in patients weighing 50 kg or more, particularly those in the 90-kg range.[67] A low energy of between 150 to 165 J was delivered to these subjects, and success in defibrillating the ventricle was good. Similar conclusions have been published by other investigators.[28,68] Ventricular defibrillation depends for its success not only on delivering an efficient electrical shock to the myocardium, but also on observing the principles of cardiopulmonary resuscitation.

Cardiac damage due to electrical current and energy is associated with morphologic changes that are easily seen by light microscopy and ultrastructural observations.[69] There is a distinct morphologic pattern when a delivered dose exceeds 1 amp/kg of body weight in an experimental animal using trapezoidal current waveforms. The higher the electrical amperage delivered, the more severe and extensive the damage. Davis and co-workers[70] showed that such cardiac lesions are discrete and are found beneath the epicardium, but they may even be transmural in their extent. There is disruption of myofilaments and of the mitochondria, which often contain lipid droplets. Areas of the myocardium that may be irreversibly damaged are replaced by fibrous scar tissue; if this is extensive, abnormal cardiac function could result. The clinical correlate of these extensive areas of myocardial damage is profound electrocardiographic changes, suggesting infarction (see Fig. 30-7),[26] and such patterns may persist for many months. In addition, they are associated with increases in serum enzyme levels.

More recently the intravenous administration of 1 mg/kg of verapamil before delivering shocks was studied in animals to see whether less myocardial damage was caused when 4000 J was passed across the chest of dogs. Prior administration of verapamil reduced the amount of damage caused, whereas propranolol, 0.4 mg/kg intravenously, had no such beneficial effect. Also demonstrated during this study was the fact that more damage was caused when the electrical energy was divided among 10 shocks than when it was applied in 20 or 40 shocks at 0.5-minute intervals. The beneficial effects of verapamil provide further evidence for the role of calcium accumulation in cardiac necrosis after high-energy electrical shocks.[71]

Thus, much more study is needed before recommending that higher-energy direct current defibrillators be universally available, lest their widespread use be associated with an increasing number of potentially serious cardiac complications following attempts at ventricular defibrillation using energy-level settings over 400 J when lower energy–level settings may well suffice.

Automatic Implantable Ventricular Defibrillator

The automatic implantable ventricular defibrillator monitors cardiac rhythm continuously, identifies ventricular fibrillation, and promptly delivers an appropriate electrical defibrillation shock.[72,73] Following animal experimental studies, encouraging preliminary use of the device was reported.[74] Subsequently, a 1-year mortality of 8.5%, a result of sudden death in 52 patients in whom the device was implanted, has been reported, compared to the expected 1-year mortality of 48% in these patients who had survived previous cardiac arrest.[75] These results indicate the demonstrated success of automatic internal defibrillation as well as the method's potential for reducing the unacceptably high mortality of patients prone to sudden death whose cardiac rhythm disturbances are not being adequately controlled by antidysrhythmic therapy or prophylactic pacemaking.

The device is now being modified to provide not only internal automatic defibrillation but overdrive and other forms of pacemaking as needed.

References

1. Hoffa, M., and Ludwig, C.: Einige neue Versuche über Herzbewegung, Z. Ration. Med., 9:107, 1850.
2. Prevost, J. L., and Batteli, F.: Quelques effets des décharges electriques sur le coeur des mammifrères. J. Physiol. Pathol. Gen. (Paris), 2:40, 1900.
3. Kouwenhoven, W. B., Hooker, D. R., and Langworthy, O. R.: The current flowing through the heart under conditions of electric shock. Am. J. Physiol., 100:344, 1932.
4. Ferris, L. P., King, B. G., Spence, P. W., and Williams, H. B.: Effects of electrical shock on the heart. Elec. Engineer., 55:498, 1936.
5. King, B. G.: The effect of electric shock on heart action with special reference to varying susceptibility in different parts of the cardiac cycle. Aberdeen, Scotland, The Aberdeen University Press, 1934.
6. Gurvich, N. L., and Yunyev, G. S.: O vosstanovlenii normalnoi deyatel'nosti fibrilliruyuschego serdtsa teplokrovnikh possedstvom kondensatornogo razryada. Biull. Eksp. Biol. Med., 8:55, 1939.
7. Lown, B., Amarasingham, R., and Neuman, J.: New method for terminating cardiac arrhythmias. Use of synchronized capacitor discharge. J.A.M.A., 182:548, 1962.
8. Hooker, D. R., Kouwenhoven, W. B., and Langworthy, O. R.: The effect of alternating electrical currents on the heart. Am. J. Physiol., 103:444, 1933.

9. Kouwenhoven, W. B., and Milnor, W. R.: Treatment of ventricular fibrillation using a capacitor discharge. J. Appl. Physiol., 7:253, 1954.
10. Yarbrough, R., Ussery, G., and Whitley, J.: A comparison of the effects of A. C. and D. C. countershock on ventricular function in thoracotomized dogs. Am. J. Cardiol., 14:504, 1964.
11. Beck, E. S., Pritchard, W. H., and Feil, H. S.: Ventricular fibrillation of long duration abolished by electric shock. J.A.M.A., 135:985, 1947.
12. McDonald, L., Resnekov, L., and Ross, D.: Resistant ventricular tachycardia a year after surgical correction of Fallot's tetralogy treated by external electric countershock. Lancet, 2:708, 1963.
13. Zoll, P. M., and Linenthal, A. J.: Termination of refractory tachycardia by external countershock. Circulation, 25:596, 1962.
14. Nachlas, M. M., Bix, H. H., Mower, M. M., and Sieband, M. P.: Observations on defibrillation and synchronized countershock. Progr. Cardiovasc. Dis., 9:64, 1966.
15. de Boer, S.: On the fibrillation of the heart. J. Physiol. (Lond.), 54:400, 1921.
16. Wiggers, C. J., and Wegria, R.: Ventricular fibrillation due to single, localized induction and condenser shocks applied during vulnerable phase of ventricular systole. Am. J. Physiol., 128:500, 1940.
17. Andrus, E. C., Carter, E. P. and Wheeler, H. A.: Refractory period of the normally beating dog's auricle, with a note on the occurrence of auricular fibrillation following a single stimulus. J. Exp. Med., 51:357, 1930.
18. Castellanos, A., Jr., Lemberg, L., and Berkovits, B. V.: Repetitive firing during synchronized ventricular stimulation (abstr.). Am. J. Cardiol., 17:119, 1966.
19. Balagot, R. C., and Bandelin, V. R.: Comparative evaluation of some DC cardiac defibrillators. Am. Heart J., 77:489, 1969.
20. Kreus, K. E., Salokannel, S. J., and Waris, E. K.: Non-synchronised and synchronised direct-current countershock in cardiac arrhythmias. Lancet, 2:405, 1966.
21. Antoni, H.: Physiologische Grundlagen der elektrischen Defibrillation des Herzens. Verch. Disch. Ges. Kreislaufforsch., 35:106, 1969.
22. Coraboeuf, E., Suekane, K., and Breton, D.: Some effects of strong stimulations on the electrical and mechanical properties of isolated heart. In Electrophysiology of the Heart. New York, Oxford Medical Publications, 1964.
23. Zoll, P. M., Linenthal, A. J., Gibson, W., et al.: Termination of ventricular fibrillation in man by externally applied countershock. N. Engl. J. Med., 254:727, 1956.
24. Resnekov, L., and McDonald, L.: Complications in 220 patients with cardiac dysrhythmias treated by phased direct current shock and indications for electroconversion. Br. Heart J., 29:926, 1967.
25. Lown, B.: Electrical reversion of cardiac arrhythmias. Br. Heart J., 29:469, 1967.
26. Resnekov, L., and McDonald, L.: Appraisal of electroconversion in treatment of cardiac dysrhythmias. Br. Heart J., 30:786, 1968.
27. McDonald, L., Resnekov, L., and O'Brien, K.: Direct current shock in treatment of drug resistant arrhythmias. Br. Med. J., 1:1468, 1964.
28. Resnekov, L.: Synchronized capacitor discharge in the management of cardiac arrhythmias with particular reference to the haemodynamic significance of atrial systole. M. D. Thesis, University of Cape Town, Cape Town, South Africa, 1965.
29. Peleška, B.: A high voltage defibrillator and the theory of high-voltage defibrillation. In Proceedings of the Third International Conference of Medical Electronics, p. 265. Springfield, Ill., Charles C Thomas, 1960.
30. Lown, B., Kleiger, R., and Wolff, G.: The technique of cardioversion. Am. Heart J., 67:282, 1964.
31. Kouwenhoven, W. B., Jude, J. R., Knickerbocker, G. G., and Chestnut, W. R.: Closed chest defibrillation of the heart. Surgery, 42:550, 1957.
32. Zoll, R. H., Zoll, P. M., Frank, H. A., and Belgard, A. H.: New defibrillation electrodes (abstr.) Med. Instrument., 2:56, 1978.
33. De Silva, R. A., Margolis, B., and Lown, B.: Determinants of success during inhospital defibrillation. Cited in Crampton, R. A.: Accepted, controversial and speculative aspects of ventricular defibrillation. Progr. Cardiovasc. Dis., 23:167, 1980.
34. Ewy, G. A., Horan, W. J., and Ewy, M. D.: Disposable defibrillator electrodes. Heart Lung, 6:127, 1977.
35. Kerber, R. E., Martins, J. B., Kelly, K. J., et al.: Self-adhesive preapplied electrode pads for defibrillation and cardioversion. Am. J. Cardiol., 3:815, 1984.
36. Rossi, M., and Lown, B.: The use of quinidine in cardioversion. Am. J. Cardiol., 19:234, 1966.
37. Resnekov, L.: Drug therapy before and after the electroversion of cardiac dysrhythmias. Prog. Cardiovasc. Dis., 16:531, 1974.
38. Goldman, J.: The management of chronic atrial fibrillation: indications for and method of conversion to sinus rhythm. Prog. Cardiovasc. Dis., 2:465, 1959–1960.
39. Storstein, D.: Cardioversion session 18. In Sandöe, E., Flensted-Jensen, E., and Olesen, K., II. (eds.): Symposium on Cardiac Arrhythmias, p. 418. Södertälje, Sweden, Astra, 1970.
40. Stock, R. J.: Cardioversion without anesthesia. N. Engl. J. Med., 269:534, 1963.
41. Lown, B.: Cardioversion without anesthesia. N. Engl. J. Med., 269:535, 1963.
42. Kahler, R. I., Burrow, G. N., and Felig, P.: Diazepam induced amnesia for cardioversion. J.A.M.A., 200:997, 1967.
43. Johnstone, M., and Nisbet, H. I. A.: Ventricular arrhythmia during halothane anaesthesia. Br. J. Anaesthesiol., 33:9, 1961.
44. Gilston, A., Fordham, R., and Resnekov, L.: Anaesthesia for direct-current shock in the treatment of cardiac dysrhythmias. Br. J. Anaesthesiol., 37:533, 1965.
45. Resnekov, L., and McDonald, L.: Electroversion of lone atrial fibrillation and flutter including haemodynamic studies at rest and on exercise. Br. Heart J., 33:339, 1971.
46. Resnekov, L.: Haemodynamic studies before and after electrical conversion of atrial fibrillation and flutter to sinus rhythm. Br. Heart J., 29:700, 1967.
47. Yang, S. S., Maranhao, V., Monheit, R., et al: Cardioversion following open-heart valvular surgery. Br. Heart J., 28:309, 1966.
48. Rabbino, M. D., Likoff, W., and Dreifus, L.: Complications and limitations of direct-current countershock. J.A.M.A., 190:417, 1964.
49. Gilston, A., and Resnekov, L.: Cardio-Respiratory Resuscitation. London, William Heinemann, 1971.
50. Lown, B.: Cardioversion of arrhythmias. II. Mod. Concepts Cardiovasc. Dis., 33:869, 1964.
51. Mandecki, T., Giec, L., and Kargal, W.: Serum enzyme activities after cardioversion. Br. Heart J., 32:600, 1970.
52. Logan, W. F. W. E., Rowlands, D. J., Howitt, G., and Holmes, A. M.: Left atrial activity following cardioversion. Lancet, 2:471, 1965.
53. Lown, B., Kleiger, R., and Williams, J.: Cardioversion and digitalis drugs: Changed threshold to electric shock in digitalized animals. Circ. Res., 17:519, 1965.
54. Gilbert, R., and Cuddy, R. P.: Digitalis intoxication following conversion to sinus rhythm. Circulation, 32:58, 1965.
55. Corwin, N. D., Klein, M. J., and Friedberg, C. K.: Countershock conversion of digitalis associated paroxysmal tachycardia with block. Am. Heart J., 66:804, 1963.
56. Sloman, G., Robinson, J. S., and McClean, K.: Propranolol in persistent ventricular fibrillation. Br. Med. J., 1:895, 1965.
57. Lown, B.: In Julian, D. G., and Oliver, M. F. (eds.): Acute Myocardial Infarction. Edinburgh, Churchill Livingstone, 1968.

58. Childers, R. W., Rothbaum, D., and Arnsdorf, M.: The effects of DC shock on the electrical properties of the heart (abstr.). Circulation, 36 (Suppl.):II-85, 1967.
59. Byrne-Quinn, E., and Wing, A. J.: Maintenance of sinus rhythm after DC reversion of atrial fibrillation. A double-blind controlled trial of long-acting quinidine bisulphate. Br. Heart J., 32:370, 1970.
60. Ehsani, A., Ewy, G. A., and Sobel, B. E.: Effects of electrical countershock on serum creatine phosphokinase (CPK) isoenzyme activity. Am. J. Cardiol., 37:12, 1976.
61. Dahl, C. F., Ewy, G. A., Warner, E. D., and Thomas, E. D.: Myocardial necrosis from direct current countershock. Effect of paddle electrode size and true interval between discharges. Circulation, 50:956, 1974.
62. Peleška, B.: Cardiac arrhythmias following condenser discharges and their dependence upon strength of current and phase of cardiac cycle. Circ. Res., 13:21, 1963.
63. Tacker, W. A., Jr., Geddes, L. A., Rosborough, J. P., et al.: Transchest ventricular defibrillation of heavy subjects using trapezoidal current waveforms. J. Electrocardiol., 8:237, 1975.
64. Geddes, L. A., Bourland, J. D., Coulter, T. W., et al.: A megawatt defibrillator for trans-chest defibrillation of heavy subjects. Med. Electron. Biol. Engineer., 11:747, 1973.
65. Geddes, L. A., Tacker, W. A., Rosborough, J., et al.: Electrical dose for ventricular defibrillation of large and small animals using precordial electrodes. J. Clin. Invest., 53:310, 1974.
66. Tacker, W. A., Galiato, F., Giuliani, E., et al.: Energy dosage for human transchest electrical ventricular defibrillation. N. Engl. J. Med., 290:214, 1974.
67. Pantridge, J., Adgey, A. A. J., and Webb, S. W.: Electrical requirements for ventricular defibrillation. Br. Med. J., 2:313, 1975.
68. Morgan, M. T., and McElroy, C. R.: Letter. Transchest electrical ventricular defibrillation. Am. Heart J., 92:674, 1976.
69. Tedeschi, C. G., and White, C. W., Jr.: A morphologic study of canine hearts subjected to fibrillation, electrical defibrillation and manual compression. Circulation, 9:916, 1954.
70. David, J. S., Lie, J. T., Bentinck, D. C., et al.: Cardiac damage due to electrical current and energy. Light microscopic and ultrastructural observations of acute and delayed myocardial cellular injuries. In Proceedings of Cardiac Defibrillation Conference, pp. 27-32. South Bend, Ind., Purdue Univerisity, 1975.
71. Patton, J. N., Allen, J. D., and Pantridge, J. F.: The effects of shock energy, propranolol and verapamil on cardiac damage caused by transthoracic countershock. Circulation, 69:357, 1984.
72. Mirowski, M., Mower, M. M., and Staewen, W. S.: Standby automatic defibrillator: An approach to prevention of sudden coronary death. Arch. Intern. Med., 126:158, 1970.
73. Bourland, J. D., Geddes, L. A., and Terry, R. S.: Automatic detection of ventricular fibrillation for an implanted defibrillator. In Frontiers in Medical Signal Processing, p. 1. Midcon, 1977.
74. Mirowski, M., Mower, M. M., Reid, P. R., et al.: The automatic implantable defibrillator. New modality for treatment of life-threatening ventricular arrhythmias. Pace, 5:58, 1982.
75. Mirowski, M., Reid, P. R., Winkle, R. A., et al.: Mortality in patients with implanted automatic defibrillators. Ann. Intern. Med., 98:52, 1983.

31

The Role of Catheter Ablation for Patients with Drug-Resistant Cardiac Arrhythmias

Melvin M. Scheinman

The introduction of catheter ablation for control of serious cardiac arrhythmias allows the clinician another important therapeutic option in the management of patients with drug-resistant cardiac arrhythmias. The basic technique involves introduction of sufficient energy through catheters to destroy myocardial tissue involved in arrhythmogenesis. Although a variety of energy sources have been used experimentally, including electricity,[1] laser,[2] and radiofrequency,[3] clinical experience to date involves only high electrical discharges delivered through standard electrode catheters. The purpose of this chapter is to review the rationale and clinical role of this new therapeutic modality.

Histologic Perspective

A number of closed-chest animal models for disruption of the atrioventricular (AV) conduction system have been described.[4-6] The described techniques generally involve injection of caustic substances in the region of the AV junction and as such are not applicable to clinical use. Beazell and colleagues[7] described a technique of closed-chest catheter ablation in dogs that involved inserting an insulated, stiff electrode wire that was positioned fluoroscopically in the region of the AV junction. Direct current shocks were delivered from the electrode to a patch positioned on the chest wall. We found it difficult to reproducibly achieve chronic complete AV block with this procedure and modified the technique.[8] The modification involved positioning the electrode catheter in proximity to the largest unipolar His bundle deflection and delivering high-energy direct current discharges to this region to electrocoagulate the AV junction. Careful pathologic studies showed disruption of the AV junction without associated perforation of the atrial septum or disruption of the AV valves.[9] The catheter technique was first used at the University of California, San Francisco Medical Center, in March 1981.

Brodman and Fisher[10] first described a technique for delivering electrical energy through the coronary sinus in dogs and showed that this could produce transmural atrial necrosis in the region of the AV ring. The same group used this technique for attempted catheter ablation of left free wall pathways in humans.[11] A number of experimental studies have described the effects of transcatheter ablative shocks delivered to ventricular myocardium.[12-14] Depending on the energy used, a hemispherical lesion of variable size and depth is produced associated with subendocardial hemorrhage and necrosis. Attempted catheter ablation of ventricular tachycardia foci in patients was first described by Hartzler.[15] More recently, Silka and associates described a technique for catheter ablation of atrial arrhythmic foci in children.[16]

Rationale for Catheter Ablative Therapy

As discussed in other chapters, cardiac arrhythmic mechanisms include disturbances in automaticity, triggered activity, or reentry. Each of the mechanisms may be operative in patients with cardiac arrhythmias. The most common mechanism for recurrent symptomatic paroxysmal supraventricular tachycardia appears to be reentry either within the AV node[17] or involving a macroreentrant circuit incorporating an extranodal bypass tract.[18] In patients with supraventricular reentrant arrhythmias involving any of the above reentrant mechanisms, the AV junction is a vital link in the reentrant circuit. If such a patient should prove to have an arrhythmia resistant to drug therapy, then alternative treatment includes attempted catheter electrocoagulation of the AV junction. Alternatively, if the accessory pathway is amenable to catheter ablation, a preferred approach is direct catheter ablation of the accessory pathway. The latter technique leaves the normal AV node–His axis intact and, in contrast to AV junctional ablation, does not commit the patient to chronic pacemaker therapy.

If the tachycardia focus can be precisely localized to a specific area in either the atrium or ventricle, then delivery of high-energy discharges may ablate the arrhythmia regardless of whether the basic mechanism is abnormal automaticity, triggered activity, or microreentry. This technique has been used in patients with either atrial or ventricular tachycardial foci.

The catheter ablative technique may also be used to control cardiac arrhythmias even without precise identification of the reentrant circuit or locus of origin of an arrhythmia. For example, in patients with atrial fibrillation, atrial flutter, or atrial tachycardia, even though the precise origin of the arrhythmia may be unknown, the AV junction acts to funnel these impulses into the ventricle. Ablation of the "funnel" will result in arrhythmia control, even though the AV junction is not a critical link in the tachycardia circuit. It must be appreciated, however, that AV junctional ablation results in complete AV block and requires permanent pacing for rate control.

In summary, the rationale for catheter ablative procedures rests on three different mechanisms. The procedure may prove effective if (1) the arrhythmic area can be precisely localized and destroyed, (2) an area that is critical to maintenance of a reentrant circuit can be ablated, or (3) an area that acts as the sole exit point from the tachycardia can be identified and destroyed.

Technique for Atrioventricular Junctional Catheter Ablation

The technique for AV junctional ablation involves percutaneous insertion of a multipolar electrode catheter into the apex of the right ventricle to allow for temporary cardiac pacing (Fig. 31-1). A small catheter is inserted into a peripheral artery to allow for continuous recording of the arterial pressure. A No. 6 or 7 French multipolar electrode catheter is then inserted through the femoral vein and positioned to allow for bipolar recording of the His bundle potential. Unipolar electrograms are then recorded from each of the electrodes, and the catheter is positioned so that the largest unipolar His potential is recorded. The patient is anesthetized with a short-acting barbiturate, and one or more shocks of 150 to 300 J is delivered from a standard direct current defibrillator. The shock is delivered from the catheter electrode (cathode) to an external patch placed over the left scapula (anode) (Fig. 31-2). Temporary pacing is achieved by the previously inserted right ventricular catheter. The patient is then transferred to an intensive care monitoring unit. If complete AV block persists for 24 to 48 hours, a permanent pacemaker is inserted.

Clinical Use

Before catheter techniques were introduced to disrupt AV conduction, patients with supraventricular tachycardia resistant to drug therapy or antitachycardia pacing were treated by direct surgical ablation of the His bundle.[19] This included patients with atrial fibrillation or flutter and those with AV junctional reciprocating tachycardia where the His bundle acts as a conduit for transmission of impulses to the ventricle. AV junctional ablation may be effective for patients with AV arrhythmias that incorporate either an extranodal or nodoventricular accessory pathway in the reentrant circuit. In patients with extranodal accessory pathways, the reentrant circuit generally involves antegrade conduction over the AV node–His pathway and retrograde conduction over the accessory pathway. Successful catheter ablation of the AV junction would prevent reentrant arrhythmias in these patients. Care must be exercised in patient selection; for example, patients with the Wolff-Parkinson-White (WPW) syndrome with accessory pathways capable of rapid antegrade conduction are not candidates for this technique, since the patient is not protected should atrial fibrillation supervene. In addition, it must be established that the AV junction is a critical part of the reentrant circuit. It is furthermore recommended that such patients undergo permanent "back-up" ventricular pacing, since the long-term stability of sole conduction over an accessory pathway has not been established. Another group of patients with accessory pathways who may benefit from AV junctional ablation are those with reentrant arrythmias involving a

A

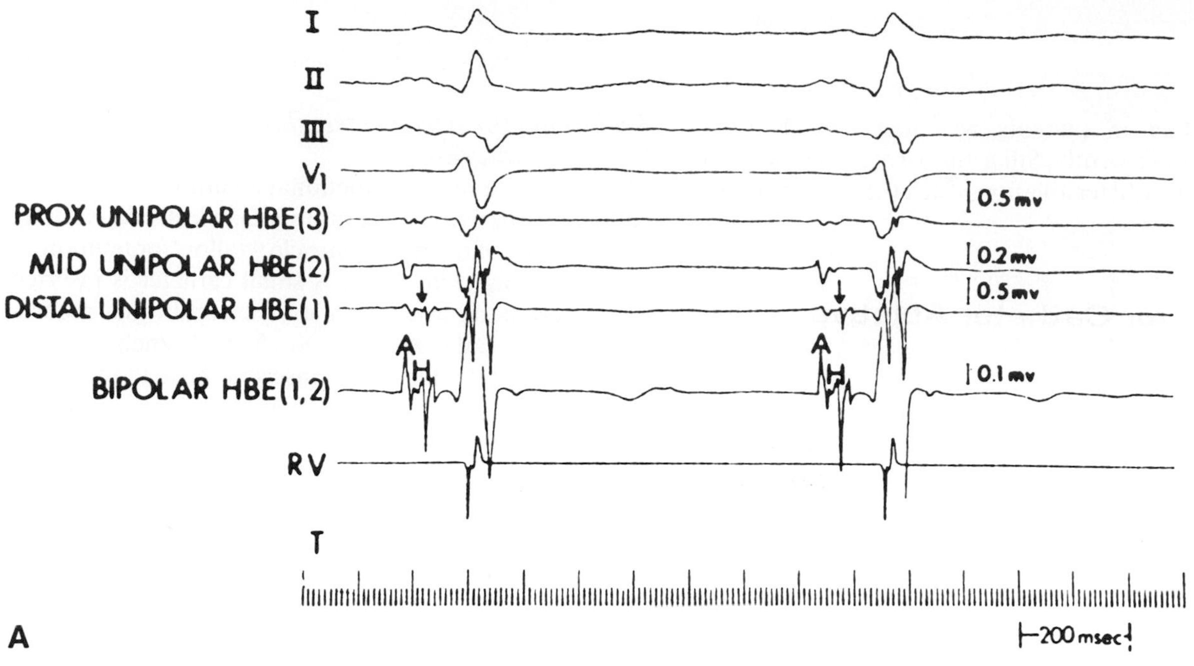

B

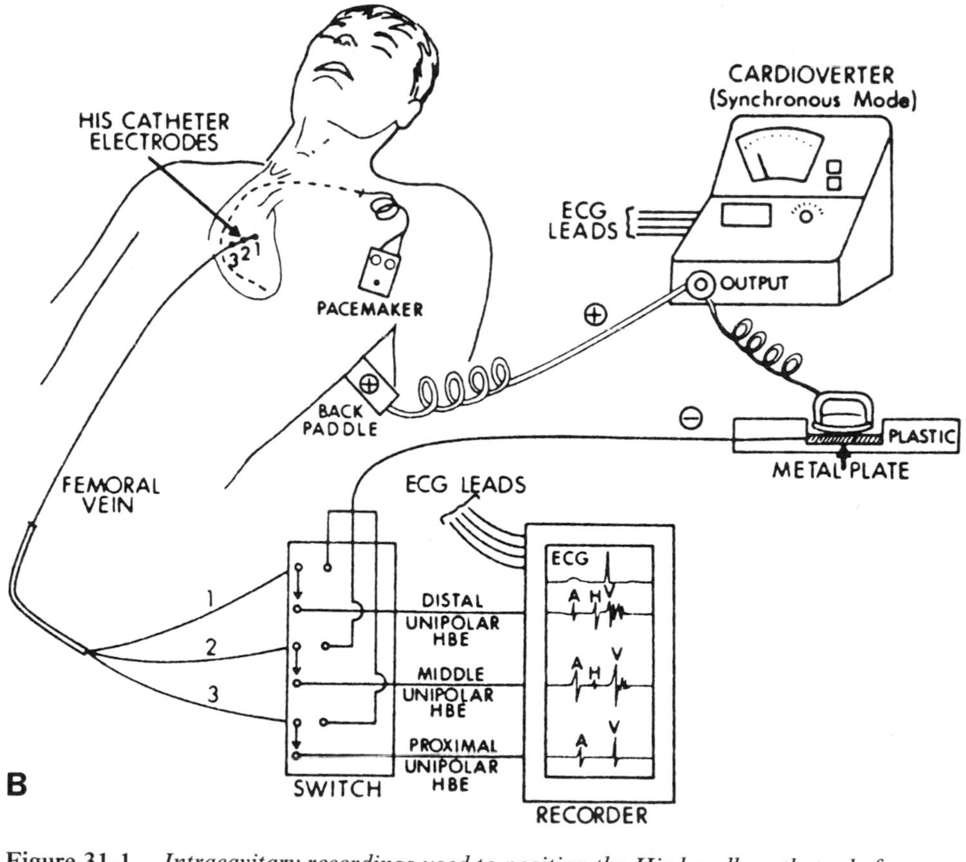

Figure 31-1. *Intracavitary recordings used to position the His bundle catheter before ablation. Recordings (from the top down) are from standard electrocardiographic leads I through III and V_1, unipolar recordings from each of the electrodes on a tripolar catheter positioned in the region of the His bundle, a bipolar recording of the His bundle obtained by a combination of the middle and distal unipolar recordings, and a bipolar electrogram from the right ventricular apex (RV). Calibration signals for the His bundle recordings appear to the right of the electrograms. An arrow on the unipolar recording obtained from the most distal electrode indicates the largest unipolar recording of the His bundle potential obtained in this patient. (PROX, the most proximal electrode of the tripolar catheter; MID, the middle electrode of the tripolar catheter; DISTAL, the most distal electrode on the tripolar electrode catheter; HBE, His bundle Electrogram; A, atrium; H, His bundle; and T, time) (Gallagher, J. J., Svenson, R. H., Kasell, J. H., et al.: Catheter technique for closed-chest ablation of the atrioventricular conduction system. N. Engl. J. Med., 306:194–200, 1982)*

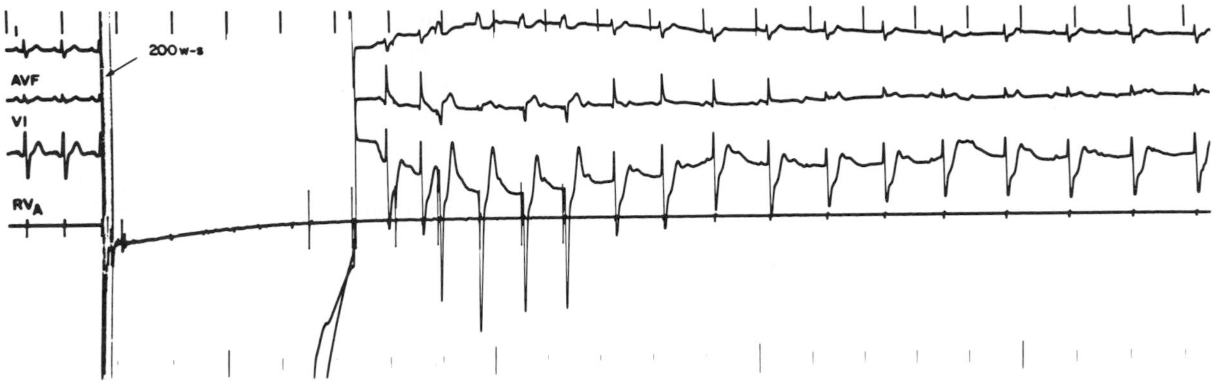

Figure 31-2. *A 200-J shock, synchronized to the QRS, is delivered during sinus rhythm. After a brief period of ventricular pacing, a junctional escape rhythm (52/min) is observed. Advanced AV block is observed with an irregular atrial at a rate of approximately 75/min being noted.*

nodoventricular bypass tract. If the mechanism of the arrhythmia involves antegrade conduction over the Mahaim tract and retrograde conduction through the AV node, the AV junctional ablation would effectively prevent reentrant arrhythmias. In some patients with nodoventricular tracts, the tachycardia mechanism is AV nodal reentry with the nodoventricular tract acting as bystander. In these patients, if the AV junction is ablated distal to the insertion site of the Mahaim tract, then tachycardia may not be prevented. In addition, preliminary experience with a small number of patients with nodoventricular tracts who have undergone AV junctional ablation suggests that permanent ventricular pacing may not be required.[20,21]

A number of reports have detailed the results of catheter ablation of the AV junction.[22-25] The largest series to date has been reported from the percutaneous mapping and ablation registry.[26] This registry was established to monitor the safety and efficacy of ablative procedures. The most recent report from the registry involved data collected from 209 patients.[27] All patients had recurrent or chronic supraventricular tachycardia and failed at least two drug trials. The types of cardiac arrhythmias for which ablative therapy was attempted are detailed in Table 31-1. Comulative energy used for ablation is shown in Figure 31-3. The most common arrhythmia requiring this form of therapy was paroxysmal or permanent atrial fibrillation or atrial flutter. The 209 patients were evaluated over a mean follow-up period of 8.4 months. Chronic complete AV block was achieved in 70%, while 8% had sufficient modification of AV conduction so that arrhythmia control was achieved without need for antiarrhythmic drugs. Thirteen percent experienced arrhythmia control with drug therapy, while the procedure was judged totally ineffective in 9%. The overall results were judged to be excellent in 78% in that arrhythmia control was achieved without need for drugs. It was deemed partially effective for the 13% who achieved arrhythmia control with drug therapy. Of the 19 patients who failed ablative therapy, six underwent surgical His bundle section.

The reported complications of this procedure have been divided into early and late adverse effects. Immediate complications are defined as those occurring within

Table 31-1. Cardiac Arrhythmias Requiring Ablation

Arrhythmia	Occurrence (%)*
Atrial fibrillation/flutter	61
AV nodal reentry	20
AV (accessory pathway)	13
Atrial tachycardia	11
Permanent junctional reentrant tachycardia	3
Other†	4

* The percentages given exceed 100% because some patients had more than one rhythm disturbance.
† Other arrhythmias include junctional ectopic tachycardia and nonparoxysmal sinus tachycardia.

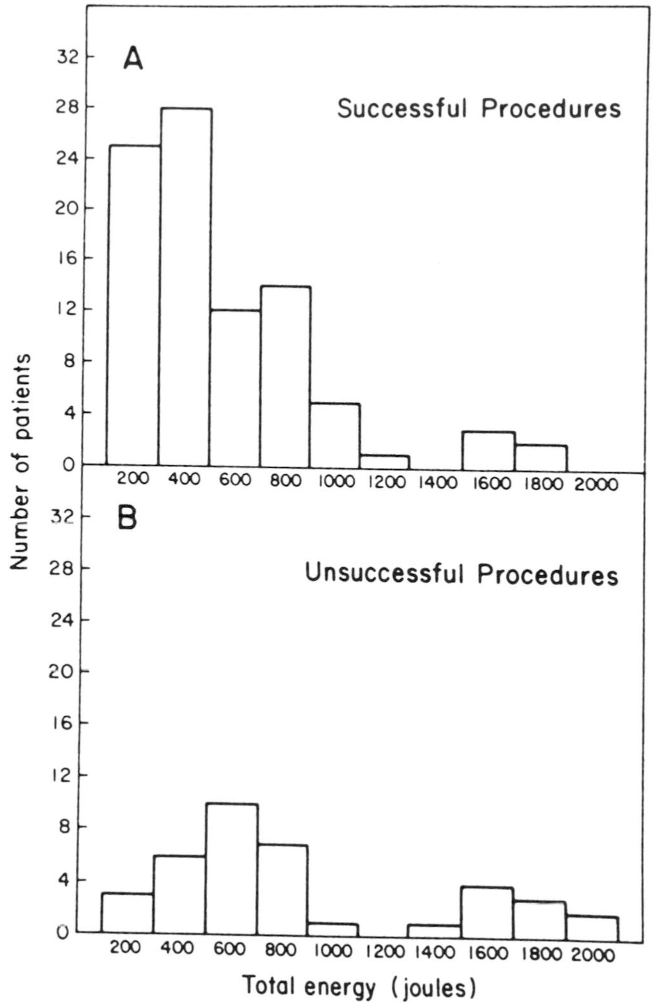

Figure 31-3. *(A) The cumulative energy (in joules) used for patients who had chronic complete AV block after attempted catheter ablation of the AV junction. (B) Similar information for those in whom AV conduction resumed.*

minutes after delivery of the shock and were usually either arrhythmic or hemodynamic. Arrhythmias included ventricular fibrillation (two patients that were successfully treated by external shock), brief episodes of self-terminating ventricular tachycardia (three patients), or junctional tachycardia (three patients). There were four episodes of hypotension requiring pressor support. The hypotension persisted for less than 40 minutes in three and persisted for several days in one patient with congenital heart disease. One instance of pericardial tamponade requiring emergent surgical drainage was reported. There were no chronic sequelae as a result of these complications.

Late complications included three episodes of ventricular tachycardia, one of which was terminated by repositioning of the right ventricular pacing electrode; the others required temporary antiarrhythmic therapy. The other late complications were related to the catheterization procedure or to insertion of the permanent pacemaker and included sepsis in four, venous thrombosis or thrombophlebitis (three patients), and pneumothorax (one patient). One patient died following overwhelming sepsis of the pacemaker pocket. There were 14 recorded deaths following attempted AV junctional ablation. In five, deaths occurred months to several years after the procedure due to progressive congestive heart failure. In these patients, congestive heart failure was present before ablation. Four deaths were noncardiac in cause. Five patients died suddenly from 1 to 5 months following ablation. All five had preexisting heart disease, and none had evidence of pacemaker failure. It is uncertain whether the sudden death was related to the procedure or occurred as part of the natural history of their heart disease.

Clinical Role

The technique of catheter ablation of the AV junction has supplanted the need for surgical ablation of the His bundle. The catheter technique has been shown to be equally effective but associated with lower mortality, morbidity, and cost.[28] The clinician must, however, carefully balance the projected benefits of this procedure against possible adverse effects. The chief limitation of this procedure is that a pacemaker-dependent state is produced. Although pacemaker technology has allowed for a remarkable safety record, the consequences of abrupt pacemaker failure may be serious or fatal. Reports of sudden death (approximately 2.5%) are disturbing, since at this point we cannot exclude the possibility that deaths resulted from malignant ventricular arrhythmias originating from a ventricular nidus induced by the ablative procedure.

Catheter Ablation of Accessory Pathways

Extranodal accessory pathways consist of muscle bundles connecting the atria and ventricles across the cardiac anulus. These pathways may be located either in the septum or across the ventricular free walls. Surgical ablation of these pathways has proved effective and safe. More recently, catheter techniques have been proposed for attempted catheter ablation of these pathways. The basic technique is similar to that described for AV junctional ablation in that shocks are delivered by catheters in close proximity to the accessory pathways. Pathway localization is achieved by endocardial mapping either during orthodromic tachycardia or ventricular pacing.[29] In addition, attempts are made to record potentials from the accessory pathway.[30] Once proper localization is achieved, one or more shocks are delivered from the electrode(s) nearest the pathway to an indifferent patch placed on the chest wall.

Free Wall Accessory Pathways

The majority of accessory pathways are located over the left free wall and travel across the AV groove. The coronary sinus lies in the AV groove in close proximity to these pathways. Fisher and coauthors[11] were the first to describe a method for attempted catheter ablation of left free wall pathways using catheters positioned within the coronary sinus. Initial reports suggest that this approach is seldom effective and carries a substantial risk of coronary sinus perforation. Only scattered reports describing small numbers of patients are available on attempted ablation of right free wall accessory pathways.[31-33]

Posteroseptal Pathways

Posteroseptal pathways are those occurring within the septum but posterior to the AV junction. Morady and Scheinman[34] recently described a technique for catheter ablation of these pathways. The technique is applicable only for those patients who show earliest atrial preexcitation in the region of the coronay sinus os and involves insertion of a quadripolar electrode catheter into the root of the coronary sinus. The catheter is positioned so that the proximal electrodes are positioned just outside the os. The proximal electrodes are electrically combined as the anode, and an indifferent chest wall patch is used as the cathode. One or more shocks are delivered from the proximal electrode pair to the external patch using a direct current defibrillator (Fig. 31-4). Our preliminary experience using this technique in eight patients has recently been described.[35] Six of these patients benefitted in that either pathway conduction was completely abolished (five patients) or sufficiently modified (one patient) so that antiarrhythmic drug therapy was not required. Our further studies have corroborated the early experience. To date, 13 patients with posteroseptal pathways have undergone attempted catheter ablation, and nine of 13 have shown either complete antegrade and retrograde block in the pathway or sufficient modification of pathway conduction so that antiarrhythmic drugs are no longer required for arrhythmia control. One of the 13 patients experienced acutc pericardial tamponade that required emergent pericardiocentesis. No other patient experienced an adverse effect.

Clinical Role

The available experience relative to catheter ablation of accessory extranodal pathways is still small. On the basis of available date, we conclude that surgical extirpation is

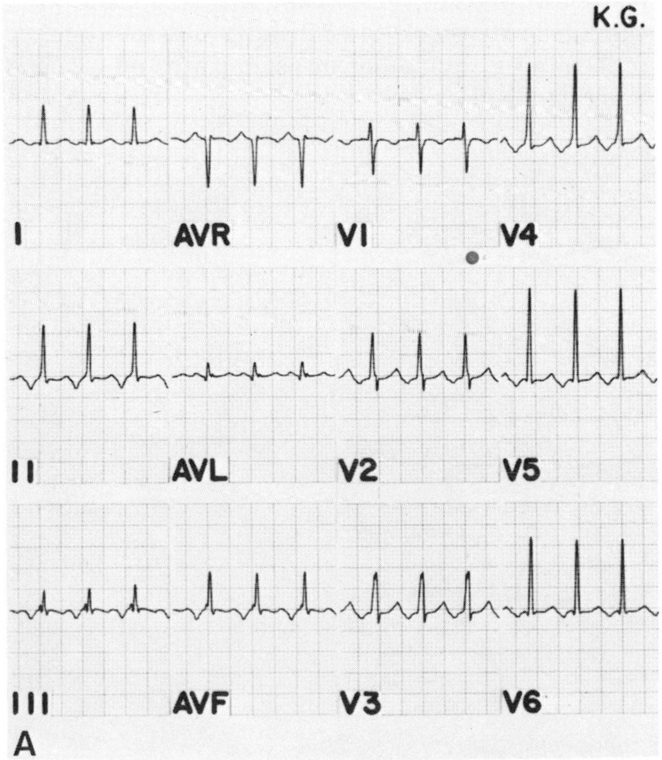

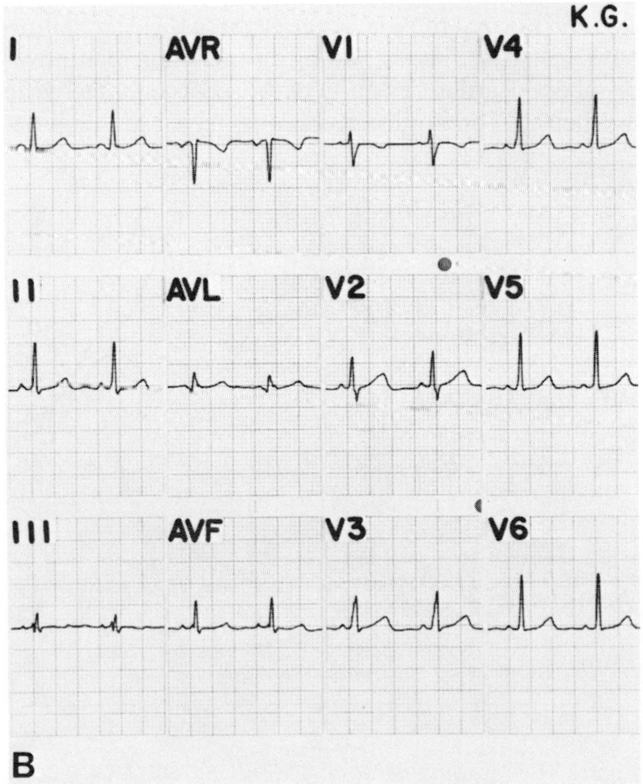

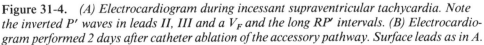

Figure 31-4. *(A) Electrocardiogram during incessant supraventricular tachycardia. Note the inverted P′ waves in leads II, III and a V_F and the long RP′ intervals. (B) Electrocardiogram performed 2 days after catheter ablation of the accessory pathway. Surface leads as in A.*

preferable to catheter ablation of free wall accessory pathways. The catheter technique has seldom proved effective and carries the associated risk of coronary sinus rupture or damage to the adjacent coronary artery. In contrast, catheter ablation of posteroseptal accessory pathways appears to hold great promise. If our early favorable experience is confirmed, this technique may supplant the surgical approach. In our own practice, we currently offer the catheter technique to those patients with posteroseptal pathways with arrhythmias refractory to drug therapy or to younger patients desirous of avoiding lifelong drug therapy for arrhythmia control.

Ventricular Tachycardia Catheter Ablation

Surgical techniques have been developed to treat patients with drug-resistant ventricular arrhythmias. The most popular technique is map-directed surgical excision of the tachycardia focus.[36] The tachycardia is induced during surgery, and the endocardium is carefully mapped with an electrode probe to define the earliest endocardial potential relative to the surface or intracardiac reference leads. The earliest breakthrough has been found to occur at the endocardium at the border between scar and normal muscle. A variety of surgical techniques have been described including an encircling myotomy[37] or subendocardial resection of the ventricular tachycardia focus.[38] The surgical techniques have been shown to be more effective than so-called blind aneurysm resection and are associated with arrhythmia control in approximately 75% to 80% of patients surviving surgery.[39,40] Patients requiring surgery for arrhythmia control often have poor ventricular function and the risk of surgery, even in very experienced surgical centers, is approximately 10%.[39,40]

The technique of catheter ablation of ventricular tachycardia foci depends on precise localization of the arrhythmic site. The latter is achieved by inserting one or more catheter electrodes into both the right and left ventricles. Standard pacing protocols are used to induce ventricular tachycardia, and the catheters are positioned to record endocardial potentials from as many ventricular sites as possible. The completeness of the endocardial catheter map depends on both the operator's technical capabilities and the patient's hemodynamic status during tachycardia. The earliest endocardial potential recorded relative to reference surface leads is taken as the exit point of the ventricular tachycardia focus. In addition, the pace-mapping technique provides further confirmation of the exit point. The latter includes recording a 12-lead electrocardiogram during ventricular endocardial pacing. The endocardial site showing a paced electrocardiogram similar or identical to the spontaneous tachycardia is felt to be near the ventricular tachycardia exit point. The catheter electrode is placed as close as possible to the putative exit point, and one or more direct current countershocks are delivered from the electrode in the heart to an indifferent patch placed on the chest wall (Fig. 31-5).

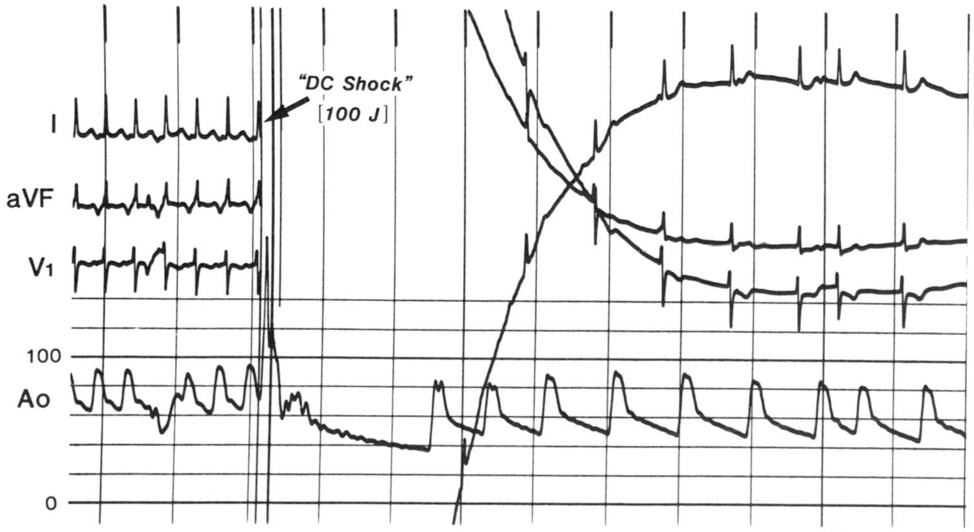

Figure 31-5. *Administration of direct current (DC) shock during supraventricular tachycardia. Surface leads I, a V_F and V_1 are displayed along with an aortic (Ao) blood pressure tracing. A synchronized shock of 100 J is followed within 2 seconds by a stable junctional rhythm. (Gang, E., Rosen, D., Rosenthal, M., et al.: Closed chest catheter ablation of an accessory pathway in a patient with permanent junctional reciprocating tachycardia. J. Am. Coll. Cardiol., 6:1167–1171, 1985)*

Our group has defined a newer technique for ablation of septal ventricular tachycardia foci.[41] This approach involves use of the right and left ventricular catheters to explore the ventricular septum. The catheters are positioned so that the earliest potentials from both right and left septum are obtained. In this technique, the shocks are delivered from the catheter electrode on the left side of the septum to its mate on the opposite side of the septum. In this fashion, the ventricular tachycardia focus is bracketed by catheters and an attempt made to electrocoagulate the abnormal zone. In either of these methods for catheter ablation, the patient is retested by ventricular programmed stimulation to determine whether the tachycardia is still inducible and additional shocks are delivered until the tachycardia is rendered noninducible. Acute complications of this procedure include myocardial perforation, deterioration of myocardial performance, and induction of more serious ventricular arrhythmias. After completion of the ablative procedure, patients are monitored in a coronary care unit and treated similar to those patients who have suffered an acute myocardial infarction. Late complications include continued hemodynamic deterioration or development of malignant ventricular arrhythmias.

Ventricular Foci

Catheter ablation has been attempted most often in patients with tachycardia foci in either the free wall of the left ventricle or the septum. The most common cause of the arrhythmia is coronary artery disease. Since the tachycardia usually arises from the diseased area of the ventricle (*i.e.,* scar, aneurysm) noninvasive techniques such as echocardiography or phase image studies[42] may help provide a general target zone. The endocardial map can then be concentrated in these areas. The clinician is often confounded by multiple ventricular tachycardia electrocardiographic forms induced at study, but primary attempt is directed at ablation of the spontaneous ventricular tachycardia form. The importance, therefore, of recording 12-lead electrocardiograms during spontaneous episodes of tachycardia cannot be overemphasized.

Catheter ablation has been used in patients with ventricular tachycardia originating from a right ventricular focus. Such tachycardias have been described in patients with cardiomyopathy,[43] arrhythmogenic right ventricular dysplasia,[44] corrected tetralogy of Fallot or ventricular septal defect repair,[45] and no structual heart disease but an arrhythmia arising from the right ventricular outflow tract.[46] Successful ablative procedures have been reported for patients with right or left ventricular foci in that either the patient is rendered free of arrhythmia without drugs or may be successfully managed with drugs that were previously ineffective.[46–49,15] Serious complications, including myocardial perforation and death, have been reported.*

Clinical Role

The accumulated experience on the use of catheter ablation for patients with ventricular tachycardia is still quite limited. Although the early published reports are quite favorable, with beneficial results varying from 60% to 90%, nevertheless, data available from the registry suggest a much lower overall success rate. In view of the potential for serious complications, it appears prudent to limit this procedure to patients who have failed medical treatment, are not candidates for automatic defibrillators, or are high-risk surgical candidates.

*Scheinman, M.M., and Evans, G.T.: Percutaneous mapping and ablation registry. Personal communication.

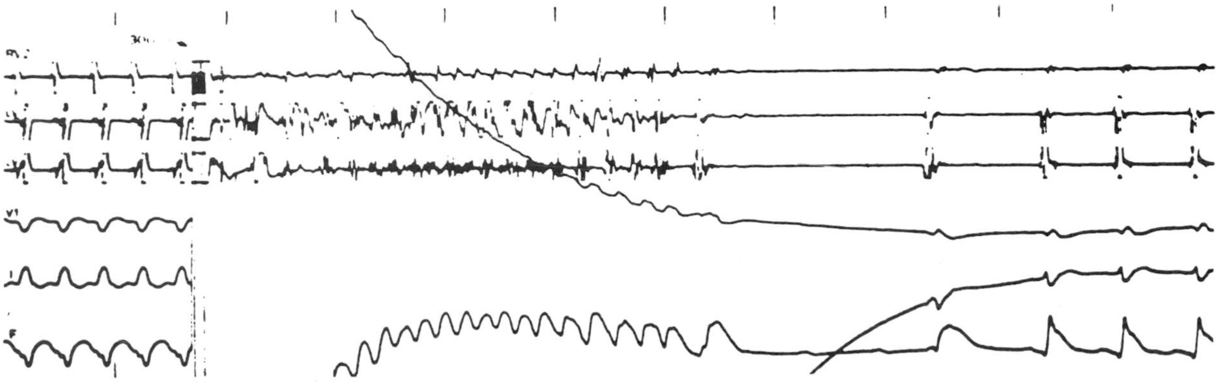

Figure 31-6. *A 300-J shock is delivered during ventricular tachycardia with discharge from the tip electrode of a quadripolar electrode catheter positioned against the mid-right ventricular septum. Induced ventricular fibrillation terminated spontaneously after 5 seconds. (RV2, right ventricular electrogram from an additional right ventricular site)*

Future of Catheter Ablative Techniques for Patients with Cardiac Arrhythmias

Future development of catheter ablative techniques depends on technical advances in catheter design and energy delivery systems. More steerable catheters and a catheter electrode array that allows for simultaneous recordings from multiple cardiac sites are needed. The ideal system would allow for ablation of discrete areas without substantial damage to surrounding normal myocardium, heart valves, or coronary vessels. Available techniques are clearly far from ideal. Perhaps more focused laser energy or radiofrequency waves will prove more effective.

Conclusion

The introduction of catheter ablative techniques for control of serious cardiac arrhythmias has initiated a new nonpharmacologic approach for arrhythmia control. Although the experience to date is still rather limited, certain conclusions can be gleaned from the available literature.

1. Catheter ablation of the AV junction is clearly superior to surgical His bundle section, since the catheter technique is as effective and is associated with lower mortality, morbidity, and cost. The use of this technique will remain limited until procedures are introduced that provide for arrhythmia control by modification of the AV junction without complete disruption of AV conduction. Total pacemaker dependency is clearly not a desirable result.

2. Surgical ablation of free wall accessory pathways is safer and more effective than presently available catheter techniques. Catheter ablation of posteroseptal accessory pathways appears to be a promising technique and, in our view, is preferable to surgery because the chance for success is approximately 75% and the risks of the procedure are acceptable. Moreover, an unsuccessful attempt at catheter ablation does not preclude the possibility of subsequent surgical interruption of this pathway.

3. Catheter ablation of ventricular tachycardia foci remains highly experimental and should be limited to those patients with drug-refractory arrhythmias who are not suitable candidates for other nonpharmacologic approaches.

References

1. Beazell, J., Tan, K., Criley, J., et al.: The electrosurgical production of heart block without thoracotomy (abstr.). Clin. Res., 24:137, 1976.
2. Narula, O. S., Boveja, B. K., Cohen, D. M., and Tarjan, D.: Laser catheter-induced A-V nodal delays and block: Acute and chronic studies. Circulation, 70:II-99, 1985.
3. Huang, S. K., Jordan, N., Graham, A., et al.: Closed chest catheter dissociation of the atrioventricular junction—a new method of catheter ablation (abstr.). Circulation, 72:III-389, 1985.
4. Randall, O. S., Westerhof, N., Van de Boss, G., and Sipkema, P.: Production of chronic heart block in closed-chest dogs: An improved technique. Am. J. Physiol., H279, 1981.
5. Steiner, C., and Kovalik, A. T. W.: A simple technique for production of chronic complete heart block in dogs. J. Appl. Physiol., 25:631, 1968.
6. Turina, M. I., Babotai, I., and Wegmann, W.: Production of chronic atrioventricular block in dogs without thoracotomy. Cardiovasc. Res., 2:389, 1968.
7. Beazell, J. W. Tan, K. S., Fewkes, J. L., et al.: Technique for productive of permanent lesions in the intracardiac conduction system (abstr.). Clin. Res., 25:141a, 1977.
8. Gonzalez, R., Scheinman, M. M., Margaretten, W., and Rubinstein, M.: Closed chest electrode catheter technique for His bundle ablation in dog. Am. J. Physiol., 241:283, 1981.
9. Gonzales, R., Scheinman, M. M., Bharati, S., and Lev, M.: Closed chest permanent atrioventricular block in dogs. Am. Heart J., 105:461, 1983.
10. Brodman, R., and Fisher, J. D.: Evaluation of a catheter technique for ablation of accessory pathways near the coronary sinus using a canine model. Circulation, 67:923, 1983.
11. Fisher, J. D., Brodman, R., Kim, S. G., et al.: Attempted nonsurgical electrical ablation of accessory pathways via the coronary sinus in the Wolff-Parkinson-White syndrome. J. Am. Coll. Cardiol., 4:685, 1984.
12. Westveer, D. C., Nelson, T., Stewart, J. R., et al.: The sequelae of left ventricular electrical ablation. J. Am. Coll. Cardiol., 5:956–960, 1985.
13. Lerman, B., Weiss, J., Bulkley, B., et al.: Myocardial injury and induction of arrhythmia by direct-current shock delivered via endocardial catheters in dogs. Circulation, 69:1006–1012, 1984.
14. Kempf, F., Falcone, R., Waxman, H., et al.: Anatomic and hemodynamic effects of electrical discharges in the ventricle. Circulation, 68:III-174, 1983.
15. Hartzler, G. O.: Electrode catheter ablation of refractory focal ventricular tachycardia. J. Am. Coll. Cardiol., 2:1107, 1983.
16. Silka, M. J., Gillette, P. C., Garson, A., Jr., and Zinner, A.: Transvenous catheter ablation of a right atrial automatic ectopic tachycardia. J. Am. Coll. Cardiol., 5:999–1001, 1985.
17. Wu, D., Denes, P., Bauernfiend, R., et al.: Effects of atropine on induction of maintenance of atrioventricular nodal reentrant tachycardia. Circulation, 59:779, 1979.
18. Sealy, W. C., Gallagher, J. J., and Wallace, A. G.: The surgical treatment of Wolff-Parkinson-White syndrome: Evaluation of improved methods for identification and interruption of the Kent bundle. Ann. Thorac. Surg., 22:443, 1976.
19. Harrison, L., Gallagher, J. J., Kasell, J., et al.: Cryosurgical ablation of the AV node-His bundle. A new method for producing AV block. Circulation, 55:463, 1977.
20. Bhandari, A., Morady, F., Shen, E. N., et al.: Catheter-induced His bundle ablation in a patient with reentrant tachycardia associated with a nodoventricular tract. J. Am. Coll. Cardiol., 4:611, 1984.
21. Ellenbogen, K., O'Callaghan, W. G., Colavita, P. G., et al.: Catheter His ablation for recurrent supraventricular tachycardia in two patients with nodoventricular fibers. J. Am. Coll. Cardiol., 55:1227–1229, 1985.
22. Nathan, A. W., Bennett, D. H., Ward, D. E., et al.: Catheter ablation of atrioventricular conduction. Lancet, 1:1280, 1984.
23. Wood, D., Hammill, S., Holmes, D. R., et al.: Catheter ablation of the atrioventricular system in patients with supraventricular tachycardia. Mayo Clin. Proc., 58:793, 1983.
24. Gillette, P. C., Garson, A., Porter, C. J., et al.: Junctional auto-

matic ectopic tachycardia: New proposed treatment by transcatheter His bundle ablation. Am. Heart J., 106:619, 1983.
25. Manz, M., Steinbeck, G., and Luderitz, B.: His-Bundel-Ablation: Eine neue methode zur behandlung bedrohlicher supraventrikularer herzrhythmusstorungen. Der Intern., 24:95, 1983.
26. Scheinman, M. M., Evans-Bell, T., and the Executive Committee of the Percutaneous Mapping and Ablation Registry: Catheter ablation of the atrioventricular junction: A report of the Percutaneous Mapping and Ablation Registry. Circulation, 70:1024, 1984.
27. Scheinman, M. M., and Evans, T.: Catheter electrocoagulation of the atrioventricular junction: A report of the Percutaneous Mapping and Ablation Registry. Proceedings of the First International Conference on Catheter Ablation, Paris, France, May 1985, in press.
28. German, L. D., Pressley, J., Smith, M. S., et al.: Comparison of cryoablation of the atrioventricular node versus catheter ablation of the His bundle (abstr.). Circulation, 70:II-412, 1984.
29. Gallagher, J. J., Svenson, R. H., Sealy, W. C., and Wallace, A. G.: The Wolff-Parkinson-White syndrome and the preexcitation dysrhythmias. Medical and surgical management. Med. Clin. North Am., 60:101, 1976.
30. Jackson, W. M., Friday, K. J., Scherlag, B. J., et al.: Direct endocardial recording from an accessory atrioventricular pathway: Localization of the site of block, effect of antiarrhythmic drugs, and attempt at nonsurgical ablation. Circulation, 68:906–916, 1983.
31. Kunz, K. P., and Kuck, K. H.: Transvenous ablation of accessory pathways in patients with incessant atrioventricular tachycardia (abstr.). Circulation, 70:II-412, 1984.
32. Nathan, A. W., Davies, D. W., Creamer, J. E., et al.: Successful catheter ablation of abnormal atrioventricular pathways in man. Circulation, 70:II-99, 1984.
33. Weber, H., Schmitz, L., and Wesselhoeft, H.: A new technique of mapping for localization and closed-chest ablation of reentry pathways. Circulation, 68:III-175, 1983.
34. Morady, E., and Scheinman, M. M.: Transvenous catheter ablation of a posteroseptal accessory pathway in a patient with the Wolff-Parkinson-White syndrome. N. Engl. J. Med., 310:705, 1984.
35. Morady, E., Scheinman, M. M., Winston, S. A., et al.: Efficacy and safety of transcatheter ablation of posteroseptal accessory pathways. Circulation, 72:170–177, 1985.
36. Kastor, J. A., Horowitz, L. N., Harken, A. H., and Josephsone, M. E.: Clinical electrophysiology of ventricular tachycardia. N. Engl. J. Med., 304:1004, 1981.
37. Guiraudon, G., Fontaine, G., Frank, R., et al: Apports de la ventriculotomie circulaire d'exclusion dan le traintment de la tachycardia ventriculaire recidivante apres infarctus du myocarde. Arch. Mal Coeur, 75:1013, 1982.
38. Miller, J. M., Kienzle, M. G., Harken, A. H., and Josephson, M. E.: Morphologically distinct sustained ventricular tachycardias in coronary artery disease: Significance and surgical results. J. Am. Coll. Cardiol., 4:1073, 1984.
39. Josephson, M. E., Harken, A. H., and Horowitz, L. N.: Long-termed results of endocardial resection for sustained ventricular tachycardia in coronary disease patients. Am. Heart J., 104:51, 1982.
40. Martin, J. L., Untereker, W. I., Harken, A. H., and Josephson, M. E.: Aneurysmectomy and endocardial resection for ventricular tachycardia: Favorable hemodynamic and antiarrhythmic results in patients with global left ventricular dysfunction. Am. Heart J., 103:960, 1982.
41. Winston, S. A., Davis, J. C., Morady, F., et al.: A new approach to electrode catheter ablation for ventricular tachycardia arising from the ventricular septum (abstr.). Circulation, 70:II-412, 1984.
42. Scheinman, M. M., Winston, S. A., Morady, F., et al.: Catheter ablation of ventricular tachycardia. Cardiology, October 1984.
43. Fontaine, G., Guiraudon, G., Frank, R., et al.: Epicardial mapping and surgical treatment in six cases of resistant ventricular tachycardia not related to coronary artery disease. In Wellens, H. J., Lie, K. I., Janse, M. J. (eds.): The Conduction System of the Heart, pp. 545–566. Philadelphia, Lea & Febiger, 1976.
44. Marcus, F. L., Fontaine, G. H., Giraudon, G., and Frank, R.: Right ventricular dysplasia: A report of 24 adult cases. Circulation, 65:384, 1982.
45. Horowitz, L. N., Vetter, V. L., Harken, A. H., and Josephson, M. E.: Electrophysiologic characteristics of sustained ventricular tachycardia occurring after repair of Tetralogy of Fallot. Am. J. Cardiol., 46:446, 1980.
46. Buxton, A. E., Waxman, H. L., Marchlinski, M. D., et al.: Right ventricular tachycardia: Clinical and electrophysiologic characteristics. Circulation, 68:917, 1983.
47. Fontaine, G., Tonet, J. L., Frank, R., et al.: La fulguration endocavitaire. Une nouvelle methode de traitment des troubles due rhythme? Ann. Cardiol. Angeol., 33:543, 1984.
48. Winston, S. A., Morady, E., Davis, J. C., et al.: Catheter ablation of ventricular tachycardia (abstr.). Circulation, 70:II-412, 1984.
49. Downar, E., Parson, I., Cameron, D., et al.: Unipolar and bipolar catheter ablation techniques for management of ventricular tachycardia—initial experience (abstr.). J. Am. Coll. Cardiol., 5:472, 1985.

32

Chronic Electrical Control of Tachyarrhythmias

Edwin G. Duffin and Douglas P. Zipes

Attempts to control arrhythmias electrically can be traced back to the 1700s, when Charles Kite created a direct current defibrillator using Leyden jars as a storage medium.[1] In the 1800s Duchenne reported treatment of tachycardias using a coil, battery, and interrupter circuit.[2] In 1884 Gaskell suppressed pacemaker activity in the tortoise using externally applied electrical stimuli.[3] Unfortunately, documentation of the results of these early attempts is sketchy.

Within the past few years a renewed interest in electrical control of tachycardias has spawned a host of devices with widely varying descriptions. Implantable devices with energy outputs ranging from 20 millionths of a joule to 40 J, using bursts, premature stimuli, scanning pulse positions at different intervals of the cardiac cycle, and synchronous or asynchronous shocks and weighing between 45 and 292 g, are available as investigational items, custom prescription devices, or fully marketed systems. Some deliver therapies automatically, while others require patient or physician intervention. Yet despite this broad menu it is estimated that uniquely antitachycardia stimulators account for less than 1% of all pulse generator implants. The primary reasons for this include availability of well-entrenched alternative therapies, fear that the devices will induce more serious arrhythmias, and design limitations in available pulse generators. Technical advances will undoubtedly reduce these barriers within the next few years, yet current state-of-the-art devices are already achieving impressive results in carefully selected patients. Table 32-l provides a brief summary of representative antitachycardia pacing systems referenced in recent literature.

In the broadest terms. electrical control of tachyarrhythmias is accomplished by one of five approaches: (1) pacing for rate support necessitated by drugs or surgery, (2) pacing to prevent the onset of tachycardia, (3) pacing to terminate tachycardia, (4) cardioversion, and (5) defibrillation. In many instances combinations of these approaches are required for effective antiarrhythmic therapy.

Pacemakers

The permanent pacemaker has become a widely used, generally accepted therapy since its first clinical application in 1959. Initially, indications for use were very narrow, with the devices intended primarily for ventricular stimulation in patients with complete AV block with Adams-Stokes seizures. In the intervening years indications broadened to the point where, worldwide, an esti-

Table 32-1. Representative Antitachycardia Pulse Generators/Systems Referenced in Recent Literature

MFG	Device	Therapy	Activity Algorithm	Brady?	Leads	Comments
Biotronik	Phylax	Burst	Auto: rate, count	SSI	Tv or Epi	Custom-built unit
Cordis	Orthocor I	PES, Burst, Scan	Manual	SSIM	Tv or Epi	Driver 1A: 1–3 PES, 170–400ms Driver IIA: 1–20 PES, 160–400ms Train 1–20, incr. or decr. int
Cordis	Orthocor II	PES, Burst, Scan	Auto or Manual	SSIM	Tv or Epi	48 one-hour event recorder
Cordis	Gemini	PES, Burst, Scan	Manual	DDDC	2 Tv or Epi	External driver triggers either chamber in DDT mode
Intec	AICD	Cardioversion, Defibrillation	Auto: rate, count, probability funct.	None	2 Tv, 1 Epi patch	2 shocks at 25 J, 3rd at 30 J
Intermedics	Cybertach-60	Burst	Auto: rate, count	SSIC	Tv or Epi	Tachycardia detection flag
Intermedics	Intertach	Burst, PES, Scan, adaptive	Auto: rate, count, acceleration, sustained high rate, rate stability	SSIC	Tv or Epi	Multiple staged therapies, multiple event monitors
Medtronic	5998-RF	Burst	Manual	None	Tv or Epi	No implanted power source
Medtronic	2404	Burst	Auto: rate, count	SSI	Tv or Epi	Custom built unit
Medtronic	Spectrax/2331	Burst	Manual	SSIM	Tv or Epi	Standard pulse generator
Medtronic	Interactive Tachycardia System	Burst, Scan, PES, Adaptive	Manual initiation with auto confirm	SSI	Tv or Epi	Associated prescription formulator allows noninvasive electrophysiologic evaluation
Medtronic	Symbios 7008	Burst, Dual Demand	Auto: rate, count	DDDC	2 Tv or Epi	Tachycardia detection flag
Medtronic	Cardioverter 7210	Cardioversion, Burst, PES	Manual or Auto: rate, count and acceleration	SSIC	Tv	0.06 to 2 J 3 shocks at programmed level, final two at 2 J
Siemens-Elema	Tachylog 651	Dual demand, PES, Scan, Burst, Adaptive	Manual or Auto: rate, count, and acceleration	SSIC	Tv or Epi	Multiple staged therapies
Siemens-Elema	668	Dual Demand	Auto: rate	SSIC	Tv or Epi	Standard pulse generator
Telectronics	PASAR 4151	Scan, PES	Auto: rate, count	None	Tv or Epi	1 or 2 PES, scans 1 or pair as set
Telectronics	PASAR 4161	Scan, PES	Auto: rate, count	None	Tv or Epi	1 or 2 PES, scans both individually
Telectronics	PASAR 4171	Scan, PES, Burst	Auto: rate, count	SSIC	Tv or Epi	Burst of 7 pulses plus scans of 4161
Telectronics	PASAR 4172	Scan, PES, Burst	Auto: rate, count	SSIC	Tv or Epi	Burst of 8 pulses plus scans of 4161
Telectronics	Optima	Dual Demand	Auto: rate	SSIC	Tv or Epi	Standard pulse generator
Vitatron	DPG1	VVI Dual Demand Adaptive overdrive	Auto: rate, count	SSIC	Tv or Epi	Sense/Pace/PVC/Tachycardia counters

PES, programmed extra stimuli; Scan, scanning of number of extra stimuli or timing of extra stimuli; Burst, a rapid sequence of stimuli, usually with unchanging coupling intervals throughout the sequence; Adaptive, coupling intervals for burst or extra stimuli set to percentages of tachycardia cycle length as measured by the device during each episode of tachycardia; Tv, transvenous; Epi, epicardial electrodes; "Brady?", antibradycardia functions of pulse generator indicated by ICHD pacemaker code.

mated 290,000 new devices were implanted in 1981. Of these, the vast majority were applied primarily to manage bradyarrhythmias. Yet as early as 1960 Zoll and colleagues reported the use of ventricular pacing to treat ventricular tachyarrhythmias in patients with complete heart block.[4] Sowton and colleagues soon extended this to patients without heart block,[5] and by 1967 Cohen and associates reported using ventricular pacing in the treatment of patients with supraventricular tachycardias associated with sick sinus syndrome.[6] Antiarrhythmic atrial pacing was also being reported in 1967 by Massumi and coauthors, Haft and colleagues, and Durrer and associates.[7-9]

In contrast to the relatively crude pioneering devices, which were not optimized to treat tachycardias, modern pacing devices are small, ranging between 40 and 95 g, offer longevities approaching 10 years, are readily adaptable to patient needs by noninvasive multiprogrammability, and are designed specifically to control tachycardias. These devices are easily accepted by patients because of their small size, minimal side-effects, and low-output energies, typically in the range of 20 to 40 mJ. Patients are usually oblivious to the effects of these devices as they accomplish their intended purpose.

Pacing for Rate Support

In patients with tachyarrhythmias that can be controlled pharmacologically or eliminated by surgical interruption, bradycardia may be a resultant side-effect. Conventional pacemakers, either single or dual chamber, can be used to restore appropriate rate. Such devices are readily available commercially and pose no unique problems in these applications. Dual-chamber DDD units may be particularly useful when a paroxysmal supraventricular tachycardia cannot be controlled, but its conduction to the ventricles can be regulated through the rate-limiting behavior of the pacemaker implanted following surgical ablation of the normal AV pathway.[10] During periods of normal sinus function the DDD pacemaker provides 1:1 conduction to the ventricles, matching appropriate rate response to patient needs. Yet during bouts of tachycardia the upper rate behavior of the pacemaker can protect the patient from excessive ventricular rates by blocking transmission of every second or every second and third atrial event.

Recent developments in antibradycardia pacing have led to the clinical introduction of rate-responsive pacemakers that do not depend on normal sinus node function for proper operation. These devices adapt their pacing rate to patients' needs by detecting changes in indicators such as QT interval,[11] *p*H,[12] respiration,[13] or physical activity.[14] Although still investigational, these devices may allow aggressive use of pharmacologic or surgical arrhythmia control while still permitting patients a relatively normal ventricular rate variability in response to physiologic demands.

Pacing to Prevent Onset of Tachycardia

Clearly the most desirable form of arrhythmia control would be an approach capable of preventing arrhythmias from occurring. Four permanent pacing techniques have been found to be effective in suppressing the onset of certain tachycardias: (1) rate support to prevent bradycardiac events that may lead to tachycardias, (2) moderately high rate suppression to prevent emergence of tachycardia ("overdrive"), (3) dual-chamber pacing to inhibit reentry, and (4) high rate atrial stimulation to induce AV block.

Patients experiencing slow heart rates (*e.g.*, sick sinus syndrome or complete AV block) may exhibit rapid "escape" rhythms due to the bradycardia.[15-19] Permanent atrial or ventricular pacing at conventional pacing rates prevents the bradycardia (Fig. 32-1) and is an acceptable method of eliminating or minimizing tachycardiac episodes.[16,20-22] It is possible that the rate support obtained by pacing maintains uniform repolarization that may prevent recurrence of the tachycardia.[23-25]

Ventricular tachyarrhythmias refractory to pharmacologic control in selected patients without coexisting bradycardia have been managed with long-term ventricular pacing. Continuous ventricular pacing at 90 to 100 pulses/min for up to 36 months,[26,27] 98 pulses/min for 14 months,[28] and 90 pulses/min for over 46 months[29] have been reported to suppress tachycardia successfully. Continuous atrial pacing at similar rates has also been shown to be effective.[29,30] The majority of patients managed in this way also had concomitant antiarrhythmic drug therapy. Several potential limitations of this technique have also been reported. In one instance a rapid rate of 104 pulses/min, although effective in controlling the spontaneous arrhythmia, produced intolerable palpitations.[28] Pacing at these rates may produce an unacceptable decrease in cardiac output.[29] In some cases, effectiveness may be hightly rate and drug specific, requiring frequent modification of each. This limitation indicates that rate-programmable pacing systems are essential in this application. (An external pacing device demonstrated by Zacouto and colleagues[31] automatically searches for an optimum rate consistent with minimal ectopic activity to minimize or prevent tachycardia episodes. This system is not available at present in an implantable form.) Finally, while moderately rapid rates in nonischemic hearts generally increase repolarization uniformity, thereby reducing ventricular arrhythmias, rapid rates in ischemic hearts may have the opposite effect. Therefore,

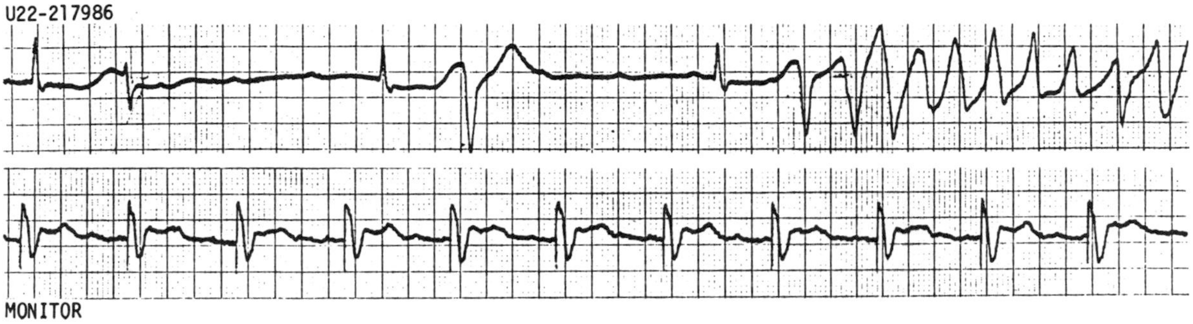

Figure 32-1. *Ventricular ectopy accompanying advanced AV block. (*Top*) Premature ventricular systoles initiate ventricular tachycardia. (*Bottom*) Ventricular pacing at 75 beats/min suppresses all ventricular arrhythmias.*

this mode of pacing must be carefully applied in patients with ischemic heart disease. In general, pacing at these rates to prevent recurrence of ventricular tachyarrhythmias in patients without accompanying bradycardia has not been very successful.

For reentry to occur, conduction pathways in one limb of the reentrant circuit must be excitable by the initiating stimulus. If the involved tissue is made refractory before the initiating stimulus arrives, the reentrant circuit will not be completed. Some patients with reentrant supraventricular tachycardias have been successfully managed with atrial synchronous[32] and AV sequential[33,34] permanent pacing systems. In each instance the pacing system was configured to ensure a shortened PR interval by initiating a premature ventricular stimulus closely coupled to the preceding atrial contraction. Because of the close coupling, conduction in the AV nodal or accessory pathway reentrant circuit might be expected to encounter refractory tissue, thereby preventing initiation of a reentrant rhythm. The principle difference between the atrial synchronous and AV sequential approaches is that in the former the premature ventricular stimuli are triggered by sensed spontaneous atrial activity, allowing the patient's ventricular rate to track the atrial rate; the latter technique stimulates both the atria and the ventricles sequentially at a preset rate, independently of the spontaneous atrial rhythm, but is inhibited in the event of ventricular activity. In applying these approaches, currently available multiprogrammable DDD pacemakers can be used. It is important, however, to select pacemaker operating parameters that will maintain the required AV relationship.[35] Careful preoperative evaluation is mandatory, since if the pacemaker loses synchrony, tachycardia may evolve and inhibit the pacemaker, thereby suppressing any further antitachycardia action. This likelihood may be addressed by the use of more sophisticated DDD pacemakers capable of terminating tachycardias.

The primary limitations in these modes of therapy are potential hemodynamic disturbances due to the less than optimal PR delay and, in the case of AV sequential pacing, loss of the normal physiologic rate control mechanism.

An approach used infrequently to limit ventricular rate has been the application of high rate atrial stimulation. The intent of this approach is either to initiate an atrial tachyarrhythmia such as atrial fibrillation, which then results in a drug-controllable, reduced ventricular rate, or to pace the atria at rates sufficiently high to induce AV block, thereby achieving a slower ventricular rate than would have occurred during supraventricular tachycardia.[36]

Recently work has been reported on the use of precisely timed subthreshold premature stimuli or trains of such stimuli[37,38] to prevent tachycardia (Fig. 32-2). Others have reported some success with the use of simultaneous multiple site stimulation of canine ventricles to prevent initiation of reentrant ventricular tachycardia[39] and temporary use of triggered simultaneous atrial and ventricular stimulation (DDT mode) to prevent the onset of supraventricular tachycardia in humans.[40] These efforts are still in the formative stage and have not yet been developed to the point where they can be considered for chronic therapy. Nevertheless, they offer great promise if practical devices can be derived.

Pacing to Terminate Tachycardias

The most commonly encountered method of controlling tachycardias electrically is that of pacing to terminate the arrhythmia once it has occurred. A wide variety of tachycardia termination techniques using permanent pacing systems have been devised and shown to be effective in carefully selected patients.

The feasibility of converting supraventricular tachycardia, with or without preexcitation syndrome, to normal sinus rhythm using an appropriately timed and po-

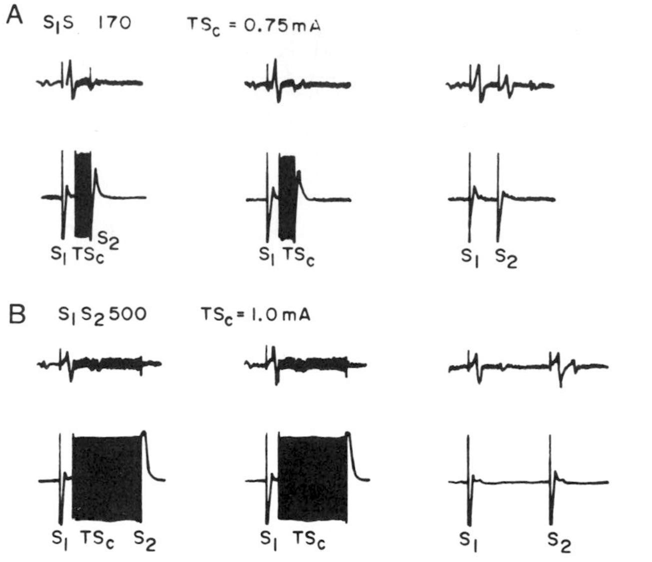

Figure 32-2. *Trains of rapid subthreshold stimuli (S_C) inhibit response to subsequent premature stimulus (S_2). (A) Premature stimulus with 170-ms coupling interval is ineffective when preceded by a train of subthreshold (0.75 mA) stimuli. Train alone provokes no response, yet single stimulus S_2 is effective when applied in the absence of the subthreshold train. (B) Same as A, except coupling interval of S_2 is increased to 500 ms and the longer subthreshold preconditioning train is 1 mA.*

sitioned stimulus has long been known.[41–43] These pacemaker-induced premature beats are presumed to cause refractoriness in the reciprocal pathway needed to sustain the tachycardia, thereby terminating the rapid rhythm.[44] This principle, using conventional permanently implanted demand pacemakers, has been employed long term after temporary pacing-initiated premature activity was shown to terminate the tachycardia effectively. During periods when the intrinsic sinus rate exceeded the preset pacemaker rate or when episodes of supraventricular tachycardia occurred, these devices were inhibited by the spontaneous rhythm. Placing a magnet placed over the pacemaker converted the device to the asynchronous mode, producing competitive stimuli at the preset rate. These stimuli were intended to "march through the cardiac cycle" until one fell into the appropriate "window," terminating the arrhythmia. This technique has been used successfully in the ventricles[45–47] and in the atria.[47,48] Magnet-induced competitive pacing has also been used to manage recurrent ventricular tachycardia.[47] While the availability of pulse generators makes this single-chamber approach attractive, it is successful on a long-term basis in only a relatively small number of patients.

More advanced systems embodying competitive underdrive pacing (*i.e.*, pacing at a rate below that of the tachycardia) have been successfully demonstrated. Automatic initiation of underdrive pacing has been used in the form of the dual demand pacemaker,[35,49–51] a single-chamber device that reverts to an asynchronous pacing rate automatically whenever sensed cardiac activity exceeds a predetermined rate. An extension of this concept is embodied in dual-chamber devices that pace asynchronously in the AV sequential mode with a short AV interval (25 to 65 ms) whenever a preselected number of ventricular events exceeds a tachycardia definition rate.[34,52] Such pacing ensures that both the atrial and ventricular segments of the reentrant pathway are rendered refractory nearly simultaneously, thereby preventing the tachycardia from being sustained.

Several limitations of these techniques have been noted. Although the arrhythmia is usually terminated rapidly, long periods of stimulation may be necessary when a single-chamber stimulus is used at a rate that allows the spontaneous and induced beats to maintain a temporally fixed relationship to each other.[47] Asynchronous pacing of the ventricles itself may produce dangerous tachyarrhythmias. Several of these approaches require active patient participation to recognize the arrhythmia, correctly apply a magnet, and perceive termination. Finally, some cases of tachycardia treated with single-chamber underdrive pacing responded well acutely but subsequently became refractory to competitive pacing.[35,53,54]

The ability of bursts of rapid atrial stimulation to terminate episodes of supraventricular tachycardia has been demonstrated.[44,55,56] Long-term application of patient-initiated rapid atrial stimulation has been effected with radiofrequency coupled pacing systems.[57–60] These systems consist of a small battery-less implanted receiver/electrode lead and an external patient-activated transmitter. Pulse frequencies up to 400/min are set by controls in the transmitter. When the patient experiences the symptoms of supraventricular tachycardia, the transmitter is placed over the implanted receiver and activated for several seconds, resulting in delivery of an asynchronous burst of stimuli. More advanced designs for patient-activated antitachycardia pacing have entered clinical trials. These systems provide a number of additional characteristics that enhance their use in dealing with the wide variability encountered with tachycardia patients. Some combine conventional multiprogrammable antibradycardia capabilities with patient-activated transmitters that generate the required antitachycardia stimulation sequences by suitable temporary programming of the implanted pulse generator.[61] Others use implantable pulse generators with two-way telemetry that signals the transmitter whenever the pacemaker senses cardiac activity. This allows the patient-activated therapy to be synchronized with the tachycardia cycle, removing the restriction to asynchronous therapies.[62] Such telemetry also makes it possible for the activating transmitter to confirm that a tachycardia does indeed exist, thereby precluding the delivery of inappropriate therapies should the patient misinterpret "symptoms."

Potential complications and limitations related to patient-initiated rapid atrial stimulation should be considered when applying this therapeutic technique. These include the following:

- Inadvertent ventricular stimulation due to either electrode placement or AV bypass tracts with the possibility of inducing malignant ventricular arrhythmias[63]
- Patient discomfort due to extracardiac stimulation[58]
- Asystole following cessation of rapid pacing
- The patient's ability to use the system correctly and to sense conversion of the rhythm[59]

The limitations imposed by patient initiation of antitachycardia therapy have been eliminated by the introduction of automatic pulse generators.[64] Newer automatic antitachycardia pacemakers incorporating single- and dual-chamber stimulation for bradycardia control have become available for clinical trial.[61,65–69] These devices can provide prophylactic antiarrhythmic therapy, protect against asystole following antitachycardia stimulation, and automatically intervene so rapidly that the patient is frequently unaware that tachycardia has occurred (Fig. 32-3).

The primary limitation of available hardware is the inability to differentiate automatically between appropriate sinus rate increases and dangerous tachycardias that have overlapping rates. This weakness makes necessary very careful patient selection or concomitant drug therapy to limit the potential for sinus rates to rise above the automatic tachycardia trip rates of the implanted device. Rapid advances in implantable microprocessor technology should eliminate this drawback.

Bursts of rapid stimuli or precisely timed sequences of stimuli delivered directly to the atria (Fig. 32-4) or to the ventricles have been used to manage episodes of ventricular tachycardia. The implanted pacemaker systems used include patient-activated devices and fully automatic pulse generators. The patient-activated systems are of two types. Some are inhibited by spontaneous ventricular activity at typical ventricular escape rates, yet during tachycardia, placing a magnet over the unit produces a preselected number of high-rate stimuli.[70] Other devices are activated by having the patient apply a "miniprogrammer" to initiate antitachycardia stimulation. The "miniprogrammer" in some cases programs by a radio or magnetic link,[61,62,71–73] while in others it "programs" the implantable generator by providing a transdermal signal that triggers the implanted device after it has been placed in a triggered mode.[74] The automatic devices combine conventional pacemakers with a circuit designed to detect tachycardia and to deliver a therapeutic stimulus sequence when appropriate.[67,75,76] Stimulation sequences vary among the devices but generally include rapid bursts and programmed extra stimuli. In an attempt to ensure long-term successful termination of the tachycardia despite rate variation or the influence of other factors, some of these systems use a scanning technique in which successive pacing sequences provide increasing numbers of stimuli or shift the position of the stimuli to different intervals in the cardiac cycle. Alternatively, these pacemakers may be

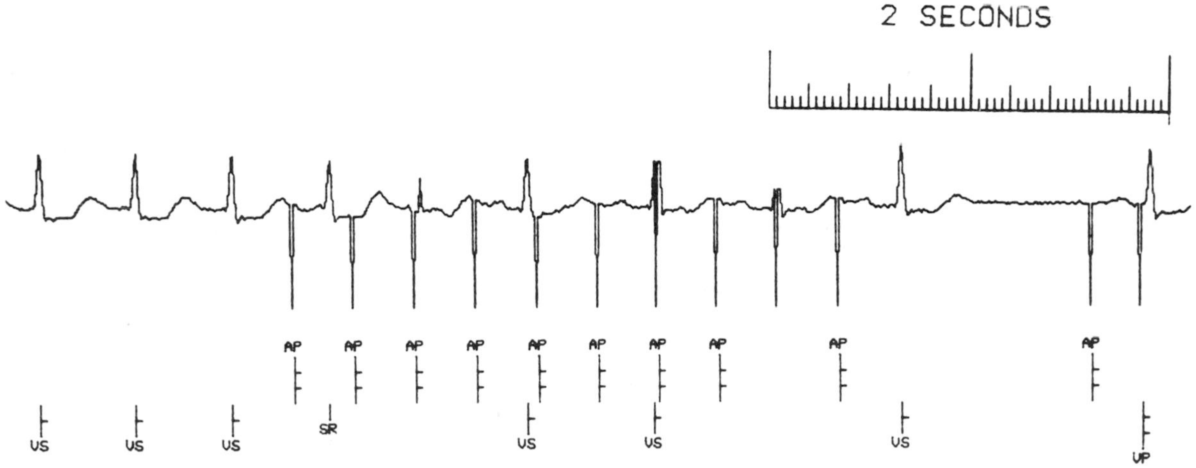

Figure 32-3. *Termination of AV nodal reentrant tachycardia by ten stimuli delivered to the atrium by an automatic-burst DDD pacemaker (Medtronic Symbios 7008). The marker channel indicates ventricular sensing (VS), atrial pacing (AP), a sensed ventricular event occurring in the refractory period of the ventricular amplifier (SR), and ventricular pacing (VP). After tachycardia termination, AV sequential pacing occurs for the last beat.*

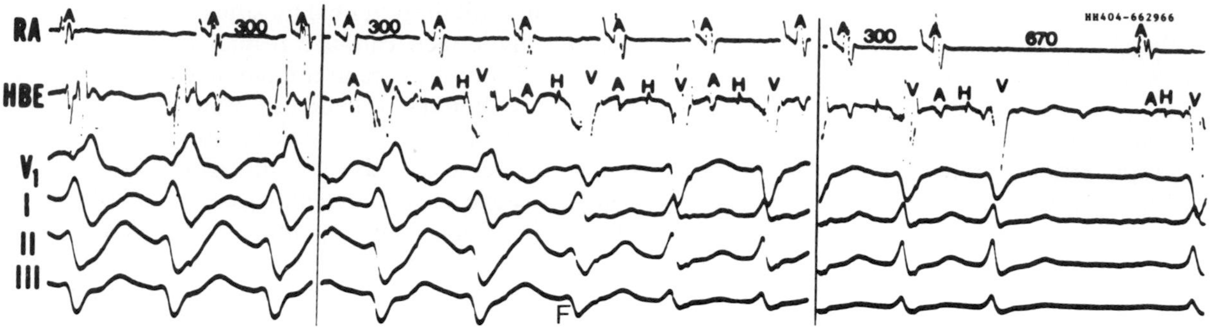

Figure 32-4. *Atrial pacing with a cycle length of 300 ms overdrives ventricular tachycardia, restoring sinus rhythm when pacing is terminated.*

able to measure the rate of the tachycardia and provide a stimulus sequence with adaptive coupling intervals (*i.e.*, intervals that vary to predetermined percentages of the tachycardia cycle length). These features may help maintain efficacy despite physiologic variations in the presumed reentrant mechanism and its associated termination zones.

Limitations of these pacing approaches to the control of ventricular tachycardia include the aforementioned problems with accurate arrhythmia detection and classification and the possibility of tachycardia acceleration even to the point of ventricular fibrillation due to device malfunction or normal electrophysiologic variability. For these reasons such systems are currently reserved for the rare, fully evaluated patient who has ventricular tachycardia refractory to other therapeutic interventions and for whom termination of ventricular tachycardia by sequenced ventricular stimulation has been repeatedly shown to be successful and uneventful.[70,71,75,77,78]

Cardioversion

Moderate doses of energy delivered in synchrony with ventricular activity are used routinely to terminate ventricular tachycardia in the acute setting. Recently it has been shown in dogs[79] and in humans[80] that ventricular tachycardia can be terminated effectively with substantially lower energies if the cardioversion shock is delivered through a suitable transvenous catheter electrode. For transthoracic cardioversion, energy levels are usually in the range of 25 to 50 J, whereas transvenous cardioversion is currently accomplished with mean energy levels of 0.5 J. (By contrast, pacemaker stimuli are typically in the range of 25 μJ. Synchronous cardioversion is attractive for several reasons, including the fact that it obviates tedious determinations of temporal sequencing of stimuli, terminates ventricular tachycardia rapidly, and is usually safe if delivered inadvertently during sinus rhythm. The transvenous approach is particularly promising in that it minimizes patient discomfort, an important fact in the fully conscious patient, and lends itself to implementation of a fully implantable automatic cardioverter suitable for chronic therapy. Such a system has been implanted in seven patients suffering from recurrent episodes of sustained monomorphic ventricular tachycardia.[81]*

The implantable cardioverter weighs 95 g and is sealed in a titanium case measuring 57 × 73 × 19 mm. The device can be programmed to cardiovert manually, on command, or automatically when tachycardia is detected. Tachycardia detection is based on rate, cardiac event count, and, optionally, rate acceleration criteria. The cardioversion pulse is delivered synchronously at the programmed energy level, 0.06 to 2 J, for as many as three attempts at tachycardia termination. If the third attempt fails, up to two additional shocks are delivered at 2 J. No further shocks are delivered unless the patient's rhythm slows to a rate below the tachycardia trigger interval, in which case the device rearms itself in preparation for subsequent arrhythmic episodes. The cardioverter also includes a multiprogrammable VVI pacemaker capable of providing antibradycardia support as well as V00 burst and premature stimulation sequences for tachycardia initiation and termination under control of the external pacemaker programmer. Bidirectional telemetry provides electrograms, program settings, battery status indications, and marker channel signals used for electrocardiographic interpretation. The current-generation device does not provide a means for defibrillation.

The implantable defibrillator was recently modified to enable it to function also as a synchronous cardioverter.[82] This device delivers substantially higher energy levels (25 J), requires three lead systems—one an epicardial type, and is substantially larger, weighing 292 g. (The system is discussed more fully later in this chapter under Defibrillation.)

*An additional 12 units have since been implanted.

Cardioversion may also have a role in chronic therapy for atrial tachyarrhythmias. It has been shown in at least one patient to terminate atrial fibrillation[83] (Fig. 32-5). In a series of canine experiments, atrial tachycardias were terminated with limited success using energy levels below 0.6 J delivered with an atrial catheter.[84]

Chronic application of the cardioversion technique is still in its infancy, and the ultimate role it may play, in conjunction with drugs, surgery or other electrical approaches, has yet to be established. Clearly it is subject to risks of tachycardia acceleration[77,81] and inadvertent induction of atrial arrhythmias,[81] as are all the tachycardia termination techniques in use. Yet as part of a staged therapeutic sequence beginning with pacing techniques and escalating to cardioversion and if required, back-up defibrillation, it may significantly improve the overall efficacy of electrical therapy for tachyarrhythmias.

Defibrillation

The goal for electrical control of arrhythmias is a small, easily implantable, fully automatic device capable of staged interventions beginning with preventive measures, progressing through increasingly aggressive pacing termination modes into cardioversion, all the while protecting the patient by providing back-up defibrillation capability in case the device fails to terminate the tachyarrhythmia or actually exacerbates the patient's arrhythmia by increasing the rate or precipitating ventricular fibrillation. No such device exists currently, but component parts are evolving. Defibrillation with a transvenous catheter has been successfully demonstrated (Fig. 32-6). Starting in the 1970s an implantable defibrillator was developed[85,86] and has now been implanted in 276 patients.[82,114] The earliest implants were restricted to survivors of recurrent sudden cardiac death, but criteria have since been relaxed, allowing trials of the device in patients experiencing single episodes of ventricular fibrillation or hemodynamically unstable ventricular tachycardia. The potential patient population for these devices is vast, given that sudden death claims the lives of an estimated 350,000 to 400,000 people each year in the United States and is thought to be predominantly the result of ventricular tachyarrhythmias.

The implantable defibrillator weighs 292 g and is sealed in a titanium case measuring approximately $112 \times 71 \times 25$ mm.[87] Powered by lithium batteries, the device has a projected longevity of 3 years or 100 shocks. Tachycardia detection is based on rate and count criteria. Detection of fibrillation is achieved using a probability density function that reflects the amount of time that the differentiated electrogram assumes amplitude values close to a narrow band around the baseline. Dur-

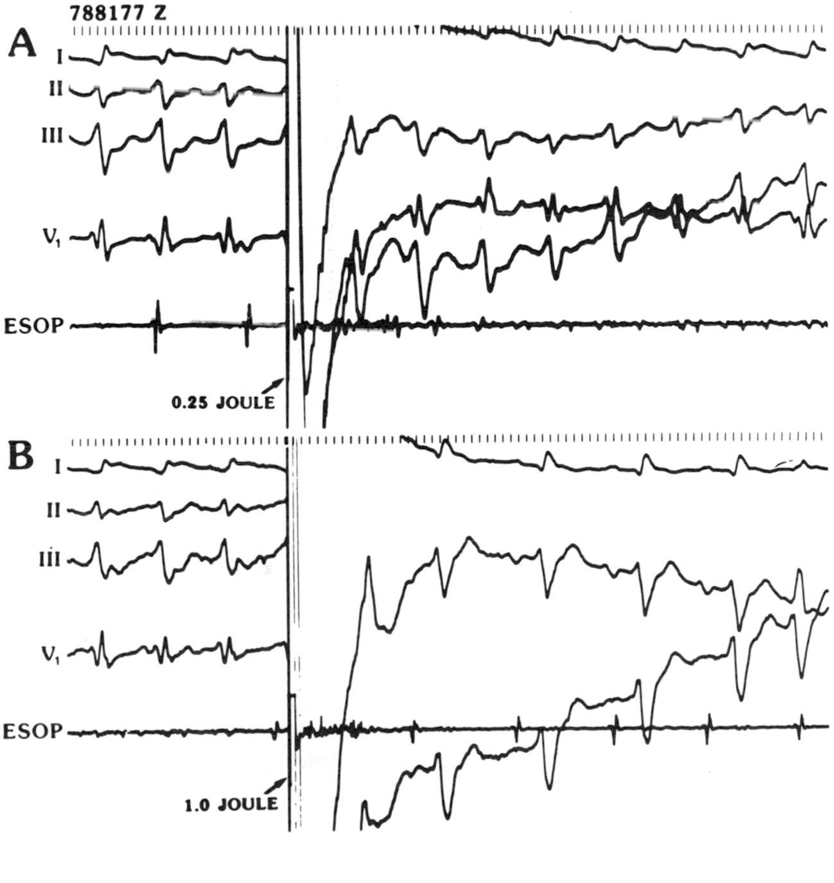

Figure 32-5. *Transvenous termination of atrial fibrillation. In A, a 0.25-J shock delivered synchronously into the QRS complex fails to convert the ventricular rhythm but induces atrial fibrillation. In B, a synchronous 1-J shock terminates both atrial fibrillation and ventricular tachycardia, restoring normal sinus rhythm.*

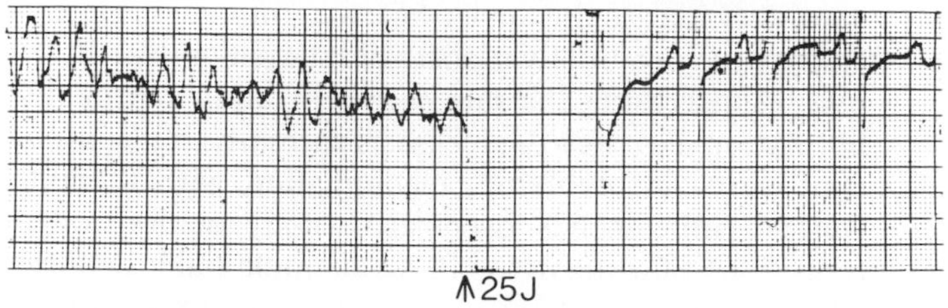

Figure 32-6. *Transvenous defibrillation. A 25-J shock* (arrow) *delivered by a transvenous catheter with electrodes in the right ventricular apex and superior vena cava terminates ventricular fibrillation.*

ing fibrillation this signal shows a paucity of baseline segments. The electrode system employed by the defibrillator includes a transvenous right ventricular bipolar lead for synchronization and tachycardia rate detection, a transvenous lead placed in the superior vena cava, and an epicardial patch electrode currently placed by a subxyphoidal approach on the ventricular apex. The latter pair of electrodes is used to detect fibrillation and to deliver the therapeutic shock. Cardioversion or defibrillation is achieved by delivery of a 25-J pulse with a 3- to 8-ms duration. Up to four attempts at termination are permitted for each tachyarrhythmic episode, with the final shock having an intensity of 30 J. The device does not provide any pacing capabilities. Should antibradycardia pacing be required, a separate pacemaker and an additional lead system must be implanted. Care must be taken to ensure that the pacemaker and defibrillator do not interact inappropriately. Unipolar pacemakers are particularly problematic in this application, since their operation causes the defibrillator arrhythmia detection algorithm great difficulty.[88]

Patient Selection and Evaluation

Current practice is to attempt pharmacologic control or surgical correction as the preferred approaches to tachyarrhythmias. There is, as yet, no convincing database to indicate that electrical control should be considered a primary therapy for any class of tachyarrhythmias except possibly recurrent ventricular fibrillation, for which an implantable defibrillator may be a viable solution. When surgical correction is not feasible and drugs are ineffective, are accompanied by intolerable side-effects, or are impractical because of patient noncompliance, then electrical approaches should be considered.

Selecting candidates for chronic electrical control of tachycardia requires a thorough understanding of the arrhythmogenic mechanism and the attendant risks of available electrical therapies.[75,88,89]

For patients in whom tachycardia has been documented electrocardiographically to be secondary to bradycardia, the prescription is relatively straightforward. Implantation of a conventional single- or dual-chamber pacemaker can be an effective and safe therapy with minimal attendant risk. Follow-up ambulatory recording may be required to determine the optimal pacing parameters for arrhythmia prevention.

Since all available electrical therapies capable of terminating tachyarrhythmias also have the potential to exacerbate such rhythms, it is imperative that appropriately thorough electrophysiologic studies precede device implantation.[75,90–93] These studies should do the following:

- Determine the specific nature and mechanism of the arrhythmia
- Determine the most appropriate site for antiarrhythmic stimulation, with due consideration to balancing efficacy with safety (*e.g.*, ventricular versus atrial stimulation)
- Develop the most effective stimulation sequence for termination
- Evaluate the degree of latitude with which the therapy maintains safety and efficacy (*e.g.*, are termination rates critically narrow or broad)
- Evaluate patient tolerance of atrial fibrillation in the event that atrial stimulation is required
- Uncover the presence of anomalous, rapidly conducting AV pathways that might result in rapid ventricular activation due to atrial stimulation
- Evaluate the potential for acceleration or induction of more malignant tachyarrhythmias.

In matching the patient with an appropriate therapeutic device, the mode of tachycardia detection employed by the system must be considered. Fully automatic devices eliminate concern for the patient's mental or psychologic condition and generally ensure rapid therapy, an important factor in patients who become rapidly disabled following onset of tachycardia. However, currently available automatic devices are not very effective in distinguishing among the pathologic arrhythmias and normal sinus acceleration; they are therefore subject to inappropriate triggering[88,89] (Fig. 32-7). This may require the use of drugs to prevent sinus rates from exceeding the tachycardia detection rate threshold of the device. Patient-initiated therapies avoid such detection problems but depend on accurate assessment of symptoms by the patient, are less rapid, and are subject to failure if the patient's external control device is lost, damaged, or misapplied; also, they cannot be used in

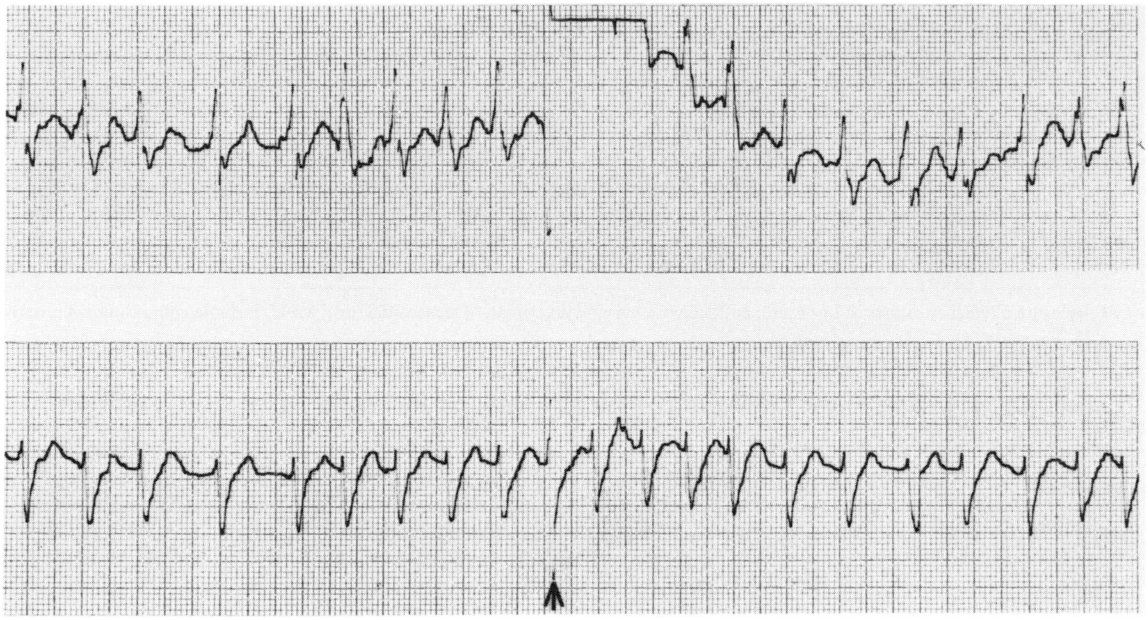

Figure 32-7. *Rapid ventricular response to atrial fibrillation is incorrectly identified as ventricular tachycardia, triggering inappropriate delivery of a cardioversion shock (*arrow*).*

patients who rapidly become incapacitated following onset of tachycardia.[93]

As with any chronic therapy it is important that patients receiving implantable antiarrhythmic devices be followed carefully. Physiologic variability, progressive disease processes, device aging, and changes in concomitant pharmacologic therapy all may impair the efficacy of the electrical system. Periodic confirmation of continued efficacy is essential.

Arrhythmias Amenable to Chronic Electrical Therapy: Current Status

Atrial Fibrillation

Atrial fibrillation is impervious to electrical approaches other than high-energy shocks.[95] There are no reports of successful chronic electrical control of atrial fibrillation, although preliminary studies suggest that techniques used in investigational implantable cardioverters may ultimately play a role in treating patients with this arrhythmia.[83]

Atrial Flutter

Many reports note the relative ease with which atrial flutter can be terminated electrically, usually with atrial bursts or entrainment sequences.[96-100] Waldo and colleagues[98] have reported that all type I flutters (rates 240 to 338 beats/min) can be interrupted by rapid atrial pacing, whereas type II flutter (rates 340 to 433 beats/min) cannot.[98] Surprisingly, very little has been published on successful chronic electrical control of atrial flutter. Table 32-2 outlines the content of two reports, only one of which deals with permanent pacing, and that is limited to a single patient. Typically half of the flutter patients treated with rapid pacing revert directly to sinus rhythm, while the remainder frequently experience transient atrial fibrillation that resolves spontaneously to sinus rhythm. Occasionally a period of asystole may follow cessation of rapid pacing, and provision must be made to deal with this. When conversion cannot be effected with pacing alone, vagal maneuvers may shorten the atrial refractory period enough to facilitate termination.[95]

Paroxysmal Supraventricular Tachycardia

Atrial, AV nodal, and AV reciprocating tachycardias are generally amenable to both pharmacologic and electrical control. Traditionally the former has been the method of choice and continues to be so in the absence of significant data showing comparative advantages of electrical alternatives. Yet as more sophisticated and functionally attractive pacing systems evolve, the approach to these supraventricular tachycardias may deserve reconsideration.

Tables 32-3 through 32-6 summarize many reports of the use of chronic electrical techniques to control supraventricular tachycardias. High degrees of success over substantial follow-up periods have been demonstrated. The most common successful method is the use of atrial

(Text continues on p. 776.)

Table 32-2. Electrical Therapy for Atrial Flutter

Reference	No. of Patients	Device	Mode	MCL	EFF	MFU	Comments
Das, G., et al.[99]	32	Temporary; Med Data MDI100A	Burst pacing with average rate 572 ppm and range 100–1500 ppm	290	0.98	N/A	1 patient required cardioversion
Wyndham, G., et al.[101]	1	Permanent; Medtronic RF 1258	Patient-initiated burst: 450 ppm	200	1	21	

EFF, measure of efficacy estimated by chapter author; MCL, mean cycle length of tachycardia (ms); MFU, mean length of follow-up study (mo).

Table 32-3. Electrical Therapy for Wolff-Parkinson-White–Related Tachycardias

Reference	No. of Patients	Device	Mode	MCL	EFF	MFU	Comments
Mandel, W., et al.[102]	1	Permanent pacemaker; American Optical custom design	Asynchronized AOO pacing with rate acceleration 165–300 ppm when magnet applied	350	1	7	Patient had frequent episodes up to 5/day, all terminated effectively
Waxman, M., et al.[59]	3	Permanent pacemaker; Medtronic 5998	Patient-initiated AOO bursts	321	1	7	
Curry, P., et al.[35]	6	Permanent pacemaker; custom modified VVI	Automatic underdrive at 70 ppm (100 ppm in one patient)	385	0.67	19.6	Leads in coronary sinus or various LV epicardial sites
Neumann, G., et al.[103]	8	Permanent pacemaker; Biotronik IDP64SD, Medtronic 2404	Automatic AOO burst, typically 230 ppm with 8 pulses	N/A	0.75	17	One patient developed chronic atrial fibrillation and one had 2 episodes not interrupted
Ringqvist, I., et al.[104]	1	Permanent pacemaker; CPI Microlith	VVI pacing at 80 ppm	428	N/A	N/A	
Medina-Ravell, V., et al.[34]	18	Permanent pacemaker; Medtronic 5992DD and 7007	Automatic AV sequential underdrive with short AV interval	N/A	1	18	DVIMN induced episodes of SVT in 1 patient; DDDMN pacing substituted
den Dulk, K., et al.[94]	5	Permanent pacemaker; Medtronic SP500/501	Patient-initiated PES, scanned, fixed, or adaptive; 1–5 PES 2 atrial, 3 ventricular	N/A	0.95	15.1	

EFF, measure of efficacy estimated by chapter author; MCL, mean cycle length of treated tachycardias (ms); MFU, mean length of follow-up study (mo).

Table 32-4. Electrical Therapy for AV Nodal Tachycardia

Reference	No. of Patients	Device	Mode	MCL	EFF	MFU
Waxman, M., et al.[59]	2	Permanent pacemaker; Medtronic 5998	Patient-initiated asynchronous AOO burst	324	1	30
Neumann, G., et al.[103]	3	Biotonik IDP64SD Medtronic 2404	Automatic AOO bursts, typically 230 ppm, 8 pulses	N/A	1	15.7
den Dulk, K., et al.[94]	3	Permanent pacemaker; Medtronic SP500/501	Patient-initiated PES, 1–6, atrial, scanned or adaptive	N/A	0.94	12.5

EFF, measure of efficacy estimated by chapter author; MCL, mean cycle length of treated tachycardias (ms); MFU, mean length of follow-up study (mo).

Table 32-5. Electrical Therapy for Concealed Bypass Supraventricular Tachycardia

Reference	No. of Patients	Device	Mode	MCL	EFF	MFU	Comments
Neumann, G., et al.[103]	4	Permanent pacemaker; Medtronic 2404	Automatic AOO burst, typically 230 ppm for 8 pulses	N/A	0.75	5	One patient had multiple episodes of atrial fibrillation
den Dulk, K., et al.[94]	4	Permanent pacemaker; Medtronic SP500/501	Patient-initiated PES, fixed (1) or scanned (3); 3 atrial and 1 ventricular	N/A	0.97	17.6	

EFF, measure of efficacy estimated by chapter author; MCL, mean cycle length of treated tachycardias (ms); MFU, mean length of follow-up study (mo).

Table 32-6. Electrical Therapy for Supraventricular Tachycardias of Mixed Etiologies

Reference	No. of Patients	Device	Mode	MCL	EFF	MFU	Comments
Fruehan, C., et al.[105]	1	Permanent pacemaker; Medtronic 1258 RF	Patient-initiated AOO burst, 300 ppm	variable	1	15	
Kahn, A., et al.	12	Permanent pacemaker; Medtronic 1258 RF	Patient-initiated asynchronous AOO burst, 200–300 ppm	N/A	0.99	26.4	1 unit explanted due to persistent pericarditis; 1 patient died, cerebral hemorrhage 1 episode in 6000 failed to terminate
Iwa, T.[106]	34	Permanent pacemaker; San-Ei Sokki Co. Atricon (RF)	Patient-initiated asynchronous burst, typically 257 ppm	364	0.91	48	
Preston, T.[107]	1	Permanent pacemaker; Medtronic 5998 RF	Continuous AOO pacing at 206 ppm	353	1	15	After 6 mo continuous pacing not needed; Occasional episodes respond to brief period of pacing
Vohra, J. et al.[108]	7	Permanent pacemaker; Medtronic 5998 (5) Medtronic 1759 (2)	Patient-activated AOO bursts (5); Patient activated pair PES, 200 and 400 ms, ventricular	N/A	0.71	18.1	PES units were not effective long term
Spurrell, R., et al[109]	13	Permanent pacemaker; Telectronics 4151	Automatic scanned PES 3 single, 7 double ventricular PES and 3 double atrial PES	334	0.99	3	1 patient had 30 sec paroxysm; 1 developed atrial fibrillation with PES (Rx: Metoprolol); 1 lost efficacy due to tachycardia cycle length change (Rx: Metoprolol)
Lerman, et al.[89]	3	Permanent pacemaker; Intermedics Cybertach-60	Automatic AOO burst	315	0.67	6	1 unit explanted—intermittent sensing induced SVT; 2 patients experienced bursts due to sinus rhythm acceleration

continued

Table 32-6. Electrical Therapy for Supraventricular Tachycardias of Mixed Etiologies *Continued*

Reference	No. of Patients	Device	Mode	MCL	EFF	MFU	Comments
Scheibelhofer, W., et al.[110]	5	Permanent pacemaker; Cordis Orthocor & Medtronic SP500	Patient-initiated automatic burst (2); PES (3)	N/A	1	17	3 SVT; 2 WPW; Almost every patient needed parameter changes
Zipes, D., et al[65]	21	Permanent pacemaker; Medtronic 7008	Automatic AOO burst (19) AV sequential underdrive (2)	N/A	N/A	4.8	6 atrial flutter and 15 SVT
Spurrell, R., et al.[66]	21	Permanent pacemaker; Telectronics 4151, 4171	Automatic scanning, 2 PES, Autoscan PES, shifting/scanning burst	N/A	0.9	N/A	9 intranodal, 12 AV reentrant; 2 sudden deaths, cause unknown
Griffin, J., et al.[68]	91	Permanent pacemaker; Intermedics Cybertach 60	Automatic bursts	N/A	0.86	22	53% AV nodal; 26% AV reentry; 15% atrial flutter; 6% atrial reentry; 11 units explanted and not replaced, 2 units not in tachycardia mode
Sowton, E., et al.[69]	16	Permanent pacemaker; Siemens Tachylog 651	Automatic bursts or complex PES searching, scanning, or adaptation 6 atrial stim., 8 vent.	273	0.88	12	12 WPW; 4 AV nodal Skeletal myopotentials triggered therapy falsely in 8 patients. 2 patients developed rapid ventricular response to atrial fibrillation so surgery performed

EFF, measure of efficacy as estimated by chapter author; MCL, mean cycle length of treated tachycardias (ms); MFU, mean length of follow-up study (mo).

bursts or programmed extra stimuli delivered by patient-activated systems. For the Wolff-Parkinson-White–related tachycardias, automatic underdrive AV sequential pacing in combination with short (25 to 65 ms) AV delay is highly successful and eliminates the possibility of rapid ventricular activation through accessory pathways, a significant concern with rapid atrial stimulation techniques.

The primary difficulties reported with use of electrical approaches to supraventricular tachycardias are induction of atrial fibrillation, false triggering of automatic devices by sensing sinus acceleration or skeletal myopotentials, and undersensing of atrial signals by demand systems with a resultant failure to deliver therapy or competitive pacing and induction of atrial arrhythmias.

Ventricular Tachycardia

Ventricular tachycardia is a vexing arrhythmia yielding at times to electrical approaches when drugs fail, yet predisposing patients to serious risks of acceleration, either due to therapy or to failure of therapy. Electrical techniques have been reported to be successful in numerous patients, as shown in Table 32-7, although the results are less convincing than are the results for supraventricular tachycardias. The most common therapeutic methods reported were bursts of ventricular stimulation, either automatic or patient initiated, and cardioversion-defibrillation.

As expected, the major complication in these studies was acceleration of the tachycardias. Also noted were numbers of unexplained sudden deaths, events that could be expected as a matter of course with such patients but that also might have been precipitated by the implanted devices. Clearly the use of pacing or cardioversion techniques in patients with ventricular tachycardia must be preceded by very thorough patient studies, and even then there remains substantial risk for physiologic variation and consequent acceleration with this mode of therapy.

Ventricular Fibrillation

The final entry in Table 32-7 summarizes the substantial current clinical experience with the implantable defibrillator. This is the only available implantable device capa-

Table 32-7. Electrical Therapy for Ventricular Tachycardia and Fibrillation

Reference	No. of Patients	Device	Mode	MCL	EFF	MFU	Comments
Johnson, R., et al.[29]	11	Permanent pacemaker; conventional design	Chronic overdrive, rates of 70–110 ppm, AOO(5) AAI(1), and VVI(5)	150–250	0.73	15.6	Most successful if prepacing rate slow; Two patients died of recurrent VT, 1 of sudden death, cause unknown
Ruskin, J., et al.[72]	3	Permanent pacemaker; Medtronic 5998 RF	Patient-initiated asynchronous burst	N/A	1	13.6	All patients doing well
Hartzler, G., et al.[71]	9	Permanent pacemaker; Medtronic 5998 RF	Patient-initiated asynchronous burst	N/A	0.67	12	3 sudden deaths, none while using pacemaker
Dunnigan, A., et al.[73]	1	Permanent pacemaker; Medtronic 5998 TDA	Patient-initiated asynchronous burst, 200 ppm	500	1	6	No hospital or ER admissions since implant; 5 admissions in 4-mo period before
Fisher, J., et al.[75]	13	Permanent pacemaker; 2 Cordis BK/M 1 Cordis 234A 1 Medtronic 5985 5 Medtronic 5998 2 Medtronic 2404 2 Intermedics 262-01	Patient-initiated asynchronous bursts, 120–295 ppm Automatic fixed or adaptive bursts, 206–232 ppm	N/A	N/A	16.3 18	Only 2 patients required emergency admissions for VT following implant, 1 because transmitter failed
Falkoff, M., et al.[76]	2	Permanent pacemaker; Intermedics Cybertach	Automatic burst	N/A	1	30	Both patients doing well
den Dulk, K., et al.[94]	6	Permanent pacemaker; Medtronic SP500/501	Patient-initiated programmed extra stimuli 1–6 PES, scanned, fixed coupling, or adaptive	N/A	0.93	14.5	
Pratap Reddy, C., et al.[111]	1	Permanent pacemaker; Telectronics 4151	Automatic scanning of two extra stimuli	400	1	6	
Brachmann, J., et al.[112]	13	Permanent pacemaker; Medtronic SP500/501	Patient-initiated burst of 4–8 pulses with CL equal to 80% of tachycardia CL	436	1	8	Drugs used to minimize VT episodes and to slow rate
Steinbach, G., et al.[113]	6	Permanent pacemaker; Cordis Orthocor	Patient-initiated burst (200 ppm); underdrive 70–90 ppm; overdrive 155–170 ppm	N/A	0.50	20.8	Accelerations at 12 mo in 2 patients; loss of efficacy at 16 mo in 1

continued

Table 32-7. Electrical Therapy for Ventricular Tachycardia and Fibrillation *Continued*

Reference	No. of Patients	Device	Mode	MCL	EFF	MFU	Comments
Griffin, J., et al.[68]	52	Permanent pacemaker; Intermedics Cybertach	Automatic bursts	N/A	0.88	12.6	58% alive and well; 4 sudden deaths, cause unknown; 2 explants
Sowton, E., et al.[69]	9	Permanent pacemaker; Siemens Tachylog 651	Automatic bursts and 1–4 PES; (ventricular)	333	0.56	N/A	4 patients with advanced coronary disease died
Zipes, D., et al.[81]	7	Permanent cardioverter; Medtronic 7210	Single synchronous shock, mean energy of 0.43 J	448	0.71	3.4	Acceleration one time each in two patients
Mirowski, M., et al.[114]	276	Permanent Defibrillator Intec AID and AICD	Automatic 25–30-J shock	N/A	See comment	9.8	Kaplan-Meier actuarial analysis: 52% reduction in mortality in first year

EFF, measure of efficacy estimated by chapter author; MCL, mean cycle length of treated tachycardias (ms); MFU, mean length of follow-up study (mo).

ble of terminating ventricular fibrillation, and it faces no competing pharmacologic approach. The study report[114] does not indicate how many of the 276 patients received the device for its primary indication, ventricular fibrillation, rather than for ventricular tachycardia. Yet despite the uncertainty regarding the study patient population, the survival analysis, indicating a 52% reduction in the anticipated incidence of death during a 1-year period following implantation of the defibrillator, is impressive.

Major reported concerns regarding use of the defibrillator include perioperative and postoperative complications due to the extensive surgery associated with implantation, lead dislodgement and fracture, and false triggering of the defibrillatory shock. Although the device has accelerated ventricular tachycardias, it can deal with such accelerations by recognizing them *de novo* and terminating them with subsequent shocks.

There is no doubt that rapidly evolving refinements in implantable defibrillators will resolve these problems, making such devices an important therapeutic tool for the treatment of patients with malignant ventricular arrhythmias.

The Future

Electrical techniques will undoubtedly become a significant factor in the chronic control of cardiac tachyarrhythmias. Effective control of supraventricular tachycardias has been amply demonstrated, and wider acceptance is hampered mainly by weaknesses in the ability of current devices to distinguish between normal and pathologic rate increases, lack of suitably controlled studies directly comparing the quality of electrical control to that achieved pharmacologically, and a firmly entrenched traditional therapeutic approach. As newly sophisticated pacing systems are introduced, there are clear signs that problems associated with tachycardia identification will be solved.

Implantable cardioversion-defibrillation devices promise to offer a safe means for treating malignant ventricular arrhythmias. Electrical control of ventricular tachycardia can frequently be achieved quickly and painlessly with pacing techniques, but widespread use has been precluded by the aforementioned detection problem and the very real risk of disastrous rhythm accelerations rather than terminations. As it becomes possible to back up pacing techniques with defibrillation capabilities in acceptably small and easily implantable devices, many ventricular tachycardias will be effectively managed with electrical devices.

The most exciting opportunity is use of the implantable defibrillator for management of patients at risk of sudden death due to fibrillation. Pharmacology has not been a notable success in managing such patients, and the electrical approach seems to offer an acceptable alternative.

The device of the near future will be a pacing system capable of antibradycardia support, staged antitachycardia therapies, cardioversion, and back-up defibrillation. The system will include patient monitoring capability, enabling physicians to verify effective device operation and helping them to titrate associated drug regimens. Ideally such a system will be comparable in size to recent pacemakers and will use transvenous electrodes to simplify operative procedures. These requirements will necessitate finding ways to reduce the energy requirements for defibrillation. Methods for achieving this are already being tested in animals.[115]

Thorough physician education will be needed to ensure that appropriate patient evaluation precedes implantation of such systems. Skillful use of these devices can potentially reduce hospitalization time for tachyarrhythmia patients and could present a meaningful cost-reduction benefit in addition to therapeutic gains. The inclusion of noninvasive electrophysiologic test facilities in antiarrhythmic devices further reinforces such gains.

Without doubt, we are rapidly approaching the day when implantable electrical devices will be commonly accepted, not just as antibradycardia instruments, but as antiarrhythmic agents.

References

1. Kite, C.: The Recovery of the Apparently Dead. London, C. Dilly, 1788.
2. Duchenne, G.: De L'Electrisation Localisee et de son Application a la Pathologie et a la Therapeutique, 3rd ed. Paris, J. B. Bailliere, 1872.
3. Gaskell, W.: On the innervation of the heart with special reference to the heart of the tortoise. J. Physiol., 4:43, 1884.
4. Zoll, P. et al.: Ventricular fibrillation: Treatment and prevention by external electric currents. N. Engl. J. Med., 262:105, 1960.
5. Sowton, E. et al.: The suppression of arrhythmias by artificial pacemaking. Lancet, 2:1098, 1964.
6. Cohen, H. et al.: Treatment of supraventricular tachycardias with catheter and permanent pacemakers. Am. J. Cardiol., 20:735, 1967.
7. Massumi, R. et al.: Termination of reciprocating, tachycardia by atrial stimulation. Circulation, 36:637, 1967.
8. Haft, J. et al.: Termination of atrial flutter by rapid electrical pacing of the atrium. Am. J. Cardiol., 20:239, 1967.
9. Durrer, D. et al.: The role of premature beats in the initiation and the termination of supraventricular tachycardia in the Wolff-Parkinson-White syndrome. Circulation, 36:644, 1967.
10. Zipes, D. et al.: Use of a new antiarrhythmic physiologic pacemaker in a patient with debilitating atrial tachyarrhythmia. Proceedings of the Sixth World Symposium on Cardiac Pacing, Montreal, 27–5, 1979.
11. Rickards, A. et al.: The use of QT interval to determine pacing rate: Early clinical experience. Pace, 6:346, 1983.
12. Cammilli, L. et al.: Results, problems and perspectives with the autoregulating pacemaker. Pace, 6:488, 1983.
13. Rossi, P. et al.: Respiratory rate as a determinant of optimal pacing rate. Pace, 6:502, 1983.
14. Humen, D. et al.: A pacemaker which automatically increases its rate with physical activity. Proceedings of the Seventh World Symposium on Cardiac Pacing, Vienna, 259, 1983.
15. Haft, J.: Treatment of arrhythmias by intracardiac electrical stimulation. Prog. Cardiovasc. Dis., 16:539, 1974.
16. Wellens, H. et al.: Electrical management of arrhythmias with emphasis on the tachycardias. Am. J. Cardiol., 41:1025, 1978.
17. Wit, A. et al.: Slow conduction and re-entry in the ventricular conducting system. l. Return extrasystole in canine Purkinje fibers. Circ. Res., 30:1, 1972.
18. Gould, L. et al.: One monitored case of sudden death. Pace, 6:238, 1983.
19. Iesaka, Y. et al.: Bradycardia dependent ventricular tachycardia facilitated by myopotential inhibition of a VVI pacemaker. Pace, 5:23, 1982.
20. Coumal, P. et al.: Treatment of tachycardias by pacing. In Proceedings of the Fifth International Symposium on Cardiac Pacing, Tokyo, 1976.
21. Sutton, R. et al.: Electrophysiological and haemodynamic basis for application of new pacemaker technology in sick sinus syndrome and atrioventricular block. Br. Heart J., 41:600, 1979.
22. LeClercq, J. et al.: Prevention of intra-atrial reentry by chronic atrial pacing. Pace, 3:162, 1980.
23. Cohen, H. et al.: Tachycardias and electrical pacing. Med. Clin. North Am., 60:343, 1976.
24. Han, H. et al.: Temporal dispersion of recovery of excitability in atrium and ventricle as a function of heart rate. Am. Heart J., 71:481, 1966.
25. Han, J. et al.: Non-uniform recovery of excitability in ventricular muscle. Circ. Res., 14:44, 1964.
26. Hyman, A.: Permanent programmable pacemakers in the management of recurrent tachycardias. Pace 2:28, 1979.
27. Hyman, A. et al.: Ventricular pacing for overdrive suppression and conversion of ventricular tachycardias. Clin. Res., 25:5A, 1977.
28. Friedberg, C. et al.: Suppression of refractory recurrent ventricular tachycardia by transvenous rapid cardiac pacing and antiarrhythmic drugs. Am. Heart J., 79:44, 1970.
29. Johnson, R. et al.: Chronic overdrive pacing in the control of refractory ventricular arrhythmias. Ann. Intern. Med., 80:380, 1974.
30. Zipes, D. et al.: Treatment of ventricular arrhythmia by permanent atrial pacemaker and cardiac sympathectomy. Ann. Intern. Med., 68:591, 1968.
31. Zacouto, F. et al.: Prevention of ventricular tachycardias by automatic rate pacing. In Levy, S., and Raymond, G. (eds): Antiarrhythmic Agents and Cardiac Pacing. London, John Libbey, 1983, pp. 415–419.
32. Spurrell, R. et al.: Pacing techniques in the management of supraventricular tachycardias. II. J. Electrocardiol., 9:89, 1976.
33. Fields, J. et al.: Surgical experience with temporary and permanent AV sequential demand pacing. J. Thorac. Cardiovasc. Surg., 66:865, 1973.
34. Medina-Ravel, V. et al.: Follow-up of twenty-five patients with implantable antitachycardia DVI, MN pulse generators. Poster presented at the Seventh World Symposium on Cardiac Pacing, Vienna, 1983.
35. Curry, P. et al.: Dual-demand pacing for refractory atrioventricular re-entry tachycardia. Pace, 2:137, 1979.
36. Davidson, R. et al.: Electrically induced atrial tachycardia with block. Circulation, 44:1014, 1971.
37. Prystowsky, E. et al.: Inhibition in the human heart. Circulation, 68:707, 1983.
38. Zipes, D. et al.: Future directions: electrical therapy for cardiac tachyarrhythmias. Pace, 7:606, 1984.
39. Mehra, R. et al.: Dual ventricular stimulation for prevention of reentrant ventricular arrhythmias (Abstr.). J. Am. Coll. Cardiol., 3:472, 1984.
40. Sung, R. et al.: Complete abolition of the reentrant supraventricular tachycardia zone using a new modality of cardiac pacing with simultaneous atrioventricular stimulation. Am. J. Cardiol., 45:72, 1980.
41. Durrer, D. et al.: Role of premature beats in the initiation and termination of supraventricular tachycardias in the Wolff-Parkinson-White syndrome. Circulation, 36:644, 1967.
42. Hunt, N. et al.: Conversion of supraventricular tachycardias with

atrial stimulation: Evidence of re-entry mechanism. Circulation, 38:1060, 1968.
43. Barold, S. et al.: Supraventricular tachycardia initiated and terminated by a single electrical stimulus. Am. J. Cardiol., 24:37, 1969.
44. Wellens, H.: Electrical Stimulation of the Heart in the Study and Treatment of Tachycardias. Baltimore, University Park Press, 1971.
45. Ryan, G. et al.: Paradoxical use of a demand pacemaker; Treatment of a supraventricular tachycardia due to the Wolff-Parkinson-White syndrome—observations on termination of a reciprocal rhythm. Circulation, 38:1037, 1968.
46. Mugica, J. et al.: Termination of ventricular and supraventricular tachycardia by an implanted stimulator triggered by the patient himself. In Thalen, 4. (ed.): Proceedings of the Fourth International Symposium on Cardiac Pacing Gronigen, Assen, The Netherlands, VanGorcum, 1973.
47. Moss, A. et al.: Termination and inhibition of recurrent tachycardias by implanted pervenous pacemakers. Circulation, 50:942, 1974.
48. Preston, T. et al.: Permanent pacing of the left atrium for treatment of WPW tachycardia. Circulation, 42:1073, 1970.
49. Krikler, D. et al.: Dual demand pacing for reciprocating atrioventricular tachycardia. Br. Med. J., 1:1114, 1976.
50. Curry, P. et al.: Dual demand pacing for refractory re-entry atrioventricular tachycardias. Br. Heart J., 39:348, 1977.
51. Rowland, E. et al.: Dual demand pacing in patients with refractory paroxysmal reentry atrioventricular tachycardia. Proceedings from the First European Symposium on Cardiac Pacing, London, 1978.
52. Berkovits, B. et al.: Double demand sequential pacing for the termination of paroxysmal reentry tachyarrhythmias. Proceedings from the Sixth World Symposium on Cardiac Pacing: 6–21,1979.
53. DeSanctis, R.: Comments to termination and inhibition of recurrent tachycardias by implanted pervenous pacemakers. Circulation, 50:947, 1974.
54. Abinader, E.: Recurrent supraventricular tachycardia: Success and subsequent failure of termination by implanted pervenous pacemaker. J. A. M. A., 236:2203, 1968.
55. Lister, J. et al.: Treatment of supraventricular tachycardias by rapid atrial stimulation. Circulation, 38:1044, 1968.
56. Lister, J. et al.: Rapid atrial stimulation in the treatment of supraventricular tachycardia. Chest, 63:995, 1973.
57. Iwa, T. et al.: Treatment of tachycardia by atrial pacing. Jpn. Circ. J., 38:82, 1974.
58. Kahn, A. et al.: Patient-initiated rapid atrial pacing to manage supraventricular tachycardia. Am. J. Cardiol., 38:200, 1976.
59. Waxman, M. et al.: Self-conversion of supraventricular tachycardia by rapid atrial pacing. Pace, 1:35, 1978.
60. Peters, R. et al.: Radiofrequency-triggered pacemakers: Uses and limitations. Ann. Intern. Med. 88:17, 1978.
61. Jenkins, J. et al.: Panel I: Present state of industrial development of devices. Pace, 7:557, 1984.
62. den Dulk, K. et al.: A versatile pacemaker system for termination of tachycardias. Am. J. Cardiol., 52:731, 1983.
63. Lister, J.: A new technology: Patient-triggered pacemakers. Ann. Intern. Med., 88:120, 1978.
64. Neumann, G. et al.: Therapie Supraventrikularer Reentry-Tachykardien durch Implantation bedarfsgesteuerter Overdrive-Schrittmacher. Herz, 9:714, 1977.
65. Zipes, D. et al.: Initial experience with Symbios model 7008 pacemaker. Pace, 7:1301, 1984.
66. Spurrell, R. et al.: Clinical experience with implantable scanning tachycardia reversion pacemakers. Pace, 7:1296, 1984.
67. Griffin, J. et al.: The treatment of ventricular tachycardia using an automatic tachycardia terminating pacemaker. Pace, 4:582, 1981.
68. Griffin, J. et al.: The management of paroxysmal tachycardias using the Cybertach-60. Pace, 7:1291, 1984.
69. Sowton, E.: Clinical results with the tachylog antitachycardia pacemaker. Pace, 7:1313, 1984.
70. Fisher, J. et al.: Termination of ventricular tachycardia with bursts of rapid ventricular pacing. Am. J. Cardiol., 41:94, 1978.
71. Hartzler, G. et al.: Patient activated transvenous cardiac stimulation for the treatment of supraventricular and ventricular tachycardia. Am. J. Cardiol., 47:903, 1981.
72. Ruskin, J. et al.: Permanent radiofrequency ventricular pacing for the management of drug resistant ventricular tachycardia. Am. J. Cardiol., 46:317, 1980.
73. Dunnigan, A. et al.: A patient-activated radio frequency pacemaker system: Therapy for recurrent ventricular tachycardia. J. Pediatr., 101:403, 1982.
74. Rothman, M. et al.: Clinical results with Omni-Orthocor, an implantable antitachycardia pacing system. Pace, 7:1306, 1984.
75. Fisher, J. et al.: Role of implantable pacemakers in control of recurrent ventricular tachycardia. Am. J. Cardiol., 49:194, 1982.
76. Falkoff, M. et al.: Implantable multiprogrammable automatic burst tachycardia-terminating pacemakers for refractory ventricular tachycardia: A 2.5 Year Follow-up. Abstract. Pace, 6:A-137, 1983.
77. Fisher, J. et al.: The sparkling joules of internal cardiac stimulation: Cardioversion, defibrillation, and ablation. Am. Heart J. 104:177, 1982.
78. Naccarelli, G. et al.: Influence of tachycardia cycle length and antiarrhythmic drugs on pacing termination and acceleration of ventricular tachycardia. Am. Heart J., 105:1, 1983.
79. Jackman, W. et al.: Low energy synchronous cardioversion of ventricular tachycardia using a catheter electrode in a canine model of subacute myocardial infarction. Circulation, 66:187, 1982.
80. Zipes, D. et al.: Clinical transvenous cardioversion of recurrent life-threatening ventricular tachyarrhythmias: Low energy synchronized cardioversion of ventricular tachycardia and termination of ventricular fibrillation in patients using a catheter electrode. Am. Heart J., 103:789, 1982.
81. Zipes, D. et al.: Early experience with an implantable cardioverter. N. Engl. J. Med., 311:485, 1984.
82. Mirowski, M. et al.: The automatic implantable cardioverter-defibrillator. Pace, 7:534, 1984.
83. Zipes, D. et al.: Synchronized low energy transvenous cardioversion. Proceedings of the Seventh World Symposium on Cardiac Pacing, Vienna, 1983.
84. Benditt, D. et al.: Cardioversion of atrial tachyarrhythmias by low-energy transvenous technique. Proceedings of the Seventh World Symposium on Cardiac Pacing, Vienna, 1983.
85. Mirowski, M. et al.: The development of the transvenous automatic defibrillator. Arch. Intern. Med., 129:773, 1972.
86. Mirowski, M. et al.: A chronically implanted system for automatic defibrillation in active conscious dogs: Experimental model for treatment of sudden death from ventricular fibrillation. Circulation, 58:90, 1978.
87. Mower, M. et al.: Automatic implantable cardioverter-defibrillator structural characteristics. Pace, 7:1331, 1984.
88. Echt, D.: Potential hazards of implanted devices for the electrical control of tachyarrhythmias. Pace, 7:580, 1984.
89. Lerman, B. et al.: Tachyarrhythmias associated with programmable automatic atrial antitachycardia pacemakers. Am. Heart J. 106:1029, 1983.
90. German, L. et al.: Electrical termination of tachyarrhythmias with discrete pulses. Pace, 7:514, 1984.

91. Reid, P. et al.: Pathophysiology of ventricular tachyarrhythmias amenable to electrical control. Pace, 7:505, 1984.
92. Horowitz, L. et al.: Selection of patients with recurrance of ventricular tachyarrhythmias for electrical studies. Pace, 7:499, 1984.
93. Brugada, P. et al.: Standard diagnostic programmed electrical stimulation protocols in patients with paroxysmal recurrent tachycardias. Pace, 7:1121, 1984.
94. den Dulk, K. et al.: Clinical experience with implantable devices for control of tachyarrhythmias. Pace, 7:548, 1984.
95. Zipes, D. et al.: The contribution of artificial pacemaking to understanding the pathogenesis of arrhythmias. Am. J. Cardiol., 28:211, 1971.
96. Haft, J.: Treatment of arrhythmias by intracardiac electrical stimulation. Prog. Cardiovasc. Dis., 16:539, 1974.
97. Pittman, D. et al.: Rapid atrial stimulation: Successful method of conversion of atrial flutter and atrial tachycardia. Am. J. Cardiol., 32:700, 1973.
98. Waldo, A. et al.: Relevance of electrograms and transient entrainment for antitachycardia devices. Pace, 7:588, 1984.
99. Das, G. et al.: Atrial pacing for cardioversion of atrial flutter in digitalized patients. Am. J. Cardiol., 41:308, 1978.
100. Waldo, A. et al.: Entrainment and interruption of atrial flutter with atrial pacing. Circulation, 56:737, 1977.
101. Wyndham, C. et al.: Self-initiated conversion of paroxysmal atrial flutter utilizing a radio-frequency pacemaker. Am. J. Cardiol., 41:1119, 1978.
102. Mandel, W. et al.: Recurrent reciprocating tachycardias in the Wolff-Parkinson-White syndrome. Control by use of a scanning pacemaker. Chest., 69:769, 1976.
103. Neumann, G. et al.: A new atrial demand pacemaker for the management of supraventricular tachycardias. Preceedings of the Sixth World Symposium on Cardiac Pacing, 1979.
104. Ringqvist, I. et al.: Long-term control of reciprocating paroxysmal tachycardia by ventricular pacing in a case of Wolff-Parkinson-White syndrome. Br. Heart J., 47:609, 1982.
105. Fruehan, C. et al.: Refractory paroxysmal supraventricular tachycardia. Am. Heart J., 87:229, 1974.
106. Iwa, T.: Surgery of supraventricular tachycardia. II. Electrical treatment of supraventricular tachycardias with implanted radiofrequency atrial pacemaker. Jpn. Circ. J., 42:294, 1978.
107. Preston, T. et al.: Permanent rapid atrial pacing to control supraventricular tachycardia. Pace, 2:331, 1979.
108. Vohra, J. et al.: Patient initiated implantable pacemakers for paroxysmal supraventricular tachycardia. Aust. N. Z. J. Med., 11:27, 1981.
109. Spurrell, R. et al.: Implantable automatic scanning pacemaker for termination of supraventricular tachycardia. Am. J. Cardiol., 49:753, 1982.
110. Scheibelhofer, W. et al.: Treatment of tachyarrhythmias by implantable devices: Patient activated pacemaker. Proceedings of the Seventh World Symposium on Cardiac Pacing, Vienna, 1983.
111. Pratap, R. et al.: Treatment of ventricular tachycardia using an automatic scanning extrastimulus pacemaker. J. Am. Coll. Cardiol., 3:225, 1984.
112. Brachmann, J. et al.: Combined treatment with patient-activated adaptive burst pacing and antiarrhythmic drugs in patients with recurrent sustained ventricular tachycardia (abstr.). Circulation, 70 (Suppl. II):810, 1984.
113. Steinbach, G. et al.: Treatment of ventricular tachyarrhythmias—pacing. Proceedings of the Seventh World Symposium on Cardiac Pacing, Vienna, 1983.
114. Mirowski, M. et al.: Clinical performance of the implantable cardioverter-defibrillator. Pace, 7:1345, 1984.
115. Zipes, D. et al.: Efficacy of sequential electrical shocks to terminate ventricular fibrillation in dogs after myocardial infarction (abstr.). Circulation, 70 (Suppl. II):407, 1984.

33

Nonpharmacologic Alternatives in the Management of Patients with Refractory Supraventricular Tachyarrhythmias Not Related to Preexcitation

Eli S. Gang

Most patients with supraventricular tachyarrhythmias that require therapeutic intervention are readily treatable with pharmacologic agents. Recent advances in clinical electrophysiology have facilitated selecting an antiarrhythmic agent in patients with tachycardias capable of being initiated in the electrophysiology laboratory.[1] Furthermore, new pharmacologic agents such as amiodarone have further enhanced the clinician's ability to deal with even the most troublesome of supraventricular arrhythmias.[2,3] Nonetheless, occasional patients who suffer from recurrent, troublesome supraventricular tachyarrhythmias unrelated to a preexcitation syndrome are either refractory to or unable to take pharmacologic agents. In such patients, nonpharmacologic alternatives must be considered. This chapter will review recent advances in the therapeutic modalities currently available to such patients. Specifically, advances in permanent electronic pacing, direct surgical approaches, and catheter ablation of the His bundle will be examined.

Permanent Pacemaker Therapy

Use of permanent pacemakers in the therapy of patients with medically refractory supraventricular tachycardias requires a knowledge of the electrophysiologic mechanism responsible for the initiation and perpetuation of the tachycardia as well as careful documentation in the clinical electrophysiology laboratory of the efficacy of a particular mode of pacing. Although permanent pacing is clearly inappropriate in the therapy of patients with some supraventricular tachyarrhythmias, for example, atrial fibrillation, other tachyarrhythmias are quite amenable to this form of therapy. For example, patient-activated radiofrequency pacemakers can be useful in providing atrial overdrive pacing to terminate AV nodal reentrant tachycardia or reentrant tachycardia using a concealed bypass tract.[4] Presumably, the tachycardia is terminated when paced impulses penetrate the reentrant pathway; although a single impulse may not penetrate a reentrant pathway, a series of impulses may shorten refractoriness of atrial tissue sufficiently to allow penetration and interruption of the reentrant circuit. Scanning pacemakers are also capable of automatically providing bursts of atrial pacing to terminate paroxysmal supraventricular tachyarrhythmias (Fig. 33-1).[5,6]

Patient-activated and scanning pacemakers that are meant to function as tachycardia-*terminating* devices are unrealistic therapeutic modalities in patients with incessant tachycardias. In such patients, tachycardia-

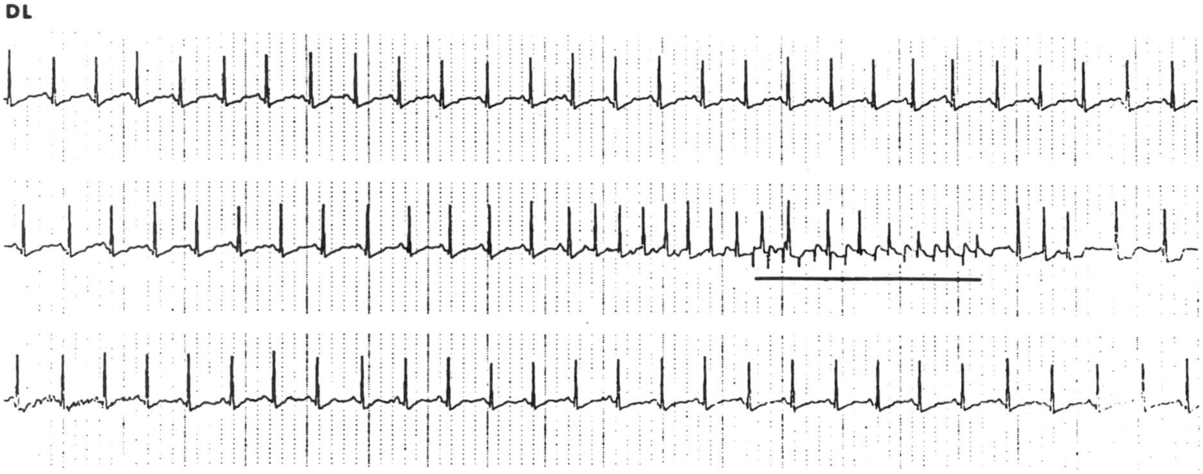

Figure 33-1. *Automatic sensing and termination of a supraventricular tachycardia (SVT). The three tracings are taken from a 24-hour Holter recording in a patient with an implanted atrial pacemaker (Cybertech-60, Intermedics). Normal sinus rhythm is recorded in the top tracing. The middle tracing shows the spontaneous onset of an SVT followed by 4 seconds of rapid atrial pacing (240 beats/min) marked by the heavy bar. The SVT is terminated, and normal sinus rhythm is restored. (Griffin, J. C., Mason, J. W., and Calfee, R. V.: Clinical use of an implantable automatic tachycardia-terminating pacemaker. Am. Heart J., 100:1093–1096, 1980)*

preventing pacemakers have been used. For example, DDT pacemakers, which provide simultaneous (or near-simultaneous) stimulation of atria and ventricles, have been shown to prevent the initiation of a sustained AV junctional reentrant tachycardia, probably by causing impulse collision in both the fast and the slow pathways incorporated in the reentrant circuit.[7,8] Permanent pacing has also been performed in a patient with a drug-resistant automatic tachycardia.[9] Previously automatic rhythms have been defined, in part, as rhythms that are not capable of being terminated or initiated by impulses delivered by an extrinsic pacemaker. In the case described by Arbel and associates,[9] a patient aged 17 years with a congestive cardiomyopathy and a persistent, drug-resistant, automatic atrial tachycardia received a permanent pacemaker that provided coupled atrial stimulation to the right atrium. In this pacing modality, impulses from the ectopic pacemaker are sensed by the atrial sensing electrode and trigger the electronic pacemaker to deliver a stimulus to the atrium at a coupling interval shorter than the effective refractory period of the AV node but longer than the effective refractory period of the paced atrium. As illustrated in Figure 33-2, the paced impulse depolarizes and resets the automatic ectopic pacemaker, thereby slowing the ventricular rate without actually terminating the tachycardia.

Permanent pacemaker therapy is, of course, not without its limitations; these include the risk of inducing atrial fibrillation or flutter as well as ventricular tachyarrhythmias in patients with dual chamber pacing. Simultaneous AV pacing of the type described above also results in the loss of atrial contribution to ventricular filling; the extent to which this hemodynamic effect is tolerated must be assessed in each patient considered for this form of pacing. In addition, patient-activated pacemakers require an alert and intelligent patient to activate them; clearly, patients who suffer significant hemodynamic deterioration during their tachycardias are not suitable for this form of pacing. (For further discussion of antitachycardia pacemakers, see Chapter 32.)

Surgical Alternatives

The surgical therapy of tachycardias related to the various preexcitation syndromes is discussed in Chapter 34. For patients with poorly responsive supraventricular tachyarrhythmias not related to preexcitation and for whom pacemaker therapy is inappropriate, three surgical methods have been devised: (1) interruption of AV conduction by destruction or transection of the AV node–His bundle conduction pathway, (2) excision or ablation of an arrhythmogenic region in the atria, and (3) surgical exclusion of an atrial arrhythmogenic area.[10–22]

Interruption of Atrioventricular Conduction

Of the three surgical approaches, interruption of AV conduction has been the most frequently employed technique.[10–16] This type of surgery has been performed

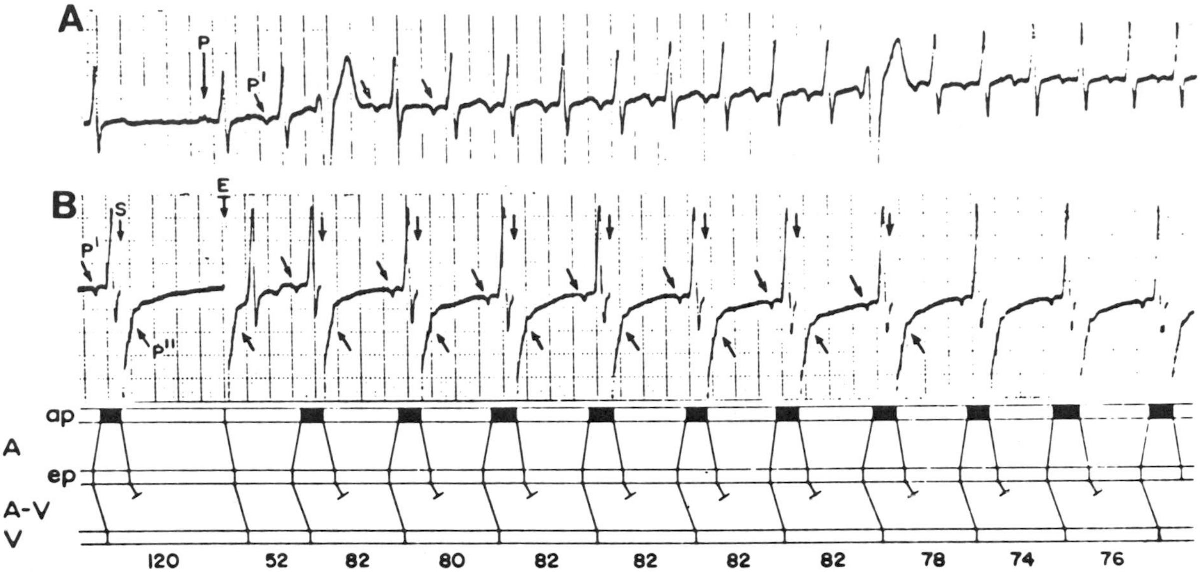

Figure 33-2. *Permanent coupled atrial pacing in a patient with a drug-resistant, automatic supraventricular tachycardia. (A) Normal sinus rhythm (P wave) followed by a run of sustained supraventricular tachycardia, each QRS complex preceded by an inverted P wave (P′). Occasional ventricular premature beats are recorded. (B) Electrocardiogram and ladder diagram illustrating ventricular slowing by the artificial pacemaker (ap). Each QRS complex contains three arrows. The first arrow shows ectopic atrial depolarization (ep) propagating to the ventricle but also triggering a coupled atrial stimulus (S), occurring after a delay of 180 msec and marked by the second arrow. The resultant atrial response depolarizes and resets the ectopic pacemaker but is blocked at the AV junction, which is still refractory (third arrow). The first ventricular complex in this panel was followed by a pause that was terminated by an escape (E) impulse generated by the atrial pacemaker at an interval of 910 msec. The ventricular rate is displayed at the bottom of the diagram; numbers are in 0.01 second. (Arbel, E. R., Cohen, H. C., Lagendorf, R., and Glick, G.: Successful treatment of drug-resistant atrial tachycardia and intractable congestive heart failure with permanent couple atrial pacing. Am. J. Cardiol., 41:336–340, 1978)*

in patients with a variety of supraventricular tachyarrhythmias, namely, patients with known Kent bundles in whom division of the pathway was unsuccessful or inadvisable; patients with drug-resistant atrial fibrillation or flutter and a rapid ventricular response; patients with an ectopic atrial pacemaking focus; patients with paroxysmal tachycardia secondary to reentry within the AV node; patients with a junctional ectopic pacemaker.

Surgical techniques for interrupting AV conduction have included suture ligation, electrocauterization, simple surgical transection, and cryoablation of the AV node–His bundle region.[12,13] Intraoperative localization of the His bundle can be performed by recording the characteristic His bundle electrogram using a hand-held probe (Fig. 33-3). Sealy advises that the incision be made across the floor of the right atrium, anterior to the os of the coronary sinus and above the tricuspid anulus.[11] The surgeon should also divide the right side of the atrial septum at its insertion into the right fibrous trigone. This approach is designed to interrupt AV conduction at the junction of the common bundle of His and the AV node, thereby preserving most of the His bundle and permitting the emergence of a stable junctional rhythm. Demand electronic pacemakers are nonetheless implanted in all patients at operation.

Currently the preferred method for interrupting impulse conduction in the AV conduction system is by cryoablation of the AV node and upper portion of the bundle of His.[10,11,14–16] Mapping of the His bundle is performed, and the area producing the most prominent His deflection is then cooled with a cryoprobe (approximately 0.5 cm in diameter) to approximately 0°C for 30 seconds. Complete temporary heart block is thereby produced, which is easily reversible with rewarming. If this test cooling does not produce satisfactory AV block, the area is mapped again for a yet greater His bundle deflection preceded by a prominent atrial deflection. When satisfactory AV block is achieved, irreversible ablation is produced by cooling the area to −60°C for 2 to 3 minutes. One or two additional freeze lesions may be produced several millimeters proximal to the first lesion and nearer to the coronary sinus. Crysosurgical ablation

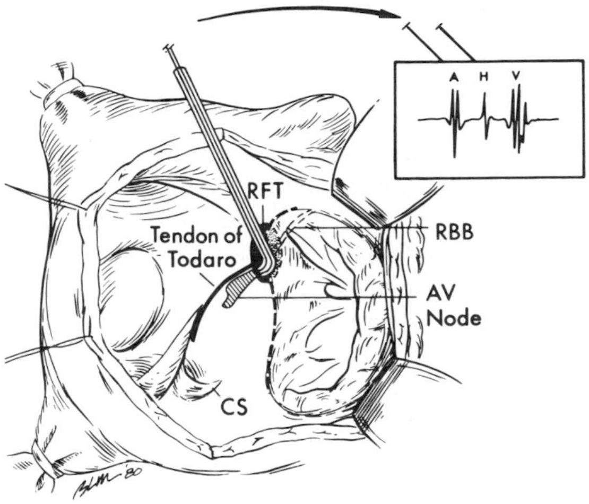

Figure 33-3. *Intraoperative localization of the His bundle. A hand-held probe electrode is positioned over the His bundle. The inset illustrates a prominent His bundle deflection on a His bundle electrogram. The dotted line shows the site of incision for interruption of AV conduction. When cryosurgery is performed, the cryoprobe is placed in the same position as the probe. (RFT, right fibrous trigone; RBB, right bundle branch; CS, coronary sinus) (Sealy, W. C.: When is surgery indicated for control of supraventricular tachycardia? Am. J. Surg., 145:711–717, 1983)*

of AV conduction offers several advantages over other surgical methods: first, it is reversible, so that permanent damage is not done to atrial structures until conduction has been definitely interrupted; second, the "ice balls" produced by cryosurgery are small (approximately 1 cm in diameter), discrete, and not arrhythmogenic; finally, these lesions do not rupture nor do they form aneurysms.[15]

Surgical Dissection, Ablation, or Excision of Arrhythmogenic Areas in the Atria

A surgical approach directed specifically at arrhythmogenic atrial foci has become a viable therapeutic alternative in recent years thanks in large measure to the experience gained by clinical electrophysiologists in the techniques of intraoperative and electrode catheter mapping. Precise localization of macroreentrant or microreentrant circuits as well as of automatic atrial foci has enabled the cardiologist to direct the surgeon to the atrial site that requires surgical excision, section, or cryoablation.

A surgical approach has been described in a small number of patients with AV junctional reentrant tachycardia in whom the tachycardia was surgically abolished but anterograde AV conduction was either unaffected or only slightly modified.[16,17,18] In the first case report, the cure of the tachycardia was, in fact, fortuitous, inasmuch as the surgical goal had been to produce complete AV block using the dissection and mapping techniques described above. Postoperatively, however, the patient maintained AV conduction (albeit with a slightly prolonged PR interval) and was free of tachycardia. Presumably, conduction in one of the limbs of the AV nodal reentrant circuit was sufficiently damaged by the operative dissection to prevent subsequent reentry within the AV node. In the second patient,[17] careful preoperative and intraoperative endocardial mapping showed earliest right atrial activation during right ventricular pacing to be low in the interatrial septum, anterior to the ostium of the coronary sinus. Selective atriotomy abolished ventriculoatrial conduction while preserving antegrade conduction (again, with slight PR interval prolongation). These preliminary results suggest that partial or total interruption of an AV nodal reentrant circuit at its atrionodal junction may be possible in selected patients.

A similar surgical approach was prospectively evaluated by Ross and his colleagues in a series of 10 patients with troublesome AV junctional reciprocating tachycardia.[18] At the preoperative electrophysiologic study, these patients were divided into two groups: those with a VA interval of 40 msec or less (7 patients) were designated as type A, and those with a VA interval greater than 40 msec as type B. All 7 type A patients demonstrated earliest atrial activation during tachycardia in the His bundle lead; in 6 of 7 patients earliest atrial activation occurred prior to or at the onset of the QRS complex, suggesting short conduction time in the retrograde limb of the tachycardia. In contrast, earliest atrial activation in 2 of the 3 type B patients was recorded at the proximal region of the coronary sinus. Intraoperative endocardial mapping performed during tachycardia (8 patients) or ventricular pacing (2 patients) confirmed the preoperative observations in that earliest atrial activation recorded in type A patients was *anterior* or anteromedial to the AV node, whereas in those with type B tachycardia earliest atrial activation was *posterior* to the AV node, near the orifice of the coronary sinus (Fig. 33-4). Surgery in these patients included (1) exposure of the wall of the left atrium, AV nodal artery, central fibrous body, and tendon of Todara; (2) dissection of the medial and anteromedial approaches to the AV node in type A patients—the posterior approaches to the AV node were preserved in this group of patients; and (3) dissection of the inferior wall of the coronary sinus with preservation of the medial approaches to the AV node in type B patients. At a mean postoperative follow-up of 8 months, no recurrences of the tachycardia had occurred. Anterograde AV conduction was normal (albeit with a slightly longer AH interval) in all patients; conduction over the anterograde "slow" pathway was abolished in 5. In addition, retrograde VA conduction was preserved in the type A patients, although a prolongation of the retrograde His to

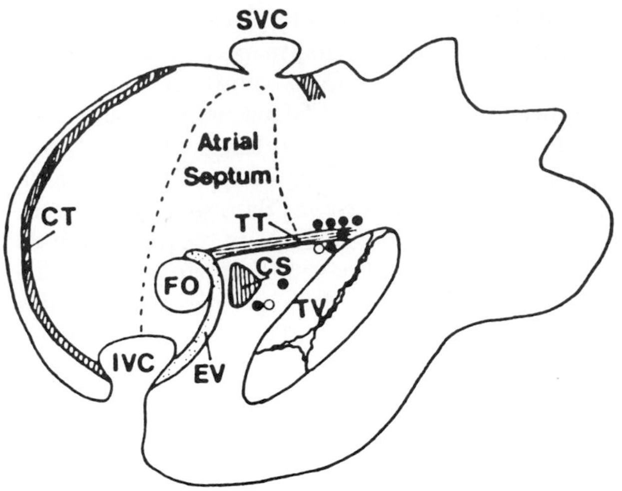

Figure 33-4. *Earliest atrial activation sites obtained with right atrial endocardial intraoperative mapping. The black dots represent earliest atrial activation during tachycardia, and the unfilled circles represent earliest activation during ventricular pacing in two patients without inducible SVT in the operating room. Earliest atrial sites from the type A patients were clustered at a site anterior or anteromedial to the AV node, whereas in the 3 type B patients earliest atrial activation was clustered near the coronary sinus. CS, coronary sinus; CT, crista terminalis; EV, eustachian valve; FO, foramen ovale; IVC, inferior vena cava; SVC, superior vena cava; TT, tendon of Todaro; TV, tricuspid valve. (Ross, D. L., Johnson, D. C., Denniss, R., et al.: Curative surgery for atrioventricular junctional [AV nodal] reentrant tachycardia. J. Am. Coll. Cardiol., 6:1383–1392, 1985.)*

atrium interval was documented in 4 of 7 patients. In contrast, VA conduction was interrupted in 2 of 3 type B patients and significantly modified in the third.

The encouraging results of these preliminary reports portend a possible curative surgical option to patients with troublesome AV junctional reciprocating tachycardia. Most importantly, and in contrast with surgical *interruption* of AV conduction, this surgical approach does *not* necessitate the implantation of a permanent ventricular pacemaker.

Recently, successful surgical excision or ablation of atrial tissue responsible for medically refractory atrial tachycardia has been performed.[19–21] Gillette and coworkers reported treatment of three children with automatic, ectopic atrial tachycardias.[19] The diagnosis of "automatic" tachycardia was based on conventional clinical electrophysiologic definitions that included inability to initiate or terminate the tachycardia with programmed electrical stimulation, "resetting" of the tachycardia following atrial premature extrastimuli, and observation of a "warm-up" phenomenon at the onset of a paroxysm of the tachycardia. Preoperative and intraoperative mapping localized two of these tachycardias to the left atrium and one to the right atrial appendage. The left atrial foci were ablated with endocardial and epicardial application of a cryoprobe during cardiopulmonary bypass; the right atrial tachycardia was cured with excision of the anterior one third of the right atrial appendage and cryoablation of the surgical margins. Cardiopulmonary bypass was not needed during the surgery performed on the right atrial tachycardia.[19]

Wyndham and associates[20] reported the surgical treatment of a patient with drug-resistant atrial tachycardia that appeared to be reentrant in mechanism in that induction and termination of the tachycardia could reliably be performed in the electrophysiology laboratory. Endocardial and epicardial mapping performed in the operating room localized the site of origin of the atrial tachycardia to the posterolateral lip of the right atrial appendage. This region was excised, and the atrial tachycardia was no longer inducible. Interestingly, microelectrode studies of the atrial tissue removed during surgery demonstrated a low resting membrane potential and, following the application of electrical stimuli, delayed afterhyperpolarization followed by delayed afterdepolarization. The latter was large enough to attain threshold and produced a sustained rhythm that was terminated with electrical stimuli.[20] This may have been the first clinical observation of triggered automaticity in humans and points to the difficulty of assigning an electrophysiologic mechanism to a tachycardia based on response to programmed electrical stimulation.

Still another example of surgical excision of an atrial tachycardia (probably automatic in mechanism) was reported by Josephson and his colleagues.[21] The site of origin of this tachycardia was at the posterior lip of the fossa ovalis (Fig. 33-5) and necessitated resection of part of the atrial septum as well as placement of a Dacron patch. Interestingly, the excised tissue contained a proliferation of mesenchymal cells, suggesting that a mesenchymal atrial tumor may have been responsible for the clinical tachycardia.

Resectable atrial tachycardias may also arise from sites of previous cardiac surgery. We have recently performed intraoperative epicardial mapping in a patient of 60 years referred because of drug-refractory, recurrent supraventricular tachycardia. Twenty-five years before the current hospital admission the patient had undergone repair of an atrial septal defect. The patient's poor response to all available antiarrhythmic medications, including amiodarone, coupled with the demonstration of a moderate-sized septal defect, prompted surgical intervention. Intraoperative epicardial mapping during the patient's atrial tachycardia (Fig. 33-6) suggested a macroreentrant circuit around the superior vena cava. Unidirectional conduction block appeared to occur at the lateral margin of the right atrium, immediately adjacent to the earliest site of atrial activation during tachycardia, and corresponded to the site of extensive scarring from the previous atriotomy. Cryoablation was performed at

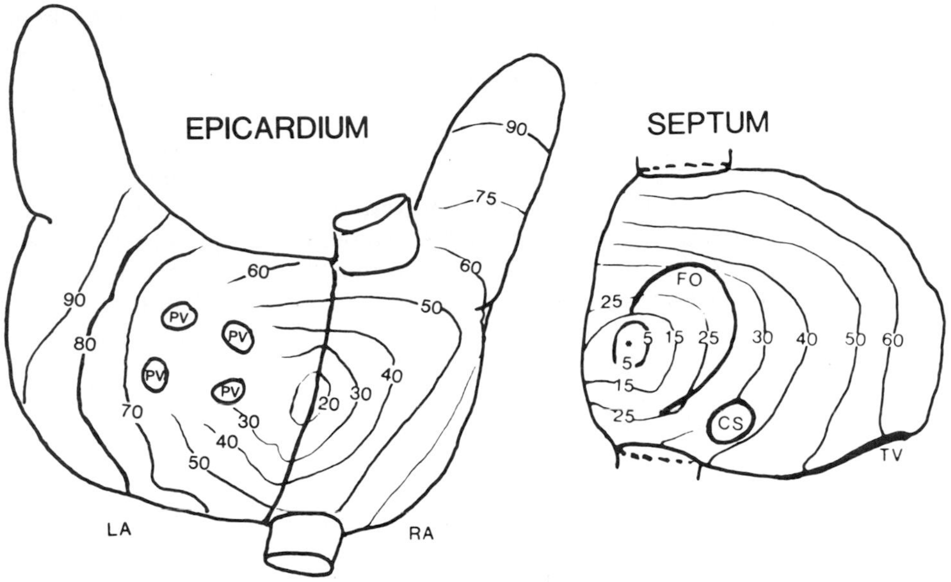

Figure 33-5. *Diagrammatic representation of the catheter technique of His bundle ablation. See text for explanation. (CS, coronary sinus; FO, fossa ovalis; LA, left atrium; PV, pulmonary veins; RA, right atrium; TV, tricuspid valve) (Josephson, M. E., Spear, J. F., Harken, A. H., et al.: Surgical excision of automatic atrial tachycardia. Am. Heart J., 104:1076, 1982.)*

the sites of earliest and latest atrial activation. Postoperatively the patient has had no recurrences of the atrial tachycardia, although episodes of atrial fibrillation have been recorded.

Surgical Exclusion of Atrial Tachycardia

Atrial tachyarrhythmias are occasionally encountered located in parts of the atria that are not resectable (*e.g.*, the left atrium near one of the pulmonary veins). Work performed by Williams and colleagues[22] in dogs suggests that the left atrium can be safely excluded surgically. While the left atrium is thereby electrically isolated from the rest of the heart (and remains either electrically silent or develops a slow intrinsic rhythm), normal AV conduction is maintained from the right atrium and no adverse hemodynamic effects are associated with loss of a synchronous left atrial contraction.

These experimental surgical principles were recently applied by Anderson and associates[23] to a patient with a paroxysmal atrial tachycardia localized to the junction of the right superior pulmonary vein and left atrium. Surgical isolation of the portion of the left atrium containing the point of earliest atrial activation and both right pulmonary veins was done by an encircling incision, with the edges then being reapproximated. Postoperatively the patient had a sinus rhythm (sinus tachycardia) with 1 : 1 AV conduction, while the isolated left

Figure 33-6. *Epicardial activation map obtained during atrial tachycardia showing a posterior unfolded view of the atria. Local epicardial activation times are shown in milliseconds. Earliest epicardial activation was 10 msec before activation of the right atrial reference electrode and was located at the posterolateral right atrium. Unidirectional block appears to occur at the recording sites caudal to the earliest site; atrial activation follows the clockwise sequence shown. Extensive atrial scarring from previous surgery was noted along the lateral margin of the right atrium. (PV, pulmonary veins; SVC, superior vena cava; IVC, inferior vena cava)*

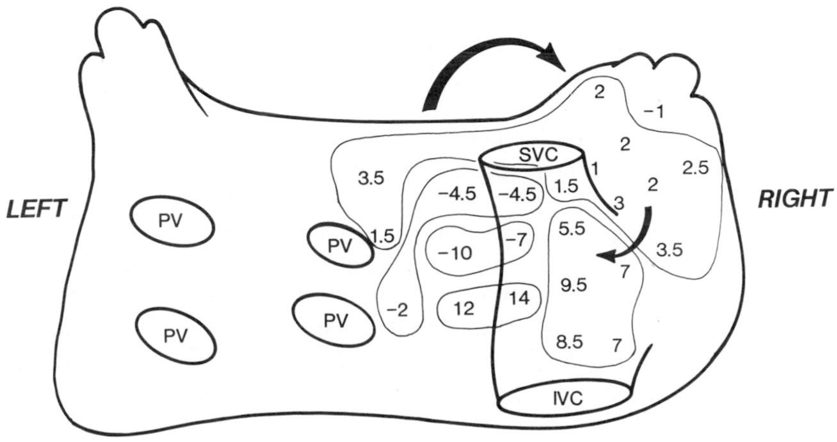

atrial tissue had a slow, independent rate that was not conducted to the right atrium or to the ventricles.

Experimental animal work has suggested that surgical exclusion of the sinus node region and a small area of surrounding tissue can be safely performed, with the postoperative emergence of a stable and reliable low right atrial pacemaker. This pacemaker, however, only becomes dominant when in contact with a large amount of right atrial tissue.[24,25] Confirmation and application of this work to humans remains to be performed.

Catheter Ablation of Atrioventricular Conduction

A recent development in clinical electrophysiology has been the introduction of closed-chest electrode catheter ablation of the AV conduction system. This technique was developed in the experimental dog laboratory by Gonzalez and colleagues, who showed that heart block can be readily induced by passing an electric current (average energy level of 35 J) through a catheter electrode positioned in the His bundle recording site.[26] Clinical application of this technique followed,[27–29] and several groups described their experience in performing closed-chest catheter ablation of the His bundle in patients with medically refractory supraventricular tachycardia. Other groups have reported a similar experience in small numbers of patients with medically refractory supraventricular tachycardia. In these studies the following technique was used: A temporary pacing wire is positioned in the apex of the right ventricle to provide demand pacing should it be required following delivery of the shock. A standard His bundle catheter is then positioned in the region of His and unipolar His bundle electrograms obtained from each lead. The catheter electrode showing the largest His deflection accompanied by the longest HV interval and an atrial electrogram amplitude of at least 0.25 mV is then connected to the cathodal output of a standard cardioversion unit. The anodal output of the cardioverter is connected to a back paddle positioned near the left scapula. The patient is then sedated and, with a stable and large His bundle deflection still evident, the chosen electrode is switched from the recording mode to the cardioversion unit. R wave synchronous countershock is then performed with a minimum of 200 J. Scheinman and colleagues recommend a higher energy shock (400 J) and have found that an additional shock is needed to maintain complete AV block.[27] A junctional escape rhythm usually emerges following the successful ablation of the proximal bundle of His. Permanent transvenous (AV sequential) pacemakers are implanted in all patients before hospital discharge.

Clinical electrophysiologists have found uses for this catheter ablative technique that extend beyond mere interruption of AV conduction. Specifically, the technique has been applied to infants with junctional automatic ectopic tachycardia,[30] children with ectopic right atrial tachycardia,[31,32] and in ablating posteroseptal accessory pathways in patients with the Wolff-Parkinson-White syndrome[33] and in a patient with "permanent" junctional reciprocating tachycardia.[34] The technique appears to be safe when performed by experienced invasive electrophysiologists. The following caveats must be borne in mind, however, when contemplating the performance of this procedure:

1. Inaccurate positioning of the catheter may result in atrial or ventricular injury, which might serve as a focus for future atrial or ventricular arrhythmias.
2. Malpositioning of the catheter might also cause a right bundle branch block *without* interrupting normal AV conduction if the catheter position is too distal.[28]
3. Patients must, of course, be aware that they may become pacemaker dependent (with all attendant risks) following ablation of the His bundle.
4. Sufficient energy must be delivered to ensure permanent heart block. Suboptimal delivery of energy may result in temporary or partial conduction disturbances.[28]

Finally, when this technique is applied to the coronary sinus, ablative procedures should be limited to the region of the *orifice* of the coronary sinus, since rupture of this structure may ensue; the potential of damage to an epicardial coronary artery in the proximity of the mid- or distal coronary sinus might also preclude the application of electric shocks to that region.[35] These caveats notwithstanding, this new catheter technique appears to carry with it an exciting nonsurgical approach to the therapy of patients with intractable supraventricular tachyarrhythmias.

Still another catheter technique for interrupting AV conduction has recently been introduced. This technique employs laser technology in the transection of the His bundle.[36] To date, it has been tried in anesthetized dogs, in which an argon laser fiber was fluoroscopically positioned near an electrode catheter recording a His bundle potential. A short burst of argon laser is reported to have caused a lesion 0.3 mm deep, completely transecting the His bundle. The clinical relevance of these experiments is likely to be determined in the next several years.

Conclusion

Significant advances have been made in recent years in the treatment of patients with refractory supraventricular tachycardias. Until new and more effective antiarrhythmic drugs become available, the therapeutic alternatives described in this chapter, namely, pacemaker therapy, direct surgical approaches, and catheter ablation, must be carefully considered in patients with disabling tachyarrhythmias.

References

1. Bauernfeind, R. A., Wyndham, C. R., Dhingra, R. C., et al.: Serial electrophysiologic testing of multiple drugs in patients with atrioventricular nodal reentrant paroxysmal tachycardia. Circulation, 62:1341-1349, 1980.
2. Marcus, F. I., Fontaine, G. H., Frank, R., and Grosgoeat, Y.: Clinical pharmacology and therapeutic applications of the antiarrhythmic agent, amiodarone. Am. Heart J., 101:480-493, 1981.
3. Haffajee, C. I., Love, J. C., Canada, A. T., et al.: Clinical pharmacokinetics and efficacy of amiodarone for refractory tachyarrhythmias. Circulation, 67:1347-1355, 1983.
4. Peters, R. W., Shafton, E., Frank, S., et al.: Radiofrequency-triggered pacemakers: Uses and limitations. Ann. Intern. Med., 88:17-11, 1978.
5. Griffin, J. C., Mason, J. W., and Calfee, R. V.: Clincial use of an implantable automatic tachycardia-terminating pacemaker. Am Heart J., 100:1093-1096, 1980.
6. Mandel, W. J., Laks, M. M., Yamaguchi, I., et al.: Control of recurrent reciprocating tachycardia in the Wolf-Parkinson-White syndrome by use of a scanning pacemaker. Chest, 69:769-774, 1976.
7. Sung, R. J., Styperefe, J. L., and Castellanos, A.: Complete abolition of reentrant supraventricular tachycardia zone using a new modality of cardiac pacing with simultaneous atrioventricular stimulation. Am. J. Cariol., 45:72-78, 1980.
8. Portillo, B., Medina-Ravell, V., Portillo-Leon, N., et al.: Treatment of drug resistant AV reciprocating tachycardias with multiprogrammable dual demand AV sequential (DVI, MN) pacemakers. Pace, 5:814-825, 1982.
9. Arbel, E. R., Cohen, H. C., Langendorf, R., and Glick, G.: Successful treatment of drug-resistant atrial tachycardia and intractable congestive heart failure with permanent couplet atrial pacing. Am. J. Cardiol. 41:336-340, 1978.
10. Sealy, W. C, Gallagher, J. J., and Kasell, J.: His bundle interruption for control of inappropriate ventricular responses to atrial arrhythmias. Ann. Thorac. Surg., 32:429-439, 1981.
11. Sealy, W. C.: When is surgery indicated for control of supraventricular tachycardia? Am. J. Surg., 145:711-717, 1983.
12. Garcia, R., and Arciniegas, E.: Recurrent atrial flutter: Treatment with a surgically induced atrioventricular block and ventricular pacing. Arch. Intern. Med., 132:754, 1973.
13. Gooch, A. S., Jan, M. A., Fernandez, J., et al.: Uncontrolled tachycardia in atrial fibrillation. Management by surgical ligature of AV bundle and pacemaker. Ann. Thorac. Surg., 17:181, 1974.
14. Harrison, L., Gallagher, J. J., Kasell, J., et al.: Cryosurgical ablation of the AV node-His bundle, a new method for producing AV block. Circulation, 55:463, 1977.
15. Klein, G. J., Sealy, W. C., Pritchett, E. L. C., et al.: Cryosurgical ablation of the atrioventricular node-His bundle: Long-term follow-up and properties of the junctional pacemaker. Circulation, 61:8, 1980.
16. Pritchett, E. L. C., Anderson, R. W., Benditt, D. G., et al.: Reentry within the atrioventricular node: Surgical cure with the atrioventricular conduction. Circulation, 60:440, 1979.
17. Marquez-Montes, J., Rufilanchas, J. J., Esteve, J. J., et al.: Paroxysmal nodal reentrant tachycardia, surgical cure. Chest, 83:690, 1983.
18. Ross, D. L., Johnson, D. C., Denniss, R., et al.: Curative surgery for atrioventricular junctional (AV nodal) reentrant tachycardia. J. Am. Coll. Cardiol., 6:1383-1392, 1985.
19. Gillette, P. C., Garson, A., Hesslein, P. S., et al.: Successful surgical treatment of atrial, junctional and ventricular tachycardia unassociated with accessory connections in infants and children. Am. Heart J., 102:984, 1981.
20. Wyndham, C. R. C., Arnsdorf, M. F., Levitsky, S., et al.: Successful surgical excision of focal paroxysmal atrial tachycardia, observations *in vivo* and *in vitro*. Circulation, 62, 1365, 1980.
21. Josephson, M. E., Spear, J. F., Harken, A. H., et al.: Surgical excision of automatic atrial tachycardia. Am. Heart J., 104:1076, 1982.
22. Williams, J. M., Ungerleider, R. M., Lofland, G. K., et al.: Left atrial isolation, new technique for the treatment of supraventricular arrhythmias. J. Thorac. Cardiovasc. Surg., 80:373, 1980.
23. Anderson, K. P., Stinson, E. B., and Mason, J. W.: Surgical exclusion of focal paroxysmal atrial tachycardia. Am. J. Cardiol., 49:869, 1982.
24. Sealy, W. C., and Seaber, A. V.: Cardiac rhythm following exclusion the sinoatrial node and most of the right atrium form the remainder of the heart. J. Thorac. Cardiovasc. Surg., 77:436, 1979.
25. Sealy, W. C., and Seaber, A. V.: Surgical isolation of the atrial septum from the atria: Identification of an atrial septal pacemaker. J. Thorac. Cardiovasc. Surg., 80:742, 1980.
26. Gonzalez, R., Scheinman, M., Margaretten, W., and Rubinstein, M.: Closed-chest electrode-catheter technique for His bundle ablation in dogs. Am. J. Physiol., 241:H283, 1981.
27. Scheinman, M. M., Morady, F., Hess, D. S., and Gonzalez, R.: Catheter-induced oblation of the atrioventricular junction to control refractory supraventricular arrhythmias. J. A. M. A., 248:851, 1982.
28. Gallagher, J. J., Suenson, R. H., Kasell, J. H., et al.: Catheter technique for a closed-chest ablation of the atrioventricular conduction system: A therapeutic alternative for the treatment of refractory supraventricular tachycardia. N. Engl. J. Med., 306:194, 1982.
29. Wood, D. L., Hammill, S. C., Homes D. R., et al.: Catheter ablation of the atrioventricular conduction system in patients with supraventricular tachycardia. Mayo Clin. Proc., 58:791, 1983.
30. Gillette, P. C., Garson, A., Porter C. J., et al.: Junctional automatic ectopic tachycardia: New proposed treatment by transcatheter His bundle oblation. Am. Heart J., 106:619, 1983.
31. Silka, M. J., Gillette, P. C., Garson, A., and Zinner, A.: Transvenous catheter ablation of a right atrial automatic ectopic tachycardia. J. Am. Coll. Cardiol., 5:999-1001, 1985.
32. Gillette, P. C., Wampler, D. G., and Garson, A.: Treatment of atrial automatic tachycardia by ablation procedures. J. Am. Coll. Cardiol., 6:405-409, 1985.
33. Morady, F., and Scheinman, M. M.: Transvenous catheter oblation of a posteroseptal accessory pathway in a patient with the Wolff-Parkinson-White syndrome. N. Engl. J. Med., 310:705, 1984.
34. Gang, E. S., Oseran, D., Rosenthal, M., et al.: Closed chest catheter ablation of an accessory pathway in a patient with permanent junctional reciprocating tachycardia. J. Am. Coll. Cardiol., 6:1167-1171, 1985.
35. Fisher, J. D., Brodman, R., Kim, S. G., et al.: Attempted nonsurgical electrical ablation of accessory pathways via the coronary sinus in the Wolff-Parkinson-White syndrome. J. Am. Coll. Cardiol., 4:685-694, 1984.
36. Narula, O. S., Bharati, S., Chan, M. C., et al.: Laser micro transection of the His bundle: A pervenous catheter technique (abstr). J. Am. Coll. Cardiol., 3:537, 1984.

34

The Wolff-Parkinson-White Syndrome: Surgical Management

Guy Fontaine, Gérard Guiraudon, Robert Frank, Christian Cabrol, and Yves Grosgogeat

Historical Background

The electrocardiographic syndrome first described by Wolff, Parkinson, and White in 1930[1] included a short PR interval and a QRS complex widened by a slurred upstroke or delta wave. These changes were found in young people prone to attacks of paroxysmal tachycardia. Thereafter, other related syndromes were described such as the association of a delta wave with a normal PR interval and a short PR interval with a normal QRS, first reported in 1938 by Clerc and associates[2] but better known as the Lown-Ganong-Levine syndrome (1952).[3]

These syndromes intrigued cardiologists from the outset. However, their exact mechanism was a mystery, with Scherf and Cohen (1964)[4] finding no fewer than 60 theories on their pathogenesis, some bordering on the fanciful.

We now know that a unique intracardiac conduction phenomenon is responsible for these syndromes, and the characteristics of this conduction phenomenon have been progressively defined. Modern clinical electrophysiologic methods using exploratory endocavitary catheters and techniques described by Scherlag and coworkers in 1969[5] and, later, epicardial mapping[6] have brought about great advances in our comprehension of these syndromes. This progress has allowed the recent development of a radical method of managing the Wolff-Parkinson-White (WPW) syndrome by surgery. The good results obtained in the majority of cases confirm unequivocally the underlying nature of the abnormality. It is interesting to review the main theories from the beginning to see how, over the years, our ideas have changed to the modern conception of this illness.

The presence of an accessory bundle has always been the most widely accepted theory. This theory was put forward in 1932 by Holzmann and Scherf[7] and intimated the existence of muscular fibers passing directly from the atrium to the ventricle. This accessory bundle was supplementary to the physiologic nodo-Hisian pathway. Not having the physiologic properties of slowing the excitation that characterizes the AV node, this bundle activated the ventricles before the normal AV conduction pathways, hence the name *preexcitation*[8] (a more widely used term than the WPW syndrome, as will be seen). The accessory pathway theory was mainly based on the work of Stanley Kent,[9] whose findings were later criticized by James.[10]

Another hypothesis, put forward by Holzmann and Scherf,[7] was that of a hyperexcitable septal focus. According to this theory, an abnormally excitable zone in the septum initiated depolarization when synchronized

This work was supported in part by grants from la Caisse Régionale d'Assurances Maladie de Paris (C.R.A.M.P.), l'Association de Recherche et d'Entraide Cardiologique et Angéiologique (A.R.E.C.A.), and la Délégation Générale à la Recherche Scientifique et Technique (D.G.R.S.T.), Grant No. 76-7-1409.

with atrial contraction. Even to its authors, this theory appeared unlikely to be true.

Prinzmetal and co-workers (1952) put forward a theory of accelerated conduction,[11] which was based on abnormal AV conduction through the physiologic pathways. The physiologic slowing effect was supressed by an abnormality of these pathways, thus causing the short PR interval. However, a longitudinal arrangement of the AV conduction pathways would be necessary for the group of fibers involved in the abnormal accelerated excitation to only activate part of the ventricular myocardium.

The results of histologic analysis were not univocally in favor of the accessory pathway theory. Although it had been possible to demonstrate abnormal conduction pathways in humans, as reported by Wood and colleagues in 1943,[12] there was no evidence to show that they were functional. Also, other histologic reports had been unable to demonstrate the same abnormal AV pathways when the WPW syndrome was obvious electrocardiographically. The probable cause of the confusion at this time was the small number of cases studied and the long and fastidious histologic technique involved in the study of the totality of the two AV rings.

Important experimental research was carried out by Butterworth and Poindexter[13] in 1942. They demonstrated the consequences of abnormal AV conduction in the cat with artificial preexcitation. An electrical circuit was constructed whereby the potentials of atrial depolarization were conducted, after electronic amplification, to the ventricle. A fusion complex was recorded on the surface electrocardiogram that resembled a delta wave, the amplitude of which varied with the precocity of the ventricular depolarization obtained with respect to the normally activated ventricular myocardium.

In a second study published in 1944,[14] the same authors inverted the atrial and ventricular electrodes so that the ventricular potentials were amplified and conducted to the atrium. With this set-up, they managed to initiate a self-sustaining tachycardia at a rate of 300 beats/min by creating a circus movement through the nodo-Hisian pathways anterogradely and through the ventricle and amplifier system retrogradely.

The 12-lead electrocardiographic changes of the WPW syndrome show important variations in the direction and amplitude of the delta wave. In 1945, Rosenbaum and co-workers[15] suggested classifying them into two groups, A and B, according to the morphology of the QRS complexes in the right precordial leads. However, a study of a large number of cases has shown that there are many intermediary forms.

Above all, in a remarkable clinical series, Durrer's group in Amsterdam in 1967[16] demonstrated the initiation and termination of paroxysmal tachycardia by properly timed atrial and ventricular electrical stimulation techniques with exploratory endocavitary catheters. This study suggested that the presence of reentry phenomena between the atrium and ventricle involving the accessory pathway was the basis of certain paroxysmal tachycardias in the WPW syndrome. It also showed that arrhythmias arising in the AV node could be another possible mechanism.

In the same year, Durrer and Roos[17] performed epicardial mapping in a patient with type B WPW syndrome and demonstrated an epicardial area situated at the junction of the right border and the right interventricular groove that was activated before the rest of the free wall of that ventricle.

The first surgical operation was performed in the same year by Burchell and co-workers.[18] They also demonstrated the origin of the abnormal activation in a case of type B WPW syndrome in a zone near to that observed by Durrer. In addition, they showed that pressure with a soft object or an injection of 1% procaine at the zone of preexcitation made the delta wave disappear. However, an attempt to section the pathway was only temporarily effective.

In 1968, Dreifus and co-workers[19] reported the first case in which deliberate section of the bundle of His successfully prevented recurrence of paroxysmal tachycardia with narrow QRS complexes that had been resistant to all medical therapy in a patient with the WPW syndrome. This case was evidence in favor of a circular pathway between the atrium and ventricle through the bundle of His and demonstrated that surgical section was capable of preventing the recurrence of attacks.

It was at Duke University in 1968[20] that the first surgical section of an accessory right anterior AV pathway in a type B WPW syndrome was performed, causing the delta wave to disappear and preventing further attacks of tachycardia. Following this, the abnormal types of AV conduction in the WPW syndrome and related syndromes were fully studied by more and more detailed electrophysiologic investigations using premature stimulus,[21] His bundle recording,[17-22] and coronary sinus pacing[23] techniques.

Boineau and Moore in 1970[24] first established the correlation between the results of electrophysiologic and histologic investigations in a dog with the WPW syndrome. An attack of atrial fibrillation was conducted to the ventricle by the abnormal pathway, thus triggering ventricular fibrillation. Epicardial mapping localized the origin of the abnormal activation, and histologic analysis of the area of preexcitation showed abnormal muscular fibers crossing the pericardial fat in the atrioventricular groove, linking the atrium directly to the ventricle (Fig. 34-1). This observation was confirmed by the same authors the following year[25] in a monkey with both right and left lateral preexcitation pathways.

At present, the theory of the accessory pathway seems

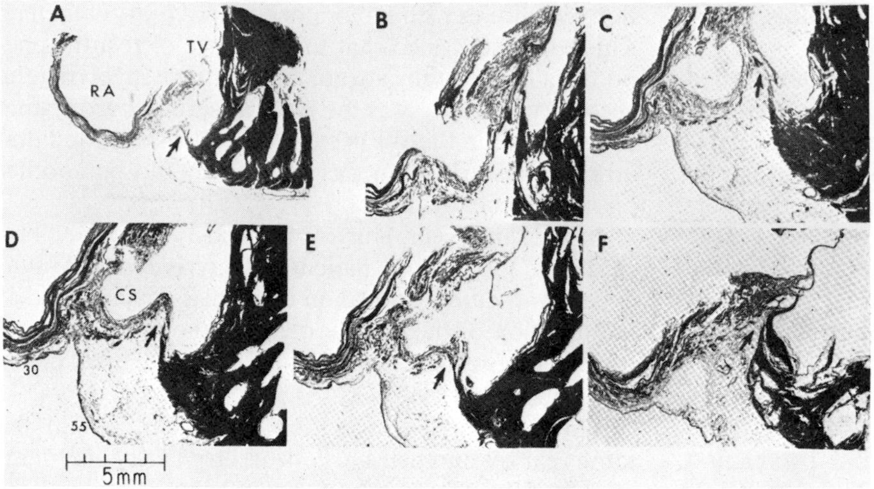

Figure 34-1. *First histologic documentation demonstrating an anatomic basis for preexcitation in a dog with type A Wolff-Parkinson-White syndrome localized by epicardial mapping. (Boineau, J. P., and Moore, E. N.: Evidence for propagation of activation across an accessory atrio-ventricular connection in types A and B pre-excitation. Circulation, 41:375, 1978. By permission of the American Heart Association, Inc.)*

to be the best explanation of this condition, and although some points still remain obscure, it forms the basis for the rest of this chapter. Somewhat contradictory results have since been published by several groups.[26-30] However, nowadays, combined medical and surgical teams, well trained in epicardial mapping, seem to have specialized in this new therapeutic approach, which increasingly demands practical knowledge of electronic and computer techniques.

The Histologic Basis of Ventricular Preexcitation Syndromes

The atria and ventricles are excitable myocardial entities separated by the fibrous tissue of the AV rings anchored to the central fibrous body and the membranous part of the interventricular septum (see Chap. 2). The only means of conduction of atrial depolarization is through the nodo-Hisian system, which is therefore the only normal activation pathway. This unique anatomic arrangement develops progressively in the embryo.[31] At birth and during the first months of life, the development of the fibrous AV rings disrupts the muscular fibers that, until then, pass quite freely from the atrium to the ventricle. If some of these fibers survive the development of the fibrous rings and are capable of conducting the depolarization, they will constitute accessory AV conduction pathways. They have been found in all regions around the rings (including the septum) except in the zone between the base of the aorta and the insertion of the anterior mitral leaflet, which seems to form a natural barrier.

Apart from these direct abnormal AV pathways, an exchange of abnormal fibers may also occur between the nodo-Hisian pathway and the nonspecific atrial or ventricular myocardium. A bridge may also cause tachycardia and should be recognized and fully explored during a correction or preoperative electrophysiologic investigation. The different types of accessory pathways may be classified anatomically as follows.[32]

Lateral Pathways

The lateral pathways are commonly called the *bundles of Kent.* They are direct AV pathways made up of muscular fibers that connect the free wall of the left or right ventricle to the adjacent atrial myocardium across the AV groove. They may cross the AV ring subendocardially or subepicardially, or they may fan out from the atrium over the shoulder of the ventricular myocardium (Fig. 34-2).[33] These pathways may be solitary or multiple and may spread over several centimeters.[34] This is an important point because of the electrophysiologic and surgical implications. The pathways may also be bilateral.[35] Sometimes the pathway may follow a long oblique course with respect to the AV ring, thus explaining the unusual electrophysiologic characteristics observed in these cases.[36]

Septal Pathways

Septal pathways are special types of Kent fibers directly connecting the atrium to the ventricle and passing through the central fibrous body without joining the bundle of His.[37] They may be isolated or may be associated with lateral AV accessory pathways.[38]

Atrio-His Pathways

The fibers of the atrio-His pathways were first described in 1974 by Brechenmacher and co-workers.[34] A similar anatomic arrangement had previously been reported by Lev,[39] but in his case, the pathway was associated with a large bundle of Mahaim fibers, which may have been responsible for the delta wave. They are often incorrectly

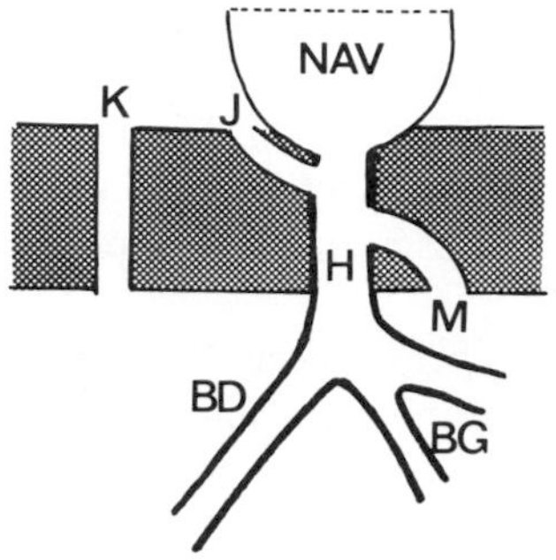

Figure 34-2. *Normal and accessory atrioventricular pathways. (NAV, atrioventricular node; K, Kent bundle; M, Mahaim fibers; H, His bundle; BD, right branch; BG, left branch)*

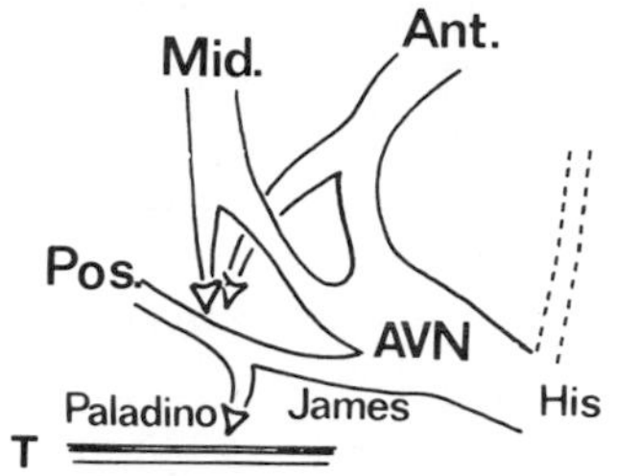

Figure 34-3. *Normal AV node, prolongating the anterior, middle, and posterior internodal atrial tracts, the latter giving normal "James fibers" and Paladino fibers. An abnormal atrio-Hisian bypass is shown by the* dotted lines. *(T, tricuspid anulus)*

referred to as the *fibers of James* (see below) and connect the atrial myocardium to the bundle of His. Therefore, the whole AV node is short-circuited. The electrocardiographic changes consist of a short PR interval with a normal QRS complex. This may also be interpreted as preexcitation of the bundle of His.

Nodoventricular and Fasciculoventricular Pathways

In 1941, Mahaim and Winston[40] described fibers branching off the penetrating part of the bundle of His to enter the upper part of the interventricular septum. These fibers, which are present normally, were thought to be part of the paraspecific septal conduction system. Since that time, however, the definition of the Mahaim fibers has been widened to include bundles passing from the inferior part of the AV node, which is therefore partially short-circuited, to the adjacent ventricular myocardium. They may be responsible for some cases of preexcitation with a delta wave and a normal PR interval.[41] However, a strict histologic and electrophysiologic correlation has not yet been established.

Paranodal Pathways

The normal anatomic connections between structures around the atrial pole of the AV node (Fig. 34-3) were suspected of acting as short-circuits in some cases.

In 1961, James[42] described fibers arising from the posterior internodal bundle joining fibers from the middle and anterior bundles and then uniting at the inferior part of the AV node. These fibers are correctly known as the *James fibers;* they are present in *all normal hearts* and do not give rise to preexcitation phenomena. A second bundle disappears over the base of the tricuspid valve and is known as the *bundle of Paladino.*[43] It was thought that these two pathways could give rise to preexcitation phenomena. The bundle of Paladino could form a circuit with the crest of the interventricular septum, or, as Scherf and James[44] proposed, the excitation crossing the inferior part of AV node could be conducted without delay directly through a bundle of fibers to preexcite the dependent zone of ventricular myocardium. This theory implied a longitudinal dissociation of the fibers of the bundle of His. Because abnormalities of ventricular depolarization have never been demonstrated by right atrial pacing in varying regions,[45] this theory seems unlikely to be true. Also, preexcitation would spread to the whole ventricular myocardium from the areas activated the earliest by the abnormal pathways. This is contrary to what is observed during electrophysiologic studies and epicardial mapping, which always show ventricular preexcitation originating at the base of the heart at the AV rings.

Other investigators[46] have suggested that branches of the posterior internodal bundle could extend from the inferior part of the atrioventricular node to bundle of His. This type of atrio-Hisian short circuit has also been incorrectly called the *James fibers.*

Histologic and electrophysiologic studies and epicardial mapping have shown the existence of accessory lateral septal and atrio-Hisian pathways. The electrophysiologic role of nodoventricular and fasciculoventricular conduction pathways in tachycardia in the WPW syndrome, apparently demonstrated in some cases,[47] merits further study.[36]

Preoperative Localization of Abnormal Pathways

Reciprocating Tachycardia Involving the Preexcitation Pathways

Electrocardiography

Preexcitation of an area of myocardium by an accessory AV conduction pathway gives rise to a fusion complex producing the delta wave. Its amplitude and direction on the electrocardiogram and vectorcardiogram (VCG) depend, among other things, on the anatomic location of the area of preexcitation around the AV rings.

Rosenbaum and co-workers[15] classified the electrocardiographic abnormalities in WPW syndrome into groups A and B according to the dominant polarity of the R wave in the precordial leads V_1 and V_2:

1. Type A is characterized by a positive or predominantly positive R wave.
2. Type B is characterized by an S, QS, or an intermediary waveform.

Rosenbaum concluded that in type A, the activation arose at the base of the ventricles and spread in a posteroanterior direction.

Puech,[48] in unipolar endocavitary studies, localized the preexcitation more precisely by investigating the delta wave rather than the whole of the QRS complex. Later, orientation of the delta wave in the frontal plane was studied to define the origin of the preexcitation.[49] However, it was only with the development of epicardial mapping that really precise topographic definition became possible because the origin of the abnormal activation could then be proved.

The delta wave, measured 40 msec after its beginning in average cases of preexcitation, can be classified in the horizontal plane of the electrocardiograms.

The origin of the abnormal activation may be located in one of four main areas situated along the left and right AV grooves and, on the one hand, corresponding to the free walls of the two ventricles and, on the other, to the two points of insertion of the interventricular septum above and anteriorly at the base of the great vessels and below and posteriorly at the crossing of the posterior interventricular and AV grooves (Fig. 34-4). These two points of insertion of the septum may activate the right or left ventricles preferentially, thus giving six locations of preexcitation.[50]

An even more detailed classification has been proposed by Gallagher,[51] distinguishing right lateral from right anterior preexcitation and left posterior from left lateral preexcitation.

It must be emphasized, however, that the electrocardiogram only gives a first approximation of the location of ventricular preexcitation and that there are limits to the deductions that can be made[50]:

1. They are only valid when, apart from preexcitation, the heart is normal, that is, free from activation problems, whether they be congenital (Ebstein's anomaly) or intramyocardial conduction defects, and, above all, free from ventricular hypertrophy. In addition, it must have a normal position in the thorax.
2. Analysis of delta wave direction on electrocardiogram, VCG, and even chest wall isopotential mapping cannot give exact information on the start of an abnormal intraseptal activation.
3. The presence of several preexcitation pathways, especially when at a distance from each other, is another cause of uncertainty.[50]

Echocardiography

Echocardiography is a recently developed method of studying parietal movement and myocardial contrac-

	I	II	III	R	L	F	1	2	3	4	5	6
1	+	−	−	−	+	−	a ± b ∓	+	+	+	+	+
2	+	+	−	−	+	+	−	+	+	+	+	+
3	+	+	+	−	±	+	− +?	+	+	+	+	+
4	−	+	+	−	−	+	+	+	+	+	+	−

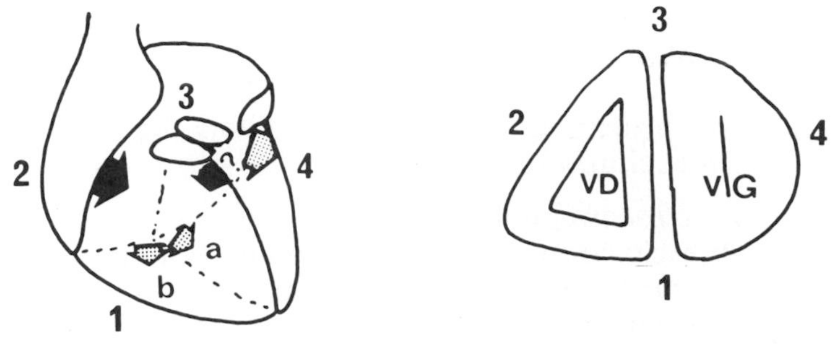

Figure 34-4. *Localization of Kent bundle according to delta vector orientation. From the frontal plan, four broad localizations may be made: (1) posterior paraseptal (right or left, according to the horizontal directions of delta wave; negative or positive in lead V_1); (2) right anterior; (3) anterior paraseptal (right or left, according to the horizontal direction of the delta wave); and (4) left lateral. (The first topographic localization was made by Boineau, J. P., et al.: In Dreifus, L. S., and Likoff, W. (eds.): Cardiac Arrhythmias, p. 421. New York, Grune & Stratton, 1973)*

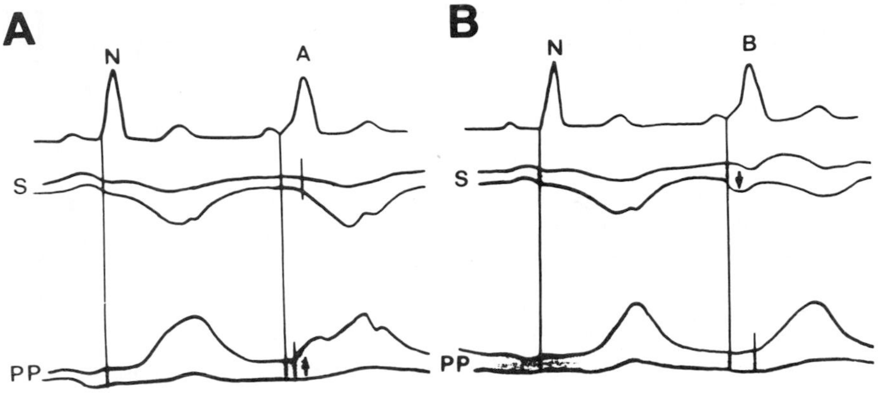

Figure 34-5. *Typical patterns of echocardiogram in preexcitation. (A) Wolff-Parkinson-White syndrome, type A: precontraction of the posterior wall of the left ventricle (PP). (B) Wolff-Parkinson-White syndrome, type B: septal precontraction (S).*

tion, and it is particularly well suited for the study of the posterior and lateral walls of the left ventricle and also of the septum in the basal region. Echocardiography has demonstrated that preexcitation corresponds to a phenomenon of ventricular pre*contraction,* and it is therefore a more direct way of localizing abnormal pathways than is the electrocardiogram. The analysis of the echocardiogram is performed in two stages, one involving morphology and the other chronology.

Morphology. The following criteria distinguish left-sided from right-sided preexcitation:

1. In left ventricular preexcitation (Fig. 34-5*A*), the echo of the endocardium of the left ventricular posterior wall exhibits an abnormal anterior movement[52] that is synchronous with the beginning of the delta wave. In some cases, this movement has two components.

   This early anterior movement seems to be specific to the WPW syndrome. The only other situation in which it occurs is when the left ventricle is paced by an endocavitary catheter positioned in the coronary sinus. It regresses simultaneously with the delta wave after the intravenous administration of a drug that blocks conduction through the accessory pathway. As a rule, the morphology of septal contraction is normal.
2. In right ventricular preexcitation (Fig. 34-5*B*), an abnormal movement of the interventricular septum is observed: the septum moves posteriorly toward the posterior wall,[53] followed by an anterior mid-systolic and another posterior end-systolic movement. This movement is similar to that observed in cases of complete left bundle branch block and disappears on pharmacologic blocking of the accessory pathway.

Chronology. The chronologic variations give some idea of the location of the area of precontraction with respect to the septum.[54,55] This is based on the study of the sequence of septal and posterior wall contraction with respect to the delta wave. In left lateral preexcitation, the beginning of septal contraction is chronologically normal; on the other hand, in left paraseptal preexcitation, the septal contraction is moderately premature, and in right posterior paraseptal preexcitation, precontraction of both posterior wall and septum may be observed.

Electrophysiologic Studies

Electrophysiologic studies with unipolar, bipolar, or multipolar endocavitary catheters combine the recording of endocavitary potentials with special techniques of atrial and ventricular pacing. These pacing techniques are carried out by electronic devices capable of programmed pacing, that is, emitting an extra stimulus of prearranged prematurity every 8 to 12 beats of the basal pacing rate. These extra stimuli can also be delivered during spontaneous sinus rhythm[16] or even during paroxysmal tachycardia, during which important information concerning the nature and the role of the accessory pathway can be obtained. The presence of an abnormal conduction pathway must be determined beforehand.[56]

The interval between the His bundle potential and the onset of ventricular depolarization is defined as the earliest potential recorded in three leads, leads I, AVF, and V_1, positioned at roughly right angles to one another. In ventricular preexcitation, the His bundle potential appears after the onset of ventricular depolarization, that is, after the delta wave (Fig. 34-6).

To understand what follows, it is important to bear in mind that the dynamic properties of AV conduction through the nodo-Hisian system and the accessory pathway are very different[21,57,58]: the accessory pathway is muscular tissue that conducts rapidly and without delay; in contrast, the conduction times through the nodo-Hisian system are physiologically delayed, and this becomes more pronounced when the pacing rate or the prematurity of the extrastimulus is increased. As a result, the His bundle potential during progressively faster atrial

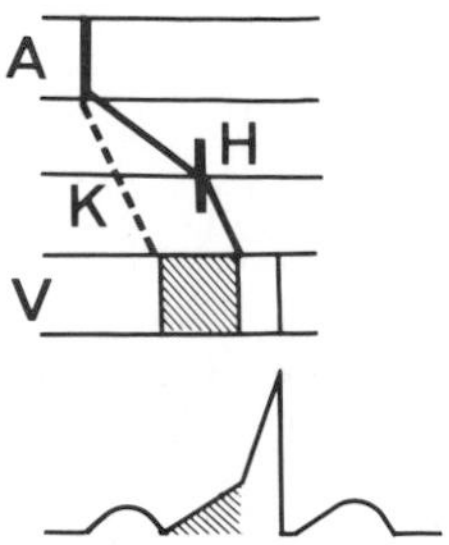

Figure 34-6. *The Wolff-Parkinson-White complex is a fusion beat between ventricular preexcitation coming from the Kent bundle (K) and the normal AV conduction system. (H, His potential)*

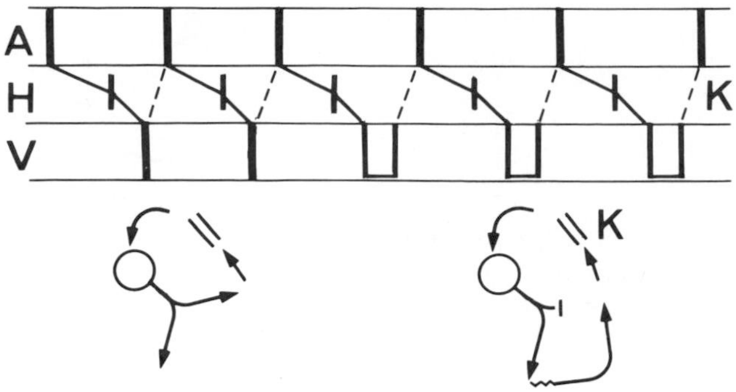

Figure 34-7. *Slowing of an orthodromic tachycardia when a bundle branch block occurs ipsilateral to the Kent bundle.*

pacing or progressively premature extra stimuli is observed to go farther and farther into thc QRS complex while the pacing artifact–Delta wave interval remains practically unchanged. During these maneuvers, the His potential tends to be masked by the large deflection produced by ventricular depolarization. This shows that the WPW complex is a fusion phenomenon between the activation conducted through the nodo-Hisian and accessory pathways because the electrical forces arising from the ventricular wall depolarized by the ventricular pole of the accessory pathway have short-circuited the nodo-Hisian system and therefore have not been subject to the physiologic delay in the AV node.

It is sometimes difficult to understand the role played by the accessory pathway in paroxysmal tachycardia. One of the characteristics of paroxysmal atrial tachycardia in the WPW syndrome is that the ventricular complexes generally do not show preexcitation. It would not appear possible to distinguish whether the tachycardia involves an accessory pathway or whether the arrhythmia originates in the atrioventricular node, in addition to and independent of the WPW syndrome. In this case, division of the accessory pathway would be of no use because the arrhythmia could recur from inside the intact nodo-Hisian system.

The solution of this problem by endocavitary electrophysiologic methods is one of the most delicate points of this investigation. Wellens, in a series of 83 cases of tachycardias initiated by stimulation techniques during electrophysiologic studies, showed the involvement of the accessory pathway in 57 patients and the AV node in 8 and was unable to determine the pathway in 15.[59]

The following arguments based on electrophysiology are in favor of paroxysmal tachycardia involving an accessory pathway.

Bundle Branch Block Slowing Down the Tachycardia. Bundle branch block is often observed during attacks of paroxysmal tachycardia, especially during electrophysiologic studies (Fig. 34-7). An important point in favor of the involvement of an accessory pathway is the appearance of bundle branch block with a slowing of the tachycardia rate.[60]

Let us take, for example, a patient with a direct left-sided AV conduction pathway. During a paroxysmal orthodromic (narrow QRS) tachycardia, the activation will pass from the atria through the AV node, the main His bundle, the left branch, the ventricular myocardium between the emergence of the left bundle, and the ventricular pole of the accessory pathway and will return to the atria through the accessory pathway. Should the left bundle become blocked because of the rapidity of the tachycardia, the narrow ventricular complexes present at the start of the tachycardia will widen and assume a left bundle branch block morphology. In addition, the activation passing through the bundle of His will have to take a longer pathway through the right bundle and across the interventricular septum to reach the ventricular pole of the accessory pathway.

The slowing effect on the tachycardia with bundle branch block only occurs if the accessory pathway is far enough away from the septum on the free wall of the ventricle whose bundle branch is blocked.

Pharmacodynamically Depressed Conduction in the Accessory Pathway. The administration of procainamide, ajmaline, or other drugs that affect the conductive properties of the abnormal pathways should either slow the tachycardia in its extranodal pathway or make it impossible to induce the tachycardia by pacing.[61,62,63]

Chronology of Paraseptal Endocavitary Excitation. When retrograde atrial activation is observed near the septum, it is difficult to distinguish whether this occurs through an accessory bundle or through the nodo-Hisian system. In this case (Fig. 34-8*C*), a premature ventricular extrasystole during the tachycardia conducts toward the atrium, with activation of the interatrial septum, before the retrograde depolarization of the bundle of His favors the tachycardia involving the accessory conduction pathway.[56]

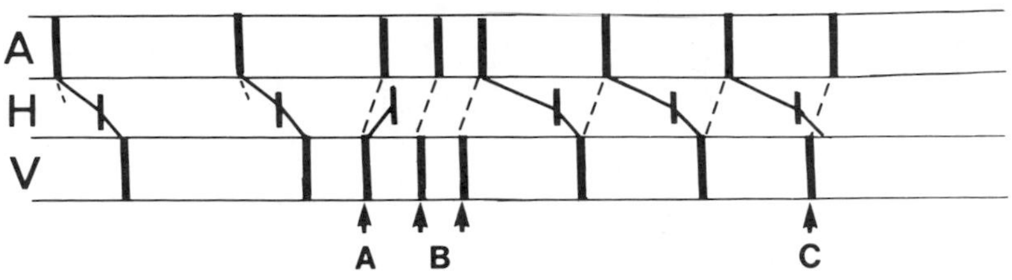

Figure 34-8. *Schematic of an electrophysiologic study in a case of latent accessory bypass tract. The laddergram shows various aspects of ventricular premature contractions in patients with bypass tracts. (A) A ventricular premature beat is conducted to the atrium before the His bundle depolarization. (B) The AV conduction time is not increased for short cycles. An orthodromic tachycardia is triggered where the impulse is able to go back to the ventricles through the His bundle. (C) During tachycardia a premature ventricular beat may capture the atrium when the His bundle is refractory. (A, atrium; H, His bundle; V, ventricle)*

Induction of Reciprocating Tachycardia. In patients whose accessory bundle has a refractory period longer than that of the nodo-Hisian pathway, applying progressively more premature extra stimuli can lead to blocking of the abnormal pathway and disappearance of the delta wave. When reciprocating orthodromic (narrow QRS) tachycardia occurs without lengthening of the AV conduction time, an accessory bundle activated retrogradely is probable. In fact, it is known that lengthening of the AV conduction time is an essential condition for reciprocating intranodal tachycardia.[64]

Retrograde Conduction During Premature Stimulation. This is shown in Figure 34-8*A* and *B*, where, after ventricular stimulation at a given basal rate, progressively more premature ventricular extra stimuli are introduced and the timing of the corresponding atrial depolarization is unchanged, especially when it is recorded before His bundle activity. The same maneuver may be simulated by ventricular pacing at a progressively more rapid rate and observing the absence of lengthening of the retrograde conduction time.[65] For this to be valid, the retrograde conduction time must be identical to that observed during spontaneous tachycardia. The sensing atrial electrode must be positioned near the atrial emergence of the accessory pathway, and the sequence of activation over the atrium must be comparable to that seen during spontaneous tachycardia.[56]

Retrograde Conduction During Tachycardia. This maneuver is performed during tachycardia. A ventricular stimulus is triggered as shown in Figure 34-8*C* before the ventricle is depolarized in the anterograde direction, and the timing of the atrial depolarization is examined.[66] The presence of an accessory pathway is suggested when atrial capture without lengthening of the ventriculoatrial conduction period is observed. However, for relatively fast tachycardias, a slightly lengthened retrograde conduction time is acceptable, being physiologic for very short coupling intervals. However, to confirm that the ventricular extra stimulus has not entered the nodo-Hisian system,[59] there must be no modification of the Hisian potential during the tachycardia.

Initiation of Antidromic Tachycardia. This is only valid in a form of paroxysmal tachycardia, which is rarely encountered in practice, with anterograde depolarization of the accessory pathway (Fig. 34-9). Ventricular pacing initiates a circus movement tachycardia with wide complexes as the accessory pathway is activated in the AV direction, giving rise to pure ventricular preexcitation.[59]

Reciprocating Tachycardia in the Atrioventricular Node

Instruction (or Triggering) of Atrial Echoes

Triggering of atrial echoes is illustrated in Figure 34-10*A*. An atrial extra stimulus with a prolonged AV conduction time leads to ventricular depolarization. However, during its conduction through the AV node, the direction of the excitation is changed and it passes back up

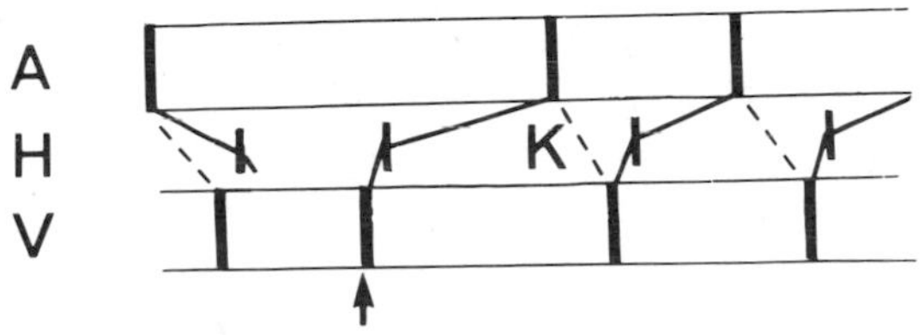

Figure 34-9. *Triggering of an antidromic tachycardia by a ventricular premature stimulation. Retrograde conduction in the Kent bundle is blocked. Activation spreads retrogradely through the His bundle to the atrium and anterogradely through the Kent bundle. (A, atrium; H, His bundle; V, ventricle)*

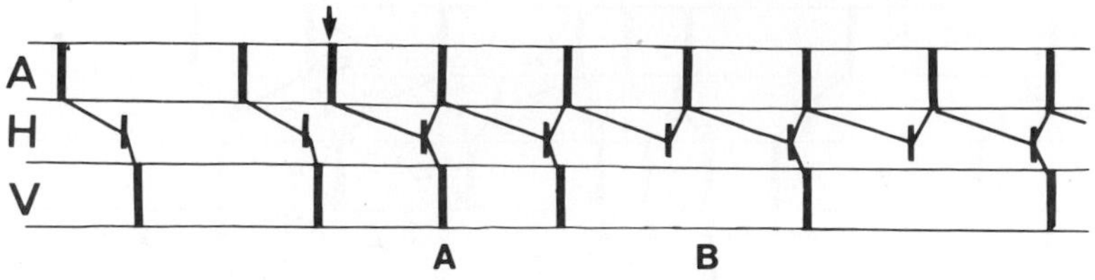

Figure 34-10. *(A) Triggering of junctional reciprocating tachycardia by an atrial extra stimulus* (arrow). *The first atrial and ventricular waves of the tachycardia occur simultaneously. (B) During tachycardia, a 2 : 1 AV block appears, demonstrating that the ventricle is not a necessary link of the circuit. (A, atrium; H, His bundle; V, ventricle)*

through the node by a second pathway. If the atrium is depolarized at the same time or earlier than the ventricle, the activation cannot have passed through an accessory conduction pathway.[59]

Dynamic Properties of Retrograde Conduction

As shown in Figure 34-11*A*, the retrograde conduction of ventricular pacing with conduction times that increase with increasing prematurity of the ventricular extra stimulus is characteristic of nodo-Hisian pathways. An accessory AV pathway can generally be excluded because its retrograde conduction, when present, is more rapid than its anterograde conduction.

Initiation of Reciprocating Tachycardia

Initiation of reciprocating tachycardia is illustrated in Figure 34-11*B*. The arrhythmia is triggered by progressively more premature ventricular stimulation with a characteristic prolongation of the retrograde ventricular conduction time, as explained above.

Reciprocating Tachycardia With Atrioventricular Block

The association of a reciprocating rhythm and a high degree of AV block excludes the participation of an accessory conduction pathway in the tachycardia circuit, except theoretically, when accessory fibers from the atrium to the upper part of the bundle of His are associated with an infra-Hisian block (see Fig. 34-10*B*).

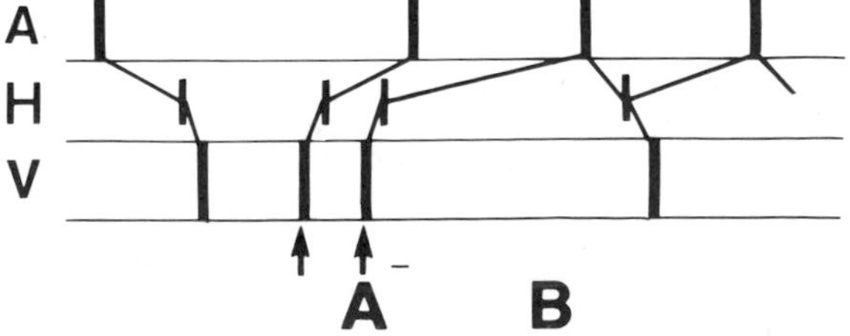

Figure 34-11. *Result of ventricular pacing in the induction of orthodromic reciprocating tachycardia. The premature extra stimulus (A, at* arrow) *is only conducted to the atrium through the AV node, as suggested by an increased retrograde conduction time. When enough prematurity is obtained, reciprocation through the accessory pathway can induce the arrhythmia. (A, atrium; H, His bundle; V, ventricle)*

Latent Preexcitation Syndromes

The absence of a delta wave in sinus rhythm in a patient with paroxysmal tachycardia with narrow QRS complexes does not in itself exclude the WPW syndrome. It is theoretically possible[67,68] for an accessory pathway[69] to conduct from the ventricle to the atrium but be blocked in the anterograde direction.[70] This is an important point because surgical section of the accessory pathway, located by *atrial* epicardial mapping, can completely cure the patient. Section of the His bundle would also be effective but would have to be associated with permanent pacemaker therapy.

Most of the previously described methods that aim to demonstrate the participation of the accessory pathway in reciprocating tachycardia in the WPW syndrome may also be used in the investigation of these cases, with the exception of the situation that involves anterograde conduction by the accessory pathway.

Anatomic Localization of the Origin of Preexcitation

Homolateral and Contralateral Stimulation

As discussed earlier, the different conduction properties of the normal and accessory pathways that show up with progressively faster atrial pacing or with premature stimuli lead generally to increased preexcitation. The degree to which this happens varies with the area paced with respect to the location of the abnormal pathway (Fig. 34-12).[23]

When the preexcitation pathway is located on the right side of the heart, low right atrial pacing will directly transmit the excitation to the right ventricle with increased preexcitation. This occurs because the atrial activation will have reached the ventricle before its conduction through the AV node and the nodo-Hisian system. When the preexcitation pathway is located on

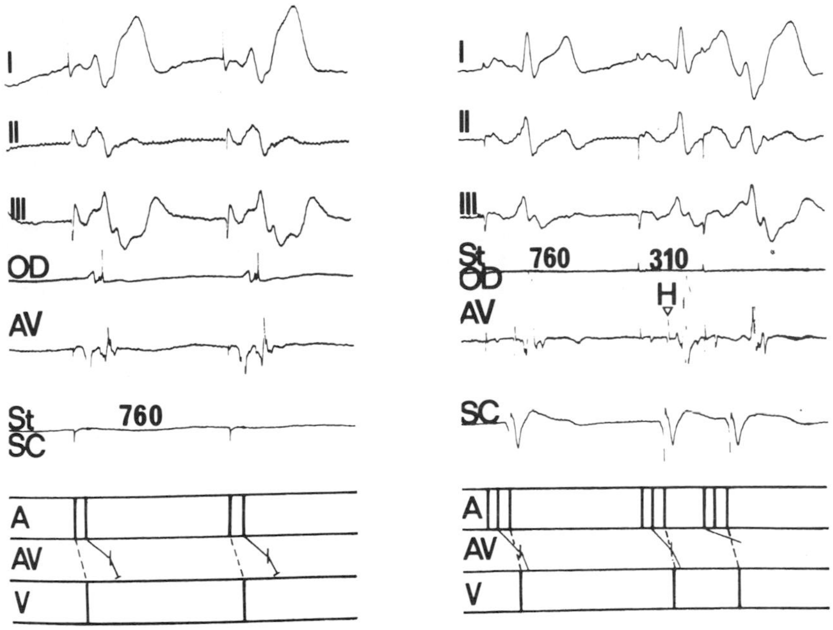

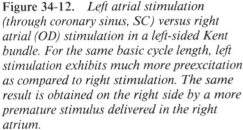

Figure 34-12. *Left atrial stimulation (through coronary sinus, SC) versus right atrial (OD) stimulation in a left-sided Kent bundle. For the same basic cycle length, left stimulation exhibits much more preexcitation as compared to right stimulation. The same result is obtained on the right side by a more premature stimulus delivered in the right atrium.*

the free wall of the left ventricle, the same maneuver will not produce such a noticeable increase in preexcitation because the activation must cross the interatrial septum to reach the atrial pole of the accessory pathway.

When the pacing catheter is in contact with the wall of the left atrium, as is possible with an atrial septal defect or with the catheter positioned in the coronary sinus, the pacing will be near the atrial pole of a left-sided accessory pathway, and increased preexcitation will be demonstrated at low pacing rates and without very premature extra stimuli. The same maneuver in right-sided preexcitation will only slightly change the amplitude of the delta wave because the excitation must follow a longer pathway from the left atrium to reach the atrial pole of the accessory pathway.

When the accessory pathway is located in the septum, these pacing techniques have little bearing on the degree of the preexcitation.

Endocardial Mapping

In endocardial mapping, a multipolar catheter or a strategic arrangement of unipolar or bipolar catheters is used to measure the endocavitary activation times of different regions of the heart. These times are then compared.

In practice, it is usually easier to locate the atrial origin of the abnormal activation than it is to locate the ventricular origin. On the left side, the anatomic relationship of the coronary sinus and vein to the inferior aspect of the AV groove enables exploration of all regions except the left anterior paraseptal area and the mitral ring. Usually it is only necessary to position a quadripolar catheter in the coronary sinus and vein to determine the activation sequences of the base of the left ventricle and atrium.[71]

On the right side, a bipolar catheter designed by Gallagher[72] is used. This catheter incorporates a curved guide wire that can be manipulated from the proximal end of the catheter, thus enabling the tip of the catheter to be positioned accurately. In this way, the circumference of the right AV ring may be explored without biplane radioscopic control. In the septal region, a supplementary endocavitary lead is used to record the His bundle potential and, thereby, the activation of the interventricular septum and the adjacent interatrial septal area. These regions are investigated during ventricular pacing, during attacks of reciprocating tachycardia, and during premature atrial stimulation triggering echo beats. The earliest point of activation recorded in the atrial endocavitary leads is then observed (Fig. 34-13):

1. When the accessory pathway is located on the left lateral wall of the heart, the distal bipolar lead of the endocavitary catheter positioned in the coronary sinus detects atrial activity immediately after ventricular depolarization. A negative P wave in lead I during tachycardia or after an atrial echo suggests, when observed, the presence of a left lateral accessory pathway.[73]
2. When the preexcitation is intraseptal, the accessory pathway may be situated in front of the bundle of His, so that the activation of the atrial mid zone is observed before the coronary sinus. The pathway may also be located behind the bundle of His, so that the coronary sinus activation is observed before, or simultaneously with, the atrial mid-zone.[56] In the latter case, it is necessary to exclude intranodal reentry by methods described above.

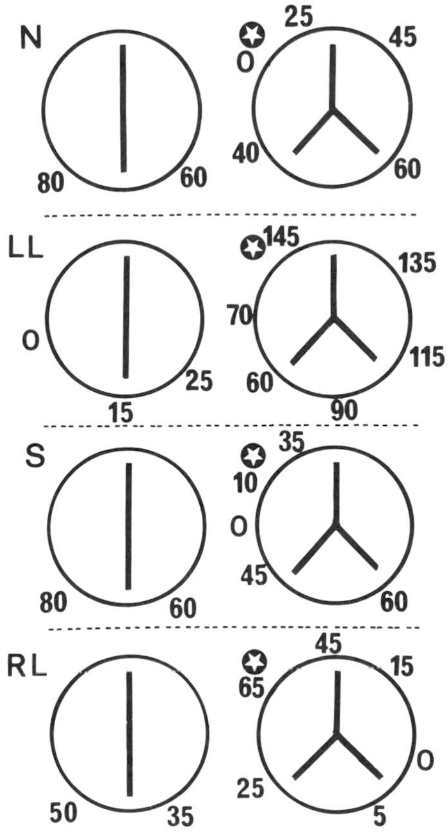

Figure 34-13. *Endocavitary retrograde conduction time at the level of mitral and tricuspid anulus during orthodromic tachycardia in normal (N), left lateral (LL), septal (S) and right lateral (RL) Kent bundle. Position of His bundle is indicated by a* star.

3. When the accessory pathway is located on the right side, the latest activation times are observed in the distal poles of the coronary sinus electrode and the earliest times are observed in the exploratory electrode positioned on the atrial aspect of the right AV ring.

Localization of Abnormal Pathway by Epicardial Mapping

Epicardial mapping is the ultimate electrophysiologic investigation, which enables a direct appraisal of preexcitation.[17,18] It consists of mapping the intrinsic deflection of ventricular epicardial activation at a number of test points. At operation, a bipolar exploratory lead, with electrodes 1 to 2 mm apart, is held by the surgeon and moved from point to point on the epicardium. The pattern of electrical activity recorded is shown in Figure 34-14.

Epicardial mapping requires special training and skills if it is to be carried out rapidly (within about 15 minutes) and with confidence, and it demands cooperation between medical and surgical teams.

Technique

At the Pitié-Salpêtrière Hospital in Paris, a basic grid is used, with at least 40 predefined points over the right ventricle and 45 over the left ventricle. In addition, intermediary points may be used.[75] The grid is defined by obvious anatomic landmarks such as the line of the left anterior descending artery from the origin of the great vessels to the apex and the line of the right border of the heart between the AV groove and the apex. Each line is divided into two equal parts, and each part is divided again, and so on, until the grid map shown in Figure 34-15 is obtained. In this way, the whole of the ventricular epicardium is represented independent of the true size of the heart. A test point is defined and codified by a letter and a number at each intersection on the grid.

The representation of the whole of the ventricular epicardium is obtained by imagining the heart as if it had been opened along the posterior interventricular groove and then spread out at the sides. The activation time at each reference point investigated by the surgeon is measured on an oscilloscope by another operator and noted on the grid against the corresponding codified point.

The first points investigated are those over the free wall of the right ventricle, followed by those over the diaphragmatic wall, which necessitates lifting the heart on its pedicle. This maneuver, which may be poorly tolerated especially during tachycardia, is minimized by the design of the exploratory electrode, which has a curved tip. Mapping is then continued over the anterolateral aspect of the left ventricle and lastly over the diaphragmatic wall of the left ventricle. In this way, the heart is given a recovery period after the investigation of each ventricle.

Because the objective of epicardial mapping is to measure the activation time at a number of points on the ventricular epicardium, a precise time reference is essential. When mapping is carried out in sinus rhythm with atrial pacing, the pacemaker stimulus triggers the sweep of the oscilloscope screen. This is a very precise method of timing provided there are no AV conduction defects (a condition that must be checked for carefully throughout the investigation). When the heart is not in sinus rhythm, such as during reciprocating rhythms or atrial fibrillation, a ventricular reference electrode is used to amplify the potential that triggers the oscilloscope time base. However, the exploratory electrode may be positioned between the origin of the activation and the reference electrode (Fig. 34-16). To overcome this problem, an electronic device such as one with magnetic tape or computer memory is used to produce an analogic time delay in the recorded potentials.

The interval between epicardial activation at each point investigated and the time base may be measured on a high-speed paper recorder or on the screen of a measuring oscilloscope with a storage space. This latter

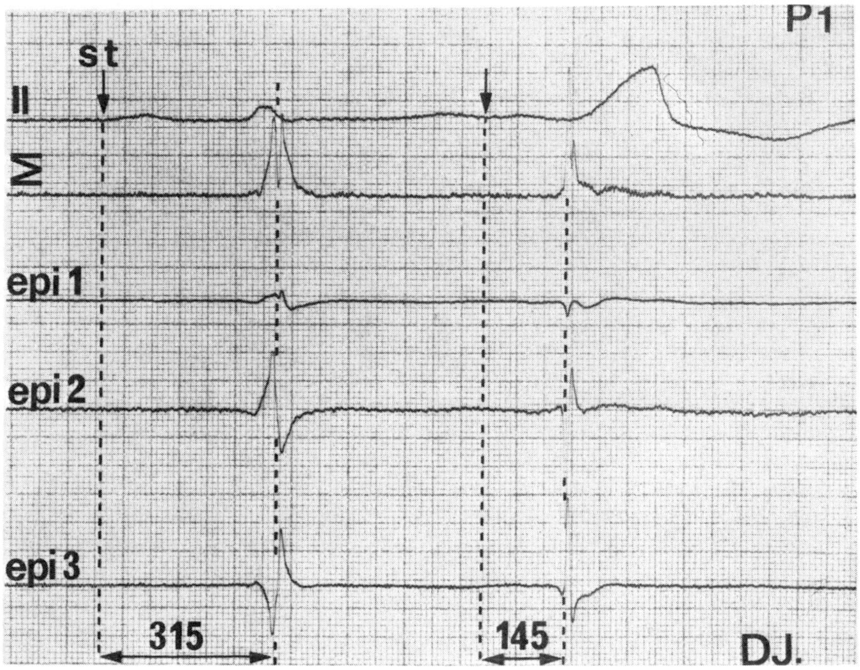

Figure 34-14. *Epicardial potentials (Epi 1-3 and summation of absolute value) at the ventricular side of the AV groove during atrial stimulation (St). In a normal beat, epicardial potentials occur at the end of the QRS (first QRS complex). In a preexcited beat, it occurs before the onset of the delta wave, being recorded near the ventricular pole of the Kent bundle (second beat). (II, standard lead II)*

method allows the superposition of several successive measurements and thus reduces the risk of recording a totally aberrant result.

The intervals are measured and recalculated with reference to their common time base corresponding to the beginning of ventricular activation. Isochrons, 5 msec apart, are then drawn by extrapolation through the points investigated. This technnique gives a clear picture of epicardial activation (Fig. 34-17).[6]

At Duke University, the ventricular epicardial activation time reference is taken as the origin of the delta wave to give a better comparison with septal activation. The time interval between the reference and epicardial electrodes is measured with a digital counter and the exploratory electrodes are slid along the AV groove as far as the point of earliest activation.[56]

Before the appearance of epicardial activation in the WPW syndrome with a lateral accessory pathway is explained, the normal epicardial map will be described.

Normal Ventricular Epicardial Map

The origin of the activation is located in the middle of the free wall of the right ventricle, close to the septum and opposite the insertion of the anterior papillary muscle of the tricuspid valve. The right AV groove, especially over the diaphragmatic wall, is the last to be depolarized, with a 60- to 70-msec delay. The left ventricular epicardium is

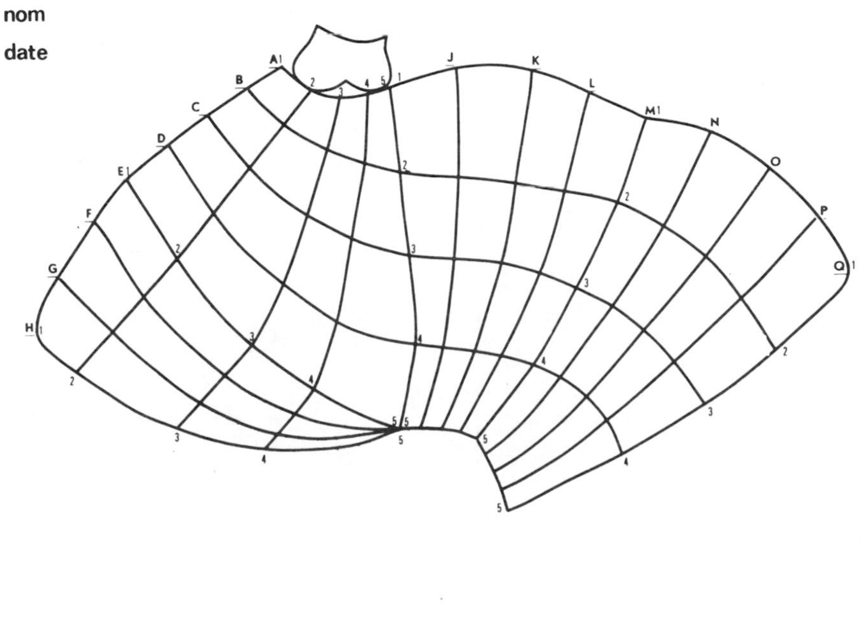

Figure 34-15. *Epicardial mapping grid designed in la Salpêtrière Hospital (Paris). The ventricles are displayed as cut along the posterior descending artery and opened. The anterior descending artery is in the middle, the right ventricular epicardium on one side, and the left ventricular epicardium on the other side. (E1–E5, acute margin of the heart line; M1–M5, left lateral coronary arteries)*

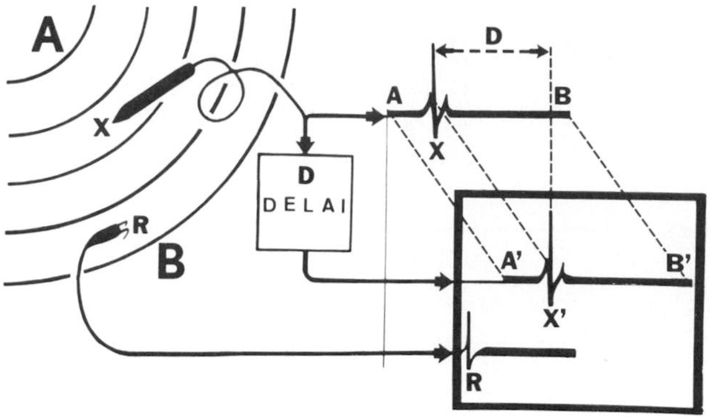

Figure 34-16. *Schematic of the equipment providing an analogic delay necessary when the exploring electrode is situated in an area (labeled X) depolarized* before *the reference electrode. (Fontaine, G., et al.: Coeur, 6:115, 1975)*

activated with a 20- to 30-msec delay because of the greater thickness of the myocardium, which slows down the conduction from the endocardium to the epicardium. The second point of emergence depolarizes the diaphragmatic wall of the left ventricle near the septum. The most-delayed activation is also situated on this side on the diaphragmatic wall of the left ventricle along the atrioventricular groove (see Fig. 34-17).

Activation on the epicardial surface gives rise to a roughly concentric pattern, except at the infundibulum and the base of the AV grooves, where the activation appears to move tangentially through nonspecific myocardium rather than directly from endocardium to epicardium.

Epicardial Mapping in the Wolff-Parkinson-White Syndrome

Whenever possible, epicardial mapping should be performed during maximal preexcitation. This is obtained by rapid atrial pacing near the predicted location of the accessory pathway. The earliest point of ventricular depolarization is observed on the ventricular aspect of the groove, which is normally the last area to be activated. The activation spreads at a relatively slow speed (as shown by the close bunching of the isochrons) over the ventricle, the insertion of the interventricular septum, and the contralateral ventricle (Fig. 34-18).

When a large degree of preexcitation is obtained, the pattern of activation is homogeneous, with the most-delayed point observed practically opposite the area of earliest activation.[50] When a moderate degree of preexcitation is obtained and the origin of the abnormal activation is situated at a distance from the nodo-Hisian system, fusion of the two activation fronts may be recorded. The contribution of the abnormal pathway to ventricular depolarization varies with the imposed atrial rhythm (Fig. 34-19) and is related to the size of the delta wave on the surface electrocardiogram.[50]

Atrial Fibrillation

When atrial fibrillation occurs at operation, either spontaneously or induced by pacing techniques, and persists during epicardial mapping, a number of problems arise. There is generally a risk of a rapid, poorly tolerated ventricular rhythm. Sinus rhythm may be reestablished by cardioverison, but this is ususally unstable, quickly reverting to atrial fibrillation. When this occurs, pharma-

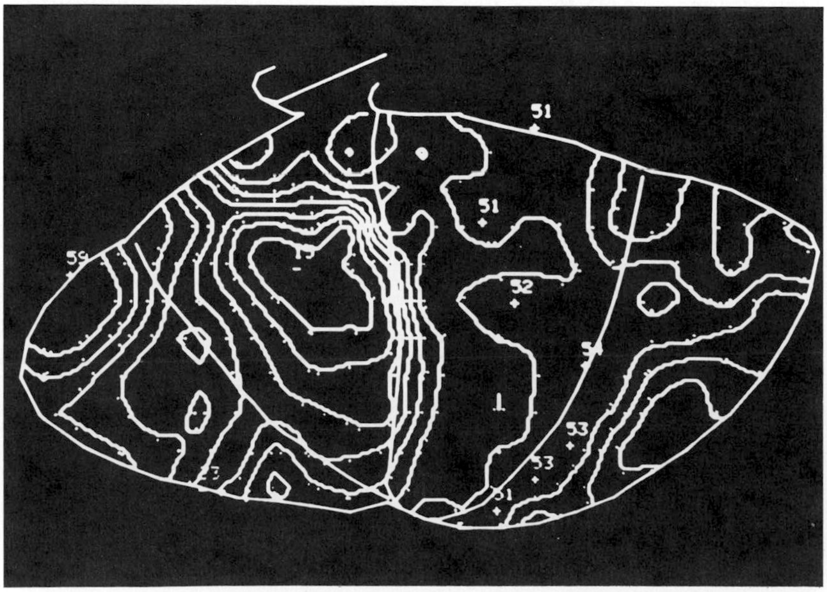

Figure 34-17. *Normal epicardial activation. (See text for explanation.) The mapping is drawn automatically by a minicomputer, the heart being displayed in a manner similar to the grid in Figure 34-15.* Dots *bordering the lines indicate the direction of depolarization.*

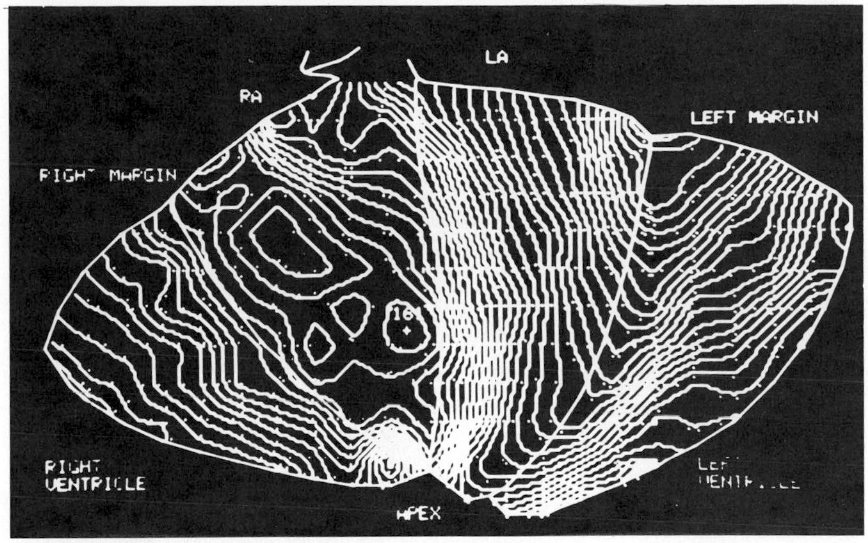

Figure 34-18. *Activation in a left lateral Kent bundle.*

logic agents such as ajmaline or procainamide, which depress abnormal (*i.e.*, bypass tract) conduction, may be given intravenously by continuous infusion until a hemodynamically acceptable ventricular rhythm is obtained. Then epicardial mapping is carried out in atrial fibrillation, and the activation times are measured in comparison to a ventricular reference electrode as previously explained. During atrial fibrillation, the morphology of the ventricular complexes may vary: there may be wide ventricular complexes of pure preexcitation; narrow ventricular complexes of nodo-Hisian depolarization; fusion complexes of these two types of activation; nodo-Hisian complexes with aberrant conduction; ventricular extrasystoles; or fusion complexes of these latter two types of activation and preexcitation.

The morphologies of the ventricular complexes may usually be distinguished by oscilloscopic analysis, the preexcitation complexes having earlier activation times and being more frequent.[75]

Reciprocating Tachycardias

Epicardial mapping during antidromic tachycardia (which is a rare situation), whether induced or spontaneous, shows pure preexcitation. The ventricular origin of the activation indicates the ventricular pole of the accessory pathway. It is always situated on the border of the AV groove, which is the most frequent situation.

During orthodromic tachycardia (which is common), ventricular activation is totally under the influence of the nodo-Hisian pathway, and the epicardial map is therefore normal. However, using a technique similar to the one for ventricular epicardial mapping, atrial epicardial mapping may demonstrate retrograde transmission of the ventricular activation to the atria through the accessory pathway and the location of its atrial pole (Fig. 34-20).[56]

Concealed Wolff-Parkinson-White Syndrome

Accessory AV pathways concealed by anterograde block but with unimpaired retrograde conduction may be demonstrated by atrial mapping. There are two situations in which this is carried out: (1) when ventricular pacing is at a rhythm faster than that of the sinus node and (2) when there is orthodromic reciprocating tachycardia.

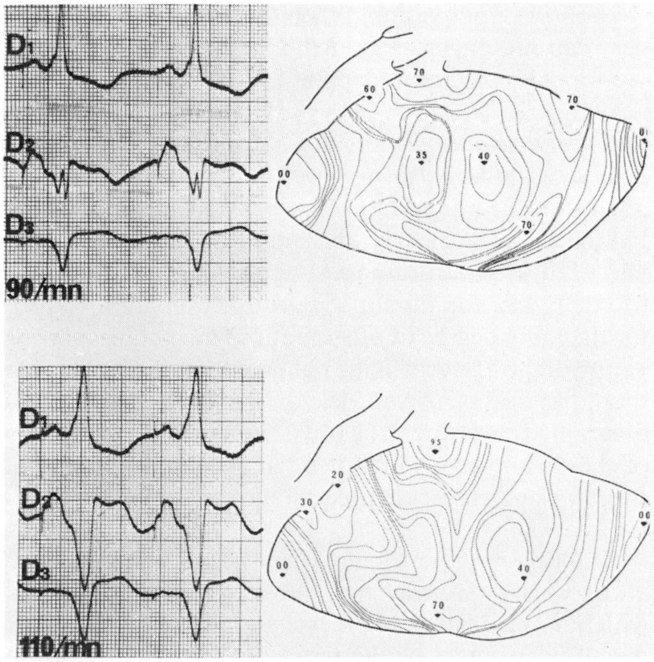

Figure 34-19. *Activation in a posterior paraseptal Kent bundle for two degrees of preexcitation at two pacing rates. Preexcitation seems to appear simultaneously at the two extremities of the representation of the epicardial surface, which are in fact adjacent.*

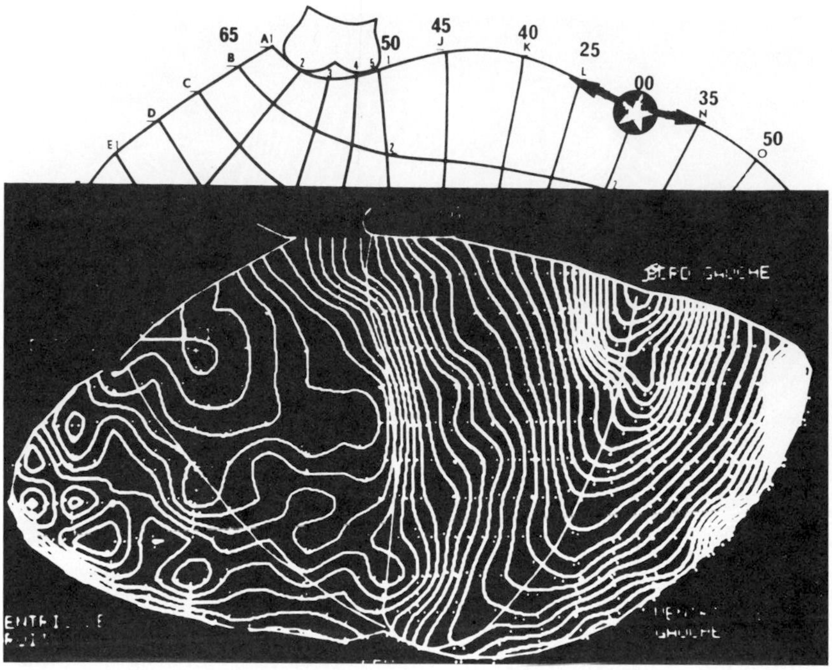

Figure 34-20. *Retrograde atrial activation time along the AV groove from a ventricular pacing site. The shortest time is located near the atrial pole of the Kent bundle. The ventricular pole of the Kent bundle has been previously localized by ventricular mapping.*

Disappearance of Preexcitation

Disappearance of preexcitation has been encountered in several patients during epicardial mapping. It may be the result of the general anesthesia or due to the operation itself. It may be very difficult to induce the preexcitation, even by ventricular pacing near the presumed origin of the abnormal activation. When this maneuver fails, surgery can no longer be guided by the results of atrial or ventricular epicardial mapping.

Interpretation of Epicardial Mapping

The ventricular origin of abnormal activation may be determined by mapping even when it is difficult to make out the delta wave (atrial fibrillation). A sufficiently large part of the myocardium must be depolarized to give rise to a delta wave on the surface electrocardiogram.[57] Also, for the same degree of preexcitation, the abnormal activation of the free wall of the right ventricle is more visible than that of the left ventricle on the surface electrocardiogram. This is due to its proximity and also to the axis of the delta wave, which is often perpendicular to the frontal plane in cases of preexcitation of the left ventricular free wall.

The origin of ventricular depolarization initiated by an accessory pathway may move several centimeters with varying degrees of preexcitation (Fig. 34-21). This phenomenon may be the result of the geometry of the accessory pathway or due to the presence of several pathways side by side, each with different conduction properties. The best method of locating the accessory pathway is by moving the exploratory and atrial pacing electrodes along the ventricular groove. The investigation is then repeated during ventricular pacing with recording of the atrial potentials.[30] In some cases, a specific activity is observed between the P and delta waves, and this is considered to be the intrinsic depolarization of the accessory pathway.[36]

When the abnormal pathway is situated in the free wall of the ventricles, the beginning of epicardial depolarization appears *before* the delta wave. However, when the abnormal pathway is located in the septum, the epicardial breakthrough appears *after* the delta wave because of the interval required for the activation to pass from the septum to the epicardium of the nearest free wall.[56] During this time, the amount of myocardium depolarized is sufficient to give rise to a delta wave. In such cases, the abnormal activation is located in the paraseptal regions as predicted by endocavitary electrophysiologic investigation.

All methods used to locate accessory pathways, electrophysiologically, in the catheter laboratory, mapping preoperatively, and probably echocardiographically, depend on the origin of the preexcitation, which imposes the direction of activation on the whole of the remaining ventricular myocardium. This origin reflects the most abnormal accessory pathway, that is, the most pronounced AV short circuit. Surgical section of this pathway may well unmask another group of accessory fibers with a smaller degree of preexcitation.

Epicardial mapping is repeated after surgical incision of the accessory pathway, and another operation using cardiopulmonary bypass may be neccessary if a second pathway is demonstrated near to or at a distance from the original accessory pathway. To avoid the necessity of

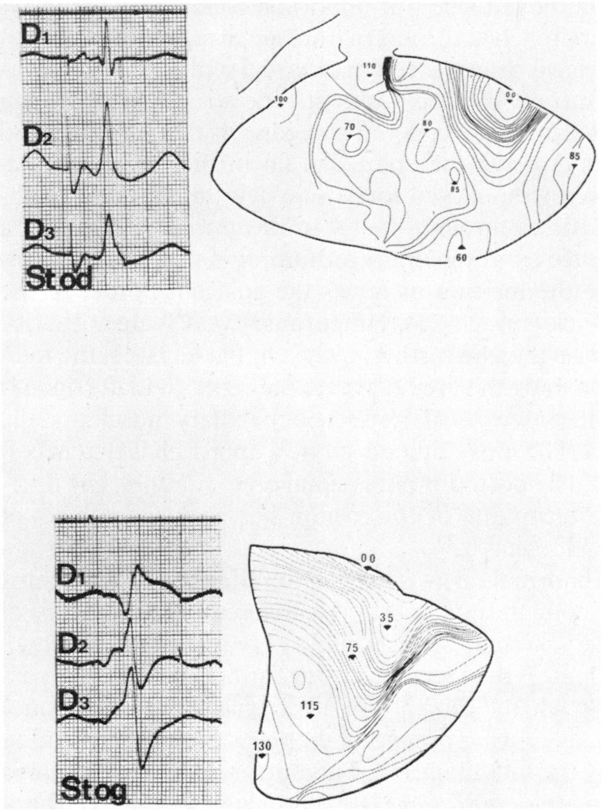

Figure 34-21. *Epicardial mapping right (St od) and left (St og) atrial pacing. The first epicardial breakthrough has moved anteriorly. Note the increased preexcitation pattern on the electrocardiogram in the* lower panel *where only the left epicardial surface has been mapped.*

reoperation, the extent of the initial surgical incision should be generous and not just limited to the area of maximal preexcitation.

However, the most rapidly conducting accessory pathway gives rise to the most severe symptoms, especially with regard to the ventricular rhythm during atrial fibrillation. Thus, an accessory pathway may even be left interrupted with a satisfactory clinical result, the eventual recurrences of arrhythmias being better tolerated. Finally, in these cases, the residual accessory pathway may be more susceptible to medical treatment.[51]

When the abnormal AV pathways or the pathways partially short-circuiting the AV node are located close to the bundle of His, this structure may inevitably be sectioned during operation, so that permanent cardiac pacing may be necessary.

Surgical Techniques

A full understanding of the basic electrophysiologic phenomena of the WPW syndrome is essential in the work-up and selection of patients for surgery when medical treatment fails. Three types of surgical procedures are possible in the WPW syndrome:

1. His bundle section
2. Accessory pathway section
3. Pacemaker therapy (see Chap. 32)

Surgical Division of the His Bundle in the Wolff-Parkinson-White Syndrome

Although surgical division of the His bundle is little used nowadays, it retains its instructive value because it was the first surgical demonstration of the interruption of a macroreentry phenomenon in the WPW syndrome.[19]

The right atrium is opened using cardiopulmonary bypass. An electrophysiologic reference is then made with a bipolar exploratory probe, with electrodes 2 mm apart, positioned along the septal insertion of the tricuspid valve.[74] Atrial pacing is used to inhibit the sinus node. The atrial response is recorded on one channel of the oscilloscope screen, and the ventricular response is recorded on another. The potentials recorded with the exploratory electrode are monitored on a third channel between the other two. In this way, the oscilloscope time base can be adjusted to display the whole of the PR interval on the screen (Fig. 34-22). The His bundle potential is soon obtained. Several surgical techniques of His bundle division are available: electrocoagulation, little used nowadays; surgical incision with suturing; and the more recent technique of cryosurgery, which is associated with a high percentage of good results.[76]

After this type of operation, all anterograde conduction is by way of the abnormal pathway, and therefore a pure preexcitation complex is observed on the surface

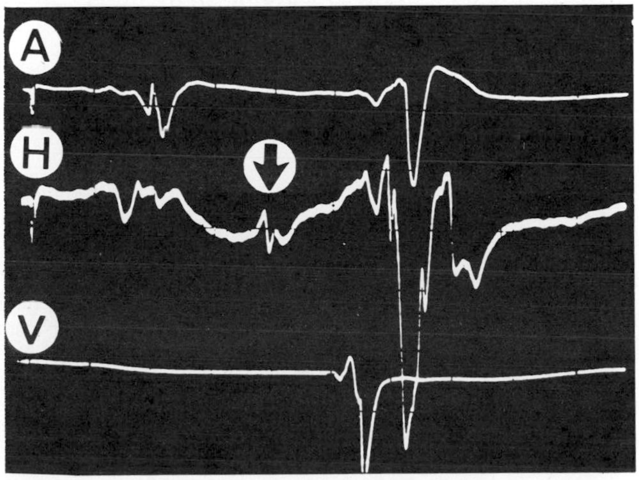

Figure 34-22. *Electrophysiologic localization of the His bundle at surgery. (A, atrial epicardial bipolar hook-shaped lead; V, ventricular bipolar hook-shaped lead; H, roving bipolar electrode recording His bundle activity)*

electrocardiogram in sinus rhythm. This sort of conduction is known to be unreliable, and spontaneous paroxysmal complete AV block may occur. Therefore, prophylactic permanent ventricular pacing is required.

The main problem with this type of operation is that it is difficult to be sure that nodo-Hisian conduction has been completely severed. Furthermore, nodo-Hisian conduction may be depressed simply by contact with the surgical instruments, so that ventricular depolarization occurs through the accessory pathway. When this occurs, the accessory pathway conduction must be depressed to ensure that the normal pathway has been completely interrupted.[19]

Even with this latter maneuver, it is not possible to be completely certain that nodo-Hisian conduction has been interrupted, and normal AV conduction may reappear several weeks postopcratively.

Surgical Division of the Accessory Pathway

Surgical division of the accessory pathway is the definitive surgical procedure in the WPW syndrome.[20,27,28,77,78] The principle of the operation is an incision through the atrial myocardium at the edge of the AV ring.

On the right side, after locating the point of maximal preexcitation on the ventricular aspect, the right atrium is opened. An incision is made with a scalpel through the atrial myocardium as far as the epicardial fat in the groove. A margin of security is thereby obtained with respect to the coronary vessels. However, the intervening structures must be destroyed completely by sliding a nerve hook or curved forceps between the two atrial edges. The length of the incision is at least 2 cm and, as previously explained, the wider the better. However, the region around the atrial septum between the coronary sinus and the membranous septum, where the AV node and bundle of His are situated, is avoided.

On the left side, the abnormal conduction pathways are approached through a transseptal atriotomy. The left AV ring is drawn through the atrial septum by sutures as for mitral valve replacement. The atrial muscle is then incised with a scalpel at the edge of the AV ring, and fibers crossing the epicardial fat in the groove are destroyed with curved forceps. When the accessory pathway passes through the fat in the groove, at times at a distance from the endocardium, it is necessary to continue the incision as far as the adjacent border of the ventricle (Fig. 34-23). The coronary vessels are not at risk because they lie further away. On the left side, the incision avoids the area between the right and left trigones and the insertion of the anterior papillary muscle and the aorta. The most difficult surgical approach is that necessitated by posterior parasseptal preexcitation. The operative technique of this region has been the subject of special research.[78]

Abnormal fibers passing from the atria to the ventricles along the epicardium are inaccessible to this type of surgery but may be sectioned by cryosurgery (scc below). Mapping is then repeated using cardiopulmonary bypass to exclude the presence of other accessory pathways not detected during preoperative electrophysiologic studies or by the first mapping. This surgery may be associated with other procedures to correct coexisting cardiopathies.

Cryosurgery

Cryosurgery is a new surgical technique that aims to destroy myocardial tissue without irreversibly damaging the collagen and fibroblastic supporting tissues.[36,76] It is performed with a probe with a 0.5-cm-diameter tip. Cooling is obtained by the expansion of nitrous oxide. The temperature of the active area is controlled by an

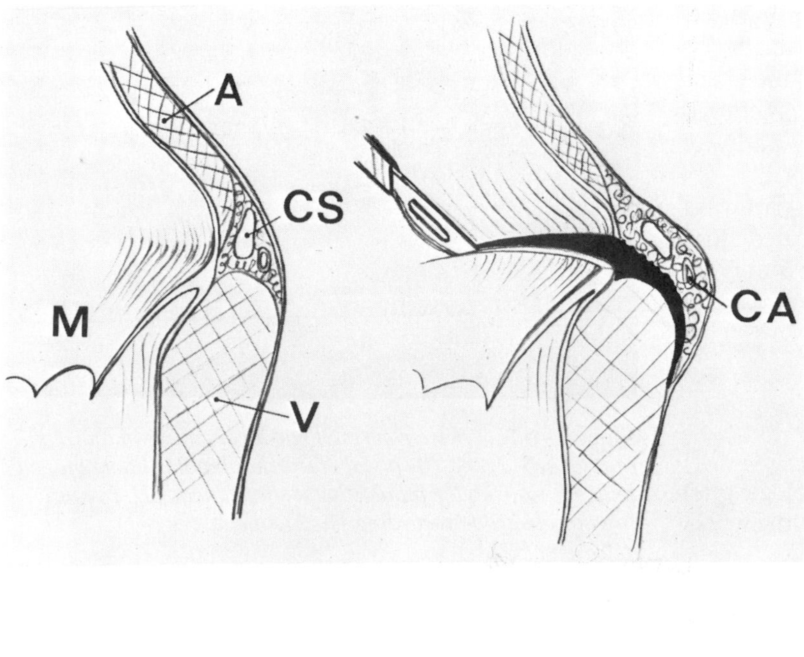

Figure 34-23. *Operation developed at Duke University by W. C. Sealy for the division of left-sided Kent bundle. (A, atrium; M, mitral leaflet; V, ventricle; CS, coronary sinus (or vein); CA, coronary artery)*

electronic device that allows cooling in two stages, first to 0°C and then to −60°C.

When the active zone of concern has been located, cooling is carried out to 0°C. The cooling blocks conduction in this zone temporarily, conduction being reestablished on rewarming. When the conduction is to be irreversibly blocked, the temperature is lowered to −60°C, thus creating a sphere of ice 1.5 cm in diameter, which selectively destroys the ventricular myocardium without creating an aneurysm or necrotic destruction.

This technique is used for two conditions:

1. The interruption of accessory epicardial fibers, in which case the epicardial potentials recorded by the exploratory unipolar probe are exclusively negative.[79]
2. In septal preexcitation or for selective His bundle section. In this latter case, better results have been reported with this method than with other methods previously reported.[76]

Cryosurgical ablation of accessory pathways has been reported from the epicardial surface, thus limited to superficial accessory pathway,[79] and from the endocardial surface, using cardiopulmonary bypass.[80] The new technique combines external dissection of the AV pad, at the site of the accessory pathway, allowing direct exposure of the anulus fibrosis, on which cryoprobe is applied. This technique has been successfully used on free wall accessory pathways. Its main advantage is to avoid cryoinjury of the coronary vessels and possible hypothetic cardiac arrest during the procedure; theoretically it could be done without cardiopulmonary bypass.[81]

Surgical Results

The largest series of WPW syndromes treated surgically is that of Gallagher and co-workers at Duke University.[82] Of the 146 patients with WPW syndrome studied by these authors in 1977, 68 were treated medically and 70 underwent surgery. Because 5 of the 70 patients had multiple accessory pathways, 72 surgical procedures were performed.

These authors showed that when the accessory pathway was situated on the free wall of the right ventricle, a good surgical result was obtained in 13 of 15 patients. In one of the failures, the accessory pathway was blocked in the anterograde direction but retrograde conduction persisted. This was, however, amenable to medical treatment. The accessory pathway was successfully interrupted in 28 out of 35 cases of left-sided preexcitation. Of the seven failures, one had an anterograde block with persistence of retrograde conduction. The greatest number of failures were observed when the accessory pathway was situated in the septum (10 out of 22), but the authors commented that a good surgical result had been obtained in their last seven consecutive patients.

Finally, of the 70 patients treated surgically, preexcitation and arrhythmias were cured in 48 patients; the His bundle was sectioned in eight patients. In 11 patients, arrhythmias recurred but responded to medical treatment. There were three postoperative deaths, two of which were due to low-output syndromes secondary to cardiomyopathy.

Indications for Surgery

Although the results of surgery in the WPW syndrome show it to be an effective therapeutic approach, success is not obtained in all patients, and in some the hemodynamic condition is too precarious for surgery to be attempted. In addition, surgery is carried out using cardiopulmonary bypass, and the risks of this procedure must also be taken into account. The surgical indications must therefore be considered at length, especially since other medical and surgical techniques are available besides direct surgery of the accessory pathway.

Assessment of Pharmacologic Treatment

In practice, surgery is considered after the documented failure of medical treatment. Recent methods of investigation have brought about undeniable progress in this field.[83] The effectiveness of medical treatment both in the choice and dose of drugs must be evaluated objectively.

Holter Monitoring

Continuous recording of the ECG on magnetic tape with rapid playback is a useful method of analyzing arrhythmias. The arrhythmias may be quantified more or less automatically by computer techniques, giving information on their number and nature and on the coupling intervals of extrasystoles or bursts of tachycardia. Repeated monitoring before and after treatment gives an objective assessment of the efficacy of antiarrhythmic therapy.

Electrophysiologic Investigation

Continuous electrocardiographic assessment is of little use when arrhythmias are infrequent. When they are associated with alarming clinical symptoms such as syncope, electrophysiologic studies are undertaken. During this investigation, the arrhythmias are induced and the clinical symptoms so produced are compared with those occurring spontaneously. The main objective, however, is the demonstration of the dynamic properties of AV conduction[17–22,57,58] (1) by measuring the Wenckebach point by progressively faster atrial pacing, thus gaining information on the maximum frequency of transmission of activation from the atria to the ventricles and (2) by measuring the refractory periods of the accessory and

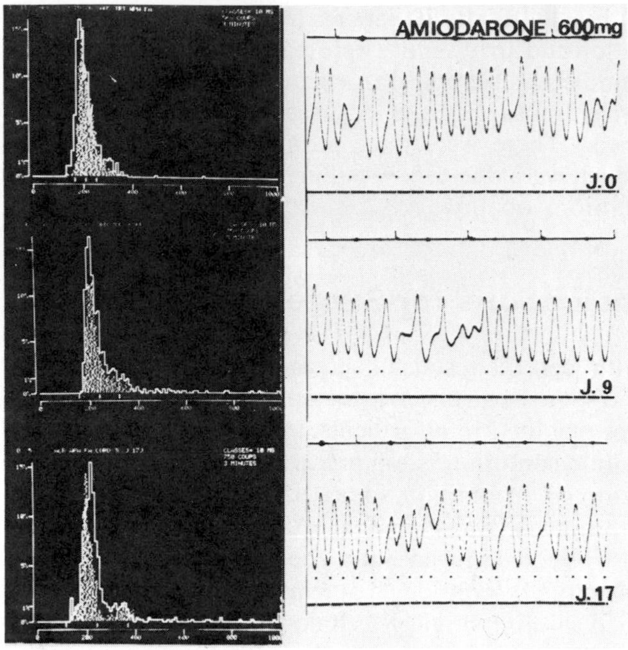

Figure 34-24. *Provoked atrial fibrillation with RR interval histograms before and after 9 and 17 days of treatment with 600 mg of amiodarone. No consistent displacement of the histogram is observed. This response is very unusual with this drug, and in such a case surgery might be considered.*

normal AV pathways by programmed pacing. There is a good correlation between these values and the risks of arrhythmias in the WPW syndrome. In addition, the rate of the ventricular rhythm during induced atrial fibrillation at rest, during exercise, and after antiarrhythmic treatment[79] (Fig. 34-24) is essential.

RR Interval Histograms

The best method of assessing arrhythmias is with interval histograms using a minicomputer.[84] When using this method to study the action of antiarrhythmic drugs, it is important to repeat the histograms over a long period because some drugs require a longer time period for myocardial binding (see Fig. 34-23).

Although it is unusual not to be able to improve a given clinical situation with drugs, in some cases their side-effects are unacceptable. The most effective drug may be difficult to obtain, and its effectiveness may gradually wear off.

Pacemaker Therapy

Pacemaker therapy may be a therapeutic alternative to drug therapy in patients with recalcitrant reciprocating tachycardia.[85,86] In any case, AV conduction must be investigated (Fig. 34-25) with reference to possible attacks of atrial fibrillation, measurement of effective refractory period, and assessment of drug therapy. Radiofrequency pacing may also be useful in some patients,[87] with the added advantage that only a minor operation is required. Atrial pacing with either a preformed J-shaped wire or a coronary sinus catheter is often used. In this way, the intracardiac conduction properties may be checked in ambulatory patients by parameters similar to those obtained in the catheter laboratory.

His Bundle Section

In extremely rare cases of patients presenting with purely orthodromic reciprocating tachycardia, His bundle section may be considered. It must be understood that, when this is undertaken, the accessory pathway is left untouched. If anterograde conduction persists, very rapid atrial flutter or fibrillation may be conducted to the unprotected ventricles.[88]

On the other hand, there may be no distal focus capable of creating an effective substitute rhythm, and, because conduction through the accessory pathway is precarious, a permanent ventricular pacemaker must be implanted. This has practical and psychologic consequences for young people.

Accessory Pathway Section

Accessory pathway section is the ultimate means of treatment when drugs are ineffective and pacemaker therapy is impracticable. It is usually reserved for very rapid reciprocating rhythms that give rise to incapacitating symptoms such as palpitations, anxiety, heart failure, and coronary insufficiency, and, above all, for rapid atrial tachycardias and flutter conducted at a ratio of 1:1, that give rise to malaise and sometimes syncopal episodes or atrial fibrillation with extremely rapid "pseudo-ventricular tachycardia," which may degenerate to life-threatening ventricular fibrillation.[88–90]

Conclusion

The surgical treatment of patients with the WPW syndrome was developed after many years of research. Understanding this disorder began with electrocardiographic interpretation and culminated in the development of surgical techniques for its definitive treatment. Surgical treatment has required the close association of electrophysiologists, cardiologists, and surgeons to develop the sophisticated electrophysiologic techniques necessary to guide the surgeon. The techniques are applicable both in the catheter laboratory and in the operating theater.

The WPW syndrome is caused by an accessory AV conduction pathway. It is an intracardiac short circuit,

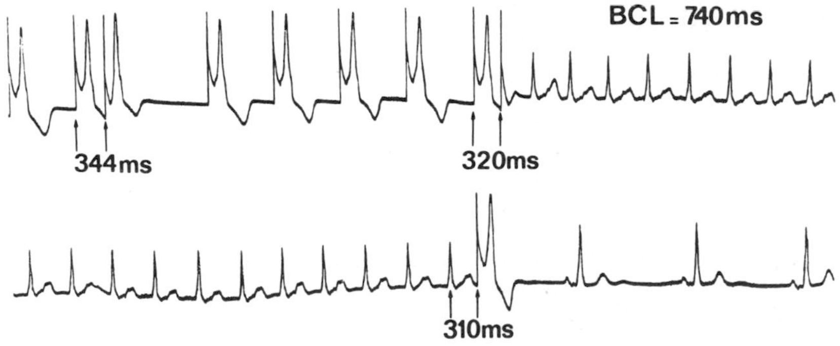

Figure 34-25. *Provocative technique to initiate (*upper panel*) and terminate (*lower panel*) an attack of orthodromic reciprocating tachycardia by a homemade radio frequency programmed stimulator. Unipolar pacing is achieved through the coronary sinus in Wolff-Parkinson-White syndrome, type A. During basic pacing, a pure preexcitation pattern is obtained. A premature stimulus generated by the external radio frequency emitter is followed by another pure preexcitation pattern for a coupling interval of 344 msec on a basic cycle length (BCL) of 740 msec. For a coupling of 320 msec, the Kent bundle is blocked and orthodromic tachycardia is initiated. A unique stimulus with a coupling interval of 310 msec exhibiting pure preexcitation pattern stops the attack.*

doubling the normal AV conduction pathway. The existence of intraseptal accessory AV conduction pathways has also been proved. It has been shown that a short PR interval with normal QRS complexes may be due to fibers passing from atrium to the infranodal region. The role of Mahaim fibers in the genesis of tachycardia cannot yet be considered to have been definitely substantiated.

It is probable that surgery for patients with the WPW syndrome will continue to improve as a result of continued research to refine techniques to localize and to sever bypass tracts, particularly in patients who have these tracts in the septum or in those who have multiple accessory pathways.

References

1. Wolff, L., Parkinson, J., and White, P. D.: Bundle branch block with short P-R interval in healthy young people prone to paroxysmal tachycardias. Am. Heart J., 5:685, 1930.
2. Clerc, A., Levy, R., and Critesco, C.: A propos du raccourcissement permanent de l'espace P-R de l'electrocardiogramme sans deformation du complexe ventriculaire. Arch. Mal. Coeur, 32:569, 1938.
3. Lown, B., Ganong, W. F., and Levine, S. A.: The syndrome of short P-R interval, normal QRS complex and paroxysmal rapid heart activation. Circulation, 5:693, 1952.
4. Scherf, D., and Cohen, J.: The atrio-ventricular node and selected cardiac arrhythmias. In Pre-excitation syndrome. p. 372. New York, Grune & Stratton, 1964.
5. Scherlag, B. J., Lau, S. H., Helfant, R. H. et al.: Catheter technique for recording His bundle activity in man. Circulation, 39:13, 1969.
6. Durrer, D., Van Dam, R. Th., Freud, G. E., et al.: Total excitation of the isolated human heart. Circulation, 41:899, 1970.
7. Holzmann, M., and Scherf, D.: Über Electrokardiogramme mit verkurzter Vorhof-Kammerdistanz und positiven P-Zacken. Z. Klin. Med., 121:404, 1932.
8. Ohnell, R. F.: Pre-excitation, a cardiac abnormality. Acta Med. Scand., 152:74, 1944.
9. Kent, A. F. S.: Researches on structure and function of mammalian heart. J. Physiol., 14:233, 1893.
10. James, T. N.: The WPW syndrome: evolving concepts of its pathogenesis. Prog. Cardiovasc. Dis., 13:159, 1970.
11. Prinzmetal, M., Kennamer, R., Corday, E., et al.: Accelerated conduction. In The WPW Syndrome and Related Conditions, p. 85, New York, Grune & Stratton, 1952.
12. Wood, F. C., Wolferth, C. G., and Geckeler, G. D.: Histologic demonstration of accessory muscular connections between auricle and ventricle in a case of short P-R interval and prolonged QRS complex. Am. Heart J., 25:454, 1943.
13. Butterworth, J. S., and Poindexter, C. A.: Short P-R interval associated with a prolonged QRS complex. A clinical and experimental study. Arch. Intern. Med., 69:437, 1942.
14. Butterworth, J. S., and Poindexter, C. A.: Fusion beats and their relation to the syndrome of short P-R interval associated with a prolonged QRS complex. Am. Heart J., 28:149, 1944.
15. Rosenbaum, F. F., Hecht, H. H., Wilson, F. N., and Johnston, F. D.: Potential variations of the thorax and the esophagus in anomalous atrioventricular excitation (W.P.W. syndrome). Am. Heart J., 29:281, 1945.
16. Durrer, D., Schoo, L., Schuilenburg, R. M., and Wellens, H. J. J.: The role of premature beats in the initiation and termination of supraventricular tachycardia in the WPW syndrome. Circulation, 36:644, 1967.
17. Durrer, D., and Roos, J. P.: Epicardial excitation of the ventricles in a patient with WPW syndrome (type B). Circulation, 35:15, 1967.
18. Burchell, H. B., Frye, R. L., Anderson, M. W., and McGoon, D. C.: Atrioventricular and ventriculoatrial excitation in WPW syndrome type B: Temporary ablation at surgery. Circulation, 36:663, 1967.
19. Dreifus, L. S., Nichols, H., Morse, D., et al.: Control of recurrent tachycardia of WPW syndrome by surgical ligature of the A-V bundle. Circulation, 38:1030, 1968.
20. Cobb, F. R., Blumenschein, S. D., Sealy, W. C., et al.: Successful

surgical interruption of the bundle of Kent in a patient with Wolff-Parkinson-White syndrome. Circulation, 38:1018, 1968.
21. Castellanos, A., Jr., Castillo, C. A., Agha, A. S., et al.: Functional properties of accessory A-V pathways during premature atrial stimulation. Br. Heart J., 35:578, 1973.
22. Castellanos, A., Jr., Chapunoff, E., Castillo, C., Maytin, O., and Lemberg, L.: His bundle electrogram in two cases of Wolff-Parkinson-White (pre-excitation) syndrome. Circulation, 41:399, 1970.
23. Touboul, P., Clement, C., Porte, J., et al.: Etude comparee des effets de la stimulation auriculaire gauche et droite dans le syndrome de WPW. Arch. Mal. Coeur, 66:1027, 1973.
24. Boineau, J. P., and Moore, E. N.: Evidence for propagation of activation across an accessory atrio-ventricular connection in types A and B pre-excitation. Circulation, 41:375, 1970.
25. Boineau, J. P., Moore, E. N., and Spear, J. F.: Biventricular pre-excitation over two accessory A-V connections in WPW. Circulation (Suppl.), 44:II-62, 1971.
26. Cole, J. S., Wills, R. E., Winterscheid, L. C., et al.: The WPW syndrome: problems in evaluation and surgical therapy. Circulation, 42:111, 1970.
27. Iwa, T.: Surgical management of WPW syndrome. In Narula, O.S. (ed.): His Bundle Electrocardiography and Clinical Electrophysiology, p. 387. Philadelphia, F. A. Davis, 1975.
28. Fontaine, G., Guiraudon, G., Bonnet, M., et al.: Section d'un faisceau de Kent dans un cas de syndrome de Wolff-Parkinson-White. II. Cartographies epicardiques. Arch. Mal. Coeur, 65:925, 1972.
29. Lindsay, A. E., Nelson, M. N., Abildskov, J. A., and Wyatt, R.: Attempted surgical division of the pre-excitation pathway in the WPW syndrome. Am. J. Cardiol., 28:581, 1971.
30. Burchell, H. B.: Surgical approach to the treatment of ventricular pre-excitation. Adv. Intern. Med., 16:43, 1970.
31. Anderson, R. H., and Taylor, J. M.: Development of atrioventricular specialized tissue in human heart. Br. Heart J., 34:1205, 1972.
32. Frank, R., Brechenmacher, C., and Fontaine, G.: Apport de l'histologie dans l'etude des syndromes de pre-excitation ventriculaire. Coeur Med. Interne, 15:337, 1976.
33. Mann, R. S., Fisher, R. S., Scherlis, S., and Hutchins, G. M.: Accessory left atrio-ventricular connection in type A WPW syndrome. Johns Hopkins Med. J., 132:242, 1973.
34. Brechenmacher, C., Laham, J., Iris, L., et al.: Etude histologique des voies anormales de conduction dans un syndrome de WPW et dans un syndrome de Lown-Ganong-Levine. Arch. Mal. Coeur, 67:507, 1974.
35. Deerhake, H. G., Kimball, J. L., Burch, G. E., and Henthorne, J. C.: WPW syndrome: histologic study of the cardiac septum and atrio-ventricular groove in one case. Ann. Intern. Med., 27:239, 1947.
36. Gallagher, J. J., Sealy, W. C., Anderson, R. W., et al.: Cryosurgical ablation of accessory atrioventricular connections: a method for correction of the pre-excitation syndrome. Circulation, 55:471, 1977.
37. Schumann, G., Jansen, H. H., and Anschutz, F.: Zur pathogenese de WPW syndroms Virehows. Arch. Pathol. Anat., 349:48, 1970.
38. Verduyin Lunel, A. A.: Significance of annulus fibrosus of heart in relation to AV conduction and ventricular activation in cases of WPW. Br. Heart J., 34:1263, 1972.
39. Lev, M.: Anatomic consideration of anomalous A-V pathways. In Dreifus, L. S. and Likeoff, W. (eds.): Mechanisms and Therapy of Cardiac Arrhythmias. New York, Grune & Stratton, 1966.
40. Mahaim, I., and Winston, M. R.: Recherches d'anatomie comparee et de pathologie experimentale sur les connexions hautes du faisceau de His-Tawarra. Cardiologia, 5:189, 1941.
41. Touboul, P., Huerta, F., Porte, J., et al.: Etude electrophysiologique de deux cas de pre-excitation ventriculaire compatibles avec la presence de fibres de mahaim. Arch. Mal. coeur, 68:841, 1975.
42. James, T. N.: Morphology of the human atrio-ventricular node with remarks pertinent to its electrophysiology. Am. Heart J., 62:756, 1961.
43. Paladino, G.: Ancora per una questione di priorita a proposito del fascio atrio-ventricular del cuore. Anat. Ang., 46:90, 1914.
44. Sherf, L., and James, T. N.: A new electrocardiographic concept of synchronized sino-ventricular conduction. Dis. Chest, 55:127, 1969.
45. Wellens, H. J. J.: Electrical stimulation of the heart in the study and treatment of tachycardias. In Wellens, H. J. J., Lie, K. I., and Janse, M. J. (eds.): The Conduction System of the Heart. Leiden, H. E. Stenfert kroese, 1971.
46. Massumi, R. A.: His bundle recording in bilateral bundle branch combined with WPW syndrome. Circulation, 42:287, 1970.
47. Tonkin, A.M., Dugan, F. A., Svenson, R. H., et al.: Coexistence of functional Kent and Mahaim-type tracts in the preexcitation syndrome. Circulation, 52:193, 1975.
48. Latour, H., and Puech, P.: Electrocardiographie Endocavitaire, p. 51. Paris, Masson, 1957.
49. Zao, Z. A., Herrmann, G. R., and Hejtmancik, M. R.: A vector study of the delta wave in non delayed conduction. Am. Heart J., 56:920, 1958.
50. Frank, R., Fontaine, G., Guiraudon, G., et al.: Correlation entre l'orientation de l'onde delta et la topographie de la pre-excitation dans le syndrome de WPW. Arch. Mal. Coeur, 5:441, 1977.
51. Gallagher, J. J., Svenson, R. H., Sealy, W. C., and Wallace, A. G.: Wolff-Parkinson-White syndrome and pre-excitation dysrhythmias. Medical and surgical management. Med. Clin. North Am., 60:101, 1975.
52. De Maria, A., Vera, Z., Neuman, A., and Mason, D. T.: Alternations in ventricular contraction pattern in the WPW Circulation, 53:249, 1976.
53. Ticzon, A. R., Damato, A. N., Caracta, A. R., et al.: Interventricular septal motion during pre-excitation and normal conduction in WPW syndrome. Echocardiographic and electrophysiologic. Am. J. Cardiol., 37:840, 1976.
54. Dohmen, X., Roelandt, X., Durrer, D., and Wellens, H. J. J.: Left ventricular wall motion in patients with Wolff-Parkinson-White syndrome studied by echocardiography. In Bom, N. (ed.): Echocardiology, p. 175, The Hague, Martinus Nijhoff, 1977.
55. Drobinski, G., Frank, R., Szymanski, C., et al.: Etude echocardiographique du syndrome de WPW. Comparaison avec les données électrocardiologiques. Arch. Mal. Coeur, 71:1209, 1978.
56. Gallagher, J. J., Gilbert, M., Svenson, R. H., et al.: WPW syndrome. The problem evaluation and surgical correction. Circulation, 51:767, 1975.
57. Frank, R.: Apport des Investigations Endocavitaires et des Cartographies Epicardiques dans l'Etude des syndromes de Pre-excitation Ventriculaire. M. D. Thesis, University of Paris, 1974.
58. Gressard, A.: Le Syndrome de WPW. Apport des Methodes d'Exploration Electrophysiologique Endocavitaire. M. D. Thesis, University of Lyon, 1976.
59. Wellens, H. J. J.: The electrophysiologic properties of the accessory pathway in the WPW syndrome. In Wellens, H. J. J., Lie, K. I., and Janse, M. J. (eds.): The Conduction System of the Heart, p. 567. Leiden, Stenfert Kroese, 1976.
60. Slama, R., Coumel, P., and Bouvrain, Y.: Les syndromes de WPW de type a inapparents ou latents en rythme sinusal Arch. Mal. Coeur, 66:639, 1973.
61. Grolleau, R., Dufoix, R., Puech, P., and Latour, H.: Les tachycardies par rythme reciproque au cours du syndrome de WPW. Physio-phathologie et traitement. Arch. Mal. Coeur, 63:74, 1970.
62. Puech, P.: L'ajmaline injectable dans les tachycardies paroxysti-

ques et le syndrome de WPW. Comparaison avec la procainamide. Arch. Mal. Coeur, 57:857, 1964.
63. Coumel, P. H., Waynberger, M., Slama, R., and Bouvrain, Y.: Interet de l'Enregistrement des potentiels Hisiens dans la comprehension de certains trobules du rythme: Bloc auriculoventriculaire, syndrome de pre-excitation, tachycardie jonctionnelle. Arch. Mal. Coeur, 63:366, 1970.
64. Goldreyer, B. N., and Damato, A. N.: The essential role of atrioventricular conduction delay in the initiation of paroxysmal supraventricular tachycardia. Circulation, 43:679, 1971.
65. Spurrell, R. A. J., Krikler, D. M., and Sowton, E.: Two or more intra AV nodal pathways in association with either a James or Kent extra-nodal bypass in 3 patients with paroxysmal supra-ventricular tachycardia. Br. Heart J., 35:113, 1973.
66. Coumel, P. H., and Attuel, P.: Localization of the circus movement during reciprocating tachycardia in WPW syndrome. In Narula, O. S. (ed.): His Bundle Electrocardiography and Clinical Electrophysiology, p. 343. Philadelphia, F. A. Davis, 1975.
67. Slama, R., Coumel, P., and Bouvrain, Y.: Les syndromes de WPW inapparents ou latents. Arch. Mal. Coeur, 65:1379, 1972.
68. Slama, R., Coumel, P., Motte, G., and Bouvrain, Y.: Tachycardies paroxystiques liees a un syndrome de WPW inapparent. Nouv. Presse Med., 4:3169, 1975.
69. De la Fuente, D., Sasyniuk, B. I., and Moe, G. K.: Conduction through a narrow isthmus in isolated canine atrial tissue. A model of the WPW syndrome. Circulation, 46:883, 1971.
70. Coumel, P. and Attuel, P.: Reciprocating tachycardia in overt and latent pre-excitation. Influence of functional bundle branch block on the rate of the tachycardia. Eur. J. Cardiol., 1:423, 1974.
71. Fontaine, G., Frank, R., Coutte, R., et al.: Rythme reciproque antidromique dans un syndrome de Wolff-Parkinson-White. Ann. Cardiol., 24:59, 1975.
72. Gallagher, J. J., Sealy, W. C., Wallace, A. G. and Kasell, J.: Correlation between catheter electrophysiologic studies and findings on mapping of ventricular excitation in the WPW syndrome. In Wellens, H. J. J., Lie, K. I., and Janse, M. J. (eds.): The Conduction System of the Heart. p. 588. Leiden, Stenfert Kroese, 1976.
73. Puech, P., and Grolleau, R.: L'onde P retrograde negative en Dl, signe de faisceau de Kent postero-lateral gauche. Arch. Mal. Coeur, 70:49, 1977.
74. Kupersmith, J.: Electrophysiologic mapping during open heart surgery. Prog. Cardiovasc. Dis., 3:167, 1976.
75. Fontaine, G., Guiraudon, G., Frank, R., et al.: Epicardial mapping in 1978. International symposium in Diagnosis and Treatment of Cardiac Arrhythmias, Barcelona, 1977.
76. Harrison, L., Gallagher, J. J., Kasell, J., et al.: Cryosurgical ablation of the AV node-His bundle: A new method for producing AV block. Circulation, 55:463, 1977.
77. Sealy, W. C., Hattler, B. J., Blumenschein, S. D., and Cobb, F. R.: Surgical treatment of WPW syndrome. Ann. Thorac. Surg., 8:1, 1969.
78. Sealy, W. C., Wallace, A. G., Ramming, K. P., Gallacher, J. J., and Svenson, R. M.: An improved operation for the definitive treatment of the Wolff-Parkinson-White syndrome. Ann. Thorac. Surg., 17:107, 1974.
79. Gallagher, J. J., Prichett, E. L. C., Sealy, W. C., et al.: The pre-excitation syndromes. Prog. Cardiovasc. Dis., 20:285, 1978.
80. Camm, J., Ward, D. E., Spurrell, R. A. J., and Rees, G. M.: Cryothermal mapping and cryoablation in the treatment of refractory cardiac arrhythmias. Circulation, 62:67, 1980.
81. Guiraudon, G., Klein, G. J., Gulamhusein, S., et al.: Section chirurgicale du faisceau de kent a coeur ferme. Arch. Mal. Coeur, 77:600–605, 1984.
82. Gallagher, J. J., Sealy, W. C., Anderson, R. W., et al.: The Surgical Treatment of Arrhythmias. In Kulbertus, H. (ed.): Reentrant Arrhythmias, p. 367. Lancaster, MTP Press, 1977.
83. Wellens, H. J. J.: Effects of drugs on WPW syndrome and its therapy. In Narula, O. S. (ed.): Clinical His bundle Electrocardiography. Philadelphia, F. A. Davis, 1974.
84. Lopes, M. G., Fitzgerald, J., Harrison, D. C., and Schroeder, J. S.: Diagnosis and quantification of arrhythmias in ambulatory patients using an improved R-R interval plotting system. Am. J. Cardiol. 35:816, 1975.
85. Mandel, W. J., Laks, M. M., Yamaguchi, I., et al.: Recurrent reciprocating tachycardias in the WPW syndrome: control by the use of a scanning pacemaker. Chest, 69:769, 1976.
86. Krikler, D., Curry, P., and Buffet, J.: Dual-demand pacing for reciprocating atrioventricular tachycardia. Br. Med. J., 1:1114, 1976.
87. Barold, S. S.: Therapeutic uses of cardiac pacing in tachyarrhythmias. In Narula, O. S. (ed.): His Bundle Electrocardiography and Clinical Electrophysiology, p. 407. Philadelphia, F. A. Davis, 1975.
88. Yahini, J. H., Zahavi, I., and Neufeld, H.: Paroxysmal atrial fibrillation in WPW syndrome simulating ventricular tachycardia. Am. J. Cardiol., 14:248, 1964.
89. Dreifus, L. S., Haiat, R. A., Watanabe, Y., et al.: Ventricular fibrillation: a possible mechanism of sudden death in patients with WPW syndrome. Circulation, 43:520, 1971.
90. Martin-Noel, P., Denis, O., Grundwald, D., and Buisson, M. Deux cas mortels de syndrome de WPW. Arch. Mal. Coeur, 63:1647, 1978.

35

Surgery for Ventricular Tachycardia

A. John Camm
and R. A. J. Spurrell

Ventricular tachyarrhythmias may cause dramatic symptoms such as presyncope and syncope. Recurrent sustained ventricular tachycardias are associated with a first-year mortality of up to 40%. Their management must therefore be approached aggressively. When the ever-increasing range of antiarrhythmic drugs fails or promises to be ineffective, alternative therapies must be considered. Implantable devices such as automatic defibrillators, cardioverters, or antitachycardia pacemakers are used to control these arrhythmias by terminating attacks of tachycardia, but they do not prevent the arrhythmia. Arrhythmia prophylaxis, or even cure, can be achieved by surgical intervention. The surgical approach is therefore an essential strategy in the management of patients with such serious arrhythmias. Indirect approaches such as sympathectomy or coronary revascularization have only limited application and success. More direct and specific methods of surgery such as ventriculotomy, tissue resection, and cryoablation have been considerably more successful, especially in the treatment of arrhythmias associated with chronic coronary disease. Increasingly, combinations of these surgical therapies or the combined application of surgery, antiarrhythmic drugs, and implantable devices have allowed successful long-term management of patients with these otherwise life-threatening arrhythmias. Although it is now apparent that surgical techniques can be successfully applied, it is not yet certain how to select patients and how to choose the most appropriate operation.

Selection of Patients for Surgery

At present the primary indication for surgical management of patients with ventricular tachycardia is failure to respond to medical therapy. Such "medical failures" may require surgery for symptomatic relief or for prognostic reasons. At present there is no valid comparison (prospective, blind, and randomized) between apparently effective medical treatment and antiarrhythmia surgery. Surgery might prove the more effective because of radical or virtually complete removal of the arrhythmia substrate and because of patients' lack of compliance with medical therapy. However, in view of the small but definite operative risk, it is not yet reasonable to offer surgical therapy as the first option without a prior trial of antiarrhythmic drugs.

With the advent of implantable automatic devices such as the defibrillator, cardiovertor, and pacemaker, which may in combination promptly and effectively terminate all varieties of ventricular tachyarrhythmia, it is now important to evaluate the relative worth of surgery and these devices.[1] This information is not currently available.

Before surgery it is important to assess the patient and the tachycardia by conventional electrophysiologic techniques and, when appropriate, by hemodynamic catheterization and coronary angiography. Because ventricular tachyarrhythmias may prove impossible to convert if very severe coronary artery disease, such as a critical left main stenosis, is present, it is advisable to perform coronary angiography on all patients with ventricular tachycardia due to coronary disease before performing an electrophysiologic study. Alternatively, coronary angiography may be limited to those who show other evidence of severe obstructive coronary disease or may be performed later if surgery is selected.

The majority of clinically symptomatic ventricular tachycardias can be provoked by programmed stimulation. This allows deductive electrophysiologic techniques to be used to ensure that the tachycardia arises in the ventricles. Recording from multiple endocavitary sites (catheter mapping) enables the approximate origin of the tachycardia to be located. It is preferable to select for surgery patients whose tachycardia may be provoked by stimulation techniques, especially if the arrhymogenic site has been determined by preoperative catheter mapping.[2,3] Tachycardias that are easily induced and well sustained are the most amenable to surgery. Those patients with ventricular tachycardia and other cardiac anomalies that require surgical attention are also obvious candidates for surgical therapy of their arrhythmias.

Indirect Surgical Methods

Sympathectomy

Although bilateral sympathectomy was employed as a form of management of medically refractory ventricular arrhythmias associated with coronary and other forms of heart disease, the technique was not particularly successful.[4,5] The advent of a wide variety of beta-blockers has virtually eliminated the need for this form of surgery. The long QT syndrome, first described by Jervell and Lange-Nielsen,[6] is associated with an imbalance in the sympathetic innervation of the heart—the sympathetic supply from the left stellate ganglion predominates. Left stallectomy leads to resolution of the malignant ventricular arrhythmias responsible for syncope and sudden death in this syndrome.[7] However, in their most recent report based on a prospective international registry that contains the histories of 196 patients with long QT syndrome, Moss and colleagues[8] report that only eight of those patients were treated by left stellate ganglionectomy. From this report it is also clear that medical treatment with adequate beta-blockade is of similar efficacy to stellectomy. Unfortunately, a stellectomy leads to unilateral Horner's syndrome, but this may be preferable to patient lack of compliance to beta-blockade therapy or the troublesome side-effects these agents produce. More specific dissection of the sympathetic nervous system may allow cardiac denervation without producing Horner's syndrome. The combination of stellectomy and beta-blockade therapy appears to be more beneficial than either treatment alone. Indeed, one recent[9] report has suggested that left stellectomy alone is thoroughly inadequate treatment for patients with the long QT syndrome. Of ten patients treated in this way, eight developed recurrent symptoms (syncope in four, presyncope in six, and cardiac arrest in three). The authors suggest that concommitant drug treatment, more extensive surgery, pacing, or implantation of an automatic defibrillator should be considered for such patients.

Mitral Valve Replacement

There is a handful of reports on the value of mitral valve replacement for the management of documented or suspected ventricular tachyarrhythmias occurring in association with mitral valve prolapse.[10-12] In most instances ventricular ectopic activity persisted after mitral valve replacement, but symptoms attributable to malignant ventricular arrhythmias did not continue. Additional antiarrhythmic therapy, sometimes unsuccessful although not always tried before surgery, was often necessary after surgery. Sustained tachyarrhythmias were not provoked before or at surgery and were therefore not usually mapped. In one instance, Cobbs and King[10] mapped spontaneously occurring ventricular ectopic beats and discovered their apparent epicardial origin close to the base of the posterior papillary muscle. Pressure at this point prevented the ectopic activity. Based on these data and the morphologic characteristics of the ventricular tachycardia, most reports have agreed that the likely mechanism of these arrhythmias in mitral valve prolapse is stretching of the mitral subvalvar structures, especially the posterior papillary muscle.

Coronary Revascularization

It has been suggested that coronary revascularization may reduce the incidence of sudden death,[13] particularly in patients without a history of ventricular tachyarrhythmias but with severe proximal and multivessel coronary stenoses. Such patients, especially those with left ventricular dysfunction, often have frequent and complex ventricular arrhythmias. Unfortunately, coronary bypass surgery does not reduce the incidence of these arrhythmias when assessed by ambulatory electrocardiographic monitoring or exercise testing[14,15] and, in some patients, may worsen the arrhythmias. The failure to improve ventricular arrhythmias by this form of surgery is presumably because the arrhythmias are not due to acute ischemia but to chronic ischemic damage and infarction that has produced the arrhythmia substrate. Because of the severity of obstructive coronary disease in victims of sudden unexpected cardiac death, it was initially expected that coronary revascularization would reduce the incidence of recurrent malignant ventricular arrhythmias in such patients. There are many hopeful reports, but long-term follow-up studies are not available.[16–18]

In some patients with exercise-induced sustained ventricular tachycardia, the relief of severe proximal coronary stenoses undoubtedly abolishes the arrhythmia as assessed by long-term follow-up study and electrophysiologic testing.[19,20] However, it is very difficult to predict which patients will benefit in this way. Certainly preoperative angiography is unhelpful, but the development of ventricular tachyarrhythmias only in the presence of ischemic repolarization changes have occurred on the electrocardiogram may be a helpful indicator, especially if the arrhythmias appear to arise from the ischemic territory.

Aneurysmectomy

In 1959 Couch[21] reported the case of a woman aged 54 years who developed drug-resistant ventricular tachycardia after suffering an anterolateral myocardial infarction. In 1956 she had undergone a ventriculoplasty (*i.e.*, excision of aneurysm), and during follow-up study she suffered no further episodes of ventricular tachycardia despite not taking antiarrhythmic drugs. Couch[21] drew attention to the association between ventricular aneurysms and ventricular arrhythmias and suggested that aneurysmectomy was successful because the irritable focus was excised with the aneurysm. There followed a host of case reports and small series of patients[22–25] testifying to the relief of ventricular tachycardia following resection of aneurysms. Buda and colleagues[26] reported a large series of 203 left ventricular aneurysmectomies, in 49 instances the surgery being performed for refractory life-threatening ventricular arrhythmias. There was a high operative mortality (20%), predominantly due to surgery closely following an acute myocardial infarction. Thirty-five of the patients who were operated for ventricular arrhythmias survived for a mean follow-up study of 41 months, and of these 13 had no recurrence of arrhythmias. However, with longer follow-up study it soon became clear that, even when combined with coronary revascularization procedures, aneurysmectomy was generally ineffective at abolishing ventricular arrhythmias. For example, in the report from Ricks and colleagues,[27] 21 patients underwent aneurysmectomy, aneurysm plication, coronary grafting for the control of life-threatening ventricular arrhythmias; 14 survived to leave hospital. There was one additional late death, three patients had recurrent documented ventricular arrhythmias, and six others had persistent, troublesome palpitations. Thus only four of the original 21 patients survived symptom free. Another study that drew attention to the inadequacy of aneurysmectomy in controlling ventricular tachyarrhythmias was that reported by Sami and colleagues.[28] Ten patients who underwent aneurysmectomy in an attempt to abolish arrhythmias were followed by ambulatory monitoring and exercise testing. Two died suddenly, and runs of ventricular tachycardia were noted in three others. The remaining five patients all had frequent multifocal extrasystoles. Similar results have been noted by other groups.[29–32]

Operative Mapping

Epicardial and endocardial mapping techniques during normal rhythms and induced arrhythmias have been used for a variety of clinical and experimental purposes since 1913.[33,34] As noted above, better surgical management of patients with ventricular tachycardia can be obtained by employing various methods of mapping to localize the origin, or likely origin, of the arrhythmia. Five different forms of "mapping" the ventricle are in use:

1. Electrogram mapping during tachycardia (endocardial, epicardial, and transmural exploration) to obtain an activation map and define the earliest activity during tachycardia or the course of a reentrant pathway critical to the perpetuation of tachycardia.
2. Electrogram mapping during sinus rhythm (endocardial, epicardial, and transmural exploration) to identify those areas of late or abnormal activation that could form the substrate for reentrant ventricular tachycardia.
3. "Cryothermal mapping during tachycardia" (epicardial and endocardial exploration) to localize a point at which freezing terminates tachycardia.
4. "Pacemapping" (epicardial and endocardial exploration) to identify a point where artificial ventricular pacing produces a QRS complex identical to that occurring during ventricular tachycardia.
5. Visual inspection "mapping" to locate abnormal tissue that might provide a substrate for tachycardia.

Electrogram recording to construct activation maps during tachycardia and cryothermal tachycardia termination mapping require that tachycardia be stimulated and sustained in the operating room. The majority of coronary-related and idiopathic tachycardias can be provoked by programmed stimulation. In the presence of anesthetic drugs and after surgery, particularly after a ventriculotomy, it may prove difficult to induce ventricular tachycardia. Elevating the blood temperature to 38°C or infusing isoprenaline may help provoke and sustain the arrhythmia. Rapid tachycardias may degenerate quickly to sinus rhythm. It is therefore essential to prepare the patient for cardiopulmonary bypass before tachycardia is stimulated. Intravenous procainamide or ajmaline[35] may slow the tachycardia sufficiently to prevent degeneration and allow accurate mapping. The induction and maintenance of tachycardia during open-chest and open-heart procedures does not seem to produce significant cardiac damage provided that the total duration of normothermic cardiopulmonary bypass with the beating heart is kept to a minimum, preferably less than 45 minutes. Some investigators have sought to minimize potential subendocardial damage during surgery by intra-aortic balloon counterpulsation during the induced arrhythmia.

Electrogram Mapping During Tachycardia

In 1975 Gallagher and colleagues[37] reported on a single patient in whom they employed epicardial mapping to guide the extent of the resection procedure. They identified an area of early activation during tachycardia on the posterior aspect of the left ventricle on the edge of, but not within, the aneurysm. This area was resected together with the aneurysm. The patient was followed for 1 year without recurrence of his arrhythmia. This report suggested that electrophysiologic guidance of tissue resection might improve the rather poor rate of success with blind aneurysmectomy. In the same year Wittig and Boineau[38] reported from their experience with the surgical treatment of three patients with ventricular tachycardia and from experimental evidence with ischaemic arrhythmias in dogs that epicardial, endocardial, and transmural mapping was necessary to locate the focus of irritability. Spielman and colleagues[39] investigated the relative value of epicardial and endocardial mapping and demonstrated that epicardial mapping alone would have missed many of the tachycardias that were correctly located with endocardial mapping.

The technique of activation mapping is as follows:

1. Stationary electrodes are fixed on the ventricle of interest or on both ventricles.
2. By pacing through one of these electrodes, tachycardia is stimulated.
3. A roving hand-held or fingertip electrode is moved over the surface of the heart using a grid reference system. This so-called mapping electrode is usually a triangular (three bipoles) arrangement to ensure that the direction of depolarization cannot be perpendicular to all three electrode pairs.
4. Electrograms are usually bipolar, band-pass filtered between approximately 50 and 500 Hz, and amplified to achieve about 1 cm/mV when recorded on paper at speeds of at least 100 mm/sec.
5. Electrograms from the mapping electrode are recorded together with several surface electrocardiographic leads and electrograms from at least one stationary electrode.

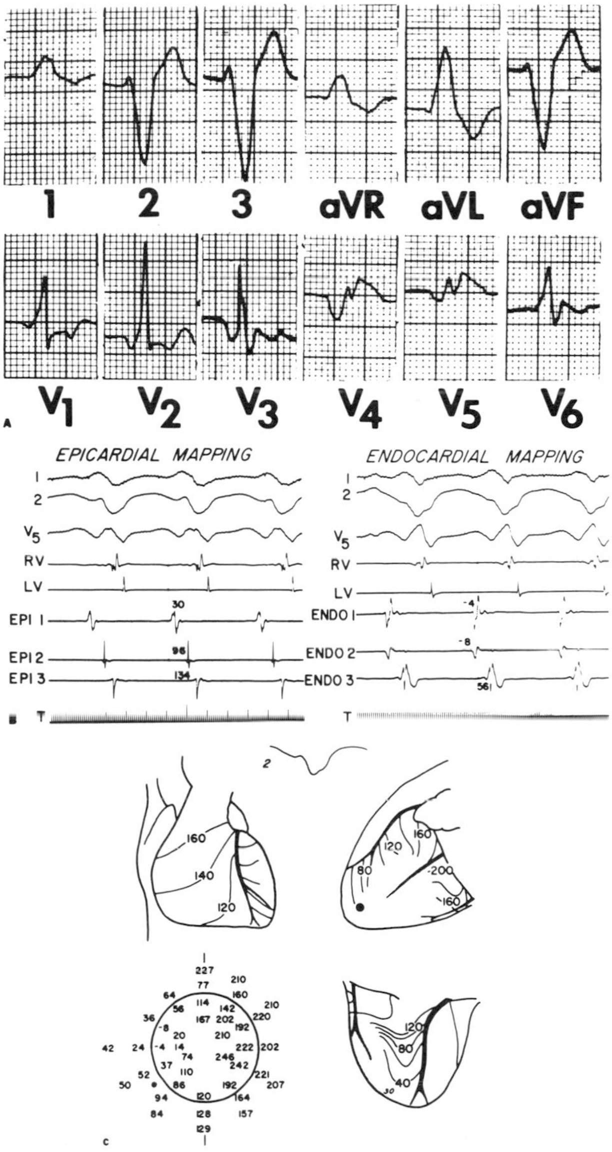

Figure 35-1. (Top panels) *A 12-lead electrocardiogram during VT.* (Middle panels, left) *epicardial mapping and* (right) *endocardial mapping.* (Bottom panel) *An epicardial isochronic map* (AP, lateral, posterior views) *and an endocardial map showing the earliest activation point (viewed from the feet toward the head). (With permission, Josephson, M. E., Harken, A. H., and Horowitz, L. N.: Endocardial excision: a new surgical technique for the treatment of recurrent ventricular tachycardia.)*

6. Each electrogram is timed in relation to a constant reference, usually the electrogram from a stationary electrode pair, and the timing is adjusted relative to the onset of the QRS complex.
7. The timing of the electrogram is related to the position from which it was recorded using a stylized grid. At this stage isochrone (equal time) contours may be calculated and drawn. This latter step is rarely necessary.
8. After the epicardial map has been performed the relevant ventricle is opened, preferably through a scar, and the endocardial surface is mapped during tachycardia (Fig. 35-1).

Since 1974 a number of comparisons between blind aneurysmectomy and electrophysiologically guided surgical therapy have been published.[40–43] All have clearly indicated that map guided surgery is vastly superior in that patients survive longer and suffer fewer recurrences of their ventricular arrhythmia. However, it is difficult to make a proper comparison because the patients treated by electrophysiologically directed resection were mostly operated on at a later date than those treated with blind aneurysmectomy, and there is no study in which patients were randomly allocated to one of the two treatment protocols. Nevertheless, the results are so convincing that this methodologic inadequacy can probably be ignored.

To construct an activation map of the endocardial or epicardial surface, electrograms must be recorded from between 50 and 100 points (Fig. 35-2). This requires that a stable rhythm must be sustained for at least 5 to 10 minutes. Ventricular tachycardias often degenerate rapidly, or several tachycardias with multiple morphologies may coexist. Therefore, it is sometimes necessary to map the ventricles very quickly. Simultaneous recording of electrograms from multiple points may allow the collection of all the data during a single beat of tachycardia. Ingenious electrode arrays and computer algorithms to collect and display the data in the form of activation

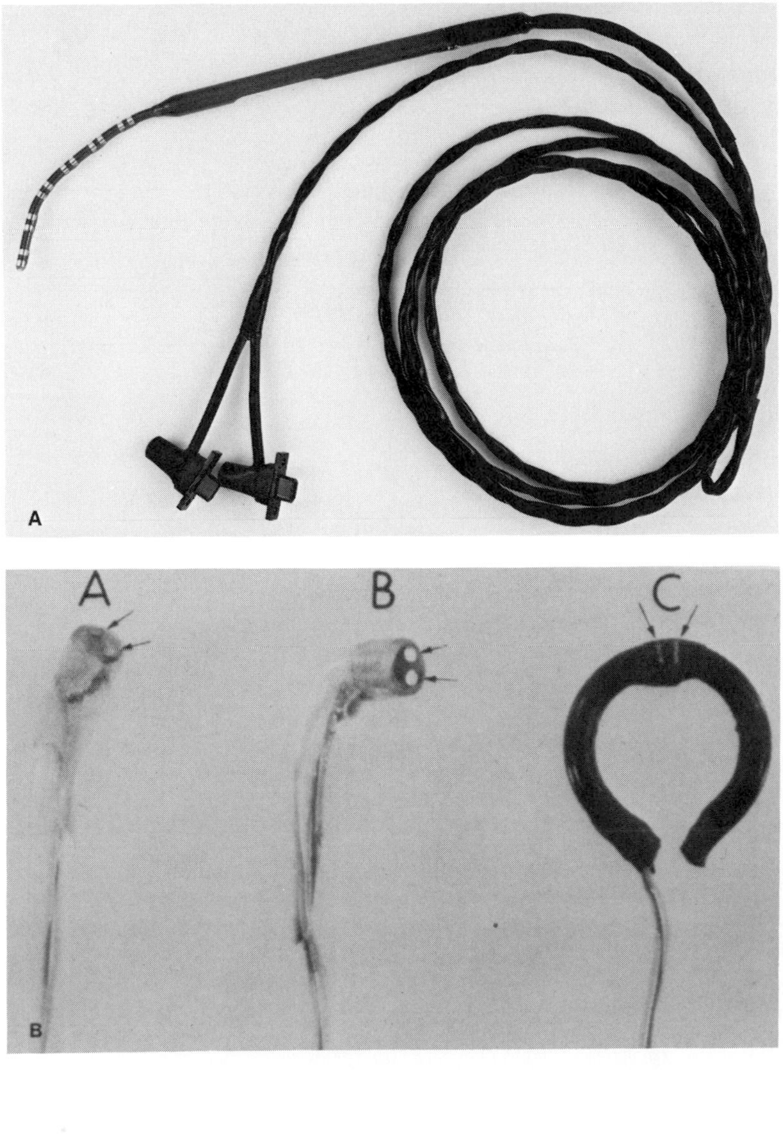

Figure 35-2. (Top) *Catheter mapping probe used in the OR to map endocardial or epicardial points. Six bipolar electrode pairs are arranged on this hand-held probe allowing rapid access to six simultaneous sites.* (Bottom) *Various bipolar probes for endocardial or epicardial mapping. In (C) a ring probe with small bipolar electrodes is shown. (With permission, Gallagher, J. J., Kasell, J. H., Cox, J. L., et al.: Techniques of intraoperative electrophysiologic mapping.)*

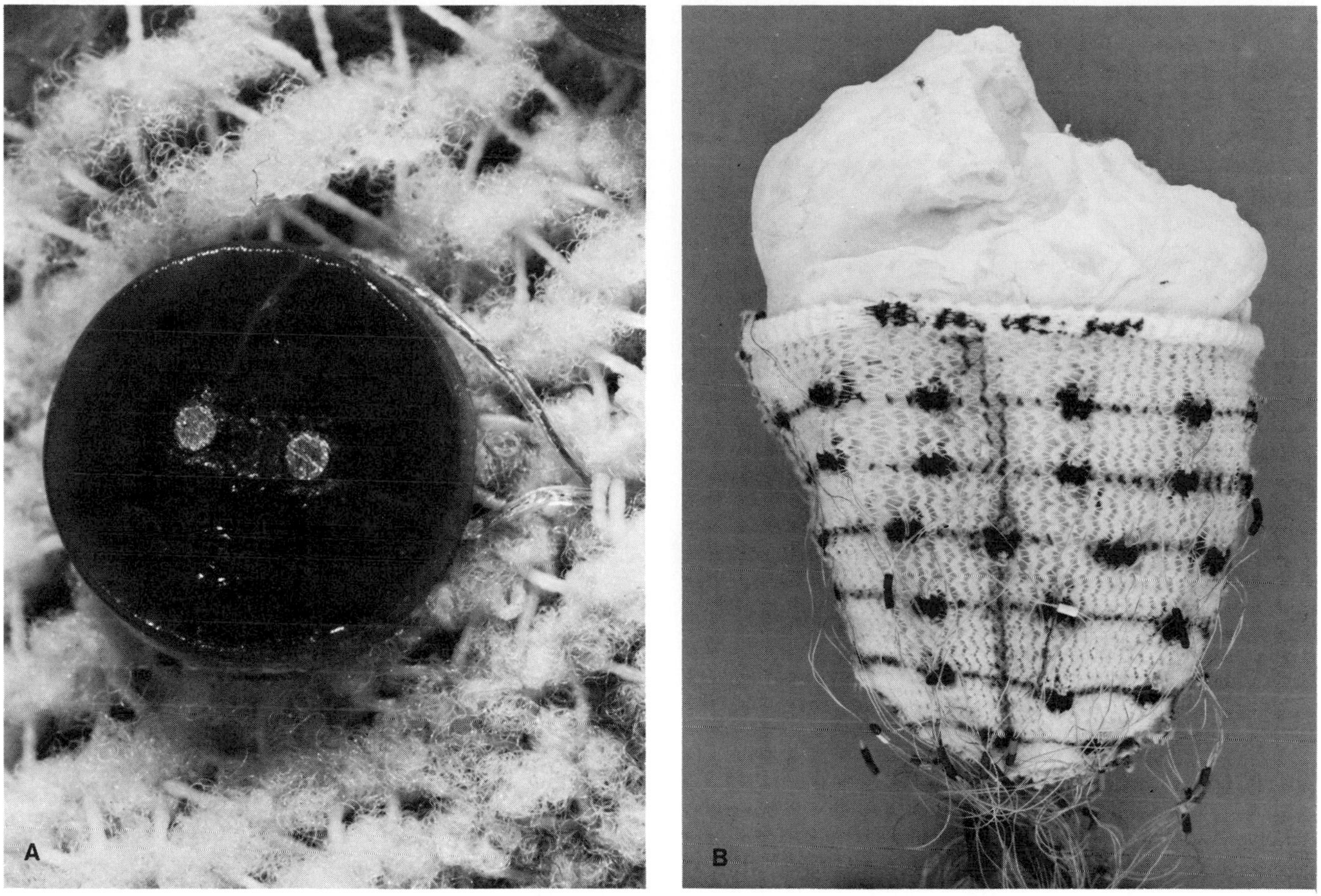

Figure 35-3. *(A) Molded epoxy bipolar snap electrode attached to the Xspan® sock. The electrode contacts are 0.7 mm in diameter and separated by 2 mm, measured center to center. The wires leading to the electrode contacts from the outside of the sock are visible to the right as they emerge from under the elastic crossmesh fibers between two longitudinal nylon fibers. The small circular indentation on the face of the electrode at 7 o'clock is from a pin used to eject the hardened epoxy from the mold. (B) The Xspan® sock electrode array applied to the latex mold of a human heart. The female snaps are sewn to the sock in six circumferential rows from base to apex. The female snaps are visible in the photograph as black circles. The top three rows have 12 snaps each, whereas the bottom three rows have eight snaps each. Each female snap supports a snap electrode on the inside of the sock. The line on the sock extending from apex to base is used to align the sock on the heart at the time of surgery. (Worley, S. J., Ideker, R. E., Mastrototaro, I., et al.: A new sock electrode for recording epicardial activation from the human heart: one size fits all. PACE vol 9, Nov 1986 [in press]).*

maps have been designed. Ideker and colleagues[44] described a triple array system. A flexible nylon mesh sock containing 27 electrodes was fitted over the epicardial surface of the heart to obtain a general activation map from which to define an approximate origin of tachycardia (Fig. 35-3). A 3-cm × 3-cm plaque containing 25 electrodes was then placed over the region of interest to allow a more detailed map of this area. Finally, a needle array, consisting of five electrodes each separated by 3 mm, was used to explore the transmural activation sequence. An electrode system designed to collect endocardial electrograms was reported by de Bakker and associates.[45] A balloon with 30 electrodes on its surface was inserted into the left ventricle through an incision usually made in an aneurysm or akinetic area. The balloon was then inflated to bring the terminals into contact with the endocardium (Fig. 35-4). With this system de Bakker and his group studied 32 patients with ventricular tachycardias and demonstrated that the endocardial site of origin of some ventricular tachycardias with iden-

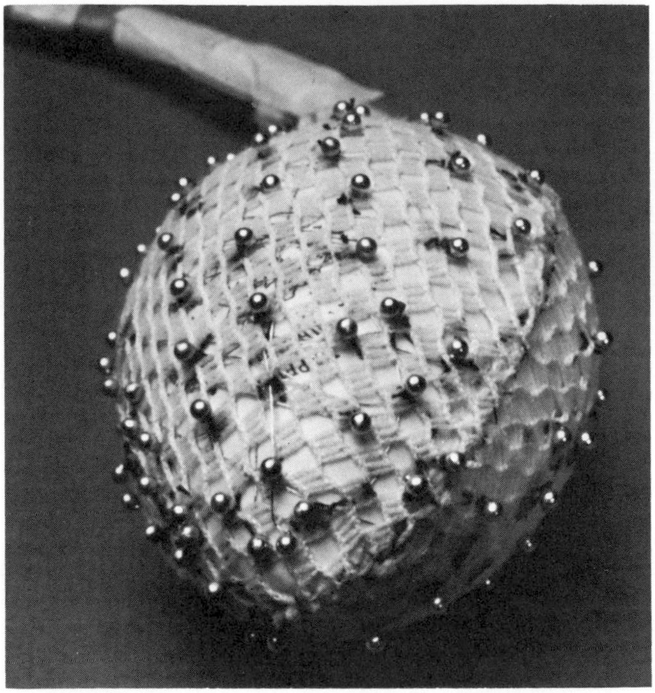

Figure 35-4. *Mapping of endocardial activation during ventricular tachycardia is done using an array of silver bead electrodes stitched on a mesh over a latex balloon. (Downar, E., et al.: Mapping of Endocardial [ENDO] Activation During Ventricular Tachycardia [VT]—A "Closed Heart" Procedure. Presented at the 35th Annual Scientific Session, American College of Cardiology, Atlanta, March 9–13, 1986.)*

tical surface QRS complexes could vary from beat to beat by up to 4 cm. Hauer and colleagues[46] have recently extended the role of the computer by developing a method whereby the site of origin of an arrhythmia in relation to anatomic landmarks can be accurately predicted from the results of catheter mapping. They performed this analysis on eight ventricular tachycardias and computed the location of the arrhythmogenic site to within 1 cm of that determined by operative mapping in seven of the eight tachycardias. In the remaining case the computed site was less than 2 cm distant from the mapped origin of tachycardia.

The development of computer-assisted mapping techniques will minimize the time taken to achieve a map and allow more accurate maps to be obtained even when arrhythmias are not sustained.

Electrogram Mapping During Sinus Rhythm

Ventricular tachycardia in association with chronic coronary artery disease or arrhythmogenic right ventricular dysplasia is thought to be due to reentry. In such cases electrical activity should continue throughout systole and diastole. If diastolic activity is confined to a small mass of tissue, it may be possible to remove that tissue and prevent further tachycardia. Diastolic potentials have been described as "late" because they occur more than 100 msec after the onset of the QRS complex[47] or are entirely outside the QRS complex.[48] Other abnormal potentials have been described in association with coronary disease. "Fractionated" potentials are continuous multicomponent electrograms longer than 50 msec and less than 1 mV in amplitude.[49] "Split" or "double" potentials have a distinct isoelectric segment between multiple discrete potentials (Fig. 35-5). Wiener and colleagues[49] demonstrated that such abnormal electrograms are often recorded from aneurysmal tissue, and in some patients, particularly those with a history of ventricular tachycardia, they may also be recorded from the epicardial or endocardial border zone surrounding an aneurysm. Klein and colleagues[47] confirmed these findings in a larger group of 38 patients, of whom 21 had serious ventricular arrhythmias associated with either a left ventricular aneurysm or an akinetic area resulting from a myocardial infarction. Although abnormal potentials could sometimes be recorded only from the endocardium, which was mapped in only 10 of the 38 patients, Klein and associates[47] found that in 21 patients with arrhythmias, 20 had late potentials, 20 had fractionated potentials, and 13 had double potentials. In the 17 patients who had no history of arrhythmia, only two had late potentials and one had both double and fractionated potentials. Thus in this study abnormal potentials were very sensitive and highly specific markers of ventricular tachycardia.

A different perspective emerged from the study reported by Kienzle and colleagues.[48] They studied 13 patients, all of whom had a history of recurrent sustained ventricular tachycardia associated with a previous extensive myocardial infarction. During sinus rhythm fractionated endocardial electrograms were recorded in all, but late potentials were only recorded in four of 13 patients. However, late electrograms were recorded from areas activated early during induced tachycardia more consistently than were fractionated or split potentials. These workers also noted that fractionated potentials were recorded from more sites (36%) than were late potentials (5%). They pointed out that if surgery were designed to remove all endocardium from which abnormal electrograms were recorded, a seemingly more extensive operation than indicated from tachycardia activation sequence mapping would be needed.

Cryothermal Mapping

Reducing the temperature of the myocardium to 0°C produces conduction block, which is relieved when the temperature is allowed to rise again. Thus if tissue that forms a critical part of the reentry circuit supporting the

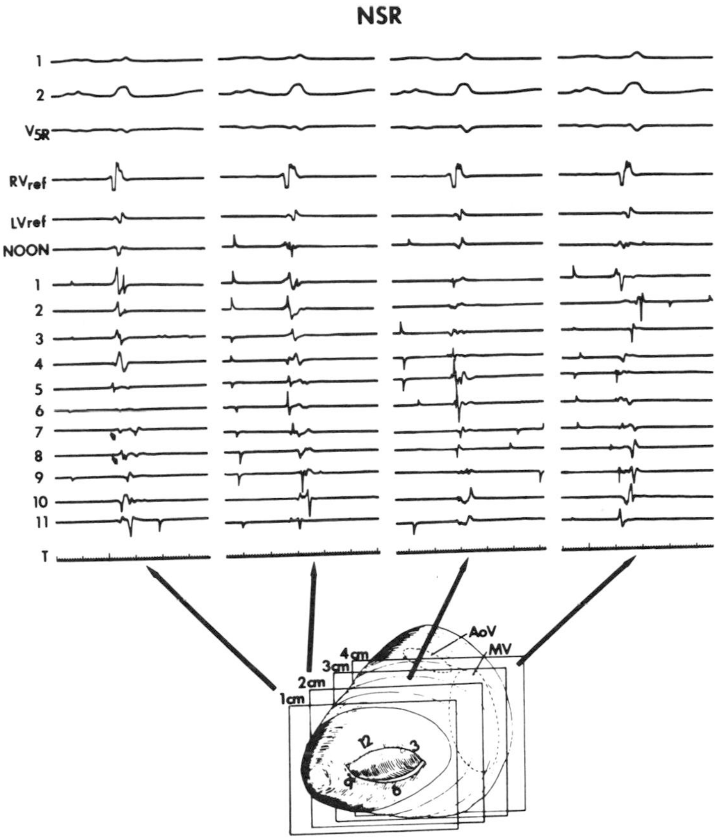

Figure 35-5. *Multiple endocardial electrograms recorded during normothermic bypass during sinus rhythm. Note the marked fractionation and reduced amplitude of some of the LV sites. (With permission, Kienzle, M. G., Miller, J., Falcone, R. A., et al.: Intraoperative endocardial mapping during sinus rhythm: relationship to site of origin of ventricular tachycardia.)*

tachycardia is cooled, the tachycardia will break and should not be reinducible until the tissue is rewarmed. Similarly, automatic mechanisms of tachycardia may be suppressed by local cooling. Therefore cooling of the myocardium with a cryoprobe may be used to confirm the origin or reentrant pathway of an arrhythmia. This technique was first applied to the localization of the His bundle or AV node[50] before attempted destruction of AV conduction. Cryomapping has been successfully used to aid in the localization of ventricular tachycardia by Gallagher and colleagues[51] and by Camm and associates.[52,53] Obviously the method requires that sustained and stable tachycardia can be initiated at surgery.

Pacemapping

When a tachycardia with a distinct morphology cannot be initiated or sustained long enough for an adequate activation map, the technique known as pacemapping[54] may be employed. This method involves pacing the ventricles with a roving electrode and attempting to match the paced QRS complex with previously recorded QRS complexes of the ventricular tachycardia (Fig. 35-6). Such recordings may have been made preoperatively or, better, during identical circumstances (e.g., chest open, during normothermic cardiopulmonary bypass) perioperatively. Pacing the ventricle from different sites results in different QRS configurations,[55] and the technique of attempting to mimic tachycardia complexes by ventricular pacing can be applied to the identification of the origin of ventricular tachycardia[56,57] and used as an aid in the direct surgical irradication of tachycardias. Initially epicardial pacing was advocated, but since the majority of coronary related tachycardias arise from the endocardium, endocardial pacing was subsequently evaluated.[58,59] Although with epicardial pacemapping O'Keefe and coauthors[60] were able to identify the tachycardia origin in a series of nine patients, it is probable that the source of some tachycardias will not be accurately identified by epicardial pacing because the epicardial breakthrough point may be many centimeters away from the true endocardial origin.

Endocardial pacing at the site of origin of ventricular tachycardia does accurately simulate the tachycardia QRS complex, but similar QRS complexes can be obtained by pacing at widely divergent points and different QRS complexes can result from pacing at closely adjacent points.[59] It may therefore take a long time to locate the tachycardia focus using pacemapping.[59] Apparently the energy and rate of pacing do not seem to influence the resultant QRS complex. Ventricular pacing may engage, drive, and entrain a reentry circuit and closely reproduce the tachycardia QRS by simply being approximately "on circuit" rather than by pacing in a critical

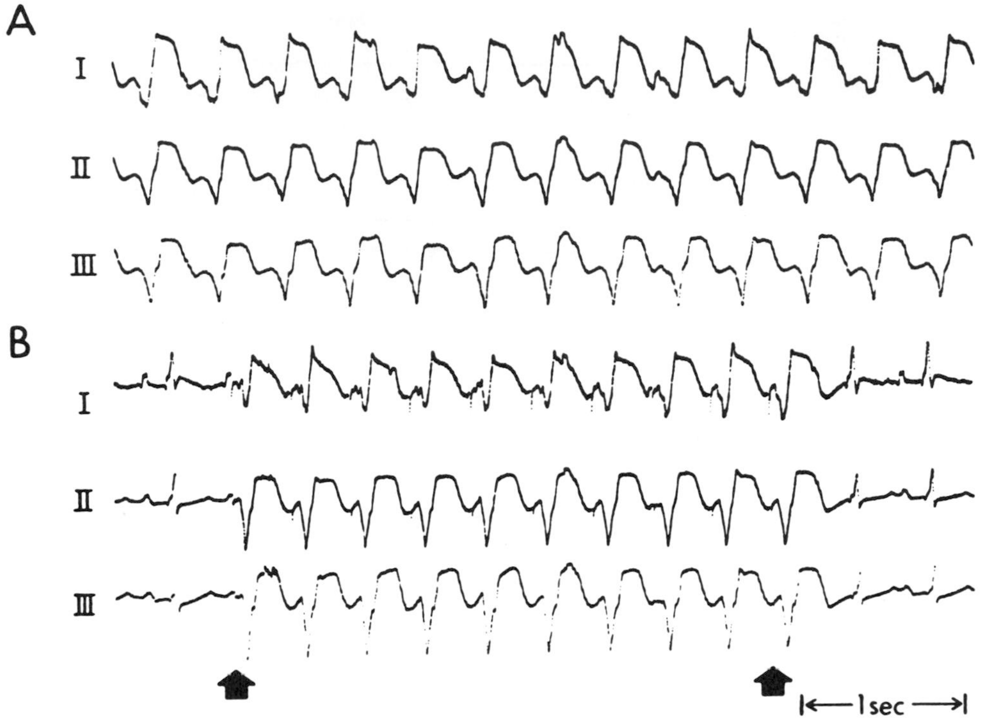

Figure 35-6. *Pace mapping techniques. (A) QRS morphology during ventricular tachycardia. (B) pacing from a site in the left ventricle produces a QRS of identical morphology. (With permission, Gallagher, J. J., Kasell, J. H., Cox, J. L., et al.: Techniques of intraoperative electrophysiologic mapping.)*

part of the circuit. Conversely, pacing from a point source may never reproduce the tachycardia QRS complex if it results from conduction over a large reentry circuit. Despite these theoretical limitations, pacemapping is very useful if tachycardia cannot be initiated in the operating room. It should not, however, be used instead of activation mapping.

Visual Inspection

For a variety of reasons, set out below, several groups of investigators have suggested that the endocardial surface of the heart should be visually inspected and that all abnormal endocardium likely to give rise to ventricular tachycardia should be removed (Fig. 35-7):

1. It may not be possible to obtain an adequate activation map or cryothermal termination point because ventricular tachyarrhythmias may not be provoked at surgery or, when successfully initiated, may not be sustained or may degenerate into ventricular fibrillation.
2. Mapping during sinus rhythm is nonspecific in that it generally reveals large areas from which abnormal electrograms are recorded. This necessitates excision of extensive areas of endocardium.
3. In some patients the endocardium cannot be mapped during any rhythm because of adherent thrombus.
4. Polymorphic (multiple distinct QRS shapes) or pleomorphic (continuously changing QRS shape) ventricular tachycardias and ventricular fibrillation are impossible to map without sophisticated multiple simultaneous recordings and computer-based algorithms to construct activation maps.
5. All mapping techniques take at least 15 minutes and may last as long as 1 hour.
6. Pacemapping may provide misleading information.

In patients with endocardial scars due to previous myocardial infarction, the abnormal (thick and white) endocardium can easily be seen. Except when the scar extends throughout the entire thickness of the free wall or septum or involves the papillary muscles or extends into the AV valve ring, it can easily and quickly be stripped away. Thus visual inspection and extensive endocardial resection has been safely and effectively used to manage patients with ventricular tachycardias and ventricular fibrillation.[61]

Comparison Between Methods of Mapping

Josephson and colleagues[62] compared preoperative endocardial mapping with operative endocardial mapping in eighteen patients undergoing surgery for the control of 24 tachycardias (right bundle branch block morphology in 12 and left bundle branch block in 12). Catheter map-

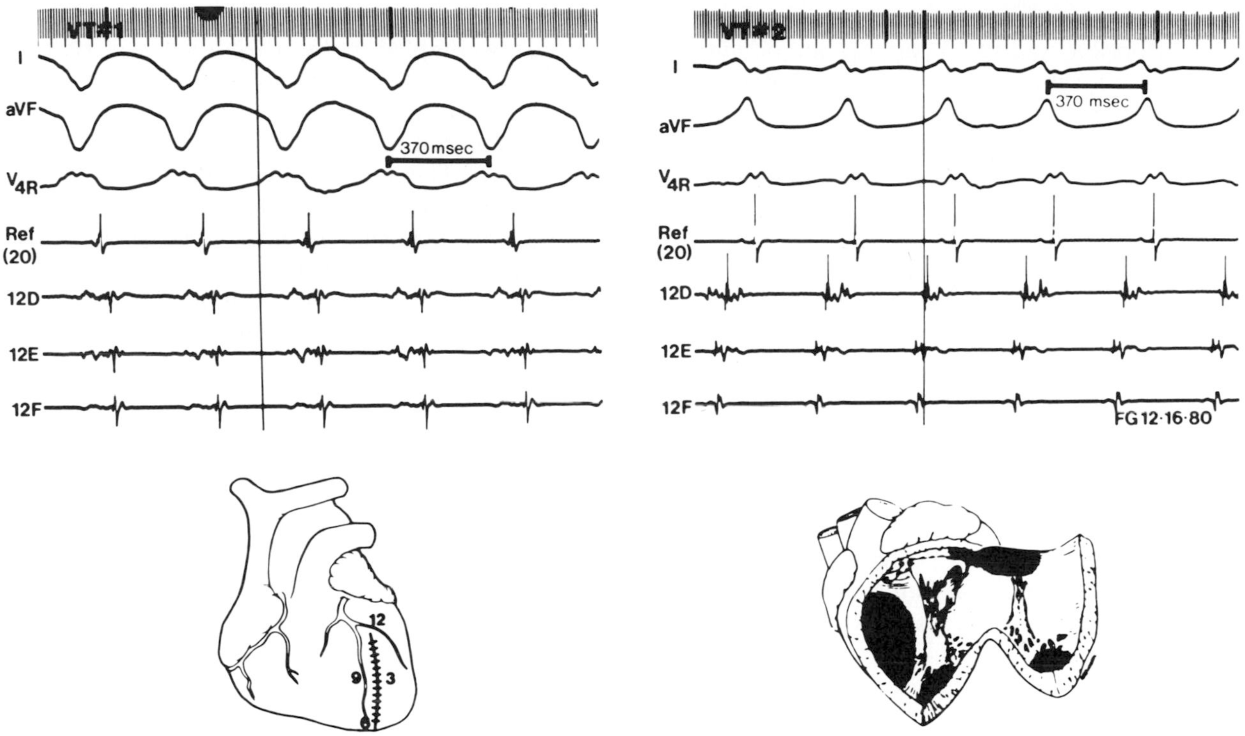

Figure 35-7. (Top panels) *LV endocardial recordings during two distinct VT morphologies.* (Bottom right panel) *Visible scar areas that were surgically resected using the incision illustrated* (bottom left panel). *(With permission, Kehoe, R. F., Loeb, J. M., Lichtenthal, P. R., et al.: Extended endocardial resection for the treatment of ventricular tachycardia and ventricular fibrillation.*

ping accurately predicted the origin of tachycardia in all 24 cases. Tachycardia origins determined by the two techniques were within 4 to 8 cm of each other. In the same paper endocardial preoperative mapping was compared with epicardial mapping. The origins of the 12 right bundle branch block morphology tachycardias were correctly localized to the left ventricle, but 11 of the 12 "left bundle branch block" morphology tachycardias were wrongly localized. One tachycardia that arose from the right ventricular outflow tract was accurately located by epicardial mapping. Otherwise, there was considerable discrepancy between epicardial breakthrough and endocardial origin because tachycardias arose from near the endocardium or within the septum. Thus endocardial activity uniformly preceded the earliest epicardial electrogram and in only one patient did epicardial activation coincide with the onset of the surface QRS. The endocardial origin was confirmed when excision of the earliest activated endocardial site led to the irradication of the tachycardias. Spielman and colleagues,[39] Wittig and Boineau,[38] and Horowitz and associates[63] also found that epicardial mapping was very inaccurate, particularly when the tachycardias arose from the interventricular septum.

The accuracy of endocardial pacemapping was evaluated against endocardial and epicardial activation mapping by Josephson and associates.[59] They found that the paced QRS complex tended to reflect the epicardial breakthrough point rather than the endocardial origin and that pacemapping could only be used to determine the gross region (e.g., anterior wall of the left ventricle) from which the tachycardia arose. They suggested that pacemapping either be corroborative or be used only when tachycardia could not be initiated at surgery.

Kienzle and colleagues[48] compared endocardial mapping in sinus rhythm with endocardial activation mapping during ventricular tachycardia in 13 patients. They noted that fractionated, split, or late electrograms during sinus rhythm were seen over large areas and were not specific to the site of tachycardia origin. Similar results with endocavitary catheter mapping during sinus rhythm were reported by Cassidy and associates.[64]

Gessman and colleagues[65] compared three methods of intraoperative mapping: tachycardia activation sequence, cryothermal termination mapping, and normal sinus rhythm late potential mapping in 14 patients undergoing surgery for the management of ventricular tachycardia. The tachycardia could be provoked and mapped in ten patients, and in eight of these a cryothermal termination site was discovered. There was an excellent correspondence between the sites of origin, identified by cryothermal and activation mapping. In all 14 patients normal sinus rhythm late potential mapping was performed, and in 13 patients late potentials were identified; in eight patients the late potentials were confined to the area from which the tachycardia arose. There was therefore a reasonable correlation between all three techniques, and they are obviously complimentary.

Direct Surgical Methods

Ventriculotomy

Fontaine and colleagues[66] first described a condition known as arrhythmogenic right ventricular dysplasia, which is characterized by ventricular tachyarrhythmias associated with thinning, fatty infiltration and aneurysmal dilatation of the right ventricle, particularly in the apical, infundibular, and posterior basal regions. Sustained ventricular arrhythmias emanate from the thinned or aneurysmal areas of the right ventricular free wall. A transmural incision through the area of epicardial breakthrough of these ventricular arrhythmias or through myocardium from which late potentials may be recorded results terminates the arrhythmia, which can then not be reinduced. In a report of 12 cases of arrhythmogenic right ventricular dysplasia, Fontaine and associates[67] found that a simple transmural ventriculotomy abolished medically refactory tachycardia in eight of the 12 patients. The ventricular tachycardia recurred in four, and there were two deaths unrelated to arrhythmias.

In arrhythmogenic right ventricular dysplasia, epicardial mapping successfully locates the arrhythmogenic site presumably because of the thinness of the abnormal right ventricle. For similar reasons reentrant activity, which supports tachycardia in arrhythmogenic right ventricular dysplasia, must conduct transversely through the myocardium rather than from endocardium to epicardium, or vice versa. Thus a simple ventriculotomy through the epicardial breakthrough point should abolish tachycardia in arrhythmogenic right ventricular dysplasia. On the other hand, in coronary patients a simple transmural ventriculotomy based on epicardial mapping has only rarely been successful.[68]

There are often multiple morphology tachycardias in patients with arrhythmogenic right ventricular dysplasia. Therefore, multiple ventriculotomies may be required. Alternatively, an encircling transmural ventriculotomy may be used to isolate several sites of origin. Such an operation was designed by Cox[69] and successfully used in three patients. In this operation a full-thickness semi-circular ventriculotomy is made between two points of the tricuspid anulus.

Guiraudon and colleagues[70] described an extensive encircling ventriculotomy to isolate the entire right ventricular free wall from the remainder of the heart. This was accomplished by a full-thickness ventriculotomy that extended along the attachment of the right ventricular free wall to the interventricular septum. The moderator band connecting the free wall to the septum was also divided. The attachments of the free wall anteriorly to the aortic anulus and posteriorly to the tricuspid anulus were divided using incision or cryoablation. The operation resulted in total electrical isolation of the right ventricular free wall. The technique was described in two patients with arrhythmogenic right ventricular dysplasia giving rise to several morphologies of ventricular tachycardia occurring from multiple sites in the right ventricular free wall. It was anticipated that a smaller exclusion procedure for discrete cryosurgery would not be sufficient because of the extensive arrhythmia substrate. The surgery was successful in the immediate postoperative period, and the patients were followed for 3 and 4 months after the operation. In one patient the right ventricular tachycardia was almost incessant but was entirely confined to the right ventricle. The patient remained asymptomatic during the arrhythmia. Although paradoxic septal motion occurred in both patients, there was no significant hemodynamic impairment.

Although right ventricular disconnection in patients with poorly contracting right ventricles produces no hemodynamic difficulties, the effect of this operation on patients with normal right ventricular function is not known. Jones and colleagues[71] reported a systematic investigation of the technique of right ventricular disconnection in the dog. No major hemodynamic disturbances were noted, but a moderate reduction of left ventricular pressure, a fall in the rate of rise of left ventricular pressure, and a reduced cardiac output occurred. This impairment of left ventricular function was almost reversed by stimulating the right ventricle synchronously with left ventricular activation.

This operation seems ideally suited for patients with arrhythmogenic ventricular dysplasia. Initial experience has been very encouraging but long-term experience is needed. In particular, the result of this operation on right ventricular diastolic function has not yet been established.

Boineau and Cox[69] have reported another rather extensive but successful exclusion procedure in which the supracristal intraventricular septum was disarticulated from the remainder of the heart to isolate a tachycardia focus in a young girl who had suffered refractory ventricular tachycardia following an episode of coxsackie B5 myocarditis 6 years previously.

Encircling Endocardial Ventriculotomy

Encircling endocardial ventriculotomy was introduced as a specific form of surgery to manage chronic ventricu-

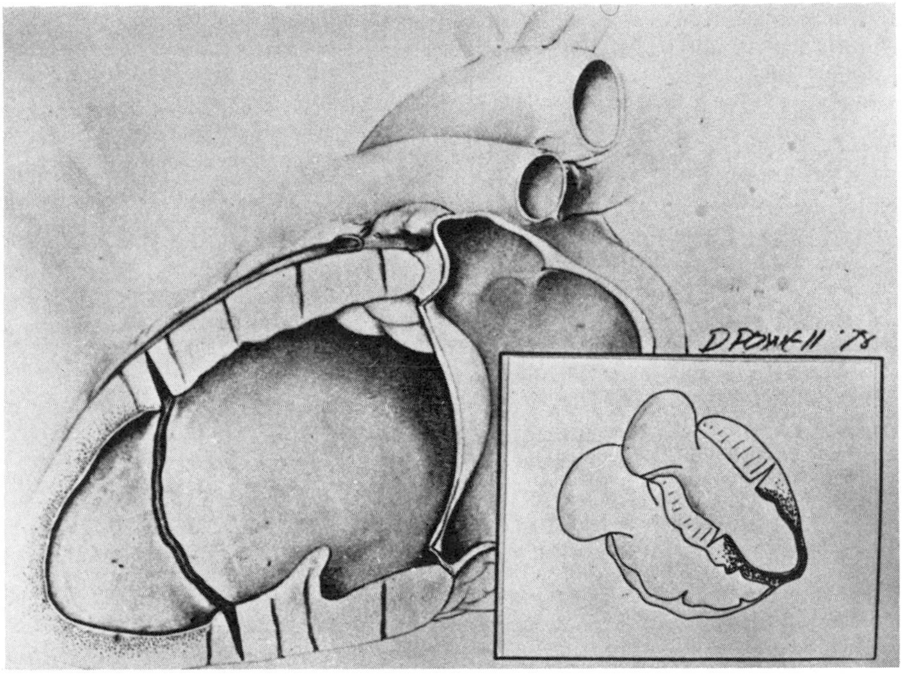

Figure 35-8. *This drawing shows the incision used for the encircling endocardial ventriculotomy. The depth of the incision is shown, as well as the need for the incision to be done above the area of endocardial fibrosis. (Guiraudon, G., Fontaine, G., Frank, R., et al.: Encircling endocardial ventriculotomy: a new surgical treatment for life-threatening ventricular tachycardias resistant to medical treatment following myocardial infarction. Ann. Thorac. Surg., 26.438, 1978)*

lar tachycardia following myocardial infarction.[72] The aim of the surgery is to exclude the origin of tachycardia from the remainder of the heart. The technique involves entering the heart through the myocardial infarction scar or aneurysm and making a vertical incision from the endocardium extending almost to the epicardium (Fig. 35-8). Theoretically such an incision conserves the epicardial blood vessels and the perpendicular penetrating branches. When the incision involves the septum it is made approximately 1-cm deep[72] or may even transect the septum completely.[73] The incision is designed to encircle the entire scar or arrhythmogenic area. It is repaired in a conventional manner with Teflon buttresses and a running suture. When the incision heals, the fibrous tissue so formed creates an insulating barrier to the spread of electrical activation, which may effectively isolate an arrhythmia mechanism or interrupt part of a reentry circuit responsible for generating the arrhythmia.[74]

The first report gave details of five patients, all of whom were successfully treated with this operation between 1975 and 1978.[72] By 1980, 21 patients had been operated on by the group in Paris; the operation was successful in 18.[75] A detailed report of the first 15 of these 22 patients[76] revealed that many had had other procedures as part of their operation (e.g., aneurysmectomy in six patients and right coronary bypass grafting in one patient). It was therefore difficult to be sure how critical the endocardial ventriculotomy was in these patients, but since other procedures do not usually abolish arrhythmias the additional specific surgery was probably responsible for the good results. In 1982, Fontaine[78] again updated the series. By then 27 patients had undergone the operation with a 1-month recurrence rate of 8% and a mortality of 15%. By 5 years after the operation there was a 24% recurrence rate and a mortality of 33%. Both the mortality and the recurrence rate were substantially less for the 16 patients operated on after December 1978[78] than for those operated on before that date. Although the original operation did not rely on perioperative electrophysiologic mapping, it was employed for later operations.

Other groups have reported their experience with encircling endocardial ventriculotomy. For example, Cox and colleagues[73] reported that nine patients underwent encircling endocardial ventriculotomy at Duke University. There were three operative deaths from low output state and two late deaths. Overall, only four patients had a successful operation, and three of these also had some endocardial resection as part of their surgery. In 1982 Ostermeyer and colleagues[79] compared the efficacy of electrophysiologically guided encircling endocardial ventriculotomy (31 patients) with simple aneurysmectomy and appropriate coronary artery bypass grafting (ten patients). Encircling endocardial ventriculotomy was clearly much more effective but possibly because of the perioperative mapping associated with the encircling ventriculotomy rather than the nature of the surgery itself. Recently, the same group[80] detailed the results of 40 patients who had undergone some form of encircling endocardial ventriculotomy guided by mapping techniques. The operation was combined with aneurysmectomy in 35 patients and coronary grafts in 30 patients. There were three operative and six late deaths. Spontaneous recurrence of tachycardia occurred in only two patients during a mean follow-up period of almost 19 months. Postoperatively, programmed ventricular stimulation provoked ventricular tachycardia in only about one quarter of the patients.

When the operation was conceived it was anticipated that the blood supply to the myocardium enclosed within the ventriculotomy would not be impaired because the epicardial and penetrating coronary arteries would not be damaged by the incision. It was therefore hoped that myocardial function in the already scarred area surrounded by the ventriculotomy would not be further compromised. This was consistent with the clinical impressions noted in earlier reports, but it soon became evident that encircling endocardial ventriculotomy was not appropriate for patients with an already badly damaged left ventricle because of further deterioration in left ventricular function following this form of surgery.[77] Ungerleider and colleagues[81] investigated the effect of encircling endocardial ventriculotomy on left ventricular function in normal dogs and demonstrated a significant decrease in diastolic compliance as well as a reduced systolic pump function. This could be attributed to the severe fall of myocardial blood flow in the area surrounded by the ventriculotomy.[82]

Several recent modifications to the technique of encircling ventriculotomy have been proposed. For example, Guiraudon and colleagues[83] have attempted in two male patients without inducible tachycardia to ablate all electrical activity in the border zone around an infarct by a series of overlapping cryolesions. Over the short follow-up period (4 months), both patients have done well with no recurrences and no need for antiarrhythmic drugs. These workers have named this technique *encircling endocardial cryoablation.*

Landymore and colleagues[61] have recently combined the concepts of encircling endocardial ventriculotomy and endocardial resection in an operation that they refer to as *encircling endocardial resection.* The authors described a simple operation consisting of the removal of all visibly diseased endocardium from the border surrounding ventricular aneurysms. The operation was performed without electrophysiologic map guidance on ten patients with drug-refactory ventricular tachycardia. Partial reimplantation of the mitral valve apparatus was needed in nine patients, an aneurysmectomy was performed in eight patients, and coronary artery bypass grafting was also carried out in nine patients. No arrhythmias recurred after the surgery, but there were two late deaths.

Endocardial Resection

Josephson,[84] Harken,[85] and their colleagues from the University of Pennsylvania introduced a surgical technique known as endocardial resection that was specifically designed to remove the anatomic substrate for this type of ventricular tachycardia. In patients with previous myocardial infarction, ventricular arrhythmias usually arise from the endocardium in the so-called twilight or border zone surrounding the infarct scar where there are islands of apparently normal myocardial cells interspersed with infarcted or ischemic tissue. It was reasoned that the arrhythmia focus could be removed by excising that endocardium. To minimize the extent of the operation, electrophysiologic mapping techniques, particularly on the endocardial surface, are used to identify the site of origin of the arrhythmia. About 10 to 25 cm^2 of endocardium is peeled off the underlying ventricular muscle. The stripping may extend 2 to 3 cm away from the scar and involve up to 40% of its circumference (Fig. 35-9).

Numerous reports have extolled endocardial resection for the management of patients with drug-refactory tachyarrhythmias.[86-90] The latest update to the series by the group from the University of Pennsylvania details the results of the first 100 patients.[91] Ninety of the 100 patients also underwent aneurysmectomy, and in 61 an average of 1.6 coronary grafts were implanted. Ninety-one patients survived surgery, and in this group 200 morphologically distinct tachycardias were mapped and managed. Sixty-four patients and 171 tachycardias could not be induced after surgery, and in ten more patients 13 more tachycardias were noninducible with the aid of antiarrhythmic drug treatment. Thus of the 89 patients who underwent postoperative electrophysiologic testing, 15 still had inducible tachycardias. The patients who were still inducible had a high rate of recurrence (4 of 15; 26%) whereas of the 64 patients who were noninducible after surgery alone, in three arrhythmia recurred and three died suddenly (10%). Similar long-term results have been reported by Rothschild and colleagues.[90] In their series 79 patients underwent endocardial resection for the treatment of ventricular tachycardia or ventricular fibrillation; ten died perioperatively. Sixty-one of the survivors had postoperative electrophysiologic testing that confirmed that 47 no longer had inducible tachycardia. Of the 14 who did, nine (64%) had recurrent arrhythmic events, whereas only two of the 47 (4%) patients with no inducible arrhythmias had such a recurrence. Similarly, 90% of the survivors of endocardial resection surgery reported by Moran and co-workers[88] were free of arrhythmias; the other 10% were responsive to antiarrhythmic drugs. Somewhat less successful results were reported by Platia and colleagues.[1] Of their small series of 28 patients with malignant ventricular arrhythmias and poor left ventricular function, 25 survived surgery; in six of these (24%) arrhythmias recurred.

On the whole this operation is successful, with an approximate perioperative mortality of 10% and a postoperative ventricular tachycardia inducibility rate of less

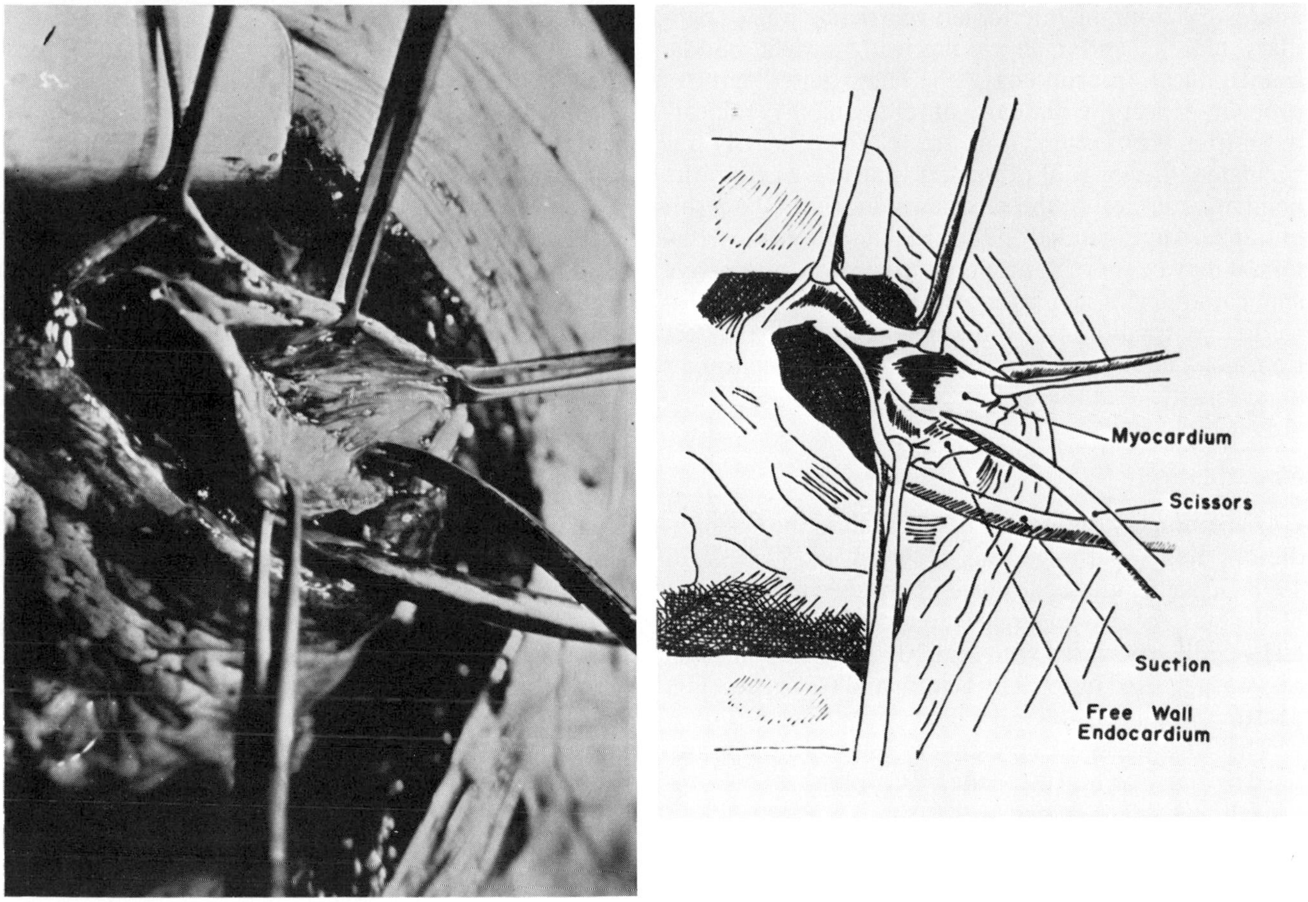

Figure 35-9. (Right) *Artist's representation of the actual surgical technique illustrated in the left-hand panel. Note the section of the endocardium from the left ventricular wall. (Harken, A. H., Josephson, M. E., and Horowitz, L. N.: Surgical endocardial resection for the treatment of malignant ventricular tachycardia. Ann. Surg., 190:456, 1979)*

than 25%. However, many of these potentially recurrent arrhythmias can then be successfully suppressed by previously ineffective antiarrhythmic medication. Thus spontaneous arrhythmia recurrences after surgery do not occur in more than 15% of patients.

The incidence of ventricular ectopic activity is uninfluenced by the endocardial resection, and frequent ventricular ectopic beats and repetitive forms of ectopic beat are seen on the 24-hour electrocardiographic recordings of patients who have neither inducible ventricular tachycardia nor spontaneous recurrences of their arrhythmia.[89,92] Serious bradyarrhythmias have not been encountered following endocardial resection. Although new bundle branch block occurs in a small proportion of patients (7%), complete heart block was not seen in the series of 82 patients reported by Kienzle and colleagues.[93]

Unlike encircling endocardial ventriculotomy, endocardial resection does not lead to noticeable hemodynamic impairment. In fact, in the 62 patients reported by Martin and colleagues,[94] there was a small but significant net increase in the ejection fraction, from 28% to 39%, and the left ventricular end diastolic pressure fell from 17 to 14 mm Hg. These favorable changes occurred predominantly in those patients with the worst preoperative left ventricular function.

In two recent reports Miller and colleagues[91,95] have analyzed the factors that predict a successful outcome from endocardial resection. Obviously preoperative left ventricular dysfunction and the patient's general health determine his or her ability to withstand surgery. For those who survive the operation the likelihood that the arrhythmias will have been effectively irradicated seems to depend predominantly on the size of the potential arrhythmia substrate. Thus patients with multiple tachycardia morphologies and widely separated sites of origin of tachycardia are less likely to escape recurrences of tachycardia. Other important predictors of failure of surgery are the absence of a discrete left ventricular aneurysm, tachycardias arising from around the mitral valve anulus and from the inferior left ventricular wall or papillary muscle, and tachycardias with a right bundle branch block morphology.[91,95] These latter features probably reflect the difficulty of removing the endocardium from the septum, from the relatively heavily trabeculated inferior wall of the left ventricle, or from the papillary muscles. In these patients, in whom the result of standard map-guided endocardial resection is less certain, it may be more appropriate to consider alternative surgical strategies such as cryoablation, encircling endocardial ventriculotomy, widespread endocardial resection,[96] or a combination of surgery and implantation of an automatic defibrillator.[1,97]

Cryoablation

Cryoablation of conduction tissue, such as the His bundle or "Kent" pathway, was reported in 1977.[50,51] In 1978 Gallagher and colleagues[51] published a case report of the successful cryosurgical treatment of ventricular tachycardia associated with scleroderma. A second success was reported in 1979 by Camm and colleagues (Fig. 35-10).[52]

The advantages of cryosurgery have been summarized by Harrison and associates.[50] Cryolesions are histologically well demarcated with a sharp border between the scar and healthy myocardium. The scar is mechanically strong because fibrous tissue, collagen, and elastic tissue are not affected by the freezing process. Hemorrhage is not produced, and cryoablation of blood vessels does not lead to hemolysis, thrombosis, or embolization. However, 6 months after the direct freezing of major epicardial canine coronary arteries there is intimal hyperplasia in most instances but in no case was the coronary vessel occluded.[98] The long-term effect of cryosurgery on human coronary vessels is unknown, but it seems a wise precaution not to freeze directly over an epicardial vessel. If possible, the coronary artery should be mobilized to allow freezing of the myocardium without injuring the coronary artery. In the experimental animal the coronary sinus is not affected by cryosurgery.

The size of the cryolesion depends on the temperature of the cryoprobe, probe size, the duration of the freeze, and the number of cryoablations performed. It also depends on the temperature of the myocardium before application of the cryoprobe. Holman and colleagues[99] created cryolesions in the left ventricular free wall of dogs. When the animals were treated during hypothermic cardioplegic cardiac arrest (6°C to 12°C), the lesions were significantly larger than those produced during normothermic arrest.

The sharp demarcation of the cryolesion from the untreated myocardium reduces the likelihood of an arrhythmia substrate being created by the cryolesion (Fig. 35-11); however, Kerr and colleagues[100] have reported a case of accelerated junctional tachycardia that appeared to arise from tissue adjacent to an area of ventricular myocardium frozen for the treatment of ventricular tachycardia. The arrhythmogenic potential of cryolesions has been systematically studied in dogs by Klein and associates.[101]

Programmed ventricular stimulation did not provoke any ventricular tachycardias, and global ventricular activation was not materially affected by the lesion. Only far-field or extrinsic electrical signals could be recorded from the cryoablated tissue. In the majority of animals, frequent ventricular ectopic activity was observed in the first few days following creation of a cryolesion. By 7 days all ectopic activity had ceased except in one animal in which ventricular premature beats had been observed

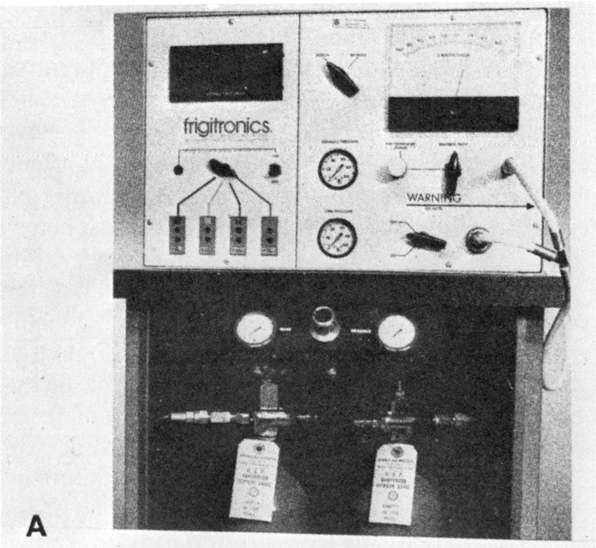

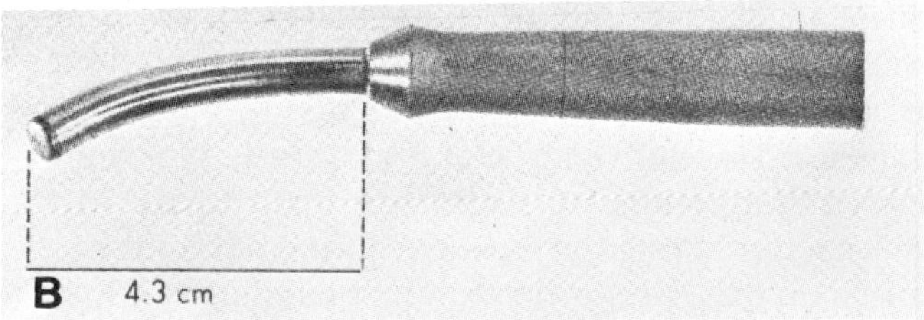

Figure 35-10. *(A) Control panel for a clinical cryoprobe unit. (B) Cryosurgical probe.*

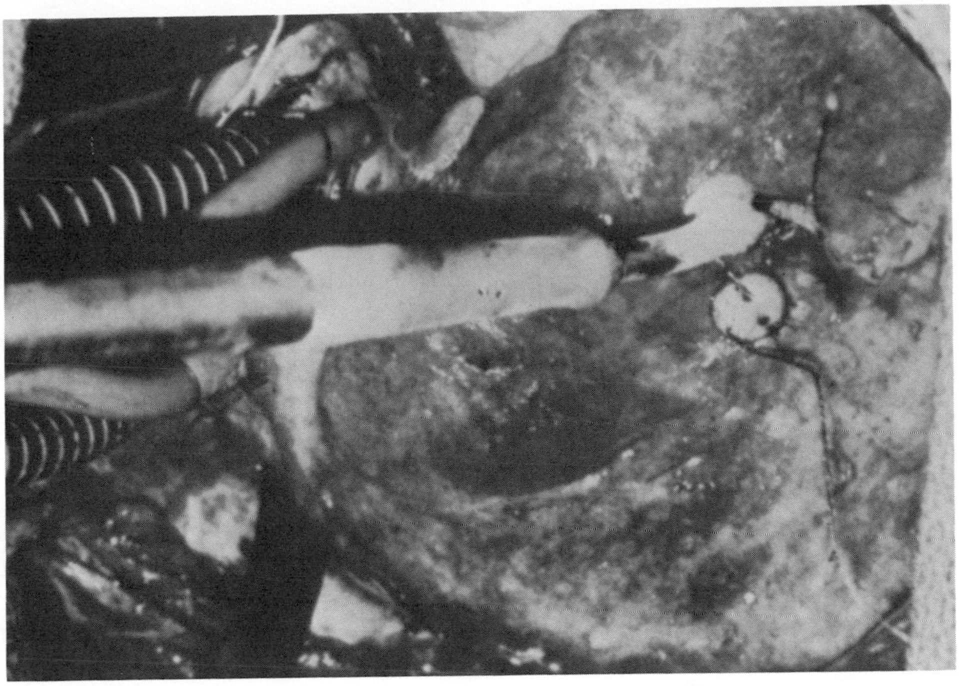

Figure 35-11. *Cryolesion* (white area) *produced with a hand-held cryosurgical probe. (With permission, Gallagher, J. J., Kasell, J. H., Cox, J. L., et al.: Techniques of intraoperative electrophysiologic mapping.)*

before the cryolesion was produced. Ectopic beats following cryosurgery appeared to arise at the edge of the cryolesion. Presumably the ventricular ectopic activity provoked by cryosurgery resulted from a thin zone of injured but not permanently ablated tissue at the edge of the lesion, or, alternatively, the arrhythmias emanated from the edge of the cryolesion, which was contracting as the scar consolidated and ceased when the demarcation became clear. The clinical importance of this finding is that arrhythmias arising in the immediate postoperative period may have a similar electrocardiographic morphology to the tachycardias treated by the cryoablation procedure.

Cryosurgery is particularly valuable for the surgical treatment of patients with ventricular tachyarrhythmias that apparently arise from a point source or that depend for their continuation on conduction through a narrow isthmus of tissue. Cryotherapy can also be used to help exclude an arrhythmogenic focus from the remainder of the ventricular myocardium. Particularly when arrhythmias arise from the base of the papillary muscles or close to a mitral or aortic anulus, cryosurgery can be used much more conveniently than methods that rely on incision or excision. Theoretically cryoablation of the free wall might be performed on the closed heart without recourse to cardiopulmonary bypass. However, the heat sink of the circulating blood volume renders it almost impossible to create a lesion large enough to reach the left ventricular endocardium.

There are no results of large series of patients with ventricular tachycardia treated with cryosurgery alone. The long-term results of this treatment are therefore largely unknown, but the treatment is almost certainly successful. The main role of cryotherapy is as an adjunct to other therapies. However, the recently introduced encircling cryolesion[83] may offer a more definitive role for cryoablation in the treatment of patients with ventricular replacement.

Miscellaneous Surgery for Ventricular Tachycardia

Very occasionally ventricular tachycardia may be excited by the presence of ventricular tumors such as rhabdomyomas and myofibromas. If the tumor can be resected, the arrhythmia may be abolished.[102] Following surgical repair of tetralogy of Fallot, sustained, potentially life-threatening ventricular tachycardias may arise from the healed ventriculotomy scar.[103] When medical and pharmacologic therapy fails to control the arrhythmia, surgical excision of the scar may successfully abolish it.[104] Thus far there are no reports of new arrhythmias arising from the excision scar. Presumably the arrhythmias, which occur relatively rarely after repair of tetralogy of Fallot, require a specific reentrant substrate that is removed but not replaced by the excision. Although fascicular tachycardia, a variety of ventricular tachycardia, usually appears to be due to triggered automaticity or reentry over a very small circuit, it has been postulated that some examples are due to reentry over a large circuit comprising the proximal His-fascicular system. In such cases division of a fascicle that forms a critical part of the reentry circuit may abolish the arrhythmia. Spurrell and associates[105] reported successful management of two patients with ventricular (fascicular) tachycardia by dividing the anterior radiation of the left bundle branch. Noncoronary, possibly congenital, or traumatic aneurysms of the left ventricle may give rise to ventricular tachycardias. Excision of these aneurysms, together with appropriate ventriculotomy or cryoablation, can successfully control the arrhythmias.[106,53] Hypertrophic cardiomyopathy is often associated with ventricular arrhythmias and sudden death. Myomectomy or myotomy has been used to reduce ventricular outflow tract obstruction and to control tachycardias but has not been uniformly successful.[107,108]

Postoperative Evaluation

Those methods used to evaluate the propensity to spontaneous ventricular tachycardia preoperatively have also been used to assess the likelihood of recurrent arrhythmic events postoperatively. Of the various techniques, inability to induce tachycardia by programmed stimulation and the loss of late potentials from the averaged surface electrocardiogram most accurately predict that postoperative tachycardia recurrence is unlikely. For example, in the study of 36 postsurgical patients reported by Kienzle and colleagues,[92] ventricular tachycardia recurred in one of seven patients whose tachycardia was still inducible and in only two of 29 in whom it was not. In another study, Page and colleagues[89] noted no recurrences in 17 patients who were noninducible after surgery compared with seven arrhythmic events (sudden death in five and sustained ventricular tachycardia in two) in the 15 patients whose tachycardia could still be provoked postoperatively. It is of practical importance to note that with a protocol that employs three premature beats, epicardial stimulation from electrodes implanted on both ventricles perioperatively is as accurate as endocardial stimulation in the right ventricular outflow tract and right ventricular apex.[109] However, the persistence of inducible tachycardia does not necessarily imply spontaneous recurrence after surgery.

Breithardt and colleagues[110] reported that tachycardia could not be induced in five patients in whom surface electrocardiographic late potentials were no longer present postoperatively, whereas in a single patient with persistent late potentials tachycardia could be provoked. Marcus and associates[111] reported similar results. Ten patients had no postoperative late potentials, and tachycardia could only be stimulated in one. Eighteen had persistent late potentials, and tachycardia could be induced in eight. Therefore, late potentials are still present in many patients who do not have inducible tachycardias postoperatively.

Thus neither the presence of late potentials nor the persistent inducibility of tachycardia prevents a good outcome from surgery; however, absence of late potentials, particularly noninducibility of tachycardia, suggests that tachycardias will not recur postoperatively.

The discovery of frequent or complex ventricular ectopic activity during 24-hour ambulatory electrocardiograms does not relate to the recurrence of arrhythmias postoperatively.[112] In the study by Kienzle and colleagues[92] there was no difference in the grade and type of rhythms recorded in patients with and without inducible tachycardia. Therefore, unless sustained ventricular tachycardia is recorded, the results of ambulatory electrocardiographic monitoring are helpful in assessing patients' likely freedom from future attacks of tachycardia.

Conclusion

The success of surgery for the abolition of ventricular tachyarrhythmias depends on left ventricular function, the accuracy with which the origin of tachycardia can be localized, the number of tachycardia morphologies and the size of the arrhythmogenic substrate, the length of the operation, and the skill of the operating team. The majority of perioperative deaths are due to heart failure, and in only a small number of patients do truly refractory arrhythmias occur. With the development of rapid data acquisition systems and the design of increasingly ingenious operations, it is anticipated that the result of surgery for ventricular tachycardia will improve still further, but the major remaining limitation will be the status of left ventricular function.

References

1. Platia, E. V., Reid, P. R., Watkins, L., et al.: Endocardial resection combined with automatic cardioverter-defibrillator implantation in patients with malignant ventricular tachycardias: Late followup. Circulation, 70 (Suppl. II): II–413, 1984.
2. Josephson, M. E., Horowitz, L. N., Farshidi, A., et al.: Recurrent sustained ventricular tachycardia. II. Endocardial mapping. Circulation, 57:440, 1978.
3. Josephson, M. E., Waxman, H. L., Cain, M. E., et al.: Ventricular activation during ventricular endocardial pacing. II. Role of pace-mapping to localize origin of ventricular tachycardia. Am. J. Cardiol., 50:11, 1982.
4. Ecker, R. R., Mullins, C. B., and Grammer, J. C.: Control of intractable ventricular tachycardia by coronary revascularisation. Circulation, 44:666, 1971.

5. Ester, E. H., and Iziar, H. L.: Recurrent ventricular tachycardia: A case successfully treated by bilateral cardiac sympathectomy. Am. J. Med., 31:493, 1961.
6. Jervell, A., and Lange-Nielson, F.: Congenital deaf mutism, functional heart disease with prolongation of the QT interval and sudden death. Am. Heart J., 54:59, 1957.
7. Moss, A. J., and McDonald, J.: Unilateral cervicothoracic sympathetic ganglionectomy for the treatment of long QT interval syndrome. N. Engl. J. Med., 285:903, 1971.
8. Moss, A. J., Schwartz, P. J., Crampton, R. S., et al.: The long QT syndrome: A prospective international study. Circulation, 71:17, 1985.
9. Bhandari, A. K., Scheinman, M. M., Morady, R., et al.: Efficacy of left cardiac sympathectomy in the treatment of patients with the long QT syndrome. Circulation, 70:1018, 1984.
10. Cobbs, B. W., and King, S. B.: Ventricular buckling: A factor in the abnormal ventriculogram and peculiar hemodynamics associated with mitral valve prolapse. Am. Heart J., 93:741, 1977.
11. Ross, A., DeWeese, J. A., and Yu, P. B.: Refractory ventricular arrhythmias in a patient with mitral valve prolapse. Successful control with mitral valve replacement. J. Electrocardiol., 11:289, 1978.
12. Missotten, A., Dotremont, G., Goddeeris, P., et al.: Acta Cardiol., 35:391, 1980.
13. Vismara, L. A., Miller, R. A., Price, J. E., et al.: Improved longevity due to reduction in sudden death by aortocoronary bypass in coronary atherosclerosis. Am. J. Cardiol., 39:919, 1977.
14. Leutenegger, F., Giger, G., Fuhr, P., et al.: Evaluation of aortocoronary venous bypass for prevention of cardiac arrhythmias. Am. J. Cardiol., 98:15, 1979.
15. de Sovza, N., Thenabadu, P. N., Murphy, M. L., et al.: Ventricular arrhythmia before and after aortocoronary bypass surgery. Int. J. Cardiol., 1:123, 1981.
16. Nordstrom, L. A., Lillehei, J. P., Adicoff, A., et al.: Coronary artery surgery for recurrent ventricular arrhythmias in patients with variant angina. Am. Heart J., 89:236, 1975.
17. Bonchek, L. I., Olinger, G. N., Keelan, M. H., et al.: Management of sudden coronary death. Ann. Thorac. Surg., 24:337, 1977.
18. Tabry, I. F., Geha, A. S., Hammond, G. L., and Baue, A. E.: Effect of surgery on ventricular tachyarrhythmia associated with coronary arterial occlusive disease. Circulation, 58:167, 1978.
19. Codini, M. A., Sommerfeldt, L., Ebel, C. E., et al.: Efficacy of coronary bypass grafting in exercise-induced ventricular tachycardia. J. Thorac. Cardiovasc. Surg., 81:502, 1981.
20. Garan, H., Ruskin, J. N., Dimarco, J. P., et al.: Electrophysiologic studies before and after myocardial revascularization in patients with life-threatening ventricular arrhythmias. Am. J. Cardiol., 51:519, 1983.
21. Couch, O. A.: Cardiac aneurysm with ventricular tachycardia and subsequent excision of aneurysm. Circulation, 55:251, 1959.
22. Basta, L. L.: Aneurysmectomy in treatment of ventricular and supraventricular tachyarrhythmias in patients with postinfarction and traumatic ventricular aneurysms. Am. J. Cardiol., 32:693, 1973.
23. Hunt, D., Sloman, G., and Westlake, G.: Ventricular aneurysmectomy for recurrent tachycardia. Br. Heart J., 31:264, 1969.
24. Magidson, O.: Resection of postmyocardial infarction ventricular aneurysms for cardiac arrhythmias. Dis. Chest, 56:211, 1969.
25. Wald, R. W.: Management of intractable ventricular tachyarrhythmias after myocardial infarction. Am. J. Cardiol., 44:329, 1979.
26. Buda, A. J., Stinson, E. B., and Harrison, D. C.: Surgery for life-threatening ventricular tachyarrhythmias. Am. J. Cardiol., 44:1171, 1979.
27. Ricks, W. B., Winkle, R. A., Shumway, N. E., and Harrison, D. C.: Surgical management of life-threatening ventricular arrhythmias in patients with coronary artery disease. Circulation, 56:38, 1977.
28. Sami, M., Chaitman, B. R., Bourassa, M. G., et al.: Long term follow-up of aneurysmectomy for recurrent ventricular tachycardia or fibrillation. Am. Heart J.,
29. Gallagher, J. J., Oldham, H. N., Wallace, A. G., et al.: Ventricular aneurysm with ventricular tachycardia. Am. J. Cardiol., 35:696, 1975.
30. Geha, A. S., Farshidi, A., Batsford, W. P., and Hammond, G. L.: Surgical treatment of ventricular aneurysms and arrhythmias associated with coronary arterial occlusive disease. Conn. Med., 44:369, 1980.
31. Brawley, R. K., Magovern, G. J., Gott, V. L., et al.: Left ventricular aneurysmectomy. J. Thorac. Cardiovasc. Surg., 85:712, 1983.
32. Loop, F. D., Effler, D. B., Navia, J. A., et al.: Aneurysms of the left ventricle. Ann. Surg., 178:399, 1973.
33. Rothberger, C. J., and Winterberg, H.: Studen uber die Bestimmung des Ausgangspunktes ventrickularer extrasystolen mit Hilfe des electrokardiogramms. Pluegers Arch. Physiol., 154:571, 1913.
34. Rothschild, L. T.: The excitatory process in the dog's heart. II. The ventricles. Proc. Trans. R. Soc. 206:181, 1915.
35. Fontaine, G., Guiraudon, G., Frank, R., et al.: Intraoperative mapping and surgery for the prevention of lethal arrhythmias after myocardial infarction. Ann. N. Y. Acad. Sci., 382:396, 1982.
36. Gallagher, J. J., Kasell, J. H., et al.: Techniques of intraoperative electrophysiologic mapping. Am. J. Cardiol., 49:221, 1982.
37. Gallagher, J. J., Oldham, H. N., Wallace, A. G., et al.: Ventricular aneurysm with ventricular tachycardia. Am. J. Cardiol., 35:696, 1975.
38. Wittig, J. H., and Boineau, J. P.: Surgical treatment of ventricular arrhythmias using epicardial, transmural, and endocardial mapping. Ann. Thorac. Surg., 20:117, 1975.
39. Spielman, S. R., Michelson, E. L., Horowitz, L. N., et al.: The limitations of epicardial mapping as a guide to the surgical therapy of ventricular tachyardia. Circulation, 57:666, 1978.
40. Harken, A. H., Horowitz, L. N., and Josephson, M. E.: Comparison of standard aneurysmectomy and aneurysmectomy with directed endocardial resection for the treatment of recurrent sustained ventricular tachycardia. J. Thorac. Cardiovasc. Surg., 8:527, 1980.
41. Mason, J. W., Stinson, E. B., Winkle, R. A., et al.: Relative efficacy of blind left ventricular aneurysm resection for the treatment of recurrent ventricular tachycardia. Am. J. Cardiol., 49:241, 1982.
42. Mason, J. W., Stinson, E. B., Winkle, R. A., et al.: Surgery for ventricular tachycardia: efficacy of left ventricular aneurysm resection compared with operation guided by electrical activation mapping. Circulation, 65:1148, 1982.
43. Ostermeyer, J., Breithardt, G., Kolvenbach, R., et al.: The surgical treatment of ventricular tachycardias. J. Thorac. Cardiovasc. Surg., 84:704, 1982.
44. Ideker, R. E., Smith, W. M., Wallace, A. G., et al.: A computerised method for the rapid display of ventricular activation during the intraoperative study of arrhythmias. Circulation, 59:449, 1979.
45. de Bakker, J. M. T., Janse, M. J., Van Capelle, F. J. L., and Durrer, D.: Endocardial mapping by simultaneous recording of endocardial electrograms during cardiac surgery for ventricular aneurysm. J. Am. Coll. Cardiol., 2:947, 1983.
46. Hauer, R. N., de Zwart, M. T., de Bakker, J. M., et al.: Wire skeleton method for representation of arrhythmogenic sites determined with catheter mapping, compared with intraoperative mapping. Circulation, 70:11, 1984.
47. Klein, H., Karp, R. B., Kouchoukos, N. T., et al.: Intraoperative

electrophysiologic mapping of the ventricles during sinus rhythm in patients with a previous myocardial infarction. Identification of the electrophysiologic substrate of ventricular arrhythmias. Circulation, 66:847, 1982.

48. Kienzle, M. G., Miller, J., Falcone, R. A., et al.: Intraoperative endocardial mapping during sinus rhythm: Relationship to site of origin of ventricular tachycardia. Circulation, 70:957, 1984.
49. Wiener, I., Mindich, B., and Pitchon, R.: Determinants of ventricular tachycardia in patients with ventricular aneurysms: Results of intraoperative epicardial and endocardial mapping. Circulation, 65:856, 1982.
50. Harrison, L., Gallagher, J. J., and Kasell, J.: Cryosurgical ablation of the A-V node-His bundle. A new method for producing A-V block. Circulation, 55:463, 1977.
51. Gallagher, J. J., Anderson, R. W., and Kasell, J.: Cryoablation of drug-resistant tachycardia in a patient with a variant of scleroderma. Circulation, 57:190, 1978.
52. Camm, J., Ward, D. E., Cory-Pearce, R., et al.: The successful cryosurgical treatment of paroxysmal ventricular tachycardia. Chest, 75:621, 1979.
53. Camm, J., Ward, D. E., Spurrell, R. A. J., and Rees, G. M.: Cryothermal mapping and cryoablation in the treatment of refractory cardiac arrhythmias. Circulation, 62:67, 1980.
54. Curry, P. V. L., O'Keefe, D. B., Pitcher, D., et al.: Localization of ventricular tachycardia by a new technique—pace-mapping (abstr.). Circulation, 60 (Suppl. II):25, 1979.
55. Lewis, T.: The mechanism and graphic registration of the heart beat. London, Shaw & Sons, 1925.
56. Kastor, J. A., Spear, J. F., and Moore, E. N.: Localisation of ventricular irritability by epicardial mapping: Origin of digitalis induced unifocal tachycardia from left ventricular Purkinje tissue. Circulation, 45:952, 1972.
57. Horowitz, L. N., Spear, J. F., and Moore, E. N.: Subendocardial origin of ventricular arrhythmias in 24 hour old experimental myocardial infarction. Circulation, 53:56, 1976.
58. Waxman, H. L., and Josephson, M. E.: Ventricular activation during ventricular endocardial pacing. I. Electrocardiographic patterns related to the site of pacing. Am. J. Cardiol., 50:1, 1982.
59. Josephson, M. E., Waxman, H. L., Cain, M. E., et al.: Ventricular activation during ventricular endocardial pacing. II. Role of pace-mapping to localize origin of ventricular tachycardia. Am. J. Cardiol., 50:11, 1982.
60. O'Keeffe, D. B., Curry, P. V. L., Prior, A. L., et al.: Surgery for ventricular tachycardia using operative pace mapping. Proc. Br. Coll. Surg., 43:116, 1980.
61. Landymore, R. W., Kinley, C. E., and Gardner, M.: Encircling endocardial resection with complete removal of endocardial scar without intraoperative mapping for the ablation of drug-resistant ventricular tachycardia. J. Thorac. Cardiovasc. Surg., 89:18, 1985.
62. Josephson, M. E., Horowitz, L. N., Spielman, S. R., et al.: Comparison of endocardial catheter mapping with intraoperative mapping of ventricular tachycardia. Circulation, 61:395, 1980.
63. Horowitz, L. N., Josephson, M. E., and Harken, A. H.: Epicardial and endocardial activation during sustained ventricular tachycardia in man. Circulation, 61:1227, 1980.
64. Cassidy, D. M., Vassallo, J. A., Buxton, A. E., et al.: The value of catheter mapping during sinus rhythm to localize site of origin of ventricular tachycardia. Circulation, 69:1103, 1984.
65. Gessman, L. J., Gallagher, J. D., Demorizi, N. M., et al.: Comparison of intraoperative activation, cryothermal and normal sinus rhythm—late potential mapping of patients with ventricular tachycardia. Pace, 8:312, 1985.
66. Fontaine, G., Guiraudon, G., Frank, R., et al.: Surgical management of ventricular tachycardia unrelated to myocardial ischaemia or infarction. Am. J. Cardiol., 49:397, 1982.
67. Fontaine, G., Guiraudon, G., and Frank, R.: Stimulation studies and epicardial mapping in ventricular tachycardia: Study of mechanisms and selection for surgery. In Kulbertus, H. E. (ed.): Reentrant Arrhythmias, pp. 334-350. Baltimore, University Park Press, 1977.
68. Spurrell, R. A. J., and Camm, A. J.: Surgical treatment of ventricular tachycardia. Br. Heart J., 40:38, 1978.
69. Boineau, J. P., and Cox, J. L.: Rationale for a direct surgical approach to control ventricular arrhythmias. Relation of specific intraoperative techniques to mechanism and location of arrhythmic circuit. Am. J. Cardiol., 49:381, 1982.
70. Guiraudon, G. M., Klein, G. J., Gulamhusein, S. S., et al.: Total disconnection of the right ventricular free wall: Surgical treatment of right ventricular tachycardia associated with right ventricular dysplasia. Circulation, 67:463, 1983.
71. Jones, D. L., Guiraudon, G. M., and Klein, G. J.: Total disconnection of the right ventricular free wall: Physiological consequences in the dog. Am. Heart J., 107:1169, 1984.
72. Guiraudon, G., Fontaine, G., Frank, R., et al.: Encircling endocardial ventriculotomy: A new surgical treatment for life-threatening ventricular tachycardias resistant to medical treatment following myocardial infarction. Ann. Thorac. Surg., 26:438, 1978.
73. Cox, J. L., Gallagher, J. J., and Ungerleider, R. M.: Encircling endocardial ventriculotomy refractory ischaemic ventricular tachycardia. J. Thorac. Cardiovasc. Surg., 83:865, 1982.
74. Ungerleider, R. M., Holman, W. L., Stanley, T. I., III, et al.: Encircling endocardial ventriculotomy for refractory ischaemic ventricular tachycardia. J. Thorac. Cardiovasc. Surg., 83:840, 1982.
75. Fontaine, G., Guiraudon, G., and Frank, R.: Ventricular resection for recurrent ventricular tachycardia. N. Engl. J. Med., 303:339, 1980.
76. Fontaine, G., Guiraudon, G., and Frank, R.: Mechanism of ventricular tachycardia with and without associated chronic myocardial ischaemia: Surgical management based on epicardial mapping. In Narula, O. S. (ed.): Cardiac Arrhythmias. Electrophysiology, Diagnosis and Management, p. 516. Baltimore, Williams & Wilkins, 1979.
77. Fontaine, G.: Surgery for ventricular tachycardia. The view from Paris. Int. J. Cardiol., 1:351, 1982.
78. Fontaine, G., Guiraudon, G., Frank, R., et al.: Intraoperative mapping and surgery for the prevention of lethal arrhythmias after myocardial infarction. Ann. N. Y. Acad. Sci., 382:396, 1982.
79. Ostermeyer, J., Breithardt, G., Kolvenbach, R., et al.: The surgical treatment of ventricular tachycardias. J. Thorac. Cardiovasc. Surg., 84:704, 1982.
80. Borggrefe, M., Breithardt, Ostermeyer, J., and Bircks, W.: Long-term efficacy of endocardial incircling ventriculotomy for ventricular tachycardia: Complete versus partial incision. Circulation, 68:176, 1983.
81. Ungerleider, R. M., Holman, W. L., Calcagno, D., et al.: Encircling endocardial ventriculotomy for refractory ischaemic ventricular tachycardia. J. Thorac. Cardiovasc. Surg., 83:857, 1982.
82. Ungerleider, R. M., Holman, W. L., Calcagno, D., et al.: Encircling endocardial ventriculotomy for refractory ischaemic ventricular tachycardia. J. Thorac. Cardiovasc. Surg., 83:850, 1982.
83. Guiraudon, G. M., Klein, G. J., Vermeulen, F. E., et al.: Encircling endocardial cryoablation: A technique for surgical treatment of ventricular tachycardia after myocardial infarction. Circulation, 68:176, 1980.
84. Josephson, M. E., Harken, A. H., and Horowitz, L. N.: Endocardial excision: A new surgical technique for the treatment of recurrent ventricular tachycardia. Circulation, 60:1430, 1979.
85. Harken, A. H., Josephson, M. E., and Horowitz, L. N.: Surgical endocardial resection for the treatment of malignant ventricular tachycardia. Ann. Surg., 190:456, 1979.
86. Josephson, M. E., Horowitz, L. N., and Harken, A. H.: Surgery

for recurrent sustained ventricular tachycardia associated with coronary artery disease: The role of subendocardial resection. Ann. N. Y. Acad. Sci., 381, 1982.

87. Horowitz, L. N., Harken, A. H., Kastor, J. A., and Josephson, M. E.: Ventricular resection guided by epicardial and endocardial mapping for treatment of recurrent ventricular tachycardia. N. Engl. J. Med., 302:590, 1980.
88. Moran, J. M., Kehoe, R. F., Loeb, J. M., et al.: Operative therapy of malignant ventricular rhythm disturbances. Ann. Surg., 198:479, 1983.
89. Page, P. L., Arciniegas, J. G., Plumb, V. J., et al.: Value of early postoperative epicardial programmed ventricular stimulation studies after surgery for ventricular tachyarrhythmias. J. Am. Coll. Cardiol., 2:1046, 1983.
90. Rothschild, M., Moran, J., Zheutlin, T., et al.: Post-operative programmed stimulation in predicting arrhythmic recurrence in patients undergoing endocardial resection. Circulation, 70:292, 1984.
91. Miller, J. M., Kienzle, M. G., Harken, A. H., and Josephson, M. E.: Subendocardial resection for ventricular tachycardia: Predictors of surgical success. Circulation, 70:624, 1984.
92. Kienzle, M. G., Doherty, J. U., Roy, D., et al.: Subendocardial resection for refractory ventricular tachycardia: Effects on ambulatory electrocardiogram, programmed stimulation and ejection fraction, and relation to outcome. J. Am. Coll. Cardiol., 2:853, 1983.
93. Kienzle, M. G., Martin, J. L., Horowitz, L. N., et al.: Electrocardiographic changes following endocardial resection for ventricular tachycardia. Am. Heart J. 104:753, 1982.
94. Martin, J. L., Untereker, W. J., Harken, A. H., et al.: Aneurysmectomy and endocardial resection for ventricular tachycardia: Favorable hemodynamic and antiarrhythmic results in patients with global left ventricular dysfunction. Am. Heart J., 103:960, 1982.
95. Miller, J. M., Kienzle, M. G., Harken, A. H., and Josephson, M. E.: Morphologically distinct sustained ventricular tachycardias in coronary artery disease: Significance and surgical results. J. Am. Coll. Cardiol., 4:1073, 1984.
96. Campbell, R. W. F., Kertes, P., Glabus, M., et al.: Origin of late potentials defined by ECG signal averaging. Br. Heart J., 53:99, 1985.
97. Watkins, L., Platia, E. V., Mower, M. M., et al.: The treatment of malignant ventricular arrhythmias with combined endocardial resection and implantation of the automatic defibrillator: Preliminary report. Ann. Thorac. Surg., 37:60, 1984.
98. Holman, W. L., Ikeshita, M., Ungerleider, R. M., et al.: Cryosurgery for cardiac arrhythmias: Acute and chronic effects on coronary arteries. Am. J. Cardiol., 51:149, 1983.
99. Holman, W. L., Ikeshita, M., Douglas, J. M., et al.: Cardiac cryosurgery: Effects of myocardial temperature on cryolesion size. Surgery, 93:268, 1983.
100. Kerr, C. R., Gallagher, J. J., Cox, J. L., et al.: Accelerated junctional tachycardia at a rate of 190 beats/minute following cryosurgery and aneurysmectomy for ventricular tachycardia: A case report. Pace, 5:442, 1982.
101. Klein, G. J., Harrison, L., Ideker, R. F., et al.: Reaction of the myocardium to cryosurgery: Electrophysiology and arrhythmogenic potential. Circulation, 59:364, 1979.
102. Engle, M. A., Ebert, P. A., and Repo, S. F.: Recurrent ventricular tachycardia due to resectable cardiac tumor. Circulation, 30:1052, 1974.
103. Horowitz, L. N., Vetter, V. L., Harken, A. H., and Josephson, M. E.: Electrophysiologic characteristics of sustained ventricular tachycardia occurring after repair of tetralogy of Fallot. Am. J. Cardiol., 46:446, 1980.
104. Harken, A. H., Horowitz, L. N., and Josephson, M. E.: Surgical correction of recurrent sustained ventricular tachycardia following complete repair of tetralogy of Fallot. J. Thorac. Cardiovasc. Surg., 80:779, 1980.
105. Spurrell, R. A. J., Sowton, E., and Deuchar, D. C.: Ventricular tachycardia in 4 patients evaluated by programmed electrical stimulation of heart and treated in 2 patients by surgical division of anterior radiation of left bundle-branch. Br. Heart J., 35:1014, 1973.
106. Boineau, J. P., Bilitch, M., Zubiate, P., et al.: Mapping cardiac excitation and surgical intervention in patients with ventricular arrhythmias (abstr.). Circulation, 52 (Suppl. II): II–138, 1975.
107. Guiraudon, G., Fontaine, G., Frank, R., et al.: Surgical treatment of ventricular tachycardia guided by ventricular mapping in 23 patients without coronary artery disease. Ann. Thorac. Surg., 32:439, 1981.
108. Beahrs, M. M., Tajik, A. J., Seward, J. B., et al.: Hypertrophic obstructive cardiomyopathy: Ten to 21 year follow-up after partial septal myomectomy. Am. J. Cardiol., 51:1160, 1983.
109. Plumb, V. J., McGiffin, D. C., Kirklin, J. K., et al.: Comparison of endocardial and epicardial stimulation for the induction of ventricular tachycardia (abstr.). Pace, 8:311, 1985.
110. Breithardt, G., Seipel, L., Ostermeyer, J., et al.: Effects of antiarrhythmic surgery on late ventricular potentials recorded by precordial signal averaging in patients with ventricular tachycardia. Am. Heart J., 104:996, 1982.
111. Marcus, N. H., Falcone, R. A., Harken, A. H., et al.: Body surface late potentials: Effects of endocardial resection in patients with ventricular tachycardia. Circulation, 70:632, 1984.
112. Herling, I. M., Horowitz, L. N., and Josephson, M. E.: Ventricular ectopic activity after medical surgical treatment for recurrent sustained ventricular tachycardia. Am. J. Cardiol., 45:633, 1980.

36

Use of the Automatic Implantable Cardioverter-Defibrillator in the Treatment of Malignant Ventricular Tachyarrhythmias

Morton M. Mower

The first clinical implantation of the automatic defibrillator (AID-R, Intec Systems, Pittsburgh) was performed on Feb. 4, 1980, at The Johns Hopkins Hospital in Baltimore.[1] Since then, over 300 defibrillators have been implanted in the United States and abroad, with The Johns Hopkins Hospital and Stanford University Hospital having over 100 patients each. After reviewing the early developmental work that led to this new therapeutic modality, this chapter will center on the current clinical use of the automatic defibrillator.

Rationale for the Automatic Defibrillator

Fully two thirds of the mortality from coronary artery disease is due to sudden cardiac death, a syndrome that occurs in patients with heart disease of other etiologies as well. There are an estimated 400,000 victims annually in the United States alone, and the incidence is no less striking in other developed nations. It has generally been accepted that sudden cardiac death usually reflects grave disturbances in cardiac electrical activity, culminating in fibrillation leading to death. Management of patients with this disorder is fraught with almost unsurmountable difficulties, since most persons die within minutes of the onset of symptoms, long before they are able to reach a medical facility.

Because of advances in clinicians' ability to identify many patients at high risk of dying suddenly, the past several years have seen a significant increase of interest in aggressive anti-arrhythmic therapy including drugs, antitachycardia pacemakers, cardiac surgery, and, recently, the automatic implantable cardioverter-defibrillator (AICD). The basic idea behind the development of the AICD is that it would provide selected high-risk patients with a means of restoring a normal rhythm within seconds, without the need for specialized medical personnel or additional equipment. Because the device obviously could not prevent arrhythmias, it would complement other treatments and serve as a back-up, or safety, mechanism. The AICD can be compared to implantable demand pacemakers, save that ventricular tachyarrhythmias rather than asystole are sensed, and the delivered discharges are a million times higher energy than pacemaker impulses.

Early Studies

The biologic and engineering feasibility of the AICD was demonstrated in 1969, when the first experimental

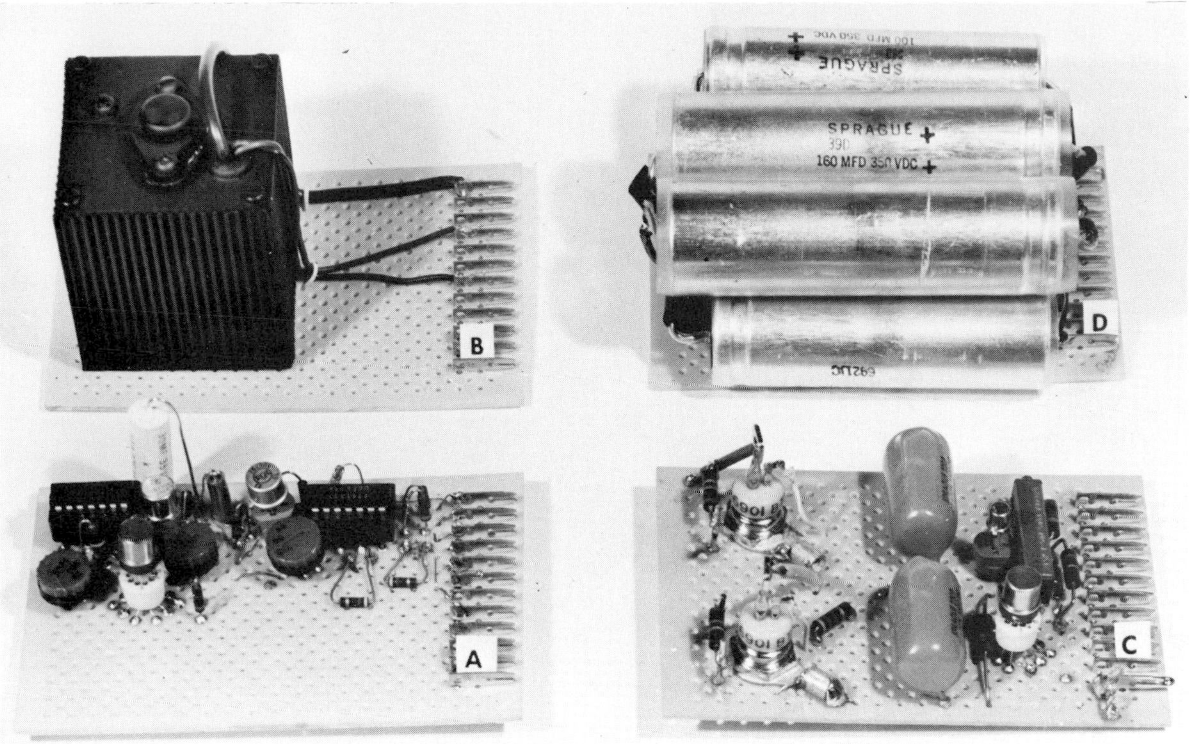

Figure 36-1. *The first experimental prototype of the automatic defibrillator on four 3 × 4-inch circuit boards. (A) Sensing circuit. (B) High-voltage converter. (C) Switching circuit. (D) Capacitor bank. The batteries, not shown, were as large as this entire array. (Mirowski, M., Mower, M. M., Staewen, W. S., et al.: Standby automatic defibrillator: An approach to prevention of sudden cardiac death. Arch. Intern. Med., 126:158, 1970)*

model was built and successfully tested in animals.[2] The initial prototype monitored the pulsatile ventricular pressure using a transducer mounted on the tip of a transvenous electrode catheter placed in the right ventricle. Ventricular fibrillation abolished the phasic nature of the pressure curve, which, if longer than 6 seconds, triggered the capacitor charging cycle. When fully charged some 20 seconds after onset of fibrillation, the device delivered an electrical shock between the right ventricular electrode and another located more proximally on the catheter at the level of the superior vena cava. In the event of unsuccessful defibrillation, the device recycled and delivered additional shocks. If at any time before the counter-shock delivery normal rhythm resumed, the discharge was inhibited. Figure 36-1 shows one of the first experimental models, and Figure 36-2 displays its functional performance. In a more advanced model (Fig. 36-3), the sensing system monitored a cardiac contraction signal and the endocardial electrogram, requiring the absence of both signals to initiate a charging cycle.[3]

The single intravascular catheter system[4-6] was shown capable of defibrillating dogs with 5 to 10 J and baboons with even less energy. Figure 36-4 shows the induction of ventricular fibrillation in an anesthetized baboon and its termination with a catheter-delivered 0.5-J countershock. Clinical studies performed during open-heart surgery for coronary bypass grafting demonstrated that catheter defibrillation was also feasible in humans, even under conditions of extreme myocardial ischemia and metabolic dysfunction.[7] The required energies ranged from 5 to 15 J, comparing favorably to those found in the animal studies.

The initial prototypes were followed by more advanced models characterized by greater miniaturization, progressive refinement of the electrode and sensing systems, increased safety, and higher reliability. As a result, the size, weight, structural characteristics, and functional performance of the units began to meet the stringent criteria required for long-term implantation in humans. Preclinical testing included analysis of the long-term bench performance of the defibrillator and the effects of exposure to various physical stresses such as vacuum, pressure, temperature cycling, mechanical vibrations, and shocks and to electromagnetic interference. Many of the test conditions exceeded the standards

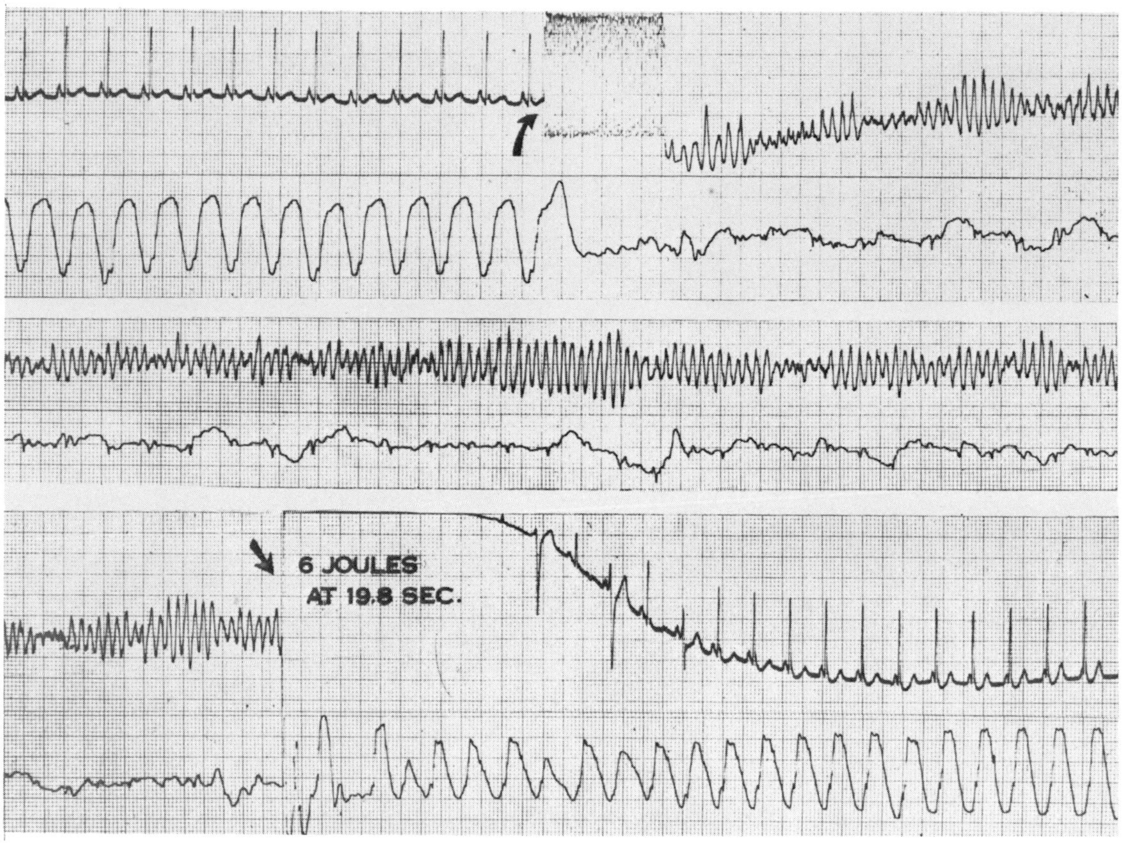

Figure 36-2. *Simultaneous electrocardiographic and right ventricular pressure curves recorded during operating cycle of the early prototype. Ventricular fibrillation is induced in a dog with low-level alternating current (*top arrow*); 19.8 seconds later, an intracardiac catheter discharge of 6 J is automatically delivered (*bottom arrow*), causing sinus rhythm to resume. The strips are continuous. (Mirowski M., Mower, M. M., Staewen, W. S., et al.: The development of the transvenous automatic defibrillator. Arch. Intern. Med., 129:773, 1972)*

required of implantable pacemakers. Anatomic effects of chronic electrode implantation and defibrillatory discharges were studied for up to 11 months and found to be minimal. Figure 36-5 shows selected frames from a film taken during a successful automatic fibrillation-defibrillation sequence in a fully conscious dog. The Applied Physics Laboratory of The Johns Hopkins University also made an independent evaluation of basic device design, provocative challenges to the sensing system, analysis of components, manufacturing and quality control procedures, and review of the preclinical test data. On the basis of the examination, the device was found suitable for use in a clinical setting.[8,9]

First Clinical Model

Because the success of catheter defibrillation depends critically on maintaining proper position of the catheter tip in the apex of the right ventricle, and because the exact energy requirements in humans were still unknown, we decided that the first clinical implants would use at least one electrode that could be precisely fixed in place surgically. Initially this was a flexible cup and later a rectangular patch containing titanium mesh. A titanium spring placed in the superior vena cava formed the second electrode (Fig. 36-6).

The first sensing system that we used clinically was based on the analysis of the probability density function and was specific for ventricular fibrillation. It identified the arrhythmia directly rather than by monitoring indirect parameters of cardiac activity such as arterial pressure, R waves, or electrical impedence.[10] The logic measured the time spent by the input electrogram between two amplitude limits located near zero potential. In essence, ventricular fibrillation is characterized by a striking absence of isoelectric potential segments (Fig. 36-7).

Truncated exponential discharges were used because

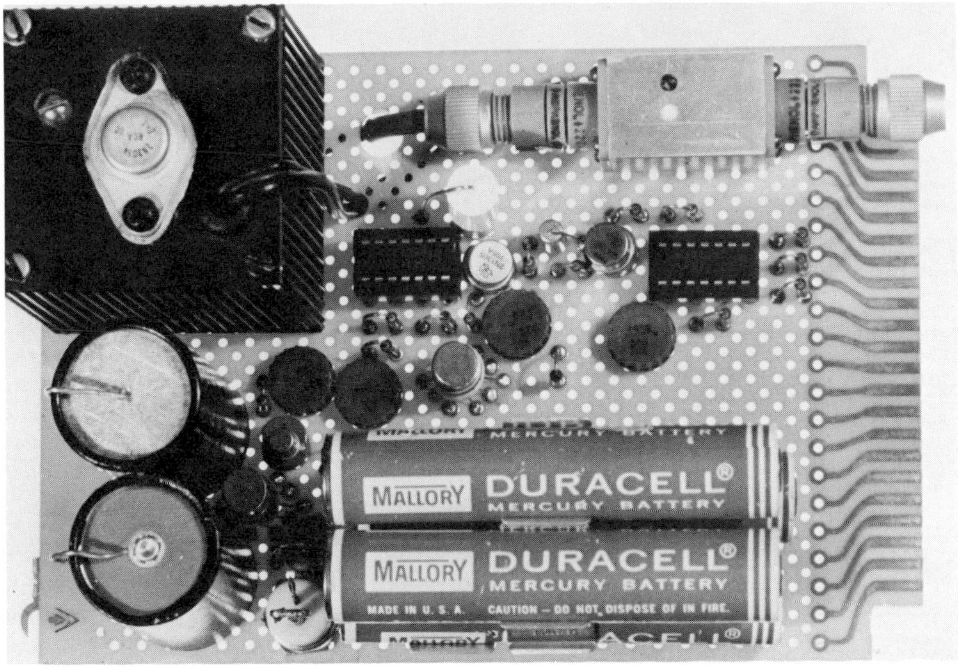

Figure 36-3. *Single-circuit board model with 10-J output capability using contraction and electrogram sensing. The 4.5- × 6.5-inch card contains a direct current–direct current converter in the* upper left-hand corner, *the capacitor bank in the* lower left, *the transducer connector and balancing network at the* upper right, *and the two AA batteries in the* lower right section. *The remaining elements form the sensing and switching circuitry. (Mirowski, M., Mower, M. M., Staewen, W. S., et al.: The development of the transvenous automatic defibrillator. Arch. Intern. Med., 129:776, 1972)*

they are simple to generate and, for a given defibrillation efficacy, require low peak voltage and current. A constant energy level was delivered by varying pulse duration between 3 and 8 msec to compensate for variations in heart-electrode resistance. Defibrillatory discharges of 25 J were delivered about 15 seconds after onset of an arrhythmia, and the device could recycle as many as three times during a single episode if needed. The strength of the third and fourth shocks was increased to 35 J. For patients with higher defibrillation energy requirements, energy output could be increased to as much as 45 J.[6]

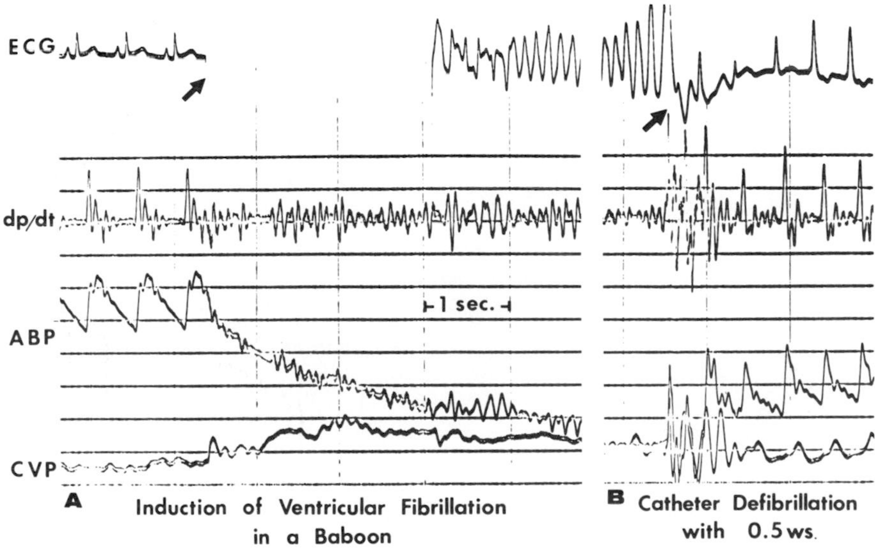

Figure 36-4. *(A) Induction of ventricular fibrillation in a baboon with low-level alternating current. (B) Restoration of normal rhythm with an 0.5-J catheter discharge. (ECG, electrocardiogram; ABP, arterial blood pressure; CVP, central venous pressure) (Mirowski, M., Mower, M. M., Reid, P. R., and Watkins, L., Jr.: Automatic implantable pacemaker. Cardiovasc. Clin., 14:197, 1983)*

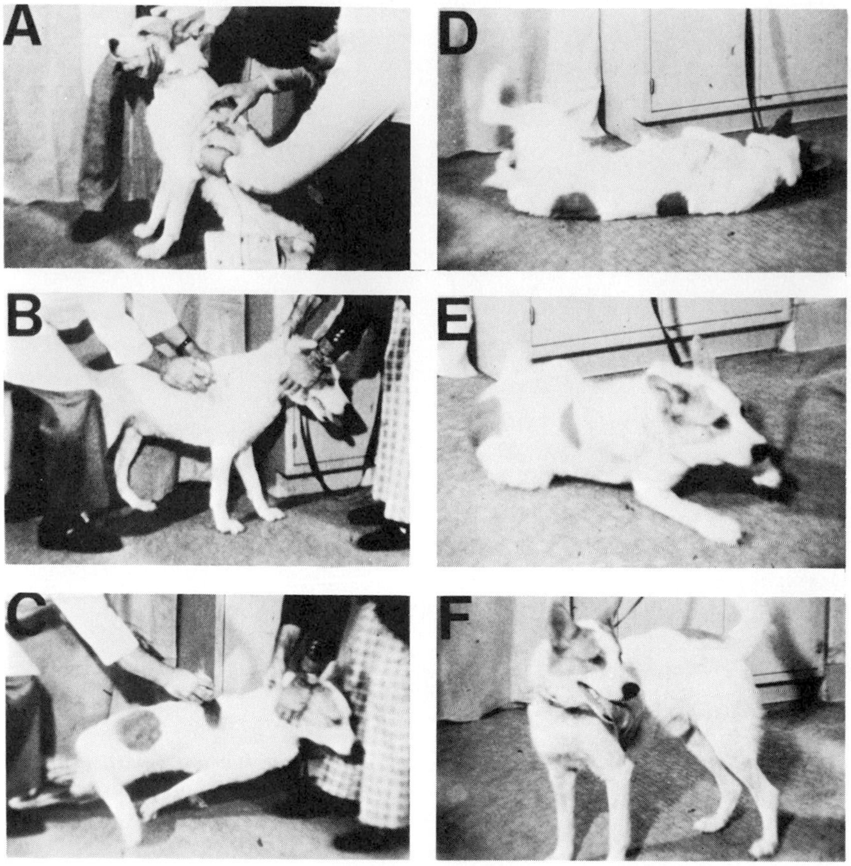

Figure 36-5. *Selected frames from a motion picture of a typical automatic defibrillation episode. (A) Defibrillator testing procedure with the external analyzer. (B) Ventricular fibrillation is induced by magnetic activation of an implanted fibrillator. (C) Loss of consciousness secondary to the arrhythmia. (D) Delivery of the defibrillatory shock, 15 seconds after the onset of fibrillation. E and F show the animal 5 and 15 seconds, respectively, after automatic defibrillation. (Mirowski, M., Mower, M. M., Langer, A.: Miniaturized Implantable Automatic Defibrillator for prevention of sudden death from ventricular fibrillation. Amsterdam, Excerpta Medica International Congress Series 458:660, 1978)*

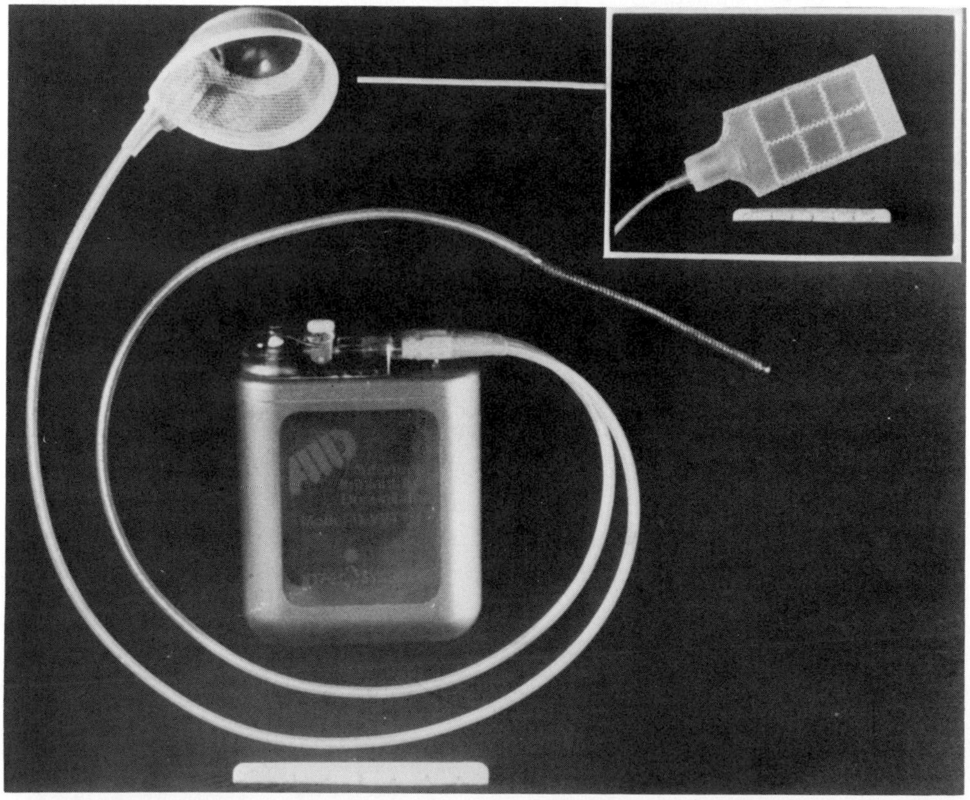

Figure 36-6. *Automatic implantable defibrillator with its two defibrillating electrodes.* **Inset,** *lower left, shows the patch electrode used as an alternative to the apical cup electrode. (Mirowski, M., Mower, M. M., and Reid, P. R.: Treatment of malignant ventricular arrhythmias in man with an implanted automatic defibrillator. Crit. Care Med., 9:388, 1981)*

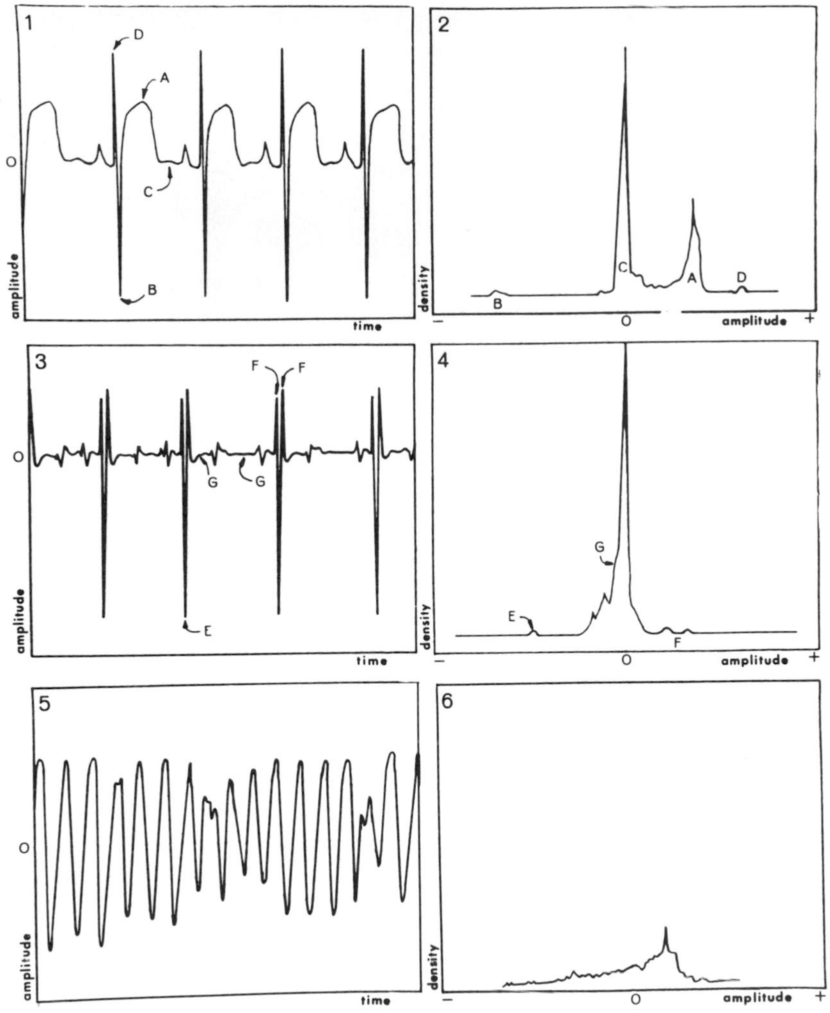

Figure 36-7. *Selected input electrograms (panels 1, 3, and 5) with their corresponding probability density function graphs (panels 2, 4, and 6). (Panel 1) Normal input electrogram. (Panel 2) The peak at zero amplitude (C) indicates that the signal spends considerable time near baseline. (Panel 3) The filtered input signal. (Panel 4) Filtering augments the peak at zero amplitude (G) and decreases the heights of secondary peaks. (Panel 5) Filtered ventricular fibrillation signal. (Panel 6) The absence of peak at zero amplitude reflects the short time the signal is near baseline and indicates the diagnosis of ventricular fibrillation. (Mirowski, M., Mower, M. M., Langer, A., and Heilman, M. S.: The automatic implantable defibrillator: A new avenue. In Bircks, W., Loogen, F., Schulte, H. D., and Seipel, L. (eds.): Medical and Surgical Management of Tachyarrhythmias, p. 77. Berlin, Springer-Verlag, 1980)*

Development of the Cardioverter-Defibrillator

Although the first clinical device was highly successful in terminating ventricular fibrillation, it soon became apparent that the majority of sudden cardiac death survivors referred for implantation suffered from hemodynamically unstable ventricular tachycardias rather than from ventricular fibrillation, which was observed only at a later stage. Consequently, significant modifications were implemented to make the system responsive to the entire range of ventricular tachyarrhythmias and to transform the original automatic defibrillator into the AICD. A bipolar right ventricular electrode was added for rate determination and R wave synchronization, and eventually for pacing as well. The AICD unit monitored heart rate as well as the probability density function. The new model was phased into the clinical study in April 1982.[11]

The AICD is physically similar to early pacemakers (Fig. 36-8). Its dimensions are 11.2 × 7.1 × 2.5 cm, and it weighs 292 g. The titanium outer can is hermetically sealed with a laser beam weld. An inner can, housing the electronic package consisting of over 300 discrete components, is located in the upper part of the device. Capacitors, lithium batteries, and a test-load resistor occupy the lower portion. A piezoelectric crystal is located near the center of the can and emits magnetically triggered coded audio signals to check the sensing function and to determine whether the unit is active or inactive (Fig. 36-9). If the device is active, the unit beeps synchronously with the QRS complexes so that one can easily ascertain that each QRS complex is being sensed and that there is no miscounting due to T wave sensing.

The magnet can activate and deactivate the device as desired. Keeping it in place for 30 seconds causes the device to change its state and different sounds to be emitted (see Fig. 36-9). In contrast to the beeping sounds of the active sensing unit, the deactivated unit has a solid, or steady, tone.

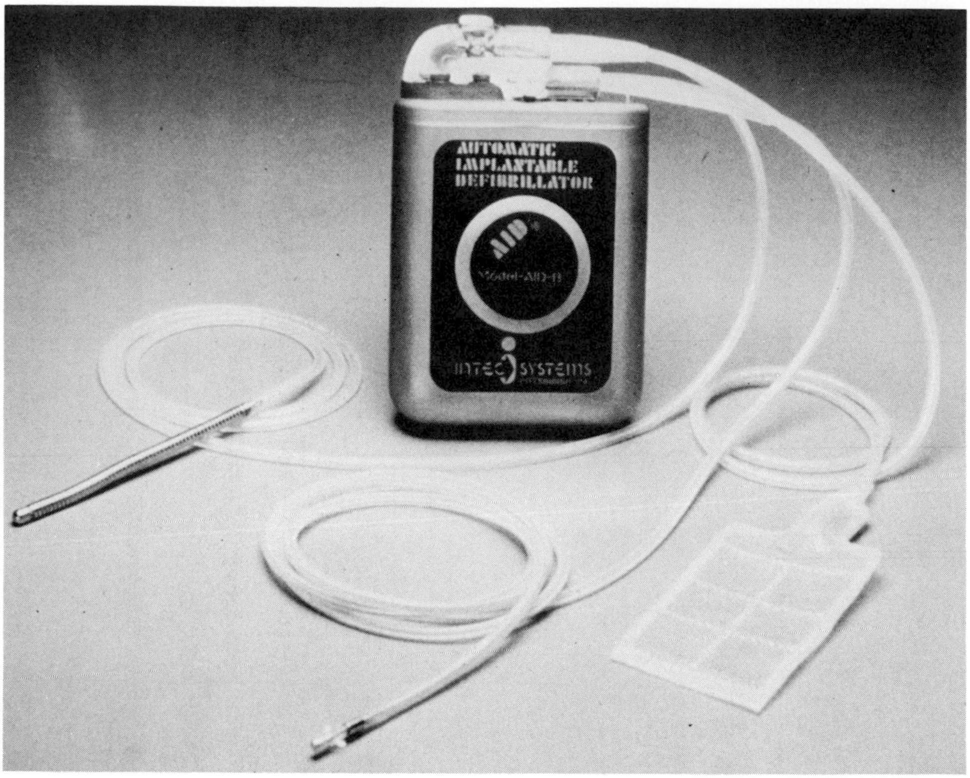

Figure 36-8. *The automatic implantable cardioverter-defibrillator with, left to right, its superior vena cava, bipolar right ventricular, and apical patch electrodes. (Mirowski, M., Reid, P. R., Mower, M. M., et al.: Use of the Automatic Implantable Cardioverter–Defibrillator in the treatment of malignant ventricular tachyarrhythmias. Herz 9:85, 1984)*

With the help of an external monitoring device, the AIDCHECK-B (Fig. 36-10), the battery strength and the cumulative number of pulses delivered through the leads to the patient can be determined. A transient application of the magnet triggers the testing cycle. As the batteries become depleted, the charge times telemetered out to the AIDCHECK-B become prolonged. When they remain elevated despite repeated testing, one should consider electively replacing the units. The magnet can also be used to divert a pulse to the internal test-load resistor if it is desired that the shock *not* be given to the patient. The AIDCHECK-B battery charger is very useful during implantation as a source of low-level alternating current to induce malignant arrhythmias for testing that the units function properly.[12]

Presently, two different versions of the sensing system are available. The conventional dual-sensing device is called AID-B. There is also an AID-BR variant (the R indicating "rate only") that is based only on the heart rate determination.[13] The precise indications for the use of the rate only and the dual-sensing versions have not yet been completely determined, but essentially the issue is one of greater sensitivity versus greater specificity. At present, the particular characteristics of a given unit with regard to the sensing parameters and energy output settings are determined during the manufacturing process.

Patient Selection

The initial patient selection criteria were quite rigorous. The patient was required to have survived at least two episodes of cardiac arrest not in the context of acute myocardial infarction; one had to occur despite presumably adequate treatment, and electro-cardiographic documentation was necessary. In fact, our implantees have been unresponsive to many conventional and investigational drug regimens as well. The average number of previous cardiac arrests in the group was four, and the average number of drugs that did not work was five. Patients were excluded if they had serious chronic or acute illness other than the heart disease that was likely to limit their lifespan significantly or if they were receiving noncardiac drugs that could in any way affect cardiac electrical activity. The criteria have since been relaxed to require only a single episode of arrhythmic cardiac arrest with evidence of incomplete protection by medical treatment as determined by continuing inducibility during electrophysiologic studies or stress testing.

In our own group of implantees, coronary artery disease has remained the dominant underlying pathophysiologic condition, being present in approximately two thirds of the group. Various types of cardiomyopathy are present in one third, with only a few patients having

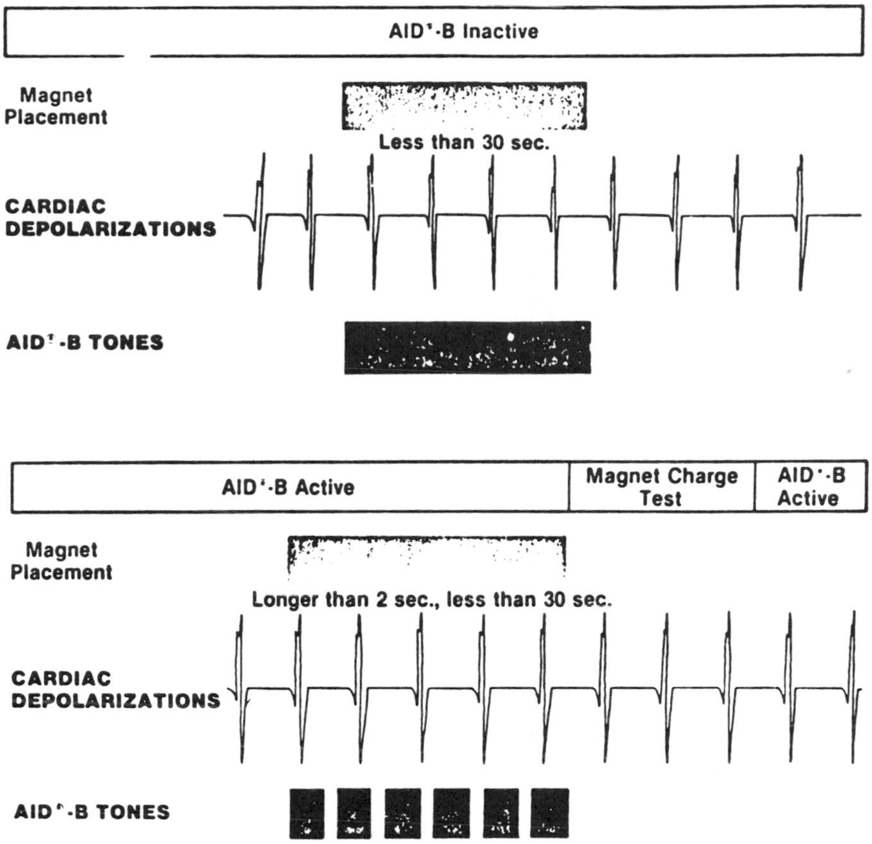

Figure 36-9. *Diagrammatic representation of the tones emitted by the automatic implantable cardioverter-defibrillator when the magnet is applied. (*Upper panel*) When the device is inactive, a steady tone is produced. After 30 seconds of continuous magnet application, the device changes to the opposite state. (*Lower panel*) When the device is active and the leads are intact, the unit beeps with each cardiac depolarization. When the magnet is removed, the unit is commanded to perform a battery strength test by charging and then discharging the capacitors through the test-load resistor. If the magnet is continuously applied for 30 seconds, the device changes to the opposite state. (AID, automatic implantable defibrillator)*

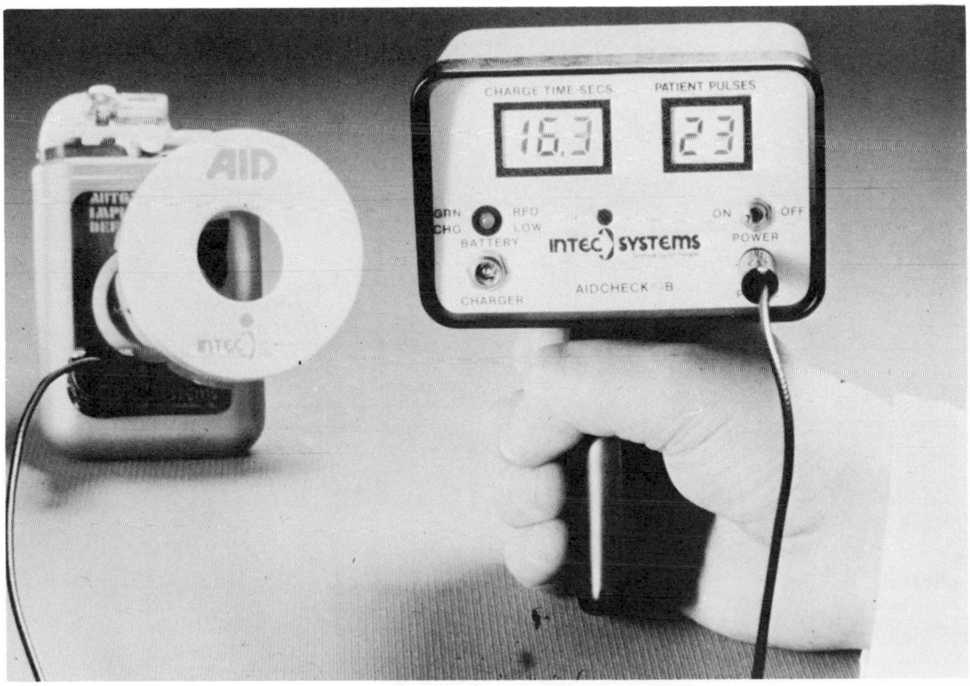

Figure 36-10. *The defibrillator analyzer with a magnet and an electromagnetic transducer placed over the pulse generator. The digital display on the left indicates the capacitor charging time, while that on the right shows the number of discharges delivered to the patient. (Mirowski, M., Reid, P. R., Mower, M. M., et al.: Use of the Automatic Implantable Cardioverter–Defibrillator in the treatment of malignant ventricular tachyarrhythmias. Herz 9:87, 1984)*

primary electrical disease in the absence of structural heart disease. The mean ejection fraction is 34%.

Implantation

Early in the clinical trials, the apical lead was always implanted through a left thoracotomy. This is still done in patients who have had previous chest surgery to avoid dissection at a previously operated site. Also, since implantation has always been considered part of an overall comprehensive strategy to combat the malignant arrhythmias, including new investigational drugs and antiarrhythmic surgery as indicated, many of the patients have undergone other cardiac surgical procedures (*e.g.,* coronary artery bypass grafting, aneurysmectomy with endocardial resection, prosthetic valve replacement, and myectomy) at implantation. Median sternotomy has thus come to be preferred for many patients. It significantly shortens the implantation procedure and minimizes postoperative discomfort.[14] More recently, subxiphoidal[15] and left subcostal techniques,* similar to pacemaker lead implantation,[16] have been developed, further simplifying the procedure and representing a significant technical and clinical advance.

*Laurie, G. M., and Griffin, J.: Personal communication.

The usual deployment of leads, consisting of an anode in the superior vena cava (SVC) and apical patch as the cathode, is shown in Figure 36-11. Alternatively, two patches can be used for the transcardiac pair. The patches come in two sizes; the smaller (model A67) has a surface area of 13.5 cm^2, and the larger (model L67) of 27 cm^2. Lower thresholds may often be achieved using larger electrodes, although they may also predispose postoperatively to greater pericardial irritation and to a higher incidence of atrial arrhythmias. The rate channel can be provided by the right ventricular endocardial lead or by a screw-in lead alternative. Other combinations are also possible. In the event, however, that an artificial pacemaker is implanted in addition to the cardioverter-defibrillator, the pacemaker must be bipolar rather than unipolar and the pacing leads must be located as far away as possible from the rate sensing leads.

The SVC catheter electrode (model C10) has a 7-cm^2 titanium spring. The rate lead consists either of a model BT 10 bipolar right ventricular endocardial catheter or of two model K57 epicardial "screw-in" electrodes placed 1 cm apart in the left ventricle. The catheter electrodes can be passed percutaneously using a No. 14 French peel-away introducer. Most often the subclavian vein is chosen, but the internal jugular vein may also serve as the entry site. Silastic anchors can be used to fix

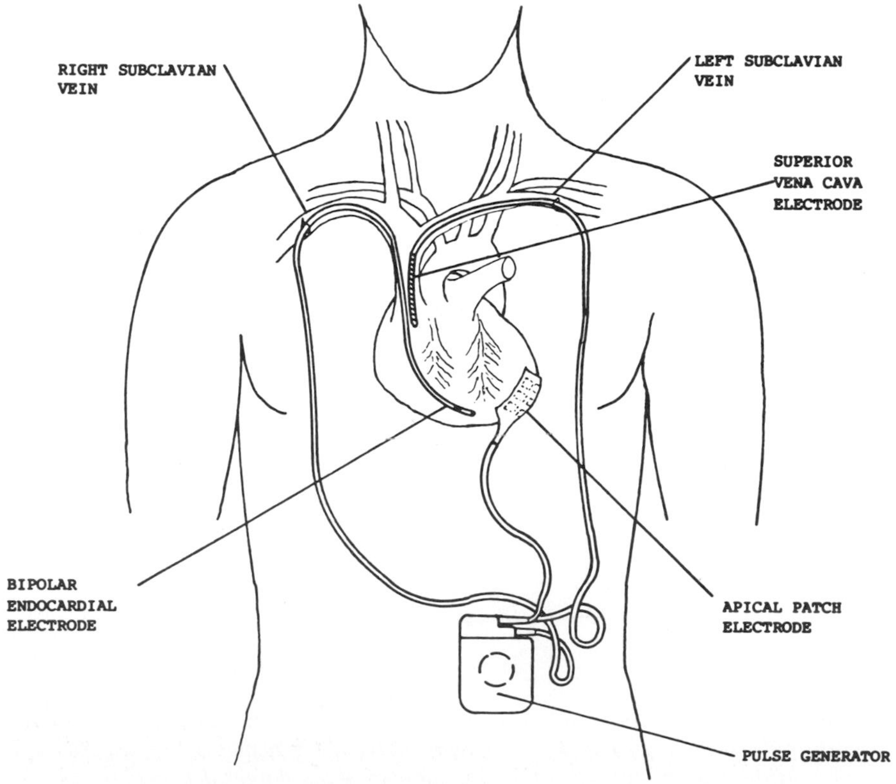

Figure 36-11. *Schematic diagram of the implanted automatic implantable cardioverter-defibrillator system. (Platia, E. V.: Internal Medicine for the Specialist. Morganville, NJ: Medical Publishing, Inc. p.97. 1984)*

the point of entry into the vein. All leads are marked with distinctive numbers and are color coded with red Teflon-coated wire in the patch leads and black Teflon coating for the catheter lead.

To assist in lead implantation, a number of measurements, including the energy requirements for defibrillation, are made at implantation. The external cardioverter-defibrillator (ECD) unit (Fig. 36-12) is connected to the implanted lead system, has an output waveform similar to that of the implantable units, and has a deliverable energy level adjustable from 1 to 40 J. The arrhythmia is provoked repeatedly with alternating current, and the amount of energy required to revert it consistently is determined. The units most suitable for the patient can thus be easily selected. The one finally chosen for implantation is then attached to the leads with temporary lead wires to the header to allow continuous recording of rate and transcardiac signals. The arrhythmia is then reinduced to ensure that the selected unit is able to recognize and correct it automatically. If so, the header lead wires are replaced with permanent nylon header caps containing O rings to cover the set screws and seal the terminals, and the implantation procedure is completed.

During the final stages of implantation, the device is often temporarily deactivated to avoid false triggering, especially when cautery is being used. Sometimes it is left off in the immediate postoperative period to minimize triggering on supraventricular arrhythmias, which are occasionally present at this time. For the long term, virtually all patients receive the most suitable antiarrhythmic regimen that can be found for them.[17]

Risks and Complications

Regarding patients' subjective reactions, internal discharges cause momentary discomfort but are generally well tolerated even in a conscious state. The sensation most frequently described by implantees has been that of a moderate blow to the chest. Since we are dealing with a very sick population, and because implantation requires extensive surgery and general anesthesia, many perioperative and postoperative problems were expected to occur. In fact, they were infrequent. Postoperatively, transient pericardial rubs have been the rule. In the patients operated on in Baltimore, infectious complications occurred in six patients and were limited to the pulse generator pocket in four. In the two cases of generalized sepsis, an antecubital cut-down site was the primary focus in one, while in the other the origin was unknown. All patients responded well to antibiotics. Lead dislodgement occurred in seven patients, requiring repositioning. There was one episode of superior vena cava thrombosis that resolved with anticoagulants. The one operative death occurred when the subclavian vein was perforated by a Swan-Ganz catheter.[18]

Functional Performance

In the electrophysiology laboratory, the diagnostic accuracy of the AICD has been 98% for both ventricular fibrillation and ventricular tachycardias, and the devices were highly effective in terminating abnormal rhythms

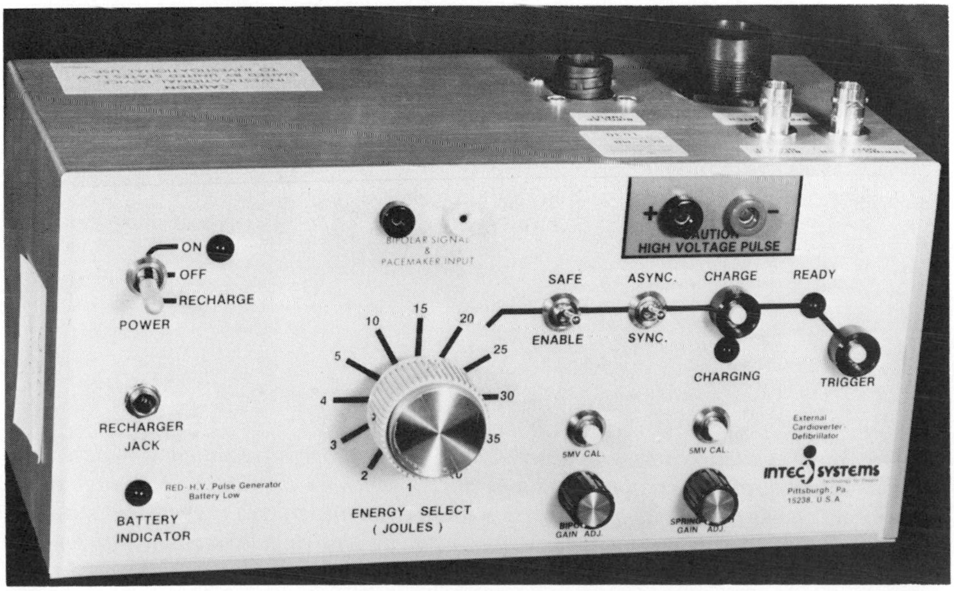

Figure 36-12. *External cardioverter-defibrillator unit. Input channels for rate and transcardiac signals are located on the top. The energy output of the device is adjustable up to 40 J, and the pulse is similar to that of implantable units.*

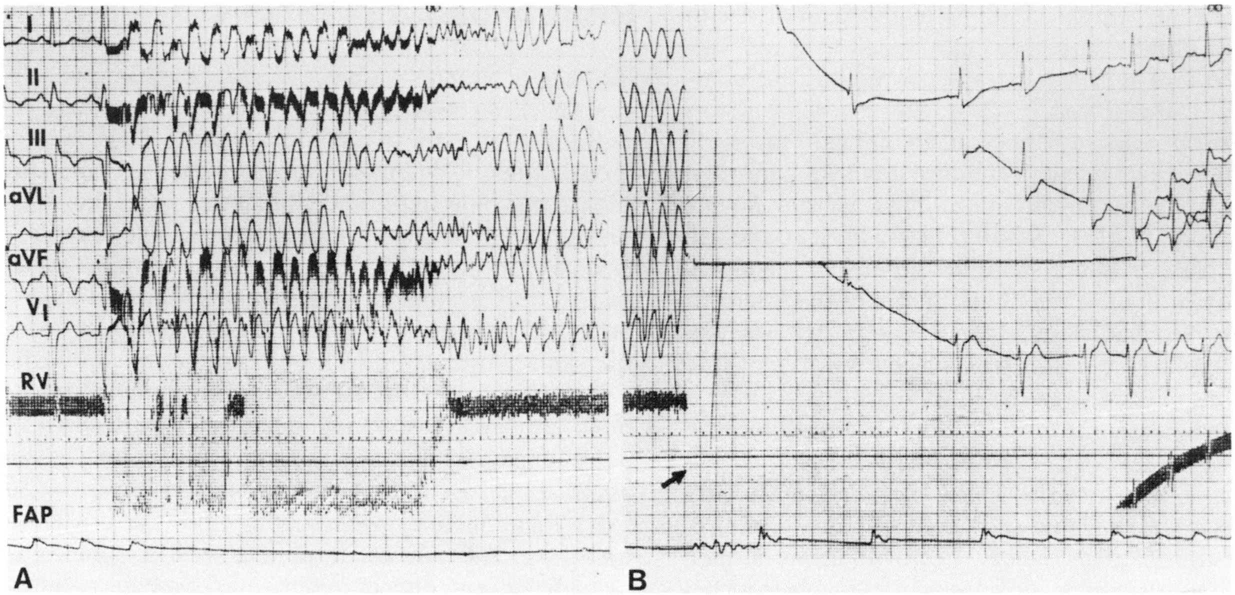

Figure 36-13. *(A) Initiation of ventricular flutter/fibrillation during an electrophysiologic study. (B,* arrow*) Unit automatically reverses the arrhythmia to normal sinus rhythm. Leads I, II, III, aV_F, and V_1 are standard electrocardiographic leads. (RV, right ventricular electrogram; FAP, femoral arterial pressure) (Mirowski, M., Mower, M. M., and Reid, P. R.: The Automatic Implantable Defibrillator. Am. Heart J., 100:1089, 1980)*

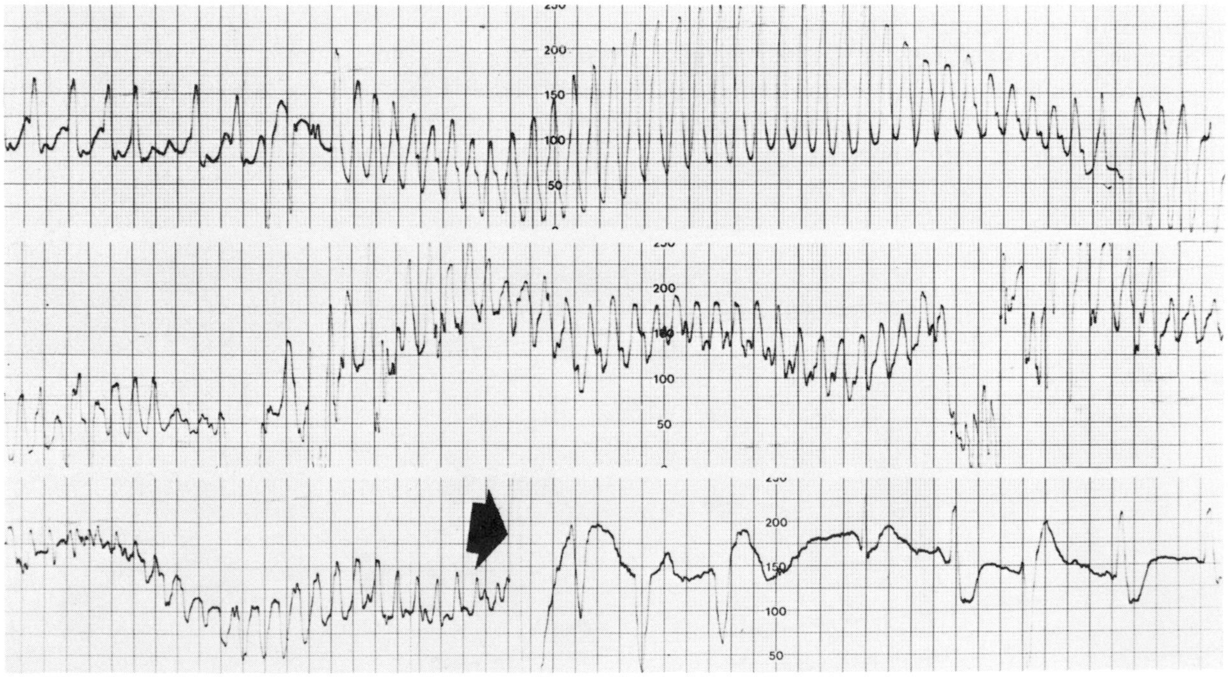

Figure 36-14. *Electrocardiographic recording in a post-operative patient who developed a well-tolerated atrial flutter 28 minutes long during which the implanted unit remained quiescent. The last few beats of this rhythm are seen in the* left part *of the* upper strip. *Two spontaneous premature ventricular contractions then occurred, followed by ventricular flutter/fibrillation; 23 seconds later (*arrow*) the malignant arrhythmia was automatically terminated by the 25-J discharge. The strips are continuous. (Mirowski, M., Reid, P. R., Watkins, L., et al.: Clinical treatment of life-threatening ventricular arrhythmias with the Automatic Implantable Defibrillator. Am. Heart J., 102:265, 1981)*

during the testing in the laboratory and for spontaneous rhythms afterward.[18] The time from onset of induced arrhythmias until their termination ranged between 11.5 and 36 seconds, with a mean of 17 seconds. Figure 36-13 is an example of a malignant arrhythmia induced in the electrophysiology laboratory with alternating current, which was automatically reverted by the implanted device. Figure 36-14 is an example of a spontaneous arrhythmia recorded on a monitor that was corrected automatically. Reversions were usually accomplished with a single internal discharge, although in some instances the device has had to recycle once or even twice to achieve this. In another spontaneous arrhythmia (Fig. 36-15), the first discharge accelerated the rhythm, but the device recycled twice and corrected it on the third shock. Postshock bradycardias have not been a problem in our experience.[18]

Conversion of Out-of-Hospital Arrhythmias

After patients had returned home following discharge, many instances of automatic termination of their malignant arrhythmias were reported.[19] These episodes have been difficult to document, and usually the diagnosis has been made on the basis of a characteristic sequence of events as reported by the patients or observed by bystanders. Palpitations and weakness were the usual initial symptoms, followed by dizziness or collapse, and then by evidence of an internal discharge consisting of a diffuse muscular contraction, followed by prompt recovery and a feeling of well-being. In several patients, however, the underlying arrhythmias were graphically documented when the patients reached a hospital after having had recurring symptoms, where, while being monitored, their arrhythmias were once again terminated automatically (Fig. 36-16).

Impact on Mortality

Kaplan-Meier survival-curve analysis was performed for the initial 52 patients from the series (Fig. 36-17). A hypothetic expected mortality statistic indicating what would have occurred in the same group of patients if the AICD had not been implanted was constructed using as endpoints either the patient's actual death or the first out-of-hospital resuscitation. Deaths were classified as sudden unless they were clearly otherwise. The 1-year

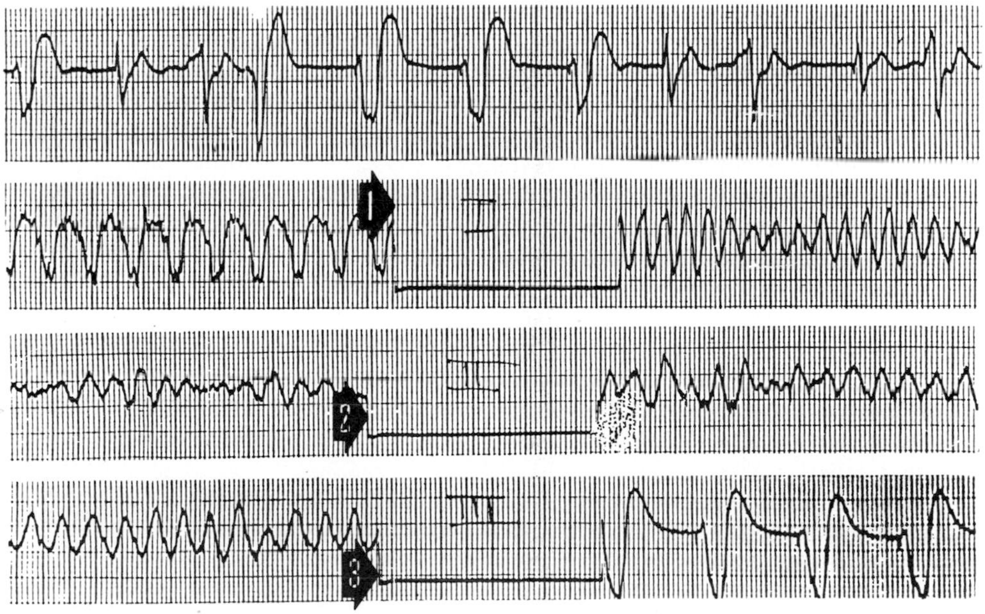

Figure 36-15. *Automatic correction of accelerated rhythm.* Upper strip *displays paced rhythm present before spontaneous ventricular tachycardia developed at a rate of 176 beats/min, shown on the* left side *of the second strip. The first discharge (*arrow 1*) accelerates the tachycardia to ventricular fibrillation. The device recycles, delivers a second discharge (*arrow 2, third strip*), which is ineffective; it then recycles again, this time restoring the patient's initial rhythm (*lower strip*). The strips are not continuous. (Mirowski, M., Reid, P. R., Mower, M. M., et al.: Use of the Automatic Implantable Cardioverter–Defibrillator in the treatment of malignant ventricular tachyarrhythmias. Herz 9:88, 1984)*

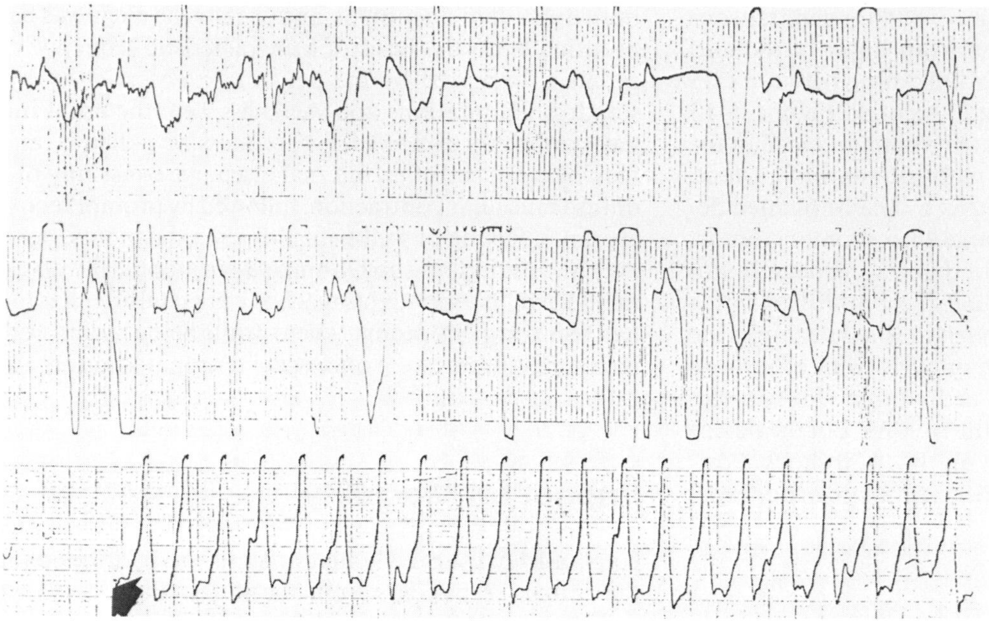

Figure 36-16. *Continuous monitoring strip recorded in the emergency room during one of the patient's episodes of hypotensive ventricular tachycardia. At* arrow, *the automatic discharge was delivered. After a short period of frequent premature ventricular contractions, the underlying sinus mechanism can be clearly seen. (Mirowski, M., Reid, P. R., Mower, M. M., and Watkins, L., Jr.: Successful conversion of out-of-hospital life-threatening ventricular arrhythmias with the implanted automatic defibrillator. Am. Heart J., 103:147, 1982)*

mortality from all causes was 22.9%, the sudden death mortality 8.5%, and the predicted mortality 48%. These figures indicated a 52% decrease in total mortality and a significant reduction in the arrhythmic component during the initial year following device implantation.[20]

Since then, with more patients enrolled, it has become possible to compare the respective effectiveness of the first- and second-generation devices used in the study. Figure 36-18 displays survival curves for the first 89 patients implanted in Baltimore, divided into two groups according to the model they received. In each panel, the arrhythmic mortality is indicated by the upper curve and the total mortality by the lower curve. Patients whose early model was subsequently replaced with the AICD were withdrawn at that time from the AID population and entered into the AICD group. The curves indicate

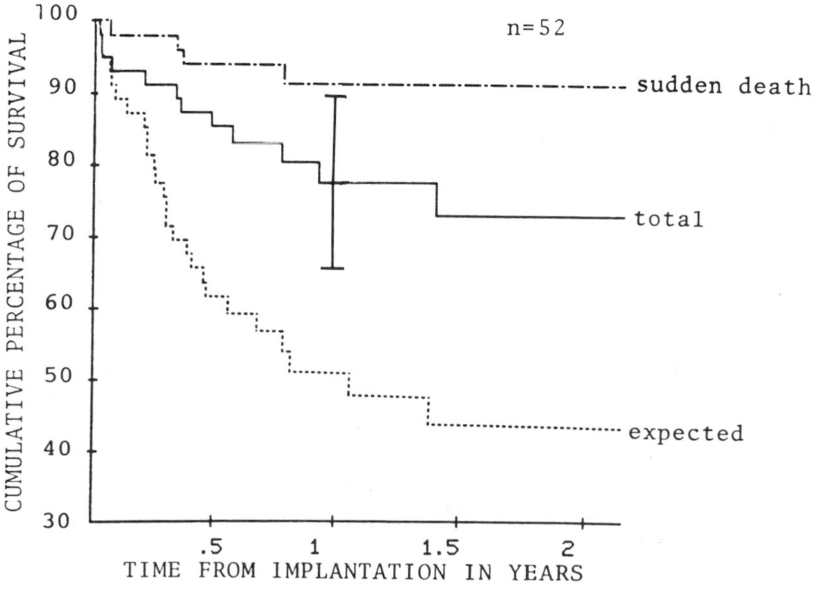

Figure 36-17. *Life-table survival analysis of the initial 52 patients with defibrillators. The upper curve (*broken line*) indicates the patients whose deaths were unwitnessed and presumably sudden and arrhythmic. The middle curve (*solid line*) shows total mortality. The lower curve (*dotted line*) estimates the mortality that would have occurred in the same group of patients without a defibrillator. The difference between identical time points on the middle and lower curves is an estimate of the improvement in survival. The 95% confidence interval at 1 year for the total survival curve is shown. (Mirowski, M., Reid, P. R., Winkle, R. A., et al.: Mortality in patients with implanted defibrillators. Ann. Intern. Med., 98:585, 1983)*

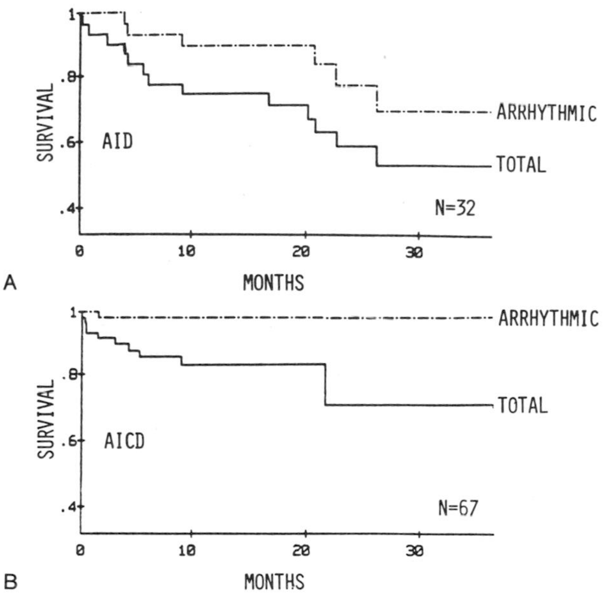

Figure 36-18. *Comparison of arrhythmic rates and total mortality in patients treated with the two different implanted models. Patients whose early automatic implantable defibrillator unit (A) was subsequently replaced with an automatic implantable cardioverter-defibrillator (B) were withdrawn from the population in A at that time and entered into the automatic implantable cardioverter-defibrillator group in B. (AID, automatic implantable defibrillator; AICD, automatic implantable cardioverter-defibrillator)*

that at 1 year, the total mortality rates were 26% and 16.6%, while the mortality due to arrhythmias was 10.6% for the early model series and only 2% for the AICD series.[18] Needless to say, the virtual abolition of arrhythmic mortality with the current model is extremely significant.

Conclusion

The ability of the AICD to diagnose ventricular fibrillation and tachycardia, and its ability to treat them, has resulted in an impressive decrease in arrhythmic mortality. The potential risks and dangers observed with this new diagnostic-therapeutic system are quite similar to those of implanted pacemakers, particularly when an epicardial implantation approach is used. The clinical benefit of the AICD system might be even greater and longer lasting for patients with less marked degrees of left ventricular dysfunction than those included so far in the study. As the clinical experience grows, the patient population that could benefit from this new intervention will most certainly be broadened.

References

1. Mirowski, M., Reid, P. R., Mower, M. M., et al.: Termination of malignant ventricular arrhythmias with an implanted automatic defibrillator in human beings. N. Engl. J. Med., 303:322–324, 1980.
2. Mirowski, M., Mower, M. M., Staewen, W. S., et al.: Standby automatic defibrillator: An approach to prevention of sudden cardiac death. Arch. Intern. Med., 126:158–161, 1970.
3. Mirowski, M., Mower, M. M., Staewen, W. S., et al.: The Development of the Transvenous Automatic Defibrillator. Arch. Intern. Med., 129:773–779, 1972.
4. Mower, M. M., Mirowski, M., Spear, J. F., and Moore, E. N.: Patterns of ventricular activity during catheter defibrillation. Circulation, 49:858–861, 1974.
5. Mirowski, M., Mower, M. M., Staewen, W. S., et al.: Ventricular defibrillation through a single intravascular catheter electrode system. Clin. Res. 19:328, 1971.
6. Mirowski, M., Mower, M. M., Reid, P. R., and Watkins, L., Jr.: Automatic implantable defibrillator. In Dreifus, L. S. (ed.): Pacemaker Therapy, pp. 195–207, Philadelphia, F. A. Davis, 1983.
7. Mirowski, M., Mower, M. M., Gott, V. L., and Brawley, R. K.: Feasibility and effectiveness of low-energy catheter defibrillation in man. Circulation, 47:79–85, 1973.
8. Mirowski, M., Mower, M. M., Langer, A., et al.: A chronically implanted system for automatic defibrillation in active conscious dogs: Experimental model for treatment of sudden death from ventricular fibrillation. Circulation, 58:90–94, 1978.
9. Mirowski, M., Mower, M. M., Bhagavan, B. S., et al.: Chronic animal and bench testing of the implantable automatic defibrillator. In Meere, C. (ed.): Proceedings of the VIIth World Symposium on Cardiac Pacing, Chap. 27-2. Montreal, Canada, Pacesymp, 1980.
10. Mirowski, M., Mower, M. M., Langer, A., and Heilman, M. S.: The automatic implantable defibrillator: A new avenue. Medical and Surgical Management of Tachyarrhythmias, In Bircks, W., Loogen, F., Schulte, H. D., and Seipel, L. (eds.) pp. 71–80. Berlin, Springer-Verlag, 1980.
11. Reid, P. R., Mirowski, M., Mower, M. M., et al.: Clinical evaluation of the internal automatic cardioverter-defibrillator in survivors of sudden cardiac death. Am. J. Cardiol., 51:1608–1613, 1983.
12. Mower, M. M., Reid, P. R., Watkins, L., Jr., and Mirowski, M.: Use of alternating current during diagnostic electrophysiologic studies. Circulation, 67:69–72, 1983.
13. Winkle, R. A., Bach, S. M., Echt, D. S., et al.: The automatic implantable defibrillator: Local ventricular bipolar sensing to detect ventricular tachycardia and fibrillation. Am. J. Cardiol., 52:265–270, 1983.
14. Watkins, L., Jr., Mirowski, M., Mower, M. M., et al.: Automatic defibrillation in man: The initial surgical experience. J. Thor. Cardiovasc. Surg., 82:492–500, 1981.
15. Watkins, L., Jr., Mirowski, M., Mower, M. M., et al.: Implantation of the automatic defibrillator: The sub-xyphoid approach. Ann. Thorac. Surg., 34:515–520, 1982.
16. Laurie, G. M., Morris, G. C., Jr., Howell, J. F., et al.: Left subcostal insertion of the sutureless myocardial electrode. Ann. Thorac. Surg., 21:350, 1976.
17. Mower, M. M., Reid, P. R., Watkins, L., Jr., et al.: Automatic implantable cardioverter-defibrillator: Structural characteristics. Pace, 7:1331–1337, 1984.
18. Mirowski, M., Reid, P. R., Mower, M. M., et al.: Automatic implantable cardioverter-defibrillator: Clinical results. Pace, 7:1345–1350, 1984.
19. Mirowski, M., Reid, P. R., Mower, M. M., and Watkins, L., Jr.: Successful conversion of out-of-hospital life-threatening ventricular tachyarrhythmias with the implanted automatic defibrillator. Am. Heart J., 103:147–148, 1981.
20. Mirowski, M., Reid, P. R., Winkle, R. A., et al.: Mortality in patients with implanted defibrillators. Ann. Intern. Med., 98:585–588, 1983.

Index

Page numbers followed by f indicate figures; numbers followed by t indicate tables.